Lymphomas and Leukemias

From
Cancer
Principles & Practice
of Oncology

10th edition

Lymphomas and Leukemias

From **Cancer** Principles & Practice of Oncology

10th edition

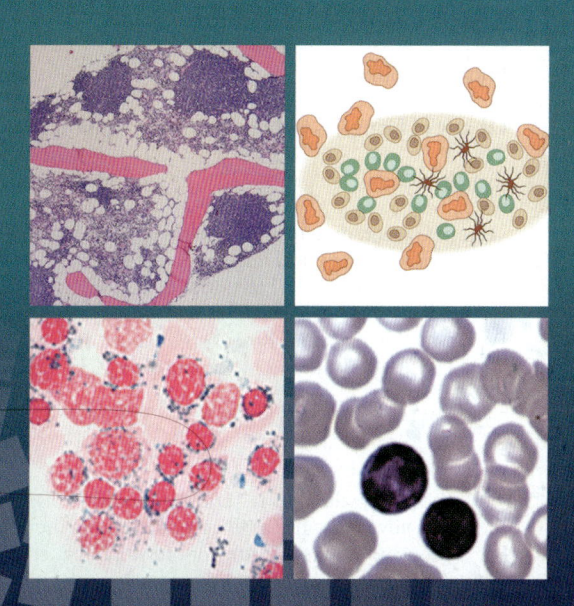

Vincent T. DeVita, Jr., MD
Amy & Joseph Perella Professor of Medicine
Yale Comprehensive Cancer Center and Smilow
Cancer Hospital at Yale-New Haven
Professor of Epidemiology and Public Health
Yale University School of Public Health
New Haven, Connecticut

Theodore S. Lawrence, MD, PhD
Isadore Lampe Professor and Chair
Department of Radiation Oncology
University of Michigan
Ann Arbor, Michigan

Steven A. Rosenberg, MD, PhD
Chief, Surgery Branch, National Cancer Institute, National Institutes of Health
Professor of Surgery, Uniformed Services University of the Health Sciences
School of Medicine
Bethesda, Maryland
Professor of Surgery
George Washington University School of Medicine
Washington, DC

Wolters Kluwer

Philadelphia · Baltimore · New York · London
Buenos Aires · Hong Kong · Sydney · Tokyo

Acquisitions Editor: Julie Goolsby
Senior Product Development Editor: Emilie Moyer
Editorial Assistant: Brian Convery
Production Project Manager: David Orzechowski
Marketing Manager: Stephanie Kindlick
Senior Designer: Stephen Druding
Illustration Coordinator: Jennifer Clements
Illustrator: Jason McAlexander, Electronic Publishing Services, Inc.
Manufacturing Coordinator: Beth Welsh
Prepress Vendor: Absolute Service, Inc.
Prepress Vendor Project Manager: Harold Medina

Copyright © 2016 Wolters Kluwer

9 8 7 6 5 4 3 2 1

Printed in China

Library of Congress Cataloging-in-Publication Data

Lymphomas and leukemias / editors, Vincent T. DeVita, Jr., Theodore S. Lawrence, Steven A. Rosenberg.
   p. ; cm.
 "From Cancer: principles & practice of oncology, 10th edition."
 Includes bibliographical references and index.
 ISBN 978-1-4963-3394-0 (alk. paper)
 I. DeVita, Vincent T., Jr., 1935- , editor. II. Lawrence, Theodore S., editor. III. Rosenberg, Steven A., editor.
IV. Devita, Hellman and Rosenberg's cancer. 10th ed. Abridgment of (expression):
 [DNLM: 1. Leukemia. 2. Lymphoma. QZ 350]
 RC643
 616.99'419--dc23

2015031784

This work is provided "as is," and the publisher disclaims any and all warranties, express or implied, including any warranties as to accuracy, comprehensiveness, or currency of the content of this work.

   This work is no substitute for individual patient assessment based on healthcare professionals' examination of each patient and consideration of, among other things, age, weight, gender, current or prior medical conditions, medication history, laboratory data, and other factors unique to the patient. The publisher does not provide medical advice or guidance, and this work is merely a reference tool. Healthcare professionals, and not the publisher, are solely responsible for the use of this work including all medical judgments and for any resulting diagnosis and treatments.

   Given continuous, rapid advances in medical science and health information, independent professional verification of medical diagnoses, indications, appropriate pharmaceutical selections and dosages, and treatment options should be made and healthcare professionals should consult a variety of sources. When prescribing medication, healthcare professionals are advised to consult the product information sheet (the manufacturer's package insert) accompanying each drug to verify, among other things, conditions of use, warnings, and side effects and identify any changes in dosage schedule or contraindications, particularly if the medication to be administered is new, infrequently used, or has a narrow therapeutic range. To the maximum extent permitted under applicable law, no responsibility is assumed by the publisher for any injury and/or damage to persons or property as a matter of products liability, negligence law or otherwise, or from any reference to or use by any person of this work.

LWW.com

CONTRIBUTORS

Gregory P. Adams, PhD
Associate Professor, Developmental
  Therapeutics Program
Director of Biological Research and
  Therapeutics
Fox Chase Cancer Center
Philadelphia, Pennsylvania

Anupriya Agarwal, PhD
Research Assistant Professor
The Knight Cancer Center
Oregon Health & Science University
Portland, Oregon

Bharat B. Aggarwal, PhD
Professor of Cancer Research
Professor of Cancer Medicine
  (Biochemistry)
Chief, Cytokine Research Laboratory
Department of Experimental
  Therapeutics
The University of Texas MD Anderson
  Cancer Center
Houston, Texas

Kenneth C. Anderson, MD
Director, Jerome Lipper Multiple
  Myeloma Center and
Lebow Institute for Myeloma
  Therapeutics
American Cancer Society
Clinical Research Professor
Kraft Family Professor of Medicine
Dana-Farber Cancer Institute
Harvard Medical School
Boston, Massachusetts

Stephen Ansell, MD, PhD
Professor, Division of Hematology
Mayo Clinic
Rochester, Minnesota

Shirin Arastu-Kapur, PhD
Associate Director
Biology at Onyx Pharmaceuticals
South San Francisco, California

Alan Ashworth, FRS
Professor and Chief Executive
The Institute of Cancer Research
London, United Kingdom

Jon C. Aster, MD, PhD
Professor, Department of Pathology
Harvard Medical School
Head, Division of Hematopathology
Brigham and Women's Hospital
Boston, Massachusetts

Sharyn D. Baker, PharmD, PhD
Associate Member
Pharmaceutical Sciences Department
St. Jude Children's Research Hospital
Memphis, Tennessee

Alberto Bardelli, MD
Laboratory of Molecular Genetics
Institute for Cancer Research and
  Treatment
University of Torino Medical School
Candiolo, Italy

Tracy T. Batchelor, MD
Giovanni Armenise—Harvard Professor of
  Neurology
Harvard Medical School
Chief, Division of Neuro-Oncology
Massachusetts General Hospital Cancer
  Center
Co-Leader, Neuro-Oncology Program
Dana-Farber/Harvard Cancer Center
Boston, Massachusetts

Susan E. Bates, MD
Head, Molecular Therapeutics Section
Developmental Therapeutics Branch
Center for Cancer Research
National Cancer Institute
Bethesda, Maryland

Stephen B. Baylin, MD
Professor of Oncology
Professor of Medicine
Johns Hopkins University School of
  Medicine
Deputy Director of the Cancer Center
Baltimore, Maryland

Andrew Berchuck, MD
Professor and Director
Gynecologic Oncology Program
Division of Gynecologic Oncology
Department of Obstetrics and
  Gynecology
Duke Cancer Institute
Duke University Medical Center
Durham, North Carolina

Leslie Bernstein, MS, PhD
Professor and Director
Division of Cancer Etiology
Department of Population Sciences
Beckman Research Institute
City of Hope Dean for Faculty Affairs
City of Hope National Medical Center
  and the Beckman Research Institute
Duarte, California

Bryan L. Betz, PhD
Assistant Professor
Department of Pathology
University of Michigan
Technical Director
Molecular Diagnostics Laboratory
University of Michigan Health System
Ann Arbor, Michigan

James S. Blachly, MD
Fellow, Division of Hematology
Department of Internal Medicine
The Ohio State University
Columbus, Ohio

Lawrence H. Boise, PhD
Professor
Winship Cancer Institute of Emory
  University
Departments of Hematology/Medical
  Oncology and Cell Biology
Emory School of Medicine
Atlanta, Georgia

Danielle C. Bonadies, MS, CGC
Director, Cancer Genetics Division
Gene Counsel, LLC
New Haven, Connecticut

Hossein Borghaei, MS, DO
Associate Professor
Chief, Thoracic Medical Oncology
Fox Chase Cancer Center
Philadelphia, Pennsylvania

Otis W. Brawley, MD, FACP
Chief Medical Officer
American Cancer Society, Inc.
Atlanta, Georgia

Dean E. Brenner, MD
Kutsche Family Professor of Internal
  Medicine
Professor of Pharmacology
University of Michigan Comprehensive
  Cancer Center
Ann Arbor, Michigan

Contributors

Christopher B. Buck, PhD
Investigator
Head, Tumor Virus Molecular Biology Section
Laboratory of Cellular Oncology
Center for Cancer Research
National Cancer Institute
Bethesda, Maryland

Tim E. Byers, MD, MPH
Associate Dean for Public Health Practice
Colorado School of Public Health
Associate Director for Cancer Prevention and Control
University of Colorado Cancer Center
Aurora, Colorado

John C. Byrd, MD
D. Warren Brown Chair of Leukemia Research
Director, Division of Hematology
Department of Internal Medicine
The Ohio State Comprehensive Cancer Center
Columbus, Ohio

A. Hilary Calvert
Professor
Gynecologic Oncology
University College Hospitals (UCLH)
London, United Kingdom

Antonino Carbone, MD
Professor and Chairman of the Department of Pathology, Centro di Riferimento Oncologico Aviano (CRO)
Instituto Nazionale dei Tumori, IRCCS
Aviano, Italy

Jan Cerny, MD, PhD
Assistant Professor of Medicine
Division of Hematology
Department of Medicine
Director, Leukemia Program
University of Massachusetts Medical School
Associate Director, Cancer Research Office
UMass Memorial Cancer Center
University of Massachusetts
Worcester, Massachusetts

Richard Champlin, MD
Professor of Medicine and Chairman
Department of Stem Cell Transplantation and Cellular Therapy
The University of Texas MD Anderson Cancer Center
Houston, Texas

Cindy H. Chau, PharmD, PhD
Scientist
Medical Oncology Branch
Center for Cancer Research
National Cancer Institute
National Institutes of Health
Bethesda, Maryland

Edward Chu, MD
Professor of Medicine and Pharmacology & Chemical Biology
Chief, Division of Hematology-Oncology
Deputy Director, University of Pittsburgh Cancer Institute
University of Pittsburgh School of Medicine
Pittsburgh, Pennsylvania

Jessica Clague, PhD, MPH
Assistant Research Professor
Division of Cancer Etiology
Department of Population Sciences
Beckman Research Institute
City of Hope National Medical Center
Duarte, California

M. Sitki Copur, MD, FACP
Medical Director of Oncology
Saint Francis Cancer Treatment Center
Grand Island, Nebraska
Professor, Department of Medicine
Division of Hematology Oncology
Adjunct Faculty
University of Nebraska Medical Center
Omaha, Nebraska

Bouthaina Dabaja, MD
Associate Professor and Section Chief, Hematology
Department of Radiation Oncology
The University of Texas MD Anderson Cancer Center
Houston, Texas

Riccardo Dalla-Favera, MD
Professor of Pathology and Cell Biology
Director, Institute for Cancer Genetics
Columbia University
New York, New York

Marcos de Lima, MD
Professor of Medicine
University Hospitals
Case Medical Center
Case Western Reserve University
Cleveland, Ohio

Hari A. Deshpande, MD
Associate Professor of Medicine
Yale University School of Medicine
Section of Medical Oncology
Yale New Haven Hospital
New Haven, Connecticut

Khanh T. Do, MD
Senior Clinical Fellow
Division of Cancer Treatment and Diagnosis
National Cancer Institute
National Institutes of Health
Bethesda, Maryland

James H. Doroshow, MD
Director, Division of Cancer Treatment and Diagnosis
Deputy Director for Clinical and Translational Research
National Cancer Institute
National Institutes of Health
Bethesda, Maryland

Brian J. Druker, MD
Director, Oregon Health & Science University
Knight Cancer Institute
JELD-WEN Chair of Leukemia Research
Oregon Health & Science University
Investigator, Howard Hughes Medical Institute
Portland, Oregon

Richard L. Edelson, MD
Aaron B. & Marguerite Lerner Professor of Dermatology
Yale School of Medicine
New Haven, Connecticut

Christopher A. Eide, BA
Research Technician III
Howard Hughes Medical Institute
Division of Hematology and Medical Oncology
Oregon Health & Science University
Knight Cancer Institute
Portland, Oregon

Charles Erlichman, MD
Professor, Department of Oncology
Deputy Director, Clinical Research
Peter and Frances Georgeson Professor of Gastroenterology Cancer Research
Mayo Clinic
Rochester, Minnesota

Elihu H. Estey, MD
Professor, Division of Hematology
University of Washington School of Medicine
Member and Director of Acute Myeloid Leukemia Clinical Research (Nontransplant)
Clinical Research Division
Fred Hutchinson Cancer Research Center
Seattle, Washington

Steven A. Feldman, PhD
Staff Scientist
Director, Surgery Branch
Vector Production Facility
National Cancer Institute
Bethesda, Maryland

William Douglas Figg, Sr., PharmD, MBA
Senior Investigator and Head of the Clinical Pharmacology Program
Clinical Director, Center for Cancer Research
Head of the Molecular Pharmacology Section
Medical Oncology Branch
Center for Cancer Research
National Cancer Institute
National Institutes of Health
Bethesda, Maryland

Antonio Tito Fojo, MD, PhD
Medical Oncology Branch and Affiliates
Head, Experimental Therapeutics Section
Senior Investigator
Center for Cancer Research
National Cancer Institute
Bethesda, Maryland

Francine M. Foss, MD
Professor of Medicine, Hematology and Bone Marrow Transplantation
Yale University School of Medicine
New Haven, Connecticut

Arnold S. Freedman, MD
Associate Professor of Medicine
Harvard Medical School
Clinical Director, Lymphoma Program
Dana-Farber Cancer Institute
Associate Physician, Brigham and Women's Hospital
Boston, Massachusetts

Larissa V. Furtado, MD
Assistant Professor
Department of Pathology
Assistant Director
Division of Genomics and Molecular Pathology
University of Chicago
Chicago, Illinois

Sheryl G. A. Gabram-Mendola, MD, MBA, FACS
Surgeon-in-Chief
Grady Memorial Hospital
Emory University School of Medicine
Deputy Director
Georgia Cancer Center for Excellence
Director, AVON Comprehensive Breast Center at Grady
Director, High Risk Assessment Program
Winship Cancer Institute of Emory University
Georgia Cancer Coalition Distinguished Cancer Scholar
Atlanta, Georgia

Jared J. Gartner, DO
Biologist, National Cancer Institute
Surgery Branch
National Institute of Health
Bethesda, Maryland

Scott Nicholas Gettinger, MD
Associate Professor of Medicine
Thoracic Oncology Program
Developmental Therapeutics
Yale Cancer Center
New Haven, Connecticut

Juliet F. Gibson, BA
Research Fellow
Dermatology and Hematology
Yale University School of Medicine
New Haven, Connecticut

Matthew P. Goetz, MD
Associate Professor of Pharmacology
Associate Professor of Oncology
Mayo Clinic
Rochester, Minnesota

Sarah B. Goldberg, MD, MPH
Assistant Professor of Internal Medicine
Medical Oncology
Yale Cancer Center
Yale University School of Medicine
New Haven, Connecticut

Steven D. Gore, MD
Yale University School of Medicine
New Haven, Connecticut

Ellen R. Gritz, PhD
Professor and Chair
Department of Behavioral Science
The University of Texas MD Anderson Cancer Center
Houston, Texas

José G. Guillem, MD, MPH
Department of Surgery
Memorial Sloan-Kettering Cancer Center
New York, New York

Douglas Hanahan, PhD
Director
Swiss Institute for Experimental Cancer Research (ISREC)
Lausanne, Switzerland

Lyndsay N. Harris, MD, FRCP(C)
Diana Hyland Chair in Breast Cancer
Director, Breast Cancer Program
Seidman Cancer Center
University Hospitals Case Medical Center
Professor of Medicine
Division of Hematology and Oncology
Case Western Reserve University
Cleveland, Ohio

James G. Herman, MD
Johns Hopkins University
Baltimore, Maryland

Jay L. Hess, MD, PhD
Professor, Department of Pathology
Carl V. Weller Professor and Chair
Professor, Department of Internal Medicine
University of Michigan Health System
Ann Arbor, Michigan

Christopher J. Hoimes, DO
Assistant Professor
UH Case Medical Center
Department of Medicine-Hematology and Oncology
Cleveland, Ohio

Vanessa W. Hui, MD
Department of Surgery
Memorial Sloan-Kettering Cancer Center
New York, New York

Caron A. Jacobson, MD, MSc
Instructor, Department of Medicine
Harvard Medical School
Brigham and Women's Hospital
Division of Medical Oncology
Hematologic Malignancies
Dana-Farber Cancer Institute
Boston, Massachusetts

Peter Johnson, MD, FRCP
Professor of Medical Oncology
Cancer Research United Kingdom Centre
University of Southampton Faculty of Medicine
Southampton, United Kingdom

Kala Y. Kamdar, MD, MS
Assistant Professor
Department of Pediatrics
Hematology/Oncology Section
Baylor College of Medicine
Associate Clinical Director
Texas Children's Cancer and Hematology Center
Houston, Texas

Partow Kebriaei, MD
Associate Professor
Division of Cancer Medicine
Department of Stem Cell Transplant and Cellular Therapy
The University of Texas MD Anderson Cancer Center
Houston, Texas

Christopher J. Kirk, MD
Vice President of Research
Onyx Pharmaceuticals, Inc.
South San Francisco, California

James N. Kochenderfer, MD
Investigator, Experimental Transplantation and Immunology Branch
National Cancer Institute
National Institutes of Health
Bethesda, Maryland

Manish Kohli, MD
Associate Professor of Oncology
Department of Oncology
College of Medicine
Mayo Clinic
Joint Appointment, Department of Urology
Mayo Clinic
Rochester, Minnesota

Rami S. Komrokji, MD
Clinical Director
Associate Member
Department of Malignant Hematology
H. Lee Moffitt Cancer Center &
 Research Institute
Tampa, Florida

Shivaani Kummar, MD, FACP
Head, Early Clinical Trials Development
Office of the Director
Division of Cancer Treatment and
 Diagnosis
National Cancer Institute
Bethesda, Maryland

John Kuruvilla, MD, FRCPC
Hematologist, Princess Margaret Cancer
 Centre
Assistant Professor Medicine
University of Toronto
Toronto, Ontario, Canada

Theodore S. Lawrence, MD, PhD
Isadore Lampe Professor and Chair
Department of Radiation Oncology
University of Michigan Health System
Ann Arbor, Michigan

Scott M. Lippman, MD
Director, Senior Associate Dean, &
 Associate Vice Chancellor
Cancer Research and Care
Chugai Pharmaceutical Chair
Professor of Medicine
University of California, San Diego
Moores Cancer Center
La Jolla, California

Alan F. List, MD
President and CEO
Senior Member
H. Lee Moffitt Cancer Center
Tampa, Florida

Mats Ljungman, PhD
Professor, Departments of Radiation
 Oncology and Environmental Health
 Sciences
Translational Oncology Program
University of Michigan Medical School
Ann Arbor, Michigan

Carlos López-Otin, PhD
Professor, Department of Biochemistry
 and Molecular Biology
Universidad de Oviedo
Principality of Asturias, Spain

Charles L. Loprinzi, MD
Regis Professor of Breast Cancer Research
Department of Oncology
Mayo Clinic
Rochester, Minnesota

Yani Lu, PhD
Assistant Research Professor
Division of Cancer Etiology
Department of Population Science
Beckman Research Institute of the City
 of Hope
Duarte, California

Xiaomei Ma, PhD
Associate Professor, Department of
 Chronic Disease Epidemiology
Yale University School of Public Health
New Haven, Connecticut

Judith F. Margolin, MD
Associate Professor
Department of Pediatrics
Baylor College of Medicine
Attending Oncologist
Texas Children's Cancer Center
Houston, Texas

David Marin, MD, DM, FRCP
Department of Stem Cell Transplantation
 and Cellular Therapy
The University of Texas MD Anderson
 Cancer Center
Houston, Texas

Ellen T. Matloff, MS, CGC
President & CEO
Gene Counsel, LLC
New Haven, Connecticut

Peter Mauch, MD
Professor of Radiation Oncology
Department of Radiation Oncology
Harvard Medical School
Boston, Massachusetts

Susan T. Mayne, PhD
C.-E.A. Winslow Professor of
 Epidemiology
Chair, Department of Chronic Disease
 Epidemiology
Yale University School of Public Health
Associate Director for Population
 Sciences
Yale Cancer Center
New Haven, Connecticut

Howard L. McLeod, PharmD
Medical Director, DeBartolo Family
 Personalized Medicine Institute
Senior Member, Division of Population
 Sciences
H. Lee Moffitt Cancer Center
Tampa, Florida

Karin B. Michels, ScD, PhD
Associate Professor
Obstetrician/Gynecologist
Epidemiology Center
Department of Obstetrics, Gynecology
 and Reproductive Biology
Brigham and Women's Hospital
Harvard Medical School
Boston, Massachusetts

Jeffrey F. Moley, MD
Chief, Section of Endocrine and
 Oncologic Surgery
Professor of Surgery
Washington University School of
 Medicine
St. Louis, Missouri

Meredith A. Morgan, PhD
Research Assistant Professor
Department of Radiation Oncology
University of Michigan
Ann Arbor, Michigan

Nikhil C. Munshi, MD
Associate Director, Jerome Lipper
 Multiple Myeloma Center
Department of Medical Oncology
Dana-Farber Cancer Institute
Associate Professor of Medicine
Harvard Medical School
Boston, Massachusetts

Jeffrey A. Norton, MD
Professor, Department of Surgery
Chief, Section of Surgical Oncology and
 Division of General Surgery
Department of Surgery
Stanford University Hospital
Stanford, California

Susan M. O'Brien, MD
Professor, Department of Leukemia
The University of Texas MD Anderson
 Cancer Center
Houston, Texas

Richard J. O'Connor, PhD
Associate Member, Department of Health
 Behavior
Division of Cancer Prevention and
 Population Sciences
Roswell Park Cancer Institute
Buffalo, New York

Peter J. O'Dwyer, MD
Professor of Medicine
Abramson Cancer Center
University of Pennsylvania
Philadelphia, Pennsylvania

Eric Padron, MD
Assistant Member
Malignant Hematology Section
Head, Genomics and Personalized
 Medicine
H. Lee Moffitt Cancer Center and
 Research Institute
Tampa, Florida

Howard L. Parnes, MD
Chief
Prostate and Urologic Cancer Research
 Group
Division of Cancer Prevention
National Cancer Institute
Rockville, Maryland

Laura Pasqualucci, MD
Associate Professor of Pathology and Cell Biology
Department of Pathology and Cell Biology
Institute for Cancer Genetics
Herbert Irving Comprehensive Cancer Center
Columbia University
New York, New York

Giao Q. Phan, MD, FACS
Associate Professor
Division of Surgical Oncology
Massey Cancer Center
Virginia Commonwealth University
Richmond, Virginia

Yves Pommier, MD, PhD
Chief, Laboratory of Molecular Pharmacology
Head, DNA Topoisomerase/Integrase Group
Center for Cancer Research
National Cancer Institute
Bethesda, Maryland

David G. Poplack, MD
Elise C. Young Professor of Pediatric Oncology
Head, Hematology-Oncology Section
Department of Pediatrics
Baylor College of Medicine
Director, Texas Children's Cancer Center
Texas Children's Hospital
Houston, Texas

Sahdeo Prasad, PhD
Cytokine Research Laboratory
Department of Experimental Therapeutics
The University of Texas MD Anderson Cancer Center
Houston, Texas

Karen R. Rabin, MD, PhD
Assistant Professor, Department of Pediatrics
Division of Pediatric Hematology and Oncology
Baylor College of Medicine
Houston, Texas

Glen D. Raffel, MD, PhD
Assistant Professor, Department of Medicine
Division of Hematology-Oncology
University of Massachusetts Medical School
Worcester, Massachusetts

Lee Ratner, MD, PhD
Professor Departments of Medicine and Molecular Microbiology
Co-Director, Medical & Molecular Oncology
Washington University School of Medicine
Barnes-Jewish Hospital
St. Louis, Missouri

Paul F. Robbins, PhD
National Institutes of Health
Bethesda, Maryland

Matthew K. Robinson, PhD
Assistant Professor, Developmental Therapeutics Program
Fox Chase Cancer Center
Philadelphia, Pennsylvania

Steven A. Rosenberg, MD, PhD
Chief, Surgery Branch, National Cancer Institute, National Institutes of Health
Professor of Surgery, Uniformed Services University of the Health Sciences
School of Medicine
Bethesda, Maryland
Professor of Surgery
George Washington University School of Medicine
Washington, District of Columbia

M. Wasif Saif, MD, MBBS
Director, Gastrointestinal Oncology Program
Leader, Experimental Therapeutics Program
Tufts Medical Center
Tufts University School of Medicine
Boston, Massachusetts

Yardena Samuels, PhD
Knell Family Professorial Chair
Department of Molecular Cell Biology
Weizmann Institute of Science
Rehovot, Israel

Charles L. Sawyers, MD
Investigator, Howard Hughes Medical Institute
Chair, Human Oncology and Pathogenesis Program
Memorial Sloan-Kettering Cancer Center
New York, New York

Peter G. Shields, MD
Deputy Director, Comprehensive Cancer Center
Professor, College of Medicine
James Cancer Hospital
The Ohio State University
Columbus, Ohio

Alex Sparreboom, PhD
Associate Member, Department of Pharmaceutical Sciences
St. Jude Children's Research Hospital
Memphis, Tennessee

Irene M. Tamí-Maury, DMD, DrPH, MSc
The University of Texas MD Anderson Cancer Center
Houston, Texas

Randall K. Ten Haken, PhD, FAAPM, FInstP, FASTRO, FACR
Professor, Associate Chair, and Physics Division Director
Department of Radiation Oncology
University of Michigan Medical School
Ann Arbor, Michigan

Kenneth D. Tew, PhD, DSc
Chairman and John C. West Chair in Cancer Research
Cell and Molecular Pharmacology
Medical University of South Carolina
Charleston, South Carolina

Benjamin A. Toll, PhD
Associate Professor of Psychiatry
Yale University School of Medicine
Yale Comprehensive Cancer Center
Program Director, Smoking Cessation Service
Smilow Cancer Hospital at Yale-New Haven
New Haven, Connecticut

Brian B. Tuch, PhD
Associate Director, Translational Genomics
Onyx Pharmaceuticals
South San Francisco, California

Christine M. Walko, PharmD, BCOP
Clinical Pharmacogenetic Scientist
DeBartolo Family Personalized Medicine Institute
Applied Clinical Scientist, Division of Population Science
H. Lee Moffitt Cancer Center and Research Institute
Tampa, Florida

Graham W. Warren, MD, PhD
Associate Professor
Vice Chair for Research in Radiation Oncology
Department of Radiation Oncology
Department of Cell and Molecular Pharmacology
Hollings Cancer Center
Medical University of South Carolina
Charleston, South Carolina

Robert A. Weinberg, PhD
Member, Whitehead Institute for Biomedical Research
Department of Biology
Massachusetts Institute of Technology
Director, Ludwig Center for Molecular Oncology
Whitehead Institute for Biomedical Research
Cambridge, Massachusetts

Louis M. Weiner, MD
Director, Lombardi Comprehensive Cancer Center
Professor and Chair, Department of Oncology
Francis L. and Charlotte G. Gragnani Chair
Georgetown University Medical Center
Washington, District of Columbia

William G. Wierda, MD, PhD
Professor, Department of Leukemia
The University of Texas MD Anderson Cancer Center
Houston, Texas

Walter C. Willett, MD, DrPH
Professor and Chair, Department of Nutrition
Harvard School of Public Health
Boston, Massachusetts

Lynn D. Wilson, MD, MPH
Professor, Vice Chairman, and Clinical Director
Department of Therapeutic Radiology
Yale University School of Medicine
New Haven, Connecticut

Anas Younes, MD
Professor, Department of Medicine
Chief, Lymphoma Service
Memorial Sloan-Kettering Cancer Center
New York, New York

Herbert Yu, MD, PhD
Professor and Director
Cancer Epidemiology Program
Associate Director for Population Sciences and Cancer Control
University of Hawaii Cancer Center
Adjunct Professor, Department of Chronic Disease Epidemiology
Yale School of Public Health
Honolulu, Hawaii

Stuart H. Yuspa, MD
Chief, Laboratory of Cancer Biology and Genetics
Center for Cancer Research
National Cancer Institute
Bethesda, Maryland

CONTENTS

Contributors v

PART I
Principles of Oncology

1. The Cancer Genome 2
Yardena Samuels, Alberto Bardelli, Jared J. Gartner, and Carlos López-Otin

2. Hallmarks of Cancer: An Organizing Principle for Cancer Medicine 24
Douglas Hanahan and Robert A. Weinberg

3. Molecular Methods in Cancer 47
Larissa V. Furtado, Jay L. Hess, and Bryan L. Betz

PART II
Etiology and Epidemiology of Cancer

SECTION 1. ETIOLOGY OF CANCER

4. Tobacco 64
Richard J. O'Connor

5. Oncogenic Viruses 73
Christopher B. Buck and Lee Ratner

6. Inflammation 88
Sahdeo Prasad and Bharat B. Aggarwal

7. Chemical Factors 95
Stuart H. Yuspa and Peter G. Shields

8. Physical Factors 102
Mats Ljungman

9. Dietary Factors 110
Karin B. Michels and Walter C. Willett

10. Obesity and Physical Activity 123
Yani Lu, Jessica Clague, and Leslie Bernstein

SECTION 2. EPIDEMIOLOGY OF CANCER

11. Epidemiologic Methods 130
Xiaomei Ma and Herbert Yu

12. Trends in United States Cancer Mortality 138
Tim E. Byers

PART III
Cancer Therapeutics

13. Essentials of Radiation Therapy 145
Meredith A. Morgan, Randall K. Ten Haken, and Theodore S. Lawrence

14. Cancer Immunotherapy 167
Steven A. Rosenberg, Paul F. Robbins, Giao Q. Phan, Steven A. Feldman, and James N. Kochenderfer

15. Pharmacokinetics and Pharmacodynamics of Anticancer Drugs 186
Alex Sparreboom and Sharyn D. Baker

16. Pharmacogenomics 196
Christine M. Walko and Howard L. McLeod

17. Alkylating Agents 203
Kenneth D. Tew

18. Platinum Analogs 214
Peter J. O'Dwyer and A. Hilary Calvert

19. Antimetabolites 223
M. Wasif Saif and Edward Chu

20. Topoisomerase Interactive Agents 233
Khanh T. Do, Shivaani Kummar, James H. Doroshow, and Yves Pommier

21. Antimicrotubule Agents 245
Christopher J. Hoimes and Lyndsay N. Harris

22. Kinase Inhibitors as Anticancer Drugs 255
Charles L. Sawyers

23. Histone Deacetylase Inhibitors and Demethylating Agents 267
Steven D. Gore, Stephen B. Baylin, and James G. Herman

24. Proteasome Inhibitors............ 279
Christopher J. Kirk, Brian B. Tuch, Shirin Arastu-Kapur, and Lawrence H. Boise

25. Poly (ADP-ribose) Polymerase Inhibitors... 285
Alan Ashworth

26. Miscellaneous Chemotherapeutic Agents.. 290
M. Sitki Copur, Scott Nicholas Gettinger, Sarah B. Goldberg, and Hari A. Deshpande

27. Hormonal Agents................. 302
Matthew P. Goetz, Charles Erlichman, Charles L. Loprinzi, and Manish Kohli

28. Antiangiogenesis Agents............ 317
Cindy H. Chau and William Douglas Figg, Sr.

29. Monoclonal Antibodies.............. 329
Hossein Borghaei, Matthew K. Robinson, Gregory P. Adams, and Louis M. Weiner

30. Assessment of Clinical Response........ 339
Antonio Tito Fojo and Susan E. Bates

PART IV
Cancer Prevention and Screening

31. Tobacco Use and the Cancer Patient...... 352
Graham W. Warren, Benjamin A. Toll, Irene M. Tamí-Maury, and Ellen R. Gritz

32. Role of Surgery in Cancer Prevention..... 368
José G. Guillem, Andrew Berchuck, Jeffrey F. Moley, Jeffrey A. Norton, Sheryl G. A. Gabram-Mendola, and Vanessa W. Hui

33. Cancer Risk–Reducing Agents.......... 384
Dean E. Brenner, Scott M. Lippman, and Susan T. Mayne

34. Cancer Screening.................. 407
Otis W. Brawley and Howard L. Parnes

35. Genetic Counseling................ 426
Ellen T. Matloff and Danielle C. Bonadies

PART V
Lymphomas and Leukemias

SECTION 1. LEUKEMIAS AND LYMPHOMAS IN CHILDREN

36. Leukemias and Lymphomas of Childhood............ 436
Karen R. Rabin, Judith F. Margolin, Kala Y. Kamdar, and David G. Poplack

SECTION 2. LYMPHOMAS IN ADULTS

37. Molecular Biology of Lymphomas........ 449
Laura Pasqualucci and Riccardo Dalla-Favera

38. Hodgkin's Lymphoma............... 469
Anas Younes, Antonino Carbone, Peter Johnson, Bouthaina Dabaja, Stephen Ansell, and John Kuruvilla

39. Non-Hodgkin's Lymphoma............ 495
Arnold S. Freedman, Caron A. Jacobson, Peter Mauch, and Jon C. Aster

40. Cutaneous Lymphomas.............. 531
Francine M. Foss, Juliet F. Gibson, Richard L. Edelson, and Lynn D. Wilson

41. Primary Central Nervous System Lymphoma................... 545
Tracy T. Batchelor

SECTION 3. LEUKEMIAS AND PLASMA CELL TUMORS

42. Molecular Biology of Acute Leukemias.... 550
Glen D. Raffel and Jan Cerny

43. Management of Acute Leukemias........ 565
Partow Kebriaei, Marcos de Lima, Elihu H. Estey, and Richard Champlin

44. Molecular Biology of Chronic Leukemias.. 589
James S. Blachly, Christopher A. Eide, John C. Byrd, and Anupriya Agarwal

45. Chronic Myelogenous Leukemia......... 598
Brian J. Druker and David Marin

46. Chronic Lymphocytic Leukemias........ 609
William G. Wierda and Susan M. O'Brien

47. Myelodysplastic Syndromes............ 627
Rami S. Komrokji, Eric Padron, and Alan F. List

48. Plasma Cell Neoplasms............... 640
Nikhil C. Munshi and Kenneth C. Anderson

Index.............................. 682

PART I

Principles of Oncology

1 The Cancer Genome

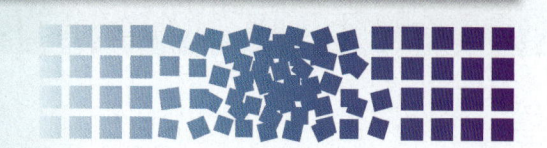

Yardena Samuels, Alberto Bardelli, Jared J. Gartner, and Carlos López-Otín

INTRODUCTION

There is a broad consensus that cancer is, in essence, a genetic disease, and that accumulation of molecular alterations in the genome of somatic cells is the basis of cancer progression (Fig. 1.1).[1] In the past 10 years, the availability of the human genome sequence and progress in DNA sequencing technologies has dramatically improved knowledge of this disease. These new insights are transforming the field of oncology at multiple levels:

1. The genomic maps are redesigning the tumor taxonomy by moving it from a histologic- to a genetic-based level.
2. The success of cancer drugs designed to target the molecular alterations underlying tumorigenesis has proven that somatic genetic alterations are legitimate targets for therapy.
3. Tumor genotyping is helping clinicians individualize treatments by matching patients with the best treatment for their tumors.
4. Tumor-specific DNA alterations represent highly sensitive biomarkers for disease detection and monitoring.
5. Finally, the ongoing analyses of multiple cancer genomes will identify additional targets, whose pharmacologic exploitation will undoubtedly result in new therapeutic approaches.

This chapter will review the progress that has been made in understanding the genetic basis of sporadic cancers. An emphasis will be placed on an introduction to novel integrated genomic approaches that allow a comprehensive and systematic evaluation of genetic alterations that occur during the progression of cancer. Using these powerful tools, cancer research, diagnosis, and treatment are poised for a transformation in the next years.

CANCER GENES AND THEIR MUTATIONS

Cancer genes are broadly grouped into oncogenes and tumor suppressor genes. Using a classical analogy, oncogenes can be compared to a car accelerator, so that a mutation in an oncogene would be the equivalent of having the accelerator continuously pressed.[2] Tumor suppressor genes, in contrast, act as brakes,[2] so that when they are not mutated, they function to inhibit tumorigenesis. Oncogene and tumor suppressor genes may be classified by the nature of their somatic mutations in tumors. Mutations in oncogenes typically occur at specific hotspots, often affecting the same codon or clustered at neighboring codons in different tumors.[1] Furthermore, mutations in oncogenes are almost always missense, and the mutations usually affect only one allele, making them heterozygous. In contrast, tumor suppressor genes are usually mutated throughout the gene; a large number of the mutations may truncate the encoded protein and generally affect both alleles, causing loss of heterozygosity (LOH). Major types of somatic mutations present in malignant tumors include nucleotide substitutions, small insertions and deletions (*indels*), chromosomal rearrangements, and copy number alterations.

IDENTIFICATION OF CANCER GENES

The completion of the Human Genome Project marked a new era in biomedical sciences.[3] Knowledge of the sequence and organization of the human genome now allows for the systematic analysis of the genetic alterations underlying the origin and evolution of tumors. Before elucidation of the human genome, several cancer genes, such as *KRAS*, *TP53*, and *APC*, were successfully discovered using approaches based on an oncovirus analysis, linkage studies, LOH, and cytogenetics.[4,5] The first curated version of the Human Genome Project was released in 2004,[3] and provided a sequence-based map of the normal human genome. This information, together with the construction of the HapMap, which contains single nucleotide polymorphisms (SNP), and the underlying genomic structure of natural human genomic variation,[6,7] allowed an extraordinary throughput in cataloging somatic mutations in cancer. These projects now offer an unprecedented opportunity: the identification of all the genetic changes associated with a human cancer. For the first time, this ambitious goal is within reach of the scientific community. Already, a number of studies have demonstrated the usefulness of strategies aimed at the systematic identification of somatic mutations associated with cancer progression. Notably, the Human Genome Project, the HapMap project, as well as the candidate and family gene approaches (described in the following paragraphs), utilized capillary-based DNA sequencing (first-generation sequencing, also known as Sanger sequencing).[8] Figure 1.2 clearly illustrates the developments in the search of cancer genes, its increased pace, as well as the most relevant findings in this field.

Cancer Gene Discovery by Sequencing Candidate Gene Families

The availability of the human genome sequence provides new opportunities to comprehensively search for somatic mutations in cancer on a larger scale than previously possible. Progress in the field has been closely linked to improvements in the throughput of DNA analysis and in the continuous reduction in sequencing costs. What follows are some of the achievements in this research area, as well as how they affected knowledge of the cancer genome.

A seminal work in the field was the systematic mutational profiling of the genes involved in the RAS-RAF pathway in multiple tumors. This candidate gene approach led to the discovery that *BRAF* is frequently mutated in melanomas and is mutated at a lower frequency in other tumor types.[9] Follow-up studies quickly revealed that mutations in *BRAF* are mutually exclusive with alterations in *KRAS*,[9,10] genetically emphasizing that these genes function in the same pathway, a concept that had been previously demonstrated in lower organisms such as *Caenorhabditis elegans* and *Drosophila melanogaster*.[11,12]

In 2003, the identification of cancer genes shifted from a candidate gene approach to the mutational analyses of gene families. The first gene families to be completely sequenced were those that

A metastatic cancer genome requires decades to develop

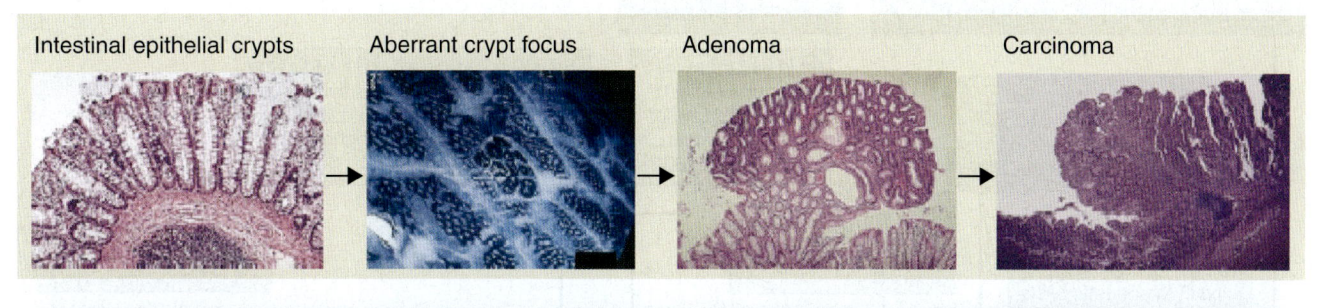

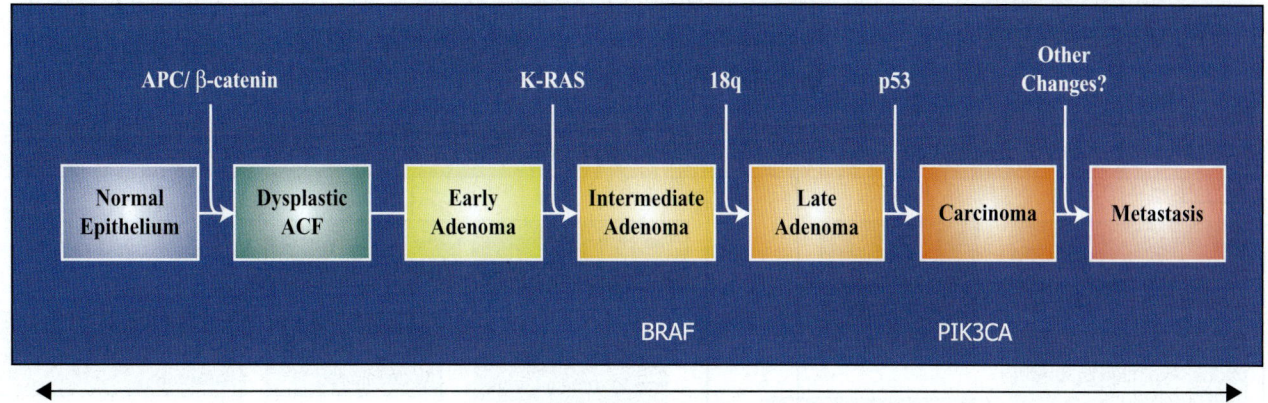

Figure 1.1 Schematic representation of the genomic and histopathologic steps associated with tumor progression: from the occurrence of the initiating mutation in the founder cell to metastasis formation. It has been convincingly shown that the genomic landscape of solid tumors such as that of pancreatic and colorectal tumors requires the accumulation of many genetic events, a process that requires decades to complete. This timeline offers an incredible window of opportunity for the early detection, which is often associated with an excellent prognosis, of this disease.

involved protein[13,14] and lipid phosphorylation.[15] The rationale for initially focusing on these gene families was threefold:

- The corresponding proteins were already known at that time to play a pivotal role in the signaling and proliferation of normal and cancerous cells.
- Multiple members of the protein kinases family had already been linked to tumorigenesis.
- Kinases are clearly amenable to pharmacologic inhibition, making them attractive drug targets.

The mutational analysis of all the tyrosine-kinase domains in colorectal cancers revealed that 30% of cases had a mutation in at least one tyrosine-kinase gene, and overall mutations were identified in eight different kinases, most of which had not previously been linked to cancer.[13] An additional mutational analysis of the coding exons of 518 protein kinase genes in 210 diverse human cancers, including breast, lung, gastric, ovarian, renal, and acute lymphoblastic leukemia, identified approximately 120 mutated genes that probably contribute to oncogenesis.[14] Because kinase activity is attenuated by enzymes that remove phosphate groups called phosphatases, the rational next step in these studies was to perform a mutation analysis of the protein tyrosine phosphatases. A mutational investigation of this family in colorectal cancer identified that 25% of cases had mutations in six different phosphatase genes (*PTPRF*, *PTPRG*, *PTPRT*, *PTPN3*, *PTPN13*, or *PTPN14*).[16] A combined analysis of the protein tyrosine kinases and the protein tyrosine phosphatases showed that 50% of colorectal cancers had mutations in a tyrosine-kinase gene, a protein tyrosine phosphatase gene, or both, further emphasizing the pivotal role of protein phosphorylation in neoplastic progression. Many of the identified genes had previously been linked to human cancer, thus validating

the unbiased comprehensive mutation profiling. These landmark studies led to additional gene family surveys.

The phosphatidylinositol 3-kinase (*PI3K*) gene family, which also plays a role in proliferation, adhesion, survival, and motility, was also comprehensively investigated.[17] Sequencing of the exons encoding the kinase domain of all 16 members belonging to this family pinpointed *PIK3CA* as the only gene to harbor somatic mutations. When the entire coding region was analyzed, *PIK3CA* was found to be somatically mutated in 32% of colorectal cancers. At that time, the *PIK3CA* gene was certainly not a newcomer in the cancer arena, because it had previously been shown to be involved in cell transformation and metastasis.[17] Strikingly, its staggeringly high mutation frequency was discovered only through systematic sequencing of the corresponding gene family.[15] Subsequent analysis of *PIK3CA* in other tumor types identified somatic mutations in this gene in additional cancer types, including 36% of hepatocellular carcinomas, 36% of endometrial carcinomas, 25% of breast carcinomas, 15% of anaplastic oligodendrogliomas, 5% of medulloblastomas and anaplastic astrocytomas, and 27% of glioblastomas.[18–22] It is known that *PIK3CA* is one of the two (the other being *KRAS*) most commonly mutated oncogenes in human cancers. Further investigation of the PI3K pathway in colorectal cancer showed that 40% of tumors had genetic alterations in one of the PI3K pathway genes, emphasizing the central role of this pathway in colorectal cancer pathogenesis.[23]

Although most cancer genome studies of large gene families have focused on the kinome, recent analyses have revealed that members of other families highly represented in the human genome are also a target of mutational events in cancer. This is the case of proteases, a complex group of enzymes consisting of at least 569 components that constitute the so-called human degradome.[24] Proteases exhibit an elaborate interplay with kinases and

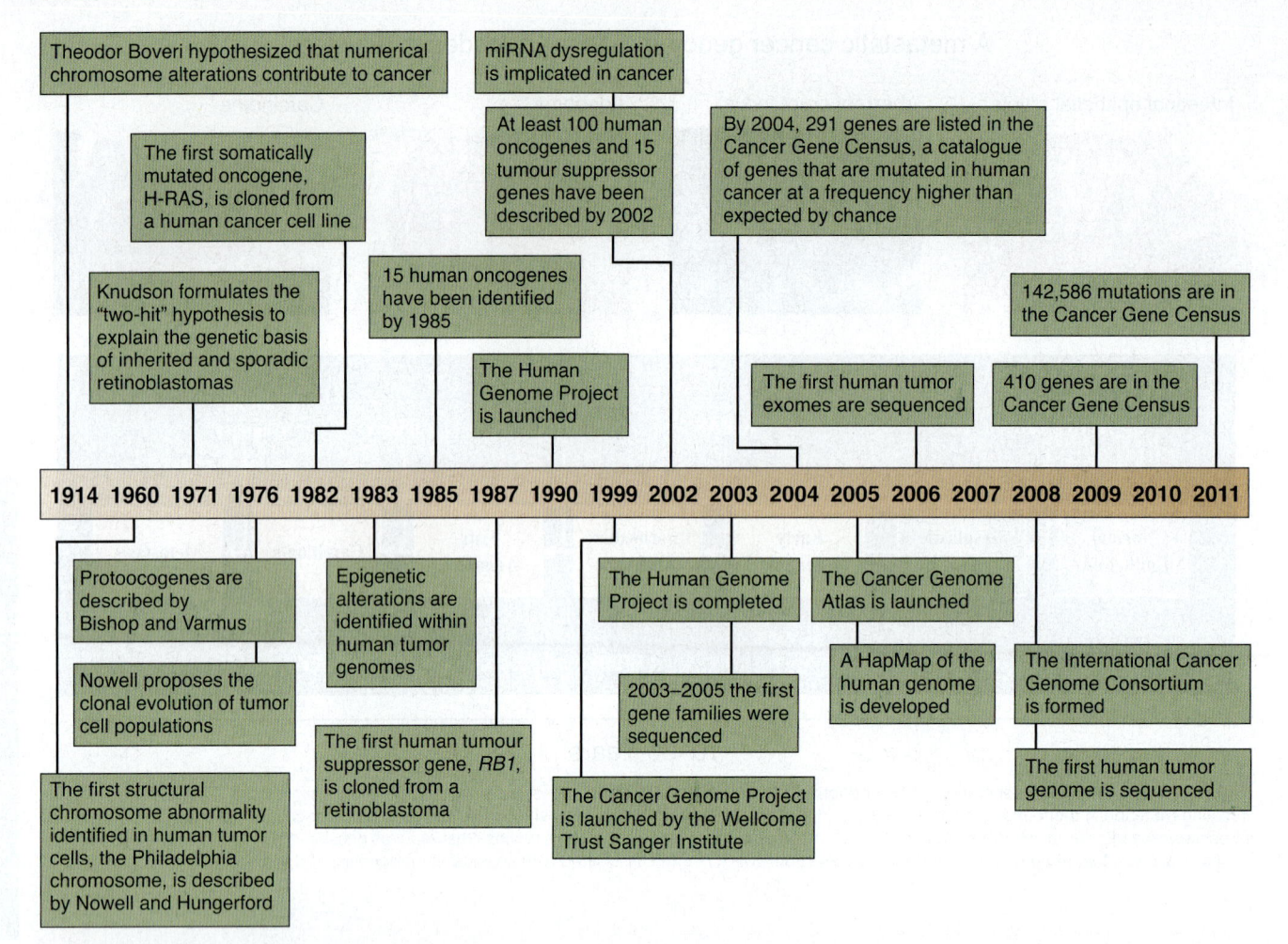

Figure 1.2 Timeline of seminal hypotheses, research discoveries, and research initiatives that have led to an improved understanding of the genetic etiology of human tumorigenesis within the past century. The consensus cancer gene data were obtained from the Wellcome Trust Sanger Institute Cancer Genome Project Web site (http://www.sanger.ac.uk/genetics/CGP). (Redrawn from Bell DW. Our changing view of the genomic landscape of cancer. *J Pathol* 2010;220:231–243.)

have traditionally been associated with cancer progression because of their ability to degrade extracellular matrices, thus facilitating tumor invasion and metastasis.[25,26] However, recent studies have shown that these enzymes hydrolyze a wide variety of substrates and influence many different steps of cancer, including early stages of tumor evolution.[27] These functional studies have also revealed that beyond their initial recognition as prometastatic enzymes, they play dual roles in cancer, as assessed by the identification of a growing number of tumor-suppressive proteases.[28]

These findings emphasized the possibility that mutational activation or inactivation of protease genes occurs in cancer. A systematic analysis of genetic alterations in breast and colorectal cancers revealed that proteases from different catalytic classes were somatically mutated in cancer.[29] These results prompted the mutational analysis of entire protease families such as matrix metalloproteinases (MMP), a disintegrin and metalloproteinase (ADAM), and ADAMs with thrombospondin domains (ADAMTS) in different tumors. These studies led to the identification of protease genes frequently mutated in cancer, such as *MMP8*, which is mutated and functionally inactivated in 6.3% of human melanomas.[30,31]

The mutational status of caspases has also been extensively analyzed in different tumors because these proteases play a fundamental role in the execution of apoptosis, one of the hallmarks of cancer.[32] These studies demonstrated that *CASP8* is deleted in neuroblastomas and inactivated by somatic mutations in a variety of human malignancies, including head and neck, colorectal, lung, and gastric carcinomas.[33–35] Other large protease families whose components are often mutated in cancer are the deubiquitinating enzymes (DUB), which catalyze the removal of ubiquitin and ubiquitin-like modifiers of their target proteins.[36] Some DUBs were initially identified as oncogenic proteins, but further work has shown that other deubiquitinases, such as CYLD, A20, and BAP1, are tumor suppressors inactivated in cancer. *CYLD* is mutated in patients with familial cylindromatosis, a disease characterized by the formation of multiple tumors of skin appendages.[37] A20 is a DUB family member encoded by the *TNFAIP3* gene, which is mutated in a large number of Hodgkin lymphomas and primary mediastinal B-cell lymphomas.[38–41] Finally, the *BAP1* gene, encoding an ubiquitin C-terminal hydrolase, is frequently mutated in metastasizing uveal melanomas[42] and in other human malignancies, such as mesothelioma and renal cell carcinoma.[43]

Mutational Analysis of Exomes Using Sanger Sequencing

Although the gene family approach for the identification of cancer genes has proven extremely valuable, it still is a candidate approach and thus biased in its nature. The next step forward in the mutational profiling of cancer has been the sequencing of exomes, which is the entire coding portion of the human genome (18,000 protein-encoding genes). The exomes of many different tumors—including breast, colorectal, pancreatic, and ovarian clear cell carcinomas; glioblastoma multiforme; and medulloblastoma—have been analyzed using Sanger sequencing. For the first time, these large-scale analyses allowed researchers to describe and understand the genetic complexity of human cancers.[29,44-48] The declared goals of these exome studies were to provide methods for exomewide mutational analyses in human tumors, to characterize their spectrum and quantity of somatic mutations, and, finally, to discover new genes involved in tumorigenesis as well as novel pathways that have a role in these tumors. In these studies, sequencing data were complemented with gene expression and copy number analyses, thus providing a comprehensive view of the genetic complexity of human tumors.[45-48] A number of conclusions can be drawn from these analyses, including the following:

- Cancer genomes have an average of 30 to 100 somatic alterations per tumor in coding regions, which was a higher number than previously thought. Although the alterations included point mutations, small insertions, deletions, or amplifications, the great majority of the mutations observed were single-base substitutions.[45,46]
- Even within a single cancer type, there is a significant intertumor heterogeneity. This means that multiple mutational patterns (encompassing different mutant genes) are present in tumors that cannot be distinguished based on histologic analysis. The concept that individual tumors have a unique genetic milieu is highly relevant for personalized medicine, a concept that will be further discussed.
- The spectrum and nucleotide contexts of mutations differ between different tumor types. For example, over 50% of mutations in colorectal cancer were C:G to T:A transitions, and 10% were C:G to G:C transversions. In contrast, in breast cancers, only 35% of the mutations were C:G to T:A transitions, and 29% were C:G to G:C transversions. Knowledge of mutation spectra is vital because it allows insight into the mechanisms underlying mutagenesis and repair in the various cancers investigated.
- A considerably larger number of genes that had not been previously reported to be involved in cancer were found to play a role in the disease.
- Solid tumors arising in children, such as medulloblastomas, harbor on average 5 to 10 times less gene alterations compared to a typical adult solid tumor. These pediatric tumors also harbor fewer amplifications and homozygous deletions within coding genes compared to adult solid tumors.

Importantly, to deal with the large amount of data generated in these genomic projects, it was necessary to develop new statistical and bioinformatic tools. Furthermore, an examination of the overall distribution of the identified mutations allowed for the development of a novel view of cancer genome landscapes and a novel definition of cancer genes. These new concepts in the understanding of cancer genetics are further discussed in the following paragraphs. The compiled conclusions derived from these analyses have led to a paradigm shift in the understanding of cancer genetics.

A clear indication of the power of the unbiased nature of the whole exome surveys was revealed by the discovery of recurrent mutations in the active site of *IDH1*, a gene with no known link to gliomas, in 12% of tumors analyzed.[46] Because malignant gliomas are the most common and lethal tumors of the central nervous system, and because glioblastoma multiforme (GBM; World Health Organization grade IV astrocytoma) is the most biologically aggressive subtype, the unveiling of *IDH1* as a novel GBM gene is extremely significant. Importantly, mutations of *IDH1* predominantly occurred in younger patients and were associated with a better prognosis.[49] Follow-up studies showed that mutations of *IDH1* occur early in glioma progression; the R132 somatic mutation is harbored by the majority (greater than 70%) of grades II and III astrocytomas and oligodendrogliomas, as well as in secondary GBMs that develop from these lower grade lesions.[49-55] In contrast, less than 10% of primary GBMs harbor these alterations. Furthermore, analysis of the associated *IDH2* revealed recurrent somatic mutations in the R172 residue, which is the exact analog of the frequently mutated R132 residue of *IDH1*. These mutations occur mostly in a mutually exclusive manner with *IDH1* mutations,[49,51] suggesting that they have equivalent phenotypic effects. Subsequently, *IDH1* mutations have been reported in additional cancer types, including hematologic neoplasias.[56-58]

Next-Generation Sequencing and Cancer Genome Analysis

In 1977, the introduction of the Sanger method for DNA sequencing with chain-terminating inhibitors transformed biomedical research.[8] Over the past 30 years, this first-generation technology has been universally used for elucidating the nucleotide sequence of DNA molecules. However, the launching of new large-scale projects, including those implicating whole-genome sequencing of cancer samples, has made necessary the development of new methods that are widely known as next-generation sequencing technologies.[59-61] These approaches have significantly lowered the cost and the time required to determine the sequence of the 3×10^9 nucleotides present in the human genome. Moreover, they have a series of advantages over Sanger sequencing, which are of special interest for the analysis of cancer genomes.[62] First, next-generation sequencing approaches are more sensitive than Sanger methods and can detect somatic mutations even when they are present in only a subset of tumor cells.[63] Moreover, these new sequencing strategies are quantitative and can be used to simultaneously determine both nucleotide sequence and copy number variations.[64] They can also be coupled to other procedures such as those involving paired-end reads, allowing for the identification of multiple structural alterations, such as insertions, deletions, and rearrangements, that commonly occur in cancer genomes.[63] Nonetheless, next-generation sequencing still presents some limitations that are mainly derived from the relatively high error rate in the short reads generated during the sequencing process. In addition, these short reads make the task of de novo assembly of the generated sequences and the mapping of the reads to a reference genome extremely complex. To overcome some of these current limitations, deep coverage of each analyzed genome is required and a careful validation of the identified variants must be performed, typically using Sanger sequencing. As a consequence, there is a substantial increase in both the cost of the process and in the time of analysis. Therefore, it can be concluded that whole-genome sequencing of cancer samples is already a feasible task, but not yet a routine process. Further technical improvements will be required before the task of decoding the entire genome of any malignant tumor of any cancer patient can be applied to clinical practice.

The number of next-generation sequencing platforms has substantially grown over the past few years and currently includes technologies from Roche/454, Illumina/Solexa, Life/APG's SOLiD3, Helicos BioSciences/HeliScope, and Pacific Biosciences/PacBio RS.[61] Noteworthy also are the recent introduction of the Polonator G.007 instrument, an open source platform with freely available software and protocols; the Ion Torrent's semiconductor sequencer; as well as those involving self-assembling DNA nanoballs or nanopore technologies.[65-67] These new machines are driving the field toward the era of third-generation sequencing, which brings enormous clinical interest because it can substantially increase the speed and accuracy of analyses at reduced costs and can facilitate the possibility of single-molecule sequencing of human genomes. A comparison of next-generation sequencing platforms is shown in Table 1.1. These various platforms differ in the method utilized for template preparation and in the nucleotide sequencing and imaging strategy, which finally result in their different performance. Ultimately, the most suitable approach depends on the specific genome sequencing projects.[61]

Current methods of template preparation first involve randomly shearing genomic DNA into smaller fragments, from which

TABLE 1.1

Comparative Analysis of Next-Generation Sequencing Platforms

Platform	Library/Template Preparation	Sequencing Method	Average Read-Length (Bases)	Run Time (Days)	Gb Per Run	Instrument Cost (U.S.$)	Comments
Roche 454 GS FLX	Fragment, mate-pair Emulsion PCR	Pyrosequencing	400	0.35	0.45	500,000	Fast run times; High reagent cost
Illumina HiSeq 2000	Fragment, mate-pair Solid phase	Reversible terminator	100–125	8 (mate-pair run)	150–200	540,000	Most widely used platform; Low multiplexing capability
Life/APG's SOLiD 5500xl	Fragment, mate-pair Emulsion PCR	Cleavable probe, sequencing by ligation	35–75	7 (mate-pair run)	180–300	595,000	Inherent error correction; Long run times
Helicos BioSciences HeliScope	Fragment, mate-pair Single molecule	Reversible terminator	32	8 (fragment run)	37	999,000	Nonbias template representation; Expensive, high error rates
Pacific Biosciences PacBio RS	Fragment Single molecule	Real-time sequencing	1,000	1	0.075	NA	Greatest potential for long reads; Highest error rates
Polonator G.007	Mate pair Emulsion PCR	Noncleavable probe, sequencing by ligation	26	5 (mate-pair run)	12	170,000	Least expensive platform; Shortest read lengths

NA, not available.
Data represent an update of information provided in Metzker ML. Sequencing technologies—the next generation. *Nat Rev Genet* 2010;11:31–46.

a library of either fragment templates or mate-pair templates are generated. Then, clonally amplified templates from single DNA molecules are prepared by either emulsion polymerase chain reaction (PCR) or solid-phase amplification.[68,69] Alternatively, it is possible to prepare single-molecule templates through methods that require less starting material and that do not involve PCR amplification reactions, which can be the source of artifactual mutations.[70] Once prepared, templates are attached to a solid surface in spatially separated sites, allowing thousands to billions of nucleotide sequencing reactions to be performed simultaneously.

The sequencing methods currently used by the different next-generation sequencing platforms are diverse and have been classified into four groups: cyclic reversible termination, single-nucleotide addition, real-time sequencing, and sequencing by ligation (Fig. 1.3).[61,71] These sequencing strategies are coupled with different imaging methods, including those based on measuring bioluminescent signals or involving four-color imaging of single molecular events. Finally, the extraordinary amount of data released from these nucleotide sequencing platforms is stored, assembled, and analyzed using powerful bioinformatic tools that have been developed in parallel with next-generation sequencing technologies.[72]

Next-generation sequencing approaches represent the newest entry into the cancer genome decoding arena and have already been applied to cancer analyses. The first research group to apply these methodologies to whole cancer genomes was that of Ley et al.,[73] who reported in 2008 the sequencing of the entire genome of a patient with acute myeloid leukemia (AML) and its comparison with the normal tissue from the same patient, using the Illumina/Solexa platform. As further described, this work allowed for the identification of point mutations and structural alterations of putative oncogenic relevance in AML and represented proof of principle of the relevance of next-generation sequencing for cancer research.

Whole-Genome Analysis Utilizing Second-Generation Sequencing

The sequence of the first whole cancer genome was reported in 2008, where AML and normal skin from the same patient were described.[73] Numerous additional whole genomes, together with the corresponding normal genomes of patients with a variety of malignant tumors, have been reported since then.[56,63,74–86]

The first available whole genome of a cytogenetically normal AML subtype M1 (AML-M1) revealed eight genes with novel mutations along with another 500 to 1,000 additional mutations found in noncoding regions of the genome. Most of the identified genes had not been previously associated with cancer. However, validation of the detected mutations did not identify novel recurring mutations in AML.[73] Concomitantly, with the expansion in the use of next-generation sequencers, many other whole genomes from a number of cancer types started to be evaluated in a similar manner (Fig. 1.4).[87]

In contrast to the first AML whole genome, the second did observe a recurrent mutation in *IDH1*, encoding isocitrate dehydrogenase.[56] Follow-up studies extended this finding and reported that mutations in *IDH1* and the related gene *IDH2* occur at a 20% to 30% frequency in AML patients and are associated with a poor prognosis in some subgroups of patients.[79,80,88] A good example illustrating the high pace at which second-generation technologies and their accompanying analytical tools are found is demonstrated by the following finding derived from a reanalysis of the first AML whole genome. Thus, when improvements in sequencing

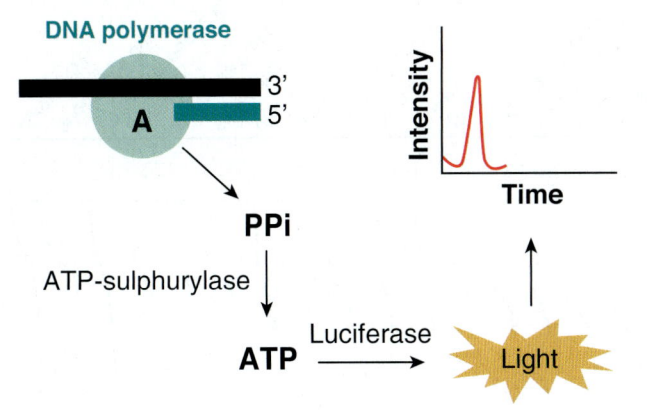

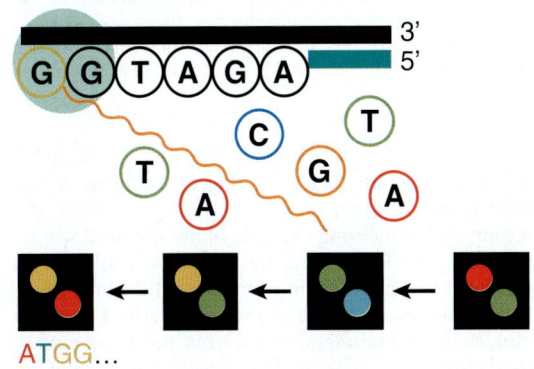

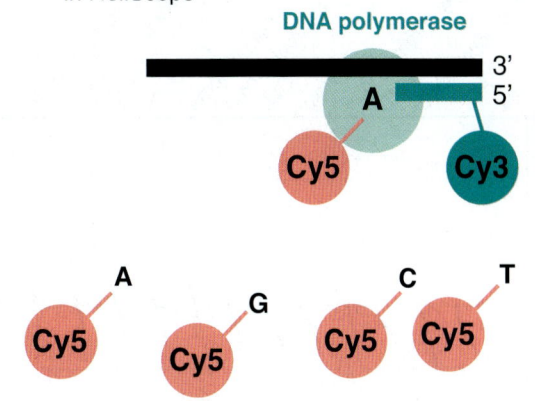

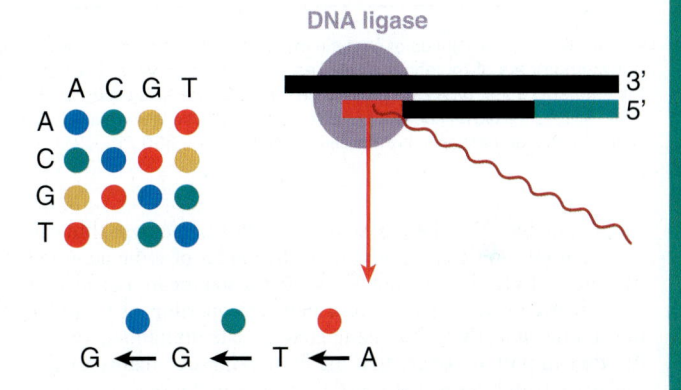

Figure 1.3 Advances in sequencing chemistry implemented in next-generation sequencers. **(A)** The pyrosequencing approach implemented in 454/Roche sequencing technology detects incorporated nucleotides by chemiluminescence resulting from PPi release. **(B)** The Illumina method utilizes sequencing by synthesis in the presence of fluorescently labeled nucleotide analogs that serve as reversible reaction terminators. **(C)** The single-molecule sequencing by synthesis approach detects template extension using Cy3 and Cy5 labels attached to the sequencing primer and the incoming nucleotides, respectively. **(D)** The SOLiD method sequences templates by sequential ligation of labeled degenerate probes. Two-base encoding implemented in the SOLiD instrument allows for probing each nucleotide position twice. (From Morozova O, Hirst M, Marra MA. Applications of new sequencing technologies for transcriptome analysis. *Annu Rev Genomics Hum Genet* 2009;10:135–151.)

techniques were available, the first AML whole genome (described previously), which identified no recurring mutations and had a 91.2% diploid coverage, was reevaluated by deeper sequence coverage, yielding 99.6% diploid coverage of the genome. This improvement, together with more advanced mutation calling algorithms, allowed for the discovery of several nonsynonymous mutations that had not been identified in the initial sequencing. This included a frameshift mutation in the DNA methyltransferase gene *DNMT3A*. Validation of *DNMT3A* in 280 additional de novo AML patients to define recurring mutations led to the significant discovery that a total of 22.1% of AML cases had mutations in *DNMT3A* that were predicted to affect translation. The median overall survival among patients with *DNMT3A* mutations was significantly shorter than that among patients without such mutations (12.3 months versus 41.1 months; p <0.001).

Shortly after this study, complete sequences of a series of cancer genomes, together with matched normal genomes of the same patients, were reported.[56,78,83,84] These works opened the way to more ambitious initiatives, including those involving large international consortia, aimed at decoding the genome of malignant tumors from thousands of cancer patients. Thus, over the last 2 years, many whole genomes of different human malignancies have been made available.[74–76]

In addition to direct applications of next-generation sequencing technologies for the mutational analysis of cancer genomes, these methods have an additional range of applications in cancer research. Thus, genome sequencing efforts have begun to elucidate the genomic changes that accompany metastasis evolution through a comparative analysis of primary and metastatic lesions from breast and pancreatic cancer patients.[77,81,82,85] Likewise, massively parallel sequencing has been used to analyze the evolution of a tongue adenocarcinoma in response to selection by targeted kinase inhibitors.[89] Detailed information of several of these whole genome projects is found in the following paragraph.

The first solid cancer to undergo whole-genome sequencing was a malignant melanoma that was compared to a lymphoblastoid cell line from the same individual.[83] Impressively, a total of 33,345 somatic base substitutions were identified, with 187 nonsynonymous substitutions in protein-coding sequences, at least one order of magnitude higher than any other cancer type. Most somatic base substitutions were C:G > T:A transitions, and of the 510 dinucleotide substitutions, 360 were CC.TT/GG.AA changes, which is consistent with ultraviolet light exposure mutation signatures previously reported in melanoma.[14] Such results from the most comprehensive catalog of somatic mutations not only provide

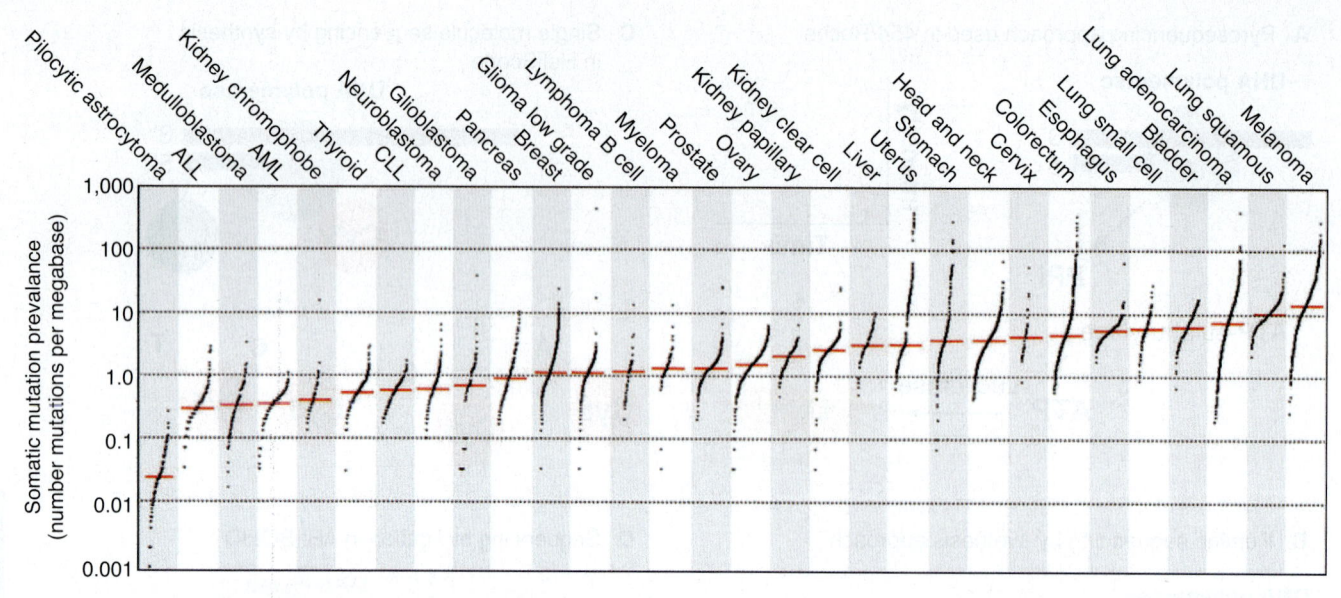

Figure 1.4 The prevalence of somatic mutations across human cancer types. Every *dot* represents a sample, whereas the *red horizontal lines* are the median numbers of mutations in the respective cancer types. The vertical axis (log scaled) shows the number of mutations per megabase, whereas the different cancer types are ordered on the horizontal axis based on their median numbers of somatic mutations. ALL, acute lymphoblastic leukemia; AML, acute myeloid leukemia; CLL, chronic lymphocytic leukemia. (Used with permission from Alexandrov LB, Nik-Zainal S, Wedge DC, et al. Signatures of mutational processes in human cancer. *Nature* 2013;500:415–421.)

insight into the DNA damage signature in this cancer type, but can also be useful in determining the relative order of some acquired mutations. Indeed, this study shows that a significant correlation exists between the presence of a higher proportion of C.A/G.T transitions in early (82%) compared to late mutations (53%). Another important aspect that the comprehensive nature of this melanoma study provided was that cancer mutations are spread out unevenly throughout the genome, with a lower prevalence in regions of transcribed genes, suggesting that DNA repair occurs mainly in these areas.

An interesting and pioneering example of the power of whole-genome sequencing in deciphering the mutation evolution in carcinogenesis was seen in a study in which a basallike breast cancer tumor, a brain metastasis, a tumor xenograft derived from the primary tumor, and the peripheral blood from the same patient were compared (Fig. 1.5).[85] This analysis showed a wide range of

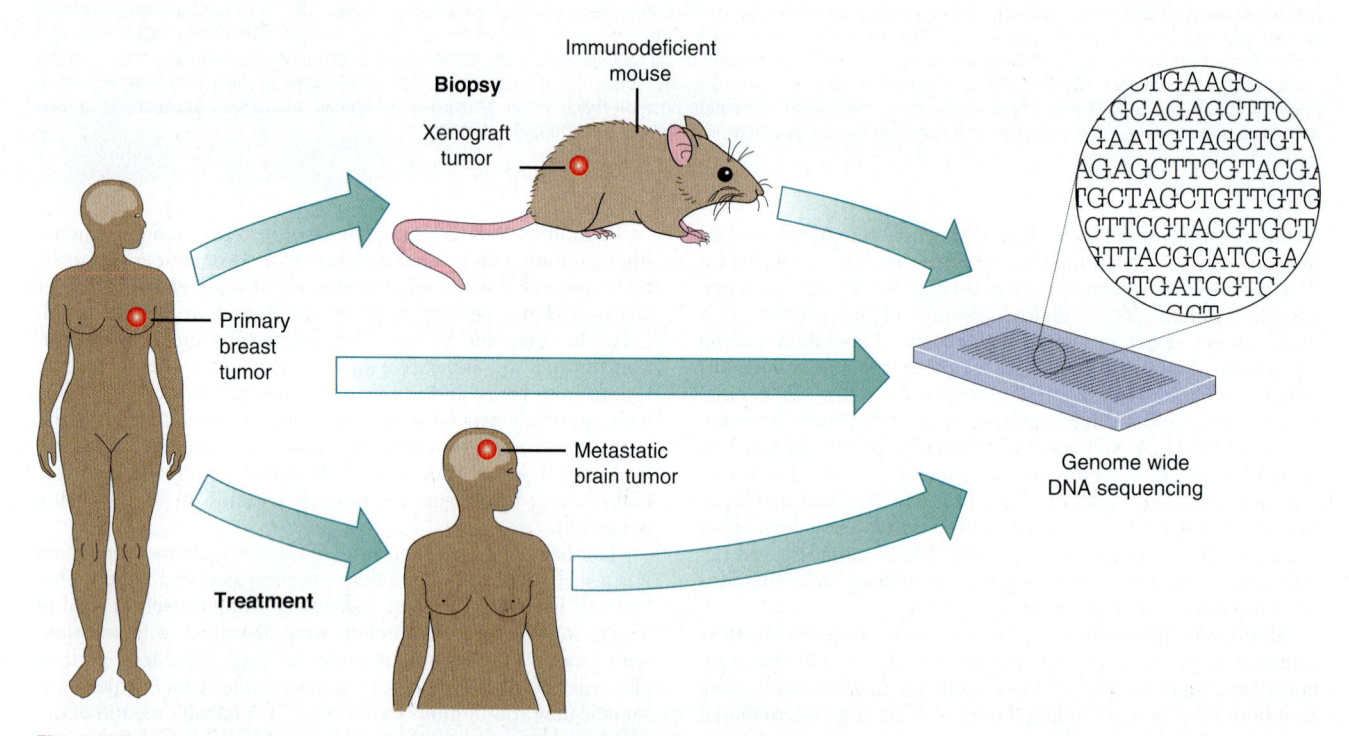

Figure 1.5 Covering all the bases in metastatic assessment. Ding et al.[85] performed a genomewide analysis on three tumor samples: a patient's primary breast tumor; her metastatic brain tumor, which formed despite therapy; and a xenograft tumor in a mouse, originating from the patient's breast tumor. They find that the primary tumor differs from the metastatic and xenograft tumors mainly in the prevalence of genomic mutations. (With permission from Gray J. Cancer: genomics of metastasis. *Nature* 2010;464:989–990.)

mutant allele frequencies in the primary tumor, which was narrowed in the metastasis and xenograft samples. This suggested that the primary tumor was significantly more heterogeneous in its cell populations compared to its matched metastasis and xenograft samples because these underwent selection processes whether during metastasis or transplantation. The clear overlap in mutation incidence between the metastatic and xenograft cases suggests that xenografts undergo similar selection as metastatic lesions and, therefore, are a reliable source for genomic analyses. The main conclusion of this whole-genome study was that, although metastatic tumors harbor an increased number of genetic alterations, the majority of the alterations found in the primary tumor are preserved. Interestingly, single-cell genome sequencing of a breast primary tumour and its liver metastasis indicated that a single clonal expansion formed the primary tumor and seeded the metastasis.[90] Further studies have confirmed and extended these findings to metastatic tumors from different types, including renal and pancreatic carcinomas.[91]

The importance of performing whole-genome sequencing has also been emphasized by the recent identification of somatic mutations in regulatory regions, which can also elicit tumorigenesis. In a study reviewing the noncoding mutations in 19 melanoma whole-genome samples, two recurrent mutations in 17 of the 19 cases studied within the *telomerase reverse transcriptase* (*TERT*) promoter region were revealed.[92] When these two mutations were investigated in an extension of 51 additional tumors and their matched normal tissues, it was observed that 33 tumors harbored one of the mutations and that the mutations occurred in a mutually exclusive manner. These two mutations generate an identical 11 bp nucleotide stretch that contains the consensus binding site for E-twenty-six (ETS) transcription factors. When cloned into a luciferase reporter assay system, it was shown that these mutations conferred a two- to fourfold increase in transcriptional activity of this promoter in five melanoma cell lines. Although this alteration is much more frequent in melanoma, it is also present in other cancer types because 16% of the cancers listed in the Cancer Cell Line Encyclopedia harbor one of the two *TERT* mutations. In combination, these *TERT* mutations are seen in a greater frequency than *BRAF*- and *NRAS*-activating mutations. They occur in a mutually exclusive manner and in regions that do not show a large background mutation rate, all suggesting that these mutations are important driver events contributing to oncogenesis. Further supporting this was another recent study that identified these same two mutations in the germ line of familial melanoma patients.[93]

As the *TERT* promoter mutation discovery shows, regions of the genome that do not code for proteins are just as vital in our understanding of the biology behind tumor development and progression. Another class of non–protein-coding regions in the genome are the noncoding RNAs. One class of noncoding RNAs are microRNAs (miRNA). Discovered 20 years ago, miRNAs are known to be expressed in a tissue or developmentally specific manner and their expression can influence cellular growth and differentiation along with cancer-related pathways such as apoptosis or stress response. miRNAs do this through either overexpression, leading to the targeting and downregulation of tumor suppressor genes, or inversely through their own downregulation, leading to increased expression of their target oncogene. miRNAs have been extensively studied in cancer and their functional effects have been noted in a wide variety of cancers like glioma[94] and breast cancer,[95] to name just a few.

Another class of noncoding RNAs (ncRNA) are the long noncoding RNAs (lncRNA). These RNAs are typically greater than 200 bp and can range up to 100 kb in size. They are transcribed by RNA polymerase II and can undergo splicing and polyadenylation. Although much less extensively studied when compared to miRNAs for their role in cancer, lncRNAs are beginning to come under much more scrutiny. A recent study of the steroid receptor RNA activator (SRA) revealed two transcripts, a lncRNA (SRA) and a translated transcript (steroid receptor RNA activator protein [SRAP]), that coexist within breast cancer cells. However, their expression varies within breast cancer cell lines with different phenotypes. It was shown that in a more invasive breast cancer line, higher relative levels of the noncoding transcript were seen.[96] Because this ncRNA acts as part of a ribonucleoprotein complex that is recruited to the promoter region of regulatory genes, it has been hypothesized that this shift in balance between both noncoding and coding transcripts may be associated with growth advantages. When this balance was shifted in vitro, it led to a large increase in transcripts associated with invasion and migration. The results of this study highlight the importance of the investigation into the roles of ncRNA in tumor development or progression and confirm again that the study of coding variants is not sufficient in determining the full genomic spectrum of cancer.

It must be also noted that the recent analysis of whole genomes of many different human tumors has provided additional insights into cancer evolution. Thus, it has been demonstrated that multiple mutational processes are operative during cancer development and progression, each of which has the capacity to leave its particular mutational signature on the genome. A remarkable and innovative study in this regard was aimed at the generation of the entire catalog of somatic mutations in 21 breast carcinomas and the identification of the mutational signatures of the underlying processes. This analysis revealed the occurrence of multiple, distinct single- and double-nucleotide substitution signatures. Moreover, it was reported that breast carcinomas harboring *BRCA1* or *BRCA2* mutations showed a characteristic combination of substitution mutation signatures and a particular profile of genomic deletions. An additional contribution of this analysis was the identification of a distinctive phenomenon of localized hypermutation, which has been termed *kataegis*, and which has also subsequently been observed in other malignancies distinct from breast carcinomas.[87]

Whole-genome sequencing of human carcinomas has also allowed for the ability to characterize other massive genomic alterations, termed *chromothripsis* and *chromoplexy*, occurring across different cancer subtypes.[97] Chromothripsis implies a massive genomic rearrangement acquired in a one-step catastrophic event during cancer development and has been detected in about 2% to 3% of all tumors, but is present at high frequency in some particular cases, such as bone cancers.[98] Chromoplexy has been originally described in prostate cancer and involves many DNA translocations and deletions that arise in a highly interdependent manner and result in the coordinate disruption of multiple cancer genes.[99] These newly described phenomena represent powerful strategies of rapid genome evolution, which may play essential roles during carcinogenesis.

Whole-Exome Analysis Utilizing Second-Generation Sequencing

Another application of second-generation sequencing involves utilizing nucleic acid "baits" to capture regions of interest in the total pool of nucleic acids. These could either be DNA, as described previously,[100,101] or RNA.[102] Indeed, most areas of interest in the genome can be targeted, including exons and ncRNAs. Despite inefficiencies in the exome-targeting process—including the uneven capture efficiency across exons, which results in not all exons being sequenced, and the occurrence of some off-target hybridization events—the higher coverage of the exome makes it highly suitable for mutation discovery in cancer samples.

Over the last few years, thousands of cancer samples have been subjected to whole-exome sequencing. These studies, combined with data from whole-genome sequencing, have provided an unprecedented level of information about the mutational landscape of the most frequent human malignancies.[74–76] In addition, whole-exome sequencing has been used to identify the somatic mutations characteristic of both rare tumors and those that are prevalent in certain geographical regions.[76]

Overall, these studies have provided very valuable information about mutation rates and spectra across cancer types and subtypes.[87,103,104] Remarkably, the variation in mutational frequency between different tumors is extraordinary, with hematologic and pediatric cancers showing the lowest mutation rates (0.001 per Mb of DNA), and melanoma and lung cancers presenting the highest mutational burden (more than 400 per Mb). Whole-exome sequencing has also contributed to the identification of novel cancer genes that had not been previously described to be causally implicated in the carcinogenesis process. These genes belong to different functional categories, including signal transduction, RNA maturation, metabolic regulation, epigenetics, chromatin remodeling, and protein homeostasis.[74] Finally, a combination of data from whole-exome and whole-genome sequencing has allowed for the identification of the signatures of mutational processes operating in different cancer types.[87] Thus, an analysis of a dataset of about 5 million mutations from over 7,000 cancers from 30 different types has allowed for the extraction of more than 20 distinct mutational signatures. Some of them, such as those derived from the activity of APOBEC cytidine deaminases, are present in most cancer types, whereas others are characteristic of specific tumors. Known signatures associated with age, smoking, ultraviolet (UV) light exposure, and DNA repair defects have been also identified in this work, but many of the detected mutational signatures are of cryptic origin. These findings demonstrate the impressive diversity of mutational processes underlying cancer development and may have enormous implications for the future understanding of cancer biology, prevention, and treatment.

SOMATIC ALTERATION CLASSES DETECTED BY CANCER GENOME ANALYSIS

Whole-genome sequencing of cancer genomes has an enormous potential to detect all major types of somatic mutations present in malignant tumors. This large repertoire of genomic abnormalities includes single nucleotide changes, small insertions and deletions, large chromosomal reorganizations, and copy number variations (Fig. 1.6).

Nucleotide substitutions are the most frequent somatic mutations detected in malignant tumors, although there is a substantial variability in the mutational frequency among different cancers.[60] On average, human malignancies have one nucleotide change per million bases, but melanomas reach mutational rates 10-fold higher, and tumors with mutator phenotype caused by DNA mismatch repair deficiencies may accumulate tens of mutations per million nucleotides. By contrast, tumors of hematopoietic origin have less than one base substitution per million. Several bioinformatic tools and pipelines have been developed to efficiently detect somatic nucleotide substitutions through comparison of the genomic information obtained from paired normal and tumor samples from the same patient. Likewise, there are a number of publicly available computational methods to predict the functional relevance of the identified mutations in cancer specimens.[60] Most of these bioinformatic tools exclusively deal with nucleotide changes in protein coding regions and evaluate the putative structural or functional effect of an amino acid substitution in a determined protein, thus obviating changes in other genomic regions, which can also be of crucial interest in cancer. In any case, current computational methods used in this regard are far from being optimal, and experimental validation is finally required to assess the functional relevance of nucleotide substitutions found in cancer genomes.

For years, the main focus of cancer genome analyses has been on identifying coding mutations that cause a change in the amino acid sequence of a gene. The rationale behind this is quite sound because any mutation that creates a novel protein or truncates an essential protein has the potential to drastically change the cellular environment. Examples of this have been shown earlier in the chapter with *BRAF* and *KRAS* along with many others. With the advancements in next-generation sequencing, larger studies are able to be conducted. These studies give the power to detect mutations occurring in the cancer genome at a lower frequency. Interesting to note is that these studies are leading to the discovery that recurrent synonymous mutations occur in cancer. Previously believed to be merely neutral mutations that maintain no functional role in tumorigenesis, these mutations were largely ignored, but a recent study shows[105] that simply dismissing these mutations as silent may be premature.

In a review of only 29 melanoma exomes and genomes, 16 recurring synonymous mutations were discovered. When these mutations were screened in additional samples, a synonymous mutation in the gene *BCL2L12* was discovered in 12 out of 285 total samples. The observed frequency of this recurrent mutation is greater than expected by chance, suggesting that it has undergone some type of selective pressure during tumor development.[105] Noting that *BCL2L12* had previously been linked to tumorigenesis, the mutation was further evaluated for its functional effect, with the finding that it led to an abrogation of the effect of a miRNA, leading to the deregulated expression of *BCL2L12*. BCL2L12 is a negative regulator of the gene p53, which functions by binding and inhibiting apoptosis in glioma.[106] Accordingly, the dysregulation observed in *BCL2L12* led to a reduction in p53 target gene expression.

Small insertions and deletions (*indels*) represent a second category of somatic mutations that can be discovered by whole-genome sequencing of cancer specimens. These mutations are about 10-fold less frequent than nucleotide substitutions, but may also have an obvious impact in cancer progression. Accordingly, specific bioinformatic tools have been created to detect these *indels* in the context of the large amount of information generated by whole-genome sequencing projects.[107]

The systematic identification of large chromosomal rearrangements in cancer genomes represents one of the most successful applications of next-generation sequencing methodologies. Previous strategies in this regard had mainly been based on the utilization of cytogenetic methods for the identification of recurrent translocations in hematopoietic tumors. More recently, a combination of bioinformatics and functional methods has allowed for the finding of recurrent translocations in solid epithelial tumors such as *TMPRSS2–ERG* in prostate cancer and *EML4–ALK* in non–small-cell lung cancer.[108,109] Now, by using a next-generation sequencing analysis of genomes and transcriptomes, it is possible to systematically search for both intrachromosomal and interchromosomal rearrangements occurring in cancer specimens. These studies have already proven their usefulness for cancer research through the discovery of recurrent translocations involving genes of the *RAF* kinase pathway in prostate and gastric cancers and in melanomas.[110] Likewise, massively parallel paired-end genome and transcriptome sequencing has already been used to detect new gene fusions in cancer and to catalog all major structural rearrangements present in some tumors and cancer cell lines.[63,111–113] The ongoing cancer genome projects involving thousands of tumor samples will likely lead to the detection of many other chromosomal rearrangements of relevance in specific subsets of cancers. It is also remarkable that whole-genome sequencing may also facilitate the identification of other types of genomic alterations, including rearrangements of repetitive elements, such as active retrotransposons, or insertions of foreign gene sequences, such as viral genomes, which can contribute to cancer development. Indeed, a next-generation sequencing analysis of the transcriptome of Merkel cell carcinoma samples has revealed the clonal integration within the tumor genome of a previously unknown polyomavirus likely implicated in the pathogenesis of this rare but aggressive skin cancer.[114]

Finally, next-generation sequencing approaches have also demonstrated their feasibility to analyze the pattern of copy number

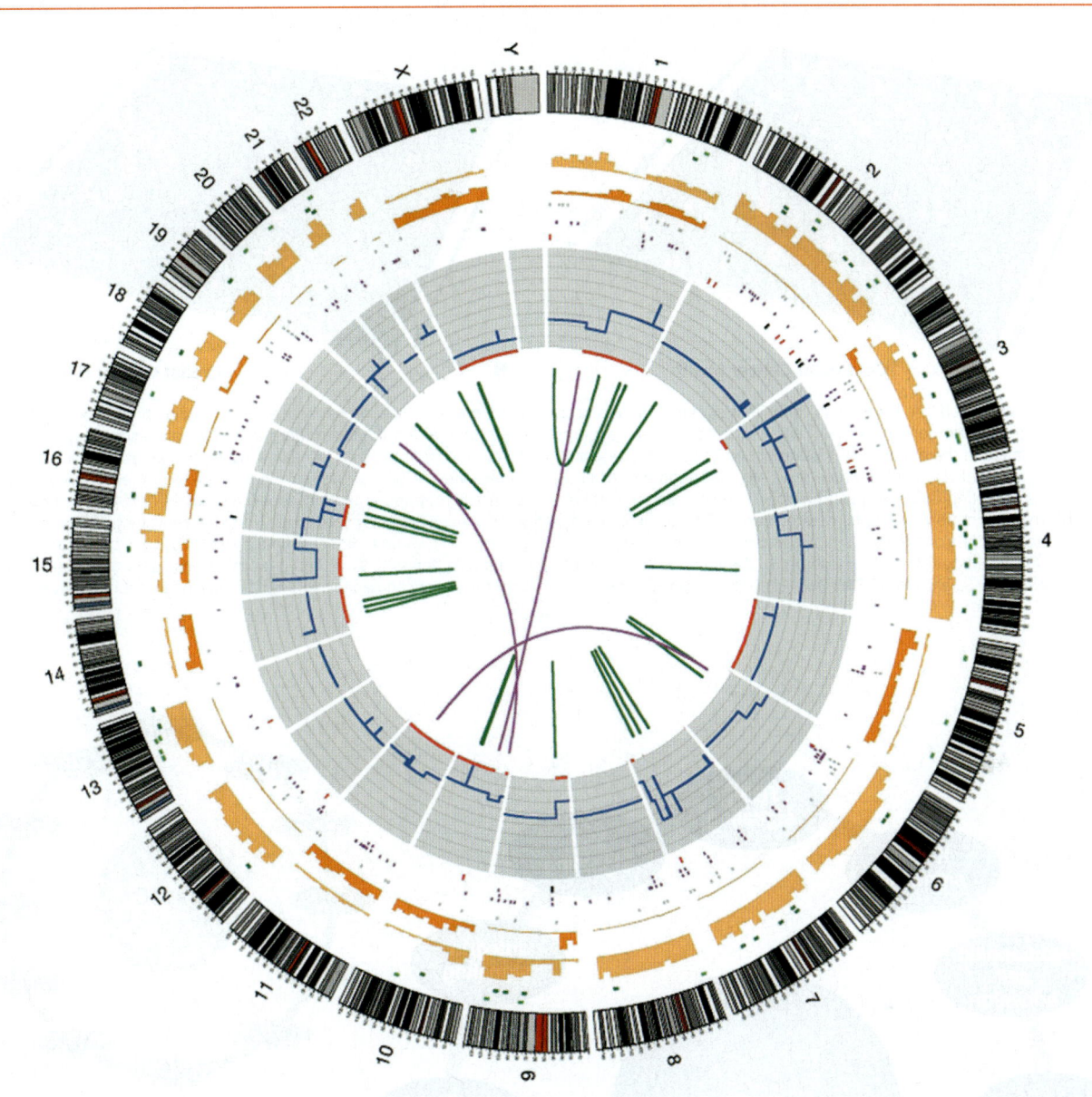

Figure 1.6 The catalog of somatic mutations in COLO-829. Chromosome ideograms are shown around the *outer ring* and are oriented pter–qter in a clockwise direction with centromeres indicated in *red*. Other tracks contain somatic alterations *(from outside to inside)*: validated insertions *(light green rectangles)*; validated deletions *(dark green rectangles)*; heterozygous *(light orange bars)*, and homozygous *(dark orange bars)* substitutions shown by density per 10 megabases; coding substitutions *(colored squares: silent in gray, missense in purple, nonsense in red, and splice site in black)*; copy number *(blue lines)*; regions of loss of heterozygosity (LOH) *(red lines)*; validated intrachromosomal rearrangements *(green lines)*; validated interchromosomal rearrangements *(purple lines)*. (From Pleasance ED, Cheetham RK, Stephens PJ, et al. A comprehensive catalogue of somatic mutations from a human cancer genome. *Nature* 2010;463:191–196.)

alterations in cancer, because they allow researchers to count the number of reads in both tumor and normal samples at any given genomic region and then to evaluate the tumor-to-normal copy number ratio at this particular region. These new methods offer some advantages when compared with those based on microarrays, including much better resolution, precise definition of the involved breakpoints, and absence of saturation, which facilitates the accurate estimation of high copy number levels occurring in some genomic loci of malignant tumors.[60]

PATHWAY-ORIENTED MODELS OF CANCER GENOME ANALYSIS

Genomewide mutational analyses suggest that the mutational landscape of cancer is made up of a handful of genes that are mutated in a high fraction of tumors, otherwise known as *mountains*, and most mutated genes are altered at relatively low frequencies, otherwise known as *hills* (Fig. 1.7).[29] The mountains probably give a high selective advantage to the mutated cell, and the hills might provide a lower advantage, making it hard to distinguish them from passenger mutations. Because the hills differ between cancer types, it seems that the cancer genome is more complex and heterogeneous than anticipated. Although highly heterogeneous, bioinformatic studies suggest that the mountains and hills can be grouped into sets of pathways and biologic processes. Some of these pathways are affected by mutations in a few pathway members and others by numerous members. For example, pathway analyses have allowed for the stratification of mutated genes in pancreatic adenocarcinomas to 12 core pathways that have at least one member mutated in 67% to 100% of the tumors analyzed (Fig. 1.8).[45] These core pathways deviated to some that harbored one single highly mutated gene,

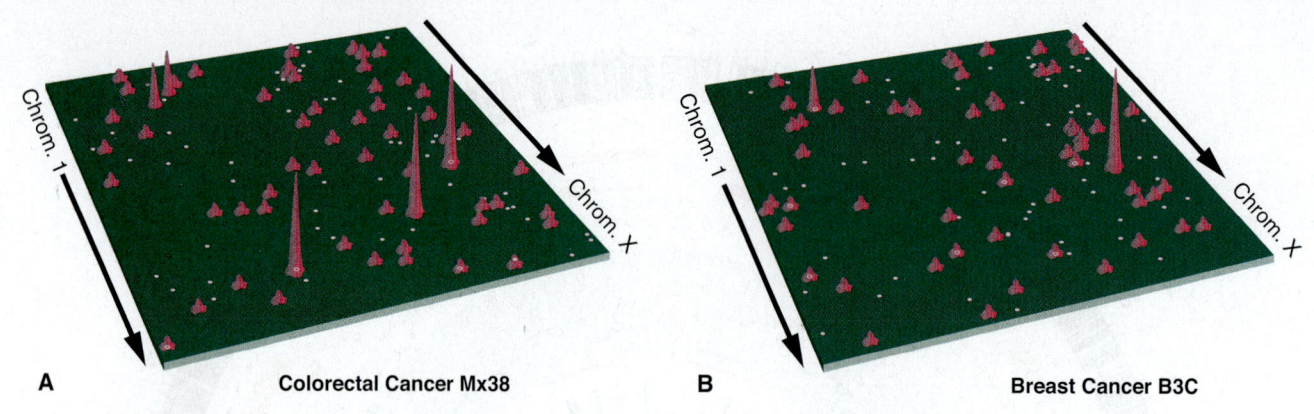

Figure 1.7 Cancer genome landscapes. Nonsilent somatic mutations are plotted in a two-dimensional space representing chromosomal positions of RefSeq genes. The telomere of the short arm of chromosome 1 is represented in the rear left corner of the *green plane* and ascending chromosomal positions continue in the direction of the arrow. Chromosomal positions that follow the front edge of the plane are continued at the back edge of the plane of the adjacent row, and chromosomes are appended end to end. Peaks indicate the 60 highest ranking CAN genes for each tumor type, with peak heights reflecting CaMP scores. The *dots* represent genes that were somatically mutated in the individual colorectal (Mx38) **(A)** or breast tumor (B3C) **(B)**. The *dots* corresponding to mutated genes that coincided with hills or mountains are black with white rims; the remaining *dots* are white with red rims. The mountain on the right of both landscapes represents *TP53* (chromosome 17), and the other mountain shared by both breast and colorectal cancers is *PIK3CA* (upper left, chromosome 3). (Redrawn from Wood LD, Parsons DW, Jones S, et al. The genomic landscapes of human breast and colorectal cancers. *Science* 2007;318:1108–1113. Reprinted with permission from the American Association for the Advancement of Science).

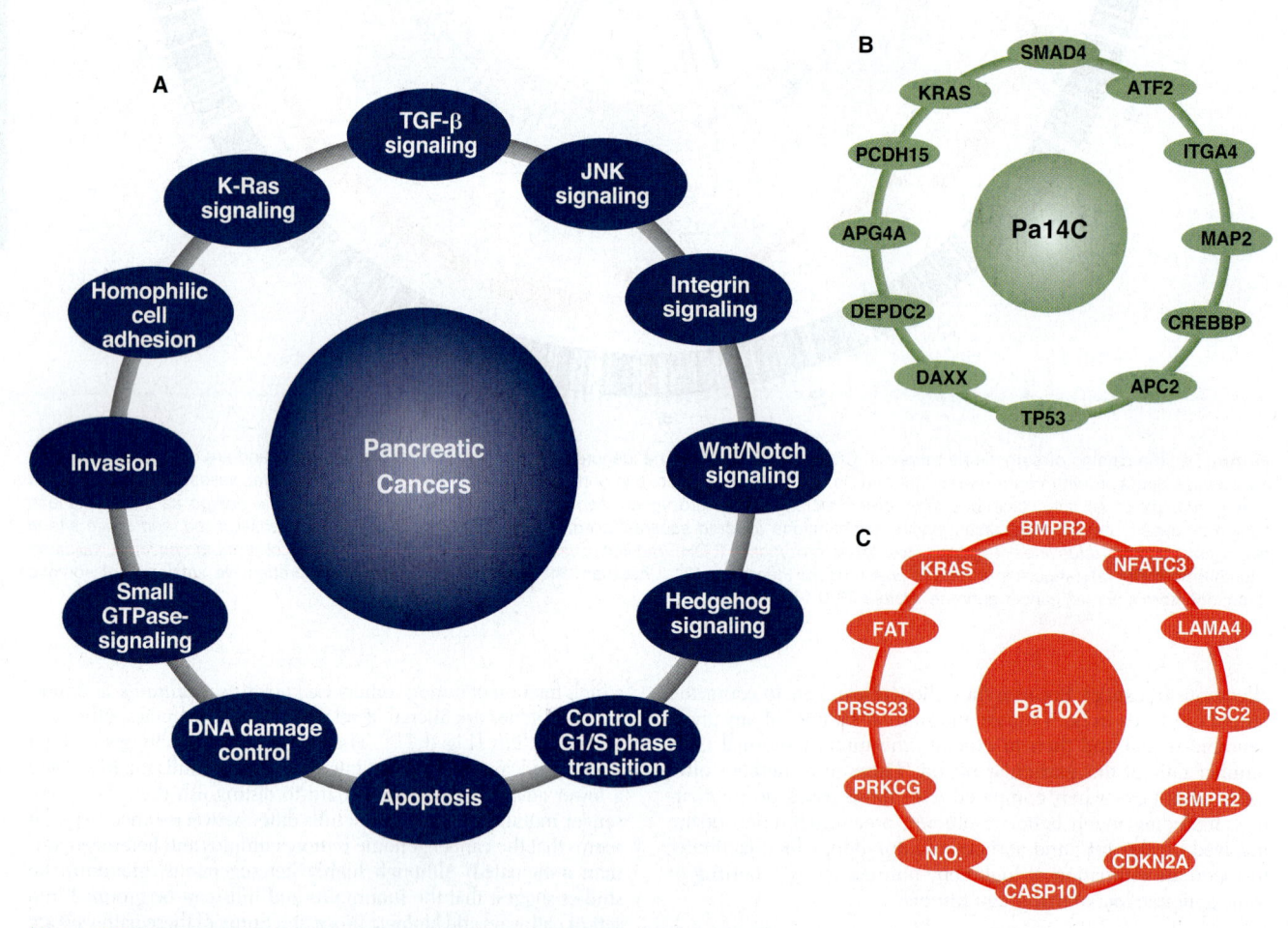

Figure 1.8 Signaling pathways and processes. **(A)** The 12 pathways and processes whose component genes were genetically altered in most pancreatic cancers. **(B,C)** Two pancreatic cancers (Pa14C and Pa10X) and the specific genes that are mutated in them. The positions around the circles in **(B)** and **(C)** correspond to the pathways and processes in **(A)**. Several pathway components overlapped, as illustrated by the BMPR2 mutation that presumably disrupted both the SMAD4 and Hedgehog signaling pathways in Pa10X. Additionally, not all 12 processes and pathways were altered in every pancreatic cancer, as exemplified by the fact that no mutations known to affect DNA damage control were observed in Pa10X. NO, not observed. (Redrawn from Jones S, Zhang X, Parsons DW, et al. Core signaling pathways in human pancreatic cancers revealed by global genomic analyses. *Science* 2008;321:1801–1806. Reprinted with permission from the American Association for the Advancement of Science).

such as in *KRAS* in the G1/S cell cycle transition pathway and pathways where a few mutated genes were found, such as the transforming growth factor (TGF-β) signaling pathway. Finally, there were pathways in which many different genes were mutated, such as invasion regulation molecules, cell adhesion molecules, and integrin signaling. Importantly, independent of how many genes in the same pathway are affected, if they are found to occur in a mutually exclusive fashion in a single tumor, they most likely give the same selective pressure for clonal expansion.

The idea of genetically analyzing pathways rather than individual genes has been applied previously, revealing the concept of mutual exclusivity. Mutual exclusivity has been shown elegantly in the case of *KRAS* and *BRAF*, where a *KRAS*-mutated cancer generally does not also harbor a *BRAF* mutation, because *KRAS* is upstream of *BRAF* in the same pathway.[9] A similar concept was applied for *PIK3CA* and *PTEN*, where both mutations do not usually occur in the same tumor.[23]

With the ever expanding amounts of genetic information being gathered, the ability to search for common pathways being affected in cancer is increasing. One new pathway that is beginning to emerge is the glutamate-signaling pathway. Glutamate dysregulation has been implicated in a number of cancers. In a study of pancreatic duct adenocarcinoma (PDAC), it was seen that glutamate levels were significantly higher in the tissue of individuals with chronic pancreatitis (CP) and PDAC when compared to normal pancreas tissue.[115] It was also observed that the increased glutamate levels led to proinvasion and antiapoptotic signaling through the activation of AMPA receptors.

Also in this regard, and through the use of whole-exome sequencing, it has been recently shown that the glutamate receptor gene *GRIN2A* is highly mutated in melanoma. The finding that many of these mutations are nonsense has suggested that *GRIN2A* is a novel tumor suppressor. Additional genes in the glutamate pathway have also found mutated in melanomas.[116] Pathway analyses and statistical testing on the whole-exome data have also revealed the glutamate signaling pathway to be dysregulated. These results have been further corroborated in another study reporting mutations in the metabotropic glutamate receptor GRM3[117,118] in melanoma. A functional analysis of mutations found in *GRM3* in melanoma tumor samples has shown an increased activation of MEK1/2 kinase, increased migration, and anchorage-independent growth.[117]

Passenger and Driver Mutations

By the time a cancer is diagnosed, it is comprised of billions of cells carrying DNA abnormalities, some of which have a functional role in malignant proliferation; however, many genetic lesions acquired along the way have no functional role in tumorigenesis.[14] The emerging landscapes of cancer genomes include thousands of genes that were not previously linked to tumorigenesis but are found to be somatically mutated. Many of these changes are likely to be *passengers*, or neutral, in that they have no functional effects on the growth of the tumor.[14] Only a small fraction of the genetic alterations are expected to drive cancer evolution by giving cells a selective advantage over their neighbors. Passenger mutations occur incidentally in a cell that later or in parallel develops a *driver* mutation, but are not ultimately pathogenic.[119] Although neutral, cataloging passengers mutations is important because they incorporate the signatures of the previous exposures the cancer cell underwent as well as DNA repair defects the cancer cell has. In many cases, the passenger and driver mutations occur at similar frequencies and the identification of drivers versus the passenger is of utmost relevance and remains a pressing challenge in cancer genetics.[120–122] This goal will eventually be achieved through a combination of genetic and functional approaches, some of which are listed as follows.

The most reliable indicator that a gene was selected for and therefore is highly likely to be pathogenic is the identification of recurrent mutations, whether at the same exact amino acid position or in neighboring amino acid positions in different patients. More than that, if somatic alterations in the same gene occur very frequently (mountains in the tumor genome landscape), these can be confidently classified as drivers. For example, cancer alleles that are identified in multiple patients and different tumors types, such as those found in *KRAS*, *TP53*, *PTEN*, and *PIK3CA*, are clearly selected for during tumorigenesis.

However, most genes discovered thus far are mutated in a relatively small fraction of tumors (hills), and it has been clearly shown that genes that are mutated in less than 1% of patients can still act as *drivers*.[123] The systematic sequencing of newly identified putative cancer genes in the vast number of specimens from cancer patients will help in this regard. However, even if examining large numbers of samples can provide helpful information to classify drivers versus passengers, this approach alone is limited by the marked variation in mutation frequency among individual tumors and individual genes. The statistical test utilized in this case calculates the probability that the number of mutations in a given gene reflects a mutation frequency that is greater than expected from the nonfunctional background mutation rate,[29,124] which is different between different cancer types. These analyses incorporate the number of somatic alterations observed, the number of tumors studied, and the number of nucleotides that were successfully sequenced and analyzed.

Another approach often used to distinguish driver from passenger mutations exploits the statistical analysis of synonymous versus nonsynonymous changes.[125] In contrast to nonsynonymous mutations, synonymous mutations do not alter the protein sequence. Therefore, they do not usually apply a growth advantage and would not be expected to be selected during tumorigenesis. This strategy works by comparing the observed-to-expected ratio of synonymous with that of nonsynonymous mutation. An increased proportion of nonsynonymous mutations from the expected 2:1 ratio implies selection pressure during tumorigenesis.

Other approaches are based on the concept that driver mutations may have characteristics similar to those causing Mendelian disease when inherited in the germ line and may be identifiable by constraints on tolerated amino acid residues at the mutated positions. In contrast, passenger mutations may have characteristics more similar to those of nonsynonymous SNPs with high minor allele frequencies. Based on these premises, supervised machine learning methods have been used to predict which missense mutations are drivers.[126] Additional approaches to decipher drivers from passengers include the identification of mutations that affect locations that have previously been shown to be cancer causing in protein members of the same gene family. Enrichment for mutations in evolutionarily conserved residues are analyzed by algorithms, such as SIFT (sorting intolerant from tolerant (SIFT),[127] which estimates the effects of the different mutations identified.

Probably the most conclusive methods to identify driver mutations will be rigorous functional studies using biochemical assays as well as model organisms or cultured cells, using knockout and knockin of individual cancer alleles.[128] Unfortunately, these methods are not well suited to the analysis of the hundreds of gene candidates that arise from every large-scale cancer genome project. In conclusion, it is fair to say that sequencing cancer genomes is only the beginning of a journey that will ultimately be completed when the thousands of the newly discovered alleles are annotated as being the drivers of this disease. A summary of the various next-generation applications and approaches for their analysis is summarized in Figure 1.9 and Table 1.2.

NETWORKS OF CANCER GENOME PROJECTS

The repertoire of oncogenic mutations is extremely heterogeneous, suggesting that it would be difficult for independent cancer genome initiatives to address the generation of comprehensive

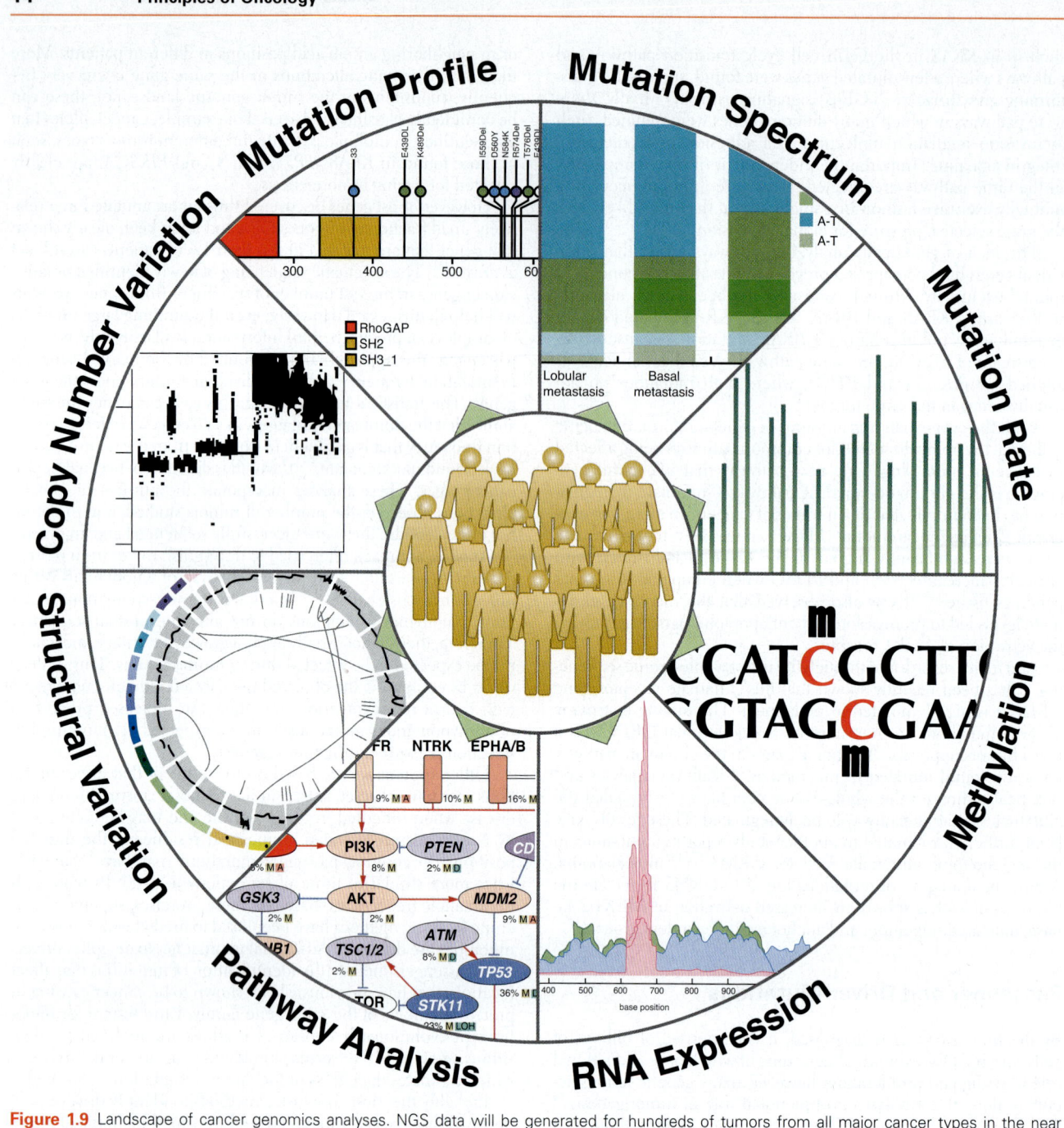

Figure 1.9 Landscape of cancer genomics analyses. NGS data will be generated for hundreds of tumors from all major cancer types in the near future. The integrated analysis of DNA, RNA, and methylation sequencing data will help elucidate all relevant genetic changes in cancers. (Used with permission from Ding L, Wendl MC, Koboldt DC, et al. Analysis of next-generation genomic data in cancer: accomplishments and challenges. *Hum Mol Genet* 2010;19:R188–R196.)

catalogs of mutations in the wide spectrum of human malignancies. Accordingly, there have been different efforts to coordinate the cancer genome sequencing projects being carried out around the world, including The Cancer Genome Atlas (TCGA) and the International Cancer Genome Consortium (ICGC). Moreover, there are other initiatives that are more focused on specific tumors, such as that led by scientists at St. Jude Children's Research Hospital in Memphis, and Washington University, which aims at sequencing multiple pediatric cancer genomes.[129]

TCGA began in 2006 in the United States as a comprehensive program in cancer genomics supported by the U.S. National Institutes of Health (NIH). The initial project focused on three tumors: GBM, serous cystadenocarcinoma of the ovary, and lung squamous carcinoma. These studies have already generated novel and interesting information regarding genes mutated in these malignancies.[134] On the basis of these positive results, the NIH announced an expansion of the TCGA program with the aim to produce genomic data sets for at least 20 to 25 cancers during the next few years.

The ICGC was formed in 2008 to coordinate the generation of comprehensive catalogs of genomic abnormalities in tumors from 50 different cancer types or subtypes that are of clinical and societal importance across the world.[130] The project aims to perform systematic studies of over 25,000 cancer genomes at the genomic level and integrate this information with epigenomic and transcriptomic studies of the same cases as well as with clinical features of patients. At present, there are a total of 69 committed projects involving at least 16 different countries coordinated by

TABLE 1.2
Computational Tools and Databases Useful for Cancer Genome Analyses

Category	Tool/Database	URL
Alignment	Maq[a]	http://maq.sourceforge.net
	Burrows-Wheeler Aligner (BWA)[b]	http://bio-bwa.sourceforge.net
Mutation calling	SNVMix[c]	http://www.bcgsc.ca/platform/bioinfo/software/SNVMix
	SAMtools[d]	http://samtools.sourceforge.net
	VarScan[e]	http://varscan.sourceforge.net
	MuTect[f]	http://www.broadinstitute.org/cancer/cga/mutect
Indel calling	Pindel[g]	http://gmt.genome.wustl.edu/pindel/current/
Copy number analysis	CBS[h]	http://www.bioconductor.org
	SegSeq[i]	http://www.broadinstitute.org/cgi-bin/cancer/publications/pub_paper.cgi?mode=view&paper_id=182
Functional effect	SIFT[j]	http://sift.jcvi.org/
	PolyPhen-2[k]	http://genetics.bwh.harvard.edu/pph2
Visualization	CIRCOS[l]	http://mkweb.bcgsc.ca/circos
	Integrative Genomics Viewer (IGV)[m]	http://www.broadinstitute.org/igv
Repository	Catalogue of Somatic Mutations in Cancer (COSMIC)[n]	http://www.sanger.ac.uk/genetics/CGP/cosmic
	Cancer Genome Project (CGP)[o]	http://www.sanger.ac.uk/genetics/CGP
	dbSNP[p]	http://www.ncbi.nlm.nih.gov/SNP
	Gene Ranker[q]	http://cbio.mskcc.org/tcga-generanker/

[a] Li H, Durbin R. Fast and accurate short read alignment with Burrows–Wheeler transform. *Bioinformatics* 2009;25:1754–1760.
[b] Li H, Durbin R. Fast and accurate long-read alignment with Burrows–Wheeler transform. *Bioinformatics* 2010;26:589–595.
[c] Goya R, Sun MG, Morin RD, et al. SNVMix: predicting single nucleotide variants from next-generation sequencing of tumors. *Bioinformatics* 2010;26:730–736.
[d] Li H, Handsaker B, Wysoker A, et al. The Sequence Alignment/Map format and SAMtools. *Bioinformatics* 2009;25:2078–2079.
[e] Koboldt DC, Chen K, Wylie T, et al. VarScan: variant detection in massively parallel sequencing of individual and pooled samples. *Bioinformatics* 2009;25:2283–2285.
[f] Cibulski K, Lawrence MS, Carter SL, et al. Sensitive detection of somatic point mutations in impure and heterogeneous cancer samples. *Nat Biotechnol* 2013;31:213–219.
[g] Ye K, Schulz MH, Long Q, et al. Pindel: a pattern growth approach to detect break points of large deletions and medium sized insertions from paired-end short reads. *Bioinformatics* 2009;25:2865–2871.
[h] Venkatraman ES, Olshen AB. A faster circular binary segmentation algorithm for the analysis of array CGH data. *Bioinformatics* 2007;23:657–663.
[i] Chiang DY, Getz G, Jaffe DB, et al. High-resolution mapping of copy-number alterations with massively parallel sequencing. *Nature Methods* 2009;6:99–103.
[j] Ng PC, Henikoff S. Predicting deleterious amino acid substitutions. *Genome Res* 2001;11:863–874.
[k] Idzhubei IA, Schmidt S, Peshkin L, et al. A method and server for predicting damaging missense mutations. *Nature Methods* 2010;7:248–249.
[l] Krzywinski M, Schein J, Birol I, et al. Circos: an information aesthetic for comparative genomics. *Genome Res* 2009;19:1639–1645.
[m] Robinson JT, Thorvaldsdóttir H, Winckler W, et al. Integrative Genomics Viewer. *Nat Biotechnol* 2011;29:24–26.
[n] Forbes SA, Bhamra S, Dawson E, et al. The catalogue of somatic mutations in cancer (COSMIC). *Curr Protoc Hum Genet* 2008;Chapter 10:Unit 10.11.
[o] Futreal PA, Coin L, Marshall M, et al. A census of human cancer genes. *Nat Rev Cancer* 2004;4:177–183.
[p] Sherry ST, Ward MH, Kholodov M, et al. dbSNP: The NCBI Database of genetic variation. *Nucleic Acids Res* 2001;29:308–311.
[q] The Cancer Genome Atlas Research Network. Comprehensive genomic characterization defines human glioblastoma genes and core pathways. *Nature* 2008;455:1061–1068.
Based on Meyerson M, Stacey G, Getz G. Advances in understanding cancer genomes through second generation sequencing. *Nature Rev Genet* 2010;11: 685–696, Table 2.

the ICGC. All of these projects deal with at least 500 samples per cancer type from cancers affecting a variety of human organs and tissues, including blood, the brain, the breast, the esophagus, the kidneys, the liver, the oral cavity, the ovaries, the pancreas, the prostate, the skin, and the stomach.[130]

All of these coordinated projects have already provided new insights into the catalog of genes mutated in cancer and have unveiled specific signatures of the mutagenic mechanisms, including carcinogen exposures or DNA-repair defects, implicated in the development of different malignant tumors.[83,84,87,131] Furthermore, these cancer genome studies have also contributed to define clinically relevant subtypes of tumors for prognosis and therapeutic management, and in some cases have identified new targets and strategies for cancer treatment.[74–76] The rapid technological advances in DNA sequencing will likely drop the costs of sequencing cancer genomes to a small fraction of the current price and will allow researchers to overcome some of the current limitations of these global sequencing efforts. Hopefully, worldwide coordination of cancer genome projects, including Pan-Cancer initiative, with those involving large-scale, functional analyses of genes in both cellular and animal models will likely provide us with the most comprehensive collection of information generated to date about the causes and molecular mechanisms of cancer.

THE GENOMIC LANDSCAPE OF CANCERS

Examining the overall distribution of the identified mutations redefined the cancer genome landscapes whereby the *mountains* are the handful of commonly mutated genes and the *hills* represent the vast majority of genes that are infrequently mutated.

One of the most striking features of the tumor genomic landscape is that it involves different sets of cancer genes that are mutated in a tissue-specific fashion.[132,133] To continue with the analogy, the scenery is very different if we observe a colorectal, a lung, or a breast tumor. This indicates that mutations in specific genes cause tumors at specific sites, or are associated with specific stages of development, cell differentiation, or tumorigenesis, despite many of those genes being expressed in various fetal and adult tissues. Moreover, different types of tumors follow specific genetic pathways in terms of the combination of genetic alterations that it must acquire. For example, no cancer outside the bowel has been shown to follow the classic genetic pathway of colorectal tumorigenesis. Additionally, *KRAS* mutations are almost always present in pancreatic cancers but are very rare or absent in breast cancers. Similarly, *BRAF* mutations are present in 60% of melanomas, but are very infrequent in lung cancers.[1] Another intriguing feature is that alterations in ubiquitous housekeeping genes, such as those involved in DNA repair or energy production, occur only in particular types of tumors.

In addition to tissue specificity, the genomic landscape of tumors can also be associated with gender and hormonal status. For example, *HER2* amplification and *PIK3C2A* mutations, two genetic alterations associated with breast cancer development, are correlated with the estrogen-receptor hormonal status.[134] The molecular basis for the occurrence of cancer mutations in tissue- and gender-specific profiles is still largely unknown. Organ-specific expression profiles and cell-specific neoplastic transformation requirements are often mentioned as possible causes for this phenomenon. Identifying tissue and gender cancer mutations patterns is relevant because it may allow for the definition of individualized therapeutic avenues.

INTEGRATIVE ANALYSIS OF CANCER GENOMICS

The implementation of novel high-throughput technologies is generating an extraordinary amount of information on cancer samples in many different ways other than those derived from whole-exome or whole-genome sequencing. Accordingly, there is a growing need to integrate genomic, epigenomic, transcriptomic, and proteomic landscapes from tumor samples, and then linking this integrated information with clinical outcomes of cancer patients. There are some examples of human malignancies in which this integrative approach has been already performed, such as for AML, glioblastoma, medulloblastoma, and renal cell, colorectal, ovarian, endometrial, prostate, and breast carcinomas.[135–142] In these cases, the integration of whole-exome and whole-genome sequencing with studies involving genomic DNA copy number arrays, DNA methylation, transcriptomic arrays, miRNA sequencing, and proteomic profiling has contributed to improving the molecular classification of complex and heterogeneous tumors. These integrative molecular analyses have also provided new insights into the mechanisms disrupted in each particular cancer type or subtype and have facilitated the association of genomic information with distinct clinical parameters of cancer patients and the discovery of novel therapeutic targets.[143] Also in this regard, there has been significant progress in the definition of the mechanisms by which the cancer genome and epigenome influence each other and cooperate to facilitate malignant transformation.[144,145] Thus, many tumor-suppressor genes are inactivated by either mutation or epigenetic silencing, and in some cases such as colorectal carcinomas, both mechanisms work coordinately to create a permissive environment for oncogenic transformation.[146] Moreover, mutations in epigenetic regulators such as DNA methyl transferases, chromatin remodelers, histones, and histone modifiers, are very frequent events in many tumors, including hepatocellular carcinomas, renal carcinomas leukemias, lymphomas, glioblastomas, and medulloblastomas. These genetic alterations of epigenetic modulators cause widespread transcriptomic changes, thereby amplifying the initial effect of the mutational event at the cancer genome level.[145]

The recent availability of different platforms for integrative cancer genome analyses will be very helpful in enabling the classification, biologic characterization, and personalized clinical management of human cancers (Table 1.3).[144,147]

THE CANCER GENOME AND THE NEW TAXONOMY OF TUMORS

Deciphering the cancer genome has already impacted clinical practice at multiple levels. On the one hand, it allowed for the identification of new cancer genes such as *IDH1*, a gene involved in glioma, which was discovered recently (see previous), and on the other hand, it is redesigning the taxonomy of tumors.

Until the genomic revolution, tumors had been classified based on two criteria: their localization (site of occurrence) and their appearance (histology). These criteria are also currently used as primary determinants of prognosis and to establish the best treatments. For many decades, it has been known that patients with histologically similar tumors have different clinical outcomes. Furthermore, tumors that cannot be distinguished based on an histologic analysis can respond very differently to identical therapies.[148]

It is becoming increasingly clear that the frequency and distribution of mutations affecting cancer genes can be used to redefine the histology-based taxonomy of a given tumor type. Lung and colorectal tumors represent paradigmatic examples. Genomic analyses led to the identification of activating mutations in the receptor tyrosine kinase *EGFR* in lung adenocarcinomas.[149] The occurrence of *EGFR* mutations molecularly defines a subtype of non–small-cell lung cancers (NSCLC) that occur mainly in non-smoking women, that tend to have a distinctly enhanced prognosis, and that typically respond to epidermal growth factor receptor (EGFR)-targeted therapies.[150–152] Similarly, the recent discovery of the *EML4-ALK* fusion identifies yet another subset of NSCLC that is clearly distinct from those that harbor *EGFR* mutations, that have distinct epidemiologic and biologic features, and that respond to ALK inhibitors.[109,153]

The second example is colorectal cancers (CRC), the tumor type for which the genomic landscape has been refined with the highest accuracy. CRCs can be clearly categorized according to the mutational profile of the genes involved in the *KRAS* pathway (Fig. 1.10). It is now known that *KRAS* mutations occur in approximately 40% of CRCs. Another subtype of CRC (approximately 10%) harbors mutations in *BRAF*, the immediate downstream effectors of *KRAS*.[10]

In CRCs and other tumor types, *KRAS* and *BRAF* mutations are known to be mutually exclusive. The mutual exclusivity pattern indicates that these genes operate in the same signaling pathway. Large epidemiologic studies have shown that the prognosis of tumors harboring wild-type *KRAS/BRAF* genes is distinct, and typically more favorable, than that of the mutated ones.[154,155] Of note, *KRAS* and *BRAF* mutations have been recently shown to impair responsiveness to the anti-EGFR monoclonal antibodies therapies in CRC patients.[156–158] Clearly distinct subgroups can be genetically identified in both NSCLCs and CRCs with respect to prognosis and response to therapy. It is likely that as soon as the genomic landscapes of other tumor types are defined, molecular subgroups like those described previously will also become defined.

Genotyping tumor tissue in search of somatic genetic alterations for *actionable* information has become routine practice in clinical oncology. The genetic profile of solid tumors is currently obtained from surgical or biopsy specimens. As the techniques

TABLE 1.3
Useful Information for the Description and Management of Cancer

Bioinformatic Tool or Webservices	Database Used	Webservice or Tool	Upload of Data Possible	Gene Search	Chromosomal Region Search	mRNA Expression	SNV	CNV	Methylation	miRNA Expression	Protein	Pathways
cBioPortal for Cancer Genomics	TCGA	Webservice	—	✓	—	✓	✓	✓	—	—	✓	✓
PARADIGM, Broad GDAC Firehose	TCGA	Webservice	✓	✓	—	✓	✓	✓	✓	—	—	✓
WashU Epigenome Browser	ENCODE	Webservice	✓	✓	✓	✓	✓	✓	✓	✓	—	✓
UCSC Cancer Genomics Browser	UCSC	Webservice	✓	✓	✓	✓	✓	✓	✓	—	—	—
The Cancer Genome Workbench	TCGA	Webservice	—	✓	✓	✓	✓	✓	✓	—	—	—
EpiExplorer	ENCODE and ROADMAP	Webservice	✓	✓	✓	—	—	—	—	—	—	—
EpiGRAPH	ENCODE	Webservice	✓	✓	✓	✓	✓	✓	✓	—	—	✓
Catalogue of Somatic Mutations in Cancer (COSMIC)	TCGA and ICGC	Webservice	—	✓	—	—	✓	✓	—	—	—	✓
PCmtl, MAGIA, miRvar, CoMeTa, etc.*	GEO and TCGA	Webservice	✓	✓	—	✓	—	—	—	✓	—	—
ICGC	ICGC	Webservice	—	✓	—	✓	✓	✓	✓	—	—	✓
Genomatix	User defined	Tool	—	✓	—	✓	✓	✓	✓	—	—	✓
Caleydo	TCGA	Tool	—	✓	✓	✓	✓	✓	✓	✓	—	✓
Integrative Genomics Viewer (IGV)	ENCODE	Tool	—	✓	✓	✓	✓	✓	✓	—	—	✓
iCluster and iCluster Plus	User defined	Tool	—	✓	—	✓	—	✓	—	—	—	—

* Web Site with links for integrated analysis of microRNA and mRNA expression.
CNV, copy-number variation; ENCODE, Encyclopedia of DNA Elements; ICGC, the International Cancer Genome Consortium; GDAC, Genomic Data Analysis Center; GEO, Gene Expression Omnibus; miRNA, microRNA; SNV, single-nucleotide variation; TCGA, The Cancer Genome Atlas; UCSC, University of California, Santa Cruz;
Based on Plass C, Pfister SM, Lindroth AM, et al. Mutations in regulators of the epigenome and their connections to global chromatin patterns in cancer. *Nat Rev Genet* 2013;14:765–780, Table 1.

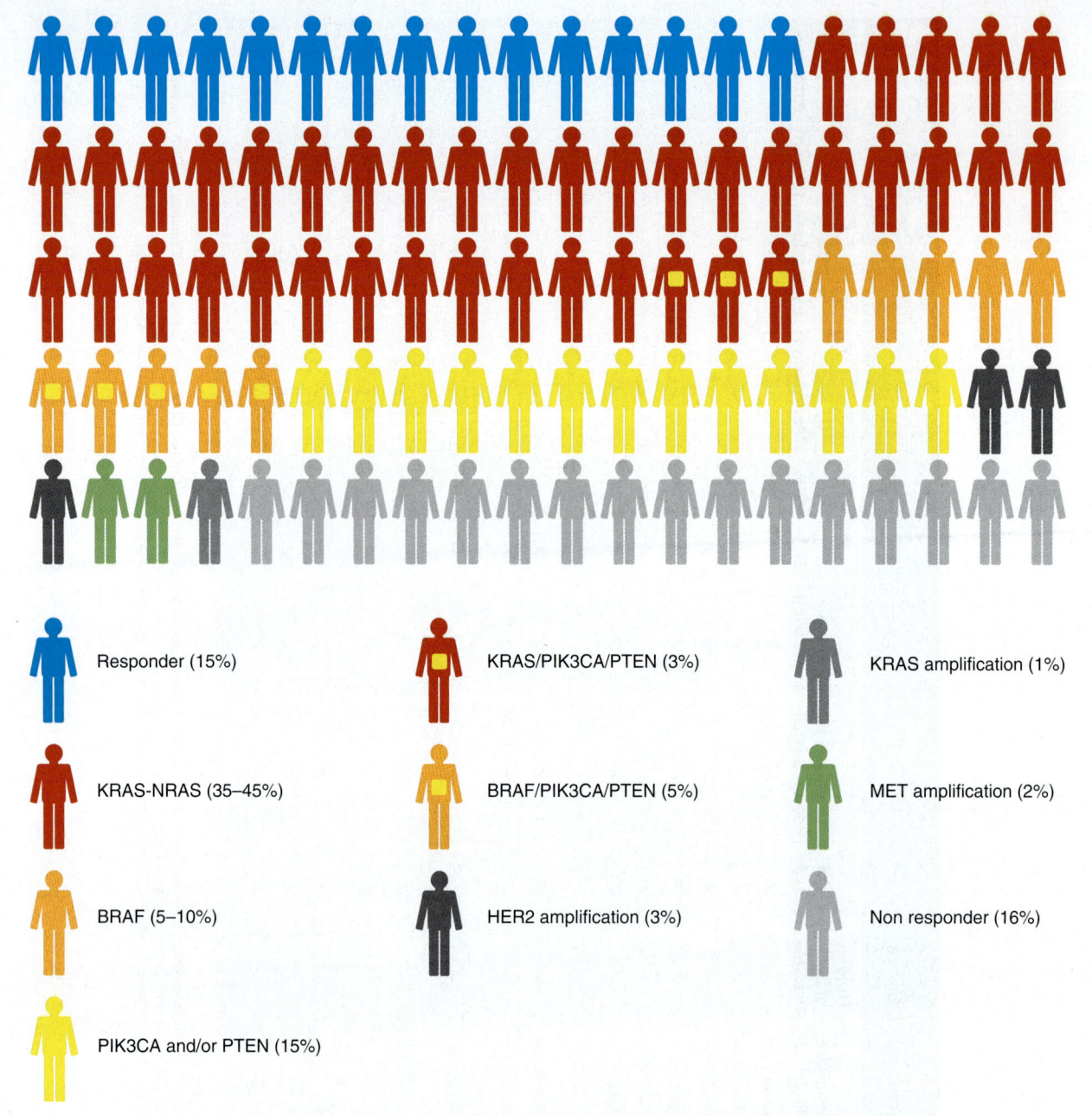

Figure 1.10 Graphic representation of a cohort of 100 patients with colorectal cancer treated with cetuximab or panitumumab. The genetic milieu of individual tumors and their impacts on the clinical response are listed. *KRAS, BRAF,* and *PIK3CA* somatic mutations as well as loss of PTEN protein expression are indicated according to different color codes. Molecular alterations mutually exclusive or coexisting in individual tumors are indicated using different color variants. The relative frequencies at which the molecular alterations occur in colorectal cancers are described. (Redrawn from Bardelli A, Siena S. Molecular mechanisms of resistance to cetuximab and panitumumab in colorectal cancer. *J Clin Oncol* 2010;28:1254–1261.)

that have enabled us to analyze tumor tissues become ever more sophisticated, we have realized the limitations of this approach. As previously discussed, cancers are heterogeneous, with different areas of the same tumor showing different genetic profiles (i.e., intratumoral heterogeneity); likewise, heterogeneity exists between metastases within the same patient (i.e., intermetastatic heterogeneity).[159] A tissue section (or a biopsy) from one part of a solitary tumor will miss the molecular intratumoral as well as intermetastatic heterogeneity. To capture tumor heterogeneity, techniques that are capable of interrogating the genetic landscapes of the overall disease in a single patient are needed.

In 1948, the publication of a manuscript describing the presence of cell-free circulating DNA (cfDNA) in the blood of humans offered—probably without realizing it—unprecedented opportunities in this area.[160] Only recently, the full potential of this seminal discovery has been appreciated. Several groups have reported that the analysis of circulating tumor DNA can, in principle, provide the same genetic information obtained from tumor tissue.[161] The levels of cfDNA are typically higher in cancer patients than healthy individuals, indicating that it is possible to screen for the presence of disease through a simple blood test. Furthermore, the specific detection of tumor-derived cfDNA has been shown to correlate with tumor burden, which changes in response to treatment or surgery.[162–164]

Although the detection of ctDNA has remarkable potential, it is also challenging for several reasons. The first is the need to discriminate DNA released from tumor cells (ctDNA) from circulating *normal* DNA. Discerning ctDNA from normal cfDNA is aided by the fact that tumor DNA is defined by the presence of mutations. These somatic mutations, commonly single base pair substitutions, are present only in the genomes of cancer cells or precancerous cells and are present in the DNA of normal cells of the same individual. Accordingly, ctDNA offers exquisite specificity as a biomarker. Unfortunately, cfDNA derived from tumor cells often represents a very small fraction (<1%) of the total cfDNA, thus limiting the applicability of the approach. The development and refinement of next-generation sequencing strategies as well as recently developed digital PCR techniques have made it possible to define rare mutant variants in complex mixtures of DNA. Using these approaches, it is possible to detect point mutations, rearrangements, and gene copy number changes in individual genes starting from a few milliliters of plasma.[165] Very recently, several groups have opened a new frontier by showing that exome analyses can also be performed from circulating DNA extracted from the blood of cancer patients.[166]

The detection of tumor-specific genetic alterations in patients' blood (often referred to as *liquid biopsies*) has several applications in the field of oncology, which are summarized as follows. Analyses of cfDNA can be used to genotype tumors when a tissue sample is not available or is difficult to obtain. Circulating tumor DNA fragments contain the identical genetic defects as the tumor themselves, thus the blood can reveal tumor point mutations (*EGFR*, *KRAS*, *BRAF*, *PIK3CA*), rearrangements (e.g., *EML4-ALK*), as well as tumor amplifications (*MET*).[167–169] *Liquid biopsies* may also be useful in monitoring tumor burden—a central aspect in the management of patients with cancer that is typically assessed with imaging. In this regard, several investigational studies have shown that ctDNA can be a surrogate for tumor burden and that, much like viral load changes (e.g., HIV viral load), levels of ctDNA correspond with clinical course. Another application of ctDNA is the detection of minimal residual disease following surgery or therapy with curative intent.[163] Finally, *liquid biopsies* can be used to monitor the genomic drift (clonal evolution) of tumors upon treatment.[166] In this setting, the analysis of ctDNA in plasma samples obtained pretreatment, during, and posttreatment can lead to an understanding of the mechanisms of primary and, especially, acquired resistance to therapies.[170,171]

Importantly, the advances in sequencing technologies have made the idea of personalized treatment of cancer a reality, which is most evident in the field of adoptive cell therapy (ACT). Although already a treatment in use, the ability to use a patient's autologous tumor-infiltrating lymphocytes (TIL) is in position to benefit greatly from advances in sequencing technologies. A recent study demonstrated this when whole-exome data, along with a major histocompatibility complex (MHC)-binding algorithm, were utilized to identify candidate tumor epitopes that are recognized by the patients' TILs.[172] This study should allow for future work in which the information obtained from the direct sequencing of a patient's tumor can quickly be used to generate tumor-reactive T cells that can then be used for a personalized treatment.

In conclusion, the taxonomy of tumors is being rewritten using the presence of genetic lesions as major criteria. Genome-based information will improve the diagnosis and will be used to determine personalized therapeutic regimens based on the genetic landscape of individual tumors.

CANCER GENOMICS AND DRUG RESISTANCE

Cancer genomics has dramatically impacted disease management, because its application is helping researchers determine which patients are likely to benefit from which drug. As discussed in great detail in Chapter 22, good examples for such treatment include targeted therapy using imatinib for chronic myeloid leukemia (CML) patients and the use of gefitinib and erlotinib for NSCLC patients.

The key to the successful development and application of anticancer agents is a better understanding of the effect of the therapeutic regimens and of resistance mechanisms that may develop. In most tumor types, a fraction of patients' tumors are refractory to therapies (intrinsic resistance). Even if an initial response to therapies is obtained, the vast majority of tumors subsequently become refractory (i.e., acquired resistance), and patients eventually succumb to disease progression. Therefore, secondary resistance should be regarded as a key obstacle to treatment progress. The analysis of the cancer genome represents a powerful tool both for the identification of chemotherapeutic signatures as well as to understand resistance mechanisms to therapeutic agents. Examples for each of these are described as follows.

An important application of systematic sequencing experiments is the identification of the effects of chemotherapy on the cancer genome. For example, gliomas that recur after temozolomide treatment have been shown to harbor large numbers of mutations with a signature typical of a DNA alkylating agent.[173,174] Because these alterations were detected using Sanger sequencing, which as described previously has limited sensitivity, the data suggested that the detected alterations were clonal. The model that unfolds from this study indicates that although temozolomide has limited efficacy, almost all of the cells in a glioma respond to the drug. However, a single cell that was resistant to the chemotherapy proliferated and formed a cell clone. Later genomic analyses of the cell clone allowed for the identification of the underlying mutated resistance genes.[173,174]

Single-molecule–targeted therapy is almost always followed by acquired drug resistance.[175–177] Genomic analyses can be successfully exploited to decipher resistance mechanisms to such inhibitors. A few paradigmatic examples are presented as follows, which will be discussed extensively in other chapters. Despite the effectiveness of gefitinib and erlotinib in EGFR mutant cases of NSCLC,[178] drug resistance develops within 6 to 12 months after the initiation of therapy. The underlying reason for this resistance was identified as a secondary mutation in *EGFR* exon 20, T790M, which is detectable in 50% of patients who relapse.[179–181] Importantly, some studies have shown the mutation to be present before the patient was treated with the drug,[182,183] suggesting that exposure to the drug selected for these cells.[184] Because the drug-resistant *EGFR* mutation is structurally analogous to the mutated gatekeeper residue T315I in BCR-ABL, T670I in c-Kit, and L1196M in EML4-ALK, which have been shown previously to confer resistance to imatinib and other kinase inhibitors,[176,185,186] this mechanism of resistance represents a general problem that needs to be overcome.

A recent elegant study, which also represents the use of genomics in understanding drug-resistance mechanisms, focused on the inhibition of activating *BRAF* (V600E) mutations, which occur in 7% of human malignancies and in 60% of melanomas.[9] Clinical trials using PLX4032, a novel class I RAF-selective inhibitor, showed an 80% antitumor response rate in melanoma patients with *BRAF* (V600E) mutations; however, cases of drug resistance were observed.[187] The use of microarray and sequencing technologies showed that, in this case, the resistance was not due to secondary mutations in *BRAF*, but due rather to either upregulation of *PDGFRB* or *NRAS* mutations.[188]

It was, however, the introduction of two anti-EGFR monoclonal antibodies, cetuximab and panitumumab, for the treatment of metastatic colorectal cancer, that provided the largest body of knowledge on the relationship between tumors' genotypes and the response to targeted therapies. The initial clinical analysis pointed out that only a fraction of metastatic CRC patients benefited from this novel treatment. Different from the NSCLC paradigm, it was found that EGFR mutations do not play a major role in the response. On the contrary, from the initial retrospective analysis, it became clear that somatic *KRAS* mutations, thought to be present in 35% to 45% of metastatic colorectal cancers, are important negative predictors of efficacy in patients who are given panitumumab or cetuximab.[156–158] Among tumors carrying wild-type *KRAS*, mutations of *BRAF* or *PIK3CA*, or a loss of phosphatase and tensin homolog (PTEN) expression may also predict resistance to EGFR-targeted monoclonal antibodies, although the latter biomarkers require further validation before they can be incorporated into clinical practice. From these few examples, it is clear that a future, deeper genomic understanding of targeted drug resistance is crucial to the effective development of additional as well as alternative therapies to overcome this resistance.

PERSPECTIVES OF CANCER GENOME ANALYSIS

The completion of the human genome project has marked a new beginning in biomedical sciences. Because human cancer is a genetic disease, the field of oncology has been one of the first to be impacted by this historic revolution. Knowledge of the sequence and organization of the human genome allows for the systematic analysis of the genetic alterations underlying the origin and evolution of tumors. High-throughput mutational profiling of common tumors, including lung, skin, breast, and colorectal cancers, and the application of next-generation sequencing to whole genome, whole exome, and whole transcriptome of cancer samples has allowed substantial advances in the understanding of this disease by facilitating the detection of all main types of somatic cancer genome alterations. These have also led to historical results, such as the identification of genetic alterations that are likely to be the major drivers of these diseases.

However, the genetic landscape of cancers is by no means complete, and what has been learned so far has raised new and exciting questions that must be addressed. There are still important technical challenges for the detection of somatic mutations.[60] Clinical tumor samples often contain large amounts of nonmalignant cells, which makes the identification of mutations in cancer genomes more challenging when compared with similar analyses of peripheral blood samples for germ-line genome studies. Moreover, the genomic instability inherent to cancer development and progression largely increases the complexity and diversity of genomic alterations of malignant tumors, making it necessary to distinguish between driver and passenger mutations. Likewise, the fact that malignant tumors are genetically heterogeneous and contain several clones simultaneously growing within the same tumor mass raises additional questions regarding the quality of the information currently derived from cancer genomes. Hopefully, in the near future, advances in third-generation sequencing technologies will make it feasible to obtain high-quality sequence data of a genome isolated from a single cell, an aspect of crucial relevance for cancer research.

One of the next imperatives is the definition of the oncogenomic profile of all tumor types. In particular, the less common—although not less lethal—ones are still largely mysterious to scientists and untreatable to clinicians. For some of these diseases, few new therapeutically amenable molecular targets have been discovered in the past years. For example, the identification of drugable genetic lesions associated with pancreatic and ovarian cancers could help define new therapeutic strategies for these aggressive diseases. To achieve this, detailed oncogenomic maps of the corresponding tumors must be drafted. The latter will hopefully be completed in the coming years, thanks to the systematic cancer genome projects that are presently being performed.

Even in the case of common cancers, a lot of genomic profiling efforts still lay ahead. For example, in a significant fraction of breast and lung tumors, the mutations that are likely to be drivers have not yet been found. This is not surprising considering that even in these tumor types only a limited number of samples have been systematically analyzed so far. Therefore, low incidence mutations that could represent potentially key therapeutic targets in a subset of tumors might have escaped detection. Consequently, the scaling up of the mutational profiling to large numbers of specimens for each tumor type is warranted.

Finally, understanding the cellular properties imparted by the hundreds of recently discovered cancer alleles is another area that must be developed. As a matter of fact, compared to the genomic discovery stage, the functional validation of putative novel cancer alleles, despite their potential clinical relevance, is substantially lagging behind. To achieve this, high-throughput functional studies in model systems that accurately recapitulate the genetic alterations found in human cancer must be developed.

To conclude, the eventual goal of profiling the cancer genome is not only to further understand the molecular basis of the disease, but also to discover novel diagnostic and drug targets. One might anticipate that the most immediate application of these new technologies will be noninvasive strategies for early cancer detection. Considering that oncogenic mutations are present only in cancer cells, screening for tumor-derived mutant DNA in patients' blood holds great potential and will progressively substitute current biomarkers, which have poor sensitivity and lack specificity.[171] Further improvements in next-generation sequencing technologies are likely to reduce their cost as well as make these analyses more facile in the future. Once this happens, most cancer patients will undergo in-depth genomic analyses as part of their initial evaluation and throughout their treatment. This will offer more precise diagnostic and prognostic information, which will affect treatment decisions. Although many challenges remain, the information gained from next-generation sequencing platforms is laying a foundation for personalized medicine, in which patients are managed with therapies that are tailored to the specific gene mutations found in their tumors. Ultimately, these should lead to therapeutic successes similar to the ones attained for CML patients with imatinib,[189,190] melanoma patients with PLX4032,[187] and NSCLC patients with gefitinib and erlotinib.[178] Clearly, this is the absolute goal for all of this work.

ACKNOWLEDGMENTS

This work was supported by the Intramural Research Programs of the National Human Genome Research Institute, National Institutes of Health, USA, YS is supported by the Henry Chanoch Krenter Institute for Biomedical Imaging and Genomics, Louis and Fannie Tolz Collaborative Research Project, Dukler Fund for Cancer Research, De Benedetti Foundation-Cherasco 1547, Peter and Patricia Gruber Awards, Gideon Hamburger, Israel, Estate of Alice Schwarz-Gardos, Estate of John Hunter and the Knell Family. YS is supported by the Israel Science Foundation grant numbers 1604/13 and 877/13 and the ERC (StG-335377). A.B. is supported by the European Communityís Seventh Framework Programme under grant agreement no. 259015 COLTHERES, Associazione Italiana per la Ricerca sul Cancro (AIRC) IG grant no. 12812 and Fondazione Piemontese per la Ricerca sul Cancro–ONLUS. C.L-O. is an Investigator of the Botin Foundation supported by grants from Ministerio de Economía y Competitividad-Spain and Instituto de Salud Carlos III (RTICC), Spain.

REFERENCES

1. Vogelstein B, Kinzler KW. Cancer genes and the pathways they control. *Nat Med* 2004;10:789–799.
2. Kinzler KW, Vogelstein B. Lessons from hereditary colon cancer. *Cell* 1996;87:159–170.
3. International Human Genome Sequencing Consortium. Finishing the euchromatic sequence of the human genome. *Nature* 2004;431:931–945.
4. Stehelin D, Varmus HE, Bishop JM, et al. DNA related to the transforming gene(s) of avian sarcoma viruses is present in normal avian DNA. *Nature* 1976;260:170–173.
5. Rous P. Transmission of a malignant new growth by means of a cell-free filtrate. *J Am Med Assoc* 1911;56:198.
6. International HapMap Consortium. The International HapMap Project. *Nature* 2003;426:89–96.
7. International HapMap Consortium. A haplotype map of the human genome. *Nature* 2005;437:1299–1320.
8. Sanger F, Nicklen S, Coulson AR. DNA sequencing with chain-terminating inhibitors. *Proc Natl Acad Sci U S A* 1977;74:5463–5467.
9. Davies H, Bignell GR, Cox C, et al. Mutations of the BRAF gene in human cancer. *Nature* 2002;417:949–954.
10. Rajagopalan H, Bardelli A, Lengauer C, et al. Tumorigenesis: RAF/RAS oncogenes and mismatch-repair status. *Nature* 2002;418:934.
11. Moodie SA, Wolfman A. The 3Rs of life: Ras, Raf and growth regulation. *Trends Genet* 1994;10:44–48.
12. Hafen E, Dickson B, Brunner D, et al. Genetic dissection of signal transduction mediated by the sevenless receptor tyrosine kinase in Drosophila. *Prog Neurobiol* 1994;42:287–292.
13. Bardelli A, Parsons DW, Silliman N, et al. Mutational analysis of the tyrosine kinome in colorectal cancers. *Science* 2003;300:949.
14. Greenman C, Stephens P, Smith R, et al. Patterns of somatic mutation in human cancer genomes. *Nature* 2007;446:153–158.
15. Samuels Y, Wang Z, Bardelli A, et al. High frequency of mutations of the PIK3CA gene in human cancers. *Science* 2004;304:554.
16. Wang Z, Shen D, Parsons DW, et al. Mutational analysis of the tyrosine phosphatome in colorectal cancers. *Science* 2004;304:1164–1166.
17. Vivanco I, Sawyers CL. The phosphatidylinositol 3-Kinase AKT pathway in human cancer. *Nat Rev Cancer* 2002;2:489–501.
18. Broderick DK, Di C, Parrett TJ, et al. Mutations of PIK3CA in anaplastic oligodendrogliomas, high-grade astrocytomas, and medulloblastomas. *Cancer Res* 2004;64:5048–5050.
19. Lee JW, Soung YH, Kim SY, et al. PIK3CA gene is frequently mutated in breast carcinomas and hepatocellular carcinomas. *Oncogene* 2005;24:1477–1480.
20. Bachman KE, Argani P, Samuels Y, et al. The PIK3CA gene is mutated with high frequency in human breast cancers. *Cancer Biol Ther* 2004;3:772–775.
21. Oda K, Stokoe D, Taketani Y, et al. High frequency of coexistent mutations of PIK3CA and PTEN genes in endometrial carcinoma. *Cancer Res* 2005;65:10669–10673.
22. Samuels Y, Waldman T. Oncogenic mutations of PIK3CA in human cancers. *Curr Top Microbiol Immunol* 2010;2:21–42.
23. Parsons DW, Wang TL, Samuels Y, et al. Colorectal cancer: mutations in a signalling pathway. *Nature* 2005;436:792.
24. Lopez-Otin C, Overall CM. Protease degradomics: a new challenge for proteomics. *Nat Rev Mol Cell Biol* 2002;3:509–519.
25. Liotta LA, Tryggvason K, Garbisa S, et al. Metastatic potential correlates with enzymatic degradation of basement membrane collagen. *Nature* 1980;284:67–68.
26. Lopez-Otin C, Hunter T. The regulatory crosstalk between kinases and proteases in cancer. *Nat Rev Cancer* 2010;10:278–292.
27. Egeblad M, Werb Z. New functions for the matrix metalloproteinases in cancer progression. *Nat Rev Cancer* 2002;2:161–174.
28. Lopez-Otin C, Matrisian LM. Emerging roles of proteases in tumour suppression. *Nat Rev Cancer* 2007;7:800–808.
29. Wood LD, Parsons DW, Jones S, et al. The genomic landscapes of human breast and colorectal cancers. *Science* 2007;318:1108–1113.
30. Palavalli LH, Prickett TD, Wunderluch JR, et al. Analysis of the matrix metalloproteinase family reveals that MMP8 is often mutated in melanoma. *Nat Genet* 2009;41:518–520.
31. Lopez-Otin C, Palavalli LH, Samuels Y. Protective roles of matrix metalloproteinases: from mouse models to human cancer. *Cell Cycle* 2009;8:3657–3662.
32. Hanahan D, Weinberg RA. The hallmarks of cancer. *Cell* 2000;100:57–70.
33. Teitz T, Wei T, Valentine MB, et al. Caspase 8 is deleted or silenced preferentially in childhood neuroblastomas with amplification of MYCN. *Nat Med* 2000;6:529–535.
34. Mandruzzato S, Brasseur F, Andry G, et al. A CASP-8 mutation recognized by cytolytic T lymphocytes on a human head and neck carcinoma. *J Exp Med* 1997;186:785–793.
35. Soung YH, Lee JW, Kim SY, et al. CASPASE-8 gene is inactivated by somatic mutations in gastric carcinomas. *Cancer Res* 2005;65:815–821.
36. Fraile JM, Quesada V, Rodríguez D, et al. Deubiquitinases in cancer: new functions and therapeutic options. *Oncogene* 2012;31:2373–2388.
37. Bignell GR, Warren W, Seal S, et al. Identification of the familial cylindromatosis tumour-suppressor gene. *Nat Genet* 2000;25:160–165.
38. Schmitz R, Hansmann ML, Bohle V, et al. TNFAIP3 (A20) is a tumor suppressor gene in Hodgkin lymphoma and primary mediastinal B cell lymphoma. *J Exp Med* 2009;206:981–989.
39. Compagno M, Lim WK, Grunn A, et al. Mutations of multiple genes cause deregulation of NF-kappaB in diffuse large B-cell lymphoma. *Nature* 2009;459:717–721.
40. Kato M, Sanada M, Kato I, et al. Frequent inactivation of A20 in B-cell lymphomas. *Nature* 2009;459:712–716.
41. Novak U, Rinaldi A, Kwee I, et al. The NF-kappa B negative regulator TNFAIP3 (A20) is inactivated by somatic mutations and genomic deletions in marginal zone lymphomas. *Blood* 2009;113:4918–4921.
42. Harbour JW, Onken MD, Roberson ED, et al. Frequent mutation of BAP1 in metastasizing uveal melanomas. *Science* 2010;330:1410–1413.
43. Carbone M, Yang H, Pass HI, et al. BAP1 and cancer. *Nat Rev Cancer* 2013;13:153–159.
44. Sjöblom T, Jones S, Wood LD, et al. The consensus coding sequences of human breast and colorectal cancers. *Science* 2006;314:268–274.
45. Jones S, Zhang X, Parsons DW, et al. Core signaling pathways in human pancreatic cancers revealed by global genomic analyses. *Science* 2008;321:1801–1806.
46. Parsons DW, Jones S, Zhang X, et al. An integrated genomic analysis of human glioblastoma multiforme. *Science* 2008;321:1807–1812.
47. Jones S, Wang TL, Shih IeM, et al. Frequent mutations of chromatin remodeling gene ARID1A in ovarian clear cell carcinoma. *Science* 2010;330:228–231.
48. Parsons DW, Li M, Zhang X, et al. The genetic landscape of the childhood cancer medulloblastoma. *Science* 2011;331:435–439.
49. Yan H, Parsons DW, Jin G, et al. IDH1 and IDH2 mutations in gliomas. *N Engl J Med* 2009;360:765–773.
50. Bleeker FE, Lamba S, Leenstra S, et al. IDH1 mutations at residue p.R132 (IDH1(R132)) occur frequently in high-grade gliomas but not in other solid tumors. *Hum Mutat* 2009;30:7–11.
51. Hartmann C, Meyer J, Balss J, et al. Type and frequency of IDH1 and IDH2 mutations are related to astrocytic and oligodendroglial differentiation and age: a study of 1,010 diffuse gliomas. *Acta Neuropathol* 2009;118:469–474.
52. Hayden JT, Frühwald MC, Hasselblatt M, et al. Frequent IDH1 mutations in supratentorial primitive neuroectodermal tumors (sPNET) of adults but not children. *Cell Cycle* 2009;8:1806–1807.
53. Ichimura K, Pearson DM, Kocialkowski S, et al. IDH1 mutations are present in the majority of common adult gliomas but rare in primary glioblastomas. *Neuro Oncol* 2009;11:341–347.
54. Kang MR, Kim MS, Oh JE, et al. Mutational analysis of IDH1 codon 132 in glioblastomas and other common cancers. *Int J Cancer* 2009;125:353–355.
55. Watanabe T, Nobusawa S, Kleihues P, et al. IDH1 mutations are early events in the development of astrocytomas and oligodendrogliomas. *Am J Pathol* 2009;174:1149–1153.
56. Mardis ER, Ding L, Dooling DJ, et al. Recurring mutations found by sequencing an acute myeloid leukemia genome. *N Engl J Med* 2009;361:1058–1066.
57. Green A, Beer P. Somatic mutations of IDH1 and IDH2 in the leukemic transformation of myeloproliferative neoplasms. *N Engl J Med* 2010;362:369–370.
58. Gross S, Cairns RA, Minden Md, et al. Cancer-associated metabolite 2-hydroxyglutarate accumulates in acute myelogenous leukemia with isocitrate dehydrogenase 1 and 2 mutations. *J Exp Med* 2010;207:339–344.
59. Mardis ER, Wilson RK. Cancer genome sequencing: a review. *Hum Mol Genet* 2009;18:R163–R168.
60. Meyerson M, Gabriel S, Getz G. Advances in understanding cancer genomes through second-generation sequencing. *Nat Rev Genet* 2010;11:685–696.
61. Metzker ML. Sequencing technologies - the next generation. *Nat Rev Genet* 2010;11:31–46.
62. Bell DW. Our changing view of the genomic landscape of cancer. *J Pathol* 2010;220:231–243.
63. Campbell PJ, Pleasance ED, Stephens PJ, et al. Subclonal phylogenetic structures in cancer revealed by ultra-deep sequencing. *Proc Natl Acad Sci U S A* 2008;105:13081–13086.
64. Kidd JM, Cooper GM, Donahue WF, et al. Mapping and sequencing of structural variation from eight human genomes. *Nature* 2008;453:56–64.
65. Drmanac R, Sparks AB, Callow MJ, et al. Human genome sequencing using unchained base reads on self-assembling DNA nanoarrays. *Science* 2010;327:78–81.
66. Clarke J, Wu HC, Jayasinghe L, et al. Continuous base identification for single-molecule nanopore DNA sequencing. *Nat Nanotechnol* 2009;4:265–270.
67. Schadt EE, Turner S, Kasarskis A. A window into third-generation sequencing. *Hum Mol Genet* 2010;19:R227–R240.
68. Dressman D, Yan H, Traverso G, et al. Transforming single DNA molecules into fluorescent magnetic particles for detection and enumeration of genetic variations. *Proc Natl Acad Sci U S A* 2003;100:8817–8822.
69. Fedurco M, Romieu A, Williams S, et al. BTA, a novel reagent for DNA attachment on glass and efficient generation of solid-phase amplified DNA colonies. *Nucleic Acids Res* 2006;34:e22.
70. Harris TD, Buzby PR, Babcock H, et al. Single-molecule DNA sequencing of a viral genome. *Science* 2008;320:106–109.
71. Morozova O, Hirst M, Marra MA. Applications of new sequencing technologies for transcriptome analysis. *Annu Rev Genomics Hum Genet* 2009;10:135–151.

72. Pop M, Salzberg SL. Bioinformatics challenges of new sequencing technology. Trends Genet 2008;24:142–149.
73. Ley TJ, Mardis ER, Ding L, et al. DNA sequencing of a cytogenetically normal acute myeloid leukaemia genome. Nature 2008;456:66–72.
74. Garraway LA, Lander ES. Lessons from the cancer genome. Cell 2013;15: 17–37.
75. Vogelstein B, Papadopoulos N, Velculescu VE, et al. Cancer genome landscapes. Science 2013;339:1546–1558.
76. Watson IR, Takahashi K, Futreal PA, et al. Emerging patterns of somatic mutations in cancer. Nat Rev Genet 2013;14:703–718.
77. Campbell PJ, Yachida S, Mudie LJ, et al. The patterns and dynamics of genomic instability in metastatic pancreatic cancer. Nature 2010;467:1109–1113.
78. Lee W, Jiang Z, Liu J, et al. The mutation spectrum revealed by paired genome sequences from a lung cancer patient. Nature 2010;465:473–477.
79. Marcucci G, Maharry K, Wu YZ, et al. IDH1 and IDH2 gene mutations identify novel molecular subsets within de novo cytogenetically normal acute myeloid leukemia: a Cancer and Leukemia Group B study. J Clin Oncol 2010;28:2348–2355.
80. Paschka P, Schlenk RF, Gaidzik VI, et al. IDH1 and IDH2 mutations are frequent genetic alterations in acute myeloid leukemia and confer adverse prognosis in cytogenetically normal acute myeloid leukemia with NPM1 mutation without FLT3 internal tandem duplication. J Clin Oncol 2010;28:3636–3643.
81. Shah SP, Morin Rd, Khattra J, et al. Mutational evolution in a lobular breast tumour profiled at single nucleotide resolution. Nature 2009;461:809–813.
82. Yachida S, Jones S, Bozic I, et al. Distant metastasis occurs late during the genetic evolution of pancreatic cancer. Nature 2010;467:1114–1117.
83. Pleasance ED, Cheetham RK, Stephens PJ, et al. A comprehensive catalogue of somatic mutations from a human cancer genome. Nature 2010;463:191–196.
84. Pleasance ED, Stephens PJ, O'Meara S, et al. A small-cell lung cancer genome with complex signatures of tobacco exposure. Nature 2010;463:184–190.
85. Ding L, Ellis MJ, Li S, et al. Genome remodelling in a basal-like breast cancer metastasis and xenograft. Nature 2010;464:999–1005.
86. Ley TJ, Ding L, Walter MJ, et al. DNMT3A mutations in acute myeloid leukemia. N Engl J Med 2010;363:2424–2433.
87. Alexandrov LB, Nik-Zainal S, Wedge DC, et al. Signatures of mutational processes in human cancer. Nature 2013;500:415–421.
88. Ward PS, Patel J, Wise DR, et al. The common feature of leukemia-associated IDH1 and IDH2 mutations is a neomorphic enzyme activity converting alpha-ketoglutarate to 2-hydroxyglutarate. Cancer Cell 2010;17:225–234.
89. Jones SJ, Laskin J, Lu YY, et al. Evolution of an adenocarcinoma in response to selection by targeted kinase inhibitors. Genome Biol 2010;11:R82.
90. Navin N, Kendall J, Troge J, et al. Tumour evolution inferred by single-cell sequencing. Nature 2011;472:90–94.
91. Vanharanta S, Massague J. Origins of metastatic traits. Cancer Cell 2013; 24:410–421.
92. Huang FW, Hodis E, Xu MJ, et al. Highly recurrent TERT promoter mutations in human melanoma. Science 2013;339:957–959.
93. Horn S, Figl A, Rachakonda PS, et al. TERT promoter mutations in familial and sporadic melanoma. Science 2013;339:959–961.
94. Ying Z, Li Y, Wu J, et al. Loss of miR-204 expression enhances glioma migration and stem cell-like phenotype. Cancer Res 2013;73:990–999.
95. Liang YJ, Wang QY, Zhou CX, et al. MiR-124 targets Slug to regulate epithelial-mesenchymal transition and metastasis of breast cancer. Carcinogenesis 2013;34:713–722.
96. Cooper C, Guo J, Yan Y, et al. Increasing the relative expression of endogenous non-coding Steroid Receptor RNA Activator (SRA) in human breast cancer cells using modified oligonucleotides. Nucleic Acids Res 2009;37:4518–4531.
97. Stephens PJ, Greenman CD, Fu B, et al. Massive genomic rearrangement acquired in a single catastrophic event during cancer development. Cell 2011; 144:27–40.
98. Korbel JO, Campbell PJ. Criteria for inference of chromothripsis in cancer genomes. Cell 2013;152:1226–1236.
99. Baca SC, Prandi D, Lawrence MS, et al. Punctuated evolution of prostate cancer genomes. Cell 2013;153:666–677.
100. Turner EH, Lee C, Ng SB, et al. Massively parallel exon capture and library-free resequencing across 16 genomes. Nat Methods 2009;6:315–316.
101. Gnirke A, Melnikov A, Maguire J, et al. Solution hybrid selection with ultra-long oligonucleotides for massively parallel targeted sequencing. Nat Biotechnol 2009;27:182–189.
102. Levin JZ, Berger MF, Adiconis X, et al. Targeted next-generation sequencing of a cancer transcriptome enhances detection of sequence variants and novel fusion transcripts. Genome Biol 2009;10:R115.
103. Lawrence MS, Stojanov P, Polak P, et al. Mutational heterogeneity in cancer and the search for new cancer-associated genes. Nature 2013;499:214–218.
104. Kandoth C, McLellan MD, Vandin F, et al. Mutational landscape and significance across 12 major cancer types. Nature 2013;502:333–339.
105. Gartner JJ, Parker SC, Prickett TD, et al. Whole-genome sequencing identifies a recurrent functional synonymous mutation in melanoma. Proc Natl Acad Sci U S A 2013;110:13481–13486.
106. Stegh AH, Brennan C, Mahoney JA, et al. Glioma oncoprotein Bcl2L12 inhibits the p53 tumor suppressor. Genes Dev 2010;24:2194–2204.
107. Mullaney JM, Mills RE, Pittard WS, et al. Small insertions and deletions (INDELs) in human genomes. Hum Mol Genet 2010;19:R131–R136.
108. Tomlins SA, Rhodes DR, Perner S, et al. Recurrent fusion of TMPRSS2 and ETS transcription factor genes in prostate cancer. Science 2005;310:644–648.
109. Soda M, Choi YL, Enomoto M, et al. Identification of the transforming EML4-ALK fusion gene in non-small-cell lung cancer. Nature 2007;448:561–566.
110. Palanisamy N, Ateeq B, Kalyana-Sundaram S, et al. Rearrangements of the RAF kinase pathway in prostate cancer, gastric cancer and melanoma. Nat Med 2010;16:793–798.
111. Leary RJ, Kinde I, Diehl F, et al. Development of personalized tumor biomarkers using massively parallel sequencing. Sci Transl Med 2010;2:20ra14.
112. Maher CA, Kumar-Sinha C, Cao X, et al. Transcriptome sequencing to detect gene fusions in cancer. Nature 2009;458:97–101.
113. Stephens PJ, McBride DJ, Lin ML, et al. Complex landscapes of somatic rearrangement in human breast cancer genomes. Nature 2009;462:1005–1010.
114. Feng H, Shuda M, Chang Y, et al. Clonal integration of a polyomavirus in human Merkel cell carcinoma. Science 2008;319:1096–1100.
115. Herner A, Sauliunaite D, Michalski CW, et al. Glutamate increases pancreatic cancer cell invasion and migration via AMPA receptor activation and Kras-MAPK signaling. Int J Cancer 2011;129:2349–2359.
116. Wei X, Walia V, Lin JC, et al. Exome sequencing identifies GRIN2A as frequently mutated in melanoma. Nat Genet 2011;43:442–446.
117. Prickett TD, Wei X, Cardenas-Navia I, et al. Exon capture analysis of G protein-coupled receptors identifies activating mutations in GRM3 in melanoma. Nat Genet 2011;43:1119–1126.
118. Krauthammer M, Kong Y, Ha BH, et al. Exome sequencing identifies recurrent somatic RAC1 mutations in melanoma. Nat Genet 2012;44:1006–1014.
119. Davies H, Hunter C, Smith R, et al. Somatic mutations of the protein kinase gene family in human lung cancer. Cancer Res 2005;65:7591–7595.
120. Bozic I, Antal T, Ohtsuki H, et al. Accumulation of driver and passenger mutations during tumor progression. Proc Natl Acad Sci U S A 2010;107:18545–18550.
121. Parmigiani G, Boca S, Lin J, et al. Design and analysis issues in genome-wide somatic mutation studies of cancer. Genomics 2009;93:17–21.
122. Kaminker JS, Zhang Y, Waugh A, et al. Distinguishing cancer-associated missense mutations from common polymorphisms. Cancer Res 2007;67:465–473.
123. Futreal PA. Backseat drivers take the wheel. Cancer Cell 2007;12:493–494.
124. Greenman C, Wooster R, Futreal PA, et al. Statistical analysis of pathogenicity of somatic mutations in cancer. Genetics 2006;173:2187–2198.
125. Baudot A, Real FX, Izarzugaza JM, et al. From cancer genomes to cancer models: bridging the gaps. EMBO Rep 2009;10:359–366.
126. Carter H, Chen S, Isik L, et al. Cancer-specific high-throughput annotation of somatic mutations: computational prediction of driver missense mutations. Cancer Res 2009;69:6660–6667.
127. Ng PC, Henikoff S. SIFT: Predicting amino acid changes that affect protein function. Nucleic Acids Res 2003;31:3812–3814.
128. Kohli M, Rago C, Lengauer C, et al. Facile methods for generating human somatic cell gene knockouts using recombinant adeno-associated viruses. Nucleic Acids Res 2004;32:e3.
129. Downing JR, Wilson RK, Zhang J, et al. The Pediatric Cancer Genome Project. Nat Genet 2012;44:619–622.
130. Hudson TJ, Anderson W, Artez A, et al. International network of cancer genome projects. Nature 2010;464:993–998.
131. Bignell GR, Greenman CD, Davies H, et al. Signatures of mutation and selection in the cancer genome. Nature 2010;463:893–898.
132. Sieber OM, Tomlinson SR, Tomlinson IP. Tissue, cell and stage specificity of (epi)mutations in cancers. Nat Rev Cancer 2005;5:649–655.
133. Benvenuti S, Frattini M, Arena S, et al. PIK3CA cancer mutations display gender and tissue specificity patterns. Hum Mutat 2008;29:284–288.
134. Karakas B, Bachman KE, Park BH. Mutation of the PIK3CA oncogene in human cancers. Br J Cancer 2006;94:455–459.
135. Brennan CW, Werhaak RG, McKenna A, et al. The somatic genomic landscape of glioblastoma. Cell 2013;155:462–477.
136. Cancer Genome Atlas Network. Comprehensive molecular characterization of human colon and rectal cancer. Nature 2012;487:330–337.
137. Cancer Genome Atlas Network. Comprehensive molecular portraits of human breast tumours. Nature 2012;490:61–70.
138. Cancer Genome Atlas Research Network. Integrated genomic analyses of ovarian carcinoma. Nature 2011;474:609–615.
139. Cancer Genome Atlas Research Network. Comprehensive molecular characterization of clear cell renal cell carcinoma. Nature 2013;499:43–49.
140. Cancer Genome Atlas Research Network. Integrated genomic characterization of endometrial carcinoma. Nature 2013;497:67–73.
141. Weischenfeldt J, Simon R, Feuerbach L, et al. Integrative genomic analyses reveal an androgen-driven somatic alteration landscape in early-onset prostate cancer. Cancer Cell 2013;23:159–170.
142. Cancer Genome Atlas Research Network. Genomic and epigenomic landscapes of adult de novo acute myeloid leukemia. N Engl J Med 2013;368:2059–2074.
143. Dawson SJ, Rueda OM, Aparicio S, et al. A new genome-driven integrated classification of breast cancer and its implications. EMBO J 2013;32:617–628.
144. Plass C, Pfister SM, Lindroth AM, et al. Mutations in regulators of the epigenome and their connections to global chromatin patterns in cancer. Nat Rev Genet 2013;14:765–780.
145. Shen H, Laird PW. Interplay between the cancer genome and epigenome. Cell 2013;153:38–55.
146. Yamamoto E, Suzuki H, Yamano HO, et al. Molecular dissection of premalignant colorectal lesions reveals early onset of the CpG island methylator phenotype. Am J Pathol 2012;181:1847–1861.
147. Gao J, Aksoy BA, Dogrusoz U, et al. Integrative analysis of complex cancer genomics and clinical profiles using the cBioPortal. Sci Signal 2013;6:pl1.

148. Bleeker FE, Bardelli A. Genomic landscapes of cancers: prospects for targeted therapies. *Pharmacogenomics* 2007;8:1629–1633.
149. Paez JG, Jänne PA, Lee JC, et al. EGFR mutations in lung cancer: correlation with clinical response to gefitinib therapy. *Science* 2004;304:1497–1500.
150. Ciardiello F, Tortora G. EGFR antagonists in cancer treatment. *N Engl J Med* 2008;358:1160–1174.
151. Janku F, Stewart DJ, Kurzrock R. Targeted therapy in non-small-cell lung cancer—is it becoming a reality? *Nat Rev Clin Oncol* 2010;7:401–414.
152. Pao W, Chmielecki J. Rational, biologically based treatment of EGFR-mutant non-small-cell lung cancer. *Nat Rev Cancer* 2010;10:760–774.
153. Gerber DE, Minna JD. ALK inhibition for non-small cell lung cancer: from discovery to therapy in record time. *Cancer Cell* 2010;18:548–551.
154. Andreyev HJ, Norman AR, Cunningham D, et al. Kirsten ras mutations in patients with colorectal cancer: the multicenter "RASCAL" study. *J Natl Cancer Inst* 1998;90:675–684.
155. Roth AD, Tejpar S, Delorenzi M, et al. Prognostic role of KRAS and BRAF in stage II and III resected colon cancer: results of the translational study on the PETACC-3, EORTC 40993, SAKK 60-00 trial. *J Clin Oncol* 2010;28:466–474.
156. Bardelli A, Siena S. Molecular mechanisms of resistance to cetuximab and panitumumab in colorectal cancer. *J Clin Oncol* 2010;28:1254–1261.
157. Siena S, Sartore-Bianchi A, Di Nicolantonio F, et al. Biomarkers predicting clinical outcome of epidermal growth factor receptor-targeted therapy in metastatic colorectal cancer. *J Natl Cancer Inst* 2009;101:1308–1324.
158. Tejpar S, Bertagnolli M, Bosman F, et al. Prognostic and predictive biomarkers in resected colon cancer: current status and future perspectives for integrating genomics into biomarker discovery. *Oncologist* 2010;15:390–404.
159. Gerlinger M, Rowan AJ, Horswell S, et al. Intratumor heterogeneity and branched evolution revealed by multiregion sequencing. *N Engl J Med* 2012;366:883–892.
160. Mandel P, Metais P. [Not Available]. *C R Seances Soc Biol Fil* 1948;142:241–243.
161. Crowley E, Di Nicolantonio F, Loupakis F, et al. Liquid biopsy: monitoring cancer-genetics in the blood. *Nat Rev Clin Oncol* 2013;10:472–484.
162. Diehl F, Li M, Dressman D, et al. Detection and quantification of mutations in the plasma of patients with colorectal tumors. *Proc Natl Acad Sci U S A* 2005;102:16368–16373.
163. Diehl F, Schmidt K, Choti MA, et al. Circulating mutant DNA to assess tumor dynamics. *Nat Med* 2008;14:985–990.
164. Frattini M, Gallino G, Signoroni S, et al. Quantitative and qualitative characterization of plasma DNA identifies primary and recurrent colorectal cancer. *Cancer Lett* 2008;263:170–181.
165. Chan KC, Jiang P, Zheng YW, et al. Cancer genome scanning in plasma: detection of tumor-associated copy number aberrations, single-nucleotide variants, and tumoral heterogeneity by massively parallel sequencing. *Clin Chem* 2013;59:211–224.
166. Murtaza M, Dawson SJ, Tsui DW, et al. Non-invasive analysis of acquired resistance to cancer therapy by sequencing of plasma DNA. *Nature* 2013;497:108–112.
167. Bardelli A, Corso S, Bertotti A, et al. Amplification of the MET receptor drives resistance to anti-EGFR therapies in colorectal cancer. *Cancer Discov* 2013;3:658–673.
168. Higgins MJ, Jelovac D, Barnathan E, et al. Detection of tumor PIK3CA status in metastatic breast cancer using peripheral blood. *Clin Cancer Res* 2012;18:3462–3469.
169. Leary RJ, Sausen M, Kinde I, et al. Detection of chromosomal alterations in the circulation of cancer patients with whole-genome sequencing. *Sci Transl Med* 2012;4:162ra154.
170. Misale S, Yaeger R, Hobor S, et al. Emergence of KRAS mutations and acquired resistance to anti-EGFR therapy in colorectal cancer. *Nature* 2012;486:532–536.
171. Diaz LA Jr, Williams RT, Wu J, et al. The molecular evolution of acquired resistance to targeted EGFR blockade in colorectal cancers. *Nature* 2012;486:537–540.
172. Robbins PF, Lu YC, El-Gamil M, et al. Mining exomic sequencing data to identify mutated antigens recognized by adoptively transferred tumor-reactive T cells. *Nat Med* 2013;19:747–752.
173. Hunter C, Smith R, Cahill DP, et al. A hypermutation phenotype and somatic MSH6 mutations in recurrent human malignant gliomas after alkylator chemotherapy. *Cancer Res* 2006;66:3987–3991.
174. Cahill DP, Levine KK, Betensky RA, et al. Loss of the mismatch repair protein MSH6 in human glioblastomas is associated with tumor progression during temozolomide treatment. *Clin Cancer Res* 2007;13:2038–2045.
175. Engelman JA, Zejnullahu K, Mitsudomi T, et al. MET amplification leads to gefitinib resistance in lung cancer by activating ERBB3 signaling. *Science* 2007;316:1039–1043.
176. Gorre ME, Mohmmed M, Ellwood K, et al. Clinical resistance to STI-571 cancer therapy caused by BCR-ABL gene mutation or amplification. *Science* 2001;293:876–880.
177. Heinrich MC, Corless CL, Blanke CD, et al. Molecular correlates of imatinib resistance in gastrointestinal stromal tumors. *J Clin Oncol* 2006;24:4764–4774.
178. Shepherd FA, Rodrigues Pereira J, Ciuleanu T, et al. Erlotinib in previously treated non-small-cell lung cancer. *N Engl J Med* 2005;353:123–132.
179. Kobayashi S, Boggon TJ, Dayaram T, et al. EGFR mutation and resistance of non-small-cell lung cancer to gefitinib. *N Engl J Med* 2005;352:786–792.
180. Kwak EL, Sordella R, Bell DW, et al. Irreversible inhibitors of the EGF receptor may circumvent acquired resistance to gefitinib. *Proc Natl Acad Sci U S A* 2005;102:7665–7670.
181. Pao W, Miller VA, Politi KA, et al. Acquired resistance of lung adenocarcinomas to gefitinib or erlotinib is associated with a second mutation in the EGFR kinase domain. *PLoS Med* 2005;2:e73.
182. Shih JY, Gow CH, Yang PC. EGFR mutation conferring primary resistance to gefitinib in non-small-cell lung cancer. *N Engl J Med* 2005;353:207–208.
183. Bell DW, Gore I, Okimoto Ra, et al. Inherited susceptibility to lung cancer may be associated with the T790M drug resistance mutation in EGFR. *Nat Genet* 2005;37:1315–1316.
184. Inukai M, Toyooka S, Ito S, et al. Presence of epidermal growth factor receptor gene T790M mutation as a minor clone in non-small cell lung cancer. *Cancer Res* 2006;66:7854–7858.
185. Daub H, Specht K, Ullrich A. Strategies to overcome resistance to targeted protein kinase inhibitors. *Nat Rev Drug Discov* 2004;3:1001–1010.
186. Choi YL, Soda M, Yamashita Y, et al. EML4-ALK mutations in lung cancer that confer resistance to ALK inhibitors. *N Engl J Med* 2010;363:1734–1739.
187. Flaherty KT, Puzanov I, Kim KB, et al. Inhibition of mutated, activated BRAF in metastatic melanoma. *N Engl J Med* 2010;363:809–819.
188. Nazarian R, Shi H, Wang Q, et al. Melanomas acquire resistance to B-RAF(V600E) inhibition by RTK or N-RAS upregulation. *Nature* 2010;468:973–977.
189. Pompetti F, Spadano A, Sau A, et al. Long-term remission in BCR/ABL-positive AML-M6 patient treated with Imatinib Mesylate. *Leuk Res* 2007;31:563–567.
190. Druker BJ, Builhot F, O'Brien SG, et al. Five-year follow-up of patients receiving imatinib for chronic myeloid leukemia. *N Engl J Med* 2006;355:2408–2417.

2 Hallmarks of Cancer: An Organizing Principle for Cancer Medicine

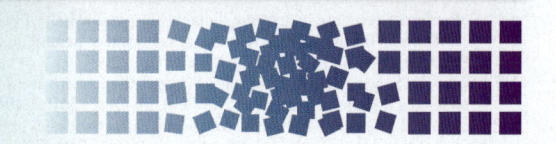

Douglas Hanahan and Robert A. Weinberg

INTRODUCTION

The hallmarks of cancer comprise eight biologic capabilities acquired by incipient cancer cells during the multistep development of human tumors. The hallmarks constitute an organizing principle for rationalizing the complexities of neoplastic disease. They include sustaining proliferative signaling, evading growth suppressors, resisting cell death, enabling replicative immortality, inducing angiogenesis, activating invasion and metastasis, reprogramming energy metabolism, and evading immune destruction. Facilitating the acquisition of these hallmark capabilities are genome instability, which enables mutational alteration of hallmark-enabling genes, and immune inflammation, which fosters the acquisition of multiple hallmark functions. In addition to cancer cells, tumors exhibit another dimension of complexity: They contain a repertoire of recruited, ostensibly normal cells that contribute to the acquisition of hallmark traits by creating the *tumor microenvironment*. Recognition of the widespread applicability of these concepts will increasingly influence the development of new means to treat human cancer.

At the beginning of the new millennium, we proposed that six *hallmarks of cancer* embody an organizing principle that provides a logical framework for understanding the remarkable diversity of neoplastic diseases.[1] Implicit in our discussion was the notion that, as normal cells evolve progressively to a neoplastic state, they acquire a succession of these hallmark capabilities, and that the multistep process of human tumor pathogenesis can be rationalized by the need of incipient cancer cells to acquire the diverse traits that in aggregate enable them to become tumorigenic and, ultimately, malignant.

We noted as an ancillary proposition that tumors are more than insular masses of proliferating cancer cells. Instead, they are complex tissues composed of multiple distinct types of neoplastic and normal cells that participate in heterotypic interactions with one another. We depicted the recruited normal cells, which form tumor-associated stroma, as active participants in tumorigenesis rather than passive bystanders; as such, these stromal cells contribute to the development and expression of certain hallmark capabilities. This notion has been solidified and extended during the intervening period, and it is now clear that the biology of tumors can no longer be understood simply by enumerating the traits of the cancer cells, but instead must encompass the contributions of the *tumor microenvironment* to tumorigenesis. In 2011, we revisited the original hallmarks, adding two new ones to the roster, and expanded on the functional roles and contributions made by recruited stromal cells to tumor biology.[2] Herein we reiterate and further refine the hallmarks-of-cancer perspectives we presented in 2000 and 2011, with the goal of informing students of cancer medicine about the concept and its potential utility for understanding the pathogenesis of human cancer, and the potential relevance of this concept to the development of more effective treatments for this disease.

HALLMARK CAPABILITIES, IN ESSENCE

The eight hallmarks of cancer—distinct and complementary capabilities that enable tumor growth and metastatic dissemination—continue to provide a solid foundation for understanding the biology of cancer (Fig. 2.1). The sections that follow summarize the essence of each hallmark, providing insights into their regulation and functional manifestations.

Sustaining Proliferative Signaling

Arguably, the most fundamental trait of cancer cells involves their ability to sustain chronic proliferation. Normal tissues carefully control the production and release of growth-promoting signals that instruct entry of cells into and progression through the growth-and-division cycle, thereby ensuring proper control of cell number and thus maintenance of normal tissue architecture and function. Cancer cells, by deregulating these signals, become masters of their own destinies. The enabling signals are conveyed in large part by growth factors that bind cell-surface receptors, typically containing intracellular tyrosine kinase domains. The latter proceed to emit signals via branched intracellular signaling pathways that regulate progression through the cell cycle as well as cell growth (that is, increase in cell size); often, these signals influence yet other cell-biologic properties, such as cell survival and energy metabolism.

Remarkably, the precise identities and sources of the proliferative signals operating within normal tissues remain poorly understood. Moreover, we still know relatively little about the mechanisms controlling the release of these mitogenic signals. In part, the study of these mechanisms is complicated by the fact that the growth factor signals controlling cell number and position within normal tissues are thought to be transmitted in a temporally and spatially regulated fashion from one cell to its neighbors; such paracrine signaling is difficult to access experimentally. In addition, the bioavailability of growth factors is regulated by their sequestration in the pericellular space and associated extracellular matrix. Moreover, the actions of these extracellular mitogenic proteins is further controlled by a complex network of proteases, sulfatases, and possibly other enzymes that liberate and activate these factors, apparently in a highly specific and localized fashion.

The mitogenic signaling operating in cancer cells is, in contrast, far better understood.[3–6] Cancer cells can acquire the capability to sustain proliferative signaling in a number of alternative ways: They may produce growth factor ligands themselves, to which they can then respond via the coexpression of cognate receptors, resulting in autocrine proliferative stimulation. Alternatively, cancer cells may send signals to stimulate normal cells within the supporting tumor-associated stroma; the stromal cells then reciprocate by supplying the cancer cells with various growth factors.[7,8] Mitogenic signaling can also be deregulated by elevating the levels of receptor proteins displayed at the cancer cell

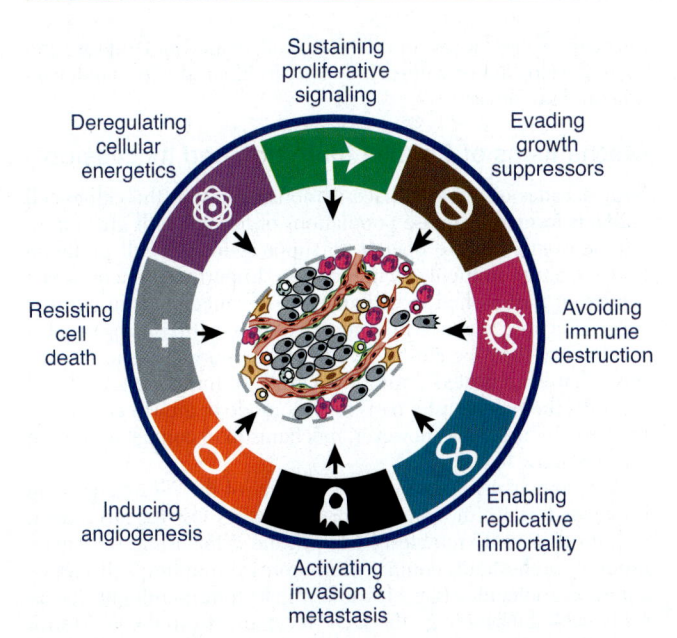

Figure 2.1 The hallmarks of cancer. Eight functional capabilities—the hallmarks of cancer—are thought to be acquired by developing cancers in the course of the multistep carcinogenesis that leads to most forms of human cancer. The order in which these hallmark capabilities are acquired and the relative balance and importance of their contributions to malignant disease appears to vary across the spectrum of human cancers. (Adapted from Hanahan D, Weinberg R. The hallmarks of cancer. *Cell* 2000;100:57–70; Hanahan D, Weinberg RA. Hallmarks of cancer: the next generation. *Cell* 2011;144:646–674.)

surface, rendering such cells hyperresponsive to otherwise limiting amounts of growth factor ligands; the same outcome can result from structural alterations in the receptor molecules that facilitate ligand-independent firing.

Independence from externally supplied growth factors may also derive from the constitutive activation of components of intracellular signaling cascades operating downstream of these receptors within cancer cells. These intracellular alterations obviate the need to stimulate cell proliferation pathways by ligand-mediated activation of cell-surface receptors. Of note, because a number of distinct downstream signaling pathways radiate from ligand-stimulated receptors, the activation of one or another of these downstream branches (e.g., the pathway responding to the Ras signal transducer) may only provide a subset of the regulatory instructions transmitted by a ligand-activated receptor.

Somatic Mutations Activate Additional Downstream Pathways

DNA sequencing analyses of cancer cell genomes have revealed somatic mutations in certain human tumors that predict constitutive activation of the signaling circuits, cited previously, that are normally triggered by activated growth factor receptors. The past 3 decades have witnessed the identification in tens of thousands of human tumors of mutant, oncogenic alleles of the *RAS* proto-oncogenes, most of which have sustained point mutations in the 12th codon, which results in RAS proteins that are constitutively active in downstream signaling. Thus, more than 90% of pancreatic adenocarcinomas carry mutant *K-RAS* alleles. More recently, the repertoire of frequently mutated genes has been expanded to include those encoding the downstream effectors of the RAS proteins. For example, we now know that ~40% of human melanomas contain activating mutations affecting the structure of the B-RAF protein, resulting in constitutive signaling through the RAF to the mitogen-activated protein (MAP)–kinase pathway.[9] Similarly, mutations in the catalytic subunit of phosphoinositide 3-kinase (PI3K) isoforms are being detected in an array of tumor types; these mutations typically serve to hyperactivate the PI3K signaling pathway, causing in turn, excess signaling through the crucial Akt/PKB signal transducer.[10,11] The advantages to tumor cells of activating upstream (receptor) versus downstream (transducer) signaling remain obscure, as does the functional impact of cross-talk between the multiple branched pathways radiating from individual growth factor receptors.

Disruptions of Negative-Feedback Mechanisms that Attenuate Proliferative Signaling

Recent observations have also highlighted the importance of negative-feedback loops that normally operate to dampen various types of signaling and thereby ensure homeostatic regulation of the flux of signals coursing through the intracellular circuitry.[12–15] Defects in these negative-feedback mechanisms are capable of enhancing proliferative signaling. The prototype of this type of regulation involves the RAS oncoprotein. The oncogenic effects of mutant RAS proteins do not result from a hyperactivation of its downstream signaling powers; instead, the oncogenic mutations affecting *RAS* genes impair the intrinsic GTPase activity of RAS that normally serves to turn its activity off, ensuring that active signal transmission (e.g., from upstream growth factor receptors) is transient; as such, oncogenic RAS mutations disrupt an autoregulatory negative-feedback mechanism, without which RAS generates chronic proliferative signals.

Analogous negative-feedback mechanisms operate at multiple nodes within the proliferative signaling circuitry. A prominent example involves phosphatase and tensin homolog (PTEN), which counteracts PI3K by degrading its product, phosphatidylinositol 3,4,5-phosphate (PIP$_3$). Loss-of-function mutations in PTEN amplify PI3K signaling and promote tumorigenesis in a variety of experimental models of cancer; in human tumors, PTEN expression is often lost by the methylation of DNA at specific sites associated with the promoter of the *PTEN* gene, resulting in the shutdown of its transcription.[10,11]

Yet another example involves the mammalian target of rapamycin (mTOR) kinase, a key coordinator of cell growth and metabolism that lies both upstream and downstream of the PI3K pathway. In the circuitry of some cancer cells, mTOR activation results, via negative feedback, in the inhibition of PI3K signaling. Accordingly, when mTOR is pharmacologically inhibited in such cancer cells (e.g., by the drug rapamycin), the associated loss of negative feedback results in increased activity of PI3K and its effector, the Akt/PKB kinase, thereby blunting the antiproliferative effects of mTOR inhibition.[16,17] It is likely that compromised negative feedback loops in this and other signaling pathways will prove to be widespread among human cancer cells, serving as important means by which cancer cells acquire the capability of signaling chronically through these pathways. Moreover, disruption of such normally self-attenuating signaling can contribute to the development of adaptive resistance toward therapeutic drugs targeting mitogenic signaling.

Excessive Proliferative Signaling Can Trigger Cell Senescence

Early studies of oncogene action encouraged the notion that ever-increasing expression of such genes and the signals released by their protein products would result in proportionately increased cancer cell proliferation and, thus, tumor growth. More recent research has undermined this notion, in that it is now apparent that excessively elevated signaling by oncoproteins, such as RAS, MYC, and RAF, can provoke counteracting (protective) responses from cells, such as induction of cell death; alternatively, cancer cells expressing high levels of these oncoproteins may be forced to enter into the nonproliferative but viable state called senescence. These responses contrast with those seen in cells expressing lower levels of these proteins, which permit cells to avoid senescence or cell death and, thus, proliferate.[18–21]

Cells with morphologic features of senescence, including enlarged cytoplasm, the absence of proliferation markers, and the expression of the senescence-induced β-galactosidase enzyme, are abundant in the tissues of mice whose genomes have been reengineered to cause overexpression of certain oncogenes[19,20]; such senescent cells are also prevalent in some cases of human melanoma.[22]

These ostensibly paradoxical responses seem to reflect intrinsic cellular defense mechanisms designed to eliminate cells experiencing excessive levels of certain types of mitogenic signaling. Accordingly, the intensity of oncogenic signaling observed in naturally arising cancer cells may represent compromises between maximal mitogenic stimulation and avoidance of these anti-proliferative defenses. Alternatively, some cancer cells may adapt to high levels of oncogenic signaling by disabling their senescence- or apoptosis-inducing circuitry.

Evading Growth Suppressors

In addition to the hallmark capability of inducing and sustaining positively acting growth-stimulatory signals, cancer cells must also circumvent powerful programs that negatively regulate cell proliferation; many of these programs depend on the actions of tumor suppressor genes. Dozens of tumor suppressors that operate in various ways to limit cell proliferation or survival have been discovered through their inactivation in one or another form of animal or human cancer; many of these genes have been validated as bona fide tumor suppressors through gain- or loss-of-function experiments in mice. The two prototypical tumor suppressor genes encode the retinoblastoma (RB)-associated and TP53 proteins; they operate as central control nodes within two key, complementary cellular regulatory circuits that govern the decisions of cells to proliferate, or alternatively, to activate growth arrest, senescence, or the cell-suicide program known as apoptosis.

The RB protein integrates signals from diverse extracellular and intracellular sources and, in response, decides whether or not a cell should proceed through its growth-and-division cycle.[23-25] Cancer cells with defects in the RB pathway function are thus missing the services of a critical gatekeeper of cell-cycle progression whose absence permits persistent cell proliferation. Whereas RB transduces growth-inhibitory signals that largely originate outside of the cell, TP53 receives inputs from stress and abnormality sensors that function within the cell's intracellular operating systems. For example, if the degree of damage to a cell's genome is excessive, or if the levels of nucleotide pools, growth-promoting signals, glucose, or oxygenation are insufficient, TP53 can call a halt to further cell-cycle progression until these conditions have been normalized. Alternatively, in the face of alarm signals indicating overwhelming or irreparable damage to such cellular systems, TP53 can trigger apoptosis. Of note, the alternative effects of activated TP53 are complex and highly context dependent, varying by cell type as well as by the severity and persistence of conditions of cell-physiologic stress and genomic damage.

Although the two canonical suppressors of proliferation—TP53 and RB—have preeminent importance in regulating cell proliferation, various lines of evidence indicate that each operates as part of a larger network that is wired for functional redundancy. For example, chimeric mice populated throughout their bodies with individual cells lacking a functional Rb gene are surprisingly free of proliferative abnormalities, despite the expectation that a loss of RB function should result in unimpeded advance through the cell division cycle by these cells and their lineal descendants; some of the resulting clusters of Rb-null cells should, by all rights, progress to neoplasia. Instead, the Rb-null cells in such chimeric mice have been found to participate in relatively normal tissue morphogenesis throughout the body; the only neoplasia observed is of pituitary tumors developing late in life.[26] Similarly, TP53-null mice develop normally, show largely normal cell and tissue homeostasis, and again develop abnormalities only later in life in the form of leukemias and sarcomas.[27]

Mechanisms of Contact Inhibition and Its Evasion

Four decades of research have demonstrated that the cell-to-cell contacts formed by dense populations of normal cells growing in 2-dimensional culture operate to suppress further cell proliferation, yielding confluent cell monolayers. Importantly, such *contact inhibition* is abolished in various types of cancer cells in culture, suggesting that contact inhibition is an in vitro surrogate of a mechanism that operates in vivo to ensure normal tissue homeostasis that is abrogated during the course of tumorigenesis. Until recently, the mechanistic basis for this mode of growth control remained obscure. Now, however, mechanisms of contact inhibition are beginning to emerge.[28]

One mechanism involves the product of the NF2 gene, long implicated as a tumor suppressor because its loss triggers a form of human neurofibromatosis. Merlin, the cytoplasmic NF2 gene product, orchestrates contact inhibition by coupling cell-surface adhesion molecules (e.g., E-cadherin) to transmembrane receptor tyrosine kinases (e.g., the EGF receptor). In so doing, Merlin strengthens the adhesiveness of cadherin-mediated cell-to-cell attachments. Additionally, by sequestering such growth factor receptors, Merlin limits their ability to efficiently emit mitogenic signals.[28-31]

Corruption of the TGF-β Pathway Promotes Malignancy

Transforming growth factor beta (TGF-β) is best known for its antiproliferative effects on epithelial cells. The responses of carcinoma cells to TGF-β's proliferation–suppressive effects is now appreciated to be far more elaborate than a simple shutdown of its signaling circuitry.[32-35] In normal cells, exposure to TGF-β blocks their progression through the G1 phase of the cell cycle. In many late-stage tumors, however, TGF-β signaling is redirected away from suppressing cell proliferation and is found instead to activate a cellular program, termed the epithelial-to-mesenchymal transition (EMT), which confers on cancer cells multiple traits associated with high-grade malignancy, as will be discussed in further detail.

Resisting Cell Death

The ability to activate the normally latent apoptotic cell-death program appears to be associated with most types of normal cells throughout the body. Its actions in many if not all multicellular organisms seems to reflect the need to eliminate aberrant cells whose continued presence would otherwise threaten organismic integrity. This rationale explains why cancer cells often, if not invariably, inactivate or attenuate this program during their development.[21,36-38]

Elucidation of the detailed design of the signaling circuitry governing the apoptotic program has revealed how apoptosis is triggered in response to various physiologic stresses that cancer cells experience either during the course of tumorigenesis or as a result of anticancer therapy. Notable among the apoptosis-inducing stresses are signaling imbalances resulting from elevated levels of oncogene signaling and from DNA damage. The regulators of the apoptotic response are divided into two major circuits, one receiving and processing extracellular death-inducing signals (the extrinsic apoptotic program, involving for example the Fas ligand/Fas receptor), and the other sensing and integrating a variety of signals of intracellular origin (the intrinsic program). Each of these circuits culminates in the activation of a normally latent protease (caspase 8 or 9, respectively), which proceeds to initiate a cascade of proteolysis involving effector caspases that are responsible for the execution phase of apoptosis. During this final phase, an apoptotic cell is progressively disassembled and then consumed, both by its neighbors and by professional phagocytic cells. Currently, the intrinsic apoptotic program is more widely implicated as a barrier to cancer pathogenesis.

The molecular machinery that conveys signals between the apoptotic regulators and effectors is controlled by counterbalancing pro- and antiapoptotic members of the Bcl-2 family of regulatory proteins.[36,37] The archetype, Bcl-2, along with its closest relatives (Bcl-XL, Bcl-W, Mcl-1, A1) are inhibitors of apoptosis, acting in large part by binding to and thereby suppressing two proapoptotic triggering proteins (Bax and Bak); the latter are embedded in the mitochondrial outer membrane. When relieved of inhibition by their antiapoptotic relatives, Bax and Bax disrupt the integrity of the outer mitochondrial membrane, causing the release into the cytosol of proapoptotic signaling proteins, the most important of which is cytochrome C. When the normally sequestered cytochrome C is released, it activates a cascade of cytosolic caspase proteases that proceed to fragment multiple cellular structures, thereby executing the apoptotic death program.[37,39]

Several abnormality sensors have been identified that play key roles in triggering apoptosis.[21,37] Most notable is a DNA damage sensor that acts through the TP53 tumor suppressor[40]; TP53 induces apoptosis by upregulating expression of the proapoptotic, Bcl-2-related Noxa and Puma proteins, doing so in response to substantial levels of DNA breaks and other chromosomal abnormalities. Alternatively, insufficient survival factor signaling (e.g., inadequate levels of interleukin (IL)-3 in lymphocytes or of insulinlike growth factors 1/2 [IGF1/2] in epithelial cells) can elicit apoptosis through another proapoptotic Bcl-2-related protein called Bim. Yet another condition triggering apoptosis involves hyperactive signaling by certain oncoproteins, such as Myc, which acts in part via Bim and other Bcl-2-related proteins.[18,21,40]

Tumor cells evolve a variety of strategies to limit or circumvent apoptosis. Most common is the loss of TP53 tumor suppressor function, which eliminates this critical damage sensor from the apoptosis-inducing circuitry. Alternatively, tumors may achieve similar ends by increasing the expression of antiapoptotic regulators (Bcl-2, Bcl-XL) or of survival signals (IGF1/2), by downregulating proapoptotic Bcl-2-related factors (Bax, Bim, Puma), or by short-circuiting the extrinsic ligand-induced death pathway. The multiplicity of apoptosis-avoiding mechanisms presumably reflects the diversity of apoptosis-inducing signals that cancer cell populations encounter during their evolution from the normal to the neoplastic state.

Autophagy Mediates Both Tumor Cell Survival and Death

Autophagy represents an important cell-physiologic response that, like apoptosis, normally operates at low, basal levels in cells but can be strongly induced in certain states of cellular stress, the most obvious of which is nutrient deficiency.[41–43] The autophagic program enables cells to break down cellular organelles, such as ribosomes and mitochondria, allowing the resulting catabolites to be recycled and thus used for biosynthesis and energy metabolism. As part of this program, intracellular vesicles (termed autophagosomes) envelope the cellular organelles destined for degradation; the resulting vesicles then fuse with lysosomes in which degradation occurs. In this fashion, low-molecular-weight metabolites are generated that support survival in the stressed, nutrient-limited environments experienced by many cancer cells. When acting in this fashion, autophagy favors cancer cell survival.

However, the autophagy program intersects in more complex ways with the life and death of cancer cells. Like apoptosis, the autophagy machinery has both regulatory and effector components.[41–43] Among the latter are proteins that mediate autophagosome formation and delivery to lysosomes. Of note, recent research has revealed intersections between the regulatory circuits governing autophagy, apoptosis, and cellular homeostasis. For example, the signaling pathway involving PI3K, AKT, and mTOR, which is stimulated by survival signals to block apoptosis, similarly inhibits autophagy; when survival signals are insufficient, the PI3K signaling pathway is downregulated, with the result that autophagy and/or apoptosis may be induced.[41,42,44,45]

Another interconnection between these two programs resides in the Beclin-1 protein, which has been shown by genetic studies to be necessary for the induction of autophagy.[41–44] Beclin-1 is a member of the Bcl-2 family of apoptotic regulatory proteins, and its BH3 domain allows it to bind the Bcl-2/Bcl-XL proteins. Stress sensor–coupled BH3-containing proteins (e.g. Bim, Noxa) can displace Beclin-1 from its association with Bcl-2/Bcl-XL, enabling the liberated Beclin-1 to trigger autophagy, much as they can release proapoptotic Bax and Bak to trigger apoptosis. Hence, stress-transducing Bcl-2–related proteins can induce apoptosis and/or autophagy depending on the physiologic state of the cell.

Genetically altered mice bearing inactivated alleles of the *Beclin-1* gene or of certain other components of the autophagy machinery exhibit increased susceptibility to cancer.[42,46] These results suggest that the induction of autophagy can serve as a barrier to tumorigenesis that may operate independently of or in concert with apoptosis. For example, excessive activation of the autophagy program may cause cells to devour too many of their own critical organelles, such that cell growth and division are crippled. Accordingly, autophagy may represent yet another barrier that needs to be circumvented by incipient cancer cells during multistep tumor development.[41,46]

Perhaps paradoxically, nutrient starvation, radiotherapy, and certain cytotoxic drugs can induce elevated levels of autophagy that apparently protect cancer cells.[45–48] Moreover, severely stressed cancer cells have been shown to shrink via autophagy to a state of reversible dormancy.[46,49] This particular survival response may enable the persistence and eventual regrowth of some late-stage tumors following treatment with potent anticancer agents. Together, observations like these indicate that autophagy can have dichotomous effects on tumor cells and, thus, tumor progression.[46,47] An important agenda for future research will involve clarifying the genetic and cell-physiologic conditions that determine when and how autophagy enables cancer cells to survive or, alternatively, causes them to die.

Necrosis Has Proinflammatory and Tumor-Promoting Potential

In contrast to apoptosis, in which a dying cell contracts into an almost invisible corpse that is soon consumed by its neighbors, necrotic cells become bloated and explode, releasing their contents into the local tissue microenvironment. A body of evidence has shown that cell death by necrosis, like apoptosis, is an organized process under genetic control, rather than being a random and undirected process.[50–52]

Importantly, necrotic cell death releases proinflammatory signals into the surrounding tissue microenvironment, in contrast to apoptosis, which does not. As a consequence, necrotic cells can recruit inflammatory cells of the immune system,[51,53,54] whose dedicated function is to survey the extent of tissue damage and remove associated necrotic debris. In the context of neoplasia, however, multiple lines of evidence indicate that immune inflammatory cells can be actively tumor-promoting by fostering angiogenesis, cancer cell proliferation, and invasiveness (discussed in subsequent sections). Additionally, necrotic cells can release bioactive regulatory factors, such as IL1α, which can directly stimulate neighboring viable cells to proliferate, with the potential, once again, to facilitate neoplastic progression.[53] Consequently, necrotic cell death, while seemingly beneficial in counterbalancing cancer-associated hyperproliferation, may ultimately do more damage to the patient than good.

Enabling Replicative Immortality

Cancer cells require unlimited replicative potential in order to generate macroscopic tumors. This capability stands in marked contrast to the behavior of the cells in most normal cell lineages in the body, which are only able to pass through a limited number of successive cell growth-and-division cycles. This limitation has been associated with two distinct barriers to proliferation: *replicative senescence*, a typically irreversible entrance into a nonproliferative but viable state, and *crisis*, which involves cell death. Accordingly, when cells are propagated in culture, repeated cycles of cell division lead first to induction of replicative senescence and then, for those cells that succeed in circumventing this barrier, to the crisis phase, in which the great majority of cells in the population die. On rare occasion, cells emerge from a population in crisis and exhibit unlimited replicative potential. This transition has been termed immortalization, a trait that most established cell lines possess by virtue of their ability to proliferate in culture without evidence of either senescence or crisis.

Multiple lines of evidence indicate that telomeres protecting the ends of chromosomes are centrally involved in the capability for unlimited proliferation.[55–58] The telomere-associated DNA, composed of multiple tandem hexanucleotide repeats, shortens progressively in the chromosomes of nonimmortalized cells propagated in culture, eventually losing the ability to protect the ends of chromosomal DNA from end-to-end fusions; such aberrant fusions generate unstable dicentric chromosomes, whose resolution during the anaphase of mitosis results in a scrambling of karyotype and entrance into crisis that threatens cell viability. Accordingly, the length of telomeric DNA in a cell dictates how many successive cell generations its progeny can pass through before telomeres are largely eroded and have consequently lost their protective functions.

Telomerase, the specialized DNA polymerase that adds telomere repeat segments to the ends of telomeric DNA, is almost absent in nonimmortalized cells but is expressed at functionally significant levels in the great majority (~90%) of spontaneously immortalized cells, including human cancer cells. By extending telomeric DNA, telomerase is able to counter the progressive telomere erosion that would otherwise occur in its absence. The presence of telomerase activity, either in spontaneously immortalized cells or in the context of cells engineered to express the enzyme, is correlated with a resistance to induction of both senescence and crisis/apoptosis; conversely, the suppression of telomerase activity leads to telomere shortening and to activation of one or the other of these proliferative barriers.

The two barriers to proliferation—replicative senescence and crisis/apoptosis—have been rationalized as crucial anticancer defenses that are hardwired into our cells and are deployed to impede the outgrowth of clones of preneoplastic and, frankly, neoplastic cells. According to this thinking, most incipient neoplasias exhaust their endowment of replicative doublings and are stopped in their tracks by either of these barriers. The eventual immortalization of rare variant cells that proceed to form tumors has been attributed to their ability to maintain telomeric DNA at lengths sufficient to avoid triggering either senescence or apoptosis, which is achieved most commonly by upregulating the expression of telomerase or, less frequently, via an alternative recombination-based (ALT) telomere maintenance mechanism.[59] Hence, telomere shortening has come to be viewed as a clocking device that determines the limited replicative potential of normal cells and, thus, one that must be overcome by cancer cells.

Reassessing Replicative Senescence

The senescent state induced by oncogenes, as described previously, is remarkably similar to that induced when cells are explanted from living tissue and introduced into culture, the latter being the replicative senescence just discussed. Importantly, the concept of replication-induced senescence as a general barrier requires refinement and reformulation. Recent experiments have revealed that the induction of senescence in certain cultured cells can be delayed and possibly eliminated by the use of improved cell culture conditions, suggesting that recently explanted primary cells may be intrinsically able to proliferate unimpeded in culture up the point of crisis and the associated induction of apoptosis triggered by critically shortened telomeres.[60–63] This result indicates that telomere shortening does not necessarily induce senescence prior to crisis. Additional insight comes from experiments in mice engineered to lack telomerase; this work has revealed that shortening telomeres can shunt premalignant cells into a senescent state that contributes (along with apoptosis) to attenuated tumorigenesis in mice genetically destined to develop particular forms of cancer.[58] Such telomerase-null mice with highly eroded telomeres exhibit multiorgan dysfunction and abnormalities that provide evidence of both senescence and apoptosis, perhaps similar to the senescence and apoptosis observed in cell culture.[58,64] Thus, depending on the cellular context, the proliferative barrier of telomere shortening can be manifested by the induction of senescence and/or apoptosis.

Delayed Activation of Telomerase May Both Limit and Foster Neoplastic Progression

There is now evidence that clones of incipient cancer cells in spontaneously arising tumors experience telomere loss-induced crisis relatively early during the course of multistep tumor progression due to their inability to express significant levels of telomerase. Thus, extensively eroded telomeres have been documented in premalignant growths through the use of fluorescence in situ hybridization (FISH), which has also revealed the end-to-end chromosomal fusions that signal telomere failure and crisis.[65,66] These results suggest that such incipient cancer cells have passed through a substantial number of successive telomere-shortening cell divisions during their evolution from fully normal cells of origin. Accordingly, the development of some human neoplasias may be aborted by telomere-induced crisis long before they have progressed to become macroscopic, frankly neoplastic growths.

A quite different situation is observed in cells that have lost the TP53-mediated surveillance of genomic integrity and, thereafter, experience critically eroded telomeres. The loss of the TP53 DNA damage sensor can enable such cells to avoid apoptosis that would otherwise be triggered by the DNA damage resulting from dysfunctional telomeres. Instead, such cells lacking TP53 continue to divide, suffering repeated cycles of interchromosomal fusion and subsequent breakage at mitosis. Such breakage-fusion-bridge (BFB) cycles result in deletions and amplifications of chromosomal segments, evidently serving to mutagenize the genome, thereby facilitating the generation and subsequent clonal selection of cancer cells that have acquired mutant oncogenes and tumor suppressor genes.[58,67] One infers, however, that the clones of cancer cells that survive this telomere collapse must eventually acquire the ability to stabilize and thus protect their telomeres via the activation of telomerase or the ALT mechanism noted previously.

These considerations present an interesting dichotomy: Although dysfunctional telomeres are an evident barrier to chronic proliferation, they can also facilitate the genomic instability that generates hallmark-enabling mutations, as will be discussed further. Both mechanisms may be at play in certain forms of carcinogenesis in the form of transitory telomere deficiency prior to telomere stabilization. Circumstantial support for this concept of transient telomere deficiency in facilitating malignant progression has come from comparative analyses of premalignant and malignant lesions in the human breast.[68,69] The premalignant lesions did not express significant levels of telomerase and were marked by telomere shortening and chromosomal aberrations. In contrast, overt carcinomas exhibited telomerase expression concordantly with the reconstruction of longer telomeres and the fixation of the aberrant karyotypes that would seem to have been acquired after telomere failure but before the acquisition of telomerase activity. When portrayed in this way, the delayed acquisition of telomerase function serves to generate tumor-promoting mutations, whereas its subsequent expression stabilizes the mutant genome and confers the unlimited replicative capacity that cancer cells require in order to generate clinically apparent tumors.

Inducing Angiogenesis

Like normal tissues, tumors require sustenance in the form of nutrients and oxygen as well as an ability to evacuate metabolic wastes and carbon dioxide. The tumor-associated neovasculature, generated by the process of angiogenesis, addresses these needs. During embryogenesis, the development of the vasculature involves the birth of new endothelial cells and their assembly into tubes (vasculogenesis) in addition to the sprouting (angiogenesis) of new vessels from existing ones. Following this morphogenesis, the normal vasculature becomes largely quiescent. In the adult, as part of physiologic processes such as wound healing and female reproductive cycling, angiogenesis is turned on, but only transiently. In contrast, during tumor progression, an *angiogenic switch* is almost always activated and remains on, causing normally quiescent vasculature to continually sprout new vessels that help sustain expanding neoplastic growths.[70]

A compelling body of evidence indicates that the angiogenic switch is governed by countervailing factors that either induce or oppose angiogenesis.[71,72] Some of these angiogenic regulators are signaling proteins that bind to stimulatory or inhibitory cell-surface receptors displayed by vascular endothelial cells. The well-known prototypes of angiogenesis inducers and inhibitors are vascular endothelial growth factor-A (VEGF-A) and thrombospondin-1 (Tsp-1), respectively.

The VEGF-A gene encodes ligands that are involved in orchestrating new blood vessel growth during embryonic and postnatal development, in the survival of endothelial cells in already-formed vessels, and in certain physiologic and pathologic situations in the adult. VEGF signaling via three receptor tyrosine kinases (VEGFR1-3) is regulated at multiple levels, reflecting this complexity of purpose. VEGF gene expression can be upregulated both by hypoxia and by oncogene signaling.[73-75] Additionally, VEGF ligands can be sequestered in the extracellular matrix in latent forms that are subject to release and activation by extracellular matrix-degrading proteases (e.g., matrix metallopeptidase 9 [MMP-9]).[76] In addition, other proangiogenic proteins, such as members of the fibroblast growth factor (FGF) family, have been implicated in sustaining tumor angiogenesis.[71] TSP-1, a key counterbalance in the angiogenic switch, also binds transmembrane receptors displayed by endothelial cells and thereby triggers suppressive signals that can counteract proangiogenic stimuli.[77]

The blood vessels produced within tumors by an unbalanced mix of proangiogenic signals are typically aberrant: Tumor neovasculature is marked by precocious capillary sprouting, convoluted and excessive vessel branching, distorted and enlarged vessels, erratic blood flow, microhemorrhaging, leaking of plasma into the tissue parenchyma, and abnormal levels of endothelial cell proliferation and apoptosis.[78,79]

Angiogenesis is induced surprisingly early during the multistage development of invasive cancers both in animal models and in humans. Histologic analyses of premalignant, noninvasive lesions, including dysplasias and in situ carcinomas arising in a variety of organs, have revealed the early tripping of the angiogenic switch.[70,80] Historically, angiogenesis was envisioned to be important only when rapidly growing macroscopic tumors had formed, but more recent data indicate that angiogenesis also contributes to the microscopic premalignant phase of neoplastic progression, further cementing its status as an integral hallmark of cancer.

Gradations of the Angiogenic Switch

Once angiogenesis has been activated, tumors exhibit diverse patterns of neovascularization. Some tumors, including highly aggressive types such as pancreatic ductal adenocarcinomas, are hypovascularized and replete with stromal deserts that are largely avascular and indeed may even be actively antiangiogenic.[81] In contrast, many other tumors, including human renal and pancreatic neuroendocrine carcinomas, are highly angiogenic and, consequently, densely vascularized.[82,83]

Collectively, such observations suggest an initial tripping of the angiogenic switch during tumor development, which is followed by a variable intensity of ongoing neovascularization, the latter being controlled by a complex biologic rheostat that involves both the cancer cells and the associated stromal microenvironment.[71,72] Of note, the switching mechanisms can vary, even though the net result is a common inductive signal (e.g., VEGF). In some tumors, dominant oncogenes operating within tumor cells, such as *Ras* and *Myc*, can upregulate the expression of angiogenic factors, whereas in others, such inductive signals are produced indirectly by immune inflammatory cells, as will be discussed.

Endogenous Angiogenesis Inhibitors Present Natural Barriers to Tumor Angiogenesis

A variety of secreted proteins have been reported to have the capability to help shut off normally transitory angiogenesis, including thrombospondin-1 (TSP-1), fragments of plasmin (angiostatin) and type 18 collagen (endostatin), along with another dozen candidate antiangiogenic proteins.[77,84-88] Most are proteins, and many are derived by proteolytic cleavage of structural proteins that are not themselves angiogenic regulators.

A number of these endogenous inhibitors of angiogenesis can be detected in the circulation of normal mice and humans. Genes that encode several endogenous angiogenesis inhibitors have been deleted from the mouse germ line without untoward developmental or physiologic effects; however, the growth of autochthonous and implanted tumors is enhanced as a consequence.[84,85,88] By contrast, if the circulating levels of an endogenous inhibitor are genetically increased (e.g., via overexpression in transgenic mice or in xenotransplanted tumors), tumor growth is impaired.[85,88] Interestingly, wound healing and fat deposition are impaired or accelerated by elevated or ablated expression of such genes.[89,90] The data suggest that, under normal conditions, endogenous angiogenesis inhibitors serve as physiologic regulators modulating the transitory angiogenesis that occurs during tissue remodeling and wound healing; they may also act as intrinsic barriers to the induction and/or persistence of angiogenesis by incipient neoplasias.

Pericytes Are Important Components of the Tumor Neovasculature

Pericytes have long been known as supporting cells that are closely apposed to the outer surfaces of the endothelial tubes in normal tissue vasculature, where they provide important mechanical and physiologic support to the endothelial cells. Microscopic studies conducted in recent years have revealed that pericytes are associated, albeit loosely, with the neovasculature of most, if not all, tumors.[91-93] More importantly, mechanistic studies (discussed subsequently) have revealed that pericyte coverage is important for the maintenance of a functional tumor neovasculature.

A Variety of Bone Marrow-Derived Cells Contribute to Tumor Angiogenesis

It is now clear that a repertoire of cell types originating in the bone marrow play crucial roles in pathologic angiogenesis.[94-97] These include cells of the innate immune system—notably, macrophages, neutrophils, mast cells, and myeloid progenitors—that assemble at the margins of such lesions or infiltrate deeply within them; the tumor-associated inflammatory cells can help to trip the angiogenic switch in quiescent tissue and sustain ongoing angiogenesis associated with tumor growth. In addition, they can help protect the vasculature from the effects of drugs targeting endothelial cell signaling.[98] Moreover, several types of bone marrow–derived *vascular progenitor cells* have been observed to have migrated into neoplastic lesions and become intercalated into the existing neovasculature, where they assumed the roles of either pericytes or endothelial cells.[92,99,100]

Activating Invasion and Metastasis

The multistep process of invasion and metastasis has been schematized as a sequence of discrete steps, often termed the invasion–metastasis cascade.[101,102] This depiction portrays a succession of cell-biologic changes, beginning with local invasion, then intravasation by cancer cells into nearby blood and lymphatic vessels, transit of cancer cells through the lymphatic and hematogenous systems, followed by the escape of cancer cells from the lumina of such vessels into the parenchyma of distant tissues (extravasation), the formation of small nests of cancer cells (micrometastases), and finally, the growth of micrometastatic lesions into macroscopic tumors, this last step being termed *colonization*. These steps have largely been studied in the context of carcinoma pathogenesis. Indeed, when viewed through the prism of the invasion–metastasis cascade, the diverse tumors of this class appear to behave in similar ways.

During the malignant progression of carcinomas, the neoplastic cells typically develop alterations in their shape as well as their attachment to other cells and to the extracellular matrix (ECM). The best-characterized alteration involves the loss by carcinoma cells of E-cadherin, a key epithelial cell-to-cell adhesion molecule. By forming adherens junctions between adjacent epithelial cells, E-cadherin helps to assemble epithelial cell sheets and to maintain the quiescence of the cells within these sheets. Moreover, increased expression of E-cadherin has been well established as an antagonist of invasion and metastasis, whereas a reduction of its expression is known to potentiate these behaviors. The frequently observed downregulation and occasional mutational inactivation of the E-cadherin–encoding gene, *CDH1*, in human carcinomas provides strong support for its role as a key suppressor of the invasion–metastasis hallmark capability.[103,104]

Notably, the expression of genes encoding other cell-to-cell and cell-to-ECM adhesion molecules is also significantly altered in the cells of many highly aggressive carcinomas, with those favoring cytostasis typically being downregulated. Conversely, adhesion molecules normally associated with the cell migrations that occur during embryogenesis and inflammation are often upregulated. For example, N-cadherin, which is normally expressed in migrating neurons and mesenchymal cells during organogenesis, is upregulated in many invasive carcinoma cells, replacing the previously expressed E-cadherin.[104]

Research into the capability for invasion and metastasis has accelerated dramatically over the past decade as powerful new research tools, and refined experimental models have become available. Although still an emerging field replete with major unanswered questions, significant progress has been made in delineating important features of this complex hallmark capability. An admittedly incomplete representation of these advances is highlighted as follows.

The Epithelial-to-Mesenchymal Transition Program Broadly Regulates Invasion and Metastasis

A developmental regulatory program, termed the EMT, has become implicated as a prominent means by which neoplastic epithelial cells can acquire the abilities to invade, resist apoptosis, and disseminate.[105–110] By co-opting a process involved in various steps of embryonic morphogenesis and wound healing, carcinoma cells can concomitantly acquire multiple attributes that enable invasion and metastasis. This multifaceted EMT program can be activated transiently or stably, and to differing degrees, by carcinoma cells during the course of invasion and metastasis.

A set of pleiotropically acting transcriptional factors (TF), including Snail, Slug, Twist, and Zeb1/2, orchestrate the EMT and related migratory processes during embryogenesis; most were initially identified by developmental genetics. These transcriptional regulators are expressed in various combinations in a number of malignant tumor types. Some of these EMT-TFs have been shown in experimental models of carcinoma formation to be causally important for programming invasion; others have been found to elicit metastasis when experimentally expressed in primary tumor cells.[105,111–114] Included among the cell-biologic traits evoked by these EMT-TFs are loss of adherens junctions and associated conversion from a polygonal/epithelial to a spindly/fibroblastic morphology, concomitant with expression of secreted matrix-degrading enzymes, increased motility, and heightened resistance to apoptosis, which are implicated in the processes of invasion and metastasis. Several of these transcription factors can directly repress E-cadherin gene expression, thereby releasing neoplastic epithelial cells from this key suppressor of motility and invasiveness.[115]

The available data suggest that EMT-TFs regulate one another as well as overlapping sets of target genes. Results from developmental genetics indicate that contextual signals received from neighboring cells in the embryo are involved in triggering expression of these transcription factors in cells that are destined to pass through an EMT[111]; in an analogous fashion, heterotypic interactions of cancer cells with adjacent tumor-associated stromal cells have been shown to induce expression of the malignant cell phenotypes that are known to be choreographed by one or more of these EMT-TFs.[116,117] Moreover, cancer cells at the invasive margins of certain carcinomas can be seen to have undergone an EMT, suggesting that these cancer cells are subject to microenvironmental stimuli distinct from those received by cancer cells located in the cores of these lesions.[118] Although the evidence is still incomplete, it would appear that EMT-TFs are able to orchestrate most steps of the invasion–metastasis cascade, except perhaps the final step of colonization, which involves adaptation of cells originating in one tissue to the microenvironment of a foreign, potentially inhospitable tissue.

We still know rather little about the various manifestations and temporal stability of the mesenchymal state produced by an EMT. Indeed, it seems increasingly likely that many human carcinoma cells only experience a *partial EMT*, in which they acquire mesenchymal markers while retaining many preexisting epithelial ones. Although the expression of EMT-TFs has been observed in certain nonepithelial tumor types, such as sarcomas and neuroectodermal tumors, their roles in programming malignant traits in these tumors are presently poorly documented. Additionally, it remains to be determined whether aggressive carcinoma cells invariably acquire their malignant capabilities through activation of components of the EMT program, or whether alternative regulatory programs can also enable expression of these traits.

Heterotypic Contributions of Stromal Cells to Invasion and Metastasis

As mentioned previously, cross-talk between cancer cells and cell types of the neoplastic stroma is involved in the acquired capabilities of invasiveness and metastasis.[94,119–121] For example, mesenchymal stem cells (MSC) present in the tumor stroma have been found to secrete CCL5/RANTES in response to signals released by cancer cells; CCL5 then acts reciprocally on the cancer cells to stimulate invasive behavior.[122] In other work, carcinoma cells secreting IL-1 have been shown to induce MSCs to synthesize a spectrum of other cytokines that proceed thereafter to promote activation of the EMT program in the carcinoma cells; these effectors include IL-6, IL-8, growth-regulated oncogene alpha (GRO-α), and prostaglandin E2.[123]

Macrophages at the tumor periphery can foster local invasion by supplying matrix-degrading enzymes such as metalloproteinases and cysteine cathepsin proteases[76,120,124,125]; in one model system, the invasion-promoting macrophages are activated by IL-4 produced by the cancer cells.[126] And in an experimental model of metastatic breast cancer, tumor-associated macrophages (TAM) supply epidermal growth factor (EGF) to breast cancer cells, while the cancer cells reciprocally stimulate the macrophages with colony stimulating factor 1 (CSF-1). Their concerted interactions facilitate intravasation into the circulatory system and metastatic dissemination of the cancer cells.[94,127]

Observations like these indicate that the phenotypes of high-grade malignancy do not arise in a strictly cell-autonomous manner, and that their manifestation cannot be understood solely through analyses of signaling occurring within tumor cells. One important implication of the EMT model, still untested, is that the ability of carcinoma cells in primary tumors to negotiate most of the steps of the invasion–metastasis cascade may be acquired in certain tumors without the requirement that these cells undergo additional mutations beyond those that were needed for primary tumor formation.

Plasticity in the Invasive Growth Program

The role of contextual signals in inducing an invasive growth capability (often via an EMT) implies the possibility of reversibility, in that cancer cells that have disseminated from a primary tumor to more distant tissue sites may no longer benefit from the activated stroma and the EMT-inducing signals that they experienced while residing in the primary tumor. In the absence of ongoing exposure to these signals, carcinoma cells may revert in their new tissue environment to a noninvasive state. Thus, carcinoma cells that underwent an EMT during initial invasion and metastatic dissemination may reverse this metamorphosis, doing so via a mesenchymal-to-epithelial transition (MET). This plasticity may result in the formation of new tumor colonies of carcinoma cells exhibiting an organization and histopathology similar to those created by carcinoma cells in the primary tumor that never experienced an EMT.[128]

Distinct Forms of Invasion May Underlie Different Cancer Types

The EMT program regulates a particular type of invasiveness that has been termed *mesenchymal*. In addition, two other distinct modes of invasion have been identified and implicated in cancer cell invasion.[129,130] *Collective invasion* involves phalanxes of cancer cells advancing en masse into adjacent tissues and is characteristic of, for example, squamous cell carcinomas. Interestingly, such cancers are rarely metastatic, suggesting that this form of invasion lacks certain functional attributes that facilitate metastasis. Less clear is the prevalence of an *amoeboid* form of invasion,[131,132] in which individual cancer cells show morphologic plasticity, enabling them to slither through existing interstices in the ECM rather than clearing a path for themselves, as occurs in both the mesenchymal and collective forms of invasion. It is presently unresolved whether cancer cells participating in the collective and amoeboid forms of invasion employ components of the EMT program, or whether entirely different cell-biologic programs are responsible for choreographing these alternative invasion programs.

Another emerging concept, noted previously, involves the facilitation of cancer cell invasion by inflammatory cells that assemble at the boundaries of tumors, producing the ECM-degrading enzymes and other factors that enable invasive growth.[76,94,120,133] These functions may obviate the need of invading cancer cells to produce these proteins through activation of EMT programs. Thus, rather than synthesizing these proteases themselves, cancer cells may secrete chemoattractants that recruit proinvasive inflammatory cells; the latter then proceed to produce matrix-degrading enzymes that enable invasive growth.

The Daunting Complexity of Metastatic Colonization

Metastasis can be broken down into two major phases: the physical dissemination of cancer cells from the primary tumor to distant tissues, and the adaptation of these cells to foreign tissue microenvironments that results in successful colonization (i.e., the growth of micrometastases into macroscopic tumors). The multiple steps of dissemination would seem to lie within the purview of the EMT and similarly acting migratory programs. Colonization, however, is not strictly coupled with physical dissemination, as evidenced by the presence in many patients of myriad micrometastases that have disseminated but never progress to form macroscopic metastatic tumors.[101,102,134–136]

In some types of cancer, the primary tumor may release systemic suppressor factors that render such micrometastases dormant, as revealed clinically by explosive metastatic growth soon after resection of the primary growth.[87,137] In others, however, such as breast cancer and melanoma, macroscopic metastases may erupt decades after a primary tumor has been surgically removed or pharmacologically destroyed. These metastatic tumor growths evidently reflect dormant micrometastases that have solved, after much trial and error, the complex problem of adaptation to foreign tissue microenvironments, allowing subsequent tissue colonization.[135,136,138] Implicit here is the notion that most disseminated cancer cells are likely to be poorly adapted, at least initially, to the microenvironment of the tissue in which they have landed. Accordingly, each type of disseminated cancer cell may need to develop its own set of ad hoc solutions to the problem of thriving in the microenvironment of one or another foreign tissue.[139]

One can infer from such natural histories that micrometastases may lack certain hallmark capabilities necessary for vigorous growth, such as the ability to activate angiogenesis. Indeed, the inability of certain experimentally generated dormant micrometastases to form macroscopic tumors has been ascribed to their failure to activate tumor angiogenesis.[135,140] Additionally, recent experiments have shown that nutrient starvation can induce intense autophagy that causes cancer cells to shrink and adopt a state of reversible dormancy. Such cells may exit this state and resume active growth and proliferation when permitted by changes in tissue microenvironment, such as increased availability of nutrients, inflammation from causes such as infection or wound healing, or other local abnormalities.[49,141] Other mechanisms of micrometastatic dormancy may involve antigrowth signals embedded in normal tissue ECM[138] and tumor-suppressing actions of the immune system.[135,142]

Metastatic dissemination has long been depicted as the last step in multistep primary tumor progression; indeed, for many tumors, that is likely the case, as illustrated by recent genome sequencing studies that provide genetic evidence for clonal evolution of pancreatic ductal adenocarcinoma to a metastatic stage.[143–145] Importantly, however, recent results have revealed that some cancer cells can disseminate remarkably early, dispersing from apparently noninvasive premalignant lesions in both mice and humans.[146,147] Additionally, micrometastases can be spawned from primary tumors that are not obviously invasive but possess a neovasculature lacking in luminal integrity.[148] Although cancer cells can clearly disseminate from such preneoplastic lesions and seed the bone marrow and other tissues, their capability to colonize these sites and develop into pathologically significant macrometastases remains unproven. At present, we view this early metastatic dissemination as a demonstrable phenomenon in mice and humans, the clinical significance of which is yet to be established.

Having developed such a tissue-specific colonizing ability, the cells in metastatic colonies may proceed to disseminate further, not only to new sites in the body, but also back to the primary tumors in which their ancestors arose. Accordingly, tissue-specific colonization programs that are evident among certain cells within a primary tumor may originate not from classical tumor progression occurring entirely within the primary lesion, but instead from immigrants that have returned home.[149] Such reseeding is consistent with the aforementioned studies of human pancreatic cancer metastasis.[143–145] Stated differently, the phenotypes and underlying gene expression programs in focal subpopulations of cancer cells within primary tumors may reflect, in part, the reverse migration of their distant metastatic progeny.

Implicit in this *self-seeding* process is another notion: The supportive stroma that arises in a primary tumor and contributes to its acquisition of malignant traits provides a hospitable site for reseeding and colonization by circulating cancer cells released from metastatic lesions.

Clarifying the regulatory programs that enable metastatic colonization represents an important agenda for future research. Substantial progress is being made, for example, in defining sets of genes (*metastatic signatures*) that correlate with and appear to facilitate the establishment of macroscopic metastases in specific tissues.[139,146,150–152] Importantly, metastatic colonization almost certainly requires the establishment of a permissive tumor microenvironment composed of critical stromal support cells. For these reasons, the process of colonization is likely to encompass a large number of cell-biologic programs that are, in aggregate, considerably more complex and diverse than the preceding steps of metastatic dissemination that allow carcinoma cells to depart from primary tumors to sites of lodging and extravasation throughout the body.

Reprogramming Energy Metabolism

The chronic and often uncontrolled cell proliferation that represents the essence of neoplastic disease involves not only deregulated control of cell proliferation but also corresponding adjustments of energy metabolism in order to fuel cell growth and division. Under aerobic conditions, normal cells process glucose, first to pyruvate via glycolysis in the cytosol and thereafter via oxidative phosphorylation to carbon dioxide in the mitochondria. Under anaerobic conditions, glycolysis is favored and relatively little pyruvate is dispatched to the oxygen-consuming mitochondria. Otto Warburg first observed an anomalous characteristic of cancer cell energy metabolism[153–155]: Even in the presence of oxygen, cancer cells can reprogram their glucose metabolism, and thus their energy production, leading to a state that has been termed *aerobic glycolysis*.

The existence of this metabolic specialization operating in cancer cells has been substantiated in the ensuing decades. A key signature of aerobic glycolysis is upregulation of glucose transporters, notably GLUT1, which substantially increases glucose import into the cytoplasm.[156–158] Indeed, markedly increased uptake and utilization of glucose has been documented in many human tumor types, most readily by noninvasively visualizing glucose uptake using positron-emission tomography (PET) with a radiolabeled analog of glucose (^{18}F-fluorodeoxyglucose [FDG]) as a reporter.

Glycolytic fueling has been shown to be associated with activated oncogenes (e.g., *RAS*, *MYC*) and mutant tumor suppressors (e.g., *TP53*),[18,156,157,159] whose alterations in tumor cells have been selected primarily for their benefits in conferring the hallmark capabilities of cell proliferation, subversion of cytostatic controls, and attenuation of apoptosis. This reliance on glycolysis can be further accentuated under the hypoxic conditions that operate within many tumors: The hypoxia response system acts pleiotropically to upregulate glucose transporters and multiple enzymes of the glycolytic pathway.[156,157,160] Thus, both the Ras oncoprotein and hypoxia can independently increase the levels of the HIF1α and HIF2α hypoxia-response transcription factors, which in turn upregulate glycolysis.[160–162]

The reprogramming of energy metabolism is seemingly counterintuitive, in that cancer cells must compensate for the ~18-fold lower efficiency of ATP production afforded by glycolysis relative to mitochondrial oxidative phosphorylation. According to one long-forgotten[163] and a recently revived and refined hypothesis,[164] increased glycolysis allows the diversion of glycolytic intermediates into various biosynthetic pathways, including those generating nucleosides and amino acids. In turn, this facilitates the biosynthesis of the macromolecules and organelles required for assembling new cells. Moreover, Warburg-like metabolism seems to be present in many rapidly dividing embryonic tissues, once again suggesting a role in supporting the large-scale biosynthetic programs that are required for active cell proliferation.

Interestingly, some tumors have been found to contain two subpopulations of cancer cells that differ in their energy-generating pathways. One subpopulation consists of glucose-dependent (Warburg-effect) cells that secrete lactate, whereas cells of the second subpopulation preferentially import and utilize the lactate produced by their neighbors as their main energy source, employing part of the citric acid cycle to do so.[165–168] These two populations evidently function symbiotically: The hypoxic cancer cells depend on glucose for fuel and secrete lactate as waste, which is imported and preferentially used as fuel by their better oxygenated brethren. Although this provocative mode of intratumoral symbiosis has yet to be generalized, the cooperation between lactate-secreting and lactate-utilizing cells to fuel tumor growth is in fact not an invention of tumors, but rather again reflects the co-opting of a normal physiologic mechanism, in this case one operative in muscle[165,167,168] and the brain.[169] Additionally, it is becoming apparent that oxygenation, ranging from normoxia to hypoxia, is not necessarily static in tumors, but instead fluctuates temporally and regionally,[170] likely as a result of the instability and chaotic organization of the tumor-associated neovasculature.

Finally, the notion of the Warburg effect needs to be refined for most if not all tumors exhibiting aerobic glycolysis. The effect does not involve a switching off oxidative phosphorylation concurrent with activation of glycolysis, the latter then serving as the sole source of energy. Rather, cancer cells become highly adaptive, utilizing both mitochondrial oxidative phosphorylation and glycolysis in varying proportions to generate fuel (ATP) and biosynthetic precursors needed for chronic cell proliferation. Finally, this capability for reprograming energy metabolism, dubbed to be an *emerging hallmark* in 2011,[2] is clearly intertwined with the hallmarks conveying deregulated proliferative signals and evasion of growth suppressors, as discussed earlier. As such, its status as a discrete, independently acquired hallmark remains unclear, despite growing appreciation of its importance as a crucial component of the neoplastic growth state.

Evading Immune Destruction

The eighth hallmark reflects the role played by the immune system in antagonizing the formation and progression of tumors. A long-standing theory of immune surveillance posited that cells and tissues are constantly monitored by an ever alert immune system, and that such immune surveillance is responsible for recognizing and eliminating the vast majority of incipient cancer cells and, thus, nascent tumors.[171,172] According to this logic, clinical detectable cancers have somehow managed to avoid detection by the various arms of the immune system, or have been able to limit the extent of immunologic killing, thereby evading eradication.

The role of defective immunologic monitoring of tumors would seem to be validated by the striking increases of certain cancers in immune-compromised individuals.[173] However, the great majority of these are virus-induced cancers, suggesting that much of the control of this class of cancers normally depends on reducing viral burden in infected individuals, in part through eliminating virus-infected cells. These observations, therefore, shed little light on the possible role of the immune system in limiting formation of the >80% of tumors of nonviral etiology. In recent years, however, an increasing body of evidence, both from genetically engineered mice and from clinical epidemiology, suggests that the immune system operates as a significant barrier to tumor formation and progression, at least in some forms of non–virus-induced cancer.[174–177]

When mice genetically engineered to be deficient for various components of the immune system were assessed for the development of carcinogen-induced tumors, it was observed that tumors arose more frequently and/or grew more rapidly in the immunodeficient mice relative to immune-competent controls. In particular, deficiencies in the development or function of either CD8+ cytotoxic T lymphocytes (CTL), CD4+ T$_H$1 helper T cells, or natural killer (NK) cells, each led to demonstrable increases in tumor incidence. Moreover, mice with combined immunodeficiencies in both T cells and NK cells were even more susceptible to cancer development. The results indicated that, at least in certain experimental models, both the innate and adaptive cellular arms of the immune system are able to contribute significantly to immune surveillance and, thus, tumor eradication.[142,178]

In addition, transplantation experiments have shown that cancer cells that originally arose in immunodeficient mice are often inefficient at initiating secondary tumors in syngeneic immunocompetent hosts, whereas cancer cells from tumors arising in immunocompetent mice are equally efficient at initiating transplanted tumors in both types of hosts.[142,178] Such behavior has been interpreted as follows: Highly immunogenic cancer cell clones are routinely eliminated in immunocompetent hosts—a process that has been referred to as *immunoediting*—leaving behind only weakly immunogenic variants to grow and generate solid tumors. Such weakly immunogenic cells can thereafter successfully colonize both immunodeficient and immunocompetent hosts. Conversely, when arising in immunodeficient hosts, the immunogenic cancer cells are not selectively depleted and can, instead, prosper along with their weakly immunogenic counterparts. When cells from such nonedited tumors are serially transplanted into syngeneic recipients, the immunogenic cancer cells are rejected when they confront, for the first time, the competent immune systems of their secondary hosts.[179] (Unanswered in these particular experiments is the question of whether the chemical carcinogens used to induce such tumors are prone to generate cancer cells that are especially immunogenic.)

Clinical epidemiology also increasingly supports the existence of antitumoral immune responses in some forms of human cancer.[180–182] For example, patients with colon and ovarian tumors that are heavily infiltrated with CTLs and NK cells have a better prognosis than those who lack such abundant killer lymphocytes.[176,177,182,183] The case for other cancers is suggestive but less compelling and is the subject of ongoing investigation. Additionally, some immunosuppressed organ transplant recipients have been observed to develop donor-derived cancers, suggesting that in ostensibly tumor-free organ donors, the cancer cells were held in check in a dormant state by a functional immune system,[184] only to launch into proliferative expansion once these *passenger cells* in the transplanted organ found themselves in immunocompromised patients who lack the physiologically important capabilities to mount immune responses that would otherwise hold latent cancer cells in check or eradicate them.

Still, the epidemiology of chronically immunosuppressed patients does not indicate significantly increased incidences of the major forms of nonviral human cancers, as noted previously. This might be taken as an argument against the importance of immune surveillance as an effective barrier to tumorigenesis and tumor progression. We note, however, that HIV and pharmacologically immunosuppressed patients are predominantly immunodeficient in the T- and B-cell compartments and thus do not present with the multicomponent immunologic deficiencies that have been produced in the genetically engineered mutant mice lacking both NK cells and CTLs. This leaves open the possibility that such patients still have residual capability for mounting an anticancer immunologic defense that is mediated by NK and other innate immune cells.

In truth, the previous discussions of cancer immunology simplify tumor–host immunologic interactions, because highly immunogenic cancer cells may well succeed in evading immune destruction by disabling components of the immune system that have been dispatched to eliminate them. For example, cancer cells may paralyze infiltrating CTLs and NK cells by secreting TGF-β or other immunosuppressive factors.[32,185,186] Alternatively, cancer cells may express immunosuppressive cell-surface ligands, such as PD-L1, that prevent activation of the cytotoxic mechanisms of the CTLs. These PD-L1 molecules serve as ligands for the PD-1 receptors displayed by the CTLs, together exemplifying a system of *checkpoint* ligands and receptors that serve to constrain immune responses in order to avoid autoimmunity.[187–189] Yet other localized immunosuppressive mechanisms operate through the recruitment of inflammatory cells that can actively suppress CTL activity, including regulatory T cells (Tregs) and myeloid-derived suppressor cells (MDSC).[174,190–193]

In summary, these eight hallmarks each contribute qualitatively distinct capabilities that seem integral to most lethal forms of human cancer. Certainly, the balance and relative importance of their respective contributions to disease pathogenesis will vary among cancer types, and some hallmarks may be absent or of minor importance in some cases. Still, there is reason to postulate their generality and, thus, their applicability to understanding the biology of human cancer. Next, we turn to the question of how these capabilities are acquired during the multistep pathways through which cancers develop, focusing on two facilitators that are commonly involved.

TWO UBIQUITOUS CHARACTERISTICS FACILITATE THE ACQUISITION OF HALLMARK CAPABILITIES

We have defined the hallmarks of cancer as acquired functional capabilities that allow cancer cells to survive, proliferate, and disseminate. Their acquisition is made possible by two *enabling characteristics* (Fig. 2.2). Most prominent is the development of genomic instability in cancer cells, which generates random mutations, including chromosomal rearrangements, among which are rare genetic changes that can orchestrate individual hallmark capabilities. A second enabling characteristic involves the inflammatory state of premalignant and frankly malignant lesions. A variety of cells of the innate and adaptive immune system infiltrate neoplasias, some of which serve to promote tumor progression through various means.

An Enabling Characteristic: Genome Instability and Mutation

Acquisition of the multiple hallmarks enumerated previously depends in large part on a succession of alterations in the genomes of neoplastic cells. Basically, certain mutant genotypes can confer selective advantage to particular subclones among proliferating nests of incipient cancer cells, enabling their outgrowth and eventual dominance in a local tissue environment. Accordingly, multistep tumor progression can be portrayed as a succession of clonal expansions, most of which are triggered by the chance acquisition of an enabling mutation.

Indeed, it is apparent that virtually every human cancer cell genome carries mutant alleles of one or several growth-regulating genes, underscoring the central importance of these genetic alterations in driving malignant progression.[194] Still, we note that many heritable phenotypes—including, notably, inactivation of tumor suppressor genes—can be acquired through epigenetic

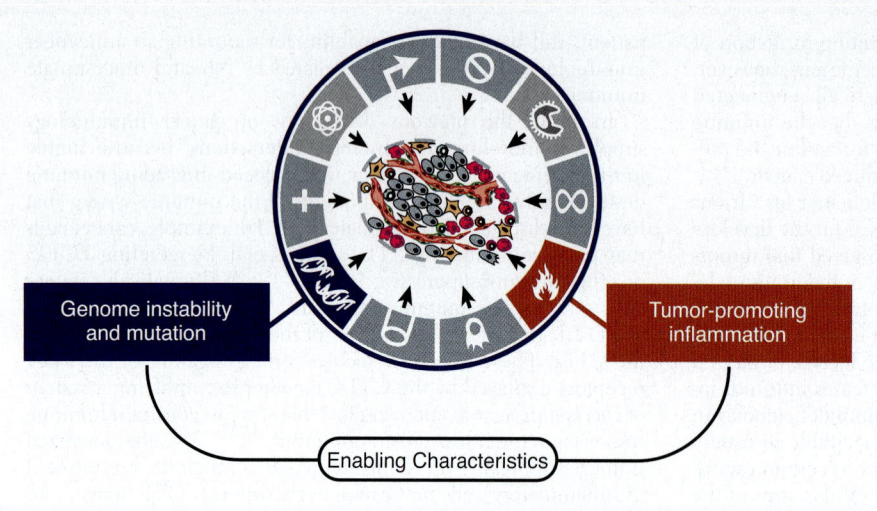

Figure 2.2 Enabling characteristics. Two ostensibly generic characteristics of cancer cells and the neoplasias they create are involved in the acquisition of the hallmark capabilities. First and foremost, the impairment of genome maintenance systems in aberrantly proliferating cancer cells enables the generation of mutations in genes that contribute to multiple hallmarks. Secondarily, neoplasias invariably attract cells of the innate immune system that are programmed to heal wounds and fight infections; these cells, including macrophages, neutrophils, and partially differentiated myeloid cells, can contribute functionally to acquisition of many of the hallmark capabilities. (Adapted from Hanahan D, Weinberg RA. Hallmarks of cancer: the next generation. *Cell* 2011;144:646–674.)

mechanisms, such as DNA methylation and histone modifications.[195–198] Thus, many clonal expansions may also be triggered by heritable nonmutational changes affecting the regulation of gene expression. At present, the relative importance of genetic versus heritable epigenetic alterations to the various clonal expansions remains unclear, and likely, varies broadly amongst the catalog of human cancer types.

The extraordinary ability of genome maintenance systems to detect and resolve defects in the DNA ensures that rates of spontaneous mutation in normal cells of the body are typically very low, both in quiescent cells and during cell division. The genomes of most cancer cells, by contrast, are replete with these alterations, reflecting loss of genomic integrity with concomitantly increased rates of mutation. This heightened mutability appears to accelerate the generation of variant cells, facilitating the selection of those cells whose advantageous phenotypes enable their clonal expansion.[199,200] This mutability is achieved through increased sensitivity to mutagenic agents, through a breakdown in one or several components of the genomic maintenance machinery, or both. In addition, the accumulation of mutations can be accelerated by aberrations that compromise the surveillance systems that normally monitor genomic integrity and force such genetically damaged cells into either quiescence, senescence, or apoptosis.[201–203] The role of TP53 is central here, leading to its being called the *guardian of the genome*.[204]

A diverse array of defects affecting various components of the DNA-maintenance machinery, referred to as the *caretakers* of the genome,[205] have been documented. The catalog of defects in these caretaker genes includes those whose products are involved in (1) detecting DNA damage and activating the repair machinery, (2) directly repairing damaged DNA, and (3) inactivating or intercepting mutagenic molecules before they have damaged the DNA.[199,201,202,206–208] From a genetic perspective, these caretaker genes behave much like tumor suppressor genes, in that their functions are often lost during the course of tumor progression, with such losses being achieved either through inactivating mutations or via epigenetic repression. Mutant copies of many of these caretaker genes have been introduced into the mouse germ line, resulting, not unexpectedly, in increased cancer incidence, thus supporting their involvement in human cancer development.[209]

In addition, research over the past decade has revealed another major source of tumor-associated genomic instability. As described earlier, the loss of telomeric DNA in many tumors generates karyotypic instability and associated amplification and deletion of chromosomal segments.[58] When viewed in this light, telomerase is more than an enabler of the hallmark capability for unlimited replicative potential. It must also be added to the list of critical caretakers responsible for maintaining genome integrity.

Advances in the molecular–genetic analysis of cancer cell genomes have provided the most compelling demonstrations of function-altering mutations and of ongoing genomic instability during tumor progression. One type of analysis—comparative genomic hybridization (CGH)—documents the gains and losses of gene copy number across the cell genome. In many tumors, the pervasive genomic aberrations revealed by CGH provide clear evidence for loss of control of genome integrity. Importantly, the recurrence of specific aberrations (both amplifications and deletions) at particular locations in the genome indicates that such sites are likely to harbor genes whose alteration favors neoplastic progression.[210]

More recently, with the advent of efficient and economical DNA sequencing technologies, higher resolution analyses of cancer cell genomes have become possible. Early studies are revealing distinctive patterns of DNA mutations in different tumor types (see: http://cancergenome.nih.gov/). In the not-too-distant future, the sequencing of entire cancer cell genomes promises to clarify the importance of ostensibly random mutations scattered across cancer cell genomes.[194] Thus, the use of whole genome resequencing offers the prospect of revealing recurrent genetic alterations (i.e., those found in multiple independently arising tumors) that in aggregate represent only minor proportions of the tumors of a given type. The recurrence of such mutations, despite their infrequency, may provide clues about the regulatory pathways playing causal roles in the pathogenesis of the tumors under study.

These surveys of cancer cell genomes have shown that the specifics of genome alteration vary dramatically between different tumor types. Nonetheless, the large number of already documented genome maintenance and repair defects, together with abundant evidence of widespread destabilization of gene copy number and nucleotide sequence, persuade us that instability of the genome is inherent to the cancer cells forming virtually all types of human tumors. This leads, in turn, to the conclusion that the defects in genome maintenance and repair are selectively advantageous and, therefore, instrumental for tumor progression, if only because they accelerate the rate at which evolving premalignant cells can accumulate favorable genotypes. As such, genome instability is clearly an *enabling characteristic* that is causally associated with the acquisition of hallmark capabilities.

An Enabling Characteristic: Tumor-Promoting Inflammation

Among the cells recruited to the stroma of carcinomas are a variety of cell types of the immune system that mediate various inflammatory functions. Pathologists have long recognized that some (but not all) tumors are densely infiltrated by cells of both the innate and adaptive arms of the immune system, thereby mirroring inflammatory conditions arising in nonneoplastic tissues.[211] With the advent of better markers for accurately identifying the distinct cell types of the immune system, it is now clear that virtually every neoplastic lesion contains immune cells present at densities ranging from subtle infiltrations detectable only with cell type–specific antibodies to gross inflammations that are apparent even by standard histochemical staining techniques.[183] Historically, such immune responses were largely thought to reflect an attempt by the immune system to eradicate tumors, and indeed, there is increasing evidence for antitumoral responses to many tumor types with an attendant pressure on the tumor to evade immune destruction,[174,176,177,183] as discussed earlier.

By 2000, however, there were also clues that tumor-associated inflammatory responses can have the unanticipated effect of facilitating multiple steps of tumor progression, thereby helping incipient neoplasias to acquire hallmark capabilities. In the ensuing years, research on the intersections between inflammation and cancer pathogenesis has blossomed, producing abundant and compelling demonstrations of the functionally important tumor-promoting effects that immune cells—largely of the innate immune system—have on neoplastic progression.[19,53,94,174,212,213] Inflammatory cells can contribute to multiple hallmark capabilities by supplying signaling molecules to the tumor microenvironment, including growth factors that sustain proliferative signaling; survival factors that limit cell death; proangiogenic factors; extracellular matrix-modifying enzymes that facilitate angiogenesis, invasion, and metastasis; and inductive signals that lead to activation of EMT and other hallmark-promoting programs.[53,94,116,212,213]

Importantly, localized inflammation is often apparent at the earliest stages of neoplastic progression and is demonstrably capable of fostering the development of incipient neoplasias into full-blown cancers.[94,214] Additionally, inflammatory cells can release chemicals—notably, reactive oxygen species—that are actively mutagenic for nearby cancer cells, thus accelerating their genetic evolution toward states of heightened malignancy.[53] As such, inflammation by selective cell types of the immune system is demonstrably an *enabling characteristic* for its contributions to the acquisition of hallmark capabilities. The cells responsible for this enabling characteristic are described in the following section.

THE CONSTITUENT CELL TYPES OF THE TUMOR MICROENVIRONMENT

Over the past 2 decades, tumors have increasingly been recognized as tissues whose complexity approaches and may even exceed that of normal healthy tissues. This realization contrasts starkly with the earlier, reductionist view of a tumor as nothing more than a collection of relatively homogeneous cancer cells, whose entire biology could be understood by elucidating the cell-autonomous properties of these cells (Fig. 2.3A). Rather, assemblages of diverse cell types associated with malignant lesions are increasingly documented to be functionally important for the manifestation of symptomatic disease (Fig. 2.3B). When viewed from this perspective, the biology of a tumor can only be fully understood by studying the individual specialized cell types within it. We enumerate as follows a set of accessory cell types recruited directly or indirectly by neoplastic cells into tumors, where they contribute in important ways to the biology of many tumors, and we discuss the regulatory mechanisms that control their individual and collective functions. Most of these observations stem from the study of carcinomas, in which the neoplastic epithelial cells constitute a compartment (the parenchyma) that is clearly distinct from the mesenchymal cells forming the tumor-associated stroma.

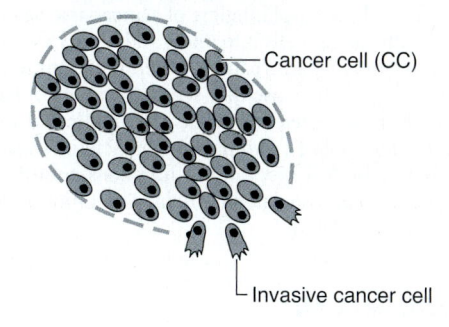

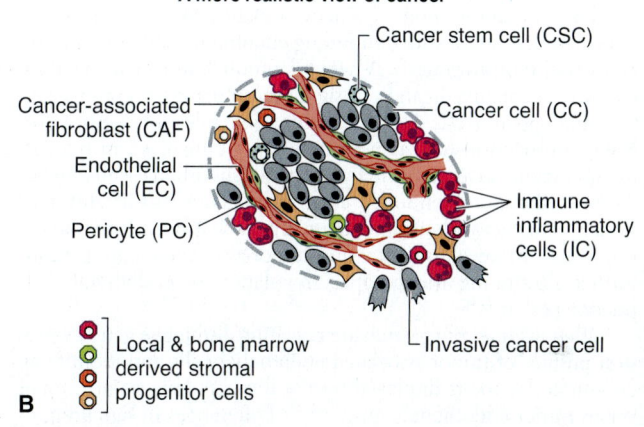

Figure 2.3 Tumors as outlaw organs. Research aimed at understanding the biology of tumors has historically focused on the cancer cells, which constitute the drivers of neoplastic disease. This view of tumors as nothing more than masses of cancer cells **(A)** ignores an important reality, that cancer cells recruit and corrupt a variety of normal cell types that form the tumor-associated stroma. Once formed, the stroma acts reciprocally on the cancer cells, affecting almost all of the traits that define the neoplastic behavior of the tumor as a whole **(B)**. The assemblage of heterogeneous populations of cancer cells and stromal cells is often referred to as the tumor microenvironment (TME). (Adapted from Hanahan D, Weinberg R. The hallmarks of cancer. *Cell* 2000;100:57–70; Hanahan D, Weinberg RA. Hallmarks of cancer: the next generation. *Cell* 2011;144:646–674.)

Cancer-Associated Fibroblasts

Fibroblasts are found in various proportions across the spectrum of carcinomas, in many cases constituting the preponderant cell population of the tumor stroma. The term *cancer-associated fibroblasts* (CAFs) subsumes at least two distinct cell types: (1) cells with similarities to the fibroblasts that create the structural foundation supporting most normal epithelial tissues, and (2) myofibroblasts, whose biologic roles and properties differ markedly from those of the widely distributed tissue-derived fibroblasts. Myofibroblasts are identifiable by their expression of α-smooth muscle actin (αSMA). They are rare in most healthy epithelial tissues, although certain tissues, such as the liver and pancreas, contain appreciable numbers of αSMA-expressing cells. Myofibroblasts transiently increase in abundance in wounds and are also found in sites of chronic inflammation. Although beneficial to tissue repair, myofibroblasts are problematic in chronic inflammation, in that they contribute to the pathologic fibrosis observed in tissues such as the lung, kidney, and liver.

Recruited myofibroblasts and variants of normal tissue-derived fibroblastic cells have been demonstrated to enhance tumor phenotypes, notably cancer cell proliferation, angiogenesis, invasion, and metastasis. Their tumor-promoting activities have largely been defined by transplantation of cancer-associated fibroblasts admixed with cancer cells into mice, and more recently by genetic and pharmacologic perturbation of their functions in tumor-prone mice.[8,121,133,215–219] Because they secrete a variety of ECM components, cancer-associated fibroblasts are implicated in the formation of the desmoplastic stroma that characterizes many advanced carcinomas. The full spectrum of functions contributed by both subtypes of cancer-associated fibroblasts to tumor pathogenesis remains to be elucidated.

Endothelial Cells

Prominent among the stromal constituents of the TME are the endothelial cells forming the tumor-associated vasculature. Quiescent tissue capillary endothelial cells are activated by *angiogenic* regulatory factors to produce a neovasculature that sustains tumor growth concomitant with continuing endothelial cell proliferation and vessel morphogenesis. A network of interconnected signaling pathways involving ligands of signal-transducing receptors (e.g., the Angiopoeitin-1/2, Notch ligands, Semaphorin, Neuropilin, Robo, and Ephrin-A/B) is now known to be involved in regulating quiescent versus activated angiogenic endothelial cells, in addition to the aforementioned counterbalancing VEGF and TSP signals. This network of signaling pathways has been functionally implicated in developmental and tumor-associated angiogenesis, further illustrating the complex regulation of endothelial cell phenotypes.[220–224]

Other avenues of research are revealing distinctive gene expression profiles of tumor-associated endothelial cells and identifying cell-surface markers displayed on the luminal surfaces of normal versus tumor endothelial cells.[78,225,226] Differences in signaling, in transcriptome profiles, and in vascular *ZIP codes* will likely prove to be important for understanding the conversion of normal endothelial cells into tumor-associated endothelial cells. Such knowledge may lead, in turn, to opportunities to develop novel therapies that exploit these differences in order to selectively target tumor-associated endothelial cells. Additionally, the activated (*angiogenic*) tumor vasculature has been revealed as a barrier to efficient intravasation and a functional suppressor of cytotoxic T cells,[227] and thus, tumor endothelial cells can contribute to the hallmark capability for evading immune destruction. As such, another emerging concept is to normalize rather than ablate them, so as to improve immunotherapy[190] as well as delivery of chemotherapy.[228]

Closely related to the endothelial cells of the circulatory system are those forming lymphatic vessels.[229] Their role in the tumor-associated stroma, specifically in supporting tumor growth, is poorly understood. Indeed, because of high interstitial pressure within solid tumors, intratumoral lymphatic vessels are typically collapsed and nonfunctional; in contrast, however, there are often functional, actively growing (*lymphangiogenic*) lymphatic vessels at the periphery of tumors and in the adjacent normal tissues that cancer cells invade. These associated lymphatics likely serve as channels for the seeding of metastatic cells in the draining lymph nodes that are commonly observed in a number of cancer types. Recent results that are yet to be generalized suggest an alternative role for the activated (i.e., lymphangiogenic) lymphatic endothelial cells associated with tumors, not in supporting tumor growth like the blood vessels, but in inducing (via VEGF-C–mediated signaling) a lymphatic tissue microenvironment that suppresses immune responses ordinarily marshaled from the draining lymph nodes.[230] As such, the real value to a tumor from activating the signaling circuit involving the ligand VEGF-C and its receptor VEGFR3 may be to facilitate the evasion of antitumor immunity by abrogating the otherwise immunostimulatory functions of draining lymphatic vessels and lymph nodes, with the collateral effect of inducing lymphatic endothelial cells to form the new lymphatic vessels that are commonly detected in association with tumors.

Pericytes

Pericytes represent a specialized mesenchymal cell type that are closely related to smooth muscle cells, with fingerlike projections that wrap around the endothelial tubing of blood vessels. In normal tissues, pericytes are known to provide paracrine support signals to the quiescent endothelium. For example, Ang-1 secreted by pericytes conveys antiproliferative stabilizing signals that are received by the Tie2 receptors expressed on the surface of endothelial cells. Some pericytes also produce low levels of VEGF that serve a trophic function in endothelial homeostasis.[93,231] Pericytes also collaborate with the endothelial cells to synthesize the vascular basement membrane that anchors both pericytes and endothelial cells and helps vessel walls to withstand the hydrostatic pressure created by the blood.

Genetic and pharmacologic perturbation of the recruitment and association of pericytes has demonstrated the functional importance of these cells in supporting the tumor endothelium.[93,217,231] For example, the pharmacologic inhibition of signaling through the platelet-derived growth factor (PDGF) receptor expressed by tumor pericytes and bone marrow–derived pericyte progenitors results in reduced pericyte coverage of tumor vessels, which in turn destabilizes vascular integrity and function.[91,217,231] Interestingly, and in contrast, the pericytes of normal vessels are not prone to such pharmacologic disruption, providing another example of the differences in the regulation of normal quiescent and tumor vasculature. An intriguing hypothesis, still to be fully substantiated, is that tumors with poor pericyte coverage of their vasculature may be more prone to permit cancer cell intravasation into the circulatory system, thereby enabling subsequent hematogenous dissemination.[91,148]

Immune Inflammatory Cells

Infiltrating cells of the immune system are increasingly accepted to be generic constituents of tumors. These inflammatory cells operate in conflicting ways: Both tumor-antagonizing and tumor-promoting leukocytes can be found in various proportions in most, if not all, neoplastic lesions. Evidence began to accumulate in the late 1990s that the infiltration of neoplastic tissues by cells of the immune system serves, perhaps counterintuitively, to promote tumor progression. Such work traced its conceptual roots back to the observed association of tumor formation with sites of chronic inflammation. Indeed, this led some to liken tumors to "wounds that do not heal."[211,232] In the course of normal wound healing and the resolution of infections, immune inflammatory cells appear transiently and then disappear, in contrast to their persistence in sites of chronic inflammation, where their presence has been associated with a variety of tissue pathologies, including fibrosis, aberrant angiogenesis, and as mentioned, neoplasia.[53,233]

We now know that immune cells play diverse and critical roles in fostering tumorigenesis. The roster of tumor-promoting inflammatory cells includes macrophage subtypes, mast cells, and neutrophils, as well as T and B lymphocytes.[96,97,119,133,212,234,235] Studies of these cells are yielding a growing list of tumor-promoting signaling molecules that they release, which include the tumor growth factor EGF, the angiogenic growth factors VEGF-A/-C, other proangiogenic factors such as FGF2, plus chemokines and cytokines that amplify the inflammatory state. In addition, these cells may produce proangiogenic and/or proinvasive matrix-degrading enzymes, including MMP-9 and other MMPs, cysteine cathepsin proteases, and heparanase.[94,96] Consistent with the expression of these diverse signals, tumor-infiltrating inflammatory cells have been shown to induce and help sustain tumor angiogenesis, to stimulate cancer cell proliferation, to facilitate tissue invasion, and to support the metastatic dissemination and seeding of cancer cells.[94,96,97,119,120,234–237]

In addition to fully differentiated immune cells present in tumor stroma, a variety of partially differentiated myeloid progenitors have been identified in tumors.[96] Such cells represent intermediaries between circulating cells of bone marrow origin and the differentiated immune cells typically found in normal and inflamed tissues. Importantly, these progenitors, like their more differentiated derivatives, have demonstrable tumor-promoting activity. Of particular interest, a class of tumor-infiltrating myeloid cells has been shown to suppress CTL and NK cell activity, having been identified as MDSCs that function to block the attack on tumors by the adaptive (i.e., CTL) and innate (i.e., NK) arms of the immune system.[94,133,193] Hence, recruitment of certain myeloid cells may be doubly beneficial for the developing tumor, by directly promoting angiogenesis and tumor progression, while at the same time affording a means of evading immune destruction.

These conflicting roles of the immune system in confronting tumors would seem to reflect similar situations that arise routinely in normal tissues. Thus, the immune system detects and targets infectious agents through cells of the adaptive immune response. Cells of the innate immune system, in contrast, are involved in wound healing and in clearing dead cells and cellular debris. The balance between the conflicting immune responses within particular tumor types (and indeed in individual patients' tumors) is likely to prove critical in determining the characteristics of tumor growth and the stepwise progression to stages of heightened aggressiveness (i.e., invasion and metastasis). Moreover, there is increasing evidence supporting the proposition that this balance can be modulated for therapeutic purposes in order to redirect or reprogram the immune response to focus its functional capabilities on destroying tumors.[133,238,239]

Stem and Progenitor Cells of the Tumor Stroma

The various stromal cell types that constitute the tumor microenvironment may be recruited from adjacent normal tissue—the most obvious reservoir of such cell types. However, in recent years, bone marrow (BM) has increasingly been implicated as a key source of tumor-associated stromal cells.[99,100,240–243] Thus, mesenchymal stem and progenitor cells can be recruited into tumors from BM, where they may subsequently differentiate into the various well-characterized stromal cell types. Some of these recent arrivals may also persist in an undifferentiated or partially differentiated state, exhibiting functions that their more differentiated progeny lack.

The BM origins of stromal cell types have been demonstrated using tumor-bearing mice in which the BM cells (and thus their disseminated progeny) have been selectively labeled with reporters such as green fluorescent protein (GFP). Although immune inflammatory cells have been long known to derive from BM, more recently progenitors of endothelial cells, pericytes, and several subtypes of cancer-associated fibroblasts have also been shown to originate from BM in various mouse models of cancer.[100,240–243] The prevalence and functional importance of endothelial progenitors for tumor angiogenesis is, however, currently unresolved.[99,242] Taken together, these various lines of evidence indicate that tumor-associated stromal cells may be supplied to growing tumors by the proliferation of preexisting stromal cells or via recruitment of BM-derived stem/progenitor cells.

In summary, it is evident that virtually all cancers, including even the *liquid tumors* of hematopoietic malignancies, depend not only on neoplastic cells for their pathogenic effects, but also on diverse cell types recruited from local and distant tissue sources to assemble specialized, supporting tumor microenvironments. Importantly, the composition of stromal cell types supporting a particular cancer evidently varies considerably from one tumor type to another; even within a particular type, the patterns and abundance can be informative about malignant grade and prognosis. The inescapable conclusion is that cancer cells are not fully autonomous, and rather depend to various degrees on stromal cells of the tumor microenvironment, which can contribute functionally to seven of the eight hallmarks of cancer (Fig. 2.4).

Heterotypic Signaling Orchestrates the Cells of the Tumor Microenvironment

Every cell in our bodies is governed by an elaborate intracellular signaling circuit—in effect, its own microcomputer. In cancer cells, key subcircuits in this integrated circuit are reprogrammed so as to activate and sustain hallmark capabilities. These changes are induced by mutations in the cells' genomes, by epigenetic alterations affecting gene expression, and by the receipt of a diverse array of signals from the tumor microenvironment. Figure 2.5A illustrates some of the circuits that are reprogrammed to enable cancer cells to proliferate chronically, to avoid proliferative brakes and cell death, and to become invasive and metastatic. Similarly, the intracellular integrated circuits that regulate the actions of stromal cells are also evidently reprogrammed. Current evidence suggests that stromal cell reprogramming is primarily affected by extracellular cues and epigenetic alterations in gene expression, rather than gene mutation.

Given the alterations in the signaling within both neoplastic cells and their stromal neighbors, a tumor can be depicted as a network of interconnected (cellular) microcomputers. This dictates that a complete elucidation of a particular tumor's biology will require far more than an elucidation of the aberrantly functioning integrated circuits within its neoplastic cells. Accordingly, the rapidly growing catalog of the function-enabling genetic mutations within cancer cell genomes[194] provides only one dimension to this problem. A reasonably complete, graphical depiction of the network of microenvironmental signaling interactions remains far beyond our reach, because the great majority of signaling molecules and their circuitry are still to be identified. Instead, we provide a hint of such interactions in Figure 2.5B. These few well-established examples are intended to exemplify a signaling network of remarkable complexity that is of critical importance to tumor pathogenesis.

Coevolution of the Tumor Microenvironment During Carcinogenesis

The tumor microenvironment described previously is not static during multistage tumor development and progression, thus creating another dimension of complexity. Rather, the abundance and functional contributions of the stromal cells populating neoplastic lesions will likely vary during progression in two respects. First, as the neoplastic cells evolve, there will be a parallel coevolution occurring in the stroma, as indicated by the shifting composition of stroma-associated cell types. Second, as cancer cells enter into different locations, they encounter distinct stromal microenvironments. Thus, the microenvironment in the interior of a primary tumor will likely be distinct both from locally invasive breakout lesions and from the one encountered by disseminated cells in distant organs (Fig. 2.6A). This dictates that the observed histopathologic progression of a tumor reflects underlying changes in heterotypic signaling between tumor parenchyma and stroma.

We envision back-and-forth reciprocal interactions between the neoplastic cells and the supporting stromal cells that change during the course of multistep tumor development and progression, as depicted in Figure 2.6B. Thus, incipient neoplasias begin the interplay by recruiting and activating stromal cell types that assemble into an initial preneoplastic stroma, which in turn responds reciprocally by enhancing the neoplastic phenotypes of the nearby cancer cells. The cancer cells, in response, may then undergo further genetic evolution, causing them to feed signals back to the stroma. Ultimately, signals originating in the stroma of primary tumors enable cancer cells to invade normal adjacent tissues and disseminate, seeding distant tissues and, with low efficiency, metastatic colonies (see Fig. 2.6B).

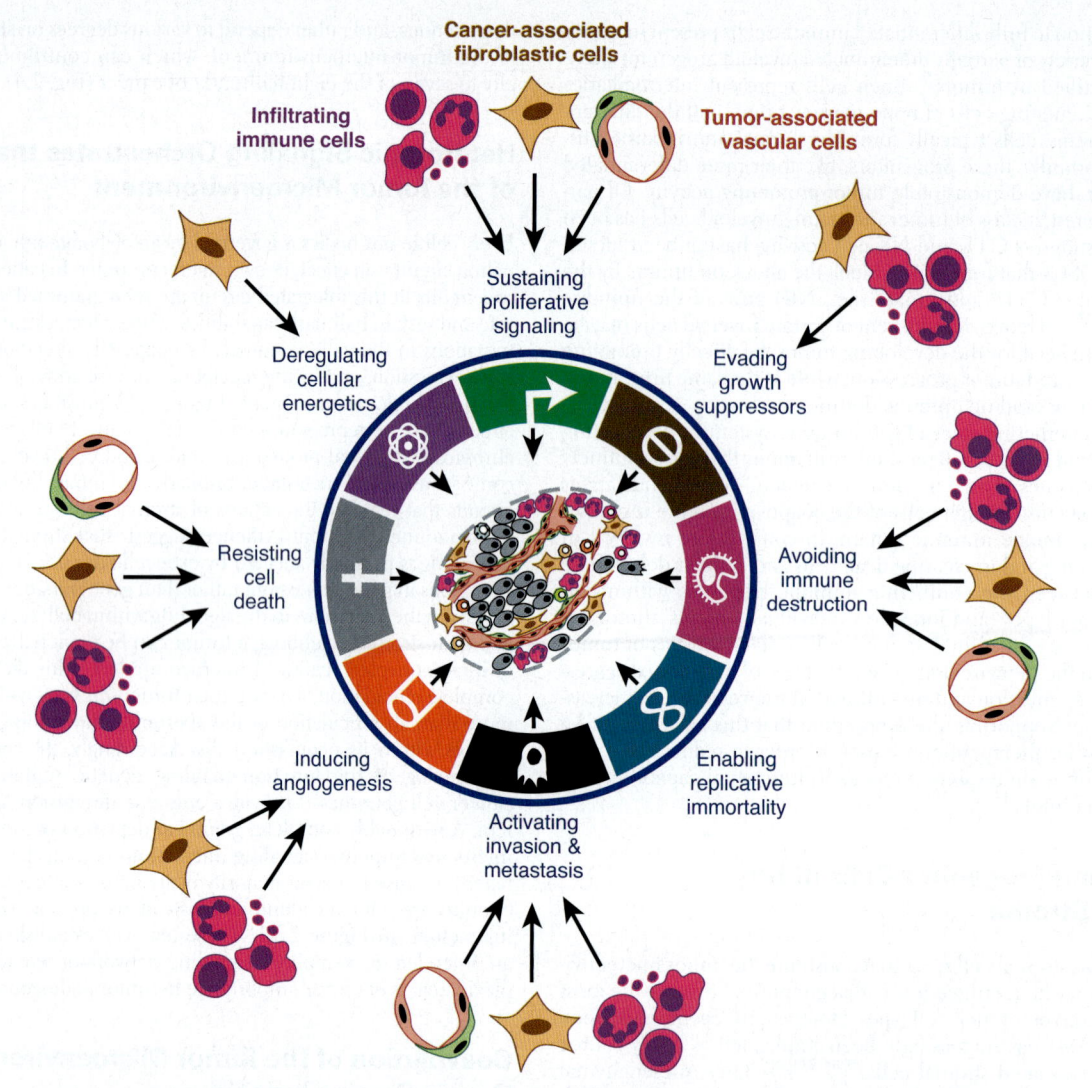

Figure 2.4 Diverse contributions of stromal cells to the hallmarks of cancer. Of the eight hallmark capabilities acquired by cancer cells, seven depend on contributions by stromal cells forming the tumor microenvironment.[2,213] The stromal cells can be divided into three general classes: infiltrating immune cells, cancer-associated fibroblastic cells, and tumor-associated vascular cells. The association of these corrupted cell types with the acquisition of individual hallmark capabilities has been documented through a variety of experimental approaches that are often supported by descriptive studies in human cancers. The relative importance of each of these stromal cell classes to a particular hallmark varies according to tumor type and stage of progression. (Adapted from Hanahan D, Coussens LM. Accessories to the crime: functions of cells recruited to the tumor microenvironment. *Cancer Cell* 2012;21:309–322.)

The circulating cancer cells that are released from primary tumors leave a microenvironment supported by this coevolved stroma. Upon landing in a distant organ, however, disseminated cancer cells must find a means to grow in a quite different tissue microenvironment. In some cases, newly seeded cancer cells must survive and expand in naïve, fully normal tissue microenvironments. In other cases, the newly encountered tissue microenvironments may already be supportive of such disseminated cancer cells, having been preconditioned prior to their arrival. Such permissive sites have been referred to as *premetastatic niches*.[146,244,245] These supportive niches may already preexist in distant tissues for various physiologic reasons,[101] including the actions of circulating factors dispatched systemically by primary tumors.[245]

The fact that signaling interactions between cancer cells and their supporting stroma are likely to evolve during the course of multistage primary tumor development and metastatic colonization clearly complicates the goal of fully elucidating the mechanisms of cancer pathogenesis. For example, this complexity poses challenges to systems biologists seeking to chart the crucial regulatory networks that orchestrate malignant progression, because much of the critical signaling is not intrinsic to cancer cells and instead operates through the interactions that these cells establish with their neighbors.

Cancer Cells, Cancer Stem Cells, and Intratumoral Heterogeneity

Cancer cells are the foundation of the disease. They initiate neoplastic development and drive tumor progression forward, having acquired the oncogenic and tumor suppressor mutations that define cancer as a genetic disease. Traditionally, the cancer cells within tumors have been portrayed as reasonably homogeneous cell populations until relatively late in the course of tumor progression, when hyperproliferation combined with increased genetic instability spawn genetically distinct clonal subpopulations. Reflecting such clonal heterogeneity, many human tumors are histopathologically diverse, containing regions demarcated by various

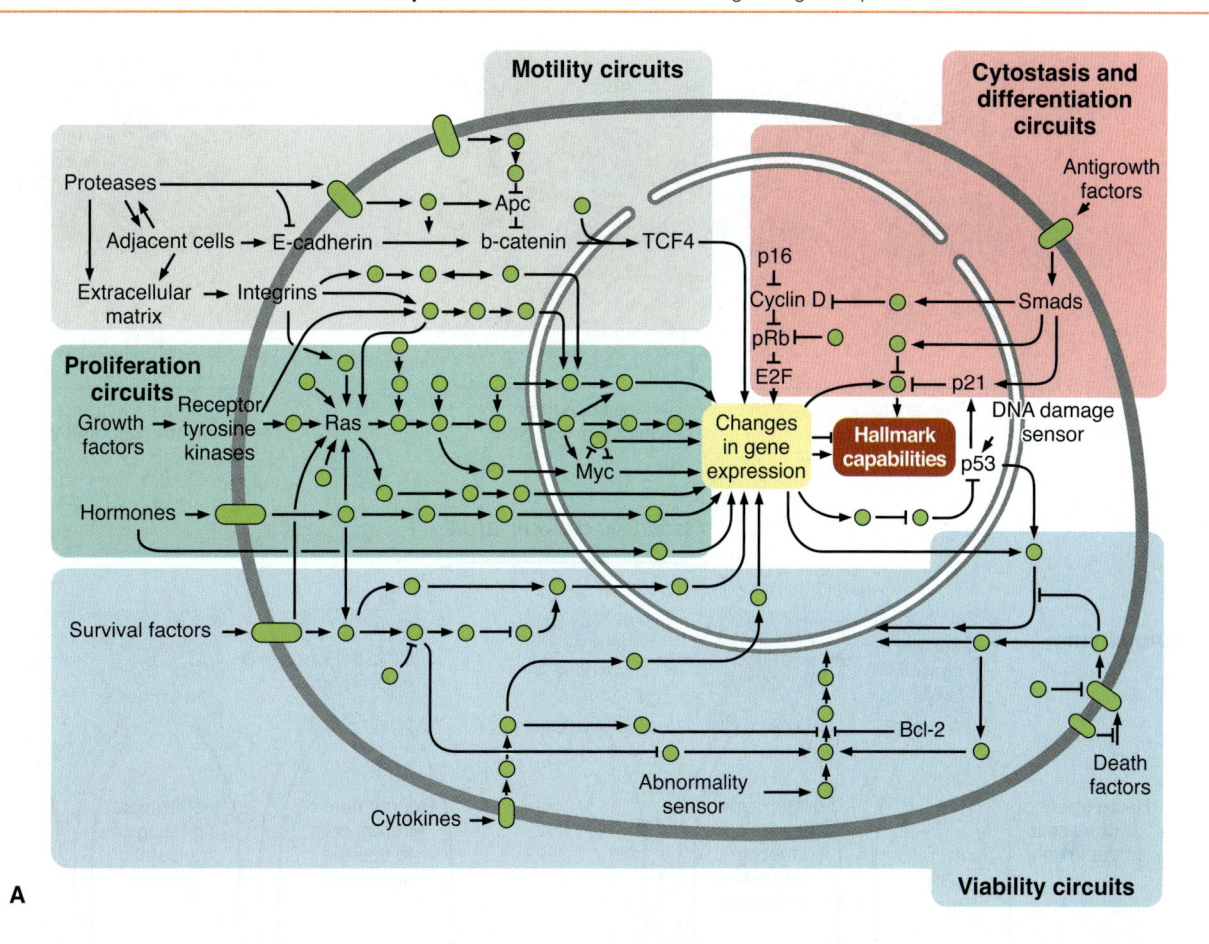

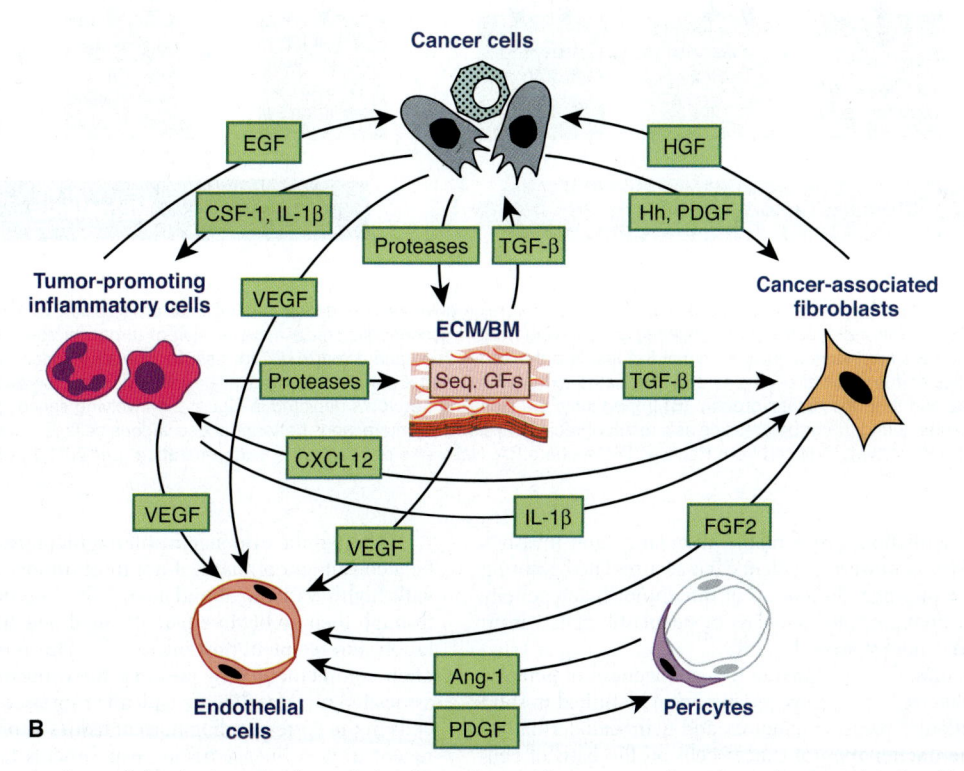

Figure 2.5 Reprogramming intracellular circuits and cell-to-cell signaling pathways dictates tumor inception and progression. An elaborate integrated circuit operating within normal cells is reprogrammed to regulate the hallmark capabilities acquired by cancer cells **(A)** and by associated stromal cells. Separate subcircuits, depicted here in differently colored fields, are specialized to orchestrate distinct capabilities. At one level, this depiction is simplistic, because there is considerable cross-talk between such subcircuits. More broadly, the integrated circuits operating inside cancer cells and stromal cells are interconnected via a complex network of signals transmitted by the various cells in the tumor microenvironment (in some cases via the extracellular matrix [ECM] and basement membranes [BM] they synthesize), of which a few signals are exemplified **(B)**. HGF, hepatocyte growth factor for the cMet receptor; Hh, hedgehog ligand for the Patched (PTCH) receptor; Seq. GF, growth factors sequestered in the ECM/BM. (Adapted from Hanahan D, Weinberg RA. Hallmarks of cancer: the next generation. *Cell* 2011;144:646–674.)

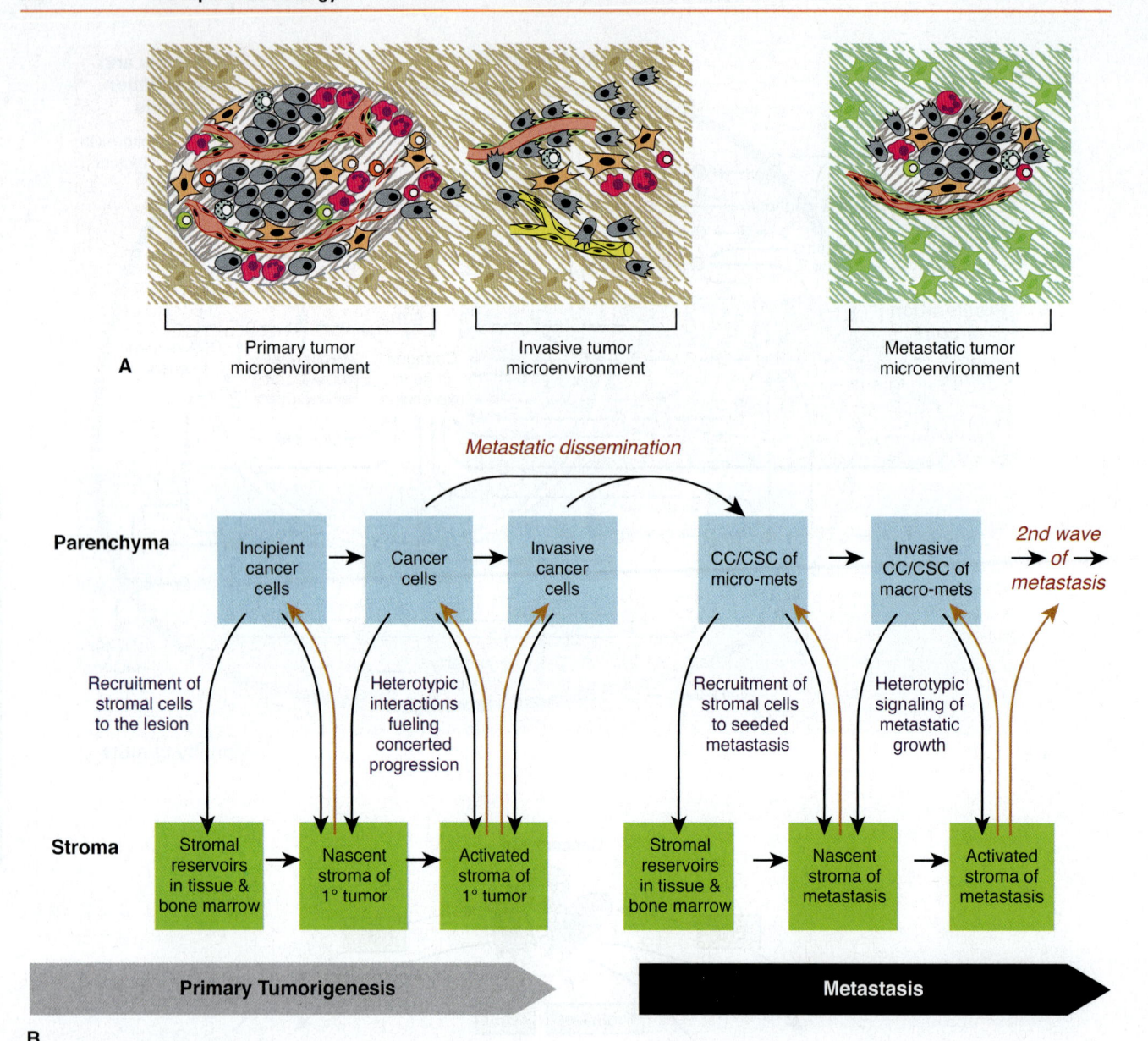

Figure 2.6 The dynamic variation and coevolution of the tumor microenvironment during the lesional progression of cancer. **(A)** Interactions between multiple stromal cell types and heterogeneously evolving mutant cancer cells create a succession of tumor microenvironments that change dynamically as tumors are initiated, invade normal tissues, and thereafter seed and colonize distant tissues. The abundance, histologic organization, and characteristics of the stromal cell types and associated extracellular matrix *(hatched background)* evolves during progression, thereby enabling primary, invasive, and then metastatic growth. **(B)** Importantly, the signaling networks depicted in Figure 2.5 involving cancer cells and their stromal collaborators change during tumor progression as a result of reciprocal signaling interactions between these various cells. CC, cancer cell; CSC, cancer stem cell; mets, metastases. (Adapted from Hanahan D, Weinberg RA. Hallmarks of cancer: the next generation. *Cell* 2011;144:646–674.)

degrees of differentiation, proliferation, vascularity, and invasiveness. In recent years, however, evidence has accumulated pointing to the existence of a new dimension of intratumor heterogeneity and a hitherto unappreciated subclass of neoplastic cells within tumors, termed cancer stem cells (CSC).

CSCs were initially implicated in the pathogenesis of hematopoietic malignancies,[246,247] and years later, were identified in solid tumors, in particular breast carcinomas and neuroectodermal tumors.[248,249] The fractionation of cancer cells on the basis of cell-surface markers has yielded subpopulations of neoplastic cells with a greatly enhanced ability, relative to the corresponding majority populations of non-CSCs, to seed new tumors upon implantation in immunodeficient mice. These, often rare, tumor-initiating cells have proven to share transcriptional profiles with certain normal tissue stem cells, thus justifying their designation as stemlike.

Although the evidence is still fragmentary, CSCs may prove to be a constituent of many, if not most tumors, albeit being present with highly variable abundance. CSCs are defined operationally through their ability to efficiently seed new tumors upon implantation into recipient host mice.[250–253] This functional definition is often complemented by profiling the expression of certain CSC-associated markers that are typically expressed by the normal stem cells in the corresponding normal tissues of origin.[249] Importantly, recent in vivo lineage-tracing experiments have provided an additional functional test of CSCs by demonstrating their ability to spawn large numbers of progeny, including non-CSCs within tumors.[250] At the same time, these experiments have provided the most compelling evidence to date that CSCs exist, and that they can be defined functionally through tests that do not depend on the implantation of tumor cells into appropriate mouse hosts.

The origins of CSCs within a solid tumor have not been clarified and, indeed, may well vary from one tumor type to another.[250,251,254] In some tumors, normal tissue stem cells may serve as the cells of origin that undergo oncogenic transformation to yield CSCs; in others, partially differentiated transit-amplifying cells, also termed progenitor cells, may suffer the initial oncogenic transformation, thereafter assuming more stemlike characters. Once primary tumors have formed, the CSCs, like their normal counterparts, may self-renew as well as spawn more differentiated derivatives. In the case of neoplastic CSCs, these descendant cells form the great bulk of many tumors and thus are responsible for creating many tumor-associated phenotypes. It remains to be established whether multiple distinct classes of increasingly neoplastic stem cells form during the inception and subsequent multistep progression of tumors, ultimately yielding the CSCs that have been described in fully developed cancers.

Recent research has interrelated the acquisition of CSC traits with the EMT transdifferentiation program discussed previously.[250,255] The induction of this program in certain model systems can induce many of the defining features of stem cells, including self-renewal ability and the antigenic phenotypes associated with both normal and cancer stem cells. This concordance suggests that the EMT program may not only enable cancer cells to physically disseminate from primary tumors, but can also confer on such cells the self-renewal capability that is crucial to their subsequent role as founders of new neoplastic colonies at sites of dissemination.[256] If generalized, this connection raises an important corollary hypothesis: The heterotypic signals that trigger an EMT, such as those released by an activated, inflammatory stroma, may also be important in creating and maintaining CSCs.

An increasing number of human tumors are reported to contain subpopulations with the properties of CSCs, as defined operationally through their efficient tumor-initiating capabilities upon xenotransplantation into mice. Nevertheless, the importance of CSCs as a distinct phenotypic subclass of neoplastic cells remains a matter of debate, as does their oft cited rarity within tumors.[254,257–259] Indeed, it is plausible that the phenotypic plasticity operating within tumors may produce bidirectional interconversion between CSCs and non-CSCs, resulting in dynamic variation in the relative abundance of CSCs.[250,260] Such plasticity could complicate a definitive measurement of their characteristic abundance. Analogous plasticity is already implicated in the EMT program, which can be engaged reversibly.[261]

These complexities notwithstanding, it is already evident that this new dimension of tumor heterogeneity holds important implications for successful cancer therapies. Increasing evidence in a variety of tumor types suggests that cells exhibiting the properties of CSCs are more resistant to various commonly used chemotherapeutic treatments.[255,262,263] Their persistence following initial treatment may help to explain the almost inevitable disease recurrence occurring after apparently successful debulking of human solid tumors by radiation and various forms of chemotherapy. Moreover, CSCs may well prove to underlie certain forms of tumor dormancy, whereby latent cancer cells persist for years or even decades after initial surgical resection or radio/chemotherapy, only to suddenly erupt and generate life-threatening disease. Hence, CSCs represent a double threat in that they are more resistant to therapeutic killing, and at the same time, are endowed with the ability to regenerate a tumor once therapy has been halted.

This phenotypic plasticity implicit in the CSC state may also enable the formation of functionally distinct subpopulations within a tumor that support overall tumor growth in various ways. Thus, an EMT can convert epithelial carcinoma cells into mesenchymal, fibroblast-like cancer cells that may well assume the duties of CAFs in some tumors (e.g., pancreatic ductal adenocarcinoma).[264] Intriguingly, several recent reports that have yet to be thoroughly validated in terms of generality, functional importance, or prevalence have documented the ability of glioblastoma cells (or possibly their associated CSC subpopulations) to transdifferentiate into endothelial-like cells that can substitute for bona fide host-derived endothelial cells in forming a tumor-associated neovasculature.[265–267] These examples suggest that certain tumors may induce some of their own cancer cells to undergo various types of metamorphoses in order to generate stromal cell types needed to support tumor growth and progression, rather than relying on recruited host cells to provide the requisite hallmark-enabling functions.

Another form of phenotypic variability resides in the genetic heterogeneity of cancer cells within a tumor. Genomewide sequencing of cancer cells microdissected from different sectors of the same tumor[145] has revealed striking intratumoral genetic heterogeneity. Some of this genetic diversity may be reflected in the long recognized histologic heterogeneity within individual human tumors. Thus, genetic diversification may produce subpopulations of cancer cells that contribute distinct and complementary capabilities, which then accrue to the common benefit of overall tumor growth, progression, and resistance to therapy, as described earlier. Alternatively, such heterogeneity may simply reflect the genetic chaos that arises as tumor cell genomes become increasingly destabilized.

THERAPEUTIC TARGETING OF THE HALLMARKS OF CANCER

We do not attempt here to enumerate the myriad therapies that are currently under development or have been introduced of late into the clinic. Instead, we consider how the description of hallmark principles is likely to inform therapeutic development at present and may increasingly do so in the future. Thus, the rapidly growing armamentarium of therapeutics directed against specific molecular targets can be categorized according to their respective effects on one or more hallmark capabilities, as illustrated in the examples presented in Figure 2.7. Indeed, the observed efficacy of these drugs represents, in each case, a validation of a particular capability: If a capability is truly critical to the biology of tumors, then its inhibition should impair tumor growth and progression.

Unfortunately, however, the clinical responses elicited by these targeted therapies have generally been transitory, being followed all too often by relapse. One interpretation, which is supported by growing experimental evidence, is that each of the core hallmark capabilities is regulated by a set of partially redundant signaling pathways. Consequently, a targeted therapeutic agent inhibiting one key pathway in a tumor may not completely eliminate a hallmark capability, allowing some cancer cells to survive with residual function until they or their progeny eventually adapt to the selective pressure imposed by the initially applied therapy. Such adaptation can reestablish the expression of the functional capability, permitting renewed tumor growth and clinical relapse. Because the number of parallel signaling pathways supporting a given hallmark must be limited, it may become possible to therapeutically cotarget all of these supporting pathways, thereby preventing the development of adaptive resistance.

Another dimension of the plasticity of tumors under therapeutic attack is illustrated by the unanticipated responses to antiangiogenic therapy, in which cancer cells reduce their dependence on this hallmark capability by increasing their dependence on another. Thus, many observers anticipated that potent inhibition of angiogenesis would starve tumors of vital nutrients and oxygen, forcing them into dormancy and possibly leading to their dissolution.[86,87,268] Instead, the clinical responses to antiangiogenic therapies have been found to be transitory, followed by relapse, implicating adaptive or evasive resistance mechanisms.[220,269–271] One such mechanism of evasive resistance, observed in certain preclinical models of antiangiogenic therapy, involves reduced dependence on continuing angiogenesis by increasing the activity of two other capabilities: invasiveness and metastasis.[269–271] By invading nearby and distant tissues, initially hypoxic cancer cells gain access to normal,

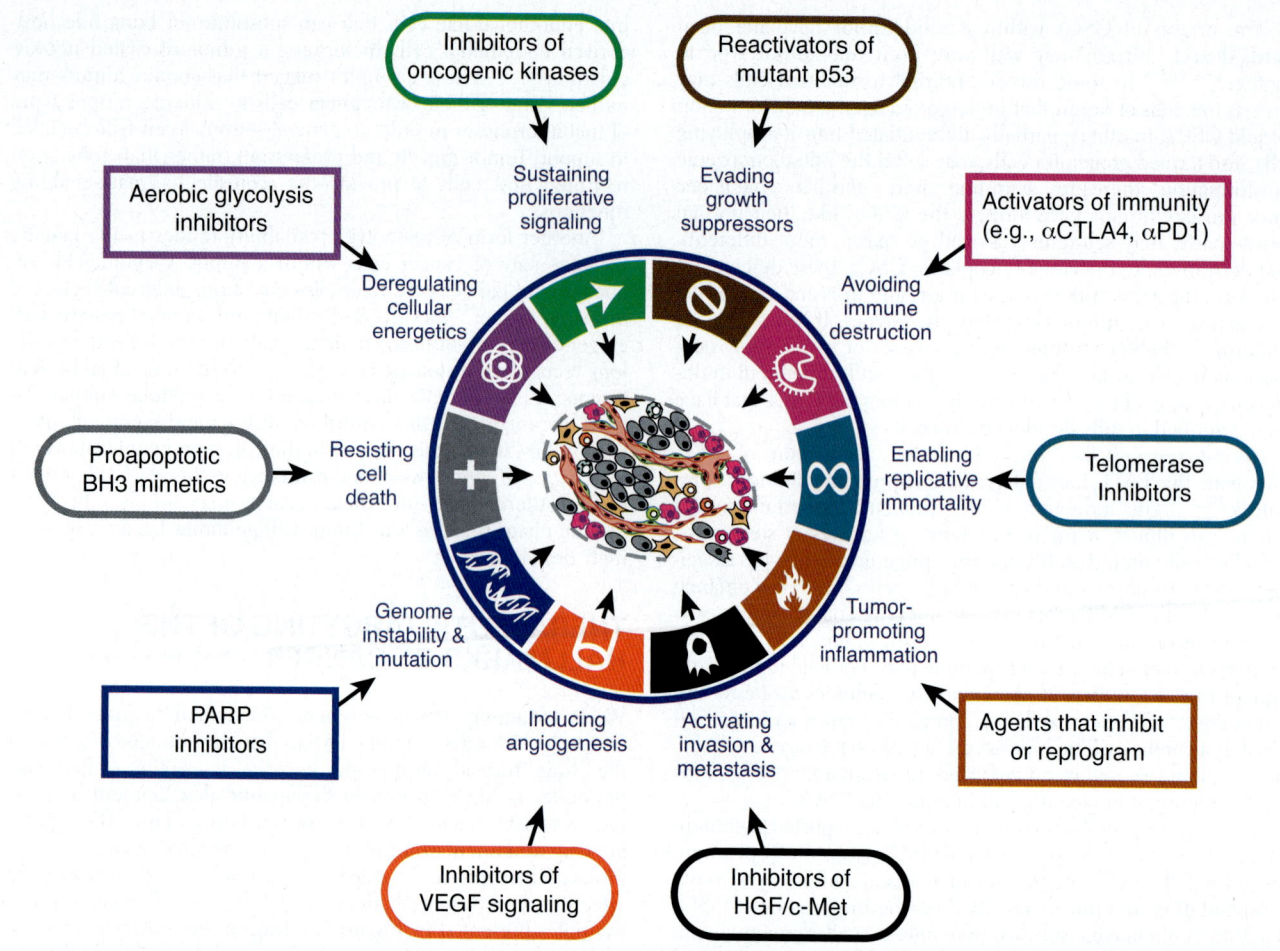

Figure 2.7 Therapeutic targeting of the hallmarks of cancer. Drugs that interfere with each of the hallmark capabilities and hallmark-enabling processes have been developed and are in preclinical and/or clinical testing, and in some cases, approved for use in treating certain forms of human cancer. A focus on antagonizing specific hallmark capabilities is likely to yield insights into developing novel, highly effective therapeutic strategies. PARP, poly ADP ribose polymerase. (Adapted from Hanahan D, Weinberg RA. Hallmarks of cancer: the next generation. *Cell* 2011;144:646–674.)

preexisting tissue vasculature. The initial clinical validation of this adaptive/evasive resistance is apparent in the increased invasion and local metastasis seen when human glioblastomas are treated with antiangiogenic therapies.[272–274] The applicability of this lesson to other human cancers has yet to be established.

Analogous adaptive shifts in dependence on other hallmark traits may also limit the efficacy of analogous hallmark-targeting therapies. For example, the deployment of apoptosis-inducing drugs may induce cancer cells to hyperactivate mitogenic signaling, enabling them to compensate for the initial attrition triggered by such treatments. Such considerations suggest that drug development and the design of treatment protocols will benefit from incorporating the concepts of functionally discrete hallmark capabilities and of the multiple biochemical pathways involved in supporting each of them. For these reasons, we envisage that attacking multiple hallmark capabilities with hallmark-targeting drugs (see Fig. 2.7), in carefully considered combinations, sequences, and temporal regimens,[275] will result in increasingly effective therapies that produce more durable clinical responses.

CONCLUSION AND A VISION FOR THE FUTURE

Looking ahead, we envision significant advances in our understanding of invasion and metastasis during the coming decade. Similarly, the role of altered energy metabolism in malignant growth will be elucidated, including a resolution of whether this metabolic reprogramming is a discrete capability separable from the core hallmark of chronically sustained proliferation. We are excited about the new frontier of immunotherapy, which will be empowered to leverage detailed knowledge about the regulation of immune responses in order to develop pharmacologic tools that can modulate them therapeutically for the purpose of effectively and sustainably attacking tumors and, most importantly, their metastases.

Other areas are currently in rapid flux. In recent years, elaborate molecular mechanisms controlling transcription through chromatin modifications have been uncovered, and there are clues that specific shifts in chromatin configuration occur during the acquisition of certain hallmark capabilities.[195,196] Functionally significant epigenetic alterations seem likely to be factors not only in the cancer cells, but also in the altered cells of the tumor-associated stroma. At present, it is unclear whether an elucidation of these epigenetic mechanisms will materially change our overall understanding of the means by which hallmark capabilities are acquired, or simply add additional detail to the regulatory circuitry that is already known to govern them.

Similarly, the discovery of hundreds of distinct regulatory microRNAs has already led to profound changes in our understanding of the molecular control mechanisms that operate in health and disease. By now, dozens of microRNAs have been implicated in various tumor phenotypes.[276,277] Still, these only scratch the surface of the true complexity, because the functions of hundreds of microRNAs known to be present in our cells and to be altered in expression levels in different forms of cancer remain total mysteries. Here again, we are unclear whether future progress will cause fundamental shifts in our understanding of the pathogenic mechanisms of cancer, or only add detail to the elaborate regulatory circuits that have already been mapped out.

Finally, the existing diagrams of heterotypic interactions between the multiple distinct cell types that collaborate to produce malignant tumors are still rudimentary. We anticipate that, in another decade, the signaling pathways describing the intercommunication between these various cell types within tumors will be charted in far greater detail and clarity, eclipsing our current knowledge. And, as before,[1,2] we continue to foresee cancer research as an increasingly logical science, in which myriad phenotypic complexities are manifestations of an underlying organizing principle.

ACKNOWLEDGMENT

This chapter is modified from Hanahan D, Weinberg RA. Hallmarks of cancer: the next generation. *Cell* 2011;144(5):646–674.

REFERENCES

1. Hanahan D, Weinberg R. The hallmarks of cancer. *Cell* 2000;100:57–70.
2. Hanahan D, Weinberg RA. Hallmarks of cancer: the next generation. *Cell* 2011;144:646–674.
3. Lemmon MA, Schlessinger J. Cell signaling by receptor tyrosine kinases. *Cell* 2010;141:1117–1134.
4. Witsch E, Sela M, Yarden Y. Roles for growth factors in cancer progression. *Physiology* 2010;25:85–101.
5. Hynes NE, MacDonald G. ErbB receptors and signaling pathways in cancer. *Curr Opin Cell Biol* 2009;21:177–184.
6. Perona T. Cell signalling: growth factors and tyrosine kinase receptors. *Clin Transl Oncol* 2006;8:77–82.
7. Franco OE, Shaw AK, Strand DW, et al. Cancer associated fibroblasts in cancer pathogenesis. *Semin Cell Dev Biol* 2010;21:33–39.
8. Bhowmick NA, Neilson EG, Moses HL. Stromal fibroblasts in cancer initiation and progression. *Nature* 2004;432:332–337.
9. Davies MA, Samuels Y. Analysis of the genome to personalize therapy for melanoma. *Oncogene* 2010;29:5545–5555.
10. Jiang BH, Liu LZ. PI3K/PTEN signaling in angiogenesis and tumorigenesis. *Adv Cancer Res* 2009;102:19–65.
11. Yuan TL, Cantley LC. PI3K pathway alterations in cancer: variations on a theme. *Oncogene* 2008;27:5497–5510.
12. Wertz IE, Dixit VM. Regulation of death receptor signaling by the ubiquitin system. *Cell Death Differ* 2010;17:14–24.
13. Cabrita MA, Christofori G. Sprouty proteins, masterminds of receptor tyrosine kinase signaling. *Angiogenesis* 2008;11:53–62.
14. Amit I, Citri A, Shay T, et al. A module of negative feedback regulators defines growth factor signaling. *Nature Genet* 2007;39:503–512.
15. Mosesson Y, Mills GB, Yarden Y. Derailed endocytosis: an emerging feature of cancer. *Nat Rev Cancer* 2008;8:835–850.
16. Sudarsanam S, Johnson DE. Functional consequences of mTOR inhibition. *Curr Opin Drug Discov Devel* 2010;13:31–40.
17. O'Reilly KE, Rojo F, She QB, et al. mTOR inhibition induces upstream receptor tyrosine kinase signaling and activates Akt. *Cancer Res* 2006;66:1500–1508.
18. Dang CV. MYC on the path to cancer. *Cell* 2012;149:22–35.
19. Collado M, Serrano M. Senescence in tumours: evidence from mice and humans. *Nat Rev Cancer* 2010;10:51–57.
20. Evan GI, d'Adda di Fagagna F. Cellular senescence: hot or what? *Curr Opin Genet Dev* 2009;19:25–31.
21. Lowe SW, Cepero E, Evan G. Intrinsic tumour suppression. *Nature* 2004;432:307–315.
22. Mooi WJ, Peeper DS. Oncogene-induced cell senescence—halting on the road to cancer. *N Engl J Med* 2006;355:1037–1046.
23. Burkhart DL, Sage J. Cellular mechanisms of tumour suppression by the retinoblastoma gene. *Nat Rev Cancer* 2008;8:671–682.
24. Deshpande A, Sicinski P, Hinds PW. Cyclins and cdks in development and cancer: a perspective. *Oncogene* 2005;24:2909–2915.
25. Sherr CJ, McCormick F. The RB and p53 pathways in cancer. *Cancer Cell* 2002;2:103–112.
26. Lipinski MM, Jacks T. The retinoblastoma gene family in differentiation and development. *Oncogene* 1999;18:7873–7882.
27. Ghebranious N, Donehower LA. Mouse models in tumor suppression. *Oncogene* 1998;17: 3385–3400.
28. McClatchey AI, Yap AS. Contact inhibition (of proliferation) redux. *Curr Opin Cell Biol* 2012;24:685–694.
29. Curto M, Cole BK, Lallemand D, et al. Contact-dependent inhibition of EGFR signaling by Nf2/Merlin. *J Cell Biol* 2007;177:893–903.
30. Okada T, Lopez-Lago M, Giancotti FG. Merlin/NF-2 mediates contact inhibition of growth by suppressing recruitment of Rac to the plasma membrane. *J Cell Biol* 2005;171:361–371.
31. Stamenkovic I, Yu Q. Merlin, a "magic" linker between the extracellular cues and intracellular signaling pathways that regulate cell motility, proliferation, and survival. *Curr Protein Pept Sci* 2010;11:471–484.
32. Pickup M, Novitskiv S, Moses HL. The roles of TGFβ in the tumour microenvironment. *Nat Rev Cancer* 2013;13:788–799.
33. Ikushima H, Miyazono K. TGFbeta signalling: a complex web in cancer progression. *Nat Rev Cancer* 2010;10:415–424.
34. Massagué J. TGF-beta in cancer. *Cell* 2008;134:215–230.
35. Bierie B, Moses HL. Tumour microenvironment: TGF-beta: the molecular Jekyll and Hyde of cancer. *Nat Rev Cancer* 2006;6:506–520.
36. Strasser A, Cory S, Adams JM. Deciphering the rules of programmed cell death to improve therapy of cancer and other diseases. *EMBO J* 2011;30:3667–3683.
37. Adams JM, Cory S. The Bcl-2 apoptotic switch in cancer development and therapy. *Oncogene* 2007;26:1324–1337.
38. Evan G, Littlewood T. A matter of life and cell death. *Science* 2004;281:1317–1322.
39. Willis SN, Adams JM. Life in the balance: how BH3-only proteins induce apoptosis. *Curr Opin Cell Biol* 2005;17:617–625.
40. Junttila MR, Evan GI. p53 — a jack of all trades but master of none. *Nat Rev Cancer* 2009;9:821–829.
41. White E. Deconvoluting the context-dependent role for autophagy in cancer. *Nat Rev Cancer* 2012;12:401–410.
42. Levine B, Kroemer G. Autophagy in the pathogenesis of disease. *Cell* 2008;132:27–42.
43. Mizushima N. Autophagy: process and function. *Genes Dev* 2007;21:2861–2873.
44. Sinha S, Levine B. The autophagy effector Beclin 1: a novel BH3-only protein. *Oncogene* 2008;27:S137–S148.
45. Mathew R, Karantza-Wadsworth V, White E. Role of autophagy in cancer. *Nat Rev Cancer* 2007;7:961–967.
46. White E, DiPaola RS. The double-edged sword of autophagy modulation in cancer. *Clin Cancer Res* 2009;15:5308–5316.
47. Apel A, Zentgraf H, Büchler MW, et al. Autophagy—A double-edged sword in oncology. *Int J Cancer* 2009;125:991–995.
48. Amaravadi RK, Thompson CB. The roles of therapy-induced autophagy and necrosis in cancer treatment. *Clin Cancer Res* 2007;13:7271–7279.
49. Lu Z, Luo RZ, Lu Y, et al. The tumor suppressor gene ARHI regulates autophagy and tumor dormancy in human ovarian cancer cells. *J Clin Invest* 2008;118:3917–3929.
50. Vanden Berghe T, Linkermann A, Jouan-Lanhouet S, et al. Regulated necrosis: the expanding network of non-apoptotic cell death pathways. *Nat Rev Mol Cell Biol* 2014;15:135–147.
51. Galluzzi L, Kroemer G. Necroptosis: a specialized pathway of programmed necrosis. *Cell* 2008;135:1161–1163.
52. Zong WX, Thompson CB. Necrotic death as a cell fate. *Genes Dev* 2006;20:1–15.
53. Grivennikov SI, Greten FR, Karin M. Immunity, inflammation, and cancer. *Cell* 2010;140:883–899.
54. White E, Karp C, Strohecker AM, et al. Role of autophagy in suppression of inflammation and cancer. *Curr Opin Cell Biol* 2010;22:212–217.
55. Blasco MA. Telomeres and human disease: ageing, cancer and beyond. *Nat Rev Genet* 2005;6:611–622.
56. Shay JW, Wright WE. Hayflick, his limit, and cellular ageing. *Nat Rev Mol Cell Biol* 2000;1:72–76.
57. Shay JW, Wright WE. Telomeres and telomerase in cancer. *Sem Cancer Biol* 2011;21:349–353.
58. Artandi SE, DePinho RA. Telomeres and telomerase in cancer. *Carcinogenesis* 2010;31:9–18.
59. Cesare AJ, Reddel RR. Alternative lengthening of telomeres: models, mechanisms and implications. *Nat Rev Genet* 2010;11:319–330.
60. Ince TA, Richardson AL, Bell GW, et al. Transformation of different human breast epithelial cell types leads to distinct tumor phenotypes. *Cancer Cell* 2007;12:160–170.
61. Passos JF, Saretzki G, von Zglinicki T. DNA damage in telomeres and mitochondria during cellular senescence: is there a connection? *Nucleic Acids Res* 2007;35:7505–7513.
62. Zhang H, Herbert BS, Pan KH, et al. Disparate effects of telomere attrition on gene expression during replicative senescence of human mammary epithelial cells cultured under different conditions. *Oncogene* 2004;23:6193–6198.
63. Sherr CJ, DePinho RA. Cellular senescence: mitotic clock or culture shock? *Cell* 2000;102:407–410.
64. Feldser DM, Greider CW. Short telomeres limit tumor progression in vivo by inducing senescence. *Cancer Cell* 2007;11:461–469.
65. Kawai T, Hiroi S, Nakanishi K, et al. Telomere length and telomerase expression in atypical adenomatous hyperplasia and small bronchioloalveolar carcinoma of the lung. *Am J Clin Pathol* 2007;127:254–262.

66. Hansel DE, Meeker AK, Hicks J. Telomere length variation in biliary tract metaplasia, dysplasia, and carcinoma. *Mod Pathol* 2006;19:772–779.
67. Artandi SE, DePinho RA. Mice without telomerase: what can they teach us about human cancer? *Nature Med* 2000;6:852–855.
68. Raynaud CM, Hernandez J, Llorca FP, et al. DNA damage repair and telomere length in normal breast, preneoplastic lesions, and invasive cancer. *Am J Clin Oncol* 2010;33:341–345.
69. Chin K, de Solorzano CO, Knowles D, et al. In situ analyses of genome instability in breast cancer. *Nature Genet* 2004;36:984–988.
70. Hanahan D, Folkman J. Patterns and emerging mechanisms of the angiogenic switch during tumorigenesis. *Cell* 1996;86:353–364.
71. Baeriswyl V, Christofori G. The angiogenic switch in carcinogenesis. *Semin Cancer Biol* 2009;19:329–337.
72. Bergers G, Benjamin LE. Tumorigenesis and the angiogenic switch. *Nat Rev Cancer* 2003;3:401–410.
73. Ferrara N. Vascular endothelial growth factor. *Arterioscler Thromb Vasc Biol* 2009;29:789–791.
74. Mac Gabhann F, Popel AS. Systems biology of vascular endothelial growth factors. *Microcirculation* 2008;15:715–738.
75. Carmeliet P. VEGF as a key mediator of angiogenesis in cancer. *Oncology* 2005;69:4–10.
76. Kessenbrock K, Plaks V, Werb Z. Matrix metalloproteinases: regulators of the tumor microenvironment. *Cell* 2010;141:52–67.
77. Kazerounian S, Yee KO, Lawler J. Thrombospondins in cancer. *Cell Mol Life Sci* 2008;65:700–712.
78. Nagy JA, Chang SH, Shih SC, et al. Heterogeneity of the tumor vasculature. *Semin Thromb Hemost* 2010;36:321–331.
79. Baluk P, Hashizume H, McDonald DM. Cellular abnormalities of blood vessels as targets in cancer. *Curr Opin Genet Dev* 2005;15:102–111.
80. Raica M, Cimpean AM, Ribatti D. Angiogenesis in pre-malignant conditions. *Eur J Cancer* 2009;45:1924–1934.
81. Olive KP, Jacobetz MA, Davidson CJ, et al. Inhibition of Hedgehog signaling enhances delivery of chemotherapy in a mouse model of pancreatic cancer. *Science* 2009;324:1457–1461.
82. Zee YK, O'Connor JP, Parker GJ, et al. Imaging angiogenesis of genitourinary tumors. *Nat Rev Urol* 2010;7:69–82.
83. Turner HE, Harris AL, Melmed S, et al. Angiogenesis in endocrine tumors. *Endocr Rev* 2003;24:600–632.
84. Xie L, Duncan MB, Pahler J, et al. Counterbalancing angiogenic regulatory factors control the rate of cancer progression and survival in a stage-specific manner. *Proc Natl Acad Sci U S A* 2011;108:9939–9944.
85. Ribatti D. Endogenous inhibitors of angiogenesis: a historical review. *Leuk Res* 2009;33:638–644.
86. Folkman J. Angiogenesis. *Annu Rev Med* 2006;57:1–18.
87. Folkman J. Role of angiogenesis in tumor growth and metastasis. *Semin Oncol* 2002;29:15–18.
88. Nyberg P, Xie L, Kalluri R. Endogenous inhibitors of angiogenesis. *Cancer Res* 2005;65:3967–3979.
89. Cao Y. Adipose tissue angiogenesis as a therapeutic target for obesity and metabolic diseases. *Nat Rev Drug Discov* 2010;9:107–115.
90. Seppinen L, Sormunen R, Soini Y, et al. Lack of collagen XVIII accelerates cutaneous wound healing, while overexpression of its endostatin domain leads to delayed healing. *Matrix Biol* 2008;27:535–546.
91. Raza A, Franklin MJ, Dudek AZ. Pericytes and vessel maturation during tumor angiogenesis and metastasis. *Am J Hematol* 2010;85:593–598.
92. Kovacic JC, Boehm M. Resident vascular progenitor cells: an emerging role for non-terminally differentiated vessel-resident cells in vascular biology. *Stem Cell Res* 2009;2:2–15.
93. Bergers G, Song S. The role of pericytes in blood-vessel formation and maintenance. *Neuro Oncol* 2005;7:452–464.
94. Qian BZ, Pollard JW. Macrophage diversity enhances tumor progression and metastasis. *Cell* 2010;141:39–51.
95. Zumsteg A, Christofori G. Corrupt policemen: inflammatory cells promote tumor angiogenesis. *Curr Opin Oncol* 2009;21:60–70.
96. Murdoch C, Muthana M, Coffelt SB, et al. The role of myeloid cells in the promotion of tumour angiogenesis. *Nat Rev Cancer* 2008;8:618–631.
97. De Palma M, Murdoch C, Venneri MA, et al. Tie2-expressing monocytes: regulation of tumor angiogenesis and therapeutic implications. *Trends Immunol* 2007;28:519–524.
98. Ferrara N. Pathways mediating VEGF-independent tumor angiogenesis. *Cytokine Growth Factor Rev* 2010;21:21–26.
99. Patenaude A, Parker J, Karsan A. Involvement of endothelial progenitor cells in tumor vascularization. *Microvasc Res* 2010;79:217–223.
100. Lamagna C, Bergers G. The bone marrow constitutes a reservoir of pericyte progenitors. *J Leukoc Biol* 2006;80:677–681.
101. Talmadge JE, Fidler IJ. AACR centennial series: the biology of cancer metastasis: historical perspective. *Cancer Res* 2010;70:5649–5669.
102. Fidler IJ. The pathogenesis of cancer metastasis: the "seed and soil" hypothesis revisited. *Nat Rev Cancer* 2003;3:453–458.
103. Berx G, van Roy F. Involvement of members of the cadherin superfamily in cancer. *Cold Spring Harb Perspect Biol* 2009;1:a003129.
104. Cavallaro U, Christofori G. Cell adhesion and signaling by cadherins and Ig-CAMs in cancer. *Nat Rev Cancer* 2004;4:118–132.
105. De Craene B, Berx G. Regulatory networks defining EMT during cancer initiation and progression. *Nat Rev Cancer* 2013;13:97–110.
106. Klymkowsky MW, Savagner P. Epithelial-mesenchymal transition: a cancer researcher's conceptual friend and foe. *Am J Pathol* 2009;174:1588–1592.
107. Polyak K, Weinberg RA. Transitions between epithelial and mesenchymal states: acquisition of malignant and stem cell traits. *Nat Rev Cancer* 2009;9:265–273.
108. Thiery JP, Acloque H, Huang RY, et al. Epithelial-mesenchymal transitions in development and disease. *Cell* 2009;139:871–890.
109. Yilmaz M, Christofori G. EMT, the cytoskeleton, and cancer cell invasion. *Cancer Metastasis Rev* 2009;28:15–33.
110. Barrallo-Gimeno A, Nieto MA. The Snail genes as inducers of cell movement and survival: implications in development and cancer. *Development* 2005;132:3151–3161.
111. Micalizzi DS, Farabaugh SM, Ford HL. Epithelial-mesenchymal transition in cancer: parallels between normal development and tumor progression. *J Mammary Gland Biol Neoplasia* 2010;15:117–134.
112. Taube JH, Herschkowitz JI, Komurov K, et al. Core epithelial-to-mesenchymal transition interactome gene-expression signature is associated with claudin-low and metaplastic breast cancer subtypes. *Proc Natl Acad Sci U S A* 2010;107:15449–15454.
113. Schmalhofer O, Brabletz S, Brabletz T. E-cadherin, beta-catenin, and ZEB1 in malignant progression of cancer. *Cancer Metastasis Rev* 2009;28:151–166.
114. Yang J, Weinberg RA. Epithelial-mesenchymal transition: at the crossroads of development and tumor metastasis. *Develop Cell* 2008;14:818–829.
115. Peinado H, Marin F, Cubillo E, et al. Snail and E47 repressors of E-cadherin induce distinct invasive and angiogenic properties in vivo. *J Cell Sci* 2004;117:2827–2839.
116. Karnoub AE, Weinberg RA. Chemokine networks and breast cancer metastasis. *Breast Dis* 2006;26:75–85.
117. Brabletz T, Jung A, Reu S, et al. Variable beta-catenin expression in colorectal cancers indicates tumor progression driven by the tumor environment. *Proc Natl Acad Sci U S A* 2001;98:10356–10361.
118. Hlubek F, Brabletz T, Budczies J, et al. Heterogeneous expression of Wnt/beta-catenin target genes within colorectal cancer. *Int J Cancer* 2007;121:1941–1948.
119. Egeblad M, Nakasone ES, Werb Z. Tumors as organs: complex tissues that interface with the entire organism. *Dev Cell* 2010;18:884–901.
120. Joyce JA, Pollard JW. Microenvironmental regulation of metastasis. *Nat Rev Cancer* 2009;9:239–252.
121. Kalluri R, Zeisberg M. Fibroblasts in cancer. *Nat Rev Cancer* 2006;6:392–401.
122. Karnoub AE, Dash AB, Vo AP, et al. Mesenchymal stem cells within tumour stroma promote breast cancer metastasis. *Nature* 2007;449:557–563.
123. Li HJ, Reinhart F, Herschman HR, et al. Cancer-stimulated mesenchymal stem cells create a carcinoma stem cell niche via prostaglandin E2 signaling. *Cancer Discov* 2012;2:840–855.
124. Palermo C, Joyce JA. Cysteine cathepsin proteases as pharmacological targets in cancer. *Trends Pharmacol Sci* 2008;29:22–28.
125. Mohamed MM, Sloane BF. Cysteine cathepsins: multifunctional enzymes in cancer. *Nat Rev Cancer* 2006;6:764–775.
126. Gocheva V, Wang HW, Gadea BB, et al. IL-4 induces cathepsin protease activity in tumor-associated macrophages to promote cancer growth and invasion. *Genes Dev* 2010;24:241–255.
127. Wyckoff JB, Wang Y, Lin EY, et al. Direct visualization of macrophage-assisted tumor cell intravasation in mammary tumors. *Cancer Res* 2007;67:2649–2656.
128. Hugo H, Ackland ML, Blick T, et al. Epithelial-mesenchymal and mesenchymal-epithelial transitions in carcinoma progression. *J Cell Physiol* 2007;213:374–383.
129. Friedl P, Wolf K. Plasticity of cell migration: a multiscale tuning model. *J Cell Biol* 2009;188:11–19.
130. Friedl P, Wolf K. Tube travel: the role of proteases in individual and collective cancer cell invasion. *Cancer Res* 2008;68:7247–7249.
131. Madsen CD, Sahai E. Cancer dissemination—lessons from leukocytes. *Dev Cell* 2010;19:13–26.
132. Sabeh F, Shimizu-Hirota R, Weiss SJ. Protease-dependent versus-independent cancer cell invasion programs: three-dimensional amoeboid movement revisited. *J Cell Biol* 2009;185:11–19.
133. Quail DF, Joyce JA. Microenvironmental regulation of tumor progression and metastasis. *Nat Med* 2013;19:1423–1437.
134. McGowan PM, Kirstein JM, Chambers AF. Micrometastatic disease and metastatic outgrowth: clinical issues and experimental approaches. *Future Oncol* 2009;5:1083–1098.
135. Aguirre-Ghiso JA. Models, mechanisms and clinical evidence for cancer dormancy. *Nat Rev Cancer* 2007;7:834–846.
136. Townson JL, Chambers AF. Dormancy of solitary metastatic cells. *Cell Cycle* 2006;5:1744–1750.
137. Demicheli R, Retsky MW, Hrushesky WJ, et al. The effects of surgery on tumor growth: a century of investigations. *Ann Oncol* 2008;19:1821–1828.
138. Barkan D, Green JE, Chambers AF. Extracellular matrix: a gatekeeper in the transition from dormancy to metastatic growth. *Eur J Cancer* 2010;46:1181–1188.
139. Gupta GP, Minn AJ, Kang,Y, et al. Identifying site-specific metastasis genes and functions. *Cold Spring Harb Symp Quant Biol* 2005;70:149–158.
140. Naumov GN, Folkman J, Straume O, et al. Tumor-vascular interactions and tumor dormancy. *APMIS* 2008;116:569–585.

141. Kenific CM, Thorburn A, Debnath J. Autophagy and metastasis: another double-edged sword. *Curr Opin Cell Biol* 2010;22:241–245.
142. Teng MW, Swann JB, Koebel CM, et al. Immune-mediated dormancy: an equilibrium with cancer. *J Leukoc Biol* 2008;84:988–993.
143. Campbell PJ, Yachida S, Mudie LJ, et al. The patterns and dynamics of genomic instability in metastatic pancreatic cancer. *Nature* 2010;467:1109–1113.
144. Luebeck EG. Cancer: genomic evolution of metastasis. *Nature* 2010;467: 1053–1055.
145. Yachida S, Jones S, Bozic I, et al. Distant metastasis occurs late during the genetic evolution of pancreatic cancer. *Nature* 2010;467:1114–1117.
146. Coghlin C, Murray GI. Current and emerging concepts in tumour metastasis. *J Pathol* 2010;222:1–15.
147. Klein CA. Parallel progression of primary tumours and metastases. *Nat Rev Cancer* 2009;9:302–312.
148. Gerhardt H, Semb H. Pericytes: gatekeepers in tumour cell metastasis? *J Mol Med* 2008;86:135–144.
149. Kim MY, Oskarsson T, Acharyya S, et al. Tumor self-seeding by circulating cancer cells. *Cell* 2009;139:1315–1326.
150. Bos PD, Zhang XH, Nadal C, et al. Genes that mediate breast cancer metastasis to the brain. *Nature* 2009;459:1005–1009.
151. Olson P, Lu J, Zhang H, et al. MicroRNA dynamics in the stages of tumorigenesis correlate with hallmark capabilities of cancer. *Genes Dev* 2009;23: 2152–2165.
152. Nguyen DX, Bos PD, Massagué J. Metastasis: from dissemination to organ-specific colonization. *Nat Rev Cancer* 2009;9:274–284.
153. Warburg OH. *The Metabolism of Tumours: Investigations from the Kaiser Wilhelm Institute for Biology, Berlin-Dahlem.* London, UK: Arnold Constable; 1930.
154. Warburg O. On the origin of cancer cells. *Science* 1956;123:309–314.
155. Warburg O. On respiratory impairment in cancer cells. *Science* 1956;124: 269–270.
156. Jones RG, Thompson CB. Tumor suppressors and cell metabolism: a recipe for cancer growth. *Genes Dev* 2009;23:537–548.
157. DeBerardinis RJ, Lum JJ, Hatzivassiliou G, et al. The biology of cancer: metabolic reprogramming fuels cell growth and proliferation. *Cell Metab* 2008;7:11–20.
158. Hsu PP, Sabatini DM. Cancer cell metabolism: Warburg and beyond. *Cell* 2008;134:703–707.
159. Ward PS, Thompson CB. Metabolic reprogramming: a cancer hallmark even warburg did not anticipate. *Cancer Cell* 2012;21:297–308.
160. Semenza GL. HIF-1: upstream and downstream of cancer metabolism. *Curr Opin Genet Dev* 2010;20:51–56.
161. Semenza GL. Defining the role of hypoxia-inducible factor 1 in cancer biology and therapeutics. *Oncogene* 2010;29:625–634.
162. Kroemer G, Pouyssegur J. Tumor cell metabolism: cancer's Achilles' heel. *Cancer Cell* 2008;13:472–482.
163. Potter V. The biochemical approach to the cancer problem. *Fed Proc* 1958; 17:691–697.
164. Vander Heiden MG, Cantley LC, Thompson CB. Understanding the Warburg effect: the metabolic requirements of cell proliferation. *Science* 2009; 324:1029–1033.
165. Semenza GL. Tumor metabolism: cancer cells give and take lactate. *J Clin Invest* 2008;118:3835–3837.
166. Nakajima EC, Van Houten B. Metabolic symbiosis in cancer: refocusing the Warburg lens. *Mol Carcinog* 2013;52:329–337.
167. Kennedy KM, Dewhirst MW. Tumor metabolism of lactate: the influence and therapeutic potential for MCT and CD147 regulation. *Future Oncol* 2010;6:127–148.
168. Feron O. Pyruvate into lactate and back: from the Warburg effect to symbiotic energy fuel exchange in cancer cells. *Radiother Oncol* 2009;92:329–333.
169. Magistretti PJ. Neuron-glia metabolic coupling and plasticity. *J Exp Biol* 2006;209:2304–2311.
170. Hardee ME, Dewhirst MW, Agarwal N, et al. Novel imaging provides new insights into mechanisms of oxygen transport in tumors. *Curr Mol Med* 2009;9:435–441.
171. Burnet FM. The concept of immunological surveillance. *Prog Exp Tumor Res* 1970;13:1–27.
172. Thomas L. On immuosurveillance in human cancer. *Yale J Biol Med* 1982;55:329–333.
173. Vajdic CM, van Leeuwen MT. Cancer incidence and risk factors after solid organ transplantation. *Int J Cancer* 2009;125:1747–1754.
174. Elinav E, Nowarski R, Thaiss CA, et al. Inflammation-induced cancer: crosstalk between tumours, immune cells and microorganisms. *Nat Rev Cancer* 2013;13:759–771.
175. Swann JB, Smyth MJ. Immune surveillance of tumors. *J Clin Invest* 2007;117: 1137–1146.
176. Fridman WH, Mlecnik B, Bindea G, et al. Immunosurveillance in human non-viral cancers. *Curr Opin Immunol* 2011;23:272–278.
177. Galon J, Angell HK, Bedognetti D, et al. The continuum of cancer immunosurveillance: prognostic, predictive, and mechanistic signatures. *Immunity* 2013;39:11–26.
178. Kim R, Emi M, Tanabe K. Cancer immunoediting from immune surveillance to immune escape. *Immunology* 2007;121:1–14.
179. Smyth MJ, Dunn GP, Schreiber RD. Cancer immunosurveillance and immune-editing: the roles of immunity in suppressing tumor development and shaping tumor immunogenicity. *Adv Immunol* 2006;90:1–50.
180. Bindea G, Mlecnik B, Fridman WH, et al. Natural immunity to cancer in humans. *Curr Opin Immunol* 2010;22:215–222.
181. Ferrone C, Dranoff G. Dual roles for immunity in gastrointestinal cancers. *J Clin Oncol* 2010;28:4045–4051.
182. Nelson BH. The impact of T-cell immunity on ovarian cancer outcomes. *Immunol Rev* 2008;222:101–116.
183. Pagès F, Galon J, Dieu-Nosjean MC, et al. Immune infiltration in human tumors: a prognostic factor that should not be ignored. *Oncogene* 2010;29: 1093–1102.
184. Strauss DC, Thomas JM. Transmission of donor melanoma by organ transplantation. *Lancet Oncol* 2010;11:790–796.
185. Yang L, Pang Y, Moses HL. TGF-beta and immune cells: an important regulatory axis in the tumor microenvironment and progression. *Trends Immunol* 2010;31:220–227.
186. Shields JD, Kourtis IC, Tomei AA, et al. Induction of lymphoidlike stroma and immune escape by tumors that express the chemokine CCL21. *Science* 2010;328:749–752.
187. Korman AJ, Peggs KS, Allison J. Checkpoint blockade in cancer immunotherapy. *Adv Immunol* 2006;90:297–339.
188. Fife BT, Pauken KE, Eagar TN, et al. Interactions between programmed death-1 and programmed death ligand-1 promote tolerance by blocking the T cell receptor-induced stop signal. *Nat Immunol* 2009;10:1185–1192.
189. Pardoll DM. The blockade of immune checkpoints in cancer immunotherapy. *Nat Rev Cancer* 2012;12:252–264.
190. Motz GT, Coukos G. Deciphering and reversing tumor immune suppression. *Immunity* 2013;39:61–73.
191. Gabrilovich DI, Nagaraj S. Myeloid-derived suppressor cells as regulators of the immune system. *Nat Rev Immunol* 2009;9:162–174.
192. Mougiakakos D, Choudhury A, Lladser A, et al. Regulatory T cells in cancer. *Adv Cancer Res* 2010;107:57–117.
193. Ostrand-Rosenberg S, Sinha P. Myeloid-derived suppressor cells: linking inflammation and cancer. *J Immunol* 2009;182:4499–4506.
194. Garraway LA, Lander ES. Lessons from the cancer genome. *Cell* 2013;153: 17–37.
195. You JS, Jones PA. Cancer genetics and epigenetics: two sides of the same coin? *Cancer Cell* 2012;22:9–20.
196. Berdasco M, Esteller M. Aberrant epigenetic landscape in cancer: how cellular identity goes awry. *Dev Cell* 2010;19:698–711.
197. Esteller M. Cancer epigenomics: DNA methylomes and histone-modification maps. *Nat Rev Genet* 2007;8:286–298.
198. Jones PA, Baylin SB. The epigenomics of cancer. *Cell* 2007;128:683–692.
199. Negrini S, Gorgoulis VG, Halazonetis TD. Genomic instability—an evolving hallmark of cancer. *Nat Rev Mol Cell Bio* 2010;11:220–228.
200. Loeb LA. A mutator phenotype in cancer. *Cancer Res* 2001;61:3230–3239.
201. Jackson SP, Bartek J. The DNA-damage response in human biology and disease. *Nature* 2009;461:1071–1078.
202. Kastan MB. DNA damage responses: mechanisms and roles in human disease. *Mol Cancer Res* 2008;6:517–524.
203. Sigal A, Rotter V. Oncogenic mutations of the p53 tumor suppressor: the demons of the guardian of the genome. *Cancer Res* 2000;60:6788–6793.
204. Lane DP. Cancer. p53, guardian of the genome. *Nature* 1992;358:15–16.
205. Kinzler KW, Vogelstein B. Cancer-susceptibility genes. Gatekeepers and caretakers. *Nature* 1997;386:761–763.
206. Ciccia A, Elledge SJ. The DNA damage response: making it safe to play with knives. *Mol Cell* 2010;40:179–204.
207. Harper JW, Elledge SJ. The DNA damage response: ten years after. *Mol Cell* 2007;28:739–745.
208. Friedberg EC, Aguilera A, Gellert M, et al. DNA repair: from molecular mechanism to human disease. *DNA Repair (Amst)* 2006;5:986–996.
209. Barnes DE, Lindahl T. Repair and genetic consequences of endogenous DNA base damage in mammalian cells. *Annu Rev Genet* 2004;38:445–476.
210. Korkola J, Gray JW. Breast cancer genomes—form and function. *Curr Opin Genet Dev* 2010;20:4–14.
211. Dvorak HF. Tumors: wounds that do not heal. Similarities between tumor stroma generation and wound healing. *N Engl J Med* 1986;315:1650–1659.
212. De Nardo DG, Andreu P, Coussens LM. Interactions between lymphocytes and myeloid cells regulate pro- versus anti-tumor immunity. *Cancer Metastasis Rev* 2010;29:309–316.
213. Hanahan D, Coussens LM. Accessories to the crime: functions of cells recruited to the tumor microenvironment. *Cancer Cell* 2012;21:309–322.
214. de Visser KE, Eichten A, Coussens LM. Paradoxical roles of the immune system during cancer development. *Nat Rev Cancer* 2006;6:24–37.
215. Servais C, Erez N. From sentinel cells to inflammatory culprits: cancer-associated fibroblasts in tumour-related inflammation. *J Pathol* 2013;229: 198–207.
216. Dirat B, Bochet L, Escourrou G, et al. Unraveling the obesity and breast cancer links: a role for cancer-associated adipocytes? *Endocr Dev* 2010;19:45–52.
217. Pietras K, Ostman A. Hallmarks of cancer: interactions with the tumor stroma. *Exp Cell Res* 2010;316:1324–1331.
218. Räsänen K, Vaheri A. Activation of fibroblasts in cancer stroma. *Exp Cell Res* 2010;316:2713–2722.
219. Shimoda M, Mellody KT, Orimo A. Carcinoma-associated fibroblasts are a rate-limiting determinant for tumour progression. *Sem Cell Dev Biol* 2010;21:19–25.
220. Welti J, Loges S, Dimmeler S, et al. Recent molecular discoveries in angiogenesis and antiangiogenic therapies in cancer. *J Clin Invest* 2013;123:3190–3200.

221. Pasquale EB. Eph receptors and ephrins in cancer: bidirectional signalling and beyond. *Nat Rev Cancer* 2010;10:165–180.
222. Ahmed Z, Bicknell R. Angiogenic signalling pathways. *Methods Mol Biol* 2009;467:3–24.
223. Dejana E, Orsenigo F, Molendini C, et al. Organization and signaling of endothelial cell-to-cell junctions in various regions of the blood and lymphatic vascular trees. *Cell Tissue Res* 2009;335:17–25.
224. Carmeliet P, Jain RK. Angiogenesis in cancer and other diseases. *Nature* 2000;407:249–257.
225. Ruoslahti E, Bhatia SN, Sailor MJ. Targeting of drugs and nanoparticles to tumors. *J Cell Biol* 2010;188:759–768.
226. Ruoslahti E. Specialization of tumour vasculature. *Nat Rev Cancer* 2002;2:83–90.
227. Motz GT, Coukos G. The parallel lives of angiogenesis and immunosuppression: cancer and other tales. *Nat Rev Immunol* 2011;11:702–711.
228. Carmeliet P, Jain RK. Principles and mechanisms of vessel normalization for cancer and other angiogenic diseases. *Nat Rev Drug Discov* 2011;10:417–427.
229. Tammela T, Alitalo K. Lymphangiogenesis: Molecular mechanisms and future promise. *Cell* 2010;140:460–476.
230. Card CM, Yu SS, Swartz MA. Emerging roles of lymphatic endothelium in regulating adaptive immunity. *J Clin Invest* 2014;124:943–952.
231. Gaengel K, Genové G, Armulik A, et al. Endothelial-mural cell signaling in vascular development and angiogenesis. *Arterioscler Thromb Vasc Biol* 2009;29:630–638.
232. Schäfer M, Werner S. Cancer as an overhealing wound: an old hypothesis revisited. *Nat Rev Mol Cell Biol* 2008;9:628–638.
233. Karin M, Lawrence T, Nizet V. Innate immunity gone awry: linking microbial infections to chronic inflammation and cancer. *Cell* 2006;124:823–835.
234. Coffelt SB, Lewis CE, Naldini L, et al. Elusive identities and overlapping phenotypes of proangiogenic myeloid cells in tumors. *Am J Pathol* 2010;176:1564–1576.
235. Johansson M, Denardo DG, Coussens LM. Polarized immune responses differentially regulate cancer development. *Immunol Rev* 2008;222:145–154.
236. Mantovani A. Molecular pathways linking inflammation and cancer. *Curr Mol Med* 2010;10:369–373.
237. Mantovani A, Allavena P, Sica A, et al. Cancer-related inflammation. *Nature* 2008;454:436-444
238. DeNardo DG, Brennan DJ, Rexhepaj E, et al. Leukocyte complexity predicts breast cancer survival and functionally regulates response to chemotherapy. *Cancer Discov* 2011;1:54–67.
239. De Palma M, Coukos G, Hanahan D. A new twist on radiation oncology: low-dose irradiation elicits immunostimulatory macrophages that unlock barriers to tumor immunotherapy. *Cancer Cell* 2013;24:559–561.
240. Koh BI, Kang Y. The pro-metastatic role of bone marrow-derived cells: a focus on MSCs and regulatory T cells. *EMBO Rep* 2012;13:412–422.
241. Bergfeld SA, DeClerck YA. Bone marrow-derived mesenchymal stem cells and the tumor microenvironment. *Cancer Metastasis Rev* 2010;29:249–261.
242. Fang S, Salven P. Stem cells in tumor angiogenesis. *J Mol Cell Cardiol* 2011;50:290–295.
243. Giaccia AJ, Schipani E. Role of carcinoma-associated fibroblasts and hypoxia in tumor progression. *Curr Top Microbiol Immunol* 2010;345:31–45.
244. Labelle M, Hynes RO. The initial hours of metastasis: the importance of cooperative host-tumor cell interactions during hematogenous dissemination. *Cancer Discov* 2012;2:1091–1099.
245. Peinado H, Lavothskin S, Lyden D. The secreted factors responsible for pre-metastatic niche formation: old sayings and new thoughts. *Semin Cancer Biol* 2011;21:139–146.
246. Reya T, Morrison SJ, Clarke MF, et al. Stem cells, cancer, and cancer stem cells. *Nature* 2001;414:105–111.
247. Bonnet D, Dick JE. Human acute myeloid leukemia is organized as a hierarchy that originates from a primitive hematopoietic cell. *Nature Med* 1997;3:730–737.
248. Gilbertson RJ, Rich JN. Making a tumour's bed: glioblastoma stem cells and the vascular niche. *Nat Rev Cancer* 2007;7:733–736.
249. al-Hajj M, Wicha M, Benito-Hernandez A, et al. Prospective identification of tumorigenic breast cancer cells. *Proc Natl Acad Sci U S A* 2003;100:3983–3988.
250. Beck B, Blanpain C. Unravelling cancer stem cell potential. *Nat Rev Cancer* 2013;13:727–738.
251. Magee JA, Piskounova E, Morrison SJ. Cancer stem cells: impact, heterogeneity, and uncertainty. *Cancer Cell* 2012;21:283–296.
252. Cho RW, Clarke MF. Recent advances in cancer stem cells. *Curr Opin Genet Devel* 2008;18:1–6.
253. Lobo NA, Shimono Y, Qian D, et al. The biology of cancer stem cells. *Annu Rev Cell Dev Biol* 2007;23:675–699.
254. Meacham CE, Morrison SJ. Tumour heterogeneity and cancer cell plasticity. *Nature* 2013;501:328–337.
255. Singh A, Settleman J. EMT, cancer stem cells and drug resistance: an emerging axis of evil in the war on cancer. *Oncogene* 2010;29:4741–4751.
256. Brabletz T, Jung A, Spaderna S, et al. Opinion: migrating cancer stem cells – an integrated concept of malignant tumor progression. *Nat Rev Cancer* 2005;5:744–749.
257. Boiko AD, Razorenova OV, van de Rijn M, et al. Human melanoma-initiating cells express neural crest nerve growth factor receptor CD271. *Nature* 2010;466:133–137.
258. Gupta P, Chaffer CL, Weinberg RA. Cancer stem cells: mirage or reality? *Nature Med* 2009;15:1010–1012.
259. Quintana E, Shackleton M, Sabel MS, et al. Efficient tumour formation by single human melanoma cells. *Nature* 2008;456:593–598.
260. Chaffer CL, Brueckmann I, Scheel C, et al. Normal and neoplastic nonstem cells can spontaneously convert to stem-like state. *Proc Natl Acad Sci U S A* 2011;108:7950–7955.
261. Thiery JP, Sleeman JR. Complex networks orchestrate epithelial-mesenchymal transitions. *Nat Rev Mol Cell Biol* 2006;7:131–142.
262. Creighton CJ, Li X, Landis M, et al. Residual breast cancers after conventional therapy display mesenchymal as well as tumor-initiating features. *Proc Natl Acad Sci U S A* 2009;106:13820–13825.
263. Buck E, Eyzaguirre A, Barr S, et al. Loss of homotypic cell adhesion by epithelial-mesenchymal transition or mutation limits sensitivity to epidermal growth factor receptor inhibition. *Mol Cancer Therap* 2007;6:532–541.
264. Rhim AD, Mirek ET, Aiello NM, et al. EMT and dissemination precede pancreatic tumor formation. *Cell* 2012;148:349–361.
265. Soda Y, Marumoto T, Friedmann-Morvinski D, et al. Transdifferentiation of glioblastoma cells into vascular endothelial cells. *Proc Natl Acad Sci U S A* 2011;108:4274–4280.
266. El Hallani S, Boisselier B, Peglion F, et al. A new alternative mechanism in glioblastoma vascularization: tubular vasculogenic mimicry. *Brain* 2010;133:973–982.
267. Wang R, Chadalavada K, Wilshire J, et al. Glioblastoma stem-like cells give rise to tumour endothelium. *Nature* 2010;468:829–833.
268. Folkman J, Kalluri R. Cancer without disease. *Nature* 2004;427:787.
269. Azam F, Mehta S, Harris AL. Mechanisms of resistance to antiangiogenesis therapy. *Eur J Cancer* 2010;46:1323–1332.
270. Ebos JM, Lee CR, Kerbel RS. Tumor and host-mediated pathways of resistance and disease progression in response to antiangiogenic therapy. *Clin Cancer Res* 2009;15:5020–5025.
271. Bergers G, Hanahan D. Modes of resistance to anti-angiogenic therapy. *Nat Rev Cancer* 2008;8:592–603.
272. Ellis LM, Reardon DA. Cancer: the nuances of therapy. *Nature* 2009;458:290–292.
273. Norden AD, Drappatz J, Wen PY. Antiangiogenic therapies for high-grade glioma. *Nat Rev Neurol* 2009;5:610–620.
274. Verhoeff JJ, van Tellingen O, Claes A, et al. Concerns about anti-angiogenic treatment in patients with glioblastoma multiforme. *BMC Cancer* 2009;9:444.
275. Hanahan D. Rethinking the war on cancer. *Lancet* 2014;383:558–563.
276. Pencheva N, Tavazoie SF. Control of metastatic progression by microRNA regulatory networks. *Nat Cell Biol* 2013;15:546–554.
277. Garzon R, Marcucci G, Croce CM. Targeting microRNAs in cancer: rationale, strategies and challenges. *Nat Rev Drug Discov* 2010;9:775–789.

3 Molecular Methods in Cancer

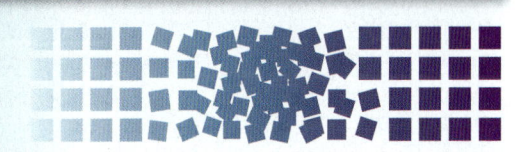

Larissa V. Furtado, Jay L. Hess, and Bryan L. Betz

APPLICATIONS OF MOLECULAR DIAGNOSTICS IN ONCOLOGY

Molecular diagnostics is increasingly impacting a number of areas of cancer care delivery including diagnosis, prognosis, in predicting response to particular therapies, and in minimal residual disease monitoring. Each of these depends on detection or measurement of one or more disease-specific molecular biomarkers representing abnormalities in genetic or epigenetic pathways controlling cellular proliferation, differentiation, or cell death (Table 3.1). In addition, molecular diagnostics is beginning to play a role in predicting host metabolism of drugs—for example, in predicting fast versus slow thiopurine metabolizers using polymorphisms in the thiopurine methyltransferase (TPMT) allele and in use in dosing patients with thiopurine drugs.[1] Molecular diagnostics has also had a major impact on assessing an engraftment after bone marrow transplantation and in tissue typing for bone marrow and solid organ transplantation.

The ideal cancer biomarker is only associated with the disease and not the normal state. The utility of the biomarker largely depends on what the clinical effect the biomarker predicts for, how large the effect is, and how strong the evidence is for the effect. For clinical application, biomarkers need a high level of *analytic validity*, *clinical validity*, and *clinical utility*. Analytic validity refers to the ability of the overall testing process to accurately detect and, in many cases, measure the biomarker. Clinical validity is the ability of a biomarker to predict a particular disease behavior or response to therapy. Clinical utility, arguably the most difficult to assess, addresses whether the information available from the biomarker is actually beneficial for patient care.

Biomarkers can take many forms including *chromosomal translocations* and *other chromosomal rearrangements*, *gene amplification*, *copy number variation*, *point mutations*, *single nucleotide polymorphisms*, *changes in gene expression* (including micro RNAs), and *epigenetic alterations*. Most biomarkers in widespread use represent either gain of function or loss of function alterations in key signaling pathways. Those that occur early and at a high frequency in tumors tend to be *driver mutations*, whose function is important for the cancer cell's proliferation and/or survival. These are particularly useful as biomarkers because they often represent important therapeutic targets. However, cancer cells accumulate many genetic alterations, called *passenger mutations*, which tend to occur at a lower frequency overall and in a subset of a heterogeneous population of tumor cells that may contribute to the cancer phenotype but are not absolutely essential.[2] Distinguishing passenger from driver mutations using various functional assays has become a major focus of translational research in cancer. The same biomarker may have utility in a variety of settings. For example, the detection of the *BCR-ABL1* translocation, pathognomonic for chronic myelogenous leukemia (CML), is used for establishing the diagnosis, for the selection of therapy, and for monitoring for minimal residual disease during and after therapy.

Some of the most heavily used genetic biomarkers in cancer, particularly in hematologic malignancies, are *chromosomal translocations*. For certain diseases such as CML, detection of the *BCR-ABL1* translocation or in Burkitt lymphoma the immunoglobulin gene-*MYC* translocation is required, according to current World Health Organization (WHO) guidelines, to make the diagnosis. Identification of translocations is important in the diagnosis and subtyping of acute leukemias (e.g., detection of *PML-RARA* and variant translocations in acute promyelocytic leukemia) and is also extremely important for the diagnosis of sarcomas such as Ewing sarcoma. The discovery of chromosomal translocations, such as the *TMPRSS-ETS* in prostate cancer and *ALK* translocations in non–small-cell lung cancer, portends an importance of detecting translocations in solid tumors.[3] Chromosomal translocations, especially for hematologic malignancies, have been traditionally detected by classical karyotyping. This approach has limitations; in particular, it requires viable, dividing cells, which are often not readily available from solid tumor biopsies. In addition, a significant proportion of chromosomal translocations are not detectable by conventional karyotyping. For example, 5% to 10% of CML cases lack detectable t(9;22) by G banding. Such "cryptic" translocations require other approaches for detection, which are to be discussed, including *fluorescent in situ hybridization (FISH)*, *polymerase chain reaction (PCR)*, as well as *nucleic acid sequencing-based methods*.

In certain settings, it can be helpful to detect if a population of cells is clonal. For example, in some lymphoid infiltrates, the cells are well differentiated and it can be difficult to determine whether these represent a reactive or neoplastic infiltrate. If dispersed, cells are available and these could be analyzed by flow cytometer to detect whether a monotypic population expressing either immunoglobulin kappa or lambda light chains is present. In theory, immunohistochemical staining (IHC) for immunoglobulin light chains could be used to assess clonality; however, in practice this is done with more sensitivity using RNA in situ hybridization for immunoglobulin kappa and lambda light chain transcripts. The most sensitive way to detect clonality in a B-cell population is to analyze the size of the break point cluster region that arises as a result of VDJ recombination by *PCR*. Reactive B cells will show a distribution in the size of the VDJ recombination for the *IGH* or *IGK* or *IGL*, whereas clonal cells will show a predominant band that represents the size of the VDJ region of the dominant clone. Similarly, sometimes it can be difficult to distinguish neoplastic from reactive T-cell infiltrates. Given the large number of T-cell antigen receptors, it is not as simple to detect clonality by IHC or flow cytometry in T-cell proliferations. One approach is to use aberrant loss of T-cell antigen expression to aid in the diagnosis of T-cell neoplasms. Another is to detect clonal rearrangement of the VDJ region of the T-cell receptor gamma (*TCRγ*) gene, which can be done by PCR on both fresh and formalin-fixed paraffin-embedded (FFPE) tissue.

Gene amplification is another important mechanism in cancer that has been found to have high utility in a subset of cancers. *MYCN* amplification occurs in approximately 40% of undifferentiated or poorly differentiated neuroblastoma subtypes,[4,5] either appearing as double minute chromosomes or homogeneously

TABLE 3.1
Genomic Alterations as Putative Predictive Biomarkers for Cancer Therapy

Genes	Pathways	Aberration Type	Disease Examples	Putative or Proven Drugs
PIK3CA,[51,52] PIK3R1,[53] PIK3R2, AKT1, AKT2, and AKT3[54,55]	Phosphoinositide 3-kinase (PI3K)	Mutation or amplification	Breast, colorectal, and endometrial cancer	■ PI3K inhibitors ■ AKT inhibitors
PTEN[56]	PI3K	Deletion	Numerous cancers	■ PI3K inhibitors
MTOR,[57] TSC1,[58] and TSC2[59]	mTOR	Mutation	Tuberous sclerosis and bladder cancer	■ mTOR inhibitors
RAS family (HRAS, NRAS, KRAS), BRAF,[60] and MEK1	RAS–MEK	Mutation, rearrangement, or amplification	Numerous cancers, including melanoma and prostate cancers	■ RAF inhibitors ■ MEK inhibitors ■ PI3K inhibitors
Fibroblast growth factor receptor 1 (FGFR1), FGFR2, FGFR3, FGFR4[36]	FGFR	Mutation, amplification, or rearrangement	Myeloma, sarcoma, and bladder, breast, ovarian, lung, endometrial, and myeloid cancers	■ FGFR inhibitors ■ FGFR antibodies
Epidermal growth factor receptor (EGFR)	EGFR	Mutation, deletion, or amplification	Lung and gastrointestinal cancer	■ EGFR inhibitors ■ EGFR antibodies
ERBB2[61]	ERBB2	Amplification or mutation	Breast, bladder, gastric, and lung cancers	■ ERBB2 inhibitors ■ ERBB2 antibodies
SMO[62,63] and PTCH1[64]	Hedgehog	Mutation	Basal cell carcinoma	■ Hedgehog inhibitor
MET[65]	MET	Amplification or mutation	Bladder, gastric, and renal cancers	■ MET inhibitors ■ MET antibodies
JAK1, JAK2, JAK3,[66] STAT1, STAT3	JAK–STAT	Mutation or rearrangement	Leukemia and lymphoma	■ JAK–STAT inhibitors ■ STAT decoys
Discoidin domain-containing receptor 2 (DDR2)	RTK	Mutation	Lung cancer	■ Some tyrosine kinase inhibitors
Erythropoietin receptor (EPOR)	JAK–STAT	Rearrangement	Leukemia	■ JAK–STAT inhibitors
Interleukin-7 receptor (IL-7R)	JAK–STAT	Mutation	Leukemia	■ JAK–STAT inhibitors
Cyclin-dependent kinases (CDKs[67]; CDK4, CDK6, CDK8), CDKN2A, and cyclin D1 (CCND1)	CDK	Amplification, mutation, deletion, or rearrangement	Sarcoma, colorectal cancer, melanoma, and lymphoma	■ CDK inhibitors
ABL1	ABL	Rearrangement	Leukemia	■ ABL inhibitors
Retinoic acid receptor-α (RARA)	RARα	Rearrangement	Leukemia	■ All-trans retinoic acid
Aurora kinase A (AURKA)[68]	Aurora kinases	Amplification	Prostate and breast cancers	■ Aurora kinase inhibitors
Androgen receptor (AR)[69]	Androgen	Mutation, amplification, or splice variant	Prostate cancer	■ Androgen synthesis inhibitors ■ Androgen receptor inhibitors
FLT3[70]	FLT3	Mutation or deletion	Leukemia	■ FLT3 inhibitors
MET	MET–HGF	Mutation or amplification	Lung and gastric cancers	■ MET inhibitors
Myeloproliferative leukemia (MPL)	THPO, JAK–STAT	Mutation	Myeloproliferative neoplasms	■ JAK–STAT inhibitors
MDM2[71]	MDM2	Amplification	Sarcoma and adrenal carcinomas	■ MDM2 antagonist
KIT[72]	KIT	Mutation	GIST, mastocytosis, and leukemia	■ KIT inhibitors
PDGFRA and PDGFRB	PDGFR	Deletion, rearrangement, or amplification	Hematologic cancer, GIST, sarcoma, and brain cancer	■ PDGFR inhibitors
Anaplastic lymphoma kinase (ALK)[9,37,73,74]	ALK	Rearrangement or mutation	Lung cancer and neuroblastoma	■ ALK inhibitors

(continued)

TABLE 3.1
Genomic Alterations as Putative Predictive Biomarkers for Cancer Therapy *(continued)*

Genes	Pathways	Aberration Type	Disease Examples	Putative or Proven Drugs
RET	RET	Rearrangement or mutation	Lung and thyroid cancers	▪ RET inhibitors
ROS1[75]	ROS1	Rearrangement	Lung cancer and cholangiocarcinoma	▪ ROS1 inhibitors
NOTCH1 and *NOTCH2*	Notch	Rearrangement or mutation	Leukemia and breast cancer	▪ Notch signalling pathway inhibitors

PIK3CA, PI3K catalytic subunit-α; *PIK3R1*, PI3K regulatory subunit 1; *PI3K*, phosphoinositide 3-kinase; *AKT*, v-akt murine thymoma viral oncogene homolog; *PTEN*, phosphatase and tensin homolog; mTOR, mechanistic target of rapamycin; *TSC1*, tuberous sclerosis 1 protein; RAS–MEK, rat sarcoma; *MEK*, MAPK/ERK (mitogen-activated protein kinase/extracellular signal-regulated kinase) kinase; RAF, v-raf murine sarcoma viral oncogene homolog; *ERBB2*, also known as HER2; *SMO*, smoothened homolog; *PTCH1*, patched homolog; *MET*, hepatocyte growth factor receptor; *JAK*, Janus kinase; *THPO*, thrombopoietin; *STAT*, signal transducer and activator of transcription; RTK, receptor tyrosine kinase; *CDKN2A*, cyclin-dependent kinase inhibitor 2A; *ABL*, Abelson murine leukemia viral oncogene homolog 1; *FLT3*, FMS-like tyrosine kinase 3; *HGF*, hepatocyte growth factor; *MDM2*, mouse double minute 2; *KIT*, v-kit Hardy-Zuckerman 4 feline sarcoma viral oncogene homolog; GIST, gastrointestinal stromal tumor; PDGFR, platelet-derived growth factor receptor; *ROS1*, v-ros avian UR2 sarcoma virus oncogene homolog.
Reprinted by permission from Macmillan Publishers Limited: Nature Reviews Drug Discovery, Simon, R. and Rowchodhury, S. 12:358–369, 2013, ©2013.

staining regions. MYCN amplification is a very strong predictor of poor outcomes, particularly in patients with localized (stage 1 or stage 2) disease or in infants with stage 4S metastatic disease, where fewer than half of patients survive beyond 5 years.[6]

Use of *other chromosome abnormalities* has been largely limited to the diagnosis and prognostication of hematologic disorders. Roughly half of all myelodysplastic disorders show cytogenetically detectable chromosomal abnormalities, such as monosomy 5 or 7, partial chromosomal loss (5q-, 7q-), or complex chromosomal abnormalities. Certain abnormalities in isolation (e.g., 5q-) have a favorable prognosis, whereas many others (e.g., "complex" karyotypes with three or more abnormalities) carry a worse prognosis. Differences in ploidy have proven to be useful predictors in pediatric acute lymphocytic leukemia (ALL), with hyperdiploid cases (>50 chromosomes) showing a distinctly more favorable course compared with hypodiploid or near diploid cases.[7] Overall, DNA ploidy can be assessed by flow cytometry. Specific chromosomal copy number alterations can be detected by *conventional karyotyping*, *array hybridization methods*, or *FISH*.

Copy number variation (CNV) represents the most common type of structural chromosomal alteration. Regions affected by CNVs range from approximately 1 kilobase to several megabases that are either amplified or deleted. It is estimated that about 0.4% of the genomes of healthy individuals differ in copy number.[8] CNVs resulting in deletion of genes such as *BRCA1*, *BRCA2*, *APC*, mismatch repair genes, and *TP53* have been implicated in a wide range of highly penetrant cancers.[9,10] CNVs can be detected by a variety of means including *FISH*, *comparative or array genomic hybridization*, or *virtual karyotyping* using *single nucleotide polymorphism* (*SNP*) *arrays*. Increasingly, CNV is detected using *next-generation sequencing*.

Large-scale sequencing of tumors has identified many *mutations* that are of potential prognostic and therapeutic significance. As will be discussed further, a wide range of strategies is available for the detection of point mutations (Fig. 3.1). It is important to

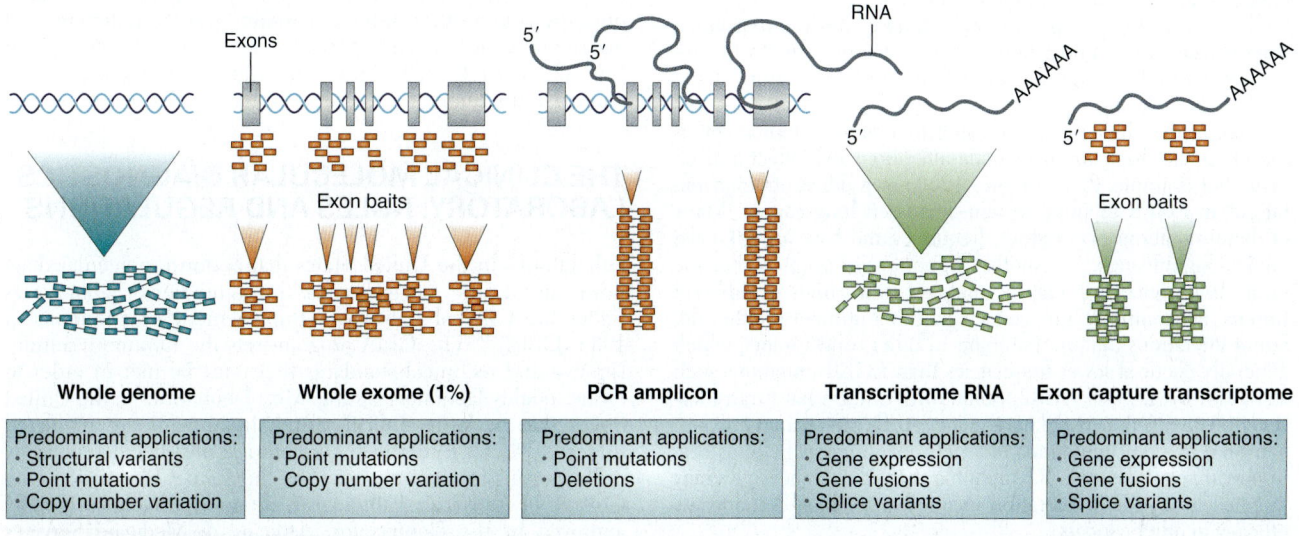

Figure 3.1 Strategies for the detection of mutations, translocations, and other structural genomic abnormalities in cancer. Whole genome sequencing, which involves determining the entire sequence of both introns and exons, is not only the most comprehensive, but also the most laborious and expensive approach. Exome sequencing uses *baits* to capture either the entire exome (roughly 20,000 genes [about 1% of the genome]) or else a subset of genes of interest. Amplicon-based sequencing uses PCR or other amplification techniques to amplify targets of interest for sequencing. Transcriptome sequencing, also known as RNAseq, is based on sequencing expressed RNA and can be used to detect not only mutations, but also translocations, other structural abnormalities, as well as differences in expression levels. This can be combined with exome capture techniques for a higher sensitivity analysis of genes of particular interest. (Reprinted by permission from Macmillan Publishers Limited: Nature Reviews Drug Discovery, Simon, R. and Rowchodhury, S. 12:358–369, 2013, ©2013.)

recognize that many nucleotide variations occur at any given allele in populations. Formally, the term *polymorphism* is used to describe genetic differences present in ≥1% of the human population, whereas *mutation* describes less frequent differences. However, in practice, *polymorphism* is often used to describe a nonpathogenic genetic change, and mutation a deleterious change, regardless of their frequencies.

Mutations can be classified according to their effect in the structure of a gene. The most common of these disease-associated alterations are single nucleotide substitutions (point mutations); however, many deletions, insertions, gene rearrangements, gene amplification, and copy number variations have been identified that have clinical significance. Point mutations may affect promoters, splicing sites, or coding regions. Coding region mutations can be classified into three kinds, depending on the impact on the codon: *missense mutation*, a nucleotide change leads to the substitution of an amino acid to another; *nonsense mutation*, a nucleotide substitution causes premature termination of codons with protein truncation; and *silent mutation*, a nucleotide change does not change the coded amino acid.

Loss of function mutations, either through point mutations or deletions in tumor suppression genes such as *APC* and *TP53*, are the most common mutations in cancers. Tumor suppression genes require two-hit (biallelic) mutations that inactivate both copies of the gene in order to allow tumorigenesis to occur. The first hit is usually an inherited or somatic point mutation, and the second hit is assumed to be an acquired deletion mutation that deletes the second copy of the tumor suppression gene. Promoter methylation of tumor suppressor genes is an alternative route to tumorigenesis that, to date, has not been commonly employed for molecular diagnostics.

Oncogenes originate from the deregulation of genes that normally encode for proteins associated with cell growth, differentiation, apoptosis, and signal transduction (proto-oncogenes, [e.g., *BRAF* and *KRAS*]). Proto-oncogenes generally require only one gain of function or activating mutation to become oncogenic. Common mutation types that result in proto-oncogene activation include point mutations, gene amplifications, and chromosomal translocations. One example is mutations in the epidermal growth factor receptor (*EGFR*) that occur in lung cancer, which are almost exclusively seen in nonmucinous bronchoalveolar carcinomas. Somatic mutations of *EGFR* constitutively activate the receptor tyrosine kinase (TK). Importantly, responsiveness of tumors harboring these mutations to the inhibitor gefitinib is highly coordinated with a mutation of the EGFR TK domain.[11,12]

One of the challenges with using mutations as biomarkers is that there can be many nucleotide alterations that affect a given gene. For example, there are over 100 known different point mutations in *EGFR* reported in non–small-cell lung cancer. Many of these mutations occur at low frequency and have an unknown clinical significance.[13,14] Another important concept is that the same driver oncogene may be mutated in a variety of different tumors. For example, lung cancers harbor a number of other different alterations that are common in other solid tumors, which generally occur at lower frequencies than *EGFR* mutations such as *KRAS*, *BRAF*, and *HER2*. Some lung cancers have translocations involving the *ALK* kinase gene. *ALK*, interestingly, is also activated by point mutations in a neuroblastoma as by translocation in anaplastic large cell lymphoma (Fig. 3.2). Hence, a therapy targeted to a genetic alteration in one cancer may demonstrate efficacy in other cancers.

The detection of mutations is also important in the evaluation of chemotherapy resistance. Roughly a third of CML patients are resistant to the frontline ABL1 kinase inhibitor imatinib, either at the time of initial treatment or, more commonly, secondarily. In cases of primary failure or secondary failure, over 100 different *ABL1* mutations have been identified, including particularly common ones such as T315I and P loop mutations. While some

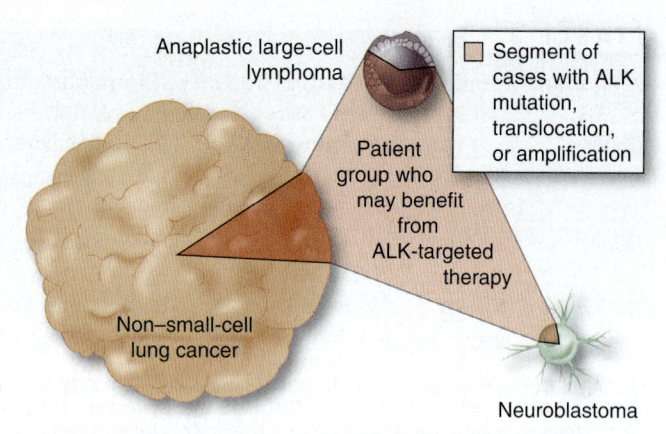

Figure 3.2 Activating genomic alterations occur in a variety of tumor types. *ALK* translocations, mutations, and amplifications occur in non–small-cell lung cancer, neuroblastomas, and in anaplastic large cell lymphomas. Such recurrent alterations in cancer, together with effective inhibitors of these pathways, are transforming oncologic therapies from organ-specific to pathway-specific interventions and are driving the use of molecular diagnostics in a wider range of tumor types. (Modified from McDermott, U. and Settleman, J. *J Clin Oncol* 2009;27:5650–5659.)

mutations, such as Y253H, respond to second generation TK inhibitors (TKI), others, such as the T315I mutation, are noteworthy because they confer resistance not only to imatinib, but also to nilotinib and dasatinib.

Mutations are also used as important predictive biomarkers (Table 3.1). Two of the most notable examples are the use of the *BRCA1* and *BRCA2* mutation analysis for women with a strong family history of breast cancer. Over 200 mutations (loss of function point mutations, small deletions, or insertions) occur in *BRCA* genes, which are distributed across the genes necessitating full sequencing for their detection. The overall prevalence of these occur in about 0.1% of the general population.[15,16] The lifetime risk of breast cancer for women carrying *BRCA1* mutations is in the range of 47% to 66%, whereas for *BRCA2* mutations, it is in the range of 40% to 57%.[17,18] In addition, the risk of other tumors including ovarian, fallopian, and pancreatic cancer is also increased. Detection of *BRCA1* and *BRCA2* mutations is, therefore, important for cancer prevention and risk reduction.

THE CLINICAL MOLECULAR DIAGNOSTICS LABORATORY: RULES AND REGULATIONS

Laboratories in the United States that perform molecular diagnostic testing are categorized as high-complexity laboratories under the Clinical Laboratory Improvement Amendments of 1988 (CLIA).[19] The CLIA program sets the minimum administrative and technical standards that must be met in order to ensure quality laboratory testing. Most laboratories in the United States that perform clinical testing in humans are regulated under CLIA. CLIA-certified laboratories must be accredited by professional organizations such as the Joint Commission, the College of American Pathologists, or another agency officially approved by the Centers for Medicare & Medicaid Services (CMS), and must comply with CLIA standards and guidelines for quality assurance. Although the regulation of laboratory services is in the U.S. Food and Drug Administration's (FDA) jurisdiction, the FDA has historically exercised enforcement discretion. Therefore, FDA approval is not currently required for clinical implementation of molecular tests as long as other regulations are met.[20,21]

SPECIMEN REQUIREMENTS FOR MOLECULAR DIAGNOSTICS

Samples typically received for molecular oncology testing include blood, bone marrow aspirates and biopsies, fluids, organ-specific fresh tissues in saline or tissue culture media such as Roswell Park Memorial Institute (RPMI), FFPE tissues, and cytology cell blocks. Molecular tests can be ordered electronically or through written requisition forms, but never through verbal requests only. All samples submitted for molecular testing need to be appropriately identified. Sample type, quantity, and specimen handling and transport requirements should conform to the laboratory's stated requirements in order to ensure valid test results.

Blood and bone marrow samples should be drawn into anticoagulated tubes. The preferred anticoagulant for most molecular assays is ethylenediaminetetraacetic acid (EDTA; lavender). Other acceptable collection tubes include ACD (yellow) solutions A and B. Heparinized tubes are not preferred for most molecular tests because heparin inhibits the polymerase enzyme utilized in PCR, which may lead to assay failure. Blood and bone marrow samples can be transported at ambient temperature. Blood samples should never be frozen prior to separation of cellular elements because this causes hemolysis, which interferes with DNA amplification. Fluids should be transported on ice. Tissues should be frozen (preferred method) as soon as possible and sent on dry ice to minimize degradation. Fresh tissues in RPMI should be sent on ice or cold packs. Cells should be kept frozen and sent on dry ice; DNA samples can be sent at ambient temperature or on ice.

For FFPE tissue blocks, typical collection and handling procedures include cutting 4 to 6 microtome sections of 10-micron thickness each on uncoated slides, air-drying unstained sections at room temperature, and staining one of the slides with hematoxylin and eosin (H&E). A board-certified pathologist reviews the H&E slides to ensure the tissue block contains a sufficient quantity of neoplastic tumor cells, and circles an area on the H&E slide that will be used as a template to guide macrodissection or microdissection of the adjacent, unstained slides. The pathologist also provides an estimate of the percentage of neoplastic cells in the area that will be tested, which should exceed the established limit of detection (LOD) of the assay.

MOLECULAR DIAGNOSTICS TESTING PROCESS

The workflow of a molecular test begins with receipt and accessioning of the specimen in the clinical molecular diagnostics laboratory followed by extraction of the nucleic acid (DNA or RNA), test setup, detection of analyte (e.g., PCR products), data analysis, and result reporting to the patient medical record (Fig. 3.3).

An extraction of intact, moderately high-quality DNA is essential for molecular assays. For DNA extraction, the preferred age for blood, bone marrow, and fluid samples is less than 5 days; for frozen or fixed tissue, it is indefinite; and for fresh tissue, it is overnight. Although there is no age limit for the use of a fixed and embedded tissue specimen for analysis, older specimens may yield a lower quantity and quality of DNA. Because RNA is significantly more labile than DNA, the preferred age for blood and bone marrow is less than 48 hours (from time of collection). Tissue samples intended for an RNA analysis should be promptly processed in fresh state, snap frozen, or preserved with RNA stabilizing agents for transport.

Dedicated areas, equipment, and materials are designated for various stages of DNA and RNA extraction procedures. DNA and RNA isolation can be done by manual or automated methods. Currently, most clinical laboratories employ commercial protocols based on liquid- or solid-phase extractions. Nucleated cells are isolated from biological samples prior to nucleic acid extraction.

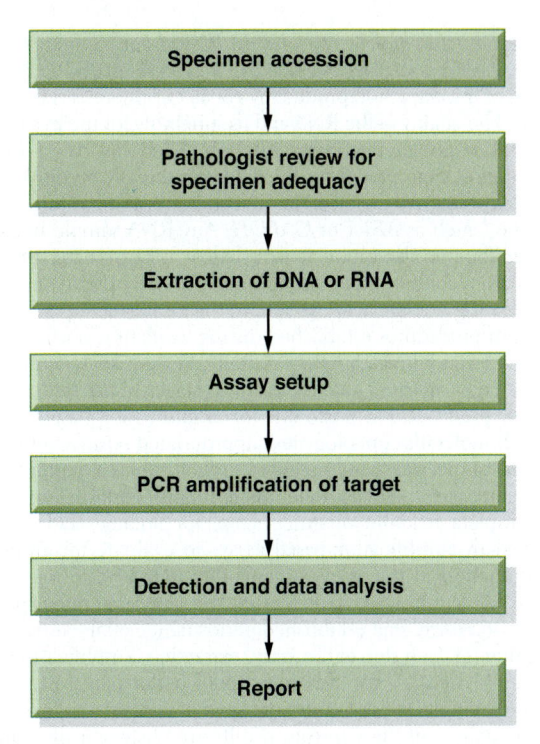

Figure 3.3 Simplified workflow of clinical molecular diagnostic testing.

White blood cells (WBC) can be isolated from blood and bone marrow samples by different methods. One method involves lysing the red blood cells with an ammonium chloride solution, which yields the total WBC population and other nucleated cells present. Another method involves a gradient preparation with a Ficoll solution, which yields the mononuclear cell population only. Sections of FFPE tissue blocks are prepared for DNA extraction by first removing the paraffin and disrupting the cell membranes with proteinase K digestion. Fresh and frozen tissues also undergo proteinase K digestion prior to nucleic acid extraction. DNA isolation protocols consist of several steps, including cell lysis, DNA purification by salting out the proteins and other debris (nonorganic method), or by solvent extractions of the proteins with phenol and chloroform solutions (organic method). The DNA is then precipitated out of the solution with isopropanol or ethanol. The pellet is washed with 70% to 80% ethanol and then solubilized in buffer, such as Tris-EDTA solution. Proteinase K can be added to assist in the disruption and to prevent nonspecific degradation of the DNA. RNase is sometimes added to eliminate contaminating RNA. The DNA yield is quantitated spectrophotometrically, and the DNA sample integrity is visually checked, if necessary, on an agarose gel followed by ethidium bromide staining. Intact DNA appears as a high–molecular-weight single band, whereas degraded DNA is identified as a smear of variably sized fragments. After extraction, the DNA is stored at 4°C prior to use in a PCR assay, and is then stored at −70°C after completion of the assay. Because the DNA extracted from formalin-fixed tissue is degraded to a variable extent, an analysis of the extraction product by gel electrophoresis is not informative. Yield and integrity of the extracted DNA is best assessed by an amplification control to ensure that the quality and quantity of input DNA is adequate to yield a valid result.

RNA isolation steps are similar to the ones described previously for DNA extraction. However, RNA is inherently less stable than DNA due to its single-strand conformation and susceptibility to degradation by RNase, which is ubiquitous in the environment. To ensure preservation of target RNA, special precautions are required, including the use of diethylpyrocarbonate (DEPC) water in all reagents used in RNA procedures, and special decontamination of work area and pipettes to prevent RNase contamination. The extracted RNA is usually degraded to a variable extent so that the analysis of the extraction product by gel electrophoresis is not informative. The quality of the RNA and its suitability for use in a reverse transcriptase polymerase chain reaction (RT-PCR)–based assay is assessed most appropriately by the demonstration of a positive result in an assay designed to detect the RNA transcripts for a "housekeeping gene," such as *ABL1* or *GAPDH*. Any RNA sample in which the 260/280-nm absorption ratio is below 1.9 or greater than 2.0 may contain contaminants and must be cleaned prior to analysis.

Following nucleic acid extraction, the assay is set up according to written procedures established during validation/verification of the assay by qualified laboratory staff. Dedicated areas, equipment, and materials are designated for various stages of the test (e.g., extraction, pre-PCR and post-PCR for amplification-based assays). For each molecular oncology test, appropriated positive and negative control specimens are included to each run as a matter of routine quality assessment. A no template (blank) control, containing the complete reaction mixture except for nucleic acids, is also included in amplification-based assays to evaluate for amplicon contamination in the assay reagents that may lead to inaccurate results. The controls are processed in the same manner as patient samples to ensure that established performance characteristics are being met for each step of the assay (extraction, amplification, and detection). All assay controls and overall performance of the run must be examined prior to interpretation of sample results. Following acceptance of the controls, results are electronically entered into reports. The final report is reviewed and signed by the laboratory director or a qualified designee who meets the same qualifications as the director, as defined by CLIA (see previous).

TECHNOLOGIES

Several traditional and emerging techniques are currently available for mutation detection in cancer (Table 3.2). In the era of personalized medicine, molecular oncology assays are rapidly moving from a mutational analysis of single genes toward a multigene panel analysis. As the number of "actionable" mutations such as *ALK*, *EGFR*, *BRAF*, and others increase, the use of next-generation sequencing platforms is expected to become much more widespread. Both traditional and emerging testing approaches have advantages and disadvantages that need to be balanced before a test platform is implemented into practice.

An important consideration when adding a new oncology test in the clinical laboratory menu is to define the intended use of the assay (e.g., diagnosis, prognosis, prediction of therapy response). The clinical utility of the assay, appropriate types of specimens, the spectrum of possible mutations that can be found in the genomic region of interest, and available methods for testing should also be determined. The laboratory director and ordering physicians should also discuss the estimated test volume, optimal reporting format, and required turnaround time for the proposed new test.[21–23]

Polymerase Chain Reaction

Polymerase chain reaction (PCR)[24,25] is widely used in all molecular diagnostics laboratories for the rapid amplification of targeted DNA sequences. The reaction includes the specimen template DNA, forward and reverse primers (18 to 24 oligonucleotides long), Taq DNA polymerase, and each of the four nucleotides bases (dATP, dTTP, dCTP, dGTP). During PCR, selected genomic sequences undergo repetitive temperature cycling (sequential heat and cooling) that allows for *denaturation* of double-stranded DNA template, *annealing* of the primers to the targeted complementary sequences on the template, and *extension* of new strands of DNA by Taq polymerase from nucleotides, using the primers as the starting point. Each cycle doubles the copy number of PCR templates for the next round of polymerase activity, resulting in an exponential amplification of the selected target sequence. The PCR products (amplicons) are detected by electrophoresis or in real-time systems simultaneously to the amplification reaction (see real-time PCR, which follows).

PCR is specifically designed to work on DNA templates because the Taq polymerase does not recognize RNA as a starting material. Nonetheless, PCR can be adapted to RNA testing by including a reverse transcription step to convert a RNA sequence into its cognate cDNA sequence before the PCR reaction is performed (see reverse-transcription PCR, which follows). Multiplex PCR reactions can also be designed with multiple primers for simultaneous amplification of multiple genomic targets. PCR is a highly sensitive and specific technique that can be employed in different capacities for the detection of point mutations, small deletions, insertions and duplications, as well as gene rearrangements and clonality assessment. Limits of detection can reach 0.1% mutant allele or lower, which is important for the detection of somatic mutations in oncology because tumor specimens are usually composed of a mixture of tumor and normal cells. Reverse transcription PCR can also be used for the relative quantification of target RNA in minimal residual disease testing, such as *BCR-ABL1* transcripts in CML. Another advantage of PCR is its ability to amplify small amounts of low quality FFPE-derived DNA. However, applications of PCR can be limited because it cannot amplify across large or highly repetitive genomic regions. Also, the PCR reaction can be inhibited by heparin or melanin if present in the extracted DNA, which may lead to assay failure. Finally, the risk of false positives due to specimen or amplicon contamination is an important issue when using PCR-based techniques; therefore, stringent laboratory procedures, as described previously, are used to minimize contamination. With the exception of hybridization assays, such as fluorescence in situ hybridization and genomic microarrays, PCR is the necessary initial step in all current molecular oncology assays.

Targeted Mutation Analysis Methods

Real-Time PCR (q-PCR)

In real-time PCR (q-PCR), the polymerase chain reaction is performed with a PCR reporter that is usually a fluorescent double-stranded DNA binding dye or a fluorescent reporter probe. The intensity of the fluorescence produced at each amplification cycle is monitored in real time, and both quantification and detection of targeted sequences is accomplished in the reaction tube as the PCR amplification proceeds.

The intensity of the fluorescent signal for a given DNA fragment (wild type or mutant) is correlated with its quantity, based on the PCR cycle in which the fluorescence rises above the background (crossing threshold [Ct] or crossing point [Cp]).[26] The Ct value can be used for qualitative or quantitative analysis. Qualitative assays use the Ct as a cutoff for determining "presence" or "absence" of a given target in the reaction. A qualitative analysis by q-PCR is particularly useful for a targeted detection of point mutations that are located in mutational hotspots. Examples include the *JAK2* V617F mutation, which is located within exon 14, and is found in several myeloproliferative neoplasms (polycythemia vera, essential thrombocythemia, and primary myelofibrosis),[27] and the *BRAF* V600E,[28] which is located within exon 15, and is found in various cancer types including melanomas and thyroid and lung cancers.

For a quantitative analysis, the Ct of standards with known template concentration is used to generate a standard curve to which Ct values of unknown samples are compared. The concentration of the unknown samples is then extrapolated from values from the standard curve. The quantity of amplicons produced in a PCR reaction is proportional to the prevalence of the targeted sequence;

TABLE 3.2
Molecular Methods in Oncology

Method	Advantages	Disadvantages	Analytic Sensitivity	Examples of Applications in Oncology
Real-time PCR (q-PCR) Allele-specific PCR (AS-PCR) Reverse transcriptase PCR (RT-PCR)	Flexible platforms that permit detection of a variety of conserved hotspot mutations including nucleotide substitutions, small length mutations (deletions, insertions), and translocations High sensitivity is beneficial for residual disease testing and specimens with limited tumor content Adaptable to quantitative assays	Detects only specific targeted mutations/chromosomal translocations Not suitable for variable mutations May not determine the exact change in nucleotide sequence	Very high	KRAS, BRAF, and EGFR mutations in solid tumors JAK2 V617F and MPL mutations in myeloproliferative neoplasms KIT D816V mutation in systemic mastocytosis and AML Quantitation of BCR-ABL1 and PML-RARA transcripts for residual disease monitoring in CML and APL, respectively
Fragment analysis	Detects small to medium insertions and deletions Detects variable insertions and deletions regardless of specific alteration Provides semiquantitative information regarding mutation level	Does not determine the exact change in nucleotide sequence Does not detect single nucleotide substitution mutations Limited multiplex capability	High	NPM1 insertion mutations in AML FLT3 internal tandem duplications in AML JAK2 exon 12 insertions and deletions in PV EGFR exon 19 deletions in NSCLC
FISH	Detects chromosomal translocation, gene amplification, and deletion Morphology of tumor is preserved, allowing for a more accurate interpretation of heterogeneous samples	High cost Unable to detect small insertions and deletions Limited multiplex capability Does not determine the exact breakpoint and change in nucleotide sequence	High	IGH/BCL2 translocation detection in follicular lymphoma and in a subset of diffuse large B-cell lymphoma ALK translocation in NSCLC EWSR1 translocation in soft tissue tumors HER2 amplification in breast cancer 1p/19q deletion in oligodendroglioma
High-resolution melting (HRM) curve analysis	Qualitative detection of variable single nucleotide substitutions and small insertions and deletions	Does not determine the exact mutation Result interpretation may require testing via an alternate technology Limited multiplex capability	Medium	KRAS and BRAF mutations in solid tumors JAK2 exon 12 mutations in PV
Sanger sequencing	Detects variable single nucleotide substitutions and small insertions and deletions Provides semiquantitative information about mutation level Current gold standard for mutation detection	Low throughput Low analytic sensitivity limits application in specimens with low tumor burden Does not detect copy number changes or large (>500 bp) insertions and deletions	Low	KIT mutations in GIST and melanoma CEBPA mutations in AML EGFR mutations in NSCLC
Pyrosequencing	Higher analytical sensitivity than Sanger sequencing Detects variable single nucleotide substitutions and small insertions and deletions Provides quantitative information about mutation level	Short read lengths limit analysis to mutational hotspots Low throughput	Medium	KRAS and BRAF mutations in solid tumors
Single nucleotide extension assay (SNaPshot)	Simultaneous detection of targeted nucleotide substitution mutations Multiplex capability	Detects only targeted mutations	High	Small gene panels (3–10) for melanoma, NSCLC, breast cancer, and metastatic colorectal cancer

(continued)

TABLE 3.2
Molecular Methods in Oncology (continued)

Method	Advantages	Disadvantages	Analytic Sensitivity	Examples of Applications in Oncology
Next-generation sequencing (NGS)	Quantitative detection of variable single nucleotide substitutions, small insertions and deletions, chromosomal translocations, and gene copy number variations Highly multiplexed High throughput	Requires costly investment in instrumentation and bioinformatics Technology is rapidly evolving Higher error rates for insertion and deletion mutations Limited ability to sequence GC-rich regions	High	Small to large gene panels (3–500) for solid tumor and hematologic malignancies
Genomic microarray	Simultaneous detection of copy number variation and LOH (SNP array)	Limited application to FFPE tissue Does not detect balanced translocations May not detect low-level mutant allele burden	Medium	Analysis of recurrent copy number variation and LOH in chronic lymphocytic leukemia and myeloproliferative neoplasms

AML, acute myelogenous leukemia; CML, chronic myelogenous leukemia; APL, acute promyelocytic leukemia; PV, polycythemia vera; NSCLC, non–small-cell lung carcinoma; GIST, gastrointestinal stromal tumor; GC, guanine-cytosine; LOH, loss of heterozygosity; FFPE, formalin-fixed paraffin-embedded.

---

therefore, samples with a higher template concentration reaches the Ct at earlier PCR cycles than one with a low concentration of the amplified target. Quantitative q-PCR has high analytical sensitivity for the detection of low mutant allele burden. For that reason, this method has been widely utilized for monitoring minimal residual disease.

Allele-Specific PCR

Allele-specific PCR (AS-PCR) is a variant of conventional PCR. The method is based on the principle that Taq polymerase is incapable of catalyzing chain elongation in the presence of a mismatch between the 3′ end of the primer and the template DNA. Selective amplification by AS-PCR is achieved by designing a forward primer that matches the mutant sequence at the 3′ end primer. A second mismatch within the primer can be introduced at the adjacent -1 or -2 position to decrease the efficiency of mismatched amplification products. This will minimize the chance of amplifying and, therefore, detecting the wild-type target. AS-PCR is usually performed as two PCR reactions: one employing a forward primer specific for the mutant sequence, the other using a forward primer specific for the correspondent wild-type sequence. In this case, a common reverse primer is used for both reactions. Following amplification, the PCR products are detected by electrophoresis (capillary or agarose gel) or in q-PCR systems. The detection of adequate PCR product in the wild-type amplification reaction is important to control for adequate specimen quality and quantity, particularly when the specimen is negative in the mutation-specific PCR reaction.

AS-PCR is particularly useful for the detection of targeted point mutations. Multiplex AS-PCR reactions can be designed for the simultaneous detection of multiple mutations by including several mutation-specific primers. The method has high analytical sensitivity and specificity and can be easily deployed in most clinical laboratories. However, an important limitation is that this approach will not detect mutations other than those for which specific primers are designed. Therefore, it is utilized for highly recurrent mutations that occur at specific locations within genes, rather than for the detection of variable mutations that may occur throughout a gene.

Examples of AS-PCR applications in oncology include the detection of *JAK2* V617F and *MPL* mutations in myeloproliferative neoplasms (primary myelofibrosis, essential thrombocythemia, and/or polycythemia vera),[29] the *BRAF* V600E mutation,[30] and *KIT* D816V mutations in cases of systemic mastocytosis and in acute myelogenous leukemia (AML).

Reverse Transcriptase PCR

RT-PCR is utilized for the detection and quantification of RNA transcripts. The first step for all amplification-based assays that use RNA as a starting material is reverse transcription of RNA into cDNA, because RNA is not a suitable substrate for Taq polymerase. In RT-PCR, RNA is isolated and reverse transcribed into cDNA by using a reverse transcriptase enzyme and one of the following: (1) random hexamer primers, which anneal randomly to RNA and reverse transcribe all RNA in the cell; (2) oligo dT primers, which anneal to the polyA tail of mRNA and reverse transcribe only mRNA; or (3) gene-specific primers that reverse transcribe only the target of interest. PCR is subsequently performed on the cDNA with forward and reverse primers specific to the gene(s) of interest. The RT-PCR products may then be analyzed by capillary electrophoresis or in real-time systems as in a standard PCR reaction.

RT-PCR is commonly used for detecting gene fusions during translocation analysis because breakpoints frequently occur within the intron of each partner gene and the precise intronic breakpoint locations may be variable. This variability complicates the design of primers used in DNA-based PCR assays. RT-PCR tests are advantageous because mature mRNA has intronic sequence spliced out, allowing for simplified primer design within the affected exon of each partner gene. In this setting, RT-PCR is useful in tests where both translocation partners are recurrent and only one or a few exons are involved in each partner gene. For instance, 95% of acute promyelocytic leukemia (APL) cases harbor the reciprocal t(15;17) chromosomal translocation and these breakpoints always occur within intron 2 of the *RARA* gene. By contrast, three distinct chromosome 15 breakpoints are involved, all occurring within the *PML* gene: intron 6, exon 6, and intron 3. Because the breakpoints in the two genes are recurrent, most of the reported *PML-RARA* fusions can be detected by targeting these three transcript isoforms.

RT-PCR is the method of choice when high sensitivity is required to detect gene translocations. For example, *PML-RARA*

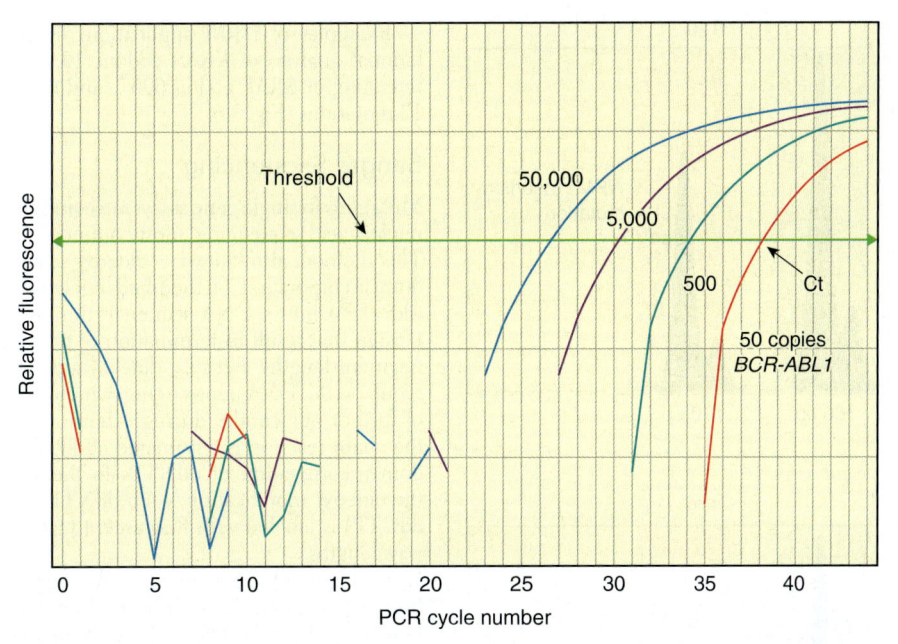

Figure 3.4 Reverse transcriptase PCR (RT-PCR) is a sensitive means to detect *BCR-ABL1* fusion transcripts in CML. RT-PCR can be combined with real-time PCR (q-PCR) to quantitate *BCR-ABL1* transcripts across four to six log range levels. Amplification products are detected during each PCR cycle using a fluorescent probe specific to the PCR product. The accumulated fluorescence in log(10) value is plotted against the number of PCR cycles. For a given specimen, the PCR cycle number is measured when the increase in fluorescence is exponential and exceeds a threshold. This point is called the Ct, which is inversely proportional to the amount of PCR target in the specimen (i.e., lower Ct values indicate a greater amount of target). Calibration standards of known quantity are used in standard curves to calculate the amount of target in a tested specimen. These are shown in the chart as different colored plots. Note that PCR increases the amount of amplification product by a factor of two with each PCR cycle. Therefore, specimens that produce a Ct value that is one cycle lower are expected to have a twofold higher concentration of target. Specimens that differ in target concentration by a factor of 10 (as shown) are expected to have a Ct value 3.3 cycles apart ($2^{3.3} = 10$).

transcript detection by RT-PCR can detect this fusion transcript down to 1 tumor cell in the background of 100,000 normal cells. Detecting low levels of fusion transcript can reveal relapse after consolidation and guide further treatment.[31] RT-PCR can also be used to quantitate the amount of expression of a gene. One major application of RT-PCR in this setting includes quantitative detection of *BCR-ABL1* fusion transcript for prognostication and minimal residual disease testing in CML (Fig. 3.4). In this setting, a three log decrease in *BCR-ABL1* levels is associated with an improved outcome.[32,33]

Fragment Analysis

A fragment analysis is a PCR amplicon-sizing technique that is relevant for the detection of small- to medium-length–affecting mutations (deletions, insertions, and duplications). This is typically performed by capillary electrophoresis, which is capable of resolving length mutations from approximately 1 to 500 base pairs in size.

Fragment analysis represents a practical strategy because it enables comprehensive detection of a wide variety of possible length mutations and has high analytic sensitivity. Further, it can provide semiquantitative information regarding the relative amount of mutated alleles. Limitations of this approach include the inability to objectively quantitate mutant allele burdens, the inability to determine the exact change in nucleotide sequence, and the inability to detect non–length-affecting mutations such as substitution mutations.

Examples of fragment analysis applications in oncology include the detection of *NPM1* insertion mutations (Fig. 3.5),[34] *EGFR* exon 19 deletions, *FLT3* internal tandem duplications, and *JAK2* exon 12 mutations.[35]

High-Resolution Melting Curve Analysis

A high-resolution melting (HRM) curve analysis is a mutation screening method that allows for the detection of DNA sequence variations based on specific sequence-related melting profiles of PCR products.[36] Because the melting property of DNA duplexes is dependent on the biophysical and chemical properties of the nucleotide sequences, mutant and wild-type DNA sequences can be differentiated from one another based on their melting characteristics.

An HRM analysis is preceded by a PCR. The reaction employs a pair of gene-specific forward and reverse primers, template DNA, and a reporter that can either be a double-stranded DNA binding dye or a fluorescent reporter probe. Following the last cycle of the PCR, the amplification products undergo a cooling step that generates homoduplexes (double-stranded molecules with perfect complementarity between alleles) and heteroduplexes (double-stranded molecules with sequence mismatch between alleles) followed by a heating step that denatures (i.e., melts) the double-stranded products. Heteroduplexes (mutant DNA) produce a melting profile different from that of wild-type samples (homoduplexes). In most cases, the reaction is performed in a q-PCR system that allows for an analysis of amplification and

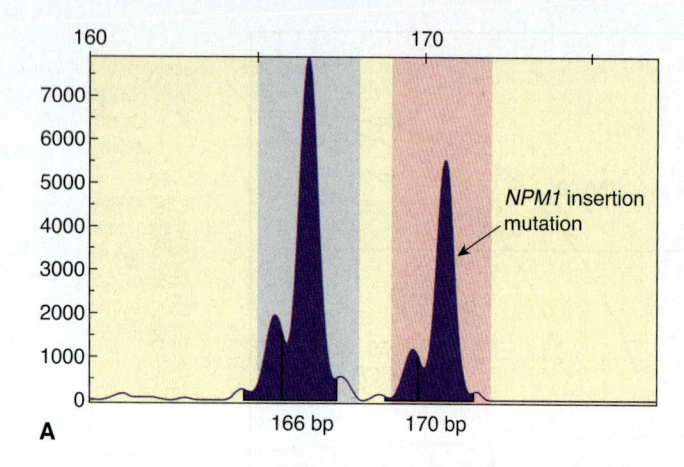

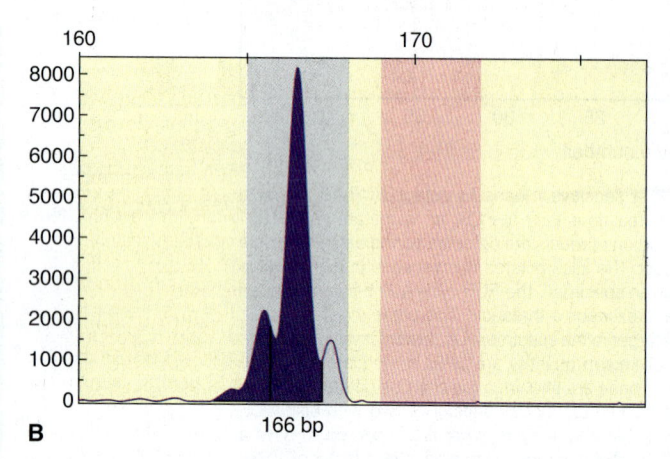

Figure 3.5 Fragment analysis. *NPM1* mutations are important prognostic markers in acute myeloid leukemia. Virtually all *NPM1* mutations result in a four nucleotide insertion within exon 12. Detection of these mutations can be accomplished by PCR utilizing primers that flank the mutation region. The amplification products are sized using capillary electrophoresis. A mutation is indicated by a PCR fragment that is 4 bp larger than the wild-type fragment. Mutation positive **(A)** and negative **(B)** cases are shown.

Examples of HRM applications in oncology include a mutational analysis of *KRAS* codons 12, 13, and 61[39]; a mutation screening of *BRAF* codon 600[39]; and the detection of *JAK2* exon 12 mutations (Fig. 3.6).[40]

Sanger Sequencing

Mutations in single gene assays are commonly analyzed by targeted nucleic acid sequencing, most commonly by Sanger sequencing.[41] This method, also known as dideoxy sequencing, is based on random incorporation of modified nucleotides (dideoxynucleotides [ddNTP]) into a DNA sequence during rounds of template extension that result in termination of the chain reaction at various fragment lengths. Because dideoxynucleotides lack a 3′ hydroxyl group on the DNA pentose ring, which is required for the addition of further nucleotides during extension of the new DNA strand, the chain reaction is terminated at different lengths with the random incorporation of ddNTPs to the sequence. In addition to the dideoxy modification, each ddNTP (ddATP, ddTTP, ddCTP, ddGTP) is labeled with fluorescent tags of different fluorescence wavelengths.

In this method, repetitive cycles of primer extension are performed using denatured PCR products (amplicons) as templates. Unlike PCR, in which both forward and reverse primers are added to the same reaction, in Sanger sequencing, the forward and reverse reactions are performed separately. Bidirectional sequencing is performed to ensure that the entire region of interest

melting data in a close-tube format, thereby minimizing the risk of amplicon contamination.

An HRM analysis is useful for the qualitative detection of variable point mutations and small length-affecting mutations that occur within mutational hotspot regions. This method has high analytical sensitivity and can detect mutations even in a small fraction of alleles in a background of wild-type DNA. However, this assay does not characterize the specific sequence alteration in the mutant allele and may be challenging to interpret, especially for cases with mutation levels that approach the detection limit of the assay. Samples with a lower abundance of mutant alleles, and consequently a decreased fraction of heteroduplexes that produced fluorescence decay during the melting analysis, usually produce a melting curve that may not differ significantly from that of wild-type samples. Likewise, the detection of duplication mutations may be hampered by the similarity between the mutant and the duplicated wild-type genome sequences, which may produce only subtle differences in the melting behavior of the DNA duplexes, especially for samples with low mutant allele burden. Therefore, both the mutant sequence and the allelic burden play in the ability of an HRM analysis to detect mutations.[37] Poor quality and impurity of genomic DNA may also lower the sensitivity of an HRM analysis.[38] In instances of patients with a low mutant allelic burden, equivocal mutations identified by this approach may not be confirmable by an alternate method such as Sanger sequencing.

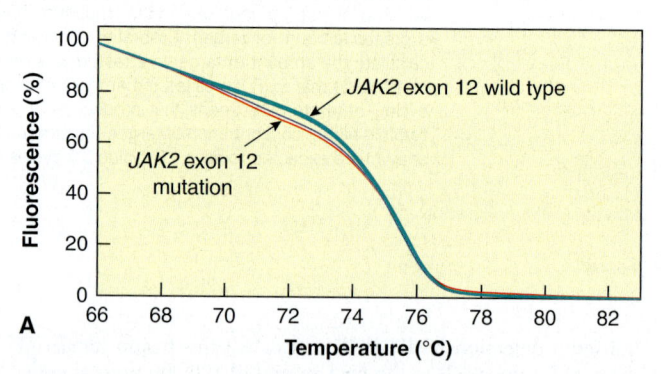

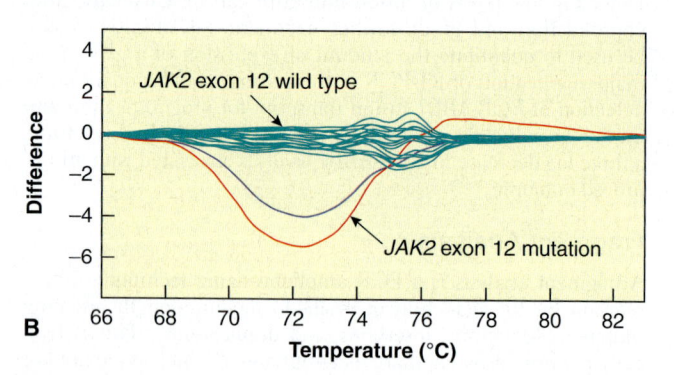

Figure 3.6 High resolution melting (HRM) curve analysis. An HRM analysis can be an efficient screening method for detecting a variety of mutations that may cluster in one or more hotspot regions, such as occurs with *JAK2* exon 12 mutations in polycythemia vera. PCR is utilized to amplify the target region in the presence of a fluorescent double-stranded DNA-binding dye. Following PCR, the product is gradually melted, and the emitted fluorescence is measured. **(A)** Plotting fluorescence versus temperature generates a melt curve characteristic of each amplicon. The presence of a mutation alters the melt profile due to mismatched double-stranded heteroduplexes of mutant and wild-type fragments. **(B)** A difference plot in which sample curves are subtracted from a wild-type control can accentuate the different melt profiles.

for each analysis is visualized adequately to produce unequivocal sequence readout. The sequencing products of increasing size are resolved by capillary electrophoresis, and the DNA sequence is determined by detection of the fluorescently labeled nucleotide sequences.

Sanger sequencing has the ability to detect a wide variety of nucleotide alterations in the DNA, including point mutations, deletions, insertions, and duplications. This technique is especially useful when mutations are scattered across the entire gene, when genes have not been sufficiently studied to determine mutational hot spots, or when it is relevant to determine the exact change in DNA sequence. Sanger sequencing can also provide semiquantitative information about mutation levels in a sample based on the evaluation of average peak drop values from forward and reverse mutant peaks on sequence chromatograms. Limitations of this approach include low throughput and limited diagnostic sensitivity. In general, heterozygous mutations at allelic levels lower than 20% may be difficult to detect by Sanger sequencing. This may be particularly problematic when testing for somatic mutations in oncogenes, such as *JAK2* exon 12 in polycythemia vera, which may occur at low levels.[35]

Examples of Sanger sequencing applications in oncology include the detection of *KIT* mutations for gastrointestinal stromal tumors (GIST) and melanomas that arise from mucosal membranes and acral skin, *EGFR* mutations for non–small-cell lung cancers, and *KRAS* mutations for colorectal and lung carcinomas (Fig. 3.7).

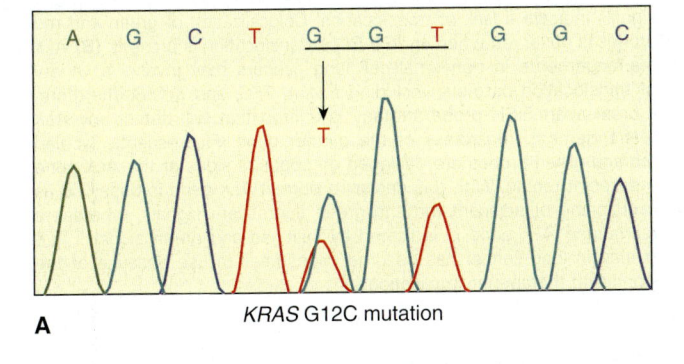

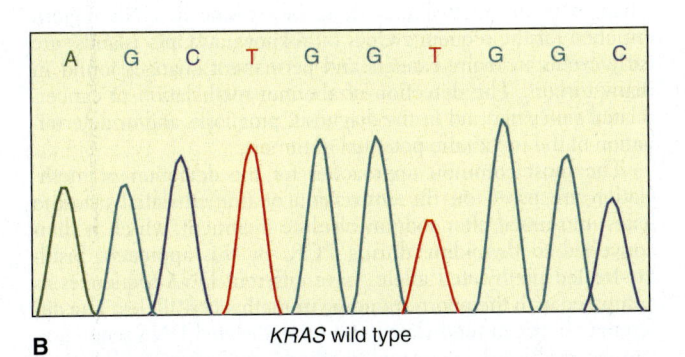

Figure 3.7 Sanger sequencing. *KRAS* mutation testing requires a technology like Sanger sequencing, which can detect the diverse variety of mutations that span multiple nucleotide sites. Overlapping peaks in the DNA sequence chromatogram indicate the presence of a mutation. The top panel **(A)** displays a G to T nucleotide substitution in codon 12. This results in a GGT to TGT codon change, leading to a glycine to cysteine (G12C) amino acid substitution. Activating mutations in *KRAS* such as G12C are associated with resistance to epidermal growth factor receptor (EGFR) targeted therapies in colon cancer. The bottom panel **(B)** displays a wild-type *KRAS* sequence.

Pyrosequencing

Pyrosequencing, also known as *sequencing by synthesis*, is based on the real-time detection of pyrophosphate release by nucleotide incorporation during DNA synthesis.[42] In the pyrosequencing reaction, as nucleotides are added to the nucleic acid chain by polymerase, pyrophosphate molecules are released and subsequently converted to ATP by ATP sulfurylase. Light is produced by an ATP-driven luciferase reaction via oxidation of a luciferin molecule. The amount of light produced is proportional to the number of incorporated nucleotides in the sequence. When a nucleotide is not incorporated into the reaction, no pyrophosphate is released and the unused nucleotide is degraded by apyrase. Light is converted into peaks in a charge-coupled device (CCD) camera. Individual dNTP nucleotides are sequentially added to the reaction, and the sequence of nucleotides that produce chemiluminescent signals allow the template sequence to be determined. Mutations appear as new peaks in the pyrogram sequence or variations of the expected peak heights.[43]

Pyrosequencing is particularly useful for the detection of point mutations and insertion/deletion mutations that occur at short stretches in mutational hotspots. This method has higher analytical sensitivity than Sanger sequencing and can provide quantitative information about mutation levels in a sample. Pyrosequencing can also be used for the detection and quantification of gene-specific DNA methylation and gene copy number assessments. A microfluidic pyrosequencing platform is available for massive parallel sequencing. However, this method is not well suited for detecting mutations that are scattered across the entire gene because pyrosequencing read lengths are limited to ~100 to 250 base pairs.[43]

Examples of pyrosequencing applications in oncology include the mutational analysis of *BRAF* (codon 600),[44,45] *KRAS* (codons 12, 13, 61),[45] *NRAS* (codon 61),[45] and the methylation analysis of *MGMT* in glioblastoma multiforme.[46,47]

Single Nucleotide Extension Assay (SNaPshot®)

The single nucleotide extension assay is a variant of dideoxy sequencing. This method consists of a single base extension of an unlabeled primer that anneals one base upstream to the relevant mutation with fluorophore-labeled dideoxynucleotides (ddNTP). Multiplexed reactions can be designed with multiple primers of differing lengths for simultaneous amplification of multiple genomic targets.[48] Mutations are identified based on amplicon size and fluorophore color via capillary electrophoresis. When a mutation is present, an alternative dideoxynucleotide triphosphate is incorporated, resulting in a different colored peak with a different amplicon length than the expected wild-type one.

The single nucleotide extension assay is particularly useful for the simultaneous detection of recurrent point mutations. Clinically, it has been employed for analyses of mutational hotspots in multiple genes involved in melanomas, non–small-cell lung cancers, breast cancers, and metastatic colorectal cancers.[49] The assay has higher analytical sensitivity than Sanger sequencing and can detect low-level mutations in FFPE-derived DNA, making it advantageous for biopsy specimens with limited tumor involvement. This assay, however, can only detect mutations that are immediately adjacent to the 3′ to the end of the primer.

Fluorescence In Situ Hybridization

FISH allows for the visualization of specific chromosome nucleic acid sequences within a cellular preparation. This method involves the annealing of a large single-stranded fluorophore-labeled oligonucleotide probe to complementary DNA target sequences within a tissue or cell preparation. The hybridization of the probe at the specific DNA region within a nucleus is visible by direct detection using fluorescence microscopy.

FISH can be used for the quantitative assessment of gene amplification or deletion and for the qualitative evaluation of gene rearrangements. Many oncologic FISH assays employ two probe types: *locus specific probes*, which are complementary to the gene of interest, and *centromeric probes*, which hybridize to the alpha-satellite regions near the centromere of a specific chromosome and help in the enumeration of the number of copies of that chromosome.

For the quantitative assessment of gene amplification, a locus-specific probe and a centromeric probe are labeled with two different fluorophores. The signals generated by each of these probes are counted and a ratio of the targeted gene to the chromosome copy number is calculated. The amount of signal produced by the locus-specific probe is proportional to the number of copies of the targeted gene in a cell. This type of gene amplification assay can be used for the detection of *HER2* gene amplification as an adjunct to existing clinical and pathologic information as an aid in the assessment of stage II, node-positive breast cancer patients for whom Herceptin treatment is being considered. It can also be used for an assessment of *MYCN* amplification in neuroblastoma.

For the detection of deletion mutations, dual-probe hybridization is usually performed using locus-specific probes. For instance, for the detection of 1p/19q codeletion in oligodendrogliomas, locus-specific probe sets for 1p36 and 19q13, and 1q25 and 19p13 (control) are used. The frequencies of signal patterns for each of these loci are evaluated. A signal pattern with 1p and 19q signals that are less than control signals is consistent with deletion of these loci.

Gene rearrangements/chromosomal translocations in hematologic or solid malignancies can be tested using locus-specific dual-fusion or break-apart probes. Dual-color, dual-fusion translocation assays employ two probes that are located in two separate genes involved in a specific rearrangement. Each gene probe is labeled in a different color. This design detects translocations by the juxtaposition of both probe signals. Dual-color, dual-fusion translocation assays are very specific for detecting a selected translocation. But, it can only be used for detecting translocations that involve consistent partners, where both partners are known. Alternate translocations with different fusion partners are not detected by this approach. Examples of application of dual-fusion probes in oncology include for the detection of the *IGH-BCL2* translocation that occurs in most follicular lymphomas and a subset of diffuse large B-cell lymphomas (Fig. 3.8) and for the detection of *IGH-CCND1* rearrangements in mantle cell lymphomas.

In break-apart FISH assays, both dual-colored probes flank the breakpoint region in a single gene that represents the constant partner in the translocation. By this approach, rearranged alleles show two split signals, whereas normal alleles show fusion signals. This design is particularly useful for genes that fuse with multiple translocation partners (e.g., *EWSR1* gene, which may undergo rearrangement with multiple partner genes, including *FLI1*, *ERG*, *ETV1*, *FEV*, and *E1AF* in Ewing sarcoma/primitive neuroectodermal tumor [PNET]; *WT1* in desmoplastic small round cell tumors; *CHN* in extraskeletal myxoid chondrosarcoma; and *ATF1* in clear cell sarcoma and angiomatoid fibrous histiocytoma).[50] The disadvantage of this approach is that break-apart FISH does not allow for the identification of the "unknown" partner in the translocation.

FISH has the advantage of being applicable to a variety of specimen types, including FFPE tissue. Because probes are hybridized to tissue in situ, the tumor morphology is preserved, which allows for an interpretation of the assay even in the context of heterogeneous samples. However, FISH is a targeted approach that will only detect specific alterations. Because most probes are large (e.g., >100 kb), small deletions or insertions will not be detected. In addition, poor tissue fixation, fixation artifacts, nuclear truncation on tissue slides, and nuclear overlaps are potential pitfalls of this technique that may hamper interpretation. Some intrachromosomal rearrangements (e.g., *RET-PTC* and *EML4-ALK*) may be challenging to interpret by FISH due to subtle rearrangements of the probe signals on the same chromosome arm.

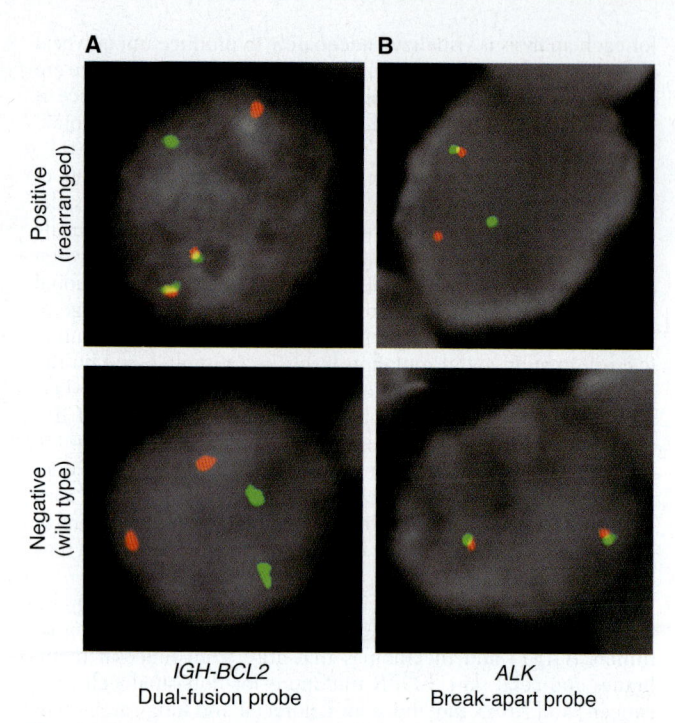

Figure 3.8 Fluorescence in situ hybridization (FISH). **(A)** Recurrent chromosomal translocations such as *IGH-BCL2* (occurring in B-cell lymphomas) can be effectively detected with a dual-fusion probe strategy. This design utilizes a green probe specific to the *IGH* locus and a red probe specific to the *BCL2* gene, with each probe spanning their respective breakpoint region. Individual green and red probe signals indicate a lack of translocation. Colocalization of green and red probes is observed when an *IGH-BCL2* translocation is present. **(B)** *ALK* rearrangements in non–small-cell lung cancers may involve a variety of translocation partners, including *EML4*, *TFG*, and *KIF5B*. Therefore, a break-apart FISH probe strategy is utilized that will detect any *ALK* rearrangement, regardless of the partner gene. Fluorescently labeled red and green probes are designed on opposite sides of the *ALK* gene breakpoint region. With this design, a normal *ALK* gene is observed as overlapping or adjacent red and green fluorescent signals, whereas a rearranged *ALK* gene is indicated by split red and green signals. *ALK* testing in lung cancer has become widespread in use because of the significant therapeutic implications.

Methylation Analysis

Changes in the methylation status of cytosine in DNA regions enriched for the sequence CpG (also known as CpG islands) are early events in many cancers and permanent changes found in many tumors. The detection of aberrant methylation of cancer-related genes may aid in the diagnosis, prognosis, and/or determination of the metastatic potential of tumors.

The most common approaches for the detection of methylation are based on the conversion of unmethylated cytosine bases into uracil after sodium bisulfite treatment, which is then converted to thymidine during PCR. By this approach, bisulfite-treated methylated alleles have different DNA sequences as compared with their corresponding unmethylated alleles. The differences between methylated and unmethylated DNA sequences can be evaluated by several methods, including methylation-sensitive restriction enzyme analysis, methylation-specific PCR, semiquantitative q-PCR, Sanger sequencing, pyrosequencing, and next-generation sequencing.

The methylation status of oncogenic genes can also be assessed by methylation-sensitive multiplex ligation-dependent probe amplification (MS-MLPA) assay.[51,52] MS-MLPA is a variant of multiplex PCR in which oligonucleotide probes hybridized to the targeted DNA samples are directly amplified using one pair of universal primers. This method is not based on bisulfite conversion of unmethylated cytosine bases into uracil. Instead, the target sequences detected by MS-MLPA probes contain a restriction site recognized by methylation-sensitive endonucleases. A probe amplification product will only be obtained if the CpG site is methylated because digested probes cannot be amplified during PCR. The level of methylation is determined by resolving PCR products by capillary electrophoresis and calculating the normalized ratio of each target probe peak area in both digested and undigested specimens. The ratio corresponds to the percentage of methylation present in the specimen.

Examples of applications of methylation analysis in oncology include an analysis of *MLH1* promoter hypermethylation in microsatellite unstable sporadic colorectal carcinomas, an analysis of *MGMT* promoter methylation status in glioblastoma multiforme patients treated with alkylating chemotherapy, and *SEPT9* promoter methylation in DNA derived from blood plasma in colorectal cancer patients.[53]

Microsatellite Instability Analysis

Microsatellites are short, tandem-repeated DNA sequences with repeating units of one to six base pairs in length. Microsatellites are distributed throughout the human genome, and individual repeat loci often vary in length from one individual to another. Microsatellite instability (MSI) is the change in length of a microsatellite allele due to either insertion or deletion of repeating units and a failure of the DNA mismatch repair (MMR) system to repair these replication errors. This genomic instability arises in a variety of human neoplasms where tumor cells have a decreased ability to faithfully replicate DNA. MSI is particularly associated with colorectal cancer, where 15% to 20% of sporadic tumors show MSI, in contrast to the more common chromosomal instability (CIN) phenotype, with MSI status being an independent prognostic indicator. MSI analysis is also clinically useful in identifying patients at increased risk of hereditary nonpolyposis colorectal cancer (HNPCC)/Lynch syndrome, where a germline mutation of an MMR gene causes a familial predisposition to colorectal cancer. MSI analysis alone is not sufficient to make a diagnosis of a germline MMR mutation given the high rate of sporadic MSI-positive colorectal tumors, but a positive result is an indication for follow-up genetic testing and counseling.

In an MSI analysis, DNA is extracted from tumor tissue and the corresponding adjacent normal mucosa. The DNA is subjected to multiplex PCR using fluorescent-labeled primers for coamplification of five mononucleotide repeat markers for MSI determination and two pentanucleotide markers for confirming tumor/normal sample identity. The resulting PCR fragments are separated and detected using capillary electrophoresis. Allelic profiles of normal versus tumor tissues are compared, and MSI is scored as the presence of novel microsatellite lengths in tumor DNA compared to normal DNA. Instability in two or more out of five mononucleotide microsatellite markers in tumor DNA compared to normal DNA is defined as MSI-H (high). MSI-L (low) is defined as instability in one out of five mononucleotide markers in tumor DNA compared to normal DNA. Tumors with no instability (zero out of five altered mononucleotide markers) are defined as microsatellite stable (MSS).[54,55]

Loss of Heterozygosity Analysis

Loss of heterozygosity (LOH) is a common event in cancer that usually occurs due to deletion of a chromosome segment and results in a loss of one copy of an allele. LOH is a common occurrence in tumor suppressor genes and may contribute to tumorigenesis when the second allele is subsequently inactivated by a second "hit" due to mutation or deletion.

LOH studies are used to identify genomic imbalance in tumors, indicating possible sites of tumor suppressor gene (TSG) deletion. LOH studies can be done by multiplex PCR analysis of microsatellites (short tandem repeats [STRs]), FISH, and genomic microarrays). By PCR, microsatellites located in the vicinity of a tumor suppressor gene are used as surrogate markers for the presence of the gene of interest. DNA is extracted from tumor tissue and corresponding adjacent normal mucosa. The DNA is subjected to multiplex PCR using fluorescent-labeled STR primers. Peak height ratio of informative (nonhomozygous) alleles at each locus is calculated from both normal and tumor tissues. LOH is defined as the decrease in peak height of one of the two alleles, relative to the allele peak heights of the normal sample.

An example of applications of LOH studies in oncology include an analysis of 1p/19q loss in oligodendrogliomas, and an analysis of 1p loss in parathyroid carcinomas.

Whole Genome Analysis Methods

Next-Generation Sequencing

Next-generation sequencing (NGS), also known as massive parallel sequencing or deep sequencing, is an emerging technology that has revolutionized the speed, throughput, and cost of sequencing and has facilitated the discovery of clinically relevant genetic biomarkers for diagnosis, prognosis, and personalized therapeutics. By way of this technology, multiple genes or the entire exome or genome can be interrogated simultaneously in multiple parallel reactions instead of a single-gene basis as in Sanger sequencing or pyrosequencing. Currently, the most common NGS approach for cancer testing in the clinical setting employs targeted sequencing of specific genes and mutation hotspot regions. This targeted approach increases sensitivity for the detection of low-level mutations by increasing the depth of sequence coverage.

Presently, there are numerous NGS platforms that employ different sequencing technologies. A comprehensive review and comparison of NGS platforms is beyond the scope of this chapter and has been reviewed elsewhere.[56,57] A generalized clinical workflow is shown (Fig. 3.9). Frequently, multiple DNA samples are individually barcoded and pooled together to leverage platform throughput. Pooled libraries are prepared and enriched, and single DNA molecules are arrayed in solid surfaces, glass slides, or beads and sequenced in situ using reversible DNA chain terminators or iterative cycles of oligonucleotide ligation. NGS signal outputs are based on luminescence, fluorescence, or changes in ion concentration. Robust bioinformatics pipelines are required for an alignment of reads to a reference genome sequence, variant calling, variant annotation, and to assist with result reporting.[58]

NGS can be used for the detection of single nucleotide variants, small insertions and deletions, translocations, inversions, alternative splicing, and copy number variations given sufficient depth of genomic DNA sequence (Fig. 3.10). Technical limitations of this technique include difficulty in sequencing guanine-cytosine (GC)–rich genomic regions, and erroneous sequencing of homologous DNA regions (e.g., pseudogenes) that may confound interpretation.

Examples of applications of NGS in oncology include small targeted panels (3 to 50 genes) for non–small-cell lung cancers, melanomas, colon cancers, and acute myeloid leukemias.[57,59–62] Larger panels (50 to 500 genes) are increasingly being utilized, particularly in both clinical trials and research.

Massively parallel sequencing of RNA (RNA-Seq) can be used for determining sequence variants, alternative splicing, gene rearrangements, and allelic expression of mutant transcripts. To date, this technique has been used primarily for discovery rather than clinical applications, but it is likely to play an increasing role in clinical diagnostics as the technology improves. For transcriptome sequencing, the RNA must first be converted to cDNA, which is then fragmented and entered into library construction. After sequencing, reads are aligned to a reference genome, compared with known transcript sequences, or assembled de novo

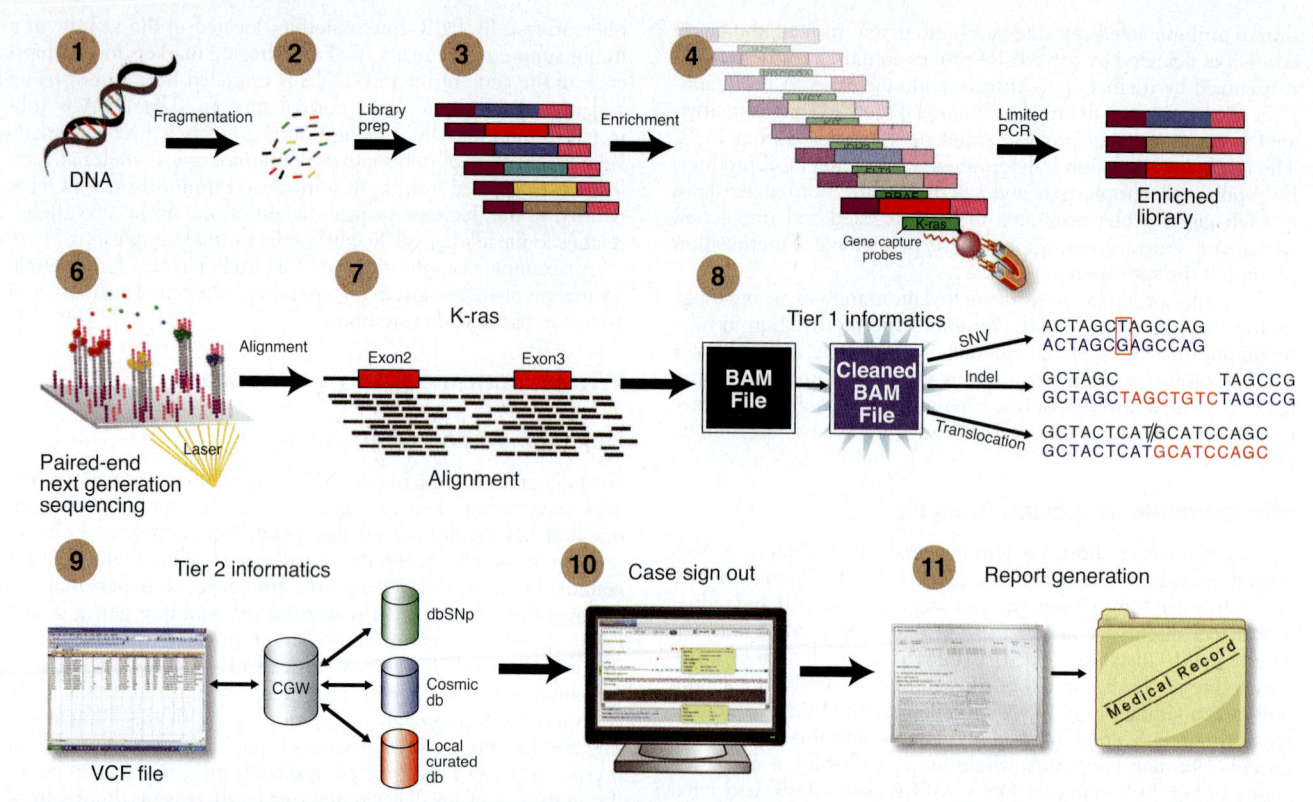

Figure 3.9 Next-generation sequencing (NGS) workflow in a clinical laboratory. Targeted-panel sequencing offers tremendous promise for cancer diagnostics due to the massive improvement in throughput, speed, and cost. NGS is a complex, multiday process that requires significant infrastructure and expertise to deploy in a clinical setting. The process begins with genomic DNA extraction, which is fragmented and to which linkers are ligated. In this targeted gene panel–based example, the sequencing libraries are enriched for the target genes, which are subjected to a limited PCR prior to sequencing. Sequence reads are mapped to a reference genome and subjected to several bioinformatics tools to provide variant calling results and variant annotation. Clinical interpretation and case sign out is performed by a physician with expertise in molecular pathology. BAM, Binary Sequence Alignment/Map; SNV, Single Nucleotide Variant; VCF, Variant Call Format; CGW, Clinical Genomicist Workstation; dbSNP, The Single Nucleotide Polymorphism Database. (Used with permission from Shashikant Kulkarni PhD and Eric Duncavage MD.)

to construct a genome-scale transcription map. Expression levels are determined from the total number of sequence reads that map to the exons of a particular gene, normalized by the length of exons that can be uniquely mapped.[56] Compared with genomic microarrays, RNA-Seq has a greater ability to distinguish RNA isoforms, determine allelic expression, and reveal sequence variants.

Chromatin immunoprecipitation with sequencing (ChIP-Seq) can be used to determine the genome-wide location of chromatin-binding transcription factors or specific epigenetic modifications of histones. This has proved to be a very powerful research tool, which to date has not been used for clinical diagnostics. Proteins in contact with genomic DNA are chemically cross-linked (usually with formaldehyde treatment) to their binding sites, the DNA is fragmented, and the proteins cross-linked with DNA are then immunoprecipitated with antibodies specific for the proteins (or specific epigenetic histone modification) of interest. The DNA harvested from the immunoprecipitate is converted into a library for NGS. The obtained reads are mapped to the reference genome of interest to generate a genome-wide protein binding map.[63,64] ChIP-Seq is rapidly replacing chromatin immunoprecipitation and microarray hybridization (ChIP-on-chip) technology[65] because of its higher sensitivity and resolution.[66]

Genomic Microarrays

High-density genomic microarrays are widely used for whole genome assessment of copy number changes, LOH, and genotyping. In array comparative genomic hybridization (aCGH), cloned genomic probes are arrayed onto glass slides and serves as targets for the competitive hybridization of normal and tumor DNA. In the aCGH reaction, tumor DNA and DNA from a normal control sample are labeled with different fluorophores. These samples are denatured and hybridized together to the arrayed single-strand probes. Digital imaging systems are used to quantify the relative fluorescence intensities of the labeled DNA probes that have hybridized to each target probe. The fluorescence ratio of the tumor and control hybridization signals is determined at different positions along the genome, which provides information on the relative copy number of sequences in the tumor genome as compared to the normal genome.[67] This method is able to detect copy number variation, such as deletions, duplications, and gene amplification, but it cannot detect polymorphic allele changes.

An SNP array has the ability to detect LOH profiles in addition to high-resolution detection of copy number aberrations, such as amplifications and deletions. This method employs thousands of unique fluorescent-labeled nucleotide probe sequences arrayed on a chip to which a fragmented single-stranded specimen DNA binds to their complementary partners. Each SNP site is interrogated by complementary sets of probes containing perfect matches and mismatches to each SNP site. Each probe is associated with one of the two alleles of an SNP (also known as A and B). Relative fluorescence intensity depends on both the amount of target DNA in the sample, as well as the affinity between target and probe. An analysis of the raw fluorescence intensity is done by computational algorithms that convert the set of probe intensities into genotypes. Deleted genomic regions are identified as having an LOH associated with copy number reduction. A copy-neutral LOH is detected when SNPs expected to be heterozygous in the normal sample are detected as homozygous in the tumor sample without copy number variation. A copy neutral LOH may arise from somatic homologous recombination of a mutated tumor suppressor allele and its surrounding DNA that replaces the other allele (uniparental disomy [UPD]). SNP microarrays are the only genomic microarrays that are able to identify UPD. Array technologies cannot detect true balanced chromosome abnormalities and low-level mosaicism.

Examples of genomic microarrays applications in oncology include the detection of copy number variations and LOH in chronic lymphocytic leukemia[68] and recurrent cytogenetic abnormalities in MDS (e.g., 5q-, -7 or 7q-, +8, 20q-).[69]

Expression Panels

Gene expression signatures of multiple cancer biomarkers are starting to be incorporated into clinical practice as an adjunct to clinical and pathologic information in diverse cancer management settings. An example of a multigene expression–based test in current use includes Oncotype DX, which is a quantitative RT-PCR–based assay that measures the expression of 21 genes in FFPE breast tumors. The test is designed to predict the potential benefit of chemotherapy and the likelihood of distant breast cancer recurrence in women with node negative or node positive, estrogen receptor (ER)-positive, and HER2-negative invasive breast cancer. This test has been in-corporated into current American Society of Clinical Oncology (ASCO) and National Comprehensive Cancer Network (NCCN) for breast cancer management.[70] Prospective trials are in progress to evaluate other multigene tests for early stage breast cancer.

With the rapid advances in molecular diagnostic technologies, it is likely that many mutation- and expression-based panels analyzing hundreds if not thousands of genes, or even the complete genome or transcriptome, will enter widespread use. Some of the many challenges to address will be to provide evidence-based, actionable reports that guide the oncologist to more effective therapies, to learn from the results of such testing to improve the algorithms guiding therapy, to handle the incidental findings in such testing in an ethically responsible way, and ultimately, with the drugs available, to provide sufficient improvements in outcomes so that society will be willing to bear the costs.

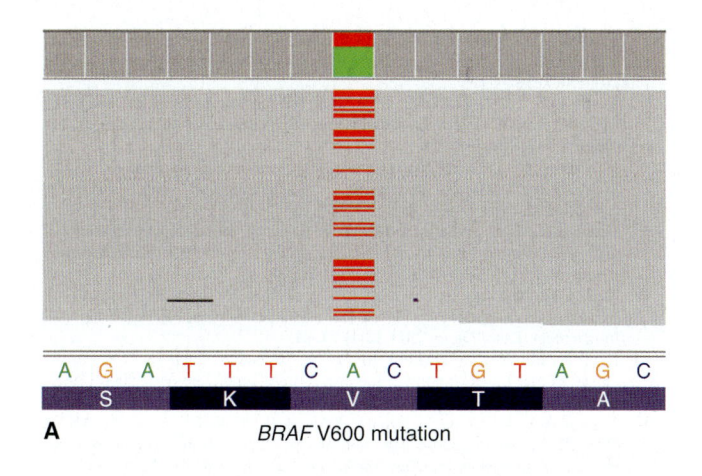

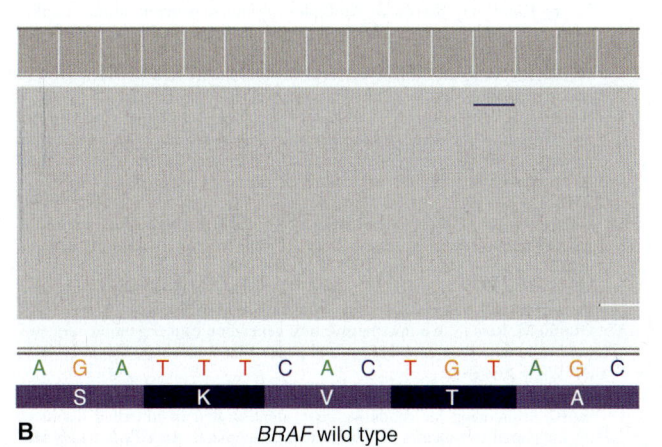

Figure 3.10 Next-generation sequencing (NGS). Hundreds to thousands of sequence reads are mapped and horizontally aligned to specific targeted regions in the reference genome (sequence shown on *bottom* of each panel). A software-assisted analysis assists in the detection of mutations, displayed as colored bars in each read above the mutation site. A wild-type sequence within each read is displayed in *gray*. Mutation frequency correlates to the number of times the mutant sequence is detected compared to the total number of reads at that nucleotide position. Shown are sequencing results from BRAF V600E mutation positive **(A)** and negative **(B)** melanomas. The A to T base substitution that leads to the V600E mutation is displayed in red. Patients with metastatic melanoma that harbors the BRAF V600E mutation are candidates for targeted therapy.

REFERENCES

1. Lennard L, Cartwright CS, Wade R, et al. Thiopurine methyltransferase genotype-phenotype discordance and thiopurine active metabolite formation in childhood acute lymphoblastic leukaemia. *Br J Clin Pharmacol* 2013;76(1):125–136.
2. Haber DA, Settleman J. Cancer: drivers and passengers. *Nature* 2007; 446(7132):145–146.
3. Hayashi T, Sudo J. Relieving effect of saline on cephaloridine nephrotoxicity in rats. *Chem Pharm Bull (Tokyo)* 1989;37(3):785–790.
4. Brodeur GM, Seeger RC, Schwab M, et al. Amplification of N-myc in untreated human neuroblastomas correlates with advanced disease stage. *Science* 1984;224(4653):1121–1124.
5. Seeger RC, Brodeur GM, Sather H, et al. Association of multiple copies of the N-myc oncogene with rapid progression of neuroblastomas. *N Engl J Med* 1985;313(18):1111–1116.
6. Weinstein JL, Katzenstein HM, Cohn SL. Advances in the diagnosis and treatment of neuroblastoma. *Oncologist* 2003;8(3):278–292.
7. Pui CH, Crist WM, Look AT. Biology and clinical significance of cytogenetic abnormalities in childhood acute lymphoblastic leukemia. *Blood* 1990;76(8):1449–1463.
8. Lee JA, Lupski JR. Genomic rearrangements and gene copy-number alterations as a cause of nervous system disorders. *Neuron* 2006;52(1):103–121.
9. Kuiper RP, Ligtenberg MJ, Hoogerbrugge N, et al. Germline copy number variation and cancer risk. *Curr Opin Genet Dev* 2010;20(3):282–289.
10. Shlien A, Malkin D. Copy number variations and cancer. *Genome Med* 2009;1(6):62.
11. Lynch TJ, Bell DW, Sordella R, et al. Activating mutations in the epidermal growth factor receptor underlying responsiveness of non–small-cell lung cancer to gefitinib. *N Engl J Med* 2004;350(21):2129–2139.
12. Paez JG, Janne PA, Lee JC, et al. EGFR mutations in lung cancer: correlation with clinical response to gefitinib therapy. *Science* 2004;304(5676): 1497–1500.
13. Forbes SA, Bindal N, Bamford S, et al. COSMIC: mining complete cancer genomes in the Catalogue of Somatic Mutations in Cancer. *Nucleic Acids Res* 2011;39(Database issue):D945–950.
14. Van Allen EM, Wagle N, Levy MA. Clinical analysis and interpretation of cancer genome data. *J Clin Oncol* 2013;31(15):1825–1833.
15. Newman B, Mu H, Butler LM, et al. Frequency of breast cancer attributable to BRCA1 in a population-based series of American women. *JAMA* 1998;279(12):915–921.
16. Ford D, Easton DF, Stratton M, et al. Genetic heterogeneity and penetrance analysis of the BRCA1 and BRCA2 genes in breast cancer families. The Breast Cancer Linkage Consortium. *Am J Hum Genet* 1998;62(3): 676–689.
17. Antoniou A, Pharoah PD, Narod S, et al. Average risks of breast and ovarian cancer associated with BRCA1 or BRCA2 mutations detected in case series unselected for family history: a combined analysis of 22 studies. *Am J Hum Genet* 2003;72(5):1117–1130.
18. Chen S, Iversen ES, Friebel T, et al. Characterization of BRCA1 and BRCA2 mutations in a large United States sample. *J Clin Oncol* 2006;24(6):863–871.

19. Bachner P, Hamlin W. Federal regulation of clinical laboratories and the Clinical Laboratory Improvement Amendments of 1988—Part II. *Clin Lab Med* 1993;13(4):987–994.
20. Halling KC, Schrijver I, Persons DL. Test verification and validation for molecular diagnostic assays. *Arch Pathol Lab Med* 2012;136(1):11–13.
21. Jennings L, Van Deerlin VM, Gulley ML, College of American Pathologists Molecular Pathology Resource C. Recommended principles and practices for validating clinical molecular pathology tests. *Arch Pathol Lab Med* 2009;133(5):743–755.
22. Jennings LJ, Smith FA, Halling KC, et al. Design and analytic validation of BCR-ABL1 quantitative reverse transcription polymerase chain reaction assay for monitoring minimal residual disease. *Arch Pathol Lab Med* 2012;136(1):33–40.
23. Pont-Kingdon G, Gedge F, Wooderchak-Donahue W, et al. Design and analytical validation of clinical DNA sequencing assays. *Arch Pathol Lab Med* 2012;136(1):41–46.
24. Saiki RK, Gelfand DH, Stoffel S, et al. Primer-directed enzymatic amplification of DNA with a thermostable DNA polymerase. *Science* 1988;239(4839):487–491.
25. Mullis KB. The unusual origin of the polymerase chain reaction. *Sci Am* 1990;262(4):56–61, 64–65.
26. Bernard PS, Wittwer CT. Real-time PCR technology for cancer diagnostics. *Clin Chem* 2002;48(8):1178–1185.
27. Bench AJ, Baxter EJ, Green AR. Methods for detecting mutations in the human JAK2 gene. *Methods Mol Biol* 2013;967:115–131.
28. Halait H, Demartin K, Shah S, et al. Analytical performance of a real-time PCR-based assay for V600 mutations in the BRAF gene, used as the companion diagnostic test for the novel BRAF inhibitor vemurafenib in metastatic melanoma. *Diagn Mol Pathol* 2012;21(1):1–8.
29. Furtado LV, Weigelin HC, Elenitoba-Johnson KS, et al. Detection of MPL mutations by a novel allele-specific PCR-based strategy. *J Mol Diagn* 2013;15(6):810–818.
30. Lang AH, Drexel H, Geller-Rhomberg S, et al. Optimized allele-specific real-time PCR assays for the detection of common mutations in KRAS and BRAF. *J Mol Diagn* 2011;13(1):23–28.
31. Wang ZY, Chen Z. Acute promyelocytic leukemia: from highly fatal to highly curable. *Blood* 2008;111(5):2505–2515.
32. O'Brien SG, Guilhot F, Larson RA, et al. Imatinib compared with interferon and low-dose cytarabine for newly diagnosed chronic-phase chronic myeloid leukemia. *N Engl J Med* 2003;348(11):994–1004.
33. Hughes TP, Kaeda J, Branford S, et al. Frequency of major molecular responses to imatinib or interferon alfa plus cytarabine in newly diagnosed chronic myeloid leukemia. *N Engl J Med* 2003;349(15):1423–1432.
34. Szankasi P, Jama M, Bahler DW. A new DNA-based test for detection of nucleophosmin exon 12 mutations by capillary electrophoresis. *J Mol Diagn* 2008;10(3):236–241.
35. Furtado LV, Weigelin HC, Elenitoba-Johnson KS, et al. A multiplexed fragment analysis-based assay for detection of JAK2 exon 12 mutations. *J Mol Diagn* 2013;15(5):592–599.
36. Reed GH, Kent JO, Wittwer CT. High-resolution DNA melting analysis for simple and efficient molecular diagnostics. *Pharmacogenomics* 2007;8(6):597–608.
37. Palais RA, Liew MA, Wittwer CT. Quantitative heteroduplex analysis for single nucleotide polymorphism genotyping. *Anal Biochem* 2005;346(1):167–175.
38. Carillo S, Henry L, Lippert E, et al. Nested high-resolution melting curve analysis is a highly sensitive, reliable, and simple method for detection of JAK2 exon 12 mutations—clinical relevance in the monitoring of polycythemia. *J Mol Diagn* 2011;13(3):263–270.
39. Ney JT, Froehner S, Roesler A, et al. High-resolution melting analysis as a sensitive prescreening diagnostic tool to detect KRAS, BRAF, PIK3CA, and AKT1 mutations in formalin-fixed, paraffin-embedded tissues. *Arch Pathol Lab Med* 2012;136(9):983–992.
40. Jones AV, Cross NC, White HE, et al. Rapid identification of JAK2 exon 12 mutations using high resolution melting analysis. *Haematologica* Oct 2008;93(10):1560–1564.
41. Sanger F, Nicklen S, Coulson AR. DNA sequencing with chain-terminating inhibitors. *Proc Natl Acad Sci U S A* 1977;74(12):5463–5467.
42. Ronaghi M, Uhlén M, Nyrén P. A sequencing method based on real-time pyrophosphate. *Science* 1998;281(5375):363, 365.
43. Ronaghi M, Shokralla S, Gharizadeh B. Pyrosequencing for discovery and analysis of DNA sequence variations. *Pharmacogenomics* 2007;8(10):1437–1441.
44. Shigaki H, Baba Y, Watanabe M, et al. KRAS and BRAF mutations in 203 esophageal squamous cell carcinomas: pyrosequencing technology and literature review. *Ann Surg Oncol* 2013;20:485–491.
45. Vaughn CP, Zobell SD, Furtado LV, et al. Frequency of KRAS, BRAF, and NRAS mutations in colorectal cancer. *Genes Chromosomes Cancer* 2011;50(5):307–312.
46. Everhard S, Tost J, El Abdalaoui H, et al. Identification of regions correlating MGMT promoter methylation and gene expression in glioblastomas. *Neuro Oncol* 2009;11(4):348–356.
47. Mikeska T, Bock C, El-Maarri O, et al. Optimization of quantitative MGMT promoter methylation analysis using pyrosequencing and combined bisulfite restriction analysis. *J Mol Diagn* 2007;9(3):368–381.
48. Dias-Santagata D, Akhavanfard S, David SS, et al. Rapid targeted mutational analysis of human tumours: a clinical platform to guide personalized cancer medicine. *EMBO Mol Med* 2010;2(5):146–158.
49. Su Z, Dias-Santagata D, Duke M, et al. A platform for rapid detection of multiple oncogenic mutations with relevance to targeted therapy in non–small-cell lung cancer. *J Mol Diagn* 2011;13(1):74–84.
50. Lazar A, Abruzzo LV, Pollock RE, et al. Molecular diagnosis of sarcomas: chromosomal translocations in sarcomas. *Arch Pathol Lab Med* 2006;130(8):1199–1207.
51. Nygren AO, Ameziane N, Duarte HM, et al. Methylation-specific MLPA (MS-MLPA): simultaneous detection of CpG methylation and copy number changes of up to 40 sequences. *Nucleic Acids Res* 2005;33(14):e128.
52. Hömig-Hölzel C, Savola S. Multiplex ligation-dependent probe amplification (MLPA) in tumor diagnostics and prognostics. *Diagn Mol Pathol* 2012;21(4):189–206.
53. Warren JD, Xiong W, Bunker AM, et al. Septin 9 methylated DNA is a sensitive and specific blood test for colorectal cancer. *BMC Med* 2011;9:133.
54. Boland CR, Thibodeau SN, Hamilton SR, et al. A National Cancer Institute Workshop on Microsatellite Instability for cancer detection and familial predisposition: development of international criteria for the determination of microsatellite instability in colorectal cancer. *Cancer Res* 1998;58(22):5248–5257.
55. Umar A, Boland CR, Terdiman JP, et al. Revised Bethesda Guidelines for hereditary nonpolyposis colorectal cancer (Lynch syndrome) and microsatellite instability. *J Natl Cancer Inst* 2004;96(4):261–268.
56. Voelkerding KV, Dames SA, Durtschi JD. Next-generation sequencing: from basic research to diagnostics. *Clin Chem* 2009;55(4):641–658.
57. Cronin M, Ross JS. Comprehensive next-generation cancer genome sequencing in the era of targeted therapy and personalized oncology. *Biomarker Med* 2011;5(3):293–305.
58. Coonrod EM, Durtschi JD, Margraf RL, et al. Developing genome and exome sequencing for candidate gene identification in inherited disorders: an integrated technical and bioinformatics approach. *Arch Pathol Lab Med* 2013;137(3):415–433.
59. Grossmann V, Kohlmann A, Klein HU, et al. Targeted next-generation sequencing detects point mutations, insertions, deletions and balanced chromosomal rearrangements as well as identifies novel leukemia-specific fusion genes in a single procedure. *Leukemia* 2011;25(4):671–680.
60. Marchetti A, Del Grammastro M, Filice G, et al. Complex mutations & subpopulations of deletions at exon 19 of EGFR in NSCLC revealed by next generation sequencing: potential clinical implications. *PLoS One* 2012;7(7):e42164.
61. McCourt CM, McArt DG, Mills K, et al. Validation of next generation sequencing technologies in comparison to current diagnostic gold standards for BRAF, EGFR and KRAS mutational analysis. *PLoS One* 2013;8(7):e69604.
62. Thol F, Kölking B, Damm F, et al. Next-generation sequencing for minimal residual disease monitoring in acute myeloid leukemia patients with FLT3-ITD or NPM1 mutations. *Genes Chromosomes Cancer* 2012;51(7):689–695.
63. Barski A, Cuddapah S, Cui K, et al. High-resolution profiling of histone methylations in the human genome. *Cell* 2007;129(4):823–837.
64. Schones DE, Zhao K. Genome-wide approaches to studying chromatin modifications. *Nat Rev Genet* 2008;9(3):179–191.
65. Ren B, Robert F, Wyrick JJ, et al. Genome-wide location and function of DNA binding proteins. *Science* 2000;290(5500):2306–2309.
66. Robertson G, Hirst M, Bainbridge M, et al. Genome-wide profiles of STAT1 DNA association using chromatin immunoprecipitation and massively parallel sequencing. *Nat Methods* 2007;4(8):651–657.
67. Shinawi M, Cheung SW. The array CGH and its clinical applications. *Drug Discov Today* 2008;13(17–18):760–770.
68. Iacobucci I, Lonetti A, Papayannidis C, Martinelli G. Use of single nucleotide polymorphism array technology to improve the identification of chromosomal lesions in leukemia. *Curr Cancer Drug Targets* 2013;13(7):791–810.
69. Ahmad A, Iqbal MA. Significance of genome-wide analysis of copy number alterations and UPD in myelodysplastic syndromes using combined CGH - SNP arrays. *Curr Med Chem* 2012;19(22):3739–3747.
70. Goncalves R, Bose R. Using multigene tests to select treatment for early-stage breast cancer. *J Natl Compr Canc Netw* 2013;11(2):174–182.

PART II

Etiology and Epidemiology of Cancer

Section 1 Etiology of Cancer

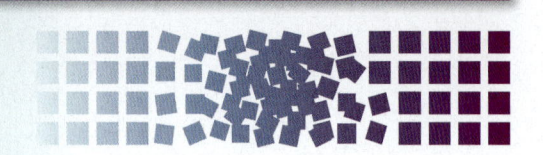

4 Tobacco

Richard J. O'Connor

INTRODUCTION

Regrettably, tobacco use remains one of the leading causes of death worldwide. It is projected to leave over 1 billion dead in the 21st century, after killing nearly 100 million during the course of the 20th century.[1] Data from the Global Adult Tobacco Survey (GATS), which conducted representative household surveys in 14 low- and middle-income countries (Bangladesh, Brazil, China, Egypt, India, Mexico, Philippines, Poland, Russia, Thailand, Turkey, Ukraine, Uruguay, and Vietnam), suggest 41% of men and 5% of women across these countries currently smoke.[2] Compare this to approximately 24% of men and 16% of women in the United States.[3] A preponderance of the death and disease associated with tobacco use is associated with its combusted forms, particularly the cigarette. However, all forms of tobacco use have negative health consequences, the severity of which can vary among products. From the introduction of the mass-manufactured, mass-marketed cigarette (e.g., Camel in 1913), smoking rates grew, first among men then among women, and peaked in Western countries in the 1960s to 1970s, before beginning a steady decline.[4] The smoking rate among US adults has dropped from its peak in 1965 of 42% to 19% in 2011.[3] Per capita consumption has been dropping almost continuously since the 1960s, although the rate of decline has slowed since the early 2000s.[5] Among youth, smoking rates have been in decline since the 1990s,[6,7] although there is some evidence of growth in use of other forms of tobacco (e.g., cigars, water pipes, electronic cigarettes) in 2011 to 2012 that may be displacing cigarette use.[8]

Tobacco control policy interventions can impact both smoking prevalence and lung cancer incidence.[9] For example, a recent analysis suggests that implementation of graphic health warnings in Canada in 1999 resulted in a significant reduction (up to 4.5 percentage points) in smoking prevalence over a decade.[10] Increases in tobacco taxes have long been shown to reduce youth smoking initiation and to prompt more attempts to quit smoking.[11] Evidence from state comparisons in the United States suggests that comprehensive tobacco control measures effectively implemented (such as in California and Massachusetts) can reduce lung cancer incidence.[12] Indeed, Holford and colleagues[13] have shown that since the seminal 1964 Report of the Surgeon General, an estimated 157 million years of life (approximately 20 years per person) have been saved by tobacco control activities in the United States over 50 years. That is, tobacco control activities are estimated to have averted 8 million premature deaths and extended mean life span by 19 to 20 years.[13] However, the marketing of cigarettes has since shifted focus to the developing world, where smoking rates are on the increase. In an attempt to head off an epidemic of smoking and associated diseases, the World Health Organization initiated a public health treaty, the Framework Convention on Tobacco Control (FCTC), to coordinate international efforts to reduce tobacco use.[14] The FCTC binds parties to enact measures to control the labeling and marketing of tobacco products, create a framework for testing and regulating product contents and emissions, combat smuggling and counterfeiting, and protect nonsmokers from secondhand smoke.[15] To date, the FCTC has been ratified by more than 150 countries. The FCTC provides governments the opportunity to regulate the marketing, labeling, and contents/emissions of tobacco products, as well as control the global trade in tobacco products. In the United States, which is currently not a party to FCTC, the U.S. Food and Drug Administration (FDA) has, since 2009, had authority to regulate tobacco products and their marketing along similar lines.[16]

EPIDEMIOLOGY OF TOBACCO AND CANCER

Linkages between tobacco use and cancers at various sites had been noted for several decades. In the late 1800s, it was believed that excessive cigar use created irritation that led to oral cancers.[17] In the 1930s, German scientists began to establish links between cigarette smoking and lung cancers.[18] However, it was not until the Doll and Hill[19] and Wynder and Graham[20] studies were published that the association was demonstrated in large samples and well-designed studies. Table 4.1 lists the cancers currently recognized by the U.S. Surgeon General as caused by smoking, along with their corresponding estimated mortality statistics.[21–23] Of these, the most well-publicized link is between smoking and lung cancer. In a recent examination of National Health and Nutrition Examination Survey (NHANES) data, Jha[24] showed a hazard ratio for lung cancer in smokers versus nonsmokers of 17.8 in women and 14.6 in men. However, smoking contributes substantially to overall cancer burden across multiple sites, including the oropharynx, cervix, and pancreas. Hazard ratios of 1.7 for women and 2.2 for men are seen for cancers other than in the lung in smokers versus nonsmokers.[24] Emerging evidence also links smoking with breast cancer, although the data are as yet insufficient to make causal conclusions.[23,25] Cancer risks associated with smoking, as well as outcomes and survival, depend on a number of factors. A common index of cancer risk is pack-years, or the number of packs of cigarettes smoked per day multiplied by the number of years smoked in the lifetime. In general, the higher the number of pack-years, the greater the cancer risk. Risks for lung cancer decline with smoking cessation, and the longer a former smoker remains off of cigarettes, the more the risk declines.[26] However, excepting those smokers who quit with relatively few pack years accumulated (typically before age 40), cancer risk rarely approaches that of a never smoker.[24,27]

A recent study using several large cohort studies examined death rates and the relative risks associated with smoking and smoking cessation for 3 epochs (1959 to 1965, 1982 to 1988, and 2000 to 2010).[27] Of most interest here is death from lung cancer. For men, the age-adjusted death rate from lung cancer increased from 1959 through 1965 to 1982 through 1988, but then fell for 2000

TABLE 4.1

Level of Evidence for Smoking-Attributable Cancers According to the United States Office of the Surgeon General by Cancer Site and Yearly Smoking-Attributable Mortality at Sites with Available Estimates, United States, 2004

	Cancer Site	Yearly Smoking-Attributable Mortality
Evidence Sufficient to Infer Causal Relationship	Bladder	4,983
	Cervix	447
	Colon and rectum	N/A
	Esophagus	8,592
	Kidney	3,043
	Larynx	3,009
	Leukemia (AML)	1,192
	Liver	N/A
	Lung	125,522
	Oral cavity and pharynx	4,893
	Pancreas	6,683
	Stomach	2,484
Evidence Suggestive but Not Sufficient to Infer Causal Relationship	Breast	
Inadequate to Infer Presence or Absence of Causal Relationship	Ovary	
Evidence Sufficient to Infer No Causal Relationship	Prostate	

N/A, not available; AML, acute myeloid leukemia.

through 2010; for women, the age-adjusted death rate continued to rise over time, with the biggest increase between 1982 through 1988 to 2000 through 2010.[27] In relative risk terms, the likelihood of dying from lung cancer given current smoking has increased from 2.73 to 12.65 to 25.66 among women, and 12.22 to 23.81 to 24.97 for men. Equivalent risks for former smokers increased from 1.3 to 3.85 to 6.7 among women, versus 3.48 to 7.41 to 6.75 for men. These and other analyses suggest that the cancer risks from smoking may have increased with time.[27,28] The histologic subtypes of lung cancer seen in the US population have also shifted with time. Into the early 1980s, squamous cell carcinomas (SCC) were the most common manifestations of lung cancer. However, a rapid rise in adenocarcinomas has been noted, and by the 1990s, had overtaken SCC as the leading type of lung cancer.[23]

Tobacco Use Behaviors

The level of tobacco exposure is ultimately driven by use behaviors, including the number of cigarettes smoked, the patterns of smoking on individual cigarettes, and the number of years smoked. The primary driver of smoking behavior is nicotine—the major addictive substance and primary reinforcer of continued smoking.[29–31] Over time, smokers learn an *acceptable* level of nicotine intake that attains the beneficial effects they seek while avoiding negative withdrawal symptoms. Smokers can affect the amount of nicotine (and accompanying toxicants) they draw from a cigarette by altering the number of puffs taken, puff size, frequency, duration, and velocity (collectively referred to as smoking topography).[32] Smokers tend to consume a relatively stable number of cigarettes per day and to smoke those cigarettes in a relatively consistent manner in order to maintain an acceptable level of nicotine in their system across the day.[33] The number of cigarettes smoked per day and the smoking pattern of an individual may be influenced by the rate of nicotine metabolism.[30] Nicotine is metabolized primarily to cotinine, which is further metabolized to trans-3′-hydroxycotinine (3HC), catalyzed by the liver cytochrome P450 2A6 enzyme.[34] Functional polymorphisms in the genes coding for these enzymes allow for the identification of *fast* metabolizers, who have more rapid nicotine clearance and show greater cigarette intake and more intensive smoking topography profiles relative to *normal* or *slow* metabolizers.[35–37] The ratio of 3HC to cotinine in plasma or saliva can be used as a reliable noninvasive phenotypic marker for CYP2A6 activity.[38,39] CYP2A6 activity is known to vary across racial/ethnic groups, with those of African or Asian descent showing slower metabolism than those of Caucasian descent.[40–42] Clinical trial data clearly show that the metabolite ratio can be used to predict success in quitting, and that the likelihood of quitting decreases as the ratio increases, such that slower metabolizers are more successful at achieving abstinence.[37,41,43] Despite their addiction to nicotine, most smokers in Western countries report that they regret ever starting to smoke and want to quit smoking, and there is evidence for similar regret in developing countries as well.[44–46] However, most smokers are unsuccessful in their attempts to quit smoking; the most effective evidence-based treatments increase the odds of quitting by 3 times, with 12-month cessation rates of approximately 40% relative to placebo.[47]

Evolution of Tobacco Products

Historically, tar was believed to be the main contributor to smoking-caused disease.[48] It is important to note that *tar* is not a specific substance, but simply the collected particulate matter from cigarette smoke, less water and nicotine (in technical reports, it is often referred to as nicotine-free dry particulate matter). Soon after the first studies were done showing that painting mice with cigarette tar caused cancerous tumors, it was theorized that reducing tar yields of cigarettes might also reduce the disease burden of smoking.[48] Concurrently, cigarette manufacturers were seeking to reassure their customers that their products were safe, that if hazardous compounds were identified they would be removed, and that product modifications could help to reduce risks.[4,49–51] Indeed, in the United States and United Kingdom, average tar levels of cigarettes dropped dramatically from the 1960s through the 1990s, and have since leveled off.[52,53] The European Union took the tar reduction mentality to heart in crafting maximum levels of tar in cigarettes that could be sold in member countries, beginning at 15 mg in 1992, then dropping to 12 mg in 1998, and 10 mg in 2005.[54] Unfortunately, these reductions in tar yields have not translated into changes in disease risks among smokers.[55] Despite initial optimism about these products, both laboratory-based and epidemiologic studies indicate neither an individual, nor a public health benefit from *low-tar* cigarettes as compared to *full-flavor* varieties.[56–58] The health consequences of mistakenly accepting the purported benefits of lower tar and nicotine products have been significant. The increases in adenocarcinoma of the lung observed in the United States over recent decades may reflect changes made to the cigarette, such as filters, filter ventilation, and tobacco-specific nitrosamines (TSNA) in smoke produced by the relatively high amount of burley tobacco used in the typical US cigarette blend.[23,59] Tobacco manufacturers engineered cigarettes be *elastic*; that is, cigarettes allow smokers to adjust their puffing patterns to regulate their intake of nicotine, regardless of how the cigarette might perform under the standard testing conditions that drove the labeling and advertising of the products.[55] Researchers have since come to determine that filter vents are the main design feature the industry relied on in creating elastic products.[54,55,60,61] Vents facilitate taking larger puffs and also contribute to sensory perceptions, because they dilute the smoke with air.[62] So, even with a larger puff, the same mass of toxins can seem less harsh and irritating because it is diluted by a proportionate amount of air, which may in turn underscore smokers' beliefs that they are smoking safer cigarettes.[62–64] Other smoke components (e.g., acetaldehyde, ammonia, minor tobacco alkaloids) and aspects of cigarette engineering (e.g., menthol, flavor additives) may further contribute to the addictiveness of cigarettes.[65]

Since the 1980s, manufacturers have introduced products that make more explicit claims about reduced health risks. Examples of modified cigarettelike products include Premier (RJ Reynolds), Eclipse (RJ Reynolds), Accord/Heatbar (Philip Morris), Omni (Vector Tobacco), and Advance (Brown and Williamson).[66] In the 2000s, as evidence of reduced lung cancer incidence and coincident increases in snus use in Sweden appeared,[67,68] manufacturers began to promote smokeless tobacco products as reduced harm alternatives. Most recently, electronic cigarettes, which vaporize a nicotine solution, have gained increasing popularity and generated concern among public health practitioners, particularly with regard to effects on youth.[8,69,70] In the United States, the FDA has authority to authorize marketing claims about reduced risk, which an Institute of Medicine panel concluded should be based on extensive testing of abuse liability, likely health effects, and effects on the whole population.[71]

CARCINOGENS IN TOBACCO PRODUCTS AND PROCESSES OF CANCER DEVELOPMENT

Cigarette smoke has been identified as carcinogenic since the 1950s, and efforts have continued to identify specific carcinogens in smoke and smokeless tobacco products. The International Agency for Research on Cancer (IARC) has classified both cigarette smoke and smokeless tobacco as Group 1 carcinogens.[72,73] IARC has also identified 72 measurable carcinogens in cigarette smoke where evidence is sufficient to classify them as Group 1 (carcinogenic to humans), 2A (probably carcinogenic to humans), or 2B (possibly carcinogenic to humans).[72] The IARC list, in addition to data from the U.S. Environmental Protection Agency (EPA), the National Toxicology Program, and the National Institute for Occupational Safety and Health (NIOSH), informed the FDA's development of a list of Harmful and Potentially Harmful Constituents (HPHC) in tobacco and tobacco smoke, which manufacturers will be required to report.[74] Table 4.2 illustrates the carcinogens listed as HPHC alongside their carcinogenicity classifications by IARC or the EPA.

Compounds of Particular Concern

Research groups have listed components of cigarette smoke theorized to impact health risk, often relying on carcinogenic potency indices and relative concentrations in smoke.[75,76] In these analyses, the N-nitrosamines, benzene, 1,3-butadiene, aromatic amines, and cadmium often rank highly. Polycyclic aromatic hydrocarbons (PAH), many of which are carcinogenic, consist of three or more fused aromatic rings resulting from incomplete combustion of organic (carbonaceous) materials, and are often found in coal tar, soot, broiled foods, and automobile engine exhaust.[77] A compound of particular concern in cigarette smoke historically has been benzo(a)pyrene (BaP), which has substantial carcinogenic activity and is considered carcinogenic to humans by the IARC.[77] In addition to PAH, other hydrocarbons found in significant quantities in cigarette smoke include benzene (a long-established cause of leukemia), 1,3-butadiene (a potent multiorgan carcinogen), naphthalene, and styrene. Carbonyl compounds, such as formaldehyde and acetaldehyde, are found in copious amounts in cigarette smoke, primarily coming from the combustion of sugars and cellulose.[78] However, there are numerous other noncigarette exposures to these compounds, including endogenous formation during metabolism. Smoke contains a number of aromatic amines, such as known bladder carcinogens 2-aminonaphthalene and 4-aminobiphenyl, heterocyclic amines, and furans. Toxic metals, including beryllium, cadmium, lead, and polonium-210, are also present in cigarette smoke in measurable quantities,[79,80] levels of which may depend in part on the region of the world where the tobacco was grown.[81] Much attention has been focused on the N-nitrosamines, primarily because they are well-established carcinogens.[82–85] Nitrosamines form through reactions of nitrite with amino groups. In tobacco, two compounds of concern are 4-(methylnitrosamino)-1-(3-pyridyl)-1-butanone (NNK), which is derived from nitrosation of nicotine, and N′-nitrosonornicotine (NNN), which is derived from nitrosation of nornicotine. Both of these compounds are tobacco specific. NNN and NNK primarily form during the curing process for tobacco, where the leaves are dried through contact with combustion gases from heat (flue) curing or microbial activity in air curing.[78] NNK is known to be a potent lung carcinogen, but also shows tumor induction activity in the nasal cavity, the pancreas, and the liver, whereas NNN has been shown to induce tumors along the respiratory tract and esophagus in various animal models. Because they are produced in the curing process and transfer into smoke, rather than being formed by combustion, it is possible to reduce nitrosamines by changing curing and storage practices.[78,86,87]

Smokeless tobacco products, although they are not burned, nonetheless contain substantial levels of carcinogens, most prominently the N-nitrosamines.[73] Here, product type and composition has an enormous effect on nitrosamine levels. For example, US moist snuff has substantially higher levels than that sold in Sweden (snus), whereas smokeless products available in India are often far higher in nitrosamines.[88] US smokeless products also can contain PAH and carbonyl compounds, likely derived from fire curing the constituent tobacco.[89] Similar to cigarettes, smokeless products would also contain toxic metals.[79,80]

Although tobacco is an exceedingly complex mixture, it is possible to use animal model and epidemiologic evidence to postulate relationships between specific components and known tobacco-induced cancers.[90–92] There is strong evidence from multiple studies to suggest that PAH and N-nitrosamines are involved in lung carcinogenesis. For example, PAH–DNA adducts are observed in lung tissues, and p53 tumor suppressor mutations in lung tumors resemble the damage created by PAH diol epoxide metabolites in vitro.[93–96] NNK appears to preferentially induce lung tumors in the rat, regardless of the route of administration, and DNA–nitrosamine adducts are detectable in lung tissues.[97,98] Most importantly, nitrosamine metabolite levels measured in smokers were prospectively related to the risk of lung cancer in cohort studies, even adjusting for other indices of smoking exposure (e.g., cotinine, pack-years).[98–102] PAH and nitrosamines are also likely to be implicated in cancers along the respiratory tract and the cervix.[103,104] Considerable evidence exist that aromatic amines such as 4-aminobiphenyl and 2-naphthylamine are potent bladder carcinogens, and smokers are known to be at an elevated risk of bladder cancer, so these are presumed to be the primary causative agents.[105–107] Similarly, as benzene is a known cause of leukemia, it is presumed that this is the link to leukemia observed in smokers.

Important to examining the role of various smoke components in cancer is the ability to measure the exposure of smokers to these components. Biomarkers of exposure may also be crucial for examining products for their potential to reduce health risks associated with tobacco use.[71,108,109] Validation of tobacco exposure biomarkers is threefold: method validation, validation with respect to product use, and validation with respect to disease risk.[71]

TABLE 4.2
Carcinogens in Tobacco and Tobacco Smoke Identified as Harmful and Potentially Harmful by the U.S. Food and Drug Administration, with International Agency for Research on Cancer Carcinogenecity (IARC) Classifications as of 2013

Compound	CAS No.	IARC Group	IARC Volume	Year
1,3-Butadiene	106-99-0	1	100F	2012
2-Aminonaphthalene	91-59-8	1	100F	2012
4-(Methylnitrosamino)-1-(3-pyridyl)-1-butanone (NNK)	64091-91-4	1	100E	2012
4-Aminobiphenyl	92-67-1	1	100F	2012
Aflatoxin B1	1162-65-8	1	100F	2012
Arsenic	7440-38-2	1	100C	2012
Benzene	71-43-2	1	100F	2012
Benzo[a]pyrene	50-32-8	1	100F	2012
Beryllium	7440-41-7	1	100C	2012
Cadmium	7440-43-9	1	100C	2012
Chromium (Hexavalent compounds)	18540-29-9	1	100C	2012
Ethylene oxide	75-21-8	1	100F	2012
Formaldehyde	50-00-0	1	100F	2012
N-Nitrosonornicotine (NNN)	16543-55-8	1	100E	2012
Nickel (compounds)		1	100C	2012
o-Toluidine	95-53-4	1	100F	2012
Polonium-210	7440-08-6	1	100D	2012
Uranium (235, 238 Isotopes)	7440-61-1	1	100D	2012
Vinyl chloride	75-01-4	1	100F	2012
Acrylamide	79-06-1	2A	60	1994
Cyclopenta[c,d]pyrene	27208-37-3	2A	92	2010
Dibenz[a,h]anthracene	53-70-3	2A	92	2010
Dibenzo[a,l]pyrene	191-30-0	2A	92	2010
Ethyl carbamate (urethane)	51-79-6	2A	96	2010
IQ (2-Amino-3-methylimidazo[4,5-f]quinoline)	76180-96-6	2A	56	1993
N-Nitrosodiethylamine	55-18-5	2A	SUP 7	1987
N-Nitrosodimethylamine (NDMA)	62-75-9	2A	SUP 7	1987
2-Nitropropane	79-46-9	2B	71	1999
2,6-Dimethylaniline	87-62-7	2B	57	1993
5-Methylchrysene	3697-24-3	2B	92	2010
A-α-C (2-Amino-9H-pyrido[2,3-b]indole)	26148-68-5	2B	SUP 7	1987
Acetaldehyde	75-07-0	2B	71	1999
Acetamide	60-35-5	2B	71	1999
Acrylonitrile	107-13-1	2B	71	1999
Benz[a]anthracene	56-55-3	2B	92	2010
Benz[j]aceanthrylene	202-33-5	2B	92	2012
Benzo[b]fluoranthene	205-99-2	2B	92	2010
Benzo[b]furan	271-89-6	2B	63	1995
Benzo[c]phenanthrene	195-19-7	2B	92	2010
Benzo[k]fluoranthene	207-08-9	2B	92	2010
Caffeic acid	331-39-5	2B	56	1993
Catechol	120-80-9	2B	71	1999
Chrysene	218-01-9	2B	92	2010
Cobalt	7440-48-4	2B	52	1991

(continued)

TABLE 4.2

Carcinogens in Tobacco and Tobacco Smoke Identified as Harmful and Potentially Harmful by the U.S. Food and Drug Administration, with International Agency for Research on Cancer Carcinogenecity (IARC) Classifications as of 2013 *(continued)*

Compound	CAS No.	IARC Group	IARC Volume	Year
Dibenzo[a,h]pyrene	189-64-0	2B	92	2010
Dibenzo[a,i]pyrene	189-55-9	2B	92	2010
Ethylbenzene	100-41-4	2B	77	2000
Furan	110-00-9	2B	63	1995
Glu-P-1 (2-Amino-6-methyldipyrido[1,2-a:3',2'-d]imidazole)	67730-11-4	2B	SUP 7	1987
Glu-P-2 (2-Aminodipyrido[1,2-a:3',2'-d]imidazole)	67730-10-3	2B	SUP 7	1987
Hydrazine	302-01-2	2B	71	1999
Indeno[1,2,3-cd]pyrene	193-39-5	2B	92	2010
Isoprene	78-79-5	2B	71	1999
Lead	7439-92-1	2B	SUP 7	1987
MeA-α-C (2-Amino-3-methyl)-9H-pyrido[2,3-b]indole)	68006-83-7	2B	SUP 7	1987
N-Nitrosodiethanolamine (NDELA)	1116-54-7	2B	77	2000
N-Nitrosomethylethylamine	10595-95-6	2B	SUP 7	1987
N-Nitrosomorpholine (NMOR)	59-89-2	2B	SUP 7	1987
N-Nitrosopiperidine (NPIP)	100-75-4	2B	SUP 7	1987
N-Nitrosopyrrolidine (NPYR)	930-55-2	2B	SUP 7	1987
N-Nitrososarcosine (NSAR)	13256-22-9	2B	SUP 7	1987
Naphthalene	91-20-3	2B	82	2002
Nickel	7440-02-0	2B	49	1990
Nitrobenzene	98-95-3	2B	65	1996
Nitromethane	75-52-5	2B	77	2000
o-Anisidine	90-04-0	2B	73	1999
PhIP (2-Amino-1-methyl-6-phenylimidazo[4,5-b]pyridine)	105650-23-5	2B	56	1993
Propylene oxide	75-56-9	2B	60	1994
Styrene	100-42-5	2B	82	2002
Trp-P-1 (3-Amino-1,4-dimethyl-5H-pyrido[4,3-b]indole)	62450-06-0	2B	SUP 7	1987
Trp-P-2 (3-Amino-1-Methyl-5H-pyrido[4,3-b]indole)	62450-07-1	2B	SUP 7	1987
Vinyl acetate	108-05-4	2B	63	1995
1-Aminonaphthalene	134-32-7	3	SUP 7	1987
Chromium	7440-47-3	3	49	1990
Crotonaldehyde	4170-30-3	3	63	1995
Dibenzo[a,e]pyrene	192-65-4	3	92	2010
Mercury	7439-97-6	3	58	1993
Quinoline	91-22-5	EPA Group B2		
Cresols (o-, m-, and p-cresol)	1319-77-3	EPA Group C		

Notes: Most recently published IARC monograph for each compound is listed.
Quinoline and cresols have not been evaluated by IARC, but have been evaluated by U.S. Environmental Protection Agency.
IARC Groups: 1, Carcinogenic to humans; 2A, Probably carcinogenic to humans; 2B, Possibly carcinogenic to humans; 3, Not classifiable as to its carcinogenicity to humans; http://monographs.iarc.fr/ENG/Classification/ClassificationsAlphaOrder.pdf
EPA Groups: B2, Likely to be carcinogenic in humans; C, Possible human carcinogen.
CAS No., Chemical Abstracts Service registry number. *CAS Registry Number is a Registered Trademark of the American Chemical Society.* EPA, Environmental Protection Agency.
Quinoline: http://www.epa.gov/iris/subst/1004.htm
Cresols: http://www.epa.gov/iris/subst/0300.htm; http://www.epa.gov/iris/subst/0301.htm; http://www.epa.gov/iris/subst/0302.htm

TABLE 4.3
Commonly Used Biomarkers of Exposure to Carcinogens in Tobacco Smoke

Biomarker	Tobacco Smoke Source	Matrices
Monohydroxy-30butenyl mercapturic acid (MHBMA)	1,3-butadiene	Urine
4-Aminobiphenyl-globin	4-aminobiphenyl	Blood
N-(2-hydroxypropyl)methacrylamide (HPMA)	Acrolein	Urine
Carbamoylethylvaline	Acrylamide	Blood
Cyanoethylvaline	Acrylonitrile	Blood
S-phenylmercapturic acid (SPMA)	Benzene	Urine
Cd	Cadmium	Urine
3-hydroxypropyl mercapturic acid (HBMA)	Crotonaldehyde	Urine
2-hydroxyethyl mercapturic acid (HEMA)	Ethylene oxide	Urine
Nicotine equivalents (nicotine, cotinine, trans-3'-hydroxycotinine, and their respective glucuronides)	Nicotine	Urine
Total 4-(methylnitrosamino)-1-(3-pyridyl)-1-butanol (NNAL) (NNAL + NNAL glucuronide)	NNK	Urine
Total NNN (NNN + NNN glucuronide)	NNN	Urine
1-Hydroxypyrene	Pyrene (representative of other PAH)	Urine

Adapted from Hecht SS, Yuan JM, Hatsukami D. Applying tobacco carcinogen and toxicant biomarkers in product regulation and cancer prevention. *Chem Res Toxicol* 2010;23:1001–1008.

Validation with respect to product use means that levels of a given biomarker differ substantially between users and nonusers, and that biomarker levels decrease substantially when product use is stopped. Validation with respect to disease risk implies that variation in biomarker levels in product users are predictive of variations in disease outcomes. Over the last decade, the development of modern high-throughput, high-resolution mass spectrometry has allowed for the measurement of multiple metabolites of tobacco carcinogens.[110–113] Commonly used biomarkers of tobacco exposure are listed in Table 4.3.

How Tobacco Use Leads to Cancer

A recent U.S. Surgeon General's report provides extensive detail on the current state of knowledge of how smoking causes cancer.[65] Therefore, only a brief overview is provided here. Hecht[101,113–116] has argued for a major pathway by which tobacco use leads to cancer: carcinogen exposure leads to the formation of carcinogen–DNA adducts, which then cause mutations that, if not repaired or removed by apoptosis, will eventually give rise to cancer. It is important to keep perspective that, whereas each cigarette may contain seemingly low levels of a given carcinogen, smoking is, for most people, a long-term addiction. Thus, a mixture of numerous carcinogens is administered multiple times per day over the course of decades. Further, compounds taken in during smokers can be metabolically activated, thus increasing their activity. Cigarette smoke compounds appear to induce the cytochrome P450 system, which facilitates the metabolic activation of carcinogens to electrophilic entities that are able to covalently bind DNA.[117,118] DNA adducts appear to be crucial to the cancer process, and numerous studies show that smoker tissues contain higher levels of DNA adducts than nonsmokers, and that DNA adduct levels are associated with cancer risk.[119,120] At the same time, other systems are involved in the detoxification and deactivation of smoke constituents, typically catalyzed by UDP-glucuronosyltransferases and glutathione-S-transferases, resulting in excretion of inactive compounds.[121,122] An individual's balance of activation and deactivation of toxicants may be an important predictor of cancer risk, although evidence for this is mixed in the literature.[123,124] Similarly, DNA repair capacity is an important consideration, because, even if adducts are formed, processes exist to remove such perturbations to normalize DNA structure. Enzymatic processes of DNA repair include alkytransferases, nucleotide excision, and mismatch repair. Polymorphisms in genes coding for these enzymes may relate to individual cancer susceptibility. Table 4.4 outlines the metabolic activation/detoxification, DNA-adduct formation, and repair processes believed to be involved for four tobacco carcinogens (nitrosamines, PAH, benzene, 4-aminobiphenyl).[65,120]

Those DNA adducts that persist can cause miscoding during DNA replication. Smoke carcinogens are known to cause G:A and G:T mutations, and mutations in the *KRAS* oncogene and the *P53* tumor suppressor gene are strongly associated with tobacco-caused cancers.[95,114,125–127] Inactivation of *P53*, together with the activation of *KRAS*, appear to reduce survival in non–small-cell lung cancer.[65] Gene mutations that do not result in apoptosis may go on to influence a number of downstream processes, which may lead to genomic instability, proliferation, and eventually, malignancy.[128–130] Some smoke constituents may also act in ways that indirectly support the development of cancer. Nicotine, although not a carcinogen in itself, is known to reduce apoptosis and increase angiogenesis and transformation processes via nuclear factor kappa B (NF-κB).[65,131] Activation of nicotinic acetylcholine receptors (nAChR) in lung epithelium by nicotine or NNK is associated with survival and proliferation of malignant cells.[65] Nitrosamines also appear to have similar activities via the activation of protein kinases A and B.[132] NNK may bind β-adrenergic receptors to stimulate the release of arachidonic acid, which is converted to prostaglandin E2 by cyclooxygenase (COX)-2. Smoke compounds appear to activate epidermal growth factor receptor (EGFR) and COX-2, both of which are found to be elevated in many cancers.[133] Ciliatoxic, inflammatory, and oxidizing compounds, such as acrolein and ethylene oxide in smoke, may also impact the likelihood of cancer development. Epigenetic changes such as hypermethylation, particularly at P16, may also play a role in lung cancer development.[65]

TABLE 4.4

Key Pathways and Processes Where Selected Smoke Constituents Are Activated and Detoxified

	NNN, NNK	PAH	Benzene	4-ABP
Metabolic Activation	Alpha hydroxylation	Diol epoxide formation	Epoxide/oxepin formation	N-oxidation
Cytochrome P450 Enzymes Involved	2A6, 2A13, 2E1	1A1, 1B1	2E1	1A2
Enzymes Involved in Detoxification/ Activation	UGT	MEH, GST, UGT	MEH, GST	UGT, NAT
DNA Adduct Formation Sites				
Lung	O6-POB-deoxyguanosine	BPDE-N2-deoxyguanosine		
Bladder				C-8 deoxyguanosine
DNA Repair Pathways	AGT, BER	NER, MMR	BER, NER, NIR	NER

UGT, uridine-5'-diphosphate-glucuronosyltransferases; MEH, microsomal epoxide hydrolases; NAT, N-Acetyltransferases; GST, glutathione-S-transferases; AGT, O6-alkylguanine–DNA alkyltransferase; BER, base excision repair; NER, nucleotide excision repair; MMR, mismatch repair; NIR, nucleotide incision repair.

REFERENCES

1. World Health Organization, Research for International Tobacco Control. *WHO Report on the Global Tobacco Epidemic, 2008: the MPOWER Package.* Geneva: World Health Organization; 2008.
2. Giovino GA, Mirza SA, Samet JM, et al. Tobacco use in 3 billion individuals from 16 countries: an analysis of nationally representative cross-sectional household surveys. *Lancet* 2012;380:668–679.
3. Centers for Disease Control and Prevention (CDC). Current cigarette smoking among adults—United States, 2011. *MMWR Morb Mortal Wkly Rep* 2012;61:889–894.
4. Proctor R. *Golden Holocaust: Origins of the Cigarette Catastrophe and the Case for Abolition.* Berkeley: University of California Press; 2011.
5. Centers for Disease Control and Prevention (CDC). Consumption of cigarettes and combustible tobacco—United States, 2000-2011. *MMWR Morb Mortal Wkly Rep* 2012;61:565–569.
6. Centers for Disease Control and Prevention (CDC). Cigarette use among high school students—United States, 1991–2009. *MMWR Morb Mortal Wkly Rep* 2010;59:797–801.
7. Centers for Disease Control and Prevention (CDC). Tobacco use among middle and high school students—United States, 2000–2009. *MMWR Morb Mortal Wkly Rep* 2010;59:1063–1068.
8. Centers for Disease Control and Prevention (CDC). Tobacco product use among middle and high school students—United States, 2011 and 2012. *MMWR Morb Mortal Wkly Rep* 2013;62:893–897.
9. Cummings KM, Fong GT, Borland R. Environmental influences on tobacco use: evidence from societal and community influences on tobacco use and dependence. *Annu Rev Clin Psychol* 2009;5:433–458.
10. Huang J, Chaloupka FJ, Fong GT. Cigarette graphic warning labels and smoking prevalence in Canada: a critical examination and reformulation of the FDA regulatory impact analysis. *Tob Control* 2014;1:i7–i12.
11. Chaloupka FJ, Yurekli A, Fong GT. Tobacco taxes as a tobacco control strategy. *Tob Control* 2012;21:172–180.
12. Centers for Disease Control and Prevention (CDC). State-specific trends in lung cancer incidence and smoking—United States, 1999-2008. *MMWR Morb Mortal Wkly Rep* 2011;60:1243–1247.
13. Holford TR, Meza R, Warner KE, et al. Tobacco control and the reduction in smoking-related premature deaths in the United States, 1964–2012. *JAMA* 2014;311:164–171.
14. Slama K. The FCTC enters into effect in 2005. *Int J Tuberc Lung Dis* 2005;9:119.
15. Liberman J. Four COPs and counting: achievements, underachievements and looming challenges in the early life of the WHO FCTC Conference of the Parties. *Tob Control* 2012;21:215–220.
16. Deyton LR. FDA tobacco product regulations: a powerful tool for tobacco control. *Public Health Rep* 2011;126:167–169.
17. Patterson JT. *The Dread Disease: Cancer and Modern American Culture.* Cambridge, MA: Harvard University Press; 1987.
18. Proctor R. *The Nazi War on Cancer.* Princeton: Princeton University Press; 1999.
19. Doll R, Hill AB. Smoking and carcinoma of the lung: a preliminary report. *BMJ* 1950;2:739–748.
20. Wynder EL, Graham EA. Tobacco smoking as a possible etiologic factor in bronchiogenic carcinoma: a study of six hundred and eighty-four proved cases. *JAMA* 1950;143:329–336.
21. US Department of Health and Human Services. *The Health Consequences of Smoking: A Report of the Surgeon General.* Atlanta: Department of Health and Human Services, Centers for Disease Control and Prevention, National Center for Chronic Disease Prevention and Health Promotion, Office on Smoking and Health; 2004.
22. Centers for Disease Control and Prevention (CDC). Smoking-attributable mortality, years of potential life lost, and productivity losses—United States, 2000-2004. *MMWR Morb Mortal Wkly Rep* 2008;57:1226–1228.
23. US Department of Health and Human Services. *The Health Consequences of Smoking—50 Years of Progress. A Report of the Surgeon General.* Atlanta: U.S. Department of Health and Human Services, Centers for Disease Control and Prevention, National Center for Chronic Disease Prevention and Health Promotion, Office on Smoking and Health; 2014.
24. Jha P, Ramasundarahettige C, Landsman V, et al. 21st-century hazards of smoking and benefits of cessation in the United States. *N Engl J Med* 2013;368:341–350.
25. Gaudet MM, Gapstur SM, Sun J, et al. Active smoking and breast cancer risk: original cohort data and meta-analysis. *J Natl Cancer Inst* 2013;105:515–525.
26. Peto R, Darby S, Deo H, et al. Smoking, smoking cessation, and lung cancer in the UK since 1950: combination of national statistics with two case-control studies. *BMJ* 2000;321:323–329.
27. Thun MJ, Carter BD, Feskanich D, et al. 50-year trends in smoking-related mortality in the United States. *N Engl J Med* 2013;368:351–364.
28. Burns DM, Anderson CM, Gray N. Has the lung cancer risk from smoking increased over the last fifty years? *Cancer Causes Control* 2011;22:389–397.
29. Benowitz NL. Clinical pharmacology of nicotine: implications for understanding, preventing, and treating tobacco addiction. *Clin Pharmacol Ther* 2008;83:531–541.
30. Benowitz NL. Pharmacology of nicotine: addiction, smoking-induced disease, and therapeutics. *Annu Rev Pharmacol Toxicol* 2009;49:57–71.
31. Benowitz NL. Nicotine addiction. *N Engl J Med* 2010;362:2295–2303.
32. Scherer G. Smoking behaviour and compensation: a review of the literature. *Psychopharmacology (Berl)* 1999;145:1–20.
33. Hammond D, Fong GT, Cummings KM, et al. Smoking topography, brand switching, and nicotine delivery: results from an in vivo study. *Cancer Epidemiol Biomarkers Prev* 2005;14:1370–1375.
34. Benowitz NL, Hukkanen J, Jacob P. Nicotine chemistry, metabolism, kinetics and biomarkers. *Handb Exp Pharmacol* 2009:29–60.
35. Benowitz NL, Swan GE, Jacob P, et al. CYP2A6 genotype and the metabolism and disposition kinetics of nicotine. *Clin Pharmacol Ther* 2006;80:457–467.
36. Johnstone E, Benowitz N, Cargill A, et al. Determinants of the rate of nicotine metabolism and effects on smoking behavior. *Clin Pharmacol Ther* 2006;80:319–330.
37. Malaiyandi V, Lerman C, Benowitz NL, et al. Impact of CYP2A6 genotype on pretreatment smoking behaviour and nicotine levels from and usage of nicotine replacement therapy. *Mol Psychiatry* 2006;11:400–409.
38. Lea RA, Dickson S, Benowitz NL. Within-subject variation of the salivary 3HC/COT ratio in regular daily smokers: prospects for estimating CYP2A6 enzyme activity in large-scale surveys of nicotine metabolic rate. *J Anal Toxicol* 2006;30:386–389.
39. St Helen G, Novalen M, Heitjan DF, et al. Reproducibility of the nicotine metabolite ratio in cigarette smokers. *Cancer Epidemiol Biomarkers Prev* 2012;21:1105–1114.

40. Benowitz NL, Dains KM, Dempsey D, et al. Racial differences in the relationship between number of cigarettes smoked and nicotine and carcinogen exposure. *Nicotine Tob Res* 2011;13:772–783.
41. Dempsey DA, St Helen G, Jacob P, et al. Genetic and pharmacokinetic determinants of response to transdermal nicotine in white, black, and asian nonsmokers. *Clin Pharmacol Ther* 2013;94:687–694.
42. Zhu AZ, Renner CC, Hatsukami DK, et al. The ability of plasma cotinine to predict nicotine and carcinogen exposure is altered by differences in CYP2A6: the influence of genetics, race, and sex. *Cancer Epidemiol Biomarkers Prev* 2013;22:708–718.
43. Schnoll RA, Patterson F, Wileyto EP, et al. Nicotine metabolic rate predicts successful smoking cessation with transdermal nicotine: a validation study. *Pharmacol Biochem Behav* 2009;92:6–11.
44. Fong GT, Hammond D, Laux FL, et al. The near-universal experience of regret among smokers in four countries: findings from the International Tobacco Control Policy Evaluation Survey. *Nicotine Tob Res* 2004;6:S341–S351.
45. Lee WB, Fong GT, Zanna MP, et al. Regret and rationalization among smokers in Thailand and Malaysia: findings from the International Tobacco Control Southeast Asia Survey. *Health Psychol* 2009;28:457–464.
46. Sansone N, Fong GT, Lee WB, et al. Comparing the experience of regret and its predictors among smokers in four Asian countries: findings from the ITC surveys in Thailand, South Korea, Malaysia, and China. *Nicotine Tob Res* 2013;15:1663–1672.
47. Tobacco Use and Dependence Guideline Panel. *Treating Tobacco Use and Dependence: 2008 Update*. Rockville, MD: U.S. Department of Health and Human Services; 2008.
48. Wynder EL, Hoffmann D. *Tobacco and Tobacco Smoke*. New York: Academic Press; 1967.
49. Cummings KM, Morley CP, Hyland A. Failed promises of the cigarette industry and its effect on consumer misperceptions about the health risks of smoking. *Tob Control* 2002;11:I110–I117.
50. Pollay RW, Dewhirst T. The dark side of marketing seemingly "Light" cigarettes: successful images and failed fact. *Tob Control* 2002;11:I18–I31.
51. Fairchild A, Colgrove J. Out of the ashes: the life, death, and rebirth of the "safer" cigarette in the United States. *Am J Public Health* 2004;94:192–204.
52. Hoffmann D, Hoffmann I. The changing cigarette, 1950–1995. *J Toxicol Environ Health*. 1997;50:307–364.
53. Jarvis MJ. Trends in sales weighted tar, nicotine, and carbon monoxide yields of UK cigarettes. *Thorax* 2001;56:960–963.
54. O'Connor RJ, Cummings KM, Giovino GA, et al. How did UK cigarette makers reduce tar to 10 mg or less? *BMJ*. 2006;332:302.
55. National Cancer Institute. *Risks Associated with Smoking Cigarettes with Low Machine-Measured Yields of Tar and Nicotine*. Bethesda, MD: The Institute; 2001.
56. Harris JE, Thun MJ, Mondul AM, et al. Cigarette tar yields in relation to mortality from lung cancer in the cancer prevention study II prospective cohort, 1982-8. *BMJ* 2004;328:72.
57. Thun MJ, Burns DM. Health impact of "reduced yield" cigarettes: a critical assessment of the epidemiological evidence. *Tob Control* 2001;10:i4–i11.
58. Benowitz NL, Jacob P, Bernert JT, et al. Carcinogen exposure during short-term switching from regular to "light" cigarettes. *Cancer Epidemiol Biomarkers Prev* 2005;14:1376–1383.
59. Burns DM, Anderson CM, Gray N. Do changes in cigarette design influence the rise in adenocarcinoma of the lung? *Cancer Causes Control* 2011;22:13–22.
60. Kozlowski LT, Mehta NY, Sweeney CT, et al. Filter ventilation and nicotine content of tobacco in cigarettes from Canada, the United Kingdom, and the United States. *Tob Control* 1998;7:369–375.
61. Kozlowski LT, O'Connor RJ, Giovino GA, et al. Maximum yields might improve public health—if filter vents were banned: a lesson from the history of vented filters. *Tob Control* 2006;15:262–266.
62. Kozlowski LT, O'Connor RJ. Cigarette filter ventilation is a defective design because of misleading taste, bigger puffs, and blocked vents. *Tob Control* 2002;11:I40–I50.
63. Kozlowski LT, Goldberg ME, Yost BA, et al. Smokers are unaware of the filter vents now on most cigarettes: results of a national survey. *Tob Control* 1996;5:265–270.
64. O'Connor RJ, Caruso RV, Borland R, et al. Relationship of cigarette-related perceptions to cigarette design features: findings from the 2009 ITC U.S. Survey. *Nicotine Tob Res* 2013;15:1943–1947.
65. Centers for Disease Control and Prevention, National Center for Chronic Disease Prevention and Health Promotion, Office on Smoking and Health. *How Tobacco Smoke Causes Disease: The Biology and Behavioral Basis for Smoking-Attributable Disease: A Report of the Surgeon General*. Rockville, MD: Centers for Disease Control and Prevetion; 2010.
66. Stratton KR. *Clearing the Smoke: Assessing the Science Base for Tobacco Harm Reduction*. Washington, DC: Institute of Medicine, National Academy Press; 2001.
67. Foulds J, Ramstrom L, Burke M, et al. Effect of smokeless tobacco (snus) on smoking and public health in Sweden. *Tob Control* 2003;12:349–359.
68. Henningfield JE, Fagerstrom KO. Swedish Match Company, Swedish snus and public health: a harm reduction experiment in progress? *Tob Control* 2001;10:253–257.
69. Pepper JK, Brewer NT. Electronic nicotine delivery system (electronic cigarette) awareness, use, reactions and beliefs: a systematic review. *Tob Control* 2013 [Epub ahead of print].
70. Schaller K, Ruppert L, Kahnert S, et al. *Electronic Cigarettes—An Overview*. Heidelberg: German Cancer Research Center (DKFZ); 2013. http://www.dkfz.de/en/presse/download/RS-Vol19-E-Cigarettes-EN.pdf
71. Institute of Medicine. *Scientific Standards for Studies on Modified Risk Tobacco Products*. Washington, DC: National Academies Press; 2012.
72. International Agency for Research on Cancer. *Tobacco Smoke and Involuntary Smoking*. Vol 83. Lyon: International Agency for Research on Cancer, World Health Organization; 2004.
73. International Agency for Research on Cancer. *Smokeless Tobacco and Tobacco-Specific Nitrosamines*. Vol 89. Lyon: International Agency for Research on Cancer, World Health Organization; 2007.
74. Center for Tobacco Products. *Reporting Harmful and Potentially Harmful Constituents in Tobacco Products and Tobacco Smoke Under Section 904(a)(3) of the Federal Food, Drug, and Cosmetic Act*. Rockville, MD: Department of Health and Human Services; 2012.
75. Fowles J, Dybing E. Application of toxicological risk assessment principles to the chemical constituents of cigarette smoke. *Tob Control* 2003;12:424–430.
76. Burns DM, Dybing E, Gray N, et al. Mandated lowering of toxicants in cigarette smoke: a description of the World Health Organization tobacco regulation proposal. *Tob Control* 2008;17:132–141.
77. Straif K, Baan R, Gosse Y, et al. Carcinogenicity of polycyclic aromatic hydrocarbons. *Lancet Oncol* 2005;6:931–932.
78. O'Connor RJ, Hurley PJ. Existing technologies to reduce specific toxicant emissions in cigarette smoke. *Tob Control* 2008;17:i39–i48.
79. Pappas RS. Toxic elements in tobacco and in cigarette smoke: inflammation and sensitization. *Metallomics* 2011;3:1181–1198.
80. Marano KM, Naufal ZS, Kathman SJ, et al. Cadmium exposure and tobacco consumption: biomarkers and risk assessment. *Regul Toxicol Pharmacol* 2012;64:243–252.
81. Stephens WE, Calder A, Newton J. Source and health implications of high toxic metal concentrations in illicit tobacco products. *Environ Sci Technol* 2005;39:479–488.
82. Hecht SS, Hoffmann D. Tobacco-specific nitrosamines, an important group of carcinogens in tobacco and tobacco smoke. *Carcinogenesis* 1988;9:875–884.
83. Hecht SS. Biochemistry, biology, and carcinogenicity of tobacco-specific N-nitrosamines. *Chem Res Toxicol* 1998;11:559–603.
84. Hoffmann D, Rivenson A, Hecht SS. The biological significance of tobacco-specific N-nitrosamines: smoking and adenocarcinoma of the lung. *Crit Rev Toxicol* 1996;26:199–211.
85. Nilsson R. The molecular basis for induction of human cancers by tobacco specific nitrosamines. *Regul Toxicol Pharmacol* 2011;60:268–280.
86. Hecht SS, Stepanov I, Hatsukami DK. Major tobacco companies have technology to reduce carcinogen levels but do not apply it to popular smokeless tobacco products. *Tob Control* 2011;20:443.
87. Stepanov I, Knezevich A, Zhang L, et al. Carcinogenic tobacco-specific N-nitrosamines in US cigarettes: three decades of remarkable neglect by the tobacco industry. *Tob Control* 2012;21:44–48.
88. Stanfill SB, Connolly GN, Zhang L, et al. Global surveillance of oral tobacco products: total nicotine, unionised nicotine and tobacco-specific N-nitrosamines. *Tob Control* 2011;20:e2.
89. Stepanov I, Villalta PW, Knezevich A, et al. Analysis of 23 polycyclic aromatic hydrocarbons in smokeless tobacco by gas chromatography-mass spectrometry. *Chem Res Toxicol* 2010;23:66–73.
90. Stanton MF, Miller E, Wrench C, et al. Experimental induction of epidermoid carcinoma in the lungs of rats by cigarette smoke condensate. *J Natl Cancer Inst* 1972;49:867–877.
91. Hoffmann D, Stepanov I, Hecht SS. *Tobacco Carcinogenesis*. New York: Academic Press; 1978.
92. Deutsch-Wenzel R, Brune H, Grimmer G. Experimental studies in rat lungs on the carcinogenicity and dose-response relationships of eight frequently occurring environmental polycyclic aromatic hydrocarbons. *J Natl Cancer Inst* 1983;71:539–544.
93. Pfeiffer GP, Denissenko MF, Olivier M, et al. Tobacco smoke carcinogens, DNA damage and p53 mutations in smoking-associated cancers. *Oncogene* 2002;21:7435–7451.
94. Boysen G, Hecht SS. Analysis of DNA and protein adducts of benzo[a]pyrene in human tissues using structure-specific methods. *Mutat Res* 2003;543:17–30.
95. Phillips DH. Smoking-related DNA and protein adducts in human tissues. *Carcinogenesis* 2002;23:1979–2004.
96. Liu Z, Muehlbauer KR, Schmeiser HH, et al. p53 Mutations in benzo[a]pyrene-exposed human p53 knock-in murine fibroblasts correlate with p53 mutations in human lung tumors. *Cancer Res* 2005;65:2583–2587.
97. Belinsky SA, Foley JF, White CM, et al. Dose-response relationship between O6-methylguanine formation in Clara cells and induction of pulmonary neoplasia in the rat by 4-(methylnitrosamino)-1-(3-pyridyl)-1-butanone. *Cancer Res* 1990;50:3772–3780.
98. Stepanov I, Sebero E, Wang R, et al. Tobacco-specific N-nitrosamine exposures and cancer risk in the Shanghai cohort study: remarkable coherence with rat tumor sites. *Int J Cancer* 2014;134:2278–2283.
99. Yuan JM, Koh WP, Murphy SE, et al. Urinary levels of tobacco-specific nitrosamine metabolites in relation to lung cancer development in two prospective cohorts of cigarette smokers. *Cancer Res* 2009;69:2990–2995.

100. Church TR, Anderson SE, Caporaso NE, et al. A prospectively measured serum biomarker for a tobacco-specific carcinogen and lung cancer in smokers. *Cancer Epidemiol Biomarkers Prev* 2009;18:260–266.
101. Hecht SS, Murphy SE, Stepanov I, et al. Tobacco smoke biomarkers and cancer risk among male smokers in the Shanghai Cohort Study. *Cancer Lett* 2012 [Epub ahead of print].
102. Yuan JM, Butler LM, Gao YT, et al. Urinary metabolites of a polycyclic aromatic hydrocarbon and volatile organic compounds in relation to lung cancer development in lifelong never smokers in the Shanghai Cohort Study. *Carcinogenesis* 2014;35:339–345.
103. Melikian AA, Sun P, Prokopczyk B, et al. Identification of benzo[a]pyrene metabolites in cervical mucus and DNA adducts in cervical tissues in humans by gas chromatography-mass spectrometry. *Cancer Lett* 1999;146: 127–134.
104. Prokopczyk B, Trushin N, Leszczynska J, et al. Human cervical tissue metabolizes the tobacco-specific nitrosamine, 4-(methylnitrosamino)-1-(3-pyridyl)-1-butanone, via alpha-hydroxylation and carbonyl reduction pathways. *Carcinogenesis* 2001;22:107–114.
105. Castelao JE, Yuan JM, Skipper PL, et al. Gender- and smoking-related bladder cancer risk. *J Natl Cancer Inst* 2001;93:538–545.
106. Sugimura T. History, present and future, of heterocyclic amines, cooked food mutagens. *Princess Takamatsu Symp* 1995;23:214–231.
107. Turesky RJ. Heterocyclic aromatic amine metabolism, DNA adduct formation, mutagenesis, and carcinogenesis. *Drug Metab Rev* 2002; 34:625–650.
108. Ashley DL, O'Connor RJ, Bernert JT, et al. Effect of differing levels of tobacco-specific nitrosamines in cigarette smoke on the levels of biomarkers in smokers. *Cancer Epidemiol Biomarkers Prev* 2010;19:1389–1398.
109. Hatsukami DK, Benowitz NL, Rennard SI, et al. Biomarkers to assess the utility of potential reduced exposure tobacco products. *Nicotine Tob Res* 2008;8: 169–191.
110. Carmella SG, Chen M, Han S, et al. Effects of smoking cessation on eight urinary tobacco carcinogen and toxicant biomarkers. *Chem Res Toxicol* 2009;22:734–741.
111. Carmella SG, Ming X, Olvera N, et al. High throughput liquid and gas chromatography-tandem mass spectrometry assays for tobacco-specific nitrosamine and polycyclic aromatic hydrocarbon metabolites associated with lung cancer in smokers. *Chem Res Toxicol* 2013;26:1209–1217.
112. Church TR, Anderson KE, Le C, et al. Temporal stability of urinary and plasma biomarkers of tobacco smoke exposure among cigarette smokers. *Biomarkers* 2010;15:345–352.
113. Hecht SS, Yuan JM, Hatsukami D. Applying tobacco carcinogen and toxicant biomarkers in product regulation and cancer prevention. *Chem Res Toxicol* 2010;23:1001–1008.
114. Hecht SS. Tobacco smoke carcinogens and lung cancer. *J Natl Cancer Inst* 1999;91:1194–1210.
115. Hecht SS. Tobacco carcinogens, their biomarkers, and tobacco-induced cancer. *Nature Rev Cancer* 2003;3:733–744.
116. Hecht SS. Lung carcinogenesis by tobacco smoke. *Int J Cancer* 2012;131: 2724–2732.
117. Guengerich FP. Common and uncommon cytochrome P450 reactions related to metabolism and chemical toxicity. *Chem Res Toxicol* 2001; 14:611–650.
118. Jalas J, Hecht SS, Murphy SE. Cytochrome P450 2A enzymes as catalysts of metabolism of 4-(methylnitrosamino)-1-(3-pyridyl)-1-butanone (NNK), a tobacco-specific carcinogen. *Chem Res Toxicol* 2005;18:95–110.
119. Nebert DW, Dalton TP, Okey AB, et al. Role of aryl hydrocarbon receptor-mediated induction of the CYP1 enzymes in environmental toxicity and cancer. *J Biol Chem* 2004;279:23847–23850.
120. Hang B. Formation and repair of tobacco carcinogen-derived bulky DNA adducts. *J Nucleic Acids* 2010;2010:709521.
121. Burchell B, McGurk K, Brierley CH, et al. *UDP-Glucuronosyltransferases*. Vol 3. New York: Elsevier Science; 1997.
122. Armstrong RN. *Glutathione-S-Transferases*. Vol 3. New York: Elsevier Science; 1997.
123. Vineis P, Veglia F, Benhamou S, et al. CYP1A1 T3801 C polymorphism and lung cancer: a pooled analysis of 2451 cases and 3358 controls. *Int J Cancer* 2003;104:650–657.
124. Carlsten C, Sagoo GS, Frodsham AJ, et al. Glutathione S-transferase M1 (GSTM1) polymorphisms and lung cancer: a literature-based systematic HuGE review and meta-analysis. *Am J Epidemiol* 2008;167:759–774.
125. Ahrendt SA, Decker PA, Alawi EA, et al. Cigarette smoking is strongly associated with mutation of the K-ras gene in patients with primary adenocarcinoma of the lung. *Cancer* 2001;92:1525–1530.
126. Ding L, Getz G, Wheeler DA, et al. Somatic mutations affect key pathways in lung adenocarcinoma. *Nature* 2008;455:1069–1075.
127. Johnson L, Mercer K, Greenbaum D, et al. Somatic activation of the K-ras oncogene causes early onset lung cancer in mice. *Nature* 2001;410:1111–1116.
128. Sekido Y, Fong KW, Minna JD. Progress in understanding the molecular pathogenesis of human lung cancer. *Biochim Biophys Acta* 1998;1378:F21–F59.
129. Bode AM, Dong A. Signal transduction pathways in cancer development and as targets for cancer prevention. *Prog Nucleic Acid Res Mol Biol* 2005;79:237–297.
130. Schuller HM. Mechanisms of smoking-related lung and pancreatic adenocarcinoma development. *Nat Rev Cancer* 2002;2:455–463.
131. Heeschen C, Jang JJ, Weis M, et al. Nicotine stimulates angiogenesis and promotes tumor growth and atherosclerosis. *Nat Med* 2001;7:833–839.
132. West KA, Brognard J, Clark AS, et al. Rapid Akt activation by nicotine and a tobacco carcinogen modulates the phenotype of normal human airway epithelial cells. *J Clin Invest* 2003;111:81–90.
133. Moraitis D, Du B, De Lorenzo MS, et al. Levels of cyclooxygenase-2 are increased in the oral mucosa of smokers: evidence for the role of epidermal growth factor receptor and its ligands. *Cancer Res* 2005;65:664–670.

5 Oncogenic Viruses

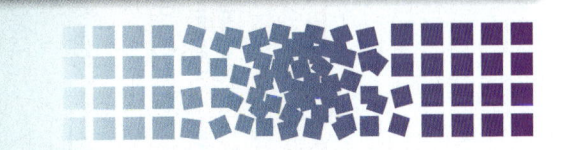

Christopher B. Buck and Lee Ratner

PRINCIPLES OF TUMOR VIROLOGY

Viral infections are estimated to play a causal role in at least 11% of all new cancer diagnoses worldwide.[1] A vast majority of cases (>85%) occur in developing countries, where poor sanitation, high rates of cocarcinogenic factors such as HIV/AIDS, and lack of access to vaccines and cancer screening all contribute to increased rates of virally induced cancers. Even in developed countries, where effective countermeasures are widely available, cancers attributable to viral infection account for at least 4% of new cases.[2,3]

Viruses thought to cause various forms of human cancer come from six distinct viral families with a range of physical characteristics (Table 5.1). All known human cancer viruses are capable of establishing durable, long-term infections and cause cancer only in a minority of persistently infected individuals. The low penetrance of cancer induction is consistent with the idea that a virus capable of establishing a durable productive infection would not benefit from inducing a disease that kills the host.[4] The slow course of cancer induction (typically over a course of many years after the initial infection) suggests that viral infection alone is rarely sufficient to cause human malignancy and that virally induced cancers arise only after additional oncogenic "hits" have had time to accumulate stochastically.

In broad terms, viruses can cause cancer through either (or both) of two broad mechanisms: direct or indirect. Direct mechanisms, in which the virus-infected cell ultimately becomes malignant, are typically driven by the effects of viral oncogene expression or through direct genotoxic effects of viral gene products. In most established examples of direct viral oncogenesis, the cancerous cell remains "addicted" to viral oncogene expression for ongoing growth and viability.

A common feature of DNA viruses that depend on host cell DNA polymerases for replication (e.g., papillomaviruses, herpesviruses, and polyomaviruses) is the expression of viral gene products that promote progression into the cell cycle. A typical mechanism of direct oncogenic effects is through the inactivation of tumor suppressor proteins, such as the guardian of the genome, p53, and retinoblastoma protein (pRB). This effectively primes the cell to express the host machinery necessary for replicating the viral DNA. The study of tumor viruses has been instrumental in uncovering the existence and function of key tumor suppressor proteins, as well as key cellular proto-oncogenes, such as Src and Myc.

In theory, viruses could cause cancer via direct hit-and-run effects. In this model, viral gene products may serve to preserve cellular viability and promote cell growth in the face of otherwise proapoptotic genetic damage during the early phases of tumor development. In principle, the precancerous cell might eventually accumulate enough additional genetic hits to allow for cell growth and survival independent of viral oncogene expression. This would allow for stochastic loss of viral nucleic acids from the nascent tumor, perhaps giving a growth advantage due to the loss of "foreign" viral antigens that might otherwise serve as targets for immune-mediated clearance of the nascent tumor. Although hit-and-run effects have been observed in animal models of virally induced cancer,[5] these effects are extremely difficult to address in humans. Currently, there are no clearly established examples of hit-and-run effects in human cancer.

In indirect oncogenic mechanisms, the cells that give rise to the malignant tumor have never been infected by the virus. Instead, the viral infection is thought to lead to cancer by attracting inflammatory immune responses that, in turn, lead to accelerated cycles of tissue damage and regeneration of noninfected cells. In some instances, virally infected cells may secrete paracrine signals that drive the proliferation of uninfected cells. At a theoretical level, it may be difficult to distinguish between indirect carcinogenesis and hit-and-run direct carcinogenesis, because, in both cases, the metastatic tumor may not contain any viral nucleic acids.

A variety of hunting approaches have been used to uncover etiologic roles for viruses in human cancer. The first clues that high-risk human papillomaviruses (HPVs), Epstein-Barr virus (EBV), Kaposi's sarcoma–associated herpesvirus (KSHV), and Merkel cell polyomavirus (MCPyV) might be carcinogenic were based on the detection of virions, viral DNA, or viral RNA in the tumors these viruses cause. A common feature of known virally induced cancers is that they are more prevalent in immunosuppressed individuals, such as individuals suffering from HIV/AIDS or patients on immunosuppressive therapy after organ transplantation. This is thought to reflect the lack of immunologic control over the cancer-causing virus. Studies focused on AIDS-associated cancers provided the first evidence for the carcinogenic potential of KSHV and MCPyV. A theoretical limitation of this approach is that some virally induced cancers may not occur at dramatically elevated rates in all types of immunosuppressed subjects, particularly if the virus causes only a fraction of cases (e.g., HPV-induced head and neck cancers). Fortunately, the unbiased analysis of nucleic acid sequences found in tumors has become substantially more tractable as deep-sequencing methods have continued to fall in price. In the coming years, it should be increasingly possible to search for viral sequences without making the starting assumption that all virally induced tumors are associated with immunosuppression.[6]

One limitation of tumor sequencing approaches is that they might miss undiscovered divergent viral species within viral families known to have extensive sequence diversity[7] and could miss viral families that have not yet been discovered.[8] Tumor-sequencing approaches might also miss viruses that cause cancer by hit-and-run or indirect mechanisms. It is conceivable that this caveat could be addressed by focusing on sequencing early precancerous lesions thought to ultimately give rise to metastatic cancer.

An additional successful approach to hunting cancer viruses involves showing that individuals who are infected with a particular virus have an increased long-term risk of developing particular forms of cancer. This approach was successful for identifying and validating the carcinogenic roles of high-risk HPV types, hepatitis B virus (HBV), hepatitis C virus (HCV), KSHV, and human T-lymphotropic virus 1 (HTLV-1). Although viruses that are extremely prevalent, such as EBV and MCPyV, are not amenable to this approach per se, it may still be possible to draw connections

TABLE 5.1
Oncogenic Viruses

Virus	Taxon	Viral Genome	Virion	Infection Rate	Site of Persistence	Diseases in Normal Hosts	Diseases in Immunocompromised Hosts	Associated Cancers
High-risk human papillomavirus types (e.g., HPV16)	*Alphapapillomavirus*	8 kb circular dsDNA	Nonenveloped	>70%	Anogenital mucosa, oral mucosa	Carcinomas of the cervix, penis, anus, vagina, vulva, tonsils, base of tongue	Increased incidence of same diseases	610,000
Hepatitis B virus (HBV)	*Hepadnaviridae*	3 kb ss/dsDNA	Enveloped	2%–8%	Hepatocytes	Cirrhosis, hepatocellular carcinoma	Same diseases, increased incidence with AIDS	380,000
Hepatitis C virus (HCV)	*Flaviviridae*	10 kb +RNA	Enveloped	~3%	Hepatocytes	Cirrhosis, hepatocellular carcinoma, splenic marginal zone lymphoma	Same diseases, increased incidence with AIDS	220,000
Epstein-Barr virus (EBV, HHV-4)	*Gammaherpesvirinae*	170 kb linear DNA	Enveloped	90%	B cells, pharyngeal mucosa	Mononucleosis, Burkitt lymphoma, other non-Hodgkin lymphoma, nasopharyngeal carcinoma	Increased incidence of same diseases, lymphoproliferative disease, other lymphomas, oral hairy leukoplakia, leiomyosarcoma	110,000
Kaposi's sarcoma herpesvirus (KSHV, HHV-8)	*Gammaherpesvirinae*	170 kb linear DNA	Enveloped	2%–60%	Oral mucosa, endothelium, B cells	Kaposi's sarcoma (KS), multicentric Castleman disease (MCD)	Increased KS, MCD incidence, primary effusion lymphoma	43,000
Merkel cell polyomavirus (MCPyV, MCV)	*Orthopolyomavirus*	5 kb circular dsDNA	Nonenveloped	75%	Skin (lymphocytes?)	Merkel cell carcinoma (MCC)	Increased MCC incidence	1,500 (US)
Human T-cell leukemia virus (HTLV-1)	*Deltaretrovirus*	9 kb +RNA (RT)	Enveloped	0.01%–6%	T and B cells	Adult T-cell leukemia/lymphoma, tropical spastic paraparesis, myelopathy, uveitis, dermatitis	Unknown	2,100

Note: Ranges for infection rates imply major variations in prevalence among populations in different world regions. *Associated cancers* indicates the annual number of new cases clearly attributable to viral infection. An estimate for the worldwide incidence of Merkel cell carcinoma is not currently available and an estimate of the annual new cases in the United States alone is given instead.

ds, double-stranded; ss, single-stranded; HHV, human herpesvirus; RT, reverse transcriptase.

Adapted from de Martel C, Ferlay J, Franceschi S, et al. Global burden of cancers attributable to infections in 2008: a review and synthetic analysis. *Lancet Oncol* 2012;13(6):607–615; Schiller JT, Lowy DR. Virus infection and human cancer: an overview. *Recent Results Cancer Res* 2014;193:1–10; Chen CJ, Hsu WL, Yang HI, et al. Epidemiology of virus infection and human cancer. *Recent Results Cancer Res* 2014;193:11–32; and Virgin HW, Wherry EJ, Ahmed R. Redefining chronic viral infection. *Cell* 2009;138(1):30–50.

between cancer risk and either unusually high serum antibody titers against viral antigens or unusually high viral load. Relatively high serologic titers reflect either comparatively poor control of the viral infection in at-risk individuals or expression of viral antigens in tumors or tumor precursor cells.[9,10]

The finding that a virus causes cancer is good news, in the sense that it can suggest possible paths to clinical intervention. These can include the development of vaccines or antiviral agents that prevent, attenuate, or eradicate the viral infection and thereby prevent cancer; the development of methods for early detection or diagnosis of cancer based on assays for viral nucleic acids or gene products; or the development of drugs or immunotherapeutics that treat cancer by targeting viral gene products. Unfortunately, establishing the carcinogenicity of a given viral species is an arduous process that must inevitably integrate multiple lines of evidence.[11] The demonstration that the virus can transform cells in culture and/or cause cancer in animal models provides circumstantial evidence of the oncogenic potential of a virus. All known human cancer viruses meet this criterion. However, it is important to recognize that viruses can theoretically coevolve to be noncarcinogenic in their native host (e.g., humans) and cause cancer only in the dysregulated environment of a nonnative host animal. This caveat may apply to human adenoviruses.

Finding that viral DNA is clonally integrated in a primary tumor and its metastatic lesions helps address the caveat that the virus might merely be a hitchhiker that finds the tumor cell a conducive environment in which to replicate (as opposed to playing a causal carcinogenic role). This caveat is also addressed by the observation that, in most instances, viruses found in tumors have lost the ability to exit viral latency and are functionally unable to produce new progeny virions. An unfortunate consequence of this is that vaccines or antiviral agents that target virion proteins (e.g., vaccines against high-risk HPVs or HBV) or gene products expressed late in the viral life cycle (e.g., herpesvirus thymidine kinase, which is the target of drugs such as ganciclovir) are rarely effective for treating existing virally induced tumors.

Demonstrating that a vaccine or antiviral agent targeting the virus either prevents or treats human cancer is by far the strongest form of evidence that a given virus causes human cancer. This type of proof has fully validated the causal role of HBV in human liver cancer. Compelling clinical trial data also show that antiherpesvirus therapeutics can prevent KSHV- or EBV-associated lymphoproliferative disorders, and that vaccination against HPV can prevent the development of precancerous lesions on the uterine cervix.

PAPILLOMAVIRUSES

History

The idea that cancer of the uterine cervix might be linked to sexual behavior was first proposed in the mid 19th century by Dominico Rigoni-Stern, who observed that nuns rarely contracted cervical cancer, whereas prostitutes suffered from cervical cancer more often than the general populace.[12] Another major milestone in cervical cancer research was Georgios Papanikolaou's development of the so-called Pap smear for early cytologic diagnosis of precancerous cervical lesions.[13] This form of screening, which allows for surgical intervention to remove precancerous lesions, has saved many millions of lives in developed countries, where public health campaigns have made testing widely available.

Although observations in the early 1980s suggested the possibility of a hit-and-run carcinogenic role for herpes simplex viruses in cervical cancer,[14] this hypothesis was abandoned in light of studies led by Harald zur Hausen. Low-stringency hybridization approaches revealed the presence of two previously unknown papillomavirus types, HPV16 and HPV18, in various cervical cancer cell lines, including the famous HeLa cell line.[15,16] There is now overwhelming evidence that a group of more than a dozen sexually transmitted HPV types, including HPV16 and HPV18, play a causal role in essentially all cases of cervical cancer. HPVs associated with a high risk of cancer also cause about half of all penile cancers, 88% of anal cancers, 43% of vulvar cancers, 70% of vaginal cancers,[2] and an increasing fraction of head and neck cancers (see the following). In 2008, zur Hausen was awarded the Nobel Prize for his groundbreaking work establishing the link between HPVs and human cancer.

The viral family *Papillomaviridae* is named for the benign skin warts (papillomas) that some members of the family cause. In the early 1930s, Richard Edwin Shope and colleagues demonstrated viral transmission of papillomas in a rabbit model system.[17] Using this system, Peyton Rous and others showed that cottontail rabbit papillomavirus-induced lesions can progress to malignant skin cancer.[18,19] This was the first demonstration of a cancer-causing virus in mammals, building on Rous' prior work demonstrating a virus capable of causing cancer in chickens (the Rous sarcoma retrovirus).

Tissue Tropism and Gene Functions

Although papillomaviruses can achieve infectious entry into a wide variety of cell types in vitro and in vivo, the late phase of the viral life cycle, during which the viral genome undergoes vegetative replication and the L1 and L2 capsid proteins are expressed, is strictly dependent on host cell factors found only in differentiating keratinocytes near the surface of the skin or mucosa. Interestingly, a majority of HPV-induced cancers appear to arise primarily at zones of transition between stratified squamous epithelia and the single-layer (columnar) epithelia of the endocervix, the inner surface of the anus, and tonsillar crypts. It is thought that the mixed phenotypic milieu in cells at squamocolumnar transition zones may cause dysregulation of the normal coupling of the HPV life cycle to keratinocyte differentiation.

There are nearly 200 known HPV types.[20] In general, each papillomavirus type is a functionally distinct serotype, meaning that serum antibodies that neutralize one HPV type do not robustly neutralize other HPV types. Various HPV types preferentially infect different skin or mucosal surfaces. Different types tend to establish either transient infections that may be cleared over the course of months, or stable infections where virions are chronically shed from the infected skin surface for the lifetime of the host. HPV infections may or may not be associated with the formation of visible warts or other lesions. High-risk HPV types, with clearly established causal links to human cancer, are preferentially tropic for the anogenital mucosa and the oral mucosa, are usually transmitted by sexual contact, rarely cause visible warts, and usually establish only transient infections in a great majority of exposed individuals. The lifetime risk of sexual exposure to a high-risk HPV type has been estimated to be >70%. Individuals who fail to clear their infection with a high-risk HPV type and remain persistently infected are at much greater risk of developing cancer. Polymerase chain reaction (PCR)-based screening for the presence of high-risk HPV types thus serves as a useful adjunct to, or even a replacement for, the traditional Pap test.[21]

A consequence of the strict tissue-differentiation specificity of the papillomavirus life cycle is that HPVs do not replicate in standard monolayer cell cultures. Papillomaviruses also seem to be highly species restricted, and there are no known examples of an HPV type capable of infecting animals.[22] Thus, the investigation of key details of papillomavirus biology has relied almost entirely on modern recombinant DNA and molecular biologic analyses.

Papillomavirus genomes are roughly 8 kb, double-stranded, closed-circular DNA molecules (essentially reminiscent of a plasmid). During the normal viral life cycle, the genome does not adopt a linear form, does not integrate into the host cell chromosome, and remains as an extrachromosomal episome or minichromosome.

All the viral protein-coding sequences are arranged on one strand of the genome. The expression of various proteins is regulated by differential transcription and polyadenylation, as well as effects at the level of RNA splicing, export from the nucleus, and translation. In addition to the late half of the viral genome, which encodes the L1 and L2 capsid proteins, all papillomaviruses encode six key early region genes: E1, E2, E4, E5, E6, and E7.

The master transcriptional regulator E2 serves as a transcriptional repressor, and loss of E2 expression (typically through integration of the viral episome into the host cell DNA) results in the upregulation of early gene expression. The most extensively studied early region proteins are the E6 and E7 oncogenes of HPV16 and HPV18. The E6 protein of high-risk HPV types triggers the destruction of p53 by recruiting a host cell ubiquitin–protein ligase, E6AP.[23-25] Another important oncogenic function of E6 is the activation of cellular telomerase.[26] A wide variety of additional high-risk E6 activities that do not involve p53 have been identified.[27]

Most E7 proteins, including those of many low-risk HPV types, contain a conserved LXCXE motif that mediates interaction with pRB and the related "pocket" proteins p107 and p130.[28] Interestingly, the LXCXE motif is present in a wide variety of other oncogenes, most notably the T antigens of polyomaviruses and the E1A oncogenes of adenoviruses. The interaction of E7 with pRB disrupts the formation of a complex between pRB and E2F transcription factors, thereby blocking the ability of pRB to trigger cell cycle arrest.[29] The E7 proteins of high-risk HPVs can also contribute to chromosomal mis-segregation and aneuploidy, which may in turn contribute to malignant progression.[30] Like E6, E7 interacts with a wide variety of additional cellular targets, the spectrum of which seems to vary with different HPV types.[27]

Some papillomavirus types express an E5 oncogene, which functions as an agonist for cell surface growth factor receptors such as platelet-derived growth factor beta (PDGF-β) and epidermal growth factor (EGF) receptor.[31] Because E5 expression is uncommon in cervical tumors, it is uncertain whether the protein plays a key role in human cancer.

Human Papilloma Virus Vaccines

Two preventive vaccines against cancer-causing HPVs, trade named Gardasil (Merck) and Cervarix (GSK), are currently marketed worldwide for the prevention of cervical cancer. Both vaccines contain recombinant L1 capsid proteins based on HPV16 and HPV18 that are assembled in vitro into virus-like particles (VLPs). Together, HPV16 and HPV18 cause about 70% of all cases of cervical cancer worldwide. Gardasil also includes VLPs based on HPV types 6 and 11, which rarely cause cervical cancer but together cause about 90% of all genital warts. The VLPs contained in the vaccines are highly immunogenic in humans, eliciting high-titer serum antibody responses against L1 that are capable of neutralizing the infectivity of the cognate HPV types represented in the vaccine. It appears that the current HPV vaccines may confer lifelong immunity against new infection with the HPV types represented in the vaccine.[32] The vaccines elicit lower titer cross-neutralizing responses against a subset of cancer-causing HPV types that are closely related to HPV16 and HPV18.[33] Although these cross-neutralizing responses can at least partially protect vaccinees against a new infection with additional high-risk types, such as HPV31 and HPV45, it remains unclear how durable the lower level cross-protection will be.[33]

Because L1 is not expressed in latently infected keratinocyte stem cells residing on the epithelial basement membrane, current HPV vaccines are very unlikely to eradicate existing infections.[34,35] Like keratinocyte stem cells, cervical cancers and precursor lesions rarely or never express L1. Thus, the existing L1-based vaccines seem unlikely to serve as therapeutic agents for treating cervical cancer.

Three types of next-generation HPV vaccines are currently in human clinical trials. Merck has recently announced that a newer version of Gardasil, which contains VLPs based on a total of nine different HPV types, remained highly effective against HPV16 and HPV18 and also prevented 97% of precancerous cervical lesions caused by a wider variety of high-risk HPV types.[36] Another class of second-generation vaccines targets the papillomavirus minor capsid protein L2. An N-terminal portion of L2 appears to represent a highly conserved "Achilles' heel", which contains conserved protein motifs required for key steps of the infectious entry process.[37] Anti-L2 antibodies can neutralize a broad range of different human and animal HPV types, and thus, L2 vaccines are hoped to offer protection against all HPVs that cause cervical cancer, all low-risk HPV types that cause abnormal Pap smear results, as well as the full range of HPV types that cause skin warts. Finally, a wide variety of vaccines that seek to elicit cell-mediated immune responses against the E6 and E7 oncoproteins are aimed at a therapeutic intervention for the treatment of cervical cancer.[38]

Oropharyngeal Cancer

It is well established that tobacco products and alcohol cause head and neck cancer. In the late 1990s, Maura Gillison and colleagues noted a surprising number of new cases of tonsillar cancer in nonsmokers.[39] Many of the tumors found in nonsmokers were found to have wild-type p53 genes, raising the possibility that the tumor might be dependent on a p53-suppressing viral oncogene (as seen in cervical cancer). Gillison and colleagues went on to show that nearly half of all tonsillar cancers contain HPV DNA, most commonly HPV16. Interestingly, HPV-positive oropharyngeal cancers tend to be less lethal than tobacco-associated HPV-negative tumors. This finding has important implications for treatment of HPV-positive head and neck cancers.[40]

Although the incidence of tobacco-associated head and neck cancer has been declining in recent decades due to decreased tobacco use, recent studies suggest an ongoing increase in the incidence of HPV-associated cancers of the tonsils and the base of the tongue. By 2025, the number of new HPV-induced head and neck cancer cases in the United States is expected to roughly equal the number of new cervical cancer cases.[39] Based in part on these observations, the U.S. Centers for Disease Control and Prevention recommends that boys, in addition to girls, should be vaccinated against high-risk HPVs.

Nonmelanoma Skin Cancer

Epidermodysplasia verruciformis (EV) is a rare immunodeficiency that is characterized by the appearance of numerous flat, wartlike lesions across wide areas of skin. The lesions typically contain genus betapapillomaviruses, such as HPV5 or HPV8. EV patients frequently develop squamous cell carcinomas (SCC) in sun-exposed skin areas (suggesting that ultraviolet [UV] light exposure is a cofactor). It is also well established that other immunosuppressed individuals, such as organ transplant recipients and HIV-infected individuals, are at increased risk of developing SCC.[41,42] Although the E6 and E7 proteins of betapapillomaviruses appear to exert a different spectrum of effects than the E6 and E7 proteins of HPV types associated with cervical cancer,[43-45] Betapapillomavirus oncogenes can transform cells in vitro.[46] Although these circumstantial lines of evidence suggest that infectious agents, such as Betapapillomaviruses, might play a causal role in SCC, recent deep sequencing studies have observed few or no viral sequences in SCC tumors.[47] Although the results argue against durable direct oncogenic effects of any known viral species in SCC, an animal model system using bovine papillomavirus type 4 strongly suggests that papillomaviruses can cause cancer by hit and run mechanisms.[5] Thus, the question of whether hit-and-run or indirect oncogenic effects of HPVs may be at play in human SCC remains open.

POLYOMAVIRUSES

History

In the early 1950s, Ludwik Gross showed that a filterable infectious agent could cause salivary gland cancer in laboratory mice.[48] Later work by Bernice Eddy and Sarah Stewart showed that the murine polyoma (Greek for "many tumors") virus caused many different types of cancer in experimentally infected mice.[49] The discovery that murine polyomavirus could be grown in cell culture helped rekindle research interest in tumor virology and interest in the question of whether viruses might cause human cancer.

Like papillomaviruses, polyomaviruses have a nonenveloped capsid assembled from 72 pentamers of a single major capsid protein (VP1). Both viral families also carry circular dsDNA genomes. These physical similarities initially led to the classification of both groups into a single family, *Papovaviridae*. When sequencing studies ultimately revealed that polyomaviruses have a unique genome organization (with early and late genes being arranged on opposing strands of the genome) and almost no sequence homology to papillomaviruses, the two groups of viruses were divided into separate families.

In the early 1960s, Bernice Eddy, Maurice Hilleman, and Benjamin Sweet reported the discovery of simian vacuolating virus 40 (SV40), a previously unknown polyomavirus that was found as a contaminant in vaccines against poliovirus.[50,51] SV40 was derived from the rhesus monkey kidney cells used to amplify poliovirus virions in culture.[52] SV40 rapidly became an important model polyomavirus, and studies of its major and minor tumor antigens (large T [LT] and small t [ST], respectively) have played an important role in understanding various aspects of carcinogenesis. Despite significant alarm about the possible risk SV40 might pose to exposed individuals, a comprehensive, decades long series of studies have failed to uncover compelling evidence that SV40 exposure is causally associated with human cancer.[53]

Two naturally human-tropic polyomaviruses, BK virus (BKV) and John Cunningham virus (JCV), were first reported in back-to-back publications in 1971.[54,55] BKV and JCV are known to cause kidney disease and a lethal brain disease called progressive multifocal leukoencephalopathy, respectively, in immunosuppressed individuals. Although both viruses can cause cancer in experimentally exposed animals, it remains unclear whether either virus plays a causal role in human cancer. Although BKV LT expression can frequently be observed in the inflammatory precursor lesions that are thought to give rise to prostate cancer,[56] there is no evidence for the persistence of BKV DNA in malignant prostate tumors.[57] There have been case studies finding BKV T-antigen expression in bladder cancer,[58] and some reports have indicated the presence of JCV DNA in colorectal tumors. The long history of conflicting evidence concerning possible roles for BKV or JCV in human cancer is reviewed elsewhere.[59,60]

Merkel Cell Polyomavirus

In 2008, Yuan Chang and Patrick Moore reported their lab's discovery of the fifth known human polyomavirus species, which they named Merkel cell polyomavirus (MCV or MCPyV) based on its presence in Merkel cell carcinoma (MCC).[61] The discovery used an RNA deep sequencing approach called digital transcriptome subtraction. Using classic Southern blotting, this report demonstrated the clonal integration of MCPyV in an MCC tumor and its distant metastases. Many other labs worldwide have independently confirmed the presence of MCPyV DNA in about 80% of MCC tumors.[11]

MCC is a rare but highly lethal form of cancer that typically presents as a fast-growing lesion on sun-exposed skin surfaces (Fig. 5.1).[62] The risk of MCC is dramatically higher in HIV/AIDS patients, offering an initial clue that MCC might be a virally induced cancer.[63] Although MCC tumors express neuroendocrine markers associated with sensory Merkel cells of the epidermis, one recent report has shown that some MCC tumors also express B-cell markers, including rearranged antibody loci.[64] Currently, there is no clear evidence for the involvement of MCPyV in other tumors with neuroendocrine features.

In 2012, the International Agency for Research on Cancer (IARC) concluded that MCPyV is a class 2A carcinogen (probably carcinogenic to humans).[10,53] It should be noted that IARC evaluations rely heavily on animal carcinogenicity studies, and the 2A designation was assigned prior to a recent report showing that MCV-positive MCC lines are tumorigenic in a mouse model system.[65]

A great majority of healthy adults have serum antibodies specific for the MCPyV major capsid protein VP1. A majority also shed MCPyV virions from apparently healthy skin surfaces, and there is a strong correlation between individual subjects' serologic titer against VP1 and the amount of MCPyV DNA they shed.[66–68] Interestingly, MCC patients tend to have exceptionally strong serologic titers against VP1.[69] MCC tumors do not express detectable amounts of VP1, so this is unlikely to reflect direct exposure to

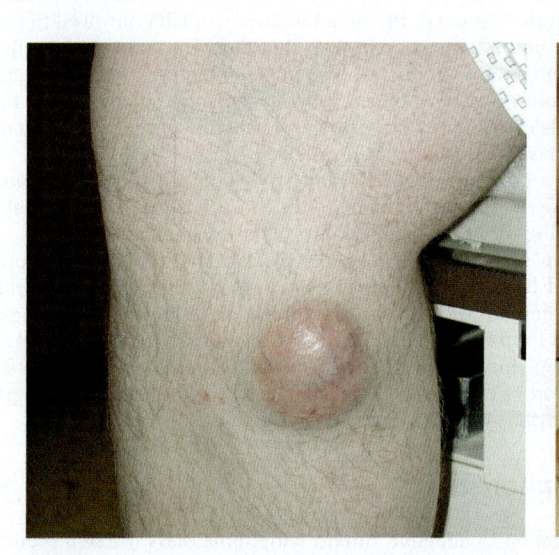

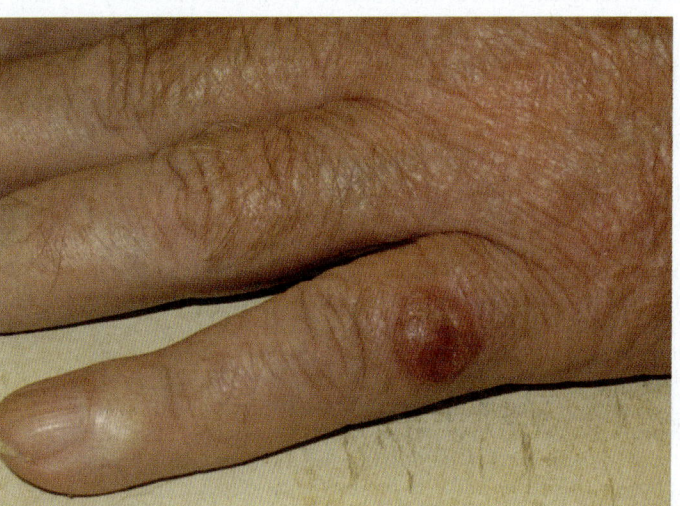

Figure 5.1 Merkel cell carcinoma (MCC). The *left panel* shows an MCC tumor on the calf. The *right panel* shows an MCC tumor on the finger. Photographs provided with permission by Dr. Paul Nghiem (University of Washington, www.merkelcell.org).

the tumor and instead likely represents a history of a high MCPyV load in MCC patients. A recent study of archived serum samples shows that unusually high serologic titers against MCPyV VP1 often precede the development of MCC by many years.[70]

Like the LT protein of SV40 (and the E7 proteins of high-risk HPVs), an N-terminal portion of the MCPyV LT protein contains an LXCXE motif that mediates inactivation of pRB function. In contrast to SV40 LT, which carries a p53-inactivation domain that overlaps the C-terminal helicase domain, MCPyV LT does not appear to inactivate p53 function.[71] Instead, the MCPyV LT helicase domain activates DNA damage responses and induces cell cycle arrest in cultured cell lines.[72] This may explain why the LT genes found in MCC tumors essentially always carry mutations that truncate LT upstream of the helicase domain. siRNA experiments indicate that most (although possibly not all) MCC tumors are "addicted" to the expression of MCPyV T antigens.[73–75] Interestingly, patients with higher levels of MCPyV DNA in their tumors, stronger T-antigen expression, and tumors that have been infiltrated by CD8+ T cells appear to have better prognoses.[76] This is consistent with the idea that cell-mediated immunity can help clear MCC tumors that express MCPyV antigens.

Recent work has shown that the pRB interacting domain of LT mediates increased expression of the cellular gene survivin. The knockdown of survivin using siRNAs results in MCC tumor cell death and YM155, a small molecule inhibitor of survivin expression, protects mice from MCC tumors in a xenograft challenge system.[77,78]

In contrast to SV40, where LT appears to be the dominant oncogene, the MCPyV ST protein appears to play a key role in cell transformation. In addition to modifying the signaling functions of the cellular proto-oncogene PP2A, ST triggers the phosphorylation of eukaryotic translation initiation factor 4E binding protein 1.[79] This results in dysregulation of cap-dependent translation and cellular transformation.

Although there is an intriguing epidemiologic correlation between MCC and chronic lymphocytic leukemia (CLL),[80] there are conflicting reports concerning the presence of MCPyV in CLL and other lymphocytic cancers.[81–83]

Other Human Polyomaviruses

In recent years, the number of known human polyomaviruses has expanded dramatically. Of the 12 currently known HPyV species, only MCPyV has been clearly linked to human cancer. One new HPyV, trichodysplasia spinulosa polyomavirus (TSV or TSPyV) has been found in association with abnormal spiny growths on the facial skin of a small number of immunocompromised individuals.

EPSTEIN-BARR VIRUS

History

In 1958, Denis Burkitt provided the first clear clinical description of an unusual B-cell–derived tumor that frequently affects the jawbones of children in equatorial Africa.[84] After hearing Burkitt give a 1961 lecture entitled "The Commonest Children's Cancer in Tropical Africa – A Hitherto Unrecognized Syndrome," Michael Epstein became interested in the idea that an insect vector-borne infection might account for the high incidence of Burkitt lymphoma in tropical Africa. Epstein, together with then PhD candidate Yvonne Barr, began examining tumor samples sent to them by Burkitt. Electron micrographs of lymphoid cells that grew out of the tumors in culture revealed viral particles with a morphology strikingly similar to herpes simplex viruses.[85] It was soon shown that Epstein-Barr herpesvirus (EBV, later designated human herpesvirus 4 [HHV-4]) can transform cultured B cells and is the agent responsible for infectious mononucleosis.[86–88]

Although the initial conjecture that tropically endemic Burkitt lymphoma depends on a geographically restricted infectious agent ultimately proved correct, it was quickly established that the EBV infection is not restricted to the tropics. It instead appears likely that the malaria parasite *Plasmodium falciparum* is a key geographically restricted cocarcinogen responsible for endemic Burkitt lymphoma.[53] In areas where children suffer repeated malaria infections, it appears that the parasite triggers abnormal B-cell responses, as well as weakened cell-mediated immune function, and these effects of recurring malaria infection in turn promote or allow the development of EBV-induced Burkitt tumors.[11]

Epstein-Barr Virus Life Cycle

EBV chronically infects nearly all humans. In a great majority of individuals, the infection is initially established in early childhood and is never associated with any noticeable symptoms. The infection is typically transmitted when virions, shed in the saliva of a chronically infected individual, come in contact with the oropharyngeal epithelium of a naïve individual. Although infected epithelial cells, such as keratinocytes, might serve to amplify the virus in some circumstances,[89] the establishment of chronic infection is ultimately dependent on mature B cells, as subjects with X-linked agammaglobulinemia (who lack mature B cells) appear to be immune to stable EBV infection.[90] Individuals who escape infection during childhood and instead first become infected during adolescence or adulthood often develop mononucleosis, which is associated with fevers and extreme fatigue lasting for weeks or sometimes months. Interestingly, late-infected individuals who experience mononucleosis and high EBV viral load are at increased risk of developing EBV-positive Hodgkin lymphoma.[91]

EBV-infected B cells can either go on to produce new virions, which are typically associated with cell lysis, or the virus can enter a nonproductive state known as latency. Viral latency is defined as a condition in which the virus expresses few (or possibly no) gene products but can, under some conditions, "reawaken" to express the full range of viral gene products and produce new progeny virions. Latently infected cells are highly resistant to immune clearance.

There are three recognized forms of EBV latency. In latency I, EBV nuclear antigen-1 (EBNA1), which is required for the stable maintenance of the circularized viral DNA minichromosome, is the only viral protein expressed. EBV-derived microRNAs (miRs) may also be expressed. At the other end of the spectrum, latency III is characterized by the expression of EBNA1–6, several latent membrane proteins (LMP1, 2A, and 2B), two noncoding RNAs (EBER1 and 2), the BCL-2 homolog BHRF1, BARF0, and multiple miRs. Although the initial discovery of EBV involved the visualization of virions, indicating that the virus had exited latency and entered the productive lytic phase of the life cycle, viral gene expression in EBV-induced cancers generally follows one of the three latent patterns. The oncogenic activities of various EBV gene products have recently been reviewed.[87,88]

In a great majority of healthy individuals, EBV exists almost exclusively in a latent state, with the occasional asymptomatic shedding of virions in the saliva. The infection is controlled, at least in part, by CD8+ T cells specific for various latency proteins. EBV, like other herpesviruses, expresses a variety of proteins that interfere with cell-mediated immune responses. Intriguingly, results from mouse model systems suggest that the chronic immunostimulatory effects of persistent gammaherpesvirus emergence (or abortive emergence) from latency in healthy hosts can nonspecifically boost immunity to other infections.[92]

Lymphomas

In addition to endemic Burkitt lymphoma, EBV is often present in sporadic cases of Burkitt lymphoma in individuals who have not been exposed to malaria. Although nearly all cases of endemic

Burkitt's lymphoma contain EBV DNA in the tumor (typically in a latency I–like state), only about 20% of sporadic cases arising in immunocompetent individuals contain EBV. Rates of Burkitt lymphoma are elevated in HIV-infected individuals, and HIV-associated Burkitt lymphomas contain EBV in about 30% of cases.

A common hallmark of all types of Burkitt's lymphomas is deregulation of the cellular Myc proto-oncogene. A classic mutation involves chromosomal translocation of the Myc gene to the antibody heavy chain locus. Burkitt's lymphoma tumors that lack detectable EBV DNA tend to carry multiple additional mutations in host cell genes, raising the possibility that an originally EBV-positive precursor cell ultimately accumulated mutations that rendered it independent of viral genes.[88,93]

In addition to Burkitt lymphoma, EBV is associated, to varying extents, with a histologically diverse range of other lymphoid cancers, including Hodgkin lymphoma, natural killer (NK)/T-cell lymphoma, primary central nervous system (CNS) lymphoma, and diffuse large B-cell lymphoma. The incidence of these various forms of lymphoma is significantly increased both in AIDS patients as well as in iatrogenically and congenitally immunosuppressed individuals.[88] In particular, the essentially universal presence of EBV in CNS lymphomas in AIDS patients makes it possible to diagnose the disease with a PCR test for EBV that, together with radiologic findings, can obviate the need for a brain biopsy.

EBV is almost invariably associated with lymphoproliferative disorders, such as plasmacytic hyperplasia and polymorphic B cell hyperplasia, which are often observed in organ transplant recipients. These polyclonal lymphoproliferative responses can, in some instances, progress to oligoclonal or monoclonal lymphomas of various types. The occurrence of EBV-associated lymphoproliferative disease in immunosuppressed patients is generally heralded by the increased detection of EBV DNA in the peripheral blood and the oral cavity. This presumably reflects the failure of cellular immune responses to drive the virus into full latency and perhaps also a failure of cell-mediated immune responses targeting latency-associated EBV gene products present in the nascent tumor.

Carcinomas

In Southern China, NPC affects 25 out of 100,000 people, accounting for 18% of all cancers in China as a whole.[94] Most other world regions have a 25- to 100-fold lower rate of NPC. EBV is present in nearly all cases of NPC, both in endemic and nonendemic regions. Although there is support for the idea that dietary intake of salted fish and other preserved foods is a factor in endemic NPC, it remains possible that genetic traits or as yet unidentified environmental cocarcinogenic factors may play a role as well. Individuals with rising or relatively high IgA antibody responses to EBNA1, DNase, and/or EBV capsid antigens have a dramatically increased risk of developing NPC, offering an early detection method for at-risk individuals.[87]

EBV is also present in a small percentage (5% to 15%) of gastric adenocarcinomas and over 90% of gastric lymphoepithelioma-like carcinomas. In contrast to NPC, the prevalence of EBV-associated gastric cancer is similar in all world regions. As with NPC, elevated antibody responsiveness to EBV antigens may offer a method for identifying individuals at greater risk of gastric cancer.

Prevention and Treatment

The reduction of immunosuppression in response to increasing EBV loads is a standard approach to preventing EBV diseases in T-cell immunosuppressed individuals. Another approach to the prevention of EBV disease relies on ganciclovir (or related antiherpesvirus drugs), which can trigger the death of cells that express the EBV thymidine kinase gene. Pretreating at-risk individuals, such as organ transplant recipients, with ganciclovir has been shown to effectively prevent the development of EBV-induced lymphoproliferative disorders.[95] However, it is important to note that thymidine kinase is only expressed in the lytic phase of the viral life cycle, and drugs of this class are not generally effective for treating existing tumors, presumably due to the fact that EBV gene expression in tumors is typically of a latent type.

Although a recently developed vaccine targeting the EBV gp350 virion surface antigen did not provide sterilizing immunity to EBV infection, vaccinees did experience lower peak EBV viral loads upon infection.[96] Given the strong correlation between high EBV loads and the development of EBV diseases, it is hoped that the vaccine's ability to merely blunt the acute infection may offer significant protection against disease.

Most forms of EBV-associated lymphoid cancers express the B-cell marker CD20, making rituximab (an anti-CD20 mAb) a potentially effective adjunct therapy.[97,98] An emerging treatment approach that has recently entered clinical trials involves stimulating T cells ex vivo against peptides based on EBV antigens or against autologous EBV-transformed B cells.

KAPOSI'S SARCOMA HERPESVIRUS

History and Epidemiology

In the late 19th century, Hungarian dermatologist Moritz Kaposi's described a relatively rare type of indolent pigmented skin sarcoma affecting older men.[99] Kaposi's sarcoma (KS) was later found to be more prevalent in the Mediterranean region and in eastern portions of sub-Saharan Africa.[100] An early clue to the emergence of the HIV/AIDS pandemic in the early 1980s was a dramatic increase in the incidence of highly aggressive forms of KS, particularly in gay men who were much younger than typical KS patients. After the discovery of HIV, it was briefly hypothesized that HIV might be a direct cause of KS. However, this hypothesis failed to explain the existence of KS long prior to the HIV pandemic and the low incidence of KS in individuals who became infected with HIV via blood products. This latter observation was more easily explained by the existence of a sexually transmitted cofactor other than HIV.[101]

Using a subtractive DNA hybridization approach known as representational difference analysis, Yuan Chang, Patrick Moore, and colleagues discovered the presence of a previously unknown herpesvirus in KS tumors.[102] The newly founded field of research rapidly established key lines of evidence supporting the conclusion that KSHV (later designated human herpesvirus-8 [HHV-8]) is a causal factor in KS.[11]

It is now clear that the rate of KSHV infection varies greatly in different world regions.[11,103] In North America and Western Europe, KSHV seroprevalence in the general population ranges from 1% to 7%. Seroprevalence among gay men in these regions is substantially higher (25% to 60%), suggesting a possible link to sexual transmission. KSHV infection is much more prevalent in the general population in central and eastern Africa, where seroprevalence ranges from 23% to 70%. In endemic areas, up to 15% of children are seropositive, suggesting either vertical transmission or transmission via nonsexual casual contact (presumably via saliva). In endemic regions, KS is estimated to be the third most common cancer among adults.[104]

Kaposi's Sarcoma-Associated Herpesvirus in Kaposi's Sarcoma

KS tumors are complex on a number of levels. In contrast to most other forms of cancer, where it is often clear that a single cell type has proliferated out of control, KS tumors are composed of cells from multiple lineages (Fig. 5.2). KSHV-infected cells in the tumor often have a spindle-shaped morphology. Interestingly,

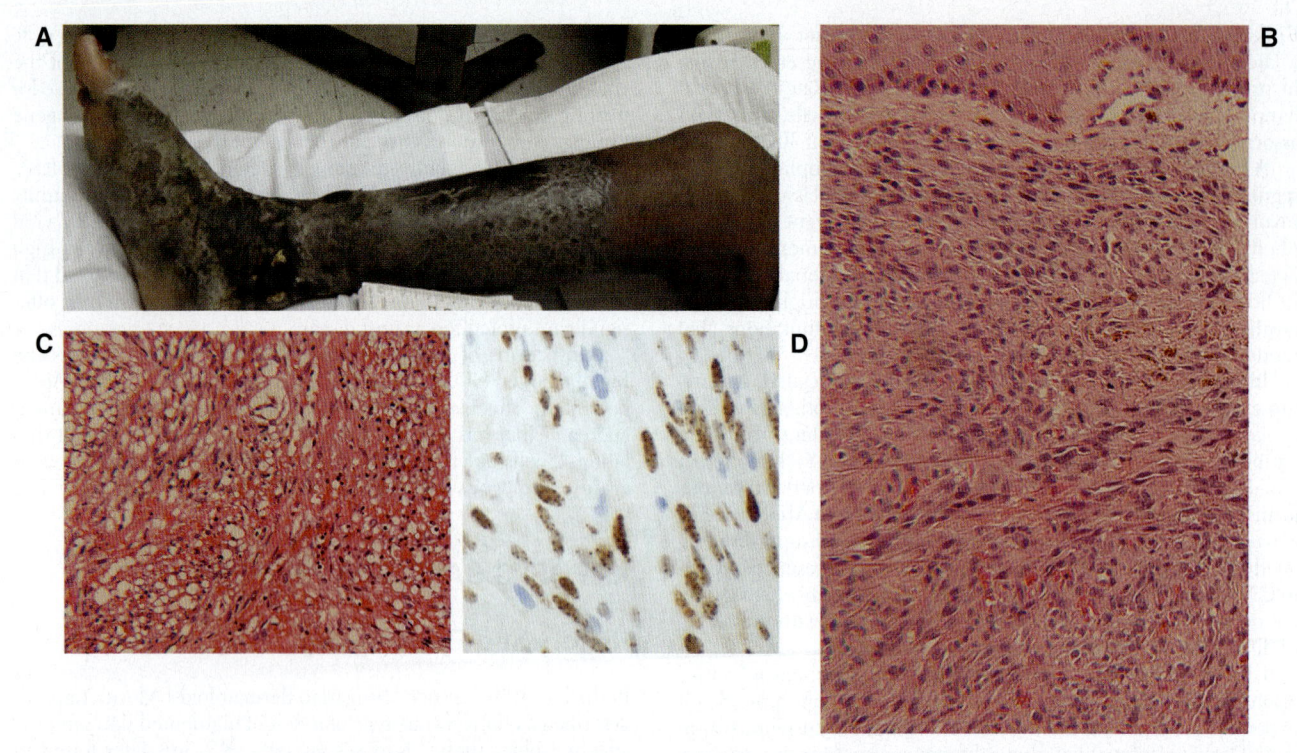

Figure 5.2 Kaposi's sarcoma (KS). **(A)** Photograph of the lower leg of an individual with severe, diffuse KS involving the lower leg. **(B)** Histology of the skin. **(C)** Lung shows a mixture of spindle to epithelioid cells, with slitlike vascular spaces intermixed with red blood cells and red blood cell fragments. **(D)** Immunohistochemical detection of KSHV LANA in the cutaneous tumor. Photographs provided with permission by Drs. Odey Ukpo and Ethel Cesarman.

spindle cells do not exhibit a highly transformed phenotype and tend to show relatively little chromosomal instability. In a culture, the cells are highly dependent on exogenous cytokines and other factors present in the tumor microenvironment in vivo. Although spindle cells express a number of markers of the endothelial lineage, it is uncertain whether they are derived from mature endothelial cells, the early precursor cells that give rise to smooth muscle and vascular endothelial cells, or cells of the lymphatic endothelial lineage. KS tumors also contain infiltrating lymphocytes and monocytes, as well as aberrant neovascular spaces lined with infected and uninfected endothelial cells. The aberrant blood vessels in KS lesion vessels rupture easily and leak red blood cells, giving KS tumors their classic dark red, brown, or purple color.

The latency status of KSHV in KS tumors is also complex, with the expression of gene products typical of latency (e.g., LANA) as well as lytic-phase genes (e.g., RTA/ORF50). Some of these gene products, such as the viral interleukin (IL)-6 homolog (vIL-6), trigger proliferation and secondary cytokine signaling in noninfected cells within the tumor. The tumorigenic effects of individual KSHV gene products have recently been reviewed.[88,103] In contrast to EBV, where tumorigenesis is driven by latency gene expression, it appears that KS pathogenesis is often dependent on lytic phase gene expression. This may explain why ganciclovir, which is not a particularly effective treatment for EBV tumors, was found to prevent the formation of new KS lesions in HIV-positive patients.[105] However, it should be noted that this outcome has more recently proven difficult to reproduce.[106] At present, there are no recommended preventive therapies for individuals at risk of KS, but this is an area of active investigation.

There are a variety of possible explanations for the need for lytic-phase KSHV gene expression during tumor development. For example, infected spindle cells may lose the viral DNA during cell division and require reinfection for ongoing tumorigenicity. Alternatively, factors secreted by a small fraction of tumor cells that enter the lytic phase may be required for tumorigenesis. An important area of current research focus is the role of KSHV gene products in the regulation of angiogenesis in KS lesions[107] and several current trials are investigating inhibitors of angiogenic pathways for the treatment of KS.

Lymphoproliferative Disorders

KSHV causes two forms of B-cell proliferative disorder: multicentric Castleman disease (MCD) and primary effusion lymphoma (PEL). Both diseases are most commonly found in association with HIV infection. In HIV-infected individuals, MCD tumors contain KSHV in nearly all cases, whereas in HIV-negative individuals, the tumor contains KSHV in only about 50% of cases.[108] KSHV in MCD tumors exhibits periodic activation of lytic replication and the expression of lytic phase genes.[109] The expression of vIL-6 during disease flare-ups appears to play a role in MCD pathogenesis, raising the possibility that tocilizumab (a mAb therapeutic that targets the IL-6 receptor) may be of therapeutic benefit.

PEL comprises about 4% of all HIV-associated non-Hodgkin lymphomas.[110] Typically, PEL tumors express markers of both plasma cells (akin to multiple myeloma tumors) and immunoblasts (similar to some EBV-induced tumors). In AIDS patients, essentially all PEL tumors are infected with KSHV and a great majority are also coinfected with EBV.[88] Although PEL is rare in HIV-negative individuals, PEL tumors in such individuals contain KSHV in about 50% of cases.

A common approach to the treatment of all KSHV-associated diseases is the restoration of immune function, either through antiretroviral therapy of HIV/AIDS or through a reduction of immunosuppressive therapy. The general success of immune reconstitution in many KSHV-associated diseases presumably involves an immune-mediated attack of cells expressing KSHV gene products, particularly the many lytic-phase gene products the virus can produce in various disease states.

ANIMAL AND HUMAN RETROVIRUSES

The first oncogenic retroviruses were discovered by Ellerman and Bang in 1908 and by Rous in 1911, but it was many years before the significance of these findings was appreciated.[111] One reason the field was stymied was the failure to identify RNA forms of the viral genome in infected cells. This led to the discovery of the reverse transcriptase independently by Baltimore and Temin in 1970. Another major development was the finding in 1976 of viral oncogenes derived from cellular genes, with the identification by Varmus and Bishop of the first dominant oncogene, *src*. With the discovery of IL-2 by Gallo in 1976, it became possible to culture the first human retrovirus, HTLV-1, from a form of adult T-cell leukemia/lymphoma (ATLL) that was first recognized by Takatsuki and coworkers.[112] These advances opened the door for Montagnier and colleagues' isolation of HIV-1 in 1983, a discovery confirmed independently by Gallo and Levy. This breakthrough led to the first licensed HIV test in 1985.

Retroviruses are positive single-strand RNA viruses that utilize transcription of their RNA genome into a DNA intermediate during virus replication.[111] This accounts for their name, retroviruses, because this is opposite to the normal flow of eukaryotic genetic information. They infect a wide range of vertebrate animal species and are distantly related to repetitive elements in the human genome, known as retrotransposons. Retroviruses are also related to hepadnaviruses, double-stranded DNA viruses, such as hepatitis B virus, which also undergo a reverse transcription step in their replication.

Retroviruses may be classified as *endogenous* or *exogenous* depending on whether they appear in the genome of the host species. There are approximately 100,000 endogenous retroviral elements in the human genome, making up nearly 8% of the genetic information, but their potential roles in disease are unclear.[113] Retroviruses may also be classified as *ecotropic*, *xenotropic*, or *polytropic* depending on whether they infect cells of the same animal species from which they are derived, infect cells of a different species, or both. *Amphotropic* retroviruses infect cells of the species of origin without producing disease, but infect cells of other species and may produce disease.

Retroviruses that produce disease after a long incubation period are termed *lentiviruses* and include human, simian, feline, ovine, caprine, and bovine immunodeficiency viruses. Another group of retroviruses that are not clearly associated with disease are known as *spumaviruses* and include human and simian foamy viruses. HTLV-1, which is classified in the genus Delta, is the only retrovirus known to be oncogenic in humans. A member of the retroviral genus Gamma identified in 2008, designated xenotropic murine leukemia virus-related virus (XMRV), was thought to be associated with human prostate cancer; however, more recent studies showed XMRV to be a lab-derived artifact.[114] A genus betaretrovirus related to the mouse mammary tumor virus has been suggested to be associated with biliary cirrhosis, but this finding requires independent validation.[115]

Retroviruses producing tumors in animals or birds are designated transforming viruses and may be classified as acute or chronic transforming retroviruses. Acute transforming retroviruses have acquired a mutated cellular gene, termed *oncogene*, and induce cancer in an animal within a few weeks. Many dominant acting proto-oncogenes in humans (e.g., *ras*, *myc*, and *erbB*), were first identified as retroviral oncogenes.

Chronic transforming retroviruses integrate almost randomly in the genome, but when integrated in the vicinity of specific genes disrupt their regulation and induce cell proliferation or resistance to apoptosis. Chronic transforming retroviruses induce malignancy only after many weeks to months of infection. The use of a murine leukemia virus vector for gene therapy in children with a form of severe combined immune deficiency syndrome characterized by defective expression of the common gamma chain of the IL-2 receptor resulted in T-cell acute lymphoblastic leukemia. This was found to be the result of persistent expression of the LIM domain only 2 (LMO2) gene triggered by the nearby integration of the retroviral vector.[116]

In addition to acute or chronic transformation mechanisms, retroviruses can transform cells through direct effects on cell physiology mediated by structural or nonstructural viral proteins. Transforming genes of HTLV-1 are nonstructural viral proteins that activate host cell signaling pathways.[117] Because the oncogenic effects of HTLV-1 transforming genes generally take many years to cause cancer, the virus does not fit the precise definition of having either an acute or a chronic oncogenic mechanism.

HIV-1 infection is also associated with a variety of malignancies, but only by indirect effects of suppressing immunity to oncogenic virus infections, such as gammaherpesviruses, high-risk human papillomaviruses, and hepatitis viruses.

Human T-Cell Leukemia Virus Epidemiology

Four species of human T-cell leukemia virus have been identified. HTLV-1 was identified in 1980 as the first human retrovirus associated with cancer, and it is the focus of the remainder of this section.[118] HTLV-2 was discovered in 1982 and shares 70% genomic homology with HTLV-1.[119] HTLV-3 and -4 were sporadically isolated from individuals who had contact with monkeys.[120] HTLV-2, -3, and -4 do not appear to be associated with disease in humans.

HTLV-1 is present in 15 to 20 million individuals worldwide, most commonly in the Caribbean Islands, South America, southern Japan, and parts of Australia, Melanesia, Africa, and Iran.[121] In the United States, Canada, and Europe, 0.01% to 0.03% of blood donors are infected with HTLV-1. It is most commonly found in individuals who emigrated from endemic regions or among African Americans. HTLV-1 is transmitted sexually, by contaminated cell-associated blood products, or by breast-feeding.[122] Only 2% to 5% of HTLV-1–infected individuals develop disease, and ATLL only occurs in individuals who acquired HTLV-1 by breast-feeding.

Human T-Cell Leukemia Virus Molecular Biology

HTLV-1, like other retroviruses, encodes Gag, Protease, Pol, and Envelope proteins.[123] Gag proteins compose the inner nucleocapsid core of the virus. The Pol proteins include the reverse transcriptase and integrase. The reverse transcriptase copies the single-stranded viral RNA into double-stranded DNA, and it is inhibited by several nucleoside analogs, but not by the nonnucleoside reverse transcriptase inhibitors approved for HIV-1.[124] The integrase is responsible for inserting the linear double-stranded DNA product of reverse transcription into the host chromosomal DNA. At least one integrase inhibitor, raltegravir, now approved for HIV-1, is active against HTLV-1.[125] Integration occurs throughout the human genome, but there is preference for integration into transcriptionally active genomic regions.[126] The viral protease proteolytically processes Gag, Protease, and Pol precursor proteins to the mature individual proteins, but it is not affected by inhibitors of HIV-1 protease. The envelope proteins include the transmembrane protein, which anchors the surface envelope protein on the virion, which mediates binding to the viral receptor.[127]

The viral genome also encodes regulatory proteins, including Tax and HTLV-1 bZIP factor (HBZ).[117] Tax is a transcriptional transactivator protein that functions as a coactivator to induce members of the cAMP response element-binding protein/activating transcription factor (CREB/ATF) family, nuclear factor kappa B (NF-κB), and serum response factor (SRF) pathways. Tax activation of the CREB/ATF pathway is responsible for upregulation of the viral promoter. Tax induction of NF-κB promotes cell proliferation and resistance to apoptosis. Tax also binds and activates cyclin-dependent kinases and inhibits cell cycle checkpoint proteins. Tax is important for tumor initiation, whereas HBZ may be important in tumor maintenance.[128]

HTLV-1 preferentially immortalizes CD4+ T lymphocytes and induces tumors in mice.[129] Tax also promotes the leukemia-initiating activity of ATLL cells in mouse models.[130] In immunodeficient mice reconstituted with human hematopoietic cells, HTLV-1 causes CD4+ lymphomas.[131]

Clinical Characteristics and Treatment of HTLV-Associated Malignancies

The diagnosis of HTLV-1 is based on serologic assays.[132] HTLV-1 is associated with various inflammatory disorders, including uveitis, polymyositis, pneumonitis, Sjögren syndrome, and myelopathy. Infected patients are susceptible to certain infectious disorders (e.g. staphylococcal dermatitis) and opportunistic infections such as pneumocystis pneumonia, disseminated cryptococcosis, strongyloidiasis, or toxoplasmosis.[133] Vaccines have not been developed for HTLV infections.

T-lymphocyte proliferative disorders develop in 1% to 5% of infected individuals and are generally CD2+, CD3+, CD4+, CD5+, CD25+, CD29+, CD45RO+, CD52+, HLA-DR+, T-cell receptor αβ+, and variably CD30+, and lack CD7, CD8, and CD26 expression. The virus is clonally integrated in the malignant cells. Complex karyotypes are often found, and cytogenetic analysis is rarely useful. The histologic features of lymph nodes in ATLL may be indistinguishable from those of other peripheral T-cell lymphomas.[134] Circulating tumor "flower cells" are helpful in the diagnosis (Fig. 5.3).

ATLL is categorized in four subtypes.[135] (1) Smoldering ATLL is defined as 5% or more abnormal T lymphocytes and lactate dehydrogenase (LDH) levels up to 1.5× the upper limit of normal, with normal lymphocyte count, calcium, and no lymph node or visceral disease other than skin or pulmonary disease. (2) Chronic ATLL is characterized by lymphocytosis, LDH up to 2× the upper limit of normal, no hypercalcemia, and no CNS, bone, pleural, peritoneal, or gastrointestinal involvement, although the lymph nodes, liver, spleen, skin, or lungs may be involved. The mean survival of these forms of ATLL is 2 to 5 years.[136] No intervention in these subtypes of ATLL has been defined that prevents progression to the more aggressive forms of ATLL. Although chronic or smoldering ATLL may respond to zidovudine and interferon, randomized studies have not been conducted.[137] (3) Lymphoma-type ATLL is characterized by ≤1% abnormal T lymphocytes and features of non-Hodgkin lymphoma. (4) Acute-type ATLL includes the remaining patients. Even with optimal therapy, the median survival of lymphoma and acute-type ATLL is less than 1 year.[138] Lymphoma and acute types of ATLL are the most common presenting subtypes. Other major prognostic factors include performance status, age, the presence of more than three involved lesions, and hypercalcemia.[139]

Combination chemotherapy for lymphoma or acute-type ATLL with the infusional etoposide, prednisone, vincristine, and doxorubicin (EPOCH) regimen or the LSG-15 regimen results in complete remission rates of 15% to 40%.[140,141] However, responses are short lived, with <10% of patients free of disease at 4 years. The addition of anti-CCR4 antibody, mogamulizumab, may improve response rates, but studies are still underway.[142]

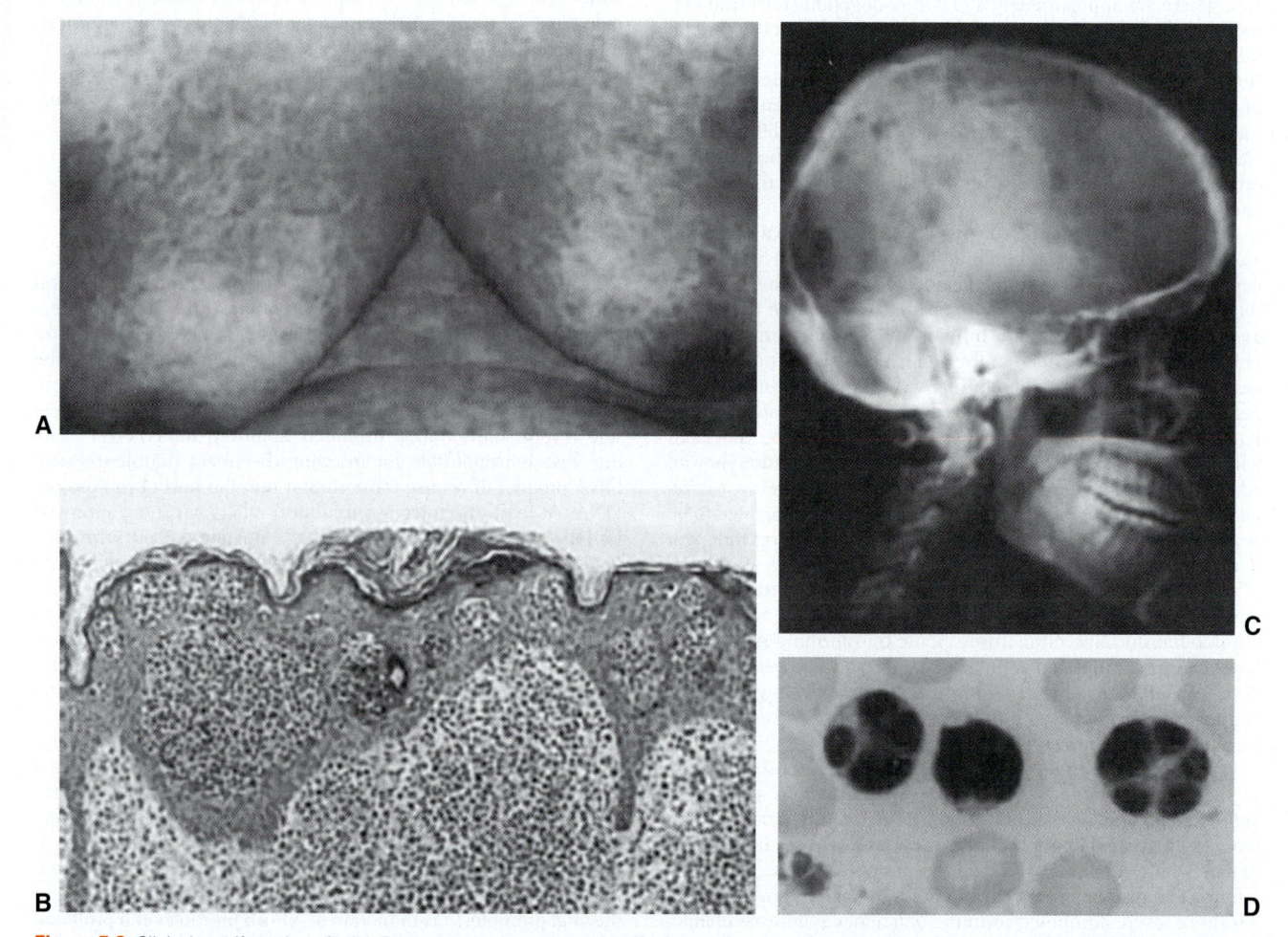

Figure 5.3 Clinical manifestation of adult T-cell leukemia/lymphoma. **(A–B)** Infiltration of malignant T lymphocytes into the skin. **(C)** Lytic bone lesions seen on lateral skull x-ray. **(D)** "Flower cells" in the blood.

The combination of interferon and zidovudine with or without arsenic may result in the remission of acute, but not lymphoma subtypes.[143] Allogenic transplantation may result in long-term, disease-free survival for patients with complete or near complete remission of disease, although infectious complications have been notable in these studies.[144]

HEPATITIS VIRUSES

The earliest record of an epidemic caused by a hepatitis virus was in 1885, occurring in individuals vaccinated for smallpox with lymph from other people.[145] The cause of the epidemic, HBV, was not identified until 1966, when Blumberg discovered the *Australian antigen* now known to be the hepatitis B surface antigen (HBsAg). This was followed by the discovery of the virus particle by Dane in 1970. In the early 1980s, the HBV genome was sequenced and the first vaccines were tested. In the mid 1970s, Alter described cases of hepatitis not due to hepatitis A or B viruses, and the suspected agent was designated non-A, non-B hepatitis virus, now known as HCV.[146] In 1987, Houghton used molecular cloning to identify the HCV genome and develop a diagnostic test, which was licensed in 1990.

Approximately 240 million people are chronically infected with HBV and 150 to 200 million people are infected with HCV worldwide, according to the World Health Organization (WHO). About 1 million deaths per year are attributed to the chronic diseases such as liver cirrhosis and hepatocellular carcinoma (HCC) that result from viral hepatitis infections. HBV and HCV are the leading cause of liver cancer in the world, accounting for almost 80% of the cases. In the United States, Europe, Egypt, and Japan, more than 60% of HCC cases are associated with HCV, and 20% are related to HBV and chronic alcoholism.[147] In Africa and Asia, 60% of HCC is associated with HBV, 20% related to HCV, and the remainder related to other risk factors, such as alcohol and aflatoxin. HCC is the sixth most common cancer worldwide and is the third most common cause of cancer death.[148]

In Asia and Africa, up to 70% of individuals have serologic evidence of current or prior HBV infection, and 8% to 15% of these subjects have a chronic active infection. Rates of HCV infection of >3.5% occur in Central and East Asia, North Africa, and the Middle East. In the United States, 0.8 to 1.4 million individuals are infected with HBV, and 3.2 million with HCV. The incidence of HCC in the United States tripled between 1975 and 2005, particularly in African American and Hispanic males.[149]

HBV is transmitted primarily through exposure to infected blood, semen, and other body fluids, whereas HCV is transmitted primarily by contact with contaminated blood. Acute HCV infection causes mild and vague symptoms in about 15% of individuals and resolves spontaneously in 10% to 50% of cases.[150] Liver enzymes are normal in 5% to 50% of individuals with chronic HCV infection.[151] After 20 years of an HCV infection, the likelihood of cirrhosis is 10% to 15% for men, and 1.5% for women.[152] Cofactors that increase the likelihood of cirrhosis are coinfection with both hepatitis viruses, persistently high levels of HBV or HCV viremia, HBeAg, certain viral genotypes, schistosoma, HIV, alcoholism, male gender, advanced age at the time of infection, diabetes, and obesity.[153,154]

Hepatitis B Virus

HBV is an enveloped DNA virus that is a member of the *Hepadnaviridae* family.[155] HBV has a strong preference for infecting hepatocytes, but small amounts of viral DNA can also be found in kidney, pancreas, and mononuclear cells, although it is not linked to extrahepatic disease. The viral genome is a relaxed circular, partially double-stranded (ds) DNA of 3.2 kb. The genome exists as an episomal covalently closed circular dsDNA (cccDNA) molecule in the nucleus of infected cells, although chromosomal integration of viral genomic sequences can occur during cycles of hepatocyte regeneration and proliferation. In addition to 40 to 42 nm virions, HBV-infected cells also produce noninfectious 20-nm spherical and filamentous particles. The viral genome encodes four open reading frames. The presurface–surface (preS-S) region encodes three proteins from different translational initiation sites; these include the S (HBsAg), M (or pre-S2), and L (or pre-S1) proteins. The L protein is responsible for receptor binding and virion assembly. The precore–core (preC-C) region encodes the HBcAg and HBeAg. The P region encodes the viral polymerase, and the X (HBx) protein modulates host-signal transduction.

After infection, the viral genome is transcribed by host RNA polymerase II, and viral proteins are translated. Nucleocapsids assemble in the cytosol, incorporating a molecule of pregenomic RNA into the viral core, where reverse transcription occurs to produce the dsDNA viral genome. Viral cores are enveloped with intracellular membranes and viral L, M, and S surface antigens, which are exported from the cells.

HBV replication is not cytotoxic. Instead, liver injury is due to the host immune response, primarily T-cell and proinflammatory cytokine responses. Chronic HBV carriers exhibit an attenuated virus-specific T-cells response, although a vigorous humoral response is still evident. About 5% of infections in adults and up to 90% of infections in neonates result in a persistent infection, which may or may not be associated with symptoms and elevated serum aminotransferase levels. About 20% of such individuals develop cirrhosis. Immunosuppressed individuals also have a higher likelihood of a persistent infection.

With acute infection, viral titers of 10^9 to 10^{10} virions per mililiter are present, whereas levels of 10^7 to 10^9 virions per mililiter and HBsAg, and in some cases, HBeAg are present in the blood of individuals with a persistent infection. The resolution of infection, which is associated with declining viral DNA titers, is observed at a rate of 5% to 10% per year in persistently infected individuals. However, even subjects who have resolved the infection continue to have very low levels of viral DNA (10^3 to 10^5 copies per mililiter) for most of their lives.

HBV infection can be managed with alpha interferon or nucleos(t)ide analogs that inhibit the viral polymerase, such as lamivudine, telbivudine, entecavir, adefovir, and tenofovir.[156] Entecavir and tenofovir are both effective at inducing viral suppression, and may be used in combination in patients with high HBV DNA load or multidrug resistance. Because these agents are all associated with some toxicity, current guidelines recommend therapy only when liver disease is clinically apparent, with continued treatment for 6 to 12 months after clearance of HBeAg or HBsAg. Although these drugs effectively control HBV, they typically fail to cure the infection due to the long-term persistence of the cccDNA form of the viral genome. Other nucleos(t)ide analogs are currently in clinical trials, as well as a novel form of interferon (IFN-λ) and an inhibitor of virus release.[157]

Hepatitis D virus (HDV) occurs only in individuals coinfected with HBV. HDV is composed a single-stranded circular viral RNA genome of 1,679 nucleotides, a central core of HDAg, and an outer coat with all three HBV envelope proteins. HDV infection results in more severe complications than infection with HBV alone, with a higher likelihood and more rapid progression to cirrhosis and HCC.

Hepatits C Virus

HCV is an enveloped RNA virus associated with cancer, primarily HCC and, rarely, splenic marginal zone lymphoma.[158] HCV is a positive-sense, single-stranded RNA virus of the *Flaviviridae* family.[159] There are seven genotypes of HCV; in the United States, about 70% of infections are caused by genotype 1.[160] HCV replicates in the cytoplasm and does not integrate into the host cell genome. The viral RNA is 9.6 kb and encodes a single polyprotein of 3,010 amino acids that is proteolytically processed into structural and nonstructural proteins. In addition to the structural roles of the core (C) protein, it has also been reported to affect various host cell functions. The envelope glycoproteins E1 and E2 mediate infectious entry through tetraspanin CD81 and other receptors on hepatocytes and B lymphocytes.

HCV non structural proteins NS2, NS3, NS4A, NS4B, NS5A, NS5B, and p7 are required for virus replication and assembly. NS2 is a membrane-associated cysteine protease. NS3 is a helicase and NTPase that unwinds RNA and DNA substrates. The complex of NS3 with NS4A forms a serine protease. NS4B induces the formation of a membranous web associated with the viral RNA replicase. NS5A is an RNA-binding phosphoprotein, whereas NS5B is the RNA-dependent RNA polymerase. The p7 protein forms a cation channel in infected cells that has a role in particle maturation and release.

Treating an HCV infection typically utilizes 24 to 48 weeks of pegylated IFN-α and ribavirin.[161] Treatment with IFN and ribavirin alone produces sustained virologic responses in 70% to 80% of subjects with genotype 2 or 3 infections. Recently approved inhibitors of the NS3-4A protease (e.g., telaprevir, boceprevir, or simeprevir) may be included in IFN-based regimens, particularly if the patient has failed prior therapy. Protease inhibitors are currently approved for use in IFN/ribavirin combination therapy for HCV genotype 1 or 4 infection. Sofosbuvir, a nucleoside analog inhibitor of the viral NS5B polymerase, has recently been approved for use in combination with ribavirin alone for genotypes 2 or 3, or in triple therapy for genotypes 1 and 4. Recently, IFN-free regimens have also been approved. Additional protease and polymerase inhibitors are currently in development. A recent meta-analysis of eight randomized controlled trials comparing antiviral therapy with placebo suggested that antiviral therapy resulted in a 50% reduced risk of HCC.[162]

Hepatitis Virus Pathogenesis

HBV and HCV depress innate immune responses by inhibiting Toll-like receptor signaling through effects of HBx and NS3-4A.[147] In addition, HCV C inhibits the Janus kinase (JAK)-signal transducer and activator of transcription (STAT) signaling, and NS5A and E2 inhibit IFN signaling. Through an undefined mechanism, HBV can inhibit JAK-STAT signaling as well.

HBV and HCV induce HCC by direct and indirect mechanisms.[147] Both HBV and HCV encode proteins that have pro- and antiapoptotic properties. High levels of HBx block activation of the NF-κB pathway, whereas HCV C and NS5A block apoptosis by the activation of AKT and NF-κB, respectively. The C and NS5A proteins may also induce epithelial–mesenchymal transition (EMT), which is important for liver fibrosis, through effects on transforming growth factor β and Src signaling. Mice transgenic for NS5A develop steatosis and HCC.

HBx and HCV C are associated with mitochondria, where they trigger oxidative stress that induces apoptosis. In addition, HBs and HBx and NS3-4A alter calcium signaling and increase reactive oxygen species, which trigger endoplasmic reticulum (ER) stress, an unfolded protein response, and the production of proinflammatory cytokines that induce collagen synthesis, which drives the development of fibrosis. Autophagy is triggered by both viruses to restore ER integrity, which promotes cell survival and viral persistence.

HBV and HCV also disrupt tumor suppressor proteins. HCV NS5B recruits an ubiquitin ligase protein to modify pRB and induce its degradation, whereas HBx and HCV C proteins both inhibit p16INK4a and p21 cell cycle inhibitors, which leads to the inactivating phosphorylation of pRB. The HBx and HCV C, NS3, and NS5A proteins deregulate p53 tumor suppressor activity, by compromising p53-mediated DNA repair. HBV and HCV also induce alterations in micro-RNAs that are partially responsible for cell cycle effects.

Although not part of the normal virus replication cycle, the tendency of HBV genomic DNA sequences to integrate within the host cell chromosomes also contributes to the pathogenesis of HBV-associated HCC. In most hepatoma cells, HBV replication is extinguished, and integration at certain sites provides a growth or survival advantage, leading to tumors that are clonal with respect to viral integration. Whole-genome sequencing studies have identified a number of cellular loci, including *TERT* and *MLL*, where HBV integration is associated with HCC.[163,164]

Both HBV and HCV promote characteristics of cancer stem cells. HBx promotes the expression of Nanog, Kruppel-like factor 4, octamer-binding transcription factor 4, and Myc. These markers are also induced by HBV and HCV-induced hypoxia and hypoxia-induced factors.

Clinical Characteristics and Treatment of Hepatitis Virus-Associated Malignancies

HBV and HCV infections are diagnosed by serologic assays, and/or antigen assays in the case of HBV.[153] Quantitative HBV DNA and HCV RNA polymerase chain reactions are utilized to measure virus load. No vaccine has been identified that protects against HCV because infections consist of a genetically heterogenous "swarm" of virus particles, some of which escape neutralization. However, a vaccine, which now utilizes a recombinant HBsAg produced in yeast cells, has been available for HBV prevention for more than 30 years. The HBV vaccine reduces the risk of infection by more than 70%.[157] Factors associated with HBV vaccination failure in adults include increased age, obesity, smoking, diabetes, end-stage renal disease, HIV infection, alcoholism, or recipients of liver or kidney transplantation. There have been recent suggestions that emerging HBV strains may be evolving to escape neutralizing antibodies elicited by the current vaccine.[165] Novel vaccine adjuvants are currently in clinical trials, as well as studies of a therapeutic HBV vaccine.

Because an early diagnosis of HCC is key to a successful treatment, there has been extensive research on surveillance techniques in HBV- and HCV-infected individuals.[166] The U.S. Centers for Disease Control and Prevention has recently recommended that all individuals born between 1945 and 1965 be tested for HCV infection. The American Association for the Study of Liver Diseases, as well as the European and Asian Pacific Associations for the Study of the Liver, endorse surveillance in HCV-infected individuals with cirrhosis using ultrasound every 6 months. Viral eradication does not fully eliminate the risk of HCC, and thus, continued surveillance is still recommended in cirrhotic patients.

Therapeutic options for HCC are determined not only by the number and size of HCC nodules as well as the presence or absence of vascular invasion and metastases, but also by liver function and the presence or absence of portal hypertension.[167] HCC amenable to liver transplantation is usually defined as either one tumor measuring ≤50 mm in diameter or two to three tumors measuring ≤30 mm in diameter without vascular extension or metastasis (Milan criteria).[168] Up to 30% of all cases of HCC present with multiple nodules of HCC, suggesting a field carcinogenesis effect of HBV and HCV.[169] HBV- and HCV-infected patients may have a lower survival than noninfected patients after liver transplantation.[170] Hepatitis B immune globulin and nucleos(t)ide analogs are recommended for reinfection prophylaxis in the posttransplant period for HBV-infected individuals.[171] Studies are underway to examine the appropriate use of antiviral therapy for HCV-infected patients undergoing liver transplantation.

Reactivation of HCV can occur with chemotherapy or monoclonal antibody-based immunosuppressive therapies, but is less frequent as compared to HBV infection.[172] Individuals who appear to have cleared an HBV infection and who have an undetectable viral load can experience HBV reactivation on rituximab therapy. Monitoring hepatic function and virus load is indicated during chemoimmunotherapy of HBV- or HCV-positive patients.[173] Although there is controversy regarding the role of virus screening for patients undergoing chemotherapy, antiviral therapy is recommended for high-risk HBV-infected patients undergoing chemoimmunotherapy, such as rituximab-based chemotherapy regimens.[174]

An association between HCV and B-cell non-Hodgkin lymphoma (NHL) has also been demonstrated in highly endemic geographic areas.[175] Lymphoproliferation has been linked to type II mixed cryoglobulinemia in many of these individuals. In addition to diffuse large B-cell lymphoma, marginal zone lymphomas and lymphoplasmacytic lymphomas are the histologic subtypes most frequently associated with HCV infection. Antiviral treatment with IFNα with or without ribavirin has been effective in the treatment of HCV-infected patients with indolent lymphoma, but rarely in individuals with aggressive lymphomas.

CONCLUSION

Oncogenic viruses are important causes of cancer, especially in less industrialized countries and in immunosuppressed individuals. They are common causes of anogenital cancers, lymphomas, oral and hepatocellular carcinomas and are associated with a variety of other malignancies. Vaccines and antiviral agents play an important role in the prevention of virus-induced cancers. Studies of virus pathogenesis will continue to establish paradigms that are critical to our understanding of cancer etiology in general.

REFERENCES

1. de Martel C, Ferlay J, Franceschi S, et al. Global burden of cancers attributable to infections in 2008: a review and synthetic analysis. *Lancet Oncol* 2012;13(6):607–615.
2. Schiller JT, Lowy DR. Virus infection and human cancer: an overview. *Recent Results Cancer Res* 2014;193:1–10.
3. Chen CJ, Hsu WL, Yang HI, et al. Epidemiology of virus infection and human cancer. *Recent Results Cancer Res* 2014;193:11–32.
4. Virgin HW, Wherry EJ, Ahmed R. Redefining chronic viral infection. *Cell* 2009;138(1):30–50.
5. Campo MS, O'Neil BW, Barron RJ, et al. Experimental reproduction of the papilloma-carcinoma complex of the alimentary canal in cattle. *Carcinogenesis* 1994;15(8):1597–1601.
6. Khoury JD, Tannir NM, Williams MD, et al. Landscape of DNA virus associations across human malignant cancers: analysis of 3,775 cases using RNA-Seq. *J Virol* 2013;87(16):8916–8926.
7. zur Hausen H, de Villiers EM. TT viruses: oncogenic or tumor-suppressive properties? *Curr Top Microbiol Immunol* 2009;331:109–116.
8. Mizutani T, Sayama Y, Nakanishi A, et al. Novel DNA virus isolated from samples showing endothelial cell necrosis in the Japanese eel, Anguilla japonica. *Virology* 2011;412(1):179–187.
9. Paulson KG, Carter JJ, Johnson LG, et al. Antibodies to merkel cell polyomavirus T antigen oncoproteins reflect tumor burden in merkel cell carcinoma patients. *Cancer Res* 2010;70:8388–8397.
10. International Agency for Research on Cancer (IARC) Working Group. IARC Monographs on the Evalation of Carcinogenic Risks to Humans. *Malaria and Some Polyomaviruses (SV40, BK, JC, and Merkel Cell Viruses)*, Vol. 104. Lyon, France: IARC; 2013.
11. Moore PS, Chang Y. The conundrum of causality in tumor virology: the cases of KSHV and MCV. *Semin Cancer Biol* 2013;26C:4–12.
12. Rigoni-Stern D. Fatti statistici relativi alle malattie cancrose. *Giornale Service Progr Pathol Terap Ser* 1842;2:507–517.
13. Lowy DR. History of papillomavirus research. In: Garcea RL, DiMaio D, eds. *The Papillomaviruses*. New York, NY: Springer; 2007:13–28.
14. zur Hausen H. Herpes simplex virus in human genital cancer. *Int Rev Exp Pathol* 1983;25:307–326.
15. Durst M, Gissmann L, Ikenberg H, et al. A papillomavirus DNA from a cervical carcinoma and its prevalence in cancer biopsy samples from different geographic regions. *Proc Natl Acad Sci U S A* 1983;80(12):3812–3815.
16. Boshart M, Gissmann L, Ikenberg H, et al. A new type of papillomavirus DNA, its presence in genital cancer biopsies and in cell lines derived from cervical cancer. *Embo J* 1984;3(5):1151–1157.
17. Christensen ND. Cottontail rabbit papillomavirus (CRPV) model system to test antiviral and immunotherapeutic strategies. *Antivir Chem Chemother* 2005;16(6):355–362.
18. Rous P, Beard J. The progression to carcinoma of virus induced rabbit papillomas (Shope). *J Exp Med* 1935;62:523–545.
19. Syverton JT, Berry GP. Carcinoma in the cottontail rabbit following spontaneous virus papilloma (Shope). *Proc Soc Exp Biol Med* 1935;33:399–400.
20. de Villiers EM. Cross-roads in the classification of papillomaviruses. *Virology* 2013;445(1–2):2–10.
21. Bosch FX, Broker TR, Forman D, et al. Comprehensive control of human papillomavirus infections and related diseases. *Vaccine* 2013;31 Suppl 8:I1–I31.
22. Van Doorslaer K. Evolution of the papillomaviridae. *Virology* 2013;445(1–2):11–20.
23. Scheffner M, Werness BA, Huibregtse JM, et al. The E6 oncoprotein encoded by human papillomavirus types 16 and 18 promotes the degradation of p53. *Cell* 1990;63(6):1129–1136.
24. Scheffner M, Huibregtse JM, Vierstra RD, Howley PM. The HPV-16 E6 and E6–AP complex functions as a ubiquitin-protein ligase in the ubiquitination of p53. *Cell* 1993;75(3):495–505.
25. Huibregtse JM, Scheffner M, Howley PM. Cloning and expression of the cDNA for E6–AP, a protein that mediates the interaction of the human papillomavirus E6 oncoprotein with p53. *Mol Cell Biol* 1993;13(2):775–784.
26. Klingelhutz AJ, Foster SA, McDougall JK. Telomerase activation by the E6 gene product of human papillomavirus type 16. *Nature* 1996;380(6569):79–82.
27. White EA, Howley PM. Proteomic approaches to the study of papillomavirus-host interactions. *Virology* 2013;435(1):57–69.
28. Dyson N, Howley PM, Munger K, et al. The human papilloma virus-16 E7 oncoprotein is able to bind to the retinoblastoma gene product. *Science* 1989;243(4893):934–937.
29. Munger K, Howley PM. Human papillomavirus immortalization and transformation functions. *Virus Res* 2002;89(2):213–228.
30. Duensing S, Lee LY, Duensing A, et al. The human papillomavirus type 16 E6 and E7 oncoproteins cooperate to induce mitotic defects and genomic instability by uncoupling centrosome duplication from the cell division cycle. *Proc Natl Acad Sci U S A* 2000;97(18):10002–10007.
31. DiMaio D, Petti LM. The E5 proteins. *Virology* 2013;445(1–2):99–114.
32. Schiller JT, Lowy DR. Understanding and learning from the success of prophylactic human papillomavirus vaccines. *Nat Rev Microbiol* 2012;10(10):681–692.
33. Kemp TJ, Safaeian M, Hildesheim A, et al. Kinetic and HPV infection effects on cross-type neutralizing antibody and avidity responses induced by Cervarix((R)). *Vaccine* 2012;31(1):165–170.
34. Haupt RM, Wheeler CM, Brown DR, et al. Impact of an HPV6/11/16/18 L1 virus-like particle vaccine on progression to cervical intraepithelial neoplasia in seropositive women with HPV16/18 infection. *Int J Cancer* 2011;129(11):2632–2642.
35. Kreuter A, Wieland U. Lack of efficacy in treating condyloma acuminata and preventing recurrences with the recombinant quadrivalent human papillomavirus vaccine in a case series of immunocompetent patients. *J Am Acad Dermatol* 2013;68(1):179–180.
36. Joura E, Team V-S, eds. Abstract SS 8–4: Efficacy and immunogenicity of a novel 9-valent HPV L1 virus-like particle vaccine in 16- to 26-year-old women. Paper presented at: Eurogin 2013 International Multidisciplinary Congress; 2013; Florence, Italy.
37. Wang JW, Roden RB. L2, the minor capsid protein of papillomavirus. *Virology* 2013;445(1–2):175–186.
38. Ma B, Maraj B, Tran NP, et al. Emerging human papillomavirus vaccines. *Expert Opin Emerg Drugs* 2012;17(4):469–492.
39. Scudellari M. HPV: sex, cancer and a virus. *Nature* 2013;503(7476):330–332.
40. Gillison ML, Alemany L, Snijders PJ, et al. Human papillomavirus and diseases of the upper airway: head and neck cancer and respiratory papillomatosis. *Vaccine* 2012;30 Suppl 5:F34–54.
41. Silverberg MJ, Leyden W, Warton EM, et al. HIV infection status, immunodeficiency, and the incidence of non-melanoma skin cancer. *J Natl Cancer Inst* 2013;105(5):350–360.
42. Kempf W, Mertz KD, Hofbauer GF, et al. Skin cancer in organ transplant recipients. *Pathobiology* 2013;80(6):302–309.
43. Wallace NA, Gasior SL, Faber ZJ, et al. HPV 5 and 8 E6 expression reduces ATM protein levels and attenuates LINE-1 retrotransposition. *Virology* 2013;443(1):69–79.
44. White EA, Kramer RE, Tan MJ, et al. Comprehensive analysis of host cellular interactions with human papillomavirus E6 proteins identifies new E6 binding partners and reflects viral diversity. *J Virol* 2012;86(24):13174–13186.
45. White EA, Sowa ME, Tan MJ, et al. Systematic identification of interactions between host cell proteins and E7 oncoproteins from diverse human papillomaviruses. *Proc Natl Acad Sci U S A* 2012;109(5):E260–267.
46. Caldeira S, Zehbe I, Accardi R, et al. The E6 and E7 proteins of the cutaneous human papillomavirus type 38 display transforming properties. *J Virol* 2003;77(3):2195–2206.
47. Arron ST, Ruby JG, Dybbro E, et al. Transcriptome sequencing demonstrates that human papillomavirus is not active in cutaneous squamous cell carcinoma. *J Invest Dermatol* 2011;131(8):1745–1753.
48. Gross L. A filterable agent, recovered from Ak leukemic extracts, causing salivary gland carcinomas in C3H mice. *Proc Soc Exp Biol Med* 1953;83(2):414–421.

49. Eddy BE, Stewart SE. Characteristics of the SE polyoma virus. *Am J Public Health Nations Health* 1959;49:1486–1492.
50. Sweet BH, Hilleman MR. The vacuolating virus, S.V. 40. *Proc Soc Exp Biol Med* 1960;105:420–427.
51. Eddy BE, Borman GS, Grubbs GE, et al. Identification of the oncogenic substance in rhesus monkey kidney cell culture as simian virus 40. *Virology* 1962;17:65–75.
52. Dang-Tan T, Mahmud SM, Puntoni R, et al. Polio vaccines, simian virus 40, and human cancer: the epidemiologic evidence for a causal association. *Oncogene* 2004;23(38):6535–6540.
53. Bouvard V, Baan RA, Grosse Y, et al. Carcinogenicity of malaria and of some polyomaviruses. *Lancet Oncol* 2012;13(4):339–340.
54. Gardner SD, Field AM, Coleman DV, et al. New human papovavirus (B.K.) isolated from urine after renal transplantation. *Lancet*.1971;1(7712): 1253–1257.
55. Padgett BL, Walker DL, ZuRhein GM, et al. Cultivation of papova-like virus from human brain with progressive multifocal leucoencephalopathy. *Lancet* 1971;1(7712):1257–1260.
56. Das D, Wojno K, Imperiale MJ. BK virus as a cofactor in the etiology of prostate cancer in its early stages. *J Virol* 2008;82(6):2705–2714.
57. Akgul B, Pfister D, Knuchel R, et al. No evidence for a role of xenotropic murine leukaemia virus-related virus and BK virus in prostate cancer of German patients. *Med Microbiol Immunol* 2012;201(2):245–248.
58. Alexiev BA, Randhawa P, Vazquez Martul E, et al. BK virus-associated urinary bladder carcinoma in transplant recipients: report of 2 cases, review of the literature, and proposed pathogenetic model. *Human Pathol* 2013;44(5):908–917.
59. Abend JR, Jiang M, Imperiale MJ. BK virus and human cancer: innocent until proven guilty. *Semin Cancer Biol* 2009;19(4):252–260.
60. Maginnis MS, Atwood WJ. JC virus: an oncogenic virus in animals and humans? *Semin Cancer Biol* 2009;19(4):261–269.
61. Feng H, Shuda M, Chang Y, et al. Clonal integration of a polyomavirus in human Merkel cell carcinoma. *Science* 2008;319(5866):1096–1100.
62. Hodgson NC. Merkel cell carcinoma: changing incidence trends. *J Surg Oncol* 2005;89(1):1–4.
63. Engels EA, Frisch M, Goedert JJ, et al. Merkel cell carcinoma and HIV infection. *Lancet* 2002;359(9305):497–498.
64. Zur Hausen A, Rennspiess D, Winnepennincks V, et al. Early B-cell differentiation in Merkel cell carcinomas: clues to cellular ancestry. *Cancer Res* 2013;73(16):4982–4987.
65. Guastafierro A, Feng H, Thant M, et al. Characterization of an early passage Merkel cell polyomavirus-positive Merkel cell carcinoma cell line, MS-1, and its growth in NOD scid gamma mice. *J Virol Methods* 2013;187(1):6–14.
66. Schowalter RM, Pastrana DV, Pumphrey KA, et al. Merkel cell polyomavirus and two previously unknown polyomaviruses are chronically shed from human skin. *Cell Host Microbe* 2010;7(6):509–515.
67. Faust H, Pastrana DV, Buck CB, et al. Antibodies to Merkel cell polyomavirus correlate to presence of viral DNA in the skin. *J Infect Dis* 2011;203(8):1096–1100.
68. Pastrana DV, Wieland U, Silling S, et al. Positive correlation between Merkel cell polyomavirus viral load and capsid-specific antibody titer. *Med Microbiol Immunol* 2011;201(1):17–23.
69. Pastrana DV, Tolstov YL, Becker JC, et al. Quantitation of human seroresponsiveness to Merkel cell polyomavirus. *PLoS Pathog* 2009;5(9):e1000578.
70. Faust H, Andersson K, Ekstrom J, et al. Prospective study of Merkel cell polyomavirus and risk of Merkel cell carcinoma. *Int J Cancer* 2014;134(4):844–848.
71. Cheng J, Rozenblatt-Rosen O, Paulson KG, et al. Merkel cell polyomavirus large T antigen has growth-promoting and inhibitory activities. *J Virol* 2013;87(11):6118–6126.
72. Li J, Wang X, Diaz J, et al. Merkel cell polyomavirus large T antigen disrupts host genomic integrity and inhibits cellular proliferation. *J Virol* 2013;87(16):9173–9188.
73. Houben R, Shuda M, Weinkam R, et al. Merkel cell polyomavirus-infected Merkel cell carcinoma cells require expression of viral T antigens. *J Virol* 2010;84(14):7064–7072.
74. Houben R, Grimm J, Willmes C, et al. Merkel cell carcinoma and Merkel cell carcinoma polyomavirus: evidence for hit-and-run oncogenesis. *J Invest Dermatol* 2012;132(1):254–256.
75. Shuda M, Chang Y, Moore PS. Merkel cell polyomavirus positive Merkel cell carcinoma requires viral small T antigen for cell proliferation. *J Invest Dermatol* 2013 [Epub ahead of print].
76. Paulson KG, Iyer JG, Tegeder AR, et al. Transcriptome-wide studies of merkel cell carcinoma and validation of intratumoral CD8+ lymphocyte invasion as an independent predictor of survival. *J Clin Oncol* 2011;29(12):1539–1546.
77. Arora R, Shuda M, Guastafierro A, et al. Survivin is a therapeutic target in Merkel cell carcinoma. *Sci Transl Med* 2012;4(133):133ra56.
78. Dresang LR, Guastafierro A, Arora R, et al. Response of merkel cell polyomavirus-positive merkel cell carcinoma xenografts to a survivin inhibitor. *PloS One* 2013;8(11):e80543.
79. Shuda M, Kwun HJ, Feng H, et al. Human Merkel cell polyomavirus small T antigen is an oncoprotein targeting the 4E-BP1 translation regulator. *J Clin Invest* 2011;121(9):3623–3634.
80. Howard RA, Dores GM, Curtis RE, et al. Merkel cell carcinoma and multiple primary cancers. *Cancer Epidemiol Biomarkers Prev* 2006;15(8): 1545–1549.
81. Pantulu ND, Pallasch CP, Kurz AK, et al. Detection of a novel truncating Merkel cell polyomavirus large T antigen deletion in chronic lymphocytic leukemia cells. *Blood* 2010;116(24):5280–5284.
82. Tolstov YL, Arora R, Scudiere SC, et al. Lack of evidence for direct involvement of Merkel cell polyomavirus (MCV) in chronic lymphocytic leukemia (CLL). *Blood* 2010;115(23):4973–4974.
83. Cimino PJ, Jr., Bahler DW, Duncavage EJ. Detection of Merkel cell polyomavirus in chronic lymphocytic leukemia T-cells. *Exp Mol Pathol* 2013;94(1):40–44.
84. Burkitt D. A sarcoma involving the jaws in African children. *Br J Surg* 1958;46(197):218–223.
85. Epstein MA, Achong BG, Barr YM. Virus particles in cultured lymphoblasts from Burkitt's lymphoma. *Lancet* 1964;1(7335):702–703.
86. Henle G, Henle W, Diehl V. Relation of Burkitt's tumor-associated herpesytpe virus to infectious mononucleosis. *Proc Natl Acad Sci U S A* 1968;59(1): 94–101.
87. Longnecker RM, Kieff E, Cohen JI. Epstein-Barr virus. In: Knipe DM, Howley PM, eds. *Fields Virology*. 6th ed. Philadelphia, PA: Lippincott Williams & Wilkins; 2013.
88. Cesarman E. Gammaherpesviruses and lymphoproliferative disorders. *Annu Rev Pathol* 2014;9:349–372.
89. Shannon-Lowe C, Rowe M. Epstein-Barr virus infection of polarized epithelial cells via the basolateral surface by memory B cell-mediated transfer infection. *PLoS Pathog* 2011;7(5):e1001338.
90. Faulkner GC, Burrows SR, Khanna R, et al. X-Linked agammaglobulinemia patients are not infected with Epstein-Barr virus: implications for the biology of the virus. *J Virol* 1999;73(2):1555–1564.
91. Hjalgrim H, Smedby KE, Rostgaard K, et al. Infectious mononucleosis, childhood social environment, and risk of Hodgkin lymphoma. *Cancer Res* 2007;67(5):2382–2388.
92. Barton ES, White DW, Cathelyn JS, et al. Herpesvirus latency confers symbiotic protection from bacterial infection. *Nature* 2007;447(7142):326–329.
93. Giulino-Roth L, Cesarman E. Molecular biology of Burkitt lymphoma. In: Robertson E, ed. *Burkitt's Lymphoma*. New York, NY: Springer; 2013: 211–226.
94. Chang ET, Adami HO. The enigmatic epidemiology of nasopharyngeal carcinoma. *Cancer Epidemiol Biomarkers Prev* 2006;15(10):1765–1777.
95. Murukesan V, Mukherjee S. Managing post-transplant lymphoproliferative disorders in solid-organ transplant recipients: a review of immunosuppressant regimens. *Drugs* 2012;72(12):1631–1643.
96. Cohen JI, Mocarski ES, Raab-Traub N, et al. The need and challenges for development of an Epstein-Barr virus vaccine. *Vaccine* 2013;31(Suppl 2): B194-196.
97. Choquet S, Leblond V, Herbrecht R, et al. Efficacy and safety of rituximab in B-cell post-transplantation lymphoproliferative disorders: results of a prospective multicenter phase 2 study. *Blood* 2006;107(8):3053–3057.
98. Barnes JA, Lacasce AS, Feng Y, et al. Evaluation of the addition of rituximab to CODOX-M/IVAC for Burkitt's lymphoma: a retrospective analysis. *Ann Oncol* 2011;22(8):1859–1864.
99. Kaposi M. Idiopathisches multiples Pigmentsarkom der Haut. *Archiv für Dermatologie und Syphilis* 1872;4(2):265–273.
100. Antman K, Chang Y. Kaposi's sarcoma. *N Engl J Med* 2000;342(14):1027–1038.
101. Beral V, Peterman TA, Berkelman RL, et al. Kaposi's sarcoma among persons with AIDS: a sexually transmitted infection? *Lancet* 1990;335(8682):123–128.
102. Chang Y, Cesarman E, Pessin MS, et al. Identification of herpesvirus-like DNA sequences in AIDS-associated Kaposi's sarcoma. *Science* 1994;266(5192): 1865–1869.
103. Damania BA, Cesarman E. Kaposi's sarcoma-associated herpesvirus. In: Knipe DM, Howley PM, eds. *Fields Virology*. 6th ed. Philadelphia, PA: Lippincott Williams & Wilkins; 2013.
104. Cook-Mozaffari P, Newton R, Beral V, et al. The geographical distribution of Kaposi's sarcoma and of lymphomas in Africa before the AIDS epidemic. *Br J Cancer* 1998;78(11):1521–1528.
105. Martin DF, Kuppermann BD, Wolitz RA, et al. Oral ganciclovir for patients with cytomegalovirus retinitis treated with a ganciclovir implant. Roche Ganciclovir Study Group. *N Engl J Med* 1999;340(14):1063–1070.
106. Krown SE, Dittmer DP, Cesarman E. Pilot study of oral valganciclovir therapy in patients with classic Kaposi sarcoma. *J Infect Dis* 2011;203(8):1082–1086.
107. Sakakibara S, Tosato G. Regulation of angiogenesis in malignancies associated with Epstein-Barr virus and Kaposi's sarcoma-associated herpes virus. *Future Microbiol* 2009;4(7):903–917.
108. Soulier J, Grollet L, Oksenhendler E, et al. Kaposi's sarcoma-associated herpesvirus-like DNA sequences in multicentric Castleman's disease. *Blood* 1995;86(4):1276–1280.
109. Polizzotto MN, Uldrick TS, Wang V, et al. Human and viral interleukin-6 and other cytokines in Kaposi sarcoma herpesvirus-associated multicentric Castleman disease. *Blood* 2013;122(26):4189–4198.
110. Simonelli C, Spina M, Cinelli R, et al. Clinical features and outcome of primary effusion lymphoma in HIV-infected patients: a single-institution study. *J Clin Oncol* 2003;21(21):3948–3954.
111. Coffin JM, Hughes SH, Varmus HE, eds. The interactions of retroviruses and their hosts. *Retroviruses*. Cold Spring Harbor, NY: Cold Spring Harbor Laboratory Press; 1997.
112. Gallo RC. History of the discovery of the first human retroviruses: HTLV-1 and HTLV-2. *Oncogene* 2005;24:5926–5930.
113. Smit AF, Riggs AD. Tiggers and DNA transposon fossils in the human genome. *Proc Natl Acad Sci U S A* 1996;93:1443–1448.
114. Delviks-Frankenberry K, Paprotka T, Cingöz O, et al. Generation of multiple replication-competent retroviruses through recombination between PreXMRV-1 and PreXMRV-2. *J Virol* 2013;87:11525–11537.

115. Mason AL, Zhang G. Linking human beta retrovirus infection with primary biliary cirrhosis. *Gastroenterol Clin Biol* 2010;34:359–366.
116. Hacein-Bey-Abina S, VonKalle C, Schmidt M, et al. LMO2-associated clonal T cell proliferation in two patients after gene therapy for SCID-X1. *Science* 2003;302:415–419.
117. Matsuoka M, Jeang K-T. Human T-cell leukaemia virus type 1 (HTLV-1) infectivity and cellular transformation. *Nat Rev Cancer* 2007;7:270–280.
118. Poiesz BJ, Ruscetti FW, Mier JW, et al. T-cell lines established from human T-lymphocytic neoplasias by direct response to T-cell growth factor. *Proc Natl Acad Sci U S A* 1980;77:6815–6819.
119. Kalyanaraman VS, Sarngadharan MG, Robert-Guroff M, et al. A new subtype of human T-cell leukemia virus (HTLV-II) associated with a T-cell variant of hairy cell leukemia. *Science* 1982;218:571–573.
120. Wolfe ND, Heneine W, Carr JK, et al. Emergence of unique primate T-lymphotropic viruses among central African bushmeat hunters. *Proc Natl Acad Sci U S A* 2005;102:7994–7999.
121. Goncalves DU, Prioietti FA, Ribas JGR, et al. Epidemiology, treatment, and prevention of human T-cell leukemia virus type 1-associated diseases. *Clin Microbiol Rev* 2010;23:577–589.
122. Hino S, Sugiyama H, Doi H, et al. Breaking the cycle of HTLV-1 transmission via carrier mothers' milk. *Lancet Oncol* 1987;2:158–159.
123. Kannian P, Green PL. Human T lymphotropic virus type 1 (HTLV-1): molecular biology and oncogenesis. *Viruses* 2010;2:2037–2077.
124. Hill SA, Lloyd PA, McDonald S, et al. Susceptibility of human T cell leukemia virus type I to nucleoside reverse transcriptase inhibitors. *J Infec Dis* 2003;188:424–427.
125. Seegulam ME, Ratner L. Integrase inhibitors effective against human T-cell leukemia virus type 1. *Antimicrob Agents Chemother* 2011;55:2011–2017.
126. Derse D, Crise B, Li Y, et al. Human T-cell leukemia virus type 1 integration target sites in the human genome: comparison with those of other retroviruses. *J Virol* 2007;81:6731–6741.
127. Jones KS, Lambert S, Bouttieer M, et al. Molecular aspects of HTLV-1 entry: functional domains of the HTLV-1 surface subunit (SU) and their relationships to the entry receptors. *Viruses* 2011;3:794–810.
128. Matsuoka M, Green PL. The HBZ gene, a key player in HTLV-1 pathogenesis. *Retrovirology* 2009;6:71.
129. Grossman WJ, Kimata JT, Wong FH, et al. Development of leukemia in mice transgenic for the tax gene of human T-cell leukemia virus type I. *Proc Natl Acad Sci U S A* 1995;92:1057–1061.
130. El Hajj H, El-Sabban M, Hasegawa H, et al. Therapy-induced selective loss of leukemia-initiating activity in murine adult T cell leukemia. *J Exp Med* 2010;207:2785–2792.
131. Villaudy J, Wencker M, Gadot N, et al. HTLV-1 propels thymic human T cell development in "human immune system" Rag2-/-IL-2Rgammac-/- mice. *PLoS Pathog* 2011;7:e1002231.
132. Costa EAS, Magri MC, Caterino-de-Arujo A. The best algorithm to confirm the diagnosis of HTLV-1 and HTLV-2 in at-risk individuals from Sao Paulo, Brazil. *J Virol Methods* 2011;173:280–286.
133. Barros N, Woll F, Watanabe L, et al. Are increased Foxp3+ regulatory T cells responsible for immunosuppression during HTLV-1 infection? Case reports and review of the literature. *BMJ Case Rep* 2012;bcr2012006574.
134. Cook LB, Rowan AG, Melamed A, et al. HTLV-1-infected T cells contain a single integrated provirus in natural infection. *Blood* 2012;120:3488–3490.
135. Shimoyama M. Diagnostic criteria and classification of clinical subtypes of adult T-cell leukemia-lymphoma: a report from the Lymphoma Study Group. *Br J Hematol* 1991;79:426–437.
136. Takasaki Y, Iwanaga M, Imaizumi Y, et al. Long-term study of indolent adult T-cell leukemia-lymphoma. *Blood* 2010;115:4337–4343.
137. Bazarbachi A, Plumelle Y, Ramos JC, et al. Meta-analysis on the use of zidovudine and interferon-alfa in adult T-cell leukemia/lymphoma showing improved survival in the leukemic subtypes. *J Clin Oncol* 2010;28:4177–4183.
138. Katsuya H, Yamanka T, Ishitsuka K, et al. Prognostic index for acute- and lymphoma-type adult T-cell leukaemia/lymphoma. *J Clin Oncol* 2012;30:1635–1640.
139. Tsukasaki K, Hermine O, Bazarbachi A, et al. Definition, prognostic factors, treatment, and reponse criteria of adult T-cell leukemia-lymphoma: a proposal from an international consensus meeting. *J Clin Oncol* 2009;27:453–459.
140. Yamada Y, Tomonaga M, Fukuda H, et al. A new G-CSF supported combination chemotherapy, LSG15, for adult T-cell leukaemia/lymphoma: Japan Clinical Oncology Group Study 9303. *Br J Hematol* 2001;113:375–382.
141. Ratner L, Harrington W, Feng X, et al. Human T cell leukemia virus reactivation with progression of adult T-cell leukemia-lymphoma. AIDS Malignancy Consortium. *PLoS One* 2009;4:e4420.
142. Tatsuro J, Ishida T, Takemoto S, et al., eds. Randomized phase II study of mogamulizumab (KW-0761) plus VCAP-AMP-VECP (mLSG15) versus mLSG15 alone for newly diagnosed aggressive adult T-cell leukemia-lymphoma (ATL). Paper presented at: 2013 ASCO Annual Meeting; 2013; Chicago, IL.
143. Bazarbachi A, Suarez F, Fields P, et al. How I treat adult T-cell leukemia/lymphoma. *Blood* 2011;118:1736–1745.
144. Utsonomiya A, Miyazaki Y, Takasuka Y, et al. Improved outcome of adult T cell leukemia/lymphoma with allogeneic hematopoietic stem cell transplanation. *Bone Marrow Transplant* 2001;27:15–20.
145. Blumberg BS. The discovery of the hepatitis B virus and the intervention of the vaccine: a scientific memoir. *J Gastroenterol Hepatol* 2002;17(Supplement s4):S502–S503.
146. Houghton M. Discovery of the hepatitis C virus. *Liver Int* 2009;29(Supplement 1):82–88.
147. Arzumanyan A, Reis HM, Feitelson MA. Pathogenic mechanisms in HBV- and HCV-associated hepatocellular carcinoma. *Nat Rev Cancer* 2013;13:123–135.
148. Soerjomataram I, Lortet-Tieulent J, Parkin DM, et al. Global burden of cancer in 2008: a systematic analysis of disability-adjusted life-years in 12 world regions. *Lancet* 2012;380:1840–1850.
149. Altekruse SF, McGlynn KA, Reichman ME. Hepatocellular carcinoma incidence, mortality, and survival trends in the United States from 1975 to 2005. *J Clin Oncol* 2009;27:1485–1491.
150. Shiffman ML, ed. *Chronic Hepatitis C Virus: Advances in Treatment, Promise for the Future*. New York: Springer Verlag; 2011.
151. Nicot F, Nassim K, Lionel R, et al. Occult hepatitis C virus infection: Where are we now? *Liver Biopsy in Modern Med* 2004;307–334.
152. Freeman AJ, Dore GJ, Law MG, et al. Estimating progression to cirrhosis in chronic hepatitis C virus infection. *Hepatology* 2001;34:809–816.
153. Wilkins T, Malcom JK, Raina D, et al. Hepatitis C: diagnosis and treatment. *Am Fam Physician* 2010;81:1351–1357.
154. Fallot G, Neuveut C, Buendia M-A. Diverse roles of hepatitis B virus in liver cancer. *Curr Opin Virol* 2012;2:467–473.
155. Ganem D, Prince AM. Hepatitis B virus infection - natural history and clinical consequences. *N Engl J Med* 2004;350:1118–1129.
156. Tujios SR, Lee WM. Update in the management of chronic hepatitis B. *Curr Opin Gastroenterol* 2013;29:250–256.
157. Seto W-K, Fung J, Yuen M-F, et al. Future prevention and treatment of chronic hepatitis B infection. *J Clin Gastroenterol* 2012;46:725–734.
158. Wang WK, Levy S. Hepatitis C virus (HCV) and lymphomagenesis. *Leuk Lymphoma* 2003;44:1113–1120.
159. Fernandez-Garcia M-D, Mazzon M, Jacobs M, et al. Pathogenesis of flavivirus infections: using and abusing the host cell. *Cell Host Microbe* 2009;318:318–328.
160. Moradpour D, Penin F, Rice CM. Replication of hepatitis c virus. *Nat Rev Microbiol* 2007;5:453–463.
161. Liang TJ, Ghany MG. Current and future therapies for hepatitis C virus infection. *N Engl J Med* 2013;368:1907–1917.
162. Kimer N, Dahl EK, Gluud LL, et al. Antiviral therapy for prevention of hepatocellular carcinoma in chronic hepatitis C: systematic review and meta-analysis of randomised controlled trials. *BMJ Open* 2012;2:e001313.
163. Fujimoto A, Totoki Y, Abe T, et al. Whole-genome sequencing of liver cancers identifies etiological influences on mutation patterns and recurrent mutations in chromatin regulators. *Nat Genet* 2012;44:760–764.
164. Sung WK, Zheng H, Li S, et al. Genome-wide survey of recurrent HBV integration in hepatocellular carcinoma. *Nat Genet* 2012;44:765–769.
165. Devi U, Locarnini S. Hepatitis B antivirals and resistance. *Curr Opin Virol* 2013;3:495–500.
166. Aghemo A, Colombo M. Hepatocellular carcinoma in chronic hepatitis C: from bench to bedside. *Semin Immunopathol* 2013;35:111–120.
167. Bruix J, Sherman M. Management of hepatocellular carcinoma: an update. *Hepatology* 2011;53:1020–1022.
168. Mazzaferro V, Regalia E, Doci R, et al. Liver transplantation for the treatment of small hepatocellular carcinomas in patients with cirrhosis. *N Engl J Med* 1996;334:693–699.
169. Mino M, Lauwers GY. Pathologic spectrum and prognostic significance of underlying liver disease in hepatocellular carcinoma. *Surg Oncol Clin N Am* 2003;12:13–24.
170. Burton JR, Everson GT. Management of the transplant recipient with chronic hepatitis C. *Clin Liver Dis* 2013;17:73–91.
171. Beckebaum S, Kabar I, Cicinnati VR. Hepatitis B and C in liver transplantation: new strategies to combat the enemies. *Rev Med Virol* 2012;23:172–193.
172. Torres HA, Davila M. Reactivation of hepatitis B virus and hepatitis C virus in patients with cancer. *Nat Rev Clin Oncol* 2012;9:156–166.
173. Huang Y-H, Hsaio L-T, Hong Y-C, et al. Randomized controlled trial of entecavir prophylaxis for rituximab-associated hepatitis B virus reactivation in patients with lymhoma and resolved hepatitis. *J Clin Oncol* 2013;31:2765–2772.
174. Artz AS, Somerfield MR, Feld JJ, et al. American Society of Clinical Oncology provisional clinical opinion: chronic hepatitis B virus infection screening in patients receiving cytotoxic chemotherapy for treatment of malignant diseases. *J Clin Oncol* 2010;28:3199–3202.
175. Forghieri F, Luppi M, Barozzi P, et al. Pathogenetic mechanisms of hepatitis C virus-induced B-cell lymphomagenesis. *Clin Dev Immunol* 2012;2012:807351.

6 Inflammation

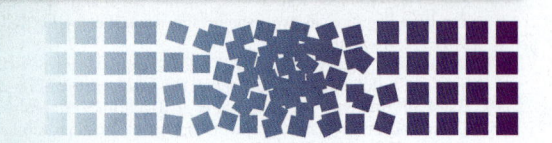

Sahdeo Prasad and Bharat B. Aggarwal

INTRODUCTION

Extensive research over the last half a century indicates that inflammation plays an important role in cancer. Although acute inflammation can play a therapeutic role, low-level chronic inflammation can promote cancer. Different inflammatory cells, the various cell signaling pathways that lead to inflammation, and biomarkers of inflammation have now been well defined. These inflammatory pathways, which are primarily mediated through the transcription factors nuclear factor kappa B (NF-κB) and signal transducer and activator of transcription 3 (STAT3), have been linked to cellular transformation, tumor survival, proliferation, invasion, angiogenesis, and metastasis of cancer. These pathways have also now been linked with chemoresistance and radioresistance. This chapter considers the role of inflammation in cancer and its potential for cancer prevention and treatment.

Inflammation is the complex biologic responses of the body to irritation, injury, or infection. The recognition of inflammation dates back to antiquity. As documented by Aulus Cornelius Celsus, a Roman of the 1st century AD, inflammation is characterized by the tissue response to injury that results in *rubor* (redness, due to hyperemia), *tumor* (swelling, caused by increased permeability of the microvasculature and leakage of protein into the interstitial space), *calor* (heat, associated with increased blood flow and the metabolic activity of the cellular mediators of inflammation), and *dolor* (pain, in part due to changes in the perivasculature and associated nerve endings). Rudolf Virchow subsequently added *functio laesa* (dysfunction of the organs involved) in the 1850s. The process includes increased blood flow with an influx of white blood cells and other chemical substances that facilitate healing. Inflammation is also considered the body's self-protective attempt to remove harmful stimuli, including damaged cells, irritants, or pathogens, and to begin the healing process.

The word inflammation is derived from the Latin *inflammo* (meaning "I set alight, I ignite"). Because inflammation is a stereotyped response, it is considered a mechanism of innate immunity, as compared with adaptive immunity. On the basis of longevity, inflammation is classified as acute or chronic. When inflammation is short term, usually appearing within a few minutes or hours and ceasing upon the removal of the injurious stimulus, it is called acute. However, if it persists longer, it is called chronic inflammation, which leads to simultaneous destruction from the inflammatory process. Inflammation is beneficial when it is acute; however, chronic inflammation leads to several diseases, including cancer. Cancer is primarily a disease of lifestyle, with 30% of all cancers having been linked to smoking, 35% to diet, 14% to 20% to obesity, 18% to infection, and 7% to environmental pollution and radiation (Fig. 6.1).[1] Smoking, obesity, infections, pollution, and radiation are all known to activate proinflammatory pathways.[2] Therefore, understanding how inflammation contributes to cancer etiology is important for both cancer prevention and treatment.[3]

MOLECULAR BASIS OF INFLAMMATION

Although it is clear that inflammation and cancer are closely related, the mechanisms underlying persistent and chronic inflammation in chronic diseases remain unclear. Numerous cytokines have been linked with inflammation, including tumor necrosis factor (TNF), interleukin (IL)-1, IL-6, IL-8, IL-17, and vascular endothelial growth factor (VEGF). Among various cytokines that have been linked with inflammation, TNF is a primary mediator of inflammation linked to cancer.[4] However, it has been shown that proinflammatory transcriptional factors (activator protein [AP]-1, STAT3, NF-κB, hypoxia-inducible factor [HIF]-1, and β-catenin/Wnt) are ubiquitously expressed and control numerous physiologic processes, including development, differentiation, immunity, and metabolism in chronic diseases. Although these transcription factors are regulated by completely different signaling mechanisms, they are activated in response to various stimuli, including stresses and cytokines, and are involved in inflammation-induced tumor development and its metastasis.[5] Interestingly, inflammation plays a role at all stages of tumor development: initiation, progression, and metastasis.[2] In initiation, inflammation induces the release of a variety of cytokines and chemokines that promote the release of inflammatory cells and associated factors. This further causes oxidative damage, DNA mutations, and other changes in the tissue microenvironment, making it more conducive to cell transformation, increased survival, and proliferation. Inflammation also contributes to tissue injury, remodeling of the extracellular matrix, angiogenesis, and fibrosis in diverse target tissues. Among all the inflammatory cell signaling pathways, NF-κB has been shown to play a major role in cancer,[6,7] and TNF is one of the most potent activators of NF-κB.[8,9]

ROLE OF INFLAMMATION IN TRANSFORMATION

Transformation is the process by which the cellular and molecular makeup of a cell is altered as it becomes malignant. Numerous factors are involved in the process of cell transformation, including inflammation. A clinical study has shown that chronic inflammation due to heavy metal deposition in lymph nodes leads to malignant transformation and, finally, to patient death.[10] More recently, chronic exposure to cigarette smoke extract[11] and arsenite[12] has been shown to induce inflammation followed by epithelial–mesenchymal transition and transformation of human bronchial epithelial (HBE) cells. Furthermore, activation of NF-κB and HIF-2α increased the levels of the proinflammatory IL-6, IL-8, and IL-1β, which are essential for the malignant progression of transformed HBE cells. Sox2, another important molecular factor, cooperates with inflammation-mediated STAT3 activation, which precedes the malignant transformation of foregut basal progenitor cells.[13] A clinical study reported that the p53 mutation is a critical event for the malignant transformation of sinonasal inverted papilloma. This p53 mutation resulted in cyclooxygenase (COX)-2–mediated inflammatory signals that contribute to the proliferation

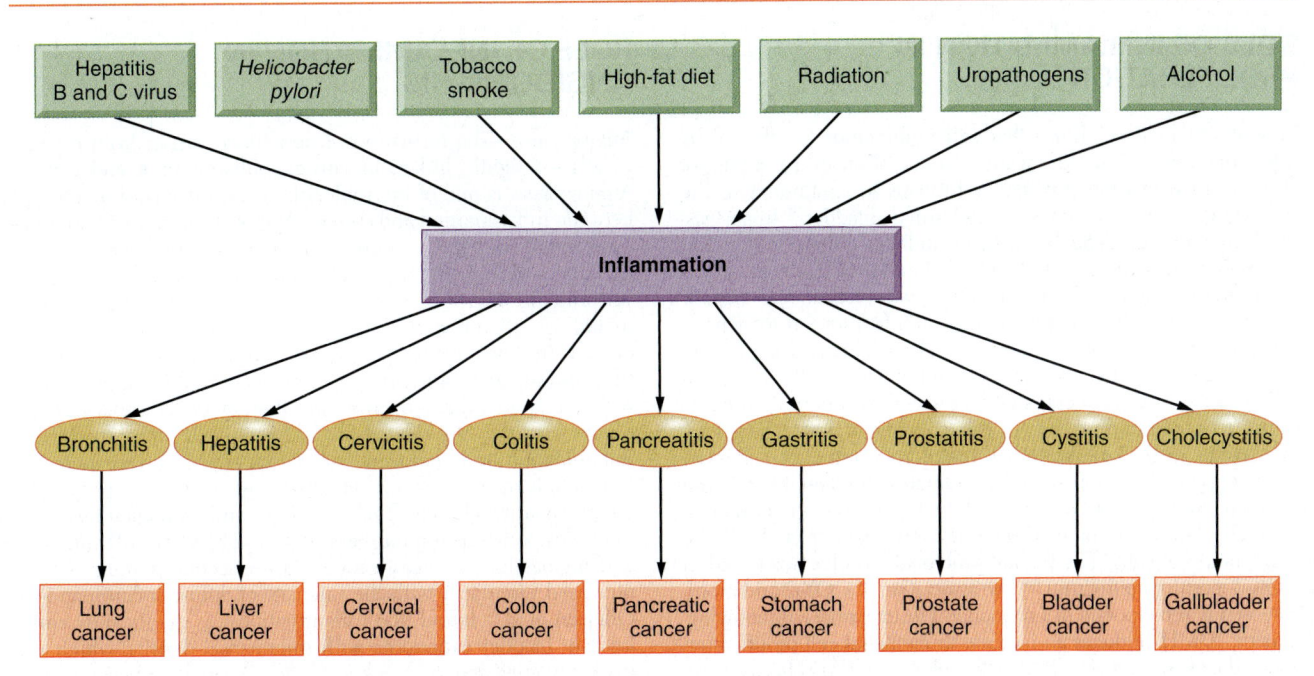

Figure 6.1 Origin of inflammation and its role in various cancers.

of advanced sinonasal inverted papilloma.[14] In another study in patients, the YKL-40 protein was found to be involved in chronic inflammation and oncogenic transformation of human breast tissues.[15] Inflammation-mediated transformation was also found to be regulated by MyD88 in a mouse model through Ras signaling.[16] In addition, inflammation contributed to the activation of the epidermal growth factor receptor (EGFR) and its subsequent interaction with PKCδ, which leads to the transformation of normal esophageal epithelia to squamous cell carcinoma.[17] Activation of Src oncoprotein triggers an inflammatory response mediated by NF-κB that directly activates Lin28 transcription and rapidly reduces let-7 microRNA levels. The inflammatory cytokine IL-6 mediates the activation of STAT3 transcription factor, which results in the transformation of cells.[18]

ROLE OF INFLAMMATION IN SURVIVAL

Numerous findings across different cancer populations have suggested that inflammation has an important role in carcinogenesis and disease progression.[19,20] The important markers of systemic inflammatory response in both in vitro findings and clinical outcomes include plasma C-reactive protein (CRP) concentration,[21,22] hypoalbuminemia,[23] and the Glasgow Prognostic Score (GPS), which combines CRP and albumin.[24,25] In addition to these, hematologic markers of systemic inflammatory response such as absolute white-cell count or its components (neutrophils, neutrophil-to-lymphocyte ratio [NLR]),[26-28] platelets, and a platelet-to-lymphocyte ratio[29,30] are also prognostic indicators for cancer clinical outcomes. Whether these inflammatory biomarkers influence the survival of cancer patients is discussed in this section.

In a study of 416 patients with renal cell carcinoma, with 362 patients included in the analysis, elevated neutrophil count, elevated platelet counts, and a high NLR were found. This inflammatory response was predictive for shorter overall patient survival.[31] Another study in unresectable malignant biliary obstruction (UMBO) found that patients with low GPS (0 and 1) had better postoperative survivals than did patients with a higher GPS. The 6-month and 1-year survival rates were 58.1% to 27.3%, respectively, for patients with low GPS and 25% to 6.2%, respectively, for patients with a higher GPS.[32] It has been also shown that prostate cancer patients with aggressive, clinically significant disease and an elevated GPS[2] had a higher risk of death overall as well as high-grade disease.[33] Other than GPS, age and gastrectomy have also been shown to independently influence the disease-specific and progression-free survival of gastric cancer patients.[34] A biomarker of systemic inflammation, the blood NLR, predicted patient survival with hepatocellular carcinoma (HCC) after transarterial chemoembolization. Patients in whom the NLR remained stable or became normalized after transarterial chemoembolization showed improved overall survival compared with patients showing a persistently abnormal index of NLR.[35]

A further study found that inflammatory transcription factors and cytokines contribute to the overall survival of patients. One study found that 97% of patients with epithelial tumors of malignant pleural mesothelioma and 95% of patients with nonepithelial tumors expressed IL-4Rα protein, and this strong IL-4Rα expression was correlated with a worse survival. In response to IL-4, human malignant pleural mesothelioma cells showed increased STAT6 phosphorylation and increased production of IL-6, IL-8, and VEGF without any effect on proliferation or apoptosis. This finding indicates that high expression of STAT6 as well as STAT3 and cytokines is inversely correlated with survival in patients.[36,37] NF-κB, along with IL-6, contributes to the survival of mammospheres in culture, because NF-κB and IL-6 were hyperactive in breast cancer-derived mammospheres.[38] In addition, elevated CRP and serum amyloid A (SAA) were associated with reduced disease-free survival of breast cancer patients.[39] In gastroesophageal cancer, proinflammatory cytokines IL-1β, IL-6, IL-8, and TNF-α and acute phase protein concentrations (CRP) were found to be elevated, and these levels were associated with reduced survival of patients.[40] Additionally, the Bcl-2 family protein COX-2, which is regulated by inflammatory transcription factors, is also involved in the survival of cancer cells.[41,42] Thus, we conclude that inflammation in general contributes to poor survival of patients.

In contrast to these findings, an in vivo study of dogs with osteosarcoma showed that survival improvement was apparent with inflammation or lymphocyte-infiltration scores >1, as well as in dogs that had apoptosis scores in the top 50th percentile.[43] Also, in patients with epithelioid malignant pleural mesothelioma, a high degree of chronic inflammatory cell infiltration in the stromal component was associated with improved overall survival.[44]

ROLE OF INFLAMMATION IN PROLIFERATION

Several studies have shown that cell proliferation is affected by inflammation.[45] More significantly, proliferation in the setting of chronic inflammation predisposes humans to carcinoma in the esophagus, stomach, colon, liver, and urinary bladder.[46] In postgastrectomy patients, Helicobacter pylori induced inflammation and was associated with increased epithelial cell proliferation.[47] Even in the mouse model, chronic infection with Helicobacter hepaticus induced hepatic inflammation, which further led to hepatic cell proliferation.[48] Other reports found an increased expression of the cell proliferative markers PCNA and Ki-67 in the linings of inflamed odontogenic keratocysts compared with noninflamed lesions.[49,50] These findings suggest the existence of greater proliferative activity in the cells with inflammation. Wang et al.[51] showed an increased expression of cell proliferative markers PCNA and Ki-67 in a sample of 45 patients with benign prostatic hyperplasia.

The inflammatory biomarker COX-2 was also associated with the proliferation of cells. The highest proliferation index was found in COX-2–positive epithelium.[51] The association of COX-2 and proliferation was also reported in a rat model. The carcinogen dimethylhydrazine (DMH) induces an increase in epithelial cell proliferation and in the expression of COX-2 in the colon of rats.[52] Erbb2, a kinase, regulates inflammation through the induction of NF-κB, Comp1, IL-1β, COX-2, and multiple chemokines in the skin by ultraviolet (UV) exposure. This inflammation has been shown to increase the proliferation of skin tissue after UV irradiation.[53]

ROLE OF INFLAMMATION IN INVASION

A characteristic of invasive cancer cells is survival and growth under nonadhesive conditions. This invasion of cancer cells causes the disease to spread, which results in poor patient survival.[54] A strong relationship has been documented between inflammation and cancer cell invasion.[55,56] In a study of 150 patients with HCC, a high GPS score was associated with a high vascular invasion of cancer cells.[57] Another study of colorectal cancer also supports the links between inflammation and the invasion of cancer cells, with a finding that a high GPS increased the invasion of colorectal cancer cells.[58] In patients with esophageal squamous cell carcinoma, a high GPS score also showed a close relationship with lymphatic and venous invasion.[59]

At the molecular level, various proteins are known to be involved in tumor cell invasion. MMP-9, a gelatinase that degrades type IV collagen—the major structural protein component in the extracellular matrix and basement membrane—is thought to play an important role in facilitating tumor invasion, as it is highly expressed in various malignant tumors.[60,61] Additionally, the high expression of HIF-1α has been proposed as being associated with a greater incidence of vascular invasion of HCC. This expression of HIF-1α was further correlated with high expression of the inflammatory molecule COX-2.[62]

Breast cancer invasion has been linked to proteolytic activity at the tumor cell surface. In inflammatory breast cancer (IBC) cells, high expression of cathepsin B, a cell surface proteolytic enzyme, has been shown to be associated with invasiveness of IBC. In addition, a high coexpression of cathepsin B and caveolin-1 was found in IBC patient biopsies. Thus, proteolytic activity of cathepsin B and its coexpression with caveolin-1 contributes to the invasiveness of IBC.[63] In IBC, RhoC GTPase is also responsible for the invasive phenotype.[64] In addition, the PI3K/Akt signaling pathway is crucial in IBC invasion. The molecules involved in cell motility are specifically upregulated in IBC patients compared with stage-matched and cell-type-of-origin–matched non-IBCs patients. Distinctively, RhoC GTPase is a substrate for Akt1, and its phosphorylation is absolutely essential for IBC cell invasion.[65]

ROLE OF INFLAMMATION IN ANGIOGENESIS

Angiogenesis—the formation of new blood vessels from existing vessels—is tightly linked to chronic inflammation and cancer. Angiogenesis is one of the molecular events that bridges the gap between inflammation and cancer. Angiogenesis results from multiple signals acting on endothelial cells. Mature vessels control exchanges of hematopoietic cells and solutes between blood and surrounding tissues by responding to microenvironmental cues, including inflammation. Although inflammation is essential to defend the body against pathogens, it has adverse effects on the surrounding tissue, and some of these effects induce angiogenesis. Inflammation and angiogenesis are thereby linked processes, but exactly how they are related has not been well understood. Both inflammation and angiogenesis are exacerbated by an increased production of chemokines/cytokines, growth factors, proteolytic enzymes, proteoglycans, lipid mediators, and prostaglandins.

A close relationship has been reported between inflammation and angiogenesis in breast cancer. Tissue section staining showed increased vascularity with the intensity of diffuse inflammation.[66] Offersen et al.[67] found that inflammation was significantly correlated in bladder carcinoma with microvessel density, which is a marker of angiogenesis. Leukocytes have been described as mediators of inflammation-associated angiogenesis. In addition, the stable expression of TNF-α in endothelial cells increased angiogenic sprout formation independently of angiogenic growth factors. Furthermore, in work using the Matrigel plug assay in vivo, increased angiogenesis was observed in endothelial TNF-α–expressing mice. Thus, chronic inflammatory changes mediated by TNF-α can induce angiogenesis in vitro and in vivo, suggesting a direct link between inflammation and angiogenesis.[68] TNF-α–induced inhibitor of nuclear factor kappa kinase (IKK)-β activation also activates the angiogenic process. IKK-β activates the mammalian target of rapamycin (mTOR) pathway and enhances angiogenesis through VEGF production.[66] In addition to TNF-α, proinflammatory cytokines IL-1 (mainly IL-1β) and IL-8 were also found to be major proangiogenic stimuli of both physiologic and pathologic angiogenesis.[69,70] Recently, another cytokine macrophage migration inhibitory factor (MIF) was found to play a role in neoangiogenesis/vasculogenesis by endothelial cell activation along with inflammation.[71]

Benest et al.[72] found that a well-known regulator of angiogenesis, angiopoietin-2 (Ang-2), can upregulate inflammatory responses, indicating a common signaling pathway for inflammation and angiogenesis. TGF-β induction was also reported in head and neck epithelia and human head and neck squamous cell carcinomas (HNSCC), with severe inflammation that leads to angiogenesis.[73] The tumor-derived cytokine endothelial monocyte-activating polypeptide II (EMAP-II) has been shown to have profound effects on inflammation as well as on the processes involved in angiogenesis.[74] NF-κB plays an important role in inflammation as well as in angiogenesis, because the suppression of NF-κB and IkB-2A blocks basic fibroblast growth factor–induced angiogenesis in vivo. NF-κB regulates the angiogenic protein VEGF promoted by α5β1 integrin, which coordinately regulates angiogenesis and inflammation.[75] It has been also reported that a coculture of cancer cells with macrophages synergistically increased the production of various angiogenesis-related factors when stimulated by the inflammatory cytokine. This inflammatory angiogenesis was mediated by the activation of NF-κB and activator protein 1 (Jun/Fos), because the administration of either NF-κB–targeting drugs or COX-2 inhibitors or the depletion of macrophages blocked inflammatory angiogenesis.[76]

In a mouse model, cigarette smoke induced the inflammatory protein 5-lipoxygenase (5-LOX), and this induction activated matrix metalloproteinase 2 (MMP-2) and VEGF to induce the angiogenic process.[77] A cellular enzyme, Tank-binding kinase 1

(TBK-1), has been proposed as a putative mediator in tumor angiogenesis. TBK-1 mediates angiogenesis through the upregulation of VEGF and exerts proinflammatory effects via the induction of inflammatory cytokines. Thus, these pathways, including TBK-1, are an important cross-link between angiogenesis and inflammation.[78]

ROLE OF INFLAMMATION IN METASTASIS

Inflammation plays a regulatory role in cancer progression and metastasis. Chronic or tumor-derived inflammation and inflammation-related stimuli within the tumor microenvironment promote blood and lymphatic vessel formation and aid in invasion and metastasis.[79,80] The association of inflammation and metastasis has been observed in several cancer types. In an immunohistochemical analysis of lung cancer tissues, a remarkably high level of metastasis was observed with severe inflammation.[81] A mouse model of breast cancer found that mammary tumors increased the frequency of lung metastases, and this effect was associated with the recruitment of inflammatory cells to the lung as well as elevated levels of IL-6 in the lung airways.[82] In another murine model, implanting human ovarian tumor cells into the ovaries of severe combined immunodeficient mice resulted in peritoneal inflammation and tumor cell dissemination from the ovaries. In addition, enhancement of the inflammatory response with thioglycolate accelerated the development of ascites and metastases, and its suppression with acetylsalicylic acid delayed metastasis.[83] Thus, it can be concluded that inflammation facilitates ovarian tumor metastasis by a mechanism largely mediated by cytokines.

It has been shown that metastatic tumor cells entering a distant organ such as the liver trigger a proinflammatory response involving the Kupffer cell–mediated release of TNF-α and the upregulation of vascular endothelial cell adhesion receptors, such as E-selectin.[84] The physiologic expression of the selectins is tightly controlled to limit the inflammatory response, but dysregulated expression of selectins contributes to inflammatory and thrombotic disorders as well as tumor metastases.[85] Using P-selectin knockout mice, the importance of P-selectin–mediated cell adhesive interactions in the pathogenesis of inflammation and metastasis of cancers has been clearly demonstrated.[86]

Tumor-associated inflammatory monocytes and macrophages are essential promoters of tumor cell migration, invasion, and metastasis.[87] Macrophages and their mediators affect the multistep process of invasion and metastasis, from interaction with the extracellular matrix to the construction of a premetastatic niche. Monocytes are attracted by cytokines and chemokines (e.g., CSF-1, GM-CSF, and MCP-1), which are released by tumor cells or cells of the tumor microenvironment. These monocytes are then induced to express proangiogenic and metastatic factors, including VEGF, fibroblast growth factor (FGF)-2, platelet-derived growth factor (PDGF), intercellular adhesion molecule (ICAM)-1, vascular cell adhesion molecule (VCAM)-1, E-selectin, P- selectin, and MMP-9.[88] Versican, a large extracellular matrix proteoglycan, has been shown to activate tumor-infiltrating myeloid cells through Toll-like receptor (TLR) 2 and its coreceptors TLR6 and CD14 and to elicit the production of proinflammatory cytokines (including TNF-α), which enhance tumor metastasis. TLR2 increases the secretion of IL-8, which potentiates metastatic growth. Ligation of TLR2 by versican induces inflammatory cytokine secretion, providing a link between inflammation and cancer metastasis.[89]

IKK-α has been shown to be important in the inflammation-associated metastasis of cancer cells. Luo et al.[90] demonstrated that activation and nuclear localization of IKK-α by tumor-infiltrating immune cells in prostatic epithelial tumor cells leads to malignant prostatic epithelial cells with a metastatic fate. Src family kinases, when inappropriately activated, promote pathologic inflammatory processes and tumor metastasis, in part through their effects on the regulation of endothelial monolayer permeability.[91] Platelet-activating factor (PAF), an inflammatory biolipid, has also been shown to increase metastasis. In particular, Melnikova et al.[92] demonstrated that PAF receptor antagonists can effectively inhibit the metastatic potential of human melanoma cells in nude mice. Mesenchymal stem cells promote HCC metastasis under the influence of inflammation through TGF-β.[93]

EPIGENETIC CHANGES AND INFLAMMATION

Epigenetics considers the heritable changes in the activity of gene expression without the alteration of DNA sequences, and such changes have been linked to many human diseases, including cancer.[94] DNA methylation and histone modification are well-known epigenetic changes that can lead to gene activation or inactivation.[94–96] DNA methylation occurs primarily at cytosine-phosphate-guanine (CpG) dinucleotides as well as at transcriptional regulatory sites on the gene promoter.[96–98] Epigenetic abnormalities result in dysregulated gene expression and function, which can further lead to cancer. Inflammation and epigenetic abnormalities in cancer are highly associated. Inflammation induces aberrant epigenetic alterations in a tissue early in the process of carcinogenesis, and accumulation of such alterations forms an epigenetic field for cancer. Yara et al.[99] have shown that increased inflammation, as evidenced by the activation of NF-κB, production of IL-6 and COX-2, as well as the decrease of IκB, leads to the promoter's methylation. However, preincubation of cells with a demethylating agent prevented inflammation.

Infectious agents also contribute to inflammation-induced epigenetic changes. Infectious agents such as *H. pylori* and hepatitis C virus as well as intrinsic mediators of inflammatory responses, including proinflammatory cytokines, induce genetic and epigenetic changes, including point mutations, deletions, duplications, recombinations, and methylation of various tumor-related genes. Interestingly, disturbances in cytokine and chemokine signals and the induction of cell proliferation are important ways that inflammation induces aberrant DNA methylation. A study has shown that infection of human gastric mucosae with *H. pylori* induces chronic inflammation and further gastric cancers.[100] This inflammation is associated with high methylation levels or high incidences of methylation.[101–103]

Furthermore, numerous reports have documented the fact that inflammation is linked with epigenetic changes in carcinogenesis. Recently, Achyut[104] reported that inflammation in stromal fibroblasts caused epigenetic silencing of p21 and further tumor progression. Chronic inflammation also led to epigenetic regulation of p16 and activation of DNA damage in a lung carcinogenesis model.[105]

A transient inflammatory signal has been shown to initiate an epigenetic switch from nontransformed cells to cancer cells via a positive feedback loop involving NF-κB, Lin28, let-7, and IL-6. This IL-6 induced STAT3, directly activated miR-21 and miR-181b-1, and further induced the epigenetic switch. Thus, STAT3 underlies the epigenetic switch of mir-21 and mir-181b-1 that links inflammation to cancer.[106] Another report also showed that transient activation of Src oncoprotein mediates an epigenetic switch from immortalized breast cells to a stably transformed line that contained cancer stem cells. Thus, inflammation activates a positive feedback loop that maintains the epigenetic transformed state for many generations in the absence of the inducing signal.[18]

DNA hypermethylation at promoter CpG islands is an important mechanism by which carcinogenesis occurs through the inactivation of tumor-suppressor genes. Aberrant CpG island hypermethylation is also frequently observed in chronic inflammation and precancerous lesions, which again suggests links between inflammation and epigenetic change.[107] In addition, inflammation induced the halogenation of cytosine nucleotide. Damage products of this inflammation-mediated halogenated cytosine interfere with normal epigenetic control by altering DNA-protein interactions that are critical for gene regulation and the heritable transmission of methylation patterns. These inflammation-mediated cytosine damage products also provide a mechanistic link between inflammation and cancer.[108]

ROLE OF INFLAMMATION IN CANCER DIAGNOSIS

Chronic inflammation plays an important role in the etiology and progression of chronic diseases, including cancer. Hence, chronic inflammation may have an important diagnostic role in cancer. Inflammation induced by inflammatory cells such as infiltrating cells and mesothelial cells is mediated via the release of various mediators and proteins, including PDGF, IL-8, monocyte chemotactic peptide (MCP-1), nitric oxide (NO), collagen, antioxidant enzymes, and the plasminogen activation inhibitor (PAI). Furthermore, several inflammatory mediators have been shown to be detected at increased concentrations, thereby aiding in the disease diagnosis.[109]

In one study, numerous inflammatory disorders were detected based on inflammation measured in gastric biopsies of patients by Fourier transform infrared spectroscopy (FT-IR). Using endoscopic samples, gastritis and gastric cancer were diagnosed.[110] Furthermore, the degree of prostate inflammation has been used to determine the level of incidental prostatitis.[111] An assessment of the expression of cytokines and other immune stimulatory molecules that drive B-cell activation provides insight into the etiology of cancers. It has been shown that the dysregulation of cytokine production precedes the diagnosis of non-Hodgkin lymphoma.[112]

Inflammation parameters have been used to diagnose cancer in patients. Inflammation parameters, including CRP, were found to differ in patients with cancer and in those without. In clinical practice, however, such parameters are considered to have modest diagnostic value for cancer.[113] In a study with 1,275 patients, granulomatous inflammation was identified in 154 patients (12.1%), of whom 12 out of 154 (7.8%) had a concurrent diagnosis of cancer.[114] In another study with 173 patients, 52% had lung adenocarcinoma. Patients with high systemic inflammation were more likely to have more than two sites of metastatic disease and to have poor performance status and less likely to receive any chemotherapy. Systemic inflammation at diagnosis is considered to be an independent marker of poor outcome in patients with advanced non-small cell lung cancer (NSCLC).[115]

INFLAMMATION AND GENOMICS

Recently, the genomic landscape of the most common forms of human cancer have been examined.[116] Almost 140 genes and 12 cell signaling pathways have been linked with most cancers. Several of these genes and pathways are directly or indirectly linked with inflammation. A cytokine pattern in patients with cancer has been identified.[117]

INFLAMMATION AND TARGETED THERAPIES

That inflammation can be used as a target for cancer prevention and treatment is indicated by the fact that several drugs approved by the U.S. Food and Drug Administration (FDA) actually modulate proinflammatory pathways. For instance, EGFR, HER2, VEGF, CXCR4, and proteasome have been shown to activate NF-κB–mediated proinflammatory pathways, and their inhibitors have been approved by the FDA for the treatment of various cancers. Similarly, steroids such as dexamethasone, nonsteroidal antiinflammatory drugs (NSAIDs), and statins that are currently used for prevention or treatment have also been found to suppress the NF-κB pathway. Thus, these observations indicate that inflammatory pathways are excellent targets for cancer.

CONCLUSIONS

According to Colditz et al.,[118] almost 50% of all cancers can be prevented based on what we know today. All the studies summarized previously suggest that inflammation is closely linked to cancer, and the incidence of most cancers can be reduced by controlling inflammation. Proinflammatory conditions such as colitis, bronchitis, hepatitis, and gastritis can all eventually lead to cancer. Thus, one must find ways to treat these conditions before the appearance of cancer. All these studies indicate that an antiinflammatory lifestyle could play an important role in both the prevention and treatment of cancer.

REFERENCES

1. Anand P, Kunnumakkara AB, Sundaram C, et al. Cancer is a preventable disease that requires major lifestyle changes. *Pharm Res* 2008;25:2097–2116.
2. Aggarwal BB, Gehlot P. Inflammation and cancer: how friendly is the relationship for cancer patients? *Curr Opin Pharmacol* 2009;9:351–369.
3. Coussens LM, Zitvogel L, Palucka AK. Neutralizing tumor-promoting chronic inflammation: a magic bullet? *Science* 2013;339:286–291.
4. Sethi G, Sung B, Aggarwal BB. TNF: a master switch for inflammation to cancer. *Front Biosci* 2008;13:5094–5107.
5. Karin M. Nuclear factor-kappaB in cancer development and progression. *Nature* 2006;441:431–436.
6. Aggarwal BB. Nuclear factor-kappaB: the enemy within. *Cancer Cell* 2004;6:203–208.
7. Chaturvedi MM, Sung B, Yadav VR, et al. NF-kappaB addiction and its role in cancer: 'one size does not fit all'. *Oncogene* 2011;30:1615–1630.
8. Aggarwal BB. Signalling pathways of the TNF superfamily: a double-edged sword. *Nat Rev Immunol* 2003;3:745–756.
9. Aggarwal BB, Gupta SC, Kim JH. Historical perspectives on tumor necrosis factor and its superfamily: 25 years later, a golden journey. *Blood* 2012;119:651–665.
10. Iannitti T, Capone S, Gatti A, et al. Intracellular heavy metal nanoparticle storage: progressive accumulation within lymph nodes with transformation from chronic inflammation to malignancy. *Int J Nanomed* 2010;5:955–960.
11. Zhao Y, Xu Y, Li Y, et al. NF-kappaB-mediated inflammation leading to EMT via miR-200c is involved in cell transformation induced by cigarette smoke extract. *Toxicol Sci* 2013;135:265–276.
12. Xu Y, Zhao Y, Xu W, et al. Involvement of HIF-2alpha-mediated inflammation in arsenite-induced transformation of human bronchial epithelial cells. *Toxicol Appl Pharmacol* 2013;272:542–550.
13. Liu K, Jiang M, Lu Y, et al. Sox2 cooperates with inflammation-mediated Stat3 activation in the malignant transformation of foregut basal progenitor cells. *Cell Stem Cell* 2013;12:304–315.
14. Yoon BN, Chon KM, Hong SL, et al. Inflammation and apoptosis in malignant transformation of sinonasal inverted papilloma: the role of the bridge molecules, cyclooxygenase-2, and nuclear factor kappaB. *Am J Otolaryngol* 2013;34:22–30.
15. Roslind A, Johansen JS. YKL-40: a novel marker shared by chronic inflammation and oncogenic transformation. *Methods Mol Biol* 2009;511:159–184.
16. Coste I, Le Corf K, Kfoury A, et al. Dual function of MyD88 in RAS signaling and inflammation, leading to mouse and human cell transformation. *J Clin Invest* 2010;120:3663–3667.
17. Parthasarathy S, Dhayaparan D, Jayanthi V, et al. Aberrant expression of epidermal growth factor receptor and its interaction with protein kinase C delta in inflammation associated neoplastic transformation of human esophageal epithelium in high risk populations. *J Gastroenterol Hepatol* 2011;26:382–390.
18. Iliopoulos D, Hirsch HA, Struhl K. An epigenetic switch involving NF-kappaB, Lin28, Let-7 MicroRNA, and IL6 links inflammation to cell transformation. *Cell* 2009;139:693–706.
19. Colotta F, Allavena P, Sica A, et al. Cancer-related inflammation, the seventh hallmark of cancer: links to genetic instability. *Carcinogenesis* 2009;30:1073–1081.
20. Hanahan D, Weinberg RA. Hallmarks of cancer: the next generation. *Cell* 2011;144:646–674.
21. Canna K, McMillan DC, McKee RF, et al. Evaluation of a cumulative prognostic score based on the systemic inflammatory response in patients undergoing potentially curative surgery for colorectal cancer. *Br J Cancer* 2004;90:1707–1709.

22. Hilmy M, Bartlett JM, Underwood MA, et al. The relationship between the systemic inflammatory response and survival in patients with transitional cell carcinoma of the urinary bladder. *Br J Cancer* 2005;92:625–627.
23. Forrest LM, McMillan DC, McArdle CS, et al. Evaluation of cumulative prognostic scores based on the systemic inflammatory response in patients with inoperable non-small-cell lung cancer. *Br J Cancer* 2003;89:1028–1030.
24. Ramsey S, Lamb GW, Aitchison M, et al. Evaluation of an inflammation-based prognostic score in patients with metastatic renal cancer. *Cancer* 2007;109:205–212.
25. Crumley AB, Stuart RC, McKernan M, et al. Comparison of an inflammation-based prognostic score (GPS) with performance status (ECOG-ps) in patients receiving palliative chemotherapy for gastroesophageal cancer. *J Gastroenterol Hepatol* 2008;23:e325–329.
26. Yamanaka T, Matsumoto S, Teramukai S, et al. The baseline ratio of neutrophils to lymphocytes is associated with patient prognosis in advanced gastric cancer. *Oncology* 2007;73:215–220.
27. Halazun KJ, Aldoori A, Malik HZ, et al. Elevated preoperative neutrophil to lymphocyte ratio predicts survival following hepatic resection for colorectal liver metastases. *Eur J Surg Oncol* 2008;34:55–60.
28. Huang ZL, Luo J, Chen MS, et al. Blood neutrophil-to-lymphocyte ratio predicts survival in patients with unresectable hepatocellular carcinoma undergoing transarterial chemoembolization. *J Vasc Interv Radiol* 2011;22:702–709.
29. Heng DY, Xie W, Regan MM, et al. Prognostic factors for overall survival in patients with metastatic renal cell carcinoma treated with vascular endothelial growth factor-targeted agents: results from a large, multicenter study. *J Clin Oncol* 2009;27:5794–5799.
30. Smith RA, Bosonnet L, Raraty M, et al. Preoperative platelet-lymphocyte ratio is an independent significant prognostic marker in resected pancreatic ductal adenocarcinoma. *Am J Surg* 2009;197:466–472.
31. Fox P, Hudson M, Brown C, et al. Markers of systemic inflammation predict survival in patients with advanced renal cell cancer. *Br J Cancer* 2013; 109:147–153.
32. Iwasaki Y, Ishizuka M, Kato M, et al. Usefulness of an inflammation-based prognostic score (mGPS) for predicting survival in patients with unresectable malignant biliary obstruction. *World J Surg* 2013;37:2222–2228.
33. Shafique K, Proctor MJ, McMillan DC, et al. Systemic inflammation and survival of patients with prostate cancer: evidence from the Glasgow Inflammation Outcome Study. *Prostate Cancer Prostatic Dis* 2012;15:195–201.
34. Kunisaki C, Takahashi M, Ono HA, et al. Inflammation-based prognostic score predicts survival in patients with advanced gastric cancer receiving biweekly docetaxel and s-1 combination chemotherapy. *Oncology* 2012;83:183–191.
35. Pinato DJ, Sharma R. An inflammation-based prognostic index predicts survival advantage after transarterial chemoembolization in hepatocellular carcinoma. *Transl Res* 2012;160:146–152.
36. Burt BM, Bader A, Winter D, et al. Expression of interleukin-4 receptor alpha in human pleural mesothelioma is associated with poor survival and promotion of tumor inflammation. *Clin Cancer Res* 2012;18:1568–1577.
37. Sethi G, Shanmugam MK, Ramachandran L, et al. Multifaceted link between cancer and inflammation. *Biosci Rep* 2012;32:1–15.
38. Papi A, Guarnieri T, Storci G, et al. Nuclear receptors agonists exert opposing effects on the inflammation dependent survival of breast cancer stem cells. *Cell Death Differ* 2012;19:1208–1219.
39. Pierce BL, Ballard-Barbash R, Bernstein L, et al. Elevated biomarkers of inflammation are associated with reduced survival among breast cancer patients. *J Clin Oncol* 2009;27:3437–3444.
40. Deans DA, Wigmore SJ, Gilmour H, et al. Elevated tumour interleukin-1beta is associated with systemic inflammation: a marker of reduced survival in gastro-oesophageal cancer. *Br J Cancer* 2006;95:1568–1575.
41. Chen LS, Balakrishnan K, Gandhi V. Inflammation and survival pathways: chronic lymphocytic leukemia as a model system. *Biochem Pharmacol* 2010;80:1936–1945.
42. Sharma-Walia N, Paul AG, Bottero V, et al. Kaposi's sarcoma associated herpes virus (KSHV) induced COX-2: a key factor in latency, inflammation, angiogenesis, cell survival and invasion. *PLoS Pathog* 2010;6:e1000777.
43. Modiano JF, Bellgrau D, Cutter GR, et al. Inflammation, apoptosis, and necrosis induced by neoadjuvant fas ligand gene therapy improves survival of dogs with spontaneous bone cancer. *Mol Ther* 2012;20:2234–2243.
44. Suzuki K, Kadota K, Sima CS, et al. Chronic inflammation in tumor stroma is an independent predictor of prolonged survival in epithelioid malignant pleural mesothelioma patients. *Cancer Immunol Immunother* 2011;60:1721–1728.
45. Hu B, Elinav E, Flavell RA. Inflammasome-mediated suppression of inflammation-induced colorectal cancer progression is mediated by direct regulation of epithelial cell proliferation. *Cell Cycle* 2011;10:1936–1939.
46. Sugar LM. Inflammation and prostate cancer. *Can J Urol* 2006;13(Suppl 1):46–47.
47. Safatle-Ribeiro AV, Ribeiro U, Jr., Clarke MR, et al. Relationship between persistence of Helicobacter pylori and dysplasia, intestinal metaplasia, atrophy, inflammation, and cell proliferation following partial gastrectomy. *Dig Dis Sci* 1999;44:243–252.
48. Ihrig M, Schrenzel MD, Fox JG. Differential susceptibility to hepatic inflammation and proliferation in AXB recombinant inbred mice chronically infected with Helicobacter hepaticus. *Am J Pathol* 1999;155:571–582.
49. de Paula AM, Carvalhais JN, Domingues MG, et al. Cell proliferation markers in the odontogenic keratocyst: effect of inflammation. *J Oral Pathol Med* 2000;29:477–482.
50. Kaplan I, Hirshberg A. The correlation between epithelial cell proliferation and inflammation in odontogenic keratocyst. *Oral Oncol* 2004;40:985–991.
51. Wang W, Bergh A, Damber JE. Chronic inflammation in benign prostate hyperplasia is associated with focal upregulation of cyclooxygenase-2, Bcl-2, and cell proliferation in the glandular epithelium. *Prostate* 2004;61:60–72.
52. Demarzo MM, Martins LV, Fernandes CR, et al. Exercise reduces inflammation and cell proliferation in rat colon carcinogenesis. *Med Sci Sports Exerc* 2008;40:618–621.
53. Madson JG, Lynch DT, Tinkum KL, et al. Erbb2 regulates inflammation and proliferation in the skin after ultraviolet irradiation. *Am J Pathol* 2006; 169:1402–1414.
54. Bondong S, Kiefel H, Hielscher T, et al. Prognostic significance of L1CAM in ovarian cancer and its role in constitutive NF-kappaB activation. *Ann Oncol* 2012;23:1795–1802.
55. Wu Y, Zhou BP. Inflammation: a driving force speeds cancer metastasis. *Cell Cycle* 2009;8:3267–3273.
56. Aggarwal BB, Vijayalekshmi RV, Sung B. Targeting inflammatory pathways for prevention and therapy of cancer: short-term friend, long-term foe. *Clin Cancer Res* 2009;15:425–430.
57. Kinoshita A, Onoda H, Imai N, et al. The Glasgow Prognostic Score, an inflammation based prognostic score, predicts survival in patients with hepatocellular carcinoma. *BMC Cancer* 2013;13:52.
58. Toiyama Y, Miki C, Inoue Y, et al. Evaluation of an inflammation-based prognostic score for the identification of patients requiring postoperative adjuvant chemotherapy for stage II colorectal cancer. *Exp Ther Med* 2011;2:95–101.
59. Kobayashi T, Teruya M, Kishiki T, et al. Inflammation-based prognostic score, prior to neoadjuvant chemoradiotherapy, predicts postoperative outcome in patients with esophageal squamous cell carcinoma. *Surgery* 2008;144:729–735.
60. Nelson AR, Fingleton B, Rothenberg ML, et al. Matrix metalloproteinases: biologic activity and clinical implications. *J Clin Oncol* 2000;18:1135–1149.
61. Clark ES, Weaver AM. A new role for cortactin in invadopodia: regulation of protease secretion. *Eur J Cell Biol* 2008;87:581–590.
62. Dai CX, Gao Q, Qiu SJ, et al. Hypoxia-inducible factor-1 alpha, in association with inflammation, angiogenesis and MYC, is a critical prognostic factor in patients with HCC after surgery. *BMC Cancer* 2009;9:418.
63. Victor BC, Anbalagan A, Mohamed MM, et al. Inhibition of cathepsin B activity attenuates extracellular matrix degradation and inflammatory breast cancer invasion. *Breast Cancer Res* 2011;13:R115.
64. van Golen KL, Bao LW, Pan Q, et al. Mitogen activated protein kinase pathway is involved in RhoC GTPase induced motility, invasion and angiogenesis in inflammatory breast cancer. *Clin Exp Metastasis* 2002;19:301–311.
65. Lehman HL, Van Laere SJ, van Golen CM, et al. Regulation of inflammatory breast cancer cell invasion through Akt1/PKBalpha phosphorylation of RhoC GTPase. *Mol Cancer Res* 2012;10:1306–1318.
66. Lee DF, Kuo HP, Chen CT, et al. IKK beta suppression of TSC1 links inflammation and tumor angiogenesis via the mTOR pathway. *Cell* 2007;130: 440–455.
67. Offersen BV, Knap MM, Marcussen N, et al. Intense inflammation in bladder carcinoma is associated with angiogenesis and indicates good prognosis. *Br J Cancer* 2002;87:1422–1430.
68. Rajashekhar G, Willuweit A, Patterson CE, et al. Continuous endothelial cell activation increases angiogenesis: evidence for the direct role of endothelium linking angiogenesis and inflammation. *J Vasc Res* 2006;43:193–204.
69. Voronov E, Carmi Y, Apte RN. Role of IL-1-mediated inflammation in tumor angiogenesis. *Adv Exp Med Biol* 2007;601:265–270.
70. Qazi BS, Tang K, Qazi A. Recent advances in underlying pathologies provide insight into interleukin-8 expression-mediated inflammation and angiogenesis. *Int J Inflam* 2011;2011:908468.
71. Asare Y, Schmitt M, Bernhagen J. The vascular biology of macrophage migration inhibitory factor (MIF). Expression and effects in inflammation, atherogenesis and angiogenesis. *Thromb Haemost* 2013;109:391–398.
72. Benest AV, Kruse K, Savant S, et al. Angiopoietin-2 is critical for cytokine-induced vascular leakage. *PLoS One* 2013;8: e70459.
73. Lu SL, Reh D, Li AG, et al. Overexpression of transforming growth factor beta1 in head and neck epithelia results in inflammation, angiogenesis, and epithelial hyperproliferation. *Cancer Res* 2004;64:4405–4410.
74. Berger AC, Tang G, Alexander HR, et al. Endothelial monocyte-activating polypeptide II, a tumor-derived cytokine that plays an important role in inflammation, apoptosis, and angiogenesis. *J Immunother* 2000;23:519–527.
75. Klein S, de Fougerolles AR, Blaikie P, et al. Alpha 5 beta 1 integrin activates an NF-kappa B-dependent program of gene expression important for angiogenesis and inflammation. *Mol Cell Biol* 2002;22:5912–5922.
76. Ono M. Molecular links between tumor angiogenesis and inflammation: inflammatory stimuli of macrophages and cancer cells as targets for therapeutic strategy. *Cancer Sci* 2008;99:1501–1506.
77. Ye YN, Liu ES, Shin VY, et al. Contributory role of 5-lipoxygenase and its association with angiogenesis in the promotion of inflammation-associated colonic tumorigenesis by cigarette smoking. *Toxicology* 2004;203:179–188.
78. Czabanka M, Korherr C, Brinkmann U, et al. Influence of TBK-1 on tumor angiogenesis and microvascular inflammation. *Front Biosci* 2008;13: 7243–7249.
79. Solinas G, Marchesi F, Garlanda C, et al. Inflammation-mediated promotion of invasion and metastasis. *Cancer Metastasis Rev* 2010;29:243–248.
80. Affara NI, Coussens LM. IKKalpha at the crossroads of inflammation and metastasis. *Cell* 2007;129:25–26.
81. Kayser K, Bulzebruck H, Ebert W, et al. Local tumor inflammation, lymph node metastasis, and survival of operated bronchus carcinoma patients. *J Natl Cancer Inst* 1986;77:77–81.

82. Hobson J, Gummadidala P, Silverstrim B, et al. Acute inflammation induced by the biopsy of mouse mammary tumors promotes the development of metastasis. *Breast Cancer Res Treat* 2013;139:391–401.
83. Robinson-Smith TM, Isaacsohn I, Mercer CA, et al. Macrophages mediate inflammation-enhanced metastasis of ovarian tumors in mice. *Cancer Res* 2007;67:5708–5716.
84. Khatib AM, Auguste P, Fallavollita L, et al. Characterization of the host proinflammatory response to tumor cells during the initial stages of liver metastasis. *Am J Pathol* 2005;167:749–759.
85. McEver RP. Selectin-carbohydrate interactions during inflammation and metastasis. *Glycoconj J* 1997;14:585–591.
86. Geng JG, Chen M, Chou KC. P-selectin cell adhesion molecule in inflammation, thrombosis, cancer growth and metastasis. *Curr Med Chem* 2004;11:2153–2160.
87. Condeelis J, Pollard JW. Macrophages: obligate partners for tumor cell migration, invasion, and metastasis. *Cell* 2006;124:263–266.
88. Siegel G, Malmsten M. The role of the endothelium in inflammation and tumor metastasis. *Int J Microcirc Clin Exp* 1997;17:257–272.
89. Wang W, Xu GL, Jia WD, et al. Ligation of TLR2 by versican: a link between inflammation and metastasis. *Arch Med Res* 2009;40:321–323.
90. Luo JL, Tan W, Ricono JM, et al. Nuclear cytokine-activated IKKalpha controls prostate cancer metastasis by repressing Maspin. *Nature* 2007;446:690–694.
91. Kim MP, Park SI, Kopetz S, et al. Src family kinases as mediators of endothelial permeability: effects on inflammation and metastasis. *Cell Tissue Res* 2009;335:249–259.
92. Melnikova V, Bar-Eli M. Inflammation and melanoma growth and metastasis: the role of platelet-activating factor (PAF) and its receptor. *Cancer Metastasis Rev* 2007;26:359–371.
93. Jing Y, Han Z, Liu Y, et al. Mesenchymal stem cells in inflammation microenvironment accelerates hepatocellular carcinoma metastasis by inducing epithelial-mesenchymal transition. *PLoS One* 2012;7:e43272.
94. Jones PA, Baylin SB. The epigenomics of cancer. *Cell* 2007;128:683–692.
95. Esteller M. Aberrant DNA methylation as a cancer-inducing mechanism. *Annu Rev Pharmacol Toxicol* 2005;45:629–656.
96. Thiagalingam S, Cheng KH, Lee HJ, et al. Histone deacetylases: unique players in shaping the epigenetic histone code. *Ann N Y Acad Sci* 2003;983:84–100.
97. Li E, Beard C, Jaenisch R. Role for DNA methylation in genomic imprinting. *Nature* 1993;366:362–365.
98. Antequera F, Bird A. Number of CpG islands and genes in human and mouse. *Proc Natl Acad Sci U S A* 1993;90:11995–11999.
99. Yara S, Lavoie JC, Beaulieu JF, et al. Iron-ascorbate-mediated lipid peroxidation causes epigenetic changes in the antioxidant defense in intestinal epithelial cells: impact on inflammation. *PLoS One* 2013;8:e63456.
100. Uemura N, Okamoto S, Yamamoto S, et al. Helicobacter pylori infection and the development of gastric cancer. *N Engl J Med* 2001;345:784–789.
101. Maekita T, Nakazawa K, Mihara M, et al. High levels of aberrant DNA methylation in Helicobacter pylori-infected gastric mucosae and its possible association with gastric cancer risk. *Clin Cancer Res* 2006;12:989–995.
102. Nakajima T, Maekita T, Oda I, et al. Higher methylation levels in gastric mucosae significantly correlate with higher risk of gastric cancers. *Cancer Epidemiol Biomarkers Prev* 2006;15:2317–2321.
103. Perri F, Cotugno R, Piepoli A, et al. Aberrant DNA methylation in non-neoplastic gastric mucosa of H. Pylori infected patients and effect of eradication. *Am J Gastroenterol* 2007;102:1361–1371.
104. Achyut BR, Bader DA, Robles AI, et al. Inflammation-mediated genetic and epigenetic alterations drive cancer development in the neighboring epithelium upon stromal abrogation of TGF-beta signaling. *PLoS Genet* 2013;9:e1003251.
105. Blanco D, Vicent S, Fraga MF, et al. Molecular analysis of a multistep lung cancer model induced by chronic inflammation reveals epigenetic regulation of p16 and activation of the DNA damage response pathway. *Neoplasia* 2007;9:840–852.
106. Iliopoulos D, Jaeger SA, Hirsch HA, et al. STAT3 activation of miR-21 and miR-181b-1 via PTEN and CYLD are part of the epigenetic switch linking inflammation to cancer. *Mol Cell* 2010;39:493–506.
107. Suzuki H, Toyota M, Kondo Y, et al. Inflammation-related aberrant patterns of DNA methylation: detection and role in epigenetic deregulation of cancer cell transcriptome. *Methods Mol Biol* 2009;512:55–69.
108. Valinluck V, Sowers LC. Inflammation-mediated cytosine damage: a mechanistic link between inflammation and the epigenetic alterations in human cancers. *Cancer Res* 2007;67:5583–5586.
109. Kroegel C, Antony VB. Immunobiology of pleural inflammation: potential implications for pathogenesis, diagnosis and therapy. *Eur Respir J* 1997;10:2411–2418.
110. Li QB, Sun XJ, Xu YZ, et al. Use of Fourier-transform infrared spectroscopy to rapidly diagnose gastric endoscopic biopsies. *World J Gastroenterol* 2005;11:3842–3845.
111. Difuccia B, Keith I, Teunissen B, et al. Diagnosis of prostatic inflammation: efficacy of needle biopsies versus tissue blocks. *Urology* 2005;65:445–448.
112. Vendrame E, Martinez-Maza O. Assessment of pre-diagnosis biomarkers of immune activation and inflammation: insights on the etiology of lymphoma. *J Proteome Res* 2011;10:113–119.
113. Baicus C, Caraiola S, Rimbas M, et al. Utility of routine hematological and inflammation parameters for the diagnosis of cancer in involuntary weight loss. *J Investig Med* 2011;59:951–955.
114. DePew ZS, Gonsalves WI, Roden AC, et al. Granulomatous inflammation detected by endobronchial ultrasound-guided transbronchial needle aspiration in patients with a concurrent diagnosis of cancer: a clinical conundrum. *J Bronchology Interv Pulmonol* 2012;19:176–181.
115. Jafri SH, Shi R, Mills G. Advance lung cancer inflammation index (ALI) at diagnosis is a prognostic marker in patients with metastatic non-small cell lung cancer (NSCLC): a retrospective review. *BMC Cancer* 2013;13:158.
116. Vogelstein B, Papadopoulos N, Velculescu VE, et al. Cancer genome landscapes. *Science* 2013;339:1546–1558.
117. Lippitz BE. Cytokine patterns in patients with cancer: a systematic review. *Lancet Oncol* 2013;14:e218–228.
118. Colditz GA, Wolin KY, Gehlert S. Applying what we know to accelerate cancer prevention. *Sci Transl Med* 2012;4(127):127rv4.

7 Chemical Factors

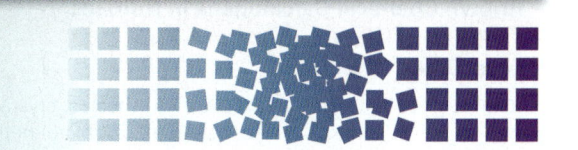

Stuart H. Yuspa and Peter G. Shields

INTRODUCTION

As early as the 1800s, initial observations of unusual cancer incidences in occupational groups provided the first indications that chemicals were a cause of human cancer, which was then confirmed in experimental animal studies during the early and mid 1900s. However, the extent to which chemical exposures contribute to cancer incidence was not fully appreciated until population-based studies documented differing organ-specific cancer rates in geographically distinct populations and in cohort studies such as those that linked smoking to lung cancer.[1] The most commonly occurring chemical exposures that increase cancer risk are tobacco, alcoholic beverages, diet, and reproductive factors (e.g., hormones). Today, it is recognized that cancer results not solely from chemical exposure (e.g., in the workplace or at home), but that a variety of biologic, social, and physical factors contribute to cancer pathogenesis.[2,3] For some common cancers, it also has been recognized that heritable factors also contribute to cancer risk from chemical exposure (e.g., genes involved in carcinogen metabolism, DNA repair, a variety of cancer pathways).[4] Twin studies show that for common cancers, nongenetic risk factors are dominant, and the best associations for genetic risks of sporadic cancers indicate that the risks for specific genetic traits are typically less than 1.5-fold.[5-7] The role of the tumor microenvironment, the cancer stem cells, and feedback signaling to and from the tumor also have been recently recognized as important contributors to carcinogenesis, although how chemicals affect these have yet been clearly demonstrated.[8-10]

The experimental induction of tumors in animals, the neoplastic transformation of cultured cells by chemicals, and the molecular analysis of human tumors have revealed important concepts regarding the pathogenesis of cancer and how laboratory studies can be used to better understand human cancer pathogenesis.[7,11,12] Chemical carcinogens usually affect specific organs, targeting the epithelial cells (or other susceptible cells within an organ) and causing genetic damage (genotoxic) or epigenetic effects regulating DNA transcription and translation. Chemically related DNA damage and consequent somatic mutations relevant to human cancer can occur either directly from exogenous exposures or indirectly by activation of endogenous mutagenic pathways (e.g., nitric oxide, oxyradicals).[13,14] The risk of developing a chemically induced tumor may be modified by nongenotoxic exogenous and endogenous exposures and factors (e.g., hormones, immunosuppression triggered by the tumor), and by accumulated exposure to the same or different genotoxic carcinogens.[7,15]

Analyses of how chemicals induce cancer in animal models and human populations has had a major impact on human health. Experimental studies have been instrumental in replicating hypotheses generated from human studies and identifying pathobiologic mechanisms. For example, animal experiments confirmed the carcinogenic and cocarcinogenic properties of cigarette smoke and identified bioactive chemical and gaseous components.[1] The transplacental carcinogenicity of diethylstilbestrol and the hazards of specific occupational carcinogens such as vinyl chloride, benzene, aromatic amines, and bis(chloromethyl)ether led to a reduction in allowable exposures of suspected human carcinogens from the workplace and a reduction in cancer rates. Dietary factors that enhance or inhibit cancer development and the contribution of obesity to specific organ sites have been identified in models of chemical carcinogenesis, and alterations in diet and obesity are expected to result in reduced cancer risk. Experimental animal studies are the mainstay of risk assessment as a screening tool to identify potential carcinogens in the workplace and the environment, although these studies do not prove specific chemical etiologies as a cause of human cancer because of interspecies differences and the use of maximally tolerated doses that do not replicate human exposure.

THE NATURE OF CHEMICAL CARCINOGENS: CHEMISTRY AND METABOLISM

The National Toxicology Program, based mostly on experimental animal studies and supported by epidemiology studies when available, lists 45 chemical, physical, and infectious agents as known human carcinogens and about 175 that are reasonably anticipated to be human carcinogens (http://ntp.niehs.nih.gov/?objectid=035E57E7-BDD9-2D9B-AFB9D1CADC8D09C1), whereas the International Agency for Research on Cancer (IARC) lists 113 agents as carcinogenic to humans and 66 that are probably carcinogenic to humans (http://monographs.iarc.fr/ENG/Classification/index.php). Table 7.1 provides a selected list of known human carcinogens, as indicated by the IARC, which are continuously updated.[16] Most chemical carcinogens first undergo metabolic activation by cytochrome P450s or other metabolic pathways so that they react with DNA and/or alter epigenetic mechanisms.[11,17] This process, evolutionarily presumed to have been developed to rid the body of foreign chemicals for excretion, inadvertently generates reactive carcinogenic intermediates that can bind cellular molecules, including DNA, and cause mutations or other alterations.[18] Recent data indicate that metabolizing enzymes also have the ability to cross-talk with transcription factors involved in the regulation of other metabolizing and antioxidant enzymes.[19] DNA is considered the ultimate target for most carcinogens to cause either mutations or gross chromosomal changes, but epigenetic effects, such as altered DNA methylation and gene transcription, also promote carcinogenesis.[20] The formation of DNA adducts, where chemicals bind directly to DNA to promote mutations, is likely necessary but not sufficient to cause cancer.

Genotoxic carcinogens may transfer simple alkyl or complexed (aryl) alkyl groups to specific sites on DNA bases.[18,21] These alkylating and aryl-alkylating agents include, but are not limited to, N-nitroso compounds, aliphatic epoxides, aflatoxins, mustards, polycyclic aromatic hydrocarbons, and other combustion products of fossil fuels and vegetable matter. Others transfer arylamine residues to DNA, as exemplified by aryl aromatic

TABLE 7.1 Known Chemical Carcinogens in Humans[a]

Target Organ	Agents	Industries	Tumor Type
Lung	Tobacco smoke, arsenic, asbestos, crystalline silica, benzo(a)pyrene, beryllium, bis(chloro)methyl ether, 1,3-butadiene, chromium VI compounds, coal tar and pitch, diesel exhaust, nickel compounds, soot, mustard gas, cobalt-tungsten carbide powders	Aluminum production, coal gasification, coke production, painting, hematite mining, painting, grinding in oil and gas	Squamous, large cell, and small cell cancer and adenocarcinoma
Pleura	Asbestos, erionite, painting	Insulation, mining	Mesothelioma
Oral cavity	Tobacco smoke, alcoholic beverages, nickel compounds, betel quid	–	Squamous cell cancer
Esophagus	Tobacco smoke, alcoholic beverages, betel quid	–	Squamous cell cancer
Gastric	Tobacco smoking	Rubber industry	Adenocarcinoma
Colon	Alcohol, tobacco smoking	–	Adenocarcinoma
Liver	Aflatoxin, vinyl chloride, tobacco smoke, alcoholic beverages	–	Hepatocellular carcinoma, hemangiosarcoma
Kidney	Tobacco smoke, trichloroethylene	–	Renal cell cancer
Bladder	Tobacco smoke, 4-aminobiphenyl, benzidine, 2-napthylamine, cyclophosphamide, phenacetin	Magenta manufacturing, auramine manufacturing, painting, rubber production	Transitional cell cancer
Prostate	Cadmium	–	Adenocarcinoma
Skin	Arsenic, benzo(a)pyrene, coal tar and pitch, mineral oils, soot, cyclosporin A, azathioprine, shale oils	–	Squamous cell cancer, basal cell cancer
Bone marrow	Benzene, tobacco smoke, ethylene oxide, antineoplastic agents, cyclosporin A, formaldehyde	Rubber workers	Leukemia, lymphoma

[a] The carcinogen designations are determined by the International Agency for Research on Cancer (http://monographs.iarc.fr/index.php). They do not imply proof of carcinogenicity in individuals. This table is not all inclusive. For additional information, the reader is referred to agency documents and publications.

amines, aminoazo dyes, and heterocyclic aromatic amines. For genotoxic carcinogens, the interaction with DNA is not random, and each class of agents reacts selectively with purine and pyrimidine targets.[7,18,21] Furthermore, targeting carcinogens to particular sites in DNA is determined by nucleotide sequence, by host cell, and by selective DNA repair processes (see later discussion), making some genetic material at risk over others. As expected from this chemistry, genotoxic carcinogens can be potent mutagens and particularly adept at causing nucleotide base mispairing or small deletions, leading to missense or nonsense mutations. Others may cause macrogenetic damage, such as chromosome breaks and large deletions. In some cases, such genotoxic damage may result in changes in transcription and translation that affect protein levels or function, which in turn alter the behavior of the specific host cell type. For example, there may be effects on cell proliferation, programmed cell death, or DNA repair. This is best typified by the signature mutations detected in the p53 gene caused by ingested aflatoxin in human liver cancer[22] and by polycyclic aromatic hydrocarbons human lung cancer caused by the inhalation of cigarette smoke.[15,23,24] Similarly, a distinct pattern of mutations is detected in pancreatic cancers from smokers when compared with pancreatic cancers from nonsmokers.[25]

Some chemicals that cause cancers in laboratory rodents are not demonstrably genotoxic. In general, these agents are carcinogenic in laboratory animals at high doses and require prolonged exposure. Synthetic pesticides and herbicides fall within this group, as do a number of natural products that are ingested. The mechanism of action by nongenotoxic carcinogens is not well understood, and may be related in some cases to toxic cell death and regenerative hyperplasia. They may also induce endogenous mutagenic mechanisms through the production of free radicals, increasing rates of depurination, and the deamination of 5-methylcytosine. In other cases, nongenotoxic carcinogens may have hormonal effects on hormone-dependent tissues. For example, some pesticides, herbicides, and fungicides have endocrine-disrupting properties in experimental models, although the relation to human cancer risk is unknown.

ANIMAL MODEL SYSTEMS AND CHEMICAL CARCINOGENESIS

Most human chemical carcinogens can induce tumors in experimental animals; however, the tumors may not be in the same organ, the exposure pathways may differ from human exposure, and the causative mechanisms may not exist in humans. In many cases, however, the cell of origin, morphogenesis, phenotypic markers, and genetic alterations are qualitatively identical to corresponding human cancers. Furthermore, animal models have revealed the constancy of carcinogen–host interaction among mammalian species by reproducing organ-specific cancers in animals with chemicals identified as human carcinogens, such as coal tar and squamous cell carcinomas, vinyl chloride and hepatic angiosarcomas, aflatoxin and hepatocellular carcinoma, and aromatic amines and bladder cancer. The introduction of genetically modified mice designed to reproduce specific human cancer syndromes and precancer models has accelerated both the understanding of the contributions of chemicals to cancer causation and the identification of potential exogenous carcinogens.[26,27] Furthermore, construction of mouse strains genetically altered to express human drug–metabolizing enzymes has added both to the relevance of mouse studies for understanding human carcinogen metabolism and the prediction of genotoxicity from suspected human carcinogens and other chemical exposures.[28] Together, these studies have indicated that carcinogenic agents can directly activate oncogenes, inactivate tumor suppressor genes, and cause the genomic changes that are associated with autonomous growth, enhanced survival, and modified gene expression profiles that are required for the malignant phenotype.[29]

Genetic Susceptibility to Chemical Carcinogenesis in Experimental Animal Models

The use of inbred strains of rodents and spontaneous or genetically modified mutant strains have led to the identification and characterization of genes that modify risks for cancer development.[30–32] For a variety of tissue sites, including the lungs, the liver, the breast, and the skin, pairs of inbred mice can differ by 100-fold in the risk for tumor development after carcinogen exposure. Genetically determined differences in the affinity for the aryl hydrocarbon hydroxylase (Ah) receptor or other differences in metabolic processing of carcinogens is one modifier that has a major impact on experimental and presumed human cancer risk.[33–35] The development of mice reconstituted with components of the human carcinogen–metabolizing genome should facilitate the extrapolation of metabolic activity by human enzymes and cancer risk.[27,28,36] Such mice also show that other loci regulate the growth of premalignant foci, the response to tumor promoters, the immune response to metastatic cells, and the basal proliferation rate of target cells.[30] In mice susceptible to colon cancer due to a carcinogen-induced constitutive mutation in the APC gene, a locus on mouse chromosome 4 confers resistance to colon cancer.[31] The identification of the phospholipase A2 gene at this locus and subsequent functional testing in transgenic mice revealed an interesting paracrine protective influence on tumor development.[31] This gene, and several other genes mapped for susceptibility to chemically induced mouse tumors (PTPRJ, a receptor type tyrosine phosphatase, and STK6/STK15, an aurora kinase), have now been shown to influence susceptibility to organ-specific cancer induction in humans.[30,31]

MOLECULAR EPIDEMIOLOGY, CHEMICAL CARCINOGENESIS, AND CANCER RISK IN HUMAN POPULATIONS

Molecular epidemiology is the application of biologically based hypotheses using molecular and epidemiologic methods and measures. New technologies continue to allow epidemiologic studies to improve the testing of biologically based hypotheses and to develop large datasets for hypothesis generation, most notably the application of various –omics technologies via next-generation sequencing (e.g., genomics, epigenomics, transcriptomics), proteomics, and metabolomics. The greatest challenge now is to develop methods that allow for analysis cutting across various technologies.[37–43] Recent advances now include the role of microRNA and long noncoding RNAs in tumor development and progression because of their impact on the regulation of gene expression.[44,45] Chemical effects on microRNAs and the resultant gene expression is currently being identified.[46] Using such technologies, emerging evidence is noting the importance of the microbiome and associated infections as a risk of human cancer.[47–50] The complexity of environmental exposure and how it interacts with humans to affect numerous biologic pathways has been characterized as the exposome, also expressed as a multidimensional complex dataset.[51] Therefore, the important goal remains: to characterize cancer risk based on gene–environment interactions. However, we remain challenged because cancer is a complex disease of diverse etiologies by multiple exposures causing damage in different genes; for example, gene^n–environment^n interactions, for which the variable n is not known.

Two fundamental principles underlie current studies of molecular epidemiology. First, carcinogenesis is a multistage process, and behind each stage are numerous genetic events that occur either due to an exogenous insult such as a chemical exposure or an endogenous insult, such as from free radicals generated via cellular processes or errors in DNA replication. Therefore, identifying a cancer risk factor can be challenging because of the multifactorial nature of carcinogenesis, given that any one risk factor occurs within a background of many risk factors. Second, wide interindividual variation in response to carcinogen exposure and other carcinogenic processes indicate that the human response is not homogeneous, so that experimental models and epidemiology (e.g., the use of a single cell clone to study a gene's effect experimentally or the assumption that the population responds similarly to the mean in epidemiology studies), might not be representative of susceptible and resistant groups within a population.

Genetic Susceptibility

In humans, the determination of genetic susceptibility can be assessed by phenotyping or genotyping methods. Phenotypes generally represent complex genotypes. Examples of phenotypes include the assessment of DNA repair capacity in cultured blood cells, mammographic breast density, or the quantitation of carcinogen-DNA adducts in a target organ. Phenotypes now also include profiles of methylation that affect gene expression, a so-called epigenetic effect, for example, identified though next-generation sequencing or other methods.[52] The contribution of genetics to cancer risk from chemical carcinogens can range from small to large, depending on its penetrance.[4] Highly penetrant cancer-susceptibility genes cause familial cancers, but account for less than 5% of all cancers. Low-penetrant genes cause common sporadic cancers, which have large public health consequences.

A genetic polymorphism (e.g., single nucleotide polymorphisms) is defined as a genetic variant present in at least 1% of the population. Because of the advent of improved genotyping methods that have reduced cost and increased high throughput, haplotyping and whole genomewide association studies are ongoing. Although haplotyping studies, facilitated through the International HapMap Project (www.hapmap.org), have not proven useful for predicting human cancers; high-density, whole genomewide, single nucleotide polymorphism association studies have shown remarkable consistency for many gene loci, although the risk estimates are only 1.0 to 1.4, which are not useful in the clinic for individual risk assessment.[6] For example, the contribution of genetic polymorphisms to cancer risk, at least for breast cancer, appears to improve risk modeling by only a few percent; known breast cancer risk factors account for about 58% of risk, and adding 10 genetic variants increases the risk prediction only to 62%.[53] Genes under study are from pathways that affect behavior, activate and detoxify carcinogens, affect DNA repair, govern cell-cycle control, trigger apoptosis, effect cell signaling, and so forth.

Biomarkers of Cancer Risk

The evaluation of dose and risk estimates in epidemiologic studies can include four components: namely, external exposure measurements, internal exposure measurements, biomarkers estimating the biologically effective dose, and biomarkers of effect or harm. The latter three measurements are biomarkers that improve on the first by quantifying exposure inside the individual and at the cellular level to characterize low-dose exposures in low-risk populations, providing a relative contribution of individual chemical carcinogens from complex mixtures, and/or estimating total burden of a particular exposure where there are many sources.[54]

Chemicals cause genetic damage in different ways, namely in the formation of carcinogen-DNA adducts leading to base mutations or gross chromosomal changes. Adducts are formed when a mutagen, or part of it, irreversibly binds to DNA so that it can cause a base substitution, insertion, or deletion during DNA replication. Gross chromosomal mutations are chromosome breaks, gaps, or translocations. The level of DNA damage is the biologically effective dose in a target organ, and reflects the net result of carcinogen exposure, activation, lack of detoxification, lack of effective DNA repair, and lack of programmed cell death. A variety of assays have been used for determining carcinogen-macromolecular adducts in human tissues; for example, for assessing risk from tobacco smoking for lung cancer and aflatoxin and liver cancer.[55,56] Important considerations for the assessment of biomarkers include sensitivity, specificity, reproducibility, accessibility for human use, and whether it represents a risk measured in a target organ or surrogate tissue. No single biomarker has been considered to be sufficiently validated for use as a cancer risk marker in an individual as it relates to chemical carcinogenesis.[57] However, there is some evidence that DNA adducts are cancer risk factors in both cohort and case-control studies.[58]

People are commonly exposed to N-nitrosamine and other N-nitroso compounds from dietary and tobacco exposures, which are associated with DNA adduct formation and cancer. Exposure can occur through endogenous formation of N-nitrosamines from nitrates in food or directly from dietary sources, cosmetics, drugs, household commodities, and tobacco smoke. Endogenous formation occurs in the stomach from the reaction of nitrosatable amines and nitrate (used as a preservative), which is converted to nitrites by bacteria. The N-nitrosamines undergo metabolic activation by cytochrome P450s (CYP2E1, CYP2A6, and CYP2D6) and form DNA adducts. Biomarkers are available to assess N-nitrosamine exposure from tobacco smoke (e.g., urinary tobacco-specific nitrosamine levels) or DNA, including in target organs such as the lungs. Recent data indicate that increasing levels of tobacco-specific nitrosamine metabolites are associated with increased lung cancer risk.[55]

Heterocyclic amines are formed from the overheating of food with creatine, such as meat, chicken, and fish.[59] Heterocyclic amines, estimated based on consumption of well-done meat, have been associated with breast and colon cancer, presumably through metabolic activation mechanisms and DNA damage.[59] Aflatoxins, another food contaminant, are considered to be a major contributor to liver cancer in China and parts of Africa, especially interacting with hepatitis viruses, and urinary aflatoxin adduct levels are predictors of liver cancer risk.[56]

Aromatic amines are another class of human carcinogens. Aryl aromatic amines have been implicated in bladder carcinogenesis, especially in occupationally exposed cohorts (e.g., dye workers) and tobacco smokers.[60] These compounds are activated by cytochrome P4501A2 and excreted via the N-acetyltransferase 2 gene. They are genotoxic, and the quantitative assessment using biomarkers has been more difficult, but some persons have studied DNA adducts as well.[61]

Polycyclic aromatic hydrocarbons (PAH) are large, aromatic (three or more fused benzene rings) compounds that are a class of more than 200 chemicals. These compounds are ubiquitous in the environment and present in the ambient air. They are formed from overcooking foods, fireplaces, charcoal barbeques, burning of coal and crude oil, tobacco smoke, and can be found in various occupational settings. In order for PAHs to exert their toxic effect, they must undergo metabolic activation via cytochromes P4501A1 and P4503A4 to form DNA adducts, or are excreted via pathways involving the glutathione-S-transferase genes. PAHs are associated with an increased risk of lung and skin cancer in the occupational setting, although risk varies by type of industry and the individual being exposed.[62,63] Benzo(a)pyrene (BaP), the most frequently studied PAH, serves as a model for chemical carcinogens. The bay region diol epoxide binds to DNA, mostly as the N2-deoxyguanosine adduct. The evidence linking BaP-deoxyguanosine adducts with a carcinogenic effect in lung cancer is very strong, including site-specific hotspot mutations in the p53 tumor suppressor gene.[64–68] Various biomarkers of exposure have been developed for assessing PAH exposure. These include measuring DNA adducts, protein adducts, and urinary 1-hydroxypyrene; only the latter is a validated biomarker of exposure and no adducts have been validated as biomarkers of cancer risk. However, recent data indicate that PAH metabolites might be risk factors for lung cancer.[58]

Air pollution has been recently classified by the IARC as a known human lung carcinogen.[69] Studies that support the conclusion include cohort studies that use biomarkers of exposure.[70] Such markers include measurements of 1-hydroxypyrene, DNA adducts, chromosomal aberrations, micronuclei, oxidative damage to nucleobases, and methylation changes.[71]

Epidemiologic and experimental studies have linked benzene to hematologic toxicity, including aplastic anemia, myelodysplastic syndrome, and acute myeloid leukemia.[72–74] Benzene is metabolized by hepatic P4502E1 (CYP2E1), yielding benzene oxide and hydroquinone, among other reactive metabolites. Circulating hydroquinones may be further metabolized to reactive benzoquinones by myeloperoxidase in bone marrow white blood cell precursors and stroma. Benzene metabolites are reported to have a variety of biologic consequences on bone marrow cells, including covalent binding to DNA and protein, alterations in gene expression, cytokine and chemokine abnormalities, and chromosomal aberrations.[75] There are well-established biomarkers of exposure to benzene, but to date, biomarkers of toxicity have not been validated (except for high-level exposure workplaces and effects of peripheral blood counts).

ARISTOLOCHIC ACID AND UROTHELIAL CANCERS AS A MODEL FOR IDENTIFYING HUMAN CARCINOGENS

Aristolochic acids come from the Aristolochia genus of plants, which have been used for herbal remedies (e.g., birthwort, Dutchman's pipe). The case of the carcinogen aristolochic acid, which is identified as a Class 1 human carcinogen by the IARC (http://monographs.iarc.fr/ENG/Monographs/vol100A/mono100A-23.pdf), presents a powerful example of how the forces of epidemiology, classical chemical carcinogenesis, and genomics collaborate to unravel the pathogenesis and prevention of a specific human cancer.[76] In the 1990s, epidemiologists independently reported on three distinct unrelated population groups that developed nephrotoxicity (interstitial fibrosis) and an extraordinary high incidence of urothelial cancer of the upper urinary track after exposure for different reasons and in different parts of the world (Belgium, the Balkans, and China). In Belgian women ingesting an extract from plants of the Aristolochia species for weight reduction, which was provided to them in a weight loss clinic, nearly 50% developed this unusual syndrome. A similar clinical picture (so-called Balkan endemic nephropathy) was reported for residents farming around the Danube River and eating home-baked bread from wheat contaminated with seeds from Aristolochia weeds grown in the same fields. In China, the Aristolochia herbs have been used for centuries in Chinese medicine and are prominently prescribed in Taiwan, a nation with the highest incidence of urothelial cancer in the world, as remedies for ailments of the heart, liver, snake bites, arthritis, gout, childbirth, and others.

Common to all Aristolochia species are one of two major nitrophenanthrene carboxylic acid toxicants, namely, aristolochic acid I and II (http://monographs.iarc.fr/ENG/Monographs/vol100A/

mono100A-23.pdf).[77,78] The oral administration of aristolochic acid to rodents is highly carcinogenic, producing predominantly forestomach cancers and lymphomas, along with cancers of the lung, kidney, and urothelium (http://monographs.iarc.fr/ENG/Monographs/vol100A/mono100A-23.pdf). The major route of excretion of aristolochic acid is through the kidneys. These clinical and experimental observations inspired further analyses of the mechanism of action of these potent human carcinogens. Studies in intact mice and mice reconstituted with humanized P450 revealed that CYP1a and CYP2a were responsible for both the activation and the detoxification of aristolochic acid I and II, and that NAD(P)H:quinone oxidoreductase produced the ultimate reactive aristolactam I nitrenium species.[78] The molecular action of the ultimate carcinogen is remarkably specific, targeting purine nucleotides in DNA to form DNA adducts and binding at the exocyclic amino group of deoxyadenosine and deoxyguanosine with a far greater affinity for dA over dG (Fig. 7.1). DNA adducts from aristolochic acids have been found in both experimental animals and humans. Furthermore, unlike any other human carcinogen, the predominant mutagenic outcome is an A:T transversion with a marked preference for the nontranscribed strand of DNA, notably in the p53 gene.[77,79] The A:T to T:A transversions are extremely uncommon among the mutation spectrum in all eukaryotes. These unique properties of aristolochic acid DNA adducts appear to elude DNA repair mechanisms that commonly focus on transcribing DNA, resulting in persistent carcinogen-DNA adducts in human tissues and surgical tumor specimens, thus confirming the association of exposure with a biologic effect.[80] In experimental models in mice where human p53 is substituted for the mouse gene, multiple sites on p53 are mutated, almost all of which are those unusual A:T transversions.[81] Modern genomic techniques have unraveled other selective properties of this unusual but potent human chemical carcinogen. Whole genome and exome sequencing of multiple aristolochic-associated kidney cancers from patients confirmed the high frequency of the unusual A:T to T:A transversion mutations. Furthermore, an unusual pattern emerges where there is selectivity for mutations at splice sites with a preferable consensus sequence of T/CAG. Among the many mutations detected, certain targets stand out, particularly in p53, MLL2, and other genes the products of which function in regulating gene expression through higher chromosome order.[82,83] This cancer story covers the gamut of all elements of chemical carcinogenesis, and its illumination has opened a door for cancer prevention.

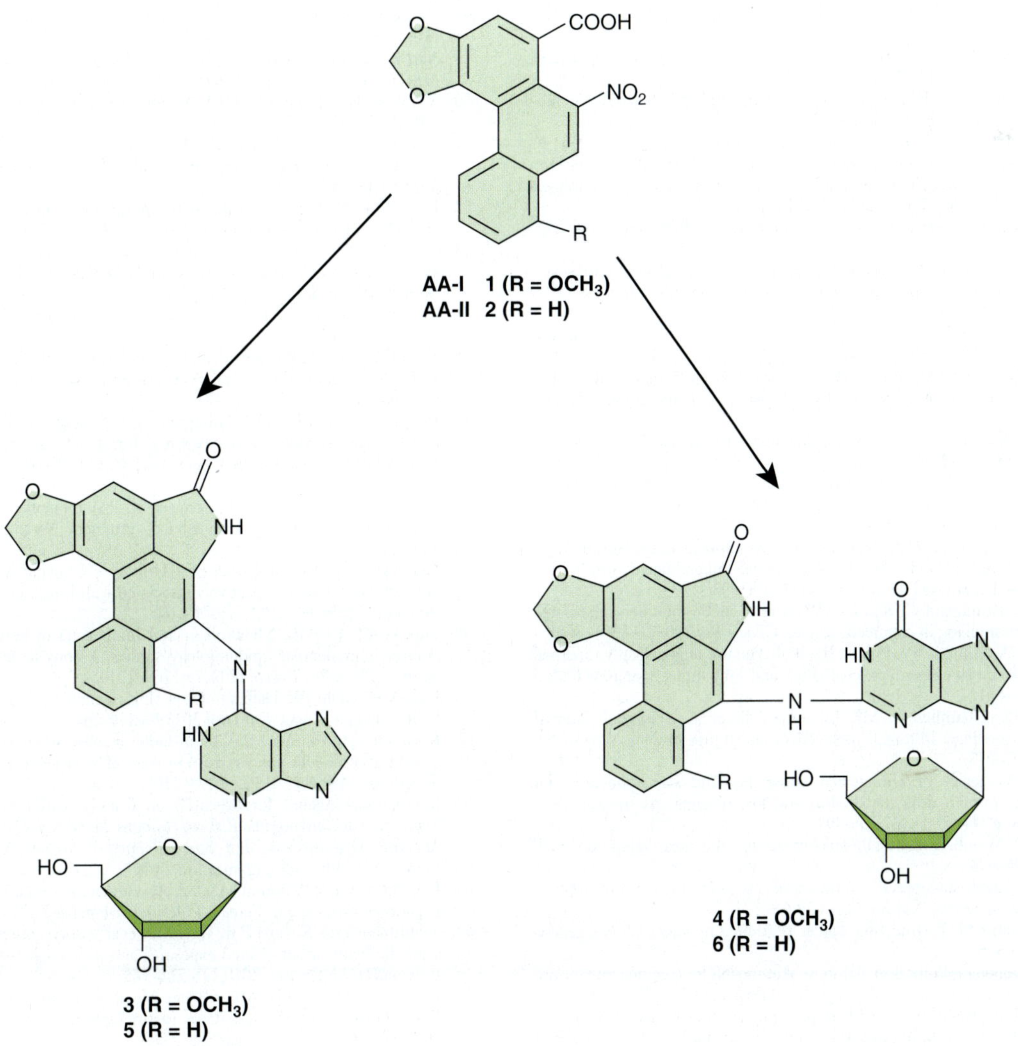

Figure 7.1 Aristolochic acid I and II form DNA adducts through the exocyclic amino group of deoxyadenosine and deoxyguanosine. The deoxyadenosine adduct is highly favored. For more detailed analysis of the complete metabolic profile, see Attaluri et al.[79]

REFERENCES

1. U.S. Department of Health and Human Services. *The Health Consequences of Smoking: 50 Years of Progress. A Report of the Surgeon General.* Atlanta: Author; 2014.
2. Colditz GA, Wei EK. Preventability of cancer: the relative contributions of biologic and social and physical environmental determinants of cancer mortality. *Annu Rev Public Health* 2012;33:137–156.
3. Lynch SM, Rebbeck TR. Bridging the gap between biologic, individual, and macroenvironmental factors in cancer: a multilevel approach. *Cancer Epidemiol Biomarkers Prev* 2013;22:485–495.
4. Rahman N. Realizing the promise of cancer predisposition genes. *Nature* 2014;505:302–308.
5. Lichtenstein P, Holm NV, Verkasalo PK, et al. Environmental and heritable factors in the causation of cancer—analyses of cohorts of twins from Sweden, Denmark, and Finland. *N Engl J Med* 2000;343:78–85.
6. Hunter DJ, Chanock SJ. Genome-wide association studies and "the art of the soluble." *J Natl Cancer Inst* 2010;102:836–837.
7. Luch A. Nature and nurture - lessons from chemical carcinogenesis. *Nat Rev Cancer* 2005;5:113–125.
8. Taddei ML, Giannoni E, Comito G, et al. Microenvironment and tumor cell plasticity: an easy way out. *Cancer Lett* 2013;341:80–96.
9. Fessler E, Dijkgraaf FE, De Sousa E Melo, et al. Cancer stem cell dynamics in tumor progression and metastasis: is the microenvironment to blame? *Cancer Lett* 2013;341:97–104.
10. Hanahan D, Coussens LM. Accessories to the crime: functions of cells recruited to the tumor microenvironment. *Cancer Cell* 2012;21:309–322.
11. Irigaray P, Belpomme D. Basic properties and molecular mechanisms of exogenous chemical carcinogens. *Carcinogenesis* 2010;31:135–148.
12. Xia HJ, Chen CS. Progress of non-human primate animal models of cancers. *Dongwuxue Yanjiu* 2011;32:70–80.
13. Yi C, He C. DNA repair by reversal of DNA damage. *Cold Spring Harb Perspect Biol* 2013;5:a012575.
14. Dizdaroglu M. Oxidatively induced DNA damage: mechanisms, repair and disease. *Cancer Lett* 2012;327:26–47.
15. Wogan GN, Hecht SS, Felton JS, et al. Environmental and chemical carcinogenesis. *Semin Cancer Biol* 2004;14:473–486.
16. Baan R, Grosse Y, Straif K, et al. A review of human carcinogens—Part F: chemical agents and related occupations. *Lancet Oncol* 2009;10:1143–1144.
17. Rendic S, Guengerich FP. Contributions of human enzymes in carcinogen metabolism. *Chem Res Toxicol* 2012;25:1316–1383.
18. Luch A. The mode of action of organic carcinogens on cellular structures. *EXS* 2006;65–95.
19. Anttila S, Raunio H, Hakkola J. Cytochrome P450-mediated pulmonary metabolism of carcinogens: regulation and cross-talk in lung carcinogenesis. *Am J Respir Cell Mol Biol* 2011;44:583–590.
20. Pogribny IP, Beland FA. DNA methylome alterations in chemical carcinogenesis. *Cancer Lett* 2012 [Epub ahead of print].
21. Shrivastav N, Li D, Essigmann JM. Chemical biology of mutagenesis and DNA repair: cellular responses to DNA alkylation. *Carcinogenesis* 2010;31:59–70.
22. Kew MC. Aflatoxins as a cause of hepatocellular carcinoma. *J Gastrointestin Liver Dis* 2013;22:305–310.
23. Feng Z, Hu W, Hu Y, et al. Acrolein is a major cigarette-related lung cancer agent: preferential binding at p53 mutational hotspots and inhibition of DNA repair. *Proc Natl Acad Sci U S A* 2006;103:15404–15409.
24. Porta M, Crous-Bou M, Wark PA, et al. Cigarette smoking and K-ras mutations in pancreas, lung and colorectal adenocarcinomas: etiopathogenic similarities, differences and paradoxes. *Mutat Res* 2009;682:83–93.
25. Blackford A, Parmigiani G, Kensler TW, et al. Genetic mutations associated with cigarette smoking in pancreatic cancer. *Cancer Res* 2009;69:3681–3688.
26. Eastmond DA, Vulimiri SV, French JE, et al. The use of genetically modified mice in cancer risk assessment: challenges and limitations. *Crit Rev Toxicol* 2013;43:611–631.
27. Boverhof DR, Chamberlain MP, Elcombe CR, et al. Transgenic animal models in toxicology: historical perspectives and future outlook. *Toxicol Sci* 2011;121:207–233.
28. Cheung C, Gonzalez FJ. Humanized mouse lines and their application for prediction of human drug metabolism and toxicological risk assessment. *J Pharmacol Exp Ther* 2008;327:288–299.
29. Hanahan D, Weinberg RA. Hallmarks of cancer: the next generation. *Cell* 2011;144:646–674.
30. Demant P. Cancer susceptibility in the mouse: genetics, biology and implications for human cancer. *Nat Rev Genet* 2003;4:721–734.
31. Klatt P, Serrano M. Engineering cancer resistance in mice. *Carcinogenesis* 2003;24:817–826.
32. Lynch D, Svoboda J, Putta S, et al. Mouse skin models for carcinogenic hazard identification: utilities and challenges. *Toxicol Pathol* 2007;35:853–864.
33. Lash LH, Hines RN, Gonzalez FJ, et al. Genetics and susceptibility to toxic chemicals: do you (or should you) know your genetic profile? *J Pharmacol Exp Ther* 2003;305:403–409.
34. Di PG, Magno LA, Rios-Santos F. Glutathione S-transferases: an overview in cancer research. *Expert Opin Drug Metab Toxicol* 2010;6:153–170.
35. Feng S, Cao Z, Wang X. Role of aryl hydrocarbon receptor in cancer. *Biochim Biophys Acta* 2013;1836:197–210.
36. Jiang XL, Gonzalez FJ, Yu AM. Drug-metabolizing enzyme, transporter, and nuclear receptor genetically modified mouse models. *Drug Metab Rev* 2011;43:27–40.
37. Tuna M, Amos CI. Genomic sequencing in cancer. *Cancer Lett* 2013;340:161–170.
38. MacConaill LE. Existing and emerging technologies for tumor genomic profiling. *J Clin Oncol* 2013;31:1815–1824.
39. Watson IR, Takahashi K, Futreal PA, et al. Emerging patterns of somatic mutations in cancer. *Nat Rev Genet* 2013;14:703–718.
40. Dumas ME. Metabolome 2.0: quantitative genetics and network biology of metabolic phenotypes. *Mol Biosyst* 2012;8:2494–2502.
41. Adamski J, Suhre K. Metabolomics platforms for genome wide association studies—linking the genome to the metabolome. *Curr Opin Biotechnol* 2013;24:39–47.
42. Verma M, Khoury MJ, Ioannidis JP. Opportunities and challenges for selected emerging technologies in cancer epidemiology: mitochondrial, epigenomic, metabolomic, and telomerase profiling. *Cancer Epidemiol Biomarkers Prev* 2013;22:189–200.
43. Edwards SL, Beesley J, French JD, et al. Beyond GWASs: illuminating the dark road from association to function. *Am J Hum Genet* 2013;93:779–797.
44. Di LG, Garofalo M, Croce CM. MicroRNAs in cancer. *Annu Rev Pathol* 2014;9:287–314.
45. Cheetham SW, Gruhl F, Mattick JS, et al. Long noncoding RNAs and the genetics of cancer. *Br J Cancer* 2013;108:2419–2425.
46. Izzotti A, Pulliero A. The effects of environmental chemical carcinogens on the microRNA machinery. *Int J Hyg Environ Health* 2014 [Epub ahead of print].
47. Kostic AD, Gevers D, Pedamallu CS, et al. Genomic analysis identifies association of Fusobacterium with colorectal carcinoma. *Genome Res* 2012;22:292–298.
48. Compare D, Nardone G. Contribution of gut microbiota to colonic and extracolonic cancer development. *Dig Dis* 2011;29:554–561.
49. Ahn J, Chen CY, Hayes RB. Oral microbiome and oral and gastrointestinal cancer risk. *Cancer Causes Control* 2012;23:399–404.
50. Schwabe RF, Jobin C. The microbiome and cancer. *Nat Rev Cancer* 2013;13:800–812.
51. Wild CP, Scalbert A, Herceg Z. Measuring the exposome: a powerful basis for evaluating environmental exposures and cancer risk. *Environ Mol Mutagen* 2013;54:480–499.
52. Brennan K, Flanagan JM. Epigenetic epidemiology for cancer risk: harnessing germline epigenetic variation. *Methods Mol Biol* 2012;863:439–465.
53. Wacholder S, Hartge P, Prentice R, et al. Performance of common genetic variants in breast-cancer risk models. *N Engl J Med* 2010;362:986–993.
54. Boffetta P, van der Hel O, Norppa H, et al. Chromosomal aberrations and cancer risk: results of a cohort study from Central Europe. *Am J Epidemiol* 2007;165:36–43.
55. Yuan JM, Gao YT, Wang R, et al. Urinary levels of volatile organic carcinogen and toxicant biomarkers in relation to lung cancer development in smokers. *Carcinogenesis* 2012;33:804–809.
56. Wogan GN, Kensler TW, Groopman JD. Present and future directions of translational research on aflatoxin and hepatocellular carcinoma. A review. *Food Addit Contam Part A Chem Anal Control Expo Risk Assess* 2012;29:249–257.
57. Hatsukami DK, Benowitz NL, Rennard SI, et al. Biomarkers to assess the utility of potential reduced exposure tobacco products. *Nicotine Tob Res* 2006;8:599–622.
58. Yuan JM, Gao YT, Murphy SE, et al. Urinary levels of cigarette smoke constituent metabolites are prospectively associated with lung cancer development in smokers. *Cancer Res* 2011;71:6749–6757.
59. Turesky RJ, Le ML. Metabolism and biomarkers of heterocyclic aromatic amines in molecular epidemiology studies: lessons learned from aromatic amines. *Chem Res Toxicol* 2011;24:1169–1214.
60. Burger M, Catto JW, Dalbagni G, et al. Epidemiology and risk factors of urothelial bladder cancer. *Eur Urol* 2013;63:234–241.
61. Besaratinia A, Tommasi S. Genotoxicity of tobacco smoke-derived aromatic amines and bladder cancer: current state of knowledge and future research directions. *FASEB J* 2013;27:2090–2100.
62. International Agency for Research on Cancer. *IARC Monographs on the Evaluation of Carcinogenic Risks to Humans: Some Non-Heterocyclic Polycyclic Aromatic Hydrocarbons and Some Related Exposures.* Volume 92. Lyon, France: World Health Organization; 2010.
63. Boffetta P, Autier P, Boniol M, et al. An estimate of cancers attributable to occupational exposures in France. *J Occup Environ Med* 2010;52:399–406.
64. Mordukhovich I, Rossner P Jr, Terry MB, et al. Associations between polycyclic aromatic hydrocarbon-related exposures and p53 mutations in breast tumors. *Environ Health Perspect* 2010;118:511–518.
65. Pfeifer GP, Denissenko MF, Olivier M, et al. Tobacco smoke carcinogens, DNA damage and p53 mutations in smoking-associated cancers. *Oncogene* 2002;21:7435–7451.
66. Pfeifer GP, Hainaut P. On the origin of G → T transversions in lung cancer. *Mutat Res* 2003;526:39–43.
67. Sjaastad AK, Jorgensen RB, Svendsen K. Exposure to polycyclic aromatic hydrocarbons (PAHs), mutagenic aldehydes and particulate matter during pan frying of beefsteak. *Occup Environ Med* 2010;67:228–232.

68. Hussain SP, Amstad P, Raja K, et al. Mutability of p53 hotspot codons to benzo(a)pyrene diol epoxide (BPDE) and the frequency of p53 mutations in nontumorous human lung. *Cancer Res* 2001;61:6350–6355.
69. Loomis D, Grosse Y, Lauby-Secretan B, et al. The carcinogenicity of outdoor air pollution. *Lancet Oncol* 2013;14:1262–1263.
70. Raaschou-Nielsen O, Andersen ZJ, Beelen R, et al. Air pollution and lung cancer incidence in 17 European cohorts: prospective analyses from the European Study of Cohorts for Air Pollution Effects (ESCAPE). *Lancet Oncol* 2013;14:813–822.
71. Demetriou CA, Raaschou-Nielsen O, Loft S, et al. Biomarkers of ambient air pollution and lung cancer: a systematic review. *Occup Environ Med* 2012;69:619–627.
72. Galbraith D, Gross SA, Paustenbach D. Benzene and human health: A historical review and appraisal of associations with various diseases. *Crit Rev Toxicol* 2010;40:1–46.
73. Vlaanderen J, Portengen L, Rothman N, et al. Flexible meta-regression to assess the shape of the benzene-leukemia exposure-response curve. *Environ Health Perspect* 2010;118:526–532.
74. Vlaanderen J, Lan Q, Kromhout H, et al. Occupational benzene exposure and the risk of chronic myeloid leukemia: a meta-analysis of cohort studies incorporating study quality dimensions. *Am J Ind Med* 2012;55:779–785.
75. Snyder R. Leukemia and benzene. *Int J Environ Res Public Health* 2012;9:2875–2893.
76. Grollman AP. Aristolochic acid nephropathy: harbinger of a global iatrogenic disease. *Environ Mol Mutagen* 2013;54:1–7.
77. Hollstein M, Moriya M, Grollman AP, et al. Analysis of TP53 mutation spectra reveals the fingerprint of the potent environmental carcinogen, aristolochic acid. *Mutat Res* 2013;753:41–49.
78. Stiborova M, Martinek V, Frei E, et al. Enzymes metabolizing aristolochic acid and their contribution to the development of aristolochic acid nephropathy and urothelial cancer. *Curr Drug Metab* 2013;14:695–705.
79. Attaluri S, Bonala RR, Yang IY, et al. DNA adducts of aristolochic acid II: total synthesis and site-specific mutagenesis studies in mammalian cells. *Nucleic Acids Res* 2010;38:339–352.
80. Sidorenko VS, Yeo JE, Bonala RR, et al. Lack of recognition by global-genome nucleotide excision repair accounts for the high mutagenicity and persistence of aristolactam-DNA adducts. *Nucleic Acids Res* 2012;40:2494–2505.
81. Nedelko T, Arlt VM, Phillips DH, et al. TP53 mutation signature supports involvement of aristolochic acid in the aetiology of endemic nephropathy-associated tumours. *Int J Cancer* 2009;124:987–990.
82. Hoang ML, Chen CH, Sidorenko VS, et al. Mutational signature of aristolochic acid exposure as revealed by whole-exome sequencing. *Sci Transl Med* 2013;5:197ra102.
83. Poon SL, Pang ST, McPherson JR, et al. Genome-wide mutational signatures of aristolochic acid and its application as a screening tool. *Sci Transl Med* 2013;5:197ra101.

8 Physical Factors

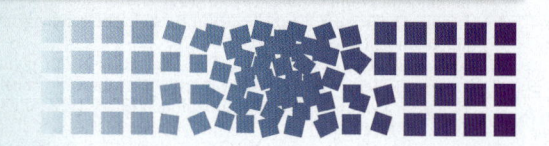

Mats Ljungman

INTRODUCTION

Ionizing radiation (IR) and ultraviolet (UV) light have challenged the genetic integrity of all living organisms throughout time. By inducing DNA damage and subsequent mutations, these physical agents have promoted diversity through natural selection, and, as a result, organisms from all kingdoms of life carry genes that encode proteins that repair damaged DNA. In higher, multicellular organisms, many additional mechanisms of genome preservation have evolved, such as cell cycle checkpoints and apoptosis. Despite the many sophisticated mechanisms to safeguard the human genome from the mutagenic actions of DNA-damaging agents, not all exposed cells successfully restore the integrity of their DNA and some cells may subsequently progress into malignant cancer cells. Furthermore, through manmade activities, we are now exposed to many new physical agents, such as radiofrequency and microwave radiation, electromagnetic fields, asbestos, and nanoparticles, for which evolution has not yet had time to deliver genome-preserving response mechanisms. This chapter will highlight the molecular mechanisms by which these physical agents affect cells and how human exposure may lead to cancer.

IONIZING RADIATION

IR is defined as radiation that has sufficient energy to ionize molecules by displacing electrons from atoms. IR can be electromagnetic, such as x-rays and gamma rays, or can consist of particles, such as electrons, protons, neutrons, alpha particles, or carbon ions. Natural sources of IR make up about 80% of human exposure and medical sources make up about 20%.[1] The increased medical use of diagnostic x-rays and computed tomography (CT) scanning procedures likely translates into higher incidences of cancer. Of the natural sources, radon exposure is the most significant exposure risk to humans. Importantly, with better and more comprehensive screening techniques, the human exposure to radon could be dramatically lowered.

Mechanisms of Damage Induction

Linear Energy Transfer

The biologic effects of IR are unique in that the induced damage is clustered due to the local deposition of energy in radiation tracks. The distance between the depositions of energy is biologically very relevant and unique to the energy and the type of radiation. The term *linear energy transfer (LET)* denotes the energy transferred per unit length of a track of radiation. Electromagnetic radiation, such as x-rays or gamma rays, are sparsely ionizing and therefore classified as low LET radiation, whereas particulate radiation, such as neutrons, protons, and alpha particles, are examples of high LET radiation.[1]

Radiation Biochemistry

Radiation-induced damage to cellular target molecules, such as DNA, proteins, and lipids, can be either direct or indirect (Fig. 8.1). The *direct action* of radiation, which is the dominant mode of action of high LET radiation, is due to the deposition of energy directly to the target molecule, resulting in one or more ionization events. The *indirect action* of radiation is due to the radiolysis of water molecules, which, after initial absorption of radiation energy, become excited and generate different types of radiolysis products where the reactive hydroxyl radical (•OH), can damage both DNA and proteins. About two-thirds of the damage induced by low LET radiation is due to the indirect action of radiation. Since the hydroxyl radical is very reactive (half-life is 10^{-9} seconds), it does not diffuse more than a few nanometers after it is formed before it reacts with other molecules, and, thus, only radicals formed in close proximity to the target molecule will contribute to the damage of that target.[2] However, by chemical recombination of the primary radiolysis products, hydrogen peroxide (H_2O_2) is formed, which in turn can produce hydroxyl radicals at a later time through the Fenton reaction, involving free metals. Because H_2O_2 is not very reactive, it can diffuse long distances away from the initial site of energy deposition.

Radical scavengers normally present in cells, such as glutathione, can protect target molecules by reacting with the hydroxyl radical (see Fig. 8.1). Even after the target molecule has been hit and ionized, glutathione can contribute to cell protection by donating a hydrogen atom to the radical, allowing the unpaired electron present in the radical to pair up with the electron from the hydrogen atom. This is considered the simplest of all types of repair and is called *chemical repair*.[3] However, if oxygen molecules are present, they will compete with scavenger molecules for the ionized molecule, and if oxygen reacts with the ionized target molecule before the hydrogen donation occurs, the damage will be solidified as a peroxide, which is not amendable to chemical repair. Instead, this lesion will require enzymatic repair for the restoration of DNA. This augmenting biologic effect of oxygen is called the *oxygen effect* and is considered an important factor for the effectiveness of radiation therapy.[1]

Damage to DNA

The direct and indirect effects of radiation induce more or less identical types of lesions in DNA. However, the density of lesions induced in a stretch of DNA is higher for high LET radiation, and this increased complexity is thought to complicate the repair of these lesions. Radiation-induced lesions consist of more than 100 chemically distinct base lesions, such as the mutagenic lesions thymine glycol and 8-hydroxyguanine.[2,4,5] Furthermore, damage to the sugar moiety in the backbone of DNA and some types of base damage can result in single-strand breaks (SSB). Because the energy deposition of radiation is clustered even for low LET radiation, it is possible that two individual strand breaks are formed in close proximity on opposite strands, resulting in the formation of a double-strand break (DSB). It has been estimated that 1 Gy of ionizing radiation gives rise to about 40 DSBs, 1,000 SSBs, 1,000 base lesions, and 150 DNA-protein cross-links per cell.[2] For a similarly lethal dose of UV light, about 400,000 lesions are required, demonstrating that the lesions induced by IR are much more toxic

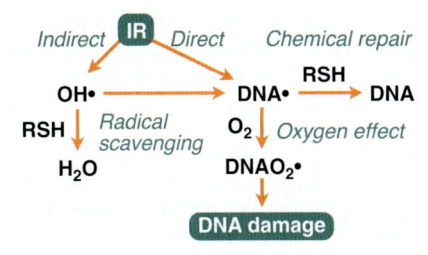

Figure 8.1 Factors affecting the induction of DNA damage by ionizing radiation (IR). Ionizing radiation can ionize DNA either by direct action or by indirect action, in which radiation energy is absorbed by neighboring molecules, such as water, leading to the generation of hydroxyl radicals that attack DNA. Sulfur-containing cellular molecules (RSH), such as glutathione, can scavenge hydroxyl radicals by hydrogen atom donations and thereby protect the DNA from the indirect action of radiation. Glutathione can also donate hydrogen atoms to ionized DNA, thereby restoring the integrity of DNA in a process termed *chemical repair*. Oxygen can compete with chemical repair in a process termed the *oxygen effect*, resulting in the enhancement of the biologic effect of ionizing radiation by the fixation of the initial DNA damage into DNA peroxides (DNAO$_2 \cdot$).

than lesions induced by UV light. It is believed that DSBs are the critical lesions that lead to cell lethality following exposure to ionizing radiation.[6]

Damage to Proteins

Although proteins and lipids are subject to damage following exposure to IR, the common belief is that DNA is the critical target for the biologic effects of radiation. Indeed, abrogation of DNA damage surveillance or repair processes in cells results in the enhanced induction of mutations and decreased cell survival following radiation.[5] However, studies of radiation-sensitive and radiation-resistant bacteria imply that mechanisms that suppress protein damage may also play important roles in radiation resistance.[7] *Deinococcus radiodurans* is a bacterium that can survive radiation exposures of up to 17,000 Gy, and its extreme radioresistance has been linked to high intracellular levels of manganese, which protect proteins from oxidation. The thought is that if a cell can limit protein oxidation, then its enzymes will remain active, and cellular functions such as DNA repair will be able to restore the integrity of DNA even after severe DNA damage.[8] It would be interesting to explore whether the concentration of manganese can be manipulated to sensitize tumor cells to radiation therapy. Furthermore, because protein damage due to reactive oxygen species (ROS) accumulate during the aging process, could supplements of manganese turn back the clock on aging?

Cellular Responses

DNA Repair

Ever since organisms started to utilize atmospheric oxygen for metabolic respiration many millions of years ago, they have been forced to deal with the cellular damage induced by ROS. Base excision repair (BER) evolved to remove many of the different types of oxidative base lesions and DNA SSBs induced by ROS. However, ROS seldom induce DSBs unless the generation of hydroxyl radicals is clustered near the DNA molecule. A more important source of intracellular generation of DSBs may instead be the process of DNA replication, and it is possible that homologous recombination (HR) repair primarily evolved to overcome DSBs sporadically induced during the replication process. The other major pathway of DSB repair is the nonhomologous end-joining (NHEJ) pathway, which is utilized by immune cells in the process of antibody generation. Although the HR pathway has high fidelity due to the utilization of homologous sister chromatids to ensure that correct DNA ends are joined, the NHEJ pathway lacks this

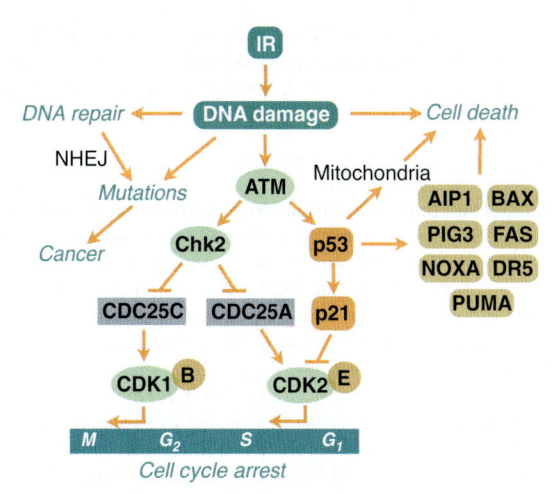

Figure 8.2 Cellular responses to ionizing radiation. Ionizing radiation induces predominantly base lesions and single- and double-strand breaks. Base lesions and single-strand breaks are repaired by base excision repair (BER), whereas double-strand breaks are repaired by nonhomologous end joining (NHEJ) and homologous recombination (HR). If DNA lesions are misrepaired by NHEJ or not repaired at all before cells enter S phase or mitosis, genomic instability is manifested as mutations or chromosome aberrations that promote carcinogenesis. In order for cells to assist DNA repair and safeguard against genetic instability and cancer, cells can induce cell cycle arrest or apoptosis. The ATM kinase is an early responder to DNA damage induced by ionizing radiation that activates the cell cycle checkpoint kinase Chk2 and the tumor suppressor p53. Chk2 inactivates the CDC25A and CDC25C phosphatases that are critical in promoting cell cycle progression by activating the cyclin-dependent kinases CDK2 or CDK1 and thereby arresting the cells at the G$_1$/S or G$_2$/M checkpoints. In addition, p53 can arrest cells at the G$_1$/S checkpoint by inducing the CDK inhibitor p21. p53 also plays a role in promoting apoptosis by inducing a number of proapoptotic proteins as well as translocating to mitochondria where it inhibits the actions of antiapoptotic factors. AIP1, actin interacting protein 1; BAX, bcl-2-like protein; PIG3, p53-inducible gene 3.

control mechanism and therefore occasionally rejoins ends incorrectly. Thus, the NHEJ pathway may contribute to the generation of mutations following radiation (Fig. 8.2). However, NHEJ is the only mechanism available for DSB repair in postmitotic cells and cells in the G$_1$ phase of the cell cycle because no sister chromatids are available in these cells to support HR repair.

Ataxia-Telangiectasia Mutated and Cell Cycle Checkpoints

Due to the enormous task of replicating the whole genome during the S phase and segregating the chromosomes during mitosis, proliferating cells are generally much more vulnerable to radiation than stationary cells. To prevent cells with damaged DNA from entering into these critical stages of the cell cycle, cells can activate cell cycle checkpoints (see Fig. 8.2). The major sensor of radiation-induced damage in cells is the ataxia-telangiectasia mutated (ATM) kinase, which, following activation, can phosphorylate more than 700 proteins in cells.[9] Two ATM substrates, p53 and Chk2, are critical for the activation of cell cycle arrests at multiple sites in the cell cycle.[10,11] The kinase p53 regulates the gene expression of specific genes such as *p21*, which inhibits cyclin-dependent kinase (CDK)2- and CDK4-mediated phosphorylation of the retinoblastoma protein, resulting in a block in the progression from the G$_1$ phase to the S phase of the cell cycle.[12,13] The Chk2 kinase promotes checkpoint activation in G$_1$ by targeting the cell division cycle 25 homolog A (CDC25A) phosphatase[14] and, in G$_2$/M, by targeting the CDC25C phosphatase.[15] The activation of a cell cycle arrest following DNA damage provides the cell with additional time to repair the DNA before entering critical cell cycle stages, which promotes genetic stability. Loss or defects in the *ATM* or *p53* genes result in abrogation of radiation-induced cell cycle checkpoints, which manifests itself as the highly cancer-prone human syndromes ataxia telangiectasia[16] or Li-Fraumeni,[17] respectively.

Radiation-Induced Cell Death

Terminally differentiated and stationary cells, such as kidney, lung, brain, muscle, and liver cells, are generally more resistant to radiation-induced killing than are cells with a high turnover rate, such as different epithelial cells, spermatogonia, and hair follicles. However, the spleen and thymus, which consist of mostly nondividing cells, are among the most radiosensitive tissues, implying that the rate of cell proliferation is not the sole determiner of the radiation sensitivity of a tissue. An important factor regulating the induction of programmed cell death (apoptosis) in tissues is the tumor suppressor p53.[18] The p53 protein is activated in cells following exposure to IR by the ATM kinase (see Fig. 8.2). When activated, it regulates the expression of multiple genes that have roles in DNA repair, cell cycle arrest, and apoptosis. p53 can also localize to mitochondria following irradiation, where it triggers apoptosis through the inactivation of antiapoptotic regulatory proteins.[19] Not all tissues induce the p53 response to the same degree after similar doses of IR, nor do they activate downstream pathways, such as DNA repair, cell cycle arrest, and apoptosis, in a similar way. For example, thymocytes have an intrinsic setting that favors apoptosis over cell cycle arrest following IR, whereas fibroblasts rarely induce apoptosis, but instead activate a strong and lasting cell cycle arrest.[18]

IR can induce cell death in tissues by many different mechanisms. Apoptosis can occur rapidly in a p53-dependent manner or later in a p53-independent manner. This later wave of radiation-induced apoptosis is often initiated by mitotic catastrophe, which occurs as a result of complications during chromosome segregation. Cell death induced by IR may in some cases be associated with autophagy, also called autophagocytosis, in which cells degrade cellular components via the lysosomal machinery. Whether autophagy is a programmed cell death or occurs in parallel with cell death is not clear. Interestingly, for some cell types, autophagy has been shown to actually protect the cells from radiation-induced death. Finally, tissue can undergo necrotic cell death following exposure to IR. Necrosis is a clinical problem following radiation therapy that can occur in normal tissues many months after treatment and can contribute to the inflammatory response.

Cancer Risks

It is clear from epidemiologic studies of radiation workers and atomic bomb and Chernobyl victims that IR can induce cancer.[20] Twenty years after the atomic bomb explosions in Japan during World War II, significant increases in the incidence of thyroid cancer and leukemia were observed. However, it took almost 50 years before solid tumors appeared in the population as a result of radiation exposure from the atomic bombs.[21] The incidences of solid tumors, such as breast, ovary, bladder, lung, and colon cancers, were estimated to have increased by a factor of 2 in the exposed group during this time period. The epidemiology studies following the nuclear power plant disaster in Chernobyl showed a clear increase in thyroid cancer as early as 4 years after the accident.[22] Young children were the most vulnerable to radiation exposure, with 1-year-old children being 237-fold more susceptible to thyroid cancer than the control group, while 10-year-old children were found to be sixfold more susceptible to thyroid cancer. Many of the thyroid cancers that developed following the Chernobyl disaster could have been prevented if the population had not consumed locally produced milk that was contaminated with radioactive iodine.

The molecular signatures of radiation-induced tumors are complex but involve point mutations that could lead to the activation of the *RAS* oncogene or inactivation of the tumor suppressor gene *p53*. Furthermore, IR induces DNA DSBs that may be unfaithfully repaired by the NHEJ pathway, leading to chromosome rearrangements. One such rearrangement found in 50% to 90% of the thyroid cancers examined following the Chernobyl accident involved the receptor tyrosine kinase c-RET, which promotes cell growth when activated.[22] Furthermore, a great majority of the thyroid cancers found in the exposed children harbored kinase fusion oncogenes affecting the mitogen-activated protein kinase (MAPK) signaling pathway.[23]

The correlation between high exposure to IR and cancer following the atomic bomb explosions and the Chernobyl accident is clear. What about the cancer risk following lower radiation exposures occurring in daily life? There are four theoretical risk models of radiation-induced cancer to consider. First, the *linear, no threshold* (LNT) *model* suggests that the induction of cancer is directly proportional to the dose of radiation, even at low doses of exposure. Second, the *sublinear* or *threshold model* suggests that below a certain threshold dose the risk of radiation-induced cancers is negligible. At these lower doses of radiation exposure, the DNA damage surveillance and repair mechanisms are thought to be fully capable of safeguarding the DNA to avoid the induction of mutations and cancer. Third, the *supralinear* or *stealth model* suggests that doses below a certain threshold or radiation with sufficiently low dose rates may not trigger the activation of DNA damage surveillance and repair mechanisms, resulting in suboptimal activation of cell cycle checkpoints and repair. This would be expected to lead to a higher rate of mutations and cancers than predicted by the LNT model, but may be balanced by a higher incident of cell death. Fourth, the *linear-quadratic model* suggest that radiation effects at low doses are due to a single track of radiation hitting multiple targets, resulting in a linear induction rate, whereas at higher doses, multiple radiation tracks hit multiple cellular targets, resulting in a quadratic induction rate.

The Biological Effects of Ionizing Radiation (BEIR) VII report, released by the Committee on Biological Effects of Ionizing Radiation of the National Academy of Sciences and commissioned by the US Environmental Protection Agency (EPA), is a review of published data regarding human health and cancer risks from exposure to low levels of IR. Although this topic is controversial and not fully settled, the BIER VII report favored the LNT model.[24] Thus, the "official" view is that no level of radiation is safe; therefore, a careful consideration of risks versus benefits is necessary to ensure that the general population only receives radiation doses as low as reasonably achievable. Furthermore, the BIER VII committee concluded that the heritable effects of radiation were not evident in the published data, indicating that an individual is not likely to develop cancer due to radiation exposure of his or her parents.

The largest source of radiation exposure to the population is radon, which is a natural radioactive gas formed as a decay product of radium in the decay chain of uranium. Radon gas can accumulate to high levels in poorly ventilated basements in houses built on rock containing uranium. The major risk with radon is that some of its radioactive decay products can attach to dust particles that accumulate in the lungs, leading to a continuous exposure of the lung tissues to high LET alpha particles. Due to this radiation exposure, the EPA claims that radon is the second leading cause of lung cancer in the United States. Another important source of human exposure to IR is medical x-ray devices, and there is a growing concern about the dramatically increased use of whole body CT scans for diagnostic purposes. For a typical CT scan, a patient will receive about 100-fold more radiation than from a typical mammogram.[24] It is recommended that the use of whole body CT scans for children be very restricted due to the elevated risk of developing radiation-induced cancer for this age group.

Cancer patients who receive radiation therapy are at risk of developing secondary tumors induced by the radiation therapy treatment.[1] This is particularly a concern for young patients since (1) children are more prone to radiation-induced cancer,

(2) children have a relatively good chance of surviving the primary cancer and would have long life expectancies so a secondary tumor would have plenty of time to develop, and (3) many childhood cancers are promoted by genetic defects in DNA damage response pathways, making these patients highly prone to the genotoxic effects of radiation and subsequent secondary cancers. The most sensitive tissues for the development of secondary cancer have been found to be bone marrow (leukemia), the thyroid, breast, and lung.[1]

ULTRAVIOLET LIGHT

Depending on the wavelength, UV light is categorized into UVA (320 to 400 nm), UVB (290 to 320 nm), and UVC (240 to 290 nm) radiation. Most of the UVC light emitted from the sun is absorbed by the ozone layer in the atmosphere, and, thus, living organisms are mostly exposed to UVA and UVB irradiation.

Mechanisms of Damage Induction

UVC light is more damaging to DNA than UVA and UVB because the absorption maximum of DNA is around 260 nm. UVB and UVC induce predominantly pyrimidine dimers and 6-4 photoproducts, which consist of covalent ring structures that link two adjacent pyrimidines on the same DNA strand.[5] The formation of these lesions results in the bending of the DNA helix, resulting in the interference with both DNA and RNA synthesis. UVA light does not induce pyrimidine dimers or 6-4 photoproducts but can induce ROS, which in turn can form SSBs and base lesions in DNA of exposed cells.

Cellular Responses

DNA Repair

The nucleotide excision repair (NER) pathway removes pyrimidine dimers and 6-4 photoproducts from cellular DNA.[5] This pathway involves proteins that recognize the DNA lesions, nucleases that excise the DNA strand that contains the lesion, a DNA polymerase that synthesizes new DNA to fill the gap, and a DNA ligase that joins the backbone in the newly synthesized strand. Genetic defects in the NER pathway result in the human syndrome xeroderma pigmentosum, with individuals more than 1,000-fold more prone to sun-induced skin cancer than normal individuals. In addition, human polymorphisms in certain NER genes are thought to predispose individuals to cancers such as lung cancer, nonmelanoma skin cancer, head and neck cancer, and bladder cancer, indicating that NER is responsible for safeguarding the genome against many types of DNA adducts in addition to UV-induced lesions.[5]

UV-induced lesions formed in the transcribed strand of active genes block the elongation of RNA polymerase II, and if a cell does not restore transcription within a certain time frame, it may undergo apoptosis (Fig. 8.3).[25,26] To rapidly restore RNA synthesis and avoid cell death, NER enzymes are recruited to the sites of blocked RNA polymerase II and the lesions are removed in a process called transcription-coupled repair (TCR).[27] Individuals with Cockayne syndrome (CS), trichiothiodystrophy, or the UV-sensitive syndrome, are unable to utilize the TCR pathway following UV irradiation.[5] Cells from these individuals do not recover RNA synthesis following UV irradiation and are therefore very prone to UV-induced apoptosis. Interestingly, despite a clear DNA repair defect, these individuals are not predisposed to UV-induced skin cancer. It is thought that the inability of CS cells to remove the toxic lesions that block transcription following UV irradiation results in the suppression of tumorigenesis by the elimination of damaged cells by apoptosis. However, while protecting against

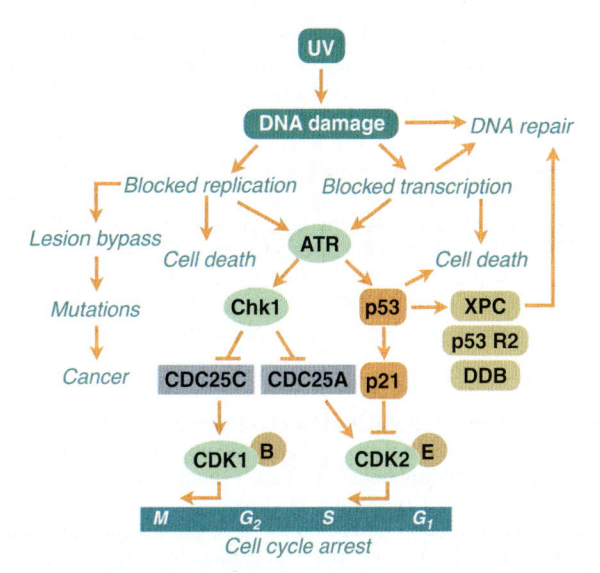

Figure 8.3 Cellular responses to ultraviolet (UV) light–induced DNA damage. UV light predominantly induces bulky DNA lesions that interfere with the processes of DNA replication and transcription. These lesions are removed from the global genome by global genomic nucleotide excision repair (GG-NER) and from transcribed DNA strands by transcription-coupled NER (TC-NER). Lesions blocking replication can be bypassed by exchanging processive DNA polymerases with less processive translesion DNA polymerases. While these polymerases allow cells to continue DNA synthesis and progress through the cell cycle, they have low fidelity, resulting in the potential induction of mutations promoting UV-induced carcinogenesis. To suppress mutations and support DNA repair efforts, the ataxia-telangiectasia and Rad3-related (ATR) kinase is activated in response to blocked replication or transcription. ATR activates the cell cycle checkpoint kinase Chk1, which, similar to Chk2, arrests cells in the G_1/S and G_2/M checkpoints by inhibiting CDC25A and CDC25C. ATR also activates p53, promoting G_1/S checkpoint activation via the induction of the Cdk-inhibitor p21. p53 also stimulates GG-NER by the transactivation of various NER genes and can promote apoptosis by the induction of proapoptotic factors and translocation to mitochondria. Finally, apoptosis is induced if cells do not recover transcription in a certain time frame, potentially due to the loss of survival factors or complications in the S phase when replication encounters stall the transcription complexes.

tumorigenesis, the elevated level of apoptosis in these cells leads to increased cell loss, which in turn may lead to neurologic degeneration.[25,28] Persistent transcription-blocking lesions in the genome have also been linked to aging.[29–31]

Translesion DNA Synthesis

Proliferating skin cells are very vulnerable to UV light because UV lesions block DNA replication (see Fig. 8.3). Cells that have entered the S phase and have initiated DNA synthesis have no choice but to finish replicating the whole genome or they will die. If DNA repair enzymes are not able to remove the blocking lesions from the template, the processive DNA polymerases may be exchanged for other, less processive DNA polymerases that can bypass the lesions. This is part of a "tolerance" mechanism, which allows cells to complete replication and eventually divide.[5] However, the translesion DNA polymerases do not have the same fidelity as the processive DNA polymerases; thus, mutations may occur. This is thought to be a major pathway by which UV light induces mutagenesis and, subsequently, cancer (see Fig. 8.3).

ATM and Rad3-Related Mediated Cell Cycle Checkpoints

In addition to utilizing the NER and BER pathways to repair UV-induced DNA damage, proliferating cells activate cell cycle checkpoints to allow more time for repair before entering critical parts of the cell cycle, such as the S phase and mitosis. The ATM and Rad3-related (ATR) kinase is activated following UV irradiation by blocked replication or transcription (see Fig. 8.3).[32] ATR phosphorylates a large number of proteins, many of which are the same as those phosphorylated by ATM after exposure to ionizing radiation.[9] Two important substrates of ATR are p53 and Chk1, which are critical in promoting cell cycle arrest. When induced by ATR, p53 transactivates the gene that encodes the cell cycle inhibitor p21, leading to the arrest of cells in the G_1 phase of the cell cycle, while Chk1 phosphorylates the CDK-activating phosphatases CDC25A and CDC25C, which targets them for degradation, resulting in an S-phase or G_2-phase arrest (see Fig. 8.3).[33]

Activation of Cell Membrane Receptors

In addition to triggering cellular stress responses by inducing DNA damage, UV light can directly induce membrane receptor signaling by receptor phosphorylation. This is thought to be due to the direct UV-mediated inhibition of protein-tyrosine phosphatases that regulate the phosphorylation levels of various membrane receptors.[34] In addition, membrane receptors may physically aggregate following UV irradiation, leading to the activation of signal transduction pathways that regulate cell growth[35] or apoptosis.[36]

Cell Death

UV light effectively induces apoptosis in skin cells. The mechanism by which UV light induces cell death is not fully understood, but failure to adequately resume RNA synthesis following UV light exposure is strongly linked to apoptosis (see Fig. 8.3).[25] Many potential mechanisms of how blocked transcription results in apoptosis have been suggested, such as a physical clash during the S phase between elongating replication machineries and transcription complexes stalled at UV lesions. Another possible mechanism involves the preferential loss of survival factors coded by highly unstable mRNAs.[37] The induction of p53 may also contribute to UV-induced apoptosis,[38] although p53 appears to protect human fibroblasts[39] and keratinocytes[40] from UV-induced apoptosis. Although complications induced by DNA damage may be the predominant mechanism by which cells die following UV irradiation, UV light may induce apoptosis in certain cell types by directly promoting the physical aggregation of the death receptor Fas/APO1.[36]

Cancer Risks

The incidence of sun-induced skin cancer, especially melanoma, is on the increase due to higher rates of sun exposure in the general population. The link between UV light exposure and skin cancer is very strong, but the role of UV light in the etiology of nonmelanoma and melanoma skin cancer differs. Although the risk of nonmelanoma cancer relates to the cumulative lifetime exposure to UV light, the risk of contracting melanoma appears to be linked to high sunlight exposure during childhood.[41] What makes UV light such a potent carcinogen is that it can initiate carcinogenesis by inducing DNA lesions as well as suppressing the immune system, resulting in a greater probability that initiated cells will survive and grow into tumors.[42,43]

Nonmelanoma Skin Cancer

Basal cell carcinoma (BCC) and squamous cell carcinoma (SCC) are the two most common skin cancer types. BCC and SCC occur predominantly in sun-exposed areas of the skin, but there are examples of these cancers forming in nonexposed areas as well. The tumor suppressor genes *p53* and *p16* are frequently inactivated in BCC and SCC, while the hedgehog-signaling pathway is activated primarily by mutations to the patched gene (percutaneous transhepatic cholangiography [*PTCH*]). This scenario promotes proliferation without the opposition of the cell cycle inhibitors p53 and p16.

Melanoma

Melanoma arises from mutations in epidermal melanocytes and is the most dangerous form of skin cancer because it has the highest propensity to metastasize. It is formed in both sun-exposed and shielded areas of the skin; therefore, the role of UV light as the major carcinogen in melanoma has been controversial.[41] Defects in the NER pathway do not seem to predispose the development of melanoma, suggesting that pyrimidine dimers or 6-4 photoproducts induced by UVB are not the initiators of melanoma carcinogenesis. Instead, ROS induced by UVA may be responsible for the development of melanoma.[41] However, a study using next-generation sequencing techniques to catalog all mutations in a melanoma cell line found a mutational spectrum of the over 33,000 mutations detected that strongly indicated that pyrimidine dimers and 6-4 photoproducts are the major mutagenic lesions in melanoma, whereas a subset of mutations may be induced by ROS.[44] The incidence of mutations in the *p16* and *ARF* genes is high, whereas *p53* and *RAS* mutations are fairly uncommon in melanoma.

Photoimmunosuppression

Studies of transplantation of mouse skin cancers into syngeneic mice revealed that prior UVB irradiation of recipient mice promoted tumor growth, whereas transplantation into naïve nonirradiated mice led to rejection.[43] These studies established that UV light has local immunosuppressing ability, and subsequent studies found that UV light preferentially depletes Langerhans cells from irradiated skin.[42] Langerhans cells play an important role in the immune response by presenting antigens to the immune cells, and, thus, depletion of these cells leads to local immunosuppression. In addition to local immunosuppression, UV light has been shown to promote systemic immunosuppression.[45] This response is complex, but it is known that UV-induced DNA lesions in skin cells contribute to the systemic immunosuppression response.[46] The secretion of the immunosuppressing cytokine interleukin (IL)-10 from irradiated keratinocytes as well as UV-induced structural alteration of the epidermal chromophore urocanic acid may mediate the long-range immunosuppressive effects of UV light.[42,45]

RADIOFREQUENCY AND MICROWAVE RADIATION

Radiofrequency radiation (RFR) is electromagnetic radiation in the frequency range 3 kHz to 300 MHz, whereas microwave radiation (MR) is in the frequency range between 300 MHz to 300 GHz. RFR and MR do not have sufficient energies to cause ionizations in target tissues. Rather, the radiation energy is converted into heat as the radiation energy is absorbed. Sources of radiofrequency and microwave radiation include mobile phones, radio transmitters of wireless communication, radars, medical devices, and kitchen appliances.

Mechanism of Damage Induction

Because human exposure to RFR has increased dramatically in recent years, it is important to know whether this type of radiation gives rise to genotoxic damage. Although there are many studies showing that RFR can induce ROS, leading to genetic damage in cell culture systems, other studies have generated conflicting results.[47] One confounding factor when assessing the genotoxic effect of RFR, and especially MR, is the heating effect that occurs in the tissue when the radiation energy is absorbed. A recent study controlling for the potential heating effect of exposure found that RFR induces ROS and DNA damage in human spermatozoa in vitro, which is an alarming finding considering the potential hereditary implications.[48] It has been suggested that MR may affect the folding of proteins in cells that promote new protein synthesis.[49] Furthermore, exposure of cells to MR has been shown to lead to the phosphorylation of numerous cellular proteins largely through the activation of the p38/MAPK stress response pathway.[50] However, the biologic consequences of these cellular changes are not clear. Epidemiology studies that monitored the genetic effects in individuals exposed to high levels of RF have revealed evidence of increased induction of chromosome aberrations in lymphocytes.[51] However, there is a level of uncertainty in these studies about exposure levels, making it difficult to come to meaningful conclusions.

Cancer Risks

Because the population's exposure to RFR and MR has dramatically increased in recent years, it is of great importance to assess the potential cancer risks of these types of radiation so that appropriate exposure limits can be implemented. A number of studies have focused on the potential cancer risks from mobile phone usage, and some of these studies indicate that long-term mobile phone usage may be associated with increased risks of developing brain tumors (see the following). Other epidemiologic studies of cancer incidences in populations living near radio towers or mobile phone base stations are inconclusive. Some studies have shown a connection between proximity to mobile phone base stations and increased cancer incidence,[52] whereas another study found no association between exposure to RFR from mobile phone base stations and early childhood cancers.[53]

ELECTROMAGNETIC FIELDS

An electromagnetic field (EMF) is a physical field produced by electrically charged objects that can affect other charged objects in the field. Typical sources of EMFs are electric power lines, electrical devices, and magnetic resonance imaging (MRI) machines.

Mechanisms of Damage Induction

A low frequency EMF does not transmit energy high enough to break chemical bonds; therefore, it is not thought to directly damage DNA or proteins in cells. The data obtained from studies to assess the potential genotoxic effects of EMF do not provide a clear conclusion. Some of the results obtained in cell culture studies suggest a harmful effect of EMFs, but the concerns are that these effects may be related to heat production induced by EMFs rather than from the magnetic field itself. A recent in vitro study detected DNA strand breaks in cells exposed to EMFs, but this induction was thought to not be the result of ROS production, but rather due to indirect effects through interference with DNA replication and induction of apoptosis in a subset of cells.[54] A study using an MRI found no evidence of an induced formation of DNA DSBs in cell cultures.[55] EMFs have been shown to induce nongenotoxic effects in cells, such as interference with cellular signaling pathways,[56] which could contribute to neurodegeneration.[57]

Cancer Risks

Studies with rodents have largely failed to detect an association between exposure to EMFs and cancer. This is also true for numerous epidemiology studies, with the only exception being the association between EMF exposure and childhood leukemia where children exposed to doses of 0.4 mcT or above may have about a twofold increased risk of developing leukemia.[58,59] There is no strong link between EMF exposure and increased risks of contracting adult leukemia, brain tumors, or breast cancer.[60,61] Furthermore, a study investigating whether EMF exposure was associated with heritable effects found no correlation between parental exposure and childhood cancer.[62]

Potential Cancer Risks from Mobile Phone Usage

Mobile phones emit RFR and generate EMFs. The biggest health concern with mobile phone usage is its potential role in the development of brain tumors. During mobile phone use, the brain tissue is exposed to doses, giving peak specific absorption rates (SAR) of 4 to 8 W/kg. At these intensities, the induction of DNA damage has been detected in laboratory studies.[63] The current epidemiologic data are largely inconclusive on the association between mobile phone usage and brain tumor incidence. Meta-analysis studies of populations who had used mobile phones for more than 10 years concluded that mobile phone usage was associated with an elevated risk for brain tumors, such as acoustic neuroma and glioma cancer.[64–66] In contrast, other large prospective studies did not observe a correlation between mobile phone usage and incidences of glioma, meningioma, or non–central nervous system (CNS) cancers.[67,68] It is important to point out that, generally, it takes 30 to 40 years for brain tumors to develop, and because mobile phones have only been in general use for about 15 years, there has not been sufficient time to fully evaluate the brain cancer risks of mobile phone usage.

ASBESTOS

Asbestos is a class of naturally occurring silicate minerals that have been widely used in building materials for its heat, sound, and electrical insulating qualities. Asbestos becomes a serious health hazard if the fibers are inhaled over a long period of time, and these health effects are increased dramatically if the exposed individual is a smoker. It was first reported in 1935 that asbestos might be an occupational health hazard that could induce cancer.[69,70] However, it was not until 1986 that the International Labor Organization recommended banning asbestos.[71] The use of asbestos products peaked in the 1970s, yet remains a major health hazard in many places around the world today.

Mechanisms of Damage Induction

Asbestos fibers can enter cells and induce ROS, especially if they contain high levels of iron.[72] In addition, ROS can be generated by "frustrated" phagocytosis, and this in turn can lead to the release of proinflammatory cytokines with subsequent inflammation of the tissue. ROS have been implicated to originate from affected mitochondria leading to induction of SSBs and base damage, such as 8-hydroxyguanine in DNA.[73] Furthermore, if not successfully repaired, asbestos-induced DNA damage has been shown to result in chromosome aberrations, micronuclei formation, and increased rates of sister chromatid exchanges.[74]

Cellular and Tissue Responses

Asbestos-induced ROS cause base lesions and DNA strand breaks, which require base excision repair for the restoration of DNA and for minimizing mutagenesis. In addition to DNA repair, a number of cellular signaling pathways are activated by asbestos. These include the epidermal growth factor receptor (EGFR) and the MAPK pathway, leading to the activation of nuclear factor kappa B

(NF-κB) and transcription factor AP-1.[72,74] Activation of the NF-κB pathway leads to the induction of proinflammatory genes such as tumor necrosis factor (TNF), *IL-6*, *IL-8*, and proliferation-promoting genes such as *c-Myc*, leading to inflammation and increased cell proliferation. Asbestos exposure also stimulates the expression of the transforming growth factor beta (TGF-β), which, in turn, stimulates fibrogenesis in exposed tissues.[74]

Cancer Risks

Lung Cancer

Epidemiologic studies have found a strong link between asbestos exposure and lung cancer.[74] It has been estimated that about 5% to 7% of all lung cancers are attributable to asbestos exposure, and asbestos and tobacco smoking act in synergy to induce lung cancer. Mutational spectra due to 8-hydroxyguanine lesions formed by ROS can be linked to asbestos exposure, and point mutations in the tumor suppressor genes *p53* and *p16/INK4A* and in the *KRAS* oncogene have been found in tumors from asbestos-exposed individuals.

Mesothelioma

After being taken up by lung tissues, asbestos fibers can translocate into the pleura, the body cavity that surrounds the lungs. The pleura are covered with a protective lining, the mesothelium, which consists of squamouslike epithelial cells. Mesothelial cells can internalize asbestos fibers, resulting in the induction of ROS and inflammatory responses, subsequently leading to the initiation and progression of malignant mesothelioma.[75] Asbestos is considered one of the major causes of malignant mesothelioma, and frequent mutations are found in the *p16/INK4A* and *NF2* genes, whereas *p53* mutations are fairly rare.

NANOPARTICLES

Nanoparticles are defined as ultrafine particles of the size range 1 to 100 nm in diameter. Nanoparticle chemistry of a certain compound is different from bulk chemistry of that compound because of the high percentage of atoms at the surface of the particle. The production of nanoparticles has increased dramatically in recent years, and they are found in many industrial and consumer products such as paint, cosmetics, and sunscreens. They also have many potential medical applications, such as delivery vehicles for specific drugs to specific target tissues or tumors.

Mechanisms of DNA Damage Induction

Many of the cellular effects of nanoparticles are similar to the effects exerted by asbestos, such as the generation of ROS and inflammation.[72] Nanoparticles have been shown to induce oxidative DNA damage, such as DNA strand breaks and 8-hydroxyguanine lesions both in cell culture[76, 77] and in vivo.[78] Nanoparticle-induced DNA lesions are manifested as histone γ-H2AX nuclear foci, chromosome deletions, and micronuclei.

Cellular Responses

Nanoparticles induce ROS either directly or indirectly, resulting in DNA lesions, such as 8-hydroxyguanine–base damage and DNA strand breaks. These lesions are repaired by the base excision repair. The phosphorylation of histone H2AX has been shown to occur following exposure of cells to nanoparticles, suggesting that the DNA lesions trigger the activation of ATM or ATR stress kinases.[79] Nanoparticles have also been found to affect the immune system[80] and can induce the release of the proinflammatory cytokine TNF-α from cells.

Cancer Risks

Some nanoparticles, such as titanium dioxide, which is used as pigments in paint, have been classified by the International Agency for Research on Cancer (IARC) as a group 2B carcinogen, "possible carcinogenic to humans." However, rigorous epidemiologic data is lacking to fully evaluate the cancer-inducing potential of nanoparticles.[81]

REFERENCES

1. Hall E, Giaccia A. *Radiobiology for the Radiologist.* Philadelphia: Lippincott Williams & Wilkins; 2012.
2. Ward JF. DNA damage produced by ionizing radiation in mammalian cells: identities, mechanisms of formation, and repairability. *Prog Nucleic Acid Res Mol Biol* 1988;35:95–125.
3. Prutz WA. 'Chemical repair' in irradiated DNA solutions containing thiols and/or disulphides. Further evidence for disulphide radical anions acting as electron donors. *Int J Radiat Biol* 1989;56:21–33.
4. Hutchinson F. Chemical changes induced in DNA by ionizing radiation. *Prog Nucleic Acid Res Mol Biol* 1985;32:115–154.
5. Friedberg E, Walker G, Siede W, et al. *DNA Repair and Mutagenesis.* 2nd ed. Washington, D.C.: ASM Press; 2006.
6. Radford IR. The level of induced DNA double-strand breakage correlates with cell killing after X-irradiation. *Int J Radiat Biol Relat Stud Phys Chem Med* 1985;48:45–54.
7. Daly MJ. A new perspective on radiation resistance based on *Deinococcus radiodurans. Nat Rev Microbiol* 2009;7:237–245.
8. Krisko A, Radman M. Biology of extreme radiation resistance: the way of *Deinococcus radiodurans. Cold Spring Harb Perspect Biol* 2013;5.
9. Matsuoka S, Ballif BA, Smogorzewska A, et al. ATM and ATR substrate analysis reveals extensive protein networks responsive to DNA damage. *Science* 2007;316:1160–1166.
10. Kastan M, Onyekwere O, Sidransky D, et al. Participation of p53 protein in the cellular response to DNA damage. *Cancer Res* 1991;51:6304–6311.
11. Matsuoka S, Huang M, Elledge SJ. Linkage of ATM to cell cycle regulation by the Chk2 protein kinase. *Science* 1998;282:1893–1897.
12. Harper J, Adami G, Wei N, et al. The p21 cdk-interacting protein Cip1 is a potent inhibitor of G1 cyclin-dependent kinases. *Cell* 1993;75:805–816.
13. El-Deiry W, Tokino T, Velculescu V, et al. WAF1, a potential mediator of p53 tumor suppression. *Cell* 1993;75:817–825.
14. Falck J, Mailand N, Syljuasen RG, et al. The ATM-Chk2-Cdc25A checkpoint pathway guards against radioresistant DNA synthesis. *Nature* 2001;410:842–847.
15. Bartek J, Falck J, Lukas J. Chk2 kinase—a busy messenger [Review]. *Nat Rev Mol Cell Biol* 2001;2:877–886.
16. Savitsky K, Bar-Shira A, Gilad S, et al. A single ataxia telangiectasia gene with a product similar to PI-3 kinase. *Science* 1995;268:1749–1753.
17. Srivastava S, Zou ZQ, Pirollo K, et al. Germ-line transmission of a mutated p53 gene in a cancer-prone family with Li-Fraumeni syndrome. *Nature*.1990;348:747–749.
18. Gudkov AV, Komarova EA. The role of p53 in determining sensitivity to radiotherapy. *Nat Rev Cancer* 2003;3:117–129.
19. Mihara M, Erster S, Zaika A, et al. p53 has a direct apoptogenic role at the mitochondria. *Mol Cell* 2003;11:577–590.
20. Williams D, Baverstock K. Chernobyl and the future: too soon for a final diagnosis. *Nature* 2006;440:993–994.
21. Thompson DE, Mabuchi K, Ron E, et al. Cancer incidence in atomic bomb survivors. Part II: Solid tumors, 1958–1987. *Radiat Res* 1994;137:S17–67.
22. Williams D. Cancer after nuclear fallout: lessons from the Chernobyl accident. *Nat Rev Cancer* 2002;2:543–549.
23. Ricarte-Filho JC, Li S, Garcia-Rendueles ME, et al. Identification of kinase fusion oncogenes in post-Chernobyl radiation-induced thyroid cancers. *J Clin Invest* 2013;123:4935–4944.
24. National Research Council. *Health Risks from Exposure to Low Levels of Ionizing Radiation: BEIR VII Phase 2.* Washington, D.C.: National Academy Press; 2006.
25. Ljungman M, Zhang F. Blockage of RNA polymerase as a possible trigger for u.v. light-induced apoptosis. *Oncogene*.1996;13:823–831.
26. Brash DE, Wikonkal NM, Remenyik E, et al. The DNA damage signal for Mdm2 regulation, Trp53 induction, and sunburn cell formation in vivo originates from actively transcribed genes. *J Invest Derm* 2001;117:1234–1240.

27. Hanawalt PC, Spivak G. Transcription-coupled DNA repair: two decades of progress and surprises. *Nat Rev Mol Cell Biol* 2008;9:958–970.
28. Lehmann AR. DNA repair-deficient diseases, xeroderma pigmentosum, Cockayne syndrome and trichothiodystrophy. *Biochimie* 2003;85:1101–1111.
29. Andressoo JO, Hoeijmakers JH. Transcription-coupled repair and premature ageing. *Mutat Res* 2005;577:179–194.
30. de Boer J, Andressoo JO, de Wit J, et al. Premature aging in mice deficient in DNA repair and transcription. *Science* 2002;296:1276–1279.
31. Garinis GA, Uittenboogaard LM, Stachelscheid H, et al. Persistent transcription-blocking DNA lesions trigger somatic growth attenuation associated with longevity. *Nat Cell Biol* 2009;11:604–615.
32. Derheimer FA, O'Hagan HM, Krueger HM, et al. RPA and ATR link transcriptional stress to p53. *Proc Natl Acad Sci U S A* 2007;104:12778–12783.
33. Kastan MB, Bartek J. Cell-cycle checkpoints and cancer. *Nature* 2004;432:316–323.
34. Gross S, Knebel A, Tenev T, et al. Inactivation of protein-tyrosine phosphatases as mechanism of UV-induced signal transduction. *J Biol Chem* 1999;274:26378–26386.
35. Sachsenmaier C, Radlerpohl A, Zinck R, et al. Involvement of growth factor receptors in the mammalian UVC response. *Cell* 1994;78:963–972.
36. Rehemtulla A, Hamilton CA, Chinnaiyan AM, et al. Ultraviolet radiation-induced apoptosis is mediated by activation of CD-95 (Fas/APO-1). *J Biol Chem* 1997;272:25783–25786.
37. Ljungman M, Lane DP. Transcription - guarding the genome by sensing DNA damage. *Nat Rev Cancer* 2004;4:727–737.
38. Ziegler A, Jonason AS, Leffell DJ, et al. Sunburn and p53 in the onset of skin cancer. *Nature* 1994;372:773–776.
39. McKay B, Ljungman M. Role for p53 in the recovery of transcription and protection against apoptosis induced by ultraviolet light. *Neoplasia* 1999;1:276–284.
40. Chaturvedi V, Sitailo LA, Qin JZ, et al. Knockdown of p53 levels in human keratinocytes accelerates Mcl-1 and Bcl-x(L) reduction thereby enhancing UV-light induced apoptosis. *Oncogene* 2005;24:5299–5312.
41. Maddodi N, Setaluri V. Role of UV in cutaneous melanoma. *Photochem Photobiol* 2008;84:528–536.
42. Murphy GM. Ultraviolet radiation and immunosuppression. *Br J Dermatol* 2009;161(Suppl 3):90–95.
43. Fisher MS, Kripke ML. Systemic alteration induced in mice by ultraviolet light irradiation and its relationship to ultraviolet carcinogenesis. *Proc Natl Acad Sci U S A* 1977;74:1688–1692.
44. Pleasance ED, Cheetham RK, Stephens PJ, et al. A comprehensive catalogue of somatic mutations from a human cancer genome. *Nature* 2010;463:191–196.
45. Schwarz T. Photoimmunosuppression. *Photodermatol Photoimmunol Photomed* 2002;18:141–145.
46. Kripke ML, Cox PA, Alas LG, et al. Pyrimidine dimers in DNA initiate systemic immunosuppression in UV-irradiated mice. *Proc Natl Acad Sci U S A* 1992;89:7516–7520.
47. Vijayalaxmi, Prihoda TJ. Genetic damage in mammalian somatic cells exposed to radiofrequency radiation: a meta-analysis of data from 63 publications (1990–2005). *Radiat Res* 2008;169:561–574.
48. De Iuliis GN, Newey RJ, King BV, et al. Mobile phone radiation induces reactive oxygen species production and DNA damage in human spermatozoa in vitro. *PLoS One* 2009;4:e6446.
49. Gerner C, Haudek V, Schandl U, et al. Increased protein synthesis by cells exposed to a 1,800-MHz radio-frequency mobile phone electromagnetic field, detected by proteome profiling. *Int Arch Occup Environ Health* 2010;83:691–702.
50. Leszczynski D, Joenvaara S, Reivinen J, et al. Non-thermal activation of the hsp27/p38MAPK stress pathway by mobile phone radiation in human endothelial cells: molecular mechanism for cancer- and blood-brain barrier-related effects. *Differentiation* 2002;70:120–129.
51. Verschaeve L. Genetic damage in subjects exposed to radiofrequency radiation. *Mutat Res* 2009;681:259–270.
52. Khurana VG, Hardell L, Everaert J, et al. Epidemiological evidence for a health risk from mobile phone base stations. *Int J Occup Environ Health* 2010;16:263–267.
53. Elliott P, Toledano MB, Bennett J, et al. Mobile phone base stations and early childhood cancers: case-control study. *BMJ* 2010;340:c3077.
54. Focke F, Schuermann D, Kuster N, et al. DNA fragmentation in human fibroblasts under extremely low frequency electromagnetic field exposure. *Mutat Res* 2010;683:74–83.
55. Schwenzer NF, Bantleon R, Maurer B, et al. Detection of DNA double-strand breaks using gammaH2AX after MRI exposure at 3 Tesla: an in vitro study. *J Magn Reson Imaging* 2007;26:1308–1314.
56. Girgert R, Hanf V, Emons G, et al. Signal transduction of the melatonin receptor MT1 is disrupted in breast cancer cells by electromagnetic fields. *Bioelectromagnetics* 2010;31:237–245.
57. Consales C, Merla C, Marino C, et al. Electromagnetic fields, oxidative stress, and neurodegeneration. *Int J Cell Biol* 2012;2012:683897.
58. Ahlbom A, Day N, Feychting M, et al. A pooled analysis of magnetic fields and childhood leukaemia. *Br J Cancer* 2000;83:692–698.
59. Malagoli C, Fabbi S, Teggi S, et al. Risk of hematological malignancies associated with magnetic fields exposure from power lines: a case-control study in two municipalities of northern Italy. *Environ Health* 2010;9:16.
60. Kheifets L, Monroe J, Vergara X, et al. Occupational electromagnetic fields and leukemia and brain cancer: an update to two meta-analyses. *J Occup Environ Med* 2008;50:677–688.
61. Chen C, Ma X, Zhong M, et al. Extremely low-frequency electromagnetic fields exposure and female breast cancer risk: a meta-analysis based on 24,338 cases and 60,628 controls. *Breast Cancer Res Treat* 2010;123:569–576.
62. Hug K, Grize L, Seidler A, et al. Parental occupational exposure to extremely low frequency magnetic fields and childhood cancer: a German case-control study. *Am J Epidemiol* 2010;171:27–35.
63. Hardell L, Sage C. Biological effects from electromagnetic field exposure and public exposure standards. *Biomed Pharmacother* 2008;62:104–109.
64. Hardell L, Carlberg M, Hansson Mild K. Mobile phone use and the risk for malignant brain tumors: a case-control study on deceased cases and controls. *Neuroepidemiology* 2010;35:109–114.
65. Hardell L, Carlberg M, Soderqvist F, et al. Meta-analysis of long-term mobile phone use and the association with brain tumours. *Int J Oncol* 2008;32:1097–1103.
66. Myung SK, Ju W, McDonnell DD, et al. Mobile phone use and risk of tumors: a meta-analysis. *J Clin Oncol* 2009;27:5565–5572.
67. Benson VS, Pirie K, Schuz J, et al. Mobile phone use and risk of brain neoplasms and other cancers: prospective study. *Int J Epidemiol* 2013;42:792–802.
68. Poulsen AH, Friis S, Johansen C, et al. Mobile phone use and the risk of skin cancer: a nationwide cohort study in Denmark. *Am J Epidemiol* 2013;178:190–197.
69. Lynch K, Smith W. Pulmonary asbestosis. III. Carcinoma of lung in asbestos-silicosis. *Am J Cancer* 1935;24:56–64.
70. Gloyne S. Two cases of squamous carcinoma of the lung occuring in asbestosis. *Tubercele* 1935;17:5–10.
71. LaDou J. The asbestos cancer epidemic. *Environ Health Perspect* 2004;112:285–290.
72. Pacurari M, Castranova V, Vallyathan V. Single- and multi-wall carbon nanotubes versus asbestos: are the carbon nanotubes a new health risk to humans? *J Toxicol Environ Health A* 2010;73:378–395.
73. Liu G, Cheresh P, Kamp DW. Molecular basis of asbestos-induced lung disease. *Annu Rev Pathol* 2013;8:161–187.
74. Nymark P, Wikman H, Hienonen-Kempas T, et al. Molecular and genetic changes in asbestos-related lung cancer. *Cancer Lett* 2008;265:1–15.
75. Jaurand MC, Renier A, Daubriac J. Mesothelioma: do asbestos and carbon nanotubes pose the same health risk? *Part Fibre Toxicol* 2009;6:16.
76. Shukla RK, Kumar A, Gurbani D, et al. TiO(2) nanoparticles induce oxidative DNA damage and apoptosis in human liver cells. *Nanotoxicology* 2013;7:48–60.
77. Horie M, Nishio K, Endoh S, et al. Chromium(III) oxide nanoparticles induced remarkable oxidative stress and apoptosis on culture cells. *Environ Toxicol* 2013;28:61–75.
78. Trouiller B, Reliene R, Westbrook A, et al. Titanium dioxide nanoparticles induce DNA damage and genetic instability in vivo in mice. *Cancer Res* 2009;69:8784–8789.
79. Prasad RY, Chastain PD, Nikolaishvili-Feinberg N, et al. Titanium dioxide nanoparticles activate the ATM-Chk2 DNA damage response in human dermal fibroblasts. *Nanotoxicology* 2013;7:1111–1119.
80. Zolnik BS, Gonzalez-Fernandez A, Sadrieh N, et al. Nanoparticles and the immune system. *Endocrinology* 2010;151:458–465.
81. Shi H, Magaye R, Castranova V, et al. Titanium dioxide nanoparticles: a review of current toxicological data. *Part Fibre Toxicol* 2013;10:15.

9 Dietary Factors

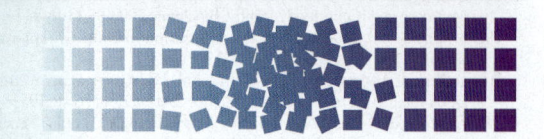

Karin B. Michels and Walter C. Willett

INTRODUCTION

Over two decades ago, Doll and Peto[1] speculated that 35% (range: 10% to 70%) of all cancer deaths in the United States may be preventable by alterations in diet. The magnitude of the estimate for dietary factors exceeded that for tobacco (30%) and infections (10%).

Studies of cancer incidence among populations migrating to countries with different lifestyle factors have indicated that most cancers have a large environmental etiology. Although the contribution of environmental influences differs by cancer type, the incidence of many cancers changes by as much as five- to tenfold among migrants over time, approaching that of the host country. The age at migration affects the degree of adaptation among first-generation migrants for some cancers, suggesting that the susceptibility to environmental carcinogenic influences varies with age by cancer type. Identifying the specific environmental and lifestyle factors most important to cancer etiology, however, has proven difficult.

Environmental factors such as diet may influence the incidence of cancer through many different mechanisms and at different stages in the cancer process. Simple mutagens in foods, such as those produced by the heating of proteins, can cause damage to DNA, but dietary factors can also influence this process by inducing enzymes that activate or inactivate these mutagens, or by blocking the action of the mutagen. Dietary factors can also affect every pathway hypothesized to mediate cancer risk–for example, the rate of cell cycling through hormonal or antihormonal effects, aiding or inhibiting DNA repair, promoting or inhibiting apoptosis, and DNA methylation. Because of the complexity of these mechanisms, knowledge of dietary influences on risk of cancer will require an empirical basis with human cancer as the outcome.

METHODOLOGIC CHALLENGES

Study Types and Biases

The association between diet and the risk of cancer has been the subject of a number of epidemiologic studies. The most prevalent designs are the case-control study, the cohort study, and the randomized clinical trial. When the results from epidemiologic studies are interpreted, the potential for confounding must be considered. Individuals who maintain a healthy diet are likely to exhibit other indicators of a healthy lifestyle, including regular physical activity, lower body weight, use of multivitamin supplements, lower smoking rates, and lower alcohol consumption. Even if the influence of these confounding variables is analytically controlled, residual confounding remains possible.

Ecologic Studies

In ecologic studies or international correlation studies, variation in food disappearance data and the prevalence of a certain disease are correlated, generally across different countries. A linear association may provide preliminary data to inform future research but, due to the high probability of confounding, cannot provide strong evidence for a causal link. Food disappearance data also may not provide a good estimate for human consumption. The gross national product is correlated with many dietary factors such as fat intake.[2] Many other differences besides dietary fat exist between the countries with low fat consumption (less affluent) and high fat consumption (more affluent); reproductive behaviors, physical activity level, and body fatness are particularly notable and are strongly associated with specific cancers.

Migrant Studies

Studies of populations migrating from areas with low incidence of disease to areas with high incidence of disease (or vice versa) can help sort out the role of environmental factors versus genetics in the etiology of a cancer, depending on whether the migrating group adopts the cancer rates of the new environment. Specific dietary components linked to disease are difficult to identify in a migrant study.

Case-Control Studies

Case-control studies of diet may be affected by recall bias, control selection bias, and confounding. In a case-control study, participants affected by the disease under study (cases) and healthy controls are asked to recall their past dietary habits. Cases may overestimate their consumption of foods that are commonly considered "unhealthy" and underestimate their consumption of foods considered "healthy." Giovannucci et al.[3] have documented differential reporting of fat intake before and after disease occurrence. Thus, the possibility of recall bias in a case-control study poses a real threat to the validity of the observed associations. Even more importantly, in contemporary case-control studies using a population sample of controls, the participation rate of controls is usually far from complete, often 50% to 70%. Unfortunately, health-conscious individuals may be more likely to participate as controls and will thus be less overweight, will consume fruits and vegetables more frequently, and will consume less fat and red meat, which can substantially distort associations observed.

Cohort Studies

Prospective cohort studies of the effects of diet are likely to have a much higher validity than retrospective case-control studies because diet is recorded by participants before disease occurrence. Cohort studies are still affected by measurement error because diet consists of a large number of foods eaten in complex combinations. Confounding by other unmeasured or imperfectly measured lifestyle factors can remain a problem in cohort studies.

Now that the results of a substantial number of cohort studies have become available, their findings can be compared with those of case-control studies that have examined the same relations. In many cases, the findings of the case-control studies have not been confirmed; for example, the consistent finding of lower risk of many cancers with higher intake of fruits and vegetables in case-control studies has generally not been seen in cohort studies.[4] These findings suggest that the concerns about biases in case-control studies of diet, and probably many other lifestyle factors, are justified, and findings from such studies must be interpreted cautiously.

Randomized Clinical Trials

The gold standard in medical research is the randomized clinical trial (RCT). In an RCT on nutrition, participants are randomly assigned to one of two or more diets; hence, the association between diet and the cancer of interest should not be confounded by other factors. The problem with RCTs of diet is that maintaining the assigned diet strictly over many years, as would be necessary for diet to have an impact on cancer incidence, is difficult. For example, in the dietary fat reduction trial of the Women's Health Initiative (WHI), participants randomized to the intervention arm reduced their fat intake much less than planned.[5] The remaining limited contrast between the two groups left the lack of difference in disease outcomes difficult to interpret. Furthermore, the relevant time window for intervention and the necessary duration of intervention are unclear, especially with cancer outcomes. Hence, randomized trials are rarely used to examine the effect of diet on cancer but have better promise for the study of diet and outcomes that require a considerably shorter follow-up time (e.g., adenoma recurrence). Also, the randomized design may lend itself better to the study of the effects of dietary supplements such as multivitamin or fiber supplements, although the control group may adopt the intervention behavior because nutritional supplements are widely available. For example, in the WHI trial of calcium and vitamin D supplementation, two-thirds of the study population used vitamin D or calcium supplements that they obtained outside of the trial, again rendering the lack of effect in the trial uninterpretable.

Diet Assessment Instruments

Observational studies depend on a reasonably valid assessment of dietary intake. Although, for some nutrients, biochemical measurements can be used to assess intake, for most dietary constituents, a useful biochemical indicator does not exist. In population-based studies, diet is generally assessed with a self-administered instrument. Since 1980, considerable effort has been directed at the development of standardized questionnaires for measuring diet, and numerous studies have been conducted to assess the validity of these methods. The most widely used diet assessment instruments are the food frequency questionnaire, the 7-day diet record, and the 24-hour recall. Although the 7-day diet record may provide the most accurate documentation of intake during the week the participant keeps a diet diary, the burden of computerizing the information and extracting foods and nutrients has prohibited the use of the 7-day diet record in most large-scale studies. The 24-hour recall provides only a snapshot of diet on one day, which may or may not be representative of the participant's usual diet and is thus affected by both personal variation and seasonal variation. The food frequency questionnaire, the most widely used instrument in large population-based studies, asks participants to report their average intake of a large number of foods during the previous year. Participants tend to substantially overreport their fruit and vegetable consumption on the food frequency questionnaire.[6] This tendency may reflect social desirability bias, which leads to overreporting healthy foods and underreporting less healthy foods. Studies of validity using biomarkers or detailed measurements of diet as comparisons have suggested that carefully designed questionnaires can have sufficient validity to detect moderate to strong associations. Validity can be enhanced by using the average of repeated assessments over time.[7]

THE ROLE OF INDIVIDUAL FOOD AND NUTRIENTS IN CANCER ETIOLOGY

Energy

The most important impact of diet on the risk of cancer is mediated through body weight. Overweight, obesity, and inactivity are major contributors to cancer risk. (A more detailed discussion is provided in Chapter 10.) In the large American Cancer Society Cohort, obese individuals had substantially higher mortality from all cancers and, in particular, from colorectal cancer, postmenopausal breast cancer, uterine cancer, cervical cancer, pancreatic cancer, and gallbladder cancer than their normal-weight counterparts.[8] Adiposity and, in particular, waist circumference are predictors of colon cancer incidence among women and men.[9,10] A weight gain of 10 kg or more is associated with a significant increase in postmenopausal breast cancer incidence among women who never used hormone replacement therapy, whereas a weight loss of comparable magnitude after menopause substantially decreases breast cancer risk.[11] Regular physical activity contributes to a lower prevalence of being overweight and obesity and consequently reduces the burden of cancer through this pathway.

The mechanisms whereby adiposity increases the risk of various cancers are probably multiple. Being overweight is strongly associated with endogenous estrogen levels, which likely contribute to the excess risks of endometrial and postmenopausal breast cancers. The reasons for the association with other cancers are less clear, but excess body fat is also related to higher circulating levels of insulin, insulin-like growth factor (IGF)-1, and C-peptide (a marker of insulin secretion), lower levels of binding proteins for sex hormones and IGF-1, and higher levels of various inflammatory factors, all of which have been hypothesized to be related to risks of various cancers.

Energy restriction is one of the most effective measures to prevent cancer in the animal model. While energy restriction is more difficult to study in humans, voluntary starvation among anorectics and situations of food rationing during famines provide related models. Breast cancer rates were substantially reduced among women with a history of severe anorexia.[12] Although breast cancer incidence was higher among women exposed to the Dutch famine during childhood or adolescence, such short-term involuntary food rationing for 9 months or less was often followed by overnutrition.[13] A more prolonged deficit in food availability during World War II in Norway was associated with a reduction in adult risk of breast cancer if it occurred during early adolescence.[14]

Alcohol

Aside from body weight, alcohol consumption is the best established dietary risk factor for cancer. Alcohol is classified as a carcinogen by the International Agency for Research on Cancer. The consumption of alcohol increases the risk of numerous cancers, including those of the liver, esophagus, pharynx, oral cavity, larynx, breast, and colorectum in a dose-dependent fashion.[15] Evidence is convincing that excessive alcohol consumption increases the risk of primary liver cancer, probably through cirrhosis and alcoholic hepatitis. At least in the developed world, about 75% of cancers of the esophagus, pharynx, oral cavity, and larynx are attributable to alcohol and tobacco, with a marked increase in risk among drinkers who also smoke, suggesting a multiplicative effect. Mechanisms may include direct damage to the cells in the upper gastrointestinal tract; modulation of DNA methylation, which affects susceptibility to DNA mutations; and an increase in acetaldehyde, the main metabolite of alcohol, which enhances the proliferation of epithelial cells, forms DNA adducts, and is a recognized carcinogen. The association between alcohol consumption and breast cancer is notable because a small but significant risk has been found even with one drink per day. Mechanisms may include an interaction with folate, an increase in endogenous estrogen levels, and an elevation of acetaldehyde. Some evidence suggests that the excess risk is mitigated by adequate folate intake possibly through an effect on DNA methylation.[16] Notably, for most cancer sites, no important difference in associations was found with the type of alcoholic beverage, suggesting a critical role of ethanol in carcinogenesis.

Dietary Fat

In recent years, reducing dietary fat has been at the center of cancer prevention efforts. In the landmark 1982 National Academy of Sciences review of diet, nutrition, and cancer, a reduction in fat intake to 30% of calories was the primary recommendation.

Interest in dietary fat as a cause of cancer began in the first half of the 20th century, when studies by Tannenbaum[17] indicated that diets high in fat could promote tumor growth in animal models. Dietary fat has a clear effect on tumor incidence in many models, although not in all; however, a central issue has been whether this is independent of the effect of energy intake. In the 1970s, the possible relation of dietary fat intake to cancer incidence gained greater attention as the large international differences in rates of many cancers were noted to be strongly correlated with apparent per capita fat consumption in ecologic studies.[2] Particularly strong associations were seen with cancers of the breast, colon, prostate, and endometrium, which include the most important cancers not due to smoking in affluent countries. These correlations were observed to be limited to animal, not vegetable, fat.

Dietary Fat and Breast Cancer

Breast cancer is the most common malignancy among women, and incidence has been increasing for decades, although a decline has been noted starting with the new millennium. Rates in most parts of Asia, South America, and Africa have been only approximately one-fifth that of the United States, but in almost all these areas rates of breast cancer are also increasing. Populations that migrate from low- to high-incidence countries develop breast cancer rates that approximate those of the new host country. However, rates do not approach those of the general US population until the second or third generation.[18] This slower rate of change for immigrants may indicate delayed acculturation; although because a similar delay in rate increase is not observed for colon cancer, it may suggest an origin of breast cancer earlier in the life course.

The results from 12 smaller case-control studies that included 4,312 cases and 5,978 controls have been summarized in a meta-analysis.[19] The pooled relative risk (RR) was 1.35 ($P < .0001$) for a 100-g increase in daily total fat intake, although the risk was somewhat stronger for postmenopausal women (RR, 1.48; $P < .001$). This magnitude of association, however, could be compatible with biases due to recall of diet or the selection of controls.

Because of the prospective design of cohort studies, most of the methodologic biases of case-control studies are avoided. In an analysis of the Nurses' Health Study that included 121,700 US female registered nurses, no association with total fat intake was observed, and there was no suggestion of any reduction in risk at intakes below 25% of energy.[20] Because repeated assessments of diet were obtained at 2- to 4-year intervals, this analysis provided a particularly detailed evaluation of fat intake over an extended period in relation to breast cancer risk. Similar observations were made in the National Institutes of Health (NIH)–American Association of Retired Persons (AARP) Diet and Health Study including 188,736 postmenopausal women[21] and in the European Prospective Investigation into Cancer and Nutrition (EPIC), which included 7,119 incident cases.[22] In a pooled analysis of seven prospective studies, which included 337,000 women who developed 4,980 incident cases of breast cancer, no overall association was seen for fat intake over the range of less than 20% to more than 45% energy (reflecting the current range observed internationally).[23] A similar lack of association was seen for specific types of fat. This lack of association with total fat intake was confirmed in a subsequent analysis of the pooled prospective studies of diet and breast cancer, which included over 7,000 cases.[24] Therefore, these cohort findings do not support the hypothesis that dietary fat is an important contributor to breast cancer incidence.

Endogenous estrogen levels have now been established as a risk factor for breast cancer. Thus, the effects of fat and other dietary factors on estrogen levels are of potential interest. Vegetarian women, who consume higher amounts of fiber and lower amounts of fat, have lower blood levels and reduced urinary excretion of estrogens, apparently due to increased fecal excretion. A meta-analysis has suggested that a reduction in dietary fat reduces plasma estrogen levels,[25] but the studies included were plagued by the lack of concurrent controls, the short duration, and the negative energy balance. In a large, randomized trial among postmenopausal women with a previous diagnosis of breast cancer, a reduction in dietary fat did not affect estradiol levels when the data were appropriately analyzed.[26]

The WHI Randomized Controlled Dietary Modification Trial similarly suggested no association between fat intake and breast cancer incidence,[5] but these results are difficult to interpret.[27] The data on biomarkers that reflect fat intake suggest little if any difference in fat intake between the intervention and control groups.[28] Even if dietary fat does truly have an effect on cancer incidence and other outcomes, this lack of adherence to the dietary intervention could explain the absence of an observed effect on total cancer incidence and total mortality. In another randomized trial in Canada that tested an intervention target of 15% of calories from fat, a small but significant difference in high-density lipoprotein (HDL) levels was observed after 8 to 9 years of follow-up suggesting a difference in fat intake in the two groups.[29] The incidence of breast cancer in the intervention and the control group did not differ significantly.

Some prospective cohort studies suggest an inverse association between monounsaturated fat and breast cancer. This is an intriguing observation because of the relatively low rates of breast cancer in southern European countries with high intakes of monounsaturated fats due to the use of olive oil as the primary fat. In case-control studies in Spain, Greece, and Italy, women who used more olive oil had reduced risks of breast cancer.

In a report of findings from the Nurses' Health Study II cohort of premenopausal women, a higher intake of animal fat was associated with an approximately 50% greater risk of breast cancer, but no association was seen with intake of vegetable fat.[30] This suggests that factors in foods containing animal fats, rather than fat per se, may account for the findings. In the same cohort, an intake of red meat and total fat during adolescence was also associated with the risk of premenopausal breast cancer.[31,32]

Dietary Fat and Colon Cancer

In comparisons among countries, rates of colon cancer are strongly correlated with a national per capita disappearance of animal fat and meat, with correlation coefficients ranging between 0.8 and 0.9.[2] Rates of colon cancer rose sharply in Japan after World War II, paralleling a 2.5-fold increase in fat intake. Based on these epidemiologic investigations and on animal studies, a hypothesis has developed that higher dietary fat increases the excretion of bile acids, which can be converted to carcinogens or act as promoters. However, evidence from many studies on obesity and low levels of physical activity increasing the risk of colon cancer suggests that at least part of the high rates in affluent countries previously attributed to fat intake is probably due to a sedentary lifestyle.

The Nurses' Health Study suggested an approximately twofold higher risk of colon cancer among women in the highest quintile of animal fat intake than in those in the lowest quintile.[33] In a multivariate analysis of these data, which included red meat intake and animal fat intake in the same model, red meat intake remained significantly predictive of colon cancer risk, whereas the association with animal fat was eliminated. Other cohort studies have supported associations of colon cancer and the consumption of red meat and processed meats but not other sources of fat or total fat.[34–36] Similar associations were also observed for colorectal adenomas. In a meta-analysis of prospective studies, red meat consumption was associated with a risk of colon cancer (RR = 1.24; 95% confidence interval [CI], 1.09 to 1.41 for an increment of 120 g per day).[37] The association with the consumption of processed meats was particularly strong (RR = 1.36; 95% CI, 1.15 to 1.61 for an increment of 30 g per day).

The apparently stronger association with red meat consumption than with fat intake in most large cohort studies needs further confirmation, but such an association could result if the fatty acids or nonfat components of meat (e.g., the heme iron or carcinogens created by cooking) were the primary etiologic factors. This issue has major practical implications because current dietary recommendations support the daily consumption of red meat as long as it is lean.[38]

Dietary Fat and Prostate Cancer

Although further data are desirable, the evidence from international correlations, case-control[39] and cohort studies[40–44] provides some support for an association between the consumption of fat-containing animal products and prostate cancer incidence. This evidence does not generally support a relation with intake of vegetable fat, which suggests that either the type of fat or other components of animal products are responsible. Some evidence also indicates that animal fat consumption may be most strongly associated with the incidence of aggressive prostate cancer, which suggests an influence on the transition from the widespread indolent form to the more lethal form of this malignancy. Data are limited on the relation of fat intake to the probability of survival after the diagnosis of prostate cancer.

Dietary Fat and Other Cancers

Rates of other cancers that are common in affluent countries, including those of the endometrium and ovary, are also correlated with fat intake internationally. In prospective studies between Iowa and Canadian women, no evidence of a relation between fat intake and risk of endometrial cancer was found. Positive associations between dietary fat and lung cancer have been observed in many case-control studies. However, in a pooled analysis of large prospective studies that included over 3,000 incident cases, no association was observed.[45] These findings provide further evidence that the results of case-control studies of diet and cancer are likely to be misleading.

Summary

Largely on the basis of the results of animal studies, international correlations, and a few case-control studies, great enthusiasm developed in the 1980s that modest reductions in total fat intake would have a major impact on breast cancer incidence. As the findings from large prospective studies have become available, however, support for this relation has greatly weakened. Although evidence suggests that a high intake of animal fat early in adult life may increase the risk of premenopausal breast cancer, this is not likely to be due to fat per se because vegetable fat intake was not related to risk. For colon cancer, the associations seen with animal fat intake internationally have been supported in numerous case-control and cohort studies, but this also appears to be explained by factors in red meat other than simply its fat content. Further, the importance of physical activity and leanness as protective factors against colon cancer indicates that international correlations probably overstate the contribution of diet to differences in colon cancer incidence. At present, the available evidence most strongly suggests an association between animal fat consumption and risk of prostate cancer, particularly the aggressive form of this disease.

As with colon cancer, the possibility remains that other factors in animal products contribute to risk.

Despite the large body of data on dietary fat and cancer that has accumulated since 1985, any conclusions should be regarded as tentative, because these are disease processes that are poorly understood and are likely to take many decades to develop. Because most of the reported literature from prospective studies is based on fewer than 20 years' follow-up, further evaluations of the effects of diet earlier in life and at longer intervals of observation are needed to fully understand these complex relations. Nevertheless, persons interested in reducing their risk of cancer could be advised, as a prudent measure, to minimize their intake of foods high in animal fat, particularly red meat. Such a dietary pattern is also likely to be beneficial for the risk of cardiovascular disease. On the other hand, unsaturated fats (with the exception of *transfatty* acids) reduce blood low-density lipoprotein cholesterol levels and the risk of cardiovascular disease, and little evidence suggests that they adversely affect cancer risk. Thus, efforts to reduce unsaturated fat intake are not warranted at this time and are likely to have adverse effects on cardiovascular disease risk. Because excess adiposity increases the risk of several cancers and cardiovascular disease, balancing calories from any source with adequate physical activity is extremely important.

Fruits and Vegetables

General Properties

Fruits and vegetables have been hypothesized to be major dietary contributors to cancer prevention because they are rich in potential anticarcinogenic substances. Fruits and vegetables contain antioxidants and minerals and are good sources of fiber, potassium, carotenoids, vitamin C, folate, and other vitamins. Although fruits and vegetables supply less than 5% of total energy intake in most countries worldwide on a population basis, the concentration of micronutrients in these foods is greater than in most others.

The comprehensive report of the World Cancer Research Fund and the American Institute for Cancer Research, published in 2007 and titled *Food, Nutrition, Physical Activity, and the Prevention of Cancer: A Global Perspective*, reached the consensus based on the available evidence: "findings from cohort studies conducted since the mid-1990s have made the overall evidence, that vegetables or fruits protect against cancers, somewhat less impressive. In no case now is the evidence of protection judged to be convincing."[15]

Fruit and Vegetable Consumption and Colorectal Cancer

The association between fruit and vegetable consumption and the incidence of colon or rectal cancer has been examined prospectively in at least six studies. In some of these prospective cohorts, inverse associations were observed for individual foods or particular subgroups of fruits or vegetables, but no consistent pattern emerged and many comparisons revealed no such links. The results from the largest studies, the Nurses' Health Study and the Health Professionals' Follow-Up Study, suggested no important association between the consumption of fruits and vegetables and the incidence of cancers of the colon or rectum during 1,743,645 person-years of follow-up.[46] In these two large cohorts, diet was assessed repeatedly during follow-up with a detailed food frequency questionnaire. Similarly, in the Pooling Project of Prospective Studies of Diet and Cancer, including 14 studies, 756,217 participants, and 5,838 cases of colon cancer, no association with overall colon cancer risk was found.[47]

Fruit and Vegetable Consumption and Stomach Cancer

At least 12 prospective cohort studies have examined the consumption of some fruits and vegetables and the incidence of stomach cancer.[15] Seven of these studies considered total vegetable intake. Three found significant protection from stomach cancer, whereas three did not. All other comparisons were made for subgroups of vegetables and produced inconsistent results. Nine prospective cohort studies investigated the association between fruit consumption and stomach cancer risk. Four studies found an inverse association of borderline statistical significance.

Fruit and Vegetable Consumption and Breast Cancer

The most comprehensive evaluation of fruit and vegetable consumption and the incidence of breast cancer was provided by a pooled analysis of all cohort studies.[48] Data were pooled from eight prospective studies that included 351,825 women, 7,377 of whom developed incident invasive breast cancer during follow-up. The pooled relative risk adjusted for potential confounding variables was 0.93 (95% CI, 0.86 to 1.0; P for trend, .08) for the highest versus the lowest quartile of fruit consumption, 0.96 (95% CI, 0.89 to 1.04; P for trend, .54) for vegetable intake, and 0.93 (95% CI, 0.86 to 1.0; P for trend, .12) for total consumption of fruits and vegetables combined. The EPIC study confirmed this lack of association.[49] In a recent analysis within the Nurses' Health Study, an inverse association was seen between vegetable intake and the risk of estrogen receptor–negative breast cancer.[50] This observation was confirmed in the pooling project of prospective studies: The pooled relative risk for the highest vs. the lowest quintile of total vegetable consumption was 0.82 (95% CI 0.74 to 0.90) for estrogen-receptor negative breast cancer.[51]

Fruit and Vegetable Consumption and Lung Cancer

The relation between fruit and vegetable consumption and the incidence of lung cancer was examined in the pooled analysis of cohort studies.[52] Overall, no association was observed, although a modest increase in lung cancer incidence was evident among participants with the lowest fruit and vegetable consumption.

Fruit and Vegetable Consumption and Total Cancer

An analysis of the Nurses' Health Study and the Health Professionals' Follow-Up Study, including over 9,000 incident cases of cancer, did not reveal a benefit of fruit and vegetable consumption for total cancer incidence.[53] Observations from the EPIC cohort were essentially consistent with these findings.[54] Although there may be no or only a very weak protection conferred for cancer from consuming an abundance of fruits and vegetables, there is a substantial benefit for protection from cardiovascular disease.

Summary

The consumption of fruits and vegetables and some of their main micronutrients appear to be less important in cancer prevention than previously assumed. With an accumulation of data from prospective cohort studies and randomized trials, a lack of association of these foods and nutrients with cancer outcomes has become apparent. A modest association cannot be excluded because of an imperfect measurement of diet, and it remains possible that a high consumption of fruits and vegetables during childhood and adolescence is more effective at reducing cancer risk than consumption in adult life due to the long latency of cancer manifestation.

Conversely, it is possible that, with the fortification of breakfast cereal, flour, and other staple foods, the frequent consumption of fruits and vegetables has become less essential for cancer prevention. Nevertheless, an abundance of fruits and vegetables as part of a healthy diet is recommended, because evidence consistently suggests that it lowers the incidence of hypertension, heart disease, and stroke.

Fiber

General Properties

Dietary fiber was defined in 1976 as "all plant polysaccharides and lignin which are resistant to hydrolysis by the digestive enzymes of men."[55] Fiber, both soluble and insoluble, is fermented by the luminal bacteria of the colon. Among the properties of fiber that make it a candidate for cancer prevention are its "bulking" effect, which reduces colonic transit time, and the binding of potentially carcinogenic luminal chemicals. Fiber may also aid in producing short-chain fatty acids that may be directly anticarcinogenic. Fiber may also induce apoptosis.

Dietary Fiber and Colorectal Cancer

In 1969, Dennis Burkitt hypothesized that dietary fiber is involved in colon carcinogenesis.[56] While working as a physician in Africa, Burkitt noticed the low incidence of colon cancer among African populations whose diets were high in fiber. Burkitt concluded that a link might exist between the fiber-rich diet and the low incidence of colon cancer. Burkitt's observations were followed by numerous case-control studies that seemed to confirm his theories. A combined analysis of 13 case-control studies[57] as well as a meta-analysis of 16 case-control studies[58] suggested an inverse association between fiber intake and the risk of colorectal cancer. The inclusion of studies was selective, however, and effect estimates unadjusted for potential confounders were used for most studies. Moreover, recall bias is a severe threat to the validity of retrospective case-control studies of fiber intake and any disease outcome.

Data from prospective cohort studies have largely failed to support an inverse association between dietary fiber and colorectal cancer incidence. Initial analyses from the Nurses' Health Study and the Health Professionals' Follow-Up Study[36] found no important association between dietary fiber and colorectal cancer. A significant inverse association between fiber intake and incidence of colorectal cancer was reported from the EPIC study. The analysis presented on dietary fiber and colorectal cancer encompassed 434,209 women and men from eight European countries.[59] The analytic model used by the EPIC investigators included adjustments for age, height, weight, total caloric intake, sex, and center assessed at baseline and identified[60] a significant inverse association between fiber intake and colorectal cancer. Applying the same analytic model used in EPIC to data from the Nurses' Health Study and the Health Professionals' Follow-Up Study encompassing 1.8 million person-years of follow-up and 1,572 cases of colorectal cancer revealed associations similar to those found in the EPIC study.[61] After a more complete adjustment for confounding variables, however, the association vanished.[61] Results from the pooled analysis of 13 prospective cohort studies, including 8,081 colorectal cancer cases diagnosed during over 7 million person-years of follow-up, suggested an inverse relation between dietary fiber and colorectal cancer incidence in age-adjusted analyses, but this association disappeared after appropriate adjustment for confounding variables, particularly other dietary factors.[62] The NIH–AARP study, which included 2,974 cases of colorectal cancer, confirmed the lack of association between total dietary fiber and colorectal cancer risk.[63]

The association between dietary fiber and colorectal cancer appears to be confounded by a number of other dietary and non-dietary factors. These methodologic considerations must be taken into account when interpreting the evidence. It is possible that other dietary factors such as folate intake are more important for colorectal cancer pathogenesis than dietary fiber.

Dietary Fiber and Colorectal Adenomas

In a few prospective cohort studies, the primary occurrence of colorectal polyps was investigated, but no consistent relation was found.

The study of fiber intake and colorectal adenoma recurrence lends itself to a randomized clinical trial design because of the relatively short follow-up necessary and because fiber can be provided as a supplement. A number of RCTs have explored the effect of fiber supplementation on colorectal adenoma recurrence. Evidence has fairly consistently indicated no effect of fiber intake.[64–68] In one RCT, an increase in adenoma recurrence was observed among participants randomly assigned to use a fiber supplement, which was stronger among those with high dietary calcium.[69]

Dietary Fiber and Breast Cancer

Investigators have speculated that dietary fiber may reduce the risk of breast cancer through a reduction in intestinal absorption of estrogens excreted via the biliary system.

Relatively few epidemiologic studies have examined the association between fiber intake and breast cancer. In a meta-analysis of 10 case-control studies, a significant inverse association was observed. However, these retrospective studies were likely affected by the aforementioned biases—selection and recall bias, in particular. Results from at least six prospective cohort studies consistently suggested no association between fiber intake and breast cancer incidence.[70–75]

Dietary Fiber and Stomach Cancer

The results from retrospective case-control studies of fiber intake and gastric cancer risk are inconsistent. In the Netherlands Cohort Study, dietary fiber was not associated with an incidence of gastric carcinoma.[76] Further investigations through prospective cohort studies must be completed before conclusions about the relation between fiber intake and stomach cancer incidence can be drawn.

Summary

The observational data presently available do not indicate an important role for dietary fiber in the prevention of cancer, although small effects cannot be excluded. The long-held perception that a high intake of fiber conveys protection originated largely from retrospectively conducted studies, which are affected by a number of biases, in particular, the potential for differential recall of diet, and from studies that were not well controlled for potential confounding variables.

OTHER FOODS AND NUTRIENTS

Red Meat

The regular consumption of red meat has been associated with an increased risk of colorectal cancer. In a recent meta-analysis, the increase in risk associated with an increase in intake of 120 g per day was 24% (95% CI, 9% to 41%).[37] The association was strongest for processed meat; the relative risk of colorectal cancer was 1.36 (95% CI, 1.15 to 1.61) for a consumption of 30 g per day.[37] No overall association has been observed between red meat consumption and breast cancer in a pooled analysis of prospective cohorts.[77] However, among premenopausal women in the Nurses' Health Study II, the risk for estrogen-receptor–positive and progesterone-receptor–positive breast cancer doubled with 1.5 servings of red meat per day compared to three or fewer servings per week.[78] No associations have been found in studies on poultry or fish.[15] Mechanisms through which red meat may increase cancer risk include anabolic hormones routinely used in meat production in the United States, heterocyclic amines, and polycyclic aromatic hydrocarbons formed during cooking at high temperatures, the high amounts of heme iron, and nitrates and related compounds in smoked, salted, and some processed meats that can convert to carcinogenic nitrosamines in the colon.

Milk, Dairy Products, and Calcium

Regular milk consumption has been associated with a modest reduction in colorectal cancer in both a pooling project[79] and a meta-analysis of cohort studies,[80] possibly due to its calcium content. In the pooling project of prospective studies of diet and cancer, a modest inverse association was also seen for calcium intake.[79] This finding is consistent with the results of a randomized trial in which calcium supplements reduced the risk of colorectal adenomas.[81] Associations with cheese and other dairy products have been less consistent.[79,80]

Conversely, in multiple studies, a high intake of calcium or dairy products has been associated with an increased risk of prostate cancer,[80,82–86] specifically fatal prostate cancer.[87,88] Similar observations were made in the NIH–AARP study, although the increase in risk there did not reach statistical significance.[89] While the Multiethnic Cohort[90] and the Prostate, Lung, Colorectal, and Ovarian Cancer Screening Trial[91] did not find an important association between dairy consumption and prostate cancer, these cohort studies did not specifically include fatal prostate cancer cases. A meta-analysis of prospective studies generated an overall relative risk of advanced prostate cancer of 1.33 (95% CI, 1.00 to 1.78) for the highest versus the lowest intake categories of dairy products.[92] In another meta-analysis, no significant association was found for cohort studies on dairy or milk consumption, but relative risk estimates suggested a positive association.[93] Thus, although the findings are not entirely consistent and are complicated by the widespread use of prostate-specific antigen (PSA) screening in the United States, the global evidence suggests a positive association between the regular consumption of dairy products and the risk of fatal prostate cancer. Consuming three or more servings of dairy products per day has been associated with endometrial cancer among postmenopausal women not using hormonal therapy.[94] A high intake of lactose from dairy products has also been associated with a modestly higher risk of ovarian cancer.[95]

These observations are particularly important in the context of national dietary recommendations to drink three glasses of milk per day.[38] Possible mechanisms include an increase in endogenous IGF-1 levels[96] and steroid hormones contained in cows' milk.[97]

Vitamin D

In 1980, Garland and Garland[98] hypothesized that sunlight and vitamin D may reduce the risk of colon cancer. Since then, substantial research has been conducted in this area supporting an inverse association between circulating 25-hydroxyvitamin D (25[OH]D) levels and colorectal cancer risk.[99–103] A meta-analysis, including five nested case-control studies with prediagnostic serum, suggested a reduction of colorectal cancer risk by about half among individuals with serum 25(OH)D levels of more than 82 nmol/L compared to individuals with less than 30 nmol/L.[104] A subsequent meta-analysis including eight studies confirmed these associations.[105] These observations are supported by similar findings for colorectal adenomas.[106] Vitamin D levels may particularly affect colorectal cancer prognosis; colorectal cancer mortality was 72% lower among individuals with 25(OH)D concentrations of 80 nmol/L or higher.[107]

The evidence for other cancers has been less consistent. High plasma levels of vitamin D have been associated with a decreased risk of several other cancers, including cancer of the breast[108–111]; prostate, especially fatal prostate cancer[112]; and ovary.[113,114] Whether vitamin D plays a role in pancreatic cancerogenesis remains to be determined with one pooling project, suggesting a positive association,[115] whereas other prospective studies[116] and a pooling project of cohort studies found inverse associations.[117]

The activation of vitamin D receptors by 1,25(OH)$_2$D induces cell differentiation and inhibits proliferation and angiogenesis.[118] Solar ultraviolet B radiation is the major source of plasma vitamin D, and dietary vitamin D without supplementation has a minor effect on plasma vitamin D. To achieve sufficient plasma levels through sun exposure, at least 15 minutes of full-body exposure to bright sunlight is necessary. Physical activity has to be considered as possible confounder of studies on plasma levels of vitamin D and cancer. Sunscreen effectively blocks vitamin D production. Populations who live in geographic areas with limited or seasonal sun exposure may benefit from a vitamin D supplementation of 1,000 IU per day.

Folate

Folate is a micronutrient commonly found in fruits and vegetables, particularly oranges, orange juice, asparagus, beets, and peas. Folate may affect carcinogenesis through various mechanisms: DNA methylation, DNA synthesis, and DNA repair. In the animal model, folate deficiency enhances intestinal carcinogenesis.[119] Folate deficiency is related to the incorporation of uracil into human DNA and to an increased frequency of chromosomal breaks. A number of epidemiologic studies suggest that a diet rich in folate lowers the risk of colorectal adenomas and colorectal cancer.[15] Because the folate content in foods is generally relatively low, is susceptible to oxidative destruction by cooking and food processing, and is not well absorbed, folic acid from supplements and fortification plays an important role. Pooled results from 13 prospective studies suggests that intake of 400 to 500 μg per day is required to minimize risk.[120]

Potential interactions among alcohol consumption, folic acid intake, and methionine intake have been described. Although alcohol consumption has been fairly consistently related to an increase in breast cancer incidence, the potential detrimental effect of alcohol seems to be eliminated in women with high folic acid intake.[16] A similar folic acid or methionine–alcohol interaction has been observed for colorectal cancer risk.[119]

Genetic susceptibility may also modify the relation between folate intake and cancer risk. A polymorphism of the *methylenetetrahydrofolate reductase (MTHFR)* gene (cytosine to thymine transition at position 677) may result in a relative deficiency of methionine. Individuals with the common C677T mutation appear to experience the greatest protection from high folic acid or methionine intake and low alcohol consumption.[121] Although the interaction between this polymorphism and dietary factors needs to be investigated further, the consistently observed association between this polymorphism and the risk of colorectal cancer supports a role of folate in the etiology of colorectal cancer.

Folate levels also affect the availability of methyl groups via S-adenosylmethionine in the one-carbon metabolism.[122] Low red blood cell folate levels are associated with low DNA methylation status among homozygous *MTHFR* 677T/T mutation carriers, whereas at high red blood cell folate levels, the amount of methylated cytosine in DNA is similar to that of the heterozygote *MTHFR* C677T genotype.[123]

Conversely, evidence from animal and human studies suggests that a high folate status may promote the progression of existing neoplasias.[122,124,125] The randomization of folic acid supplements among individuals with a history of colorectal adenoma resulted in either no effect on recurrent adenoma recurrence[126] or an increase in recurrence with over 6 to 8 years of follow-up.[127] The high proliferation rate of neoplastic cells requiring increased DNA synthesis is likely supported by folate, which is necessary for thymidine synthesis.[122,125] The effects of folate on de novo methylation and subsequent gene silencing have been insufficiently studied. An increase in colorectal cancer rates has been observed in the United States and Canada concurrent with the introduction of the folic acid fortification program, but this could be an artifact due to increased use of colonoscopies.[128] The lack of increase in mortality, but an acceleration in a long-term downward trend suggests the latter explanation (http://progressreport.cancer.gov/).

Carotenoids

Carotenoids, antioxidants prevalent in fruits and vegetables, enhance cell-to-cell communication, promote cell differentiation, and modulate immune response. In 1981, Doll and Peto[1] speculated that beta-carotene may be a major player in cancer prevention and encouraged testing its anticarcinogenic properties. Indeed, subsequent observational studies, mostly case-control investigations, suggested a reduced cancer risk—especially of lung cancer—with a high intake of carotenoids. In contrast, clinical trials randomizing the intake of beta-carotene supplements have not revealed the evidence of a protective effect of beta-carotene. In fact, beta-carotene was found to increase the risk of lung cancer and total mortality among smokers in the Finnish Alpha-Tocopherol, Beta-Carotene Cancer Prevention Study.[129] However, these adverse affects disappeared during longer periods of follow-up.[130] In a detailed analysis of prospective studies, no association was seen between the intake of beta-carotene and the risk of lung cancer.[131]

The pooled analysis of 18 cohort studies including more than 33,000 breast cancer cases suggested inverse associations between the intake of several carotenoids (beta-carotene, alpha-carotene, luteine/zeaxanthin) and estrogen-receptor–negative breast cancer incidence, whereas no association was found for estrogen-receptor–positive tumors.[132] Similarly, in a pooled analysis of data from eight prospective studies including about 3,055 breast cancer cases, blood levels of carotenoids were inversely related to estrogen-receptor–negative mammary tumor incidence.[133] Women in the highest quintile of beta-carotene levels had about half the risk of developing estrogen-receptor–negative breast cancer than women in the lowest quintile (hazard ratio [HR] = 0.52; 95% CI, 0.36 to 0.77).

The particularly pronounced antioxidant properties of lycopene, a carotenoid mainly found in tomatoes, may explain the inverse associations with some cancers. The frequent consumption of tomato-based products has been associated with a decreased risk of prostate, lung, and stomach cancers.[134] The bioavailability of lycopene from cooked tomatoes is higher than from fresh tomatoes, making tomato soup and sauce excellent sources of the carotenoid.

Selenium

Selenium has long been of interest in cancer prevention due to its antioxidative properties. Its intake is difficult to estimate because food content depends on the selenium content of the soil it is grown in. Selenium enriches in toenails, which provide an integrative measure of intake during the previous year and therefore are popular biomarkers in epidemiologic studies. Inverse associations with toenail selenium levels have been found in several prospective studies, especially for fatal protate cancer.[135-137] In a recent meta-analysis, plasma/serum selenium was also inversely correlated with prostate cancer.[138] In the Selenium and Vitamin E Cancer Prevention Trial (SELECT), no protective effect of selenium was found for prostate cancer. However, the trial was terminated prematurely after 4 years, which is a short period in which to expect a reduction in cancer.[139]

Soy Products

The role of soy products has been considered for breast carcinogenesis. In Asian countries, which traditionally have a high consumption of soy foods, breast cancer rates have been low until recently. In Western countries, soy consumption is generally low, and between-person variation may be insufficient to allow meaningful comparisons. Soybeans contain isoflavones, which are phytoestrogens that compete with estrogen for the estrogen receptor. Hence, soy consumption may affect estrogen concentrations differently depending on the endogenous baseline level. This mechanism may also contribute to the equivocal results of studies on soy foods and breast cancer risk. In a recent meta-analysis of 18 epidemiologic studies, including over 9,000 breast cancer cases, frequent soy intake was associated with a modest decrease in risk (odds ratio = 0.86; 95% CI, 0.75 to 0.99).[140] Wu et al.[141] observed that childhood intake of soy was more relevant to breast cancer prevention than adult consumption.

Carbohydrates

The Warburg hypothesis postulated in 1924 that tumor cells mainly generate energy by the nonoxidative breakdown of glucose (glucolysis) instead of pyrovate.[142] Carbohydrates with a high glycemic load increase blood glucose levels after consumption, which results in insulin spikes increasing the risk for type 2 diabetes. Several cancers, including colorectal cancer[143] and breast cancer,[144] have been associated with type 2 diabetes. The evidence on the consumption of sucrose and refined, processed flour and cancer incidence is heterogeneous.[145] Whereas in some prospective cohort studies an increase in colon cancer incidence was observed,[146] this was not found in other studies.[147] In large cohort studies, associations have been observed for pancreatic[148] and endometrial[145] cancer risk, but not for postmenopausal breast cancer.[149] Especially in obese, sedentary individuals, abnormal glucose and insulin metabolism may contribute to tumorigenesis.

DIETARY PATTERNS

Foods and nutrients are not consumed in isolation, and, when evaluating the role of diet in disease prevention and causation, it is sensible to consider the entire dietary pattern of individuals. Public health messages may be better framed in the context of a global diet than individual constituents.

The role of vegetarian diets for cancer incidence has been examined in a few studies. In the Adventist Health Study-2, vegetarians had an 8% lower incidence of cancer than nonvegetarians (95% CI, 1 to 15%).[150] The protective association was strongest for cancers of the gastrointestinal tract with 24% (95% CI, 10 to 37%). Vegans had a 16% (95%, 1 to 28%) lower incidence of cancer, with a particular protection conferred to female cancers of 34% (95% CI, 8 to 53%). A combined analysis of data from the Oxford Vegetarian Study and EPIC similarly suggest a 12% (95% CI, 4 to 19%) reduction in cancer incidence among vegetarians compared to meat eaters.[151]

During the past decade, dietary pattern analyses have gained popularity in observational studies. The most commonly employed methods are factor analyses and cluster analyses, which are largely data-driven methods, and investigator-determined methods such as dietary indices and scores. The search for associations between distinct patterns such as the "Western pattern," which is characterized by a high consumption of red and processed meats; high fat dairy products, including butter and eggs; and refined carbohydrates, such as sweets, desserts, and refined grains, and the "prudent pattern," which is defined by the frequent consumption of a variety of fruits and vegetables, whole grains, legumes, fish, and poultry, and the risk of cancer has been largely disappointing. Notable exceptions were the link between a Western dietary pattern and colon cancer incidence and an inverse relation between a prudent diet[152] and estrogen-receptor–negative breast cancer.[153] These findings were subsequently in the California Teachers Study.[154] The general lack of association between global dietary patterns and cancer supports a more modest role of nutrition during adult life in carcinogenesis than previously assumed.

DIET DURING THE EARLY PHASES OF LIFE

Some cancers may originate early in the course of life. A high birth weight is associated with an increase in the risk of childhood leukemia,[155] premenopausal breast cancer,[156] and testicular cancer.[157] Tall height is an indicator of the risk of many cancers and is in part determined by nutrition during childhood.[15] Until recently, most studies focused on the role of diet during adult life. However, the critical exposure period for nutrition to affect cancer risk may be earlier, and because the latent period for cancer may span several decades, diet during childhood and adolescence may be important. However, relating dietary information during early life and cancer outcomes prospectively is difficult because nutrition records from the remote past are not available. Studies in which recalled diet during youth is used have to be interpreted cautiously due to misclassification, although recall has been found reasonably reproducible and consistent with recalls provided by participants' mothers.[158,159] The role of early life diet has been explored in only a few studies in relation to breast cancer risk. In a study nested in the Nurses' Health Study cohorts that used data recalled by mothers, frequent consumption of french fries was associated with an increased risk of breast cancer, whereas whole milk consumption was inversely related to risk.[160] Similarly, an inverse association with milk consumption during childhood was found among younger women (30 to 39 years), but not among older premenopausal women (40 to 49 years) in a Norwegian cohort.[161] Dietary habits during high school recalled by adult participants of the Nurses' Health Study II (but before the diagnosis of breast cancer) suggested a positive association of total fat and red meat consumption.[31,32] More data are needed in this promising area of research.[162]

DIET AFTER A DIAGNOSIS OF CANCER

The role of diet in the secondary prevention of cancer recurrence and survival is generally of great interest to cancer patients because they are highly motivated to make lifestyle changes to optimize their prognosis. The compliance of cancer patients makes the RCTs a more feasible design to evaluate the role of diet than among healthy individuals. However, concurrent cancer treatments may make any effect of diet more difficult to isolate.

Most evidence is available for breast cancer, colorectal, and prostate cancer. Observational data suggest a limited role of diet in the prevention of breast cancer recurrence and survival. The Life After Cancer Epidemiology (LACE) Cohort supported a beneficial role for vitamin C and E supplement use but the effect of other health-seeking behaviors is difficult to exclude.[163] In a pooled analysis, alcohol consumption after a diagnosis did not affect survival.[164] Several randomized trials have addressed the role of diet in breast cancer prognosis. In the Women's Intervention Nutrition Study (WINS), 2,437 women with early stage breast cancer were randomized to a dietary goal of 15% of calories from fat or maintenance of their usual dietary habits.[165] The intervention group received dietary counseling by registered dieticians and, according to self-reports, a difference of 19 g in daily fat intake was maintained between the intervention and the control group after 60 months of follow-up. However, at that time, women in the intervention group were also 6 pounds lighter, making it difficult to separate an effect of dietary fat from a nonspecific effect of intensive dietary intervention, which quite consistently produces weight loss. Breast cancer recurrence was 29% lower in the intervention group (95% CI, 6% to 47%), whereas overall survival was not affected. In the Women's Healthy Eating and Living (WHEL) RCT, 3,088 early stage breast cancer patients were randomly assigned to a target of five vegetable servings, three fruit servings, 30 g fiber per day, and 15% to 20% of calories from fat.[166] After 72 months, the intervention versus control group reports were 5.8 versus 3.6 servings of vegetables, 3.4 versus 2.6 servings of fruit, 24.2 versus 18.9 g fiber per day, and 28.9% versus 32.4% of calories from fat. The total plasma carotenoid concentration, a biomarker of vegetable and fruit intake, was 43% higher in the intervention group than the comparison group after 4 years (p<0.001). Neither recurrence rates nor mortality were affected by the intervention after the 7.3-year follow-up. Overall, diet is unlikely a major factor influencing breast cancer prognosis. However, because the prognosis for breast cancer is relatively good, women diagnosed with breast cancer remain at risk for cardiovascular disease and other causes of death that affect those without breast cancer. Thus, among women in the Nurses' Health Study diagnosed with breast cancer, a higher diet quality, which was assessed by the Alternative Healthy Eating Index, was not associated with mortality due to breast cancer but was associated with substantially lower mortality due to other causes.[167] Similarly, among over 4,000 women with breast cancer, intakes of saturated and trans fat, but not of total fat, were associated with significantly greater total mortality but not specifically breast cancer mortality. Thus, there is good reason for women with breast cancer to adopt a healthy diet even if it does not affect the prognosis of breast cancer.

In a systematic review, no consistent association between individual dietary components and colorectal cancer prognosis outcome was found.[168] However, in an observational study including 1,009 patients with stage III colon cancer, a Western dietary pattern was associated with lower rates of disease-free survival, recurrence-free survival, and overall survivals.[169] In the same patient population, higher dietary glycemic load and total carbohydrate intake were significantly associated with an increased risk of recurrence and mortality.[170] These findings support a possible role of glycemic load in colon cancer progression.

In the Physician's Health Study, whole milk consumption among men with incident prostate cancer was associated with double the risk of progression to fatal disease.[171] Among men with nonmetastatic prostate cancer in the Health Professionals' Follow-up Study, replacing 10% of energy intake from carbohydrates with vegetable fat was associated with a lower risk of lethal prostate cancer.[172] A marginally increased risk of progression of localized to lethal prostate cancer among these men was also associated with postdiagnostic poultry and processed red meat consumption,[173] whereas postdiagnostic consumption of fish and tomato sauce were inversely related with a risk of progression.[174] In an intervention study, 93 patients with early stage prostate cancer (PSA = 4 to 10 ng per mililiter and Gleason score <7) were randomized to comprehensive lifestyle changes, including a vegan diet based on 10% of calories from fat and consisting predominantly of vegetables, fruit, whole grains, legumes, and soy protein.[175] Other interventions included moderate exercise, stress management, and relaxation. After 1 year, PSA values decreased 4% in the intervention group, but increased 6% in the control group. Six patients in the control group, but none in the experimental group, underwent conventional prostate cancer treatment. Although the impact of the different intervention components are difficult to separate in this study, further data on diet and the prognosis for patients with localized prostate cancer are needed.

SUMMARY

A considerable proportion of cancers are potentially preventable through lifestyle changes. Besides a curtailment of smoking, the most important strategies are maintaining a healthy body weight and regular physical activity, which contribute to a lower prevalence of being overweight and obesity. The avoidance of a positive energy balance and becoming overweight are the most important nutritional factors in cancer prevention.

Although dietary patterns, including frequent fruit and vegetable consumption, appear to play a modest role in cancer prevention, knowledge gained about some specific foods and nutrients might inform a targeted approach. Vitamin D is a strong candidate to counter carcinogenesis, thus supplementation could be a feasible and safe route to avoid several types of cancer. Although the data on vitamin D and cancer incidence are not conclusive, the prevention of bone fractures is a sufficient reason to maintain good vitamin D status.

Limiting or avoiding red meat, processed meat, and alcohol reduces the risk of breast, colorectal, stomach, esophageal, and other cancers. Although the role of dairy products and milk remains to be more fully elucidated, current evidence suggests a probable increase in the risk of prostate cancer with frequent milk consumption, and possibly endometrial cancer, which raises concern regarding current dietary recommendations of three glasses of milk per day. The relation of calcium and dairy intake to cancer is complex, as the evidence for a reduction in the risk of colorectal cancer is strong, but high intakes appear likely to increase the risk of fatal prostate cancer. The consumption of tomato-based products may contribute to the prevention of prostate cancer. Finally, diet may influence the prognosis of colorectal and prostate cancer, but more data are needed in this area. Because most people with cancer remain at risk of cardiovascular disease and other common conditions related to unhealthy diets, an overall healthy diet can be recommended while further research on diet and cancer survival is ongoing.

LIMITATIONS

Studying the role of diet in health and disease requires overcoming a number of hurdles. Because biomarkers reflecting nutrient intake with sufficient accuracy are largely lacking, assessing nutrition in a population-based study has to rely on self-reports by individuals, which inevitably leads to imprecision or error in the diet assessment. Such misclassification may produce spurious associations in case-control studies or may lead to an underestimation of true associations in prospective cohort studies. Ideally, hypotheses relating dietary factors to cancer risks would be tested in large randomized trials. Besides being extremely expensive, maintaining adherence to assigned diets has been challenging; for example, in the WHI trial that focused on dietary fat reduction, there were no differences between intervention and control groups in blood lipid fractions that are known to change with a reduction in fat intake, indicating a failure to test the hypothesis.[28]

Most observational studies are conducted within populations or countries. Although reasonable variations in nutritional habits exist within populations, allowing for the detection of substantial dietary risk factors for cardiovascular disease and diabetes, these contrasts may be too limited to detect small relative risks as they may exist for cancer. The pooled analysis of large prospective cohort studies across countries and continents attempts to overcome this limitation. Studies taking advantage of the large between-population variation in diets across developed and developing countries would appear to be advantageous, but would be plagued by confounding by other differences in lifestyle factors that might be difficult to assess and control adequately.

Few epidemiologic studies repeatedly capture dietary habits over time and thus account for potential changes in diet over time. Furthermore, the length of follow-up in prospective studies may not be sufficient to capture the impact of diets assessed at baseline. In case-control studies, a recall of dietary habits prior to the disease onset may be influenced by current disease status; moreover, the relevant time for nutrition to act may be decades earlier, which is more difficult to remember.

Most epidemiologic studies of diet and cancer have assessed intake among adults. Due to greater susceptibility to genotoxic influences earlier in life, it is possible that data on diet during childhood or early adolescence are more relevant for carcinogenesis and cancer prevention. Studies that have collected dietary data during childhood and followed the subjects for cancer incidence would be most informative but are virtually nonexistent and will be challenging to conduct.

Finally, data on special diets including organic foods, whole foods, raw foods, and a vegan diet are limited.

FUTURE DIRECTIONS

Some of the most promising research at present is in the areas of vitamin D, milk consumption, and the effect of diet early in life on cancer incidence. Recent nutrition changes in countries previously maintaining a more traditional diet such as Japan and some developing countries have already been followed by increased rates of some cancers (but declines in stomach cancer), providing a setting to study the effect of change over time. Additional insight may come from studies on gene–nutrient interaction and epigenetic changes induced by the diet. To improve observational research methods, refined dietary assessment methods, including the identification of new biomarkers, will be advantageous.

RECOMMENDATIONS

A wealth of data are available from observational studies on diet and cancer, and the current evidence supports suggestions made by Doll and Peto[1] that approximately 30% to 40% of cancers may be avoidable with changes in nutrition; however, much of this risk of cancer is related to being overweight and to inactivity. Excessive energy intake and lack of physical activity, marked by rapid growth in childhood and being overweight, have become growing threats to population health and are important contributors to risks of many cancers. Nevertheless, the cumulative incidence for many cancers has decreased over the past decade, in part due to the decreasing prevalence of smoking and use of hormone therapy.

Dietary recommendations must integrate the goal of overall avoidance of disease and maintenance of health and, thus, should not focus singularly on cancer prevention. The strength of the evidence and magnitude of the expected benefit should also be considered in recommendations. With these considerations in mind, the following recommendations are outlined, which are largely in agreement with the guidelines put forth by the American Cancer Society in 2012:[176]

1. *Engage in regular physical activity.* Physical activity is a primary method of weight control and it also reduces risk of several cancers, especially colon cancer, through independent mechanisms. Moderate to vigorous exercise for at least 30 minutes on most days is a minimum and more will provide additional benefits.
2. *Avoid being overweight and weight gain in adulthood.* A positive energy balance that results in excess body fat is one of the most important contributors to cancer risk. Staying within 10 pounds of body weight at age 20 may be a simple guide, assuming no adolescent obesity.
3. *Limit alcohol consumption.* Alcohol consumption contributes to the risk of many cancers and increases the risk of accidents and addiction, but low to moderate consumption has benefits for coronary heart disease risk. The individual family history of disease as well as personal preferences should be considered.
4. *Consume lots of fruits and vegetables.* Frequent consumption of fruits and vegetables during adult life is not likely to have a major effect on cancer incidence, but will reduce the risk of cardiovascular disease.
5. *Consume whole grains and avoid refined carbohydrates and sugars.* A regular consumption of whole grain products instead of refined flour and a low consumption of refined sugars lower the risk of cardiovascular disease and diabetes. The effect on cancer risk is less clear.
6. *Replace red meat and dairy products with fish, nuts, and legumes.* Red meat consumption increases the risk of colorectal cancer, diabetes, and coronary heart disease and should be largely avoided. Frequent dairy consumption may increase the risk of prostate cancer. Fish, nuts, and legumes are excellent sources of valuable mono- and polyunsaturated fats and vegetable proteins and may contribute to lower rates of cardiovascular disease and diabetes.
7. *Consider taking a vitamin D supplement.* A substantial proportion of the population, especially those living at higher latitudes, are vitamin D deficient. Most adults may benefit from taking 1,000 IU of vitamin D_3 per day during months of low sunlight intensity. Vitamin D supplementation will, at a minimum, reduce bone fracture rates, probably colorectal cancer incidence, and possibly other cancers.

REFERENCES

1. Doll R, Peto R. The causes of cancer: quantitative estimates of avoidable risks of cancer in the United States today. *J Natl Cancer Inst* 1981;66:1191–1308.
2. Armstrong B, Doll R. Environmental factors and cancer incidence and mortality in different countries, with special reference to dietary practices. *Int J Cancer* 1975;15:617–631.
3. Giovannucci E, Stampfer MJ, Colditz GA, et al. A comparison of prospective and retrospective assessments of diet in the study of breast cancer. *Am J Epidemiol* 1993;137:502–511.
4. Riboli E, Norat T. Epidemiologic evidence of the protective effect of fruit and vegetables on cancer risk. *Am J Clin Nutr* 2003;78:559S–569S.
5. Prentice RL, Caan B, Chlebowski RT, et al. Low-fat dietary pattern and risk of invasive breast cancer: the Women's Health Initiative Randomized Controlled Dietary Modification Trial. *JAMA* 2006;295:629–642.
6. Michels KB, Bingham SA, Luben R, et al. The effect of correlated measurement error in multivariate models of diet. *Am J Epidemiol* 2004;160:59–67.
7. Willett W. *Nutritional Epidemiology.* 3rd ed. New York: Oxford University Press; 2013.
8. Calle EE, Rodriguez C, Walker-Thurmond K, et al. Overweight, obesity, and mortality from cancer in a prospectively studied cohort of U.S. adults. *N Engl J Med* 2003;348:1625–1638.
9. Giovannucci E, Ascherio A, Rimm EB, et al. Physical activity, obesity, and risk for colon cancer and adenoma in men. *Ann Intern Med* 1995;122:327–334.
10. Martinez ME, Giovannucci E, Spiegelman D, et al. Leisure-time physical activity, body size, and colon cancer in women. Nurses' Health Study Research Group. *J Natl Cancer Inst* 1997;89:948–955.
11. Eliassen AH, Colditz GA, Rosner B, et al. Adult weight change and risk of postmenopausal breast cancer. *JAMA* 2006;296:193–201.
12. Michels KB, Ekbom A. Caloric restriction and incidence of breast cancer. *JAMA* 2004;291:1226–1230.
13. Elias SG, Peeters PH, Grobbee DE, et al. Breast cancer risk after caloric restriction during the 1944–1945 Dutch famine. *J Natl Cancer Inst* 2004;96:539–546.
14. Tretli S, Gaard M. Lifestyle changes during adolescence and risk of breast cancer: an ecologic study of the effect of World War II in Norway. *Cancer Causes Control* 1996;7:507–512.
15. World Cancer Research Fund/American Institute for Cancer Research. *Food, Nutrition, Physical Activity, and the Prevention of Cancer: A Global Perspective.* Washington, D.C.: AICR; 2007.
16. Zhang S, Hunter DJ, Hankinson SE, et al. A prospective study of folate intake and the risk of breast cancer. *JAMA* 1999;281:1632–1637.
17. Tannenbaum A. The genesis and growth of tumors. III. Effects of a high-fat diet. *Cancer Res* 1942;2:468–475.
18. Kolonel L, Hinds M, Hankin J. *Cancer Patterns Among Migrant and Native-Born Japanese in Hawaii in Relation to Smoking, Drinking, and Dietary Habits.* Tokyo: Japan Scientific Societies Press; 1980.
19. Howe GR, Hirohata T, Hislop TG, et al. Dietary factors and risk of breast cancer: combined analysis of 12 case-control studies. *J Natl Cancer Inst* 1990;82:561–569.
20. Kim EH, Willett WC, Colditz GA, et al. Dietary fat and risk of postmenopausal breast cancer in a 20-year follow-up. *Am J Epidemiol* 2006;164:990–997.
21. Thiebaut AC, Kipnis V, Chang SC, et al. Dietary fat and postmenopausal invasive breast cancer in the National Institutes of Health-AARP Diet and Health Study cohort. *J Natl Cancer Inst* 2007;99:451–462.
22. Sieri S, Krogh V, Ferrari P, et al. Dietary fat and breast cancer risk in the European Prospective Investigation into Cancer and Nutrition. *Am J Clin Nutr* 2008;88:1304–1312.
23. Hunter DJ, Spiegelman D, Adami HO, et al. Cohort studies of fat intake and the risk of breast cancer—a pooled analysis. *N Engl J Med* 1996;334:356–361.
24. Smith-Warner SA, Spiegelman D, Adami HO, et al. Types of dietary fat and breast cancer: a pooled analysis of cohort studies. *Int J Cancer* 2001;92:767–774.
25. Wu AH, Pike MC, Stram DO. Meta-analysis: dietary fat intake, serum estrogen levels, and the risk of breast cancer. *J Natl Cancer Inst* 1999;91:529–534.

26. Rose DP, Connolly JM, Chlebowski RT, et al. The effects of a low-fat dietary intervention and tamoxifen adjuvant therapy on the serum estrogen and sex hormone-binding globulin concentrations of postmenopausal breast cancer patients. *Breast Cancer Res Treat* 1993;27:253–262.
27. Michels KB. The women's health initiative—curse or blessing? *Int J Epidemiol* 2006;35:814–816.
28. Michels KB, Willett WC. The Women's Health Initiative Randomized Controlled Dietary Modification Trial: a post-mortem. *Breast Cancer Res Treat* 2009;114:1–6.
29. Martin LJ, Li Q, Melnichouk O, et al. A randomized trial of dietary intervention for breast cancer prevention. *Cancer Res* 2011;71:123–133.
30. Cho E, Spiegelman D, Hunter DJ, et al. Premenopausal fat intake and risk of breast cancer. *J Natl Cancer Inst* 2003;95:1079–1085.
31. Linos E, Willett WC, Cho E, et al. Red meat consumption during adolescence among premenopausal women and risk of breast cancer. *Cancer Epidemiol Biomarkers Prev* 2008;17:2146–2151.
32. Linos E, Willett WC, Cho E, et al. Adolescent diet in relation to breast cancer risk among premenopausal women. *Cancer Epidemiol Biomarkers Prev* 2010;19:689–696.
33. Willett WC, Stampfer MJ, Colditz GA, et al. Relation of meat, fat, and fiber intake to the risk of colon cancer in a prospective study among women. *N Engl J Med* 1990;323:1664–1672.
34. Bostick RM, Potter JD, Kushi LH, et al. Sugar, meat, and fat intake, and non-dietary risk factors for colon cancer incidence in Iowa women (United States). *Cancer Causes Control* 1994;5:38–52.
35. Goldbohm RA, van den Brandt PA, van't Veer P, et al. A prospective cohort study on the relation between meat consumption and the risk of colon cancer. *Cancer Res* 1994;54:718–723.
36. Giovannucci E, Rimm EB, Stampfer MJ, et al. Intake of fat, meat, and fiber in relation to risk of colon cancer in men. *Cancer Res* 1994;54:2390–2397.
37. Norat T, Lukanova A, Ferrari P, et al. Meat consumption and colorectal cancer risk: dose-response meta-analysis of epidemiological studies. *Int J Cancer* 2002;98:241–256.
38. Dietary Guidelines for Americans. DietaryGuidelines.gov Web site. http://www.health.gov/dietaryguidelines/.
39. Whittemore AS, Kolonel LN, Wu AH, et al. Prostate cancer in relation to diet, physical activity, and body size in blacks, whites, and Asians in the United States and Canada. *J Natl Cancer Inst* 1995;87:652–661.
40. Crowe FL, Key TJ, Appleby PN, et al. Dietary fat intake and risk of prostate cancer in the European Prospective Investigation into Cancer and Nutrition. *Am J Clin Nutr* 2008;87:1405–1413.
41. Giovannucci E, Rimm EB, Colditz GA, et al. A prospective study of dietary fat and risk of prostate cancer. *J Natl Cancer Inst* 1993;85:1571–1579.
42. Mills PK, Beeson WL, Phillips RL, et al. Cohort study of diet, lifestyle, and prostate cancer in Adventist men. *Cancer* 1989;64:598–604.
43. Park S-Y, Murphy SP, Wilkens LR, et al. Fat and meat intake and prostate cancer risk: The multiethnic cohort study. *Int J Cancer* 2007;121:1339–1345.
44. Schuurman AG, van den Brandt PA, Dorant E, et al. Association of energy and fat intake with prostate carcinoma risk: results from The Netherlands Cohort Study. *Cancer* 1999;86:1019–1027.
45. Smith-Warner SA, Ritz J, Hunter DJ, et al. Dietary fat and risk of lung cancer in a pooled analysis of prospective studies. *Cancer Epidemiol Biomarkers Prev* 2002;11:987–992.
46. Michels KB, Edward G, Joshipura KJ, et al. Prospective study of fruit and vegetable consumption and incidence of colon and rectal cancers. *J Natl Cancer Inst* 2000;92:1740–1752.
47. Koushik A, Hunter DJ, Spiegelman D, et al. Fruits, vegetables, and colon cancer risk in a pooled analysis of 14 cohort studies. *J Natl Cancer Inst* 2007;99:1471–1483.
48. Smith-Warner SA, Spiegelman D, Yaun SS, et al. Intake of fruits and vegetables and risk of breast cancer: a pooled analysis of cohort studies. *JAMA* 2001;285:769–776.
49. van Gils CH, Peeters PH, Bueno-de-Mesquita HB, et al. Consumption of vegetables and fruits and risk of breast cancer. *JAMA* 2005;293:183–193.
50. Fung TT, Hu FB, McCullough ML, et al. Diet quality is associated with the risk of estrogen receptor-negative breast cancer in postmenopausal women. *J Nutr* 2006;136:466–472.
51. Jung S, Spiegelman D, Baglietto L, et al. Fruit and vegetable intake and risk of breast cancer by hormone receptor status. *J Natl Cancer Inst* 2013;105:219–236.
52. Smith-Warner SA, Spiegelman D, Yaun SS, et al. Fruits, vegetables, and lung cancer: a pooled analysis of cohort studies. *Int J Cancer* 2003;107:1001–1011.
53. Hung HC, Joshipura KJ, Jiang R, et al. Fruit and vegetable intake and risk of major chronic disease. *J Natl Cancer Inst* 2004;96:1577–1584.
54. Boffetta P, Couto E, Wichmann J, et al. Fruit and vegetable intake and overall cancer risk in the European Prospective Investigation into Cancer and Nutrition (EPIC). *J Natl Cancer Inst* 2010;102:529–537.
55. Trowell H, Southgate DA, Waolever TM, et al. Letter: Dietary fibre redefined. *Lancet* 1976;1:967.
56. Burkitt DP. Related disease—related cause? *Lancet* 1969;2:1229–1231.
57. Howe GR, Benito E, Castelleto R, et al. Dietary intake of fiber and decreased risk of cancers of the colon and rectum: evidence from the combined analysis of 13 case-control studies. *J Natl Cancer Inst* 1992;84:1887–1896.
58. Trock B, Lanza E, Greenwald P. Dietary fiber, vegetables, and colon cancer: critical review and meta-analyses of the epidemiologic evidence. *J Natl Cancer Inst* 1990;82:650–661.
59. Bingham SA, Day NE, Luben R, et al. Dietary fibre in food and protection against colorectal cancer in the European Prospective Investigation into Cancer and Nutrition (EPIC): an observational study. *Lancet* 2003;361:1496–1501.
60. Fuchs CS, Giovannucci EL, Colditz GA, et al. Dietary fiber and the risk of colorectal cancer and adenoma in women. *N Engl J Med* 1999;340:169–176.
61. Michels KB, Fuchs CS, Giovannucci E, et al. Fiber intake and incidence of colorectal cancer among 76,947 women and 47,279 men. *Cancer Epidemiol Biomarkers Prev* 2005;14:842–849.
62. Park Y, Hunter DJ, Spiegelman D, et al. Dietary fiber intake and risk of colorectal cancer: a pooled analysis of prospective cohort studies. *JAMA* 2005;294:2849–2857.
63. Schatzkin A, Mouw T, Park Y, et al. Dietary fiber and whole-grain consumption in relation to colorectal cancer in the NIH-AARP Diet and Health Study. *Am J Clin Nutr* 2007;85:1353–1360.
64. Alberts DS, Martinez ME, Roe DJ, et al. Lack of effect of a high-fiber cereal supplement on the recurrence of colorectal adenomas. Phoenix Colon Cancer Prevention Physicians' Network. *N Engl J Med* 2000;342:1156–1162.
65. Jacobs ET, Giuliano AR, Roe DJ, et al. Intake of supplemental and total fiber and risk of colorectal adenoma recurrence in the wheat bran fiber trial. *Cancer Epidemiol Biomarkers Prev* 2002;11:906–914.
66. MacLennan R, Macrae F, Bain C, et al. Randomized trial of intake of fat, fiber, and beta carotene to prevent colorectal adenomas. The Australian Polyp Prevention Project. *J Natl Cancer Inst* 1995;87:1760–1766.
67. McKeown-Eyssen GE, Bright-See E, Bruce WR, et al. A randomized trial of a low fat high fibre diet in the recurrence of colorectal polyps. Toronto Polyp Prevention Group. *J Clin Epidemiol* 1994;47:525–536.
68. Schatzkin A, Lanza E, Corle D, et al. Lack of effect of a low-fat, high-fiber diet on the recurrence of colorectal adenomas. Polyp Prevention Trial Study Group. *N Engl J Med* 2000;342:1149–1155.
69. Bonithon-Kopp C, Kronborg O, Giacosa A, et al. Calcium and fibre supplementation in prevention of colorectal adenoma recurrence: a randomised intervention trial. European Cancer Prevention Organisation Study Group. *Lancet* 2000;356:1300–1306.
70. Graham S, Zielezny M, Marshall J, et al. Diet in the epidemiology of postmenopausal breast cancer in the New York State Cohort. *Am J Epidemiol* 1992;136:1327–1337.
71. Horn-Ross PL, Hoggatt KJ, West DW, et al. Recent diet and breast cancer risk: the California Teachers Study (USA). *Cancer Causes Control* 2002;13:407–415.
72. Jarvinen R, Knekt P, Seppanen R, et al. Diet and breast cancer risk in a cohort of Finnish women. *Cancer Lett* 1997;114:251–253.
73. Terry P, Jain M, Miller AB, et al. No association among total dietary fiber, fiber fractions, and risk of breast cancer. *Cancer Epidemiol Biomarkers Prev* 2002;11:1507–1508.
74. Verhoeven DT, Assen N, Goldbohm RA, et al. Vitamins C and E, retinol, beta-carotene and dietary fibre in relation to breast cancer risk: a prospective cohort study. *Br J Cancer* 1997;75:149–155.
75. Willett WC, Hunter DJ, Stampfer MJ, et al. Dietary fat and fiber in relation to risk of breast cancer. An 8-year follow-up. *JAMA* 1992;268:2037–2044.
76. Botterweck AA, van den Brandt PA, Goldbohm RA. Vitamins, carotenoids, dietary fiber, and the risk of gastric carcinoma: results from a prospective study after 6.3 years of follow-up. *Cancer* 2000;88:737–748.
77. Missmer SA, Smith-Warner SA, Spiegelman D, et al. Meat and dairy food consumption and breast cancer: a pooled analysis of cohort studies. *Int J Epidemiol* 2002;31:78–85.
78. Cho E, Chen WY, Hunter DJ, et al. Red meat intake and risk of breast cancer among premenopausal women. *Arch Intern Med* 2006;166:2253–2259.
79. Cho E, Smith-Warner SA, Spiegelman D, et al. Dairy foods, calcium, and colorectal cancer: a pooled analysis of 10 cohort studies. *J Natl Cancer Inst* 2004;96:1015–1022.
80. Aune D, Lau R, Chan DS, et al. Dairy products and colorectal cancer risk: a systematic review and meta-analysis of cohort studies. *Ann Oncol* 2012;23:37–45.
81. Baron JA, Beach M, Mandel JS, et al. Calcium supplements for the prevention of colorectal adenomas. Calcium Polyp Prevention Study Group. *N Engl J Med* 1999;340:101–107.
82. Allen NE, Key TJ, Appleby PN, et al. Animal foods, protein, calcium and prostate cancer risk: the European Prospective Investigation into Cancer and Nutrition. *Br J Cancer* 2008;98:1574–1581.
83. Kurahashi N, Inoue M, Iwasaki M, et al. Dairy product, saturated fatty acid, and calcium intake and prostate cancer in a prospective cohort of Japanese men. *Cancer Epidemiol Biomarkers Prev* 2008;17:930–937.
84. Chan JM, Stampfer MJ, Ma J, et al. Dairy products, calcium, and prostate cancer risk in the Physicians' Health Study. *Am J Clin Nut* 2001;74:549–554.
85. Mitrou PN, Albanes D, Weinstein SJ, et al. A prospective study of dietary calcium, dairy products and prostate cancer risk (Finland). *Int J Cancer* 2007;120:2466–2473.
86. Tseng M, Breslow RA, Graubard BI, et al. Dairy, calcium, and vitamin D intakes and prostate cancer risk in the National Health and Nutrition Examination Epidemiologic Follow-up Study cohort. *Am J Clin Nutr* 2005;81:1147–1154.
87. Giovannucci E, Liu Y, Stampfer MJ, et al. A prospective study of calcium intake and incident and fatal prostate cancer. *Cancer Epidemiol Biomarkers Prev* 2006;15:203–210.

88. Snowdon DA, Phillips RL, Choi W. Diet, obesity, and risk of fatal prostate cancer. *Am J Epidemiol* 1984;120:244–250.
89. Park Y, Mitrou PN, Kipnis V, et al. Calcium, dairy foods, and risk of incident and fatal prostate cancer: the NIH-AARP Diet and Health Study. *Am J Epidemiol* 2007;166:1270–1279.
90. Park SY, Murphy SP, Wilkens LR, et al. Calcium, vitamin D, and dairy product intake and prostate cancer risk: the Multiethnic Cohort Study. *Am J Epidemiol* 2007;166:1259–1269.
91. Ahn J, Albanes D, Peters U, et al. Dairy products, calcium intake, and risk of prostate cancer in the prostate, lung, colorectal, and ovarian cancer screening trial. *Cancer Epidemiol Biomarkers Prev* 2007;16:2623–2630.
92. Gao X, LaValley MP, Tucker KL. Prospective studies of dairy product and calcium intakes and prostate cancer risk: a meta-analysis. *J Natl Cancer Inst* 2005;97:1768–1777.
93. Huncharek M, Muscat J, Kupelnick B. Dairy products, dietary calcium and vitamin D intake as risk factors for prostate cancer: a meta-analysis of 26,769 cases from 45 observational studies. *Nutr Cancer* 2008;60:421–441.
94. Ganmaa D, Cui X, Feskanich D, et al. Milk, dairy intake and risk of endometrial cancer: a 26-year follow-up. *Int J Cancer* 2012;130:2664–2671.
95. Genkinger JM, Hunter DJ, Spiegelman D, et al. Dairy products and ovarian cancer: a pooled analysis of 12 cohort studies. *Cancer Epidemiol Biomarkers Prev* 2006;15:364–372.
96. Hoppe C, Molgaard C, Juul A, et al. High intakes of skimmed milk, but not meat, increase serum IGF-I and IGFBP-3 in eight-year-old boys. *Eur J Clin Nutr* 2004;58:1211–1216.
97. Ganmaa D, Wang PY, Qin LQ, et al. Is milk responsible for male reproductive disorders? *Med Hypotheses* 2001;57:510–514.
98. Garland CF, Garland FC. Do sunlight and vitamin D reduce the likelihood of colon cancer? *Int J Epidemiol* 1980;9:227–231.
99. Feskanich D, Ma J, Fuchs CS, et al. Plasma vitamin D metabolites and risk of colorectal cancer in women. *Cancer Epidemiol Biomarkers Prev* 2004;13:1502–1508.
100. Woolcott CG, Wilkens LR, Nomura AM, et al. Plasma 25-hydroxyvitamin D levels and the risk of colorectal cancer: the multiethnic cohort study. *Cancer Epidemiol Biomarkers Prev* 2010;19:130–134.
101. Jenab M, Bueno-de-Mesquita HB, Ferrari P, et al. Association between pre-diagnostic circulating vitamin D concentration and risk of colorectal cancer in European populations: a nested case-control study. *BMJ* 2010;340:b5500.
102. Wactawski-Wende J, Kotchen JM, Anderson GL, et al. Calcium plus vitamin D supplementation and the risk of colorectal cancer. *N Engl J Med* 2006;354:684–696.
103. Park SY, Murphy SP, Wilkens LR, et al. Calcium and vitamin D intake and risk of colorectal cancer: the Multiethnic Cohort Study. *Am J Epidemiol* 2007;165:784–793.
104. Gorham ED, Garland CF, Garland FC, et al. Optimal vitamin D status for colorectal cancer prevention: a quantitative meta analysis. *Am J Prev Med* 2007;32:210–216.
105. Yin L, Grandi N, Raum E, et al. Meta-analysis: longitudinal studies of serum vitamin D and colorectal cancer risk. *Aliment Pharmacol Ther* 2009;30:113–125.
106. Wei MY, Garland CF, Gorham ED, et al. Vitamin D and prevention of colorectal adenoma: a meta-analysis. *Cancer Epidemiol Biomarkers Prev* 2008;17:2958–2969.
107. Freedman DM, Looker AC, Chang SC, et al. Prospective study of serum vitamin D and cancer mortality in the United States. *J Natl Cancer Inst* 2007;99:1594–1602.
108. Bertone-Johnson ER, Chen WY, Holick MF, et al. Plasma 25-hydroxyvitamin D and 1,25-dihydroxyvitamin D and risk of breast cancer. *Cancer Epidemiol Biomarkers Prev* 2005;14:1991–1997.
109. McCullough ML, Rodriguez C, Diver WR, et al. Dairy, calcium, and vitamin D intake and postmenopausal breast cancer risk in the Cancer Prevention Study II Nutrition Cohort. *Cancer Epidemiol Biomarkers Prev* 2005;14:2898–2904.
110. Chen P, Hu P, Xie D, et al. Meta-analysis of vitamin D, calcium and the prevention of breast cancer. *Breast Cancer Res Treat* 2010;121:469–477.
111. Platz EA, Leitzmann MF, Hollis BW, et al. Plasma 1,25-dihydroxy- and 25-hydroxyvitamin D and subsequent risk of prostate cancer. *Cancer Causes Control* 2004;15:255–265.
112. Shui IM, Mucci LA, Kraft P, et al. Vitamin D-related genetic variation, plasma vitamin D, and risk of lethal prostate cancer: a prospective nested case-control study. *J Natl Cancer Inst* 2012;104:690–699.
113. Tworoger SS, Lee IM, Buring JE, et al. Plasma 25-hydroxyvitamin D and 1,25-dihydroxyvitamin D and risk of incident ovarian cancer. *Cancer Epidemiol Biomarkers Prev* 2007;16:783–788.
114. Toriola AT, Surcel HM, Agborsangaya C, et al. Serum 25-hydroxyvitamin D and the risk of ovarian cancer. *Eur J Cancer* 2010;46:364–369.
115. Stolzenberg-Solomon RZ, Jacobs EJ, Arslan AA, et al. Circulating 25-hydroxyvitamin D and risk of pancreatic cancer: Cohort Consortium Vitamin D Pooling Project of Rarer Cancers. *Am J Epidemiol* 2010;172:81–93.
116. Skinner HG, Michaud DS, Giovannucci E, et al. Vitamin D intake and the risk for pancreatic cancer in two cohort studies. *Cancer Epidemiol Biomarkers Prev* 2006;15:1688–1695.
117. Wolpin BM, Ng K, Bao Y, et al. Plasma 25-hydroxyvitamin D and risk of pancreatic cancer. *Cancer Epidemiol Biomarkers Prev* 2012;21:82–91.
118. Giovannucci E. Epidemiology of vitamin D and colorectal cancer: casual or causal link? *J Steroid Biochem Mol Biol* 2010;121(1–2):349–354.
119. Giovannucci E. Epidemiologic studies of folate and colorectal neoplasia: a review. *J Nutr* 2002;132:2350S–2355S.
120. Kim D, Smith-Warner S, Spiegelman D, et al. Pooled analysis of 13 prospective cohort studies on folate and colon cancer. *Cancer Causes Control* 2010;21:1919-1930.
121. Chen J, Giovannucci E, Kelsey K, et al. A methylenetetrahydrofolate reductase polymorphism and the risk of colorectal cancer. *Cancer Res* 1996;56:4862–4864.
122. Osterhues A, Holzgreve W, Michels KB. Shall we put the world on folate? *Lancet* 2009;374:959–961.
123. Friso S, Choi SW, Girelli D, et al. A common mutation in the 5,10-methylenetetrahydrofolate reductase gene affects genomic DNA methylation through an interaction with folate status. *Proc Natl Acad Sci U S A* 2002;99:5606–5611.
124. Kim YI. Folate: a magic bullet or a double edged sword for colorectal cancer prevention? *Gut* 2006;55:1387–1389.
125. Mason JB. Folate, cancer risk, and the Greek god, Proteus: a tale of two chameleons. *Nutr Rev* 2009;67:206–212.
126. Wu K, Platz EA, Willett W, et al. A randomized trial on folic acid supplementation and risk of recurrent colorectal adenoma. *Am J Clin Nutr* 2009;90:1623–1631.
127. Cole BF, Baron JA, Sandler RS, et al. Folic acid for the prevention of colorectal adenomas: a randomized clinical trial. *JAMA* 2007;297:2351–2359.
128. Mason JB, Dickstein A, Jacques PF, et al. A temporal association between folic acid fortification and an increase in colorectal cancer rates may be illuminating important biological principles: a hypothesis. *Cancer Epidemiol Biomarkers Prev* 2007;16:1325–1329.
129. The effect of vitamin E and beta carotene on the incidence of lung cancer and other cancers in male smokers. The Alpha-Tocopherol, Beta Carotene Cancer Prevention Study Group. *N Engl J Med* 1994;330:1029–1035.
130. Virtamo J, Pietinen P, Huttunen JK, et al. Incidence of cancer and mortality following alpha-tocopherol and beta-carotene supplementation: a postintervention follow-up. *JAMA* 2003;290:476–485.
131. Mannisto S, Smith-Warner SA, Spiegelman D, et al. Dietary carotenoids and risk of lung cancer in a pooled analysis of seven cohort studies. *Cancer Epidemiol Biomarkers Prev* 2004;13:40–48.
132. Zhang X, Spiegelman D, Baglietto L, et al. Carotenoid intakes and risk of breast cancer defined by estrogen receptor and progesterone receptor status: a pooled analysis of 18 prospective cohort studies. *Am J Clin Nutr* 2012;95:713–725.
133. Eliassen AH, Hendrickson SJ, Brinton LA, et al. Circulating carotenoids and risk of breast cancer: pooled analysis of eight prospective studies. *J Natl Cancer Inst* 2012;104:1905–1916.
134. Giovannucci E. Tomatoes, tomato-based products, lycopene, and cancer: review of the epidemiologic literature. *J Natl Cancer Inst* 1999;91:317–331.
135. Yoshizawa K, Willett WC, Morris SJ, et al. Study of prediagnostic selenium level in toenails and the risk of advanced prostate cancer. *J Natl Cancer Inst* 1998;90:1219–1224.
136. Amaral AF, Cantor KP, Silverman DT, et al. Selenium and bladder cancer risk: a meta-analysis. *Cancer Epidemiol Biomarkers Prev* 2010;19:2407–2415.
137. Geybels MS, Verhage BA, van Schooten FJ, et al. Advanced prostate cancer risk in relation to toenail selenium levels. *J Natl Cancer Inst* 2013;105:1394–1401.
138. Hurst R, Hooper L, Norat T, et al. Selenium and prostate cancer: systematic review and meta-analysis. *Am J Clinical Nutr* 2012;96:111–122.
139. Lippman SM, Klein EA, Goodman PJ, et al. Effect of selenium and vitamin E on risk of prostate cancer and other cancers: the Selenium and Vitamin E Cancer Prevention Trial (SELECT). *JAMA* 2009;301:39–51.
140. Trock BJ, Hilakivi-Clarke L, Clarke R. Meta-analysis of soy intake and breast cancer risk. *J Natl Cancer Inst* 2006;98:459–471.
141. Wu AH, Wan P, Hankin J, et al. Adolescent and adult soy intake and risk of breast cancer in Asian-Americans. *Carcinogenesis* 2002;23:1491–1496.
142. Warburg O, Posener K, Negelein E. Ueber den Stoffwechsel der Tumoren. *Biochemische Zeitschrift* 1924;152:319.
143. Hu FB, Manson JE, Liu S, et al. Prospective study of adult onset diabetes mellitus (type 2) and risk of colorectal cancer in women. *J Natl Cancer Inst* 1999;91:542–547.
144. Michels KB, Solomon CG, Hu FB, et al. Type 2 diabetes and subsequent incidence of breast cancer in the Nurses' Health Study. *Diabetes Care* 2003;26:1752–1758.
145. Gnagnarella P, Gandini S, La Vecchia C, et al. Glycemic index, glycemic load, and cancer risk: a meta-analysis. *Am J Clinical Nutr* 2008;87:1793–1801.
146. Slattery ML, Benson J, Berry TD, et al. Dietary sugar and colon cancer. *Cancer Epidemiol Biomarkers Prev* 1997;6:677–685.
147. Terry PD, Jain M, Miller AB, et al. Glycemic load, carbohydrate intake, and risk of colorectal cancer in women: a prospective cohort study. *J Natl Cancer Inst* 2003;95:914–916.
148. Michaud DS, Liu S, Giovannucci E, et al. Dietary sugar, glycemic load, and pancreatic cancer risk in a prospective study. *J Natl Cancer Inst* 2002;94:1293–1300.
149. Jonas CR, McCullough ML, Teras LR, et al. Dietary glycemic index, glycemic load, and risk of incident breast cancer in postmenopausal women. *Cancer Epidemiol Biomarkers Prev* 2003;12:573–577.
150. Tantamango-Bartley Y, Jaceldo-Siegl K, Fan J, et al. Vegetarian diets and the incidence of cancer in a low-risk population. *Cancer Epidemiol Biomarkers Prev* 2013;22:286–294.
151. Key TJ, Appleby PN, Spencer EA, et al. Cancer incidence in British vegetarians. *Br J Cancer* 2009;101:192–197.

152. Fung T, Hu FB, Fuchs C, et al. Major dietary patterns and the risk of colorectal cancer in women. *Arch Intern Med* 2003;163:309–314.
153. Fung TT, Hu FB, Holmes MD, et al. Dietary patterns and the risk of postmenopausal breast cancer. *Int J Cancer* 2005;116:116–121.
154. Link LB, Canchola AJ, Bernstein L, et al. Dietary patterns and breast cancer risk in the California Teachers Study cohort. *Am J Clin Nutr* 2013;98:1524–1532.
155. Caughey RW, Michels KB. Birth weight and childhood leukemia: a meta-analysis and review of the current evidence. *Int J Cancer* 2009;124:2658–2670.
156. Michels KB, Xue F. Role of birthweight in the etiology of breast cancer. *Int J Cancer* 2006;119:2007–2025.
157. Michos A, Xue F, Michels KB. Birth weight and the risk of testicular cancer: a meta-analysis. *Int J Cancer* 2007;121:1123–1131.
158. Chavarro JE, Rosner BA, Sampson L, et al. Validity of adolescent diet recall 48 years later. *Am J Epidemiol* 2009;170:1563–1570.
159. Maruti SS, Feskanich D, Colditz GA, et al. Adult recall of adolescent diet: reproducibility and comparison with maternal reporting. *Am J Epidemiol* 2005;161:89–97.
160. Michels KB, Rosner BA, Chumlea WC, et al. Preschool diet and adult risk of breast cancer. *Int J Cancer* 2006;118:749–754.
161. Hjartaker A, Laake P, Lund E. Childhood and adult milk consumption and risk of premenopausal breast cancer in a cohort of 48,844 women - the Norwegian women and cancer study. *Int J Cancer* 2001;93:888–893.
162. Michels KB, Mohllajee AP, Roset-Bahmanyar E, et al. Diet and breast cancer: a review of the prospective observational studies. *Cancer* 2007;109:2712–2749.
163. Greenlee H, Kwan ML, Kushi LH, et al. Antioxidant supplement use after breast cancer diagnosis and mortality in the Life After Cancer Epidemiology (LACE) cohort. *Cancer* 2012;118:2048–2058.
164. Kwan ML, Chen WY, Flatt SW, et al. Postdiagnosis alcohol consumption and breast cancer prognosis in the after breast cancer pooling project. *Cancer Epidemiol Biomarkers Prev* 2013;22:32–41.
165. Chlebowski RT, Blackburn GL, Thomson CA, et al. Dietary fat reduction and breast cancer outcome: interim efficacy results from the Women's Intervention Nutrition Study. *J Natl Cancer Inst* 2006;98:1767–1776.
166. Pierce JP, Natarajan L, Caan BJ, et al. Influence of a diet very high in vegetables, fruit, and fiber and low in fat on prognosis following treatment for breast cancer: the Women's Healthy Eating and Living (WHEL) randomized trial. *JAMA* 2007;298:289–298.
167. Izano MA, Fung TT, Chiuve SS, et al. Are diet quality scores after breast cancer diagnosis associated with improved breast cancer survival? *Nutr Cancer* 2013;65:820–826.
168. van Meer S, Leufkens AM, Bueno-de-Mesquita HB, et al. Role of dietary factors in survival and mortality in colorectal cancer: a systematic review. *Nutrition Rev* 2013;71:631–641.
169. Meyerhardt JA, Niedzwiecki D, Hollis D, et al. Association of dietary patterns with cancer recurrence and survival in patients with stage III colon cancer. *JAMA* 2007;298:754–764.
170. Meyerhardt JA, Sato K, Niedzwiecki D, et al. Dietary glycemic load and cancer recurrence and survival in patients with stage III colon cancer: findings from CALGB 89803. *J Natl Cancer Inst* 2012;104:1702–1711.
171. Song Y, Chavarro JE, Cao Y, et al. Whole milk intake is associated with prostate cancer-specific mortality among U.S. male physicians. *J Nutr* 2013;143:189–196.
172. Richman EL, Kenfield SA, Chavarro JE, et al. Fat intake after diagnosis and risk of lethal prostate cancer and all-cause mortality. *JAMA Intern Med* 2013;173:1318–1326.
173. Richman EL, Kenfield SA, Stampfer MJ, et al. Egg, red meat, and poultry intake and risk of lethal prostate cancer in the prostate-specific antigen-era: incidence and survival. *Cancer Prev Res (Phila)* 2011;4:2110–2121.
174. Chan JM, Holick CN, Leitzmann MF, et al. Diet after diagnosis and the risk of prostate cancer progression, recurrence, and death (United States). *Cancer Causes Control* 2006;17:199–208.
175. Ornish D, Weidner G, Fair WR, et al. Intensive lifestyle changes may affect the progression of prostate cancer. *J Urol* 2005;174:1065–1070.
176. Kushi LH, Doyle C, McCullough M, et al. American Cancer Society Guidelines on nutrition and physical activity for cancer prevention: reducing the risk of cancer with healthy food choices and physical activity. *CA Cancer J Clin* 2012;62:30–67.

10 Obesity and Physical Activity

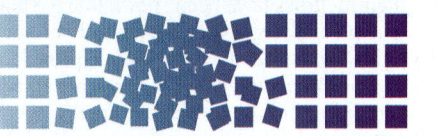

Yani Lu, Jessica Clague, and Leslie Bernstein

INTRODUCTION

Evidence showing that physical activity is associated with decreased cancer risk and that obesity is associated with increased cancer risk at certain sites is rapidly accumulating. It is not yet known whether these two factors are interrelated or independent. Physical activity may act to decrease cancer risk primarily by preventing weight gain and obesity. However, physical activity may also have independent effects on cancer risk. In this chapter, we present a summary of the current epidemiologic literature on the possible associations between physical activity and obesity and risk of cancer at several organ sites.

Physical activity is defined as any movement of the body that results in energy expenditure. In this chapter, we focus on recreational physical activity, also called leisure-time physical activity or exercise, and occupational physical activity, including household activity.[1] Occupational physical activity typically occurs over a longer period of time and generally requires less energy expenditure per hour than bouts of strenuous or moderate recreational physical activity. The distinction between recreational and occupational activity is important because increasing mechanization and technologic advances have led to decreased occupational physical activity in developed areas of the world, perhaps contributing to a decrease in overall physical activity.

Obesity is defined as the condition of being extremely overweight. In epidemiologic studies, the usual, but not necessarily the best, measure of body mass in adults is Quetelet's Index, or body mass index (BMI), which is measured as weight in kilograms (kg) divided by the square of height in meters (m^2). In the year spanning 2009 to 2010, the prevalence of obesity, defined by having a BMI of 30 kg/m^2 or greater, in the US population was 35.5% for adult men and 35.8% for adult women.[2] Physical inactivity has likely contributed to the high prevalence of obesity in the United States; data from the 2003 to 2004 National Health and Nutritional Examination Survey, a cross-sectional study of a sample of the civilian, noninstitutionalized population of the United States, has indicated that less than 5% of US adults achieve 30 minutes per day of physical activity, and that men are more physically active than women.[3]

Epidemiologic evidence on the associations of physical activity and obesity with cancer come from observational studies, including cohort studies, which follow populations forward in time after collecting exposure information, and case-control studies, which optimally identify a population-based series of newly diagnosed cases and healthy control subjects, collecting information retrospectively on exposures. In both study designs, physical activity information is usually self-reported and measures vary substantially with respect to timing and level of detail. Studies have measured lifetime or long-term physical activity, activity at defined ages or time points in life, and/or current or recent activity. Ideally, a study would capture activity by type (recreational, occupational, or other, such as an activity related to transportation), duration (minutes per session), frequency (sessions per day), and intensity (low, moderate, or strenuous as defined by examples of activity types) across the lifetime. These studies have often measured height and weight by self-report at one time point, such as at the time of study entry. Some studies have collected other or more detailed anthropometric information, such as waist circumference, hip circumference, or weight at an additional time point like at age 18. Anthropometrics are directly measured by trained study personnel in only a few studies.

Epidemiologic evidence for a role of physical activity or obesity in relation to cancer risk exists for cancers of the breast, colon, endometrium, esophagus, kidney, and pancreatic cancer. Evidence is accumulating to link at least one of these "exposures" to the incidence of gallbladder cancer, non-Hodgkin lymphoma (NHL), and advanced prostate cancer. The evidence for an association between either physical activity or obesity and lung and ovarian cancer is inconclusive.

In addition to specific biologic mechanisms pertinent to physical activity or to obesity at each specific organ site, several global mechanisms have been implicated in both relationships across a number of these organ sites. The steroid hormone and insulin/insulinlike growth factor (IGF) pathways are two such global mechanisms hypothesized to be involved in the links between physical activity or obesity and cancer.[4] The role of steroid hormones as a mediator in these relationships is perhaps best understood in the context of breast cancer and endometrial cancer, and will be discussed in those sections. The roles of the insulin and IGF pathways have been discussed in depth with respect to colon cancer and, thus, will be presented in that context. Other global mechanisms have been proposed that have more generalized anticancer impacts and may explain associations between physical activity and several cancer sites; these include heightening immune surveillance, reducing inflammation, increasing insulin sensitivity, controlling growth factor production and activation, decreasing obesity and central adiposity, optimizing DNA repair capacity, and reducing oxidative stress.[5,6] Further, obesity has been shown to produce a proinflammatory state and, thus, inflammation may mediate the relationship between obesity and cancer risk.[7] It is highly plausible that several of these mechanisms act simultaneously and that they interact synergistically to mediate the associations between physical activity, obesity, and cancer.

BREAST CANCER

Low level of physical activity is an established breast cancer risk factor among postmenopausal women and, to a lesser extent, premenopausal women.[4,8,9] The evidence for an association between physical activity and breast cancer has been classified as convincing, with a 20% to 40% reduced risk among physically active women.[10] Obesity appears to have a paradoxical relationship with breast cancer risk in that it is an established breast cancer risk factor among postmenopausal women, but may offer some protection for breast cancer among premenopausal women.[4]

The epidemiologic literature has shown with relative consistency that breast cancer risk is reduced by increasing one's amount of physical activity.[4,8,9,11–13] One of the earliest studies, a case-control study of women age 40 years or younger, showed a dramatic reduction in risk of approximately 50% among women who averaged about 4 hours of activity per week during their reproductive years.[14] Similarly, among postmenopausal women, those with higher levels of recreational physical activity during their lifetimes have been shown to have lower breast cancer risk.[15] A meta-analysis of 29 case-control studies and 19 cohort studies published between 1994 and 2006 provided strong evidence for an inverse association between physical activity and risk of breast cancer, citing that the evidence for an association between physical activity and premenopausal breast cancer was not as strong as that for postmenopausal breast cancer.[8] The conclusion of the meta-analysis was that each additional hour of physical activity per week decreases breast cancer by approximately 6%.

Epidemiologists require that a risk factor demonstrate consistency across populations before considering it as accepted. Recently, studies have been published on the association between physical activity and breast cancer risk among Japanese,[16] Chinese,[17] Mexican,[18] Tunisian,[19] and African American women.[20] All studies showed a decreased risk of breast cancer with increasing physical activity. Interestingly, both Suzuki et al.[17] and Pronk et al.[21] observed the strongest associations among "heavier" women (BMI ≥25 kg/m^2 and 23.73 kg/m^2, respectively). In the California Teachers Study (CTS), a prospective cohort study of over 133,000 female public school professionals, a variable combining strenuous and moderate long-term recreational physical activity was associated with a reduced risk of estrogen receptor (ER)-negative but not ER-positive invasive breast cancer.[11] On the contrary, the Women's Health Initiative (WHI) observed decreases in breast cancer risk associated with recreational physical activity among postmenopausal women with ER-positive breast cancer and triple negative breast cancer, with only results for ER-positive breast cancer demonstrating a 15% statistically significant reduced risk (when comparing the highest versus lowest tertile of moderate-intensity physical activity).[22] Similar but not statistically significant results were observed for strenuous recreational physical activity.[22] A major limitation to this and previous studies stratifying by hormone receptor status is the inability to comprehensively classify triple negative breast cancer due to missing HER2 status (unknown in 40% of cases in the WHI study). The use of hormone therapy did not alter the inverse association between recreational physical activity and invasive breast cancer in the Women's Contraceptive and Reproductive Experiences (CARE) Study.[23] Most recently, in the American Cancer Society Cancer Prevention Study II Nutrition Cohort, it was observed that postmenopausal women who engage in at least 7 hours of walking over the course of a week had a modest decreased risk of breast cancer, even in the absence of more vigorous exercise.[24] Further, this association did not differ by ER status, BMI, adult weight gain, postmenopausal hormone therapy use, or time spent sitting.[24]

Lastly, whether physical activity reduces breast cancer risk by impacting preinvasive disease has been studied by assessing the associations with in situ breast cancer and benign breast disease. In the CTS cohort, increasing levels of long-term strenuous recreational physical activity were associated with a decreasing risk of in situ breast cancer.[11] Furthermore, a report from the Nurses' Health Study II cohort showed that lifetime recreational physical activity was associated with a decreased risk of benign breast disease and columnar cell lesions, which may be precursors to breast cancer.[25]

In summary, epidemiologic studies investigating the association between physical activity and breast cancer risk have produced relatively consistent results showing a reduction in breast cancer risk with increasing level of physical activity. Results to date suggest that moderate-to-strenuous activity may be required for the effect between physical activity and breast cancer risk to be clear; however, clarification of other key details, such as the importance of timing and intensity of activity or variation in effects by tumor characteristics, is pending.

Adult obesity and adult weight gain have both been associated with increased breast cancer risk among postmenopausal women, especially among women who were not current users of menopausal hormone therapy.[4,26,27] Most studies among postmenopausal women show a 1.5- to 2-fold increase in risk of invasive breast cancer when comparing the most obese women or those with the largest weight gain to normal-weight women (BMI: 18.5 to 24.9 kg/m^2) or those with the least weight gain.[4] Paradoxically, overweight or obese premenopausal women have a slightly decreased risk of breast cancer compared with normal-weight or thinner women. Whether larger waist circumference is more important than BMI has been studied in order to separate overall weight gain from abdominal obesity (i.e., visceral fat, which is one element of metabolic syndrome); however, most studies have reported a null association between waist circumference, used as a surrogate for visceral fat, and risk of postmenopausal breast cancer after adjustment for BMI.[26] In contrast to the results for postmenopausal women, waist circumference and a positive association with premenopausal breast cancer was found after adjustment for BMI.[26] A recent analysis of the Nurses' Health Study suggests that self-rated body fatness during youth and BMI at age 18 years are both inversely associated with breast cancer risk, with similar results for premenopausal and postmenopausal breast cancer.[28]

Hormones are central to the discussion of biologic mechanisms linking both physical activity and obesity with breast cancer risk. Physical activity can alter menstrual cycle patterns in premenopausal women, and hormone profiles in both premenopausal and postmenopausal women. Physical activity may lower body fat among children,[29] which in turn may delay age at menarche.[30] Later age at menarche has been associated with reduced breast cancer risk.[31] Physical activity may reduce the frequency of ovulatory cycles.[32] Having less frequent and therefore fewer cumulative ovulatory cycles is likely to reduce the lifetime exposure of the breast to endogenous ovarian hormones,[31] which are proven proliferative agents.[33] Physical activity also can have a direct impact on circulating estrogen levels among postmenopausal women.[34]

In the postmenopausal period, adipose tissue is the primary source of endogenous hormones via aromatization of androstenedione to estrone.[35] Thus, heavier postmenopausal women have higher levels of circulating estrogen than women with less adipose tissue. The involvement of estrogen in the relationship between obesity and breast cancer risk is supported by the observation that obesity does not independently increase breast cancer risk among menopausal hormone therapy users[27]; the obesity-related increase in estrogen over that provided by exogenous estrogens is negligible. The breast tissue of overweight or obese perimenopausal and postmenopausal women with relatively high risk of breast cancer has been shown to have cytologic abnormalities and higher epithelial cell counts than that of normal-weight women.[36] In contrast, obese premenopausal women experience menstrual cycle disturbances, including anovulatory cycles and secondary amenorrhea, thereby lowering their cumulative exposure to estradiol and progesterone.[31] A possible explanation for the inverse association between youth body fatness and breast cancer risk is that youth body size is inversely associated with adult IGF-1 levels.[28]

Other likely mechanisms that may link physical activity[37,38] and obesity[39,40] with breast cancer risk include aspects of immune function, inflammatory mechanisms, oxidative stress and DNA repair capability, metabolic hormones, and growth factors.

COLON AND RECTAL CANCER

An inverse association between physical activity and colon cancer risk has been consistently observed among epidemiologic studies; however, the evidence for rectal cancer remains inconclusive. Historically, comprehensive reviews have estimated that physical activity may reduce colon cancer risk by 20% to 25% when comparing individuals with the highest levels to those with the lowest levels of activity.[41] Risk reductions are greater for case-control studies (24%) than for cohort studies (17%), and risk reductions for occupational activity (22%) and recreational activity (23%) are similar.[41] In cohort studies, colon cancer risk reduction associated with physical activity is greater for men than for women, which may be due to the influence of hormone therapy on colon cancer risk,[42] although case-control studies suggest similar benefits for men and women.[43]

Whether physical activity preferentially protects against proximal or distal colon cancer is of interest. A meta-analysis including 21 cohort and case-control studies that examined associations between physical activity and the risks of proximal colon and distal colon cancers produced results suggesting that physical activity is associated with a reduced risk of both proximal colon and distal colon cancers, and that the magnitude of the association does not differ by subsite.[44]

Although the majority of previous studies have not found an association between physical activity and rectal cancer,[41] the National Institutes of Health (NIH)–AARP Diet and Health Study observed a modest reduction in rectal cancer risk for men but not for women after 6.9 years of follow-up.[45] Further, in a case-control study conducted in Australia, rectal cancer risk was reduced among men but not among women who participated in vigorous recreational physical activity averaging at least 6 metabolic equivalent task (MET)-hours per week during their adult years.[46]

An emphasis has been made on trying to identify risk factors for colon adenomas, which are considered precursor lesions for colon cancer; these are detected and removed during colonoscopy or sigmoidoscopy. Wolin et al. conducted a meta-analysis of 20 studies published through April 2010 that investigated the association between recreational physical activity and colon adenomas.[47] Adenoma risk was reduced by 19% among men and by 13% among women and, when combining men and women, the inverse association with physical activity was strongest for large/advanced polyps.

Obesity is an established risk factor for colon cancer in both men and women, although the relative risks for men have been higher than those for women.[4,26] The adverse impact of being overweight or obese on colon cancer risk is stronger for distal than for proximal colon cancers. In addition, visceral adiposity appears to confer greater risk than general adiposity.[26] In the European Prospective Investigation into Cancer and Nutrition (EPIC) study, abdominal obesity as well as adult weight gain were strongly associated with colon cancer risk in both men and women.[48,49] No association between these adiposity measures and colon cancer risk was evident among postmenopausal women who had used menopausal hormone therapy, and no association was observed between any measure of adiposity and rectal cancer risk.[48] The positive association between obesity and risk of colon cancer was further supported by the findings that both general obesity and abdominal obesity increase the risk of colon adenomas[47] with one study of women indicating that the distal colon is the main target site.[50]

Given that a higher BMI and lack of physical activity are both risk factors for colon cancer, several statistical approaches have been employed to tease apart their joint and independent effects on colon cancer risk. In the Netherlands Cohort Study,[51] colorectal cancer risk was increased at each subsite among larger women in the lowest recreational activity category (<30 minutes per day) than in smaller women in the highest recreational activity category (>90 minutes per day); however, the interaction between physical activity and body size was statistically significant only for proximal tumors. Using different fatness measures for men, the only similar finding was that men with low levels of physical activity whose trouser size was below the median of that for the cohort had an increased risk of distal colon cancer; no differences in risk were noted for other subsites or for men with larger trouser sizes.[51]

The mechanisms explaining the relationship between physical activity and colon cancer are not clearly established, but include the impact on insulin sensitivity and IGF profiles, and inflammation, as well as some colon-specific mechanisms. Physical activity may stimulate stool transit in the colon, thereby decreasing the exposure of colonic mucosa to carcinogens in the stool.[6] Alternatively, physical activity–induced decreases in prostaglandin E_2 may decrease colonic cell proliferation rates and increase colonic motility.[6] In addition to steroid hormones, which have been clearly implicated as biologic modifiers of the effect of physical activity and obesity on colon cancer risk, the insulin and IGF pathways may mediate the associations between these exposures and colon cancer risk. For obesity in particular, the link can be inferred because obesity can lead to insulin resistance,[52] a syndrome characterized by high circulating insulin levels. High insulin levels appear to promote cell proliferation and tumor growth in the colon[7] and may also suppress the expression of IGF-binding proteins 1 and 2, leading to increased bioavailable IGF-1 levels.[53] Another possible mechanism is obesity-enhanced inflammation in which increases in adipose tissue macrophages lead to the secretion of inflammatory cytokines associated with colon cancer risk (e.g., tumor necrosis factor [TNF]-α, monocyte chemoattractant protein [MCP]-1, and interleukin [IL]-6).

ENDOMETRIAL CANCER

The evidence for an association between physical activity and endometrial cancer risk is accumulating[4,54-58] but is not definitive. A meta-analysis of prospective cohort studies results published through 2009 indicates that recreational physical activity lowers endometrial cancer risk by 27%, and occupational activity lowers risk by 21%.[59] Adjustments for BMI minimally change relative risk estimates, suggesting that physical activity is independently associated with endometrial cancer. Although physical activity is associated with a decreased risk of endometrial cancer in both normal-weight and obese women, two recent studies have suggested that this association is more pronounced for obese women.[54,58]

Two meta-analyses of the association between physical activity and endometrial cancer have identified some inconsistencies in dose-response relationships, indicating the importance of differences in activity type and intensity.[55,56] Little evidence exists on how long-term or lifetime physical activity and activity patterns during different life periods might influence endometrial cancer risk; it has been suggested that recent or long-term activity might be more important than activity at early ages.[56] In the CTS, higher levels of recent (at cohort formation) strenuous recreational physical activity was associated with lower levels of endometrial cancer risk; among women exercising >3 hours per week per year, risk was approximately 25% lower than that of women exercising <0.5 hour per week per year.[60] This inverse association was limited to overweight and obese women (BMI ≥25 kg/m^2). Finally, sitting time has been independently associated with increased endometrial cancer risk.[59]

Epidemiologic studies have established a strong association between obesity and endometrial cancer risk.[26] Recent studies have suggested a linear trend between increasing body weight or BMI and increasing endometrial cancer risk among postmenopausal women, whereas among premenopausal women, no trend is observed, but rather, only obese women have an increased risk.[26] Furthermore, the strong association among postmenopausal women is only observed among those who are not using hormone therapy.[26] Finally, BMI appears to exert an effect on the risk of endometrial cancer that is independent of physical activity.[55]

Physical activity and obesity are likely to influence endometrial cancer risk by altering endogenous hormone profiles.[31,53] Heavier postmenopausal women have higher circulating levels of estrogen than do lighter postmenopausal women because of the aromatization of androstenedione to estrone in adipose tissue. This is pertinent to endometrial cancer risk because this aromatization occurs in the absence of progesterone, which opposes the proliferative effects of estrogen on endometrial tissue. Physical activity may counter the proliferative effects of estrogen either directly or by restricting weight gain. Some evidence also links elevated insulin levels and diabetes to endometrial cancer risk.[61] Physical inactivity and obesity play a role in the development of insulin insensitivity and diabetes, providing another mechanism by which they may influence endometrial cancer risk.

ADENOCARCINOMA OF THE ESOPHAGUS

Several case-control studies[62-64] and one cohort study[65] have examined the association between physical activity and risk of adenocarcinoma of the esophagus. Zhang et al.[62] reported a modest association between participation in recreational physical activity more than once per week and a decreased risk of all esophageal cancer (adenocarcinomas and squamous cell tumors), although the result was not statistically significant. Lagergren et al.[63] reported no association between total, usual recreational and occupational physical activity and esophageal adenocarcinoma. Vigen et al.[64] showed that lifetime occupational physical activity was modestly associated with a lower risk of adenocarcinoma of the esophagus: the average annual level of occupational physical activity before age 65 years was associated with an approximately 40% reduction in risk of esophageal adenocarcinoma when the highest was compared with the lowest occupational physical activity category. Results from the NIH–AARP Diet and Health Study also support the hypothesis that physical activity lowers the risk of esophageal adenocarcinoma, but no association between physical activity and the risk of squamous cell esophageal cancer was found.[65]

Obesity is strongly associated with an increased risk of esophageal adenocarcinoma.[66,67] A pooled analysis of existing data showed that individuals with severe obesity (BMI ≥40 kg/m^2) had a 4.8-fold greater risk than individuals who were not overweight (BMI <25 kg/m^2), with similar risk estimates for men and women.[68] Several studies have examined the effect of abdominal adiposity, which have suggested that the risk associated with obesity is driven primarily by abdominal fatness.[26]

It is likely that obesity impacts esophageal adenocarcinoma risk because it is associated with the risk of gastroesophageal reflux disease (GERD). GERD may cause changes in the esophageal epithelium, leading to Barrett esophagus, a well-established precancerous condition for esophageal adenocarcinoma. On the other hand, obesity is associated with a systemic inflammatory state, which includes the exposure to adipocytokines and procoagulant factors released by adipocytes in central fat, which may also contribute to the development of esophageal adenocarcinoma.[67] Physical activity may influence the risk of esophageal adenocarcinoma by increasing digestive track transit time, thus reducing exposure of the esophagus to putative cancer-causing agents.

KIDNEY/RENAL CELL CANCER

Physical activity has been studied in relation to renal cell carcinoma in part because of the known deleterious effects of high BMI and hypertension on the risk of renal cell cancer; however, no association has been firmly established. A review of physical activity and risk of genitourinary cancers noted significant protective effects in 8 of 15 studies of physical activity in relation to renal cell carcinoma, with an average 8% reduction in risk when comparing individuals with the highest level of physical activity to those with the lowest level of activity.[69] Reductions in risk were greater for recreational than for other forms of activity and for activity performed later in life.

Obesity, in addition to high blood pressure and diabetes, is an established risk factor for kidney cancer.[26] It is still uncertain whether a gender difference exists, however. A meta-analysis has suggested a similar impact of BMI on kidney cancer risk among women and men, with an approximate 7% increase in risk per unit increase in BMI.[26] The effect of obesity may differ by histology; a recent study reported an increased risk observed for clear cell and chromophobe cancers, but not papillary renal cell cancer.[70]

PANCREATIC CANCER

Pancreatic cancer is generally diagnosed at an advanced stage and is associated with high mortality rates. A meta-analysis of 28 studies of pancreatic cancer showed that higher total lifetime physical activity and occupational activity were associated with a lower risk.[71] Nonsignificant reductions in risk were observed for recreational physical activity and transportation (walking and cycling as a form of commuting). Significant heterogeneity was present across the studies, making it difficult to find a definitive answer.

Evidence indicating that obesity is a risk factor for pancreatic cancer is convincing. Three large pooled analyses and three of four meta-analyses that encompass a range of well-designed, independent observational epidemiologic studies have demonstrated a positive association between obesity and pancreatic cancer risk.[72,73] Effects were relatively consistent across studies, with an approximate 10% or greater increase in risk for every 5 kg/m^2 increase in BMI. Two of the pooled analyses and one of the meta-analyses assessed measures of adiposity such as waist circumference or waist-to-hip ratio (WHR); each of the results suggested positive associations with pancreatic cancer risk.[72,74,75] The pooled analyses reported at least a 35% greater risk when the fourth quartile of WHR was compared to the first quartile. The meta-analysis study reported an 11% increase in risk associated with each 10-cm increase in waist circumference and a 19% increase in risk for each 0.1-unit increment in WHR.

GALLBLADDER CANCER

Gallbladder cancer occurs more frequently in women than in men, and the major risk factor is a history of gallstones,[10] which has been associated with the use of exogenous estrogens.[76] To date, we have found no epidemiologic literature investigating the possible association of physical activity and gallbladder cancer, although several studies have suggested a positive association between obesity and gallbladder cancer. In a meta-analysis comprised of 3,288 cases derived from eight cohort studies and three case-control studies, obesity was associated with a 66% increased risk of gallbladder cancer, and the increase in risk was larger for women than for men.[77] Further, two studies found that WHR was positively associated with gallbladder cancer risk among men and women with and without a history of gallstones, suggesting that abdominal obesity may be important in the etiology of this disease.[78,79]

NON-HODGKIN LYMPHOMA

Studies addressing physical inactivity and obesity as potential risk factors for NHL have been mixed, in part because they have not had a sufficient number of cases to assess risk by NHL subtype. Generally, studies have shown no overall association between physical activity and NHL risk.[4] The results of four cohort studies, the CTS,[80] WHI,[81] EPIC,[82] and the American Cancer Society Prevention Study-II[83] have been unconvincing, with WHI showing a nonstatistically significant positive association, whereas the other studies showed no association.

In 2008, the International Lymphoma Epidemiology Consortium (InterLymph) published a pooled analysis of 18 case-control studies with more than 10,000 cases reporting no association between BMI around the time of diagnosis and NHL risk overall, but an increased risk of diffuse NHL for severe obesity (BMI ≥40 kg/m^2).[84] The results from meta-analyses of cohort studies suggested a weak positive association overall and for diffuse NHL.[85,86] An analysis of two cohort studies has suggested that body size in early adulthood may be more predictive of NHL risk than that later in life for all NHL and for the diffuse and follicular subtypes.[87]

PROSTATE CANCER

More than 20 studies have assessed the potential association between physical activity and prostate cancer.[4,88,89] Regardless of the different approaches used, the populations studied, or the sample sizes of the studies, the majority of studies have suggested a modest reduction in risk with an increased level of physical activity.[4] In a review of the literature, Friedenreich and Orenstein[88] concluded that prostate cancer risk is reduced 10% to 30% when comparing the most active with the least active men and suggested that it may be high levels of physical activity earlier in life that are most relevant to this disease. An update to this review, based on 22 additional studies, indicates that the majority of recent research studies observed protective effects.[90] Leitzmann and Rohrmann[91] added that the associations with reduced risk may be most apparent for fatal prostate cancer. A current systematic review and meta-analysis, including 19 cohort and 24 case-control studies, agrees.[92] A pooled 19% reduction in risk was observed for occupational physical activity, and a 5% reduction was observed for recreational physical activity comparing the most physically active men to the least active.[92] An issue that somewhat reduces our confidence in these estimates is that considerable heterogeneity between studies was observed. Further, it is not yet clear whether these results reflect a true causal association or whether they are due to confounding by prostate-specific antigen testing, which may be more common among physically active men.

The early epidemiologic literature on the potential association between obesity and prostate cancer provided no consistent evidence of any relationship.[4] Recent studies have suggested that obesity may have a dual effect on prostate cancer risk. One meta-analysis reported that the risk of early-stage prostate cancer decreased by 6%, whereas the risk of advanced prostate cancer increased 9% per 5-kg/m² increase in BMI.[93] Another possibility is that obesity may decrease the likelihood of diagnosis of less aggressive prostate cancer. Proposed mechanisms include the paradoxical effects of testosterone on low-grade versus more advanced prostate cancer and alterations in insulin and circulating IGF-1.[94]

LUNG CANCER

Physical activity may reduce lung cancer risk by 30% to 40%,[88] but no definitive conclusion can be drawn because one cannot ignore potential residual confounding or effect modification due to smoking as an explanation for any observed association. Recent studies have attempted to address this issue by estimating risk within subgroups defined by smoking status. A recent review suggests an inverse relationship between heavy lifetime physical activity and lung cancer in former and current smokers that is consistent across all histologies, but is not observed among never smokers.[5] A small case-control study of current and former smokers enrolled in the Cologne Smoking Study came to a similar conclusion, observing a lower risk of lung cancer among participants who were physically active compared to those who were not.[95] In the large NIH–AARP Diet and Health Study, no associations were observed between occupational or recreation physical activity and lung cancer risk among those who never smoked.[96]

Due to sex differences in lung cancer pathology, risk factors, and prognosis, current research has also begun to investigate the association for men and women separately.[97] The recent literature consists of small case-control studies,[98] which lack statistical power to examine risks in subgroups defined by histology, smoking status, or sex, and which may be affected by survival bias in that rapidly fatal cases or those who are too ill to be interviewed are excluded from the study population.

Several studies have suggested the existence of an inverse association between increasing BMI and lung cancer risk.[99–102] Nevertheless, this inverse effect may have been due to residual confounding by smoking because the inverse association was restricted to ever smokers. One meta-analysis showed an inverse association between BMI and lung cancer in nonsmokers[103]; however, caution should be exercised when interpreting the results due to concerns about heterogeneity of risk estimates across studies, the quality of the original studies, and confounding by smoking.[104]

OVARIAN CANCER

The literature on ovarian cancer risk in relation to physical activity and obesity has been inconclusive. More than 18 studies have assessed the impact of physical activity on ovarian cancer risk. A meta-analysis of 12 studies found an approximate 20% decrease in ovarian cancer risk associated with physical activity when the highest category of exercise was compared to the lowest.[105] Four[106–109] of five[110] additional studies found no association; the fifth study found a nonsignificant 10% to 20% reduction in ovarian cancer risk for women who participated in at least 1 hour per week of recreational aerobic activity.

The evidence for an association between obesity and increased ovarian cancer risk is weak, with few studies showing a statistically significant result.[4,111] A meta-analysis of 16 studies indicated that adult obesity increases the risk for ovarian cancer; the overall pooled effect estimate was a 30% increase in ovarian cancer risk associated with adult obesity with a possible dose-response effect, but no variation in risk estimates across histologic subtypes.[111] In contrast, the results from the Ovarian Cancer Association Consortium, based on original data from 15 case-control studies, suggest that obesity only increases the risk of the less common histologic subtypes of ovarian cancer; obesity does not increase risk of high-grade invasive serous cancers, the most common subtype.[112] A pooled analysis of 12 cohort studies reported that BMI was not associated with ovarian cancer risk in postmenopausal women, but was positively associated with risk in premenopausal women.[113] Another meta-analysis, using 47 studies, showed that the positive association between BMI and ovarian cancer was restricted to women who had never used hormone therapy; among these women, risk increased by 10% with every 5 kg/m² increase in BMI.[114]

CONCLUSIONS

Table 10.1 illustrates the strength of evidence regarding increased physical activity as a protective factor and obesity as a risk factor

TABLE 10.1

Summary of the Strength of the Observational Epidemiologic Evidence for Physical Activity as a Protective Factor and Obesity as a Risk Factor for Cancer, By Type of Cancer

	Physical Activity	Overweight/Obesity
Breast, postmenopausal	+++	+++
Breast, premenopausal	++	++ (protection)
Colon	+++	+++
Endometrium	+	+++
Esophagus, adenocarcinoma	?	+++
Kidney/renal cell	?	+++
Gallbladder	?	++
Pancreas	?	+++
Non-Hodgkin lymphoma	?	+
Prostate, aggressive	+	+
Lung	+	?
Ovary	?	?

+++, evidence is convincing; ++, evidence is probable; +, evidence is possible; ?, evidence remains insufficient/inconclusive.

for cancer. The strength of evidence for each exposure is classified as convincing (+++), probable (++), possible (+), or insufficient and inconclusive (?). Overall, for physical activity, convincing evidence exists for an association with postmenopausal breast cancer and colon cancer; for obesity, the evidence is convincing for breast, colon, endometrial, esophageal, and kidney/renal cell cancer. Evidence for associations between these exposures and several other cancer sites is accumulating. Despite some convincing evidence of the effects of physical activity and obesity on the risk of certain cancers, it is difficult to make recommendations as to appropriate changes in lifestyle that will reduce a person's chances of developing cancer. We have no physical activity prescriptions to give at this time. Many questions remain to be answered: What are the ages at which physical activity will provide the most benefit? What types of activity should one do and at what intensity, frequency (times per week), and duration (hours per week)? Similarly, for BMI, is there some threshold below which the individual will not have excess cancer risk? Does purposeful weight loss during the adult years lower the risk associated with being overweight or obese? Finally, necessary research is ongoing to identify the biologic mechanisms that account for these effects and to determine whether all persons are affected equally. For instance, it is possible that genetically defined subgroups of the population respond to physical activity or obesity differently. Understanding mechanisms and population variation in these effects will illuminate appropriate prescriptions for lifestyle change.

REFERENCES

1. Caspersen CJ, Powell KE, Christenson GM. Physical activity, exercise, and physical fitness: definitions and distinctions for health-related research. *Public Health Rep* 1985;100(2):126–131.
2. Flegal KM, Carroll MD, Kit BK, et al. Prevalence of obesity and trends in the distribution of body mass index among US adults, 1999-2010. *JAMA* 2012;307(5):491–497.
3. Troiano RP, Berrigan D, Dodd KW, et al. Physical activity in the United States measured by accelerometer. *Med Sci Sports Exerc* 2008;40(1):181–188.
4. Vainio H, Bianchini F, eds. *IARC Handbooks of Cancer Prevention Volume 6: Weight Control and Physical Activity*. Lyon, France: IARC Press; 2000.
5. Anzuini F, Battistella A, Izzotti A. Physical activity and cancer prevention: a review of current evidence and biological mechanisms. *J Prev Med Hyg* 2011;52(4):174–180.
6. Hardman AE. Physical activity and cancer risk. *Proc Nutr Soc* 2001;60(1):107–113.
7. Gunter MJ, Leitzmann MF. Obesity and colorectal cancer: epidemiology, mechanisms and candidate genes. *J Nutr Biochem* 2006;17(3):145–156.
8. Monninkhof EM, Elias SG, Vlems FA, et al. Physical activity and breast cancer: a systematic review. *Epidemiol* 2007;18(1):137–157.
9. World Cancer Research Fund/American Institute for Cancer Research. *Food, Nutrition, Physical Activity, and the Prevention of Cancer: A Global Perspective*. Washington, D.C.: World Cancer Research Fund/American Institute for Cancer Research; 2007.
10. Ishiguro S, Inoue M, Kurahashi N, et al. Risk factors of biliary tract cancer in a large-scale population-based cohort study in Japan (JPHC study); with special focus on cholelithiasis, body mass index, and their effect modification. *Cancer Causes Control* 2008;19(1):33–41.
11. Dallal CM, Sullivan-Halley J, Ross RK, et al. Long-term recreational physical activity and risk of invasive and in situ breast cancer: The California Teachers Study. *Arch Intern Med* 2007;167(4):408–415.
12. Lahmann P, Friedenreich C, Schuit A, et al. Physical activity and breast cancer risk: The European Prospective Investigation into Cancer and Nutrition. *Cancer Epidemiol Biomarkers Prev* 2007;16(1):36–42.
13. Maruti SS, Willett WC, Feskanich D, et al. A prospective study of age-specific physical activity and premenopausal breast cancer. *J Natl Cancer Inst* 2008;100(10):728–737.
14. Bernstein L, Henderson BE, Hanisch R, et al. Physical exercise and reduced risk of breast cancer in young women. *J Natl Cancer Inst* 1994;86(18):1403–1408.
15. Carpenter CL, Ross RK, Paganini-Hill A, et al. Effect of family history, obesity and exercise on breast cancer risk among postmenopausal women. *Int J Cancer* 2003;106(1):96–102.
16. Iwasaki M, Tsugane S. Risk factors for breast cancer: epidemiological evidence from Japanese studies. *Cancer Sci* 2011;102(9):1607–1614.
17. Pronk A, Ji BT, Shu XO, et al. Physical activity and breast cancer risk in Chinese women. *Br J Cancer* 2011;105(9):1443–1450.
18. Sanchez-Zamorano LM, Flores-Luna L, Angeles-Llerenas A, et al. Healthy lifestyle on the risk of breast cancer. *Cancer Epidemiol Biomarkers Prev* 2011;20(5):912–922.
19. Awatef M, Olfa G, Rim C, et al. Physical activity reduces breast cancer risk: a case-control study in Tunisia. *Cancer Epidemiol* 2011;35(6):540–544.
20. Sheppard VB, Makambi K, Taylor T, et al. Physical activity reduces breast cancer risk in African American women. *Ethn Dis* 2011;21(4):406–411.
21. Suzuki R, Iwasaki M, Yamamoto S, et al. Leisure-time physical activity and breast cancer risk defined by estrogen and progesterone receptor status—the Japan Public Health Center-based Prospective Study. *Prev Med* 2011;52(3-4):227–233.
22. Phipps AI, Chlebowski RT, Prentice R, et al. Body size, physical activity, and risk of triple-negative and estrogen receptor-positive breast cancer. *Cancer Epidemiol Biomarkers Prev* 2011;20(3):454–463.
23. Dieli-Conwright CM, Sullivan-Halley J, Patel A, et al. Does hormone therapy counter the beneficial effects of physical activity on breast cancer risk in postmenopausal women? *Cancer Causes Control* 2011;22(3):515–522.
24. Hildebrand JS, Gapstur SM, Campbell PT, et al. Recreational physical activity and leisure-time sitting in relation to postmenopausal breast cancer risk. *Cancer Epidemiol Biomarkers Prev* 2013;22(10):1906–1912.
25. Jung MM, Colditz GA, Collins LC, et al. Lifetime physical activity and the incidence of proliferative benign breast disease. *Cancer Causes Control* 2011;22(9):1297–1305.
26. Boeing H. Obesity and cancer—the update 2013. *Best Pract Res Clin Endocrinol Metab* 2013;27(2):219–227.
27. Lahmann PH, Schulz M, Hoffmann K, et al. Long-term weight change and breast cancer risk: The European Prospective Investigation into Cancer and Nutrition (EPIC). *Br J Cancer* 2005;93(5):582–589.
28. Harris HR, Tamimi RM, Willett WC, et al. Body size across the life course, mammographic density, and risk of breast cancer. *Am J Epidemiol* 2011;174(8):909–918.
29. Goran MI. Energy metabolism and obesity. *Med Clin North Am* 2000;84(2):347–362.
30. Frisch R, McArthur J. Menstrual cycles: fatness as a determinant of minimum weight for height necessary for their maintenance or onset. *Science* 1974;185:949–951.
31. Bernstein L. Epidemiology of endocrine-related risk factors for breast cancer. *J Mammary Gland Biol Neoplasia* 2002;7(1):3–15.
32. Bernstein L, Ross RK, Lobo RA, et al. The effects of moderate physical activity on menstrual cycle patterns in adolescence: implications for breast cancer prevention. *Br J Cancer* 1987;55(6):681–685.
33. Anderson E, Clarke RB, Howell A. Estrogen responsiveness and control of normal human breast proliferation. *J Mammary Gland Biol Neoplasia* 1998;3(1):23–35.
34. Cauley JA, Gutai JP, Kuller LH, et al. The epidemiology of serum sex hormones in postmenopausal women. *Am J Epidemiol* 1989;129(6):1120–1131.
35. MacDonald PC, Edman CD, Hemsell DL, et al. Effect of obesity on conversion of plasma androstenedione to estrone in postmenopausal women with and without endometrial cancer. *Am J Obstet Gynecol* 1978;130(4):448–455.
36. Seewaldt FL, Goldenberg V, Jones LW, et al. Overweight and obese perimenopausal and postmenopausal women exhibit increased abnormal mammary epithelial cytology. *Cancer Epidemiol Biomarkers Prev* 2007;16:613–616.
37. Bernstein L. Exercise and breast cancer prevention. *Curr Oncol Reports* 2009;11(6):490–496.
38. Neilson HK, Friedenreich CM, Brockton NT, et al. Physical activity and postmenopausal breast cancer: proposed biologic mechanisms and areas for future research. *Cancer Epidemiol Biomarkers Prev* 2009;18(1):11–27.
39. Cleary MP, Grossmann ME. Obesity and breast cancer: the estrogen connection. *Endocrinol* 2009;150(6):2537–2542.
40. Brown KA, Simpson ER. Obesity and breast cancer: progress to understanding the relationship. *Cancer Res* 2010;70(1):4–7.
41. Friedenreich CM, Neilson HK, Lynch BM. State of the epidemiological evidence on physical activity and cancer prevention. *Eur J Cancer* 2010;46(14):2593–2604.
42. Mai PL, Sullivan-Halley J, Ursin G, et al. Physical activity and colon cancer risk among women in the California Teachers Study. *Cancer Epidemiol Biomarkers Prev* 2007;16(3):517–525.
43. Wolin KY, Yan Y, Colditz GA, et al. Physical activity and colon cancer prevention: a meta-analysis. *Br J Cancer* 2009;100(4):611–616.
44. Boyle T, Keegel T, Bull F, et al. Physical activity and risks of proximal and distal colon cancers: a systematic review and meta-analysis. *J Natl Cancer Inst* 2012;104(20):1548–1561.
45. Howard RA, Freedman DM, Park Y, et al. Physical activity, sedentary behavior, and the risk of colon and rectal cancer in the NIH-AARP Diet and Health Study. *Cancer Causes Control* 2008;19(9):939–953.
46. Boyle T, Heyworth J, Bull F, et al. Timing and intensity of recreational physical activity and the risk of subsite-specific colorectal cancer. *Cancer Causes Control* 2011;22(12):1647–1658.
47. Wolin KY, Yan Y, Colditz GA. Physical activity and risk of colon adenoma: a meta-analysis. *Br J Cancer* 2011;104(5):882–885.
48. Pischon T, Lahmann PH, Boeing H, et al. Body size and risk of colon and rectal cancer in the European Prospective Investigation Into Cancer and Nutrition (EPIC). *J Natl Cancer Inst* 2006;98(13):920–931.
49. Aleksandrova K, Pischon T, Buijsse B, et al. Adult weight change and risk of colorectal cancer in the European Prospective Investigation into Cancer and Nutrition. *Eur J Cancer* 2013;49(16):3526–3536.
50. Nimptsch K, Giovannucci E, Willett WC, et al. Body fatness during childhood and adolescence, adult height, and risk of colorectal adenoma in women. *Cancer Prev Res* 2011;4(10):1710–1718.

51. Hughes LA, Simons CC, van den Brandt PA, et al. Body size and colorectal cancer risk after 16.3 years of follow-up: an analysis from the Netherlands Cohort Study. *Am J Epidemiol* 2011;174(10):1127–1139.
52. Abate N. Insulin resistance and obesity. The role of fat distribution pattern. *Diabetes Care* 1996;19(3):292–294.
53. Calle EE, Kaaks R. Overweight, obesity and cancer: epidemiological evidence and proposed mechanisms. *Nat Rev Cancer* 2004;4(8):579–591.
54. Gierach GL, Chang SC, Brinton LA, et al. Physical activity, sedentary behavior, and endometrial cancer risk in the NIH-AARP Diet and Health Study. *Int J Cancer* 2009;124(9):2139–2147.
55. Voskuil DW, Monninkhof EM, Elias SG, et al. Physical activity and endometrial cancer risk, a systematic review of current evidence. *Cancer Epidemiol Biomarkers Prev* 2007;16(4):639–648.
56. Cust AE, Armstrong BK, Friedenreich CM, et al. Physical activity and endometrial cancer risk: a review of the current evidence, biologic mechanisms and the quality of physical activity assessment methods. *Cancer Causes Control* 2007;18(3):243–258.
57. Friedenreich C, Cust A, Lahmann PH, et al. Physical activity and risk of endometrial cancer: The European Prospective Investigation into Cancer and Nutrition. *Int J Cancer* 2007;121(2):347–355.
58. Patel AV, Feigelson HS, Talbot JT, et al. The role of body weight in the relationship between physical activity and endometrial cancer: results from a large cohort of US women. *Int J Cancer* 2008;123(8):1877–1882.
59. Moore SC, Gierach GL, Schatzkin A, et al. Physical activity, sedentary behaviours, and the prevention of endometrial cancer. *Br J Cancer* 2010;103(7):933–938.
60. Dieli-Conwright CM, Ma H, Lacey JV, Jr., et al. Long-term and baseline recreational physical activity and risk of endometrial cancer: The California Teachers Study. *Br J Cancer* 2013;109(3):761–768.
61. Kaaks R, Lukanova A, Kurzer MS. Obesity, endogenous hormones, and endometrial cancer risk: a synthetic review. *Cancer Epidemiol Biomarkers Prev* 2002;11(12):1531–1543.
62. Zhang ZF, Kurtz RC, Sun M, et al. Adenocarcinomas of the esophagus and gastric cardia: medical conditions, tobacco, alcohol, and socioeconomic factors. *Cancer Epidemiol Biomarkers Prev* 1996;5(10):761–768.
63. Lagergren J, Bergstrom R, Nyren O. Association between body mass and adenocarcinoma of the esophagus and gastric cardia. *Ann Intern Med* 1999;130(11):883–890.
64. Vigen C, Bernstein L, Wu AH. Occupational physical activity and risk of adenocarcinomas of the esophagus and stomach. *Int J Cancer* 2006;118(4):1004–1009.
65. Leitzmann MF, Koebnick C, Freedman ND, et al. Physical activity and esophageal and gastric carcinoma in a large prospective study. *Am J Prev Med* 2009;36(2):112–119.
66. Lepage C, Drouillard A, Jouve JL, et al. Epidemiology and risk factors for oesophageal adenocarcinoma. *Dig Liver Dis* 2013;45(8):625–629.
67. Ryan AM, Duong M, Healy L, et al. Obesity, metabolic syndrome and esophageal adenocarcinoma: epidemiology, etiology and new targets. *Cancer Epidemiol* 2011;35(4):309–319.
68. Hoyo C, Cook MB, Kamangar F, et al. Body mass index in relation to oesophageal and oesophagogastric junction adenocarcinomas: a pooled analysis from the International BEACON Consortium. *Int J Epidemiol* 2012;41(6):1706–1718.
69. Leitzmann MF. Physical activity and genitourinary cancer prevention. *Recent Results Cancer Res* 2011;186:43–71.
70. Purdue MP, Moore LE, Merino MJ, et al. An investigation of risk factors for renal cell carcinoma by histologic subtype in two case-control studies. *Int J Cancer* 2013;132(11):2640–2647.
71. O'Rorke MA, Cantwell MM, Cardwell CR, et al. Can physical activity modulate pancreatic cancer risk? A systematic review and meta-analysis. *Int J Cancer* 2010;126(12):2957–2968.
72. Aune D, Greenwood DC, Chan DS, et al. Body mass index, abdominal fatness and pancreatic cancer risk: a systematic review and non-linear dose-response meta-analysis of prospective studies. *Ann Oncol* 2012;23(4):843–852.
73. Bracci PM. Obesity and pancreatic cancer: overview of epidemiologic evidence and biologic mechanisms. *Mol Carcinog* 2012;51(1):53–63.
74. Arslan AA, Helzlsouer KJ, Kooperberg C, et al. Anthropometric measures, body mass index, and pancreatic cancer: a pooled analysis from the Pancreatic Cancer Cohort Consortium (PanScan). *Arch Intern Med* 2010;170(9):791–802.
75. Genkinger JM, Spiegelman D, Anderson KE, et al. A pooled analysis of 14 cohort studies of anthropometric factors and pancreatic cancer risk. *Int J Cancer* 2010;129(7):1708–1717.
76. Uhler ML, Marks JW, Judd HL. Estrogen replacement therapy and gallbladder disease in postmenopausal women. *Menopause* 2000;7(3):162–167.
77. Larsson SC, Wolk A. Obesity and the risk of gallbladder cancer: a meta-analysis. *Br J Cancer* 2007;96(9):1457–1461.
78. Hsing AW, Sakoda LC, Rashid A, et al. Body size and the risk of biliary tract cancer: a population-based study in China. *Br J Cancer* 2008;99(5):811–815.
79. Schlesinger S, Aleksandrova K, Pischon T, et al. Abdominal obesity, weight gain during adulthood and risk of liver and biliary tract cancer in a European cohort. *Int J Cancer* 2013;132(3):645–657.
80. Lu Y, Prescott J, Sullivan-Halley J, et al. Body size, recreational physical activity, and B-cell non-Hodgkin lymphoma risk among women in the California Teachers Study. *Am J Epidemiol* 2009;170(10):1231–1240.
81. Kabat GC, Kim MY, Jean Wactawski W, et al. Anthropometric factors, physical activity, and risk of non-Hodgkin's lymphoma in the Women's Health Initiative. *Cancer Epidemiol* 2012;36(1):52–59.
82. van Veldhoven CM, Khan AE, Teucher B, et al. Physical activity and lymphoid neoplasms in the European Prospective Investigation into Cancer and Nutrition (EPIC). *Eur J Cancer* 2011;47(5):748–760.
83. Teras LR, Gapstur SM, Diver WR, et al. Recreational physical activity, leisure sitting time and risk of non-Hodgkin lymphoid neoplasms in the American Cancer Society Cancer Prevention Study II Cohort. *Int J Cancer* 2012;131(8):1912–1920.
84. Willett EV, Morton LM, Hartge P, et al. Non-Hodgkin lymphoma and obesity: a pooled analysis from the InterLymph Consortium. *Int J Cancer* 2008;122(9):2062–2070.
85. Larsson SC, Wolk A. Body mass index and risk of non-Hodgkin's and Hodgkin's lymphoma: a meta-analysis of prospective studies. *Eur J Cancer* 2011;47(16):2422–2430.
86. Larsson SC, Wolk A. Obesity and risk of non-Hodgkin's lymphoma: a meta-analysis. *Int J Cancer* 2007;121(7):1564–1570.
87. Bertrand KA, Giovannucci E, Zhang SM, et al. A prospective analysis of body size during childhood, adolescence, and adulthood and risk of non-Hodgkin lymphoma. *Cancer Prev Res* 2013;6(8):864–873.
88. Friedenreich CM, Orenstein MR. Physical activity and cancer prevention: Etiologic evidence and biological mechanisms. *J Nutr* 2002;132(11 Suppl):3456S–3464S.
89. Friedenreich CM, McGregor SE, Courneya KS, et al. Case-control study of lifetime total physical activity and prostate cancer risk. *Am J Epidemiol* 2004;159(8):740–749.
90. Young-McCaughan S. Potential for prostate cancer prevention through physical activity. *World J Urol* 2012;30(2):167–179.
91. Leitzmann MF, Rohrmann S. Risk factors for the onset of prostatic cancer: age, location, and behavioral correlates. *Clin Epidemiol* 2012;4:1–11.
92. Liu Y, Hu F, Li D, et al. Does physical activity reduce the risk of prostate cancer? A systematic review and meta-analysis. *Eur Urol* 2011;60(5):1029–1044.
93. Discacciati A, Orsini N, Wolk A. Body mass index and incidence of localized and advanced prostate cancer—a dose-response meta-analysis of prospective studies. *Ann Oncol* 2012;23(7):1665–1671.
94. Rodriguez C, Freedland SJ, Deka A, et al. Body mass index, weight change, and risk of prostate cancer in the Cancer Prevention Study II Nutrition Cohort. *Cancer Epidemiol Biomarkers Prev* 2007;16(1):63–69.
95. Schmidt A, Jung J, Ernstmann N, et al. The association between active participation in a sports club, physical activity and social network on the development of lung cancer in smokers: a case-control study. *BMC Res Notes* 2012;5:2.
96. Lam TK, Moore SC, Brinton LA, et al. Anthropometric measures and physical activity and the risk of lung cancer in never-smokers: a prospective cohort study. *PLoS One* 2013;8(8):e70672.
97. Tardon A, Lee WJ, Delgado-Rodriguez M, et al. Leisure-time physical activity and lung cancer: a meta-analysis. *Cancer Causes Control* 2005;16(4):389–397.
98. Lin Y, Cai L. Environmental and dietary factors and lung cancer risk among Chinese women: a case-control study in Southeast China. *Nutr Cancer* 2012;64(4):508–514.
99. Bethea TN, Rosenberg L, Charlot M, et al. Obesity in relation to lung cancer incidence in African American women. *Cancer Causes Control* 2013;24(9):1695–1703.
100. Smith L, Brinton LA, Spitz MR, et al. Body mass index and risk of lung cancer among never, former, and current smokers. *J Natl Cancer Inst* 2012;104(10):778–789.
101. Andreotti G, Hou L, Beane Freeman LE, et al. Body mass index, agricultural pesticide use, and cancer incidence in the Agricultural Health Study cohort. *Cancer Causes Control* 2010;21(11):1759–1775.
102. Tarnaud C, Guida F, Papadopoulos A, et al. Body mass index and lung cancer risk: results from the ICARE Study, a large, population-based case-control study. *Cancer Causes Control* 2012;23(7):1113–1126.
103. Yang Y, Dong J, Sun K, et al. Obesity and incidence of lung cancer: a meta-analysis. *Int J Cancer* 2013;132(5):1162–1169.
104. El-Zein M, Parent ME, Rousseau MC. Comments on a recent meta-analysis: obesity and lung cancer. *Int J Cancer* 2012;132(8):1962–1963.
105. Olsen CM, Bain CJ, Jordan SJ, et al. Recreational physical activity and epithelial ovarian cancer: A case-control study, systematic review, and meta-analysis. *Cancer Epidemiol Biomarkers Prev* 2007;16(11):2321–2330.
106. Weiderpass E, Margolis KL, Sandin S, et al. Prospective study of physical activity in different periods of life and the risk of ovarian cancer. *Int J Cancer* 2006;118(12):3153–3160.
107. Lahmann PH, Friedenreich C, Schulz M, et al. Physical activity and ovarian cancer risk: The European Prospective Investigation into Cancer and Nutrition. *Cancer Epidemiol Biomarkers Prev* 2009;18(1):351–354.
108. Leitzmann MF, Koebnick C, Moore SC, et al. Prospective study of physical activity and the risk of ovarian cancer. *Cancer Causes Control* 2009;20(5):765–773.
109. Xiao Q, Yang HP, Wentzensen N, et al. Physical activity in different periods of life, sedentary behavior, and the risk of ovarian cancer in the NIH-AARP Diet and Health Study. *Cancer Epidemiol Biomarkers Prev* 2013;22(11):2000–2008.
110. Moorman PG, Jones LW, Akushevich L, et al. Recreational physical activity and ovarian cancer risk and survival. *Ann Epidemiol* 2011;21(3):178–187.
111. Olsen CM, Green AC, Whiteman DC, et al. Obesity and the risk of epithelial ovarian cancer: a systematic review and meta-analysis. *Eur J Cancer* 2007;43(4):690–709.
112. Olsen CM, Nagle CM, Whiteman DC, et al. Obesity and risk of ovarian cancer subtypes: evidence from the Ovarian Cancer Association Consortium. *Endocr Relat Cancer* 2013;20(2):251–262.
113. Schouten LJ, Rivera C, Hunter DJ, et al. Height, body mass index, and ovarian cancer: a pooled analysis of 12 cohort studies. *Cancer Epidemiol Biomarkers Prev* 2008;17(4):902–912.
114. Collaborative Group on Epidemiological Studies of Ovarian Cancer. Ovarian cancer and body size: individual participant meta-analysis including 25,157 women with ovarian cancer from 47 epidemiological studies. *PLoS Med* 2012;9(4):e1001200.

Section 2 Epidemiology of Cancer

11 Epidemiologic Methods

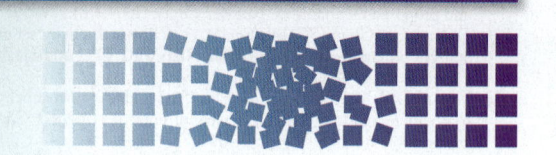

Xiaomei Ma and Herbert Yu

INTRODUCTION

Epidemiology is the study of the distribution and determinants of health-related states or events in specified populations and the application of this study to control health problems.[1] Epidemiologic principles and methods have long been applied to cancer research, with the assumptions that cancer does not occur at random and the nonrandomness of carcinogenesis can be elucidated through systematic research. An example of such applications is the lung cancer study conducted by Doll and Hill in the early 1950s, which linked tobacco smoking to an increased mortality of lung cancer in over 40,000 medical professionals in the United Kingdom.[2] The observation from this study and many other studies, in conjunction with laboratory findings regarding the underlying biologic mechanisms for the effect of tobacco smoking, helped establish the role of tobacco smoking in the etiology of lung cancer. Epidemiologic methods are also used in clinical settings, where trials are conducted to evaluate the efficacy of new treatment protocols or preventive measures and where observational studies of prognostic factors are done.

Epidemiologic studies can take different forms, but generally they can be classified into two broad categories, observational studies and experimental studies (Fig. 11.1). In experimental studies, an investigator allocates different study regimens to the subjects, usually with randomization (experimental studies without randomization are sometimes referred to as "quasi-experiments").[3] Experimental studies can be individual based or community based. An experimental study most closely resembles laboratory experiments in that the investigator has control over the study condition. Experimental studies can be used to evaluate the efficacy of a treatment protocol (e.g., low-dose compared with standard-dose chemotherapy for non-Hodgkin's lymphoma)[4] or preventive measures (e.g., tamoxifen for women at an increased risk of breast cancer).[5] Although experimental studies are often considered the "gold standard" because of well-controlled study situations, they are only suitable for the evaluation of effects that are beneficial or at least not harmful due to ethical concerns. Experimental studies are discussed in detail in other chapters of this book. This section will focus on observational studies.

Observational studies do not involve the artificial manipulation of study regimens. In an observational study, an investigator stands by to observe what happens or happened to the subjects, in terms of exposure and outcome. Observational studies can be further divided into descriptive and analytical studies (see Fig. 11.1). Descriptive studies focus on the *distribution* of diseases with respect to person, place, and time (i.e., who, where, and when), whereas analytical studies focus on the *determinants* of diseases. Descriptive studies are often used to *generate* hypotheses, whereas analytical studies are often used to *test* hypotheses. However, the two types of studies should not be considered mutually exclusive entities; rather, they are the opposite ends of a continuum. Descriptive studies are discussed in detail in other chapters of this book.

ANALYTICAL STUDIES

Ecologic Studies

As in experimental studies, the unit of analysis can be individuals or groups of people in observational studies. Studies that use groups of people as the unit of analysis are called ecologic studies, which are relatively easy to carry out when group level measures are available. However, a relationship observed between variables on a group level does not necessarily reflect the relationship that exists at an individual level. For example, the fraction of energy supply from animal products was found to be positively correlated with breast cancer mortality in a recent ecologic study, which used preexisting data on both dietary supply and breast cancer mortality rates from 35 countries.[6] Because the data were country based, no reliable inference can be made at an individual level. Within each country, it could be that the people who had a low fraction of energy supply from animal products were actually dying from breast cancer. Results from ecologic studies are useful for inference at an individual level only when the within-group variability of the exposure is low so that a group-level measure can reasonably reflect exposure at an individual level. Alternatively, if the implications for prevention or intervention are at a group level (e.g., taxation of cigarettes to reduce smoking), results from ecologic studies are very useful.

Cross-Sectional Studies

There are three main types of analytical studies in which the unit of analysis is individuals: cross-sectional, cohort, and case-control studies. In a cross-sectional study, the information on various factors is collected from the study population at a given point in time. From a public health perspective, data collected in cross-sectional studies can be of great value in assessing the general health status of a population and allocating resources. For example, the National Health and Nutrition Examination Survey has provided valuable national estimates of health and nutritional status of the US civilian, noninstitutionalized population.[7] Findings from cross-sectional studies can also help generate hypotheses that may be tested later in other types of studies. However, it should be noted that cross-sectional studies have serious methodologic limitations if the research purpose is etiologic inference. Because exposures and disease status are evaluated simultaneously, it is usually not possible to know the temporality of events unless the exposure cannot change over time (e.g., blood type, skin color, race, country of birth). If one observes that more brain cancer patients are depressed than people without brain cancer in a cross-sectional study, the correlation does not necessarily mean that depression causes brain cancer. Depression may simply have resulted from the pathogenesis and diagnosis of brain cancer, or depression may

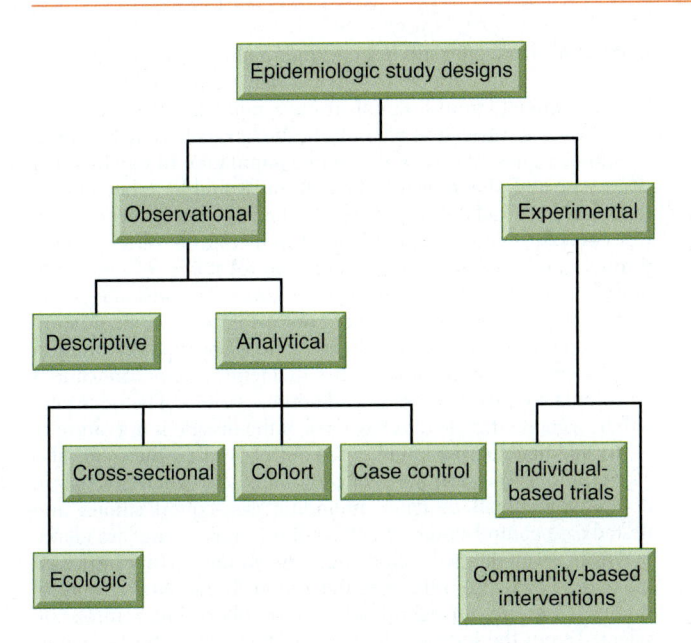

Figure 11.1 Classification of epidemiologic study designs.

have caused brain cancer in some patients and resulted from brain cancer in other patients. Without additional information on the timing of events, no conclusions can be made. Another concern in cross-sectional studies is the enrollment of prevalent cases, who survived different lengths of time after the incidence of disease. Factors that affect survival may also influence incidence. Prevalent cases may not be representative of incident cases, which makes etiologic inferences based on cross-sectional studies suspect at best.

Cohort Studies

In a cohort study, a study population free of a specific disease (or any other health-related condition) is grouped based on their exposure status and followed up for a certain period of time. Then the exposed and unexposed subjects are compared with respect to disease status at the end of the follow-up. The objective of a cohort study is usually to evaluate whether the incidence of a disease is associated with an exposure. The cohort design is fundamental in observational epidemiology and is considered "ideal" in that, if unbiased, cohort data reflect the real-life cause/effect sequence of disease.[8] Subjects in cohort studies may be a sample of the general population in a geographic area, a group of workers who are exposed to certain occupational hazards in a specific industry, or people who are considered at a high risk for a specific disease. A cohort study is considered prospective or concurrent if the investigator starts following up the cohort from the present time into the future, and retrospective or historical if the cohort is established in the past based on existing records (e.g., an occupational cohort based on employment records) and the follow-up ends before or at the time of the study. Alternatively, a cohort study can be ambidirectional in that data collection goes both directions.[9] Whether a cohort study is prospective, retrospective, or ambidirectional, the key feature is that all the subjects were free of the disease at the beginning of the follow-up and the study tracks the subjects from exposure to disease. Follow-up time, ranging from days to decades, is an essential element in cohort studies.

In a cohort study, the incidence of disease in the exposed group and the unexposed group is compared. The incidence measure can be cumulative incidence or incidence density, depending on the availability of data. When comparing the incidence in the two groups, both relative differences and absolute differences can be assessed. In cohort studies, the relative risk of developing the disease is expressed as the ratio of the cumulative incidence in the exposed group to that in the unexposed group, which is also called cumulative incidence ratio or risk ratio. If we have data on the exact person-time of follow-up for every subject, we can also calculate an incidence density ratio (also called rate ratio) in a similar way. The numeric value of the risk or rate ratio reflects the magnitude of the association between an exposure and a disease. For example, a risk ratio of 2 would be interpreted as exposed individuals have a doubled risk of developing a disease than unexposed individuals, whereas a risk ratio of 5 indicates that exposed individuals have 5 times the risk of developing a disease compared with unexposed individuals. To put in another way, a factor with a risk ratio of 5 has a stronger effect than another factor with a risk ratio of 2. In addition to risk ratio and rate ratio, another relative measure called probability odds ratio can be calculated in cohort studies. The probability odds of disease is the number of subjects who developed a disease divided by the number of subjects who did not develop the disease, and the probability odds ratio is the probability odds in the exposed group divided by the probability odds in the unexposed group. Many investigators prefer risk ratio or rate ratio to probability odds ratio in cohort studies, because the ability to directly measure the risk of developing a disease is one of the most significant advantages in cohort studies. In practice, however, a probability odds ratio is often used as an approximation for risk or rate ratio, especially when multivariate logistic regression models are employed to adjust for the effect of other factors that may influence the relationship between an exposure and a disease.

As for absolute differences, a commonly used measure is called attributable risk in the exposed, which is the incidence in the exposed group minus the incidence in the unexposed group. Attributable risk reflects the disease incidence that could be attributed to the exposure in exposed individuals and the reduction in incidence that we would expect if the exposure can be removed from the exposed individuals, provided that there is a causal relationship between the exposure and the disease. Another absolute measure called population attributable risk extends this concept to the general population; it estimates the disease incidence that could be attributed to an exposure in the general population. Because both relative and absolute differences can be assessed in cohort studies, a natural question to ask is what measures to choose. In general, the relative differences are used more often if the main research objective is etiologic inference, and they can be used for the judgment of causality. Once causality is established, or at least assumed, measures of absolute differences are more important from a public health perspective. This point can be illustrated using the following hypothetical example. Assume the following: toxin X in the environment triples the risk of bladder cancer and toxin Y doubles the risk of bladder cancer, the effects of X and Y are entirely independent of each other, the prevalence of exposure to toxin Y in the general population is 20 times higher than the prevalence of exposure to toxin X, and there are only resources available to reduce the exposure to one toxin. It would be more effective to use the resources to reduce the exposure to toxin Y instead of toxin X. This is because the population attributable risk due to Y is higher than that due to X, although the risk ratio associated with toxin Y is smaller than that associated with toxin X.

Cohort studies have many advantages. A cohort design is the best way to study the natural history of a disease.[9] There is usually a clear temporal relationship between an exposure and a disease because all the subjects are free of the disease at the beginning of the follow-up (it can be a problem if a subject has a subclinical disease such as undetected prostate cancer). Furthermore, multiple diseases can be studied with respect to the same exposure. On the other hand, cohort studies, especially prospective cohort studies, are costly in terms of both time and money. A cohort design requires the follow-up of a large number of study participants over a sometimes extremely lengthy period of time and usually extensive data collection through questionnaires, physical measurements, and/or biologic specimens at regular intervals. Participants may be "lost" during the follow-up because they became tired of the study, moved away from the study area, or died from some causes other than the disease under study. If the subjects who were lost during the follow-up are different from those who remained under observation with respect to exposure, disease, or other factors that may influence the relationship between the exposure and the disease, results from the study may be biased. To date, cohort studies have been used to study the etiology of a wide spectrum of diseases, including different types of cancer. If a cohort study is conducted to evaluate the etiology of cancer, usually the study sample size would need to be very large (such as the National Institutes of Health-AARP Diet and Health Study, which included more than half million subjects[10]) and the follow-up time would need to be long, unless the cohort selected is a high-risk population.

For simplicity, we have discussed cohort studies in which the outcome of interest is the incidence of a specific disease and there are only two exposure groups. In practice, any health-related event can be the outcome of interest, and multiple exposure groups can be compared.

Case-Control Studies

Case-control design is an alternative to cohort design for the evaluation of the relationship between an exposure and a disease (or any other health condition). A case-control approach compares the odds of past exposure between cases and noncases (controls) and uses the exposure odds ratio as an estimate for relative risk. A primary goal in a case-control study is to reach the same conclusions as what would have been obtained from a cohort study, if one had been done.[11] If appropriately designed and conducted, a case-control study can optimize speed and efficiency as the need for follow-up is avoided.[8] The starting point of a case-control study is a source population from which the cases arise. Instead of obtaining the denominators for the calculation of risks or rates in a cohort study, a control group is sampled from the entire source population. After selecting control subjects, who ideally would have become cases had they developed the disease, an investigator collects data on past exposures from both the cases and the controls and then calculates an odds ratio, which is the odds of exposure in the cases divided by the odds of exposure in the controls.

There are two main types of case-control studies: case-based case-control studies and case-control studies within defined cohorts.[8] Some variations of the case-control design also exist. For instance, if the effect of an exposure is transient, sometimes a case can be used as his/her own control (case cross-over design). In case-based case-control studies, cases and controls are selected at a given point in time from a hypothetical cohort (e.g., at the end of follow-up). A cross-sectional ascertainment of cases will result in a case group that mostly contains prevalent cases who may have survived for different lengths of time after disease incidence. Cases who died before an investigator began subject ascertainment would not be eligible to be included in the study. As a result, the cases finally included in the study may not be representative of all the cases from the entire hypothetical cohort. Another disadvantage of enrolling prevalent cases is that cases that were diagnosed a long time ago will likely have difficulties recalling exposures that occurred before the disease incidence. In case-control studies, it is preferable to ascertain incident cases as soon as they are diagnosed and to select controls as soon as cases are identified. Case-control studies that enroll only incident cases are sometimes called *prospective* case-control studies because the investigators need to wait for the incident cases to develop and get diagnosed. For cancer studies, the cases can be ascertained from population-based cancer registries or hospitals. A major advantage of using a cancer registry is the completeness of case ascertainment; however, the reporting of cancer cases to registries is usually not instantaneous. There could be a lag time of several months or even over a year, and some cases could have died during the lag time. If the cancer under study has a poor survival rate and/or clinical specimens need to be obtained in a timely manner, it may be preferable to identify cases directly from hospitals using a rapid ascertainment protocol. As for the selection of controls, the key issue is that controls should be representative of the source population from which the cases arise and, theoretically, the controls would have been ascertained as cases had they developed the disease. The most common types of controls include population-based controls (often selected through random digit dialing in case-control studies of cancer etiology), hospital controls, and friend controls. The advantages and disadvantages of different types of controls have been nicely summarized by Wacholder et al.[12] Because no follow-up is involved in case-based case-control studies, the incidence risk or rate cannot be calculated directly for case and control groups. The odds ratio will be a good estimate of relative risk if the disease is uncommon.

In addition to case-based case-control studies, there are also case-control studies within defined cohorts (also known as hybrid or ambidirectional designs), including case-cohort studies and nested case-control studies. In case-cohort studies, cases are identified from a well-defined cohort after some follow-up time, and controls are selected from the baseline cohort. In nested case-control studies, cases are also identified from a cohort, but controls are selected from the individuals at risk at the time each case occurs (i.e., incidence density sampling).[8] In these types of designs, controls are a sample of the cohort and the controls selected can theoretically become cases at some point. The possibility of selection bias in case-control studies within defined cohorts is lower than that in case-based case-control studies because the cases and the controls are selected from the same source population. Because of an increased awareness of the methodological issues inherent in the design of case-based case-control studies and the availability of a growing number of large cohorts, case-control studies within defined cohorts have become more common in recent years. The advantage of case-control studies within cohorts over traditional cohort studies is mainly the efficiency in additional data collection. For instance, a recent nested case-control study evaluated the relationship between endogenous sex hormones and prostate cancer risk.[13] Instead of measuring the serum hormones levels of the entire cohort (over 12,000 subjects), investigators chose to measure 300 cases and 300 controls selected from the cohort. Doing so not only significantly reduced the cost of measurements and the time it took to address the research question, but also helped preserve valuable serum samples for possible analyses in the future. In a case-cohort design, an odds ratio estimates risk ratio; in a nested case-control design, an odds ratio estimates rate ratio. In both designs, the disease under study does not have to be rare for the odds ratio to be a good estimate of the risk ratio or rate ratio.[8,14]

The biggest advantage of a case-control design is the speed and efficiency of obtaining data. It is claimed that investigators implement case-control studies more frequently than any other analytical epidemiologic study.[15] Because most types of cancer are uncommon and take a long time to develop, to date, most epidemiologic studies of cancer have been case-control instead of cohort in design. A case-control study can be conducted to evaluate the relationship between many different exposures and a specific disease, but the study will have limited statistical power if the exposure is rare. In general, a case-control design tends to be more susceptible to biases than a cohort design. Such biases include, but are not limited to, selection bias when choosing and enrolling subjects (especially controls) and recall bias when obtaining data from the subjects. The status of the subjects—that is, case or control—may affect how they recall and report previous exposures, some of which occurred years or even decades ago. It is important for investigators to explicitly define the diagnostic and eligibility criteria for cases, to select controls from the same population as the cases independent of the exposures of interest, to blind data collection staff to the case or control status of subjects and/or the main hypotheses of the study, to ascertain exposure in a similar manner from cases and controls, and to take into account other factors that may influence the relationship between an exposure and a disease.[15]

INTERPRETATION OF EPIDEMIOLOGIC FINDINGS

We have discussed measures of effects in various study designs. However, a risk ratio of 3 from a cohort study or an odds ratio of 2.5 from a case-control study does not necessarily mean that there is an association between an exposure and a disease. Several alternative explanations need to be assessed, including chance (random error), bias (systematic error), and confounding. Potential interaction also needs be evaluated.

Statistical methods are required to evaluate the role of chance. A usual way is to calculate the upper and lower limits of a 95% confidence interval around a point estimate for relative risk (risk ratio, rate ratio, or odds ratio). If the confidence interval does not include one, one would say that the observed association is statistically significant; if the confidence interval includes one, one would say that the observed relationship is not statistically significant. The width of a confidence interval is directly related to the number of participants in a study, which is called sample size. A larger sample size leads to less variability in the data, a tighter confidence interval, and a higher possibility in finding a statistically significant association if one truly exists. A 95% confidence interval means that if the data collection and analysis could be replicated many times, the confidence interval should include the correct value of the measure 95% of the time.[16] It is better to consider a confidence interval to be a general guide to the amount of random error in the data but not necessarily a literal measure of statistical variability.[16]

Bias can be defined as any systematic error in an epidemiologic study that results in an incorrect estimate of the association between exposure and disease, and it can occur in every type of epidemiologic study design. There are two main types of bias: selection bias and information bias. Selection bias is present when individuals included in a study are systematically different from the target population. For example, a selection bias would occur if a study aimed to generate a sample representing all women in the United States, but of the women contacted, more with a family history of breast cancer agreed to participate. This sample would be at a higher risk for breast cancer than the target population. Refusal to participate poses a constant challenge in epidemiologic studies. As individuals have become more concerned about privacy issues and as studies have become more demanding of time, biologic specimens, and other impositions, participation rates have dropped substantially in recent years. If nonparticipants are different from the participants with respect to study-related characteristics, the validity of the study is threatened. Information bias occurs when the data collected from the study subjects are erroneous. Information bias is also known as misclassification if the variable is measured on a categorical scale and the error causes a subject to be placed in a wrong category. Misclassification can happen to both exposure and disease. For example, in a case-control study of previous reproductive history and ovarian cancer, a woman who had an extremely early pregnancy loss might not even realize that she was ever pregnant and would mistakenly report no pregnancy, and another woman who has only subclinical presentations of ovarian cancer might be mistakenly selected as a control. Misclassification can be differential or nondifferential. An exposure misclassification is considered differential if it is related to disease status and nondifferential if not related to disease status. Similarly, a disease misclassification is considered differential if it is related to exposure status and nondifferential if not related to exposure status. If a binary exposure variable and a binary disease variable are analyzed, a nondifferential misclassification will result in an underestimate of the true association. Differential misclassification can either exaggerate or underestimate a true effect. Usually not much can be done to control or correct bias at the data analysis stage; therefore,

it is important to establish research protocols that are not prone to bias. The evaluation of potential bias is critical to the interpretation of study results. An invalid estimate is worse than no estimate.

Confounding refers to a situation in which the association between an exposure and a disease (or any health-related condition) is influenced by a third variable. This third variable is considered a confounding variable or confounder. A confounder must fulfill three criteria: (1) be associated with the exposure, (2) be associated with the disease independent of the exposure, and (3) not be an intermediate step between the exposure and the disease (i.e., not on the causal pathway). Unlike bias, which is primarily introduced by the investigator or study participants, confounding is a function of the complex interrelationship between various exposures and disease.[17] In a hypothetical case-control study of the effect of alcohol drinking on lung cancer, we may observe an odds ratio of 2.5 (usually called a "crude" odds ratio in the sense that no other variables were taken into account), which indicates that alcohol drinking increases the risk of lung cancer by 1.5-fold. However, if we classify all study subjects into two strata based on a history of cigarette smoking and then calculate the odds ratio in the two strata (smokers and nonsmokers) separately, we may have two stratum-specific odds ratios both equal to one, indicating that alcohol drinking is not associated with lung cancer risk. In this example, the crude odds ratio calculated to estimate the association between alcohol drinking and lung cancer without considering smoking is simply misleading. Being associated with both the exposure (i.e., alcohol drinking) and the disease (i.e., lung cancer), smoking acted as a confounder in this example. A stratified analysis is needed to evaluate the potential confounding effect of a third variable, whether it is done with pencil and paper or statistical modeling. Usually data are stratified based on the level of a third variable. If the stratum-specific effect measures are similar to each other but different from the crude effect measure, confounding is said to be present. In this section, we have illustrated basic epidemiologic principles using an overly simplified scenario and only considered a single exposure. In practice, most if not all diseases, cancer included, have a multifactorial etiology. Consequently, it is usually necessary to assess the potential confounding effect of a group of variables simultaneously using multivariate statistical models. The effect measure derived from a multivariate model will then be called an "adjusted" one in the sense that the effect of other factors was also adjusted for. Without controlling for the potential effect of other variables, an investigator cannot really judge whether an observed association between a given exposure and a specific disease is spurious.

If the effect of an exposure on the risk of a disease is not homogeneous in strata formed by a third variable, the third variable is considered an effect modifier, and the situation is called interaction or effect modification. Put in other words, interaction exists when the stratum-specific effect measures are different from each other. In the lung cancer example given previously, if the odds ratio for alcohol drinking is 1 in smokers but 3 in nonsmokers, then there is interaction and smoking is an effect modifier. The evaluation of interaction is essentially a stratified analysis, which is similar to the evaluation of confounding. Confounding and interaction can be both present in a given study. However, when interaction occurs, the stratum-specific effect measures should be reported. It is no longer appropriate to report a summary measure in the presence of interaction. Unlike confounding, which is a nuisance that an investigator hopes to remove, interaction is a more detailed description of the true relationship between an exposure and a disease.

CANCER OUTCOMES RESEARCH

The discussion of epidemiologic methods in this section focuses primarily on etiological research, which aims at identifying the risk factors of cancer. However, similar principles and methods are applicable to cancer outcomes research, which aims at studying a variety of factors related to the early identification, treatment, prognosis, health related quality of life, and cost of care. Cancer outcomes research can be experimental or observational in nature. For example, randomized clinical trials have been conducted to assess the impact of screening on prostate cancer mortality[18] and to compare the effect of radical prostatectomy versus observation in patients with localized prostate cancer.[19] Observational studies of cancer outcomes, especially those that build upon preexisting resources,[20,21] can be carried out in a large group of patients with relatively little cost to capture the patterns and cost of care and to address many other research questions that have important clinical implications. Although the findings of such observation studies are subject to bias and confounding inherent in an observational design, these studies are complementary to experimental studies and have their unique value. Given an increasing interest in improving the effectiveness and value of cancer care, more cancer outcomes research is to be expected in the future.

MOLECULAR EPIDEMIOLOGY

Molecular epidemiology involves multidisciplinary and transdisciplinary research that entails not only traditional epidemiology and biostatistics, but also genetics, molecular biology, biochemistry, cellular biology, analytical chemistry, toxicology, pharmacology, and laboratory medicine. Unlike traditional epidemiology research of cancer, which focuses on exposures or risk factors ascertained through questionnaire-based interviews or surveys, molecular epidemiology studies expand the assessment of exposure to a much broader scope that includes an analysis of biomarkers underlying internal exposure of exogenous and endogenous carcinogenic agents or risk factors, molecular alterations in response to exposure, and genetic susceptibility to cancer. The biomarkers often measured in molecular epidemiology research include DNA, RNA, proteins, chromosomes, compound molecules (e.g., DNA and protein adducts), and various metabolites as well as other endogenous and exogenous substances (e.g., steroids, nutrients, chemical or biologic toxins, and phytochemicals). Molecular markers can reflect different aspects of the tumorigenic process, which include biomarkers of internal exposure, biomarkers of molecular or cellular changes in response to exposure, and biomarkers of precursor lesions or early diseases.[22,23] Depending on the source of molecules and location of diseases, surrogates are often used in epidemiologic studies. When using a surrogate marker or tissue, the relevance of a proxy to its underlying target needs to be established or justified.[23] This justification is especially important when conducting population-based epidemiologic studies that focus on organ-specific cancers, because assessing biomarkers in target tissue is difficult for controls; molecular markers from blood samples are often used as substitutes. If a biomarker in the blood does not travel to or act on the tissue or organ of interest, an association between the circulating marker and the cancer may not be relevant. Thus, establishing a close link between a surrogate and its target is crucial in molecular epidemiology research.

Gene-environment interaction plays an essential role in cancer development.[24] Common genetic variations are considered an important determinant of host susceptibility and are a major focus of molecular epidemiology research. Depending on the biologic mechanism involved, genetic variations can influence every aspect of the carcinogenic process, ranging from external and internal exposure to carcinogens or risk factors to molecular and cellular damage, alteration, and response.[22,23] Currently, single nucleotide polymorphisms (SNPs) are the most studied genetic variations. It is believed that even if SNPs confer a small risk, they may still be important at the population level because these variations are common in the general population. It is also important that the impacts of SNPs on cancer are considered under the context of gene–gene and gene–environment interactions. As genotyping technology has advanced substantially with respect to its analytic quality, capacity, and cost, research of genetic polymorphisms has evolved rapidly from investigations of a single SNP to studies of haplotypes and tag SNPs, and from a pathway-based candidate gene approach to genome-wide association studies (GWAS).[25] A GWAS analyzes hundreds of thousands of SNPs simultaneously for hundreds or even thousands of study subjects. When these data are further combined with questionnaire information such as environmental exposures, lifestyle factors, dietary habits, and medical history, enormous information is generated, which requires a huge sample size to allow for a reliable and complete assessment of these variables individually and jointly. A single epidemiologic study can no longer provide sufficient power for this type of investigation. Multicenter investigations or study consortia that pool study information and specimens together are developed to address the sample size issue.[26] False-positive findings resulting from multiple comparisons constitute a major challenge in epidemiologic studies of genetic associations with cancer.[27] A meta-analysis or pooled analysis can be used to address this problem if sufficient studies are already published and available for evaluation. To address this issue at the time of study design, one may adopt a two- or multiphase study design in which study subjects are divided into two or multiple groups for genotyping and data analysis. Selected or genomewide SNPs are first screened in one group of the study subjects (discovery phase), and then the significant findings determined by stringent statistical criteria (usually p values less than 1×10^{-5} or 1×10^{-7}) are reanalyzed in one or several other groups of subjects for verification (validation phase). This study design also lowers the cost of genotyping. False-positive findings can also be addressed with various statistical methods, such as bootstrap, permutation test, estimate of false positive report probability, prediction of false discovery rate, and the use of a much more stringent p value to accommodate multiple comparisons. For epidemiologic studies that are not population based or not conducted strictly following epidemiology principles, population stratification is a potential source of bias that may distort genetic associations.[28]

A large number of GWAS have been completed in search for SNPs that influence host susceptibility to cancer. Considering that more than 5 million SNPs are present in the human genome, the numbers of SNPs that are found to be associated with cancer risk after rigorous validation are much fewer than what one would have anticipated. In addition, the risk associations detected are quite weak, with most of the odds ratios ranging from 1.1 to 1.5, and the functional relevance or biologic implications are unclear for most of the SNPs. Furthermore, not many SNPs associated with cancer risk are located in protein-coding regions, and even fewer are in the loci of candidate genes suspected to be involved in tumorigenesis, such as oncogenes, tumor suppressor genes, DNA repair genes, and xenobiotic metabolizing or detoxification genes. Genes where SNPs are found to be linked to cancer by GWAS include *FGFR2, MAP3K1, MRPS30, LSP1, TNRC9, TOX3, STXBP1,* and *RAD51L1* for breast cancer[29-31]; *JAZF1, HNF1B, MSMB, CTBP2,* and *KLK2/KLK3* for prostate cancer[29,32]; *SMAD7, CRAC1, EIF3H, BMP4, CDH1,* and *RHPN2* for colorectal cancer[29,33]; *CHRNA3* and *CHRNA5* for lung cancer[34,35]; *ABO* for pancreatic cancer[36]; *TACC3* and *PSCA* for bladder cancer[37,38]; and *KRT5* for basal cell carcinoma.[39] Among these genes identified by GWAS, two findings are considered especially interesting. One is the association of lung cancer with *CHRNA3* and *CHRNA5*, which encode neuronal nicotinic acetylcholine receptor subunits. Different genotypes of these receptor subunits appear to influence individual's addiction to tobacco, which further leads to different smoking exposure and lung cancer risk.[40,41] Another is the link of the *ABO* gene to pancreatic cancer. The association between pancreatic cancer risk and ABO blood type was observed 50 years ago. The GWAS finding not only confirms the relationship, but also provides new clues for understanding the underlying biologic mechanism.

Besides intragenic SNPs, GWAS also found many intergenic SNPs in association to cancer risk, which include those in the regions of 8q24, 5p15, 1p11, 1p36, 1q42, 2p15, 2q35, 3p12, 3p24,

3q28, 6p21, 6q25, 7q21, 7q32, 9p21, 9p22, 9p24, 9q22, 10p14, 11q13, 11q23, 14q13, 18q23, and 20p12.[29–31,33,39,42–48] Of these loci, SNPs in 8q24 are associated with several cancer sites, including prostate, breast, colon, and bladder.[29,31–33,47–49] Further analysis of 8q24 indicates that there are nine SNPs in five regions and each region is independently related to different types of cancer, with SNPs in regions 1, 4, and 5 associated exclusively with prostate cancer, a SNP in region 2 related to breast cancer, and SNPs in region 3 linked to prostate, colon, and ovarian cancers.[50] No known genes are located within the region of 8q24, but an oncogene c-MYC resides about 330 kb downstream of the region.[51] An initial investigation found no evidence of the SNPs' influence on c-MYC expression,[47] but a later study suggests that the SNPs in 8q24 may be distal enhancers of c-MYC, interacting with its promoter through a chromatin loop.[52] Another genomic region that is associated with the risk of multiple cancer sites is 5p15, a region involving telomerase reverse transcriptase (TERT) cleft lip and palate transmembrane protein 1–like protein (CLPTM1L). Five types of cancer are found to be linked to this region, including basal cell carcinoma, lung, bladder, prostate, and cervical cancers.[53] TERT extends the length of telomere and is associated with cell proliferation and abnormal telomere maintenance.[54] The risk alleles of TERT are associated with shorter telomere length among the elderly and with higher DNA adduct in the lungs.[53,55]

GWAS has demonstrated its value in identifying disease-related SNPs in unknown regions of the genome, which provides new clues for investigators to interrogate and understand different regions of the human genome, especially in the gene-desert areas. Despite the strength, the low yield of significant findings from the GWAS has raised concerns in several areas, including the SNP coverage in the genome (rare SNPs and SNP representativeness in unknown regions), associations with low statistical significance (p value between 0.01 and 1×10^{-5}, the GWAS cutoff), other forms of genetic variations (copy number variation and other structural variations), cancer subtypes, and genetic interplay with environmental factors (gene–environment interaction).[56,57] To address these issues, investigators propose to perform fine-mapping and resequencing to examine genetic regions more specifically and meticulously. Epidemiologists suggest that detailed environmental exposure and lifestyle factors should be included in the next wave of GWAS. Furthermore, to make the study more reliable and compelling, DNA specimens, instead of convenient samples, should come from well-designed and well-executed epidemiologic studies that pay close attention to the selection of study subjects and the measurement of environmental and lifestyle factors to eliminate or minimize selection bias and measurement errors.

As described earlier, analytical epidemiology has two major study designs: the case-control study and the cohort study. It is important that investigators choose an appropriate study design to investigate molecular markers in epidemiologic studies. Two types of molecular markers, genotypic and phenotypic markers, can be considered. Genotypic markers refer to nucleotide sequences of genomic DNA, and all other molecules are considered phenotypic markers, including most of the chemical modifications on DNA, such as cytosine methylation. The distinction between the two is a marker's status in relation to an outcome variable, usually a disease. Genotypic markers generally do not change over time and are not affected by the development of a disease, whereas phenotypic markers are likely to change over time or be influenced by the presence of a disease, either itself or the treatment associated with it. If measurements of a phenotypic marker are made from the specimens that are collected after or at the time of cancer diagnosis, investigators will have difficulties determining the status of the phenotypic marker before the cancer was diagnosed. A disease condition, however, does not affect genotypic markers such as SNPs; therefore, a temporal relationship can be easily established even if the samples are collected after the disease is diagnosed. Based on this distinction, one can evaluate genotypic markers either in case-control or cohort studies, but a case-control study would be the design of choice because of efficiency and cost-effectiveness. A prospective cohort study design is ideal for phenotypic markers. Investigators, however, may use other study designs if they can demonstrate that the disease status does not influence the phenotypic markers of interest. To reduce study cost, investigators usually use nested case-control or case-cohort designs to avoid analyzing specimens from the entire cohort. The main purpose in choosing a cohort study design for a molecular epidemiology investigation is to ensure that biospecimens are collected before the development of a disease so that a temporal relationship between a marker and disease development can be established.

The differences between molecular epidemiology and genetic epidemiology are the scope of the molecular analysis and the emphasis on heredity. Sometimes molecular and genetic epidemiology both investigate genetic factors in association with cancer risk, but each has its own emphasis. The former assesses genetic involvement, but not necessarily inheritance, whereas the latter focuses mainly on heredity. Because of the difference in focus, study populations are different between the two types of investigation. Molecular epidemiology studies unrelated individuals, whereas genetic epidemiology investigates family members in the format of pedigrees, parent–child trios, or sibling pairs. Given the different research focus between genetic and molecular epidemiology, these investigations evaluate different genetic markers. Genetic epidemiology research is designed to identify genetic markers with high penetrance (strong association with an underlying disease) but low prevalence in the general populations, whereas a molecular epidemiology investigation targets low penetrance markers that are commonly present in the general population. Given the difference in study design, the analysis of genetic marker's link to cancer is also different between the studies. Relative risks or odds ratios are calculated in molecular epidemiology studies because study participants are unrelated individuals, whereas linkage analysis is used in genetic epidemiology because individuals in the study are genetically related family members. Recently, both genetic and molecular epidemiology study designs have been considered in GWAS to improve study validity and to minimize false positive findings. Another difference between genetic and molecular epidemiology research is that molecular epidemiology also studies nongenetic molecules. Thus, the scope of molecular analysis is much broader in molecular epidemiology research than in genetic epidemiology studies.

A laboratory analysis of molecular markers is another integral part of molecular epidemiology research, which has unique features that are different from basic science research. Collecting biologic specimens is difficult and expensive in population-based epidemiologic studies. It not only increases the study cost, but also imposes constraints to multiple areas of epidemiology research. Specimen collection may adversely influence the response rate of study participants, potentially compromising study validity. For organ-specific cancer research, investigating molecular markers in target tissue is difficult. Blood is the most common and versatile specimen used in molecular epidemiology research; other specimens used include urine, stool, nail, hair, sputum, buccal cells, and saliva. Tissue samples, either fresh frozen or chemically fixed, are also used, but the availability of these samples is highly limited to patients or selected subgroups of a general study population. Comparability and generalizability are always problems in epidemiologic studies involving tissue specimens, except for those investigations that focus on cancer prognosis or treatment in which only cancer patients are involved. Attempts have been made to use special body fluids for epidemiologic research, such as nipple aspirate and breast or pulmonary lavage, but the difficulty in specimen collection and preparation makes these samples impractical in large population-based studies.

Given the research value of biologic specimens and the difficulty in collecting them for population-based studies, technical issues related to specimen collection, processing, and storage become especially important in molecular epidemiology research.

These include time and conditions for specimen transportation and processing, a sample aliquot and labeling system, a sample special treatment for storage and analysis, a sample storage and tracking system, as well as backup plans and equipment for unexpected adverse events during long-term storage (e.g., power failure, earthquake, flooding). Laboratory methods used to analyze biomarkers are also important in molecular epidemiology. Because large numbers of specimens are involved, laboratory methods are required to be robust, reproducible, high throughput, low cost, and easy to use. These requirements are often met in the analysis of nucleotide sequences that serve as genotypic markers. However, for phenotypic markers, many methods do not readily meet these requirements. Moreover, many phenotypic markers, such as proteins, require both qualitative and quantitative assessments. An ideal laboratory method should be quantitative (able to measure a wide range of values), sensitive (able to detect a small amount of analyte), specific (able to detect only the molecule of interest, no other molecules), reproducible (high precision and low variation), and versatile (easy to use). In addition, investigators need to implement appropriate quality assurance procedures during sample processing and testing as well as include appropriate quality control samples in specimen analysis.

Host–environment interaction is believed to play a key role in the etiology of most types of cancer. Genetic factors, including mutations and polymorphisms, are initially considered important host factors, but recent developments in cancer research has indicated that epigenetic factors may also play a critical role in cancer as a host factor involved in host–environment interaction. Epigenetic factors, which regulate the function of human genome without altering the physical sequences of nucleotides, include pretranscription regulation through nucleotide modification (e.g., cytosine methylation at CpG sites), chromosome modification (e.g., histone acetylation), and posttranscription regulation by noncoding small RNA (e.g., microRNAs). These epigenetic factors have two unique features that have captured the attention of cancer researchers, especially cancer epidemiologists who are interested in the gene–environment interaction. It is known that epigenetic factors are heritable, but these inherited features are readily modifiable by environmental and lifestyle factors. Monozygotic twins have an identical genome as well as epigenome at birth, but the latter undergoes substantial changes over time, resulting in distinct epigenetic profiles that depend heavily on their environmental exposures.[58] Animal studies also indicated that the maternal intake of dietary nutrients involving one-carbon metabolism could influence offsprings' growth phenotypes, which are regulated by DNA methylation.[59] As evidence mounts on epigenetic involvement in cancer, molecular epidemiologists will start to look for clues in human populations that can link epigenetic factors to both lifestyle factors and cancer risk. Given that epigenetic regulation is tissue specific and time dependent, investigators face challenges in accurately assessing these phenotypic markers in etiologic studies. However, progress in the analysis of circulating methylation markers and microRNAs may provide an alternative to study epigenetic regulation in human cancer. Furthermore, methods for a genome-wide analysis of DNA methylation have been developed and applied in epidemiologic studies, which can substantially accelerate the search for cancer-related DNA methylation. Together with the high-throughput, high-dimensional analysis of DNA methylation, two other evolving fields that will have significant impacts on molecular epidemiology of cancer research are metagenomics and metabolomics. The former focuses on environmental genomics of the microbiome that resides in our body and influences one's biologic functions and health status. The latter refers to the analysis of hundreds or thousands of metabolites in a biologic specimen, including tissue, blood, urine, body fluids, and fecal samples. These new analyses will add tremendous value to epidemiologic studies.

REFERENCES

1. Last J. *A Dictionary of Epidemiology*. 3rd ed. New York: Oxford University Press; 1995.
2. Doll R, Hill AB. Lung cancer and other causes of death in relation to smoking: a second report on the mortality of British doctors. *Br Med J* 1956;12:1071–1081.
3. Kleinbaum D, Kupper L, Morgenstern H. *Epidemiologic Research*. New York: Van Nostrand Reinhold; 1982.
4. Kaplan LD, Straus DJ, Testa MA, et al. Low-dose compared with standard-dose m-BACOD chemotherapy for non-Hodgkin's lymphoma associated with human immunodeficiency virus infection. National Institute of Allergy and Infectious Diseases AIDS Clinical Trials Group. *N Engl J Med* 1997;336:1641–1648.
5. Dunn BK, Kramer BS, Ford LG. Phase III, large-scale chemoprevention trials. Approach to chemoprevention clinical trials and phase III clinical trial of tamoxifen as a chemopreventive for breast cancer—the US National Cancer Institute experience. *Hematol Oncol Clin North Am* 1998;12:1019–1036, vii.
6. Grant WB. An ecologic study of dietary and solar ultraviolet-B links to breast carcinoma mortality rates. *Cancer* 2002;94:272–281.
7. National Center for Health Statistics. Third National Health and Nutrition Examination Survey, 1988-1994, Plan and Operations Procedures Manuals (CD-ROM). Hyattsville, MD: U.S. Department of Health and Human Services (DHHS), Centers for Disease Control and Prevention; 1996.
8. Szklo M, Nieto F. *Epidemiology: Beyond the Basics*. Gaithersburg, MD: Aspen Publishers; 2000.
9. Grimes DA, Schulz KF. Cohort studies: marching towards outcomes. *Lancet* 2002;359:341–345.
10. Schatzkin A, Subar AF, Thompson FE, et al. Design and serendipity in establishing a large cohort with wide dietary intake distributions: the National Institutes of Health-American Association of Retired Persons Diet and Health Study. *Am J Epidemiol* 2001;154:1119–1125.
11. Mantel N, Haenszel W. Statistical aspects of the analysis of data from retrospective studies of disease. *J Natl Cancer Inst* 1959;22:719–748.
12. Wacholder S, Silverman DT, McLaughlin JK, et al. Selection of controls in case-control studies. II. Types of controls. *Am J Epidemiol* 1992;135:1029–1041.
13. Chen C, Weiss NS, Stanczyk FZ, et al. Endogenous sex hormones and prostate cancer risk: a case-control study nested within the Carotene and Retinol Efficacy Trial. *Cancer Epidemiol Biomarkers Prev* 2003;12:1410–1416.
14. Pearce N. What does the odds ratio estimate in a case-control study? *Int J Epidemiol* 1993;22:1189–1192.
15. Schulz KF, Grimes DA. Case-control studies: research in reverse. *Lancet* 2002;359:431–434.
16. Rothman K. *Epidemiology: An Introduction*. New York: Oxford University Press; 2002.
17. Hennekens C, Buring J. *Epidemiology in Medicine*. Boston: Little, Brown and Company; 1987.
18. Andriole GL, Crawford ED, Grubb RL 3rd, et al. Mortality results from a randomized prostate-cancer screening trial. *N Engl J Med* 2009;360:1310–1319.
19. Wilt TJ, Brawer MK, Jones KM, et al. Radical prostatectomy versus observation for localized prostate cancer. *N Engl J Med* 2012;367:203–213.
20. Yu JB, Soulos PR, Herrin J, et al. Proton versus intensity-modulated radiotherapy for prostate cancer: patterns of care and early toxicity. *J Natl Cancer Inst* 2013;105:25–32.
21. Ma X, Wang R, Long JB, et al. The cost implications of prostate cancer screening in the Medicare population. *Cancer* 2014;120(1):96–102.
22. Rundle A, Schwartz S. Issues in the epidemiological analysis and interpretation of intermediate biomarkers. *Cancer Epidemiol Biomarkers Prev* 2003;12:491–496.
23. Shields PG. Tobacco smoking, harm reduction, and biomarkers. *J Natl Cancer Inst* 2002;94:1435–1444.
24. Hunter DJ. Gene-environment interactions in human diseases. *Nat Rev Genet* 2005;6:287–298.
25. Hirschhorn JN, Daly MJ. Genome-wide association studies for common diseases and complex traits. *Nat Rev Genet* 2005;6:95–108.
26. Breast Cancer Association Consortium. Commonly studied single-nucleotide polymorphisms and breast cancer: results from the Breast Cancer Association Consortium. *J Natl Cancer Inst* 2006;98:1382–1396.
27. Wacholder S, Chanock S, Garcia-Closas M, et al. Assessing the probability that a positive report is false: an approach for molecular epidemiology studies. *J Natl Cancer Inst* 2004;96:434–442.
28. Clayton DG, Walker NM, Smyth DJ, et al. Population structure, differential bias and genomic control in a large-scale, case-control association study. *Nat Genet* 2005;37:1243–1246.
29. Easton DF, Eeles RA. Genome-wide association studies in cancer. *Hum Mol Genet* 2008;17:R109–115.
30. Ahmed S, Thomas G, Ghoussaini M, et al. Newly discovered breast cancer susceptibility loci on 3p24 and 17q23.2. *Nat Genet* 2009;41:585–590.
31. Thomas G, Jacobs KB, Kraft P, et al. A multistage genome-wide association study in breast cancer identifies two new risk alleles at 1p11.2 and 14q24.1 (RAD51L1). *Nat Genet* 2009;41:579–584.
32. Thomas G, Jacobs KB, Yeager M, et al. Multiple loci identified in a genome-wide association study of prostate cancer. *Nat Genet* 2008;40:310–315.

33. Le Marchand L. Genome-wide association studies and colorectal cancer. *Surg Oncol Clin N Am* 2009;18:663–668.
34. Hung RJ, McKay JD, Gaborieau V, et al. A susceptibility locus for lung cancer maps to nicotinic acetylcholine receptor subunit genes on 15q25. *Nature* 2008;452:633–637.
35. Amos CI, Wu X, Broderick P, et al. Genome-wide association scan of tag SNPs identifies a susceptibility locus for lung cancer at 15q25.1. *Nat Genet* 2008;40:616–622.
36. Amundadottir L, Kraft P, Stolzenberg-Solomon RZ, et al. Genome-wide association study identifies variants in the ABO locus associated with susceptibility to pancreatic cancer. *Nat Genet* 2009;41:986–990.
37. Kiemeney LA, Sulem P, Besenbacher S, et al. A sequence variant at 4p16.3 confers susceptibility to urinary bladder cancer. *Nat Genet* 2010;42(5):415–419.
38. Wu X, Ye Y, Kiemeney LA, et al. Genetic variation in the prostate stem cell antigen gene PSCA confers susceptibility to urinary bladder cancer. *Nat Genet* 2009;41:991–995.
39. Stacey SN, Sulem P, Masson G, et al. New common variants affecting susceptibility to basal cell carcinoma. *Nat Genet* 2009;41:909–914.
40. Thorgeirsson TE, Geller F, Sulem P, et al. A variant associated with nicotine dependence, lung cancer and peripheral arterial disease. *Nature* 2008;452:638–642.
41. Spitz MR, Amos CI, Dong Q, et al. The CHRNA5-A3 region on chromosome 15q24-25.1 is a risk factor both for nicotine dependence and for lung cancer. *J Natl Cancer Inst* 2008;100:1552–1556.
42. Zheng W, Long J, Gao YT, et al. Genome-wide association study identifies a new breast cancer susceptibility locus at 6q25.1. *Nat Genet* 2009;41:324–328.
43. Gudmundsson J, Sulem P, Gudbjartsson DF, et al. Common variants on 9q22.33 and 14q13.3 predispose to thyroid cancer in European populations. *Nat Genet* 2009;41:460–464.
44. Gudmundsson J, Sulem P, Gudbjartsson DF, et al. Genome-wide association and replication studies identify four variants associated with prostate cancer susceptibility. *Nat Genet* 2009;41:1122–1126.
45. Song H, Ramus SJ, Tyrer J, et al. A genome-wide association study identifies a new ovarian cancer susceptibility locus on 9p22.2. *Nat Genet* 2009;41:996–1000.
46. Stacey SN, Gudbjartsson DF, Sulem P, et al. Common variants on 1p36 and 1q42 are associated with cutaneous basal cell carcinoma but not with melanoma or pigmentation traits. *Nat Genet* 2008;40:1313–1318.
47. Zanke BW, Greenwood CM, Rangrej J, et al. Genome-wide association scan identifies a colorectal cancer susceptibility locus on chromosome 8q24. *Nat Genet* 2007;39:989–994.
48. Haiman CA, Patterson N, Freedman ML, et al. Multiple regions within 8q24 independently affect risk for prostate cancer. *Nat Genet* 2007;39:638–644.
49. Kiemeney LA, Thorlacius S, Sulem P, et al. Sequence variant on 8q24 confers susceptibility to urinary bladder cancer. *Nat Genet* 2008;40:1307–1312.
50. Ghoussaini M, Song H, Koessler T, et al. Multiple loci with different cancer specificities within the 8q24 gene desert. *J Natl Cancer Inst* 2008;100:962–966.
51. Harismendy O, Frazer KA. Elucidating the role of 8q24 in colorectal cancer. *Nat Genet* 2009;41:868–869.
52. Wright JB, Brown SJ, Cole MD. Upregulation of c-MYC in cis through a large chromatin loop linked to a cancer risk-associated single-nucleotide polymorphism in colorectal cancer cells. *Mol Cell Biol* 2010;30:1411–1420.
53. Rafnar T, Sulem P, Stacey SN, et al. Sequence variants at the TERT-CLPTM1L locus associate with many cancer types. *Nat Genet* 2009;41:221–227.
54. Fernandez-Garcia I, Ortiz-de-Solorzano C, Montuenga LM. Telomeres and telomerase in lung cancer. *J Thorac Oncol* 2008;3:1085–1088.
55. Zienolddiny S, Skaug V, Landvik NE, et al. The TERT-CLPTM1L lung cancer susceptibility variant associates with higher DNA adduct formation in the lung. *Carcinogenesis* 2009;30:1368–1371.
56. Ioannidis JP, Thomas G, Daly MJ. Validating, augmenting and refining genome-wide association signals. *Nat Rev Genet* 2009;10:318–329.
57. Chung CC, Magalhaes WC, Gonzalez-Bosquet J, et al. Genome-wide association studies in cancer—current and future directions. *Carcinogenesis* 2010;31:111–120.
58. Fraga MF, Ballestar E, Paz MF, et al. Epigenetic differences arise during the lifetime of monozygotic twins. *Proc Natl Acad Sci U S A* 2005;102:10604–10609.
59. Dolinoy DC, Weidman JR, Waterland RA, et al. Maternal genistein alters coat color and protects Avy mouse offspring from obesity by modifying the fetal epigenome. *Environ Health Perspect* 2006;114:567–572.

12 Trends in United States Cancer Mortality

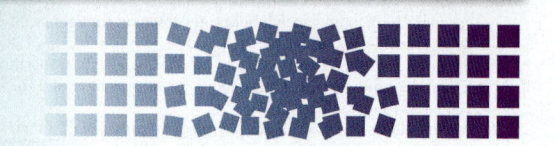

Tim E. Byers

INTRODUCTION

Cancer incidence registries now cover nearly all of the US population. State-based vital records systems and aggregate national systems regularly report trends in both cancer incidence and mortality, and national surveys routinely monitor cancer-related risk factors in the population. These surveillance systems have documented substantial changes in both risk factors for cancer and in cancer incidence and mortality rates in the United States over the past 3 decades. In 1996, the American Cancer Society (ACS) set an ambitious challenge for the United States: to reduce cancer mortality rates from their apparent peak in 1990 by 50% in the 25-year period ending in 2015.[1] In 1998, the ACS then challenged the United States to also reduce cancer incidence rates from their peak in 1992 by 25% by the year 2015.[2] In this chapter, we will examine trends in cancer risk factors as well as trends in cancer incidence and mortality rates in the United States over the 25-year period between 1990 and 2015.

CANCER SURVEILLANCE SYSTEMS

Collecting cancer incidence rates is largely a state-based activity in the United States, because cancer is a reportable disease in all states. The Centers for Disease Control and Prevention (CDC) organizes all state-based cancer registries within the National Program of Cancer Registries, which now reports collective data on cancer incidence from over 40 different state-based registries, providing data that meets strict quality standards.[3] The National Cancer Institute has supported high-quality cancer incidence and outcomes registration in selected states and cities since 1973 within the Surveillance, Epidemiology, and End Results (SEER) Program.[4] The most precise measures of long-term trends in cancer incidence come from SEER-9, a set of nine SEER registries that together include about 10% of the US population. The populations included in the SEER-9 registries document the most detailed history of cancer trends beginning in the 1970s based on highly standardized cancer case ascertainment, staging, treatment, and outcomes. Deaths from cancer are well ascertained in all states via state-based vital records, which are aggregated into annual national mortality reports by the CDC's National Center for Health Statistics.[5] Each year, the ACS, the National Cancer Institute, and the CDC publish a *Report to the Nation* on trends in cancer incidence and mortality in the United States.[6] Trends in the prevalence of behavioral factors that affect cancer risk are tracked by the Health Interview Survey, an ongoing, in-person interview of a nationally representative sample of adults, and in annual reports by the Behavioral Risk Factor Surveillance System, a continuously operating telephone-based survey operated by state departments of health and organized by the CDC.[7]

MAKING SENSE OF CANCER TRENDS

Understanding the reasons for cancer trends requires understanding trends in cancer-related risk factors. For factors like tobacco, relating trends in exposure to trends in rates is easy, because those effects are large and single. However, for many other cancer risk factors, because effects are much smaller and multifactorial, simple correlations over time are less apparent. In most situations, all that maybe possible are crude qualitative relationships between temporal trends in cancer risk factors and subsequent trends in cancer rates. Statistical methods such as linear regression joinpoint analysis can tell us when inflections in cancer trends occur, but accounting for the precise reasons for changing rates is often impaired by our incomplete knowledge about the interacting impacts of variations in cancer screening, diagnosis, and treatment, and by uncertainties about latencies between interventions and outcomes.[8]

TRENDS IN CANCER RISK FACTORS AND SCREENING

Trends in major cancer risk factors have been mixed (Table 12.1). Although the downward trends in tobacco smoking among adults that began in the 1960s slowed after 1990, there has been a continuing downward trend in the number of cigarettes smoked per day by continuing smokers.[9] Obesity trends have been adverse among both men and women since the 1970s, with more than a doubling of the prevalence of obesity between 1990 and 2010. Long-term trends in the use of hormone replacement therapy (HRT) are not routinely monitored in the Behavioral Risk Factor Surveillance System (BRFSS), but HRT use increased substantially in the last 2 decades of the 20th century. Then, following the 2002 publication of the Women's Health Initiative trial, which showed clear adverse effects of HRT, there was a rapid and substantial drop in HRT use.[10,11] The use of endoscopic screening for colorectal cancer (sigmoidoscopy or colonoscopy) has increased substantially in recent years, approximately doubling since the mid 1990s, so that, as of 2010, about two-thirds of Americans age 50 and older reported ever having had an endoscopic examination. Mammography use increased progressively through the 1990s, but mammogram rates then leveled off after 2000.[12] Widespread prostate-specific antigen (PSA) testing began in the mid to late 1980s, then increased substantially during the 1990s. By 2002, a majority of US men age 50 and older reported having been tested.

CANCER INCIDENCE AND MORTALITY

In this chapter, we describe and discuss cancer trends for the time period 1990 through 2010 using cancer incidence data from the SEER-9 registry (Table 12.2 and Fig. 12.1) and US cancer mortality data from the National Center for Health Statistics (Table 12.3).[4,5] All rates were age-adjusted to the US 2000 standard population by the direct method, using 10-year age intervals.

Lung Cancer

The lung is the second leading site for cancer incidence and the leading site for cancer death among both men and women in the

TABLE 12.1

Trends in Risk Factors and Cancer Screening Practices in the United States, 1990–2010[a]

	Men Smoking	Men PSA Screening	Women Smoking	Women Mammography	Both Genders Obesity	Both Genders CRC Screening
1990	24.9	—	21.3	58.3	11.6	—
1991	25.1	—	21.3	62.2	12.6	—
1992	24.2	—	21.0	63.1	12.6	—
1993	24.0	—	21.1	66.5	13.7	—
1994	23.9	—	21.6	66.6	14.4	—
1995	24.8	—	20.9	68.6	15.8	29.4
1996	25.5	—	21.9	69.2	16.8	—
1997	25.4	—	21.1	70.3	16.6	32.4
1998	25.3	—	20.9	72.3	18.3	—
1999	24.2	—	20.8	72.8	19.7	43.7
2000	24.4	—	21.2	76.1	20.1	—
2001	25.4	—	21.2	—	21.0	—
2002	25.7	53.9	20.8	75.9	22.1	48.1
2003	24.8	—	20.2	—	—	—
2004	23.0	52.1	19.0	74.7	23.2	53.0
2005	22.1	—	19.2	—	24.4	—
2006	22.2	53.8	18.4	76.5	25.1	57.1
2007	21.2	—	18.4	—	26.3	—
2008	20.3	54.8	16.7	76.0	26.6	61.8
2009	19.5	—	16.7	—	27.1	—
2010	18.5	53.2	15.8	75.2	27.5	65.2

CRC, colorectal cancer; PSA, prostate-specific antigen.

[a] Median percent of the population across all states in the Behavioral Risk Factor Surveillance System. The survey covered such areas as body mass index and was based on self-reported height and weight. Questions included: Are you a regular cigarette smoker? Have you ever had a sigmoidoscopy or proctoscopic examination? For women age 40 and older, the following question was included: Have you had a mammogram in the past 2 years? For men aged 50 and older, the following question was included: Have you had a PSA test in the last 2 years? (From Centers for Disease Control and Prevention. Behavioral Risk Factor Surveillance System Web site. http://cdc.gov/brfss/.)

United States.[6] There are now more deaths from lung cancer in the United States than from the sum of colorectal, breast, and prostate cancers. Trends in lung cancer incidence and mortality have been nearly identical because there are few effective treatments for lung cancer, and survival time remains short. Lung cancer trends follow historic declines in tobacco use, lagged by about 20 years.[13] Between 1965 and 1985, tobacco use among US adults dropped substantially, and more in men than in women. Lung cancer mortality rates began to decline among men in 1990, but rates increased among women throughout the 1990s. The stabilization of lung cancer incidence trends among women from 2000 to 2005 and the beginning of a decline in the period 2005 to 2010 foretells a coming persistent decline in lung cancer mortality among women in the United States.

The effectiveness of annual examinations by use of chest radiographs in reducing lung cancer mortality was studied as part of the Prostate, Lung, Colorectal, Ovary (PLCO) trial, and the effectiveness of annual screening by low-dose computed tomography (LDCT) of the lung fields was studied in the National Lung Screening Trial (NLST).[14,15] In brief, screening with standard chest radiography finds more cancers earlier but does not affect mortality, whereas screening with LDCT reduces the risk of death from lung cancer by at least 20%.[14,15] Therefore, both the ACS and the US Preventive Services Task Force have issued recommendations that favor informed decision making for lung cancer screening using LDCT.[16,17]

The major factor that will determine lung cancer incidence in the coming decade is the past history of tobacco use, but future screening will also reduce future mortality rates. Considering all factors, it is likely that over the coming decade the downward trends in mortality from lung cancer will continue at about the same rate among men, and soon will become more apparent among women.

Colorectal Cancer

The colorectum is the third leading site for cancer incidence and the second leading site for cancer death in the United States.[6] Colorectal cancer incidence rates increased until 1985, when they began to decline. The reasons for this decline are not clear, but could be related to downward trends in cigarette smoking and the increasing use of both nonsteroidal anti-inflammatory drugs (NSAIDs) and HRT.[18] The rapid decline in HRT use following the publication of the Women's Health Initiative trial results in 2002 may adversely affect colorectal trends among women in the coming years, because HRT reduces the risk for colorectal cancer among women.[11] Recent trials have demonstrated the potential for NSAIDs to reduce colorectal neoplasia, but adverse effects from these agents will limit their widespread use for that explicit purpose. Nonetheless, even the common sporadic use of NSAIDs for other indications will contribute to continuing declines in colorectal cancer incidence in the coming years.

Screening with either sigmoidoscopy or colonoscopy leads to the identification and removal of adenomas, thus preventing the development of colorectal cancer.[19,20] Medicare included

TABLE 12.2

Trends in Age-Adjusted Cancer Incidence Rates in the United States by Cancer Site, 1990–2010[a]

	Men		Women		Both Genders	
	Lung	**Prostate**	**Lung**	**Breast**	**Colorectal**	**All Sites**
1990	96.9	171.0	47.8	131.8	60.7	482.0
1991	97.2	214.8	49.6	133.9	59.5	503.0
1992	97.2	237.4	49.9	132.1	58.0	510.6
1993	94.0	209.5	49.2	129.2	56.8	493.4
1994	90.9	180.3	50.5	131.0	55.6	483.5
1995	89.8	169.3	50.4	132.6	54.0	476.9
1996	88.0	169.5	50.2	133.7	54.8	479.1
1997	86.3	173.5	52.6	138.0	56.4	486.4
1998	88.0	171.0	53.0	141.4	56.8	488.2
1999	84.6	183.4	52.4	141.5	55.5	490.4
2000	82.1	183.0	51.2	136.4	54.1	486.0
2001	81.4	184.8	51.7	138.7	53.6	489.7
2002	80.4	182.2	52.5	135.6	53.1	487.5
2003	81.0	169.6	53.0	126.8	50.8	475.2
2004	76.2	165.7	52.0	128.0	50.0	476.1
2005	75.8	156.5	53.7	126.4	47.8	471.9
2006	74.2	171.5	53.4	126.0	46.8	475.0
2007	73.5	174.3	53.4	127.9	46.3	480.5
2008	72.0	157.0	51.6	128.0	45.2	473.4
2009	70.2	153.7	51.8	130.3	43.0	470.5
2010	66.8	145.1	49.2	126.0	40.6	457.5
Average annual % change 1990–2010	−1.8	−0.5	+0.2	−0.2	−2.0	−0.2

[a] Data source is the Surveillance, Epidemiology, and End Results-9 populations for cancer incidence. Rates are age-adjusted to the year 2000 population standard. The annual percent change is the mean percent change per year across the 20-year period, 1990 to 2010. (From National Cancer Institute. Surveillance, Epidemiology, and End Results Program Web site. http://seer.cancer.gov.)

coverage for all recommended colorectal screening methods in 2001, and national publicity has substantially increased public interest in screening.[21] Colorectal screening rates have increased over time, now with about two-thirds of adults over age 50 reporting having ever been screened by lower gastrointestinal endoscopy (see Table 12.1).

Decreasing rates of colorectal cancer incidence are occurring in spite of the obesity epidemic, which is an adverse force on colorectal cancer risk, because obesity may account for as much as 20% of colorectal cancer in the United States.[22] Recently, however, obesity trends have stabilized in the United States.[23] As a result of the increased use of lower gastrointestinal endoscopy for colorectal screening and this stabilization of obesity trends, the incidence of colorectal cancer may exceed the ACS goal for 2015 of a 25% reduction, and there is a high likelihood that the rate of decline in deaths from colorectal cancer will be steep enough to reach the 2015 ACS mortality reduction goal of 50%.

Breast Cancer

The breast is the leading site of cancer incidence and the second leading site for cancer death among women in the United States.[6] Over the period 1990 to 2001, no substantial changes in incidence rates were observed, but after 2000, breast cancer incidence began to decline. The decline in breast cancer incidence observed after 2002 seems to have been the result of the sudden decline in the use of HRT following the 2002 publication of the Women's Health Initiative results.[10,11] It is likely that persisting lower rates of HRT use will cause a continued decline in breast cancer incidence in the coming years. Countering this favorable trend, however, are the adverse effects of the obesity epidemic. Obesity, a major risk factor for postmenopausal breast cancer, increased substantially between 1990 and 2005, now with over 25% of US women being obese. However, the slowing of the obesity epidemic since 2005 may have substantial beneficial effects on the future trends in breast cancer incidence.

After persistent increases in the use of mammography over a 20-year period, mammography rates declined modestly between 2000 and 2004, and then leveled off. The downgrading of the evidence recommendations by the US Preventive Services Task Force for mammography for women age 40 to 49 and recommendations for every other year mammographies for women age 50 and older have resulted in lower mammogram utilization, which is likely to continue into the coming decade.[17] This trend will have an adverse effect on breast cancer mortality, but will tend to reduce breast cancer incidence somewhat because of a lack of detection of very early stage cancers.

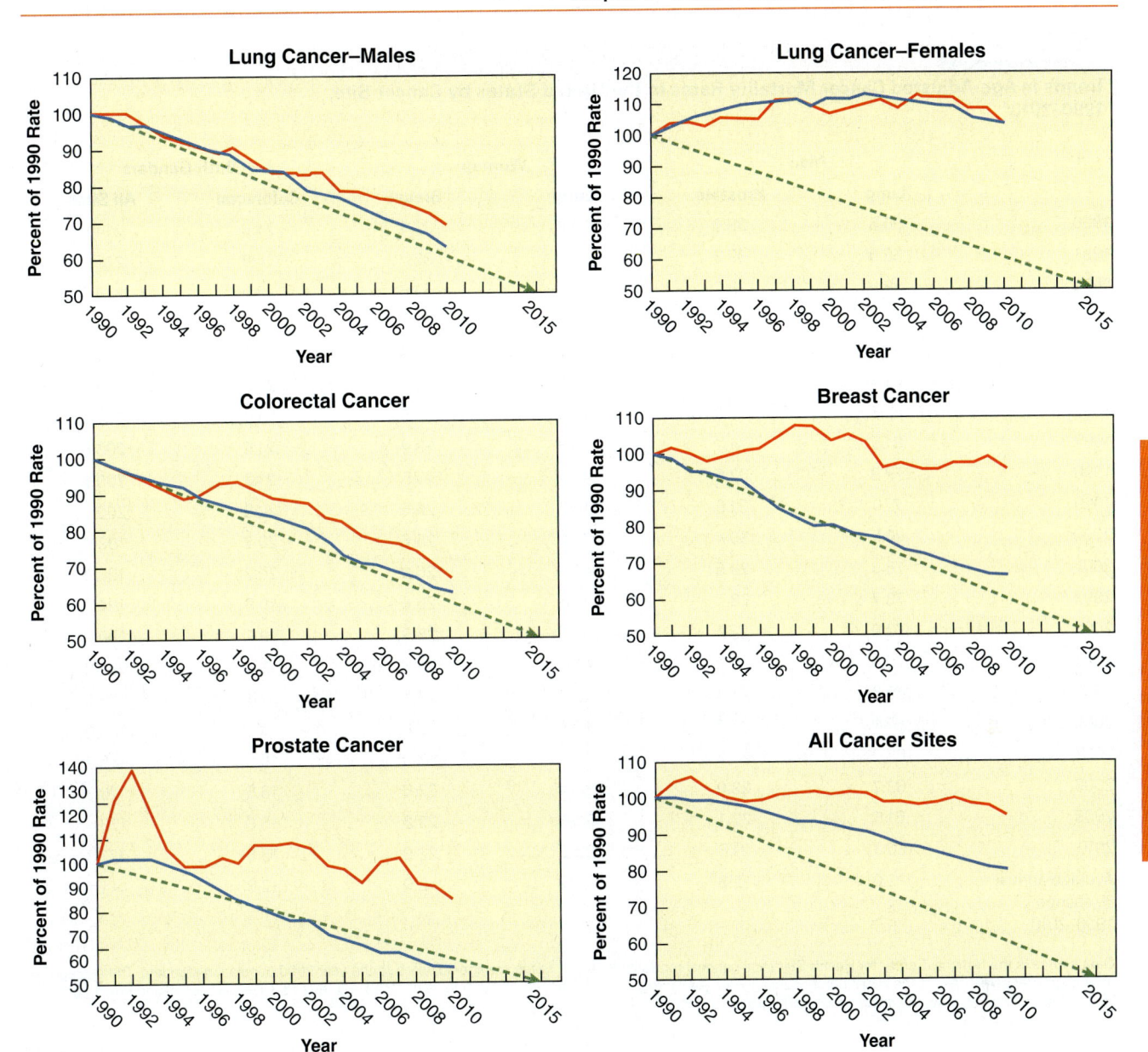

Figure 12.1 (A–F) Trends in cancer incidence and mortality between 1990 and 2010. Incidence rates are for the populations in the Surveillance, Epidemiology, and End Results Program; registries and mortality rates are for the entire United States. Rates are age-adjusted to the year 2000 standard. The y-axis rates are expressed as a percentage of the 1990 incidence and mortality rates. The *red lines* represent incidence rates, and the *blue lines* represent mortality rates. The *straight dotted green lines* represent the linear trend that would need to be followed to achieve a 50% mortality reduction between 1990 and 2015. (Data from National Cancer Institute. Surveillance, Epidemiology, and End Results Program Web site. http://seer.cancer.gov, and Centers for Disease Control and Prevention. U.S. mortality data. http://wonder.cdc.gov/ucd-icd10.html)

The antiestrogens tamoxifen and raloxifene have both been shown to reduce the risk of incident breast cancer.[24] The safety profile for tamoxifen discourages its widespread use, but there is a more favorable risk/benefit balance of raloxifene. Nonetheless, neither of these drugs is commonly used for breast cancer prevention among postmenopausal women in the United States.

The average decline in breast cancer death rates of 2% per year since 1990 is the combined result of earlier diagnosis and better treatment.[25] Progress in breast cancer treatment is continuing, especially in the development and application of hormone-targeted therapies. Aromatase inhibitors have largely replaced tamoxifen therapy for breast cancer treatment for postmenopausal women. Because all antiestrogens substantially reduce the incidence of second primary cancers in the contralateral breast, they impact both therapy and prevention. In the coming decade, the longer term effects of decreased HRT use, increased antiestrogen use, reversal of the obesity trends, and continued improvements in therapies will likely lead to continued decreases in both the incidence and mortality rates from breast cancer.

Prostate Cancer

The prostate is the leading site for cancer incidence and the second leading site for cancer death among men in the United States.[6] The incidence of prostate cancer has been extremely variable over the period 1990 to 2010. The incidence spike observed in the early 1990s actually began in the late 1980s, coincident with the advent of PSA testing. The reasons for the 2.8% annual downward trend in prostate cancer mortality since 1990 are uncertain, however, because the ongoing PSA screening trials have not yet demonstrated a mortality benefit from screening anywhere as large as the downward mortality

TABLE 12.3

Trends in Age-Adjusted Cancer Mortality Rates in the United States by Cancer Site, 1990–2010[a]

	Men		Women		Both Genders	
	Lung	Prostate	Lung	Breast	Colorectal	All Sites
1990	90.6	38.6	36.8	33.1	24.6	214.9
1991	89.9	39.3	37.6	32.7	24.0	215.1
1992	88.0	39.2	38.7	31.6	23.6	213.5
1993	87.6	39.3	39.3	31.4	23.3	213.4
1994	85.7	38.5	39.6	30.9	22.9	211.7
1995	84.4	37.3	40.3	30.6	22.6	210.0
1996	82.8	36.0	40.4	29.5	21.9	207.0
1997	81.3	34.2	40.8	28.2	21.5	203.6
1998	79.9	32.6	41.0	27.5	21.2	200.8
1999	77.0	31.6	40.2	26.6	20.9	200.7
2000	76.5	30.4	41.1	26.6	20.7	198.8
2001	75.3	29.5	41.0	26.0	20.2	196.3
2002	73.7	28.7	41.6	25.6	19.8	194.4
2003	72.0	27.2	41.3	25.3	19.1	190.9
2004	70.4	26.2	41.0	24.5	18.1	186.8
2005	69.5	25.4	40.7	24.1	17.6	185.2
2006	67.4	24.2	40.3	23.6	17.3	182.0
2007	65.2	24.2	40.1	23.0	16.9	179.3
2008	63.7	23.0	39.1	22.6	16.5	176.3
2009	61.5	22.1	38.6	22.2	15.8	173.4
2010	60.1	21.8	38.0	22.0	15.5	171.8
Average annual % change 1990–2010	−2.0	−2.8	+0.2	−2.0	−2.3	−1.1

[a] Data source is the National Center for Health Statistics national mortality data set. Rates are age-adjusted to the year 2000 population standard. The average percentage change per year is the mean percent change per year across the 20-year period, 1990 to 2010. (From Centers for Disease Control and Prevention. U.S. mortality data. http://wonder.cdc.gov/ucd-icd10.html)

decline observed since 1990.[26,27] In fact, the US trial findings suggest that there was virtually no mortality benefit within the first decade following the initiation of screening.[28] Therefore, it is not possible to know how much of this favorable trend was related to early diagnosis, how much was related to improvements in treatment, or how much might have been related to other factors, such as changes in the way cause of death has been listed on death certificates.

The Prostate Cancer Prevention Trial provided an important proof of principle that antiandrogen therapies can reduce prostate cancer risk.[29] Although the net benefits of finasteride for prevention are not clearly demonstrated from this trial, other agents that interfere with androgen effects on prostate cancer growth could prove to be useful for prostate cancer chemoprevention in the future. Prostate cancer incidence trends will likely continue to be largely driven by rates of PSA screening in the coming decade. Longer term results of a clearer benefit to mortality from either the PLCO trial in the United States or the European PSA trial would help to better specify screening recommendations.

Other Cancers

Even though mortality rates have been declining by about 2% per year from the four most common causes of cancer death (lung, colorectal, breast, and prostate), very little progress has been made in reducing death rates from the other half of all adult cancers in the United States. Continuing progress in tobacco control will have beneficial effects on many other types of cancer linked to tobacco, and stopping the obesity epidemic will have favorable effects on many obesity-related cancers that have been increasing in recent years, such as adenocarcinoma of the esophagus and renal cancer.[30] Melanoma incidence rates have been increasing substantially in recent years, likely the result of the combined effects of previous sun exposure and increased awareness and surveillance for pigmented skin lesions, but recent advances in therapy for metastatic melanoma may foretell future declines in melanoma morality. Declining rates of stomach cancer incidence and mortality over several decades may be related to the combined effects of historic improvements in nutrition and the declining prevalence of chronic infection with *Helicobacter pylori*. Liver cancer incidence has been substantially increasing in recent years, likely resulting from historic trends in chronic infection with hepatitis B and C viruses. As a result, liver cancer will likely continue to rise in the United States over the coming decade.

The incidence of thyroid cancer has been increasing in the United States for the past several decades, but thyroid cancer mortality rates have been stable, a pattern most likely due to increased detection from improved diagnostic techniques. Invasive cervical cancer is uncommon in the United States because of widespread screening using Pap smears. Although the vaccination for human papillomavirus (HPV) has been shown to be highly effective in protecting against the serotypes that together account for 70% of cervical cancer cases, so far, HPV vaccine coverage has been low among young women in the United States.[6] For many of the other cancers, such as cancers of the pancreas, brain, ovary, and the hematopoietic malignancies, risk factors are poorly understood, and there are no effective early detection methods. For these cancers, the current hope for improvement resides in the development of better methods for early cancer detection and treatment.

PREDICTING FUTURE CANCER TRENDS

In the United States, cancer is now the leading cause of death under age 85 years. Over the first half of the ACS 25-year challenge period, overall cancer incidence rates have declined by about 0.2% per year, and mortality rates have declined by about 1% per year. The trends in both incidence and mortality from the four leading cancer sites are summarized in Figure 12.1. Using simple linear extrapolation, it therefore seems that the ACS challenge goals of reducing cancer incidence by 25% and mortality by 50% over 25 years may be only half achieved.[31,32] Clearly, though, estimating future trends only by linear extrapolation is a crude way to foretell future events. Projecting cancer trends into the more distant future using complex modeling is possible, however, as knowledge about changes in major cancer risk factors can lead to reasonable predictions about the direction and approximate slope of future trends. One method to incorporate knowledge about trends in risk factors into estimates of future cancer trends is to estimate the impact of changes in the attributable risk (also called the *preventable fraction*) in the population for each risk factor. By making assumptions about latency period, then tying changes in factors to changes in cancer incidence and mortality, cancer trends resulting from risk factor changes can be predicted. For example, if there were a factor that explained 30% of a particular cancer, then cutting that exposure in half would eventually lead to a projected 15% reduction in rates (50% of 30%). This method was used to project cancer mortality trends to 2015 and seems to have projected trends that are quite similar to those observed in recent years.[33]

Progress in cancer prevention, early detection, and treatment since 1990 has been persistent, and there are many reasons to be optimistic about the future. Just how much steeper the future downward slope in cancer death rates can be driven will depend on the extent to which we can discover new factors causing cancer, and effectively deploy ways to better act on our current knowledge about how to prevent and control cancer. Especially important will be progress in reversing the epidemics of tobacco use and obesity, and ensuring that the coming improvements to health care access will lead to access to state-of-the-art cancer screening and therapy for all.

REFERENCES

1. American Cancer Society Board of Directors. ACS Challenge goals for U.S. Cancer Mortality for the Year 2015. *Proceedings of the Board of Directors.* Atlanta, GA: American Cancer Society, 1996.
2. American Cancer Society Board of Directors. ACS Challenge goals for U.S. Cancer Incidence for the Year 2015. *Proceedings of the Board of Directors.* Atlanta, GA: American Cancer Society, 1998.
3. Centers for Disease Control and Prevention. National Program of Cancer Registries (NPCR) Web site. http://cdc.gov/cancer/npcr.
4. National Cancer Institute. Surveillance, Epidemiology, and End Results Program Web site. http://seer.cancer.gov.
5. Centers for Disease Control and Prevention. U.S. mortality data. http://wonder.cdc.gov/ucd-icd10.html
6. Jemal A, Simard E, Dorell C, et al. Annual report to the nation on the status of cancer, 1975–2009, featuring the burden and trends in human papillomavirus (HPV)–associated cancers and HPV vaccination coverage levels. *J Natl Cancer Inst* 2013;105:175–201.
7. Centers for Disease Control and Prevention. Behavioral Risk Factor Surveillance System Web site. http://cdc.gov/brfss.
8. Ward E, Thun M, Hannan L, et al. Interpreting cancer trends. *Ann N Y Acad Sci* 2006;1076:29–53.
9. Centers for Disease Control and Prevention. Smoking & Tobacco Use Web site. http://cdc.gov/tobacco.
10. Rossouw JE, Anderson GL, Prentice RL, et al. Risks and benefits of estrogen plus progestin in healthy postmenopausal women: principal results from the Women's Health Initiative randomized controlled trial. *JAMA* 2002;288:321–333.
11. Hersh A, Stefanick M, Stafford R. National use of postmenopausal hormone therapy: annual trends and response to recent evidence. *JAMA* 2004;291:47–53.
12. Ryerson AB, Miller J, Eheman CR, et al. Use of mammograms among women aged ≥40 years—United States, 2000–2005. *MMWR* 2007;56:49–51.
13. Giovino GA. Epidemiology of tobacco use in the United States. *Oncogene* 2002;21:7326–7340.
14. Oken M, Hocking W, Kvale P, et al. Screening by chest radiograph and lung cancer mortality. *JAMA* 2011;306:1865–1873.
15. The National Lung Screening Trial Research Team. Reduced lung-cancer mortality with low-dose computed tomographic screening. *N Engl J Med* 2011;365:395–409.
16. Smith R, Brooks D, Cokkinides V, et al. Cancer screening in the United States, 2013: a review of current American Cancer Society guidelines, current issues in cancer screening, and new guidance on cervical cancer screening and lung cancer screening. *CA Cancer J Clin* 2013;63:88–105.
17. U.S. Preventive Services Task Force. U.S. Preventive Services Task Force Web site. http://uspreventiveservicestaskforce.org.
18. Martinez ME. Primary prevention of colorectal cancer: lifestyle, nutrition, exercise. *Recent Results Cancer Res* 2005;166:177–211.
19. Atkin W, Edwards R, Kralj-Hans I, et al. Once-only flexible sigmoidoscopy screening in prevention of colorectal cancer: a multicentre randomized controlled trial. *Lancet* 2010;375:1624–1633.
20. Schoen RE, Pinsky PF, Weissfeld JL, et al. Colorectal-cancer incidence and mortality with screening flexible sigmoidoscopy. *N Engl J Med* 2012;366:2345–2357.
21. Cram P, Fendrick A, Inadomi J, et al. The impact of celebrity promotional campaign on the use of colon cancer screening: the Katie Couric effect. *Arch Intern Med* 2003;163(13):1601–1605.
22. World Cancer Research Fund/American Institute for Cancer Prevention. *Policy and Action for Cancer Prevention. Food, Nutrition, and Physical Activity: A Global Perspective.* Washington, DC: AICR; 2009.
23. Ogden CL, Carroll MD, Curtin LR, et al. Prevalence of overweight and obesity in the United States, 1999–2004. *JAMA* 2006;295:1549–1555.
24. Vogel V, Constantino J, Wickerham D, et al. Effects of tamoxifen vs raloxifene on the risks of developing invasive breast cancer and other disease outcomes: the NSABP Study of Tamoxifen and Raloxifene (STAR) P-2 trial. *JAMA* 2006;295:2727–2741.
25. Berry D, Cronin K, Plevritis S, et al. Effect of screening and adjuvant therapy on mortality from breast cancer. *N Engl J Med* 2005;353:1784–1792.
26. Andriole GL, Crawford ED, Grubb RL 3rd, et al. Mortality results from a randomized prostate-cancer screening trial. *N Engl J Med* 2009;360(13):1310–1319.
27. Schröder FH, Hugosson J, Roobol MJ, et al. Screening and prostate-cancer mortality in a randomized European study. *N Engl J Med* 2009;360(13):1320–1328.
28. Andriole G, Crawford D, Grubb R, et al. Prostate cancer screening in the randomized Prostate, Lung, Colorectal, and Ovarian Cancer Screening Trial: mortality results after 13 years of follow-up. *J Natl Cancer Inst* 2012;104:125–132.
29. Thompson I, Goodman P, Tangen C, et al. Long-term survival of participants in the prostate cancer prevention trial. *N Engl J Med* 2013;369:603–610.
30. International Agency for Cancer Research. *Weight Control and Physical Activity. Handbook 6.* Lyon, France: IARC Press; 2002.
31. Sedjo R, Byers T, Barrera E, et al. A midpoint assessment of the American Cancer Society challenge goal to decrease cancer incidence by 25% between 1992 and 2015. *CA Cancer J Clin* 2007;57:326–340.
32. Byers T, Barrera E, Fontham E, et al. A midpoint assessment of the American Cancer Society challenge goal to halve the U.S. cancer mortality rates between the years 1990 and 2015. *Cancer* 2006;107:396–405.
33. Byers T, Mouchawar J, Marks J, et al. The American Cancer Society challenge goals. How far can cancer rates decline in the U.S. by the year 2015? *Cancer* 1999;86:715–727.

PART III

Cancer Therapeutics

13 Essentials of Radiation Therapy

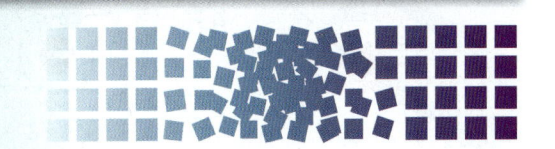

Meredith A. Morgan, Randall K. Ten Haken, and Theodore S. Lawrence

INTRODUCTION

The beneficial use of radiation was launched by the experiments of Wilhelm Roentgen, who, in 1895, found that x-rays could pass through materials that were impenetrable to light. Emil Grubbe provided one of the early examples of the therapeutic use of radiation by treating an advanced ulcerated breast cancer with x-rays in January 1896. We have made great progress since these early days, which has been strongly influenced by research in radiation chemistry, biology, and physics.

BIOLOGIC ASPECTS OF RADIATION ONCOLOGY

Radiation-Induced DNA Damage

Radiation is administered to cells either in the form of photons (x-rays and gamma rays) or particles (protons, neutrons, and electrons). When photons or particles interact with biologic material, they cause ionizations that can either directly interact with subcellular structures or they can interact with water, the major constituent of cells, and generate free radicals that can then interact with subcellular structures (Fig. 13.1).

The direct effects of radiation are the consequence of the DNA in chromosomes absorbing energy that leads to ionizations. This is the major mechanism of DNA damage induced by charged nuclei (such as a carbon nucleus) and neutrons and is termed *high linear energy transfer* (Fig. 13.2). In contrast, the interaction of photons with other molecules, such as water, results in the production of free radicals, some of which possess a lifetime long enough to be able to diffuse to the nucleus and interact with DNA in the chromosomes. This is the major mechanism of DNA damage induced by x-rays and has been termed *low linear energy transfer*.[1]

A free radical generated through the interaction of photons with other molecules that possess an unpaired electron in their outermost shell (e.g., hydroxyl radicals) can abstract a hydrogen molecule from a macromolecule such as DNA to generate damage. Cells that have increased levels of free radical scavengers, such as glutathione, would have less DNA damage induced by x-rays, but would have similar levels of DNA damage induced by a carbon nucleus that is directly absorbed by chromosomal DNA. Furthermore, a low oxygen environment would also protect cells from x-ray–induced damage because there would be fewer radicals available to induce DNA damage in the absence of oxygen, but this environment would have little impact on DNA damage induced by carbon nuclei.[2]

Cellular Responses to Radiation-Induced DNA Damage

Checkpoint Pathways

The cell cycle must progress in a specific order; checkpoint genes ensure that the initiation of late events is delayed until earlier events are complete. There are three principal places in the cell cycle at which checkpoints induced by DNA damage function: the border between G1 phase and S phase, intra-S phase, and the border between G2 phase and mitosis (Fig. 13.3). Cells with an intact checkpoint function that have sustained DNA damage stop progressing through the cycle and become arrested at the next checkpoint in the cell cycle. For example, cells with damaged DNA in G1 phase avoid replicating that damage by arresting at the G1/S interface. If irradiated cells have already passed the restriction point, a position in G1 phase that is regulated by the phosphorylation of the retinoblastoma tumor suppressor gene (*Rb*) and its dissociation from the E2F family of transcription factors, they will transiently arrest in S phase. The G1/S and intra-S phase checkpoints inhibit the replication of damaged DNA and work in a coordinated manner with the DNA repair machinery to permit the restitution of DNA integrity, thereby increasing cell survival.

The earliest response to radiation is the activation of ataxia-telangiectasia mutated (ATM), which involves a conformational change that results in the activation of its kinase domain and phosphorylation of serine 1981 (see Fig. 13.3).[3] This phosphorylation causes the ATM homodimer to dissociate into active monomers that phosphorylate a wide range of proteins such as 53BP1, the histone variant H2AX, Nbs1 (Nijmegen breakage syndrome; a member of the *MRN complex*, composed of Mre11, Rad50, and Nbs1), BRCA1, and SMC1 (structural maintenance of chromosomes), and these proteins coordinate repair with the cell cycle.[4] In response to DNA damage, H2AX is rapidly phosphorylated by ATM and localizes to sites of DNA double-strand breaks in multiprotein complexes described as foci (Fig. 13.4). Phosphorylation of H2AX by ATM results in the direct recruitment of Mdc1 and forms a complex with H2AX to recruit additional ATM molecules, forming a positive feedback loop.

The G1/S phase checkpoint is the best understood. In response to DNA damage, activated ATM can directly phosphorylate p53 and mdm2, the ubiquitin ligase that targets p53 for degradation. These phosphorylations are important for increasing the stability of the p53 protein. In addition to ATM, checkpoint kinase 2 (Chk2) also phosphorylates p53 and can enhance p53 stability. Activated p53 transcriptionally increases the expression of the $p21^{WAF1/CIP1}$ gene, which results in a sustained inhibition of G1 cyclin/Cdk, and prevents phosphorylation of pRb and progression from G1 into S.[5] Mutations in p53 that are commonly found in solid tumors result in loss of transcriptional activity and compromised checkpoint function.

Control of the S-phase checkpoint is mediated in part by the Cdc25A phosphatase inhibiting Cdk2 activity and the loading of Cdc45 onto chromatin. If Cdc45 fails to bind to chromatin, DNA polymerase α is not recruited to replication origins and replicon initiation fails to occur.[6] A more prominent mechanism for S-phase arrest is signaled through the MRN complex and the cohesin protein SMC1 by ATM.[7] Loss of ATM, MRN components, or SMC1 leads to the loss of the intra-S phase checkpoint function and increased radiosensitivity. Both the CDC45 and ATM pathways represent parallel, but seemingly independent, pathways to protect replication forks from trying to replicate through DNA strand

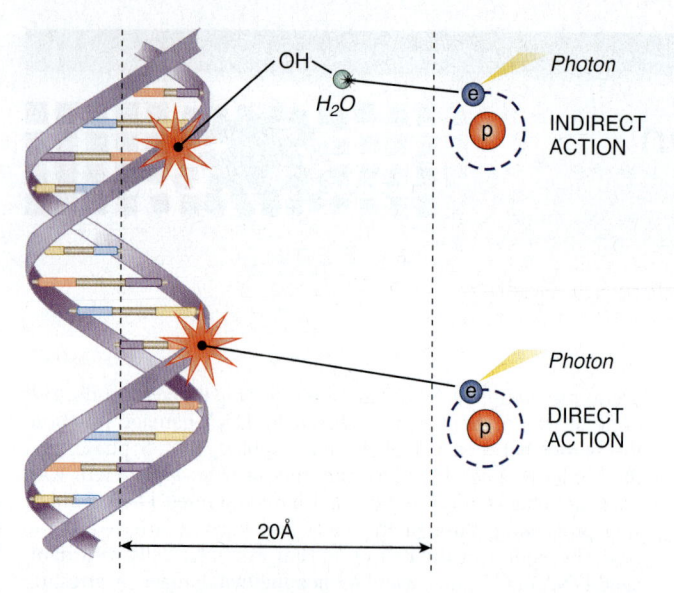

Figure 13.1 The direct and indirect effects of ionizing radiation on DNA. Incident photons transfer part of their energy to free electrons (Compton scattering). These electrons can directly interact with DNA to induce DNA damage, or they can first interact with water to produce hydroxyl radicals that can then induce damage.

breaks. Although ATM has received the lion's share of attention in signaling checkpoint activation in response to ionizing radiation, its family member ATR (ataxia telangiectasia and rad3-related) also plays a role in S-phase checkpoint responses.[8] ATM kinase activity is inducible by radiation, whereas ATR kinase activity is constitutive and does not significantly change with irradiation. (ATR is described in more detail in Chapter 19.) In contrast to Cdc45 and ATM, ATR is probably more important in monitoring

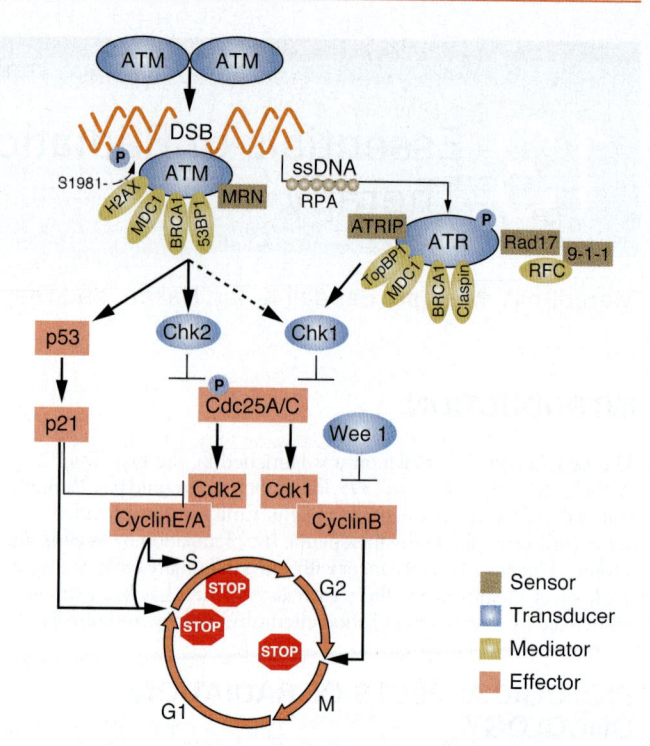

Figure 13.3 In response to DNA damage, the MRN complex—composed of MRE11, Rad50, and NBS1—together with ataxia-telangiectasia mutation (ATM) and H2AX are the earliest proteins recruited to the site of the break. ATM is released from its homodimer complex, activated by transautophosphorylation and, in turn, phosphorylates H2AX. Other members are recruited to the complex such as BRCA1 and 53BP1. As the DNA at the double-strand break (DSB) is resected, single-stranded DNA is formed and bound by replication protein A (RPA), resulting in the activation of the ataxia-telangiectasia and Rad3-related (ATR) pathway. The net result of ATM/ATR activation is the downstream activation of p53, leading to the transcription of the Cdk inhibitor, p21, and the activation of Chk1/Chk2, resulting in the degradation of Cdc25 phosphatases, Cdk-cyclin complex inactivation, and cell cycle arrest at phase G1, intra S, or G2. Note that ATM is also partially activated by changes in chromatin structure induced by DNA double-strand breaks.

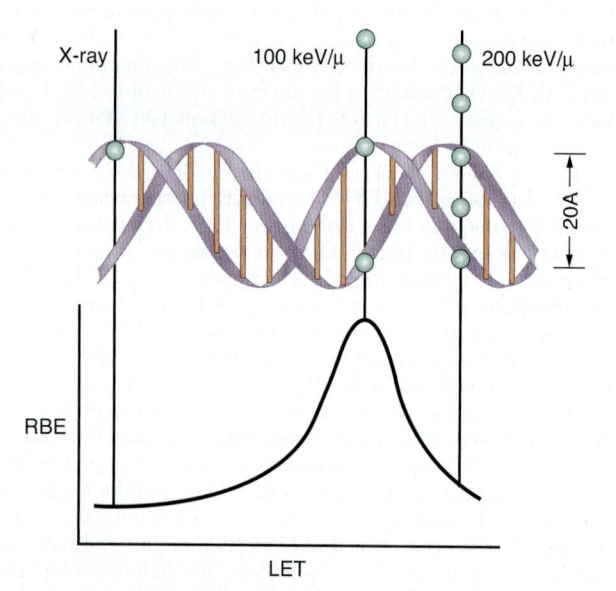

Figure 13.2 Linear energy transfer and DNA damage. Ionizing radiation deposits energy along the track (linear energy transfer [LET]), which causes DNA damage and cell killing. The most biologically potent (highest relative biologic effectiveness [RBE]) LET is 100 keV per μm because the separation between ionizing events is the same as the diameter of the DNA double helix (2 nm). (From Hall EJ, Giaccia AJ. *Radiobiology for the Radiologist*. Philadelphia: Lippincott Williams & Williams; 2012, with permission.)

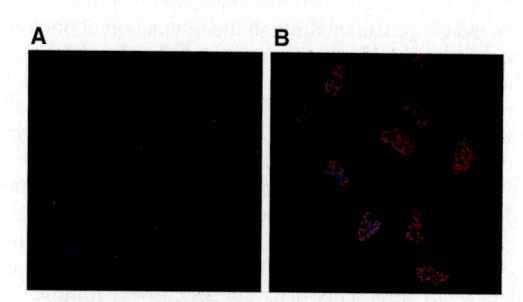

Figure 13.4 Phosphorylated histone variant H2AX as a marker of DNA damage. Phosphorylated histone variant H2AX (also called gamma H2AX) localizes to sites of DNA double-strand breaks, so that its appearance and disappearance correspond with induction and repair of breaks. The cells in panels **A** and **B** have been stained with DAPI (4′,6-diamidino-2-phenylindole) (*blue*) in order to visualize cell nuclei and stained with an antibody, which recognizes *gamma* H2AX (*red*). The cells in **A** are untreated and exhibit little to no gamma H2AX staining, whereas the cells in **B** are treated with 7.5 Gy radiation and exhibit strong gamma H2AX staining at punctate foci in the nuclei, which are thought to correlate with sites of DNA double-strand breaks. (Image provided by Dr. Leslie Parsels, University of Michigan.)

perturbations in replication that are the result of stalled replication forks to prevent the formation of DNA double-strand breaks.

The arrest of cells in the G2 phase following DNA damage is one of the most conserved evolutionary responses to ionizing radiation. It makes sense to have a final checkpoint in the G2 phase to prevent cells from entering into mitosis with damaged DNA that could be transmitted to their progeny. It follows that cells lacking the G2 checkpoint are radiosensitive because they try to divide with damaged chromosomes that cannot be aligned at metaphase to be properly apportioned to daughter cells. At the biochemical level, the regulation of the mitosis-promoting factor cyclin B/Cdk1 is the critical step in the activation of this checkpoint. At the molecular level, ATM and Chk1/2 are activated by DNA damage in the G2 phase and inhibit the activation of Cdc25A and C phosphatases, which are essential for the activation of cyclin B/Cdk1.[9,10] The pololike kinase family (Plk1 and Plk3) also responds to DNA damage and can inhibit Cdc25C activation.[11] A great deal of effort has been focused on the development of small molecules to inhibit checkpoint response proteins, such as Chk1, with the idea that they would inhibit radiation-induced G2 arrest and perhaps repair and thus be used as radiation sensitizers.[12]

DNA Repair

Ionizing radiation causes base damage, single-strand breaks, double-strand breaks, and sugar damage, as well as DNA–DNA, and DNA–protein cross-links. The critical target for ionizing radiation-induced cell inactivation and cell killing is the DNA double-strand break.[13,14] In eukaryotic cells, DNA double-strand breaks can be repaired by two processes: homologous recombination repair (HRR), which requires an undamaged DNA strand as a participant in the repair, and nonhomologous end joining (NHEJ), which mediates end-to-end joining.[15] In lower eukaryotes, such as yeast, HRR is the predominant pathway used for repairing DNA double-strand breaks, whereas mammalian cells use both HHR and non-HHR to repair their DNA. In mammalian cells, the choice of repair is biased by the phase of the cell cycle and by the abundance of repetitive DNA. HRR is used primarily in the late S phase/G2 phases of the cell-cycle, and NHEJ predominates in the G1-phase of the cell cycle (Fig. 13.5). NHEJ and HRR are not mutually exclusive, and both have been found to be active in the late S/G2 phase of the cell cycle, indicating that factors in addition to the cell-cycle phase are important in determining which mechanism will be used to repair DNA strand breaks.

Nonhomologous End Joining. In the G1-phase of the cell cycle, the ligation of DNA double-strand breaks is primarily through NHEJ because a sister chromatid does not exist to provide a template for HRR. The damaged ends of DNA double-strand breaks must first be modified before rejoining. The process of NHEJ can be divided into at least four steps: synapsis, end processing, fill-in synthesis, and ligation (Fig. 13.6).[16] Synapsis is the critical initial step where the Ku heterodimer and the DNA-dependent protein kinase catalytic subunit (DNA-PKcs) bind to the ends of the DNA double-strand break. Ku recruits not only DNA-PKcs to

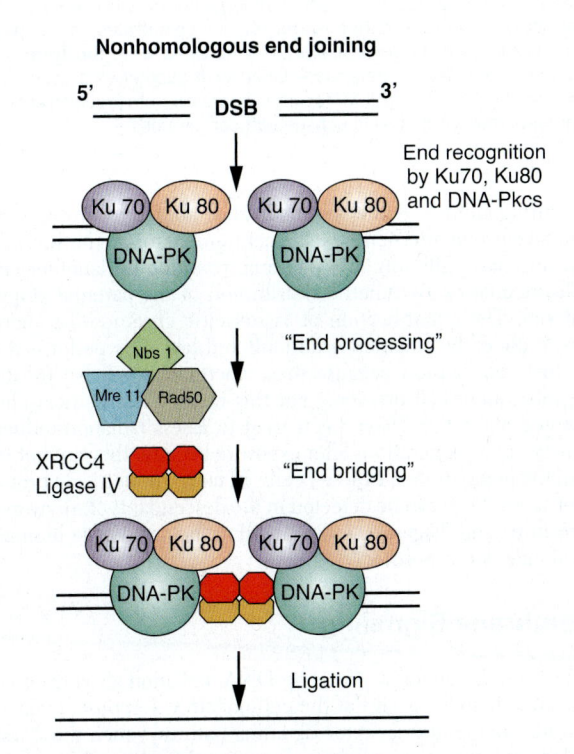

Figure 13.5 Schematic of the critical steps and proteins involved in nonhomologous end joining (NHEJ). The process of NHEJ can be divided into at least four steps: synapsis, end processing, fill-in synthesis, and ligation. DSB, double-strand break.

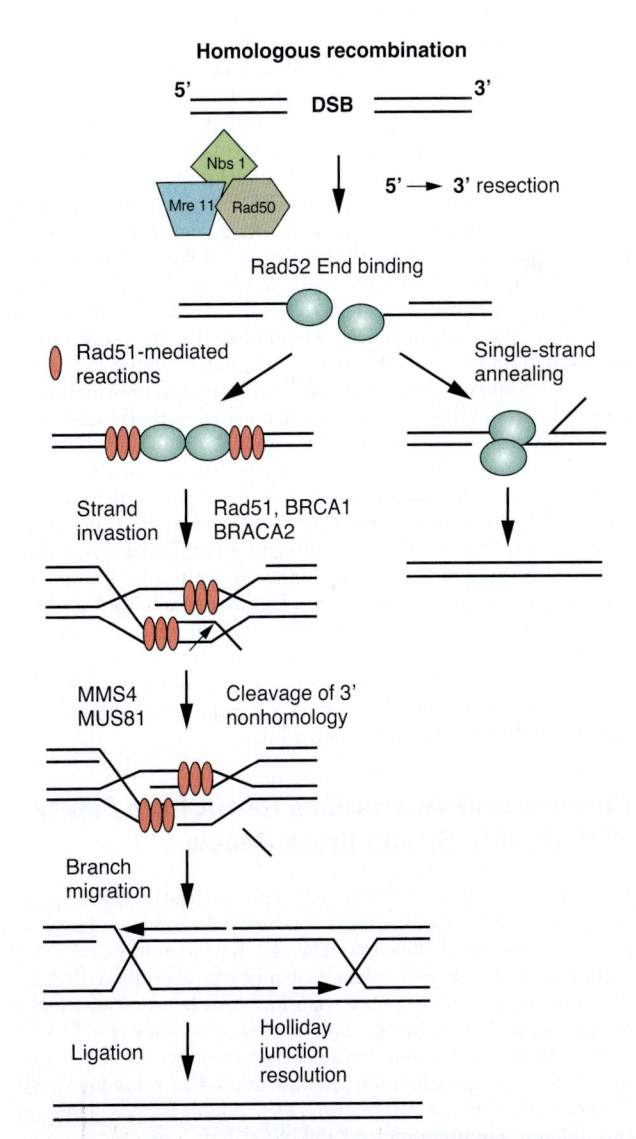

Figure 13.6 Schematic of the critical steps and proteins involved in homologous recombination repair (HRR). The process of HRR can be divided into the following steps: double-strand break (DSB) targeting by H2AX and the MRN complex, recruitment of the ataxia-telangiectasia mutation (ATM) kinase, end processing and protection, strand exchange, single-strand gap filling, and resolution into unique double-stranded molecules.

the DNA ends, but also artemis, a protein that possesses endonuclease activity for 5' and 3' overhangs as well as hairpins.[17] DNA-PKcs that is bound to the broken DNA ends phosphorylates artemis and activates its endonuclease activity for end processing. This role of artemis' endonuclease activity in NHEJ may not necessarily be required for the ligation of blunt ends or ends with compatible termini. DNA polymerase μ is associated with the Ku/DNA/XRCC4/DNA ligase IV complex, and is probably the polymerase that is used in the fill-in reaction. The actual rejoining of DNA ends is mediated by a XRCC4/DNA ligase IV complex, which is also probably recruited by the Ku heterodimer.[18,19] Although NHEJ is effective at rejoining DNA double-strand breaks, it is highly error prone. In fact, the main physiologic role of NHEJ is to generate antibodies through V(D)J rejoining, and the error-prone nature of NHEJ is essential for generating antibody diversity.

Homologous Recombination. HRR provides the mammalian genome a high-fidelity pathway of repairing DNA double-strand breaks. In contrast to NHEJ, HRR requires physical contact with an undamaged DNA template, such as a sister chromatid, for repair to occur. In response to a double-strand break, ATM as well as the complex of Mre11, Rad50, and Nbs1 proteins (MRN complex), are recruited to sites of DNA double-strand breaks (Fig. 13.6).[20] The MRN complex is also involved in the recruitment of the breast cancer tumor suppressor gene, *BRCA1*, to the site of the break.[21] In addition to recruiting *BRCA1* to the site of the DNA strand break, Mre11 and as yet unidentified endonucleases resect the DNA, resulting in a 3' single-strand DNA that serves as a binding site for Rad51. *BRCA2*, which is recruited to the double-strand break by BRCA1, facilitates the loading of the Rad51 protein onto replication protein A (RPA)-coated single-strand overhangs that are produced by endonuclease resection.[22] The Rad51 protein is a homolog of the *Escherichia coli* recombinase RecA, and possesses the ability to form nucleofilaments and catalyze strand exchange with the complementary strand of the undamaged chromatid, an essential step in HRR. Five additional paralogs of Rad51 also bind to the RPA-coated single-stranded region and recruit Rad52, which binds DNA and protects against exonucleolytic degradation.[23] To facilitate repair, the Rad54 protein uses its ATPase activity to unwind the double-stranded molecule. The two invading ends serve as primers for DNA synthesis, resulting in structures known as Holliday junctions. These Holliday junctions are resolved either by noncrossing over, in which case the Holliday junctions disengage and the DNA strands align followed by gap filling, or by crossing over of the Holliday junctions and gap filling. Because inactivation of most of the HRR genes discussed previously results in radiosensitivity and genomic instability, these genes provide a critical link between HRR and chromosome stability.

Chromosome Aberrations Result from Faulty DNA Double-Strand Break Repair

Unfaithful restitution of DNA strand breaks can lead to chromosome aberrations such as acentric fragments (no centromeres) or terminal deletions (uncapped chromosome ends). Radiation-induced DNA double-strand breaks also induce exchange-type aberrations that are the consequence of symmetric translocations between two DNA double-strand breaks in two different chromosomes (Fig. 13.7). Symmetrical chromosome translocations often do not lead to lethality, because genetic information is not lost in subsequent cell divisions. In contrast, when two DNA double-strand breaks in two different chromosomes recombine to form one chromosome with two centromeres and two fragments of chromosomes without centromeres or telomeres, cell death is inevitable. These types of chromosome aberrations are the consequence of asymmetrical chromosome translocations where the genetic material is recombined in what has been termed an *illegitimate* manner (e.g., a chromosome containing an extra centromere).

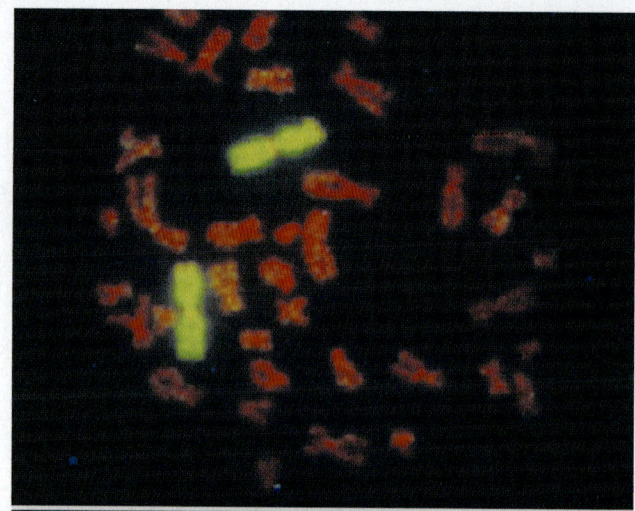

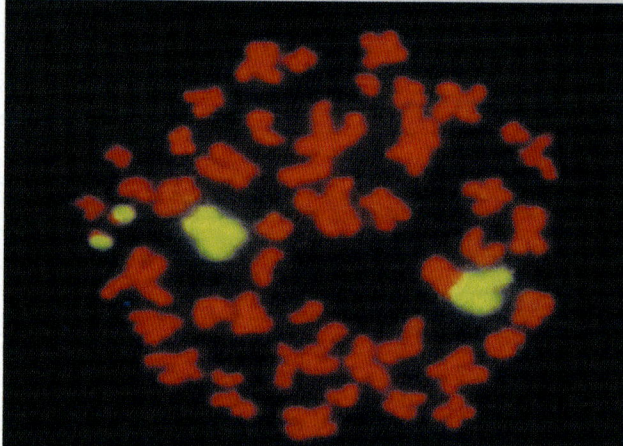

Figure 13.7 Fluorescent in situ hybridization of DNA probes that specifically recognize chromosome 4. In unirradiated cells **(top)**, two chromosome 4s are visualized. In irradiated cells **(bottom)**, one chromosome 4 illegitimately recombined with another chromosome to produce an asymmetrical chromosome aberration, with resulting acentric fragments that will be lost in subsequent cell divisions.

During mitosis, when a cell divides, aberrant chromosomes that have two centromeres, lack a centromere, or are in the shape of a ring have difficulty in separating, resulting in daughter cells with unequal or asymmetric distribution of the parental genetic material. The quantification of asymmetric chromosome aberrations induced by radiation is difficult and has to be performed by the first cell division because these aberrations will be lost during subsequent cell divisions. For this reason, symmetrical chromosome aberrations have been used to assess radiation-induced damage many generations after exposure because they are not lost from the population of exposed cells. In fact, symmetrical chromosome aberrations can be detected in the descendants of survivors of Hiroshima and Nagasaki, indicating that they are stable biomarkers of radiation exposure.[24]

Membrane Signaling

Apart from the direct of effects on DNA, radiation also affects cellular membranes. As part of the cellular stress response, radiation activates membrane receptor signaling pathways such those initiated via epidermal growth factor receptor (EGFR) and transforming growth factor β (TGF-β).[25,26] Activation of these pathways promotes overall survival in response to radiation by promoting DNA damage repair and/or cellular proliferation. In addition,

Cellular Response to Genotoxic Stress

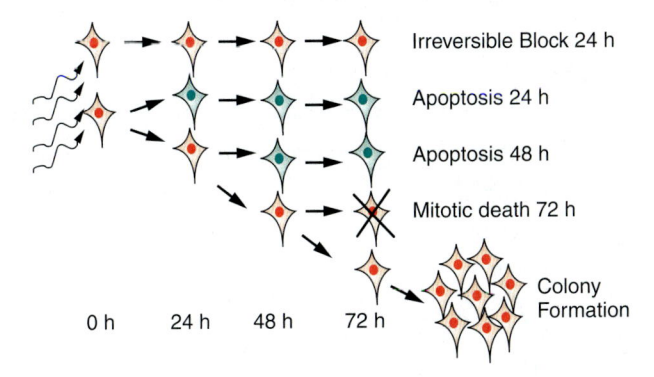

Figure 13.8 Consequences of exposure to ionizing radiation at the cellular level. Cells exposed to ionizing radiation can enter a state of senescence where they are unable to divide, but are still able to secrete growth factors. Alternatively, cells can die through apoptosis, mitotic linked cell death, or they can repair their DNA damage and produce viable progeny.

radiation also induces ceramide production at the membrane via activation of sphingomyelinases, which hydrolyze sphingomyelin to form ceramide. Ceramide production is linked to radiation-induced apoptosis.[27]

The Effect of Radiation on Cell Survival

The major potential consequences of cells exposed to ionizing radiation are normal cell division, DNA damage–induced senescence (reproductively inactive but metabolically active), apoptosis, or mitotic-linked cell death (Fig. 13.8). These manifestations of DNA damage can occur within one or two cell divisions or can manifest at later times after many cell divisions.[28] Effects that occur at later times have been termed *delayed reproductive cell death* and may also be influenced by secreted factors that are induced in response to radiation.[29]

The ability to culture cells derived from both normal and tumor tissues has allowed us to gain insight into how radiosensitivity varies between tissues by analyzing the shape of survival curves. Survival curves of tumor cells often possess a shouldered region at low doses that becomes shallower as the dose increases and eventually becomes exponential. A shoulder on a survival means that these low doses of radiation are less efficient in cell killing, presumably because cells are efficient at repairing DNA strand breaks.[13,14] Killing at low doses of radiation can be described in the form of a linear quadratic equation: $S = e^{-\alpha D - \beta D^2}$ (Fig. 13.9).[30] In this equation, S is the fraction of cells that survive a dose (D) of radiation, whereas α and β are constants. Cell killing by the linear and quadratic components are equal when $\alpha D = \beta D^2$ or $D = \alpha/\beta$. Over a larger dose range, the relationship between cell killing and dose is more complex and is described by three different components: an initial slope (D_1), a final slope (D_0), and the width of the shoulder (n, the extrapolation number) or D_q, the quasi-threshold dose (Fig. 13.10). The extrapolation number, n, defines the place where the shoulder intersects the ordinate when the dose is extrapolated to zero, and the quasithreshold dose, D_q, defines the width of the shoulder by cutting the dose axis when there is a survival fraction of unity. In contrast to photons, the shoulder on the survival curve disappears when cells are exposed to densely ionizing radiation from particles, indicating that this form of radiation is highly effective at killing cells at both low and high doses.

In Vivo Survival Determination of Normal Tissue Response to Radiation

Although much of our knowledge on the effects of radiation on cell survival has come from cell culture studies, investigators have also devised experimental approaches to assess the clonogenic survival of normal tissues. The earliest example came from McCulloch and Till,[31] who developed an assay to measure the

Figure 13.9 An analysis of survival curves for mammalian cells exposed to radiation by the linear quadratic model. The probability of hitting a critical target is proportional to dose (αD): the alpha component. The probability of hitting two critical targets will be the product of those probabilities; therefore, it will be proportional to dose^2 (βD^2): the beta component. The dose at which killing by both the alpha and beta components is equal is defined as $D = \alpha/\beta$. (From Hall EJ, Giaccia AJ. *Radiobiology for the Radiologist*. Philadelphia: Lippincott Williams & Williams; 2012, with permission.)

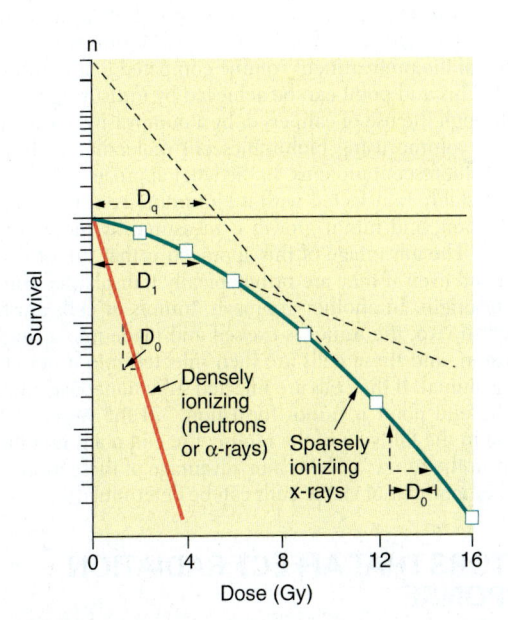

Figure 13.10 An analysis of survival curves for mammalian cells exposed to radiation by the multitarget model. This survival is described by an initial slope (D_1; dose to decreased survival to 37% on initial portion of the curve), a final slope (D_0; dose to decrease survival from starting point to 37% of that point on straight line portion of the curve), an extrapolation number (n; an estimate of the width of the shoulder), and a quasithreshold dose (D_q; a type of threshold dose below which radiation has no effect). (From Hall EJ, Giaccia AJ. *Radiobiology for the Radiologist*. Philadelphia: Lippincott Williams & Williams; 2012, with permission.)

clonogenic survival of bone marrow–derived cells in response to radiation by injecting them into a recipient mouse and quantifying the number of colonies that developed in the spleen. An analysis of these in vivo spleen assays indicated that bone marrow cells are highly radiosensitive (perhaps the most radiosensitive of all mammalian cells) in that their cell survival curve lacked a shoulder. These experiments represent two important firsts in the radiation sciences: They described the first development of an in vivo assay to assess normal tissue survival to radiation, and they demonstrated the first existence of normal tissue stem cells. Soon after, Withers and colleagues[32] developed an assay to assess the survival of skin stem cells, and Withers and Elkind[33] developed an assay to quantify the viability of small intestinal clonogens.

Because these ingenious approaches cannot be applied to all normal tissues, loss of tissue function instead of clonogenic survival has been used as an end point to assess radiation effects. Effects on tissue function can be grouped into the acute or late variety. Desquamation of skin by radiation is an example of an acute loss of function, whereas loss of spinal cord function is an example of a late functional effect. Acutely sensitive tissues such as skin, bone marrow, and intestinal mucosa possess a significant component of tissue cell division, whereas delayed sensitive tissues, such as spinal cord, breast, and bone, do not possess a significant amount of cell division or turnover and manifest radiation effects at later times.

In Vivo Determination of Tumor Response to Radiation

Assays have also been developed to assess the clonogenic survival of tumor cells in animals. Perhaps the most relevant of these assays is the tumor control dose 50% (TCD$_{50}$) assay,[34] in which the dose of radiation needed to control the growth of 50% of the tumors is determined in large cohorts of tumor-bearing animals. The TCD$_{50}$ assay in animals most closely approximates the clinical situation because tumors are irradiated in animals and the ability to kill all viable tumor cells is assessed. Unlike assays in which tumor cells are irradiated ex vivo, the TCD$_{50}$ assay takes into account the effects of the tumor microenvironment on tumor response. In contrast to the TCD$_{50}$ assay, the tumor growth delay assay reflects the time after irradiation that a transplanted tumor reaches a fixed multiple of the pretreatment volume compared to an unirradiated control. This end point can be achieved by measuring tumor volume through the use of calipers or by a noninvasive measurement of tumor volume using bioluminescent molecules such as luciferase or fluorescent proteins. In the latter approach, all the tumor cells are stably transfected with a bioluminescent marker before implantation, and tumor growth is measured by bioluminescent activity.[35] The advantage of this approach is that tumor cells can be assessed even if they are orthotopically transplanted into their tissue of origin. In another approach, tumors or cells are first irradiated in vivo, the tumor is excised and made into a single-cell suspension, and these cells are then injected into a non–tumor-bearing animal. If the cells are injected subcutaneously under the skin, the end point is tumor formation.[36] If the tumor cells are injected in the tail vein of the mouse, the end point is colony formation in the lungs.[37] The major advantage of these assays is that the actual number of viable cells can be determined.

FACTORS THAT AFFECT RADIATION RESPONSE

The Fundamental Principles of Radiobiology

Studies on split-dose repair (SDR) by Elkind et al.[38] uncovered three of what we now recognize as the most fundamental principles of fractionated radiotherapy: repair, reassortment, and repopulation (Fig. 13.11). (Reoxygenation, described in the following paragraphs, is the fourth). SDR describes the increased survival

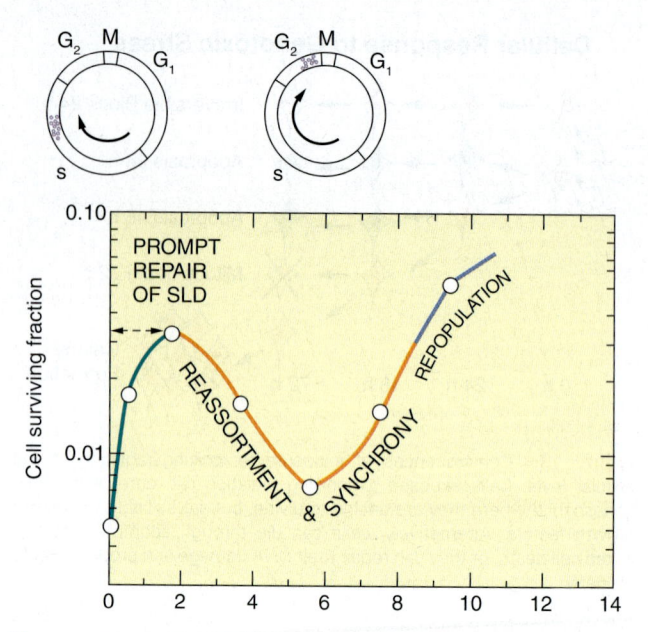

Figure 13.11 Idealized survival curve of rodent cells exposed to two fractions of x-rays. This figure illustrates how the time interval between doses alters the sensitivity of cells when exposed to multiple fractions. In this case, cells move from a resistant phase of the cell cycle (late S phase) to a sensitive phase of the cell cycle (G2 phase). This is known as *reassortment*. If longer periods of time occur between fractions of radiation, cells will undergo division. This latter process is called *repopulation*. SLD, sublethal damage. (From Hall EJ, Giaccia AJ. *Radiobiology for the Radiologist*. Philadelphia: Lippincott Williams & Williams; 2012, with permission.)

or tumor growth delay found if a dose of radiation is split into two fractions compared to the same dose administered in one fraction. This repair is likely due to DNA double-strand break rejoining. Elkind et al. found that the survival of cells increased with an increase in time between doses for up to a maximum of about 6 hours. This finding is consistent with the clinical observation that a separation of radiation treatments by 6 hours produces similar normal tissue injury as a 24-hour separation. The shoulder of a survival curve is strongly influenced by SDR: The broader the shoulder, the more SDR and the smaller α/β ratio.

Similar to repair, reassortment and repopulation are also dependent on the interval of time between radiation fractions. If cells are given short time intervals between doses, they can progress from a resistant portion of the cell cycle (e.g., S phase) to a sensitive portion of the cell cycle (e.g., G2 phase). This transit between resistant and sensitive phases of the cell cycle is termed *reassortment*. If irradiated cells are provided even longer intervals of time between doses, the survival of the population of irradiated cells will increase. This increase in split-dose survival after longer periods of time is the result of cell division and has been termed *repopulation*. Reassortment and repopulation appear to have more protracted kinetics in normal tissues than rapidly proliferating tumor cells, and thereby enhance the tumor response to fractionated radiotherapy compared to normal tissues.

Dose-Rate Effects

For sparsely ionizing radiation, dose rate plays a critical factor in cell killing. Lowering the dose rate, and thereby increasing exposure time, reduces the effectiveness of killing by x-rays because of increased SDR. A further reduction in dose rate results in more SDR and reduces the shoulder of the survival curve. Thus, if one plots the survival for individual doses in a multifraction experiment so that there is sufficient time for SDR to occur, the resulting survival curve would have little shoulder and appear almost linear.[39]

In some cell types, there is a threshold to the lowering of dose rate, and in fact, one paradoxically finds an increase, instead of a decrease, in cell killing. This increase in cell killing under these conditions of protracted dose rate is due to the accumulation of cells in a radiosensitive portion of the cell cycle. In summary, the magnitude of the dose rate effect varies between cell types because of SDR, the redistribution of cells through the cell cycle, and the time for cell division to occur.

Cell Cycle

The phase of the cell cycle at the time of radiation influences the cell's inherent sensitivity to radiation. Cells synchronized in late G1/early S and G2/M phases are most sensitive, whereas cells in G1 and mid to late S phase are more resistant to radiation.[1] These differences in sensitivity during the cell cycle are exploited by the concept of reassortment during fractioned radiotherapy as well by the use of chemotherapeutic agents, which reassort cells into more sensitive phases of the cell cycle in combination with radiation.

Tumor Oxygenation

The major microenvironmental influence on tumor response to radiation is molecular oxygen.[40] Decreased levels of oxygen (hypoxia) in tissue culture result in decreased killing after radiation, which can be expressed as an *oxygen enhancement ratio* (OER). Operationally, OER is defined as the ratio of doses to give the same killing under hypoxic and normoxic conditions. At high doses of radiation, the OER is approximately 3, whereas at low doses, it is closer to 2.[41] Oxygen must be present within 10 μs of irradiation to achieve its radiosensitizing effect. Under hypoxic conditions, damage to DNA can be repaired more readily than under oxic conditions, where damage to DNA is "fixed" because of the interaction of oxygen with free radicals generated by radiation. These changes in radiation sensitivity are detectable at oxygen ranges below 30 mm Hg. Most tumor cells exhibit a survival difference halfway between fully aerobic and fully anoxic cells when exposed to a partial pressure of oxygen between 3 and 10 mm Hg.[1] The presence of hypoxia has greater significance for single-dose fractions used in the treatment of certain primary tumors and metastases and is less important for fractionated radiotherapy, where reoxygenation occurs between fractions. Furthermore, most hypoxic cells are not actively undergoing cell division, thus impeding the efficacy of conventional chemotherapeutic agents that are targeted to actively dividing cells.

Although normal tissue and tumors vary in their oxygen concentrations, only tumors possess levels of oxygen low enough to influence the effectiveness of radiation killing. Although the variations in normal tissue oxygenation are in large part due to physiology governing acute changes in oxygen consumption, the variations in tumor oxygen can be directly attributed to abnormal vasculature that results in a more chronic condition. Thomlinson and Gray[42] observed that variations in tumor oxygen occur because there is insufficient vasculature to provide oxygen to all tumor cells. They hypothesized that oxygen is unable to reach tumor cells beyond 10 to 12 cell diameters from the lumen of a tumor blood vessel because of metabolic consumption by respiring tumor cells. This form of hypoxia caused by metabolic consumption of oxygen has been termed *chronic* or *diffusion-mediated hypoxia*. In contrast, changes in blood flow due either to interstitial pressure changes in tumor blood vessels that lack a smooth muscle component or red blood cell fluxes can cause transient occlusion of blood vessels resulting in *acute* or *transient hypoxia*. Chronically, hypoxic cells will only become reoxygenated when their distance from the lumen of a blood vessel decreases, such as during fractionated radiotherapy when tumor cords shrink. In contrast, tumor cells that are acutely hypoxic because of changes in blood flow or interstitial pressure often cycle in an unpredictable manner between oxic and hypoxic states as blood flow changes.

Based on studies demonstrating that hypoxia can alter radiation sensitivity and decrease tumor control by radiotherapy, strategies have been developed to increase tumor oxygenation. Most importantly, it appears that tumor oxygen levels increase during a course of fractionated radiation. This may be one of the most important benefits of fractionated radiation and is termed *reoxygenation* (the fourth of the four Rs of radiobiology). Tumor reoxygenation during a course of fractionated radiation may also offer an explanation for the general lack of clinical efficacy of hypoxic cell sensitizers despite the clear evidence that hypoxia causes radioresistance.

Aside from using fractionated radiation, the most direct approach to increasing tumor oxygenation is to expose patients receiving radiotherapy to hyperbaric oxygen therapy. The underlying concept is that increasing the amount of oxygen in the bloodstream should result in more oxygen being available for diffusion to the hypoxic regions of tumors. Experimentally, hyperbaric oxygen therapy increases the sensitivity of transplanted tumors to radiation. The results of clinical studies with hyperbaric oxygen therapy, when combined with radiotherapy, showed improvement for two sites—head and neck cancers, and cervix cancers—but failed to show an improvement with other sites, thus calling into question its general usefulness in radiotherapy.[43] In a related approach, erythropoietin (EPO), a hormone released by the kidney that increases red blood cell production, should also increase tumor oxygenation by increasing the delivery of hemoglobin-bound oxygen molecules. EPO has been effective at correcting anemia, but has not been successful in combination with radiation to control head and neck cancer and may, in fact, stimulate tumor growth.[44,45]

Another strategy to increase tumor oxygenation has been the combined use of nicotinamide, which increases tissue perfusion and carbogen (95% O_2 and 5% CO_2) breathing (accelerated radiotherapy with carbogen and nicotinamide [ARCON] therapy). Recently, a randomized phase III clinical trial demonstrated improved regional but not local tumor control in larynx cancer patients treated with nicotinamide, carbogen, and radiation versus radiation alone.[46] Biologics such as antivascular endothelial growth factor (anti-VEGF) therapy have also been demonstrated to increase tumor oxygenation.[47] Anti-VEGF therapy may increase tumor oxygenation by eliminating abnormal vessels that are inadequate in perfusing tumor cells—the so-called *vascular normalization hypothesis*. Although there is solid experimental evidence to support this hypothesis, there appears to be only a short window of time in which it could be effectively combined with radiotherapy.

Because the presence of hypoxia has both prognostic and potential therapeutic implications, a substantial effort has been invested in trying to image hypoxia.[48] The goal of using imaging to "paint" radiation doses to different regions of tumors, although technically possible (as described in the next section, Radiation Physics), faces the problem that changes in oxygenation are dynamic.[49] In the future, hypoxia-directed treatment may evolve from the use of hypoxic cell cytotoxins to targeted drugs that exploit cellular signaling changes induced by hypoxia such as hypoxia-inducible factor 1α (HIF-1α). However, despite the strong rationale supporting their use, at this time, there are no agents used in the clinic that target hypoxia.

Immune Response

The abscopal effects of radiation (i.e., tumor cell killing outside of the radiation field) have been attributed to the activation of antigen and cytokine release by radiation, which subsequently activates a systemic immune response against tumor cells.[50,51] This response begins with the transfer of tumor cell antigens to dendritic cells and, subsequently, the activation of tumor-specific T cells and *immunogenic tumor cell death*. It is likely that radiation dose and fractionation influence the optimal immune response with higher doses and fewer fractions of radiation than those used in conventional fractionation schemes appearing superior in experimental models. Unfortunately, abscopal effects are uncommon because immune system evasion is an inherent characteristic of cancer cells that often dominates, even in the presence of a radiation-induced immune response. Strategies to amplify radiation-induced immune responses, and thus to overcome tumor cell evasion of the immune system, are under investigation. The combination of radiation with immune *checkpoint* modulators such as ipilimumab, an antibody against cytotoxic T-lymphocyte antigen 4 (CTLA-4), have shown promising, albeit anecdotal, clinical effects.

DRUGS THAT AFFECT RADIATION SENSITIVITY

For over 30 years now, chemotherapy and radiotherapy have been administered concurrently. In order to maximize the efficacy of radiochemotherapy, it is necessary to understand the biologic mechanisms underlying radiosensitization by chemotherapeutic agents. The several classes of standard chemotherapeutic agents as well as novel molecularly targeted agents that possess radiosensitizing properties will be discussed in this section.

Antimetabolites

5-fluorouracil is among the most commonly used chemotherapeutic radiation sensitizers. Given in combination with radiation, it has led to clinical improvements in a variety of cancers, including those of the head and neck, the esophagus, the stomach, the pancreas, the rectum, the anus, and the cervix. The combination of 5-fluorouracil with radiation is now a standard therapy for cancers of the stomach (adjuvant), the pancreas (unresectable), and the rectum. For other cancers such as head and neck, esophagus, or anal, 5-fluorouracil and radiation are combined with cisplatin or mitomycin C, respectively. Being an analog of uracil, 5-flourouracil is misincorporated into RNA and DNA. However, the ability of 5-fluorouracil to radiosensitize is related to its ability to inhibit thymidylate synthase, which leads to the depletion of thymidine triphosphate (dTTP) and the inhibition of DNA synthesis. This slowed, inappropriate progression through S phase in response to 5-fluorouracil is thought to be the mechanism underlying radiosensitization.[52] Similar to 5-fluorouracil, the oral thymidylate synthase inhibitor, capecitabine, is also being increasingly used in combination with radiation.

Gemcitabine (2′, 2′-deoxyfluorocytidine [dFdCyd]) is another potent antimetabolite radiosensitizer. Preclinical studies have demonstrated that radiosensitization by gemcitabine involves the depletion of deoxyadenosine triphosphate (dATP) (related to the ability of gemcitabine diphosphate (dFdCDP) to inhibit ribonucleotide reductase) as well as the redistribution of cells into the early S phase of the cell cycle.[53] The combination of gemcitabine with radiation in clinical trials has suggested improved clinical outcomes for patients with cancers of the lung, pancreas, and bladder. Gemcitabine-based chemoradiation has developed into a standard therapy for locally advanced pancreatic cancer. However, in some clinical trials, such as those in lung and head and neck cancers, the combination of gemcitabine with radiation has led to increased mucositis and esophagitis.[54] Thus, it should be emphasized that in the presence of gemcitabine, radiation fields must be defined with great caution. Such is the case with pancreatic cancer, where the combination of full-dose gemcitabine with radiation to the gross tumor can be safely administered if clinically uninvolved lymph nodes are excluded.[55] Conversely, the inclusion of the regional lymphatics in the treatment field in combination with full-dose gemcitabine produces unacceptable toxicities.[56]

Platinums and Temozolomide

Cisplatin is likely the most commonly used chemotherapeutic agent in combination with radiation. Although cisplatin was the prototype for several other platinum analogs, carboplatin is also frequently used in combination with radiation. Cisplatin, in combination with radiation, and sometimes in conjunction with a second chemotherapeutic agent, is indicated for cancers of the head and neck, esophagus (with 5-fluorouracil), the lung, the cervix, and the anus. Radiosensitization by cisplatin is related to its ability to cause inter- and intra-strand DNA cross-links. Removal of these cross-links during the repair process results in DNA strand breaks. Although there are multiple theories to explain the mechanism(s) of radiosensitization by cisplatin, two plausible explanations are that cisplatin inhibits the repair (both homologous and nonhomologous) of radiation-induced DNA double-strand breaks and/or increases the number of lethal radiation-induced double-strand breaks.[57]

Temozolomide in combination with radiation is standard therapy for glioblastoma. Temozolomide is an alkylating agent, which forms methyl adducts at the O^6 position of guanine (as well as at N^7 and N^3-guanine) that are subsequently improperly repaired by the mismatch repair pathway. Radiosensitization by temozolomide involves the inhibition of DNA repair and/or an increase in radiation-induced DNA double-strand breaks due to radiation-induced single-strand breaks in proximity to O^6 methyl adducts. Like cisplatin, temozolomide-mediated radiosensitization does not seem to require cell cycle redistribution.

Taxanes

The taxanes, paclitaxel and docetaxel, act to stabilize microtubules resulting in the accumulation of cells in G2/M, the most radiation-sensitive phase of the cell cycle. The radiosensitizing properties of the taxanes are thought to be attributable to the redistribution of cells into G2/M. Paclitaxel, in combination with radiation (and carboplatin), has demonstrated a clinical benefit in the treatment of resectable lung carcinoma.[58]

Molecularly Targeted Agents

Molecularly targeted agents are especially appealing in the context of radiosensitization because they are generally less toxic than standard chemotherapeutic agents and need to be given in multimodality regimens (given their often inadequate efficacy as single agents). The EGFR has been intensely pursued as a target; both antibody and small molecule EGFR inhibitors, such as cetuximab and erlotinib, respectively, have been developed. The head and neck seem to be the most promising tumor sites for the combination of EGFR inhibitors with radiation therapy. Preclinical data have demonstrated that the schedule of administration of EGFR inhibitors with radiation is important; EGFR inhibition before chemoradiation may produce antagonism.[59] In a randomized phase III trial, cetuximab plus radiation produced a significant survival advantage over radiation alone in patients with locally advanced head and neck cancer.[60] In a subsequent trial, however, cetuximab in combination with concurrent, cisplatin-based chemoradiation failed to produce a survival benefit in head and neck cancer patients.[61] The combination of EGFR inhibitor with cisplatin-radiation requires further preclinical investigation.

Although EGFR inhibition, concurrent with radiation, is by far the best established combination of a molecularly targeted agent with radiation, other exciting molecularly targeted agents are being developed as radiation sensitizers. Targeting DNA damage response pathways is one approach to radiosensitization. Recently, agents that abrogate radiation-induced cell cycle checkpoints, such as Wee1 and Chk1 inhibitors, have been shown to radiosensitize tumor cells and are currently in clinical development in combination with chemotherapy, with clinical trials planned in combination with radiation.[62,63] In addition, poly(ADP-ribose) polymerase (PARP) inhibitors have been demonstrated to preclinically induce radiosensitization, and several clinical trials combining PARP inhibitors with radiation therapy are underway.[64]

Other Agents

Although the most common clinically used agents in combination with radiation have been shown to produce significant clinical benefit, as described previously, other agents with different mechanisms of action have been used as radiation sensitizers as well as radiation protectors. The vinca alkaloids, such as vincristine, possess radiosensitizing properties due to their ability to block mitotic spindle assembly and, thus, arrest cells in M phase. Although vincristine is used in combination with radiation to treat medulloblastoma, rhabdomyosarcoma, and brain stem glioma, its use is principally based on its lack of myelosuppressive side effects, which are dose limiting for radiation in these types of tumors, rather than its potential radiosensitizing properties.

Also worth mention in a discussion of modulators of radiation sensitivity are agents designed to radioprotect normal tissues. One such type of drug, amifostine, is a free radical scavenger with some selectivity toward normal tissues that express more alkaline phosphatase than tumor cells, the enzyme of which converts amifostine to a free thiol metabolite. Clinical trials in head and neck as well as lung cancers have shown a reduction in radiation-related toxicities such as xerostomia, mucositis, esophagitis, and pneumonitis, respectively.[65,66] However, further clinical investigations are necessary to conclusively demonstrate a lack of tumor protection and safety in combination with chemoradiotherapy regimens.

RADIATION PHYSICS

Physics of Photon Interactions

Tumors requiring radiation can be found at depths ranging from zero to 10s of centimeters below the skin. The goal of treatment is to deliver sufficient ionizing radiation to the tumor site, which can result in an absorbed dose. This involves both the availability of treatment beams and delivery techniques, and the methods to plan the treatments and ensure their safe delivery. This section will establish the general physical basis for the use of ionizing radiation in the treatment of tumors, briefly describe some of the treatment equipment, indicate physical qualities of the treatment beams themselves, and summarize the treatment planning process. Those who desire more in-depth details are referred to textbooks and other resources dedicated to medical physics and the technologic aspects of radiation oncology.[67] Most patients who are treated with radiation receive high-energy, external-beam photon therapy. Here, *external* indicates that the treatment beam is generated and delivered from outside of the body. High-energy (6 to 20 MV) photon beams (electromagnetic radiation) penetrate tissue, enabling the treatment of deep-seated tumors. Modern equipment generates these beams with sufficient fluence to ensure delivery of therapeutic fractions of dose in short treatment sessions. Other types of particles and beams also exist for use in treating tumors both externally and internally. They are mentioned briefly later. However, as external photon beams dominate the practice (and as common basic physics principles related to delivered dose exist among the modalities), the focus here will be on photon beam generation and interactions in tissue.

As mentioned earlier, ionizing radiation kills cells via both direct and indirect mechanisms. Radiation therapy aims to instigate those ionizations and events in the tumor cells. Photons are massless, uncharged packets of energy that primarily interact with matter via electromagnetic processes. As a consequence of those interactions, an incident photon can become either entirely absorbed (giving up its energy to the ejection of an atomic electron [photoelectric effect]), or create an energetic electron-positron pair (pair production), or scatter off an electron with a reduction in energy and a change in direction and subsequent transfer of parts of its energy to the free electron (Compton scattering). The secondary electrons generated as a consequence of these interactions have residual energy, mass, and, most importantly, electric charge. They slow down in matter through multiple interactions with (primarily) the electrons of atoms, leading to excitation and ionization of those atoms. These ionizations (hence the term *ionizing radiation*) lead to a local absorption of energy (i.e., dose = energy absorbed per unit mass) and the direct and indirect cell killing effects necessary to treat tumors.

Thus, the use of external photon beams for cancer therapy involves a two-step process: interaction (scattering) of the photons, with subsequent dose deposition via the secondary electrons. The probability of photon interactions is energy dependent. Photoelectric interactions dominate at lower photon energies. Whereas these beams are ideal for diagnostic procedures (for their preferential absorption by tissues of differing atomic number, leading to good subject contrast), they are attenuated too quickly in tissues to supply enough interactions to be useful for therapy for any but the most superficial tumors. Pair production interactions dominate at higher photon energies; however, the probability of interacting in tissues for those high-energy photons is so low as to preclude them from general use as well. In the 10s to 100s of kiloelectron volt (keV) to the few megaelectron volt (MeV) photon energy range, Compton scattering dominates. As will be shown, these beams have sufficient penetration and can be generated with sufficient intensity to be useful for tumor treatments, especially when combined in treatment plans that comprise multiple beams entering the patient from different directions but overlapping at the tumor.

It is useful to point out physical scales of reference for external photon beam therapy. A typical megavoltage photon beam may have an average photon energy near 2 MeV. Those photons primarily undergo Compton scattering with a mean free path in tissue of approximately 20 cm. An average Compton interaction results in a secondary electron with a mean energy near 0.5 MeV (and a Compton scattered photon near 1.5 MeV, which likely escapes or scatters elsewhere in the patient). A typical secondary electron of approximately 0.5 MeV will cause excitations and ionizations of atoms as it dissipates its energy over a path length of approximately 2 mm. This could be expected to lead to approximately 10,000 ionizations, or about 5 ionizations per micron of tissue. As can be seen, therapeutic damage to the DNA of cancer cells (2 nm; see Fig. 13.2) will require very many Compton scatterings with statistical interaction among the ionizations resulting from the slowing down of the secondary electrons.

Photon Beam Generation and Treatment Delivery

As previously mentioned, effective external-beam photon treatments require higher energy beams capable of reaching deep-seated tumors with sufficient fluence to make it likely that the dose deposition will kill the tumor cells. To spare normal tissues and maximize targeting, beams are arranged to enter the patient from several directions and to intersect at the center of the tumor (treatment isocenter). Although machines containing collimated beams from high-intensity radioactive sources (primarily cobalt 60 [^{60}Co]) are still in use, today's modern treatment machine accelerates electrons to high (MeV) energy and impinges them onto an x-ray production target, leading to the generation of intense beams of Bremsstrahlung x-rays. A typical photon beam treatment machine[68,69] (Fig. 13.12) consists of a high-energy (6 to 20 MeV) linear electron accelerator, electromagnetic beam steering and

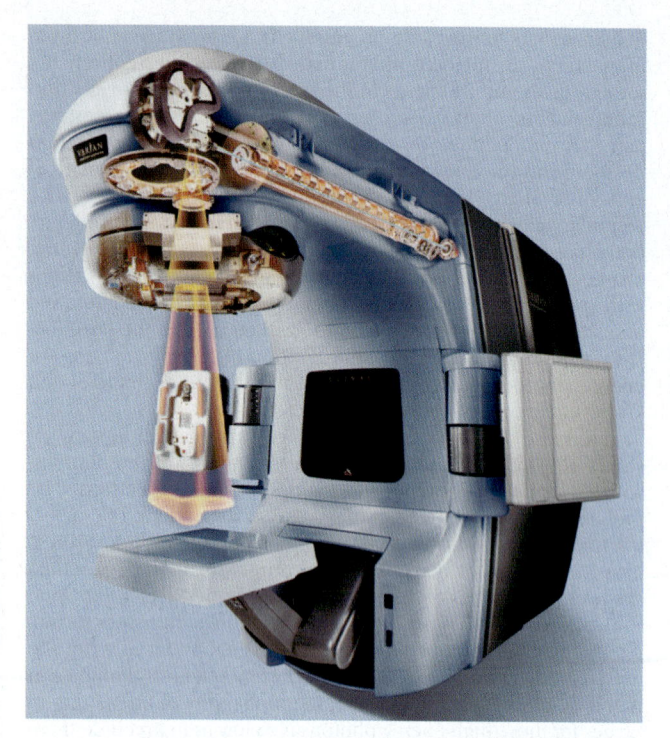

Figure 13.12 A shadow view of a C-arm linear accelerator. The electron beam (originating at upper right) is accelerated through a linear accelerator wave guide, selected for correct energy in a bending magnet, and then impinges on an x-ray production target. The x-ray beam (originating at target upper left) is flattened and collimated before leaving the treatment head. Also illustrated (downstream from the beam) is an electric portal imager that is used to measure (image) the beam exiting a patient. (From Varian Medical Systems, Palo Alto, CA, with permission.)

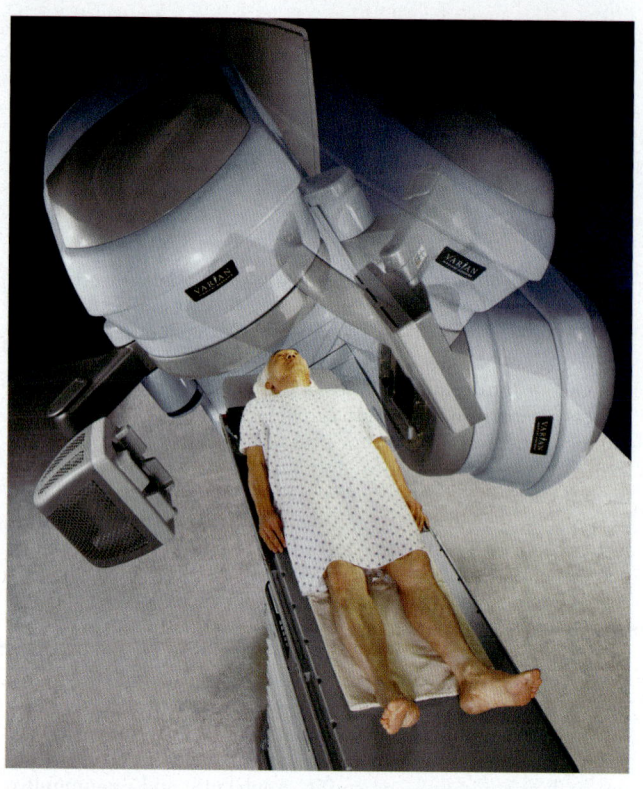

Figure 13.13 Model in treatment position on the patient support table. The treatment delivery head on the gantry's C-arm rotates about the patient, enabling the delivery of beams throughout 360 degrees of rotation. (From Varian Medical Systems, Palo Alto, CA, with permission.)

monitoring systems, x-ray generation targets, high-density treatment field-shaping devices (collimators), and up to a ton of radiation shielding on a mechanical C-arm gantry that can rotate precisely around a treatment couch (Fig. 13.13). These treatment-delivery machines routinely maintain mechanical isocenters for patient treatments to within a sphere of 1 mm radius. The development of *stereotactic radiotherapy*, which will be described in the section titled Clinical Application of Types of Radiation, depends on this level of machine precision.

X-ray production by monoenergetic high-energy electrons results in an x-ray (photon) beam that contains a continuous spectrum of energies with maximum photon energy near that of the incident electron beam. Lower energy photons appear with a much greater probability than do the highest energy ones, but they also become preferentially filtered out of the beam through the absorption in the target and the attenuation in the flattening filter. This generally results in a treatment beam energy spectrum with a mean photon energy of approximately one-third of the initial electron beam energy. In this energy range, the resulting photon beam exits the production target with a narrow angular spread focused primarily in the forward direction. These forward-peaked intensity distributions generally need to be modulated (flattened) to produce a large (up to 40 cm diameter at the patient) photon beam with uniform intensity across the beam. All modern treatment units take advantage of extensive computer control, monitoring, and feedback to produce highly stable and reproducible treatment beams.

The resulting photon beam requires beam shaping for conformal dose delivery. Some combination of primary, high-density field blocks (collimators) together with additional edge blocks generally provide the required shaping and shielding. Modern machines use computer-controlled multileaf collimators (Fig. 13.14)

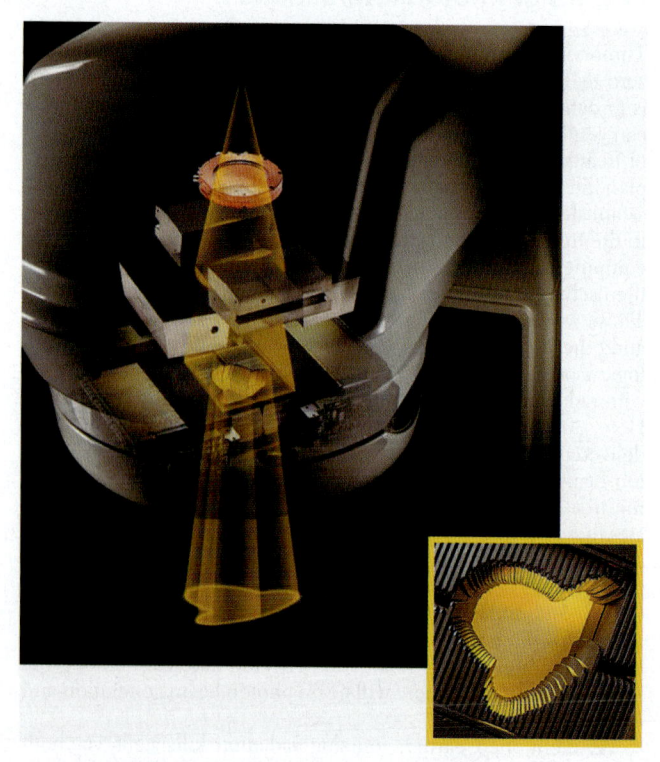

Figure 13.14 Multileaf collimator shaping of an x-ray treatment beam from a linear accelerator. *Inset* shows a view of the multileaf collimator. (From Varian Medical Systems, Palo Alto, CA, with permission.)

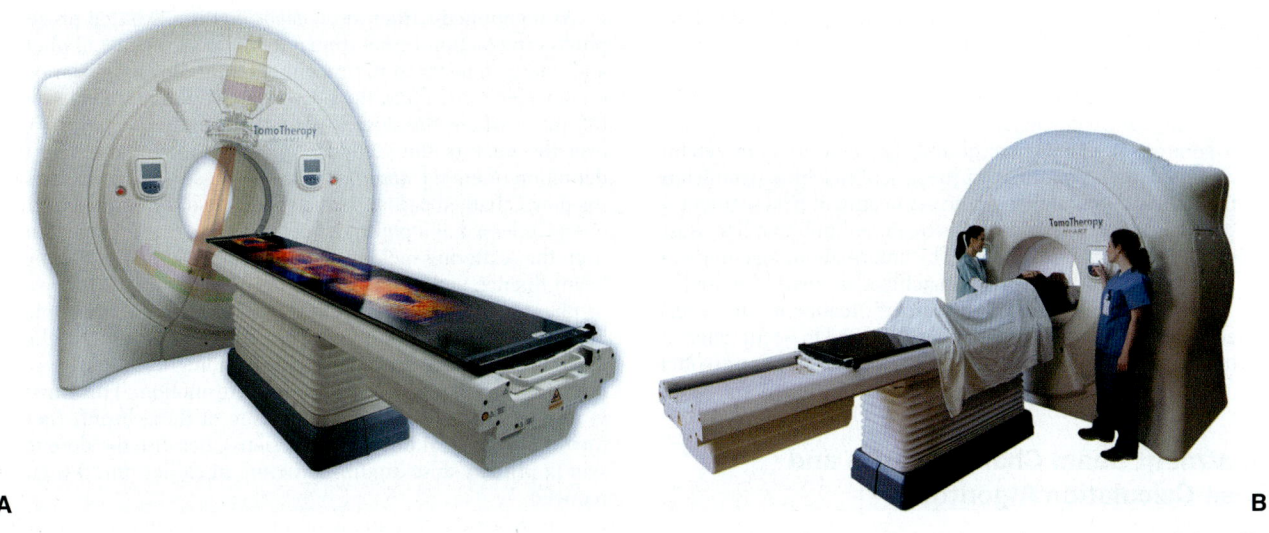

Figure 13.15 **(A)** A shadow view of linear accelerator, x-ray beam production system, and x-ray fan beam for helical tomotherapy treatment delivery. The beam production system rotates within its enclosed gantry. **(B)** The model patient on treatment table slides into the treatment unit. During treatment, the table moves as the collimated fan beam rotates about the patient, creating a modulated helical dose delivery pattern. (From TomoTherapy, Inc., Madison, WI, with permission.)

for the edge sculpting subsequent to setting the primary collimators for maximal shielding. This computer control provides high precision and reproducibility in the definition of field edges. Additionally, automation allows for a precise reshaping of the treatment beam for each angle of incidence, allowing not only conformation of irradiation to target volumes, but also modulation of the beam intensity patterns across the field (intensity-modulated radiation therapy [IMRT]).

Variations on the standard linear accelerator (linac) plus C-arm scenario that are being used for external-beam radiation treatments throughout the body include helical tomotherapy and nonisocentric miniature linac robotic delivery systems.[70] In helical tomotherapy, the accelerator, photon-production target, and collimation system are mounted on a ring gantry (similar to those found on diagnostic computed tomography [CT] scanners) (Fig. 13.15). It produces a fan beam of photons, and the intensity of each part of the fan being modulated by a binary collimator. As the gantry rotates, the patient simultaneously slides through the bore of the machine (again analogous to modern x-ray/CT imagers), which allows for the continuous delivery of intensity-modulated radiation in a helical pattern from all angles around a patient. Another delivery system uses an industrial robot to hold a miniature accelerator plus photon beam-production system (Fig. 13.16). The bulk of the system is reduced by keeping the field sizes small (spotlike). However, computer control of the robot provides flexibility in irradiating tumors from nearly any position external to the patient. The same control allows for the selection and use of many differing beam angles to build up the dose at the tumor location.

To take advantage of the precision of modern beam delivery, it is crucial to localize the patient's tumor and normal tissue.[71] This process can be divided into patient immobilization (i.e., limiting the motion of the patient) and localization (i.e., knowing the tumor and normal tissue location precisely in space). Although these concepts of immobilization and localization are related, they are not identical. Patients can be held reasonably comfortable in their treatment pose with the aid of foam molds and meshes (i.e., immobilization devices). Traditionally, localization has been achieved by indexing the immobilization device to the computer-controlled treatment couch and by using low-power laser beams aligned to skin marks. These techniques make it possible to reproducibly couple the surface of each patient with the treatment machine isocenter.

However, what is truly needed is to localize the tumor and normal tissues. The development of in-room, online x-ray, ultrasound, and infrared imaging equipment can now be used to ensure that the intended portions of each patient's internal anatomy are correctly positioned at the time of treatment. In particular, the development of rugged, low-profile, active matrix, flat-panel imaging devices, either attached to the treatment gantry or placed in the vicinity of the treatment couch, together with diagnostic x-ray generators or the patient treatment beam (see Fig. 13.13), allows the digital capture of projection x-ray images of patient anatomy with respect to the isocenter and treatment field borders. These digitized electronic images are immediately available for analysis. Software tools allow for a comparison to reference images and the generation of correction coordinates, which are in turn available for downloading to the treatment couch for automated fine adjustment of the patient's treatment position. Other precise localization systems rely on the identification of the positions of small, implanted radiopaque markers or other types of *smart* position-reporting devices. Careful use of these image-guided radiation

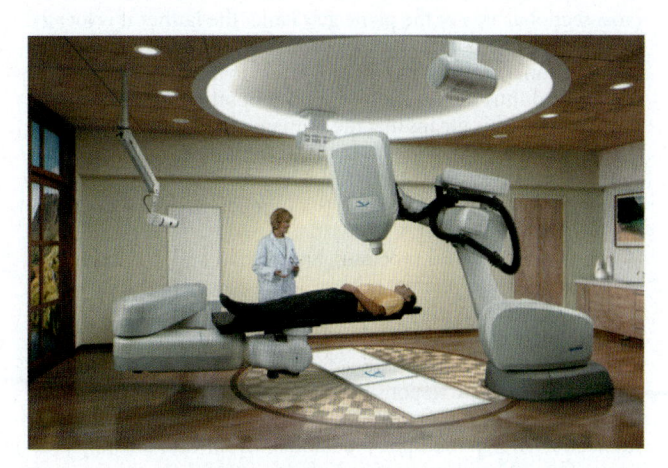

Figure 13.16 A miniature accelerator plus x-ray production system on a robotic delivery arm. Both the treatment table and the treatment head is set by a computer for multiple arbitrary angles of incidence. (From Accuray, Sunnyvale, CA, with permission.)

therapy (IGRT) systems[71,72] can result in the repeated reducibility of patient position to within a few millimeters over a 5- to 8-week course of treatment.

The final part of external-beam patient treatment is dose delivery. All modern treatment units have computer monitoring (and often control) of all mechanical and dose-delivery components. Treatment-planning information (treatment machine parameters, treatment field configurations, dose per treatment field segment) is downloaded to a work station at the treatment unit that first assists with and then records treatment. This information, together with the readbacks from the treatment machine, are used to reproducibly set up and then verify each patient's treatment parameters, which prevents many of the variations that used to occur when all treatment was performed simply by following instructions written in a treatment chart.

Treatment Beam Characteristics and Dose-Calculation Algorithms

Beyond a basic understanding of the interactions of ionizing radiation with matter lies the requirement of being able to characterize the treatment beams for purposes of planning and verifying treatments. By virtue of a few underlying principles, this generally can be accomplished via a two-step process of absolute calibration of the dose at some reference point in a phantom (i.e., measurement media representative of a patient's tissues), with relative scaling of dose values in other parts of the beam or phantom with respect to that point.

As mentioned earlier, the predominant mode of interaction for therapeutic energy photon beams in tissuelike materials is through Compton scattering. The probability of Compton scattering events is primarily proportional to the relative electron density of the media with which they interact. Because many body tissues are waterlike in composition, it has been possible to make photon beam dosimetric measurements in phantoms consisting mostly of water (water tanks) or tissue-equivalent plastic and to then scale the interactions via relative electron density values (for example, as can be derived from computed x-ray/CT) to other waterlike materials. Thus, the relative fluence of photons in a therapeutic treatment beam is attenuated as it passes through a phantom, primarily via Compton scattering.

It was stated earlier that the photon beam is generated at a small region in the head of the machine. That fluence of photons spreads out through the collimating system before reaching the patient. Thus, without any interactions (e.g., if the beam were in a vacuum), the number of photons crossing any plane perpendicular to the beam direction would remain constant. However, the cross-sectional area of the plane gets larger the farther it is located from the source point. In fact, both the width and length of the cross-sectional area increase in proportion to the distance from the source, and thus the area increases in proportion to the square of the distance. This means that the primary photon fluence per unit area in a plane perpendicular to the beam direction of a pointlike source also decreases as one over the square of the distance, the so-called $1/r^2$ reduction in fluence as a function of distance, r, from the source.

Thus, we have two processes, attenuation and $1/r^2$ reduction, which reduce the photon fluence from an external therapeutic beam as a function of depth in a patient. There is also a process that can increase the photon fluence at a point downstream. Recall that Compton scattering interactions lead not only to secondary electrons (which are responsible for deposition of dose), but also to Compton scattered photons. These photons are scattered from the interaction sites in multiple, predominantly forward-looking directions. Thus, Compton-scattered photons originating from many other places can add to the photon fluence at another point. As the irradiated area (field size) increases, the amount of scattered radiation also increases.

As mentioned earlier, dose *deposition* is a two-step process of photon interaction (proportional to the local fluence of photons) and energy transfer to the medium via the slowing down of secondary electrons. Thus, the point where a photon interacts is not the place where the dose is actually deposited, which happens over the track of the secondary electron. Dose has a very strict definition of energy *absorbed* per unit mass (i.e., due to the slowing down charged particles) and should be distinguished from the energy released at a point, defined as kerma (e.g., energy transfer from the scattering incident photon). Thus, although the photon beam fluence will always be greatest at the entrance to a patient or phantom, the actual *absorbed dose* for a megavoltage photon beam builds up over the first couple of centimeters, reaching a maximum (d-max) at a depth corresponding to the range of the higher energy Compton electrons set in motion. This turns out to be a second desirable characteristic of these beams (beyond their ability to treat deep-seated lesions), because the dose to the skin (a primary dose-limiting structure in earlier times) is greatly reduced.

The relative distributions of dose, normalized to an absolute dose measurement (using a small thimblelike air ionization chamber at a standard depth and for a standard field size according to nationally and internationally accepted protocols), are the major inputs into treatment-planning systems. The major features of these distributions are (1) the initial dose buildup up to a depth of d-max, with a more gradual drop off in dose as a function of depth into the phantom due to the attenuation and $1/r^2$ factors at deeper depths (relative depth dose), and (2) the shape of the dose in the plane perpendicular to the direction of the beams; both as a function of field size. Central axis depth dose curves for typical external photon beams are shown in Figure 13.17 for two beam energies and for both a large and smaller field size. Notice both the expected increase in penetration with increasing beam energy and the increase in dose at a particular depth with increasing field size; the latter effect due to increased numbers of secondary Compton-scattered photons for larger irradiated areas. The change in dose perpendicular to the central axis is less remarkable, because the beams are designed to be uniform across a field as a function of depth.

It is useful to also point out the depth dose characteristics of clinical external treatment beams produced using ionizing

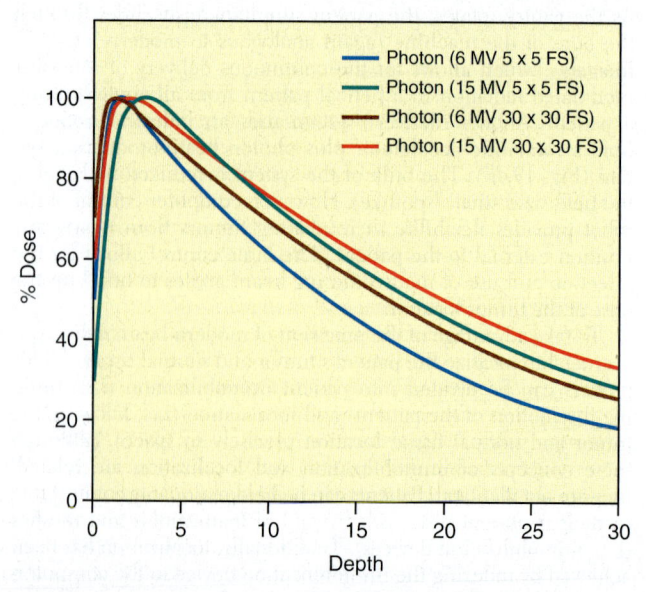

Figure 13.17 Sample depth-dose curves (change in delivered dose as a function of depth) along the central axis of some typical photon treatment beams for low (6 MV) and intermediate (15 MV) energy beams, and large (30 × 30 cm²) and smaller (5 × 5 cm²) field sizes (FS).

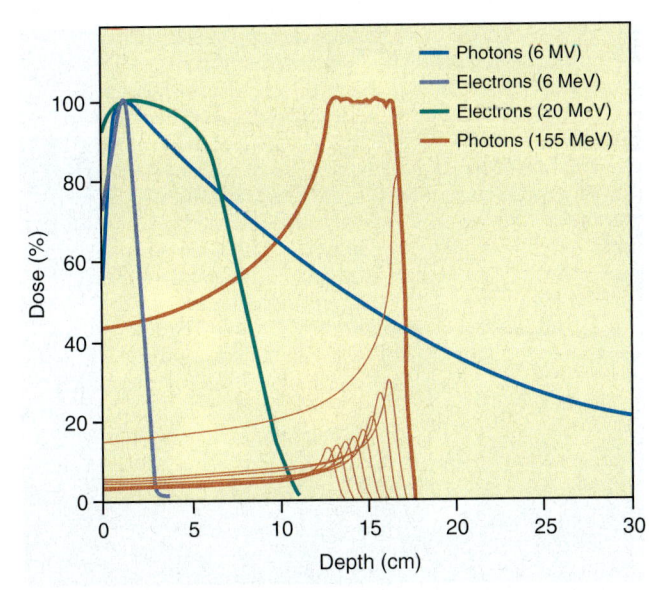

Figure 13.18 Sample depth-dose curves along the central axis of some typical charged particle treatment beams compared with that of a 6-MV proton beam. The spread out Bragg peak at the end of the 155-MeV proton beam (*thick pink curve*) is a composite dose deposition pattern from the addition of the multiple range-shifted proton curves (*thinner pink curves*).

radiations other than photons, primarily through the direct use of charged particles. Those beams (Fig. 13.18) illustrate interesting characteristics, which, when added to the options available for treatment planning (or used by themselves), can produce advantageous results. Relative to the photon beam, the direct use of electron beams leads to deposition of dose over a more localized range, but at the expense of a relative lack of penetration. Thus, electron beams are most widely used for treating, or boosting the treatment of, more superficial tumors and regions (see the section titled Clinical Application of Types of Radiation). The heavier charged particle beams (protons and carbon ions) appear to exhibit even more interesting *depth-dose* characteristics, with the advantage of both (when necessary) being highly penetrating and also lacking a significant dose beyond a certain depth (a depth that can be controlled and purposefully placed, for example, at the distal edge of a target volume).

The results of measurements such as these have been modeled so as to develop dose-calculation algorithms used in treatment-planning systems. These models all use measured beam data to set or adjust parameters used by those algorithms in their dose-distribution computations. Because most of the input data used for beam fitting come from measurements in water phantoms (or waterlike plastic phantoms), patient-specific adjustments are needed for the water phantom data to account for both geometry and tissue properties. It is the task of the dose-calculation algorithms to take those changes into account. The accuracy and precision actually realized for all dose-calculation algorithms generally need to be traded off against the time required to complete the calculation. Although the availability of ever more powerful computers has made calculation time less of a concern for broad, open-beam treatment planning, issues still remain for more specialized planning exercises that use many small beams or parts of beams such as IMRT (discussed later). Typically, relative dose distributions can be computed within patients on the scale of a few millimeters with a precision of better than a few percentage points.

An important area of research is the development of treatment-planning systems that calculate dose based on the principles of how radiation interacts with tissues, rather than simply by fitting data. These approaches use Monte Carlo techniques,[71,73] which build a dose distribution by summing the calculated paths of thousands of photons and scattered electrons. This approach is more accurate than beam-fitting algorithms in regions of differing tissue densities, such as the lung, and therefore, will ultimately replace the current generation of treatment-planning systems, particularly for complex conditions. However, the time to perform these calculations is still prohibitive for a clinic, and it is anticipated that Monte Carlo calculations will be introduced over a period of years by balancing the need for accuracy in a particular clinical situation with the need to initiate patient treatment.

TREATMENT PLANNING

As discussed in the previous section, single-treatment beams usually deposit more of the dose closer to where they enter the patient than they do at depths corresponding to where a deep-seated tumor might be located. The use of multiple beams entering the patient from different directions that overlap at the target produces more dose per unit volume throughout the tumor volume than is received by normal tissues. In fact, as noted earlier, the treatment-delivery machines are designed to make this easy to accomplish. Planning patient treatments under these circumstances should be a somewhat trivial matter of first selecting a sufficient number of beam angles to realize the desired buildup of the dose in the overlap region relative to the doses in the upstream parts of each beam, and then second, designing beam apertures that shape the edges of the beams to match the target. However, dose-limiting normal tissues often also lie in the paths of one or more of the beams. These normal tissues are often more sensitive to radiation damage than the tumor, and regardless, it is best practice to minimize the dose in any case as a general principle. Computerized treatment-planning systems function to develop patient-specific anatomic or geometric models and then use these models together with the beam-specific dose deposition properties (derived from phantom measurements, as previously described) to select beam angles, shapes, and intensities that meet an overall prescribed objective. That is, modern radiation oncology dose prescriptions contain both tumor and normal tissue objectives, and the modern computerized treatment-planning systems make it possible to design treatments that meet these objectives.

The development and use of three-dimensional (3D) models of each patient's anatomy, treatment geometry, and dose distribution led to a paradigm shift in radiation therapy treatment planning. Computerized radiation treatment planning began in the 1980s as a mainly x-ray/CT–based reconstruction of 3D geometries from information manually contoured on multiple two-dimensional (2D) transverse CT images. Today, these models often incorporate imaging data from multiple sources. Geometrically accurate anatomic information from an x-ray/CT scan still anchors these studies (as well as provides tissue density information necessary for dose calculations). However, it is now quite common to also register the CT data set with other studies such as magnetic resonance imaging (MRI), which may add anatomic detail for soft tissues, or functional MRI or positron emission tomography (PET) studies,[74,75] which provide physiologic or molecular information about tumors and normal tissues. Once registered with each other, the unique or complementary information from each data set can be fused for inspection and incorporated into the design of each patient's target and normal tissue volumes (Fig. 13.19). Beyond the ability to more fully define the extent of the primary target volume (for instance, as the encompassing envelope of disease appreciated on all the imaging studies) lies the ability to define subvolumes of the tumor volume that might be appropriate for simultaneous treatment to higher dose. For example, it should soon become possible to define different biologic components of the tumor that could potentially be targeted and then monitored for response using these same imaging techniques.[76]

Current treatment planning makes the tacit assumption that the planning image yields "the truth" about the location and condition

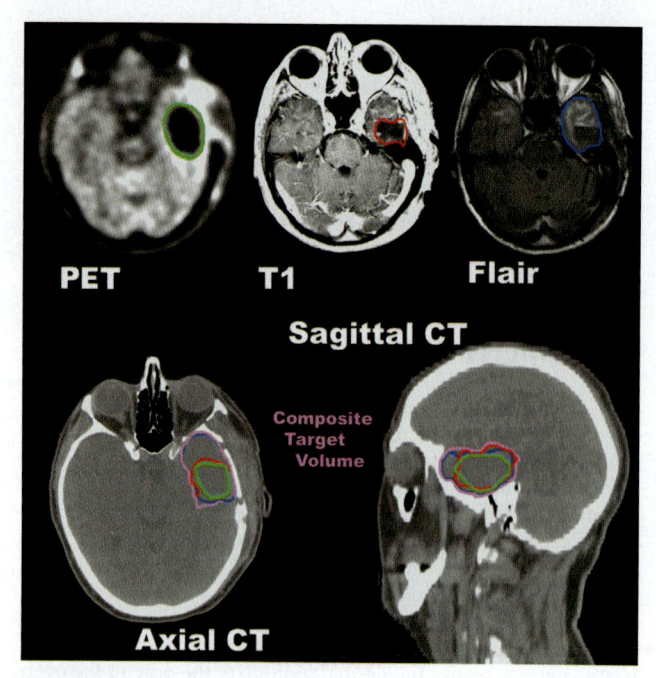

Figure 13.19 An illustration of the brain tumor target volume delineated on coregistered nuclear medicine and magnetic resonance imaging studies fused with computed tomography (CT) data for treatment planning. PET, positron emission tomography.

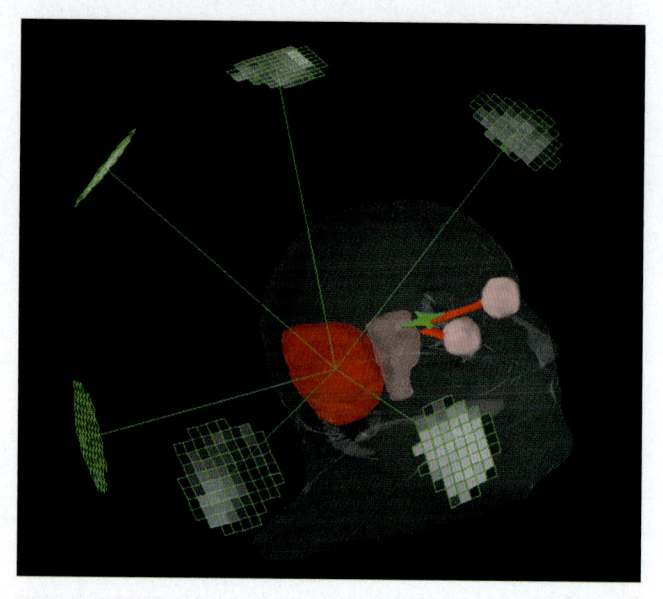

Figure 13.20 Six intensity-modulated treatment ports planned for treatment of a brain tumor (*large object in red*). Differing intensities of the 5 × 5 mm *beamlets* in each port illustrated by gray scale (brighter beamlet = higher intensity). The computer optimization of the beamlet intensities is designed to generate a delivered dose distribution that will conform to the tumor region, yet avoid critical normal tissues such as the brain stem (*dark pink*), optic chiasm (*green*), and optic nerves (*red tubular structures*).

of tumors and normal tissues throughout the course of treatment. However, this ignores the complexity inherent in attempting to build accurate 3D models from multimodality imaging for purposes of planning patient treatments. First, patients breathe and undergo other physiologic processes during a single treatment, changes that require dynamic modeling or other methods of accounting for the changes. Furthermore, the patient's condition may change over time (and hence their model). Thus, a complete design and assessment of a patient undergoing high-precision treatment requires the construction of four-dimensional (4D) patient models. Indeed, the recent ready availability of multidetector CT scanners with subsecond gantry rotations, and even more recently, the availability of cone-beam CT capabilities on the radiation therapy treatment simulators and treatment machines themselves, now makes it possible to construct 4D patient models. A very active area of physics research[72,75] deals with IGRT, including the formation of 4D patient models (including distortions and changes in anatomy) of the motion over time and the determination of the accumulated dose received by a moving tumor as well as the surrounding normal tissues such as uninvolved lung.

Complementary to the availability of these patient and dose models has come a much better understanding of the doses safely tolerated by normal tissues adjacent to a tumor volume (e.g., spinal cord) or surrounding it (e.g., brain, lung, liver).[77] Indeed, not only has knowledge of whole organ tolerances to irradiation been obtained, but it has also become possible to characterize in some detail the complex dependence of the probability of incurring a complication with respect to the highly (intentionally) inhomogeneous dose distributions these normal tissues receive as part of the planning process designed to avoid treating them. Modeling partial organ tolerances to irradiation is of great use in planning patient treatments because it enables[78] integration and manipulation of variable dose and volume distributions with respect to possible clinical outcomes.

Making the vast amount of tumor and normal tissue information useful for planning treatments requires equally sophisticated new ways of planning and delivering dose, potentially preferentially targeting subvolumes of the tumor regions or specifically avoiding selected portions of adjacent organs at risk. As mentioned earlier, modern treatment machines are capable of either varying the intensity of the radiation across each treatment port or projecting many small beams at a targeted region. This modulation of beam intensities (IMRT) from a given beam direction, together with the use of multiple beams (or parts of beams) from different directions, gives many degrees of freedom to create highly sculpted dose distributions, given that a system for designing the intensity modulation is available. Much computer programming and computational analysis has gone into the design of treatment-planning optimization systems to perform these functions.[79,80]

In IMRT, as most often applied, each treatment beam portal is broken down into simple basic components called beamlets, typically 0.5 to 1 cm × 1 cm in size, evenly distributed on a grid over the cross-section of each beam. Optimization begins with precomputation of the relative dose contribution that each of these beamlets gives to every subportion of tumor and normal tissue that the beamlet traverses as it goes through the patient model. Sophisticated optimization engines and search routines then iteratively alter the relative intensities of each beamlet in all the beams to minimize a cost function associated with target and normal tissue treatment goals. These, often hundreds of beamlets (each with its own intensity) (Fig. 13.20), provide the necessary flexibility and degrees of freedom to create dose distributions that can preferentially irradiate subportions of targets and also produce sharp dose gradients to avoid nearby organs at risk (Fig. 13.21). The cost-function approach also facilitates the ability to include factors such as the normal tissue and tumor-response models, mentioned previously in the optimization process, thus integrating the overall effects of the complex dose distributions across whole organ systems or target volumes within the planning process.

OTHER TREATMENT MODALITIES

Other types of external-beam radiation treatments use atomic or nuclear particles rather than photons. Beams of fast neutrons have been used for some cancers,[81] primarily because of the

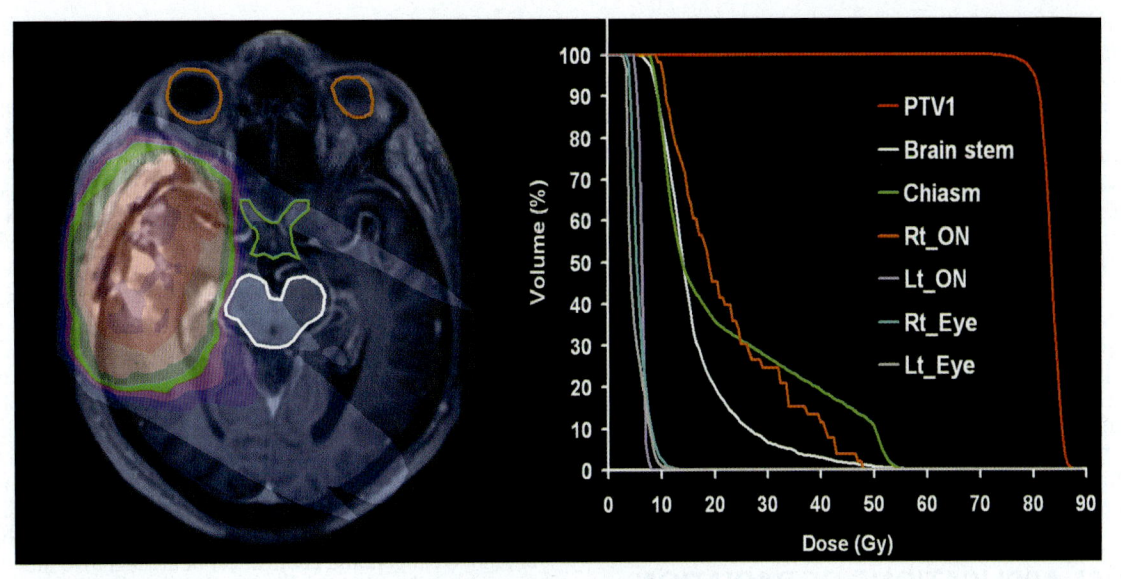

Figure 13.21 Resulting isodose distribution for an optimized intensity-modulated brain treatment. Dose-intensity pattern in the *left panel* is overlaid on the patient's magnetic resonance images used in planning. Also contoured are the optic chiasm (*green*), the brain stem (*white*), and the eyes (*orange*). In the *right panel*, the dose distribution throughout all slices of the patient's anatomy is summarized via cumulative dose-volume histograms for the various tissues and volumes that have been previously segmented. Each location on each curve represents the fraction of the volume of that tissue (%) that receives greater than or the same as the corresponding dose level.

dense ionization patterns they produce as they slow down in tissue (making cell killing less dependent on the indirect effect previously discussed). Being uncharged particles, neutron beams of therapeutic energy penetrate in tissue (have depth-dose characteristics) similar to photon beams, but with denser dose deposition in the cellular scale. Most other external-beam treatments use charged particles, primarily either electrons[82] (produced on the same machines used for photon beam treatments) or protons or heavier particles such as carbon ions.[83,84] The latter beams have desirable dose-deposition properties (see Fig. 13.18), because they can spare tissues downstream from the target volume and generally give less overall dose to normal tissue. There can also be some radiobiologic advantage to the heavier charged particle beams, similar to neutrons. The generation and delivery of proton beams and heavier charged particle beams generally requires an accelerator (in its own vault) plus a beam transport system and some sort of treatment nozzle, often located on an isocentric gantry. The cost of the accelerator is generally leveraged by having it supply beams to multiple treatment rooms, but these units still cost many times that of a standard linear accelerator.

Brachytherapy[85] is a form of treatment that uses direct placement of radioactive sources or materials within tumors (interstitial brachytherapy) or within body or surgical cavities (intracavitary brachytherapy), either permanently (allowing for full decay of short-lived radioactive materials) or temporarily (either in one extended application or over several shorter term applications). The ability to irradiate tumors from close range (even from the inside out) can lead to conformal treatments with low normal tissue doses. The radioactive isotopes most generally used for these treatments are contained within small tubelike or seedlike sealed source enclosures (which prevents direct contamination). They emit photons (gamma and x-rays) during their decay, which penetrate the source cover and interact with tissue via the same physical processes as described for external-beam treatments. The treatments have the advantage of providing a high fluence (and dose) very near each source that drops in intensity as 1 over the square of the distance from the source ($1/r^2$). Radioactive sources decay in an exponential fashion characterized by their individual half-lives. After each half-life ($T_{1/2}$) the strength of each source decreases by half. Brachytherapy treatments are further generally classified into the two broad categories of low–dose-rate and high–dose-rate treatments. Low–dose-rate treatments attempt to deliver tumoricidal doses via continuous irradiation from implanted sources over a period of several days. High–dose-rate treatments use one or more higher activity sources (stored external to the patient) together with a remote applicator or source transfer system to give one or more higher dose treatments on time scales and schedules more like external-beam treatments.

Isotopes for brachytherapy treatments are selected on the basis of a combination of specific activity (i.e., how much activity can be achieved per unit mass [i.e., to keep the source sizes small]), the penetrating ability of the decay photons (together with the $1/r^2$ fall off determines how many sources or source location will be required for treatment), and the half-life of the radioactive material (which must be accounted for in computation of dose, but also determines how often reusable sources will need to be replaced). Table 13.1 lists those isotopes most commonly used, along with some of their primary applications.

The dose-deposition patterns surrounding each type of source can be measured or computed. These data (or the parameterization

TABLE 13.1

Common Isotopes for Brachytherapy Treatment

Isotope	Form	Primary Applications
^{125}I	Implantable sealed seed	LDR: Permanent prostate implants, brain implants, tumor bed implants, eye plaques
^{192}Ir	Implantable sealed seed	LDR: Interstitial solid tumor treatments
^{192}Ir	High activity sealed source on a remote transfer wire	HDR: Intracavitary GYN treatments, intraluminal irradiations
^{137}Cs	Sealed source tubes	LDR: Intracavitary GYN treatments

LDR, low-dose rate; HDR, high-dose rate; GYN, gynecologic; ^{137}Cs, caesium-137.

of same) can be stored within a computerized treatment-planning system. Planning a brachytherapy treatment-delivery scheme (desirable source strengths and arrangements) proceeds within the planning system by distributing the sources throughout the treatment area and having the computer add up the contributions of each source to designated tumor and normal tissue locations (e.g., obtained from a CT scan). Source strengths or spacing can be adjusted until an acceptable result is obtained. Indeed, optimization systems are now routinely used to fine tune this process.

Other types of therapeutic treatments with internal sources of ionizing radiation, generally classified as systemic targeted radionuclide therapy (STaRT), use antibodies or other conjugates or carriers such as microspheres to selectively deliver radionuclides to cancer cells.[86] Computing the effective dose to tumors and normal tissues via these techniques requires information on how much of the injected activity reaches the targets (biodistribution) as well as the energy and decay properties of the radionuclide being delivered. Imaging techniques and computer models are aiding in these computations.

CLINICAL APPLICATIONS OF RADIATION THERAPY

In contrast to surgical oncology and medical oncology, which focus on early- or late-stage disease, respectively, the field of radiation oncology encompasses the 1p8.49 entire spectrum of oncology. Board certification requires 5 years of postdoctoral training, typically beginning with an internship in internal medicine or surgery, followed by 4 years of radiation oncology residency. Education, as defined by leaders in the field,[87] begins with a thorough knowledge of the biology, physics, and clinical applications of radiation. It also includes training in the theoretical and practical aspects of the administration of radiation protectors and anticancer agents used as radiation sensitizers and the management of toxicities resulting from those treatments. In addition, residents receive education in palliative care, supportive care, and symptom and pain management. This training is in preparation for a practice that, in a given week, might include patients with a 2-mm vocal cord lesion or a 20-cm soft tissue sarcoma, both of whom can be treated with curative intent, as well as a patient with widely metastatic disease who needs palliative radiation, medical care for pain and depression, and discussion of end-of-life issues. More than 50% of (nonskin) cancer patients receive radiation therapy during the course of their illness.[88]

Clinical Application of Types of Radiation

Electrons are now the most widely used form of radiation for superficial treatments. Because the depth of penetration can be well controlled by the energy of the beam, it is possible to treat, for instance, skin cancer, a small part of the breast while sparing the underlying lung, or the cervical lymph nodes but not the spinal cord, which lies several centimeters more deeply. Superficial tumors, such as of skin cancers, can also be treated very effectively with low-energy (kilovoltage) photons, but their use has decreased because a separate machine is required for their production.

The main form of treatment for deep tumors is photons. As described in the Radiation Physics section, photons spare the skin and deposit dose along their entire path until the beam leaves the body. The use of multiple beams that intersect on the tumor permit high doses to be delivered to the tumor with a relative sparing of normal tissue. The pinnacle of this concept is IMRT, which uses hundreds of beams and can treat concave shapes with relative sparing of the central region (see Figs. 13.20 and 13.21). However, as each beam continues on its path beyond the tumor, this use of multiple beams means that a significant volume of normal tissue receives a low dose. There has been considerable debate concerning the magnitude of the risk of second cancers produced by radiating large volumes with low doses of radiation.[89] Charged particle beams (proton and carbon, in this discussion) differ from photons in that they interact only modestly with tissue until they reach the end of their path, where they then deposit the majority of their energy and stop (the Bragg peak; see Fig. 13.18). This ability to stop at a chosen depth decreases the region of low dose. The chief form of charged particle used today is the proton. In the decade from 1980 to 1990, proton therapy could deliver higher doses of radiation to the target than photon therapy because protons could produce a more rapid fall off of dose between the target and the critical normal tissue (e.g., tumor and brain stem). Therefore, initially, their main application was in the treatment uveal melanomas, base-of-skull chondrosarcomas, and chordomas. In contrast, today's IMRT photons are more conformal in the high-dose region than protons due to the range uncertainty of the latter.[90] Thus, it seems unlikely that protons will permit a higher target dose to be delivered than photons. In contrast, protons have the potential to decrease regions of low dose. This would be of particular advantage in the treatment of pediatric malignancies, where low doses of radiation would tend to increase the chance of second cancers and could affect neurocognitive function in the treatment of brain tumors.

A carbon ion beam has an additional potential biologic advantage over protons. As discussed in the section Biologic Aspects of Radiation Oncology, hypoxic cells, which are found in many tumors, are up to 3 times more resistant to photon or proton radiation than well-oxygenated cells. In contrast, hypoxia does not cause resistance to a carbon beam. Whether hypoxia is a cause of clinical resistance to fractionated radiation is still debated.[91] A carbon beam is available at a few sites in Europe and Japan.

Two major issues have affected the widespread acceptance of protons. The most widely recognized is cost. Proton (approximately $120 million) and carbon beam facilities (in excess of $200 million) are substantially more expensive than a similar-sized photon facility (approximately $25 million). The operating costs appear to be significantly higher as well. Although the majority of patients who have received proton therapy have prostate cancer, there is no evidence that protons produce superior results to those obtained with IMRT planned photons.[92,93] The lack of solid evidence that protons are superior to photons for any disease site and the magnitude of these costs are of societal importance.[94] Although less expensive single gantry proton units are under construction, there are no functioning units at the time of this writing. A second, less well-appreciated issue concerns the need to develop full integration of charged particle beams with IGRT, as has already been accomplished with photons, although this feature is being incorporated into second-generation proton units.

Neutron therapy attracted significant interest in the 1980s, based on the principle that it would be more effective than photons against hypoxic cells that some have thought are responsible for radiation resistance of tumors. The effectiveness of neutron therapy has been limited by initial difficulties with collimation and targeting, although there is evidence that they have a role in the treatment of refractory parotid gland tumors.[95]

Brachytherapy refers to the placement of radioactive sources next to or inside the tumor. The chief sites where brachytherapy plays a role are in prostate and cervical cancer, although it has applications in head and neck cancers, soft tissue sarcomas, and other sites. In the case of prostate cancer, most experience is with low–dose-rate permanent implants using iodine-125 (^{125}I) or, more recently, palladium-103 (^{103}Pd). Over the last 5 years, there has been an increasing emphasis on improving the accuracy of seed placement, guided by ultrasound and confirmed by CT or MRI, and in skilled hands, outstanding results can be achieved.[96] In the case of cervical cancer, high–dose-rate treatment, which can be performed in an outpatient setting, has essentially replaced low–dose-rate treatment, which typically requires general anesthesia and a 2-day hospital stay. The results from both techniques appear to be approximately equivalent.

Yttrium microspheres represent a distinct form of brachytherapy. These spheres carry yttrium-90 (^{90}Y), a pure beta emitter with a range of about 1 cm. These have been used to treat both primary hepatocellular cancer and colorectal cancer metastatic to the liver (hepatic arterial or systemic chemotherapy) by administration through the hepatic artery.

TREATMENT INTENT

Radiation doses are chosen so as to maximize the chance of tumor control without producing unacceptable toxicity. The dose of radiation required depends on the tumor type, the volume of disease (number of tumor cells), and the use of radiation-modifying agents (such as chemotherapeutic drugs used as radiation sensitizers). Except for a subset of tumors that are exquisitely sensitive to radiation (e.g., seminoma, lymphoma), doses that are required are often close to the tolerance of the normal tissue. A key fact driving the choice of dose is that a 1-cm^3 tumor contains approximately 1 billion cells. It follows that the reduction of a tumor that is 3 cm in diameter to 3 mm, which would be called a complete response by CT scan, would still leave 1 million tumor cells. Because each radiation fraction appears to kill a fixed fraction of the tumor, the dose to cure occult disease needs to be more similar to the dose for gross disease than one might otherwise expect. Thus, radiation doses (using the standard fractionation) of 45 to 54 Gy are typically used in the adjuvant setting when there is moderate suspicion for occult disease, 60 to 65 Gy for positive margins or when there is a high suspicion for occult disease, and 70 Gy or more for gross disease.

It is common during the course of radiation to give higher doses of radiation to regions that have a higher tumor burden. For example, regions that are suspected of harboring occult disease may be targeted to receive (in once daily 2-Gy fractions) 54 Gy, whereas, to control the gross tumor, the goal may be to administer a total dose of 70 Gy. Because the gross tumor will invariably reside within the region at risk for occult disease, it has become standard practice to deliver 50 Gy to the entire region, and then an additional *boost* dose of 20 Gy to the tumor. This sequence is called the *shrinking field technique*. With the development of IMRT, it has become possible to treat both regions with a different dose each day and achieve both goals simultaneously. For example, on each of the 35 days of treatment, the gross tumor might receive 2 Gy, and the region of occult disease 1.7 Gy, for a total dose of 59.5 Gy, which is of approximately equal biologic effectiveness to 54 Gy in 1.8-Gy fractions because of the lower dose per fraction (see the section Biologic Aspects of Radiation Oncology).

Radiation therapy alone is often used with curative intent for localized tumors. The decision to use surgery or radiation therapy involves factors determined by the tumor (e.g., is it resectable without a serious compromise in function?) and the patient (e.g., is the patient a good operative candidate?). The most common tumor in this group is prostate cancer, but patients with early-stage larynx cancer often receive radiation for voice preservation, and there are many patients with early-stage lung cancer who are not operative candidates. Control rates for these early-stage lesions are in excess of 70% (and as high as 90% for early-stage larynx cancer) and are usually a function of tumor size.

Stereotactic body radiation therapy (SBRT; sometimes called *stereotactic ablative radiation*) uses many (typically more than eight) cross-firing beams and provides an improved method of curing early-stage lung cancer[97] and liver metastases.[98] This approach uses precise localization and image guidance to deliver a small number (less than five) of high doses of radiation, with the concept of ablating the tumor, rather than using fractionation to achieve a therapeutic index (see the section title Fractionation). SBRT can provide long-term, local control rates of >90% for tumors less than 4 to 5 cm with minimal side effects.

Locally advanced or aggressive cancers can be cured with radiation alone or with a combination of radiation and chemotherapy or a molecularly targeted therapy. The most common examples here are locally advanced lung cancer, head and neck, esophageal, and cervix cancers, with cure rates in the 15% to 40% range, and are discussed in detail in their own chapters. A general principle that has emerged during the last decade is that combination chemoradiation has increased the cure rates of locally advanced cancers by 5% to 10% at the cost of increased toxicity.

An important consideration in the use of radiation (with or without chemotherapy) with curative intent is the concept of organ preservation. Perhaps the best example of achieving organ preservation in the face of gross disease involves the use of chemotherapy and radiation to replace laryngectomy in the treatment of advanced larynx cancer. Combined radiation and chemotherapy does not improve overall survival compared with radical surgery; however, the organ-conservation approach permits voice preservation in approximately two-thirds of patients with advanced larynx cancer.[99] The treatment of anal cancer with chemoradiation can also be viewed in this light, with chemoradiotherapy producing organ conservation and cure rates superior to radical surgery used decades ago.[100] Multiple randomized trials have demonstrated that lumpectomy plus radiation for breast cancer produces survival rates equal to that of modified radical mastectomy, while allowing for the preservation of the breast.

In the last decade, it has become clear that some patients with metastatic disease can be cured with radiation (with or without chemotherapy). The concept underlying this approach was established by the surgical practice of resecting a limited number of liver or lung metastases. A significant fraction of patients have a limited number of liver metastases that cannot be resected because of location, but are able to undergo high-dose radiation (often combined with chemotherapy). This radical approach to *oligometastases*[101] can produce 5-year survivals in the range of 20% in selected patients.[102] Patients with a limited number of lung metastases from colorectal cancer or soft tissue sarcomas are now being approached with stereotactic body radiation with a similar concept as has been used to justify surgical resection.[102] In addition to the direct effect of radiation on metastatic tumor, there is now anecdotal but provocative evidence that radiation can stimulate the immune system so that tumors distant from the irradiated tumor can respond. Distant (abscopal) responses have been reported in patients who receive immune checkpoint inhibitors such as ipilimumab.[103]

Radiation therapy can also contribute to the cure of patients when used in an adjuvant setting. If the risk of recurrence after surgery is low or if a recurrence could be easily addressed by a second resection, adjuvant radiation therapy is not usually given. However, when a gross total resection of the tumor is still associated with a high risk of residual occult disease or if local recurrence is morbid, adjuvant treatment is often recommended. A general finding across many disease sites is that adjuvant radiation can reduce local failure rates to below 10%, even in high-risk patients, if a gross total resection is achieved. If gross disease or positive margins remain, higher doses and/or larger volumes may be required, which may be less well tolerated and are less successful in achieving tumor control.

Adjuvant therapy can be delivered before or after definitive surgery. There are some advantages to giving radiation therapy after surgery. The details of the tumor location are known and, with the surgeon's cooperation, clips can be placed in the tumor bed, permitting increased treatment accuracy. In addition, compared with preoperative therapy, postoperative therapy is associated with fewer wound complications. However, in some cases, it is preferable to deliver preoperative radiation. Radiation can shrink the tumor, diminishing the extent of the resection, or making an unresectable tumor resectable. In the case of rectal cancer, the response to treatment may carry more prognostic information than the initial TNM staging.[104] In patients who will undergo significant surgeries (particularly a Whipple procedure or an esophageal resection), preoperative (sometimes called neoadjuvant) therapy can be more reliably administered than postoperative therapy. Most importantly, after resection of abdominal or pelvic tumors (such as rectal cancers or retroperitoneal sarcomas), the small bowel may become fixed by adhesions in the region requiring treatment, thus increasing the morbidity of postoperative treatment. A randomized trial has shown that preoperative therapy produces fewer gastrointestinal side effects and has at least as good efficacy as postoperative adjuvant therapy for locally advanced rectal cancer.[105] Taken together, there appears to be a trend toward preoperative or neoadjuvant therapy in cancers of the gastrointestinal track (esophagus, stomach, pancreas, rectum), postoperative radiation seems to be favored in head and neck, lung, and breast cancer, and soft tissue sarcoma seems equally split.

The effectiveness of adjuvant therapy in decreasing local recurrence has been demonstrated in randomized trials in lung, rectal, and breast cancers. More recently, randomized trials have shown that postmastectomy radiation improved the survival for women with breast cancer and four or more positive lymph nodes, all of whom also received adjuvant chemotherapy. A fascinating analysis has revealed that, across many treatment conditions, each 4% increase in 5-year local control is associated with a 1% increase in 5-year survival.[106] It has been proposed that the long-term survival benefit of radiation in these more recent studies was revealed by the introduction of effective chemotherapy, which prevented such a high fraction of women from dying early with metastatic disease.[107] This concept has been developed into a hypothesis that the effect of adjuvant radiation on survival will depend on the effectiveness of adjuvant chemotherapy. If chemotherapy is either ineffective or very effective, adjuvant radiation may have little influence on the survival in a disease in which systemic relapse dominates survival. Radiation will have its greatest impact on survival when chemotherapy is moderately effective.[108]

In addition to these curative roles, radiation plays an important part in palliative treatment. Perhaps most importantly, emergency irradiation can begin to reverse the devastating effects of spinal cord compression and of superior vena cava syndrome. A single 8-Gy fraction is highly effective for many patients with bone pain from a metastatic lesion. There is increasing evidence of the effectiveness of body stereotactic radiation to treat vertebral body metastases in patients who have a long projected survival or who need retreatment after previous radiation.[109] Stereotactic treatment can relieve symptoms from a small number of brain metastasis, and fractionated whole-brain radiation can mitigate the effects of multiple metastases. Bronchial obstruction can often be relieved by a brief course of treatment as can duodenal obstruction from pancreatic cancer. Palliative treatment is usually delivered in a smaller number of larger radiation fractions (see the section titled Fractionation) because the desire to simplify the treatment for a patient with limited life expectancy outweighs the somewhat increased potential for late side effects.

FRACTIONATION

Two crucial features that influence the effectiveness of a physical dose of radiation are the dose given in each radiation treatment (i.e., the fraction) and the total amount of time required to complete the course of radiation. Standard fractionation for radiation therapy is defined as the delivery of one treatment of 1.8 to 2.25 Gy per day. This approach produces a fairly well-understood chance of tumor control and risk of normal tissue damage (as a function of volume). By altering the fractionation schemes, one may be able to improve the outcome for patients undergoing curative treatment or to simplify the treatment for patients receiving palliative therapy.

Two forms of altered fractionation have been tested for patients undergoing curative treatment: accelerated fractionation and hyperfractionation. Accelerated fractionation emerged from analyses of the control of head and neck cancer as a function of dose administered and total treatment time. It was found that with an increasing dose there was increasing local control, but that protraction of treatment was associated with a loss of local control that was equivalent to about 0.75 Gy per day.[110] The data were best modeled by assuming that, approximately 2 weeks into treatment, tumor cells began to proliferate more rapidly than they were proliferating early in treatment (called *accelerated repopulation*).[111] In accelerated fractionation, the goal is to complete radiation before the accelerated tumor cell proliferation occurs. The most common method of achieving accelerated fractionation is to give a standard fraction to the entire field in the morning and to give a second treatment to the boost field in the afternoon (called *concomitant boost*). As in standard radiation, the boost would be given by extending the length of the treatment course; this concomitant boost approach can shorten treatment from 7 weeks to 5 weeks in head and neck cancer.

The second approach to altering fractionation is called *hyperfractionation*. Hyperfractionation is defined as the use of more than one fraction per day separated by more than 6 hours (see the section titled Biologic Aspects of Radiation Oncology), with a dose per fraction that is less than standard. Hyperfractionation is expected to produce fewer late complications for the same acute effects against both rapidly dividing normal tissues and tumors. Pure hyperfractionation might give 1 Gy twice a day, so that the total dose per day would be 2 Gy, and thus be equal to standard fractionation. In practice, hyperfractionated treatments are usually in the range of 1.2 Gy, which means that, compared with a standard fractionation, a somewhat higher dose is administered during the same period of time (so that most hyperfractionation also includes modest acceleration). The overall effect is to increase the acute toxicity (which resolves) and tumor response, while not increasing the (dose-limiting) late toxicity, which can improve cure rate. Both accelerated fractionation and hyperfractionation have been demonstrated in a meta-analysis to be superior to standard fractionation in the treatment of head and neck cancer with radiation alone.[112] However, a recent randomized trial has shown that there is no increase in control or survival, but there is an increase toxicity using chemotherapy with hyperfractionation compared to standard chemoradiation; therefore, the use of altered fractionation schemes has decreased dramatically during the last few years.[113]

Hypofractionation refers to the administration of a smaller number of larger fractions than is standard. Hypofractionation might be expected to cause more late toxicity for the same antitumor effect than standard or hyperfractionation. In the past, this approach was reserved for palliative cases, with the sense that a modest potential for increased late toxicity was not a major concern in patients with limited life expectancy. However, more recently, it has been proposed that the ability to better exclude normal tissue by using IGRT may permit hypofractionation to be used safely and that, in the specific case of prostate cancer, hypofractionation may have beneficial effects.[114]

ADVERSE EFFECTS

Radiation produces adverse effects in normal tissues. Although these are discussed in detail in later chapters as part of comprehensive discussions of organ toxicity, it is worth making some general comments here from the perspective of how radiation biology relates to the clinical toxicities. The term *radiation toxicity* is used to describe the adverse effects caused by radiation alone and radiation plus chemotherapy. Although this latter toxicity would be better labeled as *combined modality toxicity*, the pattern typically resembles a more severe form of the toxicity produced by radiation alone. Adverse effects from radiation can be divided into acute, subacute, and chronic (or late) effects. Acute effects are common, rarely serious, and usually self-limiting. Acute effects tend to occur in organs that depend on rapid self-renewal, most commonly the skin or mucosal surfaces (oropharynx, esophagus, small intestine, rectum, and bladder). This is due to radiation-induced cell death that occurs during mitosis, so that cells that divide rapidly show the most rapid cell loss. In the treatment of head and neck cancer, mucositis becomes worse during the first 3 to 4 weeks of therapy, but then will often stabilize as the normal mucosa cell proliferation increases in response to mucosal cell loss. It seems likely that normal tissue stem cells are relatively resistant to radiation compared with the more differentiated cells, because these stem cells survive to permit the normal mucosa to reepithelialize. Acute side effects typically resolve within 1 to 2 weeks of treatment completion, although occasionally these effects are so severe that they lead to consequential late effects, as described later.

Because lymphocytes are exquisitely sensitive to radiation, there has been considerable investigation into the effects of radiation on immune function. In contrast to mucosal cell killing, which requires mitosis, radiation kills lymphocytes in all phases of the cell cycle by apoptosis, so that lymphocyte counts decrease within days of initiating treatment. These effects do not tend to put patients at risk for infection, because granulocytes, which are chiefly responsible for combating infections, are relatively unaffected.

Two acute side effects of radiation do not fit neatly into these models relating to cell kill: nausea[115,116] and fatigue.[117,118] The origin of radiation-induced nausea is not related to acute cell loss, because it can occur within hours of the first treatment. Nausea is usually associated with radiation of the stomach, but it can sometimes occur during brain irradiation or from large-volume irradiation that involves neither the brain nor the stomach. Irradiation typically produces fatigue, even if relatively small volumes are irradiated. It seems likely that the origins of both of these *abscopal* effects of radiation (i.e., effects that occur systemically or at a distance for the site of irradiation) are related to the release of cytokines, but little is known.

Radiation can also produce subacute toxicities in the form of radiation pneumonitis and radiation-induced liver disease. These typically occur 2 weeks to 3 months after radiation is completed. The risk of radiation pneumonitis and radiation-induced liver disease is proportional to the mean dose delivered.[119,120] Thus, the 3D tools that permit the calculation of dose-volume histograms (described in the physics section) are currently used to determine the maximum safe treatment that can be delivered in terms of dose and volume. These toxicities appear to be initiated subclinically during the course of radiation as a cascade of cytokines in which TGF-β, tumor necrosis factor α, interleukin 6, and other cytokines play a role.[121] High TGF-β plasma levels during a course of treatment have been found to be associated with a greater risk of radiation pneumonitis.[122] Thus, in the future, we might look toward a combination of physical dose delivery, measured by the dose-volume histogram, the functional imaging of normal tissue damage, and the detection of biomarkers of toxicity, such as TGF-β, to improve the ability to individualize therapy. Attempts to determine the genomic basis of radiation sensitivity, beyond the known rare genetic defects such as ataxia telangiectasia, have not yet been successful.[123]

Late effects, which are typically seen 6 or more months after a course of radiation, include fibrosis, fistula formation, or long-term organ damage. Two theories for the origin of late effects have been put forth: late damage to the microvasculature and direct damage to the parenchyma. Although the vascular damage theory is attractive, it does not account for the differing sensitivities of organs to radiation. Perhaps the microvasculature is unique in each organ.[124] Regardless of the mechanism of toxicity, the tolerance of whole-organ radiation is now fairly well established (Table 13.2). Late complications can also be divided into two categories: consequential and true late effects. The best example of a consequential late effect is fibrosis and dysphagia after high-dose chemoradiation for head and neck cancer. Here, late fibrosis or ulceration appears to be the result of the mucosa becoming denuded for a prolonged time period. Late consequential effects are distinct from true late effects, which can follow a normal treatment course of self-limited toxicity and a 6-month or more symptom-free period. Examples of true late effects are radiation myelitis, radiation brain necrosis, and radiation-induced bowel obstruction. In the past, radiation fibrosis was thought to be an irreversible condition. Therefore, an exciting recent development is that severe radiation-induced breast fibrosis is an active process that can be reversed by drug therapy (pentoxifylline and vitamin E).[125]

TABLE 13.2

Radiation Tolerance Doses for Normal Tissues

| | TD 5/5 (Gy)[a] | | | TD 50/5 (Gy)[b] | | | |
| | Portion of Organ Irradiated | | | Portion of Organ Irradiated | | | |
Site	1/3	2/3	3/3	1/3	2/3	3/3	Complication End Point(s)
Kidney	50	30	23	—	40	28	Nephritis
Rain	60	50	45	75	65	60	Necrosis, infarct
Brain stem	60	53	50	—	—	65	Necrosis, infarct
Spinal cord	50 (5–10 cm)	—	47 (20 cm)	70 (5–10 cm)	—	—	Myelitis, necrosis
Lung	45	30	17.5	65	40	24.5	Radiation pneumonitis
Heart	60	45	40	70	55	50	Pericarditis
Esophagus	60	58	55	72	70	68	Stricture, perforation
Stomach	60	55	50	70	67	65	Ulceration, perforation
Small intestine	50	—	40	60	—	55	Obstruction, perforation, fistula
Colon	55	—	45	65	—	55	Obstruction, perforation, fistula, ulceration
Rectum	(100 cm³ volume)		60	(100 cm³ volume)		80	Severe proctitis, necrosis, fistula
Liver	50	35	30	55	45	40	Liver failure

[a] TD 5/5, the average dose that results in a 5% complication risk within 5 years.
[b] TD 50/5, the average dose that results in a 50% complication risk within 5 years.
Adapted from Emami B, Lyman J, Brown A, et al. Tolerance of normal tissue to therapeutic irradiation. *Int J Radiat Oncol Biol Phys* 1991;21:109–122.

PRINCIPLES OF COMBINING ANTICANCER AGENTS WITH RADIATION THERAPY

Combining chemotherapy with radiation therapy has produced important improvements in treatment outcome. Randomized clinical trials show improved local control and survival through the use of concurrent chemotherapy and radiation therapy for patients with high-grade gliomas and locally advanced cancers of the head and neck, lung, esophagus, stomach, rectum, prostate, and anus. There are least two proposed reasons why chemoradiotherapy might be successful. The first is radiosensitization. In the laboratory, radiosensitization is defined as a synergistic relationship, using mathematical approaches such as isobologram or median effect analysis.[126,127] The underlying concept is that the observed effect of using chemotherapy and radiation concurrently is greater than simply adding the two together. A second proposed reason to combine radiation and chemotherapy is to realize the benefit of improved local control radiation along with the systemic effect of chemotherapy, a concept called *spatial additivity*.[128]

Clinical results show that both radiosensitization and spatial additivity contribute to varying extents in different clinical settings. In the case of head and neck cancer, radiosensitization predominates. This conclusion is supported by the meta-analysis of head and neck cancer: sequential chemotherapy and radiotherapy produces little if any improvement in survival, whereas concurrent chemoradiation produces a significant increase in survival.[129] Furthermore, in the early positive studies using concurrent chemoradiation, systemic metastases were unaffected even though survival was improved. Radiosensitization may also predominate in the success of chemoradiotherapy for locally advanced lung cancer. For instance, although initial studies indicated that sequential chemotherapy and radiation had some benefit for lung cancer,[130] more recent work indicates that concurrent therapy is superior, and it is now the standard treatment.[131] However, there are also examples of spatial additivity. For example, both radiosensitization and spatial additivity is provided by the use of chemoradiation for locally advanced cervical cancer in that both local and systemic relapses are decreased by combined therapy.[132]

By targeting the aberrant growth factor or proangiogenic pathways that are specific to cancer cells rather than all rapidly proliferating cells, molecularly targeted therapies offer the potential to improve outcome without increasing toxicity. Even a selective cytostatic effect against the tumor would be predicted to act synergistically with radiation (Fig. 13.22). Although preclinical studies (summarized in the previous biology section) have highlighted the potential therapeutic gains that could be achieved by adding EGFR inhibitors to radiation, the best validation of this combination has been from the results of clinical trials in head and neck cancer. A phase III clinical trial demonstrated that, in a cohort of 424 patients with local–regionally advanced squamous cell carcinoma of the head and neck, the addition of cetuximab nearly doubled the median survival of patients (compared to radiotherapy alone), from 28 to 54 months. This study represents the first major success

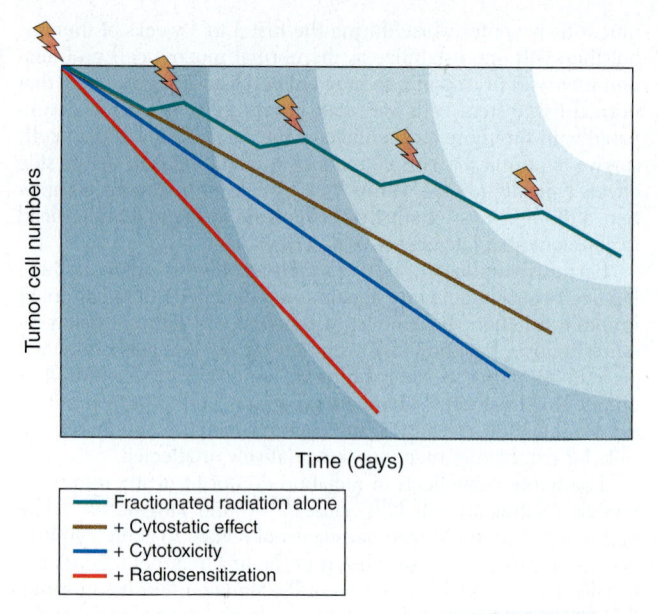

Figure 13.22 Potential mechanisms of synergy between epidermal growth factor receptor (EGFR) inhibitors and radiation. Although each daily radiation treatment kills a fraction of the cells, some cells grow back by the next day, which attenuates the effectiveness of radiation. If an EGFR inhibitor has only a selective cytostatic effect and blocks regrowth between fractions, the result would be a dramatic increase in radiation efficacy. The benefit of the inhibitor would be even greater if it caused tumor cell cytotoxicity or radiosensitization.

achieved by the addition of an EGFR antagonist to radiotherapy. This improvement was achieved without enhanced toxicity. Notably, the rates of pharyngitis and weight loss were identical in the two arms.[60] Local control was improved rather than the development of metastases, suggesting synergy rather than spatial additivity. Thus, the principle that can be derived from this study is that in tumors expressing high EGFR levels and that are likely to depend on aberrant EGF signaling, combining a true cytotoxic agent such as radiation with a cytostatic agent such as cetuximab has considerable promise.

Because of the success of chemoradiotherapy, the natural tendency has not been to substitute molecularly targeted agents such as cetuximab for chemotherapy, but to add cetuximab to chemoradiotherapy. Thus, the combination of cisplatin, cetuximab, and radiation was recently found to have the same control rate as cisplatin and radiation for patients with locally advanced head and neck cancer, but the cetuximab arm had greater toxicity. Unfortunately, the triple therapy was never evaluated preclinically, and it has been shown preclinically that when EGFR inhibitors are given prior to chemotherapy, they can produce antagonism.[133] The principles of adding molecularly targeted therapy to chemoradiation are still evolving.[63]

REFERENCES

1. Hall EJ, Giaccia AJ. *Radiobiology for the Radiologist*. Philadelphia: Lippincott Williams & Williams; 2012.
2. Fowler JF. Developing aspects of radiation oncology. *Med Phys* 1981;8:427–434.
3. Lavin MF. Ataxia-telangiectasia: from a rare disorder to a paradigm for cell signalling and cancer. *Nat Rev Mol Cell Biol* 2008;9:759–769.
4. Thompson LH. Recognition, signaling, and repair of DNA double-strand breaks produced by ionizing radiation in mammalian cells: the molecular choreography. *Mutat Res* 2012;751:158–246.
5. Sherr CJ, McCormick F. The RB and p53 pathways in cancer. *Cancer Cell* 2002;2:103–112.
6. Bartek J, Lukas J. Chk1 and Chk2 kinases in checkpoint control and cancer. *Cancer Cell* 2003;3:421–429.
7. Kitagawa R, Bakkenist CJ, McKinnon PJ, et al. Phosphorylation of SMC1 is a critical downstream event in the ATM-NBS1-BRCA1 pathway. *Genes Dev* 2004;18:1423–1438.
8. Abraham RT. Cell cycle checkpoint signaling through the ATM and ATR kinases. *Genes Dev* 2001;15:2177–2196.
9. Mailand N, Podtelejnikov AV, Groth A, et al. Regulation of G(2)/M events by Cdc25A through phosphorylation-dependent modulation of its stability. *EMBO J* 2002;21:5911–5920.
10. Donzelli M, Draetta GF. Regulating mammalian checkpoints through Cdc25 inactivation. *EMBO Rep* 2003;4:671–677.
11. Tsvetkov L. Polo-like kinases and Chk2 at the interface of DNA damage checkpoint pathways and mitotic regulation. *IUBMB Life* 2004;56:449–456.

12. Dai Y, Grant S. New insights into checkpoint kinase 1 in the DNA damage response signaling network. *Clin Cancer Res* 2010;16:376–383.
13. Giaccia A, Weinstein R, Hu J, et al. Cell cycle-dependent repair of double-strand DNA breaks in a gamma-ray-sensitive Chinese hamster cell. *Somat Cell Mol Genet* 1985;11:485–491.
14. Kemp LM, Sedgwick SG, Jeggo PA. X-ray sensitive mutants of Chinese hamster ovary cells defective in double-strand break rejoining. *Mutat Res* 1984;132:189–196.
15. Helleday T, Lo J, van Gent DC, et al. DNA double-strand break repair: from mechanistic understanding to cancer treatment. *DNA Repair (Amst)* 2007;6:923–935.
16. Hefferin ML, Tomkinson AE. Mechanism of DNA double-strand break repair by non-homologous end joining. *DNA Repair (Amst)* 2005;4:639–648.
17. Ma Y, Pannicke U, Schwarz K, et al. Hairpin opening and overhang processing by an Artemis/DNA-dependent protein kinase complex in nonhomologous end joining and V(D)J recombination. *Cell* 2002;108:781–794.
18. Grawunder U, Wilm M, Wu X, et al. Activity of DNA ligase IV stimulated by complex formation with XRCC4 protein in mammalian cells. *Nature* 1997;388:492–495.
19. Chen L, Trujillo K, Sung P, et al. Interactions of the DNA ligase IV-XRCC4 complex with DNA ends and the DNA-dependent protein kinase. *J Biol Chem* 2000;275:26196–26205.
20. Tsukuda T, Fleming AB, Nickoloff JA, et al. Chromatin remodelling at a DNA double-strand break site in Saccharomyces cerevisiae. *Nature* 2005;438:379–383.
21. Yang YG, Saidi A, Frappart PO, et al. Conditional deletion of Nbs1 in murine cells reveals its role in branching repair pathways of DNA double-strand breaks. *EMBO J* 2006;25:5527–5538.
22. Esashi F, Galkin VE, Yu X, et al. Stabilization of RAD51 nucleoprotein filaments by the C-terminal region of BRCA2. *Nat Struct Mol Biol* 2007;14:468–474.
23. Sleeth KM, Sorensen CS, Issaeva N, et al. RPA mediates recombination repair during replication stress and is displaced from DNA by checkpoint signalling in human cells. *J Mol Biol* 2007;373:38–47.
24. Littlefield LG, Kleinerman RA, Sayer AM, et al. Chromosome aberrations in lymphocytes—biomonitors of radiation exposure. *Prog Clin Biol Res* 1991;372:387–397.
25. Toulany M, Rodemann HP. Membrane receptor signaling and control of DNA repair after exposure to ionizing radiation. *Nuklearmedizin* 2010;49:S26–S30.
26. Barcellos-Hoff MH, Akhurst RJ. Transforming growth factor-beta in breast cancer: too much, too late. *Breast Cancer Res* 2009;11:202.
27. Deng X, Yin X, Allan R, et al. Ceramide biogenesis is required for radiation-induced apoptosis in the germ line of C. elegans. *Science* 2008;322:110–115.
28. Thompson LH, Suit HD. Proliferation kinetics of x-irradiated mouse L cells studied WITH TIME-lapse photography. II. *Int J Radiat Biol Relat Stud Phys Chem Med* 1969;15:347–362.
29. Sowa Resat MB, Morgan WF. Radiation-induced genomic instability: a role for secreted soluble factors in communicating the radiation response to non-irradiated cells. *J Cell Biochem* 2004;92:1013–1019.
30. Elkind MM. The initial part of the survival curve: does it predict the outcome of fractionated radiotherapy? *Radiat Res* 1988;114:425–436.
31. McCulloch EA, Till JE. The sensitivity of cells from normal mouse bone marrow to gamma radiation in vitro and in vivo. *Radiat Res* 1962;16:822–832.
32. Withers HR. Recovery and repopulation in vivo by mouse skin epithelial cells during fractionated irradiation. *Radiat Res* 1967;32:227–239.
33. Withers HR, Elkind MM. Microcolony survival assay for cells of mouse intestinal mucosa exposed to radiation. *Int J Radiat Biol Relat Stud Phys Chem Med* 1970;17:261–267.
34. Suit H, Wette R. Radiation dose fractionation and tumor control probability. *Radiat Res* 1966;29:267–281.
35. O'Neill K, Lyons SK, Gallagher WM, et al. Bioluminescent imaging: a critical tool in pre-clinical oncology research. *J Pathol* 2010;220:317–327.
36. Hewitt HB, Wilson CW. Survival curves for tumor cells irradiated in vivo. *Ann N Y Acad Sci* 1961;95:818–827.
37. Hill RP, Bush RS. A lung-colony assay to determine the radiosensitivity of cells of a solid tumour. *Int J Radiat Biol Relat Stud Phys Chem Med* 1969;15:435–444.
38. Elkind MM, Sutton-Gilbert H, Moses WB, et al. Radiation response of mammalian cells grown in culture. V. Temperature dependence of the repair of x-ray damage in surviving cells (aerobic and hypoxic). *Radiat Res* 1965;25:359–376.
39. Elkind MM, Whitmore GF. *Radiobiology of Cultured Mammalian Cells*. New York: Gordon and Breach; 1967.
40. Mottram JC. Factors of importance in radiosensitivity of tumors. *Br J Radiol* 1936;9:606.
41. Palcic B, Skarsgard LD. Reduced oxygen enhancement ratio at low doses of ionizing radiation. *Radiat Res* 1984;100:328–339.
42. Thomlinson RH, Gray LH. The histological structure of some human lung cancers and the possible implications for radiotherapy. *Br J Cancer* 1955;9:539–549.
43. Overgaard J, Horsman MR. Modification of hypoxia-induced radioresistance in tumors by the use of oxygen and sensitizers. *Semin Radiat Oncol* 1996;6:10–21.
44. Machtay M, Pajak TF, Suntharalingam M, et al. Radiotherapy with or without erythropoietin for anemic patients with head and neck cancer: a randomized trial of the Radiation Therapy Oncology Group (RTOG 99-03). *Int J Radiat Oncol Biol Phys* 2007;69:1008–1017.
45. Henke M, Laszig R, Rube C, et al. Erythropoietin to treat head and neck cancer patients with anaemia undergoing radiotherapy: randomised, double-blind, placebo-controlled trial. *Lancet* 2003;362:1255–1260.
46. Janssens GO, Rademakers SE, Terhaard CH, et al. Accelerated radiotherapy with carbogen and nicotinamide for laryngeal cancer: results of a phase III randomized trial. *J Clin Oncol* 2012;30:1777–1783.
47. Willett CG, Boucher Y, di Tomaso E, et al. Direct evidence that the VEGF-specific antibody bevacizumab has antivascular effects in human rectal cancer. *Nat Med* 2004;10:145–147.
48. Lapi SE, Voller TF, Welch MJ. Positron emission tomography imaging of hypoxia. *PET Clin* 2009;4:39–47.
49. Lee NY, Mechalakos JG, Nehmeh S, et al. Fluorine-18-labeled fluoromisonidazole positron emission and computed tomography-guided intensity-modulated radiotherapy for head and neck cancer: a feasibility study. *Int J Radiat Oncol Biol Phys* 2008;70:2–13.
50. Schaue D, Xie MW, Ratikan JA, et al. Regulatory T cells in radiotherapeutic responses. *Front Oncol* 2012;2:90.
51. Formenti SC, Demaria S. Combining radiotherapy and cancer immunotherapy: a paradigm shift. *J Natl Cancer Inst* 2013;105:256–265.
52. Lawrence TS, Davis MA, Tang HY, et al. Fluorodeoxyuridine-mediated cytotoxicity and radiosensitization require S phase progression. *Int J Radiat Biol* 1996;70:273–280.
53. Lawrence TS, Chang EY, Hahn TM, et al. Radiosensitization of pancreatic cancer cells by 2′,2′-difluoro-2′-deoxycytidine. *Int J Radiat Oncol Biol Phys* 1996;34:867–872.
54. Eisbruch A, Shewach DS, Bradford CR, et al. Radiation concurrent with gemcitabine for locally advanced head and neck cancer: a phase I trial and intracellular drug incorporation study. *J Clin Oncol* 2001;19:792–799.
55. Ben-Josef E, Schipper M, Francis IR, et al. A phase I/II trial of intensity modulated radiation (IMRT) dose escalation with concurrent fixed-dose rate gemcitabine (FDR-G) in patients with unresectable pancreatic cancer. *Int J Radiat Oncol Biol Phys* 2012;84:1166–1171.
56. Wolff RA, Evans DB, Gravel DM, et al. Phase I trial of gemcitabine combined with radiation for the treatment of locally advanced pancreatic adenocarcinoma. *Clin Cancer Res* 2001;7:2246–2253.
57. Wilson GD, Bentzen SM, Harari PM. Biologic basis for combining drugs with radiation. *Semin Radiat Oncol* 2006;16:2–9.
58. Bradley JD, Paulus R, Graham MV, et al. Phase II trial of postoperative adjuvant paclitaxel/carboplatin and thoracic radiotherapy in resected stage II and IIIA non-small-cell lung cancer: promising long-term results of the Radiation Therapy Oncology Group—RTOG 9705. *J Clin Oncol* 2005;23:3480–3487.
59. Nyati MK, Morgan MA, Feng FY, et al. Integration of EGFR inhibitors with radiochemotherapy. *Nat Rev Cancer* 2006;6:876–885.
60. Bonner JA, Harari PM, Giralt J, et al. Radiotherapy plus cetuximab for locoregionally advanced head and neck cancer: 5-year survival data from a phase 3 randomised trial, and relation between cetuximab-induced rash and survival. *Lancet Oncol* 2010;11:21–28.
61. Ang KK, Zhang QE, Rosenthal DI, et al. A randomized phase III trial (RTOG 0522) of concurrent accelerated radiation plus cisplatin with or without cetuximab for stage III-IV head and neck squamous cell carcinomas (HNC). *J Clin Oncol* 2011;29.
62. Engelke CG, Parsels LA, Qian Y, et al. Sensitization of pancreatic cancer to chemoradiation by the Chk1 inhibitor MK8776. *Clin Cancer Res* 2013;19:4412–4421.
63. Morgan MA, Parsels LA, Maybaum J, et al. Improving the efficacy of chemoradiation with targeted agents. *Cancer Discov* 2014;4:280–291.
64. Chalmers AJ, Lakshman M, Chan N, et al. Poly(ADP-ribose) polymerase inhibition as a model for synthetic lethality in developing radiation oncology targets. *Semin Radiat Oncol* 2010;20:274–281.
65. Brizel DM, Wasserman TH, Henke M, et al. Phase III randomized trial of amifostine as a radioprotector in head and neck cancer. *J Clin Oncol* 2000;18:3339–3345.
66. Winczura P, Jassem J. Combined treatment with cytoprotective agents and radiotherapy. *Cancer Treat Rev* 2010;36:268–275.
67. Van Dyk J, ed. Radiation oncology medical physics resources for working, teaching, and learning. In: *The Modern Technology of Radiation Oncology*. Volume 3. Medical Physics Publishing Web site. http://www.medicalphysics.org/vandykch16.pdf. Madison, WI: Medical Physics Publishing; 2013.
68. Karzmark C, Nunan C, Tanabe E. *Medical Electron Accelerators*. New York: McGraw-Hill Ryerson; 1993.
69. Greene D, Williams P. *Linear Accelerators for Radiation Therapy*. 2nd ed. New York: Taylor and Francis Group; 1997.
70. Fenwick JD, Tome WA, Soisson ET, et al. Tomotherapy and other innovative IMRT delivery systems. *Semin Radiat Oncol* 2006;16:199–208.
71. Curran B, Balter J, Chetty I, eds. *Integrating New Technologies into the Clinic: Monte Carlo and Image-Guided Radiation Therapy*. Madison, WI: Medical Physics Publishing; 2006.
72. Bourland J, ed. *Image-Guided Radiation Therapy*. Boca Raton, FL: Taylor & Francis; 2012.
73. Seco J, Verhaegen F, eds. *Monte Carlo Techniques in Radiation Therapy*. Boca Raton, FL: Taylor & Francis; 2013.
74. Kessler ML. Image registration and data fusion in radiation therapy. *Br J Radiol* 2006;79:S99–S108.
75. Brock K, ed. *Image Processing in Radiation Therapy*. Boca Raton, FL: Taylor & Francis Group; 2014.
76. Sovik A, Malinen E, Olsen DR. Strategies for biologic image-guided dose escalation: a review. *Int J Radiat Oncol Biol Phys* 2009;73:650–658.
77. Marks LB, Ten Haken RK, Martel MK. Guest editor's introduction to QUANTEC: a users guide. *Int J Radiat Oncol Biol Phys* 2010;76:S1–S2.

78. Li A, Alber M, Deasy JO, et al. The use and QA of biologically related models for treatment planning: short report of the TG-166 of the therapy physics committee of the AAPM. *Med Phys* 2012;39:1386–1409.
79. Bortfeld T. IMRT: a review and preview. *Phys Med Biol* 2006;51:R363–R379.
80. Webb S. *Contemporary IMRT Developing Physics and Clinical Implementation.* London: IOP Publishing; 2005.
81. Maughan R, Yudelev M. Neutron therapy. In: Van Dyk J, ed. *The Modern Technology of Radiation Oncology.* Madison, WI: Medical Physics Publishing; 1999.
82. Hogstrom KR, Almond PR. Review of electron beam therapy physics. *Phys Med Biol* 2006;51:R455–R489.
83. Schlegel W, Bortfeld T, Grosu A, eds. *New Technologies in Radiation Oncology.* Heidelberg: Springer-Verlag; 2006.
84. Ma C-MC, Lomax T, eds. *Proton and Carbon Ion Therapy.* Boca Raton, FL: Taylor & Francis Group; 2012.
85. Venselaar J, Meigooni A, Baltas D, et al., eds. *Comprehensive Brachytherapy: Physical and Clinical Aspects.* Boca Raton, FL: Taylor & Francis Group; 2012.
86. Meredith RF. Systemic targeted radionuclide therapy symposium introduction. *Int J Radiat Oncol Biol Phys* 2006;66:S7.
87. Tripuraneni P, Watson RL, Ang KK, et al. Intersociety Radiation Oncology Summit-SCOPE II. *Int J Radiat Oncol Biol Phys* 2008;72:323–326.
88. Delaney G, Jacob S, Featherstone C, et al. The role of radiotherapy in cancer treatment: estimating optimal utilization from a review of evidence-based clinical guidelines. *Cancer* 2005;104:1129–1137.
89. Zelefsky MJ, Housman D, Pei X, et al. Incidence of secondary cancer development after high-dose intensity-modulated radiotherapy and image-guided brachytherapy for the treatment of localized prostate cancer. *Int J Radiat Oncol Biol Phys* 2012;83:953–959.
90. Combs SE, Laperriere N, Brada M. Clinical controversies: proton radiation therapy for brain and skull base tumors. *Semin Radiat Oncol* 2013;23:120–126.
91. Overgaard J. Hypoxic radiosensitization: adored and ignored. *J Clin Oncol* 2007;25:4066–4074.
92. Mouw KW, Trofimov A, Zietman AL, et al. Clinical controversies: proton therapy for prostate cancer. *Semin Radiat Oncol* 2013;23:109–114.
93. Yu JB, Soulos PR, Herrin J, et al. Proton versus intensity-modulated radiotherapy for prostate cancer: patterns of care and early toxicity. *J Natl Cancer Inst* 2013;105:25–32.
94. Brada M, Pijls-Johannesma M, De Ruysscher D. Proton therapy in clinical practice: current clinical evidence. *J Clin Oncol* 2007;25:965–970.
95. Douglas JG, Koh WJ, Austin-Seymour M, et al. Treatment of salivary gland neoplasms with fast neutron radiotherapy. *Arch Otolaryngol Head Neck Surg* 2003;129:944–948.
96. Shilkrut M, Merrick GS, McLaughlin PW, et al. The addition of low-dose-rate brachytherapy and androgen-deprivation therapy decreases biochemical failure and prostate cancer death compared with dose-escalated external-beam radiation therapy for high-risk prostate cancer. *Cancer* 2013;119:681–690.
97. Iyengar P, Timmerman R. Stereotactic ablative radiotherapy for non-small cell lung cancer: rationale and outcomes. *J Natl Compr Canc Netw* 2012;10:1514–1520.
98. Lo SS, Moffatt-Bruce SD, Dawson LA, et al. The role of local therapy in the management of lung and liver oligometastases. *Nat Rev Clin Oncol* 2011;8:405–416.
99. Forastiere AA, Zhang Q, Weber RS, et al. Long-term results of RTOG 91-11: a comparison of three nonsurgical treatment strategies to preserve the larynx in patients with locally advanced larynx cancer. *J Clin Oncol* 2013;31:845–852.
100. Gunderson LL, Winter KA, Ajani JA, et al. Long-term update of US GI intergroup RTOG 98-11 phase III trial for anal carcinoma: survival, relapse, and colostomy failure with concurrent chemoradiation involving fluorouracil/mitomycin versus fluorouracil/cisplatin. *J Clin Oncol* 2012;30:4344–4351.
101. Hellman S, Weichselbaum RR. Oligometastases. *J Clin Oncol* 1995;13:8–10.
102. Hortobagyi GN. Can we cure limited metastatic breast cancer? *J Clin Oncol* 2002;20:620–623.
103. Stamell EF, Wolchok JD, Gnjatic S, et al. The abscopal effect associated with a systemic anti-melanoma immune response. *Int J Radiat Oncol Biol Phys* 2013;85:293–295.
104. Nagtegaal ID, Gosens MJ, Marijnen CA, et al. Combinations of tumor and treatment parameters are more discriminative for prognosis than the present TNM system in rectal cancer. *J Clin Oncol* 2007;25:1647–1650.
105. Sauer R, Becker H, Hohenberger W, et al. Preoperative versus postoperative chemoradiotherapy for rectal cancer. *N Engl J Med* 2004;351:1731–1740.
106. Clarke M, Collins R, Darby S, et al. Effects of radiotherapy and of differences in the extent of surgery for early breast cancer on local recurrence and 15-year survival: an overview of the randomised trials. *Lancet* 2005;366:2087–2106.
107. Hellman S. Stopping metastases at their source. *N Engl J Med* 1997;337:996–997.
108. Marks LB, Prosnitz LR. Postoperative radiotherapy for lung cancer: the breast cancer story all over again? *Int J Radiat Oncol Biol Phys* 2000;48:625–627.
109. Wang XS, Rhines LD, Shiu AS, et al. Stereotactic body radiation therapy for management of spinal metastases in patients without spinal cord compression: a phase 1-2 trial. *Lancet Oncol* 2012;13:395–402.
110. Tarnawski R, Fowler J, Skladowski K, et al. How fast is repopulation of tumor cells during the treatment gap? *Int J Radiat Oncol Biol Phys* 2002;54:229–236.
111. Peters LJ, Withers HR. Applying radiobiological principles to combined modality treatment of head and neck cancer—the time factor. *Int J Radiat Oncol Biol Phys* 1997;39:831–836.
112. Bourhis J, Overgaard J, Audry H, et al. Hyperfractionated or accelerated radiotherapy in head and neck cancer: a meta-analysis. *Lancet* 2006;368:843–854.
113. Bourhis J, Sire C, Graff P, et al. Concomitant chemoradiotherapy versus acceleration of radiotherapy with or without concomitant chemotherapy in locally advanced head and neck carcinoma (GORTEC 99-02): an open-label phase 3 randomised trial. *Lancet Oncol* 2012;13:145–153.
114. Adkison JB, McHaffie DR, Bentzen SM, et al. Phase I trial of pelvic nodal dose escalation with hypofractionated IMRT for high-risk prostate cancer. *Int J Radiat Oncol Biol Phys* 2012;82:184–190.
115. Feyer P, Maranzano E, Molassiotis A, et al. Radiotherapy-induced nausea and vomiting (RINV): antiemetic guidelines. *Support Care Cancer* 2005;13:122–128.
116. Horiot JC. Prophylaxis versus treatment: is there a better way to manage radiotherapy-induced nausea and vomiting? *Int J Radiat Oncol Biol Phys* 2004;60:1018–1025.
117. Hickok JT, Roscoe JA, Morrow GR, et al. Frequency, severity, clinical course, and correlates of fatigue in 372 patients during 5 weeks of radiotherapy for cancer. *Cancer* 2005;104:1772–1778.
118. Schwartz AL, Nail LM, Chen S, et al. Fatigue patterns observed in patients receiving chemotherapy and radiotherapy. *Cancer Invest* 2000;18:11–19.
119. Dawson LA, Ten Haken RK. Partial volume tolerance of the liver to radiation. *Semin Radiat Oncol* 2005;15:279–283.
120. Kong FM, Hayman JA, Griffith KA, et al. Final toxicity results of a radiation-dose escalation study in patients with non-small-cell lung cancer (NSCLC): predictors for radiation pneumonitis and fibrosis. *Int J Radiat Oncol Biol Phys* 2006;65:1075–1086.
121. Fleckenstein K, Gauter-Fleckenstein B, Jackson IL, et al. Using biological markers to predict risk of radiation injury. *Semin Radiat Oncol* 2007;17:89–98.
122. Hart JP, Broadwater G, Rabbani Z, et al. Cytokine profiling for prediction of symptomatic radiation-induced lung injury. *Int J Radiat Oncol Biol Phys* 2005;63:1448–1454.
123. Barnett GC, Coles CE, Elliott RM, et al. Independent validation of genes and polymorphisms reported to be associated with radiation toxicity: a prospective analysis study. *Lancet Oncol* 2012;13:65–77.
124. Fajardo LF. Is the pathology of radiation injury different in small vs large blood vessels? *Cardiovasc Radiat Med* 1999;1:108–110.
125. Delanian S, Porcher R, Rudant J, et al. Kinetics of response to long-term treatment combining pentoxifylline and tocopherol in patients with superficial radiation-induced fibrosis. *J Clin Oncol* 2005;23:8570–8579.
126. Chou TC, Talalay P. Quantitative analysis of dose-effect relationships: the combined effects of multiple drugs or enzyme inhibitors. *Adv Enzyme Regul* 1984;22:27–55.
127. Steel GG, Peckham MJ. Exploitable mechanisms in combined radiotherapy-chemotherapy: the concept of additivity. *Int J Radiat Oncol Biol Phys* 1979;5:85–91.
128. Tannock IF. Treatment of cancer with radiation and drugs. *J Clin Oncol* 1996;14:3156–3174.
129. Blanchard P, Baujat B, Holostenco V, et al. Meta-analysis of chemotherapy in head and neck cancer (MACH-NC): a comprehensive analysis by tumour site. *Radiother Oncol* 2011;100:33–40.
130. Dillman RO, Herndon J, Seagren SL, et al. Improved survival in stage III non-small-cell lung cancer: seven-year follow-up of cancer and leukemia group B (CALGB) 8433 trial. *J Natl Cancer Inst* 1996;88:1210–1215.
131. De Ruysscher D, Belderbos J, Reymen B, et al. State of the art radiation therapy for lung cancer 2012: a glimpse of the future. *Clin Lung Cancer* 2013;14:89–95.
132. Klopp AH, Eifel PJ. Chemoradiotherapy for cervical cancer in 2010. *Curr Oncol Rep* 2011;13:77–85.
133. Chun PY, Feng FY, Scheurer AM, et al. Synergistic effects of gemcitabine and gefitinib in the treatment of head and neck carcinoma. *Cancer Res* 2006;66:981–988.

14 Cancer Immunotherapy

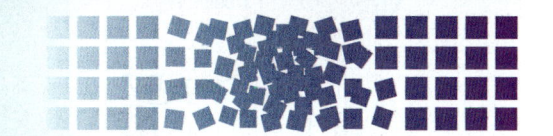

Steven A. Rosenberg, Paul F. Robbins, Giao Q. Phan, Steven A. Feldman, and James N. Kochenderfer

INTRODUCTION

Progress in understanding basic aspects of cellular immunology and tumor–host immune interactions have led to the development of immune-based therapies capable of mediating the rejection of metastatic cancer in humans. Early studies of allografts and transplanted syngeneic tumors in mice demonstrated that it was the cellular arm of the immune response rather than the action of antibodies (humoral immunity) that was responsible for tissue rejection. Thus, studies of immunotherapy have focused on enhancing antitumor immune responses of T cells that recognize cancer antigens. Antibodies that recognize growth factors on the surface of tumors can contribute to tumor regression, primarily by interfering with growth signals rather than by the direct destruction of tumor cells. The use of monoclonal antibodies in cancer treatment will be considered in Chapter 29.

Evidence for specific tumor recognition by cells of the immune system was obtained in experiments first conducted in the 1940s using murine tumors generated or induced by the mutagen methylcholanthrene (MCA). Mice that received a surgical resection of previously inoculated tumors could be protected against a subsequent tumor challenge with the immunizing tumor but not generally protected against challenge with additional MCA tumors. The observation that CD8+ cytotoxic T cells were primarily responsible for mediating the rejection of MCA-induced tumors in mice led to the identification of genes that encoded tumor rejection antigens expressed on murine tumors as well as the subsequent identification of antigens recognized by human tumor-reactive T cells. The identification of widely shared nonmutated tumor antigens led to the expectation that effective vaccine therapies could be developed for the treatment of cancer patients; however, the response rates in clinical cancer vaccine trials targeting these antigens have, to this point, been disappointingly low. Vaccination with viruslike particles expressing human papilloma virus (HPV) proteins are successful in preventing the establishment of cervical cancer and immunization with peptides derived from the oncogenic HPV E6 and E7 proteins can mediate tumor regression in woman with high vulvar neoplasia.[1] Immune-based therapies have, however, been identified that mediate the regression of large, established tumor metastases. Nonspecific immune stimulation with interleukin-2 (IL-2) administration can lead to objective clinical responses in patients with melanoma and renal cancer,[2] and inhibition of regulatory pathways mediated by CTLA-4[3] or PD-1[4] can lead to tumor regression in patients with metastatic melanoma and lung cancer. The adoptive transfer of melanoma reactive T cells can mediate objective clinical responses in 50% to 70% of patients with melanoma,[5] and the ability to genetically modify antitumor lymphocytes is expanding this cell transfer therapy approach to the treatment of patients with other cancer histologies.[6] Studies aimed at identifying potent tumor rejection antigens, as well as mechanisms that regulate immune responses to cancer, are being actively pursued.

HUMAN TUMOR ANTIGENS

To be recognized by immune lymphocytes, intracellular proteins must be digested and the resulting peptides transported to the cell surface and bound to Class I or II main histocompatibility molecules (Fig. 14.1). A variety of approaches have been used to identify the antigens that are naturally processed and presented on tumor cells. These include evaluating the ability of cells transfected with tumor cDNA library pools along with genes encoding autologous major histocompatibility complex (MHC) molecules, as well as the ability of target cells pulsed with peptides eluted from tumor cell surface MHC molecules for their ability to stimulate tumor reactive T cells. Reverse immunology approaches that involve either repeated in vitro T cell sensitization or in vivo immunization with candidate peptides or proteins have also lead to the identification of tumor antigens. Candidate epitopes identified on the basis of their ability to bind to a particular MHC molecule, however, may not necessarily be naturally processed and presented on the tumor cell surface, and there are conflicting reports on the ability of T cells generated using some candidate epitopes to recognize unmanipulated tumor targets, as discussed further.

Additional tumor antigens have been identified using antisera from cancer patients to screen tumor cell cDNA libraries, a method that has been termed serological analysis of recombinant cDNA expression (SEREX).[7] Although some of the proteins identified using this technique are expressed in a tumor-specific manner, many of these antigens are simply expressed at higher levels in tumor cells than in normal cells. This may occur due to the release of normal self-proteins from necrotic and apoptotic tumor cells leading to the generation of antibodies against intracellular proteins that are normally sequestered from the immune system.

Finally, the use of recently described approaches involving whole exomic sequencing of tumor cells has led to the identification of mutated tumor antigens. These studies will be discussed further in the section devoted to mutated tumor antigens

Cancer/Germ-Line Antigens

The first antigen identified as a target of human tumor reactive T cells was isolated by screening a melanoma genomic DNA library with an autologous cytotoxic T lymphocyte (CTL) clone.[8] The gene that was isolated, termed *MAGE-1*, was found to be a nonmutated gene that was a member of a large, previously unidentified gene family, many of whose members encode antigens recognized by tumor reactive T cells.[9] Members of this family of antigens are expressed in the testes and placenta, both of which lack an expression of MHC molecules, but often not in other normal tissues, which has led to their designation as cancer germ-line (CG) antigens. Members of the MAGE gene family are expressed in a variety of tumor types, including melanoma, breast, prostate, and esophageal cancers. The expression patterns of three

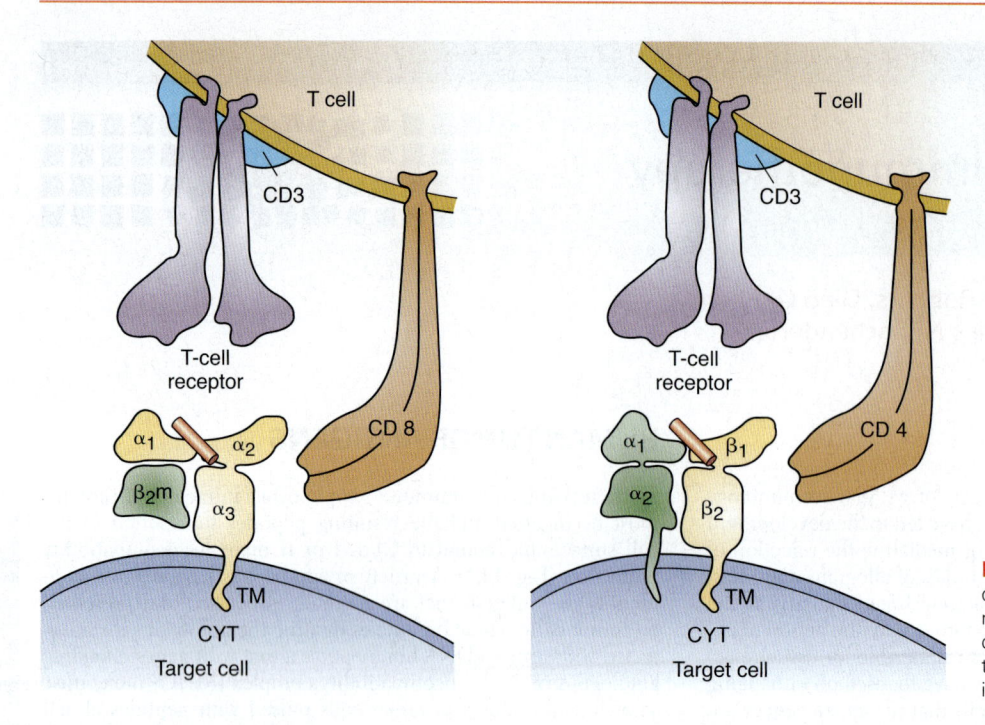

Figure 14.1 CD8 and CD4 cells use different molecules that interact with major histocompatibility complex (MHC) class I and II molecules respectively on the cell surface and serve to potentiate immune reactions.

different cancer/testes antigens in multiple tumor types is shown in Figure 14.2. The NY-ESO-1 antigen—a CG antigen that is unrelated to the MAGE family of genes—is expressed in approximately 30% of breast, prostate, and melanoma tumors, as well as between 70% and 80% of synovial cell sarcomas.[10]

Clinical adoptive immunotherapy trials targeting CG antigens have now been conducted in patients with melanoma as well as other tumor types. In a recent trial, objective clinical responses were seen in approximately 50% of patients with melanoma and 80% of patients with synovial cell sarcoma receiving autologous peripheral blood mononuclear cell (PBMC) transduced with a T-cell receptor directed against an HLA-A*02:01 restricted NY-ESO-1 epitope.[6] A trial targeting a MAGEA3 epitopes was recently carried out using a T-cell receptor (TCR) isolated from an HLA-A*02:01+ transgenic mouse immunized with the MAGEA3:112–120 peptide.[11] Objective clinical responses were observed in five of nine melanoma patients receiving the adoptively transferred PBMC that were transduced with the MAGEA3-reactive TCR.[12] Unexpectedly, neural toxicity was observed in three of the patients treated in this trial, two of whom lapsed into a coma and subsequently died. Autopsy samples of patients' brains revealed that *MAGEA12*, which encodes a cross-reactive epitope recognized by the MAGEA3 TCR, was expressed at low levels in patients' brains, which may have been responsible for the observed neurologic toxicities. In a recent trial carried out using an affinity-enhanced human TCR directed against the

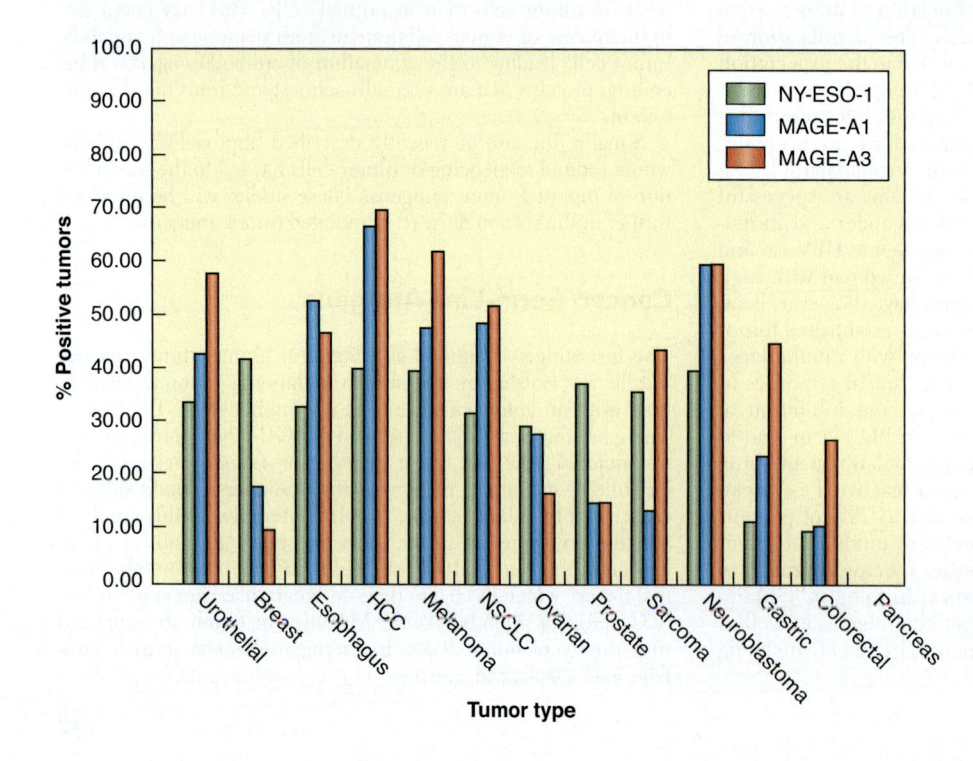

Figure 14.2 Expression of three different cancer/testes antigens in many different tumor types is shown. These data reflect reverse transcription–polymerase chain reaction measurements and is more sensitive than results obtained by immunohistochemistry. NSCLC, non–small-cell lung cancer. (Data compiled by Dr. J. Wargo. Massachusetts General Hospital.)

HLA-A*01:01-restricted, MAGEA3:168-176 epitope, the first two patients receiving TCR-transduced autologous PBMC died of cardiac arrest 4 to 5 days following infusion, which was attributed to cross-reactivity with titin, a protein expressed at high levels in cardimyocytes.[13] Taken together, these findings demonstrate the need for caution in evaluating cross-reactivity of high affinity TCRs recognizing tumor antigens.

Melanocyte Differentiation Antigens

Melanoma-reactive T cells have been frequently found to recognize gene products, termed melanocyte differentiation antigens (MDA), that are expressed in melanomas as well as in normal melanocytes present in the skin, eye, and ear but not in other normal tissues or tumor types. These include epitopes derived from gp100,[14,15] tyrosinase,[16] TRP-1,[17] and TRP-2,[18] proteins that had previously been found to play important roles in melanin synthesis. The screening of melanoma cDNA libraries with an HLA-A2–restricted tumor reactive T cells lead to the isolation of a previously unidentified gene, termed MART-1[19] or Melan-A.[20] The MART-1 antigen, which is expressed in 80% to 90% of fresh melanomas and cultured melanoma cell lines as well as normal melanocytes, represents an MDA of unknown function. The majority of melanoma reactive, HLA-A2–restricted tumor-infiltrating lymphocytes (TIL) recognize a single MART-1 epitope.[21] Studies carried out using a variety of approaches have also resulted in the identification of human leukocyte antigen (HLA) class II restricted epitopes of tyrosinase, TRP-1, TRP-2, and gp100.[9]

Overexpressed Gene Products

Gene products that are expressed at low levels in a variety of normal tissues but are overexpressed in a variety of tumor types have also been shown to be recognized by T cells. Screening of an autologous renal carcinoma cDNA library with a tumor reactive, HLA-A3–restricted T-cell clone resulted in the isolation of FGF5,[22] a protein that was expressed only at low levels in normal tissues but upregulated in multiple renal carcinomas as well as prostate and breast carcinomas. The peptide epitope recognized by FGF5-reactive T cells was generated by protein splicing, a process in which distant protein regions are joined together in the proteasome that had previously only been described in plants[23] and unicellular organisms.[24] Subsequent studies have led to the identification of multiple epitopes that result from protein splicing, suggesting that this represents a general mechanism for generating T-cell epitopes.[25-28] Screening of an autologous cDNA library led to the identification of a previously unknown gene that was termed PRAME.[29] This gene product was expressed in relatively high levels in melanomas as well as in additional tumor types but was also expressed at lower levels in a variety of normal tissues that included the testis, endometrium, ovary, and adrenals. The HLA-A24–restricted PRAME reactive T-cell clone, however, expressed the natural killer (NK) inhibitory receptor p58.2, and tumor cell recognition was dependent on the loss of expression of the HLA C*07 allele that represented the ligand for the inhibitory receptor, which may explain the lack of recognition of normal tissues that express relatively high levels of this HLA gene product.

Attempts have also been made to generate T cells directed against overexpressed candidate antigens by repeatedly stimulating PBMC in vitro with peptides that were identified as high binders for particular MHC molecules either using direct binding assays or in silico analysis carried out using peptide/MHC binding algorithms.[30,31] Using this approach, candidate epitopes have been identified from a variety of proteins that include prostate-specific antigen (PSA)[32] and prostate-specific membrane antigen (PSMA),[33] as well as Her-2/neu, a protein that is frequently overexpressed in a variety of tumor types, including breast carcinomas. Initial studies indicated that T cells derived by in vitro stimulation with a peptide that was predicted to bind with high affinity to HLA-A*02:01, Her-2/neu:369–377, recognized the appropriate natural tumor targets.[34] In one study, T cells generated following two in vitro stimulations of postvaccination PBMC from three of the four patients who were tested efficiently recognized peptide-pulsed targets but failed to recognize appropriate tumor targets.[35] Similarly, although stimulation with a peptide corresponding to amino acids 540 through 548 of the human telomerase reverse transcriptase (hTERT) catalytic subunit was initially reported to generate tumor-reactive T cells,[36] additional observations indicated that T cells generated using this peptide failed to recognize tumor targets.[37] These factors responsible for these discrepancies remain unresolved, although the in vitro stimulation of T cells with target cells pulsed with relatively high peptide concentrations could have led to the generation of low-avidity T cells that were incapable of recognizing naturally processed antigens.

Alternative screening approaches employed for tumor antigen discovery that may help to address these issues include the use of tandem mass spectrometry to sequence peptides that have been eluted from tumor cell surface MHC molecules. Use of this technique, coupled with microarray gene expression profiling, resulted in the identification of peptides derived from proteins that appeared to be overexpressed in tumor cells.[38] Peptides identified using this approach may, in many cases, not be immunogenic due to the fact that their expression in normal tissues, although lower than in tumor cells, may be high enough to lead to central or peripheral tolerance. Nevertheless, one of the peptides that were identified in this study also appeared to be recognized by human tumor reactive T cells. Recently, a similar approach was used to identify candidate peptides presented on cell surface MHC molecules that appeared to be derived from proteins that were overexpressed on glioblastomas.[39] In a clinical trial involving vaccination of patients with pools of the identified peptides, overall survival was associated with the number of peptides in the vaccine pool that elicited immune response[40]; however, this may simply reflect the fact that T cells from healthier patients can more readily generate peptide-specific responses.

Transgenic mice that express human HLA molecules have also been immunized with candidate antigens in an attempt to identify high avidity tumor-reactive T cells. Immunization of transgenic mice expressing HLA-A*0201 with the native human p53:264–272 peptide that differed from the corresponding murine p53 sequence at a single position lead to the generation of T cells that recognized tumor cells expressing high levels of p53.[41] Human T cells transduced with a murine p53 TCR isolated from an immunized mouse recognized a variety of human tumor cells; however, transduced T cells also recognized normal cells expressing lower p53 levels, indicating the dangers of targeting a normal self-protein whose expression is not strictly limited to tumor cells.[42] Similarly, a TCR that was highly reactive with HLA-A*02:01+ tumor cells expressing the human carcinoembryonic antigen (CEA), a protein that is overexpressed in colon and breast carcinomas, was isolated by immunizing HLA-A*02:01+ transgenic mice with the CEA:691–699 peptide.[43] The adoptive transfer of human PBMC transduced with the CEA-reactive TCR lead to an objective clinical response in one of the three treated patients; however, severe colitis was observed in all three of the treated patients.[44] In general, immunotherapies that target antigens present even in small amounts on normal tissues have led to normal tissue destruction and must be applied with caution.

Mutated Gene Products Recognized by CD8+ and CD4+ T Cells

A variety of mutated antigens have also been identified as targets of tumor reactive T cells. The majority of mutated antigens identified using these approaches appear to be unique or only expressed in a relatively small percentage of cancers, and so do not represent targets that are broadly applicable to the treatment of multiple patients. Nevertheless, these studies have in some cases provided insights into mechanisms involved with tumor development, as the mutations may represent drivers of the transformed phenotype. The CDK4 gene product that was cloned using a CTL clone contained a point mutation that enhanced the binding to the HLA-A2 restriction element.[45] This mutation, which was identified in 1 of an additional 28 melanomas that were analyzed, led to the inhibition of binding to the cell cycle inhibitory protein $p16^{INK4a}$ and may have played a role in the loss of growth control in this tumor cell. A point-mutated product of the β-catenin gene, containing a substitution of phenylalanine for serine at position 37, was isolated by screening a cDNA library with an HLA-24–restricted, melanoma reactive TIL.[46] This mutation was found to stabilize the β-catenin gene product by altering a critical serine phosphorylation site, and 2 of 24 additional melanoma cell lines were found to express transcripts with identical mutations.[47]

The observation that immunization against individual murine tumors did not generally cross-protect against challenge with additional syngeneic murine tumors has provided support for the hypothesis that mutant T-cell epitopes represent the predominant antigens responsible for tumor rejection.[48] Mutated epitopes also represent a foreign antigen, which may render them more immunogenic than the majority of normal self-antigens. Although many of the mutations are specific for individual tumors, T cells have been generated by carrying out in vitro sensitization with peptides encoded at mutational hot spots present in *driver* genes.[49]

Recently, novel approaches have been developed that involve the sequencing of tumor cell DNA to identify potential mutated epitopes. In one study, whole exome sequencing of the murine B16 melanoma led to the identification of mutated epitopes that elicited a T cell that appeared to specifically recognize the mutated but not the corresponding wild-type peptides.[50] In a second study, a mutated antigen was identified by screening candidate epitopes that were expressed by tumors derived from immunodeficient mice that regressed in immune-competent mice.[51] More recently, melanomas from three patients who responded to adoptive immunotherapy were subjected to whole exome sequencing, followed by *in silico* analysis using peptide/MHC binding algorithms to identify candidate epitopes that were predicted to bind to the patients' MHC molecules.[52] Using this approach, a total of seven peptides were identified as targets of the TIL that were administered to these patients. Two mutated epitopes were recently identified by whole exome sequencing of a melanoma from a patient who demonstrated a partial response to treatment with the anti–CTLA-4 antibody ipilimumab, followed by a screening of a panel of mutated candidate peptide/MHC tetramers that were predicted to bind to the patient's HLA-A and B alleles.[53] In addition, a mutated epitope expressed by a bile duct cancer was identified by screening tandem minigenes encoding all mutated epitopes that were identified by whole exome sequencing.[54] The adoptive transfer of T cells directed against this mutation-mediated regression of the patient's cancer. Mutations unique to each cancer represent ideal targets for immunotherapy and can potentially lead to the development of personalized therapies directed against these unique targets.

Antigens Identified in Viral-Associated Cancers

Viruses do not appear to play a role in the development of the majority of human cancers; however, an infection with HPV, a group of double-stranded DNA viruses that infect squamous epithelium, is highly associated with the development of a variety of genital lesions that range from warts to carcinomas, as well as the majority of oropharyngeal carcinomas. Recombinant vaccines have been produced by the generation of viruslike particles (VLP), self-assembling particles that form following the expression of the HPV L1 protein in recombinant viral and yeast systems that were initially found to be protective in animal models. The results of a phase II trial in which 2,392 women between 16 and 23 years of age were immunized with HPV-16 VLPs indicated that 100% of those who were vaccinated were protected against infection with HPV-16.[55,56] Although vaccination with VLP does not lead to the regression of established disease, some success has been seen in therapeutic vaccination trials that target the oncogenic viral proteins E6 and E7. In a trial involving the vaccination of women with HPV-16–positive high-grade vulvar intraepithelial neoplasia with synthetic long peptides that encompass both HLA class I and class II restricted epitopes from the oncogenic HPV proteins E6 and E, clinical responses were observed in 15 of the 19 vaccinated patients, and complete regression of all lesions were seen in 9 of the 19 patients in this trial.[1]

Targeting foreign antigens thus may represent a strategy that can lead to more effective immunotherapies. These include viral epitopes as well as mutated epitopes that are also foreign to the host and therefore may represent more effective targets for these therapies than normal self-antigen.

HUMAN CANCER IMMUNOTHERAPIES

A wide variety of therapies have been evaluated in model systems and are now being developed for the treatment of patients with cancer. These include nonspecific approaches, those that involve direct immunization of patients with a variety of immunogens and approaches that involve the adoptive transfer of activated effector cells (Table 14.1). Much confusion related to the effectiveness of cancer immunotherapy has resulted from the lack of proper evaluation of the results of therapy using standard, accepted oncologic criteria such as the World Health Organization or the Response Evaluation Criteria in Solid Tumors (RECIST). Many clinical trials reported a positive use of *soft* criteria such as lymphoid infiltration or tumor necrosis that can occur in the natural course of cancer growth. Because of the delayed responses seen with some immunotherapy approaches, including tumor regression after initial tumor growth, guidelines have been published suggesting the use of an alternate set of immune-related response criteria for the evaluation of immune-based cancer treatments.[57,58] Other confusion has arisen from the use of inappropriate animal models. Although animal model systems have provided important clues that may lead to improved therapies, model systems that employ artificially introduced foreign antigens or that evaluate protection from tumor challenge do not appear to be relevant to the treatment of patients with bulky metastases. Short-term lung metastasis models involve the treatment of relatively small, nonvascularized tumors and also may not be directly relevant to the majority of tumors that are the targets of current clinical trials.

TABLE 14.1

Three Main Approaches to Cancer Immunotherapy

1. Nonspecific stimulation of immune reactions
   a) Stimulate effector cells
      IL-2 (melanoma and renal cancer)
   b) Inhibit regulatory factors
      Anti-CTLA4 (melanoma)
      Anti–PD-1 (melanoma, lung cancer)
2. Active immunization to enhance antitumor reactions (cancer vaccines)
3. Passively transfer activated immune cells with antitumor activity (adoptive immunotherapy)

Nonspecific Approaches to Cancer Immunotherapy

Progress has surged in the past 10 years in the understanding and utilization of nonspecific immune stimulation for the treatment of metastatic cancers. These agents aim to activate quiescent tumor-reactive immune cells or to remove inhibitory mechanisms to allow immunosuppressed cells to function to their full capacity. Although IL-2 and ipilimumab are currently the only immune stimulants approved by the U.S. Food and Drug Administration (FDA) for the treatment of metastatic renal cell carcinoma (IL-2) and melanoma (IL-2 and ipilimumab), new immune checkpoint inhibitors such as anti–programmed cell death 1 (anti–PD-1) have shown impressive results in recent clinical trials for patients with melanoma, renal cell cancer, and also non–small-cell lung cancer (NSCLC), and will likely be approved in the near future. As expected with nonspecific immunostimulation, systemic and bystander immune-related adverse events such as colitis has been reported with all agents in varying degrees, although most side effects are controllable and reversible if addressed aggressively and promptly by experienced clinicians. Importantly, antitumor responses seen with these immune-based modalities appear to be durable for some patients and may even be potentially curative. As with many therapies for metastatic solid tumors, preliminary trials using combination therapies have suggested better than expected response rates and survival, and confirmatory trials are in process to validate and ensure that toxicities from combining agents would not be prohibitive. Overall, patients with metastatic solid tumors may soon have wider armamentarium of off-the-shelf immunotherapy options.

Interleukin-2

Morgan et al.[59] showed that a *factor* produced in the medium from stimulated normal human blood lymphocytes can allow ex vivo growth and expansion of human T lymphocytes. The identification of this soluble T-cell growth factor (IL-2)[60,61] allowed the ability to culture T cells in vitro. IL-2 is a 15-kd glycoprotein produced in minute amounts by activated peripheral blood lymphocytes, and even with using T-cell hybridomas, minimal quantities could be purified; thus, research using IL-2 was impeded by the limited amounts of purified IL-2 available. The isolation of the cDNA clone in 1983[62] enabled the development in 1984 of recombinant IL-2,[63] which permitted the ability to mass manufacture IL-2. Although murine studies demonstrated the ability of IL-2 to mediate tumor regression,[64] early phase I clinical trials did not show any antitumor response,[65] but was instructive in showing pharmacokinetics and toxicities, which led to more effective regimens. Subsequently, IL-2 was given in higher doses (up to 720,000 IU/kg intravenously every 8 hours) in a landmark trial involving 25 patients, along with nonspecific lymphokine-activated natural killer (LAK) cells, which are non-T and non-B lymphocytes.[66] This report was the first to document the regression of advanced solid cancers (melanoma, renal cell, lung, and colon) using immunotherapy in humans.[66] A follow-up trial randomizing 181 patients to either high-dose IL-2 alone (720,000 IU/kg intravenously every 8 hours) or high-dose IL-2 and LAK cells showed that the tumor response was due to IL-2 alone and not to the nonspecific LAK cells.[67] This study also narrowed the IL-2–sensitive histologies to melanoma and renal cell cancer, which had more consistent responses.

IL-2 Therapy for Metastatic Renal Cell Cancer

Subsequent to the studies discussed previously, high-dose IL-2 was tested by additional centers and in combination with other agents for renal cell cancer. A randomized phase II trial involving 99 kidney cancer patients showed no increase in antitumor responses with the addition of interferon alfa-2b (IFNα-2b). Responses were seen for 12 (17%) of 71 patients who received high-dose IL-2 alone, with 4 complete regressions.[68] A summary report of 227 patients with metastatic renal cell cancer treated with high-dose IL-2 (defined as 600,000 IU/kg or 720,000 IU/kg given intravenously every 8 hours as tolerated up to 15 doses) from 1985 to 1996 at the Surgery Branch of the National Cancer Institute (NCI) documented a total response rate of 19%, with 10% partial and 9% complete; the longest duration of a complete response was over 10 years ongoing (134+ months).[69] Another summary report from seven phase II clinical trials from multiple institutions involving 255 patients with metastatic renal cell cancer receiving high-dose IL-2 showed the overall response rate was 14%, with 9% partial and 5% complete, and responses occurred in all sites of disease, including primary kidney tumors, bone metastases, and bulking visceral tumor burdens.[70] Although the response rates were modest, the durability of the responses was remarkable, with many responses lasting over 5 years ongoing (see Fig. 14.2). Because of the striking durability of the antitumor responses, IL-2 received FDA approval for the treatment of metastatic renal cell cancer in 1992. A follow-up report in 2000 showing the response rates of the 255 renal cell patients in the seven phase II studies to be the same, with complete responses lasting over 10 years ongoing (131+ months for the longest responder), suggesting a potential cure.[71]

To ascertain whether lower doses and/or different administration routes, which would decrease toxicity and obviate the need for inpatient hospitalization for IL-2 therapy, a trial randomizing 400 patients with metastatic renal cell cancer to either standard high-dose intravenous IL-2, low-dose intravenous IL-2 (at 72,000 IU/kg), or low-dose subcutaneous IL-2 (250,000 U/kg per dose daily Monday through Friday in the first week and then 125,000 U/kg per dose daily during the next 5 weeks).[72] Although responses were seen with all three regimens, including complete responses in the low-dose subcutaneous regimen, standard high-dose IL-2 had higher overall response rates (21%) versus low-dose intravenous IL-2 (13%; p = 0.048) and low-dose subcutaneous IL-2 (10%; p = 0.033), suggesting the superiority of the high-dose intravenous regimen.[72]

The administration of IL-2 represents the only known curative treatment for patients with metastatic renal cell cancer and should be considered as front-line therapy for suitable patients.

IL-2 Therapy for Metastatic Melanoma

Between 1985 and 1993, 270 patients with metastatic melanoma enrolled into eight clinical trials in multiple centers using high-dose IL-2 (defined as 600,000 IU/kg or 720,000 IU/kg given intravenously every 8 hours as tolerated up to 15 doses). Atkins et al.[73] reported overall response rates of 16% (43 patients), with 10% partial and 6% complete; responses occurred at all tumor sites and regardless of initial tumor burden. With median follow-up at that time of 62 months, 20 responders (47%) were still alive, with 15 surviving over 5 years.[73] A follow-up report on those patients in 2000 showed that the response rates were unchanged; with the longest response duration of >12 years ongoing, disease progression was not observed in any patient responding greater than 30 months.[74] As with renal cell cancer, the flat *tail* of the Kaplan-Meier response duration and overall survival curves (Fig. 14.3), showing the potential curative nature of the antitumor responses, was the main compelling reason the FDA approved IL-2 for the treatment of metastatic melanoma in 1998.

Research in subsequent years aimed to increase the response rates of IL-2, led by increasing interests in tumor vaccinations as melanoma-associated antigens were being characterized.[75] Pilot studies suggested that vaccinations using modified melanoma differentiation antigens such as gp100:209–217(210M) could elicit immunologic responses in nearly all patients, and when combined with high-dose IL-2, could elicit potentially higher than expected clinical antitumor responses.[75] A follow-up phase III study[76] randomized 185 patients with HLA*A0201 from 21 centers to either high-dose IL-2 or high-dose IL-2 plus gp100:209–217(210M) concurrent immunization. Although the response rates for the

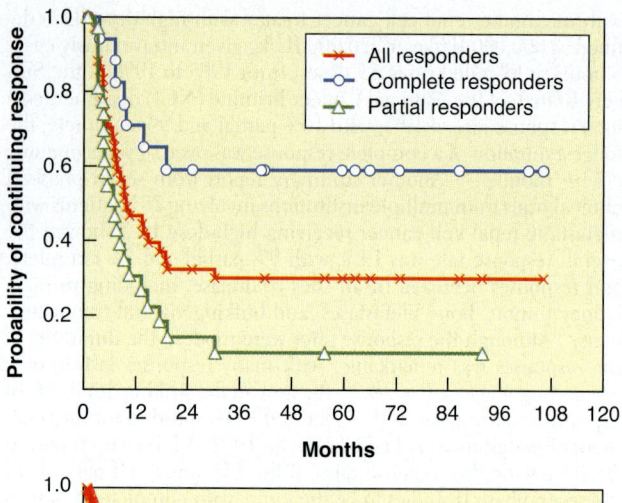

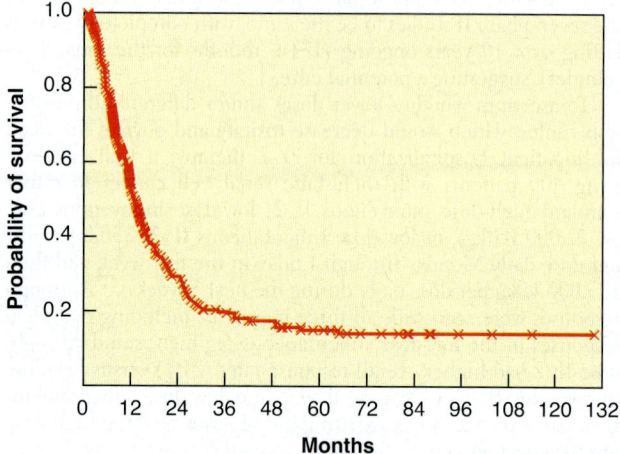

Figure 14.3 Kaplain-Meier plots of response duration (*top*) and overall survival (*bottom*) for 270 patients with metastatic melanoma who were treated with high-dose bolus IL-2 from 1985 to 1993 in eight clinical trials.[73]

IL-2 plus vaccine arm was statistically improved compared to IL-2 alone (16% versus 6%; p = 0.03), the IL-2 alone arm was notable for being much lower than in all prior studies.[76] In addition, a pilot trial of 36 melanoma patients treated high-dose IL-2 concurrently with ipilimumab (an antibody against cytotoxic T lymphocyte–associated antigen 4 discussed in the following section) gave a 25% OR rate, with 17% achieving complete response[77]; however, these data have not been further tested.

Correlative studies suggest that the total doses of IL-2 received during the first treatment course was significantly higher in patients achieving a complete response[69]; however, when limited to patients who were able to complete both cycles of the course, there was no statistical significance, suggesting that patients whose tumors progressed significantly after one cycle (and was not able to complete the second cycle of the course) accounted for some of the difference seen.[78] Responders did have a higher maximal lymphocyte count[69,78] immediately posttherapy and were more likely to develop vitiligo and thyroid dysfunction.[78] There has not been a consistent pretherapy factor that is predictive of response, although one retrospective correlative study involving 374 patients showed that patients with M1a (subcutaneous- and/or cutaneous-only disease) have a response rate of 54% compared with 12% for those with visceral M1b/c (P_2 <0.0001).[78]

Toxicities and Safe Administration of IL-2

High-dose IL-2 has been shown to be associated with adverse events that impact multiple organ systems.[73,79,80] The main component of the toxicities is due to an inflammatory response mediated by the release of cytokines such as IFNγ and tumor necrosis factor alpha (TNF-α)[81] resulting in a capillary-leak syndrome[82] and decreased systemic vascular resistance, which can lead to fever, hypotension, cardiac arrhythmia, lethargy, renal insufficiency, hepatic dysfunction, body edema, pulmonary edema, and confusion; other side effects can also include nausea, diarrhea, rash, anemia, thrombocytopenia, lymphocytosis, and neutrophil chemotactic defect[83] that predispose patients to gram-positive line infections. Since the first clinical trials with IL-2 in 1984, however, much has been learned to permit its safe dosing for appropriately screened patients[82,84,85]; importantly, if patients are appropriately supported, side effects are quickly reversible once IL-2 dosing ceases.[85] Kammula et al.[86] compared the incidences of grade 3/4 toxicities between the 155 patients treated from 1985 to 1986 to 156 patients treated from 1993 through 1997 at the NCI Surgery Branch: grade 3/4 hypotension decreased from 81% to 31%, intubations from 12% to 3%, neuropsychiatric toxicities from 19% to 8%, diarrhea from 92% to 12%, line sepsis from 18% to 4%, cardiac ischemia from 3% to 0%, and mortality from 3% to 0%. In fact, no fatality occurred strictly due to IL-2 therapy since 1989.[86] Overall strategies for the safe administration of high-dose IL-2 include careful screening for appropriately selected patients with adequate cardiopulmonary reserve, having an experienced team of physicians and nurses who are cognizant of the expected toxicities of IL-2, having routine preemptive measures such as prophylactic antibiotics to prevent line infections, and aggressive and prompt management of toxicities.

Checkpoint Modulators

Anti–Cytotoxic T Lymphocyte Antigen 4

CTLA-4 is an immunosuppressive *costimulatory* receptor found on newly activated T cells (and on regulatory T cells) that binds with costimulatory ligands B7-1 and B7-2 on antigen-presenting cells.[87,88] When CTLA-4 is engaged by B7-1 or B7-2, the T cells becomes inhibited,[89,90] suggesting that CTLA-4 likely evolved as a self-protective mechanism to prevent autoimmunity (Fig. 14.4). Thus, overcoming this *checkpoint* molecule was an aim of cancer immunotherapy. After CTLA-4 blockade in murine models led to antitumor immunity,[91,92] anti–CTLA-4 antibodies were tested in clinical trials starting in 2002.

The combination of anti–CTLA-4 blocking antibodies and vaccination worked well in murine models and led to one of the early phase II studies using ipilimumab (a fully human immunoglobulin [IgG$_1$] monoclonal antibody previously called MDX-010) with two gp100 vaccines, gp100:209–217(210M) and gp100:280–288(288V), in patients with metastatic melanoma.[93] Antitumor regressions were seen (from 11% to 22% overall response rates, with up to 8% complete response rates), along with severe autoimmune toxicities such as colitis, dermatitis, and even hypophysitis,[93–95] as would be expected based on the mechanism of CTLA-4 blockade. In fact, autoimmunity adverse events appeared to correlate with response to ipilimumab.[3] The experience with these early studies led to management strategies to screen aggressively for immune-related adverse events (IRAE), such as routine screening of endocrinopathies, and to treat IRAEs promptly, including high-dose steroids if needed for severe colitis.[96,97] Overall, ipilimumab was in some ways easier to manage for the patients than IL-2 because it was an outpatient infusion given every 3 weeks; IRAEs were unpredictable, however, and can appear suddenly many weeks after receiving a dose.

In 2010, results from a landmark phase III randomized trial comparing three treatment strategies (ipilimumab alone, gp100 peptide vaccine alone, or ipilimumab plus gp100 peptide vaccine) in 676 patients with metastatic melanoma were published showing improvement in median survival in the two arms that received ipilimumab (10 months) compared to the gp100 alone arm (6 months, p <0.001), despite showing a low response rate of 7% (among 540 patients who received ipilimumab).[98] Another

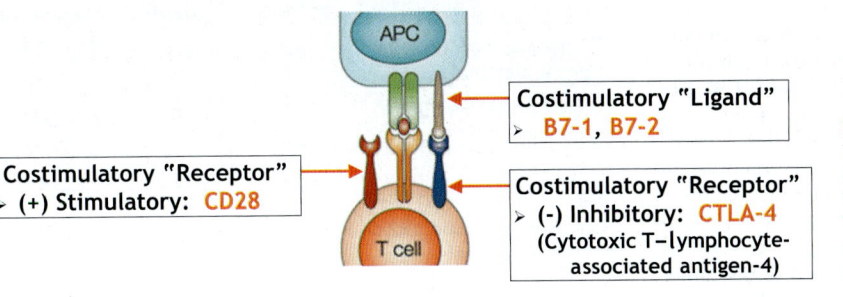

Figure 14.4 Mechanism of action of cytotoxic T-lymphocyte–associated antigen 4 (CTLA-4). When CD28 is engaged on the T cell, reactivity of the T cell is enhanced. When CTLA-4 is engaged on the T cell, reactivity of the T cell is inhibited. Blocking of CTLA-4 with a monoclonal antibody can elicit antitumor immunity but also autoimmunity.

phase III randomized trial comparing dacarbazine plus ipilimumab versus dacarbazine alone again showed improved survival in that arm containing dacarbazine (11.2 months versus 9.1 months; p <0.001).[99] These studies showing survival benefit led to FDA approval of ipilimumab for advanced melanoma in 2011.

The responses seen with ipilimumab appear to be durable.[100] A follow-up study of 177 patients with metastatic melanoma treated on the earliest trials at the NCI Surgery Branch using ipilimumab showed that response duration could last 99+ months ongoing.[77] In fact, 14 out of the 15 complete responders remain disease free 54+ to 99+ months ongoing, suggesting a potential cure for some patients. Interestingly, several patients who were deemed partial responders converted to complete responders several years later, because it took an average of 30 months to have all visible tumor marks on imaging scans to disappear.[77]

Ipilimumab was also tested on other solid tumors, and renal cell cancer again appears to be the only other type beside melanoma that had significant responses. Sixty-one patients with metastatic renal cell cancer were treated, and six developed a response (10%); however, 33% developed grade 3/4 IRAEs.[101] Subsequently, the availability of agents with lower toxicity profiles such as sunitinib and sorafenib prevented further enthusiasm to pursue this drug for renal cell cancer.

Another anti–CTLA-4 antibody, tremelimumab (previously called CP-675,206), has also demonstrated durable responses in melanoma patients.[102,103] A phase III randomized trial randomizing 655 patients with metastatic melanoma to either tremelimumab or physician's choice chemotherapy, however, failed to show a survival difference (despite a significantly different response duration favoring tremelimumab, 35.8 months versus 13.7 months; p = 0.0011), possibly due to crossover of chemotherapy patients enrolling into ipilimumab trials and expanded access programs.[103]

Anti–Programmed Death 1 and Anti–Programmed Death Ligand 1

PD-1 is another checkpoint modulator expressed on activated T cells. Although CTLA-4 appears to be involved in the early activation of T cells, PD-1 is involved in the later effector phase of T-cell activation and can function to prevent excessive damage to self by activated T cells in the periphery.[104,105] Interaction with its corresponding ligand, PD-L1 (B7-H1) and PD-L2 (B7-H2) leads to suppressed T-effector function. PD-L1 is expressed on hematopoietic and epithelial cells and is upregulated by cytokines such as IFNγ,[106] whereas PD-L1 is mainly on antigen-presenting cells. Given the clinical results with inhibiting the CTLA-4 checkpoint, recent efforts have focused on inhibiting the PD-1/PD-L1 and PD-1/PD-L2 interactions.

Nivolumab (previously known as BMS-936558, MDX-1106, and ONO-4538) is a fully human anti–PD-1 IgG4 monoclonal antibody that was initially tested in a phase I trial published in 2010 in which 39 patients with advanced solid cancers were treated in escalating doses.[107] Responses were seen in one patient with colon cancer, one with melanoma, and one with renal cell cancer; one patient developed colitis.[108] These hopeful results lead to a larger study in which 236 patients with either NSCLC (74 patients), melanoma (94 patients), or renal cell cancer (33 patients).[4] Objective responses were seen in 18% of patients with NSCLC, 28% with melanoma, and 27% with renal cell cancer.[4] Grade 3/4 adverse events occurred in 14% of patients, including those previously seen with ipilimumab (dermatitis, colitis, hepatitis, thyroiditis, hypophysitis, and pneumonitis). Nine patients developed pneumonitis, six of whom was reversible, and three (1%) with grade 3/4 died despite steroids and infliximab therapy.[4] An update on the status of 107 melanoma patients treated from 2008 to 2012 shows a 31% tumor response rate, with a median response duration of 2 years and a median overall survival of 16.8 months.[109]

Nivolumab was also tested in combination with ipilimumab in melanoma in either concurrent (53 patients) or sequenced (33 patients) regimens. The concurrent group experienced an overall response rate of 40%, whereas the sequenced group had a 20% response rate.[110] The concurrent group also experienced a higher rate of grade 3/4 adverse events (53%), compared to 18% in the sequenced group. Interestingly, 16 of 21 responders in the concurrent group experienced tumor reduction of 80% or greater by 12 weeks,[110] a tempo that is faster than was seen with ipilimumab.

Another anti–PD-1 developed independently, lambrolizumab (previously known as MK-3475, a humanized IgG4κ monoclonal antibody), was tested on 135 patients with metastatic melanoma.[111] The response rate was found to be 38% and was similar between those who had received ipilimumab and those who were ipilimumab naïve,[111] confirming that the antitumor response from lambrolizumab occurs via a different mechanism. Similar to nivolumab, 13% of patients developed grade 3/4 adverse events, with 4% developing pneumonitis, although none developed grade 3/4 pneumonitis.[111]

BMS-936559 is a fully human IgG4 monoclonal antibody that blocks PD-L1 ligation to both PD-1 and CD80. A phase I study was tested in 207 patients (75 with NSCLC, 55 with melanoma, 18 with colon cancer, and 17 with renal cell cancer, 17 with ovarian cancer, 14 with pancreatic cancer, 7 with gastric cancer, and 4 with breast cancer).[112] Among patients who were evaluated for response, objective responses were seen in 16% of melanoma patients, 17% of renal cell cancer patients, 10% of NSCLC patients, and 1 out of 17 ovarian cancer patients. Grade 3/4 toxicities were seen in 9% of patients.[112]

The advent of these checkpoint inhibitors brings additional treatment options to patients with selected advanced cancers, particularly those with histologies deemed previously to be outside the realm of immunotherapy such as NSCLC.[108,113] In addition, a new anti–PD-L1 (MPDL3280A) in clinical trials has also shown some efficacy in melanoma, renal cell cancer, and NSCLC in early reports.

Active Immunization Approaches to Cancer Therapy (Cancer Vaccines)

The molecular characterization of multiple cancer antigens led to a large number of clinical trials that attempted to actively immunize against these antigens with the expectation that cellular immune reactions would be generated capable of inhibiting the growth of established cancers. The results of these efforts have yet to produce significant vaccine efforts of value in the treatment of human cancer. There is a paucity of murine tumor models that suggests that active vaccine approaches can mediate the regression of established vascularized tumors; therefore, it is not surprising that these approaches have, with a few exceptions, shown little efficacy in humans. Enthusiasm about the effectiveness of cancer vaccines has often been grounded in surrogate and subjective end points, rather than reliable objective cancer regressions using standard oncologic criteria. In a review of the world literature, including 107 published cancer vaccine trials involving 2,242 patients, a 3.4% overall objective response rate was observed (Table 14.2).[114,115] In many cases, relatively soft criteria such as stable disease or the regression of individual metastases in the presence of progressive disease at other sites have been reported. A variety of immunizing vectors have been used, including tumor-derived peptides, proteins, whole tumor cells, recombinant viruses, dendritic cells, and heat-shock proteins.[116–122] Although many of these approaches can lead to the development of circulating T cells that can recognize the immunizing tumor antigen, these T cells rarely cause the inhibition of established tumors, a point that has led to much confusion in the field of tumor immunology. The generation of antitumor T cells in vivo is likely a necessary, but certainly not a sufficient criteria for the development of a clinically active immunotherapy. Often, T cells with weak avidity for tumor recognition are generated, and the tolerizing and inhibitory influences that exist in vivo must be overcome for an effective immune response to cause tumor destruction.

A prospective randomized trial of immunization with antigen-presenting cells was carried out by the Dendreon Corporation (Seattle, Washington). This trial used an antigen-presenting cell vaccine loaded with prostatic acid phosphatase linked to GM-CSF compared to placebo in men with hormone-refractory prostate cancer.[123] Of 330 patients who received the vaccine treatment, 1 objective partial response was seen. Only 8 patients experienced a PSA drop of at least 50%. There was no difference in the time to disease progression; however, the vaccine group had a median survival of 25.8 months compared to 21.7 months in the placebo group, and based on this statistically significant survival improvement, this treatment was approved by the FDA (Fig. 14.5).

TABLE 14.2
Experience with Therapeutic Cancer Vaccines

	Number of Trials	Number of Patients	Objective Responses
Surgery Branch, National Cancer Institute	25	541	14 (2.6%)
Published before 2005[114]	33	765	29 (4.0%)
Published 2005–2010[115]	49	936	34 (3.7%)
Total	107	2,242	77 (3.4%)

Note: Vaccines include: peptide, protein, dendritic cell, virus, plasmid DNA, and whole tumor cells.

Adoptive Cell Transfer Immunotherapy

Adoptive cellular immunotherapy refers to the transfer to the tumor-bearing host of immune lymphocytes with anticancer activity. The first successful administration of adoptive cell therapy (ACT) involving TIL, in combination with high-dose IL-2 was carried out at the National Cancer Institute Surgery Branch in 1988.[124] Studies that used cell transfer therapy in patients with metastatic melanoma have provided the clearest evidence of the power of the immune system to mediate the regression of advanced metastatic cancers in humans. Adoptive cell therapy has several theoretical as well as practical advantages.[125] Lymphocytes with antitumor activity can be expanded to very large numbers ex vivo for infusion into cancer patients. These cells can be tested in vitro for antitumor activity, and cells with appropriate properties such as high avidity for tumor recognition and a high proliferative potential

Figure 14.5 Kaplan-Meier estimate of the overall survival in patients with metastatic castration-resistant prostate cancer treated with Sipuleucel-T antigen–presenting cell immunotherapy. A modest but statistically significant improvement in survival was seen ($P = 0.03$).

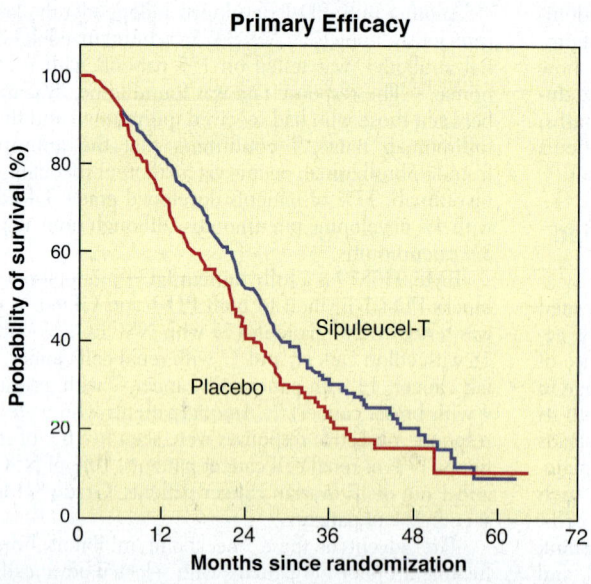

Number at risk

Sipuleucel-T	341	274	129	49	14	1
Placebo	171	123	55	19	4	1

Adoptive Transfer of Tumor Infiltrating Lymphocytes (TIL)

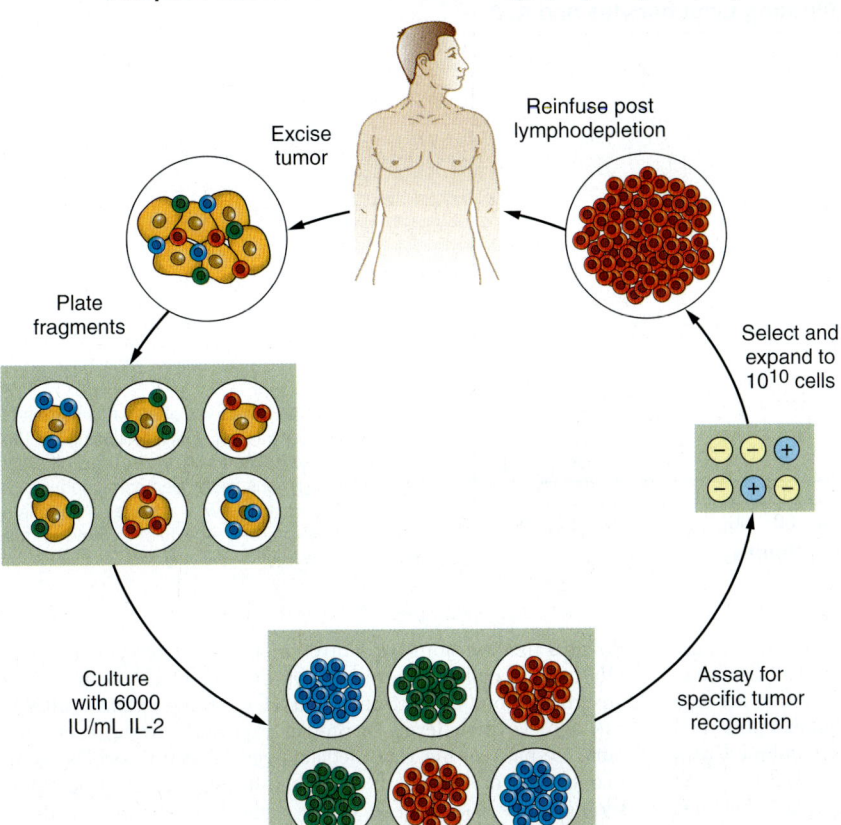

Figure 14.6 Diagram of the adoptive cell therapy of patients with metastatic melanoma. Tumors are resected and individual cultures are grown and tested for antitumor reactivity. Optimal cultures are expanded in vitro and reinfused into the autologous patient who had received a preparative lymphodepleting chemotherapy.

can be identified and selectively expanded for treatment. These cells can be activated in vitro and thus are not subjected to the tolerizing influences that exist in vivo. Perhaps, most important, the host can be manipulated prior to the transfer of the anticancer cells to provide an optimal tumor microenvironment free of in vivo suppressive factors.[125] Studies have shown that the transfer of cultured lymphocytes with antiviral activity can prevent Epstein-Barr virus (EBV) infections as well as the subsequent development of posttransplant lymphoproliferative diseases. Cultured lymphocytes have been used for the treatment of patients with established EBV-induced lymphomas.[126]

The best evidence for the ability of adoptive cell transfer to successfully treat patients with solid tumors comes from the treatment of patients with metastatic melanoma. A diagram that describes the nature of this treatment is shown in Figure 14.6. In patients with metastatic melanoma, TILs can be obtained from resected tumor deposits and individual cultures tested to identify those with optimal anticancer activity.[124,127] These cells are then expanded ex vivo and reinfused along with IL-2, which is the requisite growth factor required for the survival and persistence of these cells. The administration of a preparative lymphodepleting chemotherapy regimen, consisting of cyclophosphamide and fludarabine with or without 2 or 12 Gy total body irradiation, could substantially enhance the survival and persistence of the transferred cells and increase their in vivo antitumor effectiveness.[128,129] In a series of three pilot trials with 93 patients, objective responses were seen in 49% to 72% of patients.[5,130] Of the 93 patients, 20 (22%) experienced a complete regression of all metastatic melanoma. Only 1 of these 20 patients has recurred, and the remaining patients have ongoing complete regressions from 80 to over 104 months (Table 14.3, Fig. 14.7).

TABLE 14.3

Cell Transfer Therapy

Treatment	Total	PR	CR	OR
		Number of Patients (Percentage) (Duration in Months)		
No TBI	43	16 (37%) (84, 36, 29, 28, 14, 12, 11, 7, 7, 7, 7, 4, 4, 2, 2, 2)	5 (12%) (114+, 112+, 111+, 97+, 86+)	21 (49%)
200 TBI	25	8 (32%) (14, 9, 6, 6, 5, 4, 3, 3)	5 (20%) (101+, 98+, 93+, 90+, 70+)	13 (52%)
1,200 TBI	25	8 (32%) (21, 13, 7, 6, 6, 5, 3, 2)	10 (40%) (81+, 78+, 77+, 72+, 72+, 71+, 71+, 70+, 70+, 19)	18 (72%)

Note: 20 complete responses: 19 ongoing at 70 to 114 months.

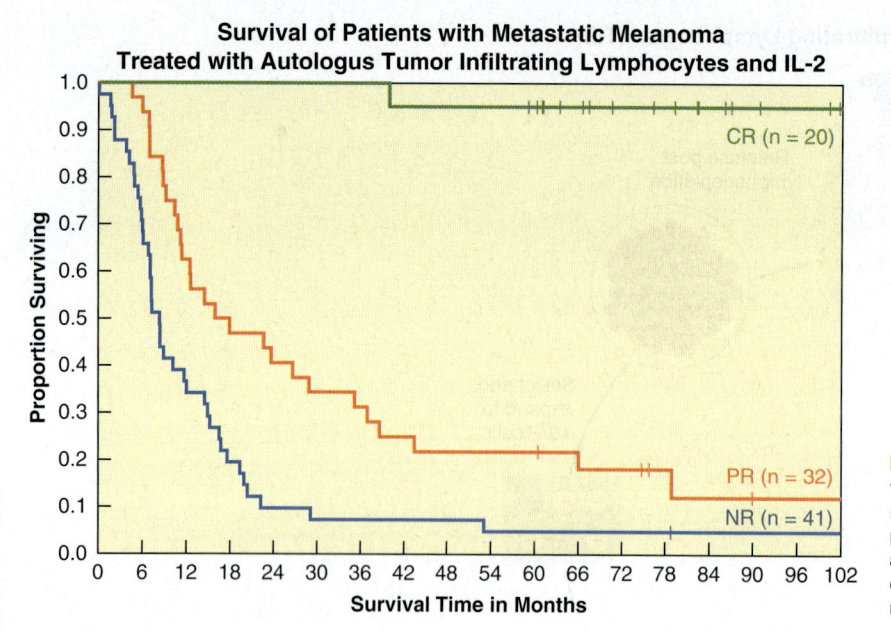

Figure 14.7 Survival curves of 93 patients treated with adoptive cell transfer using autologous TIL. The results of three consecutive trials using different preparative regimens have been combined in this analysis. Of 20 patients who achieved a complete cancer regression, only one has recurred with a median follow-up of over 8 years.[5]

The 5-year survival of these 93 patients was 29% and was similar regardless of the prior treatments that these patients had received.

Extensive genomic studies have shown that TILs that mediate complete cancer regressions recognize mutated epitopes presented by the cancer.[52] The use of exomic sequencing combined with in vitro tests of antitumor activity can be used to select for T-cell populations reactive against the cancer. This approach has now been utilized to identify T cells used to successfully treat a patient with chemotherapy-refractory cholangiocarcinoma and provides a blueprint for the application of cell transfer therapy for a variety of common epithelial cancers.[54]

The difficulty in obtaining TILs with antitumor activity from cancers other than melanoma has also led to the development of approaches using lymphocytes genetically modified using retroviral transduction to insert antitumor T-cell receptors into the normal lymphocytes of patients.[131]

Genetic Modification of Lymphocytes for Use in Adoptive Cell Therapy: Basic Principles and Applications to Solid Tumors

Efforts are in progress to genetically engineer autologous PBMCs through the introduction of exogenous high avidity receptors that specifically recognize tumor antigens (Fig. 14.8). These cells can then be expanded to large numbers in vitro and be readministered back to the patient similar to TILs in order to mediate tumor regression. The use of gene-modified cells for ACT has resulted in objective clinical responses for a variety of cancer histologies including melanoma, synovial sarcoma, and CD19-positive B-cell malignancies.[6,131–133]

There are two key requirements necessary for the use of gene-modified cells for the treatment of solid cancer. The first is the selection of an appropriate gene transfer method in order to achieve high receptor expression levels in the transferred T cells. For this discussion, we will consider both nonviral and viral-based gene delivery platforms. Generally speaking, there are two categories of nonviral gene transfer, chemical and physical. Chemical gene transfer involves the use of positively charged delivery vehicle such as calcium phosphate, cationic lipids, or polymers to form DNA complexes capable of entering a cell through endocytosis.[134] These reagents benefit from their ease of manufacture and ability to form complexes with large DNA sequences; however, low transfection efficiency of human T cells continues to be an issue.

Physical methods for gene delivery may involve direct delivery of DNA into a cell via microinjection or indirect DNA uptake via electroporation.[135] Electroporation of messenger RNA (mRNA) can achieve high levels of protein expression in cells, comparable to many of the viral-mediated gene delivery systems (gammaretroviral or lentiviral).[135,136] High-throughput electroporators should allow one to gene modify large numbers of T cells ex vivo.[137] mRNA electroporation appears to be most suited for this application, because there is significant loss of cell viability following electroporation of large amounts of DNA.[136] The electroporation of mRNA, although gaining traction as a means of redirecting T cell specificity,[137] provides for transient receptor expression because the mRNA will degrade over time. Currently, it is not clear if stable long-term receptor expression is required to mediate tumor regression. However, the main criticism of the non-viral methods described is the lack of stable gene transfer. To overcome this problem, many investigators are now using transposons such as *sleeping beauty* or *piggybac*.[138] Transposons are mobile DNA gene delivery elements encoding a gene of interest (i.e., TCR or chimeric antigen receptors [CAR]) that can randomly integrate into the genome in the presence of the transposase enzyme, thereby allowing for stable gene expression. This technology is currently being used for the ACT of CAR-modified cells targeting B-cell malignancies (see Fig. 14.8B).[139]

Viral-mediated gene delivery is currently the most common method for the genetic modification of immune cells for cancer ACT. Retroviridae is a family of RNA viruses that, upon entry into cells, undergo a process called reverse transcription whereby the viral RNA is converted into DNA as it stably integrates into the host genome. The two most common retroviral vector systems are based on the gammaretrovirus, Moloney murine leukemia virus (MLV), and the lentivirus, HIV type 1 (see Fig. 14.8B). Gammaretroviral vectors have been used in human clinical applications for over 20 years. The only reported toxicity associated with gammaretroviral engineering of human cells involved the retroviral transduction of hematopoietic stem cells for the treatment of children with severe combined immunodeficiency syndrome (X-SCID).[140] There have been no reports of clonal outgrowth following the retroviral transduction of mature T lymphocytes in adults. Highly active vectors have been generated from a variety of murine retroviruses including spleen focus forming virus (SFFV), myeloproliferative sarcoma virus (MPSV), and the murine stem cell virus (MSCV).[141–147] In most cases, these vectors are replication incompetent, but non–self-inactivating in

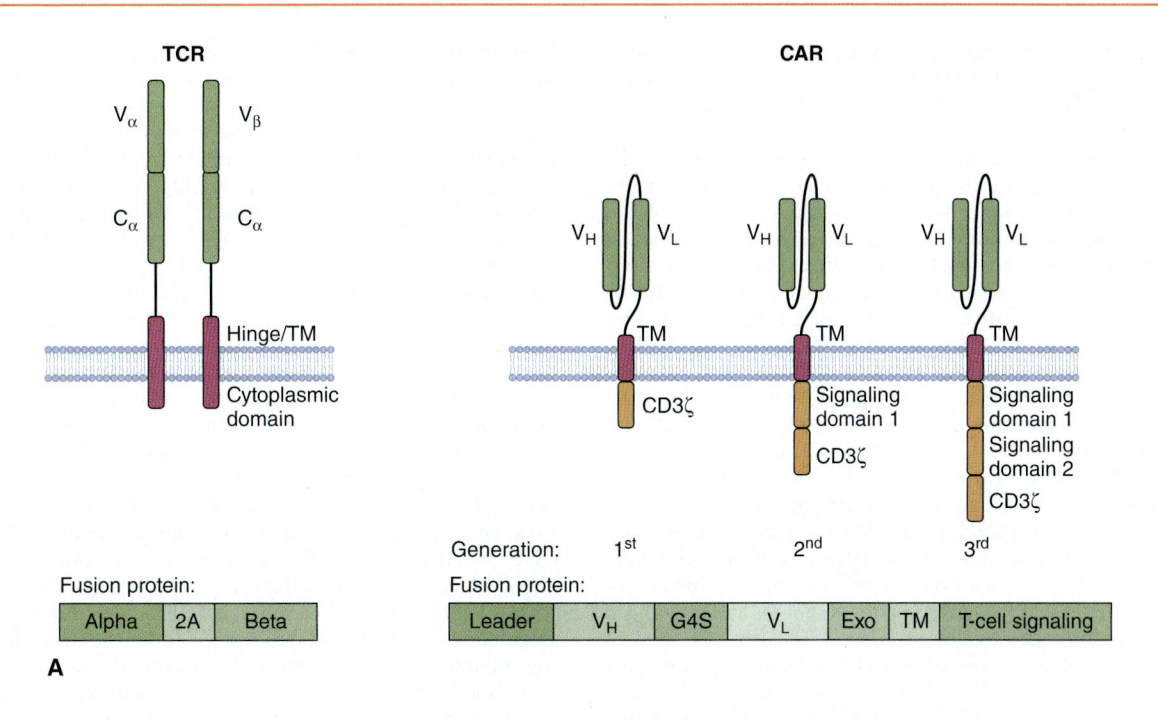

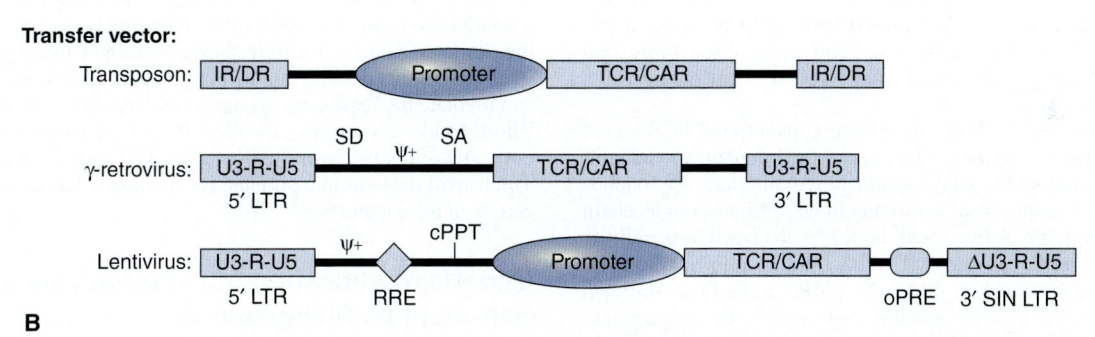

Figure 14.8 Genetic modification of T cells for the treatment of solid cancers. **(A)** In order to gene-modify T cells to confer stable tumor-specific reactivity, one can transduce T cells with an exogenous TCR derived from a naturally occurring or murine T-cell clone or a CAR derived from a tumor-specific monoclonal antibody. The TCR or CAR is synthesized as fusion proteins and inserted into the appropriate gene transfer vector. **(B)** Depending on the transfer vector selected, the T cells are then electroporated (transposon) or transduced (viral vector) to confer tumor specificity. V_α, V_β, and C_α, C_β, TCR alpha and beta chain variable and constant regions, respectively; TM, transmembrane domain; V_H and V_L, immunoglobulin variable regions; 2A and G4S, linker sequences; Exo, extracellular spacer domain; SD, splice donor; SA, splice acceptor; Ψ, packaging signal; LTR, long terminal repeat; U3, unique 3′ region; R, repeat region; U5, unique 5′ region; RRE, rev response element; cPPT, central polypurine tract; wPRE, woodchuck hepatitis virus posttranscriptional regulatory element; ΔU3, truncated unique 3′ region; SIN, self-inactivating.

that the promoter for transgene expression is derived from the viral long terminal repeat (LTR). Self-inactivating (SIN) gammaretroviral vectors have been developed that require an internal promoter to drive transgene expression. The advantage of non-SIN vectors is the ability to use a variety of retroviral packaging cell lines (PG13, Phoenix) engineered to constitutively express gag (capsid protein), pol (reverse transcriptase, integrase, and RNase H enzymes) and env (envelope protein). Transduction of these packaging lines with a non-SIN retroviral vector encoding a transgene allows for the generation of a stable packaging cell line that constitutively releases vector into the medium. This platform is easily scaled up to support large-scale vector production efforts. An alternative to the gammaretroviral vector platform is the lentiviral vector platform. There are some advantages to selecting a lentiviral vector for T-cell engineering in that one can transduce large numbers of minimally stimulated T cells,[148] transfer more complex and larger gene expression cassettes, and yield a potentially safer chromosomal integration profile as compared to gammaretroviruses. However, there has been at least one instance of clonal outgrowth following lentiviral vector transduction of CD34+ stem cells.[149] Therefore, more data will be needed to better understand the risk of insertional mutagenesis associated with the use of lentiviral vectors. The major disadvantage with using lentiviral vectors for ACT is the lack of a robust packaging cell line, which requires transient vector production and is difficult to scale up.

The first successful application ACT involved the use of autologous T cells genetically modified with a conventional αβ TCR targeting MART-1 for the treatment of patients with melanoma.[131] The success of this approach relies on the ability to identify naturally occurring TCRs with sufficiently high avidity for the tumor antigen. For this clinical trial, a tumor-specific TCR was cloned directly from melanoma TIL. Exogenous TCR can also be generated from human PBMC following a variety of in vitro sensitization techniques or immunization of transgenic mice expressing HLA molecules. A T-cell clone expressing a low avidity TCR recognizing MART-1 was isolated and the α and β chains cloned into a gammaretroviral vector. The objective response rate from this trial was 13% (2/15).[131] In a follow-up trial with a higher avidity TCR that was cloned from the same melanoma TIL, the objective response rate increased to 30% (6/20).[150] However, patients in this trial experienced significant on-target, off-tumor toxicity with the destruction of normal melanocytes in the skin, eye, and ear. These trials showed the potential to use ACT for the treatment of solid cancers, but also highlight the importance of selecting appropriate tumor antigens to target in order to minimize normal tissue toxicities. Perhaps a better class of antigen to target for ACT would be the cancer testes antigens (CTA) that are expressed only on germ cells during fetal development and then reexpressed on cancers but not other normal tissues with the exception of the testes (see Table 14.1). Because the testes do not express class I MHC molecules, they are protected from any adverse immune response.[151] NY-ESO-1 is a CTA overexpressed on melanoma, as well as a variety of solid epithelial cancers.[152–154] A high-avidity TCR was developed targeting NY-ESO-1 and patients with metastatic melanoma or synovial cell sarcoma were treated following adoptive cell transfer using autologous lymphocytes transduced with a gammaretrovirus encoding this receptor.[6] In updated results from this trial, 8 of 17 patients (47%) with melanoma showed objective tumor responses, two of which were complete responses and ongoing at 51 and 48 months after treatment. Nine of 19 patients (47%) with synovial cell sarcoma showed objective tumor response, only one of which is complete and ongoing at 12 months. Of note, no toxicities were observed in any of these trials. Thus, targeting NY-ESO-1 and other CTAs is an attractive strategy for the application of ACT for the treatment of solid cancers (see Table 14.4 for other trials conducted at the National Cancer Institute, Surgery Branch).

Redirection of T-cell specificity using conventional TCR is constrained by HLA restriction, which limits treatment only to patients expressing a particular MHC haplotype. An alternate approach is to use CAR comprised of an monoclonal antibody single chain variable fragment (scFv) fused in frame to T-cell intracellular signaling domains capable of T-cell activation following antigen-specific binding (see Fig. 14.8A).[155] CARs, unlike conventional TCRs, are not MHC restricted but are limited by the requirement for the tumor antigen to be expressed on the cell surface. CARs can also recognize carbohydrate and lipid moieties further expanding their application. To date, there has been limited success using CAR-based ACT for the treatment of solid cancers. In 2008, the first successful CAR trial targeting the disialoganglioside, GD2, for the treatment of neuroblastoma was reported.[156] In this trial, 4 out of 8 patients (50%) with evaluable tumor experienced tumor regression or necrosis with one complete responder. In that same year, a second CAR trial targeting CD20 on non-Hodgkin and mantle cell lymphomas was reported.[157] Of the 7 patients treated, one achieved a partial response. Much greater success has now been achieved using a CAR targeting CD19, a molecule expressed on normal B cells and virtually all B-cell lymphomas. In a trial conducted at the National Cancer Institute, Surgery Branch, Kochenderfer et al.[132] first reported that autologous T cells expressing a CAR targeting CD19 was able to mediate tumor regression in a patient with B-cell lymphoma (hematologic malignancies will be discussed in more detail elsewhere). Successfully expanding CAR-based ACT to other cancer histologies has been limited by the inability to identify suitable tumor antigens to target. At the National Cancer Institute, Surgery Branch, there are active clinical programs with CAR targeting the mutated epidermal growth factor receptor, EGFRvIII, expressed on approximately 40% of glioblastomas as well as head and neck cancers[158]; the vascular endothelial growth factor-2 receptor, VEGFR-2, expressed on tumor vasculature[159]; and mesothelin, expressed on the mesothelial lining of the pleura, peritoneum, and pericardium, but overexpressed on mesothelioma, pancreatic, and ovarian cancers.[160] These trials are currently accruing patients; however, no objective clinical responses have been observed to date. A summary of clinical trials at the National Cancer Institute, Surgery Branch using gene-modified autologous T cells for ACT are shown in Table 14.4. ACT can mediate the regression of large, established tumors in humans. Efforts to identify and specifically target novel tumor antigens are currently underway with the hope that ACT using gene-modified T cells will develop into an effective treatment for patients with a variety of solid cancers.

Genetic Modification of Lymphocytes to Treat Hematologic Malignancies

Immunologic therapies can be useful treatments for some hematologic malignancies as demonstrated by the effectiveness of mono-

TABLE 14.4

Surgery Branch, National Cancer Institute Program for the Application of Cell Transfer Therapy to a Wide Variety of Human Cancers

Receptor	Type	Cancers	Status
MART-1	TCR	Melanoma	Closed
gp100	TCR	Melanoma	Closed
NY-ESO-1	TCR	Epithelial & sarcomas	Accruing
CEA	TCR	Colorectal	Closed
CD19	CAR	Lymphomas	Accruing
VEGFR2	CAR	All cancers	Accruing
2G-1	TCR	Kidney	Accruing
IL-12	Cytokine	Adjuvant for all receptors	Accruing
MAGE-A3[a]	TCR	Epithelial	In development
EGFRvIII	CAR	Glioblastoma	Accruing
SSX-2	TCR	Epithelial	In development
Mesothelin	CAR	Pancreas & mesothelioma	Accruing
HPV16 (E6&7)	TCR	Cervical, oropharyngeal	In development

[a] MAGE-A3 TCRs; restricted by HLA-A2, A1, Cw7, DP4—covers 80% of patients.
EGFR, epidermal growth factor receptor; VEGFR2, vascular endothelial growth factor 2.

clonal antibodies in treating B-cell malignancies and the fact that allogeneic hematopoietic stem cell transplantation (alloHSCT) can cure a variety of hematologic malignancies.[161-167] The results with monoclonal antibodies and alloHSCT clearly prove that immunologic therapies have significant activity against hematologic malignancies, but monoclonal antibodies are not curative as single agents,[162,166] and alloHSCT has a substantial transplant-related mortality rate due to infections and an immunologic attack against normal tissues known as graft versus host disease (GVHD).[163,165] The proven curative potential of alloHSCT and the effectiveness of autologous T-cell transfer therapies for melanoma have encouraged the development of autologous T-cell therapies for hematologic malignancies.[125,129,163,165] Genetically engineering T cells to specifically recognize antigens expressed by malignant cells has emerged as a very promising strategy for cancer immunotherapy.[125,129,168]

T cells can be genetically engineered to express either of two types of receptors, CARs[168-171] or natural TCRs.[6,131,172] T cells expressing either a CAR or TCR gain the ability to specifically recognize an antigen.[171,172] CARs are artificial fusion proteins that incorporate antigen recognition domains and T-cell activation domains.[168,170,172] The antigen recognition domains are most often derived from monoclonal antibodies.[168,170,172] Antigen recognition by TCRs is major histocompatibility complex restricted.[125,128] In contrast to TCRs, recognition of antigens by CARs is not dependent on MHC molecules. An advantage of TCRs over CARs is that TCRs can recognize intracellular antigens, whereas CARs can only recognize cell-surface antigens.

Chimeric Antigen Receptors

CARs targeting hematopoietic antigens have been extensively studied in preclinical experiments and early-stage clinical trials.[168,170,172,173] For a protein to be a promising target for CAR-expressing T cells, it should be uniformly expressed on the malignant cells being targeted but not expressed on essential normal cells. Many cell-surface proteins with restricted normal tissue expression patterns have been identified on malignant hematologic cells, and CARs targeting many of these proteins are under development (Table 14.5).

Many factors can affect CAR T-cell therapies. The types of gene-therapy vectors encoding the DNA of the CAR could be an important factor. The types of vectors currently being used in clinical trials of CAR T cells are gammaretroviruses, lentiviruses, and transposon-based systems.[132,133,174-181] The design of the CAR fusion protein is another important factor. CAR fusion proteins include an antigen-recognition domain that is most often derived from an antibody, costimulatory domains such as CD28 and 4-1BB, and T-cell activation domains that are usually derived from the CD3z molecule.[168,170,171,182] Other factors that could impact the effectiveness of CAR T-cell therapies include the cell culture method used to prepare the cells and administration of chemotherapy or radiation therapy prior to the CAR T-cell infusions.[170,178,179] In mouse models, a profound enhancement of the antimalignancy activity of infused T cells occurs when the T-cell infusions are preceded by lymphocyte-depleting chemotherapy or radiation therapy.[183-185] Because chemotherapy can have a direct antimalignancy effect against hematologic malignancies, the administration of chemotherapy prior to infusions of T cells is a confounding factor that must always be kept in mind when interpreting the results of clinical trials of T-cell therapies.

Anti-CD19 Chimeric Antigen Receptors

CD19 is an appealing target antigen for CARs because CD19 is expressed on almost all malignant B cells, but CD19 is not expressed on normal cells except B cells.[186] The first preclinical studies of anti-CD19 CARs utilized either gammaretrovirus vectors[174] or plasmid electroporation[176] to insert genes encoding anti-CD19 CARs into human T cells. These studies and subsequent preclinical work by other groups showed that T cells expressing anti-CD19

TABLE 14.5

Hematologic Antigens Targeted by Genetically-Modified T-Cells

Antigen	Malignancy Expressing Antigen	Targeted by CAR or TCR	References
CD19	B-cell malignancies	CAR	17, 19, 21, 22, 23, 24, 25, 26, 34, 35, 55, 56
CD20	B-cell malignancies	CAR	36, 37, 38
CD22	B-cell malignancies	CAR	39, 40
CD23	B-cell malignancies	CAR	41
ROR1	B-cell malignancies	CAR	42
Kappa light chain	B-cell malignancies	CAR	43
B-cell maturation antigen (BCMA)	Multiple myeloma	CAR	44
Lewis Y antigen	Multiple myeloma and acute myeloid leukemia (AML)	CAR	45, 46
CD123	AML	CAR	47
CD30	Hodgkin lymphoma	CAR	48, 49
CD70	Hodgkin lymphoma	CAR	50
Wilms tumor-1 (WT1)	AML and acute lymphoid leukemia (ALL)	TCR	51
Aurora kinase-A	AML and chronic myeloid leukemia (CML)	TCR	52
Hyaluronan-mediated motility receptor (HMMR)	AML and ALL	TCR	53

CARs could specifically recognize and kill CD19-expressing malignant B cells in vitro and in vivo.[174–176,187] These preclinical studies compared many different CAR signaling moieties, which led most groups to utilize CARs with T-cell activation domains from the CD3z molecule and costimulatory molecules from either CD28 or 4-1BB (CD137).[165,180,182,187,188] Preclinical studies showed that lymphocyte-depleting radiation therapy administered before anti-CD19 CAR T-cell infusions was critical to the antimalignancy activity of CAR T cells.[183] The addition of lymphocyte-depleting radiation therapy prior to infusions of anti-CD19 CAR T cells increased the percentage of mice cured of lymphoma by the CAR T cells from 0% to 100%.[183] Preclinical experiments with anti-CD19 CARs have led to several early-phase clinical trials.

The first clinical trial to demonstrate in vivo activity of anti-CD19 CAR T cells in humans was conducted in the Surgery Branch of the National Cancer Institute.[132] The gammaretroviral vector used in this trial encoded a CAR with a CD28 costimulatory domain. Patients treated on this clinical trial received cyclophosphamide and fludarabine chemotherapy followed by an infusion of anti-CD19 CAR T cells and a short course of intravenous IL-2.[132,181] Clear antigen-specific activity of the anti-CD19 CAR T cells was demonstrated because blood B cells were selectively eliminated from four of the seven evaluable patients for several months.[181] The duration of B-cell depletion in these patients was much longer than the duration of B-cell depletion caused by the chemotherapy that the patients received.[132,181] This study also generated evidence of an antimalignancy effect by the anti-CD19 CAR T cells because six of seven evaluable patients with advanced B-cell malignancies obtained either complete remissions or partial remissions (Fig. 14.9).[181] One of these remissions is ongoing 45 months after treatment, and another remission is ongoing 31 months after treatment. Significant toxicity, including hypotension and neurologic toxicity, occurred during this clinical trial.[181] The severity of these toxicities correlated with the levels of serum inflammatory cytokines.[181] Except for one patient who died with influenza pneumonia, the toxicities were transient, with all toxicities resolving within 3 weeks of the anti-CD19 CAR T-cell infusions.[181]

Investigators at the Memorial Sloan Kettering Cancer Center treated nine patients with chronic lymphocytic leukemia (CLL) or acute lymphocytic leukemia (ALL) by infusing T cells that expressed a CAR with a CD28 costimulatory domain.[179] The gene therapy vector used in this work was a gammaretrovirus.[179] None of three patients treated with CAR T cells alone experienced a regression of leukemia, and CLL regressed in one of four evaluable patients treated with cyclophosphamide followed by an infusion of CAR T cells. Using the same CAR, the same group went on to treat five patients with ALL.[173] Patients received chemotherapy followed by an infusion of anti-CD19 CAR T cells. Four patients had detectable leukemia prior to their CAR T-cell infusions, and all of these patients became minimal residual disease negative after infusion of CAR T cells. Four of five patients on this trial rapidly underwent allogeneic stem cell transplantation after their CAR T-cell infusions.[173]

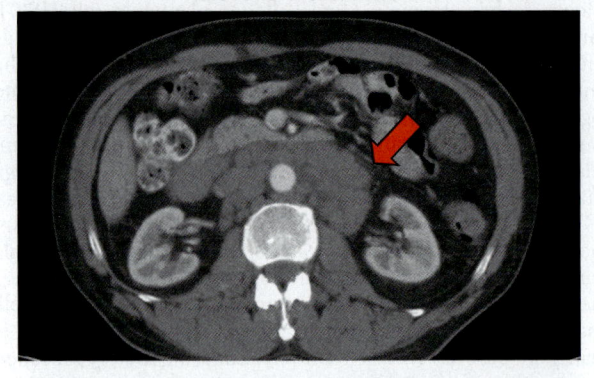

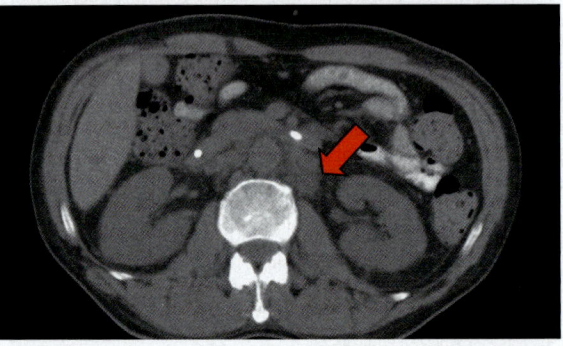

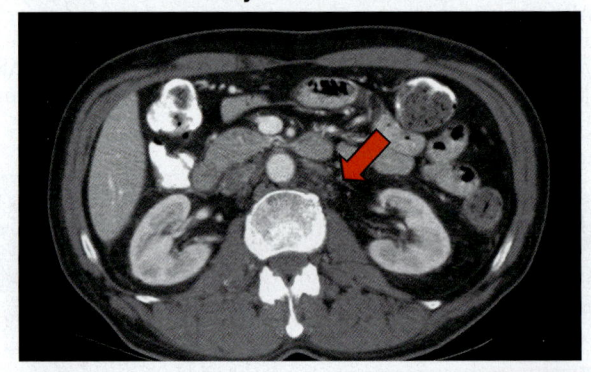

Investigators at the Baylor College of Medicine conducted clinical trials of anti-CD19 CAR T cells in which each patient simultaneously received infusions of two types of anti-CD19 CAR T cells.[189] One type of T cell expressed a CAR expressing a CD28 costimulatory domain. The other type of T cell was identical except that the CAR it expressed lacked a CD28 domain. Compared to the T cells lacking a CD28 moiety, the T cells expressing a CAR with a CD28 moiety had higher peak blood levels and longer in vivo persistence.[189] Patients on this trial did not receive chemotherapy, and there were no remissions of malignancy or long-term B-cell depletion.[189]

Investigators at the University of Pennsylvania reported results from three patients with CLL who were treated with chemotherapy followed by infusions of anti-CD19 CAR-expressing T cells.[133,180] The CAR used in this study was encoded by a lentiviral vector and contained a costimulatory domain from the 4-1BB molecule. Two

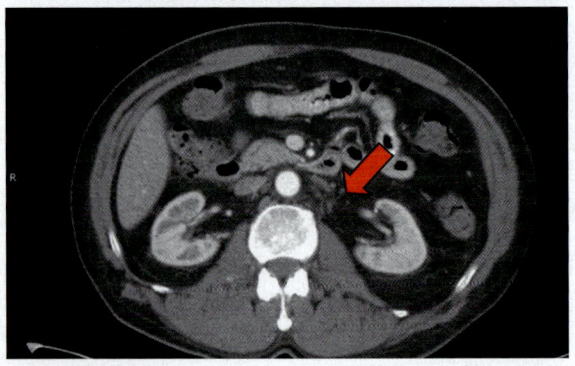

Figure 14.9 Computed tomography (CT) scans show regression of adenopathy in a patient with chronic lymphocytic leukemia (CLL) after treatment with chemotherapy followed by an infusion of autologous anti-CD19 CAR T cells. The time after the cell infusion of each CT scan is indicated. The *arrow* points to a large lymph node mass that resolved completely over time. (Reproduced from Kochenderfer JN, Rosenberg SA. Treating B-Cell cancer with T cells expressing anti-CD19 chimeric antigen receptors. *Nature Rev Clin Oncology* 2013;10:267-276, with permission.)

of the three reported patients obtained prolonged complete remissions.[180] This same CAR design was subsequently evaluated in a clinical trial enrolling patients with ALL.[190] One ALL patient obtained a prolonged complete remission but also experienced significant toxicity that was associated with elevated levels of serum cytokines.[190]

Overall, the early results with anti-CD19 CAR T cells show that this strategy holds great promise to improve the treatment of B-cell malignancies, but anti-CD19 CAR T-cell infusions are also associated with significant toxicity that is usually of short duration. Future progress will require decreasing the toxicity of anti-CD19 CAR T cells while maintaining or enhancing their antimalignancy activity. Parameters that are being studied in an effort to improve anti-CD19 CAR therapy include vector selection, CAR design, cell culture methods, and clinical application.

Chimeric Antigen Receptors and T-Cell Receptors Targeting Hematologic Antigens Other than CD19

CARs and TCRs targeting several hematologic antigens other than CD19 have been evaluated in preclinical or clinical studies. Except for CD19, the B-cell antigen CD20 has been the hematologic antigen most extensively studied as a target of CAR T cells.[191–193] Plasmid electroporation, which is not an optimal method of T-cell genetic modification, was used to transfer the anti-CD20 CAR gene to T cells in these studies. In one trial of anti-CD20 CAR T cells, patients received chemotherapy followed by infusions of T cells expressing a CAR without costimulatory domains.[192] One of seven patients obtained a partial remission that lasted 3 months. In a second trial, patients received chemotherapy followed by anti-CD20 CAR T cells expressing a CAR with both CD28 and 4-1BB costimulatory domains; in this trial, the only evaluable patient obtained a partial remission.[193]

CARs targeting other B-cell antigens including CD22,[157,194] CD23,[195] receptor tyrosine kinase–like orphan receptor-1 (ROR1),[196] and the immunoglobulin kappa light chain[197] have been evaluated in preclinical studies. CARs for treating multiple myeloma are currently being developed. B-cell maturation antigen (BCMA) is expressed on normal and malignant plasma cells, but it is not known to be expressed on other normal cells except for a small subset of mature B cells.[198] CARs targeting BCMA have undergone preclinical testing, and a clinical trial of an anti-BCMA CAR will open soon.[198] Preclinical studies have been performed on CARs targeting the Lewis Y antigen as a treatment for multiple myeloma and acute myeloid leukemia (AML),[199] and activity against AML was recently demonstrated in a phase I clinical trial of a CAR targeting the Lewis Y antigen.[200] CARs targeting the CD123 protein are undergoing preclinical testing for potential use against AML.[201] For Hodgkin lymphoma, CARs have been developed that target the CD30 protein and the CD70 protein, and anti-CD30 CARs are entering early-phase clinical trials.[202–204]

MHC-restricted TCRs targeting some antigens expressed on hematologic malignancies have undergone preclinical testing, but TCRs for treating hematologic malignancies are at a much earlier stage of development than CARs (see Table 14.1). TCRs targeting the Wilms tumor antigen-1 (WT1) are under development to treat ALL and AML.[205] Aurora kinase-A–specific TCRs and hyaluronan-mediated motility receptor (HMMR)-specific TCRs are under preclinical development as leukemia treatments.[206,207]

T-Cell Gene Therapy in the Setting of Allogeneic Hematopoietic Stem Cell Transplantation

A leading cause of death among patients undergoing alloHSCT is relapse of malignancy, and alloHSCT is often complicated by GVHD.[164,165,208] Therefore, a central goal in the field of alloHSCT is to increase the antimalignancy activity of allogeneic T cells without worsening GVHD. One way to accomplish this goal might be to genetically modify T cells to give them the ability to specifically recognize antigens expressed by malignant cells. CARs are well-suited for this task.

Two groups have recently reported promising early results treating B-cell malignancies after alloHSCT with allogeneic donor-derived T cells expressing anti-CD19 CARs.[209,210] Investigators at the National Cancer Institute treated 10 patients with B-cell malignancies that persisted despite alloHSCT and standard donor lymphocyte infusions.[209] Although patients on this trial did not receive chemotherapy before their T-cell infusions, 3 of 10 patients had objective regressions of their malignancies, and 1 patient with CLL remains in CR more than 1 year after treatment.[209] No patient developed GVHD after receiving allogeneic anti-CD19 CAR T cells on this trial.[209] Investigators at the Baylor College of Medicine reported objective antimalignancy responses in two of six patients with relapsed malignancy after infusion of donor-derived allogeneic anti-CD19 CAR T cells that were also specific for viral antigens.[210]

In an effort to improve the safety of infusions of allogeneic lymphocytes by limiting GVHD, investigators have genetically modified T cells to express *suicide genes* that cause death of the T cells containing the suicide gene when certain drugs are administered.[211–214] Suicide gene–expressing T cells are infused to treat malignancy after alloHSCT. This approach has been tested in clinical trials, and rapid abrogation of GVHD has been demonstrated.[211,213,214]

REFERENCES

1. Kenter GG, Welters MJ, Valentijn AR, et al. Vaccination against HPV-16 oncoproteins for vulvar intraepithelial neoplasia. *N Engl J Med* 2009;361:1838–1847.
2. Gaffen SL, Liu KD. Overview of interleukin-2 function, production and clinical applications. *Cytokine* 2004;28:109–123.
3. Attia P, Phan GQ, Maker AV, et al. Autoimmunity correlates with tumor regression in patients with metastatic melanoma treated with anti-cytotoxic T-lymphocyte antigen-4. *J Clin Oncol* 2005;23:6043–6053.
4. Topalian SL, Hodi FS, Brahmer JR, et al. Safety, activity, and immune correlates of anti-PD-1 antibody in cancer. *N Engl J Med* 2012;366:2443–2454.
5. Rosenberg SA, Yang JC, Sherry RM, et al. Durable complete responses in heavily pretreated patients with metastatic melanoma using T-cell transfer immunotherapy. *Clin Cancer Res* 2011;17:4550–4557.
6. Robbins PF, Morgan RA, Feldman SA, et al. Tumor regression in patients with metastatic synovial sarcoma and melanoma using genetically engineered lymphocytes reactive with NY-ESO-1. *J Clin Oncol* 2011;29:917–924.
7. Chen YT, Scanlan MJ, Sahin U, et al. A testicular antigen aberrantly expressed in human cancers detected by autologous antibody screening. *Proc Natl Acad Sci U S A* 1997;94:1914–1918.
8. Van der Bruggen P, Traversari C, Chomez P, et al. A gene encoding an antigen recognized by cytolytic T lymphocytes on a human melanoma. *Science* 1991;254:1643–1647.
9. van der Bruggen P, Stroobant V, Vigneron N, et al. Peptide database: T cell-defined tumor antigens. *Cancer Immun* 2013. https://www.cancerimmunity.org/peptide/
10. Gnjatic S, Nishikawa H, Jungbluth AA, et al. NY-ESO-1: review of an immunogenic tumor antigen. *Adv Cancer Res* 2006;95:1–30.
11. Chinnasamy N, Wargo JA, Yu Z, et al. A TCR targeting the HLA-A*0201-restricted epitope of MAGE-A3 recognizes multiple epitopes of the MAGE-A antigen superfamily in several types of cancer. *J Immunol* 2011;186:685–696.
12. Morgan RA, Chinnasamy N, Abate-Daga D, et al. Cancer regression and neurological toxicity following anti-MAGE-A3 TCR gene therapy. *J Immunother* 2013;36:133–151.
13. Linette GP, Stadtmauer EA, Maus MV, et al. Cardiovascular toxicity and titin cross-reactivity of affinity-enhanced T cells in myeloma and melanoma. *Blood* 2013;122:863–871.
14. Cox AL, Skipper J, Chen Y, et al. Identification of a peptide recognized by five melanoma-specific human cytotoxic T cell lines. *Science* 1994;264:716–719.

15. Kawakami Y, Eliyahu S, Jennings C, et al. Recognition of multiple epitopes in the human melanoma antigen gp100 by tumor infiltrating T-lymphocytes associated with in vivo tumor regression. *J Immunol* 1995;154:3961–3968.
16. Brichard V, Van Pel A, Wolfel T, et al. The tyrosinase gene codes for an antigen recognized by autologous cytolytic T lymphocytes on HLA-A2 melanomas. *J Exp Med* 1993;178:489–495.
17. Wang RF, Robbins PF, Kawakami Y, et al. Identification of a gene encoding a melanoma tumor antigen recognized by HLA-A31-restricted tumor-infiltrating lymphocytes. *J Exp Med* 1995;181:799–804.
18. Wang R-F, Appella E, Kawakami Y, et al. Identification of TRP-2 as a human tumor antigen recognized by cytotoxic T lymphocytes. *J Exp Med* 1996;184:2207–2216.
19. Kawakami Y, Eliyahu S, Delgado CH, et al. Cloning of the gene coding for a shared human melanoma antigen recognized by autologous T cells infiltrating into tumor. *Proc Natl Acad Sci U S A* 1994;91:3515–3519.
20. Coulie PG, Brichard V, Van Pel A, et al. A new gene coding for a differentiation antigen recognized by autologous cytolytic T lymphocytes on HLA-A2 melanomas. *J Exp Med* 1992;180:35–42.
21. Kawakami Y, Eliyahu S, Sakaguchi K, et al. Identification of the immunodominant peptides of the MART-1 human melanoma antigen recognized by the majority of HLA-A2-restricted tumor infiltrating lymphocytes. *J Exp Med* 1994;180:347–352.
22. Hanada K, Yewdell JW, Yang JC. Immune recognition of a human renal cancer antigen through post-translational protein splicing. *Nature* 2004;427:252–256.
23. Carrington DM, Auffret A, Hanke DE. Polypeptide ligation occurs during post-translational modification of concanavalin A. *Nature* 1985;313:64–67.
24. Paulus H. Protein splicing and related forms of protein autoprocessing. *Annu Rev Biochem* 2000;69:447–496.
25. Vigneron N, Stroobant V, Chapiro J, et al. An antigenic peptide produced by peptide splicing in the proteasome. *Science* 2004;304:587–590.
26. Warren EH, Vigneron NJ, Gavin MA, et al. An antigen produced by splicing of noncontiguous peptides in the reverse order. *Science* 2006;313:1444–1447.
27. Dalet A, Robbins PF, Stroobant V, et al. An antigenic peptide produced by reverse splicing and double asparagine deamidation. *Proc Natl Acad Sci U S A* 2011;108:E323–E331.
28. Michaux A, Larrieu P, Stroobant V, et al. A spliced antigenic peptide comprising a single spliced amino acid is produced in the proteasome by reverse splicing of a longer peptide fragment followed by trimming. *J Immunol* 2014;192:1962–1971.
29. Ikeda H, Lethe B, Lehmann F. Characterization of an antigen that is recognized on a melanoma showing partial HLA loss by CTL expressing an NK inhibitory receptor. *Immunity* 1999;6:199–208.
30. Lundegaard C, Lamberth K, Harndahl M, et al. NetMHC-3.0: accurate web accessible predictions of human, mouse and monkey MHC class I affinities for peptides of length 8-11. *Nucleic Acids Res* 2008;36:W509–W512.
31. Peters B, Sette A. Generating quantitative models describing the sequence specificity of biological processes with the stabilized matrix method. *BMC Bioinformatics* 2005;6:132.
32. Xue BH, Zhang Y, Sosman JA, et al. Induction of human cytotoxic T lymphocytes specific for prostate-specific antigen. *Prostate* 1997;30:73–78.
33. Horiguchi Y, Nukaya I, Okazawa K, et al. Screening of HLA-A24-restricted epitope peptides from prostate-specific membrane antigen that induce specific antitumor cytotoxic T lymphocytes. *Clin Cancer Res* 2002;8:3885–3892.
34. Peoples GE, Goedegeburre PS, Smith R. Breast and ovarian cancer-specific cytotoxic T lymphocytes recognize the same HER2/neu-derived peptide. *Proc Natl Acad U S A* 1995;92:432–436.
35. Zaks TZ, Rosenberg SA. Immunization with a peptide epitope (p369-377) from HER-2/neu leads to peptide-specific cytotoxic T lymphocytes that fail to recognize HER-2/neu+ tumors. *Cancer Res* 1998;58:4902–4908.
36. Vonderheide RH, Hahn WC, Schultze JL, et al. The telomerase catalytic subunit is a widely expressed tumor-associated antigen recognized by cytotoxic T lymphocytes. *Immunity* 1999;10:673–679.
37. Parkhurst MR, Riley JP, Igarashi T, et al. Immunization of patients with the hTERT:540-548 peptide induces peptide-reactive T lymphocytes that do not recognize tumors endogenously expressing telomerase. *Clin Cancer Res* 2004;10:4688–4698.
38. Weinschenk T, Gouttefangeas C, Schirle M, et al. Integrated functional genomics approach for the design of patient-individual antitumor vaccines. *Cancer Res* 2002;62: 5818–5827.
39. Dutoit V, Herold-Mende C, Hilf N, et al. Exploiting the glioblastoma peptidome to discover novel tumour-associated antigens for immunotherapy. *Brain* 2012;135:1042–1054.
40. Walter S, Weinschenk T, Stenzl A, et al. Multipeptide immune response to cancer vaccine IMA901 after single-dose cyclophosphamide associates with longer patient survival. *Nat Med* 2012;18:1254–1261.
41. Theobald M, Biggs J, Dittmer D, et al. Targeting p53 as a general tumor antigen. *Proc Natl Acad Sci U S A* 1995;92:11993–11997.
42. Theoret MR, Cohen CJ, Nahvi AV, et al. Relationship of p53 overexpression on cancers and recognition by anti-p53 T cell receptor-transduced T cells. *Hum Gene Ther* 2008;19:1219–1231.
43. Parkhurst M, Joo J, Riley JP, et al. Characterization of genetically modified T cell receptors that recognize the CEA:691-699 peptide in the context of HLA-A2.1 on human colorectal cancer cells. *Clin Cancer Res* 2009;15:169–180.
44. Parkhurst MR, Yang JC, Langan RC, et al. T cells targeting carcinoembryonic antigen can mediate regression of metastatic colorectal cancer but induce severe transient colitis. *Mol Ther* 2011;19:620–626.
45. Wolfel T, Hauer M, Schneider J, et al. A p16INK4A-insensitive CDK4 mutant targeted by cytolytic T lymphocytes in a human melanoma. *Science* 1995;269:1281–1284.
46. Robbins PF, El-Gamil M, Li YF, et al. A mutated B-catenin gene encodes a melanoma-specific antigen recognized by tumor infiltrating lymphocytes. *J Exp Med* 1996;183:1185–1192.
47. Rubinfeld B, Robbins P, El-Gamil M. Stabilization of beta-catenin by genetic defects in melanoma cell lines. *Science* 1997;275:1790–1792.
48. Mumberg D, Wick M, Schreiber H. Unique tumor antigens redefined as mutant tumor-specific antigens. *Semin Immunol* 1996;8:289–293.
49. Cheever MA, Chen W, Disis ML, et al. T-cell immunity to oncogenic proteins including mutated ras and chimeric bcr-abl. *Ann N Y Acad Sci* 1993;690: 101–112.
50. Castle JC, Kreiter S, Diekmann J, et al. Exploiting the mutanome for tumor vaccination. *Cancer Res* 2012;72:1081–1091.
51. Matsushita H, Vesely MD, Koboldt DC, et al. Cancer exome analysis reveals a T-cell-dependent mechanism of cancer immunoediting. *Nature* 2012;482: 400–404.
52. Robbins PF, Lu YC, El-Gamil M, et al. Mining exomic sequencing data to identify mutated antigens recognized by adoptively transferred tumor-reactive T cells. *Nat Med* 2013;19:747–752.
53. van Rooij N, van Buuren MM, Philips D, et al. Tumor exome analysis reveals neoantigen-specific T-cell reactivity in an ipilimumab-responsive melanoma. *J Clin Oncol* 2013;31:e439–e442.
54. Tran E, Turcotte S, Gros A, et al. Cancer immunotherapy based on mutation-specific CD4+ T cells in a patient with epithelial cancer. *Science* 2014;344:641–645.
55. Koutsky LA, Ault KA, Wheeler CM, et al. A controlled trial of a human papillomavirus type 16 vaccine. *N Engl J Med* 2002;347:1645–1651.
56. Villa LL, Costa RL, Petta CA, et al. Prophylactic quadrivalent human papillomavirus (types 6, 11, 16, and 18) L1 virus-like particle vaccine in young women: a randomised double-blind placebo-controlled multicentre phase II efficacy trial. *Lancet Oncol* 2005;6:271–278.
57. Wolchok JD, Hoos A, O'Day S, et al. Guidelines for the evaluation of immune therapy activity in solid tumors: immune-related response criteria. *Clin Cancer Res* 2009;15:7412–7420.
58. Hoos A, Eggermont AM, Janetzki S, et al. Improved endpoints for cancer immunotherapy trials. *J Natl Cancer Inst* 2010;102:1388–1397.
59. Morgan DA, Ruscetti FW, Gallo R. Selective in vitro growth of T lymphocytes from normal human bone marrows. *Science* 1976;193:1007–1008.
60. Smith KA, Gilbride KJ, Favata MF. Lymphocyte activating factor promotes T-cell growth factor production by cloned murine lymphoma cells. *Nature* 1980;287:853–855.
61. Smith KA, Lachman LB, Oppenheim JJ, et al. The functional relationship of the interleukins. *J Exp Med* 1980;151:1551–1556.
62. Taniguchi T, Matsui H, Fujita T. Structure and expression of a cloned cDNA for human interleukin-2. *Nature* 1983;302:305–307.
63. Rosenberg SA, Grimm EA, McGrogan M, et al. Biological activity of recombinant human interleukin-2 produced in *Escherichia coli*. *Science* 1984;223:1412–1414.
64. Rosenberg SA, Mule JJ, Spiess PJ, et al. Regression of established pulmonary metastases and subcutaneous tumor mediated by the systemic administration of high dose recombinant IL-2. *J Exp Med* 1985;161:1169–1188.
65. Lotze MT, Matory YL, Ettinghausen SE, et al. In vivo administration of purified human interleukin-2. II. Half life, immunologic effects and expansion of peripheral lymphoid cells in vivo with recombinant IL-2. *J Immunol* 1985;135:2865–2875.
66. Rosenberg SA, Lotze MT, Muul LM, et al. Observations on the systemic administration of autologous lymphokine-activated killer cells and recombinant interleukin-2 to patients with metastatic cancer. *N Engl J Med* 1985;313: 1485–1492.
67. Rosenberg SA, Lotze MT, Yang JC, et al. Prospective randomized trial of high-dose interleukin-2 alone or in conjunction with lymphokine-activated killer cells for the treatment of patients with advanced cancer. *J Natl Cancer Inst* 1993;85:622–632.
68. Atkins MB, Sparano J, Fisher RI, et al. Randomized phase II trial of high-dose interleukin-2 either alone or in combination with interferon alfa-2b in advanced renal cell carcinoma. *J Clin Oncol* 1993;11:661–670.
69. Rosenberg SA, Yang JC, White DE, et al. Durability of complete responses in patients with metastatic cancer treated with high-dose interleukin-2: identification of the antigens mediating response. *Ann Surg* 1998;228:307–319.
70. Fyfe G, Fisher R, Sznol M, et al. Results of treatment of 255 patients with metastatic renal cell carcinoma who received high dose proleukin interleukin-2 therapy. *J Clin Oncol* 1995;13:688–696.
71. Fisher RI, Rosenberg SA, Fyfe G. Long-term survival update for high-dose recombinant interleukin-2 in patients with renal cell carcinoma. *Cancer J Sci Am* 2000;6:S55–S57.
72. Yang JC, Sherry RM, Steinberg SM, et al. Randomized study of high-dose and low-dose interleukin-2 in patients with metastatic renal cancer. *J Clin Oncol* 2003;21:3127–3132.
73. Atkins MB, Lotze MT, Dutcher JP, et al. High-dose recombinant interleukin 2 therapy for patients with metastatic melanoma: analysis of 270 patients treated between 1985 and 1993. *J Clin Oncol* 1999;17:2105–2116.
74. Atkins MB, Kunkel L, Sznol M, et al. High-dose recombinant interleukin-2 therapy in patients with metastatic melanoma: long-term survival update. *Cancer J Sci Am* 2000;6:S11–S14.

75. Rosenberg SA, Yang JC, Schwartzentruber DJ, et al. Immunologic and therapeutic evaluation of a synthetic peptide vaccine for the treatment of patients with metastatic melanoma. *Nat Med* 1998;4:321–327.
76. Schwartzentruber DJ, Lawson DH, Richards JM, et al. gp100 peptide vaccine and interleukin-2 in patients with advanced melanoma. *N Engl J Med* 2011;364:2119–2127.
77. Prieto PA, Yang JC, Sherry RM, et al. CTLA-4 blockade with ipilimumab: long-term follow-up of 177 patients with metastatic melanoma. *Clin Cancer Res* 2012;18:2039–2047.
78. Phan GQ, Attia P, Steinberg SM, et al. Factors associated with response to high-dose interleukin-2 in patients with metastatic melanoma. *J Clin Oncol* 2001;19:3477–3482.
79. Rosenberg SA, Yang JC, Topalian SL, et al. Treatment of 283 consecutive patients with metastatic melanoma or renal cell cancer using high-dose bolus interleukin 2. *JAMA* 1994;271:907–913.
80. Rosenberg SA, Lotze MT, Yang JC, et al. Experience with the use of high-dose interleukin-2 in the treatment of 652 cancer patients. *Ann Surg* 1989;210:474–484.
81. Gemlo BT, Palladino Jr MA, Jaffe HS, et al. Circulating cytokines in patients with metastatic cancer treated with recombinant interleukin 2 and lymphokine-activated killer cells. *Cancer Res* 1988;48:5864–5867.
82. Pockaj BA, Yang JC, Lotze MT, et al. A prospective randomized trial evaluating colloid versus crystalloid resuscitation in the treatment of the vascular leak syndrome associated with interleukin-2 therapy. *J Immunother Emphasis Tumor Immunol* 1994;15:22–28.
83. Klempner MS, Noring R, Mier JW, et al. An acquired chemotactic defect in neutrophils from patients receiving interleukin-2 immunotherapy. *N Engl J Med* 1990;322:959–965.
84. Lee RE, Lotze MT, Skibber JM, et al. Cardiorespiratory effects of immunotherapy with interleukin-2. *J Clin Oncol* 1989;7:7–20.
85. Schwartzentruber DJ. Guidelines for the safe administration of high-dose interleukin-2. *J Immunother* 2001;24:287–293.
86. Kammula US, White DE, Rosenberg SA. Trends in the safety of high dose bolus interleukin-2 administration in patients with metastatic cancer. *Cancer* 1998;83:797–805.
87. Brunet JF, Denizot F, Luciani MF, et al. A new member of the immunoglobulin superfamily—CTLA-4. *Nature* 1987;328:267–270.
88. Linsley PS, Brady W, Urnes M, et al. CTLA-4 is a second receptor for the B cell activation antigen B7. *J Exp Med* 1991;174:561–569.
89. Walunas TL, Lenschow DJ, Bakker CY, et al. CTLA-4 can function as a negative regulator of T cell activation. *Immunity* 1994;1:405–413.
90. Walunas TL, Bakker CY, Bluestone JA. CTLA-4 ligation blocks CD28-dependent T cell activation. *J Exp Med* 1996;183:2541–2550.
91. van Elsas A, Hurwitz AA, Allison JP. Combination immunotherapy of B16 melanoma using anti-cytotoxic T lymphocyte-associated antigen 4 (CTLA-4) and granulocyte/macrophage colony-stimulating factor (GM-CSF)-producing vaccines induces rejection of subcutaneous and metastatic tumors accompanied by autoimmune depigmentation. *J Exp Med* 1999;190:355–366.
92. Hurwitz AA, Yu TF, Leach DR, et al. CTLA-4 blockade synergizes with tumor-derived granulocyte-macrophage colony-stimulating factor for treatment of an experimental mammary carcinoma. *Proc Natl Acad Sci U S A* 1998;95:10067–10071.
93. Phan GQ, Yang JC, Sherry RM, et al. Cancer regression and autoimmunity induced by cytotoxic T lymphocyte-associated antigen 4 blockade in patients with metastatic melanoma. *Proc Natl Acad Sci U S A* 2003;100:8372–8377.
94. Maker AV, Phan GQ, Attia P, et al. Tumor regression and autoimmunity in patients treated with cytotoxic T lymphocyte-associated antigen 4 blockade and interleukin 2: a phase I/II study. *Ann Surg Oncol* 2005;12:1005–1016.
95. Maker AV, Yang JC, Sherry RM, et al. Intrapatient dose escalation of anti-CTLA-4 antibody in patients with metastatic melanoma. *J Immunother* 2006;29:455–463.
96. Beck KE, Blansfield JA, Tran KQ, et al. Enterocolitis in patients with cancer after antibody blockade of cytotoxic T-lymphocyte-associated antigen 4. *J Clin Oncol* 2006;24:2283–2289.
97. Robinson MR, Chan CC, Yang JC, et al. Cytotoxic T lymphocyte-associated antigen 4 blockade in patients with metastatic melanoma: a new cause of uveitis. *J Immunother* 2004;27:478–479.
98. Hodi FS, O'Day SJ, McDermott DF, et al. Improved survival with ipilimumab in patients with metastatic melanoma. *N Engl J Med* 2010;363:711–723.
99. Robert C, Thomas L, Bondarenko I, et al. Ipilimumab plus dacarbazine for previously untreated metastatic melanoma. *N Engl J Med* 2011;364:2517–2526.
100. Wolchok JD, Weber JS, Maio M, et al. Four-year survival rates for patients with metastatic melanoma who received ipilimumab in phase II clinical trials. *Ann Oncol* 2013;24:2174–2180.
101. Yang JC, Hughes M, Kammula U, et al. Ipilimumab (anti-CTLA4 antibody) causes regression of metastatic renal cell cancer associated with enteritis and hypophysitis. *J Immunother* 2007;30:825–830.
102. Kirkwood JM, Lorigan P, Hersey P, et al. Phase II trial of tremelimumab (CP-675,206) in patients with advanced refractory or relapsed melanoma. *Clin Cancer Res* 2010;16:1042–1048.
103. Ribas A, Kefford R, Marshall MA, et al. Phase III randomized clinical trial comparing tremelimumab with standard-of-care chemotherapy in patients with advanced melanoma. *J Clin Oncol* 2013;31:616–622.
104. Ott PA, Hodi FS, Robert C. CTLA-4 and PD-1/PD-L1 blockade: new immunotherapeutic modalities with durable clinical benefit in melanoma patients. *Clin Cancer Res* 2013;19:5300–5309.
105. Keir ME, Butte MJ, Freeman GJ, et al. PD-1 and its ligands in tolerance and immunity. *Annu Rev Immunol* 2008;26:677–704.
106. Dong H, Strome SE, Salomao DR, et al. Tumor-associated B7-H1 promotes T-cell apoptosis: a potential mechanism of immune evasion. *Nat Med* 2002;8:793–800.
107. Brahmer JR, Drake CG, Wollner I, et al. Phase I study of single-agent anti-programmed death-1 (MDX-1106) in refractory solid tumors: safety, clinical activity, pharmacodynamics, and immunologic correlates. *J Clin Oncol* 2010;28:3167–3175.
108. Brahmer JR. Immune checkpoint blockade: the hope for immunotherapy as a treatment of lung cancer? *Semin Oncol* 2014;41:126–132.
109. Topalian SL, Sznol M, McDermott DF, et al. Survival, durable tumor remission, and long-term safety in patients with advanced melanoma receiving nivolumab. *J Clin Oncol* 2014;32:1020–1030.
110. Wolchok JD, Kluger H, Callahan MK, et al. Nivolumab plus ipilimumab in advanced melanoma. *N Engl J Med* 2013;369:122–133.
111. Hamid O, Robert C, Daud A, et al. Safety and tumor responses with lambrolizumab (anti-PD-1) in melanoma. *N Engl J Med* 2013;369:134–144.
112. Brahmer JR, Tykodi SS, Chow LQ, et al. Safety and activity of anti-PD-L1 antibody in patients with advanced cancer. *N Engl J Med* 2012;366:2455–2465.
113. Drake CG, Lipson EJ, Brahmer JR. Breathing new life into immunotherapy: review of melanoma, lung and kidney cancer. *Nat Rev Clin Oncol* 2014;11:24–37.
114. Rosenberg SA, Yang JC, Restifo NP. Cancer immunotherapy: moving beyond current vaccines. *Nat Med* 2004;10:909–915.
115. Klebanoff CA, Acquavella N, Yu Z, et al. Therapeutic cancer vaccines: are we there yet? *Immunol Rev* 2011;239:27–44.
116. Slingluff CL, Yamshchikov G, Neese P, et al. Phase I trial of a melanoma vaccine with gp100$_{280-288}$ peptide and tetanus helper peptide in adjuvant: immunologic and clinical outcomes. *Clin Cancer Res* 2001;7:3012–3024.
117. Schaed SG, Klimek VM, Panageas KS, et al. T-cell responses against tyrosinase 368-376(370D) peptide in HLA*A0201$^+$ melanoma patients: randomized trial comparing incomplete Freund's adjuvant, granulocyte macrophage colony-stimulating factor, and QS-21 as immunological adjuvants. *Clin Cancer Res* 2004;8:967–972.
118. Marshall JL, Hoyer RJ, Toomey MA, et al. Phase I study in advanced cancer patients of a diversified prime-and-boost vaccination protocol using recombinant vaccinia virus and recombinant nonreplicating avipox virus to elicit anti-carcinoembryonic antigen immune responses. *J Clin Oncol* 2000;18:3964–3973.
119. Eder JP, Kantoff PW, Roper K, et al. A phase I trial of a recombinant vaccinia virus expressing prostate-specific antigen in advanced prostate cancer. *Clin Cancer Res* 2003;6:1632–1638.
120. Lurquin C, Lethe B, De Plaen E, et al. Contrasting frequencies of antitumor and anti-vaccine T cells in metastases of a melanoma patient vaccinated with a MAGE tumor antigen. *J Exp Med* 2005;201:249–257.
121. Marincola FM, Rivoltini L, Salgaller ML, et al. Differential anti-MART-1/MelanA CTL activity in peripheral blood of HLA-A2 melanoma patients in comparison to healthy donors: evidence of in vivo priming by tumor cells. *J Immunother Emphasis Tumor Immunol* 1996;19:266–277.
122. Cormier JN, Salgaller ML, Prevette T, et al. Enhancement of cellular immunity in melanoma patients immunized with a peptide from MART-1/Melan A. *Cancer J Sci Am* 1997;3:37–44.
123. Kantoff PW, Higano CS, Shore ND, et al. Sipuleucel-T immunotherapy for castration-resistant prostate cancer. *N Engl J Med* 2010;363:422.
124. Rosenberg SA, Packard BS, Aebersold PM, et al. Use of tumor infiltrating lymphocytes and interleukin-2 in the immunotherapy of patients with metastatic melanoma. Preliminary report. *N Engl J Med* 1988;319:1676–1680.
125. Restifo NP, Dudley ME, Rosenberg SA. Adoptive immunotherapy for cancer: harnessing the T cell response. *Nat Rev Immunol* 2012;12:269–281.
126. Rooney CM, Smith CA, Ng CY, et al. Infusion of cytotoxic T cells for the prevention and treatment of Epstein-Barr virus-induced lymphoma in allogeneic transplant recipients. *Blood* 1998;92:1549–1555.
127. Rosenberg SA, Yannelli JR, Yang JC, et al. Treatment of patients with metastatic melanoma using autologous tumor-infiltrating lymphocytes and interleukin-2. *J Natl Cancer Inst* 1994;86:1159–1166.
128. Dudley ME, Wunderlich JR, Robbins PF, et al. Cancer regression and autoimmunity in patients after clonal repopulation with anti-tumor lymphocytes. *Science* 2002;298:850–854.
129. Dudley ME, Yang JC, Sherry R, et al. Adoptive cell therapy for patients with metastatic melanoma: Evaluation of intensive myeloablative chemoradiation preparative regimens. *J Clin Oncol* 2008;26:5233–5239.
130. Rosenberg SA. Cell transfer immunotherapy for metastatic solid cancer—what clinicians need to know. *Nat Rev Clin Oncol* 2011;8:577–585.
131. Morgan RA, Dudley ME, Wunderlich JR, et al. Cancer regression in patients after transfer of genetically engineered lymphocytes. *Science* 2006;314:126–129.
132. Kochenderfer JN, Wilson WH, Janik E, et al. Eradication of B-lineage cells and regression of lymphoma in a patient treated with autologous T cells genetically engineered to recognize CD19. *Blood* 2010;116:4099–4102.
133. Porter DL, Levine BL, Kalos M, et al. Chimeric antigen receptor-modified T cells in chronic lymphoid leukemia. *N Engl J Med* 2011;365:725–733.
134. Tiera MJ, Winnik FO, Fernandes JC. Synthetic and natural polycations for gene therapy: state of the art and new perspectives. *Curr Gene Ther* 2006;6:59–71.
135. Birkholz K, Hombach A, Krug C, et al. Transfer of mRNA encoding recombinant immunoreceptors reprograms CD4+ and CD8+ T cells for use in the adoptive immunotherapy of cancer. *Gene Ther* 2009;16:596–604.

136. Zhao Y, Zheng Z, Cohen CJ, et al. High-efficiency transfection of primary human and mouse T lymphocytes using RNA electroporation. *Mol Ther* 2006;13:151–159.
137. Li L, Liu LC, Feller S, et al. Expression of chimeric antigen receptors in natural killer cells with a regulatory-compliant non-viral method. *Cancer Gene Ther* 2010;17:147–154.
138. Zhao Y, Moon E, Carpenito C, et al. Multiple injections of electroporated autologous T cells expressing a chimeric antigen receptor mediate regression of human disseminated tumor. *Cancer Res* 2010;70:9053–9061.
139. Ivics Z, Izsvak Z. Transposons for gene therapy! *Curr Gene Ther* 2006;6:593–607.
140. Singh H, Huls H, Kebriaei P, et al. A new approach to gene therapy using Sleeping Beauty to genetically modify clinical-grade T cells to target CD19. *Immunol Rev* 2014;257:181–190.
141. Hacein-Bey-Abina S, von Kalle C, Schmidt M, et al. A serious adverse event after successful gene therapy for X-linked severe combined immunodeficiency. *N Engl J Med* 2003;348:255–256.
142. Riviere I, Brose K, Mulligan RC. Effects of retroviral vector design on expression of human adenosine deaminase in murine bone marrow transplant recipients engrafted with genetically modified cells. *Proc Natl Acad Sci U S A* 1995;92:6733–6737.
143. Maetzig T, Galla M, Baum C, et al. Gammaretroviral vectors: biology, technology, and application. *Viruses* 2011;3:677–713.
144. Schambach A, Swaney WP, van der Loo JC. Design and production of retro- and lentiviral vectors for gene expression in hematopoietic cells. *Methods Mol Biol* 2009;506:191–205.
145. Hughes MS, Yu YYL, Dudley ME, et al. Transfer of a TCR gene derived from a patient with a marked antitumor response conveys highly active T-cell effector functions. *Hum Gene Ther* 2005;16:457–472.
146. Zhang X, Godbey WT. Viral vectors for gene delivery in tissue engineering. *Adv Drug Deliv Rev* 2006;58:515–534.
147. Yu SS, Han E, Hong Y, et al. Construction of a retroviral vector production system with the minimum possibility of a homologous recombination. *Gene Ther* 2003;10:706–711.
148. Cavalieri S, Cazzaniga S, Geuna M, et al. Human T lymphocytes transduced by lentiviral vectors in the absence of TCR activation maintain an intact immune competence. *Blood* 2003;102:497–505.
149. Cavazzana-Calvo M, Payen E, Negre O, et al. Transfusion independence and HMGA2 activation after gene therapy of human beta-thalassaemia. *Nature* 2010;467:318–322.
150. Johnson LA, Morgan RA, Dudley ME, et al. Gene therapy with human and mouse T-cell receptors mediates cancer regression and targets normal tissues expressing cognate antigen. *Blood* 2009;114:535–546.
151. Simpson AJ, Caballero OL, Jungbluth A, et al. Cancer/testis antigens, gametogenesis and cancer. *Nat Rev Cancer* 2005;5:625.
152. Hofmann O, Caballero OL, Stevenson BJ, et al. Genome-wide analysis of cancer/testis gene expression. *Proc Natl Acad Sci U S A* 2008;105: 20422–20427.
153. Zhang Y, Wang Z, Liu H, et al. Pattern of gene expression and immune responses to Semenogelin 1 in chronic hematologic malignancies. *J Immunother* 2003;26:461–467.
154. Jungbluth AA, Antonescu CR, Busam KJ, et al. Monophasic and biphasic synovial sarcomas abundantly express cancer/testis antigen NY-ESO-1 but not MAGE-A1 or CT7. *Int J Cancer* 2001;94:252–256.
155. Gross G, Waks T, Eshhar Z. Expression of immunoglobulin-T-cell receptor chimeric molecules as functional receptors with antibody-type specificity. *Proc Natl Acad Sci U S A* 1989;86:10024–10028.
156. Pule MA, Savoldo B, Myers GD, et al. Virus-specific T cells engineered to coexpress tumor-specific receptors: persistence and antitumor activity in individuals with neuroblastoma. *Nat Med* 2008;14:1264–1270.
157. James SE, Greenberg PD, Jensen MC, et al. Antigen sensitivity of CD22-specific chimeric TCR is modulated by target epitope distance from the cell membrane. *J Immunol* 2008;180:7028–7038.
158. Morgan RA, Johnson LA, Davis JL, et al. Recognition of glioma stem cells by genetically modified T cells targeting EGFRvIII and development of adoptive cell therapy for glioma. *Hum Gene Ther* 2012;23:1043–1053.
159. Chinnasamy D, Yu Z, Theoret MR, et al. Gene therapy using genetically modified lymphocytes targeting VEGFR-2 inhibits the growth of vascularized syngenic tumors in mice. *J Clin Invest* 2010;120:3953–3968.
160. Carpenito C, Milone MC, Hassan R, et al. Control of large, established tumor xenografts with genetically retargeted human T cells containing CD28 and CD137 domains. *Proc Natl Acad Sci U S A* 2009;106:3360–3365.
161. Feugier P, Van HA, Sebban C, et al. Long-term results of the R-CHOP study in the treatment of elderly patients with diffuse large B-cell lymphoma: a study by the Groupe d'Etude des Lymphomes de l'Adulte. *J Clin Oncol* 2005;23:4117–4126.
162. Gribben JG, O'Brien S. Update on therapy of chronic lymphocytic leukemia. *J Clin Oncol* 2011;29:544–550.
163. Sorror ML, Sandmaier BM, Storer BE, et al. Long-term outcomes among older patients following nonmyeloablative conditioning and allogeneic hematopoietic cell transplantation for advanced hematologic malignancies. *JAMA* 2011;306:1874–1883.
164. Van BK. Current status of allogeneic transplantation for aggressive non-Hodgkin lymphoma. *Curr Opin Oncol* 2011;23:681–691.
165. Van BK. Stem cell transplantation for indolent lymphoma: a reappraisal. *Blood Rev* 2011;25:223–228.
166. McLaughlin P, Grillo-Lopez AJ, Link BK, et al. Rituximab chimeric anti-CD20 monoclonal antibody therapy for relapsed indolent lymphoma: half of patients respond to a four-dose treatment program. *J Clin Oncol* 1998;16:2825–2833.
167. Bacher U, Klyuchnikov E, Le-Rademacher J, et al. Conditioning regimens for allotransplants for diffuse large B-cell lymphoma: myeloablative or reduced intensity? *Blood* 2012;120:4256–4262.
168. Dotti G, Gottschalk S, Savoldo B, et al. Design and development of therapies using chimeric antigen receptor-expressing T cells. *Immunol Rev* 2014;257:107–126.
169. Eshhar Z, Waks T, Gross G, et al. Specific activation and targeting of cytotoxic lymphocytes through chimeric single chains consisting of antibody-binding domains and the gamma or zeta subunits of the immunoglobulin and T-cell receptors. *Proc Natl Acad Sci U S A* 1993;90:720–724.
170. Kochenderfer JN, Rosenberg SA. Treating B-cell cancer with T cells expressing anti-CD19 chimeric antigen receptors. *Nat Rev Clin Oncol* 2013;10:267–276.
171. Sadelain M, Brentjens R, Riviere I. The basic principles of chimeric antigen receptor design. *Cancer Discov* 2013;3:388–398.
172. Kershaw MH, Westwood JA, Darcy PK. Gene-engineered T cells for cancer therapy. *Nat Rev Cancer* 2013;13:525–541.
173. Brentjens RJ, Davila ML, Riviere I, et al. CD19-targeted T cells rapidly induce molecular remissions in adults with chemotherapy-refractory acute lymphoblastic leukemia. *Sci Transl Med* 2013;5:177ra38.
174. Brentjens RJ, Latouche JB, Santos E, et al. Eradication of systemic B-cell tumors by genetically targeted human T lymphocytes co-stimulated by CD80 and interleukin-15. *Nat Med* 2003;9:279–286.
175. Milone MC, Fish JD, Carpenito C, et al. Chimeric receptors containing CD137 signal transduction domains mediate enhanced survival of T cells and increased antileukemic efficacy in vivo. *Mol Ther* 2009;17:1453–1464.
176. Cooper LJ, Topp MS, Serrano LM, et al. T-cell clones can be rendered specific for CD19: toward the selective augmentation of the graft-versus-B lineage leukemia effect. *Blood* 2003;101:1637–1644.
177. Kebriaei P, Huls H, Jena B, et al. Infusing CD19-directed T cells to augment disease control in patients undergoing autologous hematopoietic stem-cell transplantation for advanced B-lymphoid malignancies. *Hum Gene Ther* 2012;23:444–450.
178. Wang X, Naranjo A, Brown CE, et al. Phenotypic and functional attributes of lentivirus-modified CD19-specific human CD8+ central memory T cells manufactured at clinical scale. *J Immunother* 2012;35:689–701.
179. Brentjens RJ, Rivière I, Park JH, et al. Safety and persistence of adoptively transferred autologous CD19-targeted T cells in patients with relapsed or chemotherapy refractory B-cell leukemias. *Blood* 2011;118:4817–4828.
180. Kalos M, Levine BL, Porter DL, et al. T cells with chimeric antigen receptors have potent antitumor effects and can establish memory in patients with advanced leukemia. *Sci Transl Med* 2011;3:95ra73.
181. Kochenderfer JN, Dudley ME, Feldman SA, et al. B-cell depletion and remissions of malignancy along with cytokine-associated toxicity in a clinical trial of anti-CD19 chimeric-antigen-receptor-transduced T cells. *Blood* 2011;119:2709–2720.
182. Imai C, Mihara K, Andreansky M, et al. Chimeric receptors with 4-1BB signaling capacity provoke potent cytotoxicity against acute lymphoblastic leukemia. *Leukemia* 2004;18:678–684.
183. Kochenderfer JN, Yu Z, Frasheri D, et al. Adoptive transfer of syngeneic T cells transduced with a chimeric antigen receptor that recognizes murine CD19 can eradicate lymphoma and normal B cells. *Blood* 2010;116:3875–3886.
184. North RJ. Cyclophosphamide-facilitated adoptive immunotherapy of an established tumor depends on elimination of tumor-induced suppressor T cells. *J Exp Med* 1982;155:1063–1074.
185. Gattinoni L, Finkelstein SE, Klebanoff CA, et al. Removal of homeostatic cytokine sinks by lymphodepletion enhances the efficacy of adoptively transferred tumor-specific CD8+ T cells. *J Exp Med* 2005;202:907–912.
186. Uckun FM, Jaszcz W, Ambrus JL, et al. Detailed studies on expression and function of CD19 surface determinant by using B43 monoclonal antibody and the clinical potential of anti-CD19 immunotoxins. *Blood* 1988;71:13–29.
187. Kochenderfer JN, Feldman SA, Zhao Y, et al. Construction and preclinical evaluation of an anti-CD19 chimeric antigen receptor. *J Immunother* 2009;32:689–702.
188. Brentjens RJ, Santos E, Nikhamin Y, et al. Genetically targeted T cells eradicate systemic acute lymphoblastic leukemia xenografts. *Clin Cancer Res* 2007;13:5426–5435.
189. Savoldo B, Ramos CA, Liu E, et al. CD28 costimulation improves expansion and persistence of chimeric antigen receptor-modified T cells in lymphoma patients. *J Clin Invest* 2011;121:1822–1826.
190. Grupp SA, Kalos M, Barrett D, et al. Chimeric antigen receptor-modified T cells for acute lymphoid leukemia. *N Engl J Med* 2013;368:1509–1518.
191. Jensen MC, Popplewell L, Cooper LJ, et al. Antitransgene rejection responses contribute to attenuated persistence of adoptively transferred CD20/CD19-specific chimeric antigen receptor redirected T cells in humans. *Biol Blood Marrow Transplant* 2010;16:1245–1356.
192. Till BG, Jensen MC, Wang J, et al. Adoptive immunotherapy for indolent non-Hodgkin lymphoma and mantle cell lymphoma using genetically modified autologous CD20-specific T cells. *Blood* 2008;112:2261–2271.
193. Till BG, Jensen MC, Wang J, et al. CD20-specific adoptive immunotherapy for lymphoma using a chimeric antigen receptor with both CD28 and 4-1BB domains: pilot clinical trial results. *Blood* 2012;119:3940–3950.
194. Haso W, Lee DW, Shah NN, et al. Anti-CD22-chimeric antigen receptors targeting B-cell precursor acute lymphoblastic leukemia. *Blood* 2013;121:1165–1174.
195. Giordano Attianese GM, Marin V, Hoyos V, et al. In vitro and in vivo model of a novel immunotherapy approach for chronic lymphocytic leukemia by anti-CD23 chimeric antigen receptor. *Blood* 2011;117:4736–4745.

196. Hudecek M, Schmitt TM, Baskar S, et al. The B-cell tumor-associated antigen ROR1 can be targeted with T cells modified to express a ROR1-specific chimeric antigen receptor. *Blood* 2010;116: 4532–4541.
197. Vera J, Savoldo B, Vigouroux S, et al. T lymphocytes redirected against the kappa light chain of human immunoglobulin efficiently kill mature B lymphocyte-derived malignant cells. *Blood* 2006;108:3890–3897.
198. Carpenter RO, Evbuomwan MO, Pittaluga S, et al. B-cell maturation antigen is a promising target for adoptive T-cell therapy of multiple myeloma. *Clin Cancer Res* 2013;19:2048–2060.
199. Peinert S, Prince HM, Guru PM, et al. Gene-modified T cells as immunotherapy for multiple myeloma and acute myeloid leukemia expressing the Lewis Y antigen. *Gene Ther* 2010;17:678–686.
200. Ritchie DS, Neeson PJ, Khot A, et al. Persistence and efficacy of second generation CAR T cell against the LeY antigen in acute myeloid leukemia. *Mol Ther* 2013;21:2122–2129.
201. Mardiros A, Dos SC, McDonald T, et al. T cells expressing CD123-specific chimeric antigen receptors exhibit specific cytolytic effector functions and antitumor effects against human acute myeloid leukemia. *Blood* 2013;122:3138–3148.
202. Savoldo B, Rooney CM, Di SA, et al. Epstein Barr virus specific cytotoxic T lymphocytes expressing the anti-CD30zeta artificial chimeric T-cell receptor for immunotherapy of Hodgkin disease. *Blood* 2007;110:2620–2630.
203. Hombach A, Heuser C, Sircar R, et al. An anti-CD30 chimeric receptor that mediates CD3-zeta-independent T-cell activation against Hodgkin's lymphoma cells in the presence of soluble CD30. *Cancer Res* 1998;58:1116–1119.
204. Shaffer DR, Savoldo B, Yi Z, et al. T cells redirected against CD70 for the immunotherapy of CD70-positive malignancies. *Blood* 2011;117:4304–4314.
205. Xue SA, Gao L, Hart D, et al. Elimination of human leukemia cells in NOD/SCID mice by WT1-TCR gene-transduced human T cells. *Blood* 2005;106:3062–3067.
206. Nagai K, Ochi T, Fujiwara H, et al. Aurora kinase A-specific T-cell receptor gene transfer redirects T lymphocytes to display effective antileukemia reactivity. *Blood* 2012;119:368–376.
207. Spranger S, Jeremias I, Wilde S, et al. TCR-transgenic lymphocytes specific for HMMR/Rhamm limit tumor outgrowth in vivo. *Blood* 2012;119: 3440–3449.
208. Hale GA, Shrestha S, Le-Rademacher J, et al. Alternate donor hematopoietic cell transplantation (HCT) in non-Hodgkin lymphoma using lower intensity conditioning: a report from the CIBMTR. *Biol Blood Marrow Transplant* 2012;18:1036–1043.
209. Kochenderfer JN, Dudley ME, Carpenter RO, et al. Donor-derived CD19-targeted T cells cause regression of malignancy persisting after allogeneic hematopoietic stem cell transplantation. *Blood* 2013;122:4129–4139.
210. Cruz CR, Micklethwaite KP, Savoldo B, et al. Infusion of donor-derived CD19-redirected virus-specific T cells for B-cell malignancies relapsed after allogeneic stem cell transplant: a phase 1 study. *Blood* 2013;122:2965–2973.
211. Traversari C, Marktel S, Magnani Z, et al. The potential immunogenicity of the TK suicide gene does not prevent full clinical benefit associated with the use of TK-transduced donor lymphocytes in HSCT for hematologic malignancies. *Blood* 2007;109:4708–4715.
212. Tey S, Dotti G, Rooney CM, et al. Inducible caspase 9 suicide gene to improve the safety of allodepleted T cells after haploidentical stem cell transplantation. *Biol Blood Marrow Transplant* 2007;13:924.
213. Ciceri F, Bonini C, Stanghellini MT, et al. Infusion of suicide-gene-engineered donor lymphocytes after family haploidentical haemopoietic stem-cell transplantation for leukaemia (the TK007 trial): a non-randomised phase I-II study. *Lancet Oncol* 2009;10:489–500.
214. Di Stasi A, Tey SK, Dotti G, et al. Inducible apoptosis as a safety switch for adoptive cell therapy. *N Engl J Med* 2011;365:1673–1683.

15 Pharmacokinetics and Pharmacodynamics of Anticancer Drugs

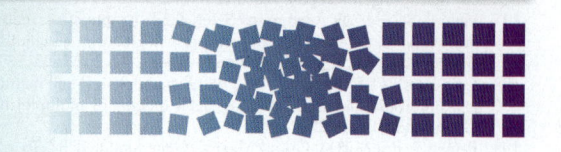

Alex Sparreboom and Sharyn D. Baker

INTRODUCTION

Drug selection and therapy considerations in oncology were originally solely based on observations of the effects produced.[1] To overcome some of the limitations of this empirical approach and to answer questions related to considerations of dose, frequency, and duration of drug treatment, it is necessary to understand the events that follow drug administration. Preclinical in vitro and in vivo studies have shown that the magnitude of antitumor response is a function of the concentration of drug,[2] and this has led to the suggestion that the therapeutic objective can be achieved by maintaining an adequate concentration at the site of action for the duration of therapy.[3] However, drugs are rarely directly administered at their sites of action. Indeed, most anticancer drugs are given intravenously or orally, and yet are expected to act in the brain, lungs, or elsewhere. Drugs must, therefore, move from the site of administration to the site of action and, moreover, distribute to all other tissues including organs that eliminate them from the body, such as the kidneys and liver. To administer drugs optimally, knowledge is needed not only of the mechanisms of drug absorption, distribution, and elimination, but also of the kinetics of these processes.[4]

The treatment of human malignancies involving drugs can be divided into two pharmacologic phases, a *pharmacokinetic* phase in which the dose, dosage form, frequency, and route of administration are related to drug level–time relationships in the body, and a *pharmacodynamic* phase in which the concentration of drug at the site(s) of action is related to the magnitude of the effect(s) produced. Once both of these phases have been defined, a dosage regimen can be designed to achieve the therapeutic objective, although additional factors need to be taken into consideration (Fig. 15.1). The clinical application of this approach allows distinctions between pharmacokinetic and pharmacodynamic causes of an unusual drug response. A basic tenet of pharmacokinetics is that the magnitude of both the desired response and toxicity are functions of the drug concentration at the site(s) of action. Accordingly, therapeutic failure results when either the concentration is too low, resulting in ineffective therapy, or is too high, producing unacceptable toxicity. Between these limits of concentrations lies a region associated with therapeutic success, the so-called *therapeutic window*.[5] Because the concentration of a drug at the site of action can rarely be measured directly, with the exception of certain hematologic malignancies, plasma or blood is commonly measured instead as a more accessible alternative.

PHARMACOKINETIC CONCEPTS

A drug's pharmacokinetic properties can be defined by two fundamental processes affecting drug behavior over time, *absorption* and *disposition*.

Absorption

Historically, most anticancer drugs have been administered intravenously; however, the use of orally administered agents is growing with the development of small-molecule targeted cancer therapeutics, such as tyrosine kinase inhibitors.[6] Moreover, drugs may also be administered regionally, for example into the pleural or peritoneal cavities,[7] the cerebrospinal fluid, or intra-arterially into a vessel leading to a cancerous tissue.[8] The process by which the unchanged drug moves from the site of administration to the site of measurement within the body is referred to as *absorption*. Loss at any site prior to the site of measurement contributes to a decrease in the apparent absorption of a drug. For an orally administered agent, this complex series of events involves disintegration of the pharmaceutical dosage form, dissolution, diffusion through gastrointestinal fluids, permeation of the gut membrane, portal circulation uptake, passage through the liver, and, finally, entry into the systemic circulation. The loss of drug as it passes for the first time through organs of elimination, such as the gastrointestinal membranes and the liver, during the absorption process is known as the *first-pass effect*.[9]

The pharmacokinetic parameter most closely associated with absorption is availability or bioavailability (F), defined as the fraction (or percent) of the administered dose that is absorbed intact. Bioavailability can be estimated by dividing the area under the plasma concentration–time curve (AUC) achieved following extravascular administration by the AUC observed after intravenous administration, and can range from 0 to 1.0 (or 0% to 100%).

Disposition

Disposition is defined as all the processes that occur subsequent to absorption of a drug; by definition, the components of disposition are *distribution* and *elimination*. Distribution is the process of reversible transfer of a drug to and from the site of measurement. Any drug that leaves the site of measurement and does not return has undergone elimination, which occurs by two processes, *excretion* and *metabolism*. Excretion is the irreversible loss of the chemically unchanged drug, whereas metabolism is the conversion of drug to another chemical species.

The extent of drug distribution can be determined by relating the concentration obtained with a known amount of drug in the body and is, in essence, a dilution space. The apparent volume into which a drug distributes in the body at equilibrium in called the volume of distribution (V_d), and may or may not correspond to an actual physiologic compartment.

The rate and extent to which a drug distributes into various tissues depend on a number of factors, including hydrophobicity, tissue permeability, tissue binding constants, binding to serum proteins, and local organ blood flow.[10] Large apparent volumes of distribution are common for agents with high tissue binding or high lipid solubility,

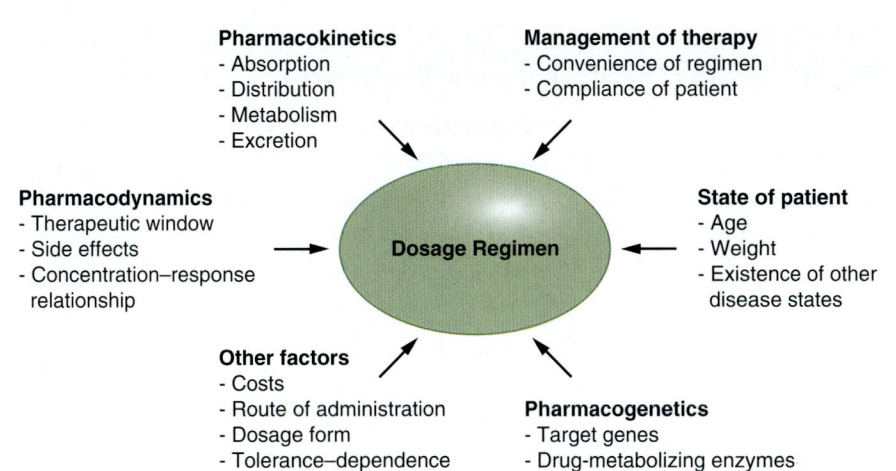

Figure 15.1 Principal determinants of dosage regimen selection for an anticancer drug

although distribution into specific body compartments may be limited by physiologic processes, such as the blood–brain barrier protecting the central nervous system[11,12] or the blood–testes barrier.[13]

Just as V_d is needed as a parameter to relate the concentration to the amount of drug in the body, there is also a need to have a parameter to relate the concentration to the rate of drug elimination, which is known as *clearance* (CL). Of all pharmacokinetic parameters, CL has the most clinical relevance because it defines the key relationship between drug dose and systemic drug exposure (AUC). Derived from V_d and CL is the parameter *elimination rate constant*, which can be regarded as the fractional rate of drug removal. It is, however, more common to refer to the half-life than to the elimination rate constant of a drug. The half-life of a drug is a useful parameter to estimate the time required to reach steady state on a multidose schedule or during a continuous intravenous drug infusion.

Dose Proportionality

When drug concentrations change in strict proportionality to the dose of drug administered, then the condition of dose proportionality (or linear pharmacokinetics) holds. If doubling the dose exactly doubles the plasma concentration or AUC, then pharmacokinetic parameters such V_d and CL are constant and remain independent of dose and concentration.[14] By strict definition, drugs with linear pharmacokinetics are dose proportional. Dose proportionality is clinically important because it means that dose adjustments will generate predictable changes in systemic drug exposure. For drugs that lack dose proportionality, V_d and CL will demonstrate concentration or time dependence, or both, making it difficult to predict the effect of dose adjustments on drug concentration (Fig. 15.2). Factors that can contribute to a lack of dose proportional pharmacokinetics include saturable oral absorption,[15] capacity-limited distribution or protein binding,[16] and/or saturable metabolism.[17] Dose proportionality of anticancer agents is typically assessed in Phase 1 dose-escalation trials in which small groups of patients are treated at a single dose level using a parallel study design, although the statistical power of such studies to detect deviations from dose proportionality is poor. An alternative, more robust study design is a crossover study in which each patient receives a low dose, an intermediate dose, and a high dose over consecutive cycles of treatment.[18] However, such studies are relatively rare in oncology because of the required use of low, potentially ineffective doses, which may raise ethical concerns for patients.

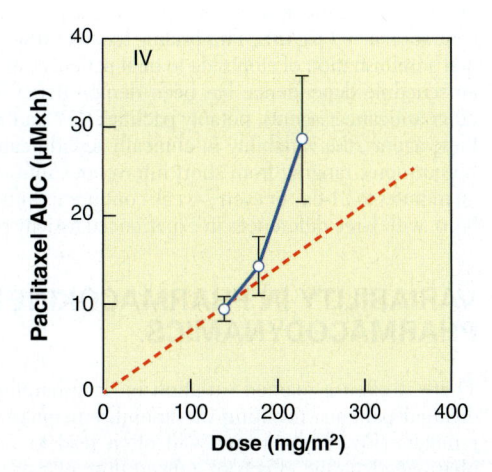

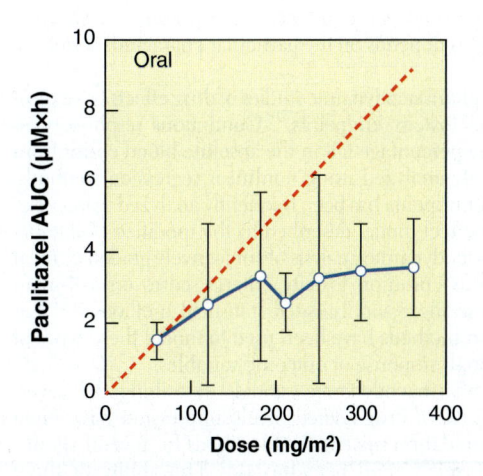

Figure 15.2 Effect of drug dose on systemic exposure to paclitaxel following intravenous (IV) or oral administration in patients with cancer. Data are expressed as mean values (symbols) and standard deviation (error bars). The *dashed line* indicates the hypothetical dose-proportional increase in the area under the plasma concentration time curve (AUC). (Data derived from van Zuylen L, Karlsson MO, Verweij J, et al. Pharmacokinetic modeling of paclitaxel encapsulation in Cremophor EL micelles. *Cancer Chemother Pharmacol* 2001;47:309–318, and Malingre MM, Terwogt JM, Beijnen JH, et al. Phase I and pharmacokinetic study of oral paclitaxel. *J Clin Oncol* 2000;18:2468–2475, respectively.)

TABLE 15.1
Examples of Systemic Exposure as a Pharmacodynamic Marker of Anticancer Drug Effects

Drug	Side Effect	Response/Survival
Carboplatin	Thrombocytopenia	Ovarian cancer
Cisplatin	Nephrotoxicity	Head and neck cancer
Cyclophosphamide	Cardiotoxicity	
Docetaxel	Neutropenia	Non–small-cell lung cancer
Doxorubicin	Neutropenia	
Epirubicin	Neutropenia	
Erlotinib	Skin rash	Non–small-cell lung and head and neck cancer
Etoposide		Non–small-cell lung cancer
5-Fluorouracil	Diarrhea, mucositis	Head and neck cancer
Imatinib		Chronic myeloid leukemia
Irinotecan	Diarrhea, neutropenia	
6-Mercaptopurine		Acute lymphoblastic leukemia
Methotrexate	Mucositis	Acute lymphoblastic leukemia
Nilotinib	Anemia, QT-interval prolongation	
Paclitaxel	Neutropenia	
Sorafenib	Hypertension, hand-foot skin reaction	Renal cell cancer
Sunitinib	Neutropenia	Renal cell cancer
Teniposide		Lymphoma

PHARMACODYNAMIC CONCEPTS

Pharmacodynamic models relate clinical drug effects with drug dose, concentration, or other pharmacokinetic parameters indicative of drug exposures (Table 15.1). In oncology, pharmacodynamic variability may account for substantial differences in clinical outcomes, even when systemic exposures are uniform. Variability in pharmacodynamic response may be heavily influenced by clinical covariates such as age, gender, prior chemotherapy, prior radiotherapy, concomitant medications, or other variables.[19] The pharmacokinetic parameters that are most often correlated with drug effects are markers of drug exposure, such as AUC. In general, the specific parameter used as the independent variable in a pharmacodynamic analysis depends on the particular characteristics of the study drug.

In oncology, pharmacodynamic studies of drug effects have most often focused on toxicity endpoints.[20] Continuous response variables, such as the percentage fall in the absolute blood count from baseline, are easily analyzed using nonlinear regression methods. Dose-limiting neutropenia has been frequently analyzed using a sigmoid maximum effect model described by the modified Hill equation. The pharmacodynamic analysis of subjectively graded clinical endpoints, such as common toxicity criteria scores on a 4-point scale, may require more sophisticated statistical methods.[21,22] Logistical regression methods have been used to model these types of categorical (ordinal) response or outcome variables.

Physiologic pharmacodynamic models describing the severity and time course of drug-related myelosuppression have been derived using population mixed-effect methods for several agents, including paclitaxel[23,24] and pemetrexed.[25] The ability of these models to predict both the severity and duration of drug-induced neutropenia substantially enhances their clinical usefulness.[26] In contrast to small-molecule therapeutics, large-molecule therapeutics such as monoclonal antibodies may not demonstrate toxicities directly related to dose levels. For these agents, a thorough understanding of the pharmacokinetic/pharmacodynamic relationships using modeling approaches may be critical for optimal dose selection.[27]

The antitumor activity of certain chemotherapeutic agents is highly schedule dependent. For such drugs, the dose fractionated over several days can produce a different antitumor response or toxicity profile compared with the same dose given over a shorter period. For example, the efficacy of etoposide in the treatment of small-cell lung cancer is markedly increased when an identical total dose of etoposide is administered by a 5-day divided-dose schedule rather than a 24-hour infusion.[28] Pharmacokinetic analysis in that study showed that both schedules produced very similar overall drug exposure (as measured by AUC), but that the divided-dose schedule produced twice the duration of exposure to an etoposide plasma concentration of >1 µg/mL. This finding has led to the use of prolonged oral administration of etoposide to treat patients with cancer.[29] Similar schedule dependence has been demonstrated for a number of other anticancer agents, notably paclitaxel[30,31] and topotecan.[32] For these agents, the variability in clinically tested treatment schedules is enormous, ranging from short intravenous infusions of less than 30 minutes to 21-day or even 7-week continuous infusion administrations, with large differences in experienced toxicity profiles.

VARIABILITY IN PHARMACOKINETICS/PHARMACODYNAMICS

There is often a marked variation in drug handling between individual patients, resulting in variability in pharmacokinetic parameters (Fig. 15.3), which will often lead to variability in the pharmacodynamic effects of a given dose of a drug.[33] That is, an identical dose of drug may result in acceptable toxicity in one patient, and unacceptable and possibly life threatening toxicity in another, or a clinical response in one individual and cancer progression in another. The principal underlying sources of this interindividual pharmacokinetic/pharmacodynamic variability are discussed in the following paragraphs.

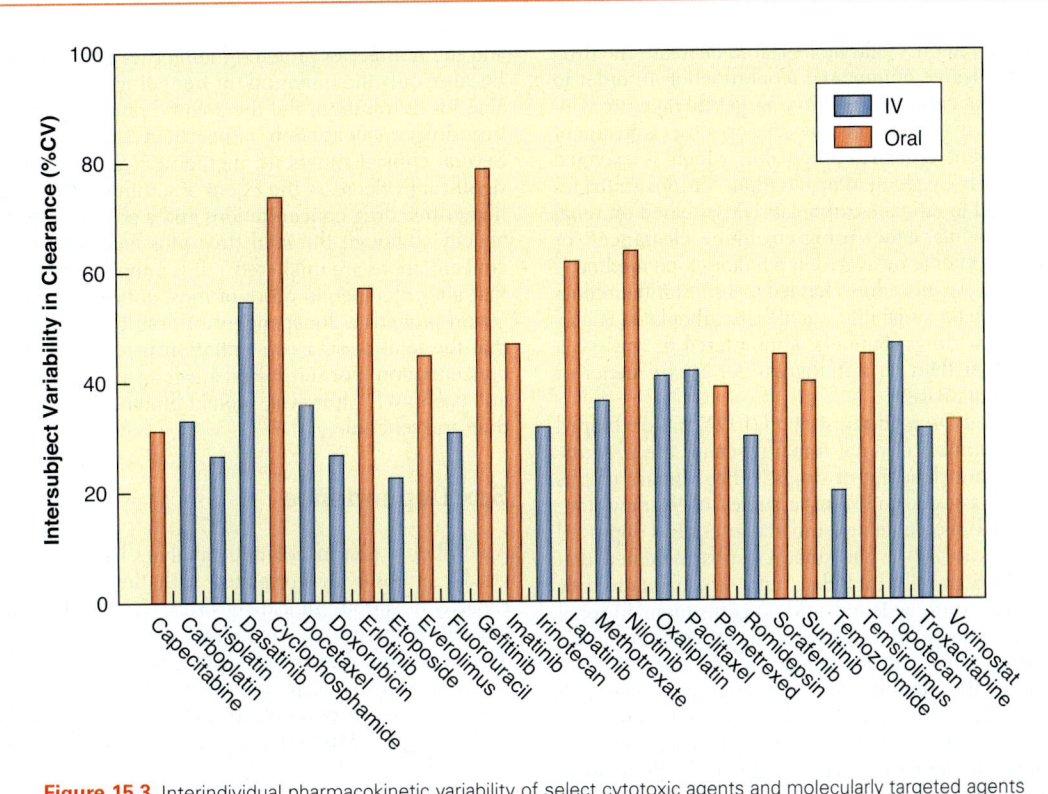

Figure 15.3 Interindividual pharmacokinetic variability of select cytotoxic agents and molecularly targeted agents expressed as a percent coefficient of variation (%CV) in apparent (oral) clearance. IV, intravenous. (Data derived from Mathijssen RH, de Jong FA, Loos WJ, et al. Flat-fixed dosing versus body surface area based dosing of anticancer drugs in adults: does it make a difference? *Oncologist* 2007;12:913–923, and publicly available prescribing information.)

Body Size and Body Composition

The traditional method of individualizing anticancer drug dosage is by using body surface area (BSA).[34] However, the usefulness of normalizing an anticancer drug dose to BSA in adults has been questioned, because, for many drugs, there is no relationship between BSA and CL.[35] Likewise, attempts to replace BSA as a size metric in dose calculation with alternate descriptors such as lean body weight, either in an average population or in individuals at the outer extremes of weight (i.e., frail, severely obese patients) have failed for many anticancer agents.[36,37] It should be pointed out that BSA is a much more important consideration in drug dose calculation for pediatric patients as compared to adults, because of the larger size range in the former population.[38] Based in part on the failure to reduce interindividual pharmacokinetic variability with the use of BSA normalization to obtain a starting dose, many of the more recently developed molecularly targeted agents are currently administered using a flat-fixed dose irrespective of an individual's BSA.[37]

Age

Changes in body composition and organ function at the extremes of age can affect both drug disposition and drug effect.[39] For example, maturational processes in infancy may alter the absorption and distribution of drugs as well as change the capacity for drug metabolism and excretion.[4] The importance of understanding the influence of age on the pharmacokinetics and pharmacodynamics of individual anticancer agents has increased steadily as treatment for the malignancies of infants,[40] adolescents,[41] and the elderly[42] has advanced. Although pediatric cancers remain rare compared with cancers in adults and the elderly population, in particular, optimizing treatment in a patient group with a high cure rate and a long expected survival becomes critical to minimize the incidence of preventable late complications while maintaining efficacy.

Pathophysiologic Changes

Effects of Disease

Pathophysiologic changes associated with particular malignancies may cause dramatic alterations in drug disposition. For example, increases in the clearance of both antipyrine and lorazepam were noted after remission induction compared with the time of diagnosis in children with acute lymphoblastic leukemia (ALL).[43] The clearance of unbound teniposide is lower in children with ALL in relapse than during first remission.[44] Because leukemic infiltration of the liver at the time of diagnosis is common, drugs metabolized by the liver may have a reduced clearance, as has been documented in preclinical models.[45]

Furthermore, in mouse models, certain tumors elicited an acute phase response that coincided with downregulation of human CYP3A4 in the liver as well as the mouse ortholog Cyp3a11.[46] The reduction of murine hepatic Cyp3a gene expression in tumor-bearing mice resulted in decreased Cyp3a protein expression and, consequently, a significant reduction in Cyp3a-mediated metabolism of midazolam. These findings support the possibility that tumor-derived inflammation may alter the pharmacokinetic and pharmacodynamic properties of CYP3A4 substrates, leading to reduced metabolism of drugs in humans.[47] This supports a possible need for disease-specific design of early clinical trials with anticancer drugs,[48] as has been recommended for docetaxel.[49]

Effects of Renal Impairment

The potential impact of pathophysiologic status on interindividual pharmacokinetic variability can be due to either the disease itself or to a dysfunction of specific organs involved in drug elimination. For example, if urinary excretion is an important elimination route for a given drug, any decrement in renal function could lead to decreased drug clearance, which may result in drug accumulation and toxicity.[50] Therefore, it would be logical to decrease the drug dose relative to the degree of impaired renal function in order to maintain plasma concentrations within a target therapeutic window. The best known example of this a priori dose adjustment of an anticancer agent remains carboplatin, which is excreted renally almost entirely by glomerular filtration. Various strategies have been developed to estimate carboplatin doses based on renal function among patients, either using creatinine clearance[51] or glomerular filtration rates as measured by a radioisotope method.[52] The application of these procedures has led to a substantial reduction in pharmacokinetic variability, such that carboplatin is currently one of the few drugs routinely administered to achieve a target exposure rather than on a milligram per square meter or milligram per kilogram basis.

The U.S. Food and Drug Administration (FDA) has developed a guidance on the impact of renal impairment on the pharmacokinetics, dosing, and labeling of drugs.[53] The impact of this guidance has been assessed following a survey of 94 new drug applications for small-molecule new molecular entities approved over the years 2003 to 2007. The survey results indicated that 41% of the applications that included renal impairment study data resulted in a recommendation of dose adjustment in renal impairment.[54] Interestingly, the survey results provided evidence that renal impairment can affect the pharmacokinetics of drugs that are predominantly eliminated by nonrenal processes such as metabolism and/or active transport. The latter finding supports the FDA recommendation to evaluate pharmacokinetic/pharmacodynamic alterations in renal impairment for those drugs that are predominantly eliminated by nonrenal processes, in addition to those that are mainly excreted unchanged by the kidneys. A striking example of a drug in the former category is imatinib, an agent that is predominantly eliminated by hepatic pathways but where predialysis renal impairment is associated with dramatically reduced drug clearance,[55] presumably due to a transporter-mediated process.[56]

Effects of Hepatic Impairment

In contrast to the predictable decline in renal clearance of drugs when glomerular filtration is impaired, it is difficult to make general predictions on the effect of impaired liver function on drug clearance. The major problem is that commonly applied criteria to establish hepatic impairment are typically not good indicators of drug-metabolizing enzyme activity and that several alternative hepatic function tests, such as indocyanine green and antipyrine, have relatively limited value in predicting anticancer drug pharmacokinetics. An alternative dynamic measure of liver function has been proposed, which is based on totaled values (scored to the World Health Organization [WHO] grading system) of serum bilirubin, alkaline phosphatase, and either alanine aminotransferase or aspartate aminotransferase to give a hepatic dysfunction score.[57] Based on pharmacokinetic studies in patients with normal and impaired hepatic function, guidelines have been proposed for dose adjustments of several agents when administered to patients with severe liver dysfunction.[58] It should be emphasized that no uniform criteria have been used in the conduct of these studies and that, ultimately, substantial advances could be made through an a priori determination of the hepatic activity of enzymes of pertinent relevance to the chemotherapeutic drug(s) of interest, as has been done for docetaxel.[59]

Effects of Serum Proteins

The binding of drugs to serum proteins, particularly those that are highly bound, may also have significant clinical implications for a therapeutic outcome.[60] Although protein binding is a major determinant of drug action, it is clearly only one of a myriad of factors that influence the disposition of anticancer drugs.[16] The extent of protein binding is a function of drug and protein concentrations, the affinity constants for the drug-protein interaction, and the number of protein-binding sites per class of binding site. Because only the unbound (or free) drug in plasma water is available for distribution, the therapeutic response will correlate with free drug concentration rather than total drug concentration. Several clinical situations, including liver and renal disease, can significantly decrease the extent of serum binding and may lead to higher free drug concentrations and a possible risk of unexpected toxicity, although the total (free plus bound forms) plasma drug concentrations are unaltered.[61] It is important to realize, however, that after therapeutic doses of most anticancer drugs, binding to serum proteins is independent of drug concentration, suggesting that the total plasma concentration is reflective of the unbound concentration. For some anticancer agents, including etoposide[62] and paclitaxel,[63] however, protein binding is highly dependent on dose and schedule.

Sex Dependence

A number of pharmacokinetic analyses have suggested that male gender is positively correlated with the maximum elimination capacity of various anticancer drugs (e.g., paclitaxel)[8] or with increased clearance (e.g., imatinib)[64] compared with female gender. These observations have added to a growing body of evidence that the pharmacokinetic profile of various anticancer drugs exhibits significant sexual dimorphism, which is rarely considered in the design of clinical trials during oncology drug development.

Drug Interactions

Coadministration of Other Chemotherapeutic Drugs

Favorable and unfavorable interactions between drugs must be considered in developing combination regimens. These interactions may influence the effectiveness of each of the components of the combination, and typically occur when the pharmacokinetic profile of one drug is altered by the other. Such interactions are important in the design of trials evaluating drug combinations because, occasionally, the outcome of concurrent drug administration is diminished therapeutic efficacy or increased toxicity of one or more of the administered agents. Although a recent survey indicated that clinically significant pharmacokinetic interactions are relatively rare in Phase I trials of oncology drug combinations,[65] interactions appear to be more common for combinations of tyrosine kinase inhibitors with cytotoxic chemotherapeutics.[66]

Coadministration of Nonchemotherapeutic Drugs

Many prescription and over-the-counter medications have the potential to cause interactions with anticancer agents by altering their pharmacokinetic characteristics and leading to clinically significant phenotypes. Most clinically relevant drug interactions in this category are due to changes in metabolic routes related to an altered expression or function of cytochrome P450 (CYP) isozymes. This class of enzymes, particularly the CYP3A4 isoform, is responsible for the oxidation of a large proportion of currently approved anticancer drugs. Elevated CYP activity (induction), translated into a more rapid metabolic rate, may result in a decrease in plasma concentrations and to a loss of therapeutic effect. For example, anticonvulsant drugs such as phenytoin, phenobarbital, and carbamazepine can induce drug-metabolizing enzymes and thereby increase the clearance of various anticancer agents.[33]

Conversely, the suppression (inhibition) of CYP activity, for example with ketoconazole,[13,67] may trigger a rise in plasma concentrations and can lead to exaggerated toxicity commensurate with overdose. It should be borne in mind that several pharmacokinetic parameters could be altered simultaneously. Especially in the development of anticancer agents given by the oral route,

TABLE 15.2
Effect of Food on Exposure to Select Oral Anticancer Agents

Drug	Food	Effect on Drug Exposure	Manufacturer's Recommendations
Abiraterone	High-fat meal	↑ AUC 1,000%	Without food
Dasatinib	High-fat meal	↑ AUC 14%	With or without food
Erlotinib	High-fat, high-calorie breakfast	Single dose, ↑ AUC 200% Multiple dose, ↑ AUC 37%–66%	Without food[a]
Gefitinib	High-fat breakfast	↓ AUC 14%, ↓ Cmax 35%	With or without food
	High-fat breakfast	↑ AUC 32%, ↑ Cmax 35%	
Imatinib	High-fat meal	No change Variability (% CV) ↓ 37%	With food and a large glass of water[b]
Lapatinib	Low-fat meal (5% fat, 500 calories)	↑ AUC 167%, ↑ Cmax 142%	Without food[c]
	High-fat meal (50% fat, 1,000 calories)	↑ AUC 325%, ↑ Cmax 203%	
Nilotinib	High-fat meal	↑ AUC 82%	Without food
Sorafenib	Moderate-fat meal (30% fat, 700 calories)	No change in bioavailability	Without food
	High-fat meal (50% fat, 900 calories)	↓ Bioavailability 29%	
Sunitinib	High-fat, high-calorie meal	↑ AUC 18%	With or without food
Everolimus	High-fat meal	↓ AUC 16%, ↓ Cmax 60%	With or without food
Vismodegib	High-fat meal	↑ AUC 74% for single dose; no effect at steady state	With or without food
Vorinostat	High-fat meal	↑ AUC 37%	With food[d]

[a] Recommended without food because the approved dose is the maximum tolerated dose.
[b] Recommended with food to reduce nausea.
[c] Recommended without food to achieve consistent drug exposure; was taken without food in clinical trials.
[d] Was taken with food in clinical trials.
AUC, area under the plasma concentration time curve; Cmax, maximum plasma concentration; CV, coefficient of variation.

oral bioavailability plays a crucial role[9]; this parameter is contingent on adequate absorption and the circumvention of intestinal and, subsequently, hepatic metabolism of the drug. It has been suggested that the prevalence of drug–drug interactions is particularly high in cancer patients receiving oral chemotherapy,[68] especially for agents that are weak bases that exhibit pH-dependent solubility.[69]

An additional consideration is related to a possible influence of food intake on the extent of drug absorption after oral administration, which can increase, decrease, or remain unchanged depending on specific physicochemical properties of the drug in question (Table 15.2). The relatively narrow therapeutic index of most of these agents means that significant inter- and intrapatient variability would predispose some individuals to excessive toxicity or, conversely, inadequate efficacy.[12]

Coadministration of Complementary and Alternative Medicine

Surveys within the past decade estimate the prevalence of complementary and alternative medicine (CAM) use in oncology patients to be as high as 87%, and in many cases the treating physician is not aware of the patients' CAM use.[70] With a larger number of participants to phase I clinical trials[71] using herbal treatments combined with allopathic therapies, the risk for herb–drug interactions is a growing concern, and there is an increasing need to understand possible adverse drug interactions in oncology at the early stages of drug development.

A number of clinically important pharmacokinetic interactions involving CAM and cancer drugs have now been recognized, although causal relationships have not always been established.[72] Most of the observed interactions point to the herbs affecting several isoforms of the CYP family, either through inhibition or induction. In the context of chemotherapeutic drugs, St. John's wort,[73] garlic,[74] milk thistle,[75] and Echinacea[11] have been formally evaluated for their pharmacokinetic drug–interaction potential in cancer patients. However, various other herbs have the potential to significantly modulate the expression and/or activity of drug-metabolizing enzymes and drug transporters (Table 15.3), including ginkgo, ginseng, and kava.[70] Because of the high prevalence of herbal medicine use, physicians should include herb usage in their routine drug histories in order to have an opportunity to outline to individual patients which potential hazards should be taken into consideration prior to participation in a clinical trial.

Inherited Genetic Factors

The discipline of pharmacogenetics describes differences in the pharmacokinetics and pharmacodynamics of drugs as a result of inherited variation in drug metabolizing enzymes, drug transporters, and drug targets between patients.[76] These inherited variations are occasionally responsible for extensive interpatient variability in drug exposure or effects. Severe toxicity might occur in the absence of a typical metabolism of active compounds, while the therapeutic effect of a drug could be diminished in the case of an absence of activation of a prodrug, such as irinotecan.[77] The importance and detectability of polymorphisms for a given enzyme or transporter depends on the contribution of the variant gene product to pharmacologic response, the availability of alternative pathways of elimination, and the frequency of occurrence of the variant allele. Although many substrates have been identified for the known polymorphic drug metabolizing enzymes

TABLE 15.3
Effects of Common Herbal Products on Exposure to Anticancer Agents

Botanical	Concurrent Chemotherapy/Condition (Suspected Effect)
Ephedra	Avoid with all cardiovascular chemotherapy (synergistic increase in blood pressure)
Ginkgo	Caution with camptothecins, cyclophosphamide, TK inhibitors, epipodophyllotoxins, taxanes, and vinca alkaloids (CYP3A4 and CYP2C19 inhibition); discourage with alkylating agents, antitumor antibiotics, and platinum analogs (free-radical scavenging)
Ginseng	Discourage in patients with estrogen-receptor–positive breast cancer and endometrial cancer (stimulation of tumor growth)
Green tea	Discourage with erlotinib and pazopanib (CYP1A2 induction)
Japanese arrowroot	Avoid with methotrexate (ABC and OAT transporter inhibition)
St. John's wort	Avoid with all concurrent chemotherapy (CYP2B6, CYP2C9, CYP2C19, CYP2E1, CYP3A4, and ABCB1 induction)
Valerian	Caution with tamoxifen (CYP2C9 inhibition), cyclophosphamide, and teniposide (CYP2C19 inhibition)
Kava-kava	Avoid in all patients with preexisting liver disease, with evidence of hepatic injury (herb-induced hepatotoxicity), and/or in combination with hepatotoxic chemotherapy; caution with camptothecins, cyclophosphamide, TK inhibitors, epipodophyllotoxins, taxanes, and Vinca alkaloids (CYP3A4 induction)

TK, tyrosine kinase; CYP, cytochrome P450; ABC, ATP-binding cassette; OAT, organic anion transporter.

and transporters, the contribution of a genetically determined source of interindividual pharmacokinetic variability has been established for only a few cancer chemotherapeutic agents. Most of these cases involve agents for which elimination is critically dependent on a rate-limiting breakdown by a polymorphic enzyme (e.g., 6-mercaptopurine by thiopurine-S-methyltransferase; 5-fluorouracil by dihydropyrimidine dehydrogenase) or when a polymorphic enzyme is involved in the formation of a toxic metabolite (e.g., tamoxifen by CYP2D6).[78]

In addition to drug metabolism, pharmacokinetic processes are highly dependent on the interplay with drug transport in organs such as the intestines, kidneys, and liver. Genetically determined variation in drug transporter function or expression is now increasingly recognized to have a significant role as a determinant of intersubject variability in response to various commonly prescribed drugs.[79] The most extensively studied class of drug transporters are those encoded by the family of ATP-binding cassette (ABC) genes, some of which also play a role in the resistance of malignant cells to anticancer agents. Among the 48 known ABC gene products, ABCB1 (P-glycoprotein), ABCC1 (multidrug-resistance associated protein-1 [MRP1]) and its homologue ABCC2 (MRP2; cMOAT), and ABCG2 (breast cancer resistance protein [BCRP]) are known to influence the oral absorption and disposition of a wide variety of drugs.[80] As a result, the expression levels of these proteins in humans have important consequences for an individual's susceptibility to certain anticancer drug–induced side effects, interactions, and treatment efficacy, for example, in the case of genetic variation in ABCG2 in relation to gefitinib-induced diarrhea.[81]

Similar to the discoveries of functional genetic variations in drug efflux transporters of the ABC family, there have been considerable advances in the identification of inherited variants in transporters that facilitate cellular drug uptake in tissues that play an important role in drug elimination, such as the liver (Fig. 15.4). Among these, members of the organic anion-transporting polypeptides (OATP), organic anion transporters (OAT), and organic cation transporters (OCT) can mediate the cellular uptake of a large number of structurally divergent compounds.[82,83] Accordingly, functionally relevant polymorphisms in these influx transporters may contribute to interindividual and interethnic variability in drug disposition and response,[84] for example, in the case of the impact of polymorphic variants in the OCT1 gene *SLC22A1* on the survival of patients with chronic myeloid leukemia receiving treatment with imatinib.[85]

DOSE-ADAPTATION USING PHARMACOKINETIC/PHARMACODYNAMIC PRINCIPLES

Therapeutic Drug Monitoring

Prolonged infusion schedules of anticancer drugs offer a very convenient setting for dose adaptation in individual patients. At the time required to achieve steady-state concentration, it is possible to modify the infusion rate for the remainder of the treatment course if a relationship is known between this steady-state concentration and a desired pharmacodynamic endpoint. This method has been successfully used to adapt the dose during continuous infusions of 5-fluorouracil and etoposide, and for repeated oral administration of etoposide or repeated intravenous administration of cisplatin.[86] Methotrexate plasma concentrations are routinely monitored to identify patients at high risk of toxicity and to adjust leucovorin rescue in patients with delayed drug excretion. This monitoring has significantly reduced the incidence of serious toxicity, including toxic death, and in fact, has improved outcome by eliminating unacceptably low systemic exposure levels.[87] Therapeutic drug monitoring has also been applied to or is currently under investigation for several more recently developed anticancer drugs, including imatinib[88–90] and sorafenib.[91]

Feedback-Controlled Dosing

It remains to be determined how information on interindividual pharmacokinetic variability can eventually be used to devise an optimal dosage regimen of a drug for the treatment of a given disease in an individual patient. Obviously, the desired objective would be most efficiently achieved if the individual's dosage requirements could be calculated prior to administering the drug. While this ideal cannot be met completely in clinical practice, with the notable exception of carboplatin, some success may be achieved by adopting feedback-controlled dosing. In the adaptive dosage with feedback control, population-based predictive models are used initially, but allow the possibility of dosage alteration based on feedback revision. In this approach, patients are first treated with standard dose and, during treatment, pharmacokinetic information is estimated by a limited-sampling strategy and compared with that predicted from the population model with which treatment was initiated. On the basis of the comparison,

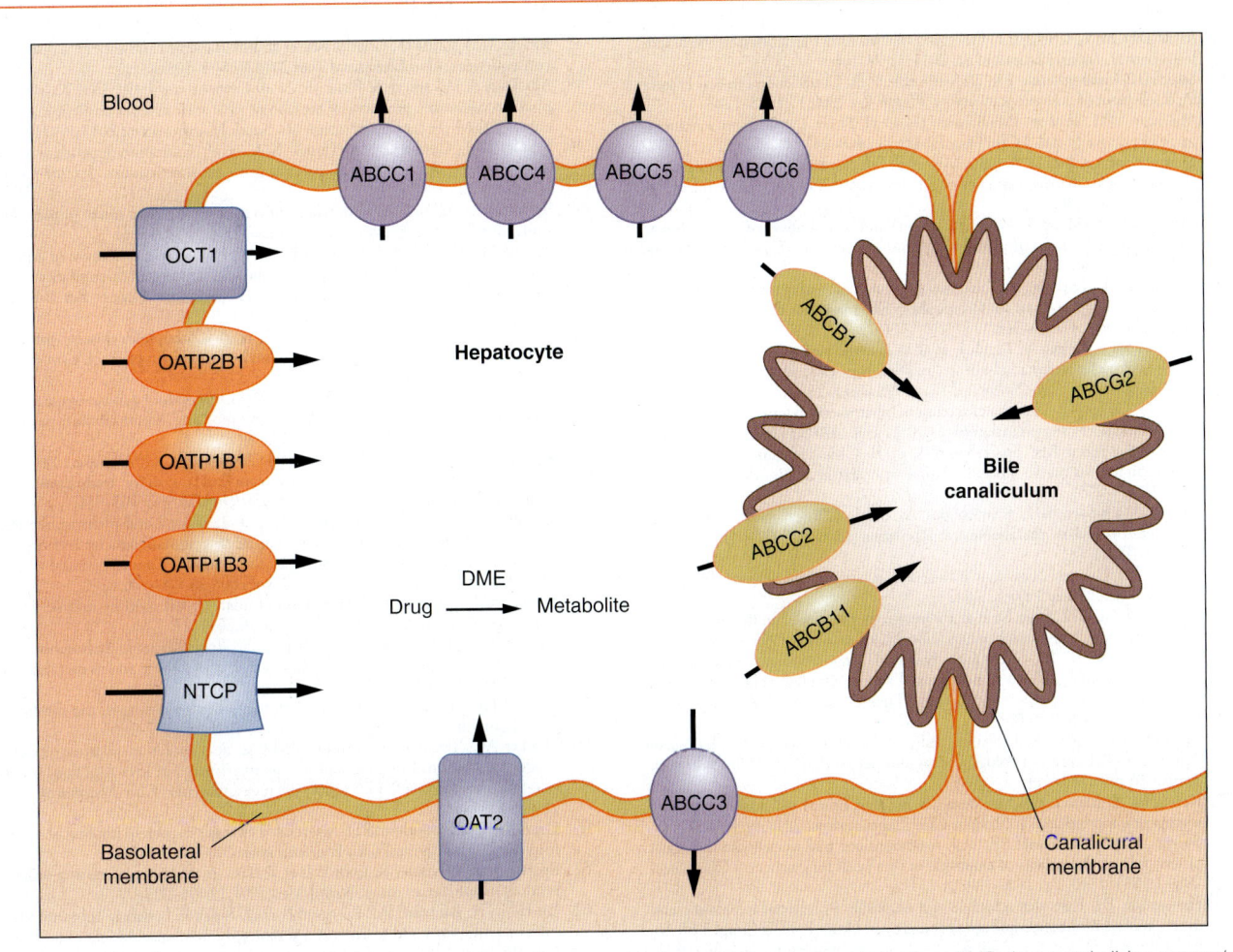

Figure 15.4 Common mechanisms for possible interactions between xenobiotics and anticancer drugs in the liver. DME, drug-metabolizing enzyme(s).

more patient-specific pharmacokinetic parameters are calculated, and dosage is adjusted accordingly to maintain the target exposure measure producing the desired pharmacodynamic effect. Despite its mathematical complexity, this approach may be the only way to deliver the desired and precise exposure of an anticancer agent.

The study of population pharmacokinetics seeks to identify the measurable factors that cause changes in the dose-concentration relationship and the extent of these alterations so that, if these are associated with clinically significant shifts in the therapeutic index, dosage can be appropriately modified in the individual patient. It is obvious that a careful collection of data during the development of drugs and subsequent analyses could be helpful to collect some essential information on the drug. Unfortunately, important information is often lost by failing to analyze this data or due to the fact that the relevant samples or data were never collected. Historically, this has resulted in the notion that tools for the identification of patient population subgroups are inadequate for most of the currently approved anticancer drugs.

However, the use of population pharmacokinetic models is increasingly studied in an attempt to accommodate as much of the pharmacokinetic variability as possible in terms of measurable characteristics. This type of analysis has been conducted for a number of clinically important anticancer drugs, including carboplatin,[92] docetaxel,[93] topotecan,[94] gefitinib,[95] and erlotinib,[96] and provided mathematical equations based on morphometric, demographic, phenotypic enzyme activity, and/or physiologic characteristics of patients, in order to predict drug clearance with an acceptable degree of precision and bias.[97]

REFERENCES

1. DeVita VT, Chu E. A history of cancer chemotherapy. *Cancer Res* 2008; 68:8643–8653.
2. Lieu CH, Tan AC, Leong S, et al. From bench to bedside: lessons learned in translating preclinical studies in cancer drug development. *J Natl Cancer Inst* 2013;105:1441–1456.
3. Sparreboom A, Verweij J. Advances in cancer therapeutics. *Clin Pharmacol Ther* 2009;85:113–117.
4. Fujita KI, Sasaki Y. Optimization of cancer chemotherapy on the basis of pharmacokinetics and pharmacodynamics: from patients enrolled in 'clinical trials' to those in the 'real world'. *Drug Metab Pharmacokin* 2014;29(1):20–28.
5. Liliemark J, Peterson C. Pharmacokinetic optimisation of anticancer therapy. *Clin Pharmacokinet* 1991;21:213–231.
6. Stuurman FE, Nuijen B, Beijnen JH, et al. Oral anticancer drugs: mechanisms of low bioavailability and strategies for improvement. *Clin Pharmacokinet* 2013;52:399–414.
7. Hasovits C, Clarke S. Pharmacokinetics and pharmacodynamics of intraperitoneal cancer chemotherapeutics. *Clin Pharmacokinet* 2012;51:203–224.
8. Cai S, Bagby TR, Forrest ML. Development of regional chemotherapies: feasibility, safety and efficacy in clinical use and preclinical studies. *Ther Deliv* 2011;2:1467–1484.
9. DeMario MD, Ratain MJ. Oral chemotherapy: rationale and future directions. *J Clin Oncol* 1998;16:2557–2567.
10. Zou P, Zheng N, Yang Y, et al. Prediction of volume of distribution at steady state in humans: comparison of different approaches. *Exp Opin Drug Metab Toxicol* 2012;8:855–872.
11. Deeken JF, Loscher W. The blood-brain barrier and cancer: transporters, treatment, and Trojan horses. *Clin Cancer Res* 2007;13:1663–1674.
12. Pitz MW, Desai A, Grossman SA, et al. Tissue concentration of systemically administered antineoplastic agents in human brain tumors. *J Neurooncol* 2011;104:629–638.

13. Mruk DD, Su L, Cheng CY. Emerging role for drug transporters at the blood-testis barrier. *Trends Pharmacol Sci* 2011;32:99–106.
14. Smith BP, Vandenhende FR, DeSante KA, et al. Confidence interval criteria for assessment of dose proportionality. *Pharm Res* 2000;17:1278–1283.
15. Malingre MM, Terwogt JM, Beijnen JH, et al. Phase I and pharmacokinetic study of oral paclitaxel. *J Clin Oncol* 2000;18:2468–2475.
16. Sparreboom A, Chen H, Acharya MR, et al. Effects of alpha1-acid glycoprotein on the clinical pharmacokinetics of 7-hydroxystaurosporine. *Clin Cancer Res* 2004;10:6840–6846.
17. Yamaoka K, Takakura Y. Analysis methods and recent advances in nonlinear pharmacokinetics from in vitro through in loci to in vivo. *Drug Metab Dispos* 2004;19:397–406.
18. van Zuylen L, Karlsson MO, Verweij J, et al. Pharmacokinetic modeling of paclitaxel encapsulation in Cremophor EL micelles. *Cancer Chemother Pharmacol* 2001;47:309–318.
19. Karlsson MO, Molnar V, Bergh J, et al. A general model for time-dissociated pharmacokinetic-pharmacodynamic relationship exemplified by paclitaxel myelosuppression. *Clin Pharmacol Ther* 1998;63:11–25.
20. Zhou Q, Gallo JM. The pharmacokinetic/pharmacodynamic pipeline: translating anticancer drug pharmacology to the clinic. *AAPS J* 2011;13:111–120.
21. Xie R, Mathijssen RH, Sparreboom A, et al. Clinical pharmacokinetics of irinotecan and its metabolites in relation with diarrhea. *Clin Pharmacol Ther* 2002;72:265–275.
22. Xie R, Mathijssen RH, Sparreboom A, et al. Clinical pharmacokinetics of irinotecan and its metabolites: a population analysis. *J Clin Oncol* 2002;20:3293–3301.
23. Kearns CM, Gianni L, Egorin MJ. Paclitaxel pharmacokinetics and pharmacodynamics. *Sem Oncol* 1995;22:16–23.
24. Minami H, Sasaki Y, Saijo N, et al. Indirect-response model for the time course of leukopenia with anticancer drugs. *Clin Pharmacol Ther* 1998;64:511–521.
25. Latz JE, Schneck KL, Nakagawa K, et al. Population pharmacokinetic/pharmacodynamic analyses of pemetrexed and neutropenia: effect of vitamin supplementation and differences between Japanese and Western patients. *Clin Cancer Res* 2009;15:346–354.
26. Karlsson MO, Anehall T, Friberg LE, et al. Pharmacokinetic/pharmacodynamic modelling in oncological drug development. *Basic Clin Pharmacol Toxicol* 2005;96:206–211.
27. Keizer RJ, Huitema AD, Schellens JH, et al. Clinical pharmacokinetics of therapeutic monoclonal antibodies. *Clin Pharmacokinet* 2010;49:493–507.
28. Slevin ML, Clark PI, Joel SP, et al. A randomized trial to evaluate the effect of schedule on the activity of etoposide in small-cell lung cancer. *J Clin Oncol* 1989;7:1333–1340.
29. Hainsworth JD. Extended-schedule oral etoposide in selected neoplasms and overview of administration and scheduling issues. *Drugs* 1999;58 Suppl 3:51–56.
30. Gelderblom H, Mross K, ten Tije AJ, et al. Comparative pharmacokinetics of unbound paclitaxel during 1- and 3-hour infusions. *J Clin Oncol* 2002;20:574–581.
31. Woodward EJ, Twelves C. Scheduling of taxanes: a review. *Curr Clin Pharmacol* 2010;5:226–231.
32. Soepenberg O, Sparreboom A, Verweij J. Clinical studies of camptothecin and derivatives. *Alkaloid Chem Biol* 2003;60:1–50.
33. Undevia SD, Gomez-Abuin G, Ratain MJ. Pharmacokinetic variability of anticancer agents. *Nat Rev Cancer* 2005;5:447–458.
34. Gurney H. Dose calculation of anticancer drugs: a review of the current practice and introduction of an alternative. *J Clin Oncol* 1996;14:2590–2611.
35. Baker SD, Verweij J, Rowinsky EK, et al. Role of body surface area in dosing of investigational anticancer agents in adults, 1991–2001. *J Natl Cancer Inst* 2002;94:1883–1888.
36. Mathijssen RH, Sparreboom A. Influence of lean body weight on anticancer drug clearance. *Clin Pharmacol Ther* 2009;85:23.
37. Sparreboom A, Wolff AC, Mathijssen RH, et al. Evaluation of alternate size descriptors for dose calculation of anticancer drugs in the obese. *J Clin Oncol* 2007;25:4707–4713.
38. Bartelink IH, Rademaker CM, Schobben AF, et al. Guidelines on paediatric dosing on the basis of developmental physiology and pharmacokinetic considerations. *Clin Pharmacokinet* 2006;45:1077–1097.
39. McLeod HL, Relling MV, Crom WR, et al. Disposition of antineoplastic agents in the very young child. *Br J Cancer* 1992;18:S23–S29.
40. Hutson JR, Weitzman S, Schechter T, et al. Pharmacokinetic and pharmacogenetic determinants and considerations in chemotherapy selection and dosing in infants. *Exp Opin Drug Metab Toxicol* 2012;8:709–722.
41. Veal GJ, Hartford CM, Stewart CF. Clinical pharmacology in the adolescent oncology patient. *J Clin Oncol* 2010;28:4790–4799.
42. Lichtman SM. Pharmacology of aging and cancer: how useful are pharmacokinetic tests? *Interdiscip Top Gerontol* 2013;38:104–123.
43. Relling MV, Crom WR, Pieper JA, et al. Hepatic drug clearance in children with leukemia: changes in clearance of model substrates during remission-induction therapy. *Clin Pharmacol Ther* 1987;41:651–660.
44. Evans WE, Rodman JH, Relling MV, et al. Differences in teniposide disposition and pharmacodynamics in patients with newly diagnosed and relapsed acute lymphocytic leukemia. *J Pharmacol Exp Ther* 1992;260:71–77.
45. Powis G, Harris RN, Basseches PJ, et al. Effects of advanced leukemia on hepatic drug-metabolizing activity in the mouse. *Cancer Chemother Pharmacol* 1986;16:43–49.
46. Charles KA, Rivory LP, Brown SL, et al. Transcriptional repression of hepatic cytochrome P450 3A4 gene in the presence of cancer. *Clin Cancer Res* 2006;12:7492–7497.
47. Moore MM, Chua W, Charles KA, et al. Inflammation and cancer: causes and consequences. *Clin Pharmacol Ther* 2010;87:504–508.
48. Albekairy A, Alkatheri A, Fujita S, et al. Cytochrome P450 3A4FNx011B as pharmacogenomic predictor of tacrolimus pharmacokinetics and clinical outcome in the liver transplant recipients. *Saudi J Gastroenterol* 2013;19:89–95.
49. Franke RM, Carducci MA, Rudek MA, et al. Castration-dependent pharmacokinetics of docetaxel in patients with prostate cancer. *J Clin Oncol* 2010;28:4562–4567.
50. Rahman A, White RM. Cytotoxic anticancer agents and renal impairment study: the challenge remains. *J Clin Oncol* 2006;24:533–536.
51. Egorin MJ, Van Echo DA, Olman EA, et al. Prospective validation of a pharmacologically based dosing scheme for the cis-diamminedichloroplatinum(II) analogue diamminecyclobutanedicarboxylatoplatinum. *Cancer Res* 1985;45:6502–6506.
52. Calvert AH, Newell DR, Gumbrell LA, et al. Carboplatin dosage: prospective evaluation of a simple formula based on renal function. *J Clin Oncol* 1989;7:1748–1756.
53. Huang SM, Temple R, Xiao S, et al. When to conduct a renal impairment study during drug development: US Food and Drug Administration perspective. *Clin Pharmacol Ther* 2009;86:475–479.
54. Zhang Y, Zhang L, Abraham S, et al. Assessment of the impact of renal impairment on systemic exposure of new molecular entities: evaluation of recent new drug applications. *Clin Pharmacol Ther* 2009;85:305–311.
55. Gibbons J, Egorin MJ, Ramanathan RK, et al. Phase I and pharmacokinetic study of imatinib mesylate in patients with advanced malignancies and varying degrees of renal dysfunction: a study by the National Cancer Institute Organ Dysfunction Working Group. *J Clin Oncol* 2008;26:570–576.
56. Franke RM, Sparreboom A. Inhibition of imatinib transport by uremic toxins during renal failure. *J Clin Oncol* 2008;26:4226–4227.
57. Twelves C, Glynne-Jones R, Cassidy J, et al. Effect of hepatic dysfunction due to liver metastases on the pharmacokinetics of capecitabine and its metabolites. *Clin Cancer Res* 1999;5:1696–1702.
58. Eklund JW, Trifilio S, Mulcahy MF. Chemotherapy dosing in the setting of liver dysfunction. *Oncology (Williston Park)* 2005;19:1057–1063.
59. Hooker AC, Ten Tije AJ, Carducci MA, et al. Population pharmacokinetic model for docetaxel in patients with varying degrees of liver function: incorporating cytochrome P4503A activity measurements. *Clin Pharmacol Ther* 2008;84:111–118.
60. Grandison MK, Boudinot FD. Age-related changes in protein binding of drugs: implications for therapy. *Clin Pharmacokinet* 2000;38:271–290.
61. Sparreboom A, Nooter K, Loos WJ, et al. The (ir)relevance of plasma protein binding of anticancer drugs. *Neth J Med* 2001;59:196–207.
62. Perdaems N, Bachaud JM, Rouzaud P, et al. Relation between unbound plasma concentrations and toxicity in a prolonged oral etoposide schedule. *Eur J Clin Pharmacol* 1998;54:677–683.
63. Sparreboom A, van ZL, Brouwer E, et al. Cremophor EL-mediated alteration of paclitaxel distribution in human blood: clinical pharmacokinetic implications. *Cancer Res* 1999;59:1454–1457.
64. Gardner ER, Burger H, van Schaik RH, et al. Association of enzyme and transporter genotypes with the pharmacokinetics of imatinib. *Clin Pharmacol Ther* 2006;80:192–201.
65. Wu K, House L, Ramirez J, et al. Evaluation of utility of pharmacokinetic studies in phase I trials of two oncology drugs. *Clin Cancer Res* 2013;19:6039–6043.
66. Hu S, Mathijssen RH, de Bruijn P, et al. Inhibition of OATP1B1 by tyrosine kinase inhibitors: in vitro-in vivo correlations. *Br J Cancer* 2014;110(4):894–898.
67. Kehrer DF, Mathijssen RH, Verweij J, et al. Modulation of irinotecan metabolism by ketoconazole. *J Clin Oncol* 2002;20:3122–3129.
68. van Leeuwen RW, Brundel DH, Neef C, et al. Prevalence of potential drug-drug interactions in cancer patients treated with oral anticancer drugs. *Br J Cancer* 2013;108:1071–1078.
69. Budha NR, Frymoyer A, Smelick GS, et al. Drug absorption interactions between oral targeted anticancer agents and PPIs: is pH-dependent solubility the Achilles heel of targeted therapy? *Clin Pharmacol Ther* 2012;92:203–213.
70. Sparreboom A, Cox MC, Acharya MR, et al. Herbal remedies in the United States: potential adverse interactions with anticancer agents. *J Clin Oncol* 2004;22:2489–2503.
71. Dy GK, Bekele L, Hanson LJ, et al. Complementary and alternative medicine use by patients enrolled onto phase I clinical trials. *J Clin Oncol* 2004;22:4810–4815.
72. Goey AK, Mooiman KD, Beijnen JH, et al. Relevance of in vitro and clinical data for predicting CYP3A4-mediated herb-drug interactions in cancer patients. *Cancer Treat Rev* 2013;39:773–783.
73. Mathijssen RH, Verweij J, De Bruijn P, et al. Effects of St. John's wort on irinotecan metabolism. *J Natl Cancer Inst* 2002;94:1247–1249.
74. Cox MC, Low J, Lee J, et al. Influence of garlic (Allium sativum) on the pharmacokinetics of docetaxel. *Clin Cancer Res* 2006;12:4636–4640.
75. van Erp NP, Baker SD, Zhao M, et al. Effect of milk thistle (*Silybum marianum*) on the pharmacokinetics of irinotecan. *Clin Cancer Res* 2005;11:7800–7806.
76. Wheeler HE, Maitland ML, Dolan ME, et al. Cancer pharmacogenomics: strategies and challenges. *Nat Rev Genet* 2013;14:23–34.
77. Fujita K, Sparreboom A. Pharmacogenetics of irinotecan disposition and toxicity: a review. *Curr Clin Pharmacol* 2010;5:209–217.
78. Huang RS, Ratain MJ. Pharmacogenetics and pharmacogenomics of anticancer agents. *CA Cancer J Clin* 2009;59:42–55.
79. Evans WE, McLeod HL. Pharmacogenomics—drug disposition, drug targets, and side effects. *N Engl J Med* 2003;348:538–549.

80. Sparreboom A, Danesi R, Ando Y, et al. Pharmacogenomics of ABC transporters and its role in cancer chemotherapy. *Drug Resist Updat* 2003;6:71–84.
81. Cusatis G, Gregorc V, Li J, et al. Pharmacogenetics of ABCG2 and adverse reactions to gefitinib. *J Natl Cancer Inst* 2006;98:1739–1742.
82. Kim RB. Organic anion-transporting polypeptide (OATP) transporter family and drug disposition. *Eur J Clin Invest* 2003;33 Suppl 2:1–5.
83. Smith NF, Figg WD, Sparreboom A. Role of the liver-specific transporters OATP1B1 and OATP1B3 in governing drug elimination. *Exp Opin Drug Metab Toxicol* 2005;1:429–445.
84. Sprowl JA, Mikkelsen TS, Giovinazzo H, et al. Contribution of tumoral and host solute carriers to clinical drug response. *Drug Resist Updat* 2012;15:5–20.
85. Kim DH, Sriharsha L, Xu W, et al. Clinical relevance of a pharmacogenetic approach using multiple candidate genes to predict response and resistance to imatinib therapy in chronic myeloid leukemia. *Clin Cancer Res* 2009;15:4750–4758.
86. Canal P, Chatelut E, Guichard S. Practical treatment guide for dose individualisation in cancer chemotherapy. *Drugs* 1998;56:1019–1038.
87. Evans WE, Relling MV, Rodman JH, et al. Conventional compared with individualized chemotherapy for childhood acute lymphoblastic leukemia. *N Engl J Med* 1998;338:499–505.
88. Blasdel C, Egorin MJ, Lagattuta TF, et al. Therapeutic drug monitoring in CML patients on imatinib. *Blood* 2007;110:1699–1701.
89. Larson RA, Druker BJ, Guilhot F, et al. Imatinib pharmacokinetics and its correlation with response and safety in chronic-phase chronic myeloid leukemia: a subanalysis of the IRIS study. *Blood* 2008;111:4022–4028.
90. Picard S, Titier K, Etienne G, et al. Trough imatinib plasma levels are associated with both cytogenetic and molecular responses to standard-dose imatinib in chronic myeloid leukemia. *Blood* 2007;109:3496–3499.
91. Blanchet B, Billemont B, Cramard J, et al. Validation of an HPLC-UV method for sorafenib determination in human plasma and application to cancer patients in routine clinical practice. *J Pharm Biomed Anal* 2009;49:1109–1114.
92. Chatelut E, Canal P, Brunner V, et al. Prediction of carboplatin clearance from standard morphological and biological patient characteristics. *J Natl Cancer Inst* 1995;87:573–580.
93. Bruno R, Hille D, Riva A, et al. Population pharmacokinetics/pharmacodynamics of docetaxel in phase II studies in patients with cancer. *J Clin Oncol* 1998;16:187–196.
94. Gallo JM, Laub PB, Rowinsky EK, et al. Population pharmacokinetic model for topotecan derived from phase I clinical trials. *J Clin Oncol* 2000;18:2459–2467.
95. Li J, Karlsson MO, Brahmer J, et al. CYP3A phenotyping approach to predict systemic exposure to EGFR tyrosine kinase inhibitors. *J Natl Cancer Inst* 2006;98:1714–1723.
96. Lu JF, Eppler SM, Wolf J, et al. Clinical pharmacokinetics of erlotinib in patients with solid tumors and exposure-safety relationship in patients with non-small cell lung cancer. *Clin Pharmacol Ther* 2006;80:136–145.
97. Mathijssen RH, de Jong FA, Loos WJ, et al. Flat-fixed dosing versus body surface area based dosing of anticancer drugs in adults: does it make a difference? *Oncologist* 2007;12:913–923.

16 Pharmacogenomics

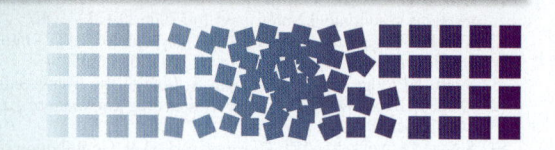

Christine M. Walko and Howard L. McLeod

INTRODUCTION

The evolution of understanding cancer biology has yielded many advances that have been translated into cancer treatment. Application of this knowledge has allowed for a shift in chemotherapeutics from traditional cytotoxic agents that worked by killing both healthy and malignant fast growing cells to chemical and biologic therapies aimed at targeting a specific gene or pathway critical to the particular cancer being treated.[1] This age of pathway-directed therapy has been made possible by the increased availability and feasibility of high throughput technology able to provide comprehensive and clinically useful molecular characterization of tumors. Translation of these efforts have resulted in improved degree to disease control for many common cancers including breast, colorectal, lung, and melanoma as well as long-term survival benefits for chronic myelogenous leukemia (CML), gastrointestinal stromal tumors (GIST), and childhood acute lymphoblastic leukemia (ALL).[2]

Pharmacogenomic-guided therapy aims the use information on DNA and RNA integrity to optimize not only the treatment choice for an individual patient, but also the dose and schedule of that treatment. The assessment of both somatic and germ-line mutations contribute to the overall individualization of cancer treatment. Somatic mutations are genetic variations found within the tumor DNA, but not DNA from the normal (germ-line) tissues, which also have functional consequences that influence disease outcomes and/or response to certain therapies. These types of mutations or biomarkers can be classified as either prognostic or predictive. Prognostic biomarkers identify subpopulations of patients with different disease courses or outcomes, independent of treatment. Predictive biomarkers identify subpopulations of patients most likely to have a response to a given therapy.[3] Germ-line mutations are heritable variations found within the individual and, in practical terms, are focused on DNA markers predictive for toxicity or therapeutic outcomes of a particular therapy as well as inheritable risk of certain cancers.[4] Pharmacogenomic mutations in the germ line provide some explanation for the interindividual and interracial variability in drug response and toxicity. For cancer chemotherapy, where cytotoxic agents are administered at doses close to their maximal tolerable dose, and therapeutic windows are relatively narrow, minor differences in individual drug handling may lead to severe toxicities. Therefore, an understanding of the sources of this variability would lead to the possibility of individualizing dosages or influencing clinical decisions that can improve patient care. Pharmacogenomics has putative utility in therapy selection, clinical study design, and as a tool to improve understanding of the pharmacology of a medication.

The term *pharmacogenetics* was initially used to define inherited differences in drug effects and typically focused on individual candidate genes. The field of pharmacogenomics now includes genomewide association studies and is used to describe genetic variations in all aspects of drug absorption, distribution, metabolism, and excretion in addition to drug targets and their downstream pathways.[5] Table 16.1 illustrates some current clinical examples of genotype-guided cancer chemotherapy. Variations in the DNA sequences encoding these proteins may take the form of deletions, insertions, repeats, frameshift mutations, nonsense mutations, and missense mutations, resulting in an inactive, truncated, unstable, or otherwise dysfunctional protein. The most common change involves single nucleotide substitutions, called single-nucleotide polymorphisms (SNP), which occur at approximately 1 per 1,000 base pairs on the human genome. Variability in toxicity or activity can also be mediated by postgenomic events, at the level of RNA, protein, or functional activity.

PHARMACOGENOMICS OF TUMOR RESPONSE

Tumor response to chemotherapy is regulated by a complex, multigenic network of genes that encompasses inherent characteristics of the tumor, differentially activated pathways of cell signaling, proliferation and DNA repair, factors that control drug delivery to the tumor cells (e.g., metabolism, transport), and cell death. These may in turn be modulated by previously administered treatment or drug exposure, which may upregulate target proteins or activate alternative pathways of drug resistance. The polygenic nature of drug response implies that a better understanding of genotype–phenotype associations would require more than the usual single-gene pharmacogenetic strategies employed to date. However, there are instances where the genomic context of a single gene within a cancer will be of high impact for specific therapeutic agents (see Table 16.1).

Pathway Directed Anticancer Therapy

One of the earliest success stories illustrating pathway-driven therapeutics is with CML. The hallmark chromosomal abnormality of this disease is the translocation of chromosomes 9 and 22 that ultimately produces the fusion gene *BCR-ABL*. This discovery in 1960 eventually led to the development of the targeted tyrosine-kinase inhibitor (TKI) imatinib and its subsequent Food and Drug Administration (FDA) approval for treatment of CML in 2001.[6] The International Randomized Study of Interferon and STI571 (IRIS) trial began enrollment in 2000 and compared imatinib with interferon and low-dose cytarabine, which was the previous standard of care for newly diagnosed patients with chronic-phase CML. All efficacy endpoints favored imatinib, including complete cytogenetic response of 76.2% with imatinib compared with 14.5% with interferon (p <0.001).[7] Overall survival (OS) after 60 months of follow-up was 89% with imatinib.[8] This example is just one of many where a once fatal disease can now be considered more akin to a chronic disease, requiring a daily medication and regular physician follow-up, similar to hypertension or diabetes. Drug development has also kept pace with these advances and now several other agents, including dasatinib, nilotinib, bosutinib, and ponatinib, have joined imatinib as treatment options for CML.

The idea of changing treatment focus from a disease-based model to a pathway-driven model is also evolving. Human epidermal

TABLE 16.1
Clinical Examples of Genotype-Guided Cancer Chemotherapy

Somatic Mutation Examples

Drug Target	Drug(s)	Malignancy
EML4-ALK	Crizotinib	Non–small-cell lung cancer
BCR-ABL	Dasatinib, imatinib, nilotinib, bosutinib, ponatinib	Chronic myelogenous leukemia
BRAF	Vemurafenib, dabrafenib	Melanoma
Epidermal growth factor receptor (EGFR)	Erlotinib, afatinib	Non–small-cell lung cancer
HER2	Trastuzumab, lapatinib, pertuzumab, Ado-trastuzumab emtansine	Breast cancer, gastric cancer
Janus kinase 2 (JAK2)	Ruxolitinib	Myelofibrosis
Kirsten rat sarcoma viral oncogene (KRAS)	Cetuximab, panitumumab	Colorectal cancer
Rearranged during transfection (RET)	Vandetanib	Medullary thyroid cancer

Germ-Line Mutation Examples

Gene Mutation	Drug	Effect
Cytochrome P450 (CYP) 2C19	Voriconazole	Decreased serum levels of active drug and potential decreased efficacy in patients with high enzyme levels (ultrarapid metabolizers)
CYP2D6	Tamoxifen, codeine, ondansetron	Decreased production of active metabolite and potential decreased efficacy in patients with low enzyme levels
Dihydropyrimidine dehydrogenase (DPYD)	5-Fluorouracil	Decreased elimination and increased risk of myelosuppression, diarrhea, and mucositis in patients with low enzyme levels
Glucose-6-phosphate dehydrogenase (G6PD)	Rasburicase	Risk of severe hemolysis in patients with G6PD deficiency
Thiopurine methyltransferase (TPMT)	Mercaptopurine, thioguanine, azathioprine	Decreased methylation of the active metabolite resulting decreased elimination and increased risk of neutropenia in patients with low enzyme levels
UDP-glucuronosyltransferase (UGT) 1A1	Irinotecan	Decreased glucuronidation of the active metabolite resulting decreased elimination and increased risk of neutropenia and diarrhea in patients with low enzyme levels

growth factor receptor 2 (HER2) is a transmembrane tyrosine kinase that is overexpressed or amplified in up to 25% of breast cancers. Trastuzumab is a humanized monoclonal antibody directed against HER2 and demonstrated improved response rates (RR) and time to disease progression in patients with metastatic HER2 positive breast cancer and improved disease-free survival (DFS) and OS in HER2-positive breast cancer patients treated with adjuvant trastuzumab.[9] Several additional agents are now available to target the HER2 pathway and vary in their pharmacology and mechanism of action. Lapatinib is an oral TKI directed against HER2 and the epidermal growth factor receptor (EGFR), pertuzumab is a humanized monoclonal antibody that binds at a different location than trastuzumab and inhibits the dimerization and subsequent activation of HER2 signaling, and ado-trastuzumab emtansine is an antibody-drug conjugate that targets HER2-positive cells and then releases the cytotoxic antimitotic agent emtansine through liposomal degradation of the linking compound. All of these agents illustrate the progress and pharmacologic diversity of pathway-directed therapy and remain as standard of care options for HER2-positive breast cancer in either the adjuvant and/or metastatic settings.[10] HER2 expression is not limited to breast cancer, however. Though less common, HER2 expression is seen in numerous solid tumors including bladder, gastric, prostate and non–small-cell lung cancer with varying degrees of incidence depending on the method of detection. Based on results from a large, open-label phase III randomized, international trial of 594 patients with gastric or gastroesophageal junction cancer expressing HER2 by either immunohistochemistry or gene amplification by fluorescence in situ hybridization, trastuzumab is also approved for treatment of metastatic gastric or gastroesophageal junction adenocarcinoma that expresses HER2. Patients randomized to chemotherapy in combination with trastuzumab had a median OS of 13.8 months compared with 11.1 months in the patients receiving chemotherapy alone (hazard ratio [HR], 0.74; 0.60 to 0.91, $p = 0.0046$).[11] Numerous examples also support that pathway-directed therapy will cross the boundaries of disease sites and that tumor genetics will become one of the biggest determining factors for treatment.

Simple expression of the drug target does not always translate into desired clinical outcomes though. Cetuximab and panitumumab are monoclonal antibodies directed against EGFR; however, it was found that colorectal cancer (CRC) patients who did not have detectable EGFR still experienced responses to these agents similar in extent to EGFR-positive patients. Kirsten rat sarcoma viral oncogene (KRAS) is a downstream effector of the EGFR pathway. Ligand binding to EGFR on the cell surface activates pathway signaling through the KRAS-RAF-mitogen-activated protein kinase (MAPK) pathway, which is thought to control cell growth, differentiation, and apoptosis.[12] Eventually it was found that CRC patients with a KRAS mutation did not derive benefit from cetuximab or panitumumab. The RR in CRC receiving either cetuximab or panitumumab who were KRAS wild type was 10% to 40% compared with near zero percent in those with KRAS mutations.[13] This finding was the result of a retrospective analysis of small group of patients and was confirmed in large, prospective trials. Additionally, it underscores the importance of tissue collection for biomarker assessment in trials with novel therapeutics. A recent clinical trial genomic analysis suggests that mutations in NRAS may also have value in predicting the utility of EGFR antibody therapy in colorectal cancer. Although the predictive value of KRAS mutation status in colorectal cancer has been well established in clinical trials, the role of KRAS in lung cancer and other malignancies is less well elucidated. Lung cancers harboring KRAS mutations have been shown to have less clinical benefit from the EGFR-targeted erlotinib in some trials, although this has not consistently been the case across all trials. Additionally, lung cancer KRAS mutation status does not appear to reproducibly predict clinical benefit from the EGFR-targeted monoclonal antibodies, as is the case in colorectal cancer.[14] Unlike the HER2 example discussed previously, the clinical application of some genetic mutations will differ between tissue of origin.

Deeper investigations and understandings of mutations driving oncogenic pathways can also elucidate mechanisms of resistance and practical therapeutic strategies for treatment and prevention. Approximately half of all cutaneous melanomas carry mutations in BRAF, with the most common being the V600E mutation. Vemurafenib is a TKI directed against mutated BRAF that demonstrated improvements in both progression-free survival (PFS) and OS when compared with the cytotoxic agent dacarbazine in previously untreated patients with metastatic melanoma carrying the BRAF V600E mutation. Vemurafenib demonstrated a 63% relative reduction in the risk of death compared with dacarbazine (p <0.001) along with a higher response rate (48% compared with 5% for dacarbazine).[15] Based on these results, vemurafenib was the first BRAF targeted TKI approved by the FDA and was soon joined by dabrafenib. Although dramatic responses to these agents have been observed, relapse almost universally occurs after a median of 6 to 8 months. Activating BRAF mutations, like V600E, result in uncontrolled activity of the MAPK pathway through activation of the downstream kinase MEK, which when phosphorylated, subsequently activates extracellular signal-regulated kinase (ERK), which ultimately translocates to the cell nucleus, resulting in cell proliferation and survival (Fig. 16.1).[16] An assessment of serial biopsies from patients treated with vemurafenib suggested numerous mechanisms for acquired resistance, including the appearance of secondary mutations in MEK.[17] This finding supports the clinical rationale for using combination therapy with a BRAF and a MEK inhibitor. The combination of dabrafenib (BRAF inhibitor) and trametinib (MEK inhibitor) was assessed in 247 metastatic melanoma patients with BRAF V600 mutations compared with dabrafenib alone. Median PFS was 9.4 months in the combination group compared with 5.8 months in the patients who received single agent therapy (HR, 0.39; 0.25 to 0.62, p <0.001). A complete or partial response was also higher in the combination therapy group (76% compared with 54%, p = 0.03). The occurrence of cutaneous squamous cell carcinoma, a known side effect of single-agent BRAF inhibitor therapy due to paradoxical activation of RAF in nonmutated cells, was also decreased in the combination therapy group (7% compared with 19%, p = 0.09), further supporting the evidence of downstream inhibition.[18] Although combination therapy does prolong the time to disease progression, resistance still occurs in patients through a variety of mechanisms. Utilization of sequential biopsies and a genetic assessment will help to inform rationale combination and sequential pathway-driven therapy trials that will ultimately aid in better understanding and mitigation of common mechanism of resistance.

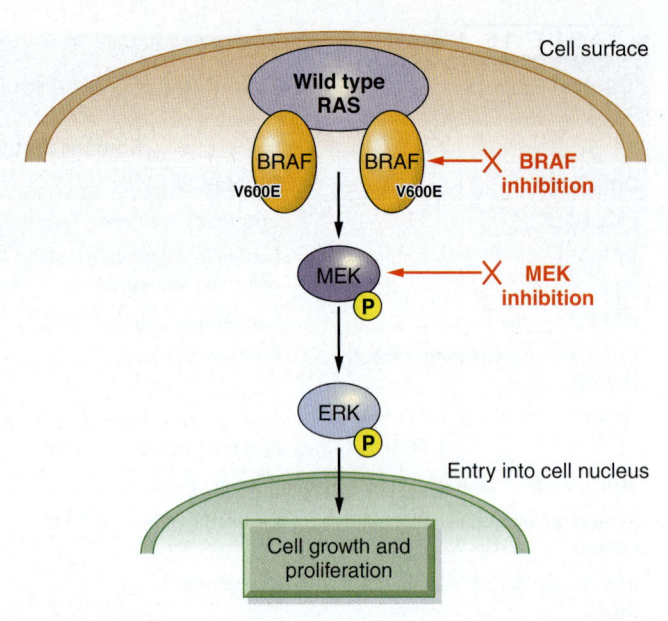

Figure 16.1 MAPK pathway in BRAF mutated melanoma. The BRAF V600E mutation results in activation of the MAPK pathway independent of growth factor binding, initially by phosphorylation (P) of MEK. MEK subsequently phosphorylates ERK. ERK then translocates to the cell nucleus and causes transcription of cellular factors, resulting in cell proliferation and survival. Because one mechanism of resistance to BRAF inhibition is through mutations in MEK, inhibition at both the upstream target of BRAF and the downstream site of MEK can prolong the clinical benefit of the BRAF inhibitor.

Although advances in basic science and drug development have translated many oncogenic driver mutations across tumor types into pathway-directed therapy, this is not the case for the majority. There are numerous examples of functionally relevant recurrent driver mutations that affect protein targets that are not currently druggable. Regardless of malignancy, one of the most commonly mutated tumor suppressors is the protein p53. Mutations can result in p53 acquiring oncogenic functions that enable proliferation, invasion, metastasis, and cell survival as well as coordinating with different proteins, such as EGFR, to enhance or inhibit its effects. However, a clinical application of p53 mutation data or directly targeting p53 has been limited, to date.[19] PIK3CA encodes a catalytic subunit of phophoinositol-3 kinase (PI3K), which includes four distinct subfamily kinases involved in regulating cell growth, motility, proliferation, and survival. Direct inhibitors of the kinase, as well as downstream targets, including AKT (protein kinase B [PKB]) and mammalian target of rapamycin (mTOR), are being assessed to target these mutations. Therapeutic challenges include understanding the complex signaling network germane to each cancer and the role of kinases in each subfamily.[20] Both the examples of p53 and PI3K illustrate the challenge of translating the multitude of somatic mutations into applications of available therapeutic agents.

Application of Genomewide Gene Expression Profiling to Guide Therapy

Single gene approaches may not reflect the overall complexity of genetic regulation of chemotherapy responses. Genomic strategies using global gene expression data are able to provide a more complete picture of the tumor through disease classification.[21] These strategies may identify subgroups of patients with early disease that need adjuvant chemotherapy, those who will not benefit from standard therapy, or help with the selection of chemotherapy from a menu of potentially active agents. Oncotype Dx is a 21-gene assay with 16 tumor-associated genes and 5 reference genes used to predict the risk of distant local recurrence in estrogen receptor (ER)-positive, HER2-negative patients with node-negative or select node-positive breast cancer. Additionally, the test also provides predictive information on which patients may benefit from the addition of chemotherapy to hormonal therapy alone. The test ultimately reports a recurrence score (RS) on a continuous scale from zero to 100. Patients with an RS <18 are considered low risk, with a 10-year distant recurrence rate (DRR) of 6.8% (95% confidence interval [CI], 4 to 9.6); RS scores of 18 to 30 are at intermediate risk, with a 10-year DRR of 14.3% (CI, 8.3 to 20.3); and RS scores ≥31 are at high risk, with a 10-year DRR of 30.5% (CI, 23.6 to 37.4).[22] Additionally, high-risk patients have the largest benefit from the addition of chemotherapy to hormonal therapy (HR, 0.26; 0.13 to 0.53), whereas low-risk patients have little benefit from the addition of chemotherapy and could consider hormonal treatment alone (HR, 1.31; 0.46 to 3.78). Intermediate risk patients are harder to classify, and clinical trials are underway to further address treatment recommendations for this group of patients.[23] These type of assays are also in development and in clinical trials for a variety of other solid tumor and hematologic malignancies.

Genetic-Guided Therapy Practical Issues in Somatic Analysis

Currently, targeted DNA capture is the most common type of somatic genetic screening and involves focusing on a few relevant candidate genes followed by deeper sequencing. These types of techniques can reveal common genes associated with a particular malignancy but also may uncover a signaling pathway that would not be obviously associated with a particular histology or tumor site. Application of a next-generation sequencing assay in 40 CRC and 24 non–small-cell lung cancer (NSCLC) tissue samples that assessed 145 cancer-relevant genes demonstrated that somatic mutations were seen in 98% of the CRC tumors and 83% of the NSCLCs (Fig. 16.2).[24] The evolution of sequencing strategies and decreasing costs has made whole genome sequencing more available in the clinical setting, and several companies offer commercially available tumor profiling services. Several limitations exist that currently restrict the broad clinical implementation of these assays, however. Although germ-line genetic assessments can be done on a peripheral blood sample or buccal swab, somatic assessments typically require biopsy tissue, which is often in limited supply and of varying quality or may not be feasible depending on the site of the cancer. Ongoing studies are assessing the value of liquid biopsies of circulating tumor DNA.[25] Optimizing and creating uniformity in quality control of gene panel or whole-genome assessment is also needed to decrease the reporting of uncertain or erroneous identification of mutations. Once sequencing is completed, a predictive analysis is needed for the 25% to 80% of instances where variants of unknown significance are identified in genes of interest. Translation of genomic sequencing into clinical practice will require a diverse team, including pathologists, medical oncologists, surgical oncologists, information technologists, geneticists, and pharmacologists.

PHARMACOGENOMICS OF CHEMOTHERAPY DRUG TOXICITY

A drug's disposition and pharmacodynamic effects can be influenced by a number of variables, including patient age, diet, concomitant medications, and underlying disease processes. However, an individual's genetic constitution is an important regulator of variability in drug effect. Differences in drug effects are more pronounced between individuals compared to within an individual. Indeed, studies in monozygotic and dizygotic twins identified that 20% to 80% of the variation in drug disposition is mediated by inheritance.[26] Drug-metabolizing enzymes, cellular transporters, and tissue receptors are governed by genetic variation.

Advances in the treatment of most common malignancies have resulted in the availability of multiple distinct combination chemotherapy regimens with similar or equal anticancer efficacy. Therefore, differences in systemic toxicity have become a major determinant in the selection of therapy. The majority of pharmacogenomic examples affecting adverse events or efficacy from cytotoxic drugs involve hepatic metabolizing enzymes that detoxify or biotransform xenobiotics.[27,28]

Thiopurine Methyltransferase

One of the best-studied pharmacogenetic syndrome involves the metabolism of the thiopurine drugs—6-mercaptopurine (6MP), 6-thioguanine, and azathioprine—which have wide applications, including maintenance therapy for childhood ALL and adult leukemias. These prodrugs must be activated to thioguanine nucleotides in order to have antiproliferative effects. However, most of the variability in the formation of active metabolites is mediated by methylation via thiopurine methyltransferase (TPMT).[29] TPMT is a cytosolic enzyme that catalyzes S-methylation of thiopurine agents, resulting in an inactive metabolite. Erythrocyte TPMT activity has a trimodal distribution, with 90% of patients having high activity, 10% intermediate activity, and 0.3% with very low or no detectable activity. TPMT deficiency results in higher intracellular activation of 6MP to form thioguanine nucleotides, resulting in severe or fatal hematologic toxicity from standard doses of therapy.[30] The variable activity results from polymorphism in the TPMT gene, located on chromosome locus 6p22.3. Genetic variants at codon 238 (TPMT*2), codon 719 (TPMT*3C), or both codons 460 and 719 (TPMT*3A) are the most clinically significant, accounting for 95% of the patients with reduced TPMT activity.[31] Heterozygotes (one wild type and one variant allele) are common (10% of patients), and have elevated levels of active metabolites (twofold more than homozygous wild type), and required more cumulative dose reductions of 6MP for maintenance ALL chemotherapy compared to homozygous wild-type patients (Fig. 16.3).[32] Patients with a homozygous variant TPMT genotype are at a fourfold risk of severe toxicity, compared with wild-type patients.[31] TPMT genotype tests are now available commercially in a Clinical Laboratory Improvement Amendments (CLIA)-certified environment. To date, patients homozygous for TPMT variant alleles appear to tolerate 10%, and heterozygotes appear to tolerate 65% of the recommended doses of 6MP, with no apparent

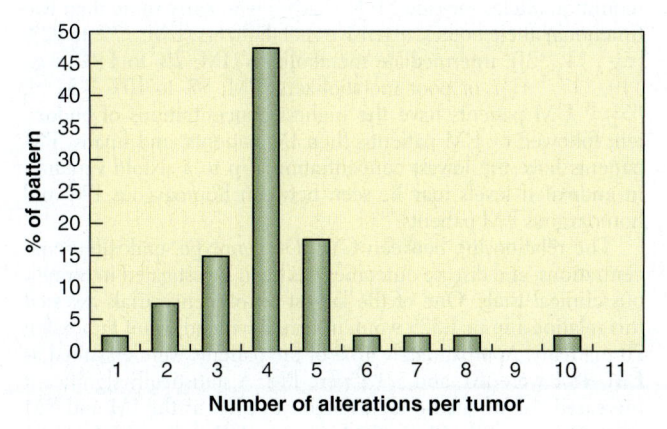

Figure 16.2 Number of alterations per tumor. Deep sequencing of 145 genes in 40 colorectal cancers found a spectrum of incidence of somatic mutations, with more than half occurring in genes that are *druggable* with medication that is either FDA approved or in late stage clinical development.

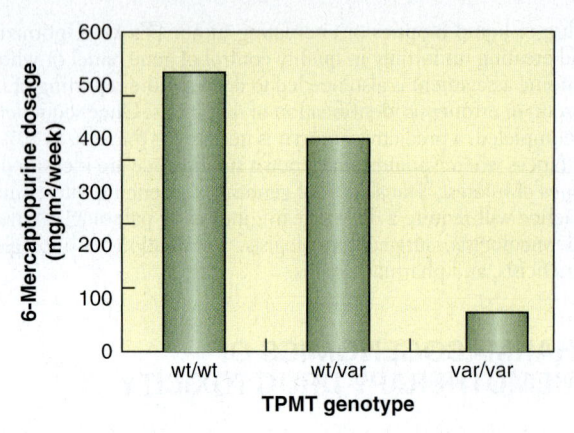

Figure 16.3 Relationship between TPMT genotype and required 6MP dose. Compared with homozygous wild-type patients, those heterozygous for a thiopurine methyltransferase (TPMT) variant allele generally require at least a 30% dose reduction in 6MP, whereas homozygous variant patients require substantial dose reductions of approximately 90% that of wild-type patients.

decrease in clinical efficacy (Fig. 16.3).[32] This has formed the basis for prospective, TPMT genotype-guided dosing of 6MP to avoid severe toxicity. Clinical Pharmacogenomics Implementation Consortium (CPIC) Guidelines recommend that homozygous wild-type patients be started at the full standard dose. Heterozygous patients should start with reduced doses at 30% to 70% of the full dose with adjustments made after 2 to 4 weeks based on myelosuppression and disease-specific guidelines. Homozygous variant patients should start with 10% of the full dose due to the extremely high levels of the active metabolite and potential for fatal toxicity at standard doses. Adjustments should be made after 4 to 6 weeks based on myelosuppression and disease-specific guidelines.[33]

Dihydropyrimidine Dehydrogenase (DPD)

Although 5-fluorouracil (5FU) has been available for over 40 years, it remains the cornerstone of colorectal cancer chemotherapy, both in the adjuvant and metastatic settings. Additionally, the oral prodrug capecitabine ultimately undergoes activation to 5FU and is commonly used in gastrointestinal and breast malignancies. 5FU is a prodrug that is activated intracellularly to 5-fluoro-2′-deoxyuridine monophosphate (5FdUMP), which inhibits thymidylate synthase (TS), among other mechanisms of action. TS inhibition results in impaired de novo pyrimidine synthesis and suppression of DNA synthesis. Approximately 85% of a 5FU dose is catabolized by dihydropyrimidine dehydrogenase (DPD) to inactive metabolites. Therefore, DPD is a primary regulator of 5FU activity. DPD deficiency has been described, resulting in higher 5FU blood levels, greater formation of active metabolites, and severe or fatal clinical toxicity, predominately myelosuppression, mucositis, and cerebellar toxicity.[34] In theory, this toxicity could be reduced or avoided by screening for DPD activity in surrogate tissues, such as peripheral mononuclear cells. However, the technical requirements for preparation of these samples make it impractical for many practice sites. Understanding the molecular basis for DPD deficiency will provide an approach for prospective identification of patients at high risk for severe 5FU toxicity. The gene encoding DPD is composed of 23 exons, and at least 23 SNPs have been found.[35] Studies in DPD-deficient patients have identified several distinct molecular variants associated with low enzyme activity. Many of these are rare, and base substitutions, splicing defects, and frame shift mutations, have been described. The prevalent variation is the splice recognition site in intron 14 (DPYD*2A), where a G to A substitution results in the skipping of exon 14, resulting in an inactive enzyme.[36–38] This polymorphism has been associated with severe DPD deficiency in heterozygous patients, with a homozygous genotype associated with a mental retardation syndrome. Patients with severe 5FU toxicity may harbor one or more variant alleles of DPD, and a recent study showed that 61% of cancer patients experiencing severe 5FU toxicities had decreased DPD activity in peripheral mononuclear cells, and DPYD*2A was commonly found.[39] In the patients with grade 4 neutropenia, 50% harbored at least one DPYD*2A. It is estimated that in the Caucasian population, homozygotes for the variant alleles have an incidence of 0.1% and heterozygotes occur at an incidence of 0.5% to 2%. There are additional DPD mutations that have been associated with impaired enzyme activity, including DPYD *3 and DPYD*13. CPIC guidelines recommend standard dosing for homozygous wild-type patients. Reducing the dose by at least 50% in heterozygous patients (*1/*2A) is recommended, followed by dose adjustment based on toxicity and/or pharmacokinetic testing. The use of an alternative agent is recommended in homozygous-variant patients (*2A/*2A).[34] There are many patients with severe 5FU toxicity that have normal DPD activity. This highlights that many factors, including multiple genes, are potential causes of 5FU toxicity, and there will not be one simple test to avoid this important clinical problem.

Cytochrome P450 2D6

Tamoxifen is a selective estrogen-receptor modulator used in ER-positive breast cancer in both the localized and metastatic settings. It is the drug of choice for premenopausal women and is a treatment option, along with aromatase inhibitors, for postmenopausal women. The low cost of tamoxifen also makes it a preferred therapy regardless of menopausal status in numerous countries. Tamoxifen metabolism is complex, with extensive metabolism through numerous phase I and II enzymes that produce several primary and secondary metabolites and their corresponding isomers, each possessing different antiestrogen effects.[40] The primary active metabolite is believed to be endoxifen, which is produced by the CYP3A4/5 mediated-conversion of tamoxifen to N-desmethyltamoxifen, which is then further converted to endoxifen (4-hydroxy-N-desmethyltamoxifen) via cytochrome P450 2D6 (CYP2D6). A direct relationship between endoxifen concentration and its antiestrogen effects has been demonstrated, potentially suggesting that a threshold concentration may be needed for optimal clinical effect.[41] CYP2D6 is highly polymorphic, with more than 80 allelic CYP2D6 variants described. These alleles vary in enzyme activity and prevalence with respect to race and ethnicity.[42] Based on genotype, patients can be classified by phenotype into ultrarapid metabolizers (UM; approximately 1% to 2% of patients [common alleles include *1xN, *2xN]) who carry more than two functional allele copies, extensive metabolizers (EM; 77% to 92% [e.g., *1, *2]), intermediate metabolizers (IM; 2% to 11% [e.g., *10, *17, *41]), or poor metabolizers (PM; 5% to 10% [*3, *4, *5]).[43] UM patients have the highest concentrations of endoxifen, followed by EM patients, then IM patients, and finally, PM patients have the lowest concentration. Up to a sixfold variation in endoxifen levels may be seen between homozygous PM and homozygous EM patients.[40]

The relationship between CYP2D6 genotype, endoxifen concentrations, and disease outcomes has been investigated in numerous clinical trials. One of the largest retrospective trials assessed this relationship in 1,325 women treated with adjuvant tamoxifen 20 mg daily. Approximately 46% of the patients were classified as EM, 48% were IM, and 5.9% were PM. A statistically significant increased risk of disease recurrence was seen in the IM and PM patients compared with the EM patients (HR, 1.40; 95% CI, 1.04 to 1.90 for IM; and HR 1.90, 95% CI, 1.10 to 3.28 for PM).[44] A large meta-analysis of 4,973 tamoxifen-treated patients across 12 international studies conducted by the International Tamoxifen Pharmacogenomics Consortium also supported this relationship.

CYP2D6 PM phenotypes were associated with decreased DFS (HR 1.25, 95% CI, 1.06 to 1.47, p = 0.009) when only considering the data from trials with postmenopausal women with ER-positive breast cancer who received tamoxifen 20 mg daily for 5 years.[45]

Not all trial results have been consistent, however, and dosing guidelines for genotype-guided therapy do not yet exist. Clinical trials do support the potential for genotype-guided therapy. IM patients who received an increased dose of 40 mg daily instead of the standard 20 mg were shown to have endoxifen concentrations similar to that of EM patients (p = 0.25).[46] This suggests that genotype-guided therapy with increased dose recommendations may be feasible, but additional prospective trials are needed to determine the clinical efficacy of this intervention.

CONCLUSIONS AND FUTURE DIRECTIONS

Genomic-driven cancer medicine is being translated into clinical practice through increased understanding of somatic mutations in a specific tumor that can be translated to pathway-directed therapeutics as well as germ-line mutations that affect the pharmacokinetics and pharmacodynamics of individual medications. For the practicing oncologist, knowledge of pharmacogenomics is necessary because therapeutic decisions of drug selection and dosage are being based on more molecularly and genetically defined variables than the current phenotypic information of tumor type, immunohistochemistry, and body surface area. Health-care policy changes preferring the bundling of care and reimbursement based on diagnosis coding may further drive individualized therapy where the goal is to optimize both treatment responses while minimizing toxicity. However, with advances always come challenges. Reimbursement for multiplex genomic testing is not universal, so deciding who and when to initiate testing is a consideration. Optimizing turnaround time, especially for referral patients who have had biopsies performed elsewhere, will require requesting this archived tissue prior to or during the initial patient visit to facilitate minimizing treatment delays. Although some variants have strong evidence supporting treatment recommendations, many currently do not yet. Multidisciplinary committees charged with reviewing the level of evidence for each genetic result and providing clinically actionable recommendations will be essential for translating these multigene tumor assay results into routine clinical practice. Decision tools and development of treatment guidelines will further assist with routine integration of this technology, especially for oncologists at smaller practice sites. Oncology fellowship training programs will also need to be expanded to ensure competence of new practitioners in the area of genomic-guided therapies.

Regardless of these challenges, the treatment paradigm of genomic-driven medicine and individualizing therapy has permitted the field of oncology to move beyond the limitations of nonselective cytotoxic therapy and toward the more optimal selection and dosing of oncology agents.

REFERENCES

1. McLeod HL. Cancer pharmacogenomics: early promise, but concerted effort needed. *Science* 2013;339:1563–1566.
2. Garraway LA. Genomics-driven oncology: framework for an emerging paradigm. *J Clin Oncol* 2013;31:1806–1814.
3. Mandrekar SJ, Sargent DJ. Predictive biomarker validation in practice: lessons from real trials. *Clin Trials* 2010;7:567–573.
4. Evans WE, Relling MV. Pharmacogenomics: translating functional genomics into rational therapeutics. *Science* 1999;286:487–491.
5. Wang L, McLeod HL, Weinshilboum RM. Genomics and drug response. *N Engl J Med* 2011;364:1144–1153.
6. Druker BJ. Translation of the Philadelphia chromosome into therapy for CML. *Blood* 2008;112:4808–4817.
7. O'Brien SG, Guilhot F, Larson RA, et al. Imatinib compared with interferon and low-dose cytarabine for newly diagnosed chronic-phase chronic myeloid leukemia. *N Engl J Med* 2003;348:994–1004.
8. Druker BJ, Guilhot F, O'Brien SG, et al. Five-year follow-up of patients receiving imatinib for chronic myeloid leukemia. *N Engl J Med* 2006;355:2408–2417.
9. Hudis CA. Trastuzumab—mechanism of action and use in clinical practice. *N Engl J Med* 2007;357:39–51.
10. Figueroa-Magalhaes MC, Jelovac D, Connolly RM, et al. Treatment of HER2-positive breast cancer. *Breast* 2014;23:128–136.
11. Bang YJ, Van Cutsem E, Feyereislova A, et al. Trastuzumab in combination with chemotherapy versus chemotherapy alone for treatment of HER2-positive advanced gastric or gastro-oesophageal junction cancer (ToGA): a phase 3, open-label, randomised controlled trial. *Lancet* 2010;76:687–697.
12. Bardelli A, Siena S. Molecular mechanisms of resistance to cetuximab and panitumumab in colorectal cancer. *J Clin Oncol* 2010;28:1254–1261.
13. Jimeno A, Messersmith WA, Hirsch FR, et al. KRAS mutations and sensitivity to epidermal growth factor receptor inhibitors in colorectal cancer: practical application of patient selection. *J Clin Oncol* 2009;27:1130–1136.
14. Roberts PJ, Stinchcombe TE, Der CJ, et al. Personalized medicine in non-small-cell lung cancer: is KRAS a useful marker in selecting patients for epidermal growth factor receptor-targeted therapy? *J Clin Oncol* 2010;28:4769–4777.
15. Chapman PB, Hauschild A, Robert C, et al. Improved survival with vemurafenib in melanoma with BRAF V600E mutation. *N Engl J Med* 2011;364:2507–2516.
16. Dhillon AS, Hagan S, Rath O, et al. MAP kinase signalling pathways in cancer. *Oncogene* 2007;26:3279–3290.
17. Trunzer K, Pavlick AC, Schuchter L, et al. Pharmacodynamic effects and mechanisms of resistance to vemurafenib in patients with metastatic melanoma. *J Clin Oncol* 2013;31:1767–1774.
18. Flaherty KT, Infante JR, Daud A, et al. Combined BRAF and MEK inhibition in melanoma with BRAF V600 mutations. *N Engl J Med* 2012;367:1694–1703.
19. Muller PA, Vousden KH. p53 mutations in cancer. *Nat Cell Biol* 2013;15:2–8.
20. Clarke PA, Workman P. Phosphatidylinositide-3-kinase inhibitors: addressing questions of isoform selectivity and pharmacodynamic/predictive biomarkers in early clinical trials. *J Clin Oncol* 2012;30:331–333.
21. Ramaswamy S, Golub T. DNA microarrays in clinical oncology. *J Clin Oncol* 2002;20:1932–1941.
22. Paik S, Shak S, Tang G, et al. A multigene assay to predict recurrence of tamoxifen-treated, node-negative breast cancer. *N Engl J Med* 2004;351:2817–2826.
23. Paik S, Tang G, Shak S, et al. Gene expression and benefit of chemotherapy in women with node-negative, estrogen receptor-positive breast cancer. *J Clin Oncol* 2006;24:3726–3734.
24. Lipson D, Capelletti M, Yelensky R, et al. Identification of new ALK and RET gene fusions from colorectal and lung cancer biopsies. *Nat Med* 2012;18:382–384.
25. Diaz LA Jr, Bardelli A. Liquid biopsies: genotyping circulating tumor DNA. *J Clin Oncol* 2014;32:579–586.
26. Watters J, McLeod H. Cancer pharmacogenomics: current and future applications. *Biochim Biophys Acta* 2003;1603:99–111.
27. Evans W, Relling M. Pharmacogenomics: translating functional genomics into rational therapeutics. *Science* 1999;286:487–491.
28. Deenen MJ, Cats A, Beijnen H, et al. Part 2: pharmacogenetic variability in drug transport and phase I anticancer drug metabolism. *Oncologist* 2011;16:820–834.
29. Krynetski E, Evans W. Drug methylation in cancer therapy: lessons from the TPMT polymorphism. *Oncogene* 2003;22:7403–7413.
30. McLeod H, Krynetski EY, Relling MV, et al. Genetic polymorphism of thiopurine methyltransferase and its clinical relevance for childhood acute lymphoblastic leukemia. *Leukemia* 2000;14:567–572.
31. Evans W, Hon YY, Bomgaars L, et al. Preponderance of thiopurine S-methyltransferase deficiency and heterozygosity among patients intolerant to mercaptopurine or azathioprine. *J Clin Oncol* 2001;19:2293–2301.
32. Relling M, Hancock ML, Rivera GK, et al. Mercaptopurine therapy intolerance and heterozygosity at the thiopurine S-methyltransferase gene locus. *J Natl Cancer Inst* 1999;91:2001–2008.
33. Relling MV, Gardner EE, Sandborn WJ, et al. Clinical pharmacogenetics implementation consortium guidelines for thiopurine methyltransferase genotype and thiopurine dosing: 2013 update. *Clin Pharmacol Ther* 2013;93:324–325.
34. Caudle KE, Thorn CF, Klein TE, et al. Clinical Pharmacogenetics Implementation Consortium guidelines for dihydropyrimidine dehydrogenase genotype and fluoropyrimidine dosing. *Clin Pharmacol Ther* 2013;94:640–645.
35. McLeod H, Collie-Duguid ES, Vreken P, et al. Nomenclature for human DPYD alleles. *Pharmacogenetics* 1998;8:455–459.
36. Wei X, Elizondo G, Sapone A, et al. Characterization of the human dihydropyrimidine dehydrogenase gene. *Genomics* 1998;51:391–400.
37. Ridge S, Sludden J, Wei X, et al. Dihydropyrimidine dehydrogenase pharmacogenetics in patients with colorectal cancer. *Br J Cancer* 1998;77:497–500.
38. Johnson M, Wang K, Diasio R. Profound dihydropyrimidine dehydrogenase deficiency resulting from a novel compound heterozygote genotype. *Clin Cancer Res* 2002;8:768–774.
39. Van Kuilenburg A, Meinsma R, Zoetekouw L, et al. Increased risk of grade IV neutropenia after administration of 5-fluorouracil due to a dihydropyrimidine dehydrogenase deficiency: high prevalence of the IVS14+1g>a mutation. *Int J Cancer* 2002;101:253–258.

40. Mürdter TE, Schroth W, Bacchus-Gerybadze L, et al. Activity levels of tamoxifen metabolites at the estrogen receptor and the impact of genetic polymorphisms of phase I and II enzymes on their concentration levels in plasma. *Clin Pharmacol Ther* 2011;89:708–717.
41. Desta Z, Ward BA, Soukhova NV, et al. Comprehensive evaluation of tamoxifen sequential biotransformation by the human cytochrome P450 system in vitro: prominent roles for CYP3A and CYP2D6. *J Pharmacol Exp Ther* 2004;310:1062–1075.
42. Bradford LD. CYP2D6 allele frequency in European Caucasians, Asians, Africans and their descendants. *Pharmacogenomics* 2002;3:229–243.
43. Crews KR, Gaedigk A, Dunnenberger HM, et al. Clinical Pharmacogenetics Implementation Consortium (CPIC) guidelines for codeine therapy in the context of cytochrome P450 2D6 (CYP2D6) genotype. *Clin Pharmacol Ther* 2012;91:321–326.
44. Schroth W, Goetz MP, Hamann U, et al. Association between CYP2D6 polymorphisms and outcomes among women with early stage breast cancer treated with tamoxifen. *JAMA* 2009;302:1429–1436.
45. Province MA, Goetz MP, Brauch H, et al. CYP2D6 genotype and adjuvant tamoxifen: meta-analysis of heterogeneous study populations. *Clin Pharmacol Ther* 2014;95:216–227.
46. Irvin WJ Jr, Walko CM, Weck KE, et al. Genotype-guided tamoxifen dosing increases active metabolite exposure in women with reduced CYP2D6 metabolism: a multicenter study. *J Clin Oncol* 2011;29:3232–3239.

17 Alkylating Agents

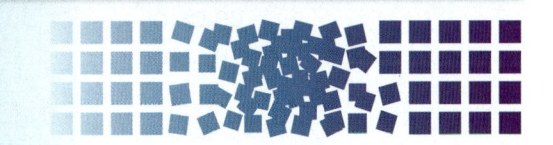

Kenneth D. Tew

PERSPECTIVES

Alkylating agents were the first anticancer molecules developed, and they are still used today. After more than 50 years of use, the basic chemistry and pharmacology of this drug family is well understood and has not changed substantially. The family contains six major classes: nitrogen mustards, aziridines, alkyl sulfonates, epoxides, nitrosoureas, and triazene compounds, although a few nonstandard agents have recently been developed. Most epoxides tend to be quite nonspecific with respect to their reactivity and, as such, few have useful clinical characteristics. This chapter provides perspective on how the limited varieties of alkylating agents continue to be useful in the therapeutic management of cancer patients.

The alkylating agents are a diverse group of anticancer agents with the commonality that they react in a manner such that an electrophilic alkyl group or a substituted alkyl group can covalently bind to cellular nucleophilic sites. Electrophilicity is achieved through the formation of carbonium ion intermediates and can result in transition complexes with target molecules. Ultimately, reactions result in the formation of covalent linkages by alkylation with a broad range of nucleophilic groups, including bases in DNA, and these are believed responsible for ultimate cytotoxicity and therapeutic effect. Although the alkylating agents react with cells in all phases of the cell cycle, their efficacy and toxicity result from interference with rapidly proliferating tissues. From a historical perspective, the vesicant properties of mustard gas used during World War I were shown to be accompanied by the suppression of lymphoid and hematologic functions in experimental animals[1] and led to the development of mechlorethamine as the first alkylating agent used in the management of human cancer.[2] Subsequently, a number of related drugs have been developed, and these have roles in the treatment of a range of leukemias, lymphomas, and solid tumors. Most of the alkylating agents cause dose-limiting toxicities to the bone marrow and, to a lesser degree, the intestinal mucosa, with other organ systems also affected contingent on the individual drug, dosage, and duration of therapy. Despite the present trend toward targeted therapies, this class of "nonspecific" drugs maintains an essential role in cancer chemotherapy.

Because of the classic nature of the drug family, there have been relatively few advances in either their use or utility since publication of the previous edition of this book.

CHEMISTRY

Alkylating reactions are generally classified through their kinetic properties as S_N1 (nucleophilic substitution, first order) or S_N2 (nucleophilic substitution, second order) (Fig. 17.1). The first-order kinetics of the S_N1 reactions depend on the concentration of the original alkylating agent. The rate-limiting step is the initial formation of the reactive intermediate, and the rate is essentially independent of the concentration of the substrate. The S_N2 alkylation reaction is a bimolecular nucleophilic displacement with second-order kinetics, where the rate depends on the concentration of both alkylating agent and target nucleophile. Reactivity of electrophiles[3] suggests that the rates of alkylation of cellular nucleophiles (including thiols, phosphates, amino and imidazole groups of amino acids, and various reactive sites in nucleic acid bases) are most dependent on their potential energy states, which can be defined as "hard" or "soft," based on the polarizability of their reactive centers.[4] Although the metabolism and metabolites of nitrogen mustards and nitrosoureas differ, the active alkylating species of each is the alkyl carbonium ion (see Fig. 17.1), a highly polarized hard electrophile as a consequence of its highly positive charge density at the electrophilic center. Alkyl carbonium ions will react most readily with hard nucleophiles (possessing a highly polarized negative charge density), where the high-energy transition state (a potential energy barrier to the reaction) is most favorable. In specific terms, an active alkylating species from a nitrogen mustard will demonstrate selectivity for cellular nucleophiles in the following order: (1) oxygen in phosphate groups of RNA and DNA, (2) oxygens of purines and pyrimidines, (3) amino groups of purine bases, (4) primary and secondary amino groups of proteins, (5) sulfur atoms of methionine, and (6) thiol groups of cysteinyl residues of protein and glutathione.[3] The least favored reactions will still occur, but at much slower rates unless they are catalyzed.

Alkylation through highly reactive intermediates (e.g., mechlorethamine) would be expected to be less selective in their targets than the less reactive S_N2 reagents (e.g., busulfan). However, the therapeutic and toxic effects of alkylating agents do not correlate directly with their chemical reactivity. Clinically useful agents include drugs with S_N1 or S_N2 characteristics, and some with both.[5] These differ in their toxicity profiles and antitumor activity, but more as a consequence of differences in pharmacokinetics, lipid solubility, penetration of the central nervous system (CNS), membrane transport, metabolism and detoxification, and specific enzymatic reactions capable of repairing alkylation sites on DNA.

CLASSIFICATION

The major classes of clinically useful alkylating agents are illustrated in Table 17.1 and summarized in the following sections. Doses and schedules of the various agents are shown in Table 17.2.

Alkyl Sulfonates

Busulfan is used for the treatment of chronic myelogenous leukemia. It exhibits S_N2 alkylation kinetics and shows nucleophilic selectivity for thiol groups, suggesting that it may exert cytotoxicity through protein alkylation rather than through DNA. In contrast to the nitrogen mustards and nitrosoureas, busulfan has a greater effect on myeloid cells than lymphoid cells, thus the reason for its use against chronic myelogenous leukemia.[6]

Aziridines

Aziridines are analogs of ring-closed intermediates of nitrogen mustards and are less chemically reactive, but they have

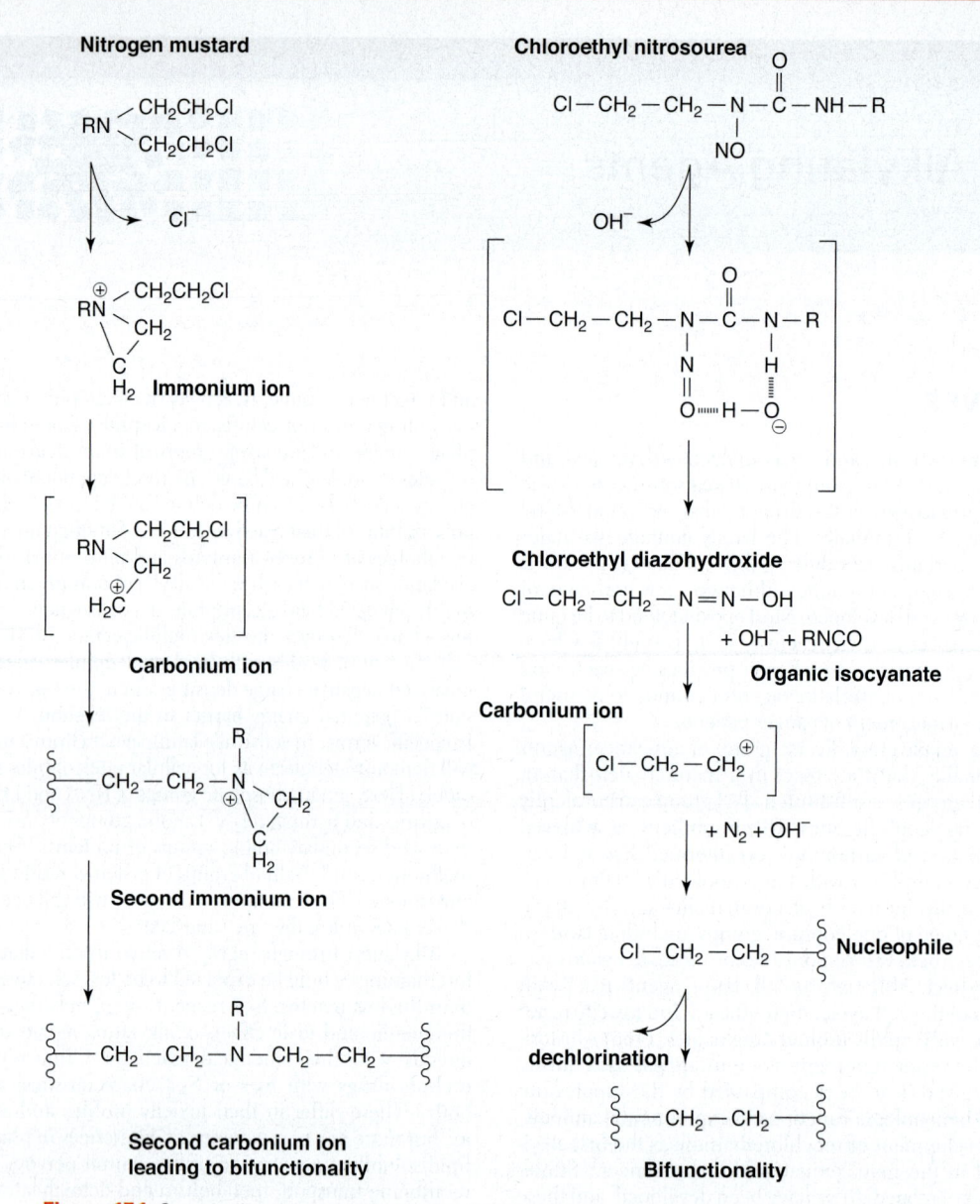

Figure 17.1 Comparative decomposition and metabolism of a typical nitrogen mustard compared to a nitrosourea. Although intermediate metabolites are distinct, the active alkylating species is a carbonium ion in each case. This electrophilic moiety reacts with target cellular nucleophiles.

equivalent therapeutic properties. Thiotepa has been used in the treatment of carcinoma of the breast, ovary, for a variety of CNS diseases, and with increasing frequency as a component of high-dose chemotherapy regimens.[7] Thiotepa and its primary desulfurated metabolite triethylenethiophosphoramide (TEPA) alkylate through aziridine ring openings, a mechanism similar to the nitrogen mustards.

Triazines

Perhaps the newest clinical development in the alkylating agent field is the emergence of temozolomide (TMZ). This agent acts as a prodrug and is an imidazotetrazine analog that undergoes spontaneous activation in solution to produce 5-(3-methyltriazen-1-yl) imidazole-4-carboxamide (MTIC), a triazine derivative. It crosses the blood–brain barrier with concentrations in the CNS approximating 30% of plasma concentrations.[8] Resistance to the methylating agent occurs quite frequently and has adversely affected the rate and durability of the clinical responses of patients. However, because of its favorable toxicity and pharmacokinetics, TMZ is being combined with numerous other classes of anticancer drugs in an effort to improve response rates in diseases such as malignant melanomas, gliomas, brain metastasis from solid tumors, and refractory leukemias. Many of these trials are currently underway.[9]

Nitrogen Mustards

Bischloroethylamines or nitrogen mustards are extensively administered in the clinic. As an initial step in alkylation, chlorine acts as a leaving group and the β-carbon reacts with the nucleophilic nitrogen atom to form the cyclic, positively charged, reactive aziridinium moiety. Reaction of the aziridinium ring with an electron-rich nucleophile creates an initial alkylation product. The remaining chloroethyl group achieves bifunctionality through the formation of a second aziridinium. Melphalan (L-phenylalanine mustard), chlorambucil, cyclophosphamide, and ifosfamide (see Table 17.1) replaced mechlorethamine as primary therapeutic agents. These derivatives have electron-withdrawing groups substituted on the nitrogen atom, reducing the nucleophilicity of the nitrogen and rendering them less reactive, but enhancing their antitumor efficacy.

TABLE 17.1
Major Classes of Clinically Useful Alkylating Agents

Drug	Main Therapeutic Uses	Clinical Pharmacology	Major Toxicities	Notes
ALKYL SULFONATES				
Busulfan	Bone marrow transplantation, especially in chronic myelogenous leukemia	Bioavailability, 80%; protein bound, 33%; $t_{1/2}$, 2.5 h	Pulmonary fibrosis, hyperpigmentation thrombocytopenia, lowered blood platelet count and activity	Oral or parenteral; high dose causes hepatic veno-occlusive disease
ETHYLENEIMINES/METHYLMELAMINES				
Altretamine		Protein bound, 94%; $t_{1/2}$, 5–10 h	Nausea, vomiting, diarrhea, and neurotoxicity	Not widely used
Thio TEPA	Breast, ovarian, and bladder cancer; also bone marrow transplant	$t_{1/2}$, 2.5 h; urinary excretion at 24 h, 25%; substrate for CYP2B6 and CYP2C11	Myelosuppression	Nadirs of leukopenia, occur 2 wk; thrombocytopenia, 3 wk (correlates with AUC of parent drug)
NITROGEN MUSTARDS				
Mechlorethamine	Hodgkin lymphoma		Nausea, vomiting, myelosuppression	Precursor for other clinical mustards
Melphalan (L-phenylalanine mustard)	Multiple myeloma and ovarian cancer, and occasionally malignant melanoma	Bioavailability 25%–90%; $t_{1/2}$, 1.5 h; urinary excretion at 24 h, 13%; clearance, 9 mL/min/kg	Nausea, vomiting, myelosuppression	Causes less mucosal damage than others in class
Chlorambucil	Chronic lymphocytic leukemia	$t_{1/2}$, 1.5 h; urinary excretion at 24 h, 50%	Myelosuppression, gastrointestinal distress, CNS, skin reactions, hepatotoxicity	Oral
Cyclophosphamide	Variety of lymphomas, leukemias, and solid tumors	Bioavailability, >75%; protein bound, >60%; $t_{1/2}$, 3–12 h; urinary excretion at 24 h, <15%	Nausea and vomiting, bone marrow suppression, diarrhea, darkening of the skin/nails, alopecia (hair loss), lethargy, hemorrhagic cystitis	IV; primary excretion route is urine
Ifosfamide	Testicular, breast cancer; lymphoma (non-Hodgkin); soft tissue sarcoma; osteogenic sarcoma; lung, cervical, ovarian, bone cancer	$t_{1/2}$, 15 h; urinary excretion at 24 h, 15%	As for cyclophosphamide	Ifosfamide is often used in conjunction with mesna to avoid cystinuria
NITROSOUREAS				
Carmustine	Glioma, glioblastoma multiforme, medulloblastoma and astrocytoma, multiple myeloma and lymphoma (Hodgkin and non-Hodgkin)	Bioavailability, 25%; protein bound, 80%; $t_{1/2}$, 30 min	Bone marrow and pulmonary toxicities are a function of lifetime cumulative dose	Clinically, nitrosoureas do not share cross-resistance with nitrogen mustards in lymphoma treatment
Streptozotocin	Cancers of the islets of Langerhans	$t_{1/2}$, 35 min; excreted in the urine (15%), feces (<1%), and in the expired air	Nausea and vomiting; nephrotoxicity can range from transient protein urea and azotemia to permanent tubular damage; can also cause aberrations of glucose metabolism	A natural product from *Streptomyces achromogenes*
TRIAZENES				
Dacarbazine	Malignant melanoma and Hodgkin lymphoma	$t_{1/2}$, 5 h; protein bound, 5% hepatic metabolism	Nausea, vomiting, myelosuppression	IV or IM
Temozolomide	Glioblastoma; astrocytoma; metastatic melanoma	Protein bound, 15%; $t_{1/2}$, 1.8 h; clearance, 5.5 l/h/m^2	Nausea, vomiting, myelosuppression	Oral; derivative of imidazotetrazine, prodrug of dacarbazine; rapidly absorbed

$t_{1/2}$, half-life; TEPA, triethylenethiophosphoramide; AUC, area under curve; CNS, central nervous system; IV, intravenous; IM, intramuscular.

TABLE 17.2
Dose and Schedules of Clinically Useful Alkylating Agents

Alkylating Agent	Disease Sites and Dose Ranges Used Clinically	Notes
BCNU (Carmustine)	General antineoplastic 150–200 mg/m² (IV, every 6 wks) Cutaneous T-cell lymphoma 200–600 mg (topical solution) Adjunct to surgical resection of brain tumor 61.6 mg (implant)	Infusion 1–2 h; in combination, dose usually reduced by 25%–50% Side effects include irritant dermatitis, telangiectasia, erythema, and bone marrow suppression Up to 8 wafers (7.7 mg of carmustine) implanted
Busulfan	Chronic myelogenous leukemia and myeloproliferative disorders 4–8 mg (daily PO) 1.8 mg/m² (daily PO) Bone marrow transplant 640 mg/m² (daily PO)	Dispensed over 3–4 d, with cyclophosphamide
Carboplatin	Advanced ovarian cancer—monotherapy 360 mg/m² (IV, every 4 wks) Ovarian cancer—combination 300 mg/m² (IV, every 4 wks for 6 cycles) Ovarian cancer—IP 200–500 mg/m² (IP, 2 L dialysis fluid) Ovarian and other sites phase 1/2 setting—high-dose therapy 800–1,600 mg/m² (IV)	With cyclophosphamide Patients usually receive marrow transplantation or peripheral stem cell support
Cisplatin	Metastatic testicular cancer: 20 mg/m²/d for 5 d of each cycle (IV) Metastatic ovarian cancer: 75–100 mg/m² (IV, once every 4 wks) Head and neck cancer: 100 mg/m² (IV) Bladder cancer: (combination prior to cystectomy) 50–70; initiate dosing at 50 mg/m² (IV, once every 3–4 wks) Metastatic breast cancer: 20 mg/m² (IV, days 1–5 every 3 wks) Cervical cancer: 70 mg/m² (IV, dosing cycled every 4 wks) Non–small-cell lung cancer: 75 mg/m² (IV, every 3 wks) Esophageal cancer: 75 mg/m² on day 1 of wks 1, 5, 8, and 11 (IV)	With other antineoplastic agents With cyclophosphamide (600 mg/m² once every 4 wks) With vincristine, bleomycin, and fluorouracil With methotrexate and fluorouracil MVAC regimen (methotrexate, vinblastine, doxorubicin, and cisplatin) used for cervical cancer Administration preceded by paclitaxel 135 mg/m² every 3 wks With radiation therapy
Cyclophosphamide	General antineoplastic 1–5 mg/kg (daily PO) 40–50 mg/kg (IV, in divided doses over 2–5 d) 40–50 mg/kg (IV, in divided doses over 2–5 d) 10–15 mg/kg (IV, every 7–10 d) 10–15 mg/kg (IV, every 7–10 d) 3–5 mg/kg (IV twice per wk) High-dose regimen in bone marrow transplantation and for other autoimmune disorders 200 mg/kg (IV) 1–2.5 mg/kg (daily PO 7–14 d/mo)	Dose used as monotherapy for patients with no hematologic toxicity
Dacarbazine	General antineoplastic 2–4.5 mg/kg/d (IV) 150 mg/m²/d (IV)	Administered for 10 d, may be repeated at 4-week intervals With other anticancer agents; treatment lasts 5 d, may be repeated every 4 wks
Etoposide	Testicular cancer 50–100 mg/m²/day (IV, slow infusion over 30–60+ min for 5 d) Small cell lung cancer 35–50 mg/m²/day (IV, slow infusion over 30–60+ min for 4–5 d)	Alternatively, 100 mg/m²/d on days 1, 3, and 5 may be used; doses for combination therapy and are repeated at 3- to 4-wk intervals after recovery from hematologic toxicity Doses are for combination therapy and repeated at 3- to 4-wk intervals after recovery from hematologic toxicity; oral dose is twice the IV, rounded to the nearest 50 mg

(continued)

TABLE 17.2
Dose and Schedules of Clinically Useful Alkylating Agents (continued)

Ifosfamide	General antineoplastic 1.2 g/m²/d (IV, for 5 consecutive days)	Repeat every 3 wks
Melphalan	Multiple myeloma: 16 mg/m² (IV, infusion over 15–20 min) 6 mg (daily PO) Epithelial ovarian cancer: 0.2 mg/kg (daily PO)	2-week intervals for 4 doses, 4-wk intervals thereafter After 2–3 wks treatment, should be discontinued for up to 4 wks, then reinstituted at 2–4 mg/d Daily dose for a 5-d course, repeated every 4–5 wks
Streptozotocin	Pancreatic tumors 500 mg/m²/d; 1,000 mg/m²/d (IV; IV)	500 mg for 5 consecutive days every 6 wks, 1,000 mg is for 2 wks, followed by an increase in weekly dose not to exceed 1,500 mg/m²/wk
Temozolomide	Brain tumors 150 mg/m² (daily PO)	Dose adjusted on the basis of blood counts
Thiotepa	General antineoplastic: 0.3–0.4 mg/kg (IV) Papillary carcinoma of the bladder: 60 mg/wk for 4 wks (bladder catheter) Control of serous effusions: 0.6–0.8 mg/kg (intracavitary)	Rapid administration given at 1- to 4-wk intervals 30 or 60 mL should be retained for 2 h, so the patient is usually dehydrated prior to administration of the drug

IV, intravenously; PO, by mouth; IP, intraperitoneal.

One distinguishing feature of melphalan is that an amino acid transporter responsible for uptake influences its efficacy across cell membranes.[10] Although a number of glutathione (GSH) conjugates of alkylating agents are effluxed through adenosine triphosphate–dependent membrane transporters,[11] specific uptake mechanisms are generally rare for cancer drugs. Cyclophosphamide and ifosfamide are prodrugs that require cytochrome P-450 metabolism to release active alkylating species. Cyclophosphamide continues to be the most widely used alkylating agent and has activity against a variety of tumors.[12] A cost saving with equivalent therapeutic activity was recently shown in a modified regimen of high-dose cyclophosphamide plus cyclosporine in patients with severe or very severe aplastic anemia.[13]

Nitrosoureas

The nitrosoureas form a diverse class of alkylating agents that have a distinct metabolism and pharmacology that separates them from others.[14] Under physiologic conditions, proton abstraction by a hydroxyl ion initiates spontaneous decomposition of the molecule to yield a diazonium hydroxide and an isocyanate (see Fig. 17.1). The chloroethyl carbonium ion generated is the active alkylating species. Through a subsequent dehalogenation step, a second electrophilic site imparts bifunctionality.[15] Thus, while cross-linking may occur similar to those lesions caused by nitrogen mustards, the chemistry leading to the endpoint is distinct. The isocyanate species generated are also electrophilic, showing nucleophilic selectivity toward sulfhydryl and amino groups that can inhibit a number of enzymes involved in nucleic acid synthesis and thiol balance.[16] Because carbamoylation is considered of minor importance to the therapeutic efficacy of clinically used nitrosoureas, chlorozotocin and streptozotocin were designed to undergo internal carbamoylation at the 1- or 3-OH group of the glucose ring, with the consequence that no carbamoylating species are produced.[17,18] Streptozotocin is also unusual in that most methylnitrosoureas have only modest therapeutic value. However, its lack of bone marrow toxicity and strong diabetogenic effect in animals led to its use in cancer of the pancreas (see Table 17.1).[19] The dose-limiting toxicities in humans are gastrointestinal and renal, but the drug has considerably less hematopoietic toxicity than the other nitrosoureas. Because of their lipophilicity and capacity to cross the blood–brain barrier, the chloroethylnitrosoureas were found to be effective against intracranially inoculated murine tumors. Indeed, early preclinical studies showed that many mouse tumors were quite responsive to nitrosoureas. The same extent of efficacy was not found in humans. Subsequent analyses demonstrated that an enzyme responsible for repair of O-6-alkyl guanine (O⁶-methylguanine-DNA methyltransferase [MGMT], or the Mer/Mex phenotype)[20] was expressed at low levels in mice, but at high levels in humans, a contributory factor in the reduced clinical efficacy of nitrosoureas in humans. In the 1980s, in particular, a number of new nitrosoureas were tested in patients in Europe and Japan, but none established a regular role in standard cancer treatment regimens.

MGMT promoter methylation is crucial in MGMT gene silencing and can predict a favorable outcome in glioblastoma patients receiving alkylating agents.[21] This biomarker is on the verge of entering clinical decision making and is currently used to stratify or even select glioblastoma patients for clinical trials. In other subtypes of glioma, such as anaplastic gliomas, the relevance of MGMT promoter methylation might extend beyond the prediction of chemosensitivity, and could reflect a distinct molecular profile. At this time, the standardization of MGMT assays will be critical in establishing prospective prognostic or predictive effects. In addition, eventual clinical trials will need to determine, for each subtype of glioma, the extent to which methylation patterns are predictive or prognostic and whether such assays could be incorporated into an individualized approach to clinical practice.[21]

CLINICAL PHARMACOKINETICS/PHARMACODYNAMICS

The pharmacokinetics of the alkylating agents are highly variable depending on the individual agent. Nevertheless, they are generally characterized by high reactivity and short half-lives. Although detailed studies on clinical pharmacology are available,[22] Table 17.1 summarizes some of the primary kinetic characteristics of the major clinically useful drugs. Mechlorethamine is unstable and is administered rapidly in a running intravenous infusion to avoid its rapid breakdown to inactive metabolites. In contrast, chlorambucil and cyclophosphamide are sufficiently stable to be given orally, and are rapidly and completely absorbed from the gastrointestinal tract, whereas others like melphalan have poor and variable

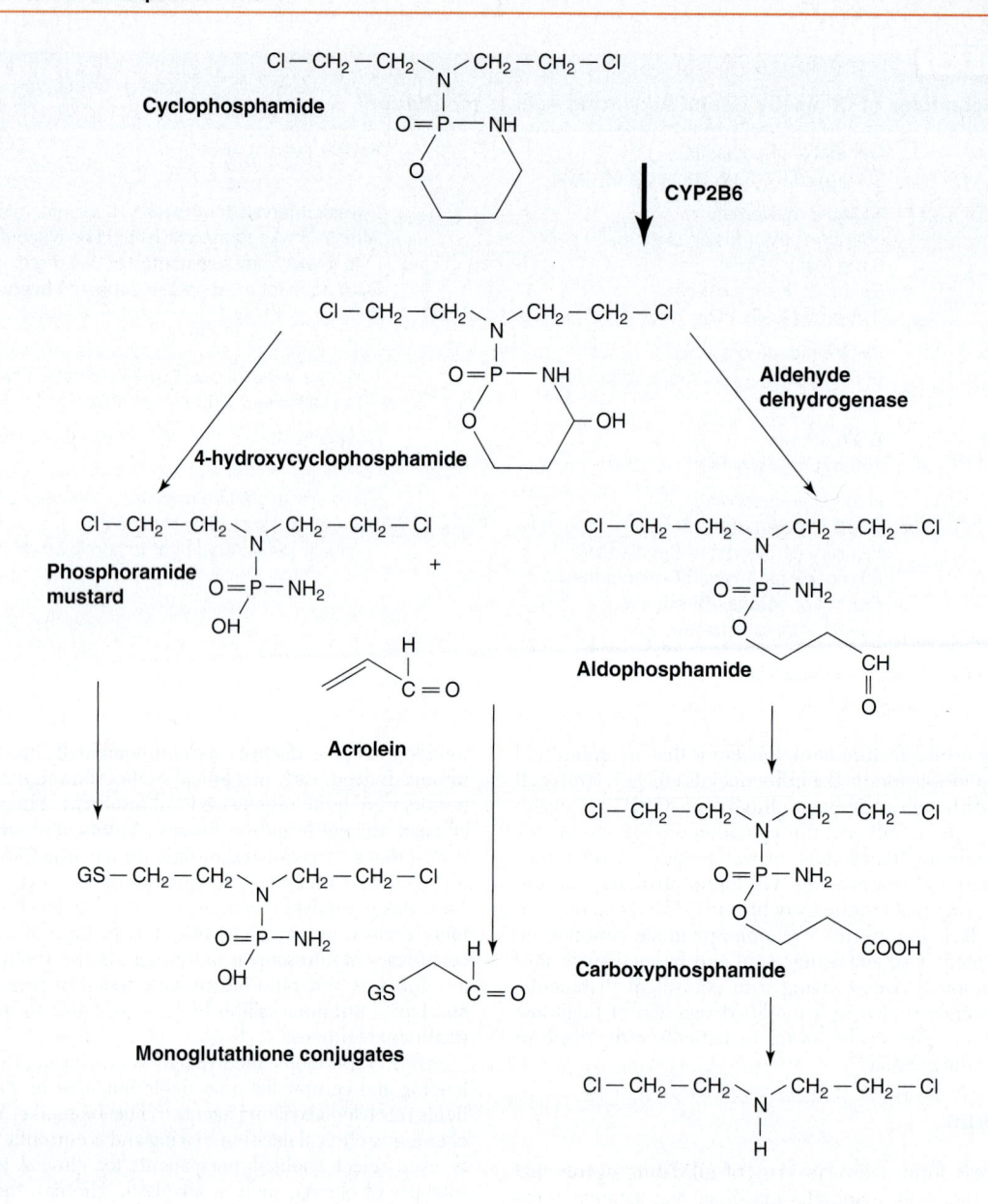

Figure 17.2 Activation and detoxification routes of metabolism for cyclophosphamide.

oral absorption. Cyclophosphamide,[23] ifosfamide, and dacarbazine are unusual in that they require activation by cytochrome P-450 in the liver before they can alkylate cellular constituents. The nitrosoureas also require activation, albeit nonenzymatic. The major route of metabolism of most alkylating agents is spontaneous hydrolysis, although many can also undergo some degree of enzymatic metabolism. This is particularly pertinent for phase II metabolic conversions where reactivity with nucleophilic thiols precedes conversion to mercapturates, with the result that most of the alkylating agents are excreted in the urine. One example of complex multistep metabolism is provided by cyclophosphamide (see Fig. 17.2). Activation by CYP2B6 is followed by the conversion of aldehyde dehydrogenase to reactive alkylating species or possible detoxification through GSH conjugation reactions. The latter is particularly important for acrolein because it is believed to contribute to the bladder toxicities associated with the drug.

The alkylating agents form covalent bonds with a number of nucleophilic groups present in proteins, RNA, and DNA (e.g., amino, carboxyl, sulfhydryl, imidazole, phosphate). Under physiologic conditions, the chloroethyl group of the nitrogen mustards undergoes cyclization, with the chloride acting as a leaving group forming an intermediate carbonium ion that attacks nucleophilic sites (see Fig. 17.1). Bifunctional alkylating agents (with two chloroethyl side chains) can undergo a subsequent cyclization to form a covalent bond with an adjacent nucleophilic group, resulting in DNA–DNA or DNA–protein cross-links. The N7 or O6 positions of guanine are particularly susceptible and may represent primary targets that determine both the cytotoxic and mutagenic consequences of therapy.[24] The nitrosoureas have a similar, but distinct, mechanism of action, spontaneously forming both alkylating and carbamoylating agents in aqueous media (see Fig. 17.1). The carbamoylating moieties are generally believed to be inconsequential to the therapeutic properties of the nitrosoureas.

THERAPEUTIC USES

The alkylating agents are frequently used in combination therapy to treat a variety of types of cancer. Perhaps the most versatile is cyclophosphamide, whereas the other alkylating agents are of more restricted clinical use. Because of early successes, many disease states are managed with drug combinations that contain several alkylating agents. Cyclophosphamide is employed to treat a variety of immune-related diseases and to purge bone marrow in autologous marrow transplant situations.[25] A general summary of the clinical uses of the primary alkylating agents is shown in Table 17.1.

TOXICITIES

The alkylating agents show significant qualitative and quantitative variability in the sites and severities of their toxicities. The primary dose-limiting toxicity is suppression of bone marrow function, with secondary limiting effects on the proliferating cells of the intestinal mucosa.

Contraindications to the use of alkylating agents would identify patients with severely depressed bone marrow function and patients with hypersensitivity to these drugs. Other listed precautions to these drugs include carcinogenic and mutagenic effects and impairment of fertility. Precaution is also advised in patients with (1) leukopenia or thrombocytopenia, (2) previous exposure to chemotherapy or radiotherapy, (3) tumor cell infiltration of the bone marrow, and (4) impaired renal or hepatic function. These drugs can also increase toxicity in adrenalectomized patients and interfere with wound healing. A brief summary of dose-limiting toxicities is shown in Table 17.1, and a narrative of each follows here.

Nausea and Vomiting

Nausea and vomiting are frequent side effects of alkylating agent therapy and are not well controlled by conventional antiemetics.[24] They are a major source of patient discomfort and a significant cause of lack of drug compliance and even discontinuation of therapy. Frequency and extent are highly variable among patients. The overall frequency of nausea and vomiting is directly proportional to the dose of alkylating agent. The onset of nausea may occur within a few minutes of the administration of the drug or may be delayed for several hours.

Bone Marrow Toxicity

Bone marrow toxicity can involve all of the blood elements, leukocytes, platelets, and red cells.[26] The extent and time course of suppression show marked interindividual fluctuation. Relative platelet sparing is a characteristic of cyclophosphamide treatment. Even at the very high doses (<200 mg/kg) of cyclophosphamide (used in preparation for bone marrow transplantation), some recovery of hematopoietic elements occurs within 21 to 28 days. This stem cell–sparing property is further reflected by the fact that cumulative damage to the bone marrow is rarely seen when cyclophosphamide is given as a single agent, and repeated high doses can be given without progressive lowering of leukocyte and platelet counts. The biochemical basis for the stem cell–sparing effect of cyclophosphamide is related to the presence of high levels of aldehyde dehydrogenase in early bone marrow progenitor cells (see Fig. 17.2). Busulfan is particularly toxic to bone marrow stem cells,[26] and treatment can lead to prolonged hypoplasia. The hematopoietic depression produced by the nitrosoureas is characteristically delayed. The onset of leukocyte and platelet depression occurs 3 to 4 weeks after drug administration and may last an additional 2 to 3 weeks.[22,26] Thrombocytopenia appears earlier and usually is more severe than leukopenia. Even if the nitrosourea is given at 6-week intervals, hematopoietic recovery may not occur between courses, and the drug dose often must be decreased when repeated courses are used.

Renal and Bladder Toxicity

Hemorrhagic cystitis is unique to the oxazaphosphorines (cyclophosphamide and ifosfamide) and may range from a mild cystitis to severe bladder damage with massive hemorrhage.[27] This toxicity is caused by the excretion of toxic metabolites (particularly acrolein) (see Fig. 17.2) in the urine, with subsequent direct irritation of the bladder mucosa. The incidence and severity can be lessened by adequate hydration and continuous irrigation of the bladder with a solution containing 2-mercaptoethane sulfonate (MESNA) and frequent bladder emptying.[26] MESNA is given in divided doses every 4 hours in dosages of 60% of those of the alkylating agent.

At high cumulative doses, all commonly used nitrosoureas can produce a dose-related renal toxicity that can result in renal failure and death.[29] In patients developing clinical evidence of toxicity, increases in serum creatinine usually appear after the completion of therapy and may be first detected up to 2 years after treatment.

Interstitial Pneumonitis and Pulmonary Fibrosis

Long-term busulfan therapy can lead to the gradual onset of fever, a nonproductive cough, and dyspnea, followed by tachypnea and cyanosis, and progressing to severe pulmonary insufficiency and death.[30] If busulfan is stopped before the onset of clinical symptoms, pulmonary function may stabilize, but if clinical symptoms are manifest, the condition may be rapidly fatal. Cyclophosphamide, bischloroethylnitrosourea, and methyl-1-(2-chloroethyl)-3-cyclohexyl-1-nitrosourea in cumulative doses exceeding 1,000 mg/m^2 may also lead to similar side effects.[31] Other alkylating agents, including melphalan, chlorambucil, and mitomycin C, can lead to pulmonary fibrosis after therapy.[32] This effect is probably caused by a direct cytotoxicity of the alkylating agent to pulmonary epithelium, resulting in alveolitis and fibrosis.

Gonadal Toxicity, Teratogenesis, and Carcinogenesis

Alkylating agents can have profound toxic effects on reproductive tissue.[33] A depletion of testicular germ (but not Sertoli) cells is accompanied by aspermia. In patients with a total absence of germ cells, an increase in plasma levels of follicle-stimulating hormone occurs. However, patients in remission and off alkylating agents for 2 to 7 years show complete spermatogenesis, indicating that testicular damage is reversible.

In women, a high incidence of amenorrhea and ovarian atrophy is associated with cyclophosphamide or melphalan therapy.[34] This seems to be age related because it developed after lower doses in older compared with younger patients, and was less likely to be reversible in the older cohort. A pathologic analysis reveals the absence of mature or primordial follicles, and endocrinology studies demonstrate decreased estrogen and progesterone levels and elevated serum follicle-stimulating hormone and luteinizing hormone levels typical of menopause.

The DNA-damaging properties of alkylating agents ensure that they are all teratogenic and carcinogenic to some degree. The administration of alkylating agents during the first trimester of pregnancy presents a definitive risk of a malformed fetus, but the administration of such drugs during the second and third trimesters does not increase the risk of fetal malformation above normal.[35]

Development of second cancer as a consequence of alkylating agent therapy has been documented. For example, a fulminant acute myeloid leukemia characterized by a preceding phase of myelodysplasia is found in some patients treated with melphalan, cyclophosphamide (which is much less leukemogenic than melphalan), chlorambucil, and the nitrosoureas.[33] This circumstance probably reflects the fact that these have been the most widely used of the alkylating agents. Also, the preponderance of patients with multiple myeloma, Hodgkin lymphoma, and carcinoma of the ovary in the reports of leukemogenesis is probably because patients with these diseases may have good responses and are often treated with alkylating agents for a number of years. The rate of occurrence of acute leukemia in patients with ovarian cancer who survive for 10 years after treatment with alkylating agents might be as high as 10%. Acute leukemia has been the most frequently described second malignancy, and it usually develops 1 to 4 years after drug exposure.[36] Other malignancies, including solid tumors, also have been reported to develop in patients treated with alkylating agents.[37]

The last four decades have yielded a significant improvement in the survival of children diagnosed with cancer (5-year survival is approximately 80%). As many as two-thirds of the survivors of childhood malignancies can experience delayed drug toxicities that may be severe or even life threatening. Such complications include impairment in growth and development, neurocognitive dysfunction, cardiopulmonary compromise, endocrine dysfunction, renal impairment, gastrointestinal dysfunction, musculoskeletal sequelae, and second cancers.[38]

Alopecia

The degree of alopecia after cyclophosphamide administration may be quite severe, especially when this drug is used in combination with vincristine sulfate or doxorubicin hydrochloride.[39] Regrowth of hair inevitably occurs after the cessation of therapy, but may be associated with a change in the color and greater curl. Use of a tourniquet or ice pack applied to the scalp during and for a short period after cyclophosphamide administration reduces the impact.

Allergic Reactions

Alkylating agents covalently bind to proteins, and these conjugates can act as haptens and produce allergic reactions.[40] An increasing number of reports of skin eruption, angioneurotic edema, urticaria, and anaphylactic reactions after the systemic administration of alkylating agents have appeared.

Immunosuppression

Alkylating agents suppress both humoral and cellular immunity in a variety of experimental systems.[41] The most immunosuppressive is cyclophosphamide, reported to cause (1) selective suppression of B-lymphocyte function, (2) depletion of B-lymphocytes, and (3) suppression of lymphocyte functions that are mediated by T cells, such as the graft-versus-host response and delayed hypersensitivity. Most intermittent antitumor regimens do not uniformly produce profound immunosuppression, and recovery is usually prompt. Sustained drug treatments can lead to severe lymphocyte depletion and profound immunosuppression and may be accompanied by an increase of viral, fungal, and protozoal infections.[41]

COMPLICATIONS WITH HIGH-DOSE ALKYLATING AGENT THERAPY

At standard doses, alkylating agents produce myelosuppression as their dose-limiting toxicity. Less severe effects on the gastrointestinal epithelium, lungs, bladder, and kidneys may become problems with long-term treatment, but rarely limit initial therapy. For this reason, and because of their steep dose response to tumor-killing curves, the alkylating agents have become a logical tool, either alone or in combination, for high-dose chemotherapy regimens in which bone marrow toxicity is expected, and is accommodated by bone marrow transplantation, stem cell reconstitution from peripheral blood monocytes, and growth factor rescue. In this high-dose setting, toxicities that affect the gut, lungs, liver, and CNS become dose limiting and life threatening.[42] The highly lipid-soluble alkylators, especially ifosfamide, busulfan, the nitrosoureas, and thiotepa, cause CNS dysfunction, including seizures, altered mental status, cerebellar dysfunction, cranial nerve palsies, and coma.[43] High-dose ifosfamide is most frequently the cause of neurotoxicity.[44] Clinical manifestations of grade 4 neurotoxicities were reported in approximately one-fourth of those patients receiving ifosfamide. The side-chain N-linked chloroethyl moiety of ifosfamide (see Table 17.1) is more likely than the bischloroethyl group of cyclophosphamide to undergo oxidation and subsequent N-deethylation and lead to the formation of chloroacetaldehyde. High-dose busulfan is also frequently used in a variety of conditioning regimens for hematopoietic cell transplantation. In this setting, busulfan causes neurotoxicity manifesting in seizures that generally are tonic–clonic in character. Phenytoin has been the preferred drug to treat busulfan-induced seizures, although some emerging clinical data support the use of benzodiazepines, most notably clonazepam and lorazepam, to prevent busulfan-induced seizures. Moreover, the second-generation antiepileptic drug levetiracetam possesses the characteristics of optimal prophylaxis for busulfan-induced seizures.[45] At least one recent study has suggested that a polymorphism in the glutathione S-transferase A2 family may be predictive of transplant-related mortality after allogeneic stem cell transplantation,[46] perhaps indicating that a pharmacogenetic approach might be possible in this disease setting. Moreover, in a preclinical setting, a proteomic analysis identified thioredoxin as a potentially important adjuvant therapy in enhancing donor cell graft enhancement in bone marrow transplantation.[47] The possibility that this approach may benefit patients following alkylating agent–based ablation remains to be tested in a clinical setting.

Cyclophosphamide at doses exceeding 100 mg/kg during a 48-hour period (preparatory to bone marrow transplantation) can cause cardiac toxicity.[48] No evidence exists for cumulative damage to the heart after repeated moderate or low doses of the drug. Cardiac toxicity occurs with greatest frequency in patients older than 50 years or in those previously treated with anthracyclines.[48]

ALKYLATING AGENT–STEROID CONJUGATES

Adapting the rationale that steroid receptors may function to localize and concentrate attached drug species intracellularly in hormone-responsive cancers, a number of synthetic conjugates of nitrogen mustards and steroids have been developed. Of these, two made the transition into clinical use.

Prednimustine is an ester-linked conjugate of chlorambucil and prednisolone designed to function as a prodrug for chlorambucil. Release of the alkylating agent occurs after cleavage by serum esterases,[49] which can release the ester link of prednimustine, producing the hormone and active alkylating drug. The elimination phase of chlorambucil in patient plasma is significantly longer after the administration of prednimustine than after chlorambucil. Estramustine is a carbamate ester–linked conjugate of nor-nitrogen mustard and estradiol. Unlike prednimustine, the pharmacology of estramustine is governed by the presence of the carbamate group in the steroid–mustard linkage. The relative resistance of the carbamate bond to enzymatic cleavage eliminates the alkylating activity of the molecule and conveys an entirely new pharmacology.[50] The crystal structural and mechanism of action studies showed that estramustine has antimitotic activity, an activity shared by some other steroids.[51] Estramustine has found a clinical niche used in combination with other antimitotic drugs in the management of hormone refractory prostate cancer.[52]

DRUG RESISTANCE AND MODULATION

As with all drugs, intrinsic or acquired resistance to alkylating agents occurs and limits the therapeutic utility of this class of anticancer drugs.[53] A plethora of preclinical studies have characterized mechanisms by which cells develop resistance and, to a lesser degree, these have been shown to occur clinically. Because alkylating agents have a narrow therapeutic index, the emergence of resistance can have a significant impact on clinical success. Some of the factors that can contribute to the expression of resistance to alkylating agents include (1) alterations in drug uptake or transport, (2) increased repair of drug-induced nucleic acid damage, (3) failure to activate alkylating agent prodrugs, (4) increased scavenging of drug species by nonessential cellular nucleophiles, (5) increased enzymatic detoxification of drug species, and (6) altered expression of genes coding for cellular commitment to apoptosis.

RECENT DEVELOPMENTS

In the era of directed targeted therapies, the lack of specificity of alkylating agents would seem to limit the likelihood that novel drugs will be forthcoming. High toxicities, narrow therapeutic indices, and chemical instabilities are all properties that consign this drug class to the lower echelons of popularity in drug-discovery platforms. Although covalent bonding to specific target sites is one approach to direct targeting, the random electrophilic attraction toward nucleic acids and proteins is not an optimal property by today's standards. Nevertheless, the relative success of the alkylating agents in gaining therapeutic responses to diseases that are difficult to treat continues to serve as an impetus to use alkylating moieties as a means to kill cells. Some novel agents are presently in development. Cyclophosphamide and ifosfamide were prodrugs synthesized in the hope that high levels of phosphoamidase in epithelial tumors would selectively activate the drugs.[27] Other efforts to improve selectivity have centered on the synthesis of antibody–enzyme conjugates that bind to tumor-specific surface antigens. Enzymes frequently associated with the cell surface include peptidases, nitroreductases, and γ-glutamyl transpeptidase; to some degree, each has been targeted to cleave circulating alkylating prodrugs, thereby in a localized fashion releasing active alkylating species. Antibody-directed enzyme prodrug therapy is exemplified by the use of an antibody linked to the peptidase carboxypeptidase G-2, which releases an active alkylator from an inactive γ-glutamyl conjugate.[54] Linkage of the peptidase to any antibody that localizes selectively to a tumor cell membrane is a viable option. Expression of the peptidase on the cell surface then leads to prodrug activation and cell kill. Such approaches have had limited clinical impact to this time; however, their development does continue.

A further rationale for enhancing tumor-specific delivery takes advantage of the observation that glutathione-S-transferase *pi* (GSTP1-1) is preferentially expressed in a number of solid tumors and some lymphomas. In this case, the prodrug consists of an unusual alkylating agent conjugated to a substituted glutathione peptidomimetic. GSTP initiates the cleavage, thereby creating a cytotoxic alkylating species.[55] The initial canfosfamide design strategy relied on the principle that proton-abstracting sites at the active site of GST could initiate a cleavage reaction that would convert an inactive prodrug into a cytotoxic species. The presence of a histidine residue in proximity to the G binding site was integral to the removal of the sulfhydryl proton from the GSH cosubstrate, resulting in the generation of a nucleophilic sulfide anion. This moiety would be more reactive with electrophiles in the absence of GSH. Unlike other standard nitrogen mustard drugs, canfosfamide contains a tetrakis (chloroethyl) phosphorodiamidate moiety. Other compounds bearing this structure have been shown to be more cytotoxic than a similar structure with a single bis-(chloroethyl) amine group.[56]

As in other nitrogen mustards, the chlorines can act as leaving groups, thus creating aziridinium ions with electrophilic characteristics. Although the exact temporal or sequential formation of the four possible chlorine leaving events is not known, the assumption is that these species possess cytotoxic properties through their capacity to alkylate target nucleophiles, such as DNA bases. Tetrafunctionality could result in the formation of cross-links with bonding distances greater than for bifunctional agents. However, a number of caveats apply to this interpretation. For example, alkylating agents, whether mono-, bi-, or putatively tetrafunctional, generally lead to some form of myelosuppression. A number of clinical trials with canfosfamide have now been completed. These include, phase 1,[57] phase 1/2a,[58] phase 2,[59] and phase 3.[60] The phase 3 study was in platinum refractory ovarian cancer patients and proved negative for enhanced survival. Nevertheless, additional trials are still in progress.

Another targeting approach delivers the gene for a cytochrome P-450 isoenzyme to tumors by viral vector, thereby enhancing specific tumor cell activation of cyclophosphamide.[61] Because this therapy has its base in gene delivery technologies, successful development in humans will await further advances in this arena.

Laromustine is in the sulfonylhydrazine class of alkylating agents. It is presently in clinical development for the treatment of malignancies such as acute myelogenous leukemia (AML).[62] Similar to nitrosoureas, laromustine is a prodrug that yields a chloroethylating and a carbamoylating (methyl isocyanate) species. As with nitrosoureas, the cytotoxicity of laromustine is attributed primarily to the chloroethylating-mediated alkylation of DNA and subsequent interstrand cross-links.[63] The carbamoylating species can inhibit DNA repair and other cellular enzyme systems. Phase 1 trials in patients with solid tumors indicated the expected myelosuppression, although few extramedullary toxicities were observed, indicating potential efficacy in the treatment of hematologic malignancies. Phase 2 trials have been completed in patients with untreated AML, high-risk myelodysplastic syndrome, and relapsed AML. The most encouraging results have been found in patients older than 60 years with poor-risk, de novo AML for which no standard treatment exists. Laromustine is currently in phase 2/3 trials for AML and phase 2 trials for myelodysplastic syndrome and solid tumors.[64] Laromustine appears to be a promising agent in elderly patients who do not respond to or are not fit for intensive chemotherapy.

Although not a new drug, bendamustine is a unique cytotoxic agent with structural similarities to alkylating agents and antimetabolites, but it lacks cross-resistance with other established alkylating agents both in vitro and in the clinic.[65] Its mechanism of action is similar to other mustards in causing DNA intra- and interstrand cross-links. In comparison with other more commonly used alkylating agents, such as cyclophosphamide or phenylalanine mustard, more DNA double-strand breaks are formed at equitoxic dosages. Treatment with bendamustine induces a concentration-dependent apoptosis as evidenced by changes in Bcl-2 and Bax expression profiles in chronic B-cell lymphocytic leukemia.[66] DNA damage produced by bendamustine is repaired via base-excision repair mechanisms, implicating an unusual mode of action, which was recently confirmed through gene expression profiling analyses. This also provided an explanation for the lack of cross-resistance with other alkylating agents, as observed in vitro with anthracycline-resistant breast cancer and cisplatin-resistant ovarian cancer.[66,67]

Clinical studies conducted in Germany more than 30 years ago suggested activity in indolent non-Hodgkin lymphoma. Subsequent American trials showed responses in more than 70% of patients with drug refractory disease, with the implication that bendamustine may be the most effective drug in this patient population. Combinations of bendamustine and rituximab elicited response rates of 90% to 92%, with complete remission in 55% to 60% in follicular and mantle cell lymphoma. Superiority over chlorambucil in previously untreated patients with chronic lymphocytic leukemia (CLL) led to its recent approval for this disease in the United States. Bendamustine is approved in Germany for the treatment of patients with indolent non-Hodgkin lymphoma, CLL, and multiple myeloma. Activity has also been noted in patients with breast cancer and non–small-cell lung cancer.

Bendamustine has been used both as a single agent and in combination with other agents, including etoposide, fludarabine, mitoxantrone, methotrexate, prednisone, rituximab, and vincristine. A multicenter phase 2 trial in lymphomas had an overall response rate of 89%; (35% complete response and 54% partial response). In previously treated patients, the overall response rate was 76% (38% complete response and 38% partial response). The estimated median progression-free survival was 19 months.[67] In CLL patients, the drug is administered at 100 mg/m^2 intravenously over 30 minutes on days 1 and 2 of a 28-day cycle, for up to six cycles. Efficacy relative to first-line therapies other than chlorambucil has not been established. It is also indicated for the treatment of patients with indolent B-cell non-Hodgkin lymphoma that has progressed during, or within, 6 months of treatment with rituximab or rituximab-containing regimens. As with most alkylating agents, the primary dose-limiting toxicity is myelosuppression; nonhematologic toxicities were mild and included fatigue, nausea, loss of appetite, and vomiting. The optimization of dose and schedule, particularly relative to other drugs, and the management of toxicities has allowed its use in combination with a range of other chemotherapeutic agents, including prednisone, methotrexate, fludarabine, etoposide, mitoxantrone, vinca alkaloids, and rituximab. The availability of bendamustine provides another effective treatment option for patients with lymphoid malignancies, frequently reducing the side effects of the more standard cyclophosphamide, hydroxy doxorubicin, Oncovin, and prednisone (CHOP) regimen.[68] Recent approval by the U.S. Food and Drug Administration has allowed Cephalon, Inc. to market bendamustine under the trade name Treanda and, in combination with mitoxantrone and rituximab, it is now standard of care in indolent lymphomas. Trial results released in 2013 indicated that this combination more than doubled the progression-free survival in this disease[69] and there is early evidence that there may be utility in relapsed or refractory multiple myeloma.[70]

REFERENCES

1. Adair FE, Bagg HJ. Experimental and clinical studies on the treatment of cancer by dichlorethylsulphide (mustard gas). *Ann Surg* 1931;93(1):190–199.
2. Rhoads C. Nitrogen mustards in treatment of neoplastic disease. *JAMA* 1946;131:656–658.
3. Coles B. Effects of modifying structure on electrophilic reactions with biological nucleophiles. *Drug Metab Rev* 1985;15:1307–1334.
4. Pearson R, Songstad J. Application of the principle of hard and soft acids and bases to organic chemistry. *J Am Chem Soc* 1967;89:1827.
5. Ross W. Alkylating agents. In: *Biological Alkylating Agents*. London: Butterworth; 1962.
6. Elson LA. Hematological effects of the alkylating agents. *Ann N Y Acad Sci* 1958;68(3):826–833.
7. Kushner BH, Kramer K, Modak S, et al. Topotecan, thiotepa, and carboplatin for neuroblastoma: failure to prevent relapse in the central nervous system. *Bone Marrow Transplant* 2006;37(3):271–276.
8. Agarwala SS, Kirkwood JM. Temozolomide, a novel alkylating agent with activity in the central nervous system, may improve the treatment of advanced metastatic melanoma. *Oncologist* 2000;5(2):144–151.
9. Tentori L, Graziani G. Recent approaches to improve the antitumor efficacy of temozolomide. *Curr Med Chem* 2009;16(2):245–257.
10. Vistica DT. Cytotoxicity as an indicator for transport mechanism: evidence that murine bone marrow progenitor cells lack a high-affinity leucine carrier that transports melphalan in murine L1210 leukemia cells. *Blood* 1980;56(3):427–429.
11. Dean M, Rzhetsky A, Allikmets R. The human ATP-binding cassette (ABC) transporter superfamily. *Genome Res* 2001;11(7):1156–1166.
12. Sensenbrenner LL, Marini JJ, Colvin M. Comparative effects of cyclophosphamide, isophosphamide, 4-methylcyclophosphamide, and phosphoramide mustard on murine hematopoietic and immunocompetent cells. *J Natl Cancer Inst* 1979;62(4):975–981.
13. Zhang F, Zhang L, Jing L, et al. (2013) High-dose cyclophosphamide compared with antithymocyte globulin for treatment of acquired severe aplastic anemia. *Exp Hematol* 2013;41:328–334.
14. Montgomery JA, James R, McCaleb GS, et al. The modes of decomposition of 1,3-bis(2-chloroethyl)-1-nitrosourea and related compounds. *J Med Chem* 1967;10(4):668–674.
15. Brundrett RB, Cowens JW, Colvin M. Chemistry of nitrosoureas: decomposition of Deuterated 1,3-bis(2-chloroethyl)-1-nitrosourea. *J Med Chem* 1976;19(7):958–961.
16. Tew KD, Kyle G, Johnson A, et al. Carbamoylation of glutathione reductase and changes in cellular and chromosome morphology in a rat cell line resistant to nitrogen mustards but collaterally sensitive to nitrosoureas. *Cancer Res* 1985;45(5):2326–2333.
17. Anderson T, Schein PS, McMenamin MG, et al. Streptozotocin diabetes: correlation with extent of depression of pancreatic islet nicotinamide adenine dinucleotide. *J Clin Invest* 1974;54(3):672–677.
18. Anderson T, McMenamin MG, Schein PS. Chlorozotocin, 2-(3-(2-chloroethyl)-3-nitrosoureido)-D-glucopyranose, an antitumor agent with modified bone marrow toxicity. *Cancer Res* 1975;35(3):761–765.
19. Schein PS, O'Connell MJ, Blom J, et al. Clinical antitumor activity and toxicity of streptozotocin (NSC-85998). *Cancer* 1974;34(4):993–1000.
20. Pieper RO. Understanding and manipulating O6-methylguanine-DNA methyltransferase expression. *Pharmacol Ther* 1997;74(3):285–297.
21. Weller M, Stupp R, Reifenberger G, et al. MGMT promoter methylation in malignant gliomas: ready for personalized medicine? *Nat Rev Neurol* 2010;6(1):39–51.
22. Tew K, Colvin OM, Jones RB. Clinical and high dose alkylating agents. In: Chabner BA, Longo DL, eds. *Cancer: Chemotherapy and Biotherapy: Principles and Practice*. Philadelphia: Lippincott-Raven; 2005: 283.
23. Brookes P, Lawley PD. The reaction of mono- and di-functional alkylating agents with nucleic acids. *Biochem J* 1961;80(3):496–503.
24. Penta JS, Poster DS, Bruno S, et al. Clinical trials with antiemetic agents in cancer patients receiving chemotherapy. *J Clin Pharmacol* 1981;21(8–9 Suppl):11S–22S.
25. Colvin M, Hilton J. Pharmacology of cyclophosphamide and metabolites. *Cancer Treat Rep* 1981;65(Suppl 3):89–95.
26. Elson L. Hematological effects of the alkylating agents. *Ann N Y Acad Sci* 1958;68:826–833.
27. Cox PJ. Cyclophosphamide cystitis—identification of acrolein as the causative agent. *Biochem Pharmacol* 1979;28(13):2045–2049.
28. Andriole GL, Sandlund JT, Miser JS, et al. The efficacy of mesna (2-mercaptoethane sodium sulfonate) as a uroprotectant in patients with hemorrhagic cystitis receiving further oxazaphosphorine chemotherapy. *J Clin Oncol* 1987;5(5):799–803.
29. Schacht RG, Feiner HD, Gallo GR, et al. Nephrotoxicity of nitrosoureas. *Cancer* 1981;48(6):1328–1334.
30. Littler WA, Ogilvie C. Lung function in patients receiving busulphan. *Br Med J* 1970;4(5734):530–532.
31. Mark GJ, Lehimgar-Zadeh A, Ragsdale BD. Cyclophosphamide pneumonitis. *Thorax* 1978;33(1):89–93.
32. Kreisman H, Wolkove N. Pulmonary toxicity of antineoplastic therapy. *Semin Oncol* 1992;19(5):508–520.
33. Kumar R, Biggart JD, McEvoy J, et al. Cyclophosphamide and reproductive function. *Lancet* 1972;1(7762):1212–1214.
34. Miller JJ 3rd, Williams GF, Leissring JC. Multiple late complications of therapy with cyclophosphamide, including ovarian destruction. *Am J Med* 1971;50(4):530–535.
35. Nicholson HO. Cytotoxic drugs in pregnancy: review of reported cases. *J Obstet Gynaecol Br Commonw* 1968;75(3):307–312.
36. Reimer RR, Hoover R, Fraumeni JF Jr, et al. Acute leukemia after alkylating-agent therapy of ovarian cancer. *N Engl J Med* 1977;297(4):177–181.
37. Penn I. Second malignant neoplasms associated with immunosuppressive medications. *Cancer* 1976;37(2 Suppl):1024–1032.
38. Bhatia S, Constine LS. Late morbidity after successful treatment of children with cancer. *Cancer J* 2009;15(3):174–180.
39. Calvert W. Alopecia and cytotoxic drugs. *Br Med J* 1966;2(5517):831.
40. Weiss RB, Bruno S. Hypersensitivity reactions to cancer chemotherapeutic agents. *Ann Intern Med* 1981;94(1):66–72.
41. Santos GW, Sensenbrenner LL, Burke PJ, et al. Marrow transplantation in man following cyclophosphamide. *Transplant Proc* 1971;3(1):400–404.
42. de Jonge ME, Huitema AD, Beijnen JH, et al. High exposures to bioactivated cyclophosphamide are related to the occurrence of veno-occlusive disease of the liver following high-dose chemotherapy. *Br J Cancer* 2006;94(9):1226–1230.
43. Baruchel S, Diezi M, Hargrave D, et al. Safety and pharmacokinetics of temozolomide using a dose-escalation, metronomic schedule in recurrent paediatric brain tumours. *Eur J Cancer* 2006;42(14):2335–2342.
44. Pratt CB, Goren MP, Meyer WH, et al. Ifosfamide neurotoxicity is related to previous cisplatin treatment for pediatric solid tumors. *J Clin Oncol* 1990;8(8):1399–1401.
45. Eberly AL, Anderson GD, Bubalo JS, et al. Optimal prevention of seizures induced by high-dose busulfan. *Pharmacotherapy* 2008;28(12):1502–1510.
46. Bonifazi F, Storci G, Bandini G, et al. Glutathione transferase-A2 S112T polymorphism predicts survival, transplant-related mortality, busulfan and bilirubin blood levels after allogeneic stem cell transplantation. *Haematologica* 2014;99(1):172–179.

47. An N, Janech MG, Bland AM, et al. Proteomic analysis of murine bone marrow niche microenvironment identifies thioredoxin as a novel agent for radioprotection and for enhancing donor cell reconstitution. *Exp Hematol* 2013;41:944–956.
48. Steinherz LJ, Steinherz PG, Mangiacasale D, et al. Cardiac changes with cyclophosphamide. *Med Pediatr Oncol* 1981;9(5):417–422.
49. Bastholt L, Johansson CJ, Pfeiffer P, et al. A pharmacokinetic study of prednimustine as compared with prednisolone plus chlorambucil in cancer patients. *Cancer Chemother Pharmacol* 1991;28(3):205–210.
50. Tew KD, Glusker JP, Hartley-Asp B, et al. Preclinical and clinical perspectives on the use of estramustine as an antimitotic drug. *Pharmacol Ther* 1992;56(3):323–339.
51. Punzi JS, Duax WL, Strong P, et al. Molecular conformation of estramustine and two analogues. *Mol Pharmacol* 1992;41(3):569–576.
52. Hudes GR, Greenberg R, Krigel RL, et al. Phase II study of estramustine and vinblastine, two microtubule inhibitors, in hormone-refractory prostate cancer. *J Clin Oncol* 1992;10(11):1754–1761.
53. Tew K, Houghton JA, Houghton PJ. *Preclinical and Clinical Modulation of Anticancer Drugs*. Boca Raton, FL: CRC Press; 1993.
54. Friedlos F, Davies L, Scanlon I, et al. Three new prodrugs for suicide gene therapy using carboxypeptidase G2 elicit bystander efficacy in two xenograft models. *Cancer Res* 2002;62(6):1724–1729.
55. Tew KD. TLK-286: a novel glutathione S-transferase-activated prodrug. *Expert Opin Investig Drugs* 2005;14(8):1047–1054.
56. Borch RF, Valente RR. Synthesis, activation, and cytotoxicity of aldophosphamide analogues. *J Med Chem* 1991;34(10):3052–3058.
57. Rosen LS, Laxa B, Boulos L, et al. Phase I study of TLK286 (Telcyta) administered weekly in advanced malignancies. *Clin Cancer Res* 2004;10(11):3689–3698.
58. Sequist LV, Fidias PM, Temel JS, et al. Phase 1–2a multicenter dose-ranging study of canfosfamide in combination with carboplatin and paclitaxel as first-line therapy for patients with advanced non-small cell lung cancer. *J Thorac Oncol* 2009;4(11):1389–1396.
59. Kavanagh JJ, Gershenson DM, Choi H, et al. Multi-institutional phase 2 study of TLK286 (TELCYTA, a glutathione S-transferase P1-1 activated glutathione analog prodrug) in patients with platinum and paclitaxel refractory or resistant ovarian cancer. *Int J Gynecol Cancer* 2005;15(4):593–600.
60. Vergote I, Finkler N, del Campo J, et al. Phase 3 randomised study of canfosfamide (Telcyta, TLK286) versus pegylated liposomal doxorubicin or topotecan as third-line therapy in patients with platinum-refractory or -resistant ovarian cancer. *Eur J Cancer* 2009;45(13):2324–2332.
61. Chase M, Chung RY, Chiocca EA. An oncolytic viral mutant that delivers the CYP2B1 transgene and augments cyclophosphamide chemotherapy. *Nat Biotechnol* 1998;16(5):444–448.
62. Vey N, Giles F. Laromustine (cloretazine). *Expert Opin Pharmacother* 2010;11(4):657–667.
63. Pigneux A. Laromustine, a sulfonyl hydrolyzing alkylating prodrug for cancer therapy. *IDrugs* 2009;12(1):39–53.
64. Schiller GJ, O'Brien SM, Pigneux A, et al. Single-agent laromustine, a novel alkylating agent, has significant activity in older patients with previously untreated poor-risk acute myeloid leukemia. *J Clin Oncol* 2010;28(5):815–821.
65. Eichbaum M, Bischofs E, Nehls K, et al. Bendamustine hydrochloride—a renaissance of alkylating strategies in anticancer medicine. *Drugs Today (Barc)* 2009;45(6):431–444.
66. Rasschaert M, Schrijvers D, Van den Brande J, et al. A phase I study of bendamustine hydrochloride administered day 1+2 every 3 weeks in patients with solid tumours. *Br J Cancer* 2007;96(11):1692–1698.
67. Weide R, Hess G, Köppler H, et al. High anti-lymphoma activity of bendamustine/mitoxantrone/rituximab in rituximab pretreated relapsed or refractory indolent lymphomas and mantle cell lymphomas: a multicenter phase II study of the German Low Grade Lymphoma Study Group (GLSG). *Leuk Lymphoma* 2007;48(7):1299–1306.
68. Cheson BD, Rummel MJ. Bendamustine: rebirth of an old drug. *J Clin Oncol* 2009;27(9):1492–1501.
69. van der Jagt R. Bendamustine for indolent non-Hodgkin lymphoma in the front-line or relapsed setting: a review of pharmacokinetics and clinical trial outcomes. *Expert Rev Hematol* 2013;6:525–537.
70. Ponisch W, Heyn S, Beck J, et al. Lenalidomide, bendamustine and prednisolone exhibits a favourable safety and efficacy profile in relapsed or refractory multiple myeloma: final results of a phase 1 clinical trial OSHO - #077. *Br J Haematol* 2013;162:202–209.

18 Platinum Analogs

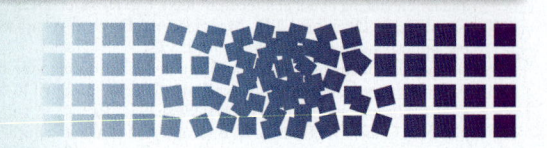

Peter J. O'Dwyer and A. Hilary Calvert

INTRODUCTION

The platinum drugs represent a unique and important class of antitumor compounds. Alone or in combination with other chemotherapeutic agents, *cis*-diamminedichloroplatinum (II) (cisplatin) and its analogs have made a significant impact on the treatment of a variety of solid tumors for nearly 40 years. The unique activity and toxicity profile observed with cisplatin in early clinical trials fueled the development of platinum analogs that are less toxic and more active against a variety of tumor types, including those that have developed resistance to cisplatin. In addition to cisplatin, two other platinum complexes are currently approved for use in the United States: *cis*-diamminecyclobutanedicarboxylate platinum (II) (carboplatin) and 1,2-diaminocyclohexaneoxalato platinum (II) (oxaliplatin). Several other analogs with unique activities are in various stages of clinical development, and nedaplatin (Japan) and lobaplatin (China) are locally registered. Progress in the development of superior analogs requires a thorough understanding of the chemical, biologic, pharmacokinetic, and pharmacodynamic properties of this important class of drugs.

HISTORY

The realization that platinum complexes exhibited antitumor activity began serendipitously in a series of experiments to investigate the effect of electromagnetic radiation on the growth of bacteria, carried out by Dr. Barnett Rosenberg and colleagues beginning in 1961.[1,2] Exposure of the bacteria to an electric field resulted in a profound change in their morphology; this effect was found not to be from the electric field, but from electrolysis products produced by the platinum electrodes. An analysis of these products resulted in the identification of the cis-isomer of a platinum coordination complex as the active compound. Tests of *cis*-diamminedichloroplatinum (II) in mice bearing several model tumor types indicated that cisplatin exhibited a broad spectrum of antitumor activity. Although early clinical trials demonstrated responses in several tumor types, particularly testicular cancers, the severe renal and gastrointestinal toxicity caused by the drug nearly led to its abandonment. Work at Memorial Sloan-Kettering[3,4] showed that these effects could be ameliorated, in part, by aggressive prehydration, which rekindled interest in its clinical use. Currently, cisplatin is curative in testicular cancer and significantly prolongs survival in combination regimens for ovarian, lung, head and neck, bladder, and upper gastrointestinal (GI) cancers. Its role is being reexamined in other tumors, too, and especially breast cancer.

PLATINUM CHEMISTRY

Platinum exists primarily in either a 2+ or 4+ oxidation state. These oxidation states dictate the stereochemistry of the ligands surrounding the platinum atom. Platinum (II) compounds exhibit a square planar geometry, in which the ammine ligands (also called carrier groups) are relatively stable, whereas the opposite, more polar ligands (leaving groups) are more easily displaced and so confer reactivity toward charged macromolecules, including DNA.[5] The stereochemistry of platinum complexes is critical to their antitumor activity as evidenced by the significantly reduced efficacy observed with *trans*-diamminedichloroplatinum (II).

In an aqueous solution, the chloride leaving groups of cisplatin are subject to mono- and diaqua substitution, particularly at chloride concentrations below 100 mmol, which characterize the intracellular environment. The administration of cisplatin in high chloride solutions (normal saline usually), therefore, contributes to stability. Intracellular formation of partially and fully aquated complexes creates the chloroaqua and hydroxoaqua cisplatin species that bind DNA.[6]

PLATINUM COMPLEXES AFTER CISPLATIN

Early in the clinical development of cisplatin, it became clear that its toxicity was a limitation to its therapeutic effectiveness, and that its activity, although striking in certain diseases, did not extend to all cancers. These observations then motivated a search for structural analogs with less toxicity and a different profile of antitumor activity. In addition, the side effects of cisplatin stimulated the development of antiemetics and other supportive care measures for use with chemotherapy. Progress in understanding the chemistry and pharmacokinetics of cisplatin has guided the development of new analogs. In general, modification of the chloride leaving groups of cisplatin results in compounds with different pharmacokinetics and reactivity towards DNA, whereas modification of the carrier ligands alters the activity of the resulting complex. The features of the more important platinum analogs that have been developed are shown in Figure 18.1.

Carboplatin

The carboplatin molecule has the same ammine carrier ligands as cisplatin. Using a murine screen for nephrotoxicity, Harrap and Calvert discovered that substituting a cyclobutanedicarboxylate moiety for the two chloride ligands of cisplatin resulted in a complex with reduced renal toxicity. This observation was translated to the clinic in the form of carboplatin, a more stable and pharmacokinetically predictable analog.[7,8] The results in humans were accurately predicted by the animal models, and marrow toxicity rather than nephrotoxicity was the principal side effect. At effective doses, carboplatin produced less nausea, vomiting, nephrotoxicity, and neurotoxicity than cisplatin. Furthermore, the myelosuppression was closely associated with the pharmacokinetics. The work of Calvert et al.[9] and Egorin and colleagues[10] showed that toxicity can be made more predictable and dose intensity less variable by dosing strategies based on the exposure. Carboplatin was shown to be indistinguishable from cisplatin in its clinical activity in all but a handful of tumor types and is the most frequently used form of platinum in current use. Cisplatin and carboplatin have almost superimposable profiles of activity in the NCI60 cell line screen, which further emphasizes the dependence of spectrum of activity on the carrier ligand.

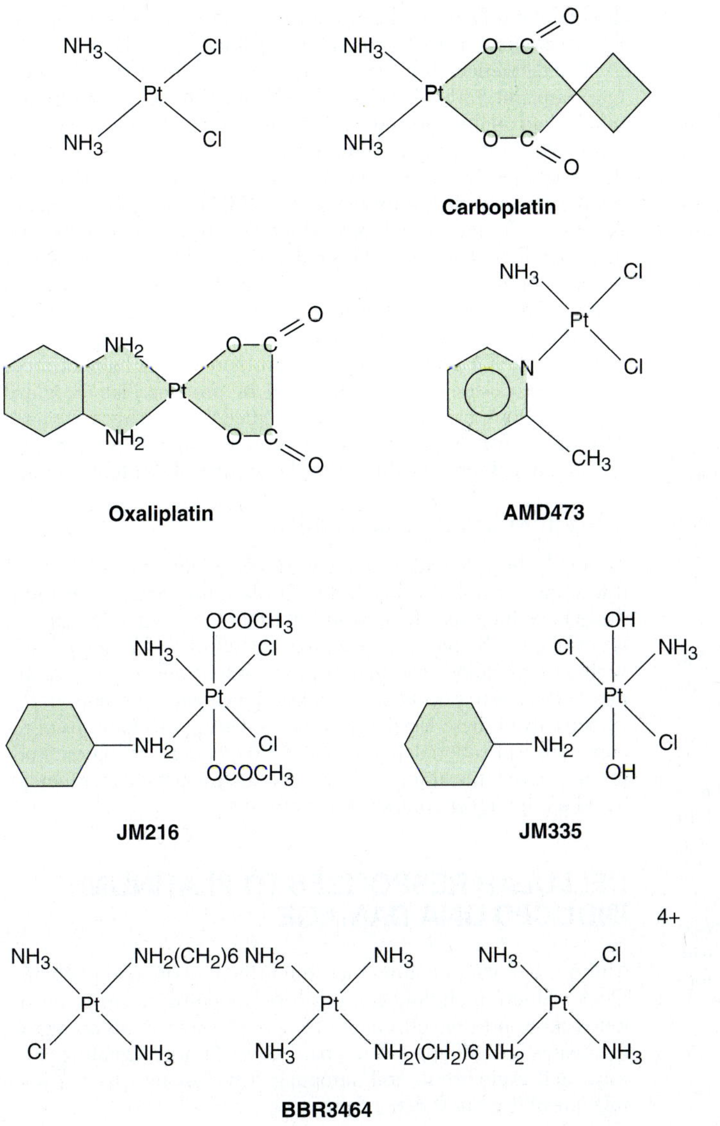

Figure 18.1 Structures of cisplatin, analogs, lobaplatin, and nedaplatin.

Oxaliplatin

Compounds with activity in cisplatin-resistant models emerged from modifications to the carrier group (see left side of the analogs in Fig. 18.1). Connors, in the late 1960s, synthesized platinum coordination compounds with varying physicochemical characteristics and found that the series that possessed a diaminocyclohexane (DACH) carrier group was active in models of cancer in vitro[11] and in vivo.[12] Subsequent studies supported the idea that DACH-based platinum complexes were non–cross-resistant with cisplatin, and DACH derivatives exhibited a unique cytotoxicity profile compared to cisplatin and carboplatin in the National Cancer Institute 60 cell line screen.[13–15] After a number of delays, a DACH analog that had been synthesized by Kidani and colleagues in the early 1970s, was developed in the clinic.[13] Oxaliplatin, a coordination compound of a DACH carrier group and an oxalato leaving group, was active in cisplatin-resistant tumor models. Like cisplatin, oxaliplatin preferentially forms adducts at the N7 position of guanine and, to a lesser extent, adenine. However, there is evidence that the three-dimensional structure of the DNA adducts and biologic response(s) they elicit are different from those of cisplatin. Oxaliplatin demonstrated activity in combination with 5-fluorouracil and leucovorin in colon cancer, a disease that is unresponsive to cisplatin. This finding validated the focus on cisplatin-resistant preclinical models to identify new active molecules. Oxaliplatin is approved for the treatment of advanced colorectal cancer, and enhances cure rates in the adjuvant setting. The therapeutic role of oxaliplatin has been found to extend to pancreatic, gastric, and esophageal cancers, in all of which it is the more active platinum derivative.

Nedaplatin and Lobaplatin

Nedaplatin is cis-diammineglycolatoplatinum, developed as a less nephrotoxic second-generation platinum analog, has been shown to be active in a range of tumors similar to that of cisplatin and carboplatin.[16] As a diammine structure, nedaplatin would fall among the cisplatin analogs analyzed in the NCI60 cell line screen,[17] and this activity is therefore anticipated. Lobaplatin is a platinum (II) complex in which the leaving group is lactic acid and the stable ammine ligand is 1,2-bis(aminomethyl)cyclobutane. In a similar way to oxaliplatin the stable ammine ligand may convey some non–cross-resistance compared to cisplatin or carboplatin. It is licensed in China for the breast cancer, small-cell lung cancer, and chronic myelogenous leukemia. It is unique among the platinum drugs for its approval for breast cancer, but there are few published clinical data and no randomized trials. It has not achieved approval in the United States or Europe.

Newer Platinum Structures

The octahedral stereochemistry adopted by platinum (IV) compounds has led investigators to speculate that they may exhibit a different spectrum of activity than that of platinum (II) drugs. Two compounds that were tested clinically without much success are ormaplatin and iproplatin. Two other platinum (IV) compounds that exhibit novel structural features, satraplatin (previously JM216) and JM335 (trans-ammine[cyclohexylamine]dichlorodihydroxo platinum [IV]), underwent more limited development. Satraplatin was the first orally active platinum compound, and showed some activity in lung and ovarian cancers, but despite promising activity in prostate cancer, a phase III trial was not successful.[18,19]

An approach based on the chemistry of the platinum-DNA interaction led to design and synthesis by Farrell et al.[20] of a novel class of compounds containing multiple platinum atoms (see Fig. 18.1). These bi- and trinuclear structures form adducts that span greater distances across the minor groove of DNA and have a profile of cell kill that differs from that of the small molecules. These compounds are unique in that their interaction with DNA is considerably different from that of cisplatin, particularly in the abundance of interstrand cross-links formed. Clinical development of candidate compounds is at a preliminary stage.

Efforts have been made to design novel platinum analogs that can circumvent putative cisplatin resistance mechanisms. An example is cis-amminedichloro(2-methylpyridine) platinum (II) (also known as AMD473 and ZD0473). This compound is a sterically hindered platinum complex that was designed to have minimal reactivity with thiols and thus avoid inactivation by molecules such as glutathione.[21,22] Responses were identified with its use in the clinic, but development was curtailed based on low levels of activity. The recent description of a monofunctional platinum (II) analog, phenanthriplatin, from the lab of Lippard is potentially of great interest, based on both potency in vitro and a mechanistic profile different from existing analogs.[23] A renewed appreciation that chemotherapeutic drugs have a continuing role in managing cancer is likely to prompt additional clinical development of novel platinum structures.

MECHANISM OF ACTION

DNA Adduct Formation

DNA has long been thought to be the major therapeutic target for platinum compounds. The cytotoxic effects are determined, in part, by the structure and relative amount of DNA adducts formed. Cisplatin and its analogs react preferentially at the N7 position of guanine and adenine residues to form a variety of monofunctional and bifunctional adducts.[24] The monoadducts may form intrastrand or interstrand cross-links. The predominant lesions that are formed when platinum compounds bind DNA are d(GpG)Pt intrastrand cross-links. Cisplatin also forms interstrand cross-links between guanine residues located on opposite strands, and these account for less than 5% of the total DNA-bound platinum. The formation of adducts and cross-links has been associated with therapeutic efficacy.[25,26] These adducts may contribute to the drug's cytotoxicity because they impede certain cellular processes that require the separation of both DNA strands, such as replication and transcription. The adducts formed in the reaction between carboplatin and DNA in cultured cells are essentially the same as those of cisplatin; however, higher concentrations of carboplatin are required (20- to 40-fold for cells) to obtain equivalent total platinum-DNA adduct levels due to its slower rate of aquation.[27] Oxaliplatin intrastrand adducts form even more slowly due to a slower rate of conversion from monoadducts; however, they are formed at similar DNA sequences and regions as cisplatin adducts. At equitoxic doses, oxaliplatin forms fewer DNA adducts than does cisplatin. This has been interpreted to mean that oxaliplatin lesions are more cytotoxic than those formed by cisplatin.

The differences observed in cytotoxicity between the diammine (e.g., cisplatin, carboplatin) and DACH platinum compounds may not depend on the type and relative amounts of the adducts formed, but on the overall three-dimensional structure of the adduct and its recognition by various cellular proteins. The major difference between them is the protrusion of the DACH moiety of oxaliplatin into the major groove of DNA, which thus produces a bulkier adduct than that of cisplatin. This bulkier, more hydrophobic adduct seems to be recognized differently by cellular proteins involved in sensing DNA damage.[28] The functional consequences are twofold: Proteins such as polymerases that recognize and participate in reactions on DNA under normal circumstances may be perturbed, whereas processes that are controlled by proteins that recognize damaged DNA may become activated (the DNA damage response). The latter group of proteins function both in the DNA repair process and in cellular signaling toward cell survival/death decisions.

DNA Interstrand Cross-Links

Although the DNA adducts are well-recognized to result in G-G interstrand cross-links, like classical alkylating agents, platinum drugs have the capacity to form intrastrand cross-links, albeit to a lesser degree. By blocking essential aspects of DNA metabolism, such as replication and transcription, intrastrand cross-links are highly cytotoxic. Recent studies have drawn attention both to the cytotoxicity of these lesions, and their differing mechanisms of repair, both replication dependent and independent.[29,30] These studies may have clinical implications in selecting patients for therapy based on the repair competence of tumors.

CELLULAR RESPONSES TO PLATINUM-INDUCED DNA DAMAGE

Multiple cellular outcomes may follow the formation of platinum-DNA adducts, including cell death by apoptosis, necrosis, or mitotic catastrophe, or cell survival by activation of various protective mechanisms including DNA repair, DNA damage signaling pathways, cell cycle arrest, and autophagy (the last may have a dual role, possibly context dependent).

Cell Fate

The cellular effects following DNA binding by platinum drugs have been analyzed. The studies of Sorenson and Eastman,[31] using DNA repair-deficient Chinese hamster ovary (CHO) cells, indicated that passage through the S phase is necessary for G2 arrest and cell death, which suggests that DNA replication on a damaged template may result in the accumulation of further damage. An aberrant mitosis was observed before apoptosis in this model.

DNA Damage Recognition

Among the initiation events that ultimately result in platinum drug–induced cell death are the binding of platinum-DNA damage recognition proteins, which then seed the accumulation of a large protein complex capable both of DNA damage signaling (as to cell cycle proteins to halt replication) and repair of the damaged DNA. Among the DNA-binding proteins are the high-mobility group proteins HMG1 and HMG2.[32–34] These proteins are capable of bending DNA as well as recognizing bent DNA structures, such as that produced by cisplatin, and different specificities for cisplatin and for oxaliplatin adducts are observed in structural studies.[35,36] Other candidate platinum-DNA damage recognition proteins include histone H1, RNA polymerase I transcription upstream binding factor (hUBF), the TATA binding protein (TBP), and proteins involved in mismatch repair (MMR). The MMR complex has been implicated in cisplatin sensitivity.[37] Studies have shown that the MSH2 and MLH1 proteins participate in the recognition of DNA adducts formed by cisplatin, but not oxaliplatin, which could contribute to differences in the cytotoxicity profiles observed between these two platinum complexes.

DNA Damage Signaling

A number of signaling events have been shown to occur after treatment of cells with platinum drugs.[38] For example, the ATM- and Rad3-related (ATR) proteins that are involved in cell-cycle checkpoint activation are activated by cisplatin. These kinases phosphorylate and activate several downstream effectors that regulate cell cycle, DNA repair, cell survival, and apoptosis, including p53, CHK2, and members of the mitogen-activated protein kinase (MAPK) pathway (extracellular signal-related kinase [ERK], c-Jun amino-terminal kinase [JNK], and p38 kinase). Recent data especially implicate signaling through the JNK pathway, and inhibition at the level of JNK seems especially relevant to platinum drug cytotoxicity in vitro and in vivo.[39,40] The pleiotropic nature of this stress response only grows, because each of these molecules subsequently controls the activity and expression of many more proteins. As a result of this complexity, acting in the context of variable genomic tumor aberrations, therapeutic strategies directed to these pathways have been slow to emerge. However, clinical trials to investigate specific inhibitors of DNA damage responses are underway and hold promise. It is also relevant to point out that these signaling pathways affect not just the tumor cell, but also may communicate to cells in the microenvironment, the responses of which may also determine the effectiveness of therapy.

IS DNA THE ONLY TARGET?

Early analyses of the action of cytotoxic drugs included a probe of whether effects on DNA were sufficient to explain drug effects. A pioneer in this field was Tritton,[41] who proposed that effects of DNA-intercalating agents on the plasma membrane could underlie the cytotoxicity of the drug. More recently, enucleated cells were shown to be susceptible to cisplatin, and a seminal paper from Voest and colleagues showed that platinum sensitivity was determined not solely by the accumulation of DNA damage in the tumor cell.[42] In analyzing the contribution of cells in the microenvironment of tumors, he showed that tumor infiltration with mesenchymal stem cells could confer drug resistance. A search for secreted factors defined platinum-induced fatty acids, metabolic products in the thromboxane synthetase, and cyclooxygenase-1 pathways as determining the effectiveness of drug therapy. A proteomic study in cisplatin-sensitive and -resistant cells confirmed the substantial effects of drug exposure on lipid metabolites and their relation to susceptibility. A current focus on therapies directed to the microenvironment, including immunologic and anti-inflammatory interventions,[43] has the potential to expand our ability to apply platinum drugs in the clinic.

MECHANISMS OF RESISTANCE

The major limitation to the successful treatment of solid tumors with platinum-based chemotherapy is the emergence of drug-resistant tumor cells.[44] Developments in tumor biology have advanced our thinking with regard to how and when these cells emerge; heterogeneity within a tumor even at its earliest diagnosis reflects the emergence of treatment-resistant clones even in advance of selection pressure and the realization that resistance may not be specific to the DNA-damaging drug. Indeed, this may be reflected clinically in the finding that after progression on initial chemotherapy, the use of second-line therapy is usually associated with a shorter duration of response.

Currently described mechanisms of platinum drug resistance (Fig. 18.2) include reduced cellular accumulation, intracellular detoxification, repair of Pt-DNA lesions, increased damage tolerance, and the activation of cellular defense mechanisms such as autophagy. In addition, we have already alluded to exogenous influences on mechanism, as may be mediated by other cells, metabolites, of physicochemical conditions (such as hypoxia) in the tumor microenvironment. It must be acknowledged, however, that our insights are very limited as to why some tumors respond and others do not to platinum chemotherapy. As genome sequencing yields increasing and often surprising revelations about the genes that drive cancers and the complexity inherent in cancers of a single histologic type, it is likely that when associated with outcomes in large patient populations, patterns will emerge to guide selection of therapies.

Reduced Accumulation

Platinum uptake in cells occurs by simple diffusion and by carrier-mediated mechanisms. Inhibition of transport mechanisms has a marked effect on intracellular platinum accumulation, and Howell's group has shown the importance of the copper transporters CTR-1 and CTR-2 in regulating the influx of various platinum analogs in eukaryotic cells.[45,46] The contribution of these mechanisms to clinical platinum drug resistance is being explored.[47] Accumulation may also be influenced by enhanced efflux, and various transport proteins are upregulated in cell lines selected for acquired resistance, and in platinum-resistant ovarian cancers.

Inactivation

Platinum complexes are highly reactive molecules and bind rapidly to multiple cellular macromolecules. Protection from such chemicals in the environment is afforded by cellular thiols, including

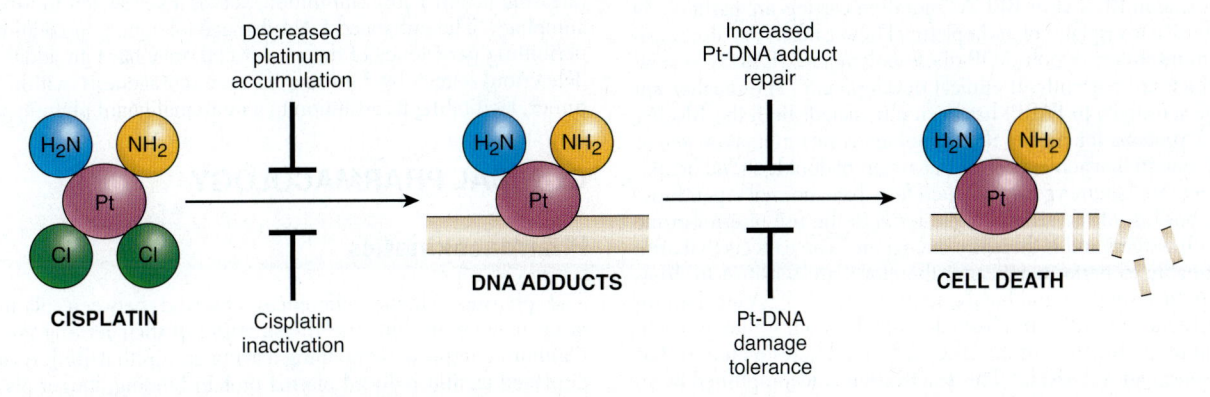

Figure 18.2 Cellular mechanisms of cisplatin resistance.

small peptides such as glutathione (GSH) and larger proteins as exemplified by metallothionein (MT). There are many reports of an association between platinum drug sensitivity and glutathione levels[48–50]; however, reducing intracellular glutathione levels with drugs such as buthionine sulfoximine has resulted in only low to modest potentiation of cisplatin sensitivity.[51] Buthionine sulfoximine was developed for clinical use, and some impact on GSH content of tumors and normal tissues was demonstrated. However, the depletion of GSH was not consistent, and ultimately, the cost of producing the active stereoisomer of the drug was judged prohibitive. Inactivation of the platinum drugs may also occur through binding to the MTs, a family of sulfhydryl-rich, low–molecular-weight proteins that participate in heavy metal binding and detoxification; however, the contribution of MT to clinical platinum drug resistance is unclear, and a therapeutic role has not emerged.

Increased DNA Repair

Once platinum-DNA adducts are formed, cells must either repair or tolerate the damage to survive. In general, the capacity to repair DNA damage seems to play a role in determining a tumor cell's sensitivity to platinum drugs and other DNA-damaging agents. For example, tumors that are unusually sensitive to cisplatin, such as testicular nonseminomatous germ cell tumors, may be deficient in their ability to repair platinum-DNA adducts.[52] The increased repair of platinum-DNA lesions in cisplatin-resistant cell lines as compared to their sensitive counterparts has been shown in several human cancer cell lines, but translation of these observations to the clinic has been difficult. The repair of platinum-DNA adducts appears to occur predominantly by nucleotide excision repair (NER), with a role for MMR under certain circumstances.[53] The molecular basis for the increased repair activity observed in cisplatin-resistant cells is not known precisely, but formation of the ERCC1/XPF protein complex may be a key step. Selvakumaran et al.[54] showed that the downregulation of ERCC-1 using an antisense approach sensitized a platinum-resistant cell line to cisplatin both in vitro and in vivo. There is substantial clinical evidence that implicates ERCC1 expression in increased NER and cisplatin resistance, and high expression of ERCC1 has been demonstrated to confer a worse outcome after cisplatin treatment in several resistant tumors. The most extensive study of this as a marker has been in non–small-cell lung cancer, results in which were summarized and analyzed by Hubner et al.[55] In gastric cancer also, high levels of ERCC1 are associated with resistance to cisplatin treatment.[56–58] However, a recent reevaluation of discrepant results questioned the reliability of the assays of ERCC1 and their relationship to function.[59] These data suggest that there is a relationship between ERCC1 expression and treatment, but that the lag in marker development precludes implementation of a predictive assay until additional studies have been performed.

Perhaps the most striking evidence that DNA repair is a determinant of platinum drug responses is that breast and ovarian cancers occurring in BRCA1 or BRCA2 mutation carriers are particularly responsive to cisplatin or carboplatin. These cancers are also sensitive to inhibitors of poly(ADP-ribose)polymerase (PARPi), several of which are currently in clinical development. The mechanism of the sensitivity to PARPi has been elucidated. Both the BRCA1 and 2 proteins form part of the homologous recombination repair (HR) system that achieves error-free repair of double strand breaks. Carriers are heterozygous and, therefore, have normal repair function, but loss of the second allele leads to the use of error-prone backup systems and is therefore oncogenic. The cancers that arise are unable to perform HR and, therefore, are sensitive to drugs that induce single strand breaks, such as PARPi.[60,61] A mechanism of resistance to PARPi has been described, which is due to reactivation of the function of the BRCA2 leading to restoration of HR and sensitivity to PARPi.[62] This reactivation is accomplished by an intragenic deletion and the restoration of an open reading frame. It has further been shown that such revertant cells are resistant to cisplatin as well as PARPi. Finally, recurrent cancers in BRCA2 mutation carriers, which have acquired platinum resistance, have been shown to have undergone reversion of the BRCA2 mutation.[63] This clearly shows that the HR system can be one cause of cisplatin resistance. However, not all cisplatin-resistant patients are also resistant to PARPi,[64] showing that there are multiple other causes of cis/carboplatin resistance.

Combinations of platinum drugs with PARPi are being actively pursued in patients with BRCA-related tumors and also in patients whose tumors are likely to have acquired loss of HR function (poorly differentiated serous ovarian cancer and triple negative breast cancer).

Autophagy

After platinum-DNA adduct formation, the cell detects the DNA damage and initiates signaling through multiple pathways, the effects of which include mobilization of repair proteins; arrest of the cell cycle; altered transcriptional programs; redirection of energy production and consumption; activation of cell death pathways and, simultaneously, of pathways that would counter a cell death decision, and so to permit survival. A process recently characterized to perform the last function is autophagy. Initially described as a mechanism of cell death, autophagy represents a regulated dissolution of cellular elements into a characteristic set of subcellular organelles detectable by electron microscopy and linked by a particular profile of gene expression changes.[65] Multiple stimuli precipitate these changes and have in common scarcity of nutrients that are required for survival, from oxygen and glucose withdrawal to less specific calorie deprivation, and inhibition of metabolic pathways. Autophagy is also a consequence of cytotoxic drug treatment and, more recently, has been appreciated as a means by which cells might survive the stress of cellular insults, and so become resistant to treatment.[66] Amaravadi and colleagues[67] demonstrated that autophagy reversal can sensitize tumors to cytotoxic drugs and several trials of platinum compounds along with the autophagy inhibitor hydroxychloroquine are in progress.

Increased DNA Damage Tolerance

The net result of DNA damage signaling in a sensitive tumor cell is engagement of cell death pathways, including apoptosis, and therapeutic benefit. In a resistant tumor cell, the cell survives as a consequence of one or many of these mechanisms, and this can result in platinum-DNA damage tolerance or multidrug resistance phenotype, or both. Contributors to the tolerance might include deficient DNA MMR (which could excise the adduct if NER failed), enhanced replicative bypass (which essentially ignores the adduct, allowing the cell to survive, but could contribute to the increase in mutation frequency observed in chemotherapy-treated cancers), and altered signaling through stress-related kinases such as JNK, which can both alter transcriptional programs and activate autophagy. Indeed JNK, by phosphorylating Bcl-2 or Bcl-XL, and releasing beclin-1 from inhibition, acts as a key switch to turn on autophagy. The enhanced DNA damage tolerance, in addition to permitting persistence of the cancer cell, may have an additional deleterious effect by fostering further mutagenesis within the tumor, facilitating its evolution to a more malignant phenotype.

CLINICAL PHARMACOLOGY

Pharmacokinetics

The pharmacokinetic differences observed between platinum drugs may be attributed to the structure of their leaving groups. Platinum complexes containing leaving groups that are less easily displaced exhibit reduced plasma protein binding, longer plasma half-lives, and higher rates of renal clearance. These features are

TABLE 18.1
Comparative Parmacokinetics of Platinum Analogs After Bolus or Short Intravenous Infusion

	Cisplatin	Carboplatin	Oxaliplatin
$T_{1/2}\alpha$			
Total platinum	14–49 min	12–98 min	26 min
Ultrafiltrate	9–30 min	8–87 min	21 min
$T_{1/2}\beta$			
Total platinum	0.7–4.6 h	1.3–1.7 h	—
Ultrafiltrate	0.7–0.8 h	1.7–5.9 h	—
$T_{1/2}\gamma$			
Total platinum	24–127 h	8.2–40.0 h	38–47 h
Ultrafiltrate	—	—	24–27 h
Protein binding	>90%	24%–50%	85%
Urinary excretion	23%–50%	54%–82%	>50%

$T_{1/2}\alpha$, half-life of first phase; $T_{1/2}\beta$, half-life of second phase; $T_{1/2}\gamma$, half-life of terminal phase.

evident in the pharmacokinetic properties of cisplatin, carboplatin, and oxaliplatin, which are summarized in Table 18.1. Platinum drug pharmacokinetics have been reviewed.[68]

Cisplatin

After intravenous infusion, cisplatin rapidly diffuses into tissues and is covalently bound to plasma protein. More than 90% of platinum is bound to plasma protein at 4 hours after infusion. The disappearance of ultrafilterable platinum is rapid and occurs in a biphasic fashion. Half-lives of 10 to 30 minutes and 0.7 to 0.8 hours have been reported for the initial and terminal phases, respectively. Cisplatin excretion is dependent on renal function, which accounts for the majority of its elimination. The percentage of platinum excreted in the urine has been reported to be between 23% and 40% at 24 hours after infusion. Only a small percentage of the total platinum is excreted in the bile.

Carboplatin

The differences in pharmacokinetics observed between cisplatin and carboplatin depend primarily on the slower rate of conversion of carboplatin to a reactive species. Thus, the stability of carboplatin results in a low incidence of nephrotoxicity. Carboplatin diffuses rapidly into tissues after infusion; however, it is considerably more stable in plasma. Only 24% of a dose was bound to plasma protein at 4 hours after infusion. The disappearance of platinum from plasma after short intravenous infusions of carboplatin has been reported to occur in a biphasic or triphasic manner. The initial half-lives for total platinum, which vary considerably among several studies, are listed in Table 18.1. The half-lives for total platinum range from 12 to 98 minutes during the first phase ($T_{1/2}\alpha$) and from 1.3 to 1.7 hours during the second phase ($T_{1/2}\beta$). Half-lives reported for the terminal phase range from 8.2 to 40 hours. The disappearance of ultrafilterable platinum is biphasic with $T_{1/2}\alpha$ and $T_{1/2}\beta$ values ranging from 7.6 to 87 minutes and 1.7 to 5.9 hours, respectively. Carboplatin is excreted predominantly by the kidneys, and cumulative urinary excretion of platinum is 54% to 82%, most as unmodified carboplatin. The renal clearance of carboplatin is closely correlated with the glomerular filtration rate (GFR).[69] This observation enabled Calvert et al.[9] to design a carboplatin-dosing formula based on the individual patient's GFR.

Oxaliplatin

After oxaliplatin infusion, platinum accumulates into three compartments: plasma-bound platinum, ultrafilterable platinum, and platinum associated with erythrocytes. When specific and sensitive mass spectrometric techniques are used, oxaliplatin itself is undetectable in plasma, even at end infusion.[70] The active forms of the drug have not been extensively characterized. Approximately 85% of the total platinum is bound to plasma protein at 2 to 5 hours after infusion.[71] Plasma elimination of total platinum and ultrafilterates is biphasic. The half-lives for the initial and terminal phases are 26 minutes and 38.7 hours, respectively, for total platinum and 21 minutes and 24.2 hours, respectively, for ultrafilterable platinum (see Table 18.1).[72] Thus, as with carboplatin, substantial differences between total and free platinum kinetics are not observed. As with cisplatin, a prolonged retention of oxaliplatin is observed in red blood cells. However, unlike cisplatin, oxaliplatin does not accumulate to any significant level after multiple courses of treatment.[71] This may explain why neurotoxicity associated with oxaliplatin is reversible. Oxaliplatin is eliminated predominantly by the kidneys, with more than 50% of the platinum being excreted in the urine at 48 hours.

Pharmacodynamics

Pharmacodynamics relates pharmacokinetic indices of drug exposure to biologic measures of drug effect, usually toxicity to normal tissues or tumor cell kill. Two issues to be addressed in such studies are whether the effectiveness of the drug can be enhanced and whether the toxicity can be attenuated by knowledge of the platinum pharmacokinetics in an individual. These questions are appropriate to the use of cytotoxic agents with relatively narrow therapeutic indices. Toxicity to normal tissues can be quantitated as a continuous variable when the drug causes myelosuppression. Thus, the early studies of carboplatin demonstrated a close relationship of changes in platelet counts to the area under the concentration-time curve (AUC) in the individual. The AUC was itself closely related to renal function, which was determined as creatinine clearance. Based on these observations, Egorin et al.,[10] Calvert et al.,[9] and Chatelut and colleagues[73] derived formulas based on creatinine clearance to predict either the percentage change in platelet count or a target AUC. Application of pharmacodynamically guided dosing algorithms for carboplatin has been widely adopted as a means of avoiding overdosage (by producing acceptable nadir platelet counts) and of maximizing dose intensity in the individual. There is good evidence that this approach can decrease the risk of unacceptable toxicity. Accordingly, a dosing strategy based on renal function is recommended for the use of carboplatin.

A key question is whether maximizing carboplatin exposure in an individual can measurably increase the probability of tumor regression or survival. In an analysis by Jodrell et al.,[74] carboplatin AUC was a predictor of response, thrombocytopenia, and leukopenia. The likelihood of a tumor response increased with increasing AUC up to a level of 5 to 7 mg × hour per milliliter, after which a plateau was reached. Similar results were obtained with carboplatin in combination with cyclophosphamide, and neither response rate nor survival was determined by the carboplatin AUC in a cohort of ovarian cancer patients.[75] As a result, most carboplatin recommended doses are based on an AUC in this range (for every 3 to 4 week schedules), and modifications of these are used for more frequent administration (as in combined chemoradiotherapy regimens).

The relationship of pharmacokinetics to response has been sought by investigating the cellular pharmacology of these agents.[76] The formation and repair of the platinum-DNA adducts in human cells are not easily measured. Schellens and colleagues[77,78] analyzed the pharmacokinetic and pharmacodynamic interactions of cisplatin administered as a single agent. In a series of patients with head and neck cancer, they found that cisplatin exposure (measured as the AUC) closely correlated with both the peak DNA adduct content in leukocytes and the area under the DNA-adduct time curve. These measures were important predictors of response, both individually and in logistic regression analysis. However, as an approach to determine who should or should not be treated with platinum drugs, it seems more likely that genomic analyses will provide guidance in the near future.

Pharmacogenomics

Variability in pharmacokinetics and pharmacodynamics of cytotoxic drugs is an important determinant of therapeutic index. This interindividual variation may be attributed in part to genetic differences among patients. Targeted analyses of germ-line DNA and, increasingly, Genome-wide association studies (GWAS) approaches, have yielded genotypic features associated with results of therapy. Detoxification pathways and DNA repair have emerged as having markers attributable to response of lack of it in response to platinum drugs. Single nucleotide polymorphisms (SNP) in genes related to glutathione metabolism and in several DNA repair genes have been identified in lung cancer, breast cancer, and various GI cancers. A concern is that larger trials have not always confirmed early findings. As yet, informative SNPs that could be used to define therapeutic strategies for individual patients have not yet been defined.

FORMULATION AND ADMINISTRATION

Cisplatin (Platinol)

Cisplatin is administered in a chloride-containing solution intravenously over 0.5 to 2.0 hours. To minimize the risk of nephrotoxicity, patients are prehydrated with at least 500 mL of salt-containing fluid. Immediately before cisplatin administration, mannitol (12.5 to 25.0 g) is given parenterally to maximize urine flow. A diuretic such as furosemide may be used also, along with parenteral antiemetics. These currently include dexamethasone together with a 5-hydroxytryptamine (5-HT$_3$) antagonist. A minimum of 1 L of posthydration fluid is usually given. The intensity of hydration varies somewhat with the dose of cisplatin. High-dose cisplatin (up to 200 mg/m^2 per course) may be administered in a formulation containing 3% sodium chloride, but this method is no longer widely used. Cisplatin may also be administered regionally to increase local drug exposure and diminish side effects. Its intraperitoneal use was defined by Ozols et al.[79] and by Howell and colleagues.[80] Measured drug exposure in the peritoneal cavity is some 50-fold higher compared to levels achieved with intravenous administration. At standard dosages in ovarian cancer patients with low-volume disease, a randomized intergroup trial suggested that intraperitoneal administration is superior to intravenous cisplatin in combination with intravenous cyclophosphamide.[81] The development of combinations of carboplatin and paclitaxel has, however, superseded this technique in the treatment of ovarian cancer, and the intraperitoneal route is now infrequently used. Regional uses also include intra-arterial delivery (as for hepatic tumors, melanoma, and glioblastoma), but none have been adopted as a standard method of treatment. There is growing interest in chemoembolization for the treatment of tumors confined to the liver, and cisplatin is a component of many popular regimens.[82]

Carboplatin (Paraplatin)

Cisplatin treatment over 3 to 6 hours is burdensome for clinical resources and tiring for cancer patients. Previously given as an in-hospital treatment, it is now usually administered in the outpatient setting. The exigencies of the modern health-care environment have contributed to the expanding use of carboplatin as an alternative to cisplatin except in circumstances in which cisplatin is clearly the superior agent. Carboplatin is substantially easier to administer. Extensive hydration is not required because of the lack of nephrotoxicity at standard dosages. Carboplatin is reconstituted in chloride-free solutions (unlike cisplatin, because chloride can displace the leaving groups) and administered over 30 minutes as a rapid intravenous infusion.

Oxaliplatin (Eloxatin)

Oxaliplatin is also uncomplicated in its clinical administration. For bolus infusion, the required dose is administered in 500 mL of chloride-free diluent over a period of 2 hours. Oxaliplatin is most frequently given as a single dose every 2 weeks (85 mg/m^2) or every 3 weeks (130 mg/m^2), alone or with other active agents. It is common to pretreat patients with active antiemetics, such as a 5-HT$_3$ antagonist, but the nausea is not as severe as with cisplatin. No prehydration is required. Besides a relatively low incidence of myelosuppression, the predominant toxicity of oxaliplatin is cumulative neurotoxicity. The development of an oropharyngeal dysesthesia, often precipitated by exposure to cold, may require prolonging the duration of administration to 6 hours. On occasion, the occurrence of hypersensitivity also requires slowing the infusion.

TOXICITY

A substantial body of literature documents the side effects of platinum compounds. As noted in the section titled History, earlier in this chapter, the toxicity of cisplatin was a driving force both in the search for less toxic analogs and for more effective treatments for its side effects, especially nausea and vomiting. The toxicities associated with cisplatin, carboplatin, and oxaliplatin are described in detail in the following sections and summarized in Table 18.2. Please review the package inserts for these drugs for full prescribing information and delineation of toxic effects.

Cisplatin

The side effects associated with cisplatin (at single doses of more than 50 mg/m^2) include nausea and vomiting, nephrotoxicity, ototoxicity, neuropathy, and myelosuppression. Rare effects include visual impairment, seizures, arrhythmias, acute ischemic vascular events, glucose intolerance, and pancreatitis. The nausea and vomiting stimulated a search for new antiemetics. These effects are currently best managed with 5-HT$_3$ antagonists, usually given with a glucocorticoid, although other combinations of agents are still widely used. In the weeks after treatment, continuous antiemetic therapy may be required. Nephrotoxicity is ameliorated but not completely prevented by hydration. The renal damage to both glomeruli and tubules is cumulative, and after cisplatin treatment, serum creatinine levels are no longer a reliable guide to GFR. An acute elevation of serum creatinine level may follow a cisplatin dose, but this index returns to normal with time. Tubule damage may be reflected in a salt-losing syndrome that also resolves with time.

Ototoxicity is a cumulative and irreversible side effect of cisplatin treatment that results from damage to the inner ear. The initial audiographic manifestation is loss of high-frequency acuity (4,000 to 8,000 Hz). When acuity is affected in the range of speech, cisplatin

TABLE 18.2
Toxicity Profiles of Platinum Analogs in Clinical Use

Toxicity	Cisplatin	Carboplatin	Oxaliplatin
Myelosuppression		X	
Nephrotoxicity	X		
Neurotoxicity	X		X
Ototoxicity	X		
Nausea and vomiting	X	X	X

should be discontinued under most circumstances and carboplatin substituted where appropriate. Peripheral neuropathy is also cumulative, although less common than with agents such as vinca alkaloids. This neuropathy is usually reversible, although recovery is often slow. A number of agents with the potential for protection from neuropathy have been developed, but none is yet used widely.

Carboplatin

Myelosuppression, which is not usually severe with cisplatin, is the dose-limiting toxicity of carboplatin. The drug is most toxic to the platelet precursors, but neutropenia and anemia are frequently observed. The lowest platelet counts after a single dose of carboplatin are observed 17 to 21 days later, and recovery usually occurs by day 28. The effect is dose dependent, but individuals vary widely in their susceptibility. As shown by Egorin et al.[10] and Calvert et al.,[9] the severity of platelet toxicity is best accounted for by a measure of the drug exposure in an individual, the AUC. Both groups derived pharmacologically based formulas to predict toxicity and guide carboplatin dosing. That of Calvert and colleagues targets a particular exposure to carboplatin:

Dose (mg) = target AUC (mg · min/mL) × (GFR mL/min + 25)

This formula has been widely used to individualize carboplatin dosing and permits targeting an acceptable level of toxicity. Patients who are elderly, have a poor performance status, or have a history of extensive pretreatment have a higher risk of toxicity even when dosage is calculated with these methods, but the safety of drug administration has been enhanced. In the combination of carboplatin and paclitaxel, AUC-based dosing has helped to maximize the dose intensity of carboplatin. Dosages some 30% higher than those using a dosing strategy based solely on body surface area may safely be used. A determination of whether this approach to dosing improves outcomes will require a randomized trial.

The other toxicities of carboplatin are generally milder and better tolerated than those of cisplatin. Nausea and vomiting, although frequent, are less severe, shorter in duration, and more easily controlled with standard antiemetics (i.e., prochlorperazine [Compazine]), dexamethasone, lorazepam) than that after cisplatin treatment. Renal impairment is infrequent, although alopecia is common, especially with the paclitaxel-containing combinations. Neurotoxicity is also less common than with cisplatin, although it is observed more frequently with the increasing use of high-dose regimens. Ototoxicity is also less common.

Oxaliplatin

The dose-limiting toxicity of oxaliplatin is sensory neuropathy, a characteristic of all DACH-containing platinum derivatives. This side effect takes two forms. First, a tingling of the extremities, which may also involve the perioral region, that occurs early and usually resolves within a few days. With repeated dosing, symptoms may last longer between cycles, but do not appear to be cumulative or of long duration. Laryngopharyngeal spasms and cold dysesthesias have also been reported but are not associated with significant respiratory symptoms and can be prevented by prolonging the duration of infusion. A second neuropathy, more typical of that seen with cisplatin, affects the extremities and increases with repeated doses. Definitive physiologic characterization of oxaliplatin-induced neuropathy has proven difficult in large studies. Electromyograms performed in six patients treated by Extra et al.[83] revealed an axonal sensory neuropathy, but nerve conduction velocities were unchanged. Specimens from peripheral nerve biopsies performed in this study showed decreased myelination and replacement with collagen pockets. The neurologic effects of oxaliplatin appear to be cumulative in that they become more pronounced and of greater duration with successive cycles; however, unlike those of cisplatin, they are reversible with drug cessation. In a review of 682 patient experiences, Brienza et al.[84] reported that 82% of patients who experienced grade 2 neurotoxicity or higher had their symptoms regress within 4 to 6 months. In a larger adjuvant trial, de Gramont et al.[85] reported that 12% of patients had grade 3 toxicity at the end of a 6-month treatment period and that the majority of these patients had relief, but not always complete resolution of the symptoms, by 1 year later. The persistence of the neurotoxicity has led to approaches to ameliorate it, including the use of protective agents. The use of calcium and magnesium salts intravenously before and after each infusion has been shown to be ineffective. Ototoxicity is not observed with oxaliplatin. Nausea and vomiting do occur and generally respond to 5-HT$_3$ antagonists. Myelosuppression is uncommon and is not severe with oxaliplatin as a single agent, but it is a feature of combinations including this drug. Oxaliplatin therapy is not associated with nephrotoxicity.

REFERENCES

1. Rosenberg B, VanCamp L, Trosko J, et al. Platinum compounds: a new class of potent antitumor agents. *Nature* 1969;222:385–386.
2. Rosenberg B. Fundamental studies with cisplatin. *Cancer* 1985;55:2303–2316.
3. Cvitkovic E, Spaulding J, Bethune V, et al. Improvement of cis-dichlorodiammineplatinum (NSC 119875): therapeutic index in an animal model. *Cancer* 1977;39:1357–1361.
4. Hayes D, Cvitkovic E, Golbey R, et al. High dose cis-platinum diamine dichloride: amelioration of renal toxicity by mannitol diuresis. *Cancer* 1977;39:1372–1381.
5. Roberts J, Thomson A. The mechanism of action of antitumor platinum compounds. *Nucleic Acids Res* 1979;22:71–133.
6. Martin R. Platinum complexes: hydrolysis and binding to N(7) and N(1) of purines. In: Lippert B, ed. *Cisplatin: Chemistry and Biochemistry of a Leading Anticancer Drug*. Zurich: Verlag Helvetica Chimica Acta; 1999:183.
7. Harrap K. Preclinical studies identifying carboplatin as a viable cisplatin alternative. *Cancer Treat Rev* 1985;12:A21–A33.
8. Harrap K. Initiatives with platinum- and quinazoline-based antitumor molecules—Fourteenth Bruce F. Cain Memorial Award Lecture. *Cancer Res* 1995;55:2761–2768.
9. Calvert A, Newell D, Gumbrell L, et al. Carboplatin dosage: prospective evaluation of a simple formula based on renal function. *J Clin Oncol* 1989;7:1748–1756.
10. Egorin M, Echo DV, Olman E, et al. Prospective validation of a pharmacologically based dosing scheme for the cis-diamminedichloroplatinum(II) analogue diamminecyclobutanedicarboxylatoplatinum. *Cancer Res* 1985;45:6502–6506.
11. Connors T, Jones M, Ross W, et al. New platinum complexes with anti-tumour activity. *Chem Biol Interact* 1972;5:415–424.
12. Burchenal J, Kalaker K, Dew K, et al. Rationale for development of platinum analogs. *Cancer Treat Rep* 1979;63:1493–1498.
13. Kidani Y, Inagaki K, Tsukagoshi S. Examination of antitumor activities of platinum complexes of 1,2-diaminocyclohexane isomers and their related complexes. *Gann* 1976;67:921–922.
14. Burchenal J, Irani G, Kern K, et al. 1,2-Diaminocyclohexane platinum derivatives of potential clinical value. *Rec Res Cancer Res* 1980;74:146–155.
15. Rixe O, Ortuzar W, Alvarez M, et al. Oxaliplatin, tetraplatin, cisplatin, and carboplatin: spectrum of activity in drug-resistant cell lines and in the cell lines of the National Cancer Institute's anticancer drug screen panel. *Biochem Pharmacol* 1996;52:1855–1865.
16. Shimada M, Itamochi H, Kigawa J. Nedaplatin: a cisplatin derivative in cancer therapy. *Cancer Manag Res* 2013;5:67–76.
17. Fojo T, Farrell N, Ortuzar W, et al. Identification of non-cross-resistant platinum compounds with novel cytotoxicity profiles using the NCI anticancer drug screen and clustered image map visualizations. *Crit Rev Oncol Hematol* 2005;53:25–34.
18. Bates SE, Amiri-Kordestani L, Giaccone G. Drug development: portals of discovery. *Clin Cancer Res* 2012;18:23–32.
19. Kelland L. The development of orally active platinum drugs. In: Lippert B, ed. *Cisplatin: Chemistry and Biochemistry of a Leading Anticancer Drug*. Zurich: Verlag Helvetica Chimica Acta; 1999:497.
20. Farrell N, Qu Y, Bierbach U, et al. Structure-activity relationships within di- and trinuclear platinum phase-I clinical anticancer agents. In: Lippert B, ed. *Cisplatin: Chemistry and Biochemistry of a Leading Anticancer Drug*. Zurich: Verlag Helvetica Chimica Acta; 1999;477–496.
21. Holford J, Sharp S, Murrer B, et al. In vitro circumvention of cisplatin resistance by the novel sterically hindered platinum complex AMD473. *Br J Cancer* 1998;77:366–373.
22. Flaherty KT, Stevenson JP, Redlinger M, et al. A phase I, dose escalation trial of ZD0473, a novel platinum analogue, in combination with gemcitabine. *Cancer Chemother Pharmacol* 2004;53:404–408.
23. Park GY, Wilson JJ, Song Y, et al. Phenanthriplatin, a monofunctional DNA-binding platinum anticancer drug candidate with unusual potency and cellular activity profile. *Proc Natl Acad Sci U S A* 2012;109:11987–11992.

24. Eastman A. The formation, isolation and characterization of DNA adducts produced by anticancer platinum complexes. *Pharmacol Ther* 1987;34:155–166.
25. Zhu G, Song L, Lippard SJ. Visualizing inhibition of nucleosome mobility and transcription by cisplatin-DNA interstrand crosslinks in live mammalian cells. *Cancer Res* 2013;73:4451–4460.
26. Martens-de Kemp SR, Dalm SU, Wijnolts FM, et al. DNA-bound platinum is the major determinant of cisplatin sensitivity in head and neck squamous carcinoma cells. *PLoS One* 2013;8:e61555.
27. Blommaert F, van Kijk-Knijnenburg H, Dijt F, et al. Formation of DNA adducts by the anticancer drug carboplatin: different nucleotide sequence preferences in vitro and in cells. *Biochemistry* 1995;34:8474–8480.
28. Scheef E, Briggs J, Howell S. Molecular modeling of the intrastrand guanine-guanine DNA adducts produced by cisplatin and oxaliplatin. *Mol Pharmacol* 1999;56:633–643.
29. Enoiu M, Jiricny J, Schärer OD. Repair of cisplatin-induced DNA interstrand crosslinks by a replication-independent pathway involving transcription-coupled repair and translesion synthesis. *Nucleic Acids Res* 2012;40:8953–8964.
30. Zhu G, Song L, Lippard SJ. Visualizing inhibition of nucleosome mobility and transcription by cisplatin-DNA interstrand crosslinks in live mammalian cells. *Cancer Res* 2013;73:4451–4460.
31. Sorenson C, Eastman A. Mechanism of cis-diamminedichloroplatinum (II)-induced cytotoxicity: role of G2 arrest and DNA double-strand breaks. *Cancer Res* 1988;48:4484–4488.
32. Toney J, Donahue B, Kellett P, et al. Isolation of cDNAs encoding a human protein that binds selectively to DNA modified by the anticancer drug cis-diamminedichloroplatinum. *Proc Natl Acad Sci U S A* 1989;86:8328–8332.
33. Bruhn S, Pil P, Essigmann J, et al. Isolation and characterization of human cDNA clones encoding a high mobility group box protein that recognizes structural distortions to DNA caused by binding of the anticancer agent cisplatin. *Proc Natl Acad Sci U S A* 1989;89:2307–2311.
34. Hughes EN, Engelsberg BN, Billings PC. Purification of nuclear proteins that bind to cisplatin-damaged DNA. Identity with high mobility group proteins 1 and 2. *J Biol Chem* 1992;267:13520–13527.
35. Ramachandran S, Temple BR, Chaney SG, et al. Structural basis for the sequence-dependent effects of platinum-DNA adducts. *Nucleic Acids Res* 2009;37:2434–2448.
36. Ramachandran S, Temple B, Alexandrova AN, et al. Recognition of platinum-DNA adducts by HMGB1a. *Biochemistry* 2012;51:7608–7617.
37. Fink D, Zheng H, Nebel S, et al. In vitro and in vivo resistance to cisplatin in cells that have lost DNA mismatch repair. *Cancer Res* 1997;57:1841–1845.
38. Kelland L. The resurgence of platinum-based cancer chemotherapy. *Nat Rev Cancer* 2007;7:573–584.
39. Vasilevskaya IA, Rakitina TV, O'Dwyer PJ. Quantitative effects on c-Jun N-terminal protein kinase signaling determine synergistic interaction of cisplatin and 17-allylamino-17-demethoxygeldanamycin in colon cancer cell lines. *Mol Pharmacol* 2004;65:235–243.
40. Vasilevskaya IA, Selvakumaran M, O'Dwyer PJ. Disruption of signaling through SEK1 and MKK7 yields differential responses in hypoxic colon cancer cells treated with oxaliplatin. *Mol Pharmacol* 2008;74:246–254.
41. Maestre N, Tritton TR, Laurent G, et al. Cell surface-directed interaction of anthracyclines leads to cytotoxicity and nuclear factor kappaB activation but not apoptosis signaling. *Cancer Res* 2001;61:2558–2561.
42. Roodhart JM, Daenen LG, Stigter EC, et al. Mesenchymal stem cells induce resistance to chemotherapy through the release of platinum-induced fatty acids. *Cancer Cell* 2011;20:370–383.
43. Beatty GL, Chiorean EG, Fishman MP, et al. CD40 regulates cancer inflammation and induces regression of pancreatic carcinoma in mice and humans. *Science* 2011;331:1612–1616.
44. Galluzzi L, Senovilla L, Vitale I, et al. Molecular mechanisms of cisplatin resistance. *Oncogene* 2012;31:1869–1883.
45. Lin X, Okuda T, Holzer A, et al. The copper transporter CTR1 regulates cisplatin uptake in Saccharomyces cerevisiae. *Mol Pharmacol* 2002;62:1154–1159.
46. Blair BG, Larson CA, Safaei R, et al. Copper transporter 2 regulates the cellular accumulation and cytotoxicity of cisplatin and carboplatin. *Clin Cancer Res* 2009;15:4312–4321.
47. Samimi G, Varki NM, Wilczynski S, et al. Increase in the expression of the copper transporter ATP7A during platinum drug-based treatment is associated with poor survival in ovarian cancer patients. *Clin Cancer Res* 2003;9:5853–5859.
48. Britten RA, Green JA, Broughton C, et al. The relationship between nuclear glutathione levels and resistance to melphalan in human ovarian tumour cells. *Biochem Pharmacol* 1991;41:647–649.
49. Mistry P, Kelland L, Abel G, et al. The relationships between glutathione, glutathione-S-transferase and cytotoxicity of platinum drugs and melphalan in eight human ovarian carcinoma cell lines. *Br J Cancer* 1991;64:215–220.
50. Godwin A, Meister A, O'Dwyer P, et al. High resistance to cisplatin in human ovarian cancer cell lines is associated with marked increase in glutathione synthesis. *Proc Natl Acad Sci U S A* 1992;89:3070–3074.
51. Hamilton T, Winker M, Louie K, et al. Augmentation of adriamycin, melphalan and cisplatin cytotoxicity in drug-resistant and -sensitive human ovarian cancer cell lines by buthionine sulfoximine mediated glutathione depletion. *Biochem Pharmacol* 1985;34:2583–2586.
52. Koberle B, Grimaldi K, Sunters A, et al. DNA repair capacity and cisplatin sensitivity of human testis tumour cells. *Int J Cancer* 1997;70:551–555.
53. Martin LP, Hamilton TC, Schilder RJ. Platinum resistance: the role of DNA repair pathways. *Clin Cancer Res* 2008;14:1291–1295.

54. Selvakumaran M, Piscarcik DA, Bao R, et al. Enhanced cisplatin cytotoxicity by disturbing the nucleotide excision repair pathway in ovarian cancer cell lines. *Cancer Res* 2003;63:1311–1316.
55. Hubner RA, Riley RD, Billingham LJ, et al. Excision repair cross-complementation group 1 (ERCC1) status and lung cancer outcomes: a meta-analysis of published studies and recommendations. *PLoS One* 2011;6:e25164.
56. De Dosso S, Zanellato E, Nucifora M, et al. ERCC1 predicts outcome in patients with gastric cancer treated with adjuvant cisplatin-based chemotherapy. *Cancer Chemother Pharmacol* 2013;72:159–165.
57. Squires MH 3rd, Fisher SB, Fisher KE, et al. Differential expression and prognostic value of ERCC1 and thymidylate synthase in resected gastric adenocarcinoma. *Cancer* 2013;119:3242–3250.
58. Yamada Y, Boku N, Nishina T, et al. Impact of excision repair cross-complementing gene 1 (ERCC1) on the outcomes of patients with advanced gastric cancer: correlative study in Japan Clinical Oncology Group Trial JCOG9912. *Ann Oncol* 2013;24:2560–2565.
59. Friboulet L, Olaussen KA, Pignon JP, et al. ERCC1 isoform expression and DNA repair in non–small-cell lung cancer. *N Engl J Med* 2013;368:1101–1110.
60. Bryant HE, Schultz N, Thomas HD, et al. Specific killing of BRCA2-deficient tumours with inhibitors of poly(ADP-ribose) polymerase. *Nature* 2005;434:913–917.
61. Farmer H, McCabe1 N, Lord C, et al. Targeting the DNA repair defect in BRCA mutant cells as a therapeutic strategy. *Nature* 2005;434:917–921.
62. Edwards SL, Brough R, Lord CJ, et al. Resistance to therapy caused by intragenic deletion in BRCA2. *Nature* 2008;451:1111–1116.
63. Sakai W, Swisher EM, Karlan BM, et al. Secondary mutations as a mechanism of cisplatin resistance in BRCA2-mutated cancers. *Nature* 2008;451:1116–1121.
64. Gelmon KA, Tischkowitz M, Mackay H, et al. Olaparib in patients with recurrent high-grade serous or poorly differentiated ovarian carcinoma or triple-negative breast cancer: a phase 2, multicentre, open-label, non-randomised study. *Lancet Oncology* 2011;12:852–861.
65. Levine B, Kroemer G. Autophagy in the pathogenesis of disease. *Cell* 2008;132:27–42.
66. Matthew R, Karantza-Wadsworth V, White E. Role of autophagy in cancer. *Nat Rev Cancer* 2007;7:961–967.
67. Amaravadi RK, Yu D, Lum JJ, et al. Autophagy inhibition enhances therapy-induced apoptosis in a Myc-induced model of lymphoma. *J Clin Invest* 2007;117:326–336.
68. Duffull S, Robinson B. Clinical pharmacokinetics and dose optimization of carboplatin. *Clin Pharmacokinet* 1997;33:161–183.
69. Harland S, Newell D, Siddik Z, et al. Pharmacokinetics of cis-diammine-1,1-cyclobutane dicarboxylate platinum(II) in patients with normal and impaired renal function. *Cancer Res* 1984;44:1693–1697.
70. Graham MA, Lockwood GF, Greenslade D, et al. Clinical pharmacokinetics of oxaliplatin: a critical review. *Clin Cancer Res* 2000;6:1205–1218.
71. Gamelin E, Bouil A, Boisdron-Celle M, et al. Cumulative pharmacokinetic study of oxaliplatin, administered every three weeks, combined with 5-fluorouracil in colorectal cancer patients. *Clin Cancer Res* 1997;3:891–899.
72. Extra JM, Marty M, Brienza S, et al. Pharmacokinetics and safety profile of oxaliplatin. *Semin Oncol* 1998;25:13–22.
73. Chatelut E, Canal P, Brunner V, et al. Prediction of carboplatin clearance from standard morphological and biological patient characteristics. *J Natl Cancer Inst* 1995;87:573–580.
74. Jodrell D, Egorin M, Canetta R, et al. Relationships between carboplatin exposure and tumor response and toxicity in patients with ovarian cancer. *J Clin Oncol* 1992;10:520–528.
75. Reyno L, Egorin M, Canetta R, et al. Impact of cyclophosphamide on relationships between carboplatin exposure and response or toxicity when used in the treatment of advanced ovarian cancer. *J Clin Oncol* 1993;11:1156–1164.
76. Shen DW, Pouliot LM, Hall MD, et al. Cisplatin resistance: a cellular self-defense mechanism resulting from multiple epigenetic and genetic changes. *Pharmacol Rev* 2012;64:706–721.
77. Ma J, Verweij J, Planting A, et al. Current sample handling methods for measurement of platinum-DNA adducts in leucocytes in man lead to discrepant results in DNA adduct levels and DNA repair. *Br J Cancer* 1995;71:512–517.
78. Schellens J, Ma J, Planting A, et al. Relationship between the exposure to cisplatin, DNA-adduct formation in leucocytes and tumour response in patients with solid tumours. *Br J Cancer* 1996;73:1569–1575.
79. Ozols R, Corden B, Jacob J, et al. High-dose cisplatin in hypertonic saline. *Ann Intern Med* 1984;100:19–24.
80. Howell S, Pfeifle C, Wung W, et al. Intraperitoneal cis-diamminedichloroplatinum with systemic thiosulfate protection. *Cancer Res* 1983;43:1426–1431.
81. Alberts D, Liu P, Hannigan E, et al. Intraperitoneal cisplatin plus intravenous cyclophosphamide versus intravenous cisplatin plus intravenous cyclophosphamide for stage III ovarian cancer. *N Engl J Med* 1996;335:1950–1955.
82. Solomon B, Soulen M, Baum R, et al. Chemoembolization of hepatocellular carcinoma with cisplatin, doxorubicin, mitomycin-C, Ethiodol, and polyvinyl alcohol: prospective evaluation of response and survival in a US population. *J Vasc Interv Radiol* 1999;10:793–798.
83. Extra J, Marty M, Brienza S, et al. Pharmacokinetics and safety profile of oxaliplatin. *Semin Oncol* 1998;25:13–22.
84. Brienza S, Vignoud J, Itzhaki M, et al. Oxaliplatin (L-OHP): global safety in 682 patients. *Proc Am Soc Clin Oncol* 1995;14:209.
85. André T, Boni C, Mounedji-Boudiaf L, et al. Oxaliplatin, fluorouracil, and leucovorin as adjuvant treatment for colon cancer. *N Engl J Med* 2004;350:2343–2351.

19 Antimetabolites

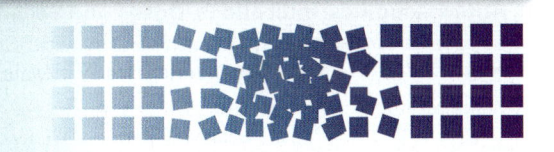

M. Wasif Saif and Edward Chu

ANTIFOLATES

Reduced folates play a key role in one-carbon metabolism, and they are essential for the biosynthesis of purines, thymidylate, and protein biosynthesis. Aminopterin was the first antimetabolite with documented clinical activity in the treatment of children with acute leukemia in the 1940s. This antifolate analog was subsequently replaced by methotrexate (MTX), the 4-amino, 10-methyl analog of folic acid, which remains the most widely used antifolate analog, with activity against a wide range of cancers (Table 19.1), including hematologic malignancies (acute lymphoblastic leukemia and non-Hodgkin's lymphoma) and many solid tumors (breast cancer, head and neck cancer, osteogenic sarcoma, bladder cancer, and gestational trophoblastic cancer).

Pemetrexed is a pyrrolopyrimidine, multitargeted antifolate analog that targets multiple enzymes involved in folate metabolism, including thymidylate synthase (TS), dihydrofolate reductase (DHFR), glycinamide ribonucleotide (GAR) formyltransferase, and aminoimidazole carboxamide (AICAR) formyltransferase.[1,2] This agent has broad-spectrum activity against solid tumors, including malignant mesothelioma and breast, pancreatic, head and neck, non–small-cell lung, colon, gastric, cervical, and bladder cancers.[3-5]

The third antifolate compound to have entered clinical practice is pralatrexate (10-propargyl-10-deazaaminopterin), a 10-deazaaminopterin antifolate that was rationally designed to bind with higher affinity to the reduced folate carrier (RFC)-1 transport protein, when compared with MTX, leading to enhanced membrane transport into tumor cells. It is also an improved substrate for the enzyme folylpolyglutamyl synthetase (FPGS), resulting in enhanced formation of cytotoxic polyglutamate metabolites.[6,7] When compared with MTX, this analog is a more potent inhibitor of multiple enzymes involved in folate metabolism, including TS, DHFR, and GAR and AICAR formyltransferases. This agent is presently approved for the treatment of relapsed or refractory peripheral T-cell lymphomas.[8]

Mechanism of Action

The antifolate compounds are tight-binding inhibitors of DHFR, a key enzyme in folate metabolism.[1] DHFR plays a pivotal role in maintaining the intracellular folate pools in their fully reduced form as tetrahydrofolates, and these compounds serve as one-carbon carriers required for the synthesis of thymidylate, purine nucleotides, and certain amino acids.

The cytotoxic effects of MTX, pemetrexed, and pralatrexate are mediated by their respective polyglutamate metabolites, with up to 5 to 7 glutamyl groups in a γ-peptide linkage. These polyglutamate metabolites exhibit prolonged intracellular half-lives, thereby allowing for prolonged drug action in tumor cells. Moreover, these polyglutamate metabolites are potent, direct inhibitors of several folate-dependent enzymes, including DHFR, TS, AICAR formyltransferase, and GAR formyltransferase.[1]

Mechanisms of Resistance

The development of cellular resistance to antifolates remains a major obstacle to its clinical efficacy.[9,10] In experimental systems, resistance to antifolates arises from several mechanisms, including an alteration in antifolate transport because of either a defect in the reduced folate carrier or folate receptor systems, decreased capacity to polyglutamate the antifolate parent compound through either decreased expression of FPGS or increased expression of the catabolic enzyme γ-glutamyl hydrolase, and alterations in the target enzymes DHFR and/or TS through increased expression of wild-type protein or overexpression of a mutant protein with reduced binding affinity for the antifolate. Gene amplification is a common resistance mechanism observed in various experimental systems, including tumor samples from patients. In in vitro and in vivo experimental model systems, the levels of DHFR and/or TS protein acutely increase after exposure to MTX and other antifolate compounds. This acute induction of target protein in response to drug exposure is mediated, in part, by a translational regulatory mechanism, which may represent a clinically relevant mechanism for the acute development of cellular drug resistance.

Clinical Pharmacology

The oral bioavailability of MTX is saturable and erratic at doses greater than 25 mg/m^2. MTX is completely absorbed from parenteral routes of administration, and peak serum levels are achieved within 30 to 60 minutes of administration.

The distribution of MTX into third-space fluid collections, such as pleural effusions and ascitic fluid, can substantially alter MTX pharmacokinetics. The slow release of accumulated MTX from these third spaces over time prolongs the terminal half-life of the drug, leading to potentially increased clinical toxicity. It is advisable to evacuate these fluid collections before treatment and monitor plasma drug concentrations closely.

Renal excretion is the main route of drug elimination, and this process is mediated by glomerular filtration and tubular secretion. About 80% to 90% of an administered dose is eliminated unchanged in the urine. Doses of MTX, therefore, should be reduced in proportion to reductions in creatinine clearance. Renal excretion of MTX is inhibited by probenecid, penicillins, cephalosporins, aspirin, and nonsteroidal anti-inflammatory drugs.

Pemetrexed enters the cell via the RFC system and, to a lesser extent, by the folate receptor protein. As with MTX, it undergoes polyglutamation within the cell to the pentaglutamate form, which is at least 60-fold more potent than the parent compound. This agent is mainly cleared by renal excretion, and in the setting of renal dysfunction, the terminal drug half-life is significantly prolonged to up to 20 hours. Pemetrexed, therefore, should be used with caution in patients with renal dysfunction. In addition, renal excretion is inhibited in the presence of other agents including probenecid, penicillins, cephalosporins, aspirin, and nonsteroidal anti-inflammatory drugs.

TABLE 19.1

Antimetabolites: Indications, Doses and Schedules, and Toxicities

Drug	Main Therapeutic Uses	Main Doses and Schedule	Major Toxicities
Methotrexate	Non-Hodgkin's lymphoma Primary CNS lymphoma Acute lymphoblastic leukemia Breast cancer Bladder cancer Osteogenic sarcoma Gestational trophoblastic cancer	Low dose: 10–50 mg/m^2 IV every 3–4 weeks Low dose weekly: 25 mg/m^2 IV weekly Moderate dose: 100–500 m/m^2 IV every 2–3 weeks High dose: 1–12 gm/m^2 IV over a 3- to 24-hour period every 1–3 weeks Intrathecal (IT): 10–15 mg IT 2 times weekly until CSF is clear, then weekly dose for 2–6 weeks, followed by monthly dose	Mucositis, diarrhea, myelosuppression, acute renal failure, transient elevations in serum transaminases and bilirubin, pneumonitis, neurologic toxicity
Pemetrexed	Mesothelioma Non–small-cell lung cancer	500 mg/m^2 IV, every 3 weeks	Myelosuppression, skin rash, mucositis, diarrhea, fatigue
Pralatrexate	Peripheral T-cell lymphoma	30 mg/m^2 IV, weekly for 6 weeks; cycles repeated every 7 weeks	Myelosuppression, skin rash, mucositis, diarrhea, elevation of serum transaminases and bilirubin, mild nausea/vomiting
5-Fluorouracil	Breast cancer Colorectal cancer Anal cancer Gastroesophageal cancer Hepatocellular cancer Pancreatic cancer Head and neck cancer	Bolus monthly schedule: 425–450 mg/m^2 IV on days 1–5 every 28 days Bolus weekly schedule: 500–600 mg/m^2 IV every week for 6 weeks every 8 weeks Infusion schedule: 2,400–3,000 mg/m^2 IV over 46 hours every 2 weeks 120-hour infusion: 1,000 mg/m^2/d IV on days 1–5 every 21–28 d Protracted continuous infusion: 200–400 mg/m^2/d IV	Nausea/vomiting, diarrhea, mucositis, myelosuppression, neurotoxicity, coronary artery vasospasm, conjunctivitis
Capecitabine	Breast cancer Colorectal cancer Gastroesophageal cancer Hepatocellular cancer Pancreatic cancer	Recommended dose for monotherapy is 1,250 mg/m^2 PO bid for 2 weeks with 1 wk rest May decrease dose of capecitabine to 850–1,000 mg/m^2 bid on days 1–14 to reduce risk of toxicity without compromising efficacy An alternative dosing schedule for monotherapy is 1,250–1,500 mg/m^2 PO bid for 1 week on and 1 week off; this schedule appears to be well tolerated, with no compromise in clinical efficacy Capecitabine should be used at lower doses (850–1,000 mg/m^2 bid on days 1–14) when used in combination with other cytotoxic agents, such as oxaliplatin and lapatinib	Diarrhea, hand-foot syndrome, myelosuppression, mucositis, nausea/vomiting, neurologic toxicity, coronary artery vasospasm
Cytarabine	Hodgkin's lymphoma Non-Hodgkin's lymphoma Acute myelogenous leukemia Acute lymphoblastic leukemia	Standard dose: 100 mg/m^2/day IV on days 1–7 as a continuous IV infusion, in combination with an anthracycline as induction chemotherapy for acute myelogenous leukemia High-dose: 1.5–3.0 gm/m^2 IV q 12 hours for 3 days as a high dose, intensification regimen for acute myelogenous leukemia SC: 20 mg/m^2 SC for 10 days per month for 6 months, associated with IFN-α for treatment of chronic myelogenous leukemia IT: 10–30 mg IT up to 3 times weekly in the treatment of leptomeningeal carcinomatosis secondary to leukemia or lymphoma.	Nausea/vomiting, myelosuppression, cerebellar ataxia, lethargy, confusion, acute pancreatitis, drug infusion reaction, hand-foot syndrome High-dose therapy: noncardiogenic pulmonary edema, acute respiratory distress and *Streptococcus viridans* pneumonia, conjunctivitis, and keratitis
Gemcitabine	Pancreatic cancer Non–small-cell lung cancer Breast cancer Bladder cancer Hodgkin's lymphoma Ovarian cancer Soft tissue sarcoma	Pancreatic cancer: 1,000 mg/m^2 IV every week for 7 weeks with 1 week rest Treatment then continues weekly for 3 weeks followed by 1 week off Bladder cancer: 1,000 mg/m^2 IV on days 1, 8, and 15 every 28 days Non–small-cell lung cancer: 1,000–1,200 mg/m^2 IV on days 1 and 8 every 21 days	Nausea/vomiting, myelosuppression, flulike syndrome, elevation of serum transaminases and bilirubin, pneumonitis, infusion reaction, mild proteinuria, and rarely, hemolytic-uremic syndrome and thrombotic thrombocytopenic purpura

(continued)

TABLE 19.1
Antimetabolites: Indications, Doses and Schedules, and Toxicities (continued)

Drug	Main Therapeutic Uses	Main Doses and Schedule	Major Toxicities
6-Mercaptopurine	Acute lymphoblastic leukemia	Induction therapy. 2.5 mg/kg PO daily Maintenance therapy: 1.5–2.5 mg/kg PO daily	Myelosuppression, nausea/vomiting, mucositis and diarrhea, hepatotoxicity, immunosuppression
6-Thioguanine	Acute myelogenous leukemia Acute lymphoblastic leukemia	Induction: 100 mg/m^2 PO every 12 hours on days 1–5, usually in combination with cytarabine Maintenance: 100 mg/m^2 PO every 12 hours on days 1–5, every 4 weeks, usually in combination with other agents Single agent: 1–3 mg/kg PO daily	Myelosuppression, nausea/vomiting, mucositis and diarrhea, hepatotoxicity, immunosuppression
Fludarabine	Chronic lymphocytic leukemia Non-Hodgkin's lymphoma	25 mg/m^2 IV on days 1–5 every 28 days For oral usage, the recommended dose is 40 mg/m^2 PO on days 1–5 every 28 days	Myelosuppression, immunosuppression with increased risk of opportunistic infections, mild nausea/vomiting, hypersensitivity reaction
Cladribine	Hairy cell leukemia Chronic lymphocytic leukemia Non-Hodgkin's lymphoma	Usual dose is 0.09 mg/kg/d IV via continuous infusion for 7 days; one course is usually administered	Myelosuppression, immunosuppression, mild nausea/vomiting, fever
Clofarabine	Acute lymphoblastic leukemia	52 mg/m^2 IV daily for 5 days every 2–6 weeks	Myelosuppression nausea/vomiting, diarrhea, systemic inflammatory response syndrome, increased risk of opportunistic infections, renal toxicity

CNS, central nervous system; IV, intravenously; CSF, cerebrospinal fluid; PO, by mouth; bid, twice daily; SC, subcutaneously; IFN-α, interferon alpha.

As with other antifolate analogs, pralatrexate is transported into the cell by the RFC carrier protein and then metabolized by FPGS to form longer chain polyglutamates, with up to four additional glutamate residues attached to the parent molecule. About 34% of the parent drug is cleared in the urine during the first 24 hours after drug administration. As such, caution is advised when using pralatrexate in patients with renal dysfunction. As with MTX and pemetrexed, the concomitant administration of other agents such as probenecid, penicillins, cephalosporins, aspirin, and nonsteroidal anti-inflammatory drugs, may inhibit renal clearance.

Toxicity

The main side effects of MTX are myelosuppression and gastrointestinal (GI) toxicity, which are usually completely reversed within 14 days, unless drug-elimination mechanisms are impaired. In patients with compromised renal function, even small doses of MTX may result in serious toxicity. MTX-induced nephrotoxicity is thought to result from the intratubular precipitation of MTX and its metabolites in acidic urine. Antifolates may also exert a direct toxic effect on the renal tubules. Vigorous hydration and urinary alkalinization have greatly reduced the incidence of renal failure in patients on high-dose regimens. Acute elevations in hepatic enzyme levels and hyperbilirubinemia are often observed during high-dose therapy, but these levels usually return to normal within 10 days. Methotrexate given concomitantly with radiotherapy may increase the risk of soft tissue necrosis and osteonecrosis.

The original rationale for high-dose MTX therapy was based on the concept of selective rescue of normal tissues by the reduced folate leucovorin (LV). However, recent data suggest that high-dose MTX may also overcome resistance mechanisms caused by impaired active transport, decreased affinity of DHFR for MTX, increased levels of DHFR resulting from gene amplification, and/or decreased polyglutamation of MTX.

The main toxicities of pemetrexed and pralatrexate include dose-limiting myelosuppression, mucositis, and skin rash, usually in the form of the hand-foot syndrome (HFS). Other toxicities include reversible transaminasemia, anorexia and fatigue syndrome, and GI toxicity. These side effects are reduced by supplementation with folic acid (350 μg orally daily) and vitamin B$_{12}$ (1,000 mg subcutaneously given at least 1 week before starting therapy, and then repeated every three cycles). To date, there is no evidence to suggest that vitamin supplementation adversely affects the clinical efficacy of pemetrexed or pralatrexate.

5-FLUOROPYRIMIDINES

The fluoropyrimidine, 5-fluorouracil (5-FU) was synthesized by Charles Heidelberger in the mid 1950s. Uracil is a normal component of RNA; as such, the rationale leading to the development of the drug was that cancer cells might be more sensitive to *decoy* molecules that mimic the natural compound than normal cells. 5-FU and its derivatives are an integral part of treatment for a broad range of solid tumors (see Table 19.1), including GI malignancies (esophageal, gastric, pancreatic, colorectal, anal, and hepatocellular cancers), breast, head and neck, and skin cancers.[11] It continues to serve as the main backbone for combination regimens used to treat metastatic colorectal cancer (mCRC) and as adjuvant therapy of early-stage colon cancer.

Mechanism of Action

5-FU enters cells via the facilitated uracil base transport mechanism and is then anabolized to various cytotoxic nucleotide forms

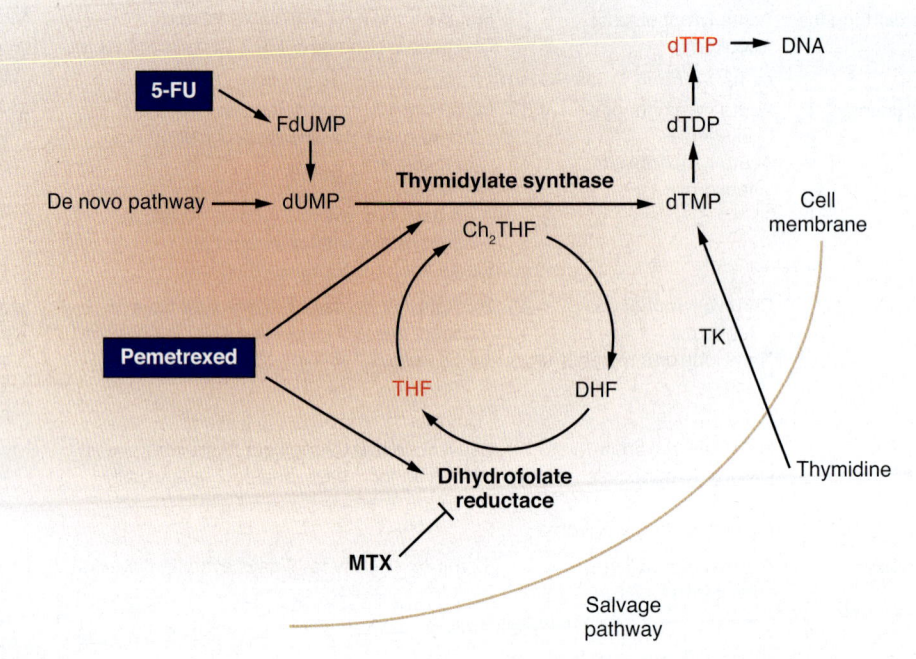

Figure 19.1 Antifolates and 5-fluorouracil (5-FU) sites of action. FdUMP, fluorodeoxyuridine monophosphate; dUMP, deoxyuridine monophosphate; dTTP, deoxythymidine triphosphate; dTDP, deoxyuridine diphosphate; dTMP, deoxythymidine monophosphate; TK, thymidine kinase; CH$_2$THF, 5,10-methylenetetrahydrofolate; THF, tetrahydrofolate; DHF, dihydrofolate.

by several biochemical pathways. It is thought that 5-FU exerts its cytotoxic effects through various mechanisms, including (1) the inhibition of TS, (2) incorporation into RNA, and (3) incorporation into DNA (Fig. 19.1). In addition to these mechanisms, the genotoxic stress resulting from TS inhibition may also activate programmed cell-death pathways in susceptible cells, which leads to the induction of parental DNA fragmentation.

Mechanisms of Resistance

Several resistance mechanisms to 5-FU have been identified in experimental and clinical settings. Alterations in the target enzyme TS represent the most commonly described mechanism of resistance. In vitro, in vivo, and clinical studies have documented a strong correlation between the levels of TS enzyme activity/TS protein and chemosensitivity to 5-FU. In this regard, cell lines and tumors with higher levels of TS are relatively more resistant to 5-FU. Mutations in the TS protein have been identified that lead to reduced binding affinity of the 5-FU metabolite fluorodeoxyuridine monophosphate (FdUMP) to the TS protein. Reduced expression and/or diminished activity of key activating enzymes may interfere with the formation of cytotoxic 5-FU metabolites. Decreased expression of mismatch repair enzymes, such as human mutL homolog 1 (hMLH1) and human mutS homolog 2 (hMSH2), and increased expression of the catabolic enzyme dihydropyrimidine dehydrogenase (DPD) are associated with fluoropyrimidine resistance. At this time, the relative contribution of each of these mechanisms in the development of cellular resistance to 5-FU in the actual clinical setting remains unclear.

Clinical Pharmacology

5-FU is not orally administered, given its erratic bioavailability resulting from high levels of the catabolic enzyme DPD present in the gut mucosa. After intravenous bolus doses, metabolic elimination is rapid, with a half-life of 8 to 14 minutes. More than 85% of an administered dose of 5-FU is enzymatically inactivated by DPD, the rate-limiting enzyme in the catabolism of 5-FU.

A pharmacogenetic syndrome has been identified in which partial or compete deficiency in the DPD enzyme is present in 3% to 5% and 0.1% of the general population, respectively. As DPD catalyzes the rate-limiting step in the catabolic pathway of 5-FU, a deficiency of DPD can result in a clinically dangerous increase in the anabolic products of 5-FU. Unfortunately, patients with DPD deficiency do not manifest a phenotype only until they are treated with 5-FU, and in that setting, they can develop severe GI toxicity in the form of mucositis and/or diarrhea, myelosuppression, neurologic toxicity, and in rare cases, death. In patients being treated with 5-FU or any other fluoropyrimidine, it is important to consider DPD deficiency in patients who present with excessive, severe toxicity.[12] It is now increasingly appreciated that DPD mutations are unable to account for all of the observed cases of excessive 5-FU toxicity, because up to 50% of patients who experience 5-FU toxicity will have no documented alterations in the *DPD* gene. Moreover, individuals with normal DPD enzyme activity may be diagnosed with high plasma levels of 5-FU, resulting in increased toxicity. Although DPD enzyme activity can be assayed from peripheral blood mononuclear cells in a specialized laboratory, routine phenotypic and genotypic screenings for DPD deficiency prior to 5-FU therapy are not yet available.

Biomodulation of 5-FU

Significant efforts have focused on enhancing the antitumor activity of 5-FU through biochemical modulation in which 5-FU is combined with various agents, including leucovorin, MTX, N-phosphonacetyl-L-aspartic acid, interferon-α, interferon-γ, and

TABLE 19.2
Toxicities of Different Forms of 5-FU

Route	Schedule	Dose	DLT
IV	Daily × 5, bolus	400–500 (mg/m²/d)	↓ BM, D, M
IV	Weekly bolus	450–500 (mg/m²/d)	↓ BM
IV	Daily × 5, CI	750–1,000 (mg/m²/d)	M, D
IV	PCI	200–400 (mg/m²/d)	M, HFS
HAI	Daily × 14–21, CI	750–1,000 (mg/m²/d)	M, D
IP	32–120 hr	5 nM	M, D
Oral (Xeloda)	14–21 d	2,000–2,500 (mg/m²/d)	HFS

DLT, dose limiting toxicity; IV, intravenous; BM, bone marrow; D, diarrhea; M, mucositis; CI, continuous infusion; PCI, protracted continuous infusion; HFS, hand-foot syndrome; HAI, hepatic artery infusion; IP, intraperitoneal.

a whole host of other agents.[13] For the past 20 to 25 years, the reduced folate LV has been the main biochemical modulator of 5-FU. An alternative approach has been to alter the schedule of 5-FU administration. Given the S-phase specificity of this agent, prolonged exposure of tumor cells to 5-FU would increase the fraction of cells being exposed to the drug. Overall response rates are significantly higher in patients treated with infusional schedules of 5-FU than in those treated with bolus 5-FU, and this improvement in response rate has translated into an improved progression-free survival. Moreover, the overall safety profile is improved with infusional regimens. A hybrid schedule of bolus and infusional 5-FU was originally developed in France, and this regimen has shown superior clinical activity compared with bolus 5-FU schedules. This hybrid schedule has now been simplified by using only the 46-hour infusion of 5-FU and completely eliminating the 5-FU bolus doses.

Toxicity

The spectrum of 5-FU toxicity is dose- and schedule-dependent (Table 19.2). The main side effects are diarrhea, mucositis, and myelosuppression. The dermatologic HFS is more commonly observed with infusional 5-FU therapy. Acute neurologic symptoms have also been reported, and they include somnolence, cerebellar ataxia, and upper motor signs. Treatment with 5-FU can, on rare occasions, cause coronary vasospasm, resulting in a syndrome of chest pain, cardiac enzyme elevations, and electrocardiographic changes. Cardiac toxicity seems to be related more to infusional 5-FU than bolus administration.[14]

CAPECITABINE

Capecitabine is an oral fluoropyrimidine carbamate that was rationally designed to allow for selective 5-FU activation in tumor tissue.[15] This oral agent was initially approved in anthracycline- and taxane-resistant breast cancer and subsequently approved for use in combination with docetaxel as second-line therapy in metastatic breast cancer and in combination with lapatinib, a tyrosine-kinase inhibitor of human epidermal growth factor receptor type 2 (HER2) and epidermal growth factor receptor (EGFR) in women with HER2-positive metastatic breast cancer following progression on trastuzumab-based therapy.[16] This agent is also approved by the U.S. Food and Drug Administration (FDA) for the first-line treatment of mCRC and as adjuvant therapy for stage III colon cancer when fluoropyrimidine therapy alone is preferred.[17] In Europe and throughout much of the world, the combination of capecitabine plus oxaliplatin (XELOX) is approved for the treatment of mCRC as well as for the adjuvant therapy of stage III colon cancer.[18] In addition, recent studies have documented the noninferiority of capecitabine to 5-FU when combined with cisplatin in the treatment of metastatic gastric cancer.

Clinical Pharmacology

Capecitabine is rapidly and extensively absorbed by the gut mucosa, with nearly 80% oral bioavailability. It is inactive in its parent form and undergoes enzymatic conversion via three successive steps. Of note, the third and final step occurs in tumor tissue and involves the conversion of 5′-deoxy-5-fluorouridine to 5-FU by the enzyme thymidine phosphorylase (TP), which is expressed at much higher levels in tumors when compared with corresponding normal tissue. Capecitabine and capecitabine metabolites are primarily excreted by the kidneys, and in contrast to 5-FU, caution must be taken in the presence of renal dysfunction, with appropriate dose modification. The use of capecitabine is absolutely contraindicated in patients whose creatinine clearance is less than 30 mL per minute. The FDA and Roche have added a black box warning and strengthened the precautions section on the capecitabine label about the drug–drug interaction between warfarin and capecitabine-based chemotherapy. It is generally recommended to do weekly monitoring of the coagulation parameters (prothrombin time/international normalized ratio [PT/INR]) for all patients receiving concomitant warfarin and capecitabine, with an appropriate adjustment of warfarin dose.

Toxicity

Similar to what is observed with infusional 5-FU, the main side effects of capecitabine include diarrhea and HFS. Of note, the incidence of myelosuppression, neutropenic fever, mucositis, alopecia, and nausea/vomiting is lower with capecitabine when compared with 5-FU. Elevations in indirect serum bilirubin can be observed, but are usually transient and clinically asymptomatic. Patients in the United States appear to be unable to tolerate as high doses of capecitabine as European patients, either as monotherapy or in combination with other cytotoxic chemotherapy.[19] Although the underlying reasons for this discrepancy are not known, it may in part be related to the increased fortification of the US diet with folate and the increased focus on vitamin and folic acid supplementation.

S-1

S-1 is an oral fluoropyrimidine that consists of tegafur (FT), a prodrug of 5-FU, combined with two 5-FU biochemical modulators: 5-chloro-2,4-dihydroxypyridine (gimeracil or CDHP), a competitive inhibitor of DPD, and oteracil potassium, which inhibits phosphorylation of 5-flurouracil in the GI tract, thereby decreasing serious GI toxicities such as nausea/vomiting, mucositis, and diarrhea.[20] As with other oral agents, S-1 offers several advantages over 5-FU, including ease of administration, no risks associated with use of central venous access such as infection, thrombosis, etc., and reduced toxicities, especially neurotoxicity. Although S-1 has yet to be approved by the FDA, it has been approved for the treatment of gastric cancer, head and neck, colorectal cancer (CRC), non–small-cell lung, breast, pancreatic, and biliary tract cancers in several countries in Asia and for the treatment of advanced gastric cancer in combination with cisplatin in a large number of European countries.

Clinical Pharmacology

S-1 was designed to provide continuous 5-FU plasma exposure comparable to the intravenous (IV) infusion. FT, the 5-FU prodrug, is absorbed in the small intestine and converted to 5-FU through the liver microsomal P-450 metabolizing enzyme system (CYP2A6). Most of the 5-FU is degraded (85%) by DPD, leading to the formation of fluoro-beta-alanine (FBAL).[21] CDHP inhibits DPD, thus allowing higher concentrations of 5-FU to enter the anabolic pathway and enhance its therapeutic effect. Additionally, the inhibition of DPD leads to a decreased amount of FBAL formation, which presumably leads to reduced neurotoxicity. Oteracil is the final component of the S-1 formulation, and it inhibits orotate phosphoribosyltransferase in the GI mucosa, which prevents the formation of fluorouridine monophosphate (FUMP), thereby decreasing GI toxicity.

The maximum tolerated dose was established at 80 mg/m^2 in two divided doses for a Japanese population and 25 mg/m^2 twice a day for a Caucasian population. This interethnic variability of S-1 pharmacokinetics and pharmacodynamics has been attributed to differences in the CYP2A6 genotypes.[22] Studies have demonstrated a high frequency of allelic variants CYP2A6*4, *7, and *9 in East Asians than in Caucasians, which might be associated with reduced enzymatic activity and decreased activation of FT. On the other hand, higher FT metabolism is seen in Caucasian patients due to higher CYP2A6 activity. However, investigators have established similar 5-FU exposure between these two ethnic groups. These findings were explained by higher CDHP exposure in Asians, resulting in increased DPD inhibition and slower catabolism of 5-FU, despite having low CYP2A6 activity, whereas Caucasians had higher CYP2A6 activity but faster 5-FU clearance.

Clinical Toxicity

Clinical studies have shown that the GI toxicities associated with S-1, such as diarrhea, nausea, vomiting, and hyperbilirubinemia, are more prominent in Western patients, whereas hematologic toxicities are more prevalent in Japanese patients. The difference in safety profile cannot be explained by differences in 5-FU exposure, because pharmacokinetic studies have shown that overall drug exposures are similar. A potential explanation might involve interethnic variations in TS promoter enhancer region polymorphisms, which are more frequently seen in Asians or in Caucasians on a higher folate diet.

CYTARABINE

Cytarabine (ara-C) is a deoxycytidine nucleoside analog isolated from the sponge *Cryptotethya crypta*, and it differs from its physiologic counterpart by virtue of a stereotypic inversion of the 2′-hydroxyl group of the sugar moiety.[23] A regimen of ara-C, combined with an anthracycline and given as a 5- or 7-day continuous infusion, is considered the standard induction treatment for acute myeloid leukemia (AML). Ara-C is active against other hematologic malignancies, such as non-Hodgkin's lymphoma, chronic myelogenous leukemia, and acute lymphocytic leukemia (see Table 19.1). However, this agent has absolutely no activity against solid tumors.

Mechanism of Action

Ara-C enters cells via nucleoside transport proteins, the most important one being the equilibrative inhibitor-sensitive (ES) receptor. Once inside the cell, ara-C requires activation for its cytotoxic effects.[23,24] The first metabolic step is the conversion of ara-C to the monophosphate form ara-cytidine monophosphate (ara-CMP) by the enzyme deoxycytidine kinase (dCK) with subsequent phosphorylation to the di- and triphosphate metabolites, respectively. Ara-cytidine triphosphate (ara-CTP) is a potent inhibitor of DNA polymerases α, β, and γ, which in turn interferes with DNA chain elongation, DNA synthesis, and DNA repair. Ara-CTP is also incorporated directly into DNA and functions as a DNA chain terminator, interfering with chain elongation. Catabolism of ara-C involves two key enzymes, cytidine deaminase and deoxycytidylate deaminase. These breakdown enzymes convert ara-C and ara-CMP into the inactive metabolites, ara-uridine (ara-U) and ara-uridine monophosphate (ara-UMP), respectively. The balance between intracellular activation and degradation is critical in determining the amount of drug that is ultimately converted to ara-CTP and, thus, its subsequent cytotoxic and antitumor activity.

Mechanisms of Resistance

Several resistance mechanisms to ara-C have been described. An impaired transmembrane transport, a decreased rate of anabolism, and an increased rate of catabolism may result in the development of ara-C resistance.[23,25,26] The level of cytidine deaminase enzyme activity has been shown to correlate with clinical response in patients with AML undergoing induction chemotherapy with ara-C–containing regimens.

Clinical Pharmacology

Ara-C has poor oral bioavailability given its extensive deamination within the GI tract. Thus, ara-C is administered intravenously via continuous infusion. After administration, ara-C undergoes extensive metabolism in the liver, plasma, and peripheral tissues. Within 24 hours, up to 80% of drug is recovered in the urine as the ara-U metabolite. Ara-C crosses the blood–brain barrier when used at high doses, with cerebrospinal fluid levels between 7% and 14% of plasma levels and reaching peak levels of up to 10 μM.

Toxicity

The toxicity profile of ara-C is highly dependent on the dose and schedule of administration. Myelosuppression is dose-limiting with a standard 7-day regimen. Leukopenia and thrombocytopenia are observed most frequently, with nadirs occurring between days 7 and 14 after drug administration. GI toxicity commonly manifests as a mild-to-moderate degree of anorexia, nausea, and vomiting along with mucositis, diarrhea, and abdominal pain. In rare cases, acute pancreatitis has been observed. The ara-C syndrome has been described in pediatric patients with hematologic malignancies, usually begins within 12 hours after the start of drug infusion, and is characterized by fever, myalgia, bone pain, maculopapular rash, conjunctivitis, malaise, and occasional chest pain.

The administration of ara-C at high doses (2 to 3 g/m^2 with each dose) is associated with profound myelosuppression.[27] Severe GI toxicity in the form of mucositis and/or diarrhea is also observed. Neurologic toxicity is significantly more common with high-dose ara-C than with standard doses, and presents with seizures, cerebral and cerebellar dysfunction, and peripheral neuropathy. Clinical signs of cerebellar dysfunction occur in up to 15% of patients and include dysarthria, dysmetria, and ataxia. Change in alertness and cognitive ability, memory loss, and frontal lobe release signs reflect cerebral toxicity. Despite discontinuation of therapy, clinical recovery is incomplete in up to 30% of affected patients. Pulmonary complications may include noncardiogenic pulmonary edema, acute respiratory distress, and pneumonia, resulting from *Streptococcus viridans* infection. Other side effects associated with high-dose ara-C include conjunctivitis (often responsive to topical corticosteroids), a painful HFS, and rarely, anaphylactic reactions.

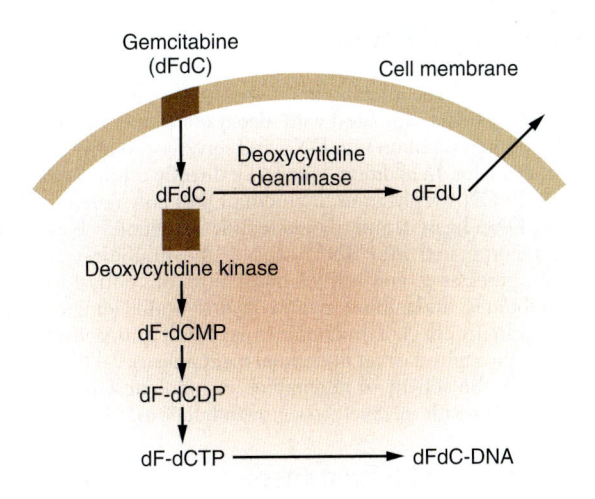

Figure 19.2 Transport and metabolism of gemcitabine. dFdC, gemcitabine; dFdU, 2′,2′-difluorodeoxyuridine; dF-dCMP, gemcitabine monophosphate; dF-dCDP, gemcitabine diphosphate; dF-dCTP, gemcitabine triphosphate.

GEMCITABINE

Gemcitabine (2′,2′-difluorodeoxycytidine) is a difluorinated deoxycytidine analog. Despite its similarity in structure, metabolism, and mechanism of action to ara-C, the spectrum of antitumor activity of gemcitabine is much broader.[23,28] This compound has significant clinical activity against several human solid tumors, including pancreatic, bile duct, gall bladder, small cell and non–small-cell lung, bladder, ovary, and breast cancers as well as hematologic malignancies, namely Hodgkin's and non-Hodgkin's lymphoma (see Table 19.1).

Mechanism of Action

The transport of gemcitabine into cells requires the nucleoside transporter system. Gemcitabine is inactive in its parent form and requires intracellular activation for its cytotoxic effects. The steps involved in the metabolic activation of gemcitabine are similar to those observed with ara-C, with both drugs being activated by the same enzymatic machinery to the active triphosphate metabolite (see Fig. 19.2). Gemcitabine triphosphate is then incorporated into DNA, resulting in chain termination and the inhibition of DNA synthesis and function, or the triphosphate form can directly inhibit DNA polymerases α, β, and γ, which in turn, interferes with DNA chain elongation, DNA synthesis, and DNA repair. The triphosphate metabolite is also a potent inhibitor of ribonucleotide reductase, which further mediates inhibition of DNA biosynthesis by reducing the levels of key deoxynucleotide pools.[29]

Mechanisms of Resistance

Several mechanisms of resistance to gemcitabine have been described in various preclinical experimental models.[30] Gemcitabine is a polar nucleoside analog that requires the activity of human equilibrative nucleoside transporter 1 (hENT1) to enter cells and exert its cytotoxic effects. Preclinical data in human pancreatic cancer cell lines showed that gemcitabine resistance is negatively correlated with hENT1 expression and can be induced by specific inhibitors of hENT1.[31] Clinical data also support the concept that a lack of hENT1 may be predictive of resistance to gemcitabine. CO-101, a lipid-drug conjugate of gemcitabine, was rationally designed to enter cells independently of hENT1. Unfortunately, two studies in pancreatic cancer failed to show any benefit of CO-101.

Additionally, several enzymes involved in the intracellular metabolism of gemcitabine have been implicated in the development of cellular drug resistance, including reduced expression and/or deficiency in dCK enzyme activity as well as increased expression and/or activity of the catabolic enzymes cytidine deaminase and dCMP deaminase. Recent studies have also identified a subset of CD44-positive cancer stem cells within pancreatic tumors that sustain tumor formation and growth, and are resistant to gemcitabine therapy.[33]

Clinical Pharmacology

Gemcitabine is administered via the intravenous route, typically over a 30-minute intravenous infusion, and it undergoes extensive metabolism by deamination to the catabolic metabolite, difluorodeoxyuridine (dFdU), with more than 90% of the metabolized drug being recovered in urine. Plasma clearance is about 30% lower in women and in elderly patients, and this pharmacokinetic difference may result in an increased risk of toxicity in these respective patient populations. The initial findings from pilot pharmacokinetic studies suggested that gemcitabine, when given at a fixed dose rate (FDR) intravenous infusion of 10 mg/m^2 per minute, produced the highest accumulation of active dFdCTP metabolites in peripheral blood mononuclear cells, which led to a randomized phase II trial that compared gemcitabine 1,500 mg/m^2 by FDR or 2,200 mg/m^2 of gemcitabine over 30 minutes. Although this phase II study suggested an improved overall survival with FDR, a subsequent phase III trial failed to confirm the survival advantage of gemcitabine by FDR over its conventional administration schedule.[34]

Toxicity

Gemcitabine is a relatively well-tolerated drug when used as a single agent. The main dose-limiting toxicity is myelosuppression, with neutropenia more commonly experienced than thrombocytopenia. Toxicity is schedule dependent, with longer infusions producing greater hematologic toxicity. Transient flulike symptoms, including fever, headache, arthralgias, and myalgias, occur in 45% of patients. Asthenia and transient transaminasemia may occur. Renal microangiopathy syndromes, including hemolytic-uremic syndrome and thrombotic thrombocytopenic purpura, have been reported rarely.

6-THIOPURINES

The development of the purine analogs in cancer chemotherapy began in the early 1950s with the synthesis of the thiopurines, 6-mercaptopurine (6-MP) and 6-thioguanine (6-TG). 6-MP has an important role in maintenance therapy for acute lymphoblastic leukemia, whereas 6-TG is active in remission induction and in maintenance therapy for AML (see Table 19.1).

Mechanism of Action

The thiopurines, 6-MP and 6-TG, act similarly with respect to their cellular biochemistry.[34] In their respective monophosphate nucleotide forms, they inhibit enzymes involved in de novo purine synthesis and purine interconversion reactions. The triphosphate nucleotide forms can get directly incorporated into either cellular RNA or DNA, leading to the inhibition of RNA and DNA synthesis and function, respectively.

Mechanisms of Resistance

The development of cellular resistance to 6-thiopurines results from a decreased level of key cytotoxic nucleotide metabolites, either through decreased formation or increased breakdown. Resistant cells have been identified that express either complete or partial deficiency of the activating enzyme hypoxanthine-guanine phosphoribosyltransferase (HGPRT). In clinical samples derived from patients with AML, drug resistance has been associated with increased concentrations of a membrane-bound alkaline phosphatase or a conjugating enzyme, 6-thiopurine methyltransferase (TPMT), the end-result being reduced formation of cytotoxic thiopurine nucleotides. Finally, the decreased expression of mismatch repair enzymes, including hMLH1 and hMSH2, has been associated with cellular drug resistance.

Clinical Pharmacology

Oral absorption of 6-MP is highly erratic, and the relatively poor oral bioavailability is mainly related to rapid first-pass metabolism in the liver. The major route of drug elimination is via metabolism by several enzymatic pathways. 6-MP is oxidized to the inactive metabolite 6-thiouric acid by xanthine oxidase. Enhanced 6-MP toxicity may result from the concomitant administration of 6-MP and the xanthine oxidase inhibitor allopurinol. In patients receiving both 6-MP and allopurinol, the 6-MP dose must be reduced by at least 50% to 75%. 6-MP also undergoes S-methylation by the enzyme TPMT to yield 6-methylmercaptopurine.[35]

6-TG is administered orally in the treatment of AML. Its oral bioavailability is erratic, with peak plasma levels occurring 2 to 4 hours after ingestion. The catabolism of 6-TG differs from 6-MP in that it is not a direct substrate for xanthine oxidase.

TPMT enzyme activity may vary considerably among patients as a result of point mutations or loss of alleles of TPMT.[36] Approximately 0.3% of the Caucasian population expresses either a homozygous deletion or a mutation of both alleles of the *TPMT* gene. In these patients, grossly elevated thiopurine nucleotides concentrations, profound myelosuppression with pancytopenia, and extensive GI symptoms are observed after only a brief course of thiopurine treatment. An estimated 10% of patients may be at increased risk for toxicity because of heterozygous loss of the gene or a mutant allele coding for a less enzymatically active TPMT.

Toxicity

The major dose-related toxicities of the thiopurines are myelosuppression and GI toxicity in the form of nausea/vomiting, anorexia, diarrhea, and stomatitis.[37] In TPMT-deficient patients, dosage reduction to 5% to 25% of the standard dosage is necessary to prevent severe excessive toxicity. Thiopurine hepatotoxicity occurs in up to 30% of adult patients and presents mainly as cholestatic jaundice, although elevations of hepatic transaminases may also be seen. Combinations of thiopurines with other known hepatotoxic agents should be avoided, and liver function should be closely monitored. The thiopurines are also potent suppressors of cell-mediated immunity, and prolonged therapy results in an increased predisposition to bacterial and parasitic infections.

FLUDARABINE

Fludarabine (9-β-D-arabinosyl-2-fluoroadenine monophosphate, F-ara-AMP) is an active agent in the treatment of chronic lymphocytic leukemia (CLL) (see Table 19.1).[38,39] It is also active against indolent non-Hodgkin's lymphoma, prolymphocytic leukemia, cutaneous T-cell lymphoma, and Waldenström macroglobulinemia. This agent has also shown promising activity in mantle cell lymphoma. In contrast to its activity in hematologic malignancies, this compound has virtually no activity against solid tumors.

Mechanism of Action

The active cytotoxic metabolite is the triphosphate metabolite F-ara-ATP, which competes with deoxyadenosine triphosphate (dATP) for incorporation into DNA and serves as a highly effective chain terminator. In addition, F-ara-ATP directly inhibits enzymes involved in DNA replication, including DNA polymerases, DNA primase, DNA ligase I, and ribonucleotide reductase.[37] F-ara-ATP is also incorporated into RNA, causing the inhibition of RNA function, processing, and mRNA translation. In contrast to other antimetabolites, fludarabine is active against nondividing cells. In fact, the primary effect of fludarabine may result from activation of apoptosis, through an as yet ill-defined mechanisms.[39] This finding may explain the activity of fludarabine in indolent lymphoproliferative diseases with relatively low growth fractions.

Mechanisms of Resistance

The decreased expression of the activating enzyme dCK resulting in diminished intracellular formation of F-ara-AMP is one of the main resistance mechanisms identified in preclinical models.[38] A high degree of cross-resistance develops to multiple nucleoside analogs, requiring activation by dCK, including cytarabine, gemcitabine, cladribine, and clofarabine. Reduced cellular transport of drug has also been identified as a resistance mechanism.

Clinical Pharmacology

Peak concentrations of F-ara-A are reached 3 to 4 hours after intravenous administration.[40] The main route of elimination is via the kidneys, with about 25% of a given dose of drug being excreted unchanged in the urine.

Toxicity

Myelosuppression and immunosuppression are the major side effects of fludarabine as highlighted by dose-limiting and possibly cumulative lymphopenia and thrombocytopenia. Suppression of the immune system affects T-cell function more than B-cell function. Fevers, often in the setting of neutropenia, occur in 20% to 30% of patients. Lymphocyte counts, specifically CD4-positive cells, decrease rapidly after the initiation of therapy, and recovery of CD4-positive cells to normal levels may take longer than 1 year. Common opportunistic pathogens include the varicella-zoster virus, *Candida*, and *Pneumocystis carinii*. In general, patients are empirically placed on sulfamethoxazole trimethoprim prophylaxis to prevent the development of *P. carinii* infection.

CLADRIBINE

Cladribine (2-CdA) is a purine deoxyadenosine analog, and it is the drug of choice for hairy cell leukemia with activity in low-grade lymphoproliferative disorders (see Table 19.1).[41,42] Salvage treatment of patients previously treated with interferon-α or splenectomy is as effective as first-line treatment. Retreatment with cladribine results in a complete response in up to 60% of relapsing patients. In addition, this agent has promising activity in patients with CLL and non-Hodgkin's lymphoma.

Mechanism of Action

Upon entry into the cell, 2-CdA undergoes an initial conversion to cladribine-monophosphate (Cd-AMP) via the reaction catalyzed by dCK, and Cd-AMP is subsequently metabolized to the active metabolite, cladribine-triphosphate. The triphosphate metabolite competitively inhibits incorporation of the normal dATP nucleotide into DNA, a process that results in the termination of chain elongation.[43] Progressive accumulation of the triphosphate metabolite leads to an imbalance in deoxyribonucleotide pools, thereby inhibiting further DNA synthesis and repair. Finally, the triphosphate metabolite is a potent inhibitor of ribonucleotide reductase, which further facilitates the inhibition of DNA biosynthesis.

Mechanisms of Resistance

Resistance to 2-CdA has been attributed to altered intracellular drug metabolism. A reduction in the activity of dCK, the enzyme responsible for generating cytotoxic nucleotide metabolites, is a major determinant of acquired resistance. The monophosphate and triphosphate metabolites are dephosphorylated by the cytoplasmic enzyme 5′-nucleotidase. Interestingly, resistant cells derived from a patient with CLL exhibited both low levels of dCK expression and high levels of 5′-nucleotidase.

Clinical Pharmacology

2-CdA is orally bioavailable, with 50% of an administered dose orally absorbed. Approximately 50% of an administered dose of drug is cleared by the kidneys, and 20% to 35% of the drug is excreted unchanged in the urine. Of note, this nucleoside can cross the blood–brain barrier with penetration into the cerebrospinal fluid.

Toxicity

At conventional doses, myelosuppression is dose limiting. After a single course of drug, recovery from thrombocytopenia usually occurs within 2 to 4 weeks, whereas recovery from neutropenia takes place in 3 to 5 weeks. GI toxicities are generally mild, with nausea/vomiting and diarrhea. Mild-to-moderate neurotoxicity occurs in 15% of patients and is at least partly reversible with discontinuation of the drug. Immunosuppression accounts for the late morbidity observed in 2-CdA–treated patients. Lymphocyte counts, particularly CD4-positive cells, decrease within 1 to 4 weeks of drug administration and may remain depressed for several years.[44] After discontinuation of 2-CdA, a median time of up to 40 months may be required for complete recovery of normal CD4-positive counts. Although opportunistic infections occur, they do so less frequently than with fludarabine therapy. Infectious complications correlate with decreases in the CD4-positive count, and they include herpes zoster, *Candida*, *Pneumocystis*, *Pseudomonas aeruginosa*, *Listeria monocytogenes*, *Cryptococcus neoformans*, *Aspergillus*, *P. carinii*, and cytomegalovirus.

CLOFARABINE

Clofarabine is a purine deoxyadenosine nucleoside analog, and it is approved for the treatment of pediatric patients with relapsed or refractory acute lymphoblastic leukemia (see Table 19.1).[45]

Ongoing studies are exploring the benefit of clofarabine alone and in combination with other agents in less heavily pretreated patients and in the use of different dose schedules for other hematologic malignancies.[46]

Mechanism of Action

Clofarabine is inactive in its parent form and, like other purine analogs, it requires intracellular activation by dCK to form the monophosphate nucleotide, which undergoes further metabolism to the cytotoxic triphosphate metabolite. Clofarabine triphosphate is then incorporated into DNA, resulting in chain termination, and inhibition of DNA synthesis and function or the triphosphate form can directly inhibit DNA polymerases α, β, and γ, which in turn, interferes with DNA chain elongation, DNA synthesis, and DNA repair. The triphosphate metabolite is also a potent inhibitor of ribonucleotide reductase, further mediating the inhibition of DNA biosynthesis by reducing the levels of key deoxyribonucleotide pools.

Mechanisms of Resistance

Several resistance mechanisms have been identified in various preclinical systems, and they include decreased activation of the drug through the reduced expression of the anabolic enzyme deoxycytidine kinase, the decreased transport of drug into cells via the nucleoside transporter protein, and the increased expression of CTP synthetase activity resulting in increased concentrations of competing physiologic nucleotide substrate dCTP. To date, the precise resistance mechanism(s) that are relevant in the clinical setting remain to be determined.

Clinical Pharmacology

Approximately 50% to 60% of an administered dose of drug is excreted unchanged in the urine, and the terminal half-life is on the order of 5 hours. To date, the pathways for nonrenal elimination have not been well defined. Caution should be exercised in patients with abnormal renal function, and concomitant use of medications known to cause renal toxicity should be avoided during drug treatment.

Toxicity

Myelosuppression is dose limiting with neutropenia, anemia, and thrombocytopenia. The capillary leak syndrome (systemic inflammatory response syndrome) presents with tachypnea, tachycardia, pulmonary edema, and hypotension.[47] In essence, this adverse event is part of the tumor lysis syndrome and results from rapid cytoreduction of peripheral leukemic cells following treatment.[47] Other side effects may include nausea/vomiting, reversible liver dysfunction (hyperbilirubinemia and elevated serum transaminases), renal dysfunction (approximately 10%), and cardiac toxicity in the form of tachycardia and acute pump dysfunction.

REFERENCES

1. Wright DL, Anderson AC. Antifolate agents: a patent review (2006–2010). *Expert Opin Ther Pat* 2011;21:1293–1308.
2. Chattopadhyay S, Moran RG, Goldman ID. Pemetrexed: biochemical and cellular pharmacology, mechanisms, and clinical applications. *Mol Cancer Ther* 2007;6:404–417.
3. Vogelzang NJ, Rusthoven JJ, Symanowski J, et al. Phase III study of pemetrexed in combination with cisplatin versus cisplatin alone in patients with malignant pleural mesothelioma. *J Clin Oncol* 2003;21:2636–2644.
4. Kindler HL. Systemic treatments for mesothelioma: standard and novel. *Curr Treat Options Oncol* 2008;9:171–179.
5. Joerger M, Omlin A, Cerny T, et al. The role of pemetrexed in advanced non small-cell lung cancer: special focus on pharmacology and mechanism of action. *Curr Drug Targets* 2010;11:37–47.
6. Zain J, O'Connor O. Pralatrexate: basic understanding and clinical development. *Expert Opin Pharmacother* 2010;11:1705–1714.
7. Sirotnak FM, DeGraw JI, Moccio DM, et al. New folate analogs of the 10-deaza-aminopterin series. Basis for structural design and biochemical and pharmacologic properties. *Cancer Chemother Pharmacol* 1984;12:18–25.
8. O'Connor OA. Pralatrexate: an emerging new agent with activity in T-cell lymphomas. *Curr Opin Oncol* 2006;18:591–597.

9. Bertino JR, Göker E, Gorlick R, et al. Resistance mechanisms to methotrexate in tumors. *Oncologist* 1996;1:223–226.
10. Zhao R, Goldman ID. Resistance to antifolates. *Oncogene* 2003;22:7431–7457.
11. Grem JL. 5-Fluorouracil: forty-plus and still ticking. A review of its preclinical and clinical development. *Invest New Drugs* 2000;18:299–313.
12. Saif MW, Ezzeldin H, Vance K, et al. DPYD*2A mutation: the most common mutation associated with DPD deficiency. *Cancer Chemother Pharmacol* 2007;60:503–507.
13. Grem JL. Biochemical modulation of 5-FU in systemic treatment of advanced colorectal cancer. *Oncology (Williston Park)* 2001;15:13–19.
14. Saif MW, Shah MM, Shah AR. Fluoropyrimidine-associated cardiotoxicity: revisited. *Expert Opin Drug Saf* 2009;8:191–202.
15. Saif MW, Eloubeidi MA, Russo S, et al. Phase I study of capecitabine with concomitant radiotherapy for patients with locally advanced pancreatic cancer: expression analysis of genes related to outcome. *J Clin Oncol* 2005;23:8679–8687.
16. Geyer CE, Forster J, Lindquist D, et al. Lapatinib plus capecitabine for HER2-positive advanced breast cancer. *N Engl J Med* 2006;355:2733–2743.
17. Saif MW, Katirtzoglou NA, Syrigos KN. Capecitabine: an overview of the side effects and their management. *Anticancer Drugs* 2008;19:447–464.
18. Van Custem E, Verslype C, Tejpar S. Oral capecitabine: bridging the Atlantic divide in colon cancer treatment. *Semin Oncol* 2005;32:43–51.
19. Haller DG, Cassidy J, Clarke SJ, et al. Potential regional differences for the tolerability profiles of fluoropyrimidines. *J Clin Oncol* 2008;26:2118–2123.
20. Saif MW, Syrigos KN, Katirtzoglou NA. S-1: a promising new oral fluoropyrimidine derivative. *Expert Opin Investig Drugs* 2009;18:335–348.
21. Saif MW, Rosen LS, Saito K, et al. A phase I study evaluating the effect of CDHP as a component of S-1 on the pharmacokinetics of 5-fluorouracil. *Anticancer Res* 2011;31:625–632.
22. Daigo S, Takahashi Y, Fujieda M, et al. A novel mutant allele of the CYP2A6 gene (CYP2A6*11) found in a cancer patient who showed poor metabolic phenotype towards tegafur. *Pharmacogenetics* 2002;12:299–306.
23. Reiter A, Hochhaus A, Berger U, et al. AraC-based pharmacotherapy of chronic myeloid leukaemia. *Expert Opin Pharmacother* 2001;2:1129–1135.
24. Braess J, Wegendt C, Feuring-Buske M, et al. Leukemic blasts differ from normal bone marrow mononuclear cells and CD34+ hematopoietic stem cells in their metabolism of cytosine arabinoside. *Br J Haematol* 1999;105:388–393.
25. Momparler RL, Laliberte J, Eliopoulos N, et al. Transfection of murine fibroblast cells with human cytidine deaminase cDNA confers resistance to cytosine arabinoside. *Anticancer Drugs* 1996;7:266–274.
26. Cai J, Damaraju VL, Groulx N, et al. Two distinct molecular mechanisms underlying cytarabine resistance in human leukemic cells. *Cancer Res* 2008;68:2349–2357.
27. Kern W, Estey EH. High-dose cytosine arabinoside in the treatment of acute myeloid leukemia: review of three randomized trials. *Cancer* 2006;107:116–124.
28. Mini E, Nobili S, Caciagli B, et al. Cellular pharmacology of gemcitabine. *Ann Oncol* 2006;17:v7–v12.
29. Saif MW, Sellers S, Li M, et al. A phase I study of bi-weekly administration of 24-h gemcitabine followed by 24-h irinotecan in patients with solid tumors. *Cancer Chemother Pharmacol* 2007;60:871–882.
30. Bergman AM, Pinedo HM, Peters GJ. Determinants of resistance to 2′,2′-difluorodeoxycytidine (gemcitabine). *Drug Resist Update* 2002;5:19–33.
31. Saif MW, Lee Y, Kim R. Harnessing gemcitabine metabolism: a step towards personalized medicine for pancreatic cancer. *Ther Adv Med Oncol* 2012;4:341–346.
32. Hong SP, Wen J, Bang S, et al. CD44-positive cells are responsible for gemcitabine resistance in pancreatic cancer cells. *Int J Cancer* 2009;125:2323–2331.
33. Poplin E, Feng Y, Berlin J, et al. Phase III, randomized study of gemcitabine and oxaliplatin versus gemcitabine (fixed-dose rate infusion) compared with gemcitabine (30-minute infusion) in patients with pancreatic carcinoma E6201: a trial of the Eastern Cooperative Oncology Group. *J Clin Oncol* 2009;27:3778–3785.
34. Hande KR. Purine antimetabolites. In: Chabner BA, Longo DL, eds. *Cancer Chemotherapy and Biotherapy: Principles and Practice*, 4th ed. Philadelphia: Lippincott–Raven; 2006: 212.
35. Evans WE. Pharmacogenetics of thiopurine S-methyltransferase and thiopurine therapy. *Ther Drug Monitor* 2004;26:186–191.
36. Wang L, Weinshilboum R. Thiopurine S-methyltransferase pharmacogenetics: insights, challenges, and future directions. *Oncogene* 2006;25:1629–1638.
37. Vora A, Mitchell CD, Lennard L, et al. Toxicity and efficacy of 6-thioguanine versus 6-mercaptopurine in childhood lymphoblastic leukaemia: a randomised trial. *Lancet* 2006;368:1339–1348.
38. Montillo M, Ricci F, Tedeschi A. Role of fludarabine in hematological malignancies. *Expert Rev Anticancer Ther* 2006;6:1141–1161.
39. Gandhi V, Plunkett W. Cellular and clinical pharmacology of fludarabine. *Clin Pharmacokinet* 2002;41:93–103.
40. van den Neste E, Cardoen S, Offner F, et al. Old and new insights into the mechanism of action of two nucleoside analogs active in lymphoid malignancies: flludarabine and cladribine. *Int J Oncol* 2005;27:1113–1124.
41. Gidron A, Tallman MS. 2-CdA in the treatment of hairy cell leukemia: a review of long-term follow-up. *Leuk Lymphoma* 2006;47:2301–2307.
42. Huang P, Robertson LE, Wright S, et al. High molecular weight DNA fragmentation: a critical event in nucleoside analog-induced apoptosis in leukemia cells. *Clin Cancer Res* 1995;1:1005–1013.
43. Grevz N, Saven A. Cladribine: from the bench to the bedside: focus on hairy cell leukemia. *Expert Rev Anticancer Ther* 2004;4:745–757.
44. Seto S, Carrera CJ, Kubota M, et al. Mechanism of deoxyadenosine and 2-chlorodeoxyadenosine toxicity to nondividing human lymphocytes. *J Clin Invest* 1985;75:377–383.
45. Bonate PL, Arthaud L, Cantrell WR Jr, et al. Discovery and development of clofarabine: a nucleoside analogue for treating cancer. *Nat Rev Drug Discov* 2006;5:855–863.
46. Faderi S, Gandhi V, Keating MJ, et al. The role of clofarabine in hematologic and solid malignancies: development of a next generation nucleoside analog. *Cancer* 2005;102:1985–1995.
47. Baytan B, Ozdemir O, Gunes AM, et al. Clofarabine-induced capillary leak syndrome in a child with refractory acute lymphoblastic leukemia. *J Pediatr Hematol Oncol* 2010;32:144–146.

20 Topoisomerase Interactive Agents

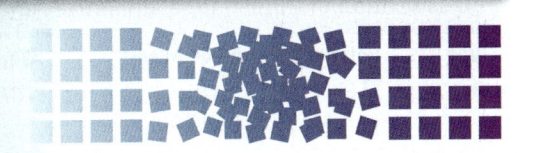

Khanh T. Do, Shivaani Kummar, James H. Doroshow, and Yves Pommier

CLASSIFICATION, BIOCHEMICAL, AND BIOLOGIC FUNCTIONS OF TOPOISOMERASES

Nucleic acids (DNA and RNA) being long polymers, topoisomerases fulfill the need for cellular DNA to be densely packaged in the cell nucleus, transcribed, replicated, and evenly distributed between daughter cells following replication without tangles. Topoisomerases are ubiquitous and essential for all organisms as they prevent and resolve DNA and RNA entanglements and resolve DNA supercoiling during transcription and replication. This chapter first summarizes the basic elements necessary to understand the mechanism of action of topoisomerases and their inhibitors. More detailed information can be found in recent reviews[1–7] and two recent books.[8,9] The second part of the chapter summarizes the use of topoisomerase inhibitors as anticancer drugs.

Classification of Topoisomerases

Human cells contain six topoisomerase genes (Table 20.1), which have been numbered historically. The commonly used abbreviations are Top1 for topoisomerases I (Top1mt being the mitochondrial topoisomerase whose gene is encoded in the cell nucleus),[10] Top2 for topoisomerases II, and Top3 for topoisomerases III. Top1 was the first eukaryotic topoisomerase discovered by Champoux and Dulbecco.[11] Topoisomerases solve DNA topologic problems by cutting the DNA backbone and religating without the assistance of any additional ligase. Top1 and Top3 act by cleaving/religating a single strand of the DNA duplex, whereas Top2 enzymes cleave and religate both strands, making a four–base pair reversible staggered cut (Fig. 20.1). It is convenient to remember that odd-numbered topoisomerases (Top1 and Top3) cleave and religate one strand, whereas the even numbered topoisomerases (Top2s) cleave and religate both strands.

Biochemical Characteristics and Cleavage Complexes of the Different Topoisomerases

The DNA cutting/relegation mechanism is common to all topoisomerases and utilizes an enzyme catalytic tyrosine residue acting as a nucleophile and becoming covalently attached to the end of the broken DNA. These catalytic intermediates are referred to as cleavage complexes (see Fig. 20.1B, E). The reverse religation reaction is carried out by the attack of the ribose hydroxyl ends toward the tyrosyl-DNA bond.

Top1 (and Top1mt) attaches to the 3′-end of the break, whereas the other topoisomerases (Top2 and Top3) have opposite polarity and covalently attach to the 5′-end of the breaks (see Table 20.1 [second column] and Fig. 20.1B, E). Topoisomerases have distinct biochemical requirements. Top1 and Top1mt are the simplest, nicking/closing, and relaxing DNA as monomers in the absence of cofactor, and even at ice temperature. Top2 enzymes, on the other hand, are the most complex topoisomerases working as dimers, requiring ATP binding and hydrolysis, and a divalent metal (Mg^{2+}) for catalysis. Top3 enzymes also require Mg^{2+} for catalysis but function as monomers without ATP requirement. Notably, the DNA substrates differ for Top3 enzymes. Whereas both Top1 and Top2 process double-stranded DNA, the Top3 substrates need to be single-stranded nucleic acids (DNA for Top3α and DNA or RNA for Top3β).[10,12,13]

Differential Topoisomerization Mechanisms: Swiveling Versus Strand Passage, DNA Versus RNA Topoisomerases

Topoisomerases use two main mechanisms to change nucleic topology. The first is by "untwisting" the DNA duplex. This mechanism is unique to Top1, which, by an enzyme-associated single-strand break, allows the broken strand to rotate around the intact strand (see Fig. 20.1B) until DNA supercoiling is dissipated. At this point, the stacking energy of adjacent DNA bases realigns the broken ends, and the 5′-hydroxyl end attacks the 3′-phosphotyrosyl end, thereby relegating the DNA. A remarkable feature of this Top1 untwisting mechanism is its extreme efficiency with a rotation speed around 6,000 rpm and relative independence from torque, thereby allowing full relaxation of DNA supercoiling.[14]

The second topologic mechanism is by "strand passage." This mechanism allows the passage of a double- or a single-stranded DNA (or RNA) through the cleavage complexes. Top2α and Top2β both act by allowing the passage of an intact DNA duplex through the DNA double-strand break generated by the enzymes. After which, Top2 religates the broken duplex. Such reactions permit DNA decatenation, unknotting, and relaxation of supercoils.[3] Top3 enzymes also act by strand passage but only pass one nucleic acid strand through the single-strand break generated by the enzymes. In the case of Top3α, the substrate is a single-stranded DNA segment (such as a double-Holliday junction), whereas in the case of Top3β, the substrate can be a single-stranded RNA segment, with Top3β acting as a RNA topoisomerase.[13,15]

TOPOISOMERASE INHIBITORS AS INTERFACIAL POISONS

Topoisomerase Inhibitors Act as Interfacial Inhibitors by Binding at the Topoisomerase–DNA Interface and Trapping Topoisomerase Cleavage Complexes

Relegation of the cleavage complexes is dependent on the structure of the ends of the broken DNA (i.e., the realignment of the broken ends). Binding the drugs at the enzyme–DNA interface misaligns the ends of the DNA and precludes relegation, resulting in the stabilization of the topoisomerase cleavage complexes (Top1cc and Top2cc). Crystal structures of drug-bound cleavage complexes have firmly established this mechanism for both Top1- and Top2-targeted drugs.[16]

TABLE 20.1
Classification of Human Topoisomerases and Topoisomerase Inhibitors

Type	Polarity	Mechanism	Genes	Proteins	Main Functions	Drugs
IB	3'-PY	Rotation/swiveling	TOP1	Top1	DNA supercoiling relaxation, replication, and transcription	Camptothecins, noncamptothecins
			TOP1MT	Top1mt		
IIA	5'-PY	Strand passage ATPase	TOP2A	Top2α	Decatenation/replication	Anthracyclines, anthracenediones, epipodophyllotoxins
			TOP2B	Top2β	Transcription	
IA	5'-PY	Strand passage	TOP3A	Top3α	DNA replication with BLM	None
			TOP3B	Top3β	RNA topoisomerase	

Top1mt, mitochondrial DNA topoisomerase; BLM, Bloom's syndrome helicare.

It is critical to understand that the cytotoxic mechanism of topoisomerase inhibitors requires the drugs to trap the topoisomerase cleavage complexes rather than block catalytic activity. This sets apart topoisomerase inhibitors from classical enzyme inhibitors such as antifolates. Indeed, knocking out Top1 renders yeast cells totally immune to camptothecin,[17,18] and reducing enzyme levels in cancer cells confers drug resistance. Conversely, in breast cancers, amplification of TOP2A, which is on the same locus as HER2, contributes to the efficacy of doxorubicin.[19] Also, cellular mutations of Top1 and Top2 that renders cells insensitive to the trapping of topoisomerase cleavage complexes produce high resistance to Top1 or Top2 inhibitors. Based on this trapping of cleavage complexes mechanism, we refer to topoisomerase inhibitors as topoisomerase cleavage complex–targeted drugs.

Top1cc-Targeted Drugs (Camptothecin and Noncamptothecin Derivatives) Kill Cancer Cells by Replication Collisions

Top1cc are cytotoxic by their conversion into DNA damage by replication and transcription fork collisions. This explains why cytotoxicity is directly related to drug exposure and why arresting DNA replication protects cells from camptothecin.[20,21] The collisions arise from the fact that the drugs, by slowing down the nicking/closing activity of Top1, uncouple the kinetics of Top1 with the polymerases and helicases, which lead polymerases to collide into Top1cc (Fig. 20.2A). Such collisions have two consequences. They generate double-strand breaks (replication and transcription runoff) and irreversible Top1–DNA adducts (see Fig. 20.2B). The replication double-strand breaks are repaired by homologous recombination, which explains the hypersensitivity of BRCA-deficient cancer cells to Top1cc-targeted drugs.[22] The Top1-covalent complexes can be removed by two pathways, the excision pathway centered around tyrosyl-DNA-phosphodiesterase 1 (TDP1)[23] and the endonuclease pathway involving 3'-flap endonucleases such as XPF-ERCC1.[24] It is also possible that drug-trapped Top1cc directly generate DNA double-strand breaks when they are within 10 base pairs on opposite strands of the DNA duplex or when they occur next to a preexisting single-strand break on the opposite strand. Finally, it is not excluded that topologic defects contribute to the cytotoxicity of Top1cc-targeted drugs (the accumulation of supercoils[25] and the formation of alternative structures such as R-loops) (see Fig. 20.2D).[26]

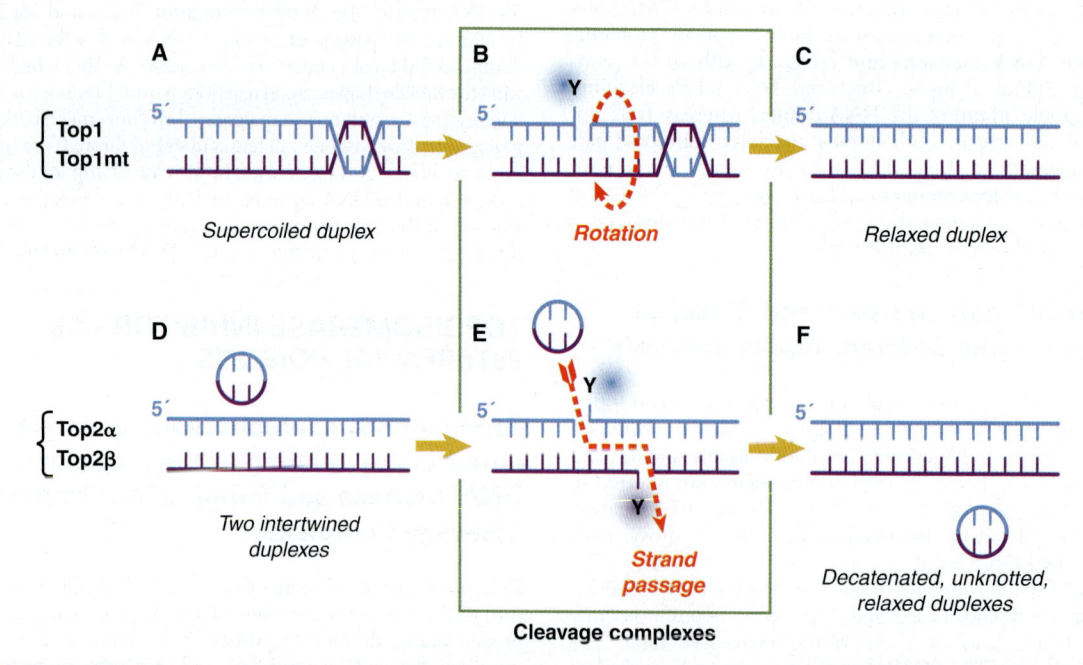

Figure 20.1 Mechanisms of action of topoisomerases. **(A–C)** Topoisomerases I (Top1 for nuclear DNA and Top1mt for mitochondrial DNA) relax supercoiled DNA **(A)** by reversibly cleaving one DNA strand, forming a covalent bond between the enzyme catalytic tyrosine and the 3' end of the nicked DNA (the Top1 cleavage complex [Top1cc]) **(B)**. This reaction allows the swiveling of the broken strand around the intact strand. Rapid religation allows the dissociation of Top1. **(D–F)** Topoisomerases II (Top2α and Top2β) act on two DNA duplexes **(A)**. They act as homodimers, cleaving both strands and forming a covalent bond between their catalytic tyrosine and the 5' end of the DNA break (Top2cc) **(E)**. This reaction allows the passage of the intact duplex through the Top2 homodimer *(red dotted arrow)* **(E)**. Top2 inhibitors trap the Top2cc and prevent the normal religation **(F)**.

Figure 20.2 Mechanisms of action of topoisomerase inhibitors beyond the trapping of topoisomerase cleavage complexes. **(A)** Stalled or slow cleavage complexes lead to collisions with replication and transcription complexes. **(B)** Collisions of replication complexes with Top1cc on the leading strand for DNA synthesis generate DNA double-strand breaks by replication runoff. Top1cc can also form DNA double-strand breaks (DSBs) when they occur opposite to another Top1cc or preexisting nick. **(C)** Top2cc, which are normally held together by Top2 homodimers, can be converted to free DSBs upon Top2cc proteolysis or dimer disjunction. **(D)** Topologic defects resulting from functional topoisomerase deficiencies play a minor role in the anticancer activity of topoisomerase cleavage complex targeted drugs.

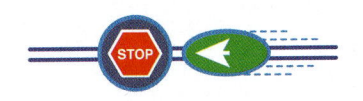

A: Collisions of polymerases and helicases (green ellipse) with trapped Top cleavage complexes (Stop sign) => Protein-DNA complexes blocking DNA metabolism

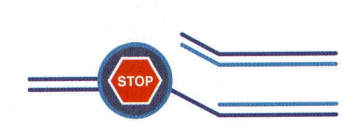

B: Conversion of Top1cc into DSB by replication "runoff"
=> Top1 needs to be removed by TDP1 and /or 3'-flap endonucleases (XPF-ERCC1)
=> DSB repaired by homologous recombination
Top1cc also form DSB when on opposite strands or opposite to a preexisting single-strand break

C: Top2cc proteolysis or mechanical disjoining
Top2cc readily form DSB when concerted cleavage on both strands and disjunction of the homodimer

D: Topologic defects resulting from Top sequestration in the cleavage complexes: accumulation of
=> Supercoils (Top1 and Top2) (1)
=> Knots (Top2) (2)
=> Catenanes (Top2) (3)

Cytotoxic Mechanisms of Top2cc-Targeted Drugs (Intercalators and Demethyl Epipodophyllotoxins)

Contrary to camptothecins, Top2 inhibitors kill cancer cells without requiring DNA replication fork collisions. Indeed, even after a 30-minute exposure, doxorubicin and other Top2cc-targeted drugs can kill over 99% of the cells, which is in vast excess of the fraction of S-phase cells in tissue culture (generally less than 50%).[27,28] The collision mechanism in the case of Top2cc-targeted drugs (see Fig. 20.2A) appears to involve transcription and proteolysis of both Top2 and RNA polymerase II.[29] Such situation would then lead to DNA double-strand breaks by disruption of the Top2 dimer interface (see Fig. 20.2C). Alternatively, the Top2 homodimer interface could be disjoined by mechanical tension (see Fig. 20.2C). Yet, it is important to bear in mind that 90% of Top2cc trapped by etoposide are not concerted and, therefore, consist in single-strand breaks,[3,30,31] which is different from doxorubicin, which traps both Top2 monomers and produces a majority of DNA double-strand breaks.[32] Finally, it is not excluded that topologic defects resulting from Top2 sequestration by the drug-induced cleavage complexes could contribute to the cytotoxicity of Top2cc-targeted drugs (see Fig. 20.2D). Such topologic defects would include persistent DNA knots and catenanes, potentially leading to chromosome breaks during mitosis.

TOPOISOMERASE I INHIBITORS: CAMPTOTHECINS AND BEYOND

Camptothecin is an alkaloid identified in the 1960s by Wall and Wani[33] in a screen of plant extracts for antineoplastic drugs. The two water-soluble derivatives of camptothecin containing the active lactone form are topotecan and irinotecan, which are approved by the U.S. Food and Drug Administration (FDA) for the treatment of several cancers. In addition, several Top1cc-targeting drugs are in clinical development, including camptothecin derivatives and formulations (including high–molecular-weight conjugates or liposomal formulations), as well as noncamptothecin compounds that exhibit greater potency or noncross resistance to irinotecan and topotecan in preclinical cancer models.[31,34–36]

Irinotecan

Irinotecan, a prodrug containing a bulky dipiperidine side chain at C-10 (Fig. 20.3), is cleaved by a carboxylesterase-converting enzyme in the liver and other tissues to generate the active metabolite, SN-38. Irinotecan is FDA approved for the treatment of colorectal cancer in the metastatic setting as first-line treatment in combination with 5-fluorouracil/leucovorin (5-FU/LV) and as a single agent in the second-line treatment of progressive colorectal cancer after 5-FU–based therapy (see Table 20.1).[37,38] Newer therapeutic uses of irinotecan include a combination with oxaliplatin and 5-FU as first-line treatment in pancreatic cancer.[39] Irinotecan is additionally used in combination with cisplatin or carboplatin in extensive-stage small-cell lung cancer[40,41] as well as refractory esophageal and gastroesophageal junction (GEJ) cancers, gastric cancer, cervical cancer, anaplastic gliomas and glioblastomas, and non–small-cell lung cancer (Table 20.2). Irinotecan is usually administered intravenously at a dose of 125 mg/m² for 4 weeks with a 2-week rest period in combination with bolus 5-FU/LV, 180 mg/m² every 2 weeks in combination with an infusion of 5-FU/LV, or 350 mg/m² every 3 weeks as a single agent.

Diarrhea and myelosuppression are the most common toxicities associated with irinotecan administration. Two mechanisms explain irinotecan-induced diarrhea. Acute cholinergic effects resulting in abdominal cramping and diarrhea occur within 24 hours of drug administration are the result of acetylcholinesterase inhibition by the prodrug, and can be treated with the administration of atropine. Direct mucosal cytotoxicity with diarrhea is typically observed after 24 hours and can result in significant morbidity. Symptoms are managed with loperamide. Hepatic metabolism and biliary excretion accounts for >70% of the elimination of the administered dose, with renal excretion accounting for the remainder of the dose. SN-38 is glucuronidated in the liver by UGT1A1, and deficiencies in this pathway increase the risk of diarrhea and myelosuppression. Dose reductions are recommended for patients who are homozygous for the UGT1A1*28 allele, for which an FDA-approved test for detection of the UGT1A1*28 allele in patients is available.[42,43] Additionally, dose reductions of irinotecan are recommended for patients with hepatic dysfunction, with bilirubin greater than 1.5 mg/mL.[44]

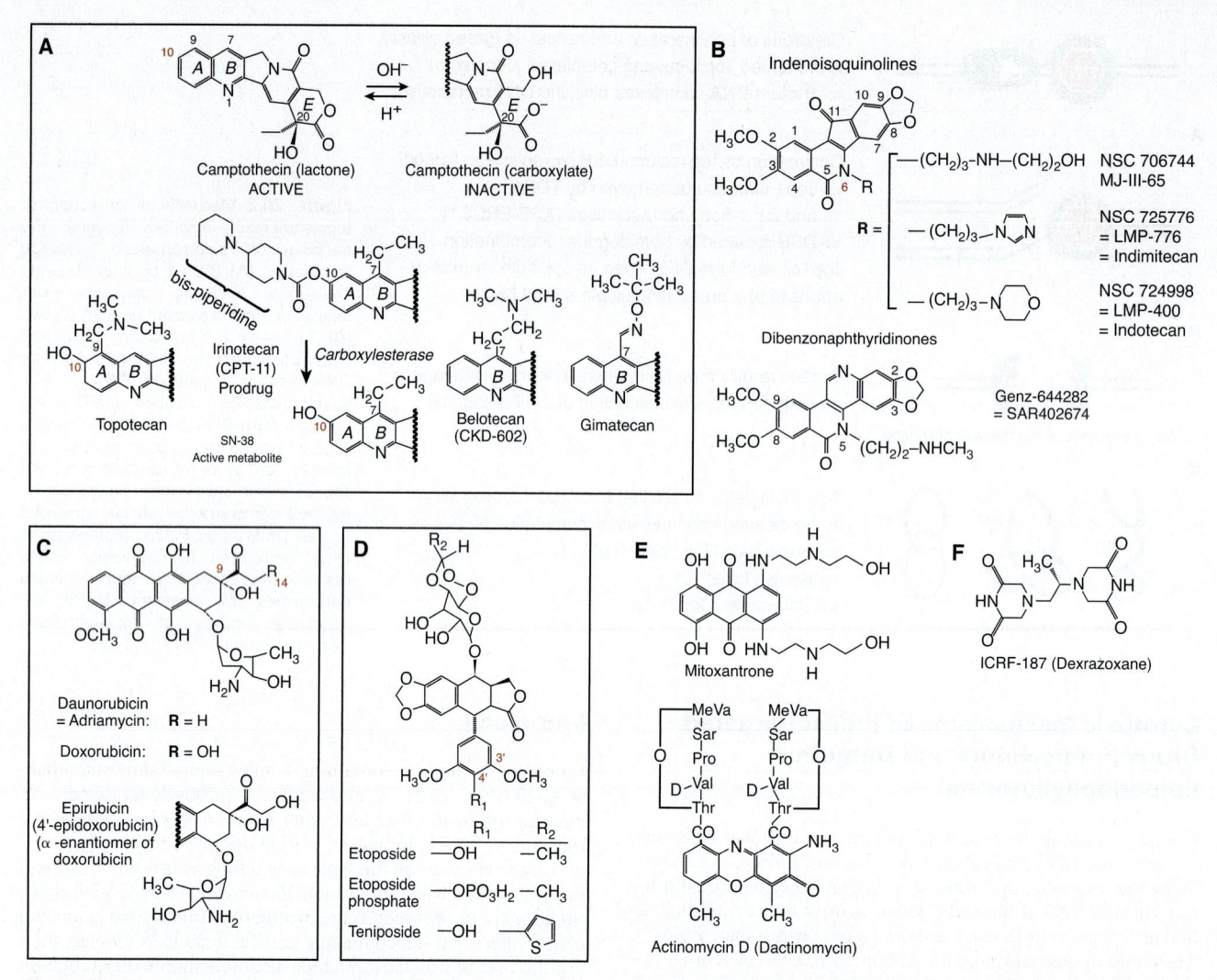

Figure 20.3 Structure of topoisomerase inhibitors. **(A)** Camptothecin derivatives are instable at physiologic pH with the formation of a carboxylate derivative within minutes. Irinotecan is a prodrug and needs to be converted to SN-38 to trap Top1cc. **(B)** Non-camptothecin derivatives in clinical trials. **(C)** Anthracycline derivatives. **(D)** Demethyl epipodophyllotoxin derivatives. **(E)** Other intercalating Top2 inhibitors acting by trapping Top2cc. **(F)** Structure of dexrazoxane, which acts as a catalytic inhibitor of Top2.

Topotecan

Topotecan contains a basic side chain at position C-9 that enhances its water solubility (see Fig. 20.3). Topotecan is approved for the treatment of ovarian cancer,[45] small-cell lung cancer,[46] and as a single agent and in combination with cisplatin for cervical cancer.[47] Additionally, it is active in acute myeloid leukemia (AML) and myelodysplastic syndrome (see Table 20.2). Topotecan is administered intravenously as a single agent at a dose of 1.5 mg/m^2 as a 30-minute infusion daily for 5 days, followed by a 2-week period of rest for the treatment of solid tumors or at a dose of 0.75 mg/m^2 as a 30-minute infusion daily for 3 days in combination with cisplatin on day 1, every 3 weeks, for the treatment of cervical cancer.

Myelosuppression is the most common dose-limiting toxicity. Extensive prior radiation or previous bone marrow–suppressive chemotherapy increases the risk of topotecan-induced myelosuppression. Other toxicities include nausea, vomiting, diarrhea, fatigue, alopecia, and transient hepatic transaminitis.

Topotecan and its metabolites are primarily cleared by the kidneys, requiring dose reduction in patients with renal dysfunction. A 50% dose reduction is recommended for patients with moderate renal impairment (creatinine clearance 20 to 39 mL per minute).

There are no formal guidelines for dose reductions in patients with hepatic dysfunction (defined as serum bilirubin >1.5 mg/dL to <10 mg/dL). Topotecan additionally penetrates the blood-brain barrier, achieving concentrations in cerebrospinal fluid that are approximately 30% that of plasma levels.[48]

Camptothecin Conjugates and Analogs

New formulations of camptothecin conjugates and analogs are currently in clinical development in an effort to improve the therapeutic index (Table 20.3). The development of camptothecin conjugates is based on the notion that the addition of a bulky conjugate would allow for a more consistent delivery system and extend the half-life of the molecule.

CRLX101, formerly IT-101, a covalent cyclodextrin-polyethylene glycol copolymer camptothecin conjugate, has plasma concentrations and area under the curve (AUC) that are approximately 100-fold higher than camptothecin, with a half-life in the range of 17 to 20 hours compared to 1.3 hours for camptothecin.[49] It has demonstrated antitumor activity in preclinical studies in irinotecan-resistant tumors with complete tumor regression in human non–small-cell lung cancer, Ewing sarcoma, and

TABLE 20.2
U.S. Food and Drug Administration–Approved Camptothecin Analogs

Irinotecan (Camptosar)	FDA approved for: Metastatic colorectal cancer	First-line therapy in combination with 5-FU/LV	Diarrhea (dose reductions are recommended for patients who are homozygous for the UGT1A1*28 allele)
		Second-line therapy as a single agent	Myelosuppression
	Category 2A[a] recommendations: Pancreatic cancer	First-line therapy in combination with oxaliplatin, 5-FU/LV	
	Extensive-stage small-cell lung cancer	First-line therapy in combination with cisplatin or carboplatin	
	Category 2B[b] recommendations: Esophageal and GEJ cancers, gastric cancer, cervical cancer, anaplastic gliomas and glioblastomas, non–small-cell lung cancer, ovarian cancer		
Topotecan (Hycamtin)	FDA approved for: Cervical cancer	Stage IVB, recurrent, or persistent carcinoma of the cervix not amenable to curative treatment with surgery and/or radiation therapy	Myelosuppression
	Ovarian cancer	After failure of initial therapy	
	Small-cell lung cancer	After failure of initial therapy	
	Class 2B recommendations: AML, MDS		

[a] Category 2A: Recommendations are based upon lower-level evidence, there is uniform National Comprehensive Cancer Network consensus that the intervention is appropriate.
[b] Category 2B: Recommendations are based upon lower-level evidence, there is National Comprehensive Cancer Network consensus that the intervention is appropriate.
MDS, myelodysplastic syndrome.

lymphoma xenograft models.[50] Preliminary data from Phase 1 studies indicate that CRLX101 is well tolerated at a dose of 15 mg/m^2 administered in a biweekly administration schedule.[51] It is currently being studied in Phase 2 studies as a single agent and in combination with chemotherapeutic agents in lung, renal cell cancer, and gynecologic malignancies.[52–54]

Etirinotecan pegol (NKTR-102), an irinotecan polymer conjugate, has a longer plasma circulation time with a lower maximum concentration of SN-38 compared with irinotecan. It was evaluated in a Phase 2 study in platinum-resistant refractory epithelial ovarian cancer at a dose of 145 mg/m^2 administered on a schedule of every 21 days; a median progression-free survival of 5.3 months and median overall survival of 11.7 months was observed.[55] Two schedules of administration, 145 mg/m^2 administered every 14 days versus every 21 days, have been tested in a Phase 2 study of NKTR-102 in patients with previously treated metastatic breast cancer.[56] Of the 70 patients evaluated in this study, 20 patients achieved an objective response (29%; 95% confidence interval [CI] 18.4 to 40.6). For both these studies, the most common adverse events on the 21-day administration schedule were dehydration and diarrhea. Etirinotecan pegol is currently being evaluated in several phase 2 studies in lung cancer, colorectal cancer, and high-grade gliomas,[57–60] with evidence of clinical activity in refractory solid tumors. A Phase 3 trial (The BEACON Study) is underway evaluating NKTR-102 against the physicians' choice in refractory breast cancer.[61]

As an alternative to macromolecular conjugates, attempts have also been made to alter the camptothecin pentacyclic ring structure with modifications of the A and B ring (see Fig. 20.3A) in an effort to improve solubility and enhance antitumor activity. Structure–activity relationship studies have shown that substitutions at the 7, 9, and 10 positions serve to enhance the antitumor activity of camptothecin.[62] Belotecan, a novel camptothecin analog, has a water-solubilizing group at the 7 position of the B ring of camptothecin (see Fig. 20.3A). Several Phase 2 studies have evaluated belotecan in combination with carboplatin in recurrent ovarian cancer[63] and in combination with cisplatin in extensive-stage small-cell lung cancer,[64] demonstrating activity in these cancers; however, these combinations were associated with prominent hematologic toxicities. Phase 2 studies evaluating belotecan as a single agent in patients with recurrent or progressive carcinoma of the uterine cervix failed to show activity.[65] Gimatecan is a lipophilic oral camptothecin analog (see Fig. 20.3A). Pharmacokinetic studies demonstrate that gimatecan is primarily present in plasma as the lactone form (>85%), and has a long half-life of 77.1 +/− 29.6 hours, with an increase in maximum concentration (Cmax) and AUC of three- to six-fold after multiple dosing.[66] Phase 2 studies show that gimatecan has demonstrated activity in previously treated ovarian cancer, with myelosuppression as the main toxicity.[67]

Newer development of analogs have attempted to modify the E-ring through introduction of an electron-withdrawing group at

TABLE 20.3
Topoisomerase I Inhibitors in Development

Camptothecin Conjugates	Camptothecin Analogs	Noncamptothecin Agents
CRLX101	Belotecan	Indenoisoquinoline
NKTR-102	Gimatecan	Indotecan (LMP-400)
MM-398	Homocamptothecin	Indimitecan (LMP-776)
	Elomotecan	Dibenzo naphthyridine Genz-644282
	Diflomotecan	

the α position in an effort to overcome the instability of the E-ring while maintaining the binding capability of the camptothecin analog to the Top1-DNA cleavage complex. Collectively called homocamptothecin analogs, two have been tested in clinical trials and include diflomotecan[68] and elomotecan.[69] The dose-limiting toxicity in the Phase I study of elomotecan was neutropenia. A five-member E-ring derivative has also been developed and has reached a Phase 1 clinical trial.[70,71]

Noncamptothecin Topoisomerase I Inhibitors

Noncamptothecin Top1 inhibitors are in clinical development, and include indenoisoquinolines and dibenzonaphthyridines (see Fig. 20.3B). Two indenoisoquinoline derivatives are currently in clinical development, indotecan (LMP400) and indimitecan (LMP776).[72,73] Early in vitro studies show enhanced potency compared with camptothecins, and persistence of Top1 cleavage complexes.[74] Genz-644282, a dibenzonaphthyridine derivative, demonstrated enhanced antitumor activity in preclinical studies[75] and is currently being evaluated in Phase 1 clinical trials.[76]

TOPOISOMERASE II INHIBITORS: INTERCALATORS AND NONINTERCALATORS

Topoisomerase II inhibitors can be classified in two main classes: DNA intercalators, which encompass different chemical classes (Fig. 20.3C, E), and nonintercalators represented by the epipodophyllotoxin derivatives (see Fig. 20.3D). Although both act by trapping Top2 cleavage complexes (Top2cc), DNA intercalators exhibit a second effect as drug concentrations increase above low micromolar values: they block the formation of Top2cc by intercalating into DNA and destabilizing the binding of Top2 to DNA. This explains why Top2α and Top2β are trapped over a relatively narrow concentration range by anthracyclines, and why intercalators have additional effects besides trapping Top2cc, namely inhibition of a broad range of DNA processing enzymes including helicases, polymerase, and even nucleosome destabilization.

Doxorubicin

Doxorubicin and daunorubicin were the first anthracyclines discovered in the 1960s and remain among the most widely used anticancer agents over a broad spectrum of malignancies. Although doxorubicin only differs by one hydroxyl substitution on position 14 (see Fig. 20.3C), doxorubicin has a much broader anticancer activity than daunorubicin. Anthracyclines are natural products derived from *Streptomyces peucetius* variation *caesius*. They were found to target Top2 well after their clinical approval.[77] Subsequent searches for less toxic drugs and formulations led to the approval of liposomal doxorubicin, idarubicin, and epirubicin.

Anthracyclines are flat, planar molecules that are relatively hydrophobic. The quinone structure of anthracyclines (see Fig. 20.3C) enhances the catalysis of oxidation-reduction reactions, thereby promoting the generation of oxygen free radicals, which may be involved in antitumor effects as well as the cardiotoxicity associated with these drugs.[78,79] Anthracyclines are also substrates for P-glycoprotein and Mrp-1, and drug efflux is thought to be a major drug resistance determinant.[80,81]

Doxorubicin is available in a standard salt form and as a liposomal formulation. FDA-labeled indications for standard doxorubicin include acute lymphocytic leukemia (ALL), AML, chronic lymphoid leukemia, Hodgkin lymphoma, non-Hodgkin lymphoma, mantle cell lymphoma, multiple myeloma, mycosis fungoides, Kaposi sarcoma, breast cancer (adjuvant therapy and advanced), advanced prostate cancer, advanced gastric cancer, Ewing sarcoma, thyroid cancer, advanced nephroblastoma, advanced neuroblastoma, advanced non–small-cell lung cancer, advanced ovarian cancer, advanced transitional cell bladder cancer, cervical cancer, and Langerhans cell tumors. Doxorubicin has activity in other malignancies as well, including soft tissue sarcoma, osteosarcoma, carcinoid, and liver cancer (Table 20.4). Doxorubicin is typically administered at a recommended dose of 30 to 75 mg/m^2 every 3 weeks intravenously.

Major acute toxicities of doxorubicin include myelosuppression, mucositis, alopecia, nausea, and vomiting. Myelosuppression is the acute dose-limiting toxicity. Other toxicities, including diarrhea, nausea, vomiting, mucositis, and alopecia, are dose and schedule related. Prophylactic antiemetics are routinely given with bolus doses of doxorubicin, and longer infusions are associated with less nausea and less cardiotoxicity. Patients should also be warned to expect their urine to redden after drug administration. Doxorubicin is a potent vesicant, and extravasation can lead to severe necrosis of skin and local tissues, requiring surgical debridement and skin grafts. Infusions via a central venous catheter are recommended. Other toxicities of doxorubicin include *radiation recall* and the risk of developing secondary leukemia. *Radiation recall* is an inflammatory reaction at sites of previous radiation and can lead to pericarditis, pleural effusion, and skin rash. Secondary leukemias are thought to be a result of balanced translocations that result from Top2 poisoning by the anthracyclines, albeit to lesser degree than other Top2 poisons, such as the epipodophyllotoxins (see the following).[82]

Anthracyclines are cleared mainly by metabolism to less active forms and by biliary excretion. Less than 10% of the administered dose is cleared by the kidneys. Dose reductions should be made in patients with elevated plasma bilirubin. Doxorubicin should be dose reduced by 50% for plasma bilirubin concentrations ranging from 1.2 to 3.0 mg/dL, by 75% for values of 3.1 to 5.0 mg/dL, and withheld for values greater than 5 mg/dL.

Liposomal Doxorubicin

Doxorubicin is also available in a polyethylene glycol (PEG)ylated liposomal form, which allows for enhancement of drug delivery. Use of liposomal doxorubicin has been associated with less cardiotoxicity even at doses exceeding 500 mg/m^2.[83] Additionally, liposomal doxorubicin produces less nausea and vomiting and relatively mild myelosuppression compared to doxorubicin. Unique to the liposomal formulation is the risk of hand–foot syndrome and an acute infusion reaction manifested by flushing, dyspnea, edema, fever, chills, rash, bronchospasm, and hypertension. These infusion reactions are related to the rate of infusion; therefore, the recommended administration schedule is set at an initial rate of 1 mg per minute for the first 10 to 15 minutes. The rate may be slowly increased to complete infusion over 60 minutes if no reaction occurs. Typical dosing schedules include 50 mg/m^2 intravenous infusion every 4 weeks for four courses in ovarian cancer, 20 mg/m^2 intravenous infusion every 3 weeks in AIDS-related Kaposi sarcoma, and 30 mg/m^2 intravenous infusion in combination with bortezomib to be given on days 1, 4, 8, and 11 every 3 weeks in multiple myeloma.

Daunorubicin

Despite its chemical similarity (see Fig. 20.3C), daunorubicin is considerably less active in solid tumors compared to doxorubicin. It is FDA approved for the treatment of ALL and AML. Daunorubicin is typically administered via intravenous push over 3 to 5 minutes at a dose of 30 to 45 mg/m^2 per day on 3 consecutive days in combination chemotherapy. For induction therapy for pediatric acute lymphoblastic leukemia, daunorubicin is dosed at 25 mg/m^2 intravenously in combination with vincristine and prednisone. In children less than 2 years of age or in those who have a body surface area less than 0.5 m^2, current recommendations are based on

TABLE 20.4
U.S. Food And Drug Administration–Approved Topoisomerase II Inhibitors in Clinical Use

Compound	Tumor Type	Clinical Indication	Major Toxicities
I. Anthracyclines			
Doxorubicin (Adriamycin)	Breast carcinoma	Adjuvant setting with axillary LN involvement following resection of primary breast cancer	Dose-dependent cardiotoxicity Myelosuppression
	ALL AML Wilms' tumor Neuroblastoma Sarcomas Ovarian cancer Transitional cell bladder cancer Thyroid cancer Gastric cancer Hodgkin lymphoma Non-Hodgkin lymphoma	In combination with other cytotoxic agents	
Pegylated liposomal doxorubicin (Doxil)	Ovarian cancer	After failure of platinum-based chemotherapy	Myelosuppression Stomatitis Hand-foot syndrome Dosage reduction recommended with hepatic dysfunction
	AIDS-related Kaposi sarcoma	After failure of prior systemic chemotherapy	
	Multiple myeloma	In combination with bortezomib	
Daunorubicin (Cerubidine)	ALL AML	Induction therapy	Dose-dependent cardiotoxicity Myelosuppression
Epirubicin (Ellence)	Breast cancer	Adjuvant therapy in patients with evidence of axillary node tumor involvement following primary resection	Dose-dependent cardiotoxicity Myelosuppression
Idarubicin (Idamycin)	AML	Induction therapy	Dose-dependent cardiotoxicity Myelosuppression
II. Anthracenediones			
Mitoxantrone (Novantrone)	Prostate cancer AML	Hormone-refractory prostate cancer	Myelosuppression
Dactinomycin (Cosmegen)	Wilms' tumor Rhabdomyosarcoma Ewing sarcoma Nonseminomatous testicular cancer Gestational trophoblastic neoplasia		Myelosuppression
III. Epipodophyllotoxins			
Etoposide (VePesid)	Small-cell lung cancer Testicular cancer	First-line in combination First-line in combination	Myelosuppression
Teniposide (Vumon)	Pediatric lymphoblastic leukemia	Refractory setting	Myelosuppression

LN, lymph node.

body mass index (1 mg/kg) rather than body surface area. A higher dose of daunorubicin at 60 mg/m² per day to 90 mg/m² per day intravenously for 3 consecutive days is currently recommended as part of the induction combination regimen for the treatment of acute myeloblastic leukemia. Daunorubicin has similar toxicities to doxorubicin, including myelosuppression, cardiac toxicity, nausea, vomiting, alopecia, and is also a vesicant. Daunorubicin is metabolized by the liver and undergoes substantial elimination by the kidneys, requiring dose reductions for both renal and hepatic dysfunction. A 50% dose reduction is recommended for either serum creatinine or bilirubin greater than 3 mg/dL, and a 25% reduction in dose for bilirubin concentrations ranging from 1.2 to 3.0 mg/dL.

Epirubicin

Epirubicin is an epimer of doxorubicin (see Fig. 20.3C) with increased lipophilicity. It is FDA approved for adjuvant therapy of breast cancer but is also used in combination for the treatment of a variety of malignancies. Epirubicin is administered intravenously at doses ranging from 60 to 120 mg/m² every 3 to 4 weeks. Epirubicin has a similar toxicity profile to doxorubicin but is overall better tolerated.

In addition to being converted to an enol by an aldose reductase, epirubicin has a unique steric orientation of the C-4 hydroxyl group that allows it to serve as a substrate for conjugation reactions mediated by liver glucuronosyltransferases and sulfatases. As such, dose adjustments are recommended in the setting of hepatic dysfunction. For patients with serum bilirubin of 1.2 to 3 mg/dL or aspartate aminotransferase of 2 to 4 times the upper limit of normal, a 50% dose reduction is recommended. For patients with bilirubin greater than 3 mg/dL or aspartate aminotransferase greater than 4 times the upper limit of normal, a dose reduction of 75% is recommended. Due to limited data, no specific dose recommendations are currently available for patients with renal impairment, although current recommendations are for consideration of dose adjustments in patients with serum creatinine greater than 5 mg/dL.

Idarubicin

Idarubicin is a synthetic derivative of daunorubicin, but lacks the 4-methoxy group (see Fig. 20.3C). It is FDA approved as part of combination chemotherapy regimen for AML and is also active in ALL. It is given intravenously at a dose of 12 mg/m² for 3 consecutive days, typically in combination with cytarabine. Idarubicin has similar toxicities as daunorubicin. Its primary active metabolite is idarubicinol, and elimination is mainly through the biliary system and, to a lesser extent, through renal excretion. A 50% dose reduction is recommended for serum bilirubin of 2.6 to 5 mg/dL and idarubicin should not be given if the bilirubin is greater than 5 mg/dL. Additionally, dose reductions in renal impairment are advised, but specific guidelines are not available.

Cardiac Toxicity of Anthracyclines

Anthracyclines are responsible for cardiac toxicities, and special considerations are necessary to minimize this severe side effect. Acute doxorubicin cardiotoxicity is reversible, and clinical signs include tachycardia, hypotension, electrocardiogram changes, and arrhythmias. It develops during or within days of anthracycline infusion, and its incidence can be significantly reduced by slowing doxorubicin infusion rates.

Chronic and delayed cardiotoxicity is more common and more severe because it is irreversible. Chronic cardiotoxicity with congestive heart failure peaks at 1 to 3 months but can occur even years after therapy. Myocardial damage has been shown to occur by several mechanisms. The classical mechanism is by the direct generation of reactive oxygen species (ROS) during the electron transfer from the semiquinone to quinone moieties of the anthracycline,[84] which leads to myocardial damage. ROS can also be generated by mitochondrial damage resulting from drug-mediated inactivation of the oxidative phosphorylation chain because doxorubicin accumulates not only in chromatin, but also in mitochondria.[78,79] A recent study has also related doxorubicin cardiotoxicity to the poisoning of Top2β cleavage complexes in myocardiocytes.[85] Endomyocardial biopsy is characterized by a predominant finding of multifocal areas of patchy and interstitial fibrosis (stellate scars) and occasional vacuolated myocardial cells (Adria cells). Myocyte hypertrophy and degeneration, loss of cross-striations, and the absence of myocarditis are also characteristic of this diagnosis.[86] The incidence of cardiomyopathy is related to both the cumulative dose and the schedule of administration, and predisposition to cardiac damage includes a previous history of heart disease, hypertension, radiation to the mediastinum, age greater than 65 years or younger than 4 years, prior use of anthracyclines or other cardiac toxins, and coadministration of other chemotherapy agents (e.g., paclitaxel, cyclophosphamide, or trastuzumab).[87,88] Sequential administration of paclitaxel followed by doxorubicin in breast cancer patients is associated with cardiomyopathy at total doxorubicin doses above 340 to 380 mg/m², whereas the reverse sequence of drug administration did not yield the same systemic toxicities at these doses.[89] When doxorubicin is given in a low-dose weekly regimen (10 to 20 mg/m² per week) or by slow continuous infusion over 96 hours, cumulative doses of more than 500 mg/m² can be given. Doses of epirubicin less than 1,000 mg/m² and daunorubicin less than 550 mg/m² are considered safe. Additionally, liposomal doxorubicin is associated with less cardiac toxicity.

Cardiac function can be monitored during treatment with anthracyclines by electrocardiography, echocardiography, or radionuclide scans. Numerous studies have established the danger of embarking on anthracycline therapy in patients with underlying cardiac disease (e.g., a baseline left ventricular ejection fraction of less than 50%) and of continuing therapy after a documented decrease in the ejection fraction by more than 10% (if this decrease falls below the lower limit of normal). Because anthracycline-induced cardiotoxicity has been related to the generation of free radicals, efforts have been aimed at attenuating this effect through the targeting of redox response and reduction in oxidative stress. Dexrazoxane is a metal chelator that decreases the myocardial toxicity of doxorubicin in breast cancer patients. In two multicenter, double-blind studies, advanced breast cancer patients were randomized to chemotherapy with dexrazoxane or a placebo; dexrazoxane was shown to have a cardioprotective effect based on serial, noninvasive cardiac testing during the course of the trial and is approved for that use by the FDA.[90] Dexrazoxane chelates iron and copper, thereby interfering with the redox reactions that generate free radicals and damage myocardial lipids. Notably, dexrazoxane is also a Top2 catalytic inhibitor (see Fig. 20.3F), which potentially might minimize the therapeutic activity of anthracyclines by interfering with the trapping of Top2 cleavage complexes by anthracyclines.[2,3,91] Other agents currently in use include β-blockers and statins. A recent meta-analysis of 12 randomized controlled trials and 2 observational studies involving the use of agents to prevent the cardiotoxicity associated with anthracyclines demonstrated relatively similar efficacy regardless of which prophylactic treatment was used.[92]

Anthracenediones

Mitoxantrone (see Fig. 20.3E) is currently the only clinically approved anthracenedione. Compared to anthracyclines, mitoxantrone is less cardiotoxic owing to a decreased ability to undergo oxidation-reduction reactions and form free radicals.

Mitoxantrone is FDA approved for the treatment of advanced hormone-refractory prostate cancer[93] and AML.[94] It is typically administered intravenously at a dose of 12 to 14 mg/m² every 3 weeks in the treatment of prostate cancer, and at a dose of 12 mg/m² in combination with cytosine arabinoside for 3 days in the treatment of AML.

Toxicities are generally less severe compared to doxorubicin and include myelosuppression, nausea, vomiting, alopecia, and mucositis. Cardiac toxicity can be seen at cumulative doses greater than 160 mg/m².[95] Mitoxantrone is rapidly cleared from the plasma and is highly concentrated in tissues. The majority of the drug is eliminated in the feces, with a small amount undergoing renal excretion. Dose adjustments for hepatic dysfunction are recommended, but formal guidelines are currently not available.

Dactinomycin

Dactinomycin was the first antibiotic shown to have antitumor activity[96] and consists of a planar phenoxazone ring attached to two peptide side chains. This unique structure allows for tight intercalation into DNA between adjacent guanine–cytosine bases, leading to Top2 and Top1 poisoning and transcription inhibition.[97] Dactinomycin was one of the first drugs shown to be transported by P-glycoprotein, and represents the major mechanism of resistance.[98]

Dactinomycin is FDA approved for Ewing sarcoma,[99] gestational trophoblastic neoplasm,[100] metastatic nonseminomatous testicular cancer,[101] nephroblastoma,[102] and rhabdomyosarcoma.[103] Typically, it is administered intravenously at doses of 15 μg/kg for 5 days in combination with other chemotherapeutic agents for the treatment of nephroblastoma, rhabdomyosarcoma, and Ewing sarcoma; at does of 12 μg/kg intravenously as a single agent in the treatment of gestational trophoblastic neoplasias; and at doses of 1,000 μg/m² intravenously on day 1 as part of a combination regimen with cyclophosphamide, bleomycin, vinblastine, and cisplatin in the treatment of metastatic nonseminomatous testicular cancer. Toxicities include myelosuppression, veno-occlusive disease of the liver, nausea, vomiting, alopecia, erythema, and acne. Additionally, similar to doxorubicin, dactinomycin can cause radiation recall and severe tissue necrosis in cases of extravasation. Dactinomycin is largely excreted unchanged in the feces and urine. Guidelines for dosing in patients with impaired renal or liver function are currently not available.

Epipodophyllotoxins

Epipodophyllotoxins are glycoside derivatives of podophyllotoxin, an antimicrotubule agent extracted from the mandrake plant. Two derivatives, demethylated on the pendant ring (see R1 in Fig. 20.3D), etoposide and teniposide were shown to primarily function as Top2 poisons rather than through antimicrotubule mechanisms.[104,105] Epipodophyllotoxins poison Top2 through a mechanism distinct from that of anthracyclines and other DNA intercalators,[106] without intercalating into normal DNA in the absence of Top2. Therefore, they are "cleaner" Top2 inhibitors than the anthracyclines, anthracenediones, and dactinomycin. However, etoposide and teniposide trap Top2 cleavage complexes by base stacking in a ternary complex at the interface of the DNA and the Top2 homodimer. Mechanisms that have been implicated in resistance to etoposide include drug efflux, because epipodophyllotoxins are substrates for P-glycoprotein[107]; altered localization of Top2α; decreased cellular expression of Top2α[108]; and impaired phosphorylation of Top2.[109]

Etoposide

Etoposide (see Fig. 20.3D) is available in intravenous and oral forms. It is FDA approved for the treatment of small-cell lung cancer[110] and refractory testicular cancer.[111] It also has activity in hematologic malignancies and various solid tumors. The intravenous form is generally administered at doses of 35 to 50 mg/m² for 4 to 5 days every 3 to 4 weeks in combination therapy for small-cell lung cancer, and 50 to 100 mg/m² for 5 days every 3 to 4 weeks in combination therapy for refractory testicular cancer. The dose of oral etoposide is usually twice the intravenous dose. Oral bioavailability is highly variable due to dependence on intestinal P-glycoprotein.[112]

The dose-limiting toxicity for etoposide is myelosuppression, with white blood cell count nadirs typically occurring on days 10 to 14. Thrombocytopenia is less common than leukopenia. Additionally, mild to moderate nausea, vomiting, diarrhea, mucositis, and alopecia are associated with etoposide. Among topoisomerase inhibitors, epipodophyllotoxins have the greatest association with secondary malignancies, with etoposide having the highest risk, with an estimated 4% 6-year cumulative risk.[113] The majority of etoposide is cleared unchanged by the kidneys, and a 25% dose reduction is recommended in patients with a creatinine clearance of 15 to 50 mL per minute. A 50% dose reduction is recommended in patients with a creatinine clearance less than 15 mL per minute. Because the unbound fraction of etoposide is dependent on albumin and bilirubin concentrations, dose adjustments for hepatic dysfunction are advised, but consensus guidelines are currently not available.

Teniposide

Teniposide contains a thiophene group in place of the methyl group on the glucose moiety of etoposide (Fig. 20.3D). Teniposide is FDA approved for refractory pediatric ALL.[114,115] In pediatric ALL studies, doses ranged from 165 mg/m² intravenously in combination with cytarabine to 250 mg/m² intravenously weekly in combination with vincristine and prednisone. Similar to etoposide, the dose-limiting toxicity of teniposide is myelosuppression. Additional toxicities include mild-to-moderate nausea, vomiting, diarrhea, alopecia, and secondary leukemia. Teniposide is associated with greater frequency of hypersensitivity reactions compared to etoposide.

Teniposide is 99% bound to albumin and, as compared to etoposide, undergoes hepatic metabolism more extensively and renal clearance less extensively. No specific guidelines are currently available on dose adjustments for renal or hepatic dysfunction.

THERAPY-RELATED SECONDARY ACUTE LEUKEMIA

One of the major complications of Top2 inhibitor therapies, especially for etoposide and mitoxantrone, is acute secondary leukemia, which occurs in approximately 5% of patients. Therapy-related AMLs (t-AML) are characterized by their relatively rapid onset (they can occur only a few months after therapy) and the presence of recurrent balanced translocations involving the mixed lineage leukemia (MLL) locus on 11q23 and over 50 partner genes.[116] The molecular mechanism is likely from the disjoining of two drug-trapped Top2 cleavage complexes on different chromosomes (see Fig. 20.2C) in relationship with transcription collisions and illegitimate relegation.[117] Top2β, rather than Top2α, has been implicated in the generation of these disjoined cleavage complexes.[117,118]

FUTURE DIRECTIONS

Current challenges in the development of topoisomerase inhibitors lie in the inherent chemical instability of current and established agents. In addition to recent developments designed to enhance the stability with semisynthetic analogs and the development of novel delivery systems in an effort to achieve higher intratumoral concentrations, attention is also being focused on targeting other topoisomerase isoenzymes. Driving this trend has been the recent elucidation of the role of Top2β inhibition in the development of treatment-related cardiotoxicity and secondary AML.[86,117,118] In addition to combination chemotherapy regimens already in use, attempts have also been made for the sequential inhibition of Top1 and Top2. Based on early preclinical models suggesting synergy with sequential inhibition of Top1 and Top2,[120] phase 1 studies have evaluated the sequential administration of topotecan and etoposide in extensive-stage small-cell lung cancer and ovarian cancer, with significant myelosuppression as the dose-limiting toxicity.[121,122] Future rational drug combinations include targeting DNA repair pathways in combination with Top1 inhibition, although further characterization is needed of the specific DNA repair and stress response pathways invoked in response to DNA damage as a result of Top1 inhibition. However, one such attempt of combining topotecan with veliparib, a small molecule inhibitor of poly (ADP-ribose) polymerase, was poorly tolerated due to significant myelosuppression, thus limiting the doses of topotecan that could be safely administered.[123]

Molecular characterization of tumors to better define patient selection and the development of pharmacodynamic biomarkers to monitor the response to treatment and to optimize the combination dose and schedules is needed for the further clinical development of topoisomerase inhibitors. Validated assays have been developed to evaluate topoisomerase 1 levels and levels of phosphorylated histone H2AX (gamma-H2AX) as a marker of DNA damage response to topoisomerase inhibition,[124,125] and are being incorporated in current phase I studies of indenoisoquinolines.[72,73]

REFERENCES

1. Nitiss JL. DNA topoisomerase II and its growing repertoire of biological functions. *Nat Rev Cancer* 2009;9(5):327–337.
2. Nitiss JL. Targeting DNA topoisomerase II in cancer chemotherapy. *Nat Rev Cancer* 2009;9(5):338–350.
3. Pommier Y, Leo E, Zhang H, et al. DNA topoisomerases and their poisoning by anticancer and antibacterial drugs. *Chem Biol* 2010;17(5):421–433.
4. Fortune JM, Osheroff N. Topoisomerase II as a target for anticancer drugs: when enzymes stop being nice. *Prog Nucleic Acid Res Mol Biol* 2000;64:221–253.
5. Wang JC. A journey in the world of DNA rings and beyond. *Annu Rev Biochem* 2009;78:31–54.
6. Wang JC. Cellular roles of DNA topoisomerases: a molecular perspective. *Nat Rev Mol Cell Biol* 2002;3(6):430–440.
7. Champoux JJ. DNA topoisomerases: structure, function, and mechanism. *Annu Rev Biochem* 2001;70:369–413.
8. Wang JC. *Untangling the Double Helix: DNA Entanglements and the Action of DNA Topoisomerases*. Cold Spring Harbor, NY: Cold Spring Harbor Laboratory Press; 2009.
9. Pommier Y. DNA Topoisomerases and cancer. In: Teicher BA, ed. *Cancer Discovery and Development*. New York: Springer & Humana Press; 2012.
10. Zhang H, Barceló JM, Lee B, et al. Human mitochondrial topoisomerase I. *Proc Natl Acad Sci U S A* 2001;98(10):10608–10613.
11. Champoux JJ, Dulbecco R. An activity from mammalian cells that untwists superhelical DNA—a possible swivel for DNA replication (polyoma-ethidium bromide-mouse-embryo cells-dye binding assay). *Proc Natl Acad Sci U S A* 1972;69(1):143–146.
12. Chen SH, Wu CH, Plank JL, et al. Essential functions of C terminus of Drosophila Topoisomerase IIIα in double Holliday junction dissolution. *J Biol Chem* 2012;287(23):19346–19353.
13. Xu D, Shen W, Guo R, et al. Top3β is an RNA topoisomerase that works with fragile X syndrome protein to promote synapse formation. *Nat Neurosci* 2013;16(9):1238–1247.
14. Seol Y, Gentry AC, Osheroff N, et al. Chiral discrimination and writhe-dependent relaxation mechanism of human topoisomerase IIα. *J Biol Chem* 2013;288(19):13695–13703.
15. Stoll G, Pietiläinen OP, Linder B, et al. Deletion of TOP3b, a component of FMRP-containing mRNPs, contributes to neurodevelopmental disorders. *Nat Neurosci* 2013;16(9):1228–1237.
16. Pommier Y, Marchand C. Interfacial inhibitors: targeting macromolecular complexes. *Nat Rev Drug Discov* 2011;11(1):25–36.
17. Nitiss J, Wang JC. DNA topoisomerase-targeting antitumor drugs can be studied in yeast. *Proc Natl Acad Sci U S A* 1988;85(20):7501–7505.
18. Bjornsti MA, Benedetti P, Vigilanti GA, et al. Expression of human DNA topoisomerase I in yeast cells lacking yeast DNA topoisomerase I: restoration of sensitivity of the cells to the antitumor drug camptothecin. *Cancer Res* 1989;49(22):6318–6323.
19. Dressler LG, Berry DA, Broadwater G, et al. Comparison of HER2 status by fluorescence in situ hybridization and immunohistochemistry to predict benefit from dose escalation of adjuvant doxorubicin-based therapy in node-positive breast cancer patients. *J Clin Oncol* 2005;23(19):4287–4297.
20. Holm C, Covey JM, Kerrigan D, et al. Differential requirement of DNA replication for the cytotoxicity of DNA topoisomerase I and II inhibitors in Chinese hamster DC3F cell. *Cancer Res* 1989;49(22):6365–6368.
21. Hsiang YH, Lihou MG, Liu LF. Arrest of DNA replication by drug-stabilized topoisomerase I-DNA cleavable complexes as a mechanism of cell killing by camptothecin. *Cancer Res* 1989;49(18):5077–5082.
22. Maede Y, Shimizu H, Fukushima T, et al. Differential and common DNA repair pathways for topoisomerase I- and II-targeted drug in a genetic DT40 repair screen panel. *Mol Cancer Ther* 2014;13(1):214–220.
23. Huang SN, Pommier Y, Marchand C. Tyrosyl-DNA Phosphodiesterase 1(Tdp1) inhibitors. *Expert Opinion Ther Pat* 2011;21(9):1285–1292.
24. Zhang YW, Regairaz M, Seiler JA, et al. Poly(ADP-ribose) polymerase and XPF-ERCC1 participate in distinct pathways for the repair of topoisomerase I-induced DNA damage in mammalian cells. *Nucleic Acids Res* 2011;39(9):3607–3620.
25. Koster DA, Palle K, Bot ES, et al. Antitumor drugs impede DNA uncoiling by topoisomerase I. *Nature* 2007;448(7150):213–217.
26. Sordet O, Redon CE, Guirouilh-Barbat J, et al. Ataxia telangiectasia mutated activation by transcription- and topoisomerase I-induced DNA double-strand breaks. *EMBO Rep* 2009;10(8):887–893.
27. Pommier Y, Zwelling LA, Mattern MR, et al. Effects of dimethyl sulfoxide and thiourea upon intercalator-induced DNA single-strand breaks in mouse leukemia (L1210) cells. *Cancer Res* 1983;43(12 Pt 1):5718–5724.
28. Long BH, Musial ST, Brattain MG. Comparison of cytotoxicity and DNA breakage activity of congeners of podophyllotoxin including VP16-213 and VM26: a quantitative structure-activity relationship. *Biochemistry* 1984;23(6):1183–1188.
29. Ban Y, Ho CW, Lin RK, et al. Activation of a novel ubiquitin-independent proteasome pathway when RNA polymerase II encounters a protein roadblock. *Mol Cell Biol* 2013;33(20):4008–4016.
30. Long BH, Musial ST, Brattain MG. Single- and double-strand DNA breakage and repair in human lung adenocarcinoma cells exposed to etoposide and teniposide. *Cancer Res* 1985;45(7):3106–3112.
31. Pommier Y. Drugging topoisomerases: lessons and challenges. *ACS Chem Biol* 2013;8(1):82–95.
32. Zwelling LA, Michaels S, Erickson LC, et al. Protein-associated deoxyribonucleic acid strand breaks in L1210 cells treated with the deoxyribonucleic acid intercalating agents 4′-(9-acridinylamino) methanesulfon-m-anisidide and adriamycin. *Biochemistry* 1981;20(23):6553–6563.
33. Wall ME, Wani MC. Camptothecin and taxol: discovery to clinic—thirteenth Bruce F. Cain Memorial Award Lecture. *Cancer Res* 1995;55:753–760.
34. Pommier Y. Topoisomerase I inhibitors: camptothecins and beyond. *Nat Rev Cancer* 2006;6(10):789–802.
35. Teicher BA. Next generation topoisomerase I inhibitors: rationale and biomarker strategies. *Biochem Pharmacol* 2008;75(6):1262–1271.
36. Pommier Y, Cushman M. The indenoisoquinoline noncamptothecin topoisomerase I inhibitors: update and perspectives. *Mol Cancer Ther* 2009;8(5):1008–1014.
37. Douillard JY, Cunningham D, Roth AD, et al. Irinotecan combined with fluorouracil compared with fluorouracil alone as first-line treatment for metastatic colorectal cancer: a multicentre randomised trial. *Lancet* 2000;355:1041–1047.
38. Saltz LB, Cox JV, Blanke C, et al. Irinotecan plus fluorouracil and leucovorin for metastatic colorectal cancer. Irinotecan Study Group. *N Engl J Med* 2000;343:905–914.
39. Conroy T, Desseigne F, Tchou M, et al. FOLFIRINOX versus gemcitabine for metastatic pancreatic cancer. *N Engl J Med* 2011;364:1817–1825.
40. Hanna N, Bunn PA Jr, Langer C, et al. Randomized phase III trial comparing irinotecan/cisplatin with etoposide/cisplatin in patients with previously untreated extensive-stage disease small-cell lung cancer. *J Clin Oncol* 2006;24:2038–2043.
41. Schmittel A, Fischer von Weikersthal L, Sebastian M, et al. A randomized phase II trial of irinotecan plus carboplatin versus carboplatin treatment in patients with extended disease small-cell lung cancer. *Ann Oncol* 2006;17:663–667.
42. Iyer L, King CD, Whitington PF, et al. Genetic predisposition to the metabolism of irinotecan (CPT-11). Role of uridine diphosphate glucuronosyltransferase isoform 1A1 in the glucuronidation of its active metabolite (SN-38) in human liver microsomes. *J Clin Invest* 1998;101:847–854.
43. Innocenti F, Undevia SD, Iyer L, et al. Genetic variants in the UDP-glucuronosyltransferase 1A1 gene predict the risk of severe neutropenia of irinotecan. *J Clin Oncol* 2004;22:1382–1388.
44. Schaaf LJ, Hammond LA, Tipping SJ, et al. Phase 1 and pharmacokinetic study of intravenous irinotecan in refractory solid tumor patients with hepatic dysfunction. *Clin Cancer Res* 2006;12:3782–3791.
45. ten Bokkel Huinink W, Gore M, Carmichael J, et al. Topotecan versus paclitaxel for the treatment of recurrent epithelial ovarian cancer. *J Clin Oncol* 1997;15:2183–2193.
46. Ardizzoni A, Hansen H, Dombernowsky P, et al. Topotecan, a new active drug in the second-line treatment of small-cell lung cancer: a phase II study in patients with refractory and sensitive disease. The European Organization for Research and Treatment of Cancer Early Clinical Studies Group and New Drug Development Office, and the Lung Cancer Cooperative Group. *J Clin Oncol* 1997;15:2090–2096.
47. Long HJ 3rd, Bundy BN, Grendys EC Jr, et al. Randomized phase III trial of cisplatin with or without topotecan in carcinoma of the uterine cervix: a Gynecologic Oncology Group Study. *J Clin Oncol* 2005;23:4626–4633.
48. Baker SD, Heideman RL, Crom WR, et al. Cerebrospinal fluid pharmacokinetics and penetration of continuous infusion topotecan in children with central nervous system tumors. *Cancer Chemother Pharmacol* 1996;37:195–202.
49. Schluep T, Cheng J, Khin KT, et al. Pharmacokinetics and biodistribution of the camptothecin-polymer conjugate IT-101 in rats and tumor-bearing mice. *Cancer Chemother Pharmacol* 2006;57:654–662.
50. Young C, Schluep T, Hwang J, et al. CRLX101 (formerly IT-101)-A novel nanopharmaceutical of camptothecin in clinical development. *Curr Bioact Compd* 2011;7:8–14.
51. Weiss GJ, Chao J, Neidhart JD, et al. First-in-human phase 1/2a trial of CRLX101, a cyclodextrin-containing polymer-camptothecin nanopharmaceutical in patients with advanced solid tumor malignancies. *Invest New Drugs* 2013;31:986–1000.
52. University of Chicago. A randomized phase II study of IV Topotecan versus CRLX101 in the second line treatment of recurrent small cell lung cancer. ClinicalTrials.gov Identifier: NCT01803269.
53. Cerulean Pharma Inc. A randomized, phase 2, study to assess the safety and activity of CRLX101, a nanoparticle formulation of camptothecin, in patients with advanced non-small cell lung cancer who have failed one or two previous regimens of chemotherapy. ClinicalTrials Identifier: NCT01380769.
54. Massachusetts General Hospital. A Phase II, 2-stage Trial of CRLX101-202 in recurrent ovarian, tubal and peritoneal cancer. ClinicalTrials.gov Identifier: NCT01652079.
55. Vergote IB, Garcia A, Micha J et al. Randomized multicentre phase II trial comparing two schedules of etirinotecan pegol (NKTR-102) in women with recurrent platinum-resistant/refractory epithelial ovarian cancer. *J Clin Oncol* 2013;31(32):4060–4066.
56. Awada A, Garcia AA, Chan S et al. Two schedules of etirinotecan pegol (NKTR-102) in patients with previously treated metastatic breast cancer: a randomized phase 2 study. *Lancet Oncol* 2013;14(12):1216–1225.
57. Roswell Park Cancer Institute. A phase II study of single agent topoisomerase-I inhibitor polymer conjugate, Etirinotecan Pegol (NKTR-102), in patients with relapsed small cell lung cancer. ClinicalTrials Identifier: NCT01876446.
58. Abramson Cancer Center of the University of Pennsylvania. Phase 2 study of Etirinotecan Pegol (NKTR-102) in the treatment of patients with metastatic and recurrent non-small cell lung cancer (NSCLC) after failure of 2nd line treatment. ClinicalTrials Identifier: NCT01773109.

59. Nektar Therapeutics. A multicentre, open-label, randomized, phase 2 study to evaluate the efficacy and safety of NKTR-102 versus irinotecan in patients with second-line, irinotecan-naive, KRAS-mutant, metastatic colorectal cancer (mCRC). ClinicalTrials Identifier: NCT00856375.
60. Lawrence Recht. A phase II, single arm, open label study of NKTR-102 in bevacizumab-resistant high-grade glioma. ClinicalTrials Identifier: NCT01663012.
61. Nektar Therapeutics. The BEACON study (breast cancer outcomes with NKTR-102): a phase 3 open-label, randomized, multicenter study of NKTR-102 versus treatment of physician's choice (TPC) in patients with locally recurrent or metastatic breast cancer previously treated with an anthracycline, a taxane and capecitabine. ClinicalTrials Identifier: NCT01492101.
62. Basili S, Moro S. Novel camptothecin derivatives as topoisomerase I inhibitors. *Expert Opin Ther Pat* 2009;19:555–574.
63. Choi CH, Lee YY, Song TJ, et al. Phase II study of belotecan, a camptothecin analogue, in combination with carboplatin for the treatment of recurrent ovarian cancer. *Cancer* 2011;117:2104–2111.
64. Rhee CK, Lee SH, Kim JS, et al. A multicentre phase II study of belotecan, a new camptothecin analogue, as a second-line therapy in patients with small cell lung cancer. *Lung Cancer* 2011;72(1):64–67.
65. Hwang JH, Lim MC, Seo SS, et al. Phase II study of belotecan (CKD 602) as a single agent in patients with recurrent or progressive carcinoma of the uterine cervix. *Jpn J Clin Oncol* 2011;41:624–629.
66. Frapolli R, Zucchetti M, Sessa C, et al. Clinical pharmacokinetics of the new oral camptothecin gimatecan: the inter-patient variability is related to alpha1-acid glycoprotein plasma levels. *Eur J Cancer* 2010;46:505–516.
67. Pecorelli S, Ray-Coquard I, Tredan O, et al. Phase II of oral gimatecan in patients with recurrent epithelial ovarian, fallopian tube or peritoneal cancer, previously treated with platinum and taxanes. *Ann Oncol* 2010;21:759–765.
68. Graham JS, Falk S, Samuel LM et al. A multi-centre dose escalation and pharmacokinetic study of diflomotecan in patients with advanced malignancy. *Cancer Chemother Pharmacol* 2009;63:945–952.
69. Trocóniz IF, Cendrós JM, Soto E, et al. Population pharmacokinetic/pharmacodynamics modeling of drug-induced adverse effects of a novel homocamptothecin analog, elomotecan (BN80927), in a Phase I dose finding study in patients with advanced solid tumors. *Cancer Chemother Pharmacol* 2012;70:239–250.
70. Takagi K, Dexheimer TS, Redon C, et al. Novel E-ring camptothecin keto analogues (S38809 and S39625) are stable, potent, and selective topoisomerase I inhibitors without being substrates of drug efflux transporters. *Mol Cancer Ther* 2007;6(12 Pt 1):3229–3238.
71. Lansiaux A, Léonce S, Kraus-Berthier L, et al. Novel stable camptothecin derivatives replacing the E-ring lactone by a ketone function are potent inhibitors of topoisomerase I and promising antitumor drugs. *Mol Pharmacol* 2007;72(2):311–319.
72. National Cancer Institute. A Phase I Study of Indenoisoquinolines LMP400 and LMP776 in Adults With Relapsed Solid Tumors and Lymphomas. ClinicalTrials Identifier: NCT01051635.
73. National Cancer Institute. A phase I trial of weekly Indenoisoquinolines LMP400 in adults with relapsed solid tumors and lymphomas. ClinicalTrials Identifier: NCT01794104.
74. Antony S, Agama KK, Miao ZH, et al. Novel indenoisoquinolines NSC 725776 and NSC 724998 produce persistent topoisomerase I cleavage complexes and overcome multidrug resistance. *Cancer Res* 2007;67:10397–10405.
75. Kurtzberg LS, Roth S, Krumbholz R, et al. Genz-644282, a novel non-camptothecin topoisomerase I inhibitor for cancer treatment. *Clin Cancer Res* 2011;17:2777–2787.
76. Genzyme, a Sanofi Company. Dose Escalation Study to Assess the Safety and Tolerability of Genz-644282 in Patients With Solid Tumors. ClinicalTrials Identifier: NCT00942799.
77. Capranico G, Zunino F, Kohn KW, et al. Sequence-selective topoisomerase II inhibition by anthracycline derivatives in SV40 DNA: relationship with DNA binding affinity and cytotoxicity. *Biochemistry* 1990;29(2):562–569.
78. Davies KJ, Doroshow JH. Redox cycling of anthracyclines by cardiac mitochondria. I. Anthracycline radical formation by NADH dehydrogenase. *J Biol Chem* 1986;261(7):3060–3067.
79. Doroshow JH, Davies KJ. Redox cycling of anthracyclines by cardiac mitochondria. II. Formation of superoxide anion, hydrogen peroxide, and hydroxyl radical. *J Biol Chem* 1986;261:3068–3074.
80. Schneider E, Cowan KH. Multiple drug resistance in cancer therapy. *Med J Aust* 1994;160(6):371–373.
81. Alvarez M, Paull K, Monks A, et al. Generation of a drug resistance profile by quantitation of mdr-1/P-glycoprotein in the cell lines of the National Cancer Institute Anticancer Drug Screen. *J Clin Invest* 1995;95(5):2205–2214.
82. Felix CA, Kolaris CP, Osheroff N. Topoisomerase II and the etiology of chromosomal translocations. *DNA Repair* 2006;5:1093–1108.
83. O'Brien ME, Wigler N, Inbar M, et al. Reduced cardiotoxicity and comparable efficacy in a phase III trial of pegylated liposomal doxorubicin HCl (CAELYX/Doxil) versus conventional doxorubicin for first-line treatment of metastatic breast cancer. *Ann Oncol* 2004;15(3):440–449.
84. Doroshow JH. Effect of anthracycline antibiotics on oxygen radical formation in rat heart. *Cancer Res* 1983;43(2):460–472.
85. Zhang S, Liu X, Bawa-Khalfe T, et al. Identification of the molecular basis of doxorubicin-induced cardiotoxicity. *Nat Med* 2012;18:1639–1642.
86. Speyer J, Wasserheit C. Strategies for reduction of anthracycline cardiac toxicity. *Sem Oncol* 1998;25:525–537.
87. Chanan-Khan A, Srinivasan S, Czuczman MS. Prevention and management of cardiotoxicity from antineoplastic therapy. *J Support Oncol* 2004;2:251–256.
88. Von Hoff DD, Layard MW, Basa P, et al. Risk factors for doxorubicin-induced congestive heart failure. *Ann Intern Med* 1979;91:710–717.
89. Shan K, Lincoff AM, Young JB. Anthracycline-induced cardiotoxicity. *Ann Intern Med* 1996;125:47–58.
90. Swain SM, Whaley FS, Gerber MC, et al. Cardioprotection with dexrazoxane for doxorubicin-containing therapy in advanced breast cancer. *J Clin Oncol* 15(4):1318–1332.
91. Andoh T, Ishida R. Catalytic inhibitors of DNA topoisomerase II. *Biochim Biophys Acta* 1998;1400(1–3):155–171.
92. Kalam K, Marwick TH. Role of cardioprotective therapy for prevention of cardiotoxicity with chemotherapy: a systematic review and meta-analysis. *Eur J Cancer* 2013;49:2900–2909.
93. Tannock IF, Osoba D, Stockler MR, et al. Chemotherapy with mitoxantrone plus prednisone or prednisone alone for symptomatic hormone-resistant prostate cancer: a Canadian randomized trial with palliative end points. *J Clin Oncol* 1996;14:1756–1764.
94. Reece DE, Elmongy MB, Barnett MJ, et al. Chemotherapy with high-dose cytosine arabinoside and mitoxantrone for poor-prognosis myeloid leukemias. *Cancer Invest* 1993;11:509–516.
95. Shenkenberg TD, Von Hoff DD. Mitoxantrone: a new anticancer drug with significant clinical activity. *Ann Intern Med* 1986;105:67–81.
96. Hollstein U. Actinomycin. Chemistry and mechanism of action. *Chem Rev* 1974;74(6):625–652.
97. Wassermann K, Markovits J, Jaxel C, et al. Effects of morpholinyl doxorubicins, doxorubicin, and actinomycin D on mammalian DNA topoisomerases I and II. *Mol Pharmacol* 1990;38(1):38–45.
98. Biedler JL, Riehm H. Cellular resistance to actinomycin D in Chinese hamster cells in vitro: cross-resistance, radioautographic, and cytogenetic studies. *Cancer Res* 1970;30:1174–1184.
99. Jaffe N, Paed D, Traggis D, et al. Improved outlook for Ewing's sarcoma with combination chemotherapy (vincristine, actinomycin D and cyclophosphamide) and radiation therapy. *Cancer* 1976;38(5):1925–1930.
100. Turan T, Karacay O, Tulunay G, et al. Results of EMA/CO (etoposide, methotrexate, actinomycin D, cyclophosphamide, vincristine) chemotherapy in gestational trophoblastic neoplasia. *Int J Gynecol Cancer* 2006;16(3):1432–1438.
101. Early KS, Albert DJ. Single agent chemotherapy (actinomycin D) in the treatment of metastatic testicular carcinoma. *South Med J* 1976;69(8):1017–1021.
102. Fernbach DJ, Martyn DT. Role of dactinomycin in the improved survival of children with Wilm's tumor. *JAMA* 1966;195(1222):1005–1009.
103. Maurer HM, Moon T, Donaldson M, et al. The intergroup rhabdomyosarcoma study: a preliminary report. *Cancer* 1977;40(5):2015–2026.
104. Chen GL, Yang L, Rowe TC, et al. Nonintercalative antitumor drugs interfere with the breakage-reunion reaction of mammalian DNA topoisomerase. *J Biol Chem* 1984;259(21):13560–13566.
105. Long BH, Musial ST, Brattain MG. Comparison of cytotoxicity and DNA breakage activity of cogeners of podophyllotoxin including VP16-213 and VM26: a quantitative structure-activity relationship. *Biochemistry* 1984;23(6):1183–1188.
106. Ross W, Rowe T, Glisson B, et al. Role of topoisomerase II in mediating epipodophyllotoxin-induced DNA cleavage. *Cancer Res* 1984;44:5857–5860.
107. Meresse P, Dechaux E, Monneret C, et al. Etoposide: discovery and medicinal chemistry. *Curr Med Chem* 2004;11:2443–2466.
108. Valkov NI, Gump JL, Engel R, et al. Cell density-dependent VP-16 sensitivity of leukaemic cells is accompanied by the translocation of topoisomerase IIalpha from the nucleus to the cytoplasm. *Br J Haematol* 2000;108:331–345.
109. Takano H, Kohno K, Ono M, et al. Increased phosphorylation of DNA topoisomerase II in etoposide-resistant mutants of human cancer KB cells. *Cancer Res* 1991;51:3951–3957.
110. Sundstrøm S, Bremnes RM, Kaasa S, et al. Cisplatin and etoposide regimen is superior to cyclophosphamide, epirubicin, and vincristine regimen in small-cell lung cancer: results from a randomized phase III trial with 5 years' follow-up. *J Clin Oncol* 2002;20:4665–4672.
111. Nichols CR, Catalano PJ, Crawford ED, et al. Randomized comparison of cisplatin and etoposide and either bleomycin or ifosfamide in treatment of advanced disseminated germ cell tumors: an Eastern Cooperative Oncology Group, Southwest Oncology Group, and Cancer and Leukemia Group B Study. *J Clin Oncol* 1998;16:1287–1293.
112. Leu BL, Huang JD. Inhibition of intestinal P-glycoprotein and effects on etoposide absorption. *Cancer Chemother Pharmacol* 1995;35:432–436.
113. Smith MA, Rubinstein L, Anderson JR, et al. Secondary leukemia or myelodysplastic syndrome after treatment with epipodophyllotoxins. *J Clin Oncol* 1999;17:569–577.
114. Maluf PT, Odone Filho V, Cristofani LM, et al. Teniposide plus cytarabine as intensification therapy and in continuation therapy for advanced nonlymphoblastic lymphomas of childhood. *J Clin Oncol* 1994;12:1963–1968.
115. Rivera G, Bowman WP, Murphy SB, et al. VM-26 with prednisone and vincristine for treatment of refractory acute lymphocytic leukemia. *Med Pediatr Oncol* 1982;10:439–446.
116. Lovett BD, Lo Nigro L, Rappaport EF, et al. Near-precise interchromosomal recombination and functional DNA topoisomerase II cleavage sites at MLL and AF-4 genomic breakpoints in treatment-related acute lymphoblastic leukemia with t(4;11) translocation. *Proc Natl Acad Sci U S A* 2001;98(17):9802–9807.
117. Cowell IG, Sondka Z, Smith K, et al. Model for MLL translocations in therapy-related leukemia involving topoisomerase IIb-mediated DNA strand breaks and gene proximity. *Proc Natl Acad Sci U S A* 2012;109(23):8989–8994.

118. Azarova AM, Lyu YL, Lin CP, et al. Roles of DNA topoisomerases II isozymes in chemotherapy and secondary malignancies. *Proc Natl Acad Sci U S A* 2007;104:11014–11019.
119. Changela A, DiGate RJ, Mondragón A. Structural studies of E. Coli topoisomerase III-DNA complexes reveal a novel type IA topoisomerase-DNA conformational intermediate. *J Mol Biol* 2007;368:105–118.
120. Bertrand R, O'Connor PM, Kerrigan D, et al. Sequential administration of camptothecin and etoposide circumvents the antagonistic cytotoxicity of simultaneous drug administration in slowly growing human colon carcinoma HT-29 cells. *Eur J Cancer* 1992;28A(4–5):743–748.
121. Miller AA, Al Omari A, Murry DJ, et al. Phase I and pharmacologic study of sequential topotecan-carboplatin-etoposide in patients with extensive stage small cell lung cancer. *Lung Cancer* 2006;54:379–385.
122. Rose PG, Markham M, Bell JG, et al. Sequential prolonged oral topotecan and prolonged oral etoposide as second-line therapy in ovarian or peritoneal carcinoma: a phase I Gynecologic Oncology Study Group study. *Gynecol Oncol* 2006;102:236–239.
123. Kummar S, Chen A, Ji J, et al. Phase I study of PARP inhibitor ABT-888 in combination with topotecan in adults with refractory solid tumors and lymphomas. *Cancer Res* 2011;71(17):5626–5634.
124. Pfister TD, Hollingshead M, Kinders RJ, et al. Development and validation of an immunoassay for quantification of topoisomerase I in solid tumor tissues. *PLoS One* 2012;7:e50494.
125. Kinders RJ, Hollingshead M, Lawrence S, et al. Development of a validated immunofluorescence assay for gH2AX as a pharmacodynamics marker of topoisomerase I inhibitor activity. *Clin Cancer Res* 2010;16:5447–5457.

21 Antimicrotubule Agents

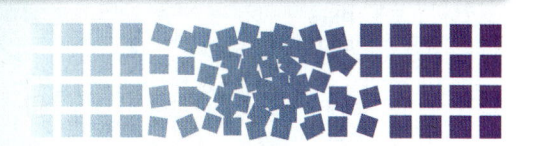

Christopher J. Hoimes and Lyndsay N. Harris

MICROTUBULES

Microtubules are vital and dynamic cytoskeletal polymers that play a critical role in cell division, signaling, vesicle transport, shape, and polarity, which make them attractive targets in anticancer regimens and drug design.[1] Microtubules are composed of 13 linear protofilaments of polymerized α/β-tubulin heterodimers arranged in parallel around a cylindrical axis and associated with regulatory proteins such as microtubule-associated proteins, tau, and motor proteins kinesin and dynein.[2] The specific biologic functions of microtubules are due to their unique polymerization dynamics. Tubulin polymerization is mediated by a nucleation-elongation mechanism. One end of the microtubules, termed the *plus end*, is kinetically more dynamic than the other end, termed the *minus end* (Fig. 21.1). Microtubule dynamics are governed by two principal processes driven by guanosine 5′-triphosphate (GTP) hydrolysis: *treadmilling* or *poleward flux* is the net growth at one end of the microtubule and the net shortening at the opposite end, and *dynamic instability*, which is a process in which the microtubule ends switch spontaneously between states of slow sustained growth and rapid depolymerization.[2] Antimicrotubule agents are tubulin-binding drugs that directly bind tubules, inhibitors of tubulin-associated scaffold kinases, or inhibitors of their associated mitotic motor proteins to, ultimately, disrupt microtubule dynamics. They are broadly classified as microtubule stabilizing or microtubule destabilizing agents according to their effects on tubulin polymerization.

TAXANES

Taxanes were the first-in-class microtubule stabilizing drugs. Ancient medicinal attempts at cardiac pharmacotherapy using material from the toxic coniferous yew tree, *Taxus* spp., were likely related to the plant's alkaloid *taxine* effect on sodium and calcium channels. Taxane compounds are the result of a drug screening of 35,000 plant extracts in 1963 that led to the identification of activity from the bark extract of the Pacific yew tree, *Taxus brevifolia*. Paclitaxel was identified as the active constituent with a report of its activity in carcinoma cell lines in 1971.[3] Motivation to identify taxanes derived from the more abundant and available needles of *Taxus baccata* led to the development of docetaxel, which is synthesized by the addition of a side chain to 10-deacetylbaccatin III, an inactive taxane precursor.[4] The taxane rings of paclitaxel and docetaxel are linked to an ester side chain attached to the C13 position of the ring, which is essential for antimicrotubule and antitumor activity. Nanoparticle albumin-bound paclitaxel (nab-paclitaxel) is a formulation that avoids the solvent related side effects of non–water-soluble paclitaxel and docetaxel. Overcoming docetaxel and paclitaxel's susceptibility to the P-glycoprotein efflux pump led to the development of cabazitaxel.[5] Cabazitaxel is synthesized by adding two methoxy groups to the 10-deacetylbaccatin III, which results in the inhibition of the 5′-triphosphate–dependent efflux pump of P-glycoprotein.

Paclitaxel initially received regulatory approval in the United States in 1992 for the treatment of patients with ovarian cancer after failure of first-line or subsequent chemotherapy (Table 21.1).[1,4] Subsequently, it has been approved for several other indications, including advanced breast cancer after anthracycline-based regimens[6]; combination chemotherapy of lymph node–positive breast cancer in the adjuvant setting[7]; advanced ovarian cancer in combination with a platinum compound; second-line treatment of AIDS-related Kaposi sarcoma; and first-line treatment of non–small-cell lung cancer (NSCLC) in combination with cisplatin[8] (see Table 21.1). In addition to the U.S. Food and Drug Administration (FDA) on-label indications, paclitaxel is widely used for several other tumor types, such as cancers of unknown origin, bladder, esophagus, gastric, head and neck, and cervical cancers. The U.S. patent for paclitaxel expired in 2002, and a generic form of paclitaxel is now available.

Docetaxel was first approved for use in the United States in 1996 for patients with metastatic breast cancer that progressed or relapsed after anthracycline-based chemotherapy, which was later broadened to a general second-line indication (see Table 21.1).[4,6] Subsequently, it received regulatory approval in adjuvant chemotherapy of stage II breast cancer in combination with Adriamycin and cyclophosphamide (TAC)[9], and first-line treatment for locally advanced or metastatic breast cancer.[10] In addition, docetaxel has indications in nonresectable, locally advanced, or metastatic NSCLC after failure of or in combination with cisplatin therapy; metastatic castration-resistant prostate cancer in combination with prednisone[11]; first-line treatment of gastric adenocarcinoma, including gastroesophageal junction adenocarcinoma in combination with cisplatin and 5-fluorouracil (5-FU)[12]; and inoperable locally advanced squamous cell cancer of the head and neck in combination with cisplatin and 5-FU (see Table 21.1). Docetaxel came off patent in 2010 and a generic form is available.

Mechanism of Action

The unique mechanism of action for paclitaxel was initially defined by Schiff et al.[13] in 1979, who showed that it bound to the interior surface of the microtubule lumen at binding sites completely distinct from those of exchangeable GTP, colchicine, podophyllotoxin, and the vinca alkaloids.[14] The taxanes profoundly alter the tubulin dissociation rate constants at both ends of the microtubule, suppressing treadmilling and dynamic instability. Dose-dependent taxane β-tubular binding induces mitotic arrest at the G2/M transition and induces cell death. By stabilizing microtubules, they also can stall ligand-dependent intracellular trafficking, as shown in sequestration of the androgen receptor to the cytosol in metastatic prostate cancer patients treated with docetaxel, and is associated with decreased androgen-regulated gene expression, such as prostate-specific antigen (PSA).[15,16] Peripheral neuropathy is a common dose-limiting toxicity across the antimicrotubule agents and likely is a result of their direct effect on microtubules. Studies

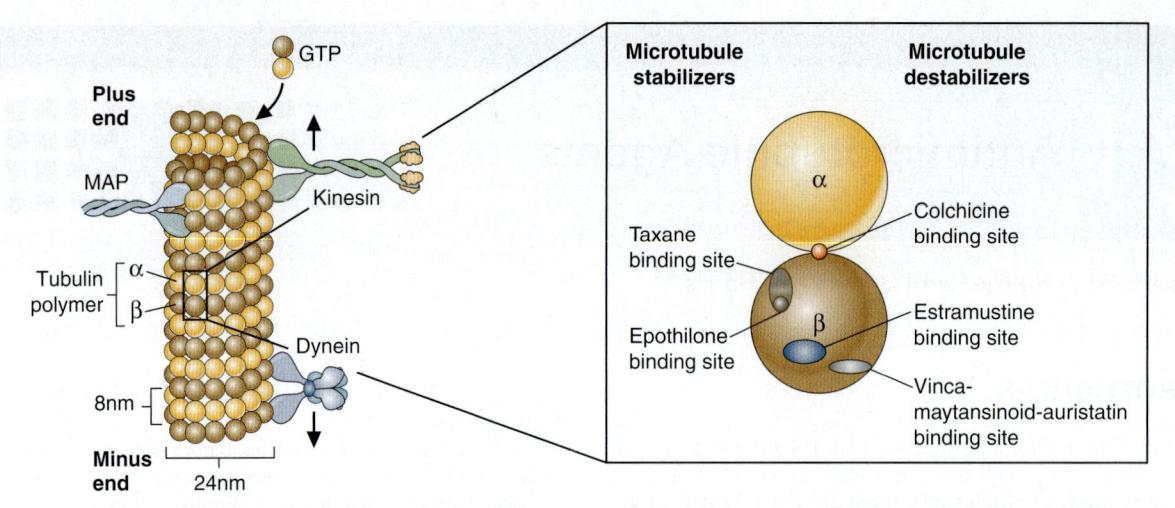

Figure 21.1 Antimicrotubule agents bind tubulin directly or inhibit its associated proteins. Taxanes and epothilones have distinct binding pockets within the same site on the interior surface of the tubule. Estramustine has a distinct site on β-tubulin, although it also directly binds microtubule-associated proteins (MAP). (Adapted from Lieberman M, Marks A. *Mark's Basic Medical Biochemistry: A Clinical Approach.* 3rd ed. Philadelphia: Lippincott Williams & Wilkins; 2009.)

have shown that they inhibit anterograde and/or retrograde fast axonal transport and can explain the demyelinating "dying back" pattern seen and the vulnerability of sensory neurons with the longest axonal projections.[17]

Recent evidence suggests that microtubule inhibitors have collateral effects during interphase that lead to cell death. For instance, paclitaxel-stabilized microtubules serve as a scaffold for the binding of the death-effector domain of pro-caspase-8, and thereby enabling a caspase-8 downstream proteolytic cascade.[18,19] This caspase-8–dependent mechanism also serves as an important basis for the understanding of the loss of function and/or low expression of the breast cancer 1, early onset gene (*BRCA1*) association with resistance to taxane therapy.[20]

Another mechanism of the anticancer effect of taxanes is currently being elaborated and is tied to the B-cell lymphoma-2 (Bcl-2) antiapoptosis family of proteins. Paclitaxel has been shown to cause the phosphorylation of Bcl-2 and the sequestration of Bak and Bim; however, this seemingly cancer-protective phosphorylation needs to be reconciled and likely correlates with Bcl-2–expression levels.[21–23] Interestingly, neutralizing Bcl-2 homology 3 (BH3) domains with compounds such as ABT-737 is synergistic with docetaxel.[24]

Clinical Pharmacology

Paclitaxel

With prolonged infusion schedules (6 and 24 hours), drug disposition is a biphasic process with values for alpha and beta half-lives averaging approximately 20 minutes and 6 hours, respectively.[4] When administered as a 3-hour infusion, the pharmacokinetics are nonlinear and may lead to unexpected toxicity with a small dose escalation, or a disproportionate decrease in drug exposure and loss of tumor response with a dose reduction. Approximately 71% of an administered dose of paclitaxel is excreted in the stool via the enterohepatic circulation over 5 days as either the parent compound or metabolites in humans. Renal clearance of paclitaxel and metabolites is minimal, accounting for 14% of the administered dose. In humans, the bulk of drug disposition is metabolized by cytochrome P-450 mixed-function oxidases—specifically, the isoenzymes CYP2C8 and CYP3A4, which metabolize paclitaxel to hydroxylated 3′p-hydroxypaclitaxel (minor) and 6α-hydroxypaclitaxel (major), as well as dihydroxylated metabolites.

Nanoparticle Albumin-Bound Paclitaxel

Nab-paclitaxel is a solvent-free colloidal suspension made by homogenizing paclitaxel with 3% to 4% albumin under high pressure to form nanoparticles of ~130 nm that disperse in plasma to ~10 nm (see Table 21.1).[25] It received regulatory approval in the United States in 2005 based on results in patients with metastatic breast cancer, and is now also approved in combination with carboplatin for first-line treatment of locally advanced or metastatic NSCLC, and in combination with gemcitabine for first-line treatment of metastatic pancreatic adenocarcinoma.[26–28] The improved responses seen with nab-paclitaxel, when compared to solvent-based paclitaxel, are not fully understood. Nab-paclitaxel likely capitalizes on several mechanisms, which include an improved pharmacokinetic profile with a larger volume of distribution and a higher maximal concentration of circulating, unbound, free drug; improved tumor accumulation by the enhanced permeability and retention (EPR) effect; and receptor-mediated transcytosis via an albumin-specific receptor (gp60) for endothelial transcytosis and binding of secreted protein acidic and rich in cysteine (SPARC) in the tumor interstitium.[29,30] In contrast to cremophor/ethanol (CrEL) solvent-based paclitaxel, nab-paclitaxel exhibits an extensive extravascular volume of distribution exceeding that of water, indicating extensive tissue and extravascular protein distribution. Some studies show that nab-paclitaxel achieves 33% higher drug concentration over CrEL-paclitaxel.[31] Additionally, the maximum concentration (Cmax), the mean plasma half-life of 15 to 18 hours, the area under curve (AUC), and the dose-independent plasma clearance correspond to linear pharmacokinetics over 80 to 300 mg/m^2.[29,32] The improved deposition of a nanoparticle, such as nab-paclitaxel in a tumor tissue, can occur passively through an EPR effect in areas of leaky vasculature, sufficient vascular pore size, and decreased lymphatic flow.[25,33] Once in the tissue, the nab-paclitaxel nanovehicle can deliver the drug locally or benefit from further receptor-mediated targeting to SPARC, which has been shown to be overexpressed, and correlates with disease progression in many tumor types.[34–38] Although preclinical models, as well as one clinical trial, have shown how nanoparticle therapy can benefit from this targeted approach,[39,40] correlative data for nab-paclitaxel is limited. The high stromal SPARC level was associated with longer survival in patients treated with nab-paclitaxel in the phase I/II study of patients with pancreatic cancer; however, this correlative analysis was not included in the phase III trial report and requires validation.[28,41]

TABLE 21.1

Antimicrotubule Agents: Dosages and Toxicities

Chemotherapeutic Agent	Dosage	Indications	Common Toxicities
Paclitaxel	135–200 mg/m² IV over 3 h or 135 mg/m² IV over 24 h every 3 wk; or 80 mg/m² IV over 1 h weekly	Adjuvant therapy of node-positive breast cancer; metastatic breast, ovarian, non–small-cell lung, bladder, esophagus, cervical, gastric, and head and neck cancer; AIDS-related Kaposi sarcoma; cancer of unknown origin	Myelosuppression, hypersensitivity, nausea and vomiting, alopecia, arthralgia, myalgia, peripheral neuropathy
Docetaxel	60–100 mg/m² IV over 1 h every 3 wk	Adjuvant therapy of node-positive breast cancer; metastatic breast, gastric, head and neck, prostate, non–small-cell lung, and ovarian cancer	Myelosuppression, hypersensitivity, edema, alopecia, nail damage, rash, diarrhea, nausea, vomiting, asthenia, neuropathy
Cabazitaxel	25 mg/m² IV every 3 wk over 1 h	Docetaxel-refractory metastatic castration resistant prostate cancer	Neutropenia, infections, myelosuppression, diarrhea, nausea, vomiting, constipation, abdominal pain, asthenia
Nab-paclitaxel	260 mg/m² IV over 30 min every 3 wk; or 125 mg/m² IV weekly on days 1, 8, and 15 every 28 d	Metastatic breast cancer, non–small-cell lung cancer, pancreatic cancer	Myelosuppression, nausea, vomiting, alopecia, myalgia, peripheral neuropathy
Ixabepilone	40 mg/m² IV over 3 h every 3 wk	Metastatic and locally advanced breast cancer	Myelosuppression, fatigue/asthenia, myalgia/arthralgia, alopecia, nausea, vomiting, stomatitis/mucositis, diarrhea, musculoskeletal pain
Vincristine	0.5–1.4 mg/m²/wk IV (maximum 2 mg per dose); or 0.4 mg/d continuous infusion for 4 d	Lymphoma, acute leukemia, neuroblastoma, rhabdomyosarcoma, AIDS-related Kaposi sarcoma, multiple myeloma, testicular cancer	Constipation, nausea, vomiting, alopecia, diplopia, myelosuppression
Vinblastine	6 mg/m² IV on days 1 and 15 as part of the ABVD regimen; 0.15 mg/kg IV on days 1 and 2 as part of the PVB regimen; 3 mg/m² IV as part of days 2, 15, 22 MVAC regimen	Hodgkin and non-Hodgkin lymphoma; Kaposi sarcoma; breast, testicular, bladder, prostate, and renal cell cancer	Myelosuppression, constipation, alopecia, malaise, bone pain
Vinorelbine	25–30 mg/m² IV weekly	Non–small-cell lung, breast, cervical, and ovarian cancer	Alopecia, diarrhea, nausea, vomiting, asthenia, neuromyopathy
Estramustine	14 mg/kg PO daily in 3 or 4 divided doses	Metastatic prostate cancer	Nausea, vomiting, gynecomastia, fluid retention
Ado-trastuzumab emtansine	3.6 mg/kg IV every 3 wk	Metastatic breast cancer	Thrombocytopenia, nausea, constipation or diarrhea, peripheral neuropathy, fatigue, increased AST/ALT
Brentuximab vedotin	1.8 mg/kg every 3 wk, maximum dose 180 mg	Refractory Hodgkin lymphoma, refractory systemic anaplastic large cell lymphoma	Neutropenia, anemia, thrombocytopenia, fatigue, fever, peripheral neuropathy

ABVD, doxorubicin (Adriamycin), bleomycin, vinblastine, dacarbazine; PVB, cisplatin, vinblastine, bleomycin; MVAC, methotrexate, vinblastine, doxorubicin (Adriamycin), cisplatin; IV, intravenous; PO, by mouth; AST/ALT, aspartate amniotransferase–alanine amniotransferase.

Docetaxel

The pharmacokinetics of docetaxel on a 1-hour schedule is tri-exponential and linear at doses of 115 mg/m² or less.[4] Terminal half-lives ranging from 11.1 to 18.5 hours has been reported. The most important determinants of docetaxel clearance were the body surface area (BSA), hepatic function, and plasma α_1-acid glycoprotein concentration. Plasma protein binding is high (greater than 80%), and binding is primarily to α_1-acid glycoprotein, albumin, and lipoproteins. The hepatic cytochrome P-450 mixed-function oxidases, particularly isoforms CYP3A4 and CYP3A5, are principally involved in biotransformation. The principal pharmacokinetic determinants of toxicity, particularly neutropenia, are drug exposure and the time that plasma concentrations exceed biologically relevant concentrations. The baseline level of α_1-acid glycoprotein may be elevated as an acute phase reactant in advanced disease and is an independent predictor of response and a major objective prognostic factor of survival in patients with non–small-cell lung cancer treated with docetaxel chemotherapy.

Cabazitaxel

Cabazitaxel is a semisynthetic derivative of the natural taxoid 10-deacetylbaccatin III. It binds to and stabilizes the β-tubulin subunit, resulting in the inhibition of microtubule depolymerization and cell division, cell cycle arrest in the G_2/M phase, and the inhibition of tumor cell proliferation.[5] It is active against diverse cancer cell lines and tumor models that are sensitive and resistant to docetaxel, including prostate, mammary, melanoma, kidney, colon, pancreas, lung, gastric, and head and neck.[5] Cabazitaxel is a poor substrate for the membrane-associated, multidrug resistance P-glycoprotein efflux pump; therefore, is useful for treating docetaxel-refractory prostate cancer for which it gained FDA approval in 2010.[5] In addition, it penetrates the blood–brain barrier.[42] Pharmacokinetics of cabazitaxel is similar to docetaxel; however, cabazitaxel has a larger volume of distribution and a longer terminal half-life (mean 77.3 hours versus 11.2 hours for docetaxel).[43,44]

Tesetaxel

Tesetaxel (DJ-927, XRP6258) is a semisynthetic, orally bioavailable taxane currently in clinical trials in breast, gastric, and prostate cancer. Administration in phase I and II trials has been once per week or every 3 weeks and not associated with hypersensitivity and possibly less neurotoxicity compared to other taxanes. Dose-limiting toxicity has been neutropenia. Overall responses in phase II studies have been 50% and 38% in patients treated for first- and second-line breast cancer, respectively. A phase I/II study in advanced NSCLC showed an overall response rate of 5.6%. Tesetaxel activity is independent of P-glycoprotein expression.[45] Pharmacokinetics on a schedule of every 3 weeks have an AUC of ~1,750 ng/mL per hour, a half life of ~170 hours, and no drug interactions that have been noted.[46]

Drug Interactions

Sequence-dependent pharmacokinetic and toxicologic interactions between paclitaxel and several other chemotherapy agents have been noted. The sequence of cisplatin followed by paclitaxel (on a 24-hour schedule) induces more profound neutropenia than the reverse sequence, which is explained by a 33% reduction in the clearance of paclitaxel after cisplatin.[47] Treatment with paclitaxel on either a 3- or 24-hour schedule followed by carboplatin has been demonstrated to produce equivalent neutropenia and less thrombocytopenia as compared to carboplatin as a single agent, which is not explained by pharmacokinetic interactions. Neutropenia and mucositis are more severe when paclitaxel is administered on a 24-hour schedule before doxorubicin, compared to the reverse sequence, which is most likely due to an approximately 32% reduction in the clearance rates of doxorubicin and doxorubicinol when doxorubicin is administered after paclitaxel. Several agents that inhibit cytochrome P-450 mixed-function oxidases interfere with the metabolism of paclitaxel and docetaxel in human microsomes in vitro; however, the clinical relevance of these findings is not known.[47]

Toxicity

Paclitaxel

The micelle-forming CrEL vehicle, which is required for suspension and intravenous delivery of paclitaxel, causes its nonlinear pharmacokinetics and thereby impacts its therapeutic index. CrEL causes hypersensitivity reactions, with major reactions usually occurring within the first 10 minutes after the first treatment and resolving completely after stopping the treatment. All patients should be premedicated with steroids, diphenhydramine, and an H2 antagonist, although up to 3% will still have reactions. Those who have major reactions have been rechallenged successfully after receiving high doses of corticosteroids.

Neuropathy is the principal toxicity of paclitaxel. Paclitaxel induces a peripheral neuropathy that presents in a symmetric stocking glove distribution, at first transient and then persistent.[48] A neurologic examination reveals sensory loss, and neurophysiologic studies reveal axonal degeneration and demyelination.[48] Compared with cisplatin, a loss of deep tendon reflexes occurs less commonly; however, autonomic and motor changes can occur. Severe neurotoxicity is uncommon when paclitaxel is given alone at doses below 200 mg/m² on a 3- or 24-hour schedule every 3 weeks, or below 100 mg/m² on a continuous weekly schedule. There is no convincing evidence that any specific measure is effective at ameliorating existing manifestations or preventing the development or worsening of neurotoxicity.[48]

Neutropenia is also frequent with paclitaxel. The onset is usually on days 8 to 11, and recovery is generally complete by days 15 to 21 with an every 3 weeks dosing regimen. Neutropenia is noncumulative, and the duration of severe neutropenia—even in heavily pretreated patients—is usually brief. Severity of neutropenia is related to the duration of exposure above the biologically relevant levels of 0.05 to 0.10 μM/L, and paclitaxel's nonlinear pharmacokinetics should be considered whenever adjusting dose.[49]

The most common cardiac rhythm disturbance, a transient sinus bradycardia, can be observed in up to 30% of patients. Routine cardiac monitoring during paclitaxel therapy is not necessary but is advisable for patients who may not be able to tolerate bradyarrhythmias. Drug-related gastrointestinal effects, such as vomiting and diarrhea, are uncommon. Severe hepatotoxicity and pancreatitis have also been noted rarely. Pulmonary toxicities, including acute bilateral pneumonitis, have been reported. Extravasation of large volumes can cause moderate soft tissue injury. Paclitaxel also induces reversible alopecia of the scalp in a dose-related fashion. Nail disorders have also been reported with paclitaxel use and include ridging, nail bed pigmentation, onychorrhexis, and onycholysis. These side effects have been reported more commonly with dose-intensified paclitaxel regimens.

Recent studies have suggested a role for the adenosine triphosphatase (ATP)-binding cassette (ABC) transporter polymorphisms in the development of neuropathy and neutropenia. Sissung et al.[50] reported that patients carrying two reference alleles for the *ABCB1* (P-glycoprotein, MDR1) 3435C greater than T polymorphism had a reduced risk to develop neuropathy as compared to patients carrying at least one variant allele ($P = .09$). Data from a large controlled trial to evaluate these and other candidate polymorphisms failed to detect a significant association between genotype and outcome or toxicity for any of the genes analyzed, although the correlative studies were retrospective and the sample size was inadequate to rule out smaller differences.[51] A large randomized trial of the CALGB 40101 using an integrated genomewide associate study found two polymorphisms associated with paclitaxel-induced polyneuropathy.[52] Both are involved in nerve development and maintenance, including the hereditary peripheral neuropathy Charcot-Marie-Tooth disease gene, *FGD4*. Further studies are required to adequately assess the role of these variants in predicting toxicity from taxane therapy.

Nab-paclitaxel

Hypersensitivity reactions have not been observed during the infusion period and, therefore, steroid premedications are not necessary. The main dose-limiting toxicities are neutropenia and sensory neuropathy. In a trial comparing weekly paclitaxel 90 mg/m² to nab-paclitaxel 150 mg/m² to ixabepilone in patients with metastatic breast cancer, there was more hematologic toxicity and peripheral neuropathy in the nab-paclitaxel arm compared to the paclitaxel arm, although median progression-free survival was not significantly different at the 12-month follow-up.[53] This led to dose reductions in 45% of patients in the nab-paclitaxel arm compared with 15% for the paclitaxel arm.[53] Other toxicities include alopecia, diarrhea, nausea and vomiting, elevations in liver enzymes, arthralgia, myalgia, and asthenia.

Docetaxel

Neutropenia is the main toxicity of docetaxel.[4] When docetaxel is administered on an every 3 weeks schedule, the onset of neutropenia is usually noted on day 8, with complete resolution by days 15 to 21. Neutropenia is significantly less when low doses are administered weekly. FDA black box warnings include increased toxicity in patients with abnormal liver function and, in select NSCLC patients that received prior platinum, severe hypersensitivity reactions and severe fluid retention despite dexamethasone at-home premedication.

Hypersensitivity reactions were noted in approximately 31% of patients who received the drug without premedications in early studies.[4] Symptoms include flushing, rash, chest tightness, back pain, dyspnea, and fever or chills. Severe hypotension, bronchospasm, generalized rash, and erythema may also occur.[54] Major reactions usually occur during the first two courses and within minutes after the start of treatment. Signs and symptoms generally resolve within 15 minutes after cessation of treatment, and docetaxel can usually be reinstituted without sequelae after treatment with diphenhydramine and an H2-receptor antagonist. Docetaxel induces a unique fluid retention syndrome characterized by edema, weight gain, and third-space fluid collection. Fluid retention is cumulative and is due to increased capillary permeability. Prophylactic treatment with corticosteroids has been demonstrated to reduce the incidence of fluid retention. Aggressive and early treatment with diuretics has been successfully used to manage fluid retention. Skin toxicity may occur in as many as 50% to 75% of patients; however, premedication may reduce the overall incidence of this effect.[4] Other cutaneous effects include palmar–plantar erythrodysesthesia and onychodystrophy. Docetaxel produces neurotoxicity, which is qualitatively similar to that of paclitaxel; however, neurosensory and neuromuscular effects are generally less frequent and less severe than with paclitaxel. Mild-to-moderate peripheral neurotoxicity occurs in approximately 40% of untreated patients.[55] Asthenia has been a prominent complaint in patients who have been treated with large cumulative doses. Stomatitis appears to occur more frequently with docetaxel than with paclitaxel. Other reported toxicities of note include necrotizing enterocolitis, interstitial pneumonitis, and organizing pneumonia.[56,57]

Cabazitaxel

A phase III multi-institutional study of men with metastatic castration-resistant prostate cancer who had failed docetaxel improved overall median survival on cabazitaxel compared to mitoxantrone.[58] Cabazitaxel was approved by the FDA in June 2010 to treat metastatic castration-resistant prostate cancer in those who had received prior chemotherapy. This was despite a higher rate of adverse deaths (4.9%), a third of which were due to neutropenic sepsis. Cabazitaxel was associated with more grade 3 or 4 neutropenia (82%) than mitoxantrone (58%). Side effects reported in more than 20% of patients treated with cabazitaxel included myelosuppression, diarrhea, nausea, vomiting, constipation, abdominal pain, or asthenia. FDA black box warnings are similar to those for docetaxel.

VINCA ALKALOIDS

The vinca alkaloids have been some of the most active agents in cancer chemotherapy since their introduction 40 years ago. The naturally occurring members of the family, vinblastine (VBL) and vincristine (VCR), were isolated from the leaves of the periwinkle plant *Catharanthus roseus* G. Don. In the late 1950s, their antimitotic and, therefore, cancer chemotherapeutic potential was discovered by groups both at Eli Lilly Research Laboratories and at the University of Western Ontario, and they came into widespread use for the single-agent treatment of childhood hematologic and solid malignancies and, shortly after, for adult hematologic malignancies (see Table 21.1).[1] Their clinical efficacy in several combination therapies has led to the development of various novel semisynthetic analogs, including vinorelbine (VRL), vindesine (VDS), and vinflunine (VFL).

Mechanism of Action

In contrast to the taxanes, the vinca alkaloids depolymerize microtubules and destroy mitotic spindles.[1] At low but clinically relevant concentrations, VBL does not depolymerize spindle microtubules, yet it powerfully blocks mitosis. This has been suggested to occur as a result of the suppression of microtubule dynamics rather than microtubule depolymerization. This group of compounds binds to the β subunit of tubulin dimers at a distinct region called the vinca-binding domain. Importantly, VBL binding induces a conformational change in tubulin in connection with tubulin self-association. In mitotic spindles, the slowing of the growth and shortening or treadmilling dynamics of the microtubules block mitotic progression. Disruption of the normal mitotic spindle assembly leads to delayed cell cycle progress with chromosomes stuck at the spindle poles and unable to pass from metaphase into anaphase, which eventually induces to apoptosis. The naturally occurring vinca alkaloids VCR and VBL, the semisynthetic analog VRL, and a novel bifluorinated analog VFL have similar mechanisms of action.

Tissue and tumor sensitivities to the vinca alkaloids, which, in part, relate to differences in drug transport and accumulation, also vary. Intracellular or extracellular concentration ratios range from five- to 500-fold depending on the individual cell type, lipophilicity, tissue-specific factors such as tubulin isotype composition, and tissue-specific microtubule-associated proteins (MAP).[59–61] Although the vinca alkaloids are retained in cells for long periods of time and thus may have prolonged cellular effects, intracellular retention is markedly different among the various vinca alkaloids. For instance, VBL appears to be retained in lipophilic tissue much more than either VCR or VDS.[59] Newer theories of antimicrotubule agents' mechanism of action have emerged, suggesting that the more important target of these drugs may be the tumor vasculature, as reviewed in the next section.

Clinical Pharmacology

The vinca alkaloids are usually administered intravenously as a brief infusion, and their pharmacokinetic behavior in plasma has generally been explained by a three-compartment model. The vinca alkaloids share many pharmacokinetic properties, including large volumes of distribution, high clearance rates, and long terminal half-lives that reflect the high magnitude and avidity of drug binding in peripheral tissues. VCR has the longest terminal half-life and the lowest clearance rate; VBL has the shortest terminal half-life and the highest clearance rate; and VDS has intermediate characteristics. Although prolonged infusion schedules may avoid excessively toxic peak concentrations and increase the duration of drug exposure in plasma above biologically relevant threshold concentrations, there is little evidence to support the notion that prolonged infusions are more effective than bolus schedules. The longest half-life and lowest clearance rate of VCR may account for its greater propensity to induce neurotoxicity, but there are many other nonpharmacokinetic determinants of tissue sensitivity, as discussed in the previous section.

Vincristine

After conventional doses of VCR (1.4 mg/m^2) given as brief infusions, peak plasma levels approach 0.4 μmol. Plasma clearance is slow, and terminal half-lives that range from 23 to 85 hours have been reported. VCR is metabolized and excreted primarily by the hepatobiliary system. The nature of the VCR metabolites identified to date, as well as the results of metabolic studies in vitro, indicate that VCR metabolism is mediated principally by hepatic cytochrome P-450 CYP3A5.

Vinblastine

The clinical pharmacology of VBL is similar to that of VCR. VBL binding to plasma proteins and formed elements of blood is extensive.[62,63] Peak plasma drug concentrations are approximately 0.4 μm after rapid intravenous injections of VBL at standard doses. Distribution is rapid, and terminal half-lives range from 20 to 24 hours. Like VCR, VBL disposition is principally through the hepatobiliary system with excretion in feces (approximately 95%); however, fecal excretion of the parent compound is low, indicating that hepatic metabolism is extensive.[59]

Vinorelbine

The pharmacologic behavior of VRL is similar to that of the other vinca alkaloids, and plasma concentrations after rapid intravenous administration have been reported to decline in either a biexponential or triexponential manner.[64] After intravenous administration, there is a rapid decay of VRL concentrations followed by a much slower elimination phase (terminal half-life, 18 to 49 hours). Plasma protein binding, principally to α_1-acid glycoprotein, albumin, and lipoproteins, has been reported to range from 80% to 91%, and drug binding to platelets is extensive.[64] VRL is widely distributed, and high concentrations are found in virtually all tissues, except the central nervous system.[64] The wide distribution of VRL reflects its lipophilicity, which is among the highest of the vinca alkaloids. As with other vinca alkaloids, the liver is the principal excretory organ, and up to 80% of VRL is excreted in the feces, whereas urinary excretion represents only 16% to 30% of total drug disposition, the bulk of which is unmetabolized VRL. Studies in humans indicate that 4-O-deacetyl-VRL and 3,6-epoxy-VRL are the principal metabolites, and several minor hydroxy-VRL isomer metabolites have been identified. Although most metabolites are inactive, the deacetyl-VRL metabolite may be as active as VRL. The cytochrome P-450 CYP3A isoenzyme appears to be principally involved in biotransformation.

Vinflunine

VFL is a novel semisynthetic microtubule inhibitor with a fluorinated catharanthine moiety, which translates into lower affinity for the vinca binding site on tubulin and, therefore, different quantitative effects on microtubule dynamics.[65] The low affinity for tubulin may be responsible for its reduced clinical neurotoxicity. Despite this lower affinity, it is more active in vivo than other vinca alkaloids, and resistance develops more slowly. VFL is a new vinca and still under clinical development. Its volume of distribution is large, and has a terminal half-life of nearly 40 hours.[65] The only active metabolite is 4-O-deacetylvinflunine, which has a terminal half-life approximately 5 days longer than that of the parent compound.[65]

Drug Interactions

Methotrexate accumulation in tumor cells is enhanced in vitro by the presence of VCR or VBL, an effect mediated by a vinca alkaloid–induced blockade of drug efflux; however, the minimal concentrations of VCR required to achieve this effect occur only transiently in vivo.[66] The vinca alkaloids also inhibit the cellular influx of the epipodophyllotoxins in vitro, resulting in less cytotoxicity. However, the clinical implications of this potential interaction are unknown. L-asparaginase may reduce the hepatic clearance of the vinca alkaloids, which may result in increased vinca-related toxicity. To minimize the possibility of this interaction, the vinca alkaloids should be given 12 to 24 hours before L-asparaginase. The combined use of mitomycin C and the vinca alkaloids has been associated with acute dyspnea and bronchospasm. The onset of these pulmonary toxicities has ranged from within minutes to hours after treatment with the vinca alkaloids, or up to 2 weeks after mitomycin C.

Treatment with the vinca alkaloids has precipitated seizures associated with subtherapeutic plasma phenytoin concentrations.[66] Reduced plasma phenytoin levels have been noted from 24 hours to 10 days after treatment with VCR and VBL. Because of the importance of the cytochrome P-450 CYP3A isoenzyme in vinca alkaloid metabolism, administration of the vinca alkaloids with erythromycin and other inhibitors of CYP3A may lead to severe toxicity.[67] Concomitantly administered drugs, such as pentobarbital and H_2-receptor antagonists, may also influence VCR clearance by modulating hepatic cytochrome P-450 metabolic processes.[66]

Toxicity

Despite close similarities in structure, the vinca alkaloids differ in their safety profiles. Neutropenia is the principal dose-limiting toxicity of VBL and VRL. Thrombocytopenia and anemia occur less commonly. The onset of neutropenia is usually day 7 to 11, with recovery by day 14 to 21, and can be potentiated by hepatic dysfunction. Gastrointestinal autonomic dysfunction, as manifested by bloating, constipation, ileus, and abdominal pain, occur most commonly with VCR or high doses of the other vinca alkaloids. Mucositis occurs more frequently with VBL than with VRL and is least common with VCR. Nausea, vomiting, diarrhea,[31,43,45] and pancreatitis[53,54] also occur to a lesser extent.

VCR principally induces neurotoxicity characterized by a peripheral, symmetric mixed sensory motor and autonomic polyneuropathy.[68,69] Toxic manifestations include constipation, abdominal cramps, paralytic ileus, urinary retention, orthostatic hypotension, and hypertension. Its primary neuropathologic effects are due to interference with axonal microtubule function. Early symmetric sensory impairment and paresthesias can progress to neuritic pain and loss of deep tendon reflexes with continued treatment, which may be followed by foot drop, wrist drop, motor dysfunction, ataxia, and paralysis. Cranial nerves are rarely affected because the uptake of VCR into the central nervous system is low. Severe neurotoxicity occurs infrequently with VBL and VDS. VRL has been shown to have a lower affinity for axonal microtubules than either VCR or VBL, which seems to be confirmed by clinical observations.[70] Mild-to-moderate peripheral neuropathy, principally characterized by sensory effects, occurs in 7% to 31% of patients, and constipation and other autonomic effects are noted in 30% of patients, whereas severe toxicity occurs in 2% to 3%.

In adults, neurotoxicity may occur after treatment with cumulative doses as little as 5 to 6 mg, and manifestations may be profound after cumulative doses of 15 to 20 mg. Patients with delayed biliary excretion or hepatic dysfunction, and those with antecedent neurologic disorders, such as Charcot-Marie-Tooth disease, hereditary and sensory neuropathy type 1, and Guillain-Barré syndrome, are predisposed to neurotoxicity.

The vinca alkaloids are potent vesicants. To decrease the risk of phlebitis, the vein should be adequately flushed after treatment. If extravasation is suspected, treatment should be discontinued, aspiration of any residual drug remaining in the tissues should be attempted, and prompt application of heat (*not* ice) for 1 hour four times daily for 3 to 5 days can limit tissue damage.[71] Hyaluronidase, 150 to 1,500 U (15 U/mL in 6 mL 0.9% sodium chloride solution) subcutaneously, through six clockwise injections in a circumferential manner using a 25-gauge needle (changing the needle with each new injection) into the surrounding tissues may minimize discomfort and latent cellulitis. A surgical consultation to consider early debridement is also recommended. Mild and reversible alopecia occurs in approximately 10% and 20% of patients treated with VLR and VCR, respectively. Acute cardiac ischemia, chest pains without evidence of ischemia, fever, Raynaud syndrome, hand–foot syndrome, and pulmonary and liver toxicity (transaminitis and hyperbilirubinemia) have also been reported with use of the vinca alkaloids. All of the vinca alkaloids can cause a syndrome of inappropriate secretion of antidiuretic hormone (SIADH), and patients who are receiving intensive hydration are particularly prone to severe hyponatremia secondary to SIADH.

MICROTUBULE ANTAGONISTS

Estramustine Phosphate

Estramustine is a conjugate of nor-nitrogen mustard linked to 17β-estradiol by a carbamate ester bridge. Estramustine phosphate received regulatory approval in the United States in 1981 for treating patients with castration-resistant prostate cancer (CRPC). Although the recommended daily dose of estramustine phosphate is 14 mg/kg per day, patients are usually treated in the daily dosing range of 10 to 16 mg/kg in three to four divided daily doses (see Table 21.1). Estramustine has significant activity in CRPC and had been used in combination with VBL or docetaxel. However, phase III trials in patients with CRPC showed that when combined with docetaxel, there is no added benefit to overall survival compared to docetaxel alone.[72,73]

Estramustine binds to β-tubulin at a site distinct from the colchicine and vinca alkaloid binding sites. This agent depolymerizes microtubules and microfilaments, binds to and disrupts MAPs, and inhibits cell growth at high concentrations, resulting in mitotic arrest and apoptosis in tumor cells. The selective accumulation and actions of estramustine phosphate and its metabolite, estromustine, in specific tissues appear to be dependent on the expression of the estramustine-binding protein (EMBP). The disposition of estramustine is principally by rapid oxidative metabolism of the parent compound to estromustine. Estromustine concentrations in plasma are maximal within 2 to 4 hours after oral administration, and the mean elimination half-life of estromustine is 14 hours. Estromustine and estramustine are principally excreted in the feces, with only small amounts of conjugated estrone and estradiol detected in the urine (less than 1%).

In general, this agent has a manageable safety profile. Nausea and vomiting are the principal toxicities encountered. In contrast to the taxanes and the vinca alkaloids, myelosuppression is rarely clinically relevant. Common estrogenic side effects include gynecomastia, nipple tenderness, and fluid retention. Thromboembolic complications may occur in up to 10% of patients.

Epothilones

The epothilones are macrolide compounds that were initially isolated from the mycobacterium *Sorangium cellulosum*. They exert their cytotoxic effects by promoting tubulin polymerization and inducing mitotic arrest.[74] In general, the epothilones are more potent than the taxanes. In contrast to the taxanes and vinca alkaloids, overexpression of the efflux protein P-glycoprotein minimally affects the cytotoxicity of epothilones. Epothilones include the natural epothilone B (patupilone; EPO906) and several semisynthetic epothilone compounds such as aza-epothilone B (ixabepilone; BMS-247550), epothilone D (deoxyepothilone B, KOS-862), and a fully synthetic analog, sagopilone (ZK-EPO).[75]

Ixabepilone has been evaluated in several schedules using a cremophor-based formulation and is FDA approved for the treatment of patients with breast cancer.[75] It is active in breast cancer previously treated with paclitaxel or docetaxel. The principal toxicities observed include neutropenia and peripheral neuropathy, in addition to fatigue, nausea, emesis, and diarrhea.[55,74] It also has been evaluated in other solid tumors such as ovarian, prostate, and renal cell carcinomas.[75] Epothilones are still undergoing evaluations in several clinical trials. Pharmacokinetic studies based on patupilone have shown large volume of distribution (41-fold the total body water) and low body clearance (13% of hepatic blood flow).[76] There do not appear to be active metabolites once the parent drug is hydrolyzed, which is the main elimination pathway.[76]

Maytansinoids and Auristatins: DM1, MMAE

Antibody drug conjugates (ADC) were first attempted with delivery of doxorubicin. Although tissue localization seemed promising, it became clear that the delivery of more potent chemotherapeutics was necessary.[77,78] One of the major advances for the promise of ADC came with the discovery and development of highly potent anticancer compounds such as calicheamicins, maytansinoids, and auristatins.[78] The next necessary advance was a linker that released the drug only when intended, and avoiding, or in some cases capitalizing on, in vivo proteases, oxidizing, or reducing environments. Gemtuzumab ozogamicin was the first ADC using calicheamicin, a potent DNA minor groove binder (and not a microtubule agent), approved in 2000 although withdrawn from the market in 2013 due to failed confirmatory studies. Maytansinoids and auristatins are unrelated, although are both tubulin-binding agents of the vinca binding site and inhibit tubulin polymerization.[78] They are 100- to 1,000-fold more cytotoxic that most cancer chemotherapeutics.[79]

Drug maytansinoid-1 (DM1) is the chemotherapeutic delivered using a thioether linker in the ADC ado-trastuzumab emtansine (T-DM1) that was FDA approved for patients with HER2- positive metastatic breast cancer previously treated with trastuzumab and taxane chemotherapy.[80,81] In the international phase III study, there was a 3.2-month improved progression-free survival among patients that received T-DM1 compared to those receiving standard treatment with capecitabine and lapatinib.[81] Despite a potent chemotherapeutic, the tolerability was much better in the experimental arm, which was dosed at 3.6 mg/kg intravenously every 21 days. The most common side effects in the trial were thrombocytopenia (12.8%), transient transaminitis (4.3%), as well as nausea, fatigue, myalgias, and arthralgias.[81]

Monomethyl auristatin E (MMAE) is linked to a monoclonal antibody against CD30 as an ADC (brentuximab vedotin, SGN35) and approved for refractory Hodgkin lymphoma or anaplastic large cell lymphoma. The linker is a peptide-based substrate for cathepsin-B and thereby designed to detect the lysosome/endosome compartment for drug release.[82,83] Dose-limiting toxicities include thrombocytopenia, hyperglycemia, diarrhea, and vomiting, and the most common side effects in this heavily pretreated population (including autologous stem cell transplant) includes peripheral neuropathy (42%), nausea (35%), and fatigue (34%).[84] The FDA black box warning includes contraindicated use with bleomycin due to increased pulmonary toxicity and the risk of John Cunningham (JC) virus–induced progressive multifocal leukoencephalopathy. Reports of severe pancreatitis are also emerging.[85]

MITOTIC MOTOR PROTEIN INHIBITORS

Aurora Kinase and Pololike Kinase Inhibitors

Aurora kinases are serine/threonine kinases crucial for mitosis in their recruitment of mitotic motor proteins for spindle formation. They are particularly overexpressed in high growth rate tumors. Aurora A and B kinases are expressed globally throughout all tissues, and Aurora C kinase is expressed in testes and participates in meiosis. Aurora A kinase is expressed and frequently amplified in many epithelial tumors and implicated in the microtubule-targeted agent-resistant phenotype.[86] Aurora A kinase interacts with p53, and there is evidence that p53 wild-type tumors are more sensitive to aurora A kinase inhibitors than p53 mutant tumors.[87] MLN-8237 has an IC_{50} of 1 nm for aurora A kinase and >200 nm for aurora B kinase and is in clinical development for treatment-related neuroendocrine prostate cancer.[86,88] The main dose-limiting toxicity of these agents is neutropenia. Pololike kinases (PLKs) are serine or threonine kinases crucial for cell cycle process. Overexpression of PLKs has been shown to be related to histologic grading and poor prognosis in several types of cancer. BI-2536 and ON01910 are PLK inhibitors in early clinical development.[89]

Kinesin Spindle Protein Inhibitor

Ispinesib

Kinesin spindle protein (KSP; also known as EG5) is a kinesin motor protein required to establish mitotic-spindle bipolarity.[90] Several KSP inhibitors have been evaluated in early phase clinical trials. SB-715992 (ispinesib) is a small-molecule inhibitor of KSP ATPase and has been evaluated in two different schedules.[89] The dose-limiting toxicity is neutropenia. Ispinesib was found to be inactive in phase 2 studies evaluating efficacy in patients with castration-resistant and largely docetaxel-resistant prostate cancer, advanced renal cancer, and head and neck cancer.[90–92]

MECHANISMS OF RESISTANCE TO MICROTUBULE INHIBITORS

Drug resistance is often complex and multifaceted and can involve diverse mechanisms such as (1) factors that reduce the ability of drugs to reach their cellular target (e.g., activation of detoxification pathways and decreased drug accumulation); (2) modifications in the drug target; and (3) events downstream of the target (e.g., decreased sensitivity to, or defective, apoptotic signals). Many tubulin binding agents are substrates for multidrug transporters such as P-glycoprotein and the multidrug resistance gene (MDR1).[93,94]

The MDR1-encoded gene product MDR1 (ABC subfamily B1; ABCB1) and MDR2 (ABC subfamily ABCB4) are the best-characterized ABC transporters thought to confer drug resistance to taxanes.[94,95] MDR-related taxane resistance can be reversed by many classes of drugs, including the calcium channel blockers, cyclosporin A, and antiarrhythmic agents.[94,95] However, the clinical utility of this approach has never been proven, despite several clinical trials. The role of ABC transporters in resistance to microtubule inhibitors remains to be determined.[96]

An increasing number of studies suggest that the expression of individual tubulin isotypes are altered in cells resistant to antimicrotubule drugs and may confer drug resistance.[93,97] Inherent differences in microtubule dynamics and drug interactions have been observed with some isotypes in vitro and in vivo.[98] Several taxane-resistant mutant cell lines that have structurally altered α- and β-tubulin proteins and an impaired ability to polymerize into microtubules have also been identified.[99] Mutations of tubulin isotype genes, gene amplifications, and isotype switching have also been reported in taxane-resistant cell lines.[99] In patients, levels of class III β-tubulin have been shown to correlate with response—those with high RNA levels have poor response—and immunohistochemical stains can correlate and may be predictive.[96,100,101] As opposed to taxanes, resistance to vinca alkaloids has been associated with decreased class II β-tubulin expression.[97,98]

MAPs are important structural and regulatory components of microtubules that act in concert to remodel the microtubule network by stabilizing or destabilizing microtubules during mitosis or cytokinesis. Alterations in the activity and/or balance of stabilizing or destabilizing MAPs can profoundly affect microtubule function.[99,102] The overexpression of stathmin, a destabilizing protein, has been reported to decrease sensitivity to paclitaxel and vinblastine.[1] An analysis of predictive or prognostic factors in a large phase 3 study (National Surgical Adjuvant Breast and Bowel Project NSABP-B 28) in patients with node-positive breast cancer showed that MAP-tau, a stabilizing protein, was a prognostic factor; however, it was not predictive for benefit from paclitaxel-based chemotherapy.[1,93] In a separate randomized controlled trial in breast cancer (TAX 307), where the only variable was docetaxel, MAP-tau was also shown to be prognostic, but not predictive of taxane benefit.[103]

Additional studies have shown a correlation with BRCA1 loss measured by gene or protein expression, or gene signatures, with resistance to taxane and sensitivity to DNA-damaging agents (such as cisplatin and anthracyclines).[104–107] BRCA1 is a tumor-suppressor gene with DNA damage response and repair, as well as cell cycle checkpoint activation, which explains why its loss leads to enhanced cisplatin sensitivity.[20] BRCA1 also indirectly regulates microtubule dynamics and stability and can favorably control how microtubules respond to paclitaxel treatment via their association with pro-caspase-8. The loss of BRCA1 can lead to impaired taxane-induced activation of apoptosis due to microtubules that are more dynamic and less susceptible to taxane-induced stabilization and proximity-induced activation of caspase-8 signaling.[20]

In addition to resistance, certain tumor subtypes may be sensitive to the taxane dosing schedule. In two randomized trials of low-dose, weekly paclitaxel, the luminal breast cancer subtype was found to have a better outcome compared with the control arm. This suggests that not only the drug, but also the schedule may influence the response to therapy and that genomic approaches may reveal these insights.[108]

REFERENCES

1. Kavallaris M. Microtubules and resistance to tubulin-binding agents. *Nat Rev Cancer* 2010;10:194–204.
2. Nogales E. Structural insights into microtubule function. *Ann Rev Biophys Biomol Struct* 2001;30:397–420.
3. Wani MC, Taylor HL, Wall ME, et al. Plant antitumor agents. VI. Isolation and structure of taxol, a novel antileukemic and antitumor agent from Taxus brevifolia. *J Am Chem Soc* 1971;93:2325–2327.
4. Rowinsky E, Donehower R. Antimicrotubule agents. In: DeVita VT, Hellmann S, Rosenberg SA, eds. *Cancer: Principles and Practice of Oncology.* 5th ed. Philadelphia: Lippincott-Raven;1997.
5. Vrignaud P, Sémiond D, Lejeune P, et al. Preclinical antitumor activity of cabazitaxel, a semisynthetic taxane active in taxane-resistant tumors. *Clin Cancer Res* 2013;19:2973–2983.
6. Sparano JA. Taxanes for breast cancer: an evidence-based review of randomized phase II and phase III trials. *Clin Breast Cancer* 2000;1:32–40.
7. Mamounas E, Leinbersky B, Bryant J, et al. Paclitaxel after doxorubicin plus cyclophosphamide as adjuvant chemotherapy for node-positive breast cancer: results from NSABP B-28. *J Clin Oncol* 2005;23:3686–3696.
8. Bonomi P, Kim KM, Fairclough D, et al. Comparison of survival and quality of life in advanced non-small-cell lung cancer patients treated with two dose levels of paclitaxel combined with cisplatin versus etoposide with cisplatin: results of an Eastern Cooperative Oncology Group trial. *J Clin Oncol* 2000;18:623–631.
9. Martin M, Pienkowski T, Mackey J, et al. Adjuvant docetaxel for node-positive breast cancer. *N Engl J Med* 2005;352:2302–2313.
10. Jones SE, Erban J, Overmoyer B, et al. Randomized phase III study of docetaxel compared with paclitaxel in metastatic breast cancer. *J Clin Oncol* 2005;23:5542–5551.
11. Tannock IF, de Wit R, Berry WR, et al. Docetaxel plus prednisone or mitoxantrone plus prednisone for advanced prostate cancer. *N Engl J Med* 2004;351:1502–1512.
12. Van Cutsem E, Moiseyenko V, Tjulandin S, et al. Phase III study of docetaxel and cisplatin plus fluorouracil compared with cisplatin and fluorouracil as first-line therapy for advanced gastric cancer: a report of the V325 Study Group. *J Clin Oncol* 2006;24:4991–4997.
13. Schiff PB, Fant J, Horwitz SB. Promotion of microtubule assembly in vitro by taxol. *Nature* 1979;277:665–667.

14. Nogales E. Structural insight into microtubule function. *Annu Rev Biophys Biomol Struct* 2001;30:397–420.
15. Darshan MS, Loftus MS, Thadani-Mulero M, et al. Taxane-induced blockade to nuclear accumulation of the androgen receptor predicts clinical responses in metastatic prostate cancer. *Cancer Res* 2011;71:6019–6029.
16. Hoimes CJ, Kelly WK. Redefining hormone resistance in prostate cancer. *Ther Adv Med Oncol* 2010;2:107–123.
17. LaPointe NE, Morfini G, Brady ST, et al. Effects of eribulin, vincristine, paclitaxel and ixabepilone on fast axonal transport and kinesin-1 driven microtubule gliding: Implications for chemotherapy-induced peripheral neuropathy. *Neurotoxicology* 2013;37:231–239.
18. Mielgo A, Torres VA, Clair K, et al. Paclitaxel promotes a caspase 8-mediated apoptosis through death effector domain association with microtubules. *Oncogene* 2009;28:3551–3562.
19. Komlodi-Pasztor E, Sackett D, Wilkerson J, et al. Mitosis is not a key target of microtubule agents in patient tumors. *Nat Rev Clin Oncol* 2011;8:244–250.
20. Sung M, Giannakakou P. BRCA1 regulates microtubule dynamics and taxane-induced apoptotic cell signaling. *Oncogene* 2014;33(11):1418–1428.
21. Strobel T, Kraeft SK, Chen LB, et al. BAX expression is associated with enhanced intracellular accumulation of paclitaxel: a novel role for BAX during chemotherapy-induced cell death. *Cancer Res* 1998;58:4776–4781.
22. Srivastava RK, Mi QS, Hardwick JM, et al. Deletion of the loop region of Bcl-2 completely blocks paclitaxel-induced apoptosis. *Proc Natl Acad Sci U S A* 1999;96:3775–3780.
23. Dai H, Ding H, Meng XW, et al. Contribution of Bcl-2 phosphorylation to Bak binding and drug resistance. *Cancer Res* 2013;73(23):6998–7008.
24. Oakes SR, Vaillant F, Lim E, et al. Sensitization of BCL-2–expressing breast tumors to chemotherapy by the BH3 mimetic ABT-737. *Proc Natl Acad Sci* 2012;109:2766–2771.
25. Chauhan VP, Stylianopoulos T, Martin JD, et al. Normalization of tumour blood vessels improves the delivery of nanomedicines in a size-dependent manner. *Nat Nanotechnol* 2012;7:383–388.
26. Gradishar W, Tjulandin S, Davidson N, et al. Phase III trial of nanoparticle albumin-bound paclitaxel compared with polyethylated castor oil-based paclitaxel in women with breast cancer. *J Clin Oncol* 2005;23:7794–7803.
27. Socinski MA, Bondarenko I, Karaseva NA, et al. Weekly nab-paclitaxel in combination with carboplatin versus solvent-based paclitaxel plus carboplatin as first-line therapy in patients with advanced non–small-cell lung cancer: final results of a Phase III trial. *J Clin Oncol* 2012;30:2055–2062.
28. Von Hoff DD, Ervin T, Arena FP, et al. Increased survival in pancreatic cancer with nab-paclitaxel plus gemcitabine. *N Engl J Med* 2013;369:1691–1703.
29. Sparreboom A, Scripture CD, Trieu V, et al. Comparative preclinical and clinical pharmacokinetics of a cremophor-free, nanoparticle albumin-bound paclitaxel (ABI-007) and paclitaxel formulated in cremophor (Taxol). *Clin Cancer Res* 2005;11:4136–4143.
30. Yardley DA. nab-Paclitaxel mechanisms of action and delivery. *J Control Release* 2013;170:365–372.
31. Desai N, Trieu V, Yao Z, et al. Increased antitumor activity, intratumor paclitaxel concentrations, and endothelial cell transport of cremophor-free, albumin-bound paclitaxel, ABI-007, compared with cremophor-based paclitaxel. *Clin Cancer Res* 2006;12:1317–1324.
32. Nyman DW, Campbell KJ, Hersh E, et al. Phase I and pharmacokinetics trial of ABI-007, a novel nanoparticle formulation of paclitaxel in patients with advanced nonhematologic malignancies. *J Clin Oncol* 2005;23:7785–7793.
33. Cheng CJ, Saltzman WM. Nanomedicine: downsizing tumour therapeutics. *Nat Nanotechnol* 2012;7:346–347.
34. Infante JR, Matsubayashi H, Sato N, et al. Peritumoral fibroblast SPARC expression and patient outcome with resectable pancreatic adenocarcinoma. *J Clin Oncol* 2007;25:319–325.
35. Kato Y, Nagashima Y, Baba Y, et al. Expression of SPARC in tongue carcinoma of stage II is associated with poor prognosis: an immunohistochemical study of 86 cases. *Int J Mol Med* 2005;16:263–268.
36. Lau CPY, Poon RTP, Cheung ST, et al. SPARC and Hevin expression correlate with tumour angiogenesis in hepatocellular carcinoma. *J Pathol* 2006;210:459–468.
37. Thomas R, True LD, Bassuk JA, et al. Differential expression of osteonectin/SPARC during human prostate cancer progression. *Clin Cancer Res* 2000;6:1140–1149.
38. Watkins G, Douglas-Jones A, Bryce R, et al. Increased levels of SPARC (osteonectin) in human breast cancer tissues and its association with clinical outcomes. *Prostaglandins Leukot Essent Fatty Acids* 2005;72:267–272.
39. Cheng CJ, Saltzman WM. Enhanced siRNA delivery into cells by exploiting the synergy between targeting ligands and cell-penetrating peptides. *Biomaterials* 2011;32:6194–6203.
40. Davis ME, Zuckerman JE, Choi CH, et al. Evidence of RNAi in humans from systemically administered siRNA via targeted nanoparticles. *Nature* 2010;464:1067–1070.
41. Von Hoff DD, Ramanathan RK, Borad MJ, et al. Gemcitabine Plus nab-paclitaxel is an active regimen in patients with advanced pancreatic cancer: a Phase I/II trial. *J Clin Oncol* 2011;29:4548–4554.
42. Mita A, Denis L, Rowinsky E, et al. Phase I and pharmacokinetic study of XRP6258 (RPR 116258A), a novel taxane, administered as a 1-hour infusion every 3 weeks in patients with advanced solid tumors. *Clin Cancer Res* 2009;15:723–730.
43. Diéras V, Lortholary A, Laurence V, et al. Cabazitaxel in patients with advanced solid tumours: results of a Phase I and pharmacokinetic study. *Eur J Cancer* 2013;49:25–34.
44. Mita AC, Denis LJ, Rowinsky EK, et al. Phase I and pharmacokinetic study of XRP6258 (RPR 116258A), a novel taxane, administered as a 1-hour infusion every 3 weeks in patients with advanced solid tumors. *Clin Cancer Res* 2009;15:723–730.
45. Yared JA, Tkaczuk KH. Update on taxane development: new analogs and new formulations. *Drug Des Devel Ther* 2012;6:371–384.
46. Baas P, Szczesna A, Albert I, et al. Phase I/II study of a 3 weekly oral taxane (DJ-927) in patients with recurrent, advanced non-small cell lung cancer. *J Thorac Oncol* 2008;3:745–750.
47. Vigano L, Locatelli A, Grasselli G, et al. Drug interactions of paclitaxel and docetaxel and their relevance for the design of combination therapy. *Invest New Drugs* 2001;19:179–196.
48. Kudlowitz D, Muggia F. Defining risks of taxane neuropathy: insights from randomized clinical trials. *Clin Cancer Res* 2013;19:4570–4577.
49. Henningsson A, Karlsson MO, Viganò L, et al. Mechanism-based pharmacokinetic model for paclitaxel. *J Clin Oncol* 2001;19:4065–4073.
50. Sissung T, Mross K, Steinberg S, et al. Association of ABCB1 genotypes with paclitaxel-mediated peripheral neuropathy and neutropenia. *Eur J Cancer* 2006;42:2893–2896.
51. Marsh S, Paul J, King C, et al. Pharmacogenetic assessment of toxicity and outcome after platinum plus taxane chemotherapy in ovarian cancer: the Scottish Randomised Trial in Ovarian Cancer. *J Clin Oncol* 2007;25:4528–4535.
52. Baldwin RM, Owzar K, Zembutsu H, et al. A genome-wide association study identifies novel loci for paclitaxel-induced sensory peripheral neuropathy in CALGB 40101. *Clin Cancer Res* 2012;18:5099–5109.
53. Rugo H, Barry W, Moreno Aspitia A, et al. CALGB 40502/NCCTG N063H: Randomized phase III trial of weekly paclitaxel (P) compared to weekly nanoparticle albumin bound nab-paclitaxel (NP) or ixabepilone (Ix) with or without bevacizumab (B) as first-line therapy for locally recurrent or metastatic breast cancer (MBC). *J Clin Oncol* 2012;30.
54. Baker J, Ajani J, Scotté F, et al. Docetaxel-related side effects and their management. *Eur J Oncol Nurs* 2009;13:49–59.
55. Lee J, Swain S. Peripheral neuropathy induced by microtubule-stabilizing agents. *J Clin Oncol* 2006;24:1633–1642.
56. Alsamarai S, Charpidou AG, Matthay RA, et al. Pneumonitis related to docetaxel: case report and review of the literature. *In Vivo* 2009;23:635–637.
57. Dumitra S, Sideris L, Leclerc Y, et al. Neutropenic enterocolitis and docetaxel neoadjuvant chemotherapy. *Ann Oncol* 2009;20:795–796.
58. de Bono JS, Oudard S, Ozguroglu M, et al. Prednisone plus cabazitaxel or mitoxantrone for metastatic castration-resistant prostate cancer progressing after docetaxel treatment: a randomised open-label trial. *Lancet* 2010;376:1147–1154.
59. Zhou JY, Placidi M, Rahmani R. Uptake and metabolism of vinca alkaloids by freshly isolated human hepatocytes in suspension. *Anticancer Res* 1994;14:1017–1022.
60. Zhou J, Giannakakou P. Targeting microtubules for cancer chemotherapy. *Curr Med Chem Anticancer Agents* 2005;5:65–71.
61. Jordan MA, Wilson L. Microtubules as a target for anticancer drugs. *Nat Rev Cancer* 2004;4:253–265.
62. Bender RA, Castle MC, Margileth DA, et al. The pharmacokinetics of [3H]-vincristine in man. *Clin Pharmacol Ther* 1977;22:430–435.
63. Zhou XJ, Martin M, Placidi M, et al. In-vivo and in-vitro pharmacokinetics and metabolism of vinca alkaloids in rat. II. Vinblastine and vincristine. *Eur J Drug Metab Pharmacokinet* 1990;15:323–332.
64. Rowinsky EK, Noe DA, Trump DL, et al. Pharmacokinetic, bioavailability, and feasibility study of oral vinorelbine in patients with solid tumors. *J Clin Oncol* 1994;12:1754–1763.
65. Fumoleau P, Guiu S. New vinca alkaloids in clinical development. *Curr Breast Cancer Rep* 2013;5:69–72.
66. Chan JD. Pharmacokinetic drug interactions of vinca alkaloids: summary of case reports. *Pharmacotherapy* 1998;18:1304–1307.
67. Tobe SW, Siu LL, Jamal SA, et al. Vinblastine and erythromycin: an unrecognized serious drug interaction. *Cancer Chemother Pharmacol* 1995;35:188–190.
68. Peltier A, Russell J. Recent advances in drug-induced neuropathies. *Curr Opin Neurol* 2002;15:633–638.
69. Quasthoff S, Hartung H. Chemotherapy-induced peripheral neuropathy. *J Neurol* 2002;249:9–17.
70. Lobert S, Vulevic B, Correia JJ. Interaction of vinca alkaloids with tubulin: a comparison of vinblastine, vincristine, and vinorelbine. *Biochemistry* 1996;35:6806–6814.
71. Schrijvers DL. Extravasation: a dreaded complication of chemotherapy. *Ann Oncol* 2003;14:iii26–iii30.
72. Petrylak D, Hussain MHA, Tangen C, et al. Docetaxel and estramustine compared with mitoxantrone and prednisone for advanced refractory prostate cancer. *N Engl J Med* 2004;351:1513–1520.
73. Tannock IF, de Wit R, Berry WR, et al. Docetaxel plus prednisone or mitoxantrone plus prednisone for advanced prostate cancer. *N Engl J Med* 2004;351:1502–1512.
74. Lee JJ, Kelly WK. Epothilones: tubulin polymerization as a novel target for prostate cancer therapy. *Nat Clin Pract Oncol* 2009;6:85–92.
75. Kelly WK. Epothilones in prostate cancer. *Urol Oncol* 2011;29:358–365.
76. Kelly K, Zollinger M, Lozac'h F, et al. Metabolism of patupilone in patients with advanced solid tumor malignancies. *Invest New Drugs* 2013;31:605–615.
77. Trail PA, Willner D, Lasch SJ, et al. Cure of xenografted human carcinomas by BR96-doxorubicin immunoconjugates. *Science* 1993;261:212–215.

78. Carter PJ, Senter PD. Antibody-drug conjugates for cancer therapy. *Cancer J* 2008;14:154–169.
79. Doronina SO, Toki BE, Torgov MY, et al. Development of potent monoclonal antibody auristatin conjugates for cancer therapy. *Nat Biotechnol* 2003;21:778–784.
80. Lewis Phillips GD, Li G, Dugger DL, et al. Targeting HER2-positive breast cancer with trastuzumab-DM1, an antibody–cytotoxic drug conjugate. *Cancer Res* 2008;68:9280–9290.
81. Verma S, Miles D, Gianni L, et al. Trastuzumab emtansine for HER2-positive advanced breast cancer. *N Engl J Med* 2012;367:1783–1791.
82. Okeley NM, Miyamoto JB, Zhang X, et al. Intracellular activation of SGN-35, a potent anti-CD30 antibody-drug conjugate. *Clin Cancer Res* 2010;16:888–897.
83. Younes A, Bartlett NL, Leonard JP, et al. Brentuximab vedotin (SGN-35) for relapsed CD30-positive lymphomas. *N Engl J Med* 2010;363:1812–1821.
84. Younes A. Brentuximab vedotin for the treatment of patients with Hodgkin lymphoma. *Hematol Oncol Clin North Am* 2014;28:27–32.
85. Gandhi M, Evens AM, Fenske TS, et al. Pancreatitis in patients treated with brentuximab vedotin: a previously unrecognized serious adverse event. *Blood* 2013;122:4380.
86. Mosquera JM, Beltran H, Park K, et al. Concurrent AURKA and MYCN gene amplifications are harbingers of lethal treatment-related neuroendocrine prostate cancer. *Neoplasia* 2013;15:1–10.
87. Ujhazy P, Stewart D. DNA Repair. *J Thorac Oncol* 2009;4:S1068–S1070.
88. Green MR, Woolery JE, Mahadevan D. Update on aurora kinase targeted therapeutics in oncology. *Expert Opin Drug Discov* 2011;6:291–307.
89. Jackson JR, Patrick DR, Dar MM, et al. Targeted anti-mitotic therapies: can we improve on tubulin agents? *Nat Rev Cancer* 2007;7:107–117.
90. Tang PA, Siu LL, Chen EX, et al. Phase II study of ispinesib in recurrent or metastatic squamous cell carcinoma of the head and neck. *Invest New Drugs* 2008;26:257–264.
91. Beer TM, Goldman B, Synold TW, et al. Southwest oncology group phase II study of ispinesib in androgen-independent prostate cancer previously treated with taxanes. *Clin Genitourin Cancer* 2008;6:103–109.
92. Lee RT, Beekman KE, Hussain M, et al. A university of chicago consortium phase II trial of SB-715992 in advanced renal cell cancer. *Clin Genitourin Cancer* 2008;6:21–24.
93. Perez EA. Microtubule inhibitors: differentiating tubulin-inhibiting agents based on mechanisms of action, clinical activity, and resistance. *Mol Cancer Ther* 2009;8:2086–2095.
94. Gottesman MM, Fojo T, Bates SE. Multidrug resistance in cancer: role of ATP-dependent transporters. *Nat Rev Cancer* 2002;2:48–58.
95. Fojo AT, Menefee M. Microtubule targeting agents: basic mechanisms of multidrug resistance (MDR). *Semin Oncol* 2005;32:S3–S8.
96. Mozzetti S, Ferlini C, Concolino P, et al. Class III beta-tubulin overexpression is a prominent mechanism of paclitaxel resistance in ovarian cancer patients. *Clin Cancer Res* 2005;11:298–305.
97. Drukman S, Kavallaris M. Microtubule alterations and resistance to tubulin-binding agents (review). *Int J Oncol* 2002;21:621–628.
98. Verrills NM, Kavallaris M. Improving the targeting of tubulin-binding agents: lessons from drug resistance studies. *Curr Pharm Des* 2005;11:1719–1733.
99. Orr GA, Verdier-Pinard P, McDaid H, et al. Mechanisms of Taxol resistance related to microtubules. *Oncogene* 2003;22:7280–7295.
100. Monzó M, Rosell R, Sánchez JJ, et al. Paclitaxel resistance in non-small-cell lung cancer associated with beta-tubulin gene mutations. *J Clin Oncol* 1999;17:1786–1793.
101. Seve P, Mackey J, Isaac S, et al. Class III beta-tubulin expression in tumor cells predicts response and outcome in patients with non-small lung cancer receiving paclitaxel. *Mol Cancer Ther* 2005;4:2001–2007.
102. Baquero MT, Hanna JA, Neumeister V, et al. Stathmin expression and its relationship to microtubule-associated protein tau and outcome in breast cancer. *Cancer* 2012;118:4660–4669.
103. Baquero MT, Lostritto K, Gustavson MD, et al. Evaluation of prognostic and predictive value of microtubule associated protein tau in two independent cohorts. *Breast Cancer Res* 2011;13(5):R85.
104. Quinn JE, James CR, Stewart GE, et al. BRCA1 mRNA expression levels predict for overall survival in ovarian cancer after chemotherapy. *Clin Cancer Res* 2007;13:7413–7420.
105. Byrski T, Gronwald J, Huzarski T, et al. Response to neo-adjuvant chemotherapy in women with BRCA1-positive breast cancers. *Breast Cancer Res Treat* 2008;108:289–296.
106. Font A, Taron M, Gago JL, et al. BRCA1 mRNA expression and outcome to neoadjuvant cisplatin-based chemotherapy in bladder cancer. *Ann Oncol* 2011;22:139–144.
107. Reguart N, Cardona AF, Carrasco E, et al. BRCA1: a new genomic marker for non-small-cell lung cancer. *Clin Lung Cancer* 2008;9:331–339.
108. Martin M, Prat A, Rodriguez-Lescure A, et al. PAM50 proliferation score as a predictor of weekly paclitaxel benefit in breast cancer. *Breast Cancer Res Treat* 2013;138:457–466.

22 Kinase Inhibitors as Anticancer Drugs

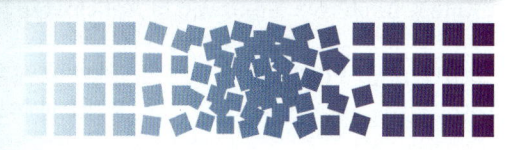

Charles L. Sawyers

INTRODUCTION

In 2001, the first tyrosine-kinase inhibitor imatinib was approved for clinical use in chronic myeloid leukemia. The spectacular success of this first-in-class agent ushered in a transformation in cancer drug discovery from efforts that were largely based on novel cytotoxic chemotherapy agents to an almost exclusive focus on molecularly targeted agents across the pharmaceutical and biotechnology industry and academia. This chapter summarizes this remarkable progress in this field over ~15 years, with the focus on the concepts underlying this paradigm shift as well as the considerable challenges that remain (Table 22.1). Readers in search of more specific details on individual drugs and their indications should consult the relevant disease-specific chapters elsewhere in this volume as well as references cited within this chapter. Readers should also note that the epidermal growth factor receptor (EGFR) and human epidermal growth factor receptor 2 (HER2) receptor tyrosine kinases covered here have also been successfully targeted by monoclonal antibodies that engage these proteins at the cell surface. These drugs, referred to as biologics rather than small molecule inhibitors, are covered in other chapters. The chapter is organized around kinase targets rather than diseases and, intentionally, has a historical flow to make certain thematic points and to illustrate the broad lessons that have been and continue to be learned through the clinical development of these exciting agents.

Perhaps the most stunning discovery from the clinical trials of the Abelson murine leukemia (ABL) kinase inhibitor imatinib was the recognition that tumor cells acquire exquisite dependence on the breakpoint cluster region protein BCR-ABL fusion oncogene, created by the Philadelphia chromosome translocation.[1] Although this may seem intuitive at first glance, consider the fact that the translocation arises in an otherwise normal hematopoietic stem cell, the survival of which is regulated by a complex array of growth factors and interactions with the bone marrow microenvironment. Although BCR-ABL clearly gives this cell a growth advantage that, over years, results in the clinical phenotype of chronic myeloid leukemia, there was no reason to expect that these cells would depend on BCR-ABL for their survival when confronted with an inhibitor. In the absence of BCR-ABL, these tumor cells could presumably rely on the marrow microenvironment, just like their normal, nontransformed neighbors. Thus, it seemed more likely that, by shutting down the driver oncogene, BCR-ABL inhibitors might halt the progression of chronic myeloid leukemia but not eliminate the preexisting tumor cells. In fact, chronic myeloid leukemia (CML) progenitors are eliminated after just a few months of anti–BCR-ABL therapy, indicating they are dependent on the driver oncogene for their survival and have "forgotten" how to return to normal. This phenomenon, subsequently documented in a variety of human malignancies, is colloquially termed *oncogene addiction*.[2] Although the molecular basis for this addiction still remains to be defined, the notion of finding an Achilles' heel for each cancer continues to captivate the cancer research community and has spawned a broad array of efforts to elucidate the molecular identity of these targets and discover relevant inhibitors.

EARLY SUCCESSES: TARGETING CANCERS WITH WELL-KNOWN KINASE MUTATIONS (BCR-ABL, KIT, HER2)

From the beginning, clinical trials of imatinib were restricted to patients with Philadelphia chromosome–positive chronic myeloid leukemia. For what seem like obvious reasons, there was never any serious discussion about treating patients with Philadelphia chromosome–negative leukemia because the assumption was that only patients with the BCR-ABL fusion gene would have a chance of responding. This was clearly a wise decision because hematologic response rates approached 90% and cytogenetic remissions were seen in nearly half of the patients in the early phase studies.[3] It was obvious that the drug worked, and imatinib was approved in record time. Unwittingly, the power of genome-based patient selection was demonstrated in the clinical development of the very first kinase inhibitor. As we will see, it took nearly a decade for this lesson to be fully learned. Today, the much larger clinical experience, with an array of different kinase inhibitors across many tumor types, has led to a much better understanding of the principles that dictate oncogene addiction that, in retrospect, were staring us in the face. Foremost among them is the notion that tumors with a somatic mutation or amplification of a kinase drug target are much more likely to be dependent on that target for survival. Hence, a patient whose tumor has such a mutation is much more likely to respond to treatment with the appropriate inhibitor. This has also led to a new paradigm at the regulatory level of drug approval requiring codevelopment of a *companion diagnostic* (a molecularly based diagnostic test that reliably identifies patients with the mutation) with the new drug.

After chronic myeloid leukemia, the next example to illustrate this principle was gastrointestinal stromal tumor (GIST), which is associated with mutations in the KIT tyrosine-kinase receptor or, more rarely, in the platelet-derived growth factor (PDGF) receptor.[4,5] Serendipitously, imatinib inhibits both KIT and the PDGF receptor; therefore, the clinical test of KIT inhibition in GIST followed quickly on the heels of the success in CML.[6] In retrospect, the rapid progress made in these two diseases was based, in part, on the fact that the driver molecular lesion (BCR-ABL or KIT mutation, respectively) is present in nearly all patients who are diagnosed with these two diseases. The molecular analysis merely confirmed the diagnosis that was made using standard clinical and histologic criteria. Consequently, clinicians could identify the patients most likely to respond based on clinical criteria rather than rely on an elaborate molecular profiling infrastructure to prescreen patients. Consequently, clinical trials evaluating kinase inhibitors in CML and GIST accrued quickly, and the therapeutic benefit became clear almost immediately.

The notion that molecular alteration of a driver kinase determines sensitivity to a cognate kinase inhibitor was further validated during the development of the dual EGFR/HER2 kinase inhibitor lapatinib. Clinical trials of this kinase inhibitor were conducted in women with advanced HER2-positive breast cancer based on earlier success in these same patients with the monoclonal antibody trastuzumab, which targets the extracellular domain of the HER2

TABLE 22.1
Kinase Inhibitors: Approved or Anticipated Approval In 2014

Target	Drug	Approved Indications	Anticipated Future Indications
ALK	Crizotinib Ceritinib	ALK mutant lung cancer	ALK mutant neuroblastoma, anaplastic lymphoma
BCR-ABL	Imatinib Dasatinib Nilotinib Bosutinib Ponatinib	Chronic myeloid leukemia Philadelphia chromosome–positive acute lymphoid leukemia T315 mutation only (ponatinib)	
BRAF	Vemurafenib Dabrafenib	BRAF mutant melanoma	Other BRAF mutant tumors
BTK	Ibrutinib	Chronic lymphocytic leukemia Mantle cell lymphoma	
EGFR	Gefitinib Erlotinib Afatinib	Lung adenocarcinoma with EGFR mutation	
HER2	Lapatinib	Her2$^+$ breast cancer	
JAK2	Ruxolitinib	JAK2 mutant myelofibrosis	
KIT	Imatinib Sunitinib	Gastrointestinal stromal tumor	
MEK	Trametinib	BRAF mutant melanoma	
PI3K delta[a]	Idelalisib	Chronic lymphocytic leukemia Indolent non-Hodgkin lymphoma	
PDGFR-α/β	Imatinib	Chronic myelomonocytic leukemia (with TEL-PDGFR-β fusion) hypereosinophilic syndrome (with PDGFR-β fusion) Dermatofibrosarcoma protuberans	
RET	Vandetanib Sorafenib Cabozantinib	Medullary thyroid cancer	
TORC1 (mTOR)	Sirolimus (rapamycin) Everolimus Temsirolimus	Kidney cancer Breast cancer Tuberous sclerosis	
VEGF Receptor	Sorafenib Sunitinib Axitinib Pazopanib	Kidney cancer Hepatocellular carcinoma (sorafenib only) Pancreatic neuroendocrine tumors (sunitinib)	

[a] Approval is anticipated based on positive phase 3 data and announcement of accepted Food and Drug Administration submission by the sponsor.

kinase. Lapatinib was initially approved in combination with the cytotoxic agent capecitabine for women with resistance to trastuzumab,[7] and then was subsequently approved for frontline use in metastatic breast cancer in combination with chemotherapy or hormonal therapy, depending on estrogen receptor status. A key ingredient that enabled the clinical development of lapatinib was the routine use of HER2 gene amplification testing in the diagnosis of breast cancer, pioneered during the development of trastuzumab several years earlier. This widespread clinical practice allowed for the rapid identification of those patients most likely to benefit. If lapatinib trials had been conducted in unselected patients, the clinical signal in breast cancer would likely have been missed.

The Serendipity of Unexpected Clinical Responses: EGFR in Lung Cancer

In contrast to the logical development of imatinib and lapatinib in molecularly defined patient populations, the EGFR kinase inhibitors gefitinib and erlotinib entered the clinic without the benefit of such a focused clinical development plan. Although considerable preclinical data implicated EGFR as a cancer drug target, there was little insight into which patients were most likely to benefit. The first clue that EGFR inhibitors would have a role in lung cancer came from the recognition by several astute clinicians of remarkable responses in a small fraction of patients with lung adenocarcinoma.[8] Further studies revealed the curious clinical circumstance that those patients most likely to benefit tended to be those who never smoked, women, and those of Asian ethnicity.[9] Clearly, there was a strong clinical signal in a subgroup of patients, who could perhaps be enriched based on these clinical features, but it seemed that a unifying molecular lesion must be present. Three academic groups simultaneously converged on the answer. Mutations in the EGFR gene were detected in the 10% to 15% of patients with lung adenocarcinoma who had radiographic responses.[10–12] It may seem surprising that mutations in a gene as highly visible as EGFR and in such a prevalent cancer had not been detected earlier. But the motivation to search aggressively for EGFR mutations was not there until the clinical responses were seen. Perhaps even more surprising was the failure of the pharmaceutical company sponsors of the two most advanced compounds, gefitinib and erlotinib, to embrace this important discovery and refocus future clinical development plans on patients with EGFR mutant lung adenocarcinoma.

But that was 2004, when the prevailing approach to cancer drug development was an empiric one originally developed (with great success) for cytotoxic agents. Typically, small numbers of patients with different cancers were treated in *all comer* phase I studies (no enrichment for subgroups) with the goal of eliciting a clinical signal in at least one tumor type. A single-agent response rate of 20% to 30% in a disease-specific phase II trial would justify a randomized phase III registration trial, where the typical endpoint for drug approval is time to progression or survival. Cytotoxics were also typically evaluated in combination with existing standard of care treatment (typically approved chemotherapy agents) with the goal of increasing the response rate or enhancing the duration of response. (Note: The use of the past tense here is intentional. As we will see later in this chapter, nearly all cancer drug development today is based on selecting patients with a certain molecular profile.)

The clinical development of gefitinib and erlotinib followed the cytotoxic model. Both drugs had similarly low but convincing single-agent response rates (10% to 15%) in chemotherapy-refractory, advanced lung cancer. Indeed, gefitinib was originally granted accelerated approval by the U.S. Food and Drug Administration (FDA) in 2003 based on the impressive nature of these responses, contingent on the completion of formal phase III studies with survival endpoints.[13] The sponsors of both drugs, therefore, conducted phase III registration studies in patients with chemotherapy-refractory, advanced stage lung cancer but without pre-screening patients for EGFR mutation status. (In fairness, these trials were initiated prior to the discovery of EGFR mutations in lung cancer but study amendments could have been considered.) Erlotinib was approved in 2004 on the basis of a modest survival advantage over placebo (the BR.21 trial); however, gefitinib failed to demonstrate a survival advantage in essentially the same patient population.[14,15] This difference in outcome was surprising because the two drugs have highly similar chemical structures and biologic properties. Perhaps the most important difference was drug dose. Erlotinib was given at the maximum tolerated dose, which produces a high frequency of rash and diarrhea. Both side effects are presumed *on target* consequences of EGFR inhibition because EGFR is highly expressed in skin and gastrointestinal epithelial cells. In contrast, gefitinib was dosed slightly lower to mitigate these toxicities, with the rationale that responses were clearly documented at lower doses.

In parallel with the single-agent phase III trials in chemotherapy-refractory patients, both gefitinib and erlotinib were studied as an upfront therapy for advanced lung cancer to determine if either would improve the efficacy of standard *doublet* (carboplatin/paclitaxel or gemcitabine/cisplatin) chemotherapy when all three drugs were given in combination. These trials, termed INTACT-1 and INTACT-2 (gefitinib with either gemcitabine/cisplatin or with carboplatin/paclitaxel) and TRIBUTE (erlotinib with carboplatin/paclitaxel), collectively enrolled over 3,000 patients.[16-18] Excitement in the oncology community was high based on the clear single-agent activity of both EGFR inhibitors. But, both trials were spectacular failures; neither drug showed any benefit over chemotherapy alone. The fact that EGFR mutations are present in only 10% to 15% of patients (i.e., those likely to benefit) provided a logical explanation. The clinical signal from those whose tumors had EGFR mutations was likely diluted out by all the patients whose tumors had no EGFR alterations, many of whom benefited from chemotherapy.

The convergence of the EGFR mutation discovery with these clinical trial results will be remembered as a remarkable time in the history of targeted cancer therapies, not just for the important role of these agents as lung cancer therapies, but also for missteps in deciding that the EGFR genotype should drive treatment selection. Perhaps the most egregious error came from a retrospective analysis of tumors from patients treated on the BR.21 trial, which concluded that EGFR mutations did *not* predict for a survival advantage.[19] (EGFR gene amplification *was* associated with survival, but only in a univariate analysis.) This conclusion was concerning because less than 30% of patients on the trial had tissue available for EGFR mutation analysis, raising questions about the adequacy of the sample size. Furthermore, the EGFR mutation assay used by the authors was subsequently criticized because a significant number of the EGFR mutations reported in these patients were in residues not previously found by others, who had sequenced thousands of tumors. Many of these mutations were suspected to be an artifact of working from formalin-fixed biopsies. Fortunately, recent advances in DNA mutation detection, using massively parallel next-generation sequencing technology, have largely eliminated this concern. These new platforms are now being used in the clinical setting.

Clinical investigators in Asia, where a greater fraction of lung cancers (roughly 30%) are positive for EGFR mutations, addressed the question of whether mutations predict for clinical benefit in a prospective trial. In this study known as IPASS, gefitinib was clearly superior to standard doublet chemotherapy as frontline therapy for patients with advanced EGFR mutation–positive lung adenocarcinoma.[20] Conversely, EGFR mutation–negative patients fared much worse with gefitinib and benefited from chemotherapy. In addition, EGFR mutation–positive patients had a more favorable overall prognosis regardless of treatment, indicating that EGFR mutation is also a prognostic biomarker. The IPASS trial serves as a compelling example of a properly designed (and executed) biomarker-driven clinical trial. Although the rationale for this clinical development strategy had been demonstrated years earlier with BCR-ABL in leukemia, KIT in GIST, and HER2 in breast cancer, it was difficult to derail the empiric approach that had been used for decades in developing cytotoxic agents.

A Mix of Science and Serendipity: PDGF Receptor–Driven Leukemias and Sarcoma

The discovery of EGFR mutations in lung cancer (motivated by dramatic clinical responses in a subset of patients treated with EGFR kinase inhibitors) is the most visible example of the power of bedside-to-bench science, but it is not the only (or the first) such example from the kinase inhibitor era. Shortly after the approval of imatinib for CML in 2001, two case reports documented dramatic remissions in patients with hypereosinophilic syndrome (HES), a blood disorder characterized by prolonged elevation of eosinophil counts and subsequent organ dysfunction from eosinophil infiltration, when treated with imatinib.[21,22] Although HES resembles myeloproliferative diseases such as CML, the molecular pathogenesis of HES was completely unknown at the time. Reasoning that these clinical responses must be explained by inhibition of a driver kinase, a team of laboratory-based physician/scientists quickly searched for mutations in the three kinases known to be inhibited by imatinib (ABL, KIT, and PDGF receptor). ABL and KIT were quickly excluded, but the PDGF receptor α (PDGFR-α) gene was targeted by an interstitial deletion that fused the upstream FIP1L1 gene to PDGFR-α.[23] FIP1L1-PDGFR-α is a constitutively active tyrosine kinase, analogous to BCR-ABL, and is also inhibited by imatinib. As with EGFR-mutant lung cancer, the molecular pathophysiology of HES was discovered by dissecting the mechanism of response to the drug used to treat it.

The HES/FIP1L1-PDGFR-α story serves as a nice bookend to an earlier discovery that the t(5;12) chromosome translocation, found rarely in patients with chronic myelomonocytic leukemia, creates the TEL-PDGFR-β fusion tyrosine kinase.[24] Similar to HES, treatment of patients with t(5;12) translocation-positive leukemias with imatinib has also proven successful.[25] A third example comes from dermatofibrosarcoma protuberans, a sarcoma characterized by a t(17;22) translocation that fuses the COL1A gene to the PDGFB *ligand* (not the receptor). COL1A-PDGFB is oncogenic through autocrine stimulation of the normal PDGF receptor in these tumor cells. Patients with dermatofibrosarcoma protuberans respond to imatinib therapy because it targets the PDGF receptor, just one step downstream from the oncogenic lesion.[26]

Exploiting the New Paradigm: Searching for Other Kinase-Driven Cancers

The benefits of serendipity notwithstanding, the growing number of examples of successful kinase inhibitor therapy in tumors with a mutation or amplification of the drug target begged for a more rational approach to drug discovery and development. In 2002, the list of human tumors known to have mutations in kinases was quite small. Due to advances in automated gene sequencing, it became possible to ask whether a much larger fraction of human cancers might also have such mutations through a brute force approach. To address this question comprehensively, one would have to sequence all of the kinases in the genome in hundreds of samples of each tumor type. Several early pilot studies demonstrated the potential of this approach by revealing important new targets for drug development. Perhaps the most spectacular was the discovery of mutations in the BRAF kinase in over half of patients with melanoma, as well as in a smaller fraction of colon and thyroid cancers.[27] Another was the discovery of mutations in the JAK2 kinase in nearly all patients with polycythemia vera, as well as a significant fraction of patients with myelofibrosis and essential thrombocytosis.[28–30] A third example was the identification of PIK3CA mutations in a variety of tumors, with the greatest frequencies in breast, endometrial, and colorectal cancers.[31] PIK3CA encodes a lipid kinase that generates the second messenger phosphatidyl inositol 3-phosphate (PIP3). PIP3 activates growth and survival signaling through the AKT family of kinases as well as other downstream effectors. Coupled with the well-established role of the phosphatase and tensin homolog (PTEN) lipid phosphatase in dephosphorylating PIP3, the discovery of PIK3CA mutations focused tremendous attention on developing inhibitors at multiple levels of this pathway, as discussed further in the follow paragraphs.

Each of these important discoveries—BRAF, JAK2, and PIK3CA—came from relatively small efforts (less than 100 tumors) and generally focused on resequencing only those exons that coded for regions of kinases where mutations had been found in other kinases (typically, the juxtamembrane and kinase domains). These restricted searches were largely driven by the high cost of DNA sequencing using the Sanger method. In 2006, a comprehensive effort to sequence all of the exons in all kinases in 100 tumors could easily exceed several million dollars. Financial support for such projects could not be obtained easily through traditional funding agencies because the risk/reward was considered too high. Furthermore, substantial infrastructure for sample acquisition, microdissection of the tumors from normal tissue, nucleic acid preparation, high throughput automated sequencing, and computational analysis of the resulting data was essential. Few institutions were equipped to address these challenges. In response, the National Cancer Institute in the United States (in partnership with the National Human Genome Research Institute) and an international group known as the International Cancer Genome Consortium (ICGC) launched large-scale efforts to sequence the complete genomes of thousands of cancers. In parallel, next-generation sequencing technologies resulted in massive reductions in cost, allowing a more comprehensive analysis of much larger numbers of tumors. At the time of this writing, the US effort (called The Cancer Genome Atlas [TCGA]) had reported data on 29 different tumor types (https://tcga-data.nci.nih.gov/tcga/). The international consortium has committed to sequencing 25,000 tumors representing 50 different cancer subtypes.[32] Both groups have enforced immediate release of all sequence information to the research community free of charge so that the entire scientific community can learn from the data. This policy enabled *pan cancer* mutational analyses that give an overall view of the genomic landscape of cancer, serving as a blueprint for the community of cancer researchers and drug developers.[33,34]

Rounding Out the Treatment of Myeloproliferative Disorders: JAK2 and Myelofibrosis

Taken together with the BCR-ABL translocation in CML and FIP1L1-PDGFR-α in HES, the discovery of JAK2 mutations in polycythemia, essential thrombocytosis, and myelofibrosis provided a unifying understanding of myeloproliferative disorders as diseases of abnormal kinase activation. The JAK family kinases are the primary effectors of signaling through inflammatory cytokine receptors and, therefore, had been considered compelling targets for anti-inflammatory drugs. But the JAK2 mutation discovery immediately shifted these efforts toward developing JAK2 inhibitors for myeloproliferative disorders. Because most patients have a common JAK2 V617F mutation, these efforts could rapidly focus on screening for activity against a single genotype. Progress has been rapid. Myelofibrosis was selected as the initial indication (instead of essential thrombocytosis or polycythemia vera) because the time to registration is expected to be the shortest. Currently, ruxolitinib is approved for myelofibrosis based on shrinkage in spleen size as the primary endpoint. Clinical trials in essential thrombocytosis and polycythemia vera (versus hydroxyurea) are ongoing. Other JAK2 inhibitors are also in clinical development.

BRAF Mutant Melanoma: Several Missteps Before Finding the Right Inhibitor

As with JAK2 mutations in myeloproliferative disorders, the discovery of BRAF mutations in patients with melanoma launched widespread efforts to find potent BRAF inhibitors. One early candidate was the drug sorafenib, which had been optimized during drug discovery to inhibit RAF kinases. (Sorafenib also inhibits vascular endothelial growth factor (VEGF) receptors, which led to its approval in kidney cancer, as discussed later in this chapter.) Despite the compelling molecular rationale for targeting BRAF, clinical results of sorafenib in melanoma were extremely disappointing and reduced enthusiasm for pursuing BRAF as a drug target.[35] In hindsight, this concern was completely misguided. Sorafenib dosing is limited by toxicities that preclude achieving serum levels in patients that potently inhibit RAF, but are sufficient to inhibit VEGF receptors. In addition, patients were enrolled without screening for BRAF mutations in their tumors. Although the frequency of BRAF mutations in melanoma is high, the inclusion of patients without the BRAF mutation diluted the chance of seeing any clinical signal. In short, the clinical evaluation of sorafenib in melanoma was poorly designed to test the hypothesis that BRAF is a therapeutic target. The danger is that negative data from such clinical experiments can slow subsequent progress. It is critical to know the pharmacodynamic properties of the drug and the molecular phenotype of the patients being studied when interpreting the results of a negative study.

The fact that RAF kinases are intermediate components of the well-characterized RAS/ mitogen-activated protein (MAP) kinase pathway (transducing signals from RAS to RAF to MEK to ERK) raised the possibility that tumors with BRAF mutations might respond to inhibitors of one of these downstream kinases (Fig. 22.1). Preclinical studies revealed that tumor cell lines with BRAF mutation were exquisitely sensitive to inhibitors of the downstream kinase MEK.[36] (Sorafenib, in contrast, does not show this profile of activity.[37] Thus, proper preclinical screening would have revealed the shortcomings of sorafenib as a BRAF inhibitor.) Curiously, cell lines with a mutation or amplification of EGFR or HER2, which

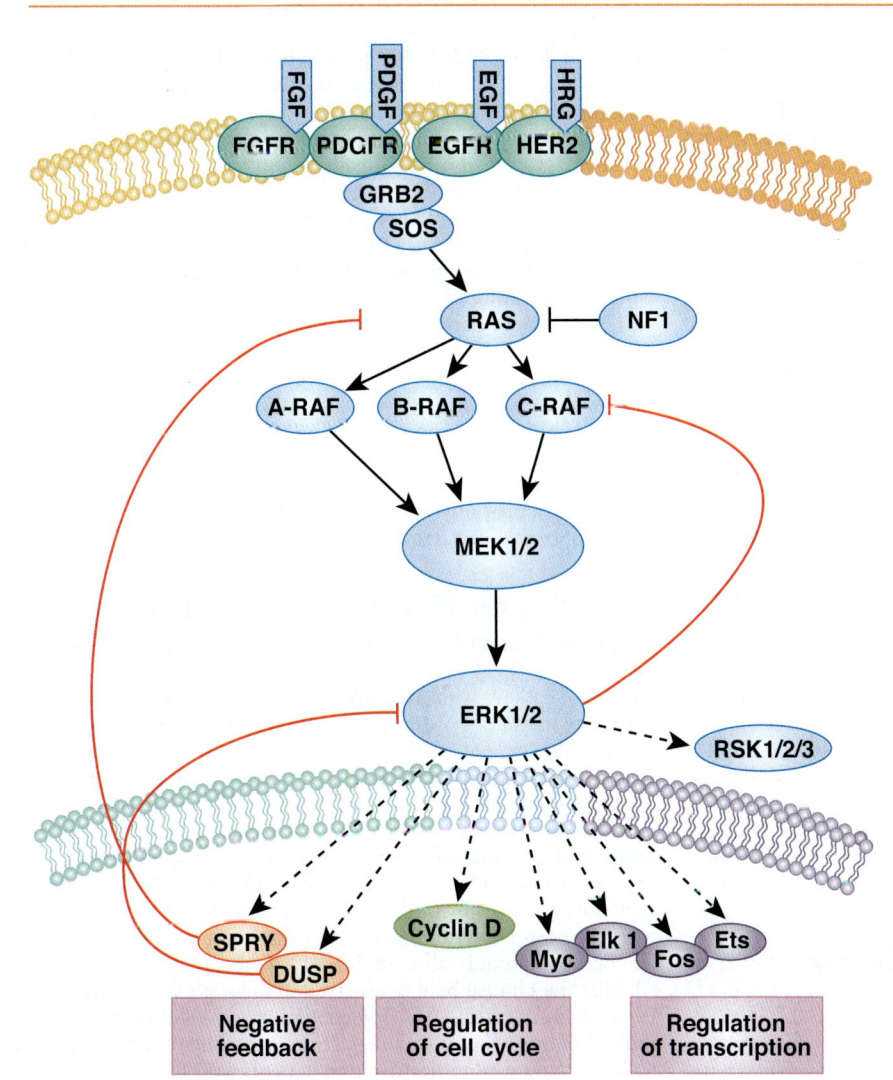

Figure 22.1 The RAS–RAF–MEK–ERK signaling pathway. The classical mitogen-activated protein kinase (MAPK) pathway is activated in human tumors by several mechanisms, including the binding of ligand to receptor tyrosine kinases (RTK), the mutational activation of an RTK, by loss of the tumor suppressor NF1, or by mutations in RAS, BRAF, and MEK1. Phosphorylation and, thus, activation of ERK regulates the transcription of target genes that promote cell cycle progression and tumor survival. The ERK pathway contains a classical feedback loop in which the expression of feedback elements such as SPRY and DUSP family proteins are regulated by the level of ERK activity. Loss of expression of SPRY and DUSP family members due to promoter methylation or deletion is thus permissive for persistently elevated pathway output. In the case of tumors with mutant BRAF, pathway output is enhanced by impaired upstream feedback regulation. FGF, fibroblast growth factor; HRG, heregulin; NF1, neurofibromatosis 1. (From Bernt KM, Zhu N, Sinha AU, et al. MLL-rearranged leukemia is dependent on aberrant H3K79 methylation by DOT1L. *Cancer Cell* 2011;20(1):66–78, with permission.)

function upstream in the pathway, were insensitive to MEK inhibition. Even tumor lines with RAS mutations were variably sensitive. In short, the preclinical data made a strong case that MEK inhibitors should be effective in BRAF mutant melanoma, but not in other subtypes. The reason that HER2, EGFR, and RAS mutant tumors were not sensitive to MEK inhibitors is explained, at least in part, by the existence of negative feedback loops that modulate the flux of signal transduction through MEK.[38]

In parallel with the generation of these preclinical findings, clinical trials of several MEK inhibitors were initiated. Patients with various cancers were enrolled in the early studies, but there was a strong bias to include melanoma patients. Significant efforts were made to demonstrate MEK inhibition in tumor cells by measuring the phosphorylation status of the direct downstream substrate ERK using an immunohistochemical analysis of biopsies from patients with metastatic disease. Phase I studies of the two earliest compounds in clinical development (PD325901 and AZD6244) documented reduced phospho-ERK staining at multiple dose levels in several patients for whom baseline and treatment biopsies were obtained.[39,40] (In the following, we will learn that these pharmacodynamic studies, while well intentioned, were not quantitative enough to document the magnitude of MEK inhibition in these patients.) Furthermore, clinical responses were observed in a few patients with BRAF mutant melanoma. Armed with this confidence, a randomized phase II clinical trial of AZD6244 was conducted in advanced melanoma, with the chemotherapeutic agent temozolomide (which is approved for glioblastoma) as the comparator arm. (The clinical development of PD325901 was discontinued because of safety concerns about ocular and neurologic toxicity.) Disappointingly, patients receiving AZD6244 had no benefit in progression-free survival when compared to temozolomide-treated patients, raising further concerns about the viability of BRAF as a drug target.[41] A closer examination of the data revealed that clinical responses were, indeed, seen in patients receiving AZD6244. The fact that BRAF mutation status was not required for study entry likely diminished the clinical signal in the AZD6244 arm, a lesson learned from the EGFR inhibitor trials in lung cancer. Indeed, a different MEK inhibitor, trametinib, received FDA approval in 2013 based on activity in melanoma patients with the BRAF mutation.[42]

All doubts about BRAF as a target vanished in 2009 to 2010 when dramatic clinical responses were observed with a novel BRAF inhibitor vemurafenib (PLX4032). Like sorafenib, this compound was optimized to inhibit RAF, but with an additional focus on mutant BRAF. Vemurafenib differs dramatically from sorafenib because it potently inhibits BRAF without the additional broad range of activities that sorafenib has against other kinases like the VEGF receptor.[43] The greater selectivity of vemurafenib relative to sorafenib resulted in a much greater tolerability, such that it could be given at high doses while avoiding significant toxicity. The early days of vemurafenib clinical development were plagued by challenges in maximizing the oral bioavailability of the drug.[44] Consequently, the initial phase I clinical trial was temporarily halted to develop a novel formulation (i.e., the coingredients in the drug capsule or tablet that improve solubility and absorption through the gastrointestinal tract). Much higher serum levels were obtained in patients who received the new vemurafenib formulation and, shortly thereafter, complete and partial responses were observed in about 80% of the melanoma patients with B-RAF mutant tumors. Strikingly, no activity was observed in patients whose tumors were wild type for BRAF.[45,46] The data were so compelling that vemurafenib was immediately advanced to a phase III registration trial. Similarly impressive responses in BRAF mutant melanoma patients were observed with a second potent RAF inhibitor dabrafenib,[47] providing further proof that BRAF is a important cancer target.

The vemurafenib and dabrafenib data also provide insight into why sorafenib and the early MEK inhibitor trials failed to demonstrate activity. One lesson is the critical importance of achieving adequate target inhibition. Clinical responses with vemurafenib were observed only after the drug was reformulated to achieve substantially higher serum levels. Reductions in phospho-ERK staining (as documented by immunohistochemistry) were documented in the earlier trials but, in retrospect, the assays were not sensitive enough to distinguish between modest (~50%) kinase inhibition versus more complete BRAF or MEK inhibition. Efficacy in preclinical models is significantly improved using doses that give >80% inhibition, and the human trial data suggest that this degree of pathway blockade is also required for a high clinical response rate.[46] Collectively, these experiences illustrate the critical need for quantitative pharmacodynamic assays to measure target inhibition early in clinical development. A second lesson is the importance of genotyping all patients for mutation or amplification of the relevant drug target. Not only does this ensure that a sufficient number of patients with the biomarker of interest are included in the study, but also that the results provide compelling evidence early in clinical development in support (or not) of the preclinical hypothesis.

Getting It Right: ALK and Lung Cancer

The development of the ALK inhibitor crizotinib (PF-02341066) illustrates how an unexpected signal obtained in a small number of patients can quickly shift a program in an entirely new direction with a high probability of success. The key ingredient is this story is a familiar one—a strong molecular hypothesis backed up by clinical response data in a small number of carefully selected patients. Crizotinib emerged from a drug discovery program at Pfizer that was focused on finding inhibitors of the MET receptor tyrosine kinase and entered the clinic with this target as its lead indication.[48] As we previously learned with imatinib, essentially all kinase inhibitors have activity against other targets (so called *off-target* activities), which can sometimes prove to be advantageous. Off-target activities are typically discovered by screening compounds against a large panel of kinases to establish profiles of relative selectivity against the intended target. Off-target activity, potency, and pharmaceutical properties (bioavailability, half-life) are all factors that influence the decision of which compound to advance to clinical development. The primary off-target activity of crizotinib is against the ALK tyrosine kinase.

ALK was first identified as a candidate driver oncogene in 1994 through the cloning of the t(2,5) chromosomal translocation associated with anaplastic large cell lymphoma, which creates the nucleophosmin/anaplastic lymphoma kinase (NPM-ALK) fusion gene.[49] This discovery, together with the demonstration that NPM-ALK causes lymphoma in mice, made a compelling case for ALK as a drug target in this disease. But there was limited interest in developing ALK inhibitors because this particular lymphoma subtype is rare and most commonly found in children. (Companies are generally reluctant to develop drugs solely for pediatric indications because of complexities related to dose selection and additional regulatory guidelines. Efforts to streamline this development process are underway, such as the Creating Hope Act, which provides new incentives for companies to pursue pediatric indications.) In 2007, a different ALK fusion gene called EML4-ALK was discovered in a small fraction of patients with lung adenocarcinoma, with an estimated frequency of 1% to 5%.[50] This discovery did not immediately capture the attention of drug developers, but several academic groups who had already begun testing lung cancer patients seen at their institutions for EGFR mutations simply added an EML4-ALK fusion test to the screening panel. Astute clinical investigators participating in the phase I trial of crizotinib, which was designed to include patients with a broad array of advanced cancers, were aware of the off-target ALK activity and enrolled several lung cancer patients with EML4-ALK fusions in the study. These patients had remarkably dramatic responses.[51] This serendipitous finding in a few ALK-positive patients was confirmed in a larger cohort, resulting in a strongly positive pivotal phase III study in ALK-positive lung cancer, just 2 years after the discovery of the EML4-ALK fusion.[52] Crizotinib is also being evaluated in other diseases associated with genomic alterations in ALK, including large-cell anaplastic lymphoma, neuroblastoma,[53] and inflammatory myofibroblastic sarcoma.[54]

Extending the Model to RET Mutations in Thyroid Cancer: Clinical Responses, But Why?

Subsets of patients with papillary or medullary thyroid cancer have activating mutations or translocations targeting the RET tyrosine-kinase receptor, raising the question of whether RET inhibitors might have a role in this disease.[55] Although no drugs specifically designed to inhibit RET have entered the clinic, four compounds with off-target activity against RET (vandetanib, sorafenib, motesanib, and cabozantinib) have all shown single-agent activity in thyroid cancer studies.[56–60] Vandetanib and cabozantinib are currently approved in medullary thyroid cancer based on improved progression-free survival in phase III registration trials.[61,62] Because all four compounds also inhibit VEGF receptor, it is unclear whether the clinical benefit observed in these studies is explained by inhibition of RET, VEGF receptor, or both. Unlike the crizotinib trials in ALK-positive lung cancer, enrollment in these registration studies was not restricted to patients with RET mutations. In addition to the fact that thyroid cancer patients are not routinely screened for these mutations, the primary reason for including all comers in these studies is that clinical responses are observed in a larger fraction of patients than can be accounted for based on the suspected frequency of an RET mutation. Responses in patients without RET mutation (if they occur) might be explained by mutations in other genes in the RAS-MAP kinase pathway such as BRAF or HRAS, which are found in a substantial fraction of patients and typically do not overlap with RET alterations.[55] Clearly, detailed genotype/response correlations, as demonstrated in lung cancer and melanoma, will clarify the role of these mutations in predicting the response to these drugs. Thyroid cancer is also a compelling indication for the BRAF and MEK inhibitors discussed previously in melanoma.

FLT3 Inhibitors in Acute Myeloid Leukemia: Did the Genomics Mislead Us?

Shortly after the success of imatinib, the receptor tyrosine–kinase FLT3 emerged as a compelling drug candidate based on the presence of activating mutations in about one-third of patients with acute myeloid leukemia.[63] Laboratory studies documented that FLT3 alleles bearing these mutations, which occur as internal tandem duplications (ITD) of the juxtamembrane domain or a point mutation in the kinase domain, function as driver oncogenes in mouse models, giving phenotypes analogous to BCR-ABL.[64] As with RET in thyroid cancer, no compounds had been specifically optimized to target FLT3, but several drugs with off-target FLT3 activity were redirected to acute myeloid leukemia (AML).

Disappointingly, the first three of the compounds tested (midostaurin, lestaurtinib, and sunitinib) showed only marginal single-agent activity in relapsed AML patients, even in those with FLT3 mutations.[65-67] Despite the strong molecular rationale for FLT3 as a driver lesion, questions were raised about the viability of FLT3 as a drug target. Pharmacodynamic studies showed evidence of FLT3 kinase inhibition in tumor cells, but the magnitude and duration of these effects were difficult to quantify, raising the possibility of inadequate target inhibition.[65] Indeed, the dose of all three compounds was limited by toxicities believed to be independent of FLT3. A more pessimistic interpretation was that FLT3, although presumably important for the initiation of AML, was no longer required for tumor maintenance due to the accumulation of additional driver genomic alterations. If true, even a complete FLT3 blockade with a highly selective inhibitor would be expected to fail. But this view was not supported by the fact that clinical responses were observed in the somewhat analogous situation of single-agent ABL kinase inhibitor treatment of CML in blast crisis, where BCR-ABL is just one of many additional genomic alterations that contribute to disease progression, yet complete remissions are observed in many patients.

Despite this pessimism about FLT3 as a viable drug target, several drugs are now advancing toward drug registration trials. Midostaurin, one of the early compounds that showed disappointing single-agent activity in relapsed AML, is being evaluated in a randomized phase III trial in newly diagnosed AML combined with standard induction chemotherapy. A single-arm phase II study showed higher and more durable remission rates in FLT3 mutant patients when compared to historical controls.[68] The second compound, quizartinib (AC220), is a next-generation FLT3 inhibitor with greater potency and specificity and with single-agent activity in FLT3 mutant relapsed AML—precisely the population where midostaurin and others failed.[69,70] The fact that some responder patients have relapsed with drug-resistant gatekeeper mutations in the FLT3 kinase domain provides formal proof that FLT3 is the relevant target.[71] Assuming these compounds prove successful in AML, it will be important to examine their activity in the rare cases of pediatric acute lymphoid leukemia associated with FLT3 mutation. Although the jury is still out on FLT3 inhibitors, the failure of early compounds in AML is reminiscent of the failures of early RAF and MEK inhibitors in melanoma. Collectively, these examples emphasize the importance of using optimized compounds to test a molecularly based hypothesis in patients and to focus enrollment on those patients with the relevant molecular lesion.

Kidney Cancer: Targeting the Tumor and the Host With Mammalian Target of Rapamycin and VEGF Receptor Inhibitors

A recurring theme in this chapter is the critical role of driver kinase mutations in guiding the development of kinase inhibitors. Ironically, several kinase inhibitors have been approved for kidney cancer over the past 5 years in a tumor type with no known kinase mutations. The most common molecular alteration in kidney cancer is a loss of function in the Von Hippel-Lindau (VHL) tumor suppressor gene, resulting in the activation of the hypoxia inducible factor[68] pathway.[72] As a consequence of VHL loss, which normally targets hypoxia-inducible factor (HIF) proteins for proteasomal degradation, HIF-1α and HIF-2α are constitutively active transcription factors that function as oncogenes through activation of an array of downstream target genes. Among these is the angiogenesis factor VEGF, which is secreted by HIF-expressing cells and promotes the development and maintenance of tumor neovasculature. HIF-mediated secretion of VEGF by tumor cells likely explains the highly vascular histopathology of clear cell renal carcinoma. All three currently approved angiogenesis inhibitors (the monoclonal antibody bevacizumab targeting VEGF and the kinase inhibitors sorafenib and sunitinib targeting or its receptor VEGF receptor) have single-agent clinical activity in clear cell carcinoma.[73-75] The high specificity of bevacizumab for VEGF leaves little doubt that the activity of this drug is explained by antiangiogenic effects. In contrast, the off-target activities of sorafenib and sunitinib include several kinases expressed in kidney tumor cells, stroma, and inflammatory cells (PDGFR, RAF, RET, FLT3, and others). Interestingly, the primary effect of bevacizumab in kidney cancer is disease stabilization, whereas sorafenib and sunitinib have substantial partial response rates. This raises the question of whether the superior antitumor activity of the VEGF receptor kinase inhibitors is due to the concurrent inhibition of other kinases. However, partial responses rates with next-generation VEGF receptor inhibitors (axitinib, pazopanib, and tivozanib), all of which have greater potency and selectivity for the VEGF receptor, are similarly high, and reinforce the importance of the VEGF receptor as the critical target in kidney cancer.[76-78] Pazopanib is approved for advanced kidney cancer, whereas axitinib is approved as second-line therapy.

Two inhibitors of the mammalian target of rapamycin (mTOR) kinase (temsirolimus and everolimus) are also approved for advanced renal cell carcinoma.[79,80] Both temsirolimus and everolimus are known as rapalogs because both are chemical derivatives of the natural product sirolimus (rapamycin). Sirolimus was approved more than 10 years ago to prevent graft rejection in transplant recipients based on its immunosuppressive properties against T cells. Sirolimus also has potent antiproliferative effects against vascular endothelial cells and, on that basis, is incorporated into drug-eluting cardiac stents to prevent coronary artery restenosis following angioplasty.[81] Rapalogs differ from all the other kinase inhibitors discussed in this chapter in that they inhibit the kinase through an allosteric mechanism rather than by targeting the mTOR kinase domain. Because rapalogs also inhibit the growth of cancer cell lines from different tissues of origin, clinical trials were initiated to study their potential role as anticancer agents in a broad range of tumor types. Based on responses in a few phase I patients with different tumor types (including kidney cancer), exploratory phase II studies were conducted in several diseases. Single-agent activity of temsirolimus was observed in a phase II kidney cancer study,[82] then confirmed in a phase III registration trial.[79] The phase III everolimus trial, which was initiated after temsirolimus, was noteworthy because clinical benefit was demonstrated in patients who had progressed on the VEGF receptor inhibitors sorafenib or sunitinib.[80]

In parallel with the empirical clinical development of rapalogs, various laboratories explored the molecular basis for mTOR dependence in cancer cells. mTOR functions at the center of a complex network that integrates signals from growth factor receptors and nutrient sensors to regulate cell growth and size (Fig. 22.2). It does so, in part, by controlling the translation of various mRNAs with complex 5′ untranslated regions into protein. mTOR exists in two distinct complexes known as TOR complex 1 (TORC1) and TORC2. Rapalogs only inhibit the TORC1 complex, which is largely responsible for downstream phosphorylation of targets such as S6K1/2 and 4EBP1/2 that regulate protein translation.[83] The TORC2 complex contributes to the activation of AKT by phosphorylating the important regulatory serine residue S473 and is unaffected by rapalogs.

Two hypotheses have emerged to explain the clinical activity of rapalogs in kidney cancer. The antiproliferative activity of these compounds against endothelial cells suggests an antiangiogenic mechanism, which is consistent with the clinical activity of the VEGF receptor inhibitors. But rapalogs also inhibit the growth of kidney cancer cell lines in laboratory models where the effects on tumor angiogenesis have been eliminated. Interestingly, mRNAs for HIF1/2 are among those whose translation is impaired by rapalogs, and this effect has been implicated as the primary mechanism of rapalog activity in kidney cancer xenograft models.[84] As with the VEGF receptor inhibitors, a detailed molecular annotation of tumors from responders and nonresponders will shed light on these issues.

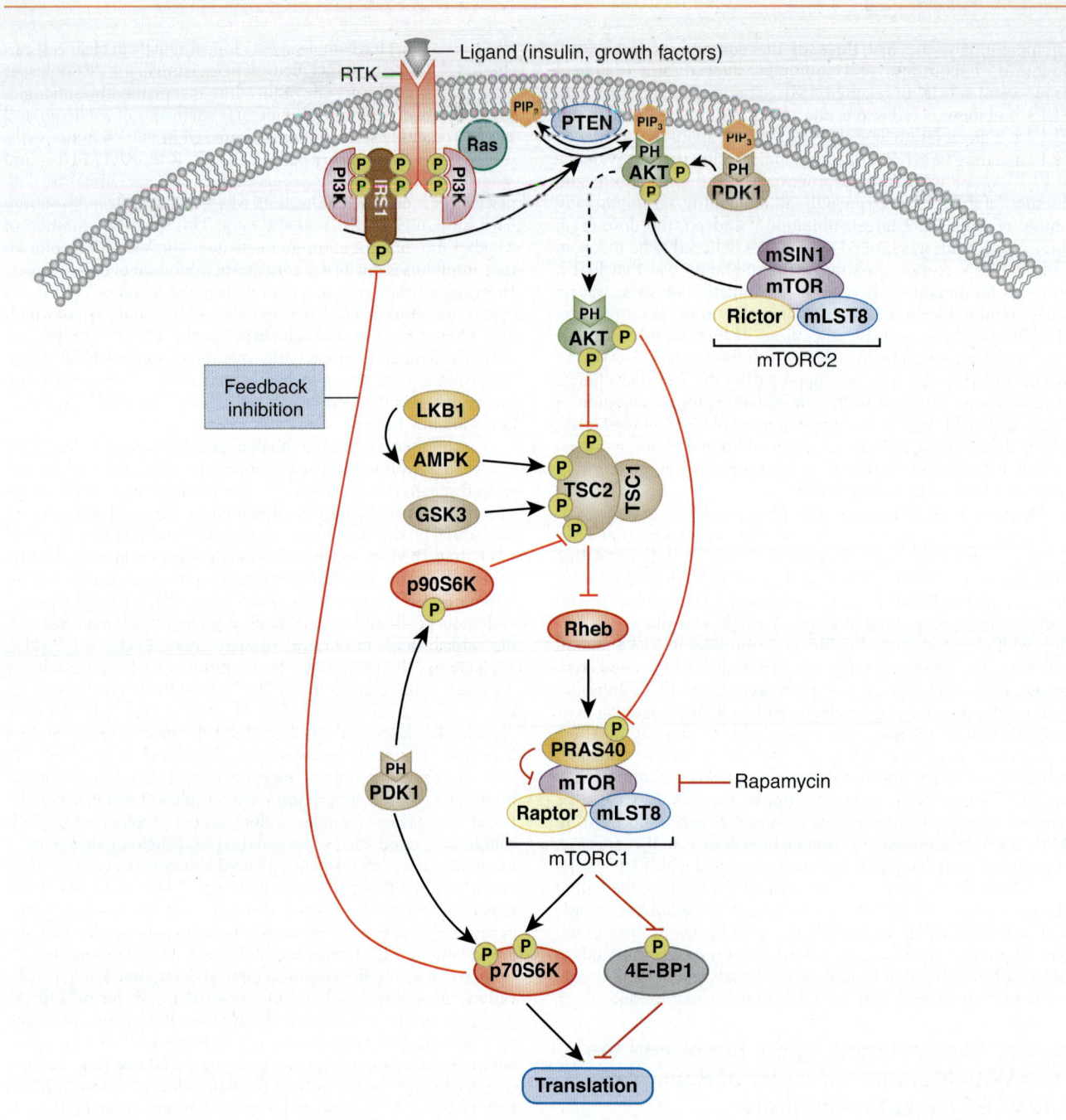

Figure 22.2 Feedback inhibition of the phosphatidylinositol 3-kinase (PI3K) pathway. Activated AKT regulates cellular growth through mammalian target of rapamycin (mTOR), a key player in protein synthesis and translation. mTOR forms part of two distinct complexes known as mTORC1, which contains mTOR, Raptor, mLST8, and PRAS40, and mTORC2, which contains mTOR, Rictor, mLST8, and mSIN1. mTORC1 is sensitive to rapamycin and controls protein synthesis and translation, at least in part, through p70S6K and eukaryotic translation initiation factor 4E–binding protein 1 (4E-BP1). AKT phosphorylates and inhibits tuberous sclerosis complex 2 (TSC2), resulting in increased mTORC1 activity. AKT also phosphorylates PRAS40, thus relieving the PRAS40 inhibitory effect on mTOR and the mTORC1 complex. mTORC2 and 3-phosphoinositide–dependent kinase (PDK1) phosphorylate AKT on Ser473 and Thr308, respectively, rendering it fully active. mTORC1-activated p70S6K can phosphorylate insulin receptor substrate 1 (IRS1), resulting in inhibition of PI3K activity. In addition, PDK1 phosphorylates and activates p70S6K and p90S6K. The latter has been shown to inhibit TSC2 activity through direct phosphorylation. Conversely, LKB1-activated AMP-activated protein kinase (AMPK) and glycogen synthase kinase 3 (GSK3) activate the TSC1/TSC2 complex through direct phosphorylation of TSC2. Thus, signals through PI3K as well as through LKB1 and AMPK converge on mTORC1. Inhibition of mTORC1 can lead to increased insulin receptor–mediated signaling, and inhibition of PDK1 may lead to activation of mTORC1 and may, paradoxically, promote tumor growth. (From Daigle SR, Olhava EJ, Therkelsen CA, et al. Selective killing of mixed lineage leukemia cells by a potent small-molecule DOT1L inhibitor. *Cancer Cell* 2011;20(1):53–65, with permission.)

Other Indications for mTOR Inhibitors: Breast Cancer and Tuberous Sclerosis Complex Mutant Cancers

Two other indications for mTOR have emerged, both based on fundamental insights from laboratory studies but from quite different angles. Preclinical studies of estrogen receptor (ER) therapy in breast cancer suggested that phosphatidylinositol 3-kinase (PI3K) pathway activation may be a mechanism of resistance and that this resistance could be prevented or overcome by combined treatment with ER-based drugs and rapalogs such as everolimus. Based on evidence that some women with progressive disease while receiving the aromatase inhibitor letrozole have clinical benefit from the addition of everolimus, randomized trials were initiated comparing everolimus + exemestane to exemestane alone (called BOLERO-2), or everolimus + tamoxifen to tamoxifen alone (called TAMRAD). Both studies demonstrated substantial improvements in time to progression in women with metastatic breast cancer who had already failed one aromatase inhibitor,[85,86] resulting in FDA approval of the everolimus/exemestane combination. Evidence of cross-talk between the PI3K pathway and hormone receptor signaling (ER in breast cancer, androgen receptor in prostate cancer) provides a molecular rationale for the clinical benefit of combination therapy and is currently under investigation in metastatic prostate cancer.[87]

Yet another indication for rapalog therapy emerged from the genetics of children with tuberous sclerosis caused by a loss of function mutations in tuberous sclerosis complex 1 (TSC1) or TSC2, which encode the proteins hamartin and tuberin that function in the PI3K signaling pathway just upstream of mTOR. Based on laboratory studies showing that TSC1- or TSC2-deficient cells are exquisitely sensitive to rapalogs, a clinical trial was conducted in tuberous sclerosis patients with benign subependymal giant-cell astrocytomas (SEGA) that showed tumor shrinkage in 21 of 28 patients.[88] This genetic dependence on mTOR in tumors with tuberous sclerosis complex (TSC) loss has also been observed in bladder cancer. In a remarkable example of the power of comprehensive DNA sequencing to provide insight into rare clinical phenotypes, investigators examined the tumor genome of the single complete responder patient on a phase II trial of everolimus in bladder cancer and discovered somatic mutations in TSC2 as well as a second gene, NF2, that also controls mTOR activity.[89] This plus other examples of how a retrospective genomic analysis of *extraordinary responders* has led to a national effort to capture these cases, as well as prospective clinical trials of patients with the relevant tumor genotype regardless of histology (called *basket* trials).

It is unclear why rapalogs have failed in other tumor types. One explanation is the concurrence of PI3K pathway mutations with alterations in other pathways that mitigate sensitivity to rapalogs. Another possibility is the disruption of negative feedback loops regulated by mTOR that inhibit signaling from upstream receptor tyrosine kinases. Rapalogs paradoxically *increase* signaling through PI3K due to loss of this negative feedback. A primary consequence is *increased* AKT activation, which signals to an array of downstream substrates that can enhance cell proliferation and survival (other than TORC1, which remains inhibited by rapalog) (see Fig. 22.2). This problem might be overcome by combining rapalogs with an inhibitor of an upstream kinase in the feedback loop, such as HER kinases or the insulinlike growth factor receptor (IGFR), to block this undesired effect of rapalogs on PI3K activation.[90]

DIRECTLY TARGETING THE PI3K PATHWAY

Mutations or copy number alterations (e.g., amplification or deletion of oncogenes or tumor suppressor genes) in PI3K pathway genes (PIK3CA, PIK3R1, PTEN, AKT1, and others) are among the most common abnormalities in cancer. Consequently, intensive efforts at many pharmaceutical companies have been devoted to the discovery of small-molecule inhibitors targeting kinases in the PI3K pathway. Inhibitors of PI3K, AKT, and ATP-competitive (rather than allosteric) inhibitors of mTOR that target both the TORC1 and TORC2 complex are all in clinical development. Phase I clinical trials have, in general, established that the pathway can be efficiently targeted without serious toxicity other than easily manageable effects on glucose metabolism (which is anticipated based on the importance of PI3K signaling in insulin signaling). Unfortunately, there has been no evidence to date of dramatic single-agent clinical activity with any of these agents, although early results with PI3K alpha selective inhibitor BYL719 in PIK3CA mutant breast cancer appear promising.[91]

However, the first approval of a direct PI3K inhibitor in cancer is likely to come in chronic lymphocytic leukemia and in lymphoma, but not on the basis of tumor genomics. Normal and malignant B cells are dependent on PI3K delta as well as Bruton tyrosine kinase (BTK) for proliferation and survival, raising the possibility that inhibitors of these kinases might be broadly active in B-cell malignancies. Concerns about toxicity on normal B cells were alleviated, in part, by the earlier clinical success of the CD20 antibody rituximab in lymphoma, which also eliminates normal circulating B cells, but without significant clinical sequelae. The first such PI3K delta inhibitor, idelalisib, has shown impressive activity in indolent non-Hodgkin lymphoma as a single agent and in relapsed chronic lymphocytic leukemia when given in combination with rituximab. The BTK inhibitor ibrutinib, following a similar clinical development path, was recently approved as second-line therapy for chronic lymphocytic leukemia and for mantle cell lymphoma.[92,93]

COMBINATIONS OF KINASE INHIBITORS TO INDUCT RESPONSE AND PREVENT RESISTANCE

Preclinical studies indicate that combinations of kinase inhibitors are required to realize their full potential as anticancer agents. The most common rationale is to address the problem of concurrent mutations in different pathways that alleviate dependence on a single-driver oncogene. The best examples are cancers with mutations in both the RAS/MAP kinase pathway (RAS or BRAF) and the PI3K pathway (PIK3CA or PTEN). In mouse models, such doubly mutant tumors fail to respond to single-agent treatment with either an AKT inhibitor or a MEK inhibitor. However, combination treatment can give dramatic regressions.[94] Similarly, genetically engineered mice that develop KRAS-driven lung cancer respond only to combination therapy with a PI3K inhibitor and a MEK inhibitor.[95] To date, clinical trials combining different PI3K pathway and RAS/MAP kinase pathway inhibitors have been challenging due to toxicities associated with continuous, concurrent PI3K and RAS/MAP kinase pathway inhibition.

Many of the tumor types discussed in this chapter *do* respond to treatment with a single-agent kinase, but relapse despite continued inhibitor therapy. Research into the causes of "acquired" kinase inhibitor resistance has revealed two primary mechanisms: (1) novel mutations in the kinase domain of the drug target that preclude inhibition, or (2) *bypass* of the driver kinase signal by activation of a parallel kinase pathway. In both cases, the solution is combination therapy to prevent the emergence of resistance. An elegant demonstration of this approach comes from CML where resistance to imatinib is primarily caused by mutations in the BCR-ABL kinase domain.[96,97] The second-generation ABL inhibitors dasatinib and nilotinib are effective against most imatinib-resistant BCR-ABL mutants and were initially approved as single-agent therapy for imatinib-resistant CML.[98,99] Very recently, both drugs have proven superior to imatinib in the upfront treatment of CML due to increased potency and fewer mechanisms of acquired resistance.[100–102] However, one BCR-ABL mutation called T315I is resistant to all three drugs. The third-generation ABL kinase inhibitor ponatinib blocks T315I and showed activity in a phase II clinical trial that included CML patients with the T315I mutation,[103] resulting in FDA approval. However, subsequent reports of severe vascular occlusive events, such as stroke and heart failure, led to withdrawal from the market, followed by approval for restricted use in T315I-mutant patients. Analogous approaches are ongoing in other diseases such as EGFR-mutant lung cancer, where acquired resistance to the frontline kinase inhibitor is also associated with mutations in the target kinase.[104,105] Promising clinical results have been reported with irreversible EGFR inhibitors such as CO-1686 and AZD9291.

The clinical development of kinase inhibitor combinations to prevent acquired resistance is relatively straightforward. Because the frontline drug is already approved, success would be determined by an improvement in response duration using the combination. The situation is more complex when two experimental compounds (e.g., a PI3K pathway inhibitor and a MEK inhibitor) are combined, neither of which shows significant single-agent activity. Older regulatory guidelines required a four-arm study that compared each single agent to the combination and to a control group in order to obtain approval of the combination. Recognizing that this design could discourage drug developers as well as patients from moving forward because it requires a large sample size, the FDA has issued new guidelines for the development of novel combinations that require a two-arm registration study comparing the combination to standard of care http://www.fda.gov/downloads/Drugs/GuidanceComplianceRegulatoryInformation/Guidances/UCM236669.pdf. A more challenging issue may be dose optimization and dose schedule that is needed to safely combine two investigational drugs. Much like the development of combination chemotherapy several decades ago, it may be important to select compounds with nonoverlapping toxicities to allow for sufficient doses of each drug to be achieved.

SPECULATIONS ON THE FUTURE ROLE OF KINASE INHIBITORS IN CANCER MEDICINE

The role of genomics in predicting a response to kinase inhibitor therapy is now irrefutable. As the number of kinase driver mutations continues to grow, the field is likely to move away from the current strategy of a *companion diagnostic* for each drug. Rather, comprehensive mutational profiling platforms that query each tumor for hundreds of potential cancer mutations are more likely to emerge as the diagnostic platform. The number of directly *actionable* mutations (meaning the presence of a mutation defines a treatment decision supported by clinical trial data) remains low, but this number will undoubtedly grow. In addition, it is becoming apparent that many patients have rare mutations (defined as rare in that histologic tumor type) but are, in theory, actionable. Because these examples are unlikely to be formally evaluated in clinical trials, many centers have opened *basket* studies (with eligibility based solely on mutation profile) to capture these cases with some reports of remarkable success.

More effort must be devoted to manipulating the dose and schedule of kinase inhibitor therapy to maximize efficacy and minimize toxicity. To date, all kinase inhibitors have been developed based on the assumption that a 24/7 coverage of the target is required for efficacy. Consequently, most compounds are optimized to have a long serum half-life (12 to 24 hours). Phase II doses are then selected based on the maximum tolerated dose determined with daily administration. But a recent clinical of the ABL inhibitor dasatinib in CML indicates that equivalent antitumor activity can be achieved with intermittent therapy.[106] By giving larger doses intermittently, higher peak drug concentrations were achieved that resulted in equivalent and possibly superior efficacy.[107] Similar results were observed in laboratory studies of EGFR inhibitors in EGFR-mutant lung cancer. Clinically robust, quantitative assays of target inhibition are needed to hasten progress in this area.

Although the focus of this chapter is kinase inhibitors, the themes developed here should apply broadly to inhibitors of other cancer targets. Inhibitors of the G-protein coupled receptor smoothened (SMO) in patients with metastatic basal cell carcinoma or medulloblastoma establish that the driver mutation hypothesis extends beyond kinase inhibitors. SMO is a component in the Hedgehog pathway, which is constitutively activated in subsets of patients with basal cell carcinoma and medulloblastoma due to mutations in the Hedgehog ligand-binding receptor Patched-1. Treatment with the SMO inhibitor vismodegib led to impressive responses in basal cell carcinoma and medulloblastoma patients whose tumors had Patched-1 mutations,[108,109] resulting in FDA approval. Other novel cancer targets are emerging from cancer genome sequencing projects. Somatic mutations in the Krebs cycle enzyme isocitrate dehydrogenase (IDH1/2) were found in subsets of patients with glioblastoma, AML, chondrosarcoma, and cholangiocarcinoma,[110–112] and the first IDH2 inhibitor has entered clinical trials in leukemia. Mutations in enzymes involved in chromatin remodeling, such as the histone methyltransferase EZH2, have been reported in lymphoma and have spurred the ongoing development of EZH2 inhibitors.[113,114] Inhibitors of another histone methyltransferase DOT1L, which is required for the maintenance of mixed lineage leukemia (MLL) fusion leukemias, are also in clinical development.[115,116] Kinase inhibitors are just the first wave of molecularly targeted drugs ushered in by our understanding of the molecular underpinnings of cancer cells. There is much more to follow.

REFERENCES

1. Sawyers CL. Shifting paradigms: the seeds of oncogene addiction. *Nat Med* 2009;15(10):1158–1161.
2. Weinstein IB. Cancer. Addiction to oncogenes—the Achilles heal of cancer. *Science* 2002;297(5578):63–64.
3. Druker BJ, Talpaz M, Resta DJ, et al., Efficacy and safety of a specific inhibitor of the BCR-ABL tyrosine kinase in chronic myeloid leukemia. *N Engl J Med* 2001;344(14):1031–1037.
4. Hirota S, Isozaki K, Moriyama Y, et al. Gain-of-function mutations of c-kit in human gastrointestinal stromal tumors. *Science* 1998;279(5350):577–580.
5. Heinrich MC, Corless CL, Duensing A, et al. PDGFRA activating mutations in gastrointestinal stromal tumors. *Science* 2003;299(5607):708–710.
6. Demetri GD, von Mehren M, Blanke CD, et al. Efficacy and safety of imatinib mesylate in advanced gastrointestinal stromal tumors. *N Engl J Med* 2002;347(7):472–480.
7. Geyer CE, Forster J, Lindquist D, et al. Lapatinib plus capecitabine for HER2-positive advanced breast cancer. *N Engl J Med* 2006;355(26):2733–2743.
8. Kris MG, Natale RB, Herbst RS, et al. Efficacy of gefitinib, an inhibitor of the epidermal growth factor receptor tyrosine kinase, in symptomatic patients with non-small cell lung cancer: a randomized trial. *JAMA* 2003;290(16):2149–2158.
9. Miller VA, Kris MG, Shah N, et al. Bronchioloalveolar pathologic subtype and smoking history predict sensitivity to gefitinib in advanced non-small-cell lung cancer. *J Clin Oncol* 2004;22(6):1103–1109.
10. Paez JG, Jänne PA, Lee JC, et al. EGFR mutations in lung cancer: correlation with clinical response to gefitinib therapy. *Science* 2004;304(5676):1497–1500.
11. Lynch TJ, Bell DW, Sordella R, et al. Activating mutations in the epidermal growth factor receptor underlying responsiveness of non-small-cell lung cancer to gefitinib. *N Engl J Med* 2004;350(21):2129–2139.
12. Pao W, Miller V, Zakowski M, et al. EGF receptor gene mutations are common in lung cancers from "never smokers" and are associated with sensitivity of tumors to gefitinib and erlotinib. *Proc Natl Acad Sci U S A* 2004;101(36):13306–13311.
13. Cohen MH, Williams GA, Sridhara R, et al. FDA drug approval summary: gefitinib (ZD1839) (Iressa) tablets. *Oncologist* 2003;8(4):303–306.
14. Shepherd FA, Rodrigues Pereira J, Ciuleanu T, et al. Erlotinib in previously treated non-small-cell lung cancer. *N Engl J Med* 2005;353(2):123–132.

15. Thatcher N, Chang A, Parikh P, et al. Gefitinib plus best supportive care in previously treated patients with refractory advanced non-small-cell lung cancer: results from a randomised, placebo-controlled, multicentre study (Iressa Survival Evaluation in Lung Cancer). *Lancet* 2005;366(9496):1527–1537.
16. Herbst RS, Giaccone G, Schiller JH, et al. Gefitinib in combination with paclitaxel and carboplatin in advanced non-small-cell lung cancer: a phase III trial—INTACT 2. *J Clin Oncol* 2004;22(5):785–794.
17. Giaccone G, Herbst RS, Manegold C, et al. Gefitinib in combination with gemcitabine and cisplatin in advanced non-small-cell lung cancer: a phase III trial—INTACT 1. *J Clin Oncol* 2004;22(5):777–784.
18. Herbst RS, Prager D, Hermann R, et al. TRIBUTE: a phase III trial of erlotinib hydrochloride (OSI-774) combined with carboplatin and paclitaxel chemotherapy in advanced non-small-cell lung cancer. *J Clin Oncol* 2005;23(25):5892–5899.
19. Tsao MS, Sakurada A, Cutz JC, et al. Erlotinib in lung cancer - molecular and clinical predictors of outcome. *N Engl J Med* 2005;353(2):133–144.
20. Mok TS, Wu YL, Thongprasert S, et al. Gefitinib or carboplatin-paclitaxel in pulmonary adenocarcinoma. *N Engl J Med* 2009;361(10):947–957.
21. Schaller JL, Burkland GA. Case report: rapid and complete control of idiopathic hypereosinophilia with imatinib mesylate. *MedGenMed* 2001;3(5):9.
22. Ault P, Cortes J, Koller C, et al. Response of idiopathic hypereosinophilic syndrome to treatment with imatinib mesylate. *Leuk Res* 2002;26(9):881–884.
23. Cools J, DeAngelo DJ, Gotlib J, et al. A tyrosine kinase created by fusion of the PDGFRA and FIP1L1 genes as a therapeutic target of imatinib in idiopathic hypereosinophilic syndrome. *N Engl J Med* 2003;348(13):1201–1214.
24. Golub TR, Barker GF, Lovett M, et al. Fusion of PDGF receptor beta to a novel ets-like gene, tel, in chronic myelomonocytic leukemia with t(5;12) chromosomal translocation. *Cell* 1994;77(2):307–316.
25. Apperley JF, Gardembas M, Melo JV, et al. Response to imatinib mesylate in patients with chronic myeloproliferative diseases with rearrangements of the platelet-derived growth factor receptor beta. *N Engl J Med* 2002;347(7):481–487.
26. Rutkowski P, Van Glabbeke M, Rankin CJ, et al. Imatinib mesylate in advanced dermatofibrosarcoma protuberans: pooled analysis of two phase II clinical trials. *J Clin Oncol* 2010;28(10):1772–1779.
27. Davies H, Bignell GR, Cox C, et al. Mutations of the BRAF gene in human cancer. *Nature* 2002;417(6892):949–954.
28. Baxter EJ, Scott LM, Campbell PJ, et al., Acquired mutation of the tyrosine kinase JAK2 in human myeloproliferative disorders. *Lancet* 2005;365(9464):1054–1061.
29. James C, Ugo V, Le Couédic JP, et al. A unique clonal JAK2 mutation leading to constitutive signalling causes polycythaemia vera. *Nature* 2005;434(7037):1144–1148.
30. Levine RL, Wadleigh M, Cools J, et al. Activating mutation in the tyrosine kinase JAK2 in polycythemia vera, essential thrombocythemia, and myeloid metaplasia with myelofibrosis. *Cancer Cell* 2005;7(4):387–397.
31. Samuels Y, Wang Z, Bardelli A, et al. High frequency of mutations of the PIK3CA gene in human cancers. *Science* 2004;304(5670):554.
32. International Cancer Genome Consortium, Hudson TJ, Anderson W, et al. International network of cancer genome projects. *Nature* 2010;464(7291):993–998.
33. Vogelstein B, Papadopoulos N, Velculescu VE, et al. Cancer genome landscapes. *Science* 2013;339(6127):1546–1558.
34. Lawrence MS, Stojanov P, Mermel CH, et al. Discovery and saturation analysis of cancer genes across 21 tumour types. *Nature* 2014;505(7484):495–501.
35. Eisen T, Ahmad T, Flaherty KT, et al. Sorafenib in advanced melanoma: a Phase II randomised discontinuation trial analysis. *Br J Cancer* 2006;95(5):581–586.
36. Solit DB, Garraway LA, Pratilas CA, et al. BRAF mutation predicts sensitivity to MEK inhibition. *Nature* 2006;439(7074):358–362.
37. McDermott U, Sharma SV, Dowell L, et al. Identification of genotype-correlated sensitivity to selective kinase inhibitors by using high-throughput tumor cell line profiling. *Proc Natl Acad Sci U S A* 2007;104(50):19936–19941.
38. Pratilas CA, Taylor BS, Ye Q, et al. (V600E)BRAF is associated with disabled feedback inhibition of RAF-MEK signaling and elevated transcriptional output of the pathway. *Proc Natl Acad Sci U S A* 2009;106(11):4519–4524.
39. LoRusso PM, Krishnamurthi SS, Rinehart JJ, et al. Phase I pharmacokinetic and pharmacodynamic study of the oral MAPK/ERK kinase inhibitor PD-0325901 in patients with advanced cancers. *Clin Cancer Res* 2010;16(6):1924–1937.
40. Adjei AA, Cohen RB, Franklin W, et al. Phase I pharmacokinetic and pharmacodynamic study of the oral, small-molecule mitogen-activated protein kinase kinase 1/2 inhibitor AZD6244 (ARRY-142886) in patients with advanced cancers. *J Clin Oncol* 2008;26(13):2139–2146.
41. Dummer R, Chapman PB, Sosman JA, et al. AZD6244 (ARRY-142886) vs temozolomide (TMZ) in patients (pts) with advanced melanoma: An open-label, randomized, multicenter, phase II study. *J Clin Oncol* 2008;26(May 20 suppl):9033.
42. Flaherty KT, Robert C, Hersey P, et al. Improved survival with MEK inhibition in BRAF-mutated melanoma. *N Engl J Med* 2012;367(2):107–114.
43. Joseph EW, Pratillas CA, Poulikakos PI, et al. The RAF inhibitor PLX4032 inhibits ERK signaling and tumor cell proliferation in a V600E BRAF-selective manner. *Proc Natl Acad Sci U S A* 2010;107(33):14903–14908.
44. Flaherty K, Puzanov I, Sosman J, et al. Phase I study of PLX4032: proof of concept for V600E BRAF mutation as a therapeutic target in human cancer. *J Clin Oncol* 2009;27(15s):abstract 9000.
45. Flaherty KT, Puzanov I, Kim KB, et al. Inhibition of mutated, activated BRAF in metastatic melanoma. *N Engl J Med* 2010;363(9):809–819.
46. Bollag G, Hirth P, Tsai J, et al. Clinical efficacy of a RAF inhibitor needs broad target blockade in BRAF-mutant melanoma. *Nature* 2010;467(7315):596–599.
47. Hauschild A, Grob JJ, Demidov LV, et al. Dabrafenib in BRAF-mutated metastatic melanoma: a multicentre, open-label, phase 3 randomised controlled trial. *Lancet* 2012;380(9839):358–365.
48. Kwak EL, Camidge DR, Clark J, et al. Clinical activity observed in a phase I dose escalation trial of an oral c-MET and ALK inhibitor, PF-02341066. *J Clin Oncol* 2009;27(Suppl):148s.
49. Morris SW, Kirstein MN, Valentine MB, et al. Fusion of a kinase gene, ALK, to a nucleolar protein gene, NPM, in non-Hodgkin's lymphoma. *Science* 1994;263(5151):1281–1284.
50. Soda M, Choi YL, Enomoto M, et al. Identification of the transforming EML4-ALK fusion gene in non small cell lung cancer. *Nature* 2007;448(7153):561–566.
51. Bang Y, Kwak EL, Shaw AT, et al. Clinical activity of the oral ALK inhibitor PF-02341066 in ALK-positive patients with non-small cell lung cancer (NSCLC). *J Clin Oncol* 2010;28:18s.
52. Shaw AT, Kim DW, Nakagawa K, et al. Crizotinib versus chemotherapy in advanced ALK-positive lung cancer. *N Engl J Med* 2013;368(25):2385–2394.
53. Chen Y, Takita J, Choi YL, et al. Oncogenic mutations of ALK kinase in neuroblastoma. *Nature* 2008;455(7215):971–974.
54. Sirvent N, Hawkins AL, Moeglin D, et al. ALK probe rearrangement in a t(2;11;2)(p23;p15;q31) translocation found in a prenatal myofibroblastic fibrous lesion: toward a molecular definition of an inflammatory myofibroblastic tumor family? *Genes Chromosomes Cancer* 2001;31(1):85–90.
55. Fagin JA, Mitsiades N. Molecular pathology of thyroid cancer: diagnostic and clinical implications. *Best Pract Res Clin Endocrinol Metab* 2008;22(6):955–969.
56. Wells SA Jr, Gosnell JE, Gagel RF, et al. Vandetanib for the treatment of patients with locally advanced or metastatic hereditary medullary thyroid cancer. *J Clin Oncol* 28(5):767–772.
57. Lam ET, Ringel MD, Kloos RT, et al. Phase II clinical trial of sorafenib in metastatic medullary thyroid cancer. *J Clin Oncol* 28(14):2323–2330.
58. Kloos RT, Ringel MD, Knopp MV, et al. Phase II trial of sorafenib in metastatic thyroid cancer. *J Clin Oncol* 2009;27(10):1675–1684.
59. Schlumberger MJ, Elisei R, Bastholt L, et al. Phase II study of safety and efficacy of motesanib in patients with progressive or symptomatic, advanced or metastatic medullary thyroid cancer. *J Clin Oncol* 2009;27(23):3794–3801.
60. Kurzrock R, Cohen EE, Sherman SI, et al. Long-term results in a cohort of medullary thyroid cancer (MTC) patients (pts) in a phase I study of XL184 (BMS 907351), an oral inhibitor of MET, VEGFR2, and RET. *J Clin Oncol* 2010;28(Suppl):15s.
61. Wells SA Jr, Robinson BG, Gagel RF, et al. Vandetanib in patients with locally advanced or metastatic medullary thyroid cancer: a randomized, double-blind phase III trial. *J Clin Oncol* 2012;30(2):134–141.
62. Elisei R, Schlumberger MJ, Müller SP, et al. Cabozantinib in progressive medullary thyroid cancer. *J Clin Oncol* 2013;31(29):3639–3646.
63. Sawyers CL. Finding the next Gleevec: FLT3 targeted kinase inhibitor therapy for acute myeloid leukemia. *Cancer Cell* 2002;1(5):413–415.
64. Kelly LM, Qing L, Jeffery L, et al. FLT3 internal tandem duplication mutations associated with human acute myeloid leukemias induce myeloproliferative disease in a murine bone marrow transplant model. *Blood* 2002;99(1):310–318.
65. Stone RM, DeAngelo DJ, Klimek V, et al. Patients with acute myeloid leukemia and an activating mutation in FLT3 respond to a small-molecule FLT3 tyrosine kinase inhibitor, PKC412. *Blood* 2005;105(1):54–60.
66. Knapper S, Burnett AK, Littlewood T, et al. A phase 2 trial of the FLT3 inhibitor lestaurtinib (CEP701) as first-line treatment for older patients with acute myeloid leukemia not considered fit for intensive chemotherapy. *Blood* 2006;108(10):3262–3270.
67. Fiedler W, Serve H, Döhner H, et al. A phase 1 study of SU11248 in the treatment of patients with refractory or resistant acute myeloid leukemia (AML) or not amenable to conventional therapy for the disease. *Blood* 2005;105(3):986–993.
68. Stone RM, Fischer T, Paquette R, et al. A Phase 1b study of midostaurin (PKC412) in combination with daunorubicin and cytarabine induction and high-dose cytarabine consolidation in patients under age 61 with newly diagnosed de novo acute myeloid leukemia: overall survival of patients whose blasts have FLT3 mutations is similar to those with wild-type FLT3. Paper presented at: 2009 American Society of Hematology Annual Meeting; 2009; New Orleans, LA.
69. Zarrinkar PP, Gunawardane RN, Cramer MD, et al. AC220 is a uniquely potent and selective inhibitor of FLT3 for the treatment of acute myeloid leukemia (AML). *Blood* 2009;114(14):2984–2992.
70. Cortes J, et al. AC220, a potent, selective, second generation FLT3 receptor tyrosine kinase (RTK) inhibitor, in a first-in-human (FIH) phase 1 AML study. Paper presented at: 2009 American Society of Hematology Annual Meeting; 2009; New Orleans, LA.
71. Smith CC, Wang Q, Chin CS, et al. Validation of ITD mutations in FLT3 as a therapeutic target in human acute myeloid leukaemia. *Nature* 2012;485(7397):260–263.
72. Kaelin WG Jr. The von Hippel-Lindau tumour suppressor protein: O2 sensing and cancer. *Nat Rev Cancer* 2008;8(11):865–873.
73. Yang JC, Haworth L, Sherry RM, et al. A randomized trial of bevacizumab, an anti-vascular endothelial growth factor antibody, for metastatic renal cancer. *N Engl J Med* 2003;349(5):427–434.

74. Escudier B, Eisen T, Stadler WM, et al. Sorafenib in advanced clear-cell renal-cell carcinoma. *N Engl J Med* 2007;356(2):125–134.
75. Motzer RJ, Hutson TE, Tomczak P, et al. Sunitinib versus interferon alfa in metastatic renal-cell carcinoma. *N Engl J Med* 2007;356(2):115–124.
76. Rini BI, Wilding G, Hudes G, et al. Phase II study of axitinib in sorafenib refractory metastatic renal cell carcinoma. *J Clin Oncol* 2009;27(27):4462–4468.
77. Sonpavde G, Hutson TE, Sternberg CN. Pazopanib, a potent orally administered small-molecule multitargeted tyrosine kinase inhibitor for renal cell carcinoma. *Expert Opin Investig Drugs* 2008;17(2):253–261.
78. Bhargava P, Esteves B, Al-Adhami M, et al. Activity of tivozanib (AV-951) in patients with renal cell carcinoma (RCC): Subgroup analysis from a phase II randomized discontinuation trial (RDT). *J Clin Oncol* 2010;28(suppl):15s.
79. Hudes G, Carducci M, Tomczak P, et al. Temsirolimus, interferon alfa, or both for advanced renal-cell carcinoma. *N Engl J Med* 2007;356(22):2271–2281.
80. Motzer RJ, Escudier B, Oudard S, et al. Efficacy of everolimus in advanced renal cell carcinoma: a double-blind, randomised, placebo-controlled phase III trial. *Lancet* 2008;372(9637):449–456.
81. McKeage K, Murdoch D, Goa FL. The sirolimus-eluting stent: a review of its use in the treatment of coronary artery disease. *Am J Cardiovasc Drugs* 2003;3(3):211–230.
82. Atkins MB, Hidalgo M, Stadler WM, et al. Randomized phase II study of multiple dose levels of CCI-779, a novel mammalian target of rapamycin kinase inhibitor, in patients with advanced refractory renal cell carcinoma. *J Clin Oncol* 2004;22(5):909–918.
83. Guertin DA, Sabatini DM. Defining the role of mTOR in cancer. *Cancer Cell* 2007;12(1):9–22.
84. Thomas GV, Tran C, Mellinghoff IK, et al. Hypoxia-inducible factor determines sensitivity to inhibitors of mTOR in kidney cancer. *Nat Med* 2006;12(1):122–127.
85. Bachelot T, Bourgier C, Cropet C, et al. Randomized phase II trial of everolimus in combination with tamoxifen in patients with hormone receptor-positive, human epidermal growth factor receptor 2-negative metastatic breast cancer with prior exposure to aromatase inhibitors: a GINECO study. *J Clin Oncol* 2012;30(22):2718–2724.
86. Baselga J, Campone M, Piccart M, et al. Everolimus in postmenopausal hormone-receptor-positive advanced breast cancer. *N Engl J Med* 2012;366(6):520–529.
87. Carver BS, Chapinski C, Wongvipat J, et al. Reciprocal feedback regulation of PI3K and androgen receptor signaling in PTEN-deficient prostate cancer. *Cancer Cell* 2011;19(5):575–586.
88. Krueger DA, Care MM, Holland K, et al. Everolimus for subependymal giant-cell astrocytomas in tuberous sclerosis. *N Engl J Med* 2010;363(19):1801–1811.
89. Iyer G, Hanrahan AL, Milowsky MI, et al. Genome sequencing identifies a basis for everolimus sensitivity. *Science* 2012;338(6104):221.
90. O'Reilly KE, Rojo F, She QB, et al. mTOR inhibition induces upstream receptor tyrosine kinase signaling and activates Akt. *Cancer Res* 2006;66(3):1500–1508.
91. Gonzalez-Angulo AM, Juric D, Argilis G, et al. Safety, pharmacokinetics, and preliminary activity of the alpha-specific PI3K inhibitor BYL719: results from the first-in-human study. *J Clin Oncol* 2013;31(15 Suppl):2531.
92. Byrd JC, Furman RR, Coutre SE, et al. Targeting BTK with ibrutinib in relapsed chronic lymphocytic leukemia. *N Engl J Med* 2013;369(1):32–42.
93. Wang ML, Rule S, Martin P, et al. Targeting BTK with ibrutinib in relapsed or refractory mantle-cell lymphoma. *N Engl J Med* 2013;369(6):507–516.
94. She QB, Halilovic E, Ye Q, et al. 4E-BP1 is a key effector of the oncogenic activation of the AKT and ERK signaling pathways that integrates their function in tumors. *Cancer Cell* 18(1):39–51.
95. Engelman JA, Chen L, Tan X, et al. Effective use of PI3K and MEK inhibitors to treat mutant Kras G12D and PIK3CA H1047R murine lung cancers. *Nat Med* 2008;14(12):1351–1356.
96. Gorre ME, Mohammed M, Ellwood K, et al. Clinical resistance to STI-571 cancer therapy caused by BCR-ABL gene mutation or amplification. *Science* 2001;293(5531):876–880.
97. Shah NP, Nicoll JM, Nagar B, et al. Multiple BCR-ABL kinase domain mutations confer polyclonal resistance to the tyrosine kinase inhibitor imatinib (STI571) in chronic phase and blast crisis chronic myeloid leukemia. *Cancer Cell* 2002;2(2):117–125.
98. Shah NP, Tran C, Lee FY, et al. Overriding imatinib resistance with a novel ABL kinase inhibitor. *Science* 2004;305(5682):399–401.
99. Talpaz M, Shah NP, Kantarjian H, et al. Dasatinib in imatinib-resistant Philadelphia chromosome-positive leukemias. *N Engl J Med* 2006;354(24):2531–2541.
100. Kantarjian H, Shah NP, Hochhaus A, et al. Dasatinib versus imatinib in newly diagnosed chronic-phase chronic myeloid leukemia. *N Engl J Med* 2010;362(24):2260–2270.
101. Sawyers CL. Even better kinase inhibitors for chronic myeloid leukemia. *N Engl J Med* 2010;362(24):2314–2315.
102. Saglio G, Kim DW, Issaragrisil S, et al. Nilotinib versus imatinib for newly diagnosed chronic myeloid leukemia. *N Engl J Med* 362(24):2251–2259.
103. Cortes JE, Kim DW, Pinilla-Ibarz J, et al. A phase 2 trial of ponatinib in Philadelphia chromosome-positive leukemias. *N Engl J Med* 2013;369(19):1783–1796.
104. Pao W, Miller VA, Politi KA, et al. Acquired resistance of lung adenocarcinomas to gefitinib or erlotinib is associated with a second mutation in the EGFR kinase domain. *PLoS Med* 2005;2(3):e73.
105. Antonescu CR, Besmer P, Guo T, et al. Acquired resistance to imatinib in gastrointestinal stromal tumor occurs through secondary gene mutation. *Clin Cancer Res* 2005;11(11):4182–4190.
106. Shah NP, Kantarjian HM, Kim DW, et al. Intermittent target inhibition with dasatinib 100 mg once daily preserves efficacy and improves tolerability in imatinib-resistant and -intolerant chronic-phase chronic myeloid leukemia. *J Clin Oncol* 2008;26(19):3204–3212.
107. Shah NP, Kasap C, Weier C, et al. Transient potent BCR-ABL inhibition is sufficient to commit chronic myeloid leukemia cells irreversibly to apoptosis. *Cancer Cell* 2008;14(6):485–493.
108. Von Hoff DD, LoRusso PM, Rudin CM, et al. Inhibition of the hedgehog pathway in advanced basal-cell carcinoma. *N Engl J Med* 2009;361(12):1164–1172.
109. Rudin CM, Hann CL, Laterra J, et al. Treatment of medulloblastoma with hedgehog pathway inhibitor GDC-0449. *N Engl J Med* 2009;361(12):1173–1178.
110. Parsons DW, Jones S, Zhang X, et al. An integrated genomic analysis of human glioblastoma multiforme. *Science* 2008;321(5897):1807–1812.
111. Mardis ER, Ding L, Dooling DJ, et al. Recurring mutations found by sequencing an acute myeloid leukemia genome. *N Engl J Med* 2009;361(11):1058–1066.
112. Ward PS, Patel J, Wise DR, et al. The common feature of leukemia-associated IDH1 and IDH2 mutations is a neomorphic enzyme activity converting alpha-ketoglutarate to 2-hydroxyglutarate. *Cancer Cell* 2010;17(3):225–234.
113. McCabe MT, Ott HM, Ganji G, et al. EZH2 inhibition as a therapeutic strategy for lymphoma with EZH2-activating mutations. *Nature* 2012;492(7427):108–112.
114. Morin RD, Johnson NA, Severson TM, et al. Somatic mutations altering EZH2 (Tyr641) in follicular and diffuse large B-cell lymphomas of germinal-center origin. *Nat Genet* 2010;42(2):181–185.
115. Bernt KM, Zhu N, Sinha AU, et al. MLL-rearranged leukemia is dependent on aberrant H3K79 methylation by DOT1L. *Cancer Cell* 2011;20(1):66–78.
116. Daigle SR, Olhava EJ, Therkelsen CA, et al. Selective killing of mixed lineage leukemia cells by a potent small-molecule DOT1L inhibitor. *Cancer Cell* 2011;20(1):53–65.

23 Histone Deacetylase Inhibitors and Demethylating Agents

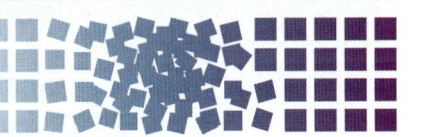

Steven D. Gore, Stephen B. Baylin, and James G. Herman

INTRODUCTION

The past decade has seen an explosive growth, especially at a genome-wide level, in our understanding of the role of chromatin in the normal regulation of gene expression and in the concept of the *epigenome*.[1–3] Concomitant with these advances has been the increasing appreciation of the role of epigenetic abnormalities in the progression of cancer[4–7] and the concept of the *cancer epigenome*. The translational consequences of this research include the possibilities for developing therapies in cancer that target epigenetic abnormalities. These are being explored in clinical trials and several have entered clinical practice.[4,5,7,8] Of these epigenetic abnormalities, the most thoroughly examined is the occurrence of abnormal cytosine guanine (CpG) promoter region DNA methylation and associated altered chromatin involving histone modifications, in the transcriptional silencing of genes, including a group of well-defined tumor suppressor genes.[4,5,7,8] However, targeting epigenetic processes to downregulate the action of overexpressed genes is also an emerging area of research.[9,10] This chapter describes the basis of epigenetic changes in cancer and discusses some of the latest approaches that target epigenetic abnormalities in cancer,[11] including those designed to induce the reexpression of silenced genes, for cancer therapy. The two approaches most mature in development are the inhibition of DNA methyltransferases, which mediate the abnormal promoter DNA methylation, and the inhibition of histone deacetylases, which remove histone modifications associated with active chromatin that alone, or in association with DNA methylation, are associated with transcriptional repression.[4,5,7,8] However, several exciting newer approaches are now in clinical trials and these will be mentioned.

Aberrant gene function and altered patterns of gene expression are key features of cancer.[4] Although genetic alterations remain the best characterized in the development and progression of cancer, increasingly it is appreciated that epigenetic abnormalities cooperate with genetic alterations in multiple ways to cause dysfunction of key regulatory pathways. Through genomic approaches to mutation discovery, there is growing recognition of the frequency of mutations in genes encoding for proteins that regulate the epigenome.[12] This chapter will outline the understanding of how each of these epigenetic alterations contribute to cancer and how derivation of therapeutic approaches may depend on understanding the biology of these changes.

EPIGENETIC ABNORMALITIES AND GENE EXPRESSION CHANGES IN CANCER

Epigenetic changes are defined as heritable alterations of gene expression patterns and cell phenotypes, which are not accompanied by changes in DNA sequence.[13] This definition clearly delineates the two key features of epigenetic regulation important for an understanding of therapies described in this chapter. Specifically, in contrast to genetic alterations (point mutations, deletions, or translocations), epigenetic changes do not alter the coding sequence of targeted genes. Thus, reversal of epigenetic changes can potentially restore the normal function of affected genes and their encoded proteins. Second, the heritable nature of epigenetic changes—that is, the ability of a cell to pass on regulation of gene expression through DNA replication—suggests that such changes, while relatively stable, can be reversed. Thus, therapeutic reprogramming of patterns of gene expression could theoretically result in a long-term change in the cancer cell phenotype, even after the inducing drugs are removed, although to date, this has not been accomplished.

The fundamental unit that determines epigenetic states is the nucleosome that contains an octamer of histone proteins around which approximately 160 base pairs of DNA are wrapped.[13] It is the positioning of these structures, and the three-dimensional aspects of their spacing, and the regulation of this process by posttranslational modifications of the constituent histones that underpins the functions of the epigenome.[13,14]

Abnormal Gene Silencing

One key alteration in cancer, which can be associated with altered epigenetic control, is abnormal gene silencing. Normally, such silencing is fundamental and required at the level of chromatin and DNA methylation regulation for the life of multicellular eukaryotic organisms. The silencing is critical for regulating important biologic processes, including all aspects of development, differentiation, imprinting, and silencing of large chromosomal domains, including the X chromosome of female mammals.[13] For example, the diversity of structure and function of cells derived from epithelial or mesenchymal origin, ultimately differentiating into cells lining the intestine or lung or forming mature granulocytes and myocytes, result from heritable changes in gene expression that are not the result of a change in DNA sequence. Although in many species, silencing can be initiated and maintained solely by processes involving the covalent modifications of histones and other chromatin components, vertebrates utilize an additional layer of gene regulation. This process involves the only natural covalent modification of DNA in humans and is characterized by DNA cytosine methylation that occurs nearly exclusively at the fifth position of the cytosine ring in cytosines preceding guanine, the so-called CpG dinucleotide (Fig. 23.1).[13,15]

Like most biologic processes, the normal patterns of silencing can be altered, resulting in the development of disease states. Thus, activation of genes normally not expressed, or silencing of a gene that should be expressed, can contribute to the dysregulation of gene function that characterizes cancer and, when stably present, represent epigenetic alterations.[4–7] Most studies have focused on the silencing of normally expressed genes. For the purposes of understanding the rationale behind epigenetic therapy, it is important to understand the mechanisms through which such silencing occurs. Alterations in gene expression associated with epigenetic changes that give rise to a growth advantage would be expected to be selected for in the host tissue, leading to progressive dysregulated

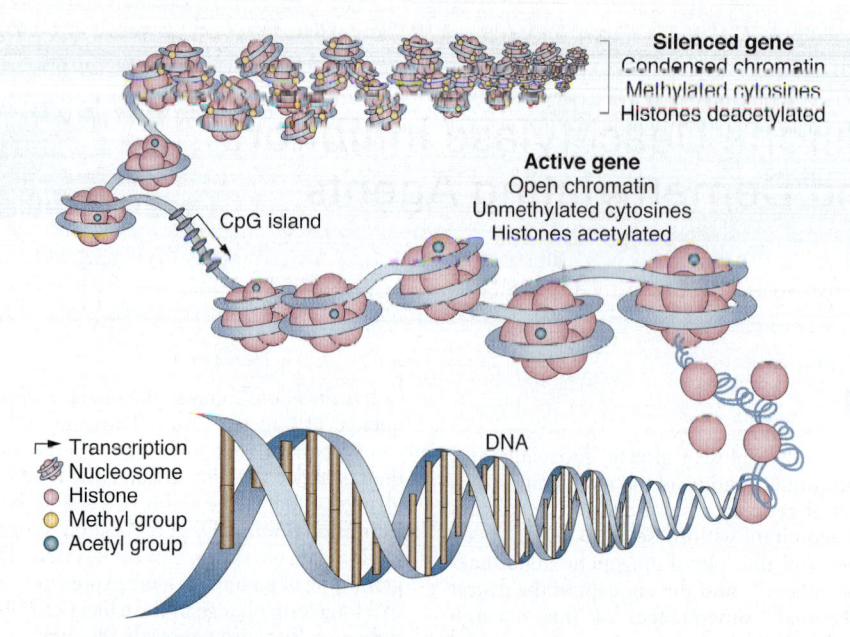

Figure 23.1 Epigenetic regulation of gene expression. In the promoter region, gene expression is controlled by a combination of DNA methylation and chromatin configuration. In normal cells, gene expression is silenced by condensing chromatin, methylating DNA, and deacetylating histones. By contrast, active genes are those with open nucleosome spacing around the transcription start site, are unmethylated, and are associated with acetylated histones. In cancer cells, CpG islands that are rich in cytosine and guanine—and are typically unmethylated to promote gene expression—can be epigenetically silenced by hypermethylation. (Redrawn with permission from Azad N, Zahnow CA, Rudin CM, et al. The future of epigenetic therapy in solid tumours—lessons from the past. *Nat Rev Clin Oncol* 2013;10:256–266.)

growth of the tumor. Such dysregulation is commonly associated with increases in promoter region DNA methylation and is associated with repressive chromatin changes.

Changes in DNA Methylation

The importance of abnormal cytosine methylation and gene silencing has been clearly established in the past 2 decades and been shown convincingly to be involved in cancer development.[4-7] The CpG dinucleotide, usually underrepresented in the genome, is clustered in the promoter regions of approximately 50% of human genes in regions termed *CpG islands*. These regions are largely protected from DNA methylation in normal cells, with the exception of genes on the inactive X chromosome and imprinted genes.[16] This protection is critical, because the methylation of promoter region CpG islands is associated with a loss of gene expression.[4-7] Abnormal de novo DNA methylation of gene promoter CpG islands is a very frequent abnormality in virtually all cancer types and is associated with a process that can serve as an alternative mechanism for loss of tumor suppressor gene function.[4-7] Although a limited number of classic tumor suppressor genes can be affected by this process, a patient's individual cancer may harbor hundreds of such genes.[4-7] Which of these latter genes are drivers of cancer, individually or in groups, versus those which are passengers reflecting only the widespread effects of a global epigenetic abnormality is a leading question in the field and the target of much research.[5,6] A clue to the importance of at least groups of the previous DNA hypermethylated genes may come from the fact that an inordinate number of them are involved in holding normal embryonic and adult stem cells in the self-renewal state and/or rendering such cells refractory to differentiation cues.[17,18] Normally, these genes are then in a poised expression state and can be induced to be activated or repressed as needed for changes in cell state.[18] Abnormal promoter DNA methylation of such genes renders them more repressed and could be a factor in the fact that cancers inevitably exhibit cell populations with enhanced self-renewal or refractoriness to full differentiation.[18]

Recent studies have also suggested that DNA regions other than promoter CpG islands may undergo changes of DNA methylation in cancer. For example, non–CpG-rich sequences surrounding promoter CpG islands, termed CpG island shores, are abnormally methylated in cancers[19] and may be altered in stem cell populations.[20] Thus, the relative cancer specificity of changes of DNA methylation in multiple CpG regions makes reversal of these changes by targeting DNA methyltransferases, the enzymes that catalyze DNA methylation, logical for cancer therapeutics.

As a key example of the previous points, perhaps the most studied tumor suppressor gene for promoter hypermethylation is the *p16* gene, currently designated *CDKN2A*, a cyclin-dependent kinase inhibitor that functions in the regulation of the phosphorylation of the Rb protein. Hypermethylation associated with loss of expression of the *CDKN2A* gene has been found to be one of the most frequent alterations in neoplasia being common in the lung, head and neck, gliomas, colorectal, and breast carcinomas[21,22] and other cancer types. A member of the same gene family, *p15* or *CDKN2B*, also regulates Rb and is silenced in association with promoter methylation in many forms of leukemia and in the chronic myeloid neoplasm myelodysplastic syndrome (MDS).[23] These two previous changes are of much relevance for the clinical uses of epigenetic therapies discussed later.

As mentioned, many hundreds of genes may be inactivated in a single cancer by promoter methylation,[5,6,18,24] providing potential targets for gene reactivation using epigenetic therapies.[25-27] The latter represents one of the potential ways in which epigenetic therapy may be effective: Multiple genes and gene pathways, all

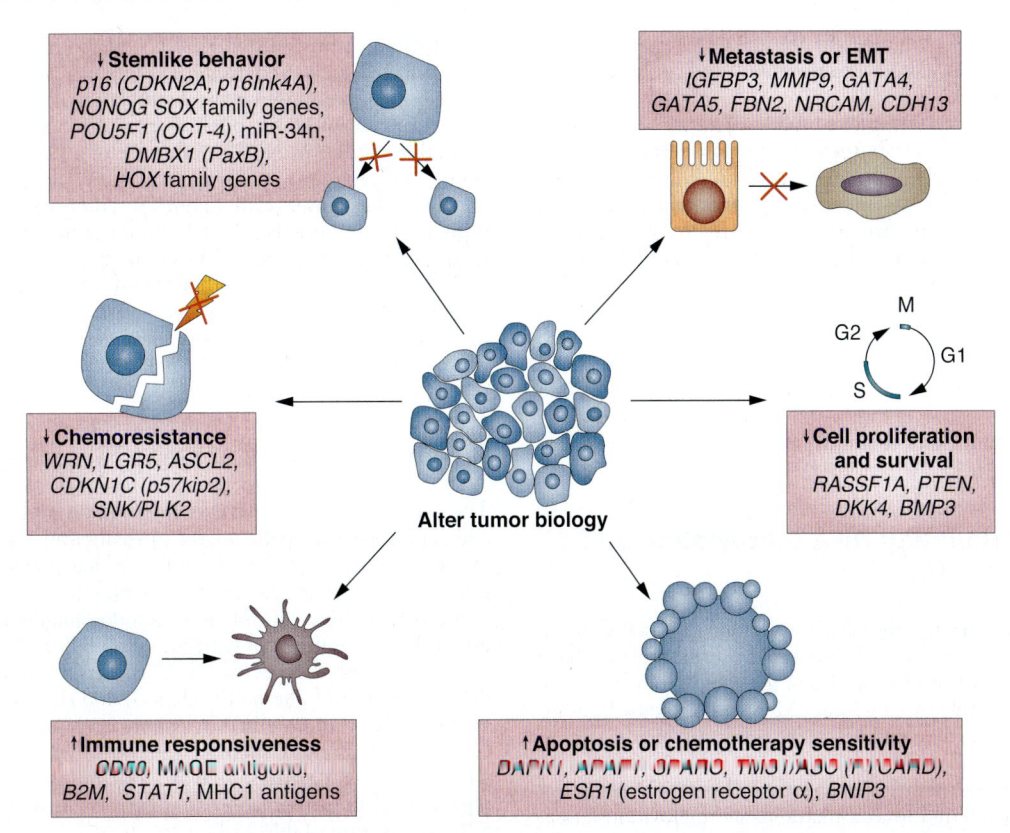

Figure 23.2 Concurrent widespread changes in gene expression with epigenetic therapy. Anticancer efficacy of treatment with epigenetic-modulating agents is associated with extensive changes in gene expression that influence several biologic processes. Gene expression is increased through the direct reversal of epigenetic modifications of genomic DNA, whereas for cancer-promoting genes, gene expression is reduced by the regression of their regulatory genes. EMT, epithelial-membrane transition. (Redrawn with permission from Azad N, Zahnow CA, Rudin CM, et al. The future of epigenetic therapy in solid tumours—lessons from the past. *Nat Rev Clin Oncol* 2013;10:256–266.)

repressed by changes in DNA methylation and chromatin modification, can be reactivated by DNA methyltransferase inhibitors and histone deacetylase (HDAC) inhibitors (HDACi), thereby restoring normal cell cycle control, differentiation, and apoptotic signaling (Fig. 23.2).[8,26,28] In general, methylated CpG islands are not capable of the initiation of transcription unless the methylation signal can be overridden by alterations in factors that modulate chromatin, such as the removal of methylated cytosine-binding proteins. However, reversal of DNA methylation with secondary changes in histone modification or directed reversal of repressive histone modifications represent a target for epigenetic therapies.[8,26,28]

Most studies of DNA methylation, particularly in the study of cancer, have focused on CpG island promoter methylation. However, about 40% of human genes do not contain bona fide CpG islands in their promoters.[29] The primary focus on CpG islands has resulted from the clear demonstration that CpG-island promoter methylation permanently silences genes both physiologically and pathologically in mammalian cells. However, recent work has shown correlations between tissue-specific expression and methylation of non-CpG islands, including, for example, the maspin gene,[30] and as mentioned previously, regions near CpG islands,[19,20] suggesting that many additional genes could be regulated, either normally or abnormally, by changes in DNA methylation.

An exciting new area of DNA methylation research involves the role of this change in regulating gene enhancers: small DNA regions that regulate the expression of multiple target genes.[31–33] The presence of DNA methylation in these areas, which can reside considerable distances from the genes that are being regulated, generally works together with histone modifications to mediate a repressive state for that enhancer.[31–33] The status of enhancers is also emerging as important for cancer risk states.[34]

Chromatin in Gene Regulation

Heritable gene silencing involves the interplay between DNA methylation and histone covalent modifications. Complexes of proteins that can regulate how nucleosomes are positioned perform nucleosomal remodeling.[35–37] What was initially termed the *histone code*, with reference to how histones are modified, has emerged to be much more complex than originally envisioned. An explosion of research findings during the last several years now allows for an appreciation of how the epigenome is controlled by a complex interplay between a myriad of posttranslational histone modifications that occur on key amino acid residues of these proteins.[37] Acetylation, deacetylation, methylation, phosphorylation, and other modifications all modify chromatin structure and thereby alter gene expression.[38] Some of the enzymes that catalyze these modifications include HDACs, histone methyltransferases (HMT), and most recently, histone demethylases.[13,14,39,40] These modifications help establish heritable states at the start site of genes, but also at enhancers and other transcribed DNA regions not encoding for canonical genes. The latter areas contain noncoding RNAs (ncRNAs) and micro-RNAs (miRNAs), which play key modulatory roles for overall gene expression and protein patterns that can be altered in cancer.[41–43] Again, much research is being focused on epigenetic changes in these DNA regions, which may be important to cancer development and, potentially, to cancer management.

A link between covalent histone modifications and DNA methylation has been clearly established.[44-46] In this interaction, cytosine methylation attracts methylated DNA-binding proteins and HDACs to methylated CpG sites during chromatin compaction and gene silencing.[46,47] In addition, the DNA methylation binding protein (MBD2) interacts with the nucleosomal remodeling complex (NuRD) and directs the complex to methylated DNA.[48] This complex also binds HDACs and has recently been identified as a central player for the abnormal silencing of genes associated with promoter DNA hypermethylation in cancer.[47] Thus, the three processes of DNA cytosine methylation, histone modification, and nucleosomal remodeling are intimately linked, and alterations in these processes can result in abnormalities of gene expression in cancer-relevant genes.

Enzymes Regulating DNA Methylation and Histone Acetylation

DNA methylation involves the covalent addition of a methyl group to the 5′ position of cytosine. In mammals, three enzymes have been shown to catalyze this transfer of a methyl group from the methyl donor S-adenosylmethionine. Most of the methyltransferase activity present in differentiated cells is derived from the expression of DNMT1.[49] This enzyme is thought to be most important in maintaining DNA methylation patterns following DNA replication and thus is referred to as a maintenance methyltransferase. However, the enzyme does possess the ability to methylate previously unmethylated DNA sequences (de novo activity).[50] In contrast, the other enzymes, DNMT3a and DNMT3b, are efficient at methylating previously unmethylated DNA and thus are considered de novo methyltransferases. Each of these enzymes possesses a similar catalytic site,[51] a fact important for the inhibition of DNMT enzymes by nucleoside analogs, discussed later in this chapter.

DNA methylation is closely associated with changes in the histone modifications. As previously discussed, histone proteins are the central components of the nucleosome, and modifications of the histone tails of core histones are associated with active or repressed chromatin.[52] Although it is beyond the scope of this chapter to fully discuss the complex series of modifications to the histone tails of histone H3 and H4, a few well-characterized modifications should be mentioned that are relevant to therapies designed to target epigenetic abnormalities in cancer. In reference to currently investigated epigenetic therapies, changes in histone acetylation are of importance. Acetylation of histones H3 and H4 at key amino acids is associated with the active chromatin present at the promoters of transcribed genes, whereas the absence of histone acetylation is associated with repressed, silenced genes.[13,14,53] Histone acetyltransferases (HAT) HDACs have opposing functions to maintain the proper level of histone acetylation for gene expression.[13,14,53] HDACs specifically deacetylate the lysine residues of the histone tails, and this deacetylation is associated with condensation of nucleosome positions in what is termed a closed chromatin formation. This scenario is key to transcriptional repression. There are four classes of HDACs.[53] Class I HDACs are characterized by their similarity to the yeast Rpd3 HDAC. In humans, this class of enzymes includes HDAC1, -2, -3, and -8. These HDACs are thought to be ubiquitously expressed in tissue throughout the body. In contrast, class II HDACs are similar to yeast Hda1 and include HDAC4, -5, -6, -7, -9, and -10, and they have a greater degree of tissue specificity. Class III HDACs are similar to yeast Sir2 and are set apart from the other classes by their dependence on nicotinamide adenine dinucleotide (NAD+) as a cofactor. Finally, class IV includes HDAC11.[53]

Of the previously listed HDACs, class I and 2 HDACs have been most closely tied to gene silencing associated with abnormal promoter DNA hypermethylation.[48] These are bound to the nucleosome remodeling complex, NuRD.[48,49] Experimental decreases in NURD, after use of a DNA demethylating agent, can augment reactivation of many abnormally silenced and DNA hypermethylated genes in colon cancer cells.[48] Manipulation of these HDACs is under study in clinical trials, with and without the use of DNA methyltransferase inhibitors, and is discussed later. Another HDAC, SIRT1 in the class III of these proteins, is also involved with gene silencing.[54,55] This deacetylase has been linked to silencing of DNA hypermethylated genes, and blocking its activity can be associated with reactivation of such genes.[55]

Reversal of Layers of Gene Silencing

The interaction between DNA methylation and HDAC activity and repressive chromatin marks in maintaining aberrant silencing of hypermethylated genes in cancer has therapeutic implications for epigenetic therapies. Experimental evidence suggests that DNA methylation functions as a dominant event that stably establishes transcriptional repression. Inhibition of HDAC activity alone, by potent and specific HDACis, does not generally result in the reactivation of aberrantly silenced and densely hypermethylated genes in tumor cells.[56] In contrast, treatment with HDACis can reactivate densely silenced genes if the cells are first treated with demethylating drugs, such as 5-azacitidine.[56] The clinical implications of this observation are discussed in more detail in the following section (Table 23.1).

DNA Methyltransferase Inhibitors

Originally synthesized as cytotoxic antimetabolite drugs in the 1960s,[57] azacytosine nucleosides were recognized as inhibitors of DNA methylation in the early 1980s. The inhibitors 5-azacitidine (5AC) and 2′-deoxy-5-azacytidine induced muscle, fat, and chondrocyte differentiation in mouse embryo cells, in association with a reversal of DNA methylation.[58,59] The incorporation of azacytosine nucleosides into DNA in lieu of cytosine residues was shown to be associated with inhibition of DNMT activity.[59,60] DNMT inhibition requires the incorporation of decitabine triphosphate into DNA. The incorporated azacytosine nucleoside forms an irreversible inactive adduct with DNMT. The sequential reversal of DNA methylation then results when DNA replication proceeds in the absence of active DNMT.[61] The inhibitor 5AC must be phosphorylated and converted to decitabine diphosphate by ribonucleotide reductase before it can be activated through triphosphorylation, whereas decitabine does not require ribonucleotide reductase. The inhibitor 5AC can also be incorporated into RNA. DNMT2, a misnamed protein that is actually an RNA-specific methyltransferase,[62] becomes inhibited, leading to the depletion of methylated tRNA.[60] This may contribute to the inhibition of protein synthesis and is a potential difference between azacitidine and decitabine.[63] The previous DNA methyltransferase inhibitors not only block the catalytic activities of DNMTs, but also trigger degradation of these proteins, especially DNMTs 1 and 3B.[64-68] This latter activity is potentially important for their activities for gene reexpression because each of these two proteins, experimentally, possess transcriptional repression properties independent of their DNA methylation catalytic sites.[69,70]

The azacytosine nucleosides exhibit complex dose–response characteristics. At low concentrations (0.2 to 1 μM), the *epigenetic* activities of these drugs predominate, with dose-dependent reversal of DNA methylation[71,72] and induction of terminal differentiation in some systems.[28,71] As concentrations are increased, DNA damage and apoptosis become more prominent.[28,72] Cell lines with 30-fold resistance to the cytotoxic effects of doxifluridine,

TABLE 23.1
Small Molecules Targeting Epigenetic Abnormalities in Clinical Development

Drug	Class	Target	Dose Range	Schedule	Route of Administration
5-Azacitidine	Nucleoside	DNA methyl-transferase	30–75 mg/m^2/d	Daily × 7–14 d/28 d	Subcutaneous or intravenous
2'-Deoxy-5-azacytidine	Nucleoside	DNA methyl-transferase	10–45 mg/m^2/d	Daily × 3–5 d/4–6 wk	Intravenous
SGI10	Nucleoside	DNA methyl-transferase	Being determined	Being determined	Subcutaneous
Valproic acid	Small chain fatty acid	Histone deacetylase (class I and II)	25–50 mg/kg/d	Daily	Oral or intravenous
Vorinostat	Hydroxamic acid	Histone deacetylase (class I and II)	400–600 mg/d	Divided doses	Oral
Entinostat	Benzamide	Histone deacetylase (class I)	2–8 mg/m^2	Weekly	Oral
Belinostat	Hydroxamic acid	Histone deacetylase (class I and II)	600–1,000 mg/m^2	Daily × 5/28 d	Intravenous
Romidepsin	Cyclic tetrapeptide	Histone deacetylase (class I and II)	13–18 mg/m^2	Weekly	Intravenous
LBH-589	Hydroxamic acid	Histone deacetylase (class I and II)	5–11 mg/m^2	Daily × 3	Intravenous
MGCD-0103	Benzamide	Histone deacetylase (class I)	40–125 mg/m^2	Twice weekly	Oral
CI-994	Benzamide	Histone deacetylase (class I)	5–8 mg/m^2	Daily	Oral

adriamycin, cyclophosphamide (DAC) continue to reverse methylation in response to this nucleoside, suggesting that the methylation reversing and cytotoxic activities of this compound can be separated.[73] The ability of these drugs to inhibit the cell cycle, at least in part through induction of p21$^{WAF1/CIP1}$ expression, complicates the goal of reversing DNA methylation, because the latter requires DNA replication with the azacytosine nucleoside incorporated into the DNA.

The importance of low doses of the two azacytosine nucleosides to achieve a targeted therapeutic effect has been recently explored in a series of laboratory observations. Transient exposure of both leukemia and solid tumor cells to submicromolar doses induce such cells to undergo cellular reprogramming, accompanied by decreases in ability to clone in long-term self-renewal assays and to grow as explants in immune-incompetent mice.[28] These effects occur with partial genome-wide DNA demethylation and changes in gene expression in multiple pathways potentially key for driving tumorigenesis.

The pharmacokinetic properties of the two azacytosine nucleosides are also very important to consider for their clinical use. In this regard, a major potential challenge for their usage is the fact that these drugs are highly unstable in an aqueous solution, resulting in their rapid hydrolysis and resultant inactivation.[74] In clinical practice, the drugs must be administered shortly after reconstitution. The drugs are also metabolized by cytidine deaminase,[74] leading to a short half-life in plasma. When injected subcutaneously, 5AC reaches a maximal plasma concentration at 30 minutes, with a terminal half-life of 1.5 to 2.3 hours.[75,76] At the U.S. Food and Drug Administration (FDA) approved dose of 5AC (75 mg/m^2 administered subcutaneously daily for 7 days), peak plasma concentrations were 3 to 5 µM, which is well within the range of DNMT inhibitory concentrations.[75,76] Intravenous (IV) administration of the same dose has led to higher peak plasma concentrations (11 µM) with a shorter half-life (approximately 22 minutes).[75] DAC given over 1 hour IV at 15 to 20 mg/m^2 produced plasma concentrations of 1.1 to 1.6 µM during the infusion,[77] whereas in a phase 1 study in patients with thoracic malignancies, patients were treated with escalating doses of decitabine for 72-hour IV infusions for two 35-day cycles. The maximum tolerated total dose was 60 to 75 mg/m^2 with neutropenia as the dose-limiting toxicity. Steady-state plasma concentrations ranged from 25 to 40 nM, which is less than those usually used to induce expression of methylated genes in tissue culture models.[78] An oral formulation of 5AC has also been studied. The oral bioavailability of oral azacitidine ranged from 6% to 20%. Nonetheless, MDS and acute myelogenous leukemia (AML) patients receiving oral azacitidine developed clinical responses similar to patients receiving parenteral azacitidine. Oral azacitidine has also been safely administered on 14-daily and 21-daily schedules repeated monthly. The extended administration of lower daily doses may provide favorable pharmacodynamics of DNA methylation reversal given the need for ongoing cell cycling to effect methylation reversal.[79]

SGI-110 is a dinucleoside that acts as a prodrug for decitabine. This drug is being studied in myelodysplasia and AML.[80]

HISTONE DEACETYLASE INHIBITORS

The increasing recognition of the critical importance of histone modifications in regulating the transcriptional permissivity of chromatin has led to intense interest in compounds that can inhibit the activity of HDAC proteins, facilitating the acetylation of lysines associated with transcriptional activation of genes. As with the DNMT inhibitors discussed previously, there are multiple, sometimes dose-dependent, effects of HDACis in preclinical studies. Some of these may truly be epigenetic, others strictly cytotoxic, and others a combination of both.[9,81–84] Some actions of HDACis may relate to altering how chromatin is central to the repair of DNA. Thus, at especially high doses, these compounds can blunt efficient repair and even induce DNA breaks.[84,85] These effects may underlie cell cycle arrest and induction of cell death as is often observed in preclinical studies of HDACis.[81–84]

Perhaps novel uses of these drugs may be inferred by results from recent studies suggesting they could be extremely powerful epigenetic therapy agents when used in proper doses, for targeted purposes, and at key time intervals. Recent studies by Settleman and colleagues[86] suggest that histone acetylation changes, and thus epigenetic mechanisms, could be a key factor for cancer therapy resistance to both targeted therapy agents and conventional chemotherapy. The mechanisms involved may involve the emergence of drug-tolerant stem-like cells.[86] In such cells, gene expression studies suggest that a protein upregulated in resistance is a histone demethylase, which diminishes a key histone modification for active transcription, H3K4methyl.[86] A very similar enzyme has been shown in other studies to be central to self-renewal of stem-like melanoma cells.[87] Key to the therapies under discussion is that, in the previous drug-resistance studies, low doses of HDACis, could reversibly reduce drug-resistant cells induced by the various anticancer drugs.[86] It is essential going forward to sort out which of these effects are dose-related off-target effects and which are desired on-target effects that can be optimized for efficacious therapy strategies.

Types of Histone Deacetylase Inhibitors

Small Chain Fatty Acids

The earliest report of the use of an HDACi to treat leukemia described the treatment of a child with refractory AML with intravenous sodium butyrate, with a concomitant clearance of peripheral blood blast cells and a decrement in bone marrow blasts.[88] No responses developed in a subsequent study of nine AML patients who were treated with intravenous butyrate.[89] Phase 1 studies of sodium phenylbutyrate (NaPB) in MDS and AML explored 7-day continuous infusions administered monthly or biweekly, and 21-day continuous infusions administered monthly.[90,91] At the maximum tolerated dose (375 mg per kilogram per day), the mean steady-state plasma concentration was 0.3 mM, within the range of HDAC inhibition.[90–92] Isolated patients developed hematologic improvement in response to NaPB.

Similar to NaPB, valproic acid (VPA) requires near millimolar concentrations to effectively inhibit HDACs. Of 18 patients with MDS or AML with trilineage dysplasia treated with VPA to target plasma concentrations of 0.3 to 0.7 mM, 6 patients developed hematologic improvement.[93] Of 20 elderly patients with AML treated with VPA, only 11 could remain in control long enough to be considered evaluable for response. Five had improvement in platelet counts.[94] VPA induced hematologic improvement in combination with all-transretinoic acid in two of eight patients treated with AML; a fluorescence in situ hybridization analysis showed definitive evidence of terminal differentiation of the malignant cells.[95] A larger study of this combination induced hematologic response in only 2 of 26 elderly patients with AML.[96] It appears unlikely that the small chain fatty acids will develop an important role in the treatment of malignancy given the availability of HDACis with vastly greater potency.

Hydroxamic Acids

The FDA approved vorinostat as the first commercially available HDACi. The approval was based on activity of this agent in cutaneous T-cell lymphoma (CTCL). Thirty-three patients with a median number of five prior systemic therapy regimens received one of three dose schedules of vorinostat in a single institution study.[97] Eight patients achieved a partial response, with a median time to response of 12 weeks and a median duration of response of 15 weeks. Overall, 45% of patients had relief of pruritus. Fatigue, diarrhea, nausea, and thrombocytopenia were common toxicities. In a multicenter phase 2 trial, 74 patients with relapsed or refractory CTCL were treated with 400 mg daily.[98] Similar to the prior study, 29% of patients responded, consisting almost entirely of partial responses. Median time to response was 56 days, and median duration of response was greater than 6 months. In phase 1 trials, responses to vorinostat have developed in other non-Hodgkin's and Hodgkin's lymphoma cases.[99] More recently, in a trial combining vorinostat with carboplatin and paclitaxel in patients with untreated, advanced, non–small-cell lung cancer (NSCLC), response rates increased significantly from 12.5% to 34%, and a trend to improved progression-free survival and overall survival was observed.[100]

Panobinostat (LBH589), a cinnamic hydroxamic acid HDACi, reduced peripheral blood blast percentage but did not induce remissions in a phase 1 trial of daily times 7 oral dosing in patients with a variety of relapsed hematologic malignancies.[101] Asymptomatic changes in electrocardiographic T waves developed in 80% of treated patients. Gastrointestinal symptoms and thrombocytopenia were common. Panobinostat has recently been approved by the FDA for the treatment of multiple myeloma.[102]

Cyclic Tetrapeptides

Romidepsin is FDA approved for the treatment of CTCL[103] and peripheral T-cell lymphoma.[104,105] Antitumor activity, including tumor lysis syndrome, was demonstrated in a phase 1 study that enrolled patients with chronic lymphocytic leukemia and AML, but no complete or partial remissions were seen.[75] The administration of romidepsin induces electrocardiographic changes, including T-wave flattening and ST-T wave depression in greater than half of the posttreatment tracings; however, no changes in serum cardiac troponin levels or left ventricular ejection fraction have been reported.[106]

Benzamides

Entinostat, formerly known as MS-275, was administered weekly times four to patients with relapsed and refractory AML in a phase 1 study. Infections, unsteady gate, and somnolence were dose-limiting toxicities. No clinical responses developed, although improvements in neutrophil counts were observed.[107] Entinostat did not increase the response rate in patients with higher risk MDS and AML with MDS-related changes when combined with azacitidine compared to azacitidine alone.[108] Most recently, however, studies NSCLC suggest that entinostat could be a valuable therapeutic agent in solid tumors when used with established therapies. When combined with the epidermal growth factor inhibitor erlotinib, in a randomized phase 2 trial for patients with recurrent advanced NSCLC, entinostat was not efficacious alone but appeared to combine with erlotinib to benefit a group of patients whose tumors contained baseline high E-cadherin levels. Overall survival in these latter patients yielded an increased survival benefit of 9.4 versus 5.4 months.[109] Finally, entinostat significantly increased survival when combined with an aromatase inhibitor in a phase 2 trial for patients with breast cancer.[110]

Pharmacodynamic Properties

The administration of oral vorinostat was associated with a transient increase in acetylation of histone H3 in peripheral blood lymphocytes, which peaked at 2 hours post dosing and reverted to baseline by 8 hours; similar changes were observed in the lymph node of a treated patient with lymphoma.[99] Treatment with vorinostat was associated with translocation of phosphorylated signal transducer and activator of transcription 3 (STAT-3) from nucleus to cytoplasm in responding patients and with reduced microvessel density.[97]

Similar changes in the acetylation of histones 2B and 3 were observed in peripheral blood cells from patients treated with LBH589.[101] Romidepsin induced acetylation of H3 and H4 in peripheral blood tumor cells within 4 hours of dosing[111]; of interest, p21$^{WAF1/CIP1}$ protein levels also increased, associated with an increase in acetylation of H4 at the p21 promoter (using chromatin immunoprecipitation). Treatment with entinostat led to increased acetylation of H3 and H4 in both peripheral blood and bone marrow. This increase was detectable within 8 hours and remained above baseline throughout the treatment cycle. Thus, this compound may provide the most prolonged inhibition of protein deacetylation of HDACis and is under current investigation.[107] Increases in p21$^{WAF1/CIP1}$ and activation of caspase 3 were also demonstrated in these samples.

EPIGENETIC THERAPY FOR HEMATOLOGIC MALIGNANCIES

DNA Methyltransferase Inhibitors

Epigenetic therapy has seen the most widespread use to date and achieved the greatest efficacy in hematologic malignancies. The therapeutic efficacy of 5AC and DAC for patients with the chronic myeloid neoplasm myelodysplasia (MDS) and AML has been well reviewed.[26,27] Their FDA approval for MDS/AML emerged only after doses were reduced, with resultant diminishing toxicities for patients. The successful development of 5AC for the treatment of MDS can be credited largely to Silverman et al.[25,112,114] in the Cancer and Leukemia Group B (CALGB). The inhibitor 5AC had successfully induced the expression of hemoglobin F in patients with sickle cell anemia.[25,112] Viewing this compound as a potential inducer of terminal differentiation, Silverman et al. conducted a series of phase 2 trials of 5AC administered as a continuous intravenous infusion or as subcutaneous injections for the treatment of MDS.[113,114] Based on significant hematologic responses, the group performed a phase 2 trial (CALGB 9221) in which patients with low- and high-risk MDS with significant hematopoietic compromise were randomly assigned to receive subcutaneous 5AC (75 mg/m^2 per day daily for 7 days, repeated on a 28-day cycle) or observation. Patients on the observation arm with progressive disease could cross over to receive 5AC. This study firmly established the ability of 5AC to induce hematologic improvement, and, less frequently, complete and partial responses.[113,115] The median time to development of AML (defined by 30% bone marrow blast cells) or death was greater in the 5AC arm by 9 months (21 versus 12 months); of note, the observation arm included patients who subsequently crossed over to 5AC treatment.

In a subsequent phase 3 trial (AZA001),[116] patients with higher risk myelodysplastic syndromes were randomly assigned one-to-one to receive 5AC (75 mg/m^2 per day for 7 days every 28 days) or conventional care (best supportive care, low-dose cytarabine, or intensive chemotherapy as selected by investigators before randomization). Three hundred fifty-eight patients were randomly assigned to receive 5AC (n = 179) or conventional care regimens (n = 179). After a median follow-up of 21.1 months (interquartile range [IQR] 15.1 to 26.9), median overall survival was 24.5 months (9.9 not reached) for the azacitidine group versus 15.0 months (5.6 to 24.1) for the conventional care group (hazard ratio [HR] 0.58; 95% confidence interval [CI], 0.43 to 0.77; $p = 0.0001$). At 2 years, on the basis of Kaplan-Meier estimates, 50.8% (95% CI, 42.1 to 58.8) of patients in the 5AC group were alive compared with 26.2% (95% CI, 18.7 to 34.3) in the conventional care group ($p < 0.0001$). Median time to AML transformation was 17.8 months (IQR 8.6 to 36.8; 95% CI, 13.6 to 23.6) in the 5AC group compared with 11.5 months (4.9 not reached; 8.3 to 14.5) in the conventional care group (HR 0.50; 95% CI, 0.35 to 0.70; $p < 0.0001$). Subsequent unplanned analyses of AZA001 included an examination of elderly patients with what would now be classified as AML (blast count 20% to 30%). In these 113 patients, there remains a statistically significant improvement in survival of 24.5 months versus 16.0 months (HR 0.47; 95% CI; $p = 0.0001$).[117]

The early development of decitabine in MDS took place primarily in Europe under the leadership of Wijermans et al.[118,119] These investigators pursued intravenous scheduling of decitabine administered three times daily for 3 days (45 mg/m^2 per day total dose). This cycle was repeated every 6 weeks. Phase 2 studies suggested a response rate of approximately 50% in MDS patients. In a randomized trial of DAC versus observation, patients with International Prognostic Score risk categories intermediate 1 to high received the previously listed schedule of decitabine or observation. No crossover was allowed in this trial. Response rates reported were: complete response: 9%, partial response: 8%, and hematologic improvement: 13%.[120] A 10% induction death rate occurred, suggesting that this schedule of DAC may be more toxic than the CALGB schedule of 5AC (1% induction mortality). DAC has also been investigated in low-dose daily intravenous dosing[121] and in daily-times-five schedules. The latter appears convenient and well tolerated. A daily-times-five schedule (20 mg/m^2 per day) has been FDA approved[121]; 99 patients with MDS (de novo or secondary) of any French-American-British (FAB) subtype and an International Prognostic Scoring System (IPSS) score equal to or greater than 0.5 were treated, with an overall response rate of 32% (17 complete responses [CR] plus 15 marrow CRs [mCR]).[122] Among patients who improved, 82% demonstrated responses by the end of cycle two. This well-tolerated regimen allows outpatient administration and, as noted previously, provides plasma levels of decitabine that inhibit DNMTs.

The 3-day intravenous schedule of DAC has been studied in two randomized trials compared to supportive care in patients with higher risk MDS. The first trial confirmed the hematologic activity of decitabine in this patient population but failed to show an improvement in survival in the DAC-treated patients.[123] Survival was also not increased in the subsequent trial, performed by the European Organization for Research and Treatment of Cancer (EORTC).[124] The failure of the randomized decitabine trials to show a survival benefit may be partially due to study design. Both randomized trials of 5AC continued treatment until disease progression for patients who did not achieve complete remission; in fact, this meant that most patients received maintenance therapy. In contrast, both randomized trials of decitabine allowed a maximum of eight cycles of treatment. The need for maintenance therapy in patients treated with DNMT inhibitors has not been tested in prospective randomized trials. An additional difference in the conduct of the two sets of DNMT inhibitor trials involves the duration of therapy administered. The median number of cycles of treatment administered in the two randomized trials of decitabine was three, compared to nine in the azacytidine trials. This may reflect greater toxicity of the originally 3-day schedule of decitabine compared to that of the approved schedule of 5AC. Although the differences in survival may reflect differences in trial design and trial conduct, emerging data suggests that despite similarities in methylation reversal, the two drugs differ in other potentially important biologic parameters, which may contribute to clinical outcomes.[62,63,125]

Two randomized phase 3 trials have been published treating elderly AML patients (greater than 20% blasts) with decitabine, both demonstrating improvement in survival that was not statistically significant. In the European study, 233 patients received either

DAC at 15 mg/m² × 9 doses over 3 days on 42 day cycles or best supportive care. The patients received a median of 4 cycles (0 to 9), and the overall survival was improved in the decitabine-treated patients, but did not reach statistical significance (median overall survival [OS], 10.1 versus 8.5 months, respectively; HR, 0.88; 95% CI, 0.66 to 1.17; two-sided, log-rank p = 0.38).[126] In the M.D. Anderson Cancer Center–led multicenter trial,[127] 485 patients 65 years or older were randomly assigned to receive decitabine 20 mg/m² per day as a 1-hour intravenous infusion for 5 consecutive days every 4 weeks or best supportive care or low-dose cytarabine (20 mg/m² per day for 10 days every 4 weeks). There was a similar improvement in OS with decitabine (7.7 months; 95% CI, 6.2 to 9.2) versus the control group (5.0 months; 95% CI, 4.3 to 6.3; p = 0.108; HR, 0.85; 95% CI, 0.69 to 1.04).[127]

The azacytosine nucleosides require prolonged administration to demonstrate hematologic improvement in MDS. Median time to development of first clinical response in the CALGB studies of 5AC was three cycles; 90% of responses developed by cycle six.[114] In the phase 3 trial of decitabine, the median time to response was two cycles,[123] as also seen in the alternative regimen of decitabine.[122] It is, therefore, extremely important when treating patients with azacytosine nucleosides to commit to administering between four and six cycles of therapy before determining whether a patient is responding to treatment. Furthermore, survival benefit is seen even in patients not showing bone marrow improvement for 5AC, perhaps related to decreased transfusion requirements or delayed progression to AML.[116]

Because AML in the context of MDS is arbitrarily defined based on marrow blast count, activity of the azanucleoside analogs in AML should not be surprising. In CALGB 9221, 20 patients were reclassified upon central pathology review as meeting criteria for AML (greater than 30% blasts). Their outcomes were comparable to the overall population in the study.[115] In all three CALGB studies among patients meeting current World Health Organization (WHO) criteria for AML (greater than 20% blasts), a complete response was achieved in 9% and hematologic improvement in 26%.[114] A retrospective review of 20 patients with AML, including 8 patients with bone marrow blasts greater than 29% treated with 5AC, reported a complete remission in 4 patients, a partial response in 5, and a hematologic improvement in 3. The median duration of response was 8 months (range: 3 to 33 months).[128] DAC induced a complete hematologic response in 2 of 20 patients treated who had the blastic phase of chronic myeloid leukemia.[129] These studies suggest activity of the azacytosine nucleosides in the treatment of a subset of AML patients. Current studies do not allow for the determination of whether this subset is limited to MDS-associated AML (AML with MDS-related changes), which tends to have low white blood cell counts and have a low proliferative rate, or whether these compounds are also active for those with AML without a history of antecedent hematologic disorder. Several reports describe the sensitivity MDS and AML, characterized by abnormalities of chromosome 7 and associated with poor outcomes in response to cytarabine-based therapy to azanucleosides. In one nonrandomized retrospective study, survival of such patients following the administration of DNMT inhibitors surpassed survival in response to conventional cytotoxic chemotherapy, similar to the outcomes of AZA001.[130–132]

Although the mechanisms underlying the clinical activity of azacytosine analogs may involve reversal of gene methylation, other actions need to be considered. The administration of DAC has been shown to induce transient decrements of methylation in noncoding regions, including long interspersed nuclear element (LINE) and ALU elements.[133] Early studies that examined methylation reversal of the target gene p15^{INK4B} in response to DAC showed no correlation between methylation reversal and clinical response.[134,135] Clinical responders to DAC developed significantly higher expression of this gene following treatment, and certainly key biologic roles for this gene and its low basal expression are probable. Moreover, in one study, the clinical response was closely associated with the reversal of methylation of p15 or CDH-1 during the first cycle of treatment with 5AC followed by the HDACi NaPB.[25] In that study, it was noteworthy that the administration of 5AC prior to the addition of an HDACi was associated with the induction of histone acetylation. Although the mechanism underlying this activity is unknown, histone acetylation has been observed following DNA damage due to gamma irradiation.[136] Subsequent studies have found demethylation following treatment with either DAC or 5AC[137–140] but not consistently associated with response.[137,138,140] More work will be required to answer the important mechanistic question underpinning the clinical activity of azacytosine analogs.

Combining Inhibitors in the Treatment of Hematologic Malignancies

It is almost certain that the biggest promise of epigenetic therapy lies in strategies to combine existing and newer drugs with each other and with current chemotherapies and targeted therapies. To date, the example for existing agents is the combination of DNMT inhibitors and HDAC inhibitors based on the hypothesis from the laboratory that this paradigm leads to optimal reexpression of transcriptionally silenced genes with promoter methylation.[56,141] This in vitro treatment paradigm has led to a variety of clinical studies that have attempted to apply this concept to the treatment of hematologic malignancies. Much remains to be determined with regard to its efficacy and precisely what determines this. The first study of sequential DNMT/HDAC inhibitors administered a variety of doses of 5AC for 5 to 14 days followed by 7 days of NaPB by continuous infusion at its maximum tolerated dose to patients with MDS and AML.[25] The combination was well tolerated, and clinical responses were frequent in patients receiving 5AC at 50 mg/m² per day daily for 10 days and 25 mg/m² per day daily for 14 days, with 5 of 14 patients at those dose schedules achieving complete or partial response.

In a pilot study, 10 patients with MDS or AML were treated with 5AC at 75 mg/m² per day daily times seven followed by 5 days of NaPB given at 200 mg per kilogram per day as a 1- to 2-hour infusion. Three patients developed a partial response.[142]

In a similar study, investigators at the M.D. Anderson Cancer Center treated leukemic patients with decitabine (15 mg/m² per day IV daily times 10) and concomitant VPA at a variety of doses. Of 54 patients, 12 achieved complete remission or complete remission with incomplete platelet recovery.[143] The inhibitors 5AC, VPA, and all-transretinoic acid have been administered to patients with AML and MDS. Of 33 previously untreated patients, 14 over the age of 60 years developed a complete remission or a complete remission with inadequate platelet recovery.[144] A subsequent study of 5AC and VPA suggests increased efficacy of this combination in high-risk MDS.[145]

Entinostat has been successfully combined with azacytidine in patients with myeloid malignancies.[140] The US Leukemia Intergroup recently completed a randomized phase 2 trial of this combination compared with 5AC alone. In this study, of 149 patients, the primary endpoint of hematologic normalization was statistically similar, with 32% (95% CI, 22% to 44%) of the 5AC group reaching hematologic normalization (HN) versus 27% (95% CI, 17% to 39%) in the AZA + entinostat group. Median overall survivals were 18 months for the AZA group and 13 months for the AZA + entinostat group, but were also not statistically significant.[108] In the latter study, the administration of the combination was associated with less DNA methylation reversal compared to azacitidine monotherapy, likely due to cell cycle inhibitory effects of the HDACi. This highlights the complexity of effectively targeting epigenetic gene regulation.

It remains to be established whether combination therapies are more effective than single-agent demethylating therapies.

Epigenetically Targeted Therapy in Nonhematologic Malignancies

The efficacies that have emerged in the application of epigenetically targeted drugs to hematologic malignancies has spurred interest in using epigenetic therapy for other types of cancer. As outlined as follows, laboratory studies and clinical trials support this approach. Studies in the lab have been directed by lessons learned from therapy in hematologic malignancies, suggesting that low doses of drugs like DAC and 5AC, in the nanomolar range, may avoid excess toxicities due to off-target effects of the drugs and may maximize epigenetic effects of the agents.[28] The desired effects may require minimizing initial cellular cytotoxicity, giving tumor cells time to accrue maximal cellular reprogramming responses to the inhibition of DNMTs.[28] DAC and 5AC are effective only when they have been incorporated into DNA, after which they irreversibly inhibit DNMT catalytic activity and target these proteins for degradation.[64-68] In cell culture and mouse explants, low nanomolar doses appear to induce both human leukemic and solid tumor cells to exhibit blunting of self-renewal and tumorigenic activity of tumor stem-like cells.[28] These preclinical results suggest a key possibility that use of epigenetic therapies might inhibit these latter cell populations, which often are difficult to eradicate and are a factor in resistance to many standard cancer therapies.[146] Exhaustion of such cells over time during therapy with DAC or 5AC might explain the observation that most patients with MDS/AML take several months to reach best response.[147] Leukemic stem cells were not eliminated in one study in MDS and AML patients treated with 5AC in combination with VPA, although their frequency decreased in clinical responders.[148]

Clinical trials for common solid tumors, informed through the previous laboratory studies, have been initiated including phase 2 designs using low-dose strategies with 5AC often combined with use of histone deacetylase inhibitors. Sixty-five patients with advanced, multiply treated NSCLCs were treated with 5AC plus entinostat.[149] Only 3% of patients developed Response Evaluation Criteria (RECIST)-measureable responses; however, these two patients had durable responses, with survival of 3 to 4 years.[149] Upregulation of immunogenic pathways in NSCLC and other solid tumor cells, observed in laboratory studies, suggest a potential for sequencing DNMT inhibitors with immune checkpoint inhibitors.[150] This drug is also reported to induce antitumor responses and immune recognition in a model of pancreatic cancer.[151] Other laboratory results and emerging clinical trials also suggest the promise of combining epigenetic therapy approaches to sensitize cancers other than NSCLC to subsequent therapies. Low-dose DAC appears able to upregulate a key mediator of 5-fluorouracil (5FU) action, uridine monophosphate (UMP) kinase, in colorectal cancer cell lines.[152] These increases correlated with a reversal of 5FU resistance. Similar to studies discussed previously, DAC plus the HDACi, trichostatin A, decreased marker identified self-renewal populations in ovarian cancer while simultaneously inducing increased sensitivity to cisplatin.[153] In advanced ovarian cancer, 5AC or DAC plus carboplatin have yielded durable responses and induced stable disease in ovarian cancer patients.[154,155] These early results are being extrapolated for verification in larger, ongoing clinical trials.

NEW APROACHES TO EPIGENETIC THERAPY

As we have outlined previously, the emerging promise for epigenetic therapy and the future of the approaches may lie in combinatorial drug strategies. Although this is already being explored with older agents, new drugs for new targets are now entering the picture.[9,11,156-158] In these efforts, several themes we have introduced in this chapter will likely dominate.

Most epigenetic therapies will not induce, when used at truly targeting doses, immediate cytotoxic effects. Therapeutic efficacy based on cellular reprogramming may require significant time to manifest. Clinical trial designs may need adaptation so that effective therapies are not discarded due to premature response evaluations. Finally, the ultimate promise for epigenetic therapy may lie with newer drugs now entering clinical trials. Outcomes with DNMT inhibitors may be improved with alternative scheduling of oral azacitidine or through prolonged pharmacokinetics of the decitabine prodrug SGI110.[79] Also, drugs targeting other proteins including BET family bromodomain proteins are generating much excitement.[9,82,156-159] BET inhibitors may interfere with localization of the oncogene C-MYC to acetylated lysines in regulatory regions of target genes.[9,82,156-159] These inhibitors are now entering clinical trials. Other promising approaches include the use of inhibitors of EZH2, the enzyme in the PcG system, which catalyzes the repressive histone mark H3K27me3.[9,82,156-159] Another clinical trial underway employs targeting of the translocation in which the protein mixed lineage leukemia (MLL) is fused with several targets, such as in infant leukemias. These translocations result in abnormal recruitment of the histone methyltransferase, DOT1L, to target genes like *HOXA9*.[158] This fusion induces hypermethylation of H3K79 and abnormal activation of MLL target genes.[158,160] Very selective inhibitors of DOT1L are now in clinical trials.

Epigenetically targeted therapies continue to hold great promise that reprogramming of malignant cells could alter approaches to cancer management. Strategies to merge older drugs, which we have focused on in this chapter, with the newer agents briefly discussed in this section, will underpin future trials to test this approach.

REFERENCES

1. Bernstein BE, Meissner A, Lander ES. The mammalian epigenome. *Cell* 2007;128:669–681.
2. Young RA. Control of the embryonic stem cell state. *Cell* 2011;144:940–954.
3. Suva ML, Riggi N, Bernstein BE. Epigenetic reprogramming in cancer. *Science* 2013;339:1567–1570.
4. Herman JG, Baylin SB. Gene silencing in cancer in association with promoter hypermethylation. *N Engl J Med* 2003;349:2042–2054.
5. Jones PA, Baylin SB. The epigenomics of cancer. *Cell* 2007;128:683–692.
6. Baylin SB, Jones PA. A decade of exploring the cancer epigenome — biological and translational implications. *Nat Rev Cancer* 2011;11:726–734.
7. Esteller M. Cancer epigenomics: DNA methylomes and histone-modification maps. *Nat Rev Genet* 2007;8:286–298.
8. Yoo CB, Jones PA. Epigenetic therapy of cancer: past, present and future. *Nat Rev Drug Discov* 2006;5:37–50.
9. Dawson MA, Kouzarides T. Cancer epigenetics: from mechanism to therapy. *Cell* 2012;150:12–27.
10. Dawson MA, Kouzarides T, Huntly BJ. Targeting epigenetic readers in cancer. *N Engl J Med* 2012;367:647–657.
11. Bradner J. New targets for hematologic malignancies. *Clin Adv Hematol Oncol* 2013;11:375–376.
12. You JS, Jones PA. Cancer genetics and epigenetics: two sides of the same coin? *Cancer Cell* 2012;22:9–20.
13. Allis C, Jenuwein T, Reinberg D. *Epigenetics*, Vol. 1. Cold Spring Harbor, NY: Cold Spring Harbor Laboratory Press; 2007.

14. Kouzarides T. Chromatin modifications and their function. *Cell* 2007;128: 693–705.
15. Baylin SB, Jones PA. Epigenetic determinants of cancer. In: Allis CD, Jenuwein T, Reinberg D, eds. *Epigenetics*. Cold Spring Harbor, NY: Cold Spring Harbor Laboratory Press, 2006. 457–476.
16. Bird AP. CpG-rich islands and the function of DNA methylation. *Nature* 1986;321:209–213.
17. Morey L, Pascual G, Cozzuto L, et al. Nonoverlapping functions of the Polycomb group Cbx family of proteins in embryonic stem cells. *Cell Stem Cell* 2012;10:47–62.
18. Easwaran H, Johnstone SE, Van Neste L, et al. A DNA hypermethylation module for the stem/progenitor cell signature of cancer. *Genome Res* 2012;22: 837–849.
19. Irizarry RA, Ladd-Acosta C, Wen B, et al. The human colon cancer methylome shows similar hypo- and hypermethylation at conserved tissue-specific CpG island shores. *Nat Genet* 2009;41:178–186.
20. Doi A, Park IH, Wen B, et al. Differential methylation of tissue- and cancer-specific CpG island shores distinguishes human induced pluripotent stem cells, embryonic stem cells and fibroblasts. *Nat Genet* 2009;41:1350–1353.
21. Herman JG, Merlo A, Mao L, et al. Inactivation of the CDKN2/p16/MTS1 gene is frequently associated with aberrant DNA methylation in all common human cancers. *Cancer Res* 1995;55:4525–4530.
22. Merlo A, Herman JG, Mao L, et al. 5′ CpG island methylation is associated with transcriptional silencing of the tumour suppressor p16/CDKN2/MTS1 in human cancers. *Nat Med* 1995;1:686–692.
23. Herman JG, Civin CI, Issa JP, et al. Distinct patterns of inactivation of p15INK4B and p16INK4A characterize the major types of hematological malignancies. *Cancer Res* 1997;57:837–841.
24. Costello JF, Fruhwald MC, Smiraglia DJ, et al. Aberrant CpG-island methylation has non-random and tumour-type-specific patterns. *Nat Genet* 2000;24:132–138.
25. Gore SD, Baylin S, Sugar E, et al. Combined DNA methyltransferase and histone deacetylase inhibition in the treatment of myeloid neoplasms. *Cancer Res* 2006;66:6361–6369.
26. Azad N, Zahnow CA, Rudin CM, et al. The future of epigenetic therapy in solid tumours—lessons from the past. *Nat Rev Clin Oncol* 2013;10:256–266.
27. Issa JP, Kantarjian HM. Targeting DNA methylation. *Clin Cancer Res* 2009;15:3938–3946.
28. Tsai HC, Li H, Van Neste L, et al. Transient low doses of DNA-demethylating agents exert durable antitumor effects on hematological and epithelial tumor cells. *Cancer Cell* 2012;21:430–446.
29. Takai D, Jones PA. Comprehensive analysis of CpG islands in human chromosomes 21 and 22. *Proc Natl Acad Sci U S A* 2002;99:3740–3745.
30. Futscher BW, Oshiro MM, Wozniak RJ, et al. Role for DNA methylation in the control of cell type specific maspin expression. *Nat Genet* 2002;31:175–179.
31. Feldmann A, Ivanek R, Murr R, et al. Transcription factor occupancy can mediate active turnover of DNA methylation at regulatory regions. *PLoS Genet* 2013;9:e1003994.
32. Aran D, Hellman A. Unmasking risk loci: DNA methylation illuminates the biology of cancer predisposition: analyzing DNA methylation of transcriptional enhancers reveals missed regulatory links between cancer risk loci and genes. *Bioessays* 2014;36:184–190.
33. Ziller MJ, Gu H, Muller F, et al. Charting a dynamic DNA methylation landscape of the human genome. *Nature* 2013;500:477–481.
34. Akhtar-Zaidi B, Cowper-Sal-lari R, Corradin O, et al. Epigenomic enhancer profiling defines a signature of colon cancer. *Science* 2012;336:736–739.
35. Kingston R, Tamkun JW. Transcriptional regulation by trithorax group. In: Allis CD, Jenuwein T, Reinberg D, eds. *Epigenetics*. Cold Spring Harbor, NY: Cold Spring Harbor Laboratory Press; 2006: 231–248.
36. Becker PB, Workman JL. Nucleosome remodeling and epigenetics. *Cold Spring Harb Perspect Biol* 2013;5.
37. Petty E, Pillus L. Balancing chromatin remodeling and histone modifications in transcription. *Trends Genet* 2013;29:621–629.
38. Jones PA. Functions of DNA methylation: islands, start sites, gene bodies and beyond. *Nat Rev Genet* 2012;13:484–492.
39. Bannister AJ, Kouzarides T. Reversing histone methylation. *Nature* 2005; 436:1103–1106.
40. Bannister AJ, Kouzarides T. Regulation of chromatin by histone modifications. *Cell Res* 2011;21:381–395.
41. Di Leva G, Garofalo M, Croce CM. MicroRNAs in cancer. *Annu Rev Pathol* 2014;9:287–314.
42. Han BW, Chen YQ. Potential pathological and functional links between long noncoding RNAs and hematopoiesis. *Sci Signal* 2013;6:re5.
43. Xi JJ. MicroRNAs in Cancer. *Cancer Treat Res* 2013;158:119–137.
44. Nan X, Ng HH, Johnson CA, et al. Transcriptional repression by the methyl-CpG-binding protein MeCP2 involves a histone deacetylase complex. *Nature* 1998;393:386–389.
45. Jones PL, Veenstra GJ, Wade PA, et al. Methylated DNA and MeCP2 recruit histone deacetylase to repress transcription. *Nat Genet* 1998;19:187–191.
46. Parry L, Clarke AR. The Roles of the Methyl-CpG Binding Proteins in Cancer. *Genes Cancer* 2011;2:618–630.
47. Lopez-Serra L, Esteller M. Proteins that bind methylated DNA and human cancer: reading the wrong words. *Br J Cancer* 2008;98:1881–1885.
48. Cai Y, Geutjes EJ, de Lint K, et al. The NuRD complex cooperates with DNMTs to maintain silencing of key colorectal tumor suppressor genes. *Oncogene* 2014;33:2157–2168.

49. Bestor TH. Cloning of a mammalian DNA methyltransferase. *Gene* 1998; 74:9–12.
50. Jair KW, Bachman KE, Suzuki H, et al. De novo CpG island methylation in human cancer cells. *Cancer Res* 2006;66:682–692.
51. Rius M, Lyko F. Epigenetic cancer therapy: rationales, targets and drugs. *Oncogene* 2012;31:4257–4265.
52. Jenuwein T, Allis CD. Translating the histone code. *Science* 2001;293: 1074–1080.
53. Bolden JE, Peart MJ, Johnstone RW. Anticancer activities of histone deacetylase inhibitors. *Nat Rev Drug Discov* 2006;5:769–784.
54. Vaquero A, Scher M, Erdjument-Bromage H, et al. SIRT1 regulates the histone methyl-transferase SUV39H1 during heterochromatin formation. *Nature* 2007;450:440–444.
55. Pruitt K, Zinn RL, Ohm JE, et al. Inhibition of SIRT1 reactivates silenced cancer genes without loss of promoter DNA hypermethylation. *PLoS Genet* 2006;2:344–352.
56. Cameron EE, Bachman KE, Myöhanen S, et al. Synergy of demethylation and histone deacetylase inhibition in the re-expression of genes silenced in cancer. *Nat Genet* 1999;21:103–107.
57. Sorm F, Piskala A, Cihak A, et al. 5-Azacytidine, a new, highly effective cancerostatic. *Experientia* 1964;20:202–203.
58. Taylor SM, Jones PA. Multiple new phenotypes induced in 10T1/2 and 3T3 cells treated with 5-azacytidine. *Cell* 1979;17:771–779.
59. Jones PA, Taylor SM. Hemimethylated duplex DNAs prepared from 5-azacytidine-treated cells. *Nucleic Acids Res* 1981;9:2933–2947.
60. Lu SH, Ohshima H, Bartsch H. Recent studies on N-nitroso compounds as possible etiological factors in oesophageal cancer. *IARC Sci Publ* 1984;947–953.
61. Taylor SM, Jones PA. Mechanism of action of eukaryotic DNA methyltransferase. Use of 5-azacytosine-containing DNA. *J Mol Biol* 1982;162:679–692.
62. Schaefer M, Hagemann S, Hanna K, et al. Azacytidine inhibits RNA methylation at DNMT2 target sites in human cancer cell lines. *Cancer Res* 2009; 69:8127–8132.
63. Hollenbach PW, Nguyen AN, Brady H, et al. A comparison of azacitidine and decitabine activities in acute myeloid leukemia cell lines. *PLoS One* 2010; 5:e9001.
64. Kelly TK, De Carvalho DD, Jones PA. Epigenetic modifications as therapeutic targets. *Nat Biotechnol* 2010;28:1069–1078.
65. Ferguson AT, Vertino PM, Spitzner JR, et al. Role of estrogen receptor gene demethylation and DNA methyltransferase. DNA adduct formation in 5-aza-2′deoxycytidine-induced cytotoxicity in human breast cancer cells. *J Biol Chem* 1997;272:32260–32266.
66. Gabbara S, Bhagwat AS. The mechanism of inhibition of DNA (cytosine-5-)-methyltransferases by 5-azacytosine is likely to involve methyl transfer to the inhibitor. *Biochem J* 1995;307:87–92.
67. Santi DV, Norment A, Garrett CE. Covalent bond formation between a DNA-cytosine methyltransferase and DNA containing 5-azacytosine. *Proc Natl Acad Sci U S A* 1984;81:6993–6997.
68. Ghoshal K, Datta J, Majumder S, et al. 5-Aza-deoxycytidine induces selective degradation of DNA methyltransferase 1 by a proteasomal pathway that requires the KEN box, bromo-adjacent homology domain, and nuclear localization signal. *Mol Cell Biol* 2005;25:4727–4741.
69. Rountree MR, Bachman KE, Baylin SB. DNMT1 binds HDAC2 and a new co-repressor, DMAP1, to form a complex at replication foci. *Nat Genet* 2000;25:269–277.
70. Bachman KE, Rountree MR, Baylin SB. Dnmt3a and Dnmt3b are transcriptional repressors that exhibit unique localization properties to heterochromatin. *J Biol Chem* 2001;276:32282–32287.
71. Jones PA, Taylor SM. Cellular differentiation, cytidine analogs and DNA methylation. *Cell* 1980;20:85–93.
72. Berg T, Guo Y, Abdelkarim M, et al. Reversal of p15/INK4b hypermethylation in AML1/ETO-positive and -negative myeloid leukemia cell lines. *Leuk Res* 2007;31:497–506.
73. Flatau E, Gonzales FA, Michalowsky LA, et al. DNA methylation in 5-aza-2′-deoxycytidine-resistant variants of C3H 10T1/2 C18 cells. *Mol Cell Biol* 1984;4:2098–2102.
74. Chan KK, Giannini DD, Staroscik JA, et al. 5-Azacytidine hydrolysis kinetics measured by high-pressure liquid chromatography and 13C-NMR spectroscopy. *J Pharm Sci* 1979;68:807–812.
75. Gore SD, Weng LJ, Figg WD, et al. Impact of prolonged infusions of the putative differentiating agent sodium phenylbutyrate on myelodysplastic syndromes and acute myeloid leukemia. *Clin Cancer Res* 2002;8:963–970.
76. Yu L, Liu C, Vandeusen J, et al. Global assessment of promoter methylation in a mouse model of cancer identifies ID4 as a putative tumor-suppressor gene in human leukemia. *Nat Genet* 2005;37:265–274.
77. Blum W, Klisovic RB, Hackanson B, et al. Phase I study of decitabine alone or in combination with valproic acid in acute myeloid leukemia. *J Clin Oncol* 2007;25:3884–3891.
78. Schrump DS, Fischette MR, Nguyen DM, et al. Phase I study of decitabine-mediated gene expression in patients with cancers involving the lungs, esophagus, or pleura. *Clin Cancer Res* 2006;12:5777–5785.
79. Garcia-Manero G, Gore SD, Cogle C, et al. Phase I study of oral azacitidine in myelodysplastic syndromes, chronic myelomonocytic leukemia, and acute myeloid leukemia. *J Clin Oncol* 2011;29:2521–2527.
80. Issa JP, Roboz G, Rizzieri D, et al. Abstract LB-214: Interim results from a randomized Phase 1-2 first-in-human (FIH) study of PK/PD guided escalating doses of SGI-110, a novel subcutaneous (SQ) second generation hypomethylating

agent (HMA) in relapsed/refractory MDS and AML. *Cancer Res* 2012;72: LB-214.
81. Mund C, Lyko F. Epigenetic cancer therapy: Proof of concept and remaining challenges. *Bioessays* 2010;32:949–957.
82. Popovic R, Licht JD. Emerging epigenetic targets and therapies in cancer medicine. *Cancer Discov* 2012;2:405–413.
83. Verbrugge I, Johnstone RW, Bots M. Promises and challenges of anticancer drugs that target the epigenome. *Epigenomics* 2011;3:547–565.
84. Robert C, Rassool FV. HDAC inhibitors: roles of DNA damage and repair. *Adv Cancer Res* 2012;116:87–129.
85. Kachhap SK, Rosmus N, Collis SJ, et al. Downregulation of homologous recombination DNA repair genes by HDAC inhibition in prostate cancer is mediated through the E2F1 transcription factor. *PLoS One* 2010;5:e11208.
86. Sharma SV, Lee DY, Li B, et al. A chromatin-mediated reversible drug-tolerant state in cancer cell subpopulations. *Cell* 2010;141:69–80.
87. Villanueva J, Vultur A, Lee JT, et al. Acquired resistance to BRAF inhibitors mediated by a RAF kinase switch in melanoma can be overcome by cotargeting MEK and IGF-1R/PI3K. *Cancer Cell* 2010;18:683–695.
88. Novogrodsky A, Dvir A, Ravid A, et al. Effect of polar organic compounds on leukemic cells. Butyrate-induced partial remission of acute myelogenous leukemia in a child. *Cancer* 1983;51:9–14.
89. Miller AA, Kurschel E, Osieka R, et al. Clinical pharmacology of sodium butyrate in patients with acute leukemia. *Eur J Cancer Clin Oncol* 1987; 23:1283–1287.
90. Gore SD, Weng LJ, Zhai S, et al. Impact of the putative differentiating agent sodium phenylbutyrate on myelodysplastic syndromes and acute myeloid leukemia. *Clin Cancer Res* 2001;7:2330–2339.
91. Gore SD, Weng LJ, Figg WD, et al. Impact of prolonged infusions of the putative differentiating agent sodium phenylbutyrate on myelodysplastic syndromes and acute myeloid leukemia. *Clin Cancer Res* 2002;8:963–970.
92. DiGiuseppe JA, Weng LJ, Yu KH, et al. Phenylbutyrate-induced G1 arrest and apoptosis in myeloid leukemia cells: structure-function analysis. *Leukemia* 1999;13:1243–1253.
93. Kuendgen A, Strupp C, Aivado M, et al. Treatment of myelodysplastic syndromes with valproic acid alone or in combination with all-trans retinoic acid. *Blood* 2004;104:1266–1269.
94. Pilatrino C, Cilloni D, Messa E, et al. Increase in platelet count in older, poor-risk patients with acute myeloid leukemia or myelodysplastic syndrome treated with valproic acid and all-trans retinoic acid. *Cancer* 2005;104:101–109.
95. Fizzotti M, Cimino G, Pisegna S, et al. Detection of homozygous deletions of the cyclin-dependent kinase 4 inhibitor (p16) gene in acute lymphoblastic leukemia and association with adverse prognostic features. *Blood* 1995; 85:2685–2690.
96. Xu GL, Bestor TH, Bourc'his D, et al. Chromosome instability and immunodeficiency syndrome caused by mutations in a DNA methyltransferase gene. *Nature* 1999;402:187–191.
97. Duvic M, Talpur R, Ni X, et al. Phase 2 trial of oral vorinostat (suberoylanilide hydroxamic acid, SAHA) for refractory cutaneous T-cell lymphoma (CTCL). *Blood* 2007;109:31–39.
98. Olsen EA, Kim YH, Kuzel TM, et al. Phase IIb multicenter trial of vorinostat in patients with persistent, progressive, or treatment refractory cutaneous T-cell lymphoma. *J Clin Oncol* 2007;25:3109–3115.
99. O'Connor OA, Heaney ML, Schwartz L, et al. Clinical experience with intravenous and oral formulations of the novel histone deacetylase inhibitor suberoylanilide hydroxamic acid in patients with advanced hematologic malignancies. *J Clin Oncol* 2006;24:166–173.
100. Ramalingam SS, Maitland ML, Frankel P, et al. Carboplatin and Paclitaxel in combination with either vorinostat or placebo for first-line therapy of advanced non-small-cell lung cancer. *J Clin Oncol* 2010;28:56–62.
101. Giles F, Fischer T, Cortes J, et al. A phase I study of intravenous LBH589, a novel cinnamic hydroxamic acid analogue histone deacetylase inhibitor, in patients with refractory hematologic malignancies. *Clin Cancer Res* 2006; 12:4628–4635.
102. Richardson PG, Hungria VTM, Yoon S-S, et al. Panorama 1: A randomized, double-blind, phase 3 study of panobinostat or placebo plus bortezomib and dexamethasone in relapsed or relapsed and refractory multiple myeloma. *ASCO Meeting Abstracts* 2014;32:8510.
103. Piekarz RL, Robey R, Sandor V, et al. Inhibitor of histone deacetylation, depsipeptide (FR901228), in the treatment of peripheral and cutaneous T-cell lymphoma: a case report. *Blood* 2001;98:2865–2868.
104. Coiffier B, Pro B, Prince HM, et al. Romidepsin for the treatment of relapsed/refractory peripheral T-cell lymphoma: pivotal study update demonstrates durable responses. *J Hematol Oncol* 2014;7:11.
105. Coiffier B, Pro B, Prince HM, et al. Results from a pivotal, open-label, phase II study of romidepsin in relapsed or refractory peripheral T-cell lymphoma after prior systemic therapy. *J Clin Oncol* 2012;30:631–636.
106. Piekarz RL, Frye AR, Wright JJ, et al. Cardiac studies in patients treated with depsipeptide, FK228, in a phase II trial for T-cell lymphoma. *Clin Cancer Res* 2006;12:3762–3773.
107. Gojo I, Jiemjit A, Trepel JB, et al. Phase 1 and pharmacologic study of MS-275, a histone deacetylase inhibitor, in adults with refractory and relapsed acute leukemias. *Blood* 2007;109:2781–2790.
108. Prebet T, Sun JP, Figueroa ME, et al. Prolonged administration of azacitidine with or without entinostat for myelodysplastic syndrome and acute myeloid leukemia with myelodysplasia-related changes: results of the US Leukemia Intergroup Trial E1905. *J Clin Oncol* 2014;32:1242–1248.
109. Witta SE, Jotte RM, Konduri K, et al. Randomized phase II trial of erlotinib with and without entinostat in patients with advanced non-small-cell lung cancer who progressed on prior chemotherapy. *J Clin Oncol* 2012;30:2248–2255.
110. Yardley DA, Ismail-Khan RR, Melichar B, et al. Randomized phase II, double-blind, placebo-controlled study of exemestane with or without entinostat in postmenopausal women with locally recurrent or metastatic estrogen receptor-positive breast cancer progressing on treatment with a nonsteroidal aromatase inhibitor. *J Clin Oncol* 2013;31:2128–2135.
111. Byrd JC, Marcucci G, Parthun MR, et al. A phase 1 and pharmacodynamic study of depsipeptide (FK228) in chronic lymphocytic leukemia and acute myeloid leukemia. *Blood* 2005;105:959–967.
112. Charache S, Dover G, Smith K, et al. Treatment of sickle cell anemia with 5-azacytidine results in increased fetal hemoglobin production and is associated with nonrandom hypomethylation of DNA around the gamma-delta-beta-globin gene complex. *Proc Natl Acad Sci U S A* 1983;80:4842–4846.
113. Silverman LR, Holland JF, Weinberg RS, et al. Effects of treatment with 5-azacytidine on the in vivo and in vitro hematopoiesis in patients with myelodysplastic syndromes. *Leukemia* 1993;7:21–29.
114. Silverman LR, McKenzie DR, Peterson BL, et al. Further analysis of trials with azacitidine in patients with myelodysplastic syndrome: studies 8421, 8921, and 9221 by the Cancer and Leukemia Group B. *J Clin Oncol* 2006;24:3895–3903.
115. Silverman LR, Demakos EP, Peterson BL, et al. Randomized controlled trial of azacitidine in patients with the myelodysplastic syndrome: a study of the Cancer and Leukemia Group B. *J Clin Oncol* 2002;20:2429–2440.
116. Fenaux P, Mufti GJ, Hellstrom-Lindberg E, et al. Efficacy of azacitidine compared with that of conventional care regimens in the treatment of higher-risk myelodysplastic syndromes: a randomised, open-label, phase III study. *Lancet Oncol* 2009;10:223–232.
117. Fenaux P, Mufti GJ, Hellstrom-Lindberg E, et al. Azacitidine prolongs overall survival compared with conventional care regimens in elderly patients with low bone marrow blast count acute myeloid leukemia. *J Clin Oncol* 2010;28: 562–569.
118. Wijermans P, Lubbert M, Verhoef G, et al. Low-dose 5-aza-2'-deoxycytidine, a DNA hypomethylating agent, for the treatment of high-risk myelodysplastic syndrome: a multicenter phase II study in elderly patients. *J Clin Oncol* 2000;18:956–962.
119. Wijermans PW, Krulder JW, Huijgens PC, et al. Continuous infusion of low-dose 5-Aza-2'-deoxycytidine in elderly patients with high-risk myelodysplastic syndrome. *Leukemia* 1997;11:1–5.
120. Kantarjian HM, O'Brien S, Cortes J, et al. Results of decitabine (5-aza-2'deoxycytidine) therapy in 130 patients with chronic myelogenous leukemia. *Cancer* 2003;98:522–528.
121. Kantarjian H, Oki Y, Garcia-Manero G, et al. Results of a randomized study of 3 schedules of low-dose decitabine in higher-risk myelodysplastic syndrome and chronic myelomonocytic leukemia. *Blood* 2007;109:52–57.
122. Steensma DP, Baer MR, Slack JL, et al. Multicenter study of decitabine administered daily for 5 days every 4 weeks to adults with myelodysplastic syndromes: the alternative dosing for outpatient treatment (ADOPT) trial. *J Clin Oncol* 2009;27:3842–3848.
123. Kantarjian H, Issa JP, Rosenfeld CS, et al. Decitabine improves patient outcomes in myelodysplastic syndromes: results of a phase III randomized study. *Cancer* 2006;106:1794–1803.
124. WijerMans P, Suciu S, Baila L, et al. Low-dose decitabine versus best supportive care in elderly patients with intermediate or high risk MDS not eligible for intensive chemotherapy: final results of the randomized phase III study (06011) of the EORTC Leukemia and German MDS Study Groups. *ASH Annual Meeting Abstracts* 2008;112:226.
125. Flotho C, Claus R, Batz C, et al. The DNA methyltransferase inhibitors azacitidine, decitabine and zebularine exert differential effects on cancer gene expression in acute myeloid leukemia cells. *Leukemia* 2009;23:1019–1028.
126. Lübbert M, Suciu S, Baila L, et al. Low-dose decitabine versus best supportive care in elderly patients with intermediate- or high-risk myelodysplastic syndrome (MDS) ineligible for intensive chemotherapy: final results of the randomized phase III study (06011) of the European Organisation for Research and Treatment of Cancer Leukemia Group and the German MDS Study Group. *J Clin Oncol* 2011;29:1987–1996.
127. Kantarjian HM, Thomas XG, Dmoszynska A, et al. Multicenter, randomized, open-label, phase III trial of decitabine versus patient choice, with physician advice, of either supportive care or low-dose cytarabine for the treatment of older patients with newly diagnosed acute myeloid leukemia. *J Clin Oncol* 2012;30:2670–2677.
128. Sudan N, Rossetti JM, Shadduck RK, et al. Treatment of acute myelogenous leukemia with outpatient azacitidine. *Cancer* 2006;107:1839–1843.
129. Kantarjian HM, O'Brien SM, Keating M, et al. Results of decitabine therapy in the accelerated and blastic phases of chronic myelogenous leukemia. *Leukemia* 1997;11:1617–1620.
130. Ruter B, Wijermans P, Claus R, et al. Preferential cytogenetic response to continuous intravenous low-dose decitabine (DAC) administration in myelodysplastic syndrome with monosomy 7. *Blood* 2007;110:1080–1082.
131. Raj K, John A, Ho A, et al. CDKN2B methylation status and isolated chromosome 7 abnormalities predict responses to treatment with 5-azacytidine. *Leukemia* 2007;21:1937–1944.
132. Ravandi F, Issa JP, Garcia-Manero G, et al. Superior outcome with hypomethylating therapy in patients with acute myeloid leukemia and high-risk myelodysplastic syndrome and chromosome 5 and 7 abnormalities. *Cancer* 2009;115:5746–5751.

133. Yang AS, Doshi KD, Choi SW, et al. DNA methylation changes after 5-aza-2'-deoxycytidine therapy in patients with leukemia. *Cancer Res* 2006;66:5495–5503.
134. Yang AS, Estecio MR, Doshi K, et al. A simple method for estimating global DNA methylation using bisulfite PCR of repetitive DNA elements. *Nucleic Acids Res* 2004;32:e38.
135. Daskalakis M, Nguyen TT, Nguyen C, et al. Demethylation of a hypermethylated P15/INK4B gene in patients with myelodysplastic syndrome by 5-Aza-2'-deoxycytidine (decitabine) treatment. *Blood* 2002;100:2957–2964.
136. Bakkenist CJ, Kastan MB. DNA damage activates ATM through intermolecular autophosphorylation and dimer dissociation. *Nature* 2003;421:499–506.
137. Borthakur G, Ahdab SE, Ravandi F, et al. Activity of decitabine in patients with myelodysplastic syndrome previously treated with azacitidine. *Leuk Lymphoma* 2008;49:690–695.
138. Shen L, Kantarjian H, Guo Y, et al. DNA methylation predicts survival and response to therapy in patients with myelodysplastic syndromes. *J Clin Oncol* 2010;28:605–613.
139. Figueroa ME, Skrabanek L, Li Y, et al. MDS and secondary AML display unique patterns and abundance of aberrant DNA methylation. *Blood* 2009;114:3448–3458.
140. Fandy TE, Herman JG, Kerns P, et al. Early epigenetic changes and DNA damage do not predict clinical response in an overlapping schedule of 5-azacytidine and entinostat in patients with myeloid malignancies. *Blood* 2009;114:2764–2773.
141. Schuebel KE, Chen W, Cope L, et al. Comparing the DNA hypermethylome with gene mutations in human colorectal cancer. *PLoS Genet* 2007;3:1709–1723.
142. Maslak P, Chanel S, Camacho LH, et al. Pilot study of combination transcriptional modulation therapy with sodium phenylbutyrate and 5-azacytidine in patients with acute myeloid leukemia or myelodysplastic syndrome. *Leukemia* 2006;20:212–217.
143. Garcia-Manero G, Kantarjian HM, Sanchez-Gonzalez B, et al. Phase I/II study of the combination of 5-aza-2'-deoxycytidine with valproic acid in patients with leukemia. *Blood* 2006;108:3271–3279.
144. Soriano AO, Yang H, Faderl S, et al. Safety and clinical activity of the combination of 5-azacytidine, valproic acid, and all-trans retinoic acid in acute myeloid leukemia and myelodysplastic syndrome. *Blood* 2007;110:2302–2308.
145. Voso MT, Santini V, Finelli C, et al. Valproic acid at therapeutic plasma levels may increase 5-azacytidine efficacy in higher risk myelodysplastic syndromes. *Clin Cancer Res* 2009;15:5002–5007.
146. Sharma S, Kelly TK, Jones PA. Epigenetics in cancer. *Carcinogenesis* 2010;31:27–36.
147. Silverman LR, Fenaux P, Mufti GJ, et al. Continued azacitidine therapy beyond time of first response improves quality of response in patients with higher-risk myelodysplastic syndromes. *Cancer* 2011;117:2697–2702.
148. Craddock C, Quek L, Goardon N, et al. Azacitidine fails to eradicate leukemic stem/progenitor cell populations in patients with acute myeloid leukemia and myelodysplasia. *Leukemia* 2013;27:1028–1036.
149. Juergens RA, Wrangle J, Vendetti FP, et al. Combination epigenetic therapy has efficacy in patients with refractory advanced non-small cell lung cancer. *Cancer Discov* 2011;1:598–607.
150. Wrangle J, Wang W, Koch A, et al. Alterations of immune response of Non-Small Cell Lung Cancer with Azacytidine. *Oncotarget* 2013;4:2067–2079.
151. Shakya R, Gonda TA, Quante M, et al. Hypomethylating therapy in an aggressive stroma rich model of pancreatic carcinoma. *Cancer Res* 2013;73:885–896.
152. Humeniuk R, Menon LG, Mishra PJ, et al. Decreased levels of UMP kinase as a mechanism of fluoropyrimidine resistance. *Mol Cancer Ther* 2009;8:1037–1044.
153. Meng F, Sun G, Zhong M, et al. Anticancer efficacy of the combination of low-dose cisplatin and trichostatin A or 5-aza-2'-deoxycytidine in ovarian cancer cells. Paper presented at: 2012 ASCO Annual Meeting; 2012; Chicago, IL.
154. Matei D, Fang F, Shen C, et al. Epigenetic resensitization to platinum in ovarian cancer. *Cancer Res* 2012;72:2197–2205.
155. Fu S, Hu W, Iyer R, et al. Phase 1b-2a study to reverse platinum resistance through use of a hypomethylating agent, azacitidine, in patients with platinum-resistant or platinum-refractory epithelial ovarian cancer. *Cancer* 2011;117:1661–1669.
156. Chung CW, Coste H, White JH, et al. Discovery and characterization of small molecule inhibitors of the BET family bromodomains. *J Med Chem* 2011;54:3827–3838.
157. Bernt KM, Zhu N, Sinha AU, et al. MLL-rearranged leukemia is dependent on aberrant H3K79 methylation by DOT1L. *Cancer Cell* 2011;20:66–78.
158. Daigle SR, Olhava EJ, Therkelsen CA, et al. Selective killing of mixed lineage leukemia cells by a potent small-molecule DOT1L inhibitor. *Cancer Cell* 2011;20:53–65.
159. Spannhoff A, Hauser AT, Heinke R, et al. The emerging therapeutic potential of histone methyltransferase and demethylase inhibitors. *ChemMedChem* 2009;4:1568–1582.
160. Okada Y, Feng Q, Lin Y, et al. hDOT1L links histone methylation to leukemogenesis. *Cell* 2005;121:167–178.

24 Proteasome Inhibitors

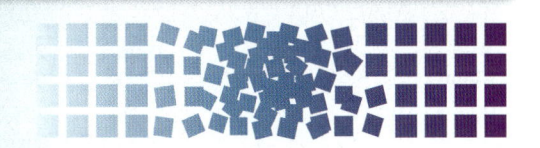

Christopher J. Kirk, Brian B. Tuch, Shirin Arastu-Kapur, and Lawrence H. Boise

BIOCHEMISTRY OF THE UBIQUITIN-PROTEASOME PATHWAY

The ubiquitin proteasome system is involved in the degradation of more than 80% of cellular proteins, including those that control cell-cycle progression, apoptosis, DNA repair, and the stress response.[1] A key step in this process is the *tagging* of proteins targeted for degradation with multiple copies of ubiquitin, a 76–amino acid protein whose primary sequence and structure is highly conserved in organisms ranging from yeasts to mammals.[2,3] Once polyubiquitinated, proteins targeted for degradation bind to the 26S proteasome, a holoenzyme composed of two 19S regulatory complexes capping a central 20S proteolytic core. The 20S core is a hollow "barrel" consisting of four stacked heptameric rings. The subunits of the rings are classified as either β subunits (outer two rings) or β subunits (inner two rings). The 19S regulatory complex consists of a lid that recognizes ubiquitinated protein substrates with high fidelity, and a base that contains six adenosine triphosphatases, unfolds protein substrates, removes the polyubiquitin tag, and threads them into the catalytic chamber of the 20S particle in an adenosine triphosphate–dependent manner.[4,5] Unlike typical proteases, the 20S proteasome in eukaryotic cells contains multiple proteolytic activities resulting in the cleavage of protein targets after many different amino acids. In most cells, the 20S core particle contains the catalytic subunits β5 (PSMB5), β1 (PSMB1), and β2 (PSMB2), accounting for chymotrypsin-like (CT-L), caspaselike (C-L), and trypsinlike (T-L) activities, respectively, each differing in their substrate preference.[6] However, in cells of hematopoietic origin, such as lymphocytes and monocytes, the proteasome catalytic subunits are encoded by homologous gene products: LMP7 (PSMB8), LMP2 (PSMB9), and MECL-1 (PSMB10).[7] These immunoproteasome subunits are also induced in nonhematopoietic cells following exposure to inflammatory cytokines such as interferon-γ (IFN-γ) and tumor necrosis factor alpha (TNF-α).[8] In the immunoproteasome, the 19S regulatory complex can be replaced with proteasome activators such as PA28, whose expression is also induced in cells following exposure to IFN-γ. Hybrid proteasomes, both for the catalytic subunits and regulatory particles, have been described.[9]

Given its key role in maintaining cellular homeostasis, the ubiquitin proteasome system appeared to be an unlikely target for pharmaceutical intervention. However, a variety of groundbreaking studies in the 1990s suggested that inhibitors of proteasome function might prove to be viable therapeutic agents.[10] Initial studies used substrate-related peptide aldehydes to investigate the proteolytic functions and specificity of the proteasome.[11] In vitro and in vivo studies with these inhibitors demonstrated their ability to induce apoptosis as well as inhibit tumor growth.[12–15] It was subsequently discovered that several natural products with antitumor activity exert their action via proteasome inhibition, providing additional rationale for the development of selective proteasome inhibitors (PIs).[16,17]

PROTEASOME INHIBITORS

Chemical Classes of Proteasome Inhibitors in Clinical Development

As of the writing of this overview, six different proteasome inhibitors comprising three distinct chemical classes have been tested in clinical trials (Table 24.1) and include: (1) dipeptide boronic acids, (2) peptide epoxy ketones, and (3) β-lactones.[18,19] Bortezomib (PS-341, Velcade), a dipeptide boronic acid, was developed by Millennium Pharmaceuticals (Cambridge, MA) and was the first PI approved for clinical use.[20] Two additional dipeptide boronic acids have entered clinical development, ixazomib/MLN 9708 (Millennium), currently in phase III studies, and delanzomib/CEP-18770 (Teva Pharmaceuticals; Frazer, PA), the clinical development of which has been halted. Carfilzomib (Onyx Pharmaceuticals; San Francisco, CA), a tetrapeptide epoxy ketone, received U.S. Food and Drug Administration (FDA) approval in 2012.[21] A second peptide epoxy ketone proteasome inhibitor, oprozomib (Onyx), entered clinical study in 2010. The third class of proteasome inhibitors, β-lactones, is represented by NPI-0052 (salinosporamide A [Marizomib]) and is currently being developed by Nereus Pharmaceuticals, Inc. (San Diego, CA). The initial approvals for both bortezomib and carfilzomib were in multiple myeloma (MM), a plasma cell neoplasm and the second most common hematologic cancer. However, the activity of PIs in other B-cell neoplasms has resulted in an expansion of the clinical utilization of this drug class.

Preclinical Activity of Proteasome Inhibitors

Each of the three classes of inhibitors has a distinct chemical mechanism of proteasome inhibition.[22] Peptide boronates form stable but reversible tetrahedral intermediates with the γ-hydroxyl (γ-OH) group of the catalytic N-terminal threonine of the proteasome active sites.[23,24] β-lactones also interact with this γ-OH, but form a completely irreversible interaction.[25] Similarly, peptide epoxy ketones form irreversible covalent adducts with the active site threonine but do so via a dual covalent adduction of γ-OH group and the free amine.[26] This interaction is highly specific for N-terminal threonine-containing hydrolases and renders peptide epoxy ketones the most selective proteasome inhibitors yet described.[27,28]

The primary targets of these PIs within the constitutive and immunoproteasomes are the CT-L subunits, β5 and LMP7, respectively. Despite accounting for less than 50% of total protein turnover by the proteasome, these subunits are essential for cell survival.[29] In MM cell lines, inhibiting both subunits (β5 and LMP7) is necessary and sufficient for tumor cell death.[30] Cytotoxicity of other tumor cell types requires the inhibition of multiple active sites beyond the CT-L activity. The combination of inhibitors specific for either the T-L or C-L activities, which have no cytotoxic activity on their own, augments the cytotoxic potential of the CT-L–specific inhibitors.[31,32]

TABLE 24.1 Proteasome Inhibitors in Clinical Development

Agent	Other Names	Drug Class	Stage of Development	Tumor Types	Route of Administration	Dose Levels	Schedule of Administration
Bortezomib	Velcade PS-341	Peptide boronate	FDA/EMEA approved	Multiple myeloma, mantle cell lymphoma	Intravenous, subcutaneous	1.3 mg/m^2	Days 1, 4, 8, & 11 (21-day cycle)
Ixazomib	MLN 9708 MLN 2238	Peptide boronate	Phase III	Multiple myeloma, AL amyloidosis	Oral	4 mg	Once weekly (21-day cycle)
Delanzomib	CEP-18770	Peptide boronate	Phase I (discontinued)	Multiple myeloma	Intravenous	0.1–1.8 mg/m^2	Days 1, 4, 8, & 11 (21-day cycle)
Carfilzomib	Kyprolis PR-171	Peptide epoxy ketone	FDA approved, phase III	Multiple myeloma	Intravenous	20/27 mg/m^2	Days 1, 2, 8, 9, 15, & 16 (28-day cycle)
Oprozomib	ONX 0912 PR-047	Peptide epoxy ketone	Phase I/II	Multiple myeloma	Oral	150–240 mg (dose escalation ongoing)	Days 1, 2, 8, & 9 (14-day cycle) Days 1–5 (14-day cycle)
Marizomib	NPI-0052 Salinosporamide A	β-lactone	Phase II	Multiple myeloma	Intravenous	0.075–0.6 mg/m^2	Days 1, 4, 8, & 11 (21-day cycle)

EMEA, European Medicines Agency; AL, amyloid light chain.

Given its status as the first proteasome inhibitor approved for marketed use, the antitumor potential and preclinical activity of other proteasome inhibitors have generally been compared to bortezomib.[19] Carfilzomib showed equivalent antitumor activity to bortezomib in vitro against a panel of tumor cell lines under standard culture conditions but was >10-fold more potent at inducing tumor cell death when cells were exposed to drug for a 1-hour pulse, which mimics the pharmacokinetics of both compounds.[33] MLN2238 (the active agent of ixazomib) was active in the same mouse models of human tumors as bortezomib, but demonstrated greater levels of proteasome inhibition in the tumors.[34] In biochemical assays of proteasome activity, delanzomib had an identical potency and subunit activity profile to bortezomib, but in tumor cytotoxicity assays, potency relative to bortezomib was 2- to 10-fold less.[35] In addition, delanzomib appeared to be less cytotoxic than bortezomib to normal cells and had a differential effect on cytokine release in bone marrow stromal cells, suggesting a different pharmacologic activity. Oprozomib is 10-fold less potent than carfilzomib in proteasome activity assays, but showed similar antitumor activity in mouse tumor models.[36,37] Marizomib displayed greater potency against the non–CT-L active sites of the proteasome than bortezomib.[38] Interestingly, this agent synergized with bortezomib in killing tumor cells in vitro.[39] All of the second-generation inhibitors have shown activity in tumor cells made resistant to bortezomib and/or MM cells isolated from patients relapsed from bortezomib-based therapies.[35,36,40–42]

The inhibition of tumor cells with proteasome inhibitors induces cell death via the induction of apoptosis through death effector caspase activation.[10] Although the mechanism underlying the induction of cell death remains to be fully elucidated, extensive research suggests a complex interplay of multiple pathways. PIs have been shown to affect the half-life of the *BH3-only* members of the Bcl-2 family, specifically BH3–interacting-domain death agonist (Bid) and Bcl-2 interacting killer (Bik).[43] Moreover the BH3-only protein NOXA is upregulated at the transcription level by PIs.[44–48] Proteasome inhibition also upregulates the expression of several key cell-cycle checkpoint proteins that include p53 (an inducer of G0/G1 cell-cycle arrest through accumulation of the cyclin-dependent kinase [CDK] inhibitor p27); the CDK inhibitor p21; mammalian cyclins A, B, D, and E; and transcription factors E2F and Rb.[49,50] The transcription factor nuclear factor kappa B (NF-κB), an important regulator of cell survival and cytokine/growth factor production,[51] is also affected by proteasome inhibition in multiple ways. The net effect on NF-κB signaling is not consistent across various assays and cell lines, and its relative importance in the antitumor effects of PIs remains unclear. Although it is interesting to note that patients whose myeloma harbor NF-κB–activating mutations (~20%) respond better to bortezomib than those without NF-κB–activating mutations.[52–54] In MM cell lines, there is growing evidence that the major determinant of sensitivity to proteasome inhibition is the relative load of protein flux to the proteasome.[55–57] These data suggest that induction of the terminal unfolded protein response may drive cell death. Whether proteotoxic stress induced cell death reflects sensitivity to proteasome inhibitors in other tumor types remains to be determined.

Pharmacokinetics and Pharmacodynamics of Proteasome Inhibitors in Animals

Following intravenous (IV) administration to animals and humans, proteasome activity is inhibited in a dose-dependent fashion within minutes; however, PIs such as bortezomib and carfilzomib are also rapidly cleared from circulation.[55,56,58–61] Recovery of proteasome activity in animals occurs in tissues with a half-life of approximately 24 hours, mirroring the recovery time of cells exposed to sublethal concentrations of PIs in vitro and likely reflecting new protein synthesis.[33,62]

PROTEASOME INHIBITORS IN CANCER

Clinical Activity of Bortezomib

Bortezomib is typically administered on days 1, 4, 8, and 11 of a 3-week cycle either as an IV bolus or subcutaneous administration. Increasing doses of bortezomib inhibit proteasome activity in blood in a dose-dependent fashion, reaching a maximum of 74% inhibition at a dose of 1.38 mg/m^2. Daily dosing schedules in animal studies have been associated with severe toxicity and have not been attempted in humans. In clinical trials, thrombocytopenia and peripheral neuropathy (PN) were common adverse events.[20,63,64] Bortezomib has shown remarkable single-agent antitumor activity in a wide range of B-cell neoplasms, including MM, non Hodgkin lymphoma (NHL), and Waldenström macroglobulinemia (WM). In 2003, bortezomib was approved by the FDA for use as a single agent for the treatment of patients with MM following two prior therapies and who demonstrated disease progression with their most recent therapy. The primary efficacy data for this approval was derived from the SUMMIT trial in which 202 patients with heavily pretreated disease were treated with bortezomib at 1.3 mg/m^2.[65] In this trial, the overall response rate (ORR), defined as patients achieving at least a 50% reduction in serum or urine levels of the myeloma M protein, was 35%. This clinical trial was supported by the CREST trial, in which the activity of 1.3 mg/m^2 dose was determined to be superior to a dose of 1.0 mg/m^2.[66] Bortezomib is also active as a single agent in earlier stage MM patient populations. A single-agent ORR of 38%, with a 6% complete response (CR) rate, was seen in the phase III APEX study in early relapsed MM, with a time to progression (TTP) of 6.2 months and a median duration of response of 8 months.[67] In this study, the major grade 3 and 4 toxicities were PN, 12%; dysesthesia and related symptoms, 8% to 10%; anemia, 8%; diarrhea, 8%; neutropenia, 14%; and fatigue, 12%. In the frontline setting, bortezomib demonstrated a single-agent response rate of 41% (5% CR rate).[68]

Bortezomib is also approved for newly diagnosed MM in combination with velcade, melphalan and prednisone (VMP). The phase III VISTA trial evaluated VMP in patients with untreated MM who were ineligible for high-dose therapy.[69] The addition of bortezomib to the melphalan prednisone (MP) backbone significantly improved response rates in this setting with an ORR of 71% for VMP (including 30% CR) versus 35% (with only 4% CR) for MP.[52] VMP was associated with a TTP of ~24 months, compared with ~16.6 months with MP. After a 5-year follow-up, there was a 31% reduced risk of death for the VMP group versus MP-treated patients.[70]

Bortezomib has also shown promise when combined with other agents in relapsed and refractory MM patients. The combination of bortezomib with pegylated doxorubicin (Doxil, Centocor Ortho Biotech Products, L.P.; Horsham, PA) resulted in an ORR of 79% in relapsed patients, and toxicities were similar to those observed with each agent administered separately.[71] A phase III study in 646 patients with relapsed and refractory MM compared this treatment with bortezomib alone; the combination produced a 44% ORR and extended the TTP from 6 to 9.3 months.[72,73] The combination of bortezomib with revlimid, lenalidomide and dexamethasone (Rd), a standard of care in the treatment of MM, resulted in an ORR of 64% and a median duration of response of 8.7 months.[74] This activity is striking given that 53% of patients had received prior bortezomib and 75% of patients had received prior thalidomide, a closely related analog of lenalidomide. Other agents tested in combination with bortezomib include vorinostat, the anti-CS1 mAb, elotuzumab, the Hsp90 inhibitor tanespimycin, and the Akt inhibitor perifosine.[75]

Frontline combinations with bortezomib in MM patients have shown high ORRs with a notable improvement in CR rates. In longer term studies, CR rates with bortezomib-based combinations have been shown to be associated with improved clinical outcomes.[63,64] A community-based phase IIIb study evaluating bortezomib + dexamethasone (VD) versus bortezomib + thalidomide + dexamethasone (VTD) versus VMP found similar ORR (60%, 70%, and 52%, respectively) and CR rates (13%, 18%, and 15%, respectively).[63] Bortezomib + melphalan + prednisone + thalidomide (VMPT) followed by bortezomib + thalidomide (VT) maintenance resulted in a superior CR rate compared with VMP with no maintenance (34% versus 21%) and improved 2-year progression-free survival (70% versus 58.2%).[64] A protocol modification in this trial involved changing from twice weekly to weekly bortezomib administration, which yielded similar TTP but reduced the incidence (21% versus 43%) and severity of PN (2% grade 3/4 versus 14%).[64] The bortezomib, lenalidomide, and dexamethasone combination in newly diagnosed MM resulted in a ORR of 100% in 66 patients, 29% of whom achieved a CR.[76]

Bortezomib has also shown activity in other hematologic cancers, most notably mantle cell lymphoma (MCL).[77,78] As a single agent in 155 relapsed and refractory MCL patients, bortezomib yielded an ORR of 33% (8% CR), a median duration of response of 9.2 months, and a TTP of 6.2 months.[78] Toxicities observed were similar to those seen in patients with MM and included thrombocytopenia, PN, and fatigue. When bortezomib was used to treat both newly diagnosed and refractory MCL, a response rate of 46% was observed in both populations,[77] leading to FDA approval late in 2006.

Bortezomib has been tested in a variety of solid tumors in phase I and II studies.[79] Partial responses (PR) were reported in 8% of patients with refractory non–small-cell lung cancer (NSCLC), although the TTP was 1.5 months.[80] Exacerbation of PN was common. Bortezomib was subsequently tested in combination with paclitaxel, irinotecan, and gemcitabine/carboplatin; however, results have not been encouraging. Bortezomib continues to be tested in combination with other agents in a variety of tumor types.[81,82]

Recent clinical activity and preclinical data suggest that proteasome inhibition may extend to nononcology applications. Single-agent bortezomib therapy in kidney transplant patients undergoing antibody-mediated rejection resulted in a reduction of donor-specific antibodies and improved renal function.[83] In mouse models of lupus nephritis, bortezomib resulted in a reduction of pathogenic plasma cells and the prevention of disease progression.[84] These data suggest that PIs may be useful in a wide range of B-cell–mediated diseases. However, toxicities with bortezomib, particularly PN, may prevent wider application of this particular agent.

Carfilzomib

Parallel phase I studies of carfilzomib have been conducted in patients with multiple tumor types, and two phase I dose-finding studies targeting B-cell malignancies have been completed. The first study used daily IV bolus dosing with doses up to 20 mg/m^2 for 5 consecutive days followed by 9 days of rest and resulted in substantial inhibition of proteasome activity.[85] In the second study, carfilzomib was administered daily for 2 days for 3 consecutive weeks (days 1, 2, 8, 9, 15, and 16), followed by 12 days of recovery.[86] Hematologic toxicities were the most frequent adverse events, observed along with transient, noncumulative elevations in serum creatinine, usually with increases in serum urea nitrogen and consistent with a *prerenal* etiology. New onset PN was infrequent. Among 20 evaluable patients (including bortezomib-refractory patients), 4 PRs and 1 minor response were seen. Responses were also durable, lasting more than 1 year in some cases. Although the maximum tolerated dose of carfilzomib was not established in this study, a dose of 20 mg/m^2 was initially selected for the phase II studies.

Based on the phase I studies, an open-label, single-arm, phase II study of single-agent carfilzomib in relapsed and refractory MM was initiated in 2007.[87,88] Carfilzomib was administered as an IV bolus on the twice-weekly dose schedule. Patients enrolled in the initial phase of the study (003-A0) had received a median of five prior therapies, and 78% of patients had grade 1/2 PN at entry.[87] Among 39 evaluable patients in 003-A0, 10 (26%) achieved a minor response or better, including 5 PRs, and 16 additional patients with stable disease. Based on new safety information from phase I studies, the protocol was amended and the carfilzomib dose was escalated to 27 mg/m^2 after the first cycle (003-A1).[89] In this trial, 266 patients were enrolled and all patients had previously been treated with an immunomodulatory agent (IMiD) and bortezomib and were refractory to their last therapy. An ORR of 24% with a median duration of response of 8 months was reported. Adverse events were predominantly hematopoietic (thrombocytopenia, lymphopenia, and anemia) and there was a <1% rate of grade 3 PN, despite 77% having a history of PN. Based on these findings, carfilzomib was granted conditional approval by the FDA in 2012 for the treatment of patients with relapsed and refractory myeloma who had received prior bortezomib and IMiD therapy.

The parallel PX-171-004 trial enrolled patients with relapsed MM following one to three prior treatments and who may have been refractory to one or more of these therapies.[90,91] Of the 155 patients enrolled in this trial, 120 had not received prior bortezomib-based therapy. In patients with relapsed disease, non-hematologic and hematologic toxicity profiles were similar. Despite high rates of baseline PN, reports of worsening neuropathic symptoms were infrequent (2% incidence of grade 3 and no grade 4 events). Carfilzomib demonstrated considerable activity in bortezomib-naïve patients, inducing PR or better in 46% of 54 evaluable patients at 20 mg/m^2 and 53% of patients at 27 mg/m^2.[91] The response rate in patients previously exposed to bortezomib was lower (18%).[90] Responses across groups are durable, typically 8 to 9 months.[90,91]

Based on findings in animal studies in which a 30-minute infusion of carfilzomib resulted in reduced toxicities,[61] the effect of infusional administration was tested in patients with relapsed and refractory myeloma. In a dose escalation study, PX-171-007, the MTD dose of carfilzomib was determined to be 56 mg/m^2, more than twice the dose used in the studies described previously. In a cohort of 24 patients receiving this dose and who had received a median of five prior lines of therapy (including two prior bortezomib-containing regimens), the ORR was 60%.[92] This enhanced efficacy also correlated with a greater level of inhibition of all three subunits of the immunoproteasome measured in isolated peripheral blood mononuclear cells (Lee S, et al., unpublished).[93] This same dose and infusion time is currently being explored in a phase III trial of nearly 900 patients comparing carfilzomib plus low-dose dexamethasone (Cd) to bortezomib plus low-dose dexamethasone (Vd) in MM patients with relapsed disease.

Trials of carfilzomib in combination with other agents in MM have been initiated, including a phase Ib/II safety and efficacy study of carfilzomib in combination with lenalidomide and low-dose dexamethasone (CRd) in relapsed and/or refractory MM. At the maximum planned dose, the ORR was 77% with a median duration of response of 22 months.[94] The CRd combination is now being tested in an international, multicenter, randomized, open-label phase III study in comparison with lenalidomide and low-dose dexamethasone (Rd) in approximately 780 patients with relapsed MM following one to three prior therapies. The CRd regimen has also been explored in newly diagnosed MM patients.[95] When carfilzomib is combined with Rd at a dose of 36 mg/m^2, 62% of the 53 patients treated achieved a CR. In addition, 20 of 21 patients analyzed for signs of minimal residual disease (MRD), utilizing multiparameter flow cytometry were determined to be free of MRD.

Ixazomib

Initial clinical studies of ixazomib involved dose escalation studies in patients with hematologic malignancies and explored both weekly and twice weekly dosing schedules.[96,97] Oral administration resulted in potent proteasome inhibition of ~65%. Clinical activity in patients with relapsed MM was 16%.[98] In patients with newly diagnosed MM, ixazomib plus lenalidomide and low-dose dexamethasone resulted in an ORR of 93% with 24% achieving a CR.[99] This combination is also being investigated in a phase III trial comparing this to Rd in patients with relapsed MM.

Oprozomib

Initial clinical testing of oprozomib in patients with solid tumors investigated a dosing schedule consisting of a 14-day cycle with once daily administration for 5 consecutive days.[100] In patients with relapsed and/or refractory B-cell neoplasms, two dosing schedules are being utilized: the schedule described previously and one involving 2 consecutive days of dosing repeated weekly.[101] Proteasome inhibition following the administration of oprozomib reached >80% and clinical activity was noted in patients with MM and WM. In patients receiving the 5 consecutive day schedule, 5 of 19 MM patients (26%) and 8 of 10 WM patients (80%) achieved a partial response or better. Exploration of the dose and schedule continues as a single agent and in combination with other anti-MM therapies.

Biomarkers for Proteasome Inhibitors

As described previously, PI-based therapies have proven highly effective in the treatment of MM and other B-cell neoplasms. Given that response rates in single agent trials are generally <50%, there would be a distinct clinical benefit to identify those patients most likely to respond to proteasome inhibition prior to treatment initiation. Gene expression analysis from bone marrow–derived MM tumor cells from 169 bortezomib-treated patients and 70 dexamethasone-treated patients revealed a 100-gene signature that provided a stratification for patients likely to respond that performed better than standard staging systems.[102] However, this signature provided only a modest increase in predictive power for treatment with bortezomib versus dexamethasone. More recently, Keats et al.[54] reanalyzed this dataset based on a pathway analysis of NF-κB and the realization that TRAF3, a key regulatory of the noncanonical NF-κB pathway, is a tumor suppressor in MM cell lines. They found a dramatic enrichment for response to bortezomib in patients with low levels of TRAF3 expression. However, these data remain to be validated in a separate sample set. A transcriptomic analysis of samples derived from single-agent carfilzomib trials suggest that patients with the highest level of immunoglobulin heavy chain expression were the most sensitive to carfilzomib therapy.[103] Similar findings were noted in the expression data from bortezomib-treated patients described previously.[103] These data are supported by phenotypic data from patients progressing on bortezomib-based therapy, in which resistance to bortezomib was associated with a dedifferentiated (and lower immunoglobulin expressing) B-cell phenotype.[104] Taken together, these findings suggest that biomarkers, potentially those involving an analysis of protein load of immunoglobulin expression, may be developed to predict those patients most likely to respond to PIs.

REFERENCES

1. Ciechanover A. Intracellular protein degradation: from a vague idea thru the lysosome and the ubiquitin proteasome system and onto human diseases and drug targeting. *Biochim Biophys Acta* 2012;1824:3–13.
2. Kopp F, Hendil KB, Dahlmann B, et al. Subunit arrangement in the human 20S proteasome. *Proc Natl Acad Sci U S A* 1997;94:2939–2944.
3. Wilkinson KD. Ubiquitination and deubiquitination: targeting of proteins for degradation by the proteasome. *Semin Cell Dev Biol* 2000;11:141–148.
4. Braun BC, Glickman M, Kraft R, et al. The base of the proteasome regulatory particle exhibits chaperone-like activity. *Nat Cell Biol* 1999;1:221–226.
5. Groll M, Ditzel L, Lowe J, et al. Structure of 20S proteasome from yeast at 2.4 A resolution. *Nature* 1997;386:463–471.
6. Borissenko L, Groll M. 20S proteasome and its inhibitors: crystallographic knowledge for drug development. *Chem Rev* 2007;107:687–717.
7. Kloetzel PM, Ossendorp F. Proteasome and peptidase function in MHC-class-I-mediated antigen presentation. *Curr Opin Immunol* 2004;16:76–81.
8. Griffin TA, Nandi D, Cruz M, et al. Immunoproteasome assembly: cooperative incorporation of interferon gamma (IFN-gamma)-inducible subunits. *J Exp Med* 1998;187:97–104.

9. Tanahashi N, Murakami Y, Minami Y, et al. Hybrid proteasomes. Induction by interferon-gamma and contribution to ATP-dependent proteolysis. *J Biol Chem* 2000;275:14336–14345.
10. Adams J. The proteasome: a suitable antineoplastic target. *Nat Rev Cancer* 2004;4:349–360.
11. Vinitsky A, Michaud C, Powers JC, et al. Inhibition of the chymotrypsin-like activity of the pituitary multicatalytic proteinase complex. *Biochemistry* 1992;31:9421–9428.
12. Orlowski RZ, Eswara JR, Lafond-Walker A, et al. Tumor growth inhibition induced in a murine model of human Burkitt's lymphoma by a proteasome inhibitor. *Cancer Res* 1998;58:4342–4348.
13. Imajoh-Ohmi S, Kawaguchi T, Sugiyama S, et al. Lactacystin, a specific inhibitor of the proteasome, induces apoptosis in human monoblast U937 cells. *Biochem Biophys Res Commun* 1995;217:1070–1077.
14. Shinohara K, Tomioka M, Nakano H, et al. Apoptosis induction resulting from proteasome inhibition. *Biochem J* 1996;317:385–388.
15. Delic J, Masdehors P, Omura S, et al. The proteasome inhibitor lactacystin induces apoptosis and sensitizes chemo- and radioresistant human chronic lymphocytic leukaemia lymphocytes to TNF-alpha-initiated apoptosis. *Br J Cancer* 1998;77:1103–1107.
16. Meng L, Mohan R, Kwok BH, et al. Epoxomicin, a potent and selective proteasome inhibitor, exhibits in vivo antiinflammatory activity. *Proc Natl Acad Sci U S A* 1999;96:10403–10408.
17. Meng L, Kwok BH, Sin N, et al. Eponemycin exerts its antitumor effect through the inhibition of proteasome function. *Cancer Res* 1999;59:2798–2801.
18. Dick LR, Fleming PE. Building on bortezomib: second-generation proteasome inhibitors as anti-cancer therapy. *Drug Discov Today* 2010;15:243–249.
19. Kirk CJ. Discovery and development of second-generation proteasome inhibitors. *Semin Hematol* 2012;49:207–214.
20. Bross PF, Kane R, Farrell AT, et al. Approval summary for bortezomib for injection in the treatment of multiple myeloma. *Clin Cancer Res* 2004;10:3954–3964.
21. Herndon TM, Deisseroth A, Kaminskas E, et al. U.S. Food and Drug Administration approval: carfilzomib for the treatment of multiple myeloma. *Clin Cancer Res* 2013;19:4559–4563.
22. Bennett MK, Kirk CJ. Development of proteasome inhibitors in oncology and autoimmune diseases. *Curr Opin Drug Discov Devel* 2008;11:616–625.
23. Adams J, Behnke M, Chen S, et al. Potent and selective inhibitors of the proteasome: dipeptidyl boronic acids. *Bioorg Med Chem Lett* 1998;8:333–338.
24. Groll M, Berkers CR, Ploegh HL, et al. Crystal structure of the boronic acid-based proteasome inhibitor bortezomib in complex with the yeast 20S proteasome. *Structure* 2006;14:451–456.
25. Groll M, Huber R, Potts BC. Crystal structures of Salinosporamide A (NPI-0052) and B (NPI-0047) in complex with the 20S proteasome reveal important consequences of beta-lactone ring opening and a mechanism for irreversible binding. *J Am Chem Soc* 2006;19:5136–5141.
26. Groll M, Kim KB, Kairies N, et al. Crystal structure of epoxomicin: 20S proteasome reveals a molecular basis for selectivity of a' b'-epoxyketone proteasome inhibitors. *J Am Chem Soc* 2000;122:1237–1238.
27. Kisselev AF, van der Linden WA, Overkleeft HS. Proteasome inhibitors: an expanding army attacking a unique target. *Chem Biol* 2012;19:99–115.
28. Arastu-Kapur S, Anderl JL, Kraus M, et al. Nonproteasomal targets of the proteasome inhibitors bortezomib and carfilzomib: a link to clinical adverse events. *Clin Cancer Res* 2011;17:2734–2743.
29. Kisselev AF, Callard A, Goldberg AL. Importance of the different proteolytic sites of the proteasome and the efficacy of inhibitors varies with the protein substrate. *J Biol Chem* 2006;281:8582–8590.
30. Parlati F, Lee SJ, Aujay M, et al. Carfilzomib can induce tumor cell death through selective inhibition of the chymotrypsin-like activity of the proteasome. *Blood* 2009;114:3439–3447.
31. Britton M, Lucas MM, Downey SL, et al. Selective inhibitor of proteasome's caspase-like sites sensitizes cells to specific inhibition of chymotrypsin-like sites. *Chem Biol* 2009;16:1278–1289.
32. Mirabella AC, Pletnev AA, Downey SL, et al. Specific cell-permeable inhibitor of proteasome trypsin-like sites selectively sensitizes myeloma cells to bortezomib and carfilzomib. *Chem Biol* 2011;18:608–618.
33. Demo SD, Kirk CJ, Aujay MA, et al. Antitumor activity of PR-171, a novel irreversible inhibitor of the proteasome. *Cancer Res* 2007;67:6383–6391.
34. Kupperman E, Lee EC, Cao Y, et al. Evaluation of the proteasome inhibitor MLN9708 in preclinical models of human cancer. *Cancer Res* 2010;70:1970–1980.
35. Piva R, Ruggeri B, Williams M, et al. CEP-18770: A novel, orally active proteasome inhibitor with a tumor-selective pharmacologic profile competitive with bortezomib. *Blood* 2008;111:2765–2775.
36. Chauhan D, Singh AV, Aujay M, et al. A novel orally active proteasome inhibitor ONX 0912 triggers in vitro and in vivo cytotoxicity in multiple myeloma. *Blood* 2010;116:4906–4915.
37. Zhou HJ, Aujay MA, Bennett MK, et al. Design and synthesis of an orally bioavailable and selective peptide epoxyketone proteasome inhibitor (PR-047). *J Med Chem* 2009;52:3028–3038.
38. Chauhan D, Catley L, Li G, et al. A novel orally active proteasome inhibitor induces apoptosis in multiple myeloma cells with mechanisms distinct from Bortezomib. *Cancer Cell* 2005;8:407–419.
39. Chauhan D, Singh A, Brahmandam M, et al. Combination of proteasome inhibitors bortezomib and NPI-0052 trigger in vivo synergistic cytotoxicity in multiple myeloma. *Blood* 2008;111:1654–1664.
40. Chauhan D, Tian Z, Zhou B, et al. In vitro and in vivo selective antitumor activity of a novel orally bioavailable proteasome inhibitor MLN9708 against multiple myeloma cells. *Clin Cancer Res* 2011;17:5311–5321.
41. Kuhn DJ, Chen Q, Voorhees PM, et al. Potent activity of carfilzomib, a novel, irreversible inhibitor of the ubiquitin-proteasome pathway, against preclinical models of multiple myeloma. *Blood* 2007;110:3281–3290.
42. Suzuki E, Demo S, Deu E, et al. Molecular mechanisms of bortezomib resistant adenocarcinoma cells. *PLoS One* 2011;6:e27996.
43. Zhang HG, Wang J, Yang X, et al. Regulation of apoptosis proteins in cancer cells by ubiquitin. *Oncogene* 2004;23:2009–2015.
44. Fernandez Y, Verhaegen M, Miller TP, et al. Differential regulation of noxa in normal melanocytes and melanoma cells by proteasome inhibition: therapeutic implications. *Cancer Res* 2005;65:6294–6304.
45. Nikiforov MA, Riblett M, Tang WH, et al. Tumor cell-selective regulation of NOXA by c-MYC in response to proteasome inhibition. *Proc Natl Acad Sci U S A* 2007;104:19488–19493.
46. Qin JZ, Ziffra J, Stennett L, et al. Proteasome inhibitors trigger NOXA-mediated apoptosis in melanoma and myeloma cells. *Cancer Res* 2005;65:6282–6293.
47. Wang Q, Mora-Jensen H, Weniger MA, et al. ERAD inhibitors integrate ER stress with an epigenetic mechanism to activate BH3-only protein NOXA in cancer cells. *Proc Natl Acad Sci U S A* 2009;106:2200–2205.
48. Mannava S, Zhuang D, Nair JR, et al. KLF9 is a novel transcriptional regulator of bortezomib- and LBH589-induced apoptosis in multiple myeloma cells. *Blood* 2012;119:1450–1458.
49. Koepp DM, Harper JW, Elledge SJ. How the cyclin became a cyclin: regulated proteolysis in the cell cycle. *Cell* 1999;97:431–434.
50. Pagano M, Tam SW, Theodoras AM, et al. Role of the ubiquitin-proteasome pathway in regulating abundance of the cyclin-dependent kinase inhibitor p27. *Science* 1995;269:682–685.
51. Wan F, Lenardo MJ. The nuclear signaling of NF-kappaB: current knowledge, new insights, and future perspectives. *Cell Res* 2010;20:24–33.
52. Annunziata CM, Davis RE, Demchenko Y, et al. Frequent engagement of the classical and alternative NF-kappaB pathways by diverse genetic abnormalities in multiple myeloma. *Cancer Cell* 2007;12:115–130.
53. Chapman MA, Lawrence MS, Keats JJ, et al. Initial genome sequencing and analysis of multiple myeloma. *Nature* 2011;471:467–472.
54. Keats JJ, Fonseca R, Chesi M, et al. Promiscuous mutations activate the noncanonical NF-kappaB pathway in multiple myeloma. *Cancer Cell* 2007;12:131–144.
55. Meister S, Schubert U, Neubert K, et al. Extensive immunoglobulin production sensitizes myeloma cells for proteasome inhibition. *Cancer Res* 2007;67:1783–1792.
56. Obeng EA, Carlson LM, Gutman DM, et al. Proteasome inhibitors induce a terminal unfolded protein response in multiple myeloma cells. *Blood* 2006;107:4907–4916.
57. Shabaneh TB, Downey SL, Goddard AL, et al. Molecular basis of differential sensitivity of myeloma cells to clinically relevant bolus treatment with bortezomib. *PLoS One* 2013;8:e56132.
58. Papadopoulos KP, Burris HA III, Gordon M, et al. A phase I/II study of carfilzomib 2-10-min infusion in patients with advanced solid tumors. *Cancer Chemother Pharmacol* 2013;72:861–868.
59. Papandreou CN, Daliani DD, Nix D, et al. Phase I trial of the proteasome inhibitor bortezomib in patients with advanced solid tumors with observations in androgen-independent prostate cancer. *J Clin Oncol* 2004;22:2108–2121.
60. Wang Z, Yang J, Kirk C, et al. Clinical pharmacokinetics, metabolism, and drug-drug interaction of carfilzomib. *Drug Metab Dispos* 2013;41:230–237.
61. Yang J, Wang Z, Fang Y, et al. Pharmacokinetics, pharmacodynamics, metabolism, distribution, and excretion of carfilzomib in rats. *Drug Metab Dispos* 2011;39:1873–1882.
62. Meiners S, Heyken D, Weller A, et al. Inhibition of proteasome activity induces concerted expression of proteasome genes and de novo formation of mammalian proteasomes. *J Biol Chem* 2003;278:21517–21525.
63. Lonial S, Waller EK, Richardson PG, et al. Risk factors and kinetics of thrombocytopenia associated with bortezomib for relapsed, refractory multiple myeloma. *Blood* 2005;106:3777–3784.
64. Richardson PG, Briemberg H, Jagannath S, et al. Frequency, characteristics, and reversibility of peripheral neuropathy during treatment of advanced multiple myeloma with bortezomib. *J Clin Oncol* 2006;24:3113–3120.
65. Richardson PG, Barlogie B, Berenson J, et al. A phase 2 study of bortezomib in relapsed, refractory myeloma. *N Engl J Med* 2003;348:2609–2617.
66. Jagannath S, Barlogie B, Berenson J, et al. A phase 2 study of two doses of bortezomib in relapsed or refractory myeloma. *Br J Haematol* 2004;127:165–172.
67. Richardson PG, Sonneveld P, Schuster MW, et al. Bortezomib or high-dose dexamethasone for relapsed multiple myeloma. *N Engl J Med* 2005;352:2487–2498.
68. Jagannath S, Brian D, Wolf JL, et al. A phase 2 study of bortezomib as first-line therapy in patients with multiple myeloma. *Blood* 2004;104:333.
69. San Miguel JF, Schlag R, Khuageva NK, et al. Bortezomib plus melphalan and prednisone for initial treatment of multiple myeloma. *N Engl J Med* 2008;359:906–917.
70. San Miguel JF, Schlag R, Khuageva NK, et al. Persistent overall survival benefit and no increased risk of second malignancies with bortezomib-melphalan-prednisone versus melphalan-prednisone in patients with previously untreated multiple myeloma. *J Clin Oncol* 2013;31:448–455.
71. Orlowski RZ, Voorhees PM, Garcia RA, et al. Phase 1 trial of the proteasome inhibitor bortezomib and pegylated liposomal doxorubicin in patients with advanced hematologic malignancies. *Blood* 2005;105:3058–3065.

72. Orlowski RZ, Nagler A, Sonneveld P, et al. Randomized phase III study of pegylated liposomal doxorubicin plus bortezomib compared with bortezomib alone in relapsed or refractory multiple myeloma: combination therapy improves time to progression. *J Clin Oncol* 2007;25:3892–3901.
73. Sonneveld P, Hajek R, Nagler A, et al. Combined pegylated liposomal doxorubicin and bortezomib is highly effective in patients with recurrent or refractory multiple myeloma who received prior thalidomide/lenalidomide therapy. *Cancer* 2008;112:1529–1537.
74. Richardson PG, Xie W, Jagannath S, et al. A phase II trial of lenalidomide, bortezomib and dexamethasone in patients with relapsed and relapsed/refractory myeloma. *Blood* 2014;123:1461–1469.
75. Kapoor P, Ramakrishnan V, Rajkumar SV. Bortezomib combination therapy in multiple myeloma. *Semin Hematol* 2012;49:228–242.
76. Richardson PG, Weller E, Lonial S, et al. Lenalidomide, bortezomib, and dexamethasone combination therapy in patients with newly diagnosed multiple myeloma. *Blood* 2010;116.679–686.
77. Belch A, Kouroukis CT, Crump M, et al. A phase II study of bortezomib in mantle cell lymphoma: the National Cancer Institute of Canada Clinical Trials Group trial IND.150. *Ann Oncol* 2007;18:116–121.
78. Fisher RI, Bernstein SH, Kahl BS, et al. Multicenter phase II study of bortezomib in patients with relapsed or refractory mantle cell lymphoma. *J Clin Oncol* 2006;24:4867–4874.
79. Milano A, Iaffaioli RV, Caponigro F. The proteasome: a worthwhile target for the treatment of solid tumours? *Eur J Cancer* 2007;43:1125–1133.
80. Fanucchi MP, Fossella FV, Belt R, et al. Randomized phase II study of bortezomib alone and bortezomib in combination with docetaxel in previously treated advanced non-small-cell lung cancer. *J Clin Oncol* 2006;24:5025–5033.
81. Ramaswamy B, Phelps MA, Baiocchi R, et al. A dose-finding, pharmacokinetic and pharmacodynamic study of a novel schedule of flavopiridol in patients with advanced solid tumors. *Invest New Drugs* 2012;30:629–638.
82. Luu T, Chow W, Lim D, et al. Phase I trial of fixed-dose rate gemcitabine in combination with bortezomib in advanced solid tumors. *Anticancer Res* 2010;30:167–174.
83. Everly MJ, Everly JJ, Susskind B, et al. Bortezomib provides effective therapy for antibody- and cell-mediated acute rejection. *Transplantation* 2008;86:1754–1761.
84. Neubert K, Meister S, Moser K, et al. The proteasome inhibitor bortezomib depletes plasma cells and protects mice with lupus-like disease from nephritis. *Nat Med* 2008;14:748–755.
85. O'Connor OA, Stewart AK, Vallone M, et al. A phase 1 dose escalation study of the safety and pharmacokinetics of the novel proteasome inhibitor carfilzomib (PR-171) in patients with hematologic malignancies. *Clin Cancer Res* 2009;15:7085–7091.
86. Alsina M, Trudel S, Furman RR, et al. A phase I single-agent study of twice-weekly consecutive-day dosing of the proteasome inhibitor carfilzomib in patients with relapsed or refractory multiple myeloma or lymphoma. *Clin Cancer Res* 2012;18:4830–4840.
87. Jagannath S, Vij R, Stewart AK, et al. An open-label single-arm pilot phase II study (PX-171-003-A0) of low-dose, single-agent carfilzomib in patients with relapsed and refractory multiple myeloma. *Clin Lymphoma Myeloma Leuk* 2012;12:310–318.
88. Siegel DS, Martin T, Wang M, et al. A phase 2 study of single-agent carfilzomib (PX-171-003-A1) in patients with relapsed and refractory multiple myeloma. *Blood* 2012;120:2817–2825.
89. Siegel DS, Martin T, Wang M, et al. Results of PX-171-003-A1, an open-label, single-arm, phase 2 (Ph 2) study of carfilzomib (CFZ) in patients (pts) with relapsed and refractory multiple myeloma (MM). *Blood* 2012;120:2817–2825.
90. Vij R, Siegel DS, Jagannath S, et al. An open-label, single-arm, phase 2 study of single agent carfilzomib in patients with relapsed and/or refractory multiple myeloma who have been previously treated with bortezomib. *Br J Haematol* 2012;158:739–748.
91. Vij R, Wang M, Kaufman JL, et al. An open-label, single-arm, phase 2 (PX-171-004) study of single-agent carfilzomib in bortezomib-naive patients with relapsed and/or refractory multiple myeloma. *Blood* 2012;119:5661–5670.
92. Papadopoulos K, Capua Siegel DS, Singhal SB, et al. Phase 1b evaluation of the safety and efficacy of a 30-minute IV infusion of carfilzomib in patients with relapsed and/or refractory multiple myeloma. *Blood* 2010;116:3024.
93. Lee SJ, Levitsky K, Parlati F, et al. Clinical activity of carfilzomib correlates with inhibition of multiple proteasome subunits: application of a novel pharmacodynamics assay. (In press).
94. Wang M, Martin T, Bensinger W, et al. Phase 2 dose-expansion study (PX-171-006) of carfilzomib, lenalidomide, and low-dose dexamethasone in relapsed or progressive multiple myeloma. *Blood* 2013;122:3122–3128.
95. Jakubowiak AJ, Dytfeld D, Griffith KA, et al. A phase 1/2 study of carfilzomib in combination with lenalidomide and low-dose dexamethasone as a frontline treatment for multiple myeloma. *Blood* 2012;120:1801–1809.
96. Richardson PG, Baz R, Wang L, et al. Investigational agent MLN9708, an oral proteasome inhibitor, in patients (Pts) with relapsed and/or refractory multiple myeloma (MM): results from the expansion cohorts of a phase 1 dose-escalation study. *Blood* 2011;118:301.
97. Richardson PG, Spencer A, Cannell P, et al. Phase 1 clinical evaluation of twice-weekly marizomib (NPI-0052), a novel proteasome inhibitor, in patients with relapsed/refractory multiple myeloma (MM). *Blood* 2011;118:302.
98. Roy V, Reeder C, LaPlant BR, et al. Phase 2 trial Of single agent MLN9708 in patients with relapsed multiple myeloma not refractory to bortezomib. *Blood* 2013;122:1944.
99. Hofmeister CC, Rosenbaum CA, Htut M, et al. Twice-weekly oral MLN9708 (ixazomib citrate), an investigational proteasome inhibitor, in combination with lenalidomide (len) and dexamethasone (dex) in patients (pts) with newly diagnosed multiple myeloma (MM): final phase 1 results and phase 2 data. *Blood* 2013;122:535.
100. Papadopoulos KP, Mendelson DS, Tolcher AW, et al. A phase I, open-label, dose-escalation study of the novel oral proteasome inhibitor (PI) ONX 0912 in patients with advanced refractory or recurrent solid tumors. *Blood* 2011;29:3075.
101. Kaufman JL, Siegel DS, Vij R, et al. Clinical profile of single-agent modified-release oprozomib tablets in patients (pts) with hematologic malignancies: updated results from a multicenter, open-label, dose escalation phase 1b/2 study. *Blood* 2013;122:3184.
102. Mulligan G, Mitsiades C, Bryant B, et al. Gene expression profiling and correlation with outcome in clinical trials of the proteasome inhibitor bortezomib. *Blood* 2007;109:3177–3188.
103. Loehr A, Degenhardt JD, Kwei KA, et al. Immunoglobulin expression is a major determinant of patient sensitivity to proteasome inhibitors. *Blood* 2013;122:1903.
104. Leung-Hagesteijn C, Erdmann N, Cheung G, et al. Xbp1s-negative tumor B cells and pre-plasmablasts mediate therapeutic proteasome inhibitor resistance in multiple myeloma. *Cancer Cell* 2013;24:289–304.

25 Poly (ADP-ribose) Polymerase Inhibitors

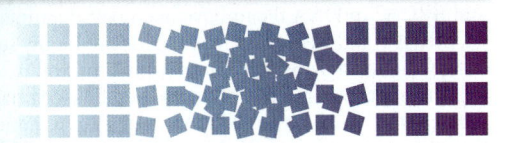

Alan Ashworth

INTRODUCTION

Cancer cells may harbor defects in DNA repair pathways leading to genomic instability. This can foster tumorigenesis but also provides a weakness that can be exploited therapeutically. Tumors with compromised ability to repair double-strand DNA breaks by homologous recombination, including those with defects in the *BRCA1* and *BRCA2* genes, are highly sensitive to blockade of the repair of DNA single-strand breaks, via the inhibition of the enzyme poly(ADP-ribose) (PARP). This provides the basis for a *synthetic lethal* approach to cancer therapy, which is showing considerable promise in the clinic.

CELLULAR DNA REPAIR PATHWAYS

DNA is continually damaged by environmental exposures and endogenous activities, such as DNA replication and cellular free-radical generation, which cause diverse lesions including base modifications, double-strand breaks (DSB), single-strand breaks (SSB), and intrastrand and interstrand cross-links.[1] These aberrations are repaired by distinct repair pathways, which are coordinated to maintain the stability and integrity of the genome. This faithful repair of DNA damage is an essential prerequisite for the maintenance of genomic integrity and cellular and organismal viability. Where one DNA strand is affected and the intact complementary strand is available as a template, the base-excision repair (BER), nucleotide-excision repair, or mismatch repair pathways are used and these pathways are highly efficient at repairing damage. DSBs, more problematic than SSBs because the complementary strand is not available as a template, are repaired by the homologous recombination (HR) or nonhomologous end-joining (NHEJ) pathways.[1]

Endogenous base damage, including SSBs, is the most common DNA aberration and it has been estimated that the average cell may repair 10,000 such lesions every day. BER is an important pathway for the repair of SSBs and involves the sensing of the lesion followed by the recruitment of a number of other proteins. PARP-1 (poly[ADP]ribose polymerase) is a critical component of the major "short-patch" BER pathway. PARP is an enzyme, discovered over 40 years ago,[2] that produces large branched chains of poly(ADP) ribose (PAR) from NAD^+. In humans, there are 17 members of the PARP gene family but most of these are poorly characterized.[3,4] The abundant nuclear protein PARP-1 senses and binds to DNA nicks and breaks, resulting in activation of catalytic activity causing poly(ADP)ribosylation of PARP-1 itself as well as other acceptor proteins including histones. This modification may signal the recruitment of other components of DNA repair pathways as well as modify their activity. The highly negatively charged PAR that is produced around the site of damage may also serve as an antirecombinogenic factor. In addition to the BER pathway PARP enzymes have been implicated in numerous cellular pathways.[3,4]

Two main DSB repair pathways are available within eukaryotic cells: NHEJ and HR.[5,6] HR can be further subdivided into the gene conversion (GC) and single-strand annealing (SSA) subpathways.[1] Both GC and SSA rely on sequence homology for repair whereas NHEJ uses no, or little, homology.[2,3] NHEJ is the most important pathway for the repair of DSBs during G_0, G_1, and early S phases of the cell cycle, although it is likely active throughout the cell cycle.[7,8] This form of DSB repair usually results in changes in DNA sequence at the break site and, occasionally, in the joining of previously unlinked DNA molecules, potentially resulting in gross chromosomal rearrangements such as translocations.[9] GC uses a homologous sequence, preferably the sister chromatid, as a template to resynthesize the DNA surrounding the DSB, and therefore generally results in accurate repair of the break. Repair by GC is critically dependent on the recombinase function of RAD51 and is facilitated by a number of other proteins. SSA also involves the use of homologous sequences for the repair of DSBs, but unlike GC, SSA is RAD51-independent and involves the annealing of DNA strands formed after resection at the DSB. The detailed mechanism of SSA is still obscure but it frequently results in the loss of one of the homologous sequences and deletion of the intervening sequence.[9] SSA is a potentially important pathway of mutagenesis because a significant fraction of mammalian genomes consist of repetitive elements. GC and SSA are cell-cycle regulated and are most active in $S-G_2$ phases of the cell cycle.[10]

THE DEVELOPMENT OF PARP INHIBITORS

PARP inhibitors were originally developed as chemopotentiators, which are agents that enhance the effects of DNA damage—a common mechanism of action of drugs used to treat cancer. The rationale was that inhibition of the repair of chemotherapy-induced DNA damage might give greater efficacy. Early studies using relatively nonspecific PARP inhibitors such as 3-aminobenzamide, demonstrated potential synergy with alkylating agents.[11] Subsequent studies with more potent PARP inhibitors demonstrated synergy with temozolomide, an observation that was taken into a clinical trial with AG014699,[12] a PARP inhibitor developed by Pfizer. This agent is now being developed by Clovis. Although the major focus of this chapter is the use of PARP inhibitors in synthetic lethal therapeutic strategies, their use in chemopotentiation in combination with chemotherapy remains under active investigation, as described later.

BRCA1 AND *BRCA2* MUTATIONS AND DNA REPAIR

Heterozygous germline mutations in the *BRCA1* and *BRCA2* genes confer a high risk of breast (up to 85% lifetime risk) and ovarian (10% to 40%) cancer in addition to a significantly increased risk of pancreatic, prostate, and male breast cancer.[13] The genes have been classified as tumor suppressors, because the wild-type *BRCA* allele is frequently lost in tumors, a phenomenon that occurs by a variety of mechanisms. The *BRCA1* and *BRCA2* genes encode large proteins that likely function in multiple cellular pathways, including transcription, cell-cycle regulation, and the maintenance of genome integrity. However, the roles of BRCA1 and BRCA2 in DNA repair have been best documented.[14]

BRCA1- and BRCA2-deficient cells are highly sensitive to ionizing radiation and display chromosomal instability, which is likely to be a direct consequence of unrepaired DNA damage.[14] The similar genomic instability in BRCA1- and BRCA2-deficient cells and the interaction of both BRCA1 and BRCA2 with RAD51 suggested a functional link between the three proteins in the RAD51-mediated DNA damage repair process. However although BRCA2 is directly involved in RAD51-mediated repair, affecting the choice between GC and SSA, BRCA1 acts upstream of these pathways[15]; both GC and SSA are reduced in BRCA1 deficient cells, placing BRCA1 before the branch point of GC and SSA.[15]

BRCA1 has a role in signaling DNA damage and cell-cycle checkpoint regulation,[14,15] whereas BRCA2 has a more direct role in DNA repair itself. BRCA2 is thought to promote genomic stability through a role in the error-free repair of DSBs by GC via association with RAD51. Aberrations in BRCA2-deficient cells arise at least in part by the use of the SSA pathway. NHEJ, however, is apparently unaffected in BRCA2-deficient cells.[14,15] Loss of BRCA2, therefore, results in the repair of DSBs by preferential utilization of an error-prone mechanism, which potentially explains the apparent chromosome instability associated with BRCA2 deficiency.[15]

The physical interaction between BRCA2 and RAD51 is essential for error-free DSB repair. BRCA2 is required for the localization of RAD51 to sites of DNA damage, where RAD51 forms the nucleoprotein filament required for recombination. The foci of the RAD51 protein are apparent in the nucleus after certain forms of DNA damage and these likely represent sites of repair by HR; BRCA2-deficient cells do not form RAD51 foci in response to DNA damage.[15] Two different domains within BRCA2 interact with RAD51, the eight BRC repeats in the central part of the protein and a distinct domain, TR2, at the C-terminus.[16]

PARP-1 INHIBITION AS A SYNTHETIC LETHAL THERAPEUTIC STRATEGY FOR THE TREATMENT OF BRCA-DEFICIENT CANCERS

Synthetic lethality is defined as the situation when a mutation in either of two genes individually has no effect, but combining the mutations leads to death.[17] This effect was first described and studied in genetically tractable organisms such as Drosophila and yeast.[17,18] This effect can arise because of a number of different gene–gene interactions. Examples include two genes in separate semiredundant or cooperating pathways, and two genes acting in the same pathway where loss of both critically affects flux through the pathway. The implication is that targeting one of these genes in a cancer where the other is defective should be selectively lethal to the tumor cells but not toxic to the normal cells. In principle, this should lead to a large therapeutic window.[19] The original suggestion that the concept of synthetic lethality could be used in the selection or development of cancer therapeutics came from Hartwell et al.,[18] and from experiments performed in yeast. Synthetic lethal screens have now been performed in a number of model organisms[20] and in human cells,[21] and these have revealed multiple potential gene–gene interactions, some of which could be exploited clinically. However, synthetic lethal therapies have not been clinically used until recently, when evidence has been provided for PARP-1 inhibition as a potential synthetic lethal approach for the treatment of BRCA-mutation–associated cancers.

PARP-1 inhibition causes failure of the repair of SSB lesions but does not affect DSB repair.[22] However, a persistent DNA SSB encountered by a DNA replication fork will cause stalling of the fork and may result in either fork collapse or the formation of a DSB.[23] Therefore, the loss of PARP-1 increases the formation of DNA lesions that might be repaired by GC. As a loss of function of either BRCA1 or BRCA2 impairs GC,[14,15] a loss of PARP-1 function in a BRCA1- or BRCA2-defective background could result in the generation of replication-associated DNA lesions normally repaired by sister chromatid exchange. If so, this might lead to cell cycle arrest and/or cell death. Therefore, PARP inhibitors could be selectively lethal to cells lacking functional BRCA1 or BRCA2 but might be minimally toxic to normal cells. This would indicate a synthetic lethal interaction between PARP and BRCA1 or BRCA2. Exemplifying this principle, potent inhibitors of PARP were applied to cells deficient in either BRCA1 or BRCA2. Cell survival assays showed that cell lines lacking wild-type BRCA1 or BRCA2 were extremely sensitive to these agents compared with heterozygous mutant or wild-type cells.[24,25]

To explain these observations, a model was proposed whereby persistent single-strand gaps in DNA caused by PARP inhibition when encountered by a replication fork might trigger fork arrest, collapse, and/or a DSB.[26] Alternatively, PARP-1 trapped on DNA by the inhibition of enzyme activity might also cause a fork collapse. Normally, these DSBs would be repaired by RAD51-dependent GC.[14,15] However, in the absence of BRCA1 or BRCA2, the replication fork cannot be restarted and collapses, causing persistent chromatid breaks. When repaired by the alternative error-prone DSB repair mechanisms of SSA or NHEJ, large numbers of chromatid aberrations would be induced, leading to cell lethality.[26] The idea that the defect in GC is being targeted in BRCA-deficient cells is supported by the demonstration that deficiency in other genes implicated in HR also confers sensitivity to PARP inhibitors.[27] This further suggests that this approach may be more widely applicable in the treatment of sporadic cancers with impairments of the HR pathway or BRCAness[28] (see the following).

INITIAL CLINICAL RESULTS TESTING SYNTHETIC LETHALITY OF PARP INHIBITORS AND BRCA MUTATION

Phase I studies[29] established that olaparib (AstraZeneca, London, UK; formerly KU-0059436, KuDOS Pharmaceuticals, Cambridge, UK) could be administered safely as a single agent at a dose of 400 mg twice per day. Side effects were classified as mild and were unlike those typically experienced with cytotoxic chemotherapy. Significant and durable responses were observed in patients with germ-line BRCA1 or BRCA2 mutations and breast ovary or prostate cancer. Of the 19 mutation carriers enrolled, 9 had an objective response defined by Response Evaluation Criteria in Solid Tumors (RECIST) criteria and 12 had stable disease for more than 4 months in duration. A similar magnitude of clinical responses was observed in an expanded cohort.[30] These observations are impressive because the cohort had been heavily pretreated and most were resistant to a wide range of chemotherapies.[29,30]

Phase II studies were subsequently performed in advanced breast and ovarian cancers arising in BRCA1 and BRCA2 mutation carriers.[31,32] The reported response rate was 41% in the breast study and 52% in the ovarian group; both groups had been heavily pretreated. Again, the drug was well tolerated. Another study of BRCA1/2 carriers with ovarian cancer compared olaparib with pegylated liposomal doxorubicin (PLD).[33] There was no significant difference in the response rates, but there were some differences in the patient characteristics and an unexpectedly high rate of response to PLD.

There are also reports of responses to PARP inhibitors in BRCA2 mutation carriers with prostate[34] and pancreatic[35] cancer. A number of other PARP inhibitors are in clinical development (Table 25.1), and some of these have shown efficacy in the treatment of cancers arising in BRCA1 or BRCA2 mutation carriers.[36,37]

TABLE 25.1
PARP Inhibitors in Late Stage Clinical Development

Agent	Company	Phase III Trials
Olaparib	AstraZeneca (formerly KuDOS)	BRCA-mutant ovarian cancer
Niraparib	Tesaro (formerly Merck)	Platinum sensitive ovarian cancer; BRCA-mutant breast cancer
Rucaparib	Clovis (formerly Pfizer)	Platinum sensitive ovarian cancer
Veliparib	AbbVie (formerly Abbot)	Undisclosed
BMN673	BioMarin (formerly Lead)	BRCA-mutant breast cancer

Adapted from Garber, K. PARP inhibitors bounce back. *Nat Rev Drug Discov* 2013;12:725–727.

THE USE OF PARP INHIBITORS IN SPORADIC CANCERS

Germline mutations in *BRCA1* or *BRCA2* are relatively common in hereditary breast and ovarian cancer. However, inactivation of *BRCA* genes by mutation in sporadic cancers is rare, at least in breast cancer, which may seem to limit the application of PARP inhibitors to a wider range of patients. However, many tumors display features in common with BRCA-deficient tumors, including similar defects in DNA repair due to either epigenetic mutation of *BRCA1*, such as promoter methylation, or mutation of other components of BRCA-associated pathways.[28] This *BRCA*-ness may make these tumors also susceptible to PARP inhibition.[28] For example, phosphatase and tensin homolog (PTEN) mutations, which occur with a frequency estimated at 50% to 80% in sporadic tumors,[38] may cause PARP inhibitor sensitivity in preclinical models, possibly because PTEN-null cells display BRCAness phenotypes, such as the inability to efficiently repair certain forms of DNA damage.[39]

Traditional histopathologic methods and, more recently, gene expression profiling approaches have shown the phenotypic overlap between triple-negative breast cancers, basal-like breast cancers, and *BRCA1* familial breast cancers.[40,41] In gene expression profiling studies, it has been observed that *BRCA1* familial cancers strongly segregate with basal-like tumors and share features such as high-grade and pushing margins.[28,40,41] Although the overlap is not absolute, it leads to the hypothesis that there may be a subset of sporadic breast cancers that exhibits features of BRCAness, including deficiencies in HR and that may be susceptible to treatment with drugs such as PARP inhibitors.[26]

There have been several studies of PARP inhibitors in sporadic ovarian cancer. A study by Lederman[42] showed in a maintenance study following the response to platinum therapy a significant benefit in terms of progression-free survival (PFS) of olaparib compared to placebo. This was even more pronounced when the subgroup of BRCA mutation carriers were examined.[43] In both cases, the overall survival (OS) advantage was less than the PFS, but in the case of the BRCA mutation group, this reached statistical significance. Gelmon[44] also showed activity in sporadic ovarian cancer. In contrast, a study in sporadic triple-negative breast cancer failed to observe any benefit, although the study was small and the patients were heavily pretreated.[44]

Iniparib (initially reported as a PARP inhibitor) showed an overall survival benefit in a Phase II trial of triple-negative breast cancer in combination with gemcitabine and carboplatin compared with chemotherapy alone.[45] However, a subsequent Phase III study showed no improvement in PFS.[45] The reasons for this are uncertain, but significant questions have been raised about whether iniparib is indeed a bona fide PARP inhibitor. Therefore, it is now generally conceded that studies of iniparib have no implications for PARP inhibitors as a drug class.[46]

Which population of patients lacking a *BRCA1* or *BRCA2* mutation might benefit from PARP inhibitors remains unclear. This is likely to require the development of a clinical test to identify prospectively tumors with intrinsic sensitivity. Presently, most efforts are directed at developing assays of DNA repair deficiency.[47]

MECHANISMS OF RESISTANCE TO PARP INHIBITORS

Resistance to targeted therapy frequently occurs, but it was unclear how resistance might arise to a synthetic lethal therapy.[48] Potential mechanisms of resistance to PARP inhibitors have, however, been elucidated both directly in vitro, in mouse models, and in the clinic.[48] An in vitro model for resistance was developed by producing cells from the highly PARP inhibitor–sensitive BRCA2-deficient cell line CAPAN1, which carries a c.6174delT *BRCA2* frameshift mutation. CAPAN1 cells cannot form damage-induced RAD51 foci, are defective for HR, and are extremely sensitive to treatment with PARP inhibitors.[49] PARP inhibitor–resistant clones were highly resistant (over 1,000-fold) to the drug and were also cross-resistant to the DNA cross-linking agent cisplatin, but not to the microtubule-stabilizing drug docetaxel. PARP inhibitors and cisplatin both exert their effects on BRCA-deficient cells by increasing the frequency of misrepaired DSBs in the absence of effective HR. Therefore, this observation indicates that the resistance of PARP inhibitor–resistant clones to PARP inhibitors might be because of restored HR. This contention was supported by the acquisition in PARP inhibitor–resistant clone cells of the ability to form RAD51 foci after PARP inhibitor treatment or exposure to irradiation.

DNA sequencing of PARP inhibitor–resistant clones revealed the unexpected presence of novel *BRCA2* alleles that resulted in the elimination of the c.6174delT mutation and restoration of an open reading frame.[49] Therefore, in this case, resistance arises because of gain of function mutations in the synthetic lethal partner (BRCA2) rather than the direct drug target (PARP). Alternative mechanisms of PARP inhibitor resistance have also been described.[48] A mouse model of *BRCA1*-associated mammary gland cancer demonstrated the efficacy of olaparib in vivo and was used to study mechanisms of resistance.[50] Resistance seemed to be caused by the upregulation of *ABCB1a/b*, which encode P-glycoprotein pumps; this effect could be reversed with the P-glycoprotein inhibitor tariquidar. In addition, other alterations in DNA repair pathways have been proposed to compensate for BRCA1 deficiency resulting in PARP inhibitor deficiency.[48]

Studies of the mechanisms of resistance to PARP inhibitors in patient material are still at an early stage. Initial studies addressed the mechanism of resistance to platinum salts in BRCA mutation carriers. Cisplatin and carboplatin are part of the standard of care for the treatment of ovarian cancer, including individuals with *BRCA1* or *BRCA2* mutations. Platinum salts are thought to exert their BRCA-selective effects by a similar mechanism to PARP inhibitors.[15] Clinical observations suggest that BRCA mutation carriers with ovarian cancer usually respond better to these agents than patients without BRCA mutations[51,52]; however, resistance does eventually occur. To investigate this effect, *BRCA1* and *BRCA2* have been sequenced in tumor material from mutation carriers.[49,53] These studies revealed mutations in *BRCA1* or *BRCA2* that restored the open reading frame and likely contributed to platinum resistance. These observations suggest that specific mutations in *BRCA1* or *BRCA2* and sensitivity to therapeutics in cell lines and patients can be suppressed by intragenic deletion. Presumably, these mutations occur randomly and are then selected for by differential drug sensitivity. Therefore, the best use of these agents is likely to be earlier in the disease process when the disease burden is smaller, which will reduce the probability of resistance based on stochastic genetic reversion. Recently, similar observations of revertant *BRCA* alleles were made in two patients who became resistant after an initial response to olaparib.[54] Although preliminary, these results suggest that this mechanism is responsible for at least some of the clinical resistance observed. Doubtless, as with other targeted therapies, multiple resistance mechanisms will be implicated as further patients are studied.[48]

PROSPECTS

Currently, the treatments for cancers arising in carriers of *BRCA1* or *BRCA2* mutations are the same as those that occur sporadically matched for tumor pathology and age of onset. However, tumors in *BRCA1* or *BRCA2* mutation carriers lack wild-type *BRCA1* or *BRCA2*, but normal tissues retain a single wild-type copy of the relevant gene. This is a potentially targetable alteration that provides the basis for new mechanism-based approaches to the treatment of cancer. The biochemical difference in capacity to carry out HR between the tumor and normal tissues, in a *BRCA1* or *BRCA2* carrier, provides the rationale for this approach. Inhibiting the DNA repair protein PARP results in the generation of specific DNA lesions that require BRCA1 and BRCA2 specialized repair function(s) for their removal. Preclinical data indicate that tumors defective in wild-type BRCA1 or BRCA2 could be much more sensitive to PARP inhibition than unaffected heterozygous tissues, providing a potentially large therapeutic window. The safety and efficacy of this approach is currently being tested in clinical trials, which, if successful, may lead to registration for routine clinical use of one or more PARP inhibitors.[57]

Synthetic lethality by combinatorial targeting of DNA repair pathways may have usefulness as a therapeutic approach beyond familial cancers. The majority of solid tumors also exhibit genomic instability and aneuploidy. This suggests that pathways involved in the maintenance of genomic stability are dysfunctional in a significant proportion of neoplastic disorders.[47] Understanding which specialized DNA damage response and repair pathways are abrogated in sporadic tumor subtypes may allow for the development of therapies that target the residual repair pathways on which the cancer, but not normal tissue, is now completely dependent. These potential therapies may significantly improve response rates while causing fewer treatment-related toxicities. However, these approaches may be associated with mechanism-associated resistance, and careful consideration of their optimal use will be required.

REFERENCES

1. Hoeijmakers JH. Genome maintenance mechanisms for preventing cancer. *Nature* 2001;411:366–374.
2. Chambon P, Weill JD, Mandel P. Nicotinamide mononucleotide activation of new DNA-dependent polyadenylic acid synthesizing nuclear enzyme. *Biochem Biophys Res Commun* 1963;11:39–43.
3. Amé JC, Spenlehauer C, de Murcia G. The PARP superfamily. *Bioessays* 2004;26:882–893.
4. Otto H, Reche PA, Bazan F, et al. In silico characterization of the family of PARP-like poly(ADP-ribosyl)transferases (pARTs). *BMC Genomics* 2005;6:139.
5. van Gent DC, Hoeijmakers JH, Kanaar R. Chromosomal stability and the DNA double-stranded break connection. *Nat Rev Genet* 2001;2:196–206.
6. Shin DS, Chahwan C, Huffman JL, et al. Structure and function of the double-strand break repair machinery. *DNA Repair (Amst)* 2004;3:863–873.
7. Takata M, Sasaki MS, Sonoda E, et al. Homologous recombination and non-homologous end-joining pathways of DNA double-strand break repair have overlapping roles in the maintenance of chromosomal integrity in vertebrate cells. *EMBO J* 1998;17:5497–5508.
8. Rothkamm K, Krüger I, Thompson LH, et al. Pathways of DNA double-strand break repair during the mammalian cell cycle. *Mol Cell Biol* 2003;23:5706–5715.
9. Stark JM, Pierce AJ, Oh J, et al. Genetic steps of mammalian homologous repair with distinct mutagenic consequences. *Mol Cell Biol* 2004;24:9305–9316.
10. Elliott B, Richardson C, Jasin M. Chromosomal translocation mechanisms at intronic alu elements in mammalian cells. *Mol Cell* 2005;17:885–894.
11. Durkacz BW, Omidiji O, Gray DA, et al. (ADP-ribose)n participates in DNA excision repair. *Nature* 1980;283(5747):593–596.
12. Tentori L, Graziani G. Chemosensitisation by PARP inhibitors in cancer therapy. *Pharmacol Res* 2005;52:25–33.
13. Wooster R, Weber BL. Breast and ovarian cancer. *N Engl J Med* 2003;348:2339–2347.
14. Gudmundsdottir K, Ashworth A. The roles of BRCA1 and BRCA2 and associated proteins in the maintenance of genomic stability. *Oncogene* 2006;25:5864–5874.
15. Tutt AN, Lord CJ, McCabe N, et al. Exploiting the DNA repair defect in BRCA mutant cells in the design of new therapeutic strategies for cancer. *Cold Spring Harb Symp Quant Biol* 2005;70:139–148.
16. Lord CJ, Ashworth A. RAD51, BRCA2 and DNA repair: a partial resolution. *Nat Struct Mol Biol* 2007;14:461–462.
17. Dobzhansky T. Genetics of natural populations: Xiii. Recombination and variability in populations of Drosophila pseudoobscura. *Genetics* 1946;31:269–290.
18. Hartwell LH, Szankasi P, Roberts CJ, et al. Integrating genetic approaches into the discovery of anticancer drugs. *Science* 1997;278:1064–1068.
19. Kaelin WG Jr. The concept of synthetic lethality in the context of anticancer therapy. *Nat Rev Cancer* 2005;5:689–698.
20. Ooi SL, Pan X, Peyser BD, et al. Global synthetic-lethality analysis and yeast functional profiling. *Trends Genet* 2006;22:56–63.
21. Iorns E, Lord CJ, Turner N, et al. Utilizing RNA interference to enhance cancer drug discovery. *Nat Rev Drug Discov* 2007;6:556–568.
22. Noël G, Giocanti N, Fernet M, et al. Poly(ADP-ribose) polymerase (PARP-1) is not involved in DNA double-strand break recovery. *BMC Cell Biol* 2003;4:7.
23. Haber JE. DNA recombination: the replication connection. *Trends Biochem Sci* 1999;24:271–275.
24. Farmer H, McCabe N, Lord CJ, et al. Targeting the DNA repair defect in BRCA mutant cells as a therapeutic strategy. *Nature* 2005;434:917–921.
25. Bryant HE, Schultz N, Thomas HD, et al. Specific killing of BRCA2-deficient tumours with inhibitors of poly(ADP-ribose) polymerase. *Nature* 2005;434:913–917.
26. Ashworth A. A synthetic lethal therapeutic approach: PARP inhibitors for the treatment of cancers deficient in double-strand break repair. *J Clin Oncol* 2008;26:3785–3790.
27. McCabe N, Turner NC, Lord CJ, et al. Deficiency in the repair of DNA damage by homologous recombination and sensitivity to poly(ADP-ribose) polymerase inhibition. *Cancer Res* 2006;66:8109–8115.
28. Turner N, Tutt A, Ashworth A. Hallmarks of 'BRCAness' in sporadic cancers. *Nat Rev Cancer* 2004;4:814–819.
29. Fong PC, Boss DS, Yap TA, et al. Inhibition of poly(ADP-ribose) polymerase in tumors from BRCA mutation carriers. *N Engl J Med* 2009;361:123–134.
30. Fong PC, Yap TA, Boss DS, et al. Poly(ADP)-ribose polymerase (PARP) inhibition: frequent durable responses in BRCA carrier ovarian cancer correlating with platinum-free interval. *J Clin Oncol* 2010;28:2512–2519.
31. Audeh MW, Carmichael J, Penson RT, et al. Oral poly(ADP-ribose) polymerase inhibitor olaparib in patients with BRCA1 or BRCA2 mutations and recurrent ovarian cancer: a proof-of-concept trial. *Lancet* 2010;376:245–251.
32. Tutt A, Robson M, Garber JE, et al. Oral poly(ADP-ribose) polymerase inhibitor olaparib in patients with BRCA1 or BRCA2 mutations and advanced breast cancer: a proof-of-concept trial. *Lancet* 2010;376:235–244.
33. Kaye SB, Lubinski J, Matulonis U, et al. Phase II, open-label, randomized, multicenter study comparing the efficacy and safety of olaparib, a poly (ADP-ribose) polymerase inhibitor, and pegylated liposomal doxorubicin in patients with BRCA1 or BRCA2 mutations and recurrent ovarian cancer. *J Clin Oncol* 2012;30:372–379.
34. Sandhu SK, Omlin A, Hylands L et al. Poly (ADP-ribose) polymerase (PARP) inhibitors for the treatment of advanced germline BRCA2 mutant prostate cancer. *Ann Oncol* 2013;24:1416–1418.
35. Fogelman DR, Wolff RA, Kopetz S, et al. Evidence for the efficacy of Iniparib, a PARP-1 inhibitor, in BRCA2-associated pancreatic cancer. *Anticancer Res* 2011;31:1417–1420.
36. Maxwell KN, Domchek SM. Cancer treatment according to BRCA1 and BRCA2 mutations *Nat Rev Clin Oncol* 2012;9:520–528.
37. Garber K. PARP inhibitors bounce back. *Nat Rev Drug Discov* 2013;12:725–727.
38. Salmena L, Carracedo A, Pandolfi PP. Tenets of PTEN tumor suppression. *Cell* 2008;133:403–414.
39. Mendes-Pereira AM, Martin SA, Brough R, et al. Synthetic lethal targeting of PTEN mutant cells with PARP inhibitors. *EMBO Mol Med* 2009;1:315–322.
40. Foulkes WD, Stefansson IM, Chappuis PO, et al. Germline BRCA1 mutations and a basal epithelial phenotype in breast cancer. *J Natl Cancer Inst* 2003;95:1482–1485.

41. Turner NC, Reis-Filho JS. Basal-like breast cancer and the BRCA1 phenotype. *Oncogene* 2006;25:5846–5853.
42. Ledermann J, Harter P, Gourley C, et al. Olaparib maintenance therapy in platinum-sensitive relapsed ovarian cancer. *N Engl J Med* 2012;366:1382–1392.
43. Ledermann JA, Harter P, Gourley C. Olaparib maintenance therapy in patients with platinum-sensitive relapsed serous ovarian cancer (SOC) and a BRCA mutation (BRCAm). *J Clin Oncol* 2013;31 (suppl; abstr 5505).
44. Gelmon KA, Tischkowitz M, Mackay H, et al. Olaparib in patients with recurrent high-grade serous or poorly differentiated ovarian carcinoma or triple-negative breast cancer: a phase 2, multicentre, open-label, non-randomised study. *Lancet Oncol* 2011;12:852–861.
45. O'Shaughnessy J, Osborne C, Pippen J, et al. Iniparib plus chemotherapy in metastatic triple-negative breast cancer. *N Engl J Med* 2011;3:205–214.
46. Mateo J, Ong M, Tan DS, et al. Appraising iniparib, the PARP inhibitor that never was—what must we learn? *Nat Rev Clin Oncol* 2013;10:688–696.
47. Lord CJ, Ashworth A. The DNA damage response and cancer therapy. *Nature* 2012;481:287–294.
48. Lord CJ, Ashworth A. Mechanisms of resistance to therapies targeting BRCA-mutant cancers. *Nat Med* 2013;19:1381–1388.
49. Edwards S, Brough R, Lord CJ, et al. Resistance to therapy caused by intragenic deletion in BRCA2. *Nature* 2008;451(7182):1111–1115.
50. Rottenberg S, Jaspers JE, Kersbergen A, et al. High sensitivity of *BRCA1*-deficient mammary tumors to the PARP inhibitor AZD2281 alone and in combination with platinum drugs. *Proc Natl Acad Sci U S A* 2008;105: 17079–17084.
51. Cass I, Baldwin RL, Varkey T, et al. Improved survival in women with BRCA-associated ovarian carcinoma. *Cancer* 2003;97:2187–2195.
52. Pal T, Permuth-Wey J, Kapoor R, et al. Improved survival in BRCA2 carriers with ovarian cancer. *Fam Cancer* 2007;6:113–119.
53. Sakai W, Swisher EM, Karlan BY, et al. Secondary mutations as a mechanism of cisplatin resistance in BRCA2-mutated cancers. *Nature* 2008;451: 1116–1120.
54. Barber LJ, Sandhu S, Chen L, et al. Secondary mutations in BRCA2 associated with clinical resistance to a PARP inhibitor. *J Pathol* 2013;229:422–429.

26 Miscellaneous Chemotherapeutic Agents

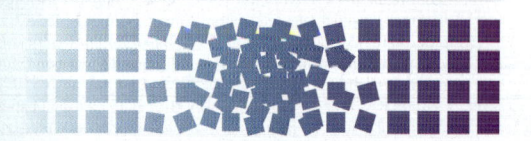

M. Sitki Copur, Scott Nicholas Gettinger, Sarah B. Goldberg, and Hari A. Deshpande

HOMOHARRINGTONINE AND OMACETAXINE

Homoharringtonine and its congener, harringtonine, are cephalotaxine esters isolated from the evergreen tree *Cephalotaxus hainanensis*, which are distributed throughout southern and northeastern China. The two differ only by a single methylene group, but both have a similar activity against murine leukemia.[1] The primary action of homoharringtonine appears to be the inhibition of protein synthesis and chain elongation through binding to 80S ribosome in eukaryotic cells.[2] DNA effects may also be important, involving a block in progression of cells from G1 phase into S phase and from G2 phase into M phase.[3] Homoharringtonine exhibits a triphasic plasma decay with a terminal half-life of 65.3 hours and apparent volume of distribution of 2.4 L/kg.[4] In early phase I studies, homoharringtonine was administered as a 10 to 360 minute infusion daily for 10 days.[5] Dose-limiting cardiovascular toxicity with hypotension began 4 or more hours after drug administration, which was alleviated by interrupting the infusion or by fluid administration and prolonging the duration of administration. Initial clinical studies with homoharringtonine in China showed activity against acute myeloid leukemia (AML) and chronic phase chronic myeloid leukemia (CML).[6] Variable activity was observed in the initial series of phase II trials in pediatric and adult patients with acute leukemia. In early studies of homoharringtonine, a continuous intravenous (IV) infusion at 2.5 mg/m² per day for 10 to 14 days per month induced complete hematologic and cytogenetic responses in 72% and 31% of patients, respectively, with chronic phase CML.[7]

The greater availability of homoharringtonine led to its further testing and the development of a semisynthetic cephalotaxine ester, omacetaxine mepesuccinate.[2] The mechanism of action of omacetaxine includes inhibition of protein synthesis and is independent of direct Bcr-Abl binding. In vitro, it reduces protein levels of the Bcr-Abl oncoprotein and Mcl-1, an antiapoptotic B-cell lymphoma 2 (Bcl-2) family member. The antileukemic effect of omacetaxine is not affected by the presence of mutations in Bcr-Abl.[8] Omacetaxine is absorbed following subcutaneous administration of 1.25 mg/m² twice daily for 11 days with a mean half-life of 6 hours, and a volume of distribution of 141 +/−93.4 L. A phase 2 trial assessed the efficacy of omacetaxine in CML patients with T315I and tyrosine–kinase inhibitor failure. Patients received subcutaneous omacetaxine 1.25 mg/m² twice daily on days 1 through 14, every 28 days until hematologic response or a maximum of 6 cycles, and then days 1 through 7 every 28 days as maintenance. Complete hematologic response was achieved in 77%, with a median response duration of 9.1 months. Of patients, 23% achieved a major cytogenetic response, including a complete cytogenetic response in 16%. Hematologic toxicity included thrombocytopenia (76%), neutropenia (44%), and anemia (39%) and was typically manageable by dose reduction. Nonhematologic adverse events were mostly grade 1/2 and included infection, diarrhea, and nausea.[9]

L-ASPARAGINASE

L-Asparaginase (L-asparagine aminohydrolase, EC 3.5.1.1), which catalyzes the hydrolysis of the essential amino acid L-asparagine to L-aspartic acid and ammonia, is a naturally occurring enzyme in some microorganisms.[10,11] Although cancer cells depend on an exogenous source of L-asparagine for survival, normal cells can synthesize asparagine. In addition to the depletion of L-asparagine, it may exert its antitumor activity through a glutaminase effect, depleting essential glutamine stores and leading to the inhibition of DNA biosynthesis. It comes in three preparations, two of which are native forms purified from bacterial sources, *Escherichia coli* and *Erwinia carotovora*. A third preparation, pegylated (PEG)-L-asparaginase, is a chemically modified form of the enzyme in which native *E. coli* L-asparaginase has been covalently conjugated to polyethylene glycol.[12]

After an intramuscular (IM) injection, peak plasma levels, approximately one-half of those achieved with IV administration, are reached within 14 to 24 hours. Plasma protein binding is 30%. The pharmacokinetics vary depending on the source of the enzyme.[13] Pharmacokinetic studies in newly diagnosed children with acute lymphocytic leukemia (ALL) have shown peak serum concentrations in the range of 1 to 10 IU/mL in 24 to 48 hours of a single dose of 2,500 to 25,000 IU/m² of the enzyme derived from *E. coli*. After a single dose of 25,000 IU/m², peak serum levels are reached within 24 hours. PEG-L-asparaginase, when administered at a dose of 2,500 IU/m², achieves peak drug levels at 72 to 96 hours and has a significantly longer half-life (5.7 days) than the *E. coli* L-asparaginase preparation.[13] Clinical trials have demonstrated the efficacy, safety, and tolerability of PEG-L-asparaginase administered intramuscularly, subcutaneously, or intravenously as part of multiagent chemotherapy regimens in the management of newly diagnosed and relapsed pediatric and adult ALL. L-Asparaginase can antagonize antineoplastic effects of methotrexate if given concurrently or immediately before. These two drugs should be administered sequentially at least 24 hours apart. L-Asparaginase has also been shown to inhibit the metabolic clearance of vincristine and can result in increased neurotoxicity. Toxicity is less pronounced if L-asparaginase is administered after vincristine. Hypersensitivity reactions occur in up to 25% of patients as a skin rash and urticaria or serious anaphylactic reactions. The risk increases with repeat exposure, and as a single-agent use without steroids. PEG-L-asparaginase is less immunogenic than the native nonpegylated forms of the enzyme. A number of other side effects are observed that are secondary to the inhibitory effects of L-asparaginase on cellular protein synthesis. Decreased serum levels of insulin, key lipoproteins, and albumin have been reported. L-Asparaginase can cause alterations in thyroid function tests as early as 2 days after an administered dose, possibly secondary to a reduction in the serum levels of thyroxine-binding globulin. Alterations in coagulation parameters with prolonged thrombin time, prothrombin time, and partial thromboplastin time have been observed. Patients treated with L-asparaginase are at an increased risk for bleeding or thromboembolic events.[14] L-Asparaginase is contraindicated in patients with a prior history of pancreatitis, because there is a 10% incidence of acute pancreatitis. Neurologic toxicity includes lethargy, confusion, agitation, hallucinations, and/or coma. In contrast to the other anticancer agents used to treat ALL, myelosuppression is rare.

BLEOMYCIN

Bleomycin is a glycopeptide antibiotic produced by the bacterium *Streptomyces verticillus*. The most active chemotherapeutical forms are bleomycin A_2 and B_2.[15] The effect of bleomycin is cell cycle specific, because its main effects are mediated in the G_2 and M phases of the cell cycle.[16] The exact mechanism for DNA strand scission has been suggested to be due to bleomycin's chelating of metal ions (primarily iron) and producing a pseudoenzyme that reacts with oxygen to produce superoxide- and hydroxide-free radicals, thus cleaving DNA. Alternatively, bleomycin may bind at specific sites in the DNA strand and induce scission by abstracting the hydrogen atom from the base, resulting in strand cleavage as the base undergoes a Criegee-type rearrangement, or bleomycin may form an alkali-labile lesion.[17] Bleomycin is used in the treatment of Hodgkin lymphoma (as a component of the ABVD and BEACOPP regimens), squamous cell carcinomas, and testicular cancer; in the treatment of plantar warts,[18] as a means of effecting pleurodesis,[19] as well as an intralesional agent with electrochemotherapy in the management of cutaneous malignancies.[20]

The oral bioavailability is poor. It must be administered via IV or IM routes. The initial distribution half-life is 10 to 20 minutes with a terminal half-life of 3 hours. Bleomycin can be administered via the intracavitary route to control malignant pleural effusions or ascites, or both. Approximately 45% to 55% of an administered intracavitary dose of bleomycin is absorbed into the systemic circulation. Elimination is primarily via the kidneys, and approximately 60% to 70% of an administered dose is excreted unchanged in the urine. Dose reductions are required if creatinine clearance is less than 25 mL per minute.

Bleomycin-induced pneumonitis, the dose-limiting toxicity of the drug, occurs in 10% of patients, and is dependent on the cumulative dose.[21] The risk increases in patients older than 70 years and in those who receive a total cumulative dose greater than 400 U. In addition, patients with an underlying lung disease, prior irradiation to the chest or mediastinum, and exposure to high concentrations of inspired oxygen are at increased risk. Increased use of granulocyte colony-stimulating factor (G-CSF) has been paralleled by an increased incidence of bleomycin-induced pulmonary toxicity. The exacerbating effects of G-CSFs seem to be associated with a marked infiltration of activated neutrophils along with the lung injury caused by the direct effects of bleomycin.[22,23] In a retrospective review, 18% of a total of 141 patients with Hodgkin lymphoma treated with a bleomycin-containing regimen developed pulmonary toxicity. G-CSF use was one of the key factors associated with the development of this complication, and omission of bleomycin had no impact on clinical outcomes.[24] Similarly the combination of brentuximab vedotin and ABVD was associated with excessive pulmonary toxicity, indicating that brentuximab vedotin and bleomycin should not be used together.[25]

Patients with bleomycin-induced pulmonary toxicity may present with cough, dyspnea, dry inspiratory crackles, and infiltrates on chest radiograph. Pulmonary function testing is the most sensitive approach to monitor patients, and pulmonary function tests should be obtained at baseline and before each cycle of therapy, with a specific focus on the carbon monoxide diffusion capacity and vital capacity. A decrease greater than 15% in either diffusion capacity of carbon monoxide or vital capacity should mandate immediate discontinuation of bleomycin. Early clinical trials and isolated case reports suggest that bleomycin-induced acute hypersensitivity reactions occur in 1% of patients with lymphoma and less than 0.5% of those with solid tumors. The reactions are mainly characterized by high-grade fever, chills, hypotension, and, in a few cases, cardiovascular collapse, which can lead to death. The exact mechanism of these reactions is unclear, but is thought to be related to the release of endogenous pyrogens from the host cells. Supportive care, including hydration, steroids, antipyretics, and antihistamines, may resolve the symptoms.

Clinicians should monitor their patients for any signs and symptoms of acute hyperpyrexic reactions during bleomycin administration. Because the onset of the reactions can occur with any dose of bleomycin and at any time, routine test dosing does not seem to predict when drug reactions may occur.[26] Mucocutaneous toxicity presents as mucositis, erythema, hyperpigmentation, induration, hyperkeratosis, and skin peeling, which may progress to ulceration, and usually develops in the 2nd and 3rd week of treatment and after a cumulative dose of 150 to 200 U of the drug. Levels of bleomycin hydrolase are relatively low in lung and skin tissue, perhaps offering an explanation as to why these normal tissues are more adversely affected by bleomycin. Myelosuppression and immunosuppression are relatively mild. In rare cases, vascular events, including myocardial infarction, stroke, and Raynaud phenomenon, have been reported.

PROCARBAZINE

Originally prepared as a monoamine oxidase inhibitor, procarbazine is a prodrug, which after oxidation of the hydrazine in the liver, undergoes a complex enzymatic and chemical breakdown to its alkylating and methylating species.[27,28] The precise mechanism of action is uncertain, but may involve damaging the DNA, RNA or transfer RNA, and the inhibition of protein synthesis. Procarbazine is a cell-cycle phase-nonspecific antineoplastic agent. This agent was initially approved by the U.S. Food and Drug Administration (FDA) in 1969 as part of the MOPP (mechlorethamine, vincristine, procarbazine, and prednisone) regimen for the treatment of Hodgkin lymphoma. Since then, it has also demonstrated clinical activity in non-Hodgkin lymphoma, cutaneous T-cell lymphoma, and brain tumors.

Procarbazine is rapidly and completely absorbed from the gastrointestinal tract. Following oral administration, peak drug levels are reached within 10 to 15 minutes. Procarbazine crosses the blood–brain barrier and rapidly equilibrates between plasma and cerebrospinal fluid after oral administration. Peak cerebrospinal fluid drug concentrations are reached within 30 to 90 minutes after drug administration. The biologic half-life of procarbazine hydrochloride in both plasma and cerebrospinal fluid is approximately 1 hour. Procarbazine is metabolized to active and inactive metabolites by chemical breakdown in an aqueous solution and the liver microsomal P-450 system. Approximately 70% of procarbazine is excreted in urine within 24 hours, and less than 5% to 10% of the drug is eliminated in an unchanged form.[29,30]

A careful food and drug history is required before starting a patient on procarbazine therapy, because there are several potential drug–drug and drug–food interactions. Patients should avoid tyramine-containing foods, such as dark beer, wine, cheese, yogurt, bananas, and smoked foods. Procarbazine produces a disulfiramlike reaction with concurrent use of alcohol. Acute hypertensive reactions may occur with coadministration of tricyclic antidepressants and sympathomimetic drugs. Concurrent use of procarbazine with antihistamines and other central nervous system (CNS) depressants can result in CNS and/or respiratory depression.

Dose-limiting toxicity is myelosuppression, more commonly thrombocytopenia, and the nadir in platelet count is generally observed at 4 weeks. Patients with glucose-6-phosphate dehydrogenase deficiency can develop hemolytic anemia while receiving procarbazine therapy. Stepwise dose increments over the first few days of drug administration may minimize gastrointestinal intolerance. On rare occasions, procarbazine may induce interstitial pneumonitis, which mandates the discontinuation of therapy. Azoospermia and infertility after treatment with MOPP can be attributed, in part, to procarbazine. Procarbazine is associated with an increased risk of secondary malignancies, especially acute leukemia.

VISMODEGIB

Vismodegib (Erivedge, GDC-0449, Genentech) is a first-in-class small-molecule inhibitor of the Hedgehog pathway. It binds to and inhibits smoothened, a transmembrane protein that is involved in Hedgehog signaling.[31] Pharmacodynamic downmodulation in the Hedgehog pathway was shown by a 90% decrease in transcription factor Gli1 mRNA in basal-cell carcinoma biopsy specimens of patients treated for a month. One-month vismodegib treatment also significantly reduced tumor proliferation, as assessed by Ki 67 expression, but did not change apoptosis, as assessed by cleaved caspase 3. The extent of Gli1 downmodulation does not seem to correlate with pharmacokinetic levels of vismodegib in individual patients. Vismodegib is absorbed from the gastrointestinal tract, with an oral bioavailability of 32%. Food does not affect drug exposure. Elimination is mainly hepatic, with excretion in feces. The median steady-state concentration is not changed by increasing the dose from 150 mg to 270 mg, and the median time to steady state is 14 days. The half-life is estimated at 8 days after a single dose. Intermittent doses (e.g., three times per week or once per week) were associated with a decrease of 50% and 80% in effective plasma levels of unbound drug, respectively, thus reinforcing the recommended dose and schedule of 150 mg orally daily.[32] Vismodegib is approved for the treatment of adults with metastatic basal-cell carcinoma that has recurred following surgery or in those who are not candidates for surgery and who are not candidates for radiation.[33]

No dose-limiting toxic effects or grade 5 events have been observed. However, 54% of patients receiving vismodegib discontinued the medication owing to side effects, and only one out of five eligible patients was able to continue vismodegib for 18 months. Abdominal pain, fatigue, weight loss, dysgeusia, and anorexia were reasons for discontinuation of the drug. When vismodegib was withdrawn, dysgeusia and muscle cramps ceased within 1 month, and scalp and body hair started to regrow within 3 months. Other side effects reported include hyponatremia, dyspnea, muscle spasm, atrial fibrillation, aspiration, back pain, corneal abrasion, dehydration, keratitis, lymphopenia, pneumonia, urinary tract infection, and a prolonged QT interval.[34]

ADO-TRASTUZUMAB EMTANSINE

Ado-trastuzumab emtansine (T-DM1), is a HER2-targeted antibody-drug conjugate (ADC). It is a novel compound composed of trastuzumab, a stable thioether linker, and DM1. DM1, a derivative of maytansine, is a microtubule polymerization inhibitor with activity similar to that of vinca alkaloids. T-DM1 is taken up into cells after binding to HER2, allowing for cytotoxic drug delivery specifically to cells overexpressing HER2. It has a drug-to-antibody ratio of approximately 3.5:1. T-DM1 is administered intravenously every 3 weeks and has been tested in a phase I trial at doses ranging from 0.3 to 4.8 mg/kg. The maximally tolerated dose is 3.6 mg/kg, which was the dose used in further phase II–III trials. T-DM1 is metabolized by the liver, via CYP3A4/5, and has a half-life of 3.5 days.[35]

T-DM1 is approved for use in patients with metastatic HER2-positive breast cancer who have received prior trastuzumab and a taxane. This approval was based on the results of the EMILIA trial, which randomized 991 patients with HER2-positive unresectable, locally advanced or metastatic breast cancer to T-DM1 3.6 mg/kg IV every 21 days or lapatinib 1,250 mg daily plus capecitabine 1,000 mg/m^2 on days 1 through 14 every 21 days. All patients were previously treated with trastuzumab and a taxane. T-DM1 resulted in a progression-free survival of 9.6 months compared to 6.4 months for lapatinib plus capecitabine (hazard ratio [HR] 0.65; 95% confidence interval [CI] 0.55 to 0.77; p <0.001). The response rate and overall survival was also higher with T-DM1 compared to lapatinib plus capecitabine.[36]

Although maytansine itself is associated with significant toxicity, T-DM1 is very well tolerated overall, which is likely due to the targeted nature of the compound. Side effects from T-DM1 include thrombocytopenia, hepatotoxicity, hypersensitivity/infusion reactions, and cardiotoxicity. Nausea, fatigue, headaches, and anemia are also common. The left ventricular ejection fraction should be monitored prior to and at least every 3 months during therapy because of the potential for cardiac dysfunction.

SIROLIMUS AND TEMSIROLIMUS

Sirolimus (rapamycin) was isolated from the soil bacteria *Streptomyces hygroscopicus*, in the mid 1970s.[37] This bacterial macrolide later became the preferred immunosuppressant for kidney transplantation, because it was mildly immunosuppressive; however, in contrast to cyclosporine A, it did not enhance tumor incidence.[38] Sirolimus is the prototypic inhibitor of the mammalian target of rapamycin (mTOR), a serine/threonine protein kinase that is a highly conserved regulatory protein involved in cell-cycle progression, proliferation, and angiogenesis.[39] Signaling pathways both upstream and downstream of mTOR have been shown to be commonly dysregulated in cancer. mTOR functions through two main mechanisms, depending on the presence and activity of the mTOR-associated protein complexes, mTORC1 and mTORC2. Sirolimus and its analog compounds, temsirolimus and everolimus, form a complex with the FK-binding protein (FKBP) and inhibit activation of a subset of mTOR proteins residing within mTORC1. In contrast, mTORC2 holds mTOR in a form that is not as readily inhibited by these rapamycin analogs, and upregulation of mTORC2 may represent a mechanism by which resistance can develop to this class of compounds.

Temsirolimus (CCI-779), a novel functional ester of sirolimus, is a water-soluble dihydroxymethyl propionic acid compound that rapidly undergoes hydrolysis to sirolimus after IV administration, reaching peak concentrations within 0.5 to 2.0 hours.[40] This drug is widely distributed in tissues, and steady-state drug levels are reached in 7 to 8 days. Temsirolimus is metabolized primarily in the liver by CYP3A4 microsomal enzymes to yield sirolimus as the main metabolite. The terminal half-life of temsirolimus is 17 hours, whereas that of sirolimus is approximately 55 hours. When bound to temsirolimus, mTOR is unable to phosphorylate the key protein translation factors, such as 4E-BP1 and S6K1, leading to translational inhibition of several critical regulatory proteins involved in cell-cycle control. Several other cellular proteins involved in the regulation of angiogenesis, such as hypoxia-inducible factor-1α (HIF-1α) and vascular endothelial growth factor (VEGF), are suppressed through mTOR inhibition by temsirolimus.

Phase I studies of temsirolimus have investigated various schedules and doses, ranging from 7.5 mg to 220 mg given as weekly 30-minute infusions.[40] A phase II study in patients with cytokine-refractory renal cell cancer (RCC) investigated the efficacy and safety of three different dose levels (25 mg, 75 mg, and 250 mg, respectively) administered on a weekly schedule. This study showed promising antitumor activity for all three dose levels with no significant difference in efficacy or toxicity.[41] As a result, the 25-mg dose was eventually selected as the monotherapy dose for further study. A phase III randomized trial compared interferon, temsirolimus, and the combination of the two agents in previously untreated patients with advanced RCC who had at least three of six poor prognostic features.[42] Once-weekly IV temsirolimus, 25 mg, prolonged the median overall survival of patients with poor prognostic features by 49% from 7.3 months (95% CI, 6.1 to 8.8 months) in the interferon arm to 10.9 months (95% CI, 8.6 to 12.7 months) in the temsirolimus arm ($P = .008$). The temsirolimus arm also had a prolonged median progression-free survival of 5.5 months compared to 3.1 months in the interferon arm ($P <.001$). Moreover, temsirolimus was effective for both clear cell and non–clear cell histologies.[43,44]

Mantle cell lymphoma was the first hematologic malignancy in which mTOR inhibition was explored as a treatment strategy. The rationale for this approach was that mantle cell lymphoma is characterized by overexpression of cyclin D1, which is a cyclin whose expression appears to be tightly regulated by mTOR signaling. The early-phase clinical trials of temsirolimus showed promising activity against non-Hodgkin lymphomas, multiple myeloma, and myeloid leukemias, with some evidence of success thus far.[45]

In terms of the safety profile, the most common adverse events associated with temsirolimus were asthenia and fatigue, dry skin with acneiform skin rash, nausea/vomiting, mucositis, and anorexia. Hyperlipidemia with increased serum triglycerides and/or cholesterol as well as hyperglycemia occur in up to 90% of patients. Allergic, hypersensitivity reactions have been observed in about 10% of patients, and pulmonary toxicity, presenting as increased cough, dyspnea, fever, and pulmonary infiltrates, is a relatively rare event, occurring in less than 1% of patients. However, the risk of pulmonary toxicity increases in patients with an underlying pulmonary disease.[46]

EVEROLIMUS

Everolimus (RAD001) is an orally active hydroxyethyl ether analog of rapamycin that contains a 2-hydroxyethyl chain substitution. This molecule is significantly more water soluble than sirolimus. As with sirolimus and temsirolimus, everolimus targets mTOR by forming a complex with mTOR and FKBP, resulting in inhibition of mTOR activity. Few data are available regarding the actual differences in the ability of temsirolimus and everolimus to inhibit mTOR. One preclinical in vitro study showed that the binding of everolimus to FKBP was approximately threefold weaker than that of sirolimus.[47] In vivo studies, however, have documented similar efficacy of the two agents in terms of immunosuppressive activity as well as antitumor activity. In preclinical models, the administration of everolimus results in the inhibition of mTOR, similar to what has been observed with the other rapamycin analogs.[48] In terms of clinical pharmacology, peak drug levels are achieved within 1 to 2 hours after oral administration, and food with a high fat content reduces oral bioavailability by up to 20%. This compound is metabolized in the liver, mainly by the CYP3A4 system, and six main metabolites have been identified. In general, these metabolites are less active than the parent compound. Elimination is mainly hepatic with excretion in feces, and caution should be used in patients with moderate liver impairment (Child-Pugh class B).[49] In this setting, the daily dose of drug should be reduced to 5 mg. In patients with severe liver dysfunction (Child-Pugh class C), the use of this drug is contraindicated.

Encouraging clinical activity was initially observed in phase 1/2 trials in patients with non–small-cell lung, gastric, and esophageal cancers, sarcomas, pancreatic neuroendocrine tumors, as well as hematologic malignancies.[50–53] Presently, everolimus is indicated and approved for the treatment of adults with advanced RCC after failure with sunitinib or sorafenib; advanced hormone receptor-positive, HER2-negative breast cancer in combination with exemestane; and progressive unresectable, locally advanced, or metastatic neuroendocrine tumors of pancreatic origin (PNET).[54,55] The recommended dose of everolimus for these indications is 10 mg taken orally once daily.

The safety profile of everolimus is similar to what has been observed with temsirolimus. The most common adverse events include asthenia and fatigue, dry skin with acneiform skin rash, nausea/vomiting, mucositis, and anorexia. Hyperlipidemia with increased serum triglycerides and/or cholesterol as well as hyperglycemia occur in up to 90% of patients. Allergic, hypersensitivity reactions have been observed in about 10% of patients, and pulmonary toxicity, presenting as increased cough, dyspnea, fever, and pulmonary infiltrates, are a relatively rare event, occurring in less than 1% of patients. However, the risk of pulmonary toxicity increases in patients with an underlying pulmonary disease.

THALIDOMIDE, LENALIDOMIDE, AND POMALIDOMIDE

Thalidomide and its amino-substituted analogs, lenalidomide and pomalidomide, are small-molecule glutamic acid derivatives that possess a wide range of biologic properties, including immunomodulating, antiangiogenic, and epigenetic effects. They are classified as class I (non–phosphodiesterase-4 inhibitory) immunomodulatory drugs (IMiDs). Although their primary mechanism of activity against malignancy is uncertain, it is believed that IMiDs exert their anticancer effects both directly on cancer cells and indirectly via effects on the tumor microenvironment and host antitumor immunity. Specific mechanisms include the inhibition of nuclear factor kappa B (NF-κB) transcriptional activity in malignant cells with a resultant decrease in the production of antiapoptotic molecules; the inhibition of surface adhesion molecule expression on both multiple myeloma cells and bone marrow stromal cells; the inhibition of the production and release of various growth factors (including vascular endothelial growth factor, basic fibroblast growth factor, tumor necrosis factor alpha, and interleukin [IL] 6) that regulate angiogenesis and tumor cell proliferation; and costimulation of IL-2 and interferon gamma (IFN-γ) release with T-helper 1 subset skewing and augmentation of cytotoxic T-cell and natural killer cell effector function.[56,57] Unlike thalidomide, both lenalidomide and pomalidomide result in cell cycle arrest and apoptosis of myeloma cells in vitro, believed in part to be related to epigenetic effects.[58] They are also more potent stimulators of IL-2 and INF-γ production and T-cell proliferation than thalidomide, and appear to additionally inhibit T-regulatory cells.[57] Clinically, lenalidomide has activity in patients with thalidomide-resistant multiple myeloma, and pomalidomide has additional activity in patients with lenalidomide-resistant disease.[59,60] Recently, the protein cereblon (cerebral protein with lon protease), a highly conserved E3 ligase, was recognized as a primary target of IMiDs teratogenic effect, and appears to be an important target of IMiD anticancer activity.[61–63] Efforts are currently under way to evaluate the expression of Cereblon as a predictive biomarker of response to IMiDs.[63] Due to the potential risk of significant teratogenicity, thalidomide, lenalidomide, and pomalidomide can only be prescribed by licensed prescribers who are registered in restricted distribution programs.

Thalidomide

Thalidomide (2-[2,6-dioxopiperidin-3-yl]-2,3-dihydro-1H-isoindole-1,3-dione; Thalomid) is a synthetic glutamic acid derivative that was initially synthesized in 1953. It was used widely in Europe between 1956 and 1962 as a sleeping aid and antiemetic for pregnant women before it was discovered to cause severe congenital malformations. Initial reports of its efficacy in multiple myeloma were published in 1999, and the 200-mg daily dose combined with pulse dexamethasone (40-mg daily dose on days 1 through 4, 9 through 12, and 17 through 20 on a 28-day schedule) was approved by the FDA in 2006 for newly diagnosed multiple myeloma. The use of thalidomide has dropped precipitously in the United States with the FDA approval of more efficacious and less toxic therapies for myeloma. Thalidomide is poorly soluble, and it is absorbed slowly from the gastrointestinal tract, reaching peak plasma concentration in 3 to 6 hours, with 55% to 66% bound to plasma proteins. The exact metabolic route and fate of thalidomide is not known. Thalidomide does not appear to be hepatically metabolized, but rather undergoes spontaneous nonenzymatic hydrolysis in plasma to multiple metabolites, with a half-life of elimination ranging from 5 to 7 hours. These metabolites are believed to be responsible for the antitumor effects of thalidomide. Less than 1% is excreted into the urine as unchanged drug.[64]

Thalidomide frequently causes drowsiness, constipation, and fatigue. Peripheral neuropathy is a common and potentially severe and irreversible side effect occurring in up to 30% of patients. Increased incidences of venous thromboembolic events, such as deep venous thrombosis and pulmonary embolus, have also been observed with thalidomide, particularly when used in combination with dexamethasone or anthracycline-based chemotherapy. Patients who are appropriate candidates may benefit from concurrent prophylactic anticoagulation or aspirin treatment.[65] Other side effects of thalidomide include rash, nausea, dizziness, orthostatic hypotension, bradycardia, and mood changes. In 2013, additional alerts were released linking thalidomide to an increased risk of developing second primary malignancies (both acute myelogenous leukemia and myelodysplastic syndrome) and arterial thromboembolic events.

Lenalidomide

Lenalidomide (3-[4-amino-1-oxo-2,3-dihydro-1H-isoindol-2-yl]piperidine-2,6-dione; Revlimid) is a thalidomide derivative that shares the immunomodulatory and antineoplastic properties of its parent compound. However, lenalidomide appears to be more potent in vitro with less nonhematologic toxicities in clinical studies. It initially received FDA approval (10-mg daily dose) in 2005 for the treatment of patients with transfusion dependent anemia secondary to low or intermediate risk myelodysplastic syndromes associated with a deletion 5q cytogenetic abnormality, with or without additional cytogenetic abnormalities. In 2006, lenalidomide (25-mg daily dose on days 1 through 21 of a 28-day cycle) in combination with dexamethasone (40-mg daily dose on days 1 through 4, 9 through 12, and 17 through 20 on each 28-day cycle for the first four cycles, then 40 mg daily on days 1 through 4 every 28 days) was approved by the FDA for the treatment of patients with multiple myeloma who had received at least one prior therapy for multiple myeloma. In 2013, lenalidomide 25 mg daily (days 1 through 21 on repeated 28-day cycles) was additionally approved for use in refractory mantle cell lymphoma (after relapse/ progression on two lines of therapy, one of which contained bortezomid). Lenalidomide is administered orally and is rapidly absorbed from the gastrointestinal tract. Maximum plasma concentration is reached 0.625 to 1.5 hours after dosing, with approximately 30% bound to plasma proteins. The half-life of elimination is approximately 3 hours, with little information currently available concerning metabolism. Approximately 70% of an administered dose is excreted unchanged by the kidneys.[66]

Compared with thalidomide, lenalidomide is associated with less sedation, constipation, and peripheral neuropathy. However, myelosuppression in the form of neutropenia and thrombocytopenia can be dose limiting. As with thalidomide, the incidence of thromboembolic events is significant with the combination of dexamethasone and lenalidomide. A pooled analysis of 691 patients enrolled in two randomized studies reported a 12% incidence of thrombotic or thromboembolic events with the combination, compared with 4% with dexamethasone alone.[67]

Pomalidomide

Pomalidomide (4-amino-2-[2,6-dioxopiperidin-3-yl]-2,3-dihydro-1H-isoindole-1,3-dione; Pomalyst) is another thalidomide derivative designed to be more potent and less toxic than both thalidomide and lenalidomide. It is currently FDA approved (4-mg once daily dose orally on days 1 through 21 of a 28 day cycle, with or without dexamethasone) for use in patients with progressive multiple myeloma who have received at least two prior therapies, including lenalidomide and bortezomid. Pomalidomide is administered orally and is rapidly absorbed. Maximum plasma concentration is reached 2 to 3 hours after ingestion, with approximately 12% to 44% protein binding.[68] The half-life of elimination is between 7.5 and 9.5 hours. Pomalidomide is metabolized in the liver, via CYP1A2/CYP3A4 (major) and CYP2C19/CYP2D6 (minor), and excretion occurs primarily through the kidneys (73%; 2% as unchanged drug).

Like lenalidomide, pomalidomide is better tolerated than thalidomide at approved doses with less constipation, fatigue, and neuropathy.[69] The primary toxicity appreciated in myeloma trials has been myelosuppression, particularly neutropenia, which can be dose limiting. The risk of thromboembolic events is similar to that seen with thalidomide and lenalidomide. Unlike thalidomide or lenalidomide, dermatologic toxicity is rare with pomalidomide. A summary of the characteristics of the miscellaneous drugs mentioned in this chapter is provided in Table 26.1. A summary of all hematology oncology drug approvals since the last edition of the textbook can be viewed in Table 26.2.

TABLE 26.1
Miscellaneous Chemotherapeutic Agents

	Main Therapeutic Uses	Clinical Pharmacology	Major Toxicities	Notes
Omacetaxine	CML	Mean half-life of 6 h after subcutaneous injection	Thrombocytopenia, anemia, nausea, diarrhea	Efficacy shown in Bcr-Abl–mutated CML
L-Asparaginase	Pediatric and adult ALL	Peak concentration 7–12 h after IV administration; 30% plasma protein binding; PEG form has longer half-life of 5.7 days; antagonize effects of methotrexate if given before or concurrently	Hypersensitivity reactions, alterations in thyroid function, prolonged PT/PTT, decreased levels of vitamin K–dependent factors, acute pancreatitis	Myelosuppression is rare; hypersensitivity reaction risk increases with repeated exposure and when used as single agent; PEG form is less immunogenic
Bleomycin	Hodgkin disease, neoplastic pleural effusion, non-Hodgkin lymphoma, squamous cell carcinoma of cervix, squamous cell carcinoma of nasopharynx, squamous cell carcinoma of penis, squamous cell carcinoma of the head and neck, squamous cell carcinoma of vulva, testicular cancer	Terminal half-life of 3h; can be given intracavitary; 45%–55% of intracavitary dose absorbed systemically; elimination via kidneys if CrCl <25–35 mL/min dose reduction required	Pulmonary toxicity dose-limiting; more if age >70 y; cumulative dose >400 U; acute hypersensitivity reactions rare (1%); mucositis, erythema, hyperpigmentation	Not myelosuppressive; immunosuppressive; metabolizing enzyme; bleomycin hydrolase enzyme low in lung and skin tissue; G-CSF use seems to exacerbate pulmonary toxicity

(continued)

TABLE 26.1
Miscellaneous Chemotherapeutic Agents (continued)

	Main Therapeutic Uses	Clinical Pharmacology	Major Toxicities	Notes
Procarbazine	Hodgkin lymphoma	Rapid complete oral absorption; peak concentration, 10–15 min; crosses blood–brain barrier; half-life 1 h; several drug–drug and food–drug interactions; metabolized by hepatic microsomal P-450 system; 70% excreted in urine	Dose-limiting toxicity is myelosuppression, more commonly thrombocytopenia nadir at 4 wk; G-6PD–deficient patients can develop hemolytic anemia, nausea, vomiting, diarrhea, flulike symptoms, peripheral neuropathy, hypersensitivity reactions	Avoid tyramine-containing foods; disulfiramlike reaction with concurrent alcohol use; hypertensive reaction with concurrent tricyclic antidepressant use; increased risk for azoospermia/infertility and secondary malignancy
Vismodegib	Basal cell carcinoma of the skin	Oral bioavailability 32%; not affected by food	No dose limiting toxicity; abdominal pain, fatigue, weight loss, dysgeusia	Hedgehog-signaling pathway inhibitor
Ado-trastuzumabemtansine	Advanced HER2-positive breast cancer	Peak concentration near the end of infusion metabolized by CYP3A4/5; half-life, 3.5 days	Thrombocytopenia, hepatotoxicity, cardiac toxicity fatigue, nausea	Monitor cardiac function
Temsirolimus	Advanced renal cancer	Peak concentration, 0.5–2 h; widely distributed in tissues; steady-state levels reached in 7–8 d; half-life, 17 h	Asthenia, fatigue, dry skin, acneiform skin rash, mucositis, anorexia, hyperlipidemia, hyperglycemia	Efficacy shown for both clear cell and non–clear-cell histologies; efficacy in hematologic malignancies (mantle cell lymphoma, non-Hodgkin lymphoma, multiple myeloma)
Everolimus	Advanced renal cell carcinoma, breast cancer, pancreatic neuroendocrine tumor	Peak concentration, 1–2 hr; reduced bioavailability with high fat content food; metabolized by CYP3A4 system; mainly hepatic excretion	Asthenia, dry skin, nausea, vomiting, mucositis, hyperlipidemia, hyperglycemia, allergic hypersensitivity reaction, pulmonary toxicity	Contraindicated in Child-Pugh class C patients; encouraging activity in gastric, non–small-cell, lung, esophageal cancers, sarcomas; approved for organ rejection prophylaxis
Thalidomide	Multiple myeloma, erythema nodosum leprosum	Oral absorption slow; peak concentration, 3–6 h; 55%–66% bound to plasma proteins; half-life, 5–7 h; spontaneous nonenzymatic hydrolysis in plasma	Drowsiness, constipation, fatigue, skin rash, increased risk for thromboembolic complications	Pregnancy category X; may be present in semen; serious skin reactions including Stevens-Johnson syndrome
Lenalidomide	Low-to-intermediate risk myelodysplastic syndrome associated with 5q deletion, multiple myeloma	Rapid oral absorption; peak concentration, 0.6–1.5 h; half-life, 3 h; 70% excreted unchanged by kidneys	Less sedation, drowsiness, constipation than thalidomide; myelosuppression; thromboembolic events; peripheral neuropathy	Pregnancy category X; caution in patients with renal function impairment; neutropenia; thrombocytopenia may be dose limiting
Pomalidomide	Multiple myeloma who have received at least two prior therapies	Rapid oral absorption; peak concentration, 2–3 h; half-life, 7.5 h	Myelosuppression; thromboembolic events; skin toxicity rare	Better tolerated than thalidomide; effective in prior bortezomib- and lenalidomide-receiving patients

PT, prothrombin time; PTT, partial thromboplastin time; CrCl, creatinine clearance.

TABLE 26.2
U.S. Food And Drug Administration Hematology Oncology Drug Approvals 2010–2013

Drug/Manufacturer	Indication	Approval Date
Sorafenib (NEXAVAR tablets, Bayer Healthcare Pharmaceuticals Inc.)	For the treatment of locally recurrent or metastatic, progressive, differentiated thyroid carcinoma (DTC) refractory to radioactive iodine treatment.	November 22, 2013
Crizotinib (Xalkori, Pfizer, Inc.) capsules	For the treatment of patients with metastatic non–small-cell lung cancer (NSCLC) whose tumors are anaplastic lymphoma kinase (ALK) positive as detected by an FDA-approved test.	November 20, 2013
Ibrutinib (IMBRUVICA, Pharmacyclics, Inc.)	For the treatment of patients with mantle cell lymphoma (MCL) who have received at least one prior therapy.	November 13, 2013
Obinutuzumab (GAZYVA injection, for intravenous use, Genentech, Inc.; previously known as GA101)	For use in combination with chlorambucil for the treatment of patients with previously untreated chronic lymphocytic leukemia (CLL).	November 1, 2013
Pertuzumab injection (PERJETA, Genentech, Inc.)	For use in combination with trastuzumab and docetaxel for the neoadjuvant treatment of patients with HER2-positive, locally advanced, inflammatory, or early stage breast cancer (either greater than 2 cm in diameter or node positive) as part of a complete treatment regimen for early breast cancer.	September 30, 2013
Paclitaxel protein-bound particles (albumin-bound) (Abraxane for injectable suspension, Abraxis BioScience, LLC, a wholly owned subsidiary of Celgene Corporation)	In combination with gemcitabine for the first-line treatment of patients with metastatic adenocarcinoma of the pancreas.	September 6, 2013
Afatinib (Gilotrif tablets, Boehringer Ingelheim Pharmaceuticals, Inc.)	For the first-line treatment of patients with metastatic NSCLC whose tumors have epidermal growth factor receptor (EGFR) exon 19 deletions or exon 21 (L858R) substitution mutations as detected by an FDA-approved test. The safety and efficacy of afatinib have not been established in patients whose tumors have other EGFR mutations.	July 12, 2013
Denosumab (Xgeva injection, for subcutaneous use, Amgen Inc.)	For the treatment of adults and skeletally mature adolescents with a giant cell tumor of bone that is unresectable or where surgical resection is likely to result in severe morbidity.	June 13, 2013
Lenalidomide capsules (REVLIMID, Celgene Corporation)	For the treatment of patients with MCL whose disease has relapsed or progressed after two prior therapies, one of which included bortezomib.	June 5, 2013
Trametinib (MEKINIST tablet, GlaxoSmithKline, LLC)	For the treatment of patients with unresectable or metastatic melanoma with BRAF V600E or V600K mutation as detected by an FDA-approved test.	May 29, 2013
Dabrafenib (TAFINLAR capsule, GlaxoSmithKline, LLC)	For the treatment of patients with unresectable or metastatic melanoma with BRAF V600E mutation as detected by an FDA-approved test.	May 29, 2013
Radium Ra 223 dichloride (Xofigo Injection, Bayer HealthCare Pharmaceuticals Inc.)	For the treatment of patients with castration-resistant prostate cancer, symptomatic bone metastases, and no known visceral metastatic disease.	May 15, 2013
Erlotinib (Tarceva, Astellas Pharma Inc.)	For the first-line treatment of metastatic NSCLC patients whose tumors have EGFR exon 19 deletions or exon 21 (L858R) substitution mutations.	May 14, 2013
Ado-trastuzumab emtansine (KADCYLA for injection, Genentech, Inc.)	For use as a single agent for the treatment of patients with HER2-positive, metastatic breast cancer who previously received trastuzumab and a taxane, separately or in combination.	February 22, 2013
Pomalidomide (POMALYST capsules, Celgene Corporation)	For the treatment of patients with multiple myeloma who have received at least two prior therapies, including lenalidomide and bortezomib, and have demonstrated disease progression on or within 60 days of completion of the last therapy.	February 8, 2013

(continued)

TABLE 26.2

U.S. Food And Drug Administration Hematology Oncology Drug Approvals 2010–2013 *(continued)*

Drug/Manufacturer	Indication	Approval Date
Doxorubicin hydrochloride liposome injection (Sun Pharma Global FZE), a generic version of DOXIL Injection (doxorubicin hydrochloride liposome; Janssen Products, L.P.)	For the treatment of ovarian cancer in patients whose disease has progressed or recurred after platinum-based chemotherapy and for AIDS-related Kaposi sarcoma after failure of prior systemic chemotherapy or intolerance to such therapy.	February 4, 2013
Bevacizumab (Avastin, Genentech U.S., Inc.)	For use in combination with fluoropyrimidine–irinotecan- or fluoropyrimidine–oxaliplatin-based chemotherapy for the treatment of patients with metastatic colorectal cancer (mCRC) whose disease has progressed on a first-line bevacizumab-containing regimen.	January 23, 2013
Ponatinib (Iclusig tablets, ARIAD Pharmaceuticals, Inc.)	For the treatment of adult patients with chronic phase, accelerated phase, or blast phase chronic myeloid leukemia (CML) that is resistant or intolerant to prior tyrosine–kinase inhibitor (TKI) therapy or Philadelphia chromosome–positive acute lymphoblastic leukemia (Ph+ ALL) that is resistant or intolerant to prior TKI therapy.	December 17, 2012
Abiraterone acetate (Zytiga Tablets, Janssen Biotech, Inc.)	In combination with prednisone for the treatment of patients with metastatic castration-resistant prostate cancer.	December 10, 2012
Cabozantinib (COMETRIQ capsules, Exelixis, Inc.)	For the treatment of patients with progressive metastatic medullary thyroid cancer (MTC). Cabozantinib is a small molecule that inhibits the activity of multiple tyrosine kinases, including RET, MET, and VEGF receptor 2.	November 29, 2012
Omacetaxine mepesuccinate (SYNRIBO for injection, for subcutaneous use, Teva Pharmaceutical Industries Ltd.)	For the treatment of adult patients with chronic or accelerated phase CML with resistance and/or intolerance to two or more TKIs.	October 26, 2012
Paclitaxel protein-bound particles for injectable suspension, albumin-bound (ABRAXANE for injectable suspension; Abraxis Bioscience a wholly owned subsidiary of Celgene Corporation)	For use in combination with carboplatin for the initial treatment of patients with locally advanced or metastatic NSCLC who are not candidates for curative surgery or radiation therapy.	October 11, 2012
Regorafenib (Stivarga tablets, Bayer HealthCare Pharmaceuticals, Inc.)	For the treatment of patients with mCRC who have been previously treated with fluoropyrimidine-, oxaliplatin-, and irinotecan-based chemotherapy, an anti-VEGF therapy, and, if KRAS wild-type, an anti-EGFR therapy.	September 27, 2012
Bosutinib tablets (Bosulif, Pfizer, Inc.)	for the treatment of chronic, accelerated, or blast phase Ph+ CML in adult patients with resistance or intolerance to prior therapy.	September 4, 2012
Enzalutamide (XTANDI Capsules, Medivation, Inc., and Astellas Pharma US, Inc.)	For the treatment of patients with metastatic castration-resistant prostate cancer who have previously received docetaxel.	August 31, 2012
Everolimus tablets for oral suspension (Afinitor Disperz, Novartis Pharmaceuticals Corp.)	For the treatment of pediatric and adult patients with tuberous sclerosis complex (TSC) who have subependymal giant cell astrocytoma (SEGA) that requires therapeutic intervention, but that cannot be curatively resected.	August 30, 2012
Vincristine sulfate LIPOSOME injection (Marqibo, Talon Therapeutics, Inc.)	For the treatment of adult patients with Ph- ALL in second or greater relapse or whose disease has progressed following two or more antileukemia therapies.	August 9, 2012
Ziv-aflibercept injection (ZALTRAP, Sanofi U.S., Inc.)	For use in combination with 5-fluorouracil, leucovorin, irinotecan (FOLFIRI) for the treatment of patients with mCRC that is resistant to or has progressed following an oxaliplatin-containing regimen.	August 3, 2012
Everolimus tablets (Afinitor, Novartis Pharmaceuticals Corporation)	For the treatment of postmenopausal women with advanced hormone receptor–positive, HER2-negative breast cancer in combination with exemestane, after failure of treatment with letrozole or anastrozole.	July 20, 2012

(continued)

TABLE 26.2
U.S. Food And Drug Administration Hematology Oncology Drug Approvals 2010–2013 *(continued)*

Drug/Manufacturer	Indication	Approval Date
Carfilzomib injection (Kyprolis, Onyx Pharmaceuticals)	For the treatment of patients with multiple myeloma who have received at least two prior therapies, including bortezomib and an immunomodulatory agent, and have demonstrated disease progression on or within 60 days of the completion of the last therapy.	July 20, 2012
Cetuximab (Erbitux, ImClone LLC, a wholly owned subsidiary of Eli Lilly and Co.)	For use in combination with FOLFIRI for first-line treatment of patients with K-ras mutation-negative (wild type), EGFR expressing mCRC as determined by FDA-approved tests for this use.	July 9, 2012
Pertuzumab injection (PERJETA, Genentech, Inc.)	For use in combination with trastuzumab and docetaxel for the treatment of patients with HER2-positive metastatic breast cancer who have not received prior anti-HER2 therapy or chemotherapy for metastatic disease.	June 8, 2012
Pazopanib tablets (VOTRIENT, a registered Trademark of GlaxoSmithKline)	For the treatment of patients with advanced soft tissue sarcoma (STS) who have received prior chemotherapy.	April 26, 2012
Everolimus (Afinitor tablets, Novartis)	For the treatment of adults with renal angiomyolipoma, associated with TSC who do not require immediate surgery.	April 26, 2012
Imatinib mesylate tablets (Gleevec, Novartis Pharmaceuticals)	For the adjuvant treatment of adult patients following complete gross resection of Kit (CD117)-positive gastrointestinal stromal tumors (GIST).	January 31, 2012
Vismodegib (ERIVEDGE Capsule, Genentech, Inc.)	For the treatment of adults with metastatic basal cell carcinoma or with locally advanced basal cell carcinoma that has recurred following surgery or who are not candidates for surgery and who are not candidates for radiation.	January 30, 2012
Axitinib tablets (Inlyta, Pfizer, Inc.)	For the treatment of advanced renal cell carcinoma after failure of one prior systemic therapy.	January 27, 2012
Glucarpidase injection (Voraxaze, BTG International Inc.)	For the treatment of toxic plasma methotrexate concentrations (> 1 µmol/L) in patients with delayed methotrexate clearance due to impaired renal function.	January 17, 2012
Asparaginase *Erwinia chrysanthemi* (Erwinaze, injection, EUSA Pharma [USA], Inc.)	As a component of a multiagent chemotherapeutic regimen for the treatment of patients with ALL who have developed hypersensitivity to *E. coli*–derived asparaginase.	November 18, 2011
Ruxolitinib (Jakafi oral tablets, Incyte Corporation)	For the treatment of intermediate and high risk myelofibrosis, including primary myelofibrosis, postpolycythemia vera myelofibrosis, and postessential thrombocythemia myelofibrosis.	November 16, 2011
Cetuximab (Erbitux, ImClone LLC, a wholly owned subsidiary of Eli Lilly and Company)	In combination with platinum-based therapy plus 5-fluorouracil (5-FU) for the first-line treatment of patients with recurrent locoregional disease and/or metastatic squamous cell carcinoma of the head and neck (SCCHN).	November 7, 2011
Eculizumab (Soliris, Alexion, Inc.)	For the treatment of pediatric and adult patients with atypical hemolytic uremic syndrome (aHUS).	September 23, 2011
Denosumab (Prolia, Amgen Inc.)	As a treatment to increase bone mass in patients at high risk for fracture receiving androgen-deprivation therapy (ADT) for nonmetastatic prostate cancer or adjuvant aromatase inhibitor (AI) therapy for breast cancer.	September 16, 2011
Crizotinib (XALKORI Capsules, Pfizer Inc.)	For the treatment of patients with locally advanced or metastatic NSCLC that is ALK-positive as detected by an FDA-approved test.	August 26, 2011

(continued)

TABLE 26.2

U.S. Food And Drug Administration Hematology Oncology Drug Approvals 2010–2013 *(continued)*

Drug/Manufacturer	Indication	Approval Date
Brentuximab vedotin (Adcetris for injection, Seattle Genetics, Inc.)	For treatment of patients with Hodgkin lymphoma after failure of autologous stem cell transplant (ASCT) or after failure of at least two prior multiagent chemotherapy regimens in patients who are not ASCT candidates and treatment of patients with systemic anaplastic large cell lymphoma (ALCL) after failure of at least one prior multiagent chemotherapy regimen.	August 19, 2011
Vemurafenib tablets (ZELBORAF, Hoffmann-La Roche Inc.)	For the treatment of patients with unresectable or metastatic melanoma with the BRAFV600E mutation as detected by an FDA-approved test.	August 17, 2011
Sunitinib (Sutent capsules, Pfizer, Inc.)	For the treatment of progressive, well-differentiated pancreatic neuroendocrine tumors (pNET) in patients with unresectable, locally advanced, or metastatic disease.	May 20, 2011
Everolimus (Afinitor tablets, Novartis Pharmaceuticals Corporation)	For the treatment of progressive PNET in patients with unresectable, locally advanced, or metastatic disease.	May 5, 2011
Abiraterone acetate (Zytiga tablets, Centocor Ortho Biotech, Inc.)	For use in combination with prednisone for the treatment of patients with metastatic castration-resistant prostate cancer (mCRPC) who have received prior chemotherapy containing docetaxel.	April 28, 2011
Vandetanib tablets (Vandetanib tablets, AstraZeneca Pharmaceuticals LP)	For the treatment of symptomatic or progressive medullary thyroid cancer in patients with unresectable, locally advanced, or metastatic disease.	April 6, 2011
Peginterferon alfa-2b (Sylatron, Schering Corporation, Kenilworth, NJ 07033)	For the treatment of patients with melanoma with microscopic or gross nodal involvement within 84 days of definitive surgical resection including complete lymphadenectomy.	March 29, 2011
Ipilimumab injection (YERVOY, Bristol-Myers Squibb Company)	For the treatment of unresectable or metastatic melanoma.	March 25, 2011
Rituximab (Rituxan, Genentech, Inc.)	For maintenance therapy in patients with previously untreated follicular, CD-20 positive, B-cell non-Hodgkin lymphoma who achieve a response to rituximab in combination with chemotherapy.	January 28, 2011
Eribulin mesylate (Halaven injection, Eisai Inc.)	For the treatment of patients with metastatic breast cancer who have previously received an anthracycline and a taxane in either the adjuvant or metastatic setting, and at least two chemotherapeutic regimens for the treatment of metastatic disease.	November 15, 2010
Everolimus (Afinitor, Novartis), an mTOR inhibitor	For patients with SEGA associated with tuberous sclerosis (TS) who require therapy but who are not candidates for surgical resection.	October 29, 2010
Dasatinib (Sprycel, Bristol-Myers Squibb)	For the treatment of newly diagnosed adult patients with Ph+ CML in chronic phase (CP-CML).	October 28, 2010
Trastuzumab (Herceptin, Genentech, Inc.)	In combination with cisplatin and a fluoropyrimidine (capecitabine or 5-FU), for the treatment of patients with HER2-overexpressing metastatic gastric or gastroesophageal (GE) junction adenocarcinoma, who have not received prior treatment for metastatic disease.	October 20, 2010
Nilotinib (Tasigna capsules, Novartis Pharmaceuticals Corporation)	For the treatment of adult patients with newly diagnosed Ph+ CP-CML.	June 17, 2010
Cabazitaxel (Jevtana injection, Sanofi-Aventis)	For use in combination with prednisone for treatment of patients with metastatic hormone-refractory prostate cancer (mHRPC) previously treated with a docetaxel-containing regimen.	June 17, 2010

REFERENCES

1. Powell RG, Weisleder D, Smith CR, et al. Antitumor alkaloids from Cephalotaxus harringtonia structure and activity. *J Pharm Sci* 1972;61:1227–1230.
2. Huang MT. Harringtonine, an inhibitor of initiation of protein biosynthesis. *Mol Pharmacol* 1975;11:511–519.
3. Baaske DM, Heinstein P. Cytotoxicity and cell cycle specificity of homoharringtonine. *Antimicrob Agents Chemother* 1977;12:298–300.
4. Savaraj N, Lu K, Dimery I, et al. Clinical pharmacology of homoharringtonine. *Cancer Treat Rep* 1986;70:1403–1407.
5. Neidhart JA, Young DC, Derocher D, et al. Phase I trial of homoharringtonine. *Cancer Treat Rep* 1983;67:801–804.
6. Grem JL, Cheson BD, King SA, et al. Cephalotaxine esters: antileukemic advance of therapeutic failure. *J Natl Cancer Inst* 1988;80:1095–1103.
7. O'Brien S, Kantarjian H, Keating M, et al. Homoharringtonine therapy induces responses in patients with chronic myelogenous leukemia in late chronic phase. *Blood* 1995;86:3322–3326.
8. Legros L, Hayette S, Nicolini FE, et al. BCR-ABL(T315I) transcript disappearance in an imatinib-resistant CML patient treated with homoharringtonine: a new therapeutic challenge? *Leukemia* 2007;21(10):2204–2206.
9. Jorge Cortes J, Lipton JF, Rea D, et al. Phase 2 study of subcutaneous omacetaxine mepesuccinate after TKI failure in patients with chronic-phase CML with T315I mutation. *Blood* 2012;120:2573–2580.
10. Labrou NE, Papageorgiou AC, Avramis VI. Structure-function relationships and clinical applications of L-Asparaginases. *Curr Med Chem* 2010;17:2183–2195.
11. Verma N, Kumar K, Kaur G, et al. L-Asparaginase: a promising chemotherapeutic agent. *Crit Rev Biotechnol* 2007;27:45–62.
12. Zeidan A, Wang ES, Wetzler M. Pegasparaginase: where do we stand? *Expert Opin Biol Ther* 2009;9:111–119.
13. Avramis VI, Panosyan EH. Pharmacokinetic/pharmacodynamic relationships of asparaginase formulations: the past, the present and recommendations for the future. *Clin Pharmacokinet* 2005;44:367–393.
14. Appel IM, Hop WC, Pieters R. Changes in hypercoagulability by asparaginase: a randomized study between two asparaginases. *Blood Coagul Fibrinolysis* 2006;17:139–146.
15. Evans WE, Yee CC, Crom WR, et al. Clinical pharmacology of bleomycin and cisplatin. *Head Neck Surg* 1981;4:98–110.
16. Chen J, Stubbe J. Bleomycins: towards better therapeutics. *Nat Rev Cancer* 2005;2:102–112.
17. Hecht SM. Bleomycin: new perspectives on the mechanism of action. *J Nat Prod* 2000;63:158–168.
18. Lewis TG, Nydorf ED. Intralesional bleomycin for warts: a review. *J Drugs Dermatol* 2006;5:499–504.
19. Shaw P, Agarwal R. Pleurodesis for malignant pleural effusions. *Cochrane Database Syst Rev* 2004;(1):CD002916.
20. Good LM, Miller MD, High WA. Intralesional agents in the management of cutaneous malignancy: a review. *J Am Acad Dermatol* 2011;64:413–422.
21. Kawai K, Akaza H. Bleomycin-induced pulmonary toxicity in chemotherapy for testicular cancer. *Expert Opin Drug Saf* 2003;2:587–596.
22. Azulay E, Herigault S, Levame M, et al. Effect of granulocyte colony-stimulating factor on bleomycin-induced acute lung injury and pulmonary fibrosis. *Crit Care Med* 2003;31:1442–1448.
23. Adachi M, Suzuki M, Sugimoto T, et al. Effects of granulocyte colony-stimulating factor on the kinetics of inflammatory cells in the peripheral blood and pulmonary lesions during the development of bleomycin-induced lung injury in rats. *Exp Toxicol Pathol* 2003;55:21–32.
24. Martin WG, Ristow KM, Habermann TM, et al. Bleomycin pulmonary toxicity has a negative impact on the outcome of patients with Hodgkin's lymphoma. *J Clin Oncol* 2005;23:7614–7620.
25. Younes A, Connors JM, Park SI et al. Brentuximab vedotin combined with ABVD or AVD for patients with newly diagnosed Hodgkin's lymphoma: a phase 1, open-label, dose-escalation study. *Lancet Oncol* 2013;14:1348–1356.
26. Lam MS. The need for routine bleomycin test dosing in the 21st century. *Ann Pharmacother* 2005;39:1897–1902.
27. Swaffar DS, Horstman MG, Jaw JY, et al. Methylazoxyprocarbazine, the active metabolite responsible for the anticancer activity of procarbazine against L1210 leukemia. *Cancer Res* 1989;49:2442–2447.
28. Patterson LH, Murray GI. Tumour cytochrome P450 and drug activation. *Curr Pharm Des* 2002;8:1335–1347.
29. Swaffar DS, Pomerantz SC, Harker WG, et al. Non-enzymatic activation of procarbazine to active cytotoxic species. *Oncol Res* 1992;4:49–58.
30. Preiss R, Baumann F, Regenthal R, et al. Plasma kinetics of procarbazine and azo-procarbazine in humans. *Anticancer Drugs* 2006;17:75–80.
31. Von Hoff DD, LoRusso PM, Rudin CM, et al. Inhibition of the hedgehog pathway in advanced basal-cell carcinoma. *N Engl J Med* 2009;361:1164–1172.
32. Rudin CM. Vismodegib. *Clin Cancer Res* 2012;18:1–5
33. U.S. Food and Drug Administration. News & Events: FDA News Release: FDA approves new treatment for most common types of skin cancer. http://www.fda.gov/NewsEvents/Newsroom/PressAnnouncements/ucm289545.htm. Published January 30, 2012. Updated January 31, 2012.
34. Tang JY, Mackay-Wiggan JM, Aszterbaum M, et al. Inhibiting the Hedgehog pathway in patients with the basal-cell nevus syndrome. *N Engl J Med* 2012;366:2180–2188.
35. Krop IE, Beeram M, Modi S, et al. Phase I study of trastuzumab DM1, an HER2 antibody-drug conjugate, given every 3 weeks to patients with HER2-positive metastatic breast cancer. *J Clin Oncol* 2010;28:2698–2704.
36. Verma S, Miles D, Gianni L, et al. Trastuzumab emtansine for HER2 positive advanced breast cancer. *N Engl J Med* 2012;367:1783–1791.
37. Sehgal SN, Baker H, Vézina C. Rapamycin (AY-22,989), a new antifungal antibiotic. II. Fermentation, isolation and characterization. *J Antibiot (Tokyo)* 1975;28:727–732.
38. Sehgal SN, Molnar-Kimber K, Ocain TD, et al. Rapamycin: a novel immunosuppressive macrolide. *Med Res Rev* 1994;14:1–22.
39. Wullschleger S, Loewith R, Hall MN. TOR signaling in growth and metabolism. *Cell* 2006;124:471–484.
40. Raymond E, Alexandre J, Faivre S, et al. Safety and pharmacokinetics of escalated doses of weekly intravenous infusion of CCI-779, a novel mTOR inhibitor in patients with cancer. *J Clin Oncol* 2004;22:2336–2347.
41. Zeng Z, Sarbassov dos D, Samudio IJ, et al. Rapamycin derivatives reduce mTORC2 signaling and inhibit AKT activation in AML. *Blood* 2007;109:3509–3512.
42. Kapoor A, Figlin RA. Targeted inhibition of mammalian target of rapamycin for the treatment of advanced renal cell carcinoma. *Cancer* 2009;115:3618–3630.
43. Atkins MB, Hidalgo M, Stadler WM, et al. Randomized phase II study of multiple dose levels of CCI-779, a novel mammalian target of rapamycin kinase inhibitor, in patients with advanced refractory renal cell carcinoma. *J Clin Oncol* 2004;22:909–918.
44. Hudes G, Carducci M, Tomczak P, et al. Temsirolimus, interferon alfa, or both for advanced renal-cell carcinoma. *N Engl J Med* 2007;356:2271–2281.
45. Smith SM, van Besien K, Karrison T, et al. Temsirolimus has activity in non-mantle cell non-Hodgkin's lymphoma subtypes: The University of Chicago phase II consortium. *J Clin Oncol* 2010;28:4740–4746.
46. Duran I, Siu LL, Oza AM, et al. Characterization of the lung toxicity of the cell cycle inhibitor temsirolimus. *Eur J Cancer* 2006;42:1875–1880.
47. Schuler W, Sedrani R, Cottens S, et al. SDZ RAD, a new rapamycine derivative: pharmacological properties in vitro and in vivo. *Transplantation* 1997;64:36–42.
48. Dudkin L, Dilling MB, Cheshire PJ, et al. Biochemical correlates of mTOR inhibition by the rapamycin ester CCI-779 and tumor growth inhibition. *Clin Cancer Res* 2001;7:1758–1764.
49. Kirchner GI, Meier-Wiedenbach I, Manns MP. Clinical pharmacokinetics of everolimus. *Clin Pharmacokinet* 2004;43:83–95.
50. Doi T, Muro K, Boku N, et al. Multicenter phase II study of everolimus in patients with previously treated metastatic gastric cancer. *J Clin Oncol* 2010;28:1904–1910.
51. Yao JC, Lombard-Bohas C, Baudin E, et al. Daily oral everolimus activity in patients with metastatic pancreatic neuroendocrine tumors after failure of cytotoxic chemotherapy: a phase II trial. *J Clin Oncol* 2010;28:69–76.
52. Yee KW, Zeng Z, Konopleva M, et al. Phase I/II study of the mammalian target of rapamycin inhibitor everolimus(RAD001) in patients with relapsed or refractory hematological malignancies. *Clin Cancer Res* 2008;12:5165–5173.
53. Okuno S. Mammalian target of rapamycin inhibitors in sarcomas. *Curr Opin Oncol* 2006;18:360–362.
54. Yao JC, Shah MH, Ito T, et al. Everolimus for advanced pancreatic neuroendocrine tumors. *N Engl J Med* 2011;364:514–523.
55. Baselga J, Campone M, Piccart M, et al. Everolimus in postmenopausal hormone-receptor-positive advanced breast cancer. *N Engl J Med* 2012;366:520–529.
56. Shortt J, Hsu AK, Johnstone RW. Thalidomide-analogue biology: immunological, molecular and epigenetic targets in cancer therapy. *Oncogene* 2013;32:4191–4202.
57. Zhu YX, Kortuem KM, Stewart AK. Molecular mechanism of action of immune-modulatory drugs thalidomide, lenalidomide and pomalidomide in multiple myeloma. *Leuk Lymphoma* 2013;54:683–687.
58. Escoubet-Lozach L, Lin IL, Jensen-Pergakes K, et al. Pomalidomide and lenalidomide induce p21 WAF-1 expression in both lymphoma and multiple myeloma through a LSD1-mediated epigenetic mechanism. *Cancer Res* 2009;69:7347–7356.
59. Madan S, Lacy MQ, Dispenzieri A, et al. Efficacy of retreatment with immunomodulatory drugs (IMiDs) in patients receiving IMiDs for initial therapy of newly diagnosed multiple myeloma. *Blood* 2011;118:1763–1765.
60. Lacy MQ, Tefferi A. Pomalidomide therapy for multiple myeloma and myelofibrosis: an update. *Leuk Lymphoma* 2011;52:560–566.
61. Ito T, Ando H, Suzuki T, et al. Identification of a primary target of thalidomide teratogenicity. *Science* 2010;327:1345–1350.
62. Zhu YX, Braggio E, Shi CX, et al. Cereblon expression is required for the antimyeloma activity of lenalidomide and pomalidomide. *Blood* 2011;118:4771–4779.
63. Lopez-Girona A, Mendy D, Ito T, et al. Cereblon is a direct protein target for immunomodulatory and antiproliferative activities of lenalidomide and pomalidomide. *Leukemia* 2012;26:2326–2335.
64. Schuster SR, Kortuem KM, Zhu YX, et al. Cereblon expression predicts response, progression free and overall survival after pomalidomide and

dexamethasone therapy in multiple myeloma. *ASH Ann Meeting Abstracts* 2012;120:194.
65. Bennett CL, Angelotta C, Yarnold PR, et al. Thalidomide- and lenalidomide-associated thromboembolism among patients with cancer. *JAMA* #2006;296: 2558–2560.
66. Rao KV. Lenalidomide in the treatment of multiple myeloma. *Am J Health Syst Pharm* 2007;64:1799–1807.
67. Lenalidomide. Drugs@FDA. Food and Drug Administration Web site. http://www.accessdata.fda.gov/drugsatfda_docs/label/2009/021880s006s016s017lbl.pdf. Published December 2008.
68. Pomalidomide. Drugs@FDA. Food and Drug Administration Web site. http://www.accessdata.fda.gov/drugsatfda_docs/label/2013/204026lbl.pdf. Revised February 2013.
69. Lacy MQ, McCurdy AR. Pomalidomide. *Blood* 2013;122:2305–2309.

27 Hormonal Agents

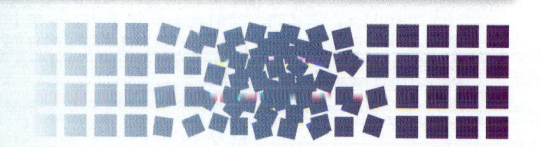

Matthew P. Goetz, Charles Erlichman, Charles L. Loprinzi, and Manish Kohli

INTRODUCTION

Hormonal agents are commonly used as a treatment of hormonally responsive cancers, such as breast, prostate, or endometrial carcinomas. Other uses for some hormonal therapies include the treatment of paraneoplastic syndromes, such as carcinoid syndrome, and symptoms caused by cancer, including anorexia. This chapter discusses the major hormonal agents for such therapy, first with an overview of their use in practice, then with more detailed pharmacologic information regarding them (Table 27.1).

SELECTIVE ESTROGEN RECEPTOR MODULATORS

Tamoxifen

Tamoxifen continues to be an important hormonal therapy for the prevention and treatment of breast cancer worldwide. The continued importance of tamoxifen is reflected in the fact that it is the only hormonal agent approved by the U.S. Food and Drug Administration (FDA) for the prevention of premenopausal breast cancer,[1] the treatment of ductal carcinoma in situ (DCIS),[2] and the treatment of surgically resected premenopausal estrogen receptor (ER)–positive breast cancer.[3]

The standard daily dose of tamoxifen is 20 mg, and the optimal duration depends on the underlying clinical setting. Although the recommended duration in the prevention and DCIS settings is 5 years, recently published prospective studies have demonstrated that for the adjuvant treatment of invasive breast cancer, a duration of 10 years (compared to 5 years) further reduced the risk of breast cancer mortality and improved overall survival.[4]

The most common toxicity from tamoxifen is hot flashes, affecting approximately 50% of treated women. These hot flashes are of varying intensity and duration. Tamoxifen-induced hot flashes appear to increase over the first 3 months of therapy and then plateau. They appear to be more prominent in women with a history of hot flashes or estrogen replacement use. Tamoxifen-induced hot flashes can be ameliorated by a number of different pharmacotherapies, including low doses of megestrol[5]; antidepressants such as venlafaxine,[6] desvenlafaxine,[7] citalopram,[8] escitalopram,[9] and paroxetine[10]; and the anticonvulsant drugs gabapentin[11] and pregabalin.[12] There is evidence that drugs that inhibit CYP2D6 (e.g., paroxetine) alter the metabolic activation of tamoxifen to endoxifen, a critical metabolite associated with in vivo tamoxifen efficacy.[13]

The estrogenic properties of tamoxifen are responsible for both beneficial and deleterious side effects. Tamoxifen increases the incidence of endometrial cancer in postmenopausal (but not premenopausal) women, with the increase in the annual incidence of endometrial cancer being approximately 2.58 (ratio of incidence rates).[14] The absolute risk depends on the duration of tamoxifen administration. For women who receive 10 years of adjuvant tamoxifen, the cumulative risk is 3.1% (mortality, 0.4%) versus 1.6% (mortality, 0.2%) for 5 years of tamoxifen.[4] The incidence of a rarer form of uterine cancer, uterine sarcoma, is also increased after tamoxifen use.[15] This form of endometrial cancer comprises approximately 15% of all uterine malignancies that develop after tamoxifen use.[15] Beneficial estrogenic effects from tamoxifen include a decrease in total cholesterol[16] and the preservation of bone density in postmenopausal women.[17] In premenopausal women, however, tamoxifen has a negative effect on bone density.[18] Although most patients do not complain of vaginal symptoms, a few complain of vaginal dryness, whereas others have increased vaginal secretions and discharge, the latter of which is an indication of the estrogenic activity of tamoxifen on the vagina. In the Arimidex, Tamoxifen, Alone or in Combination (ATAC) trial, a commonly observed tamoxifen side effect was vaginal bleeding, leading to a higher hysterectomy rate for patients randomized to tamoxifen (5%) compared to anastrozole (1%).[19] An uncommon effect from tamoxifen is retinal toxicity. This drug can also increase the risk of cataracts. However, no difference in the rate of vision threatening ocular toxicity has been seen among prospectively treated tamoxifen patients.[20] Tamoxifen predisposes patients to thromboembolic phenomena, especially if used with concomitant chemotherapy. Depression has also been described, but the association with tamoxifen is not clear. Although liver cancers have been noted in laboratory animals, there is no established association between tamoxifen and liver cancers in humans.

Pharmacology

Tamoxifen acts by blocking estrogen stimulation of breast cancer cells, inhibiting both translocation and nuclear binding of the ER. This alters transcriptional and posttranscriptional events mediated by this receptor.[21] Tamoxifen has agonistic, partial agonistic, or antagonistic effects depending on the species, tissue, or endpoints that have been assessed. Additionally, there are marked differences between the antiproliferative properties of tamoxifen and its metabolites.[22]

Resistance to tamoxifen can be intrinsic or acquired, and the potential mechanisms for this resistance are reviewed in the following paragraphs. At each step of the signal transduction pathway with which tamoxifen or its metabolites interferes, there is the potential for an alteration in response. The most important factor appears to be the level of ER, which is highly predictive for a response to tamoxifen. Tamoxifen is ineffective in ER-negative breast cancer. Although decreased or absent expression of the progesterone receptor (PR) is associated with a worse prognosis, the relative risk reduction in tamoxifen-treated patients is the same regardless of the presence or absence of the PR.

Following binding to the ER, subsequent translocation of the tamoxifen/ER complex to the nucleus and binding to an estrogen-response element may occur. This binding prevents transcriptional activation of estrogen-responsive genes. Laboratory and clinical data have demonstrated that ER-positive breast cancers that overexpress HER2 may be less responsive to tamoxifen and

TABLE 27.1
Overview of Major Hormonal Agents Used in Cancer

Class of Drug	Individual Drug	Dose	Route of Delivery	Frequency of Delivery
Selective estrogen receptor modulator	Tamoxifen Toremifene Raloxifene	20 mg 60 mg 60 mg	Oral Oral Oral	Once daily Once daily Once daily
Aromatase inhibitor	Anastrozole Letrozole Exemestane	1 mg 2.5 mg 25 mg	Oral Oral Oral	Once daily Once daily Once daily
Estrogen receptor downregulator	Fulvestrant	500 mg	IM	Once monthly
Luteinizing hormone releasing hormone agonist	Goserelin Leuprolide	7.5 3.6	IM IM	Once monthly[a] Once monthly[a]
GnRH antagonist	Degarelix	240 mg loading dose	SC	80 mg SC monthly maintenance dose
Antiandrogen	Flutamide Bicalutamide Nilutamide	250 mg 50 mg 300 mg for 30 d then 150 mg	Oral Oral Oral	Three times daily Once daily Once daily
Cytochrome P45017 alpha inhibitors	Abiraterone Acetate	1,000 mg (four 250 mg capsules)	Oral	Once Daily
AR "super antagonists"	Enzalutamide	160–240 mg	Oral	Daily
Androgen	Fluoxymesterone	10 mg	Oral	Twice daily
Estrogen	Estradiol	10 mg	Oral	Up to three times daily
Somatostatin analog	Octreotide	Varies	SC or IV	Up to three times daily[b]
Progestational agents	Megestrol Medroxyprogesterone acetate	Varies Varies	Oral Oral or IM	Once daily Varies

[a] Longer acting depot preparations (every 3 months) are available.
[b] Depot formulations are available.
IM, intramuscular; SC, subcutaneous; GnRH, gonadotropin-releasing hormone; CYP, cytochrome P-450; AR, androgen receptor.

to hormonal therapy in general.[23–26] In these tumors, ligand-independent activation of the ER by mitogen-activated protein kinase (MAPK) pathways may contribute to resistance.[27–29] In addition, the expression of AIB1, an estrogen-receptor coactivator, has been associated with tamoxifen resistance in patients whose breast cancers overexpress HER2.[30] In some cases, resistance may result from a decrease or loss of ER expression.[31,32] Although mutations in the ER ligand binding domain (LBD) are rare in newly diagnosed breast cancer, ER mutations are present in up to 20% of recurrent breast cancers.[33–36] These mutations lead to a conformational change in the LBD, which mimics the conformation of activated ligand-bound receptor and constitutive, ligand-independent transcriptional activity, resulting in resistance to hormonal therapy. Preclinical studies suggest that some of these mutations, although insensitive to aromatase inhibitors, retain sensitivity to higher dose selective estrogen-receptor modulators (SERM), such as endoxifen, as well as fulvestrant.[35]

The carcinogenic potential of tamoxifen has been recognized in rat studies[37–39] and in humans (endometrial cancer).[40] It has been proposed that the generation of reactive intermediates that bind covalently to macromolecules underlies the process. Such reactive intermediates have been demonstrated in vitro.[40–43] In addition, the induction of covalent DNA adducts in rat livers treated with tamoxifen has been reported.[44] Both constitutive and inducible cytochrome P-450 (CYP) enzymes have been implicated in the formation of metabolites with tamoxifen,[45,46] and the flavone-containing monooxygenase has been implicated in the formation of the N-oxide of tamoxifen. Reactive intermediates from such metabolic steps are being evaluated for their carcinogenic potential in vitro and in vivo.

Multiple studies to evaluate tumor gene expression profiling have identified gene expression patterns or specific genes associated with resistance to tamoxifen therapy. A commonly utilized gene expression assay, Oncotype DX 21 gene assay (Genomic Health, Redwood City, California), measures the expression of genes known to be involved in estrogen signaling (e.g., ER, PR), HER2, proliferation (e.g., Ki-67), and others. In multiple different data sets, the recurrence score has been associated with a higher risk of breast cancer recurrence in patients treated with hormonal therapy (e.g., tamoxifen or aromatase inhibitors) without concomitant chemotherapy.[47–49]

The pharmacokinetics of tamoxifen is complex. The chemical structure and metabolic pathway of tamoxifen are shown in Figure 27.1. Metabolic activation of tamoxifen is associated with greater pharmacologic activity. The two most active tamoxifen metabolites are 4-hydroxytamoxifen (4-OH tamoxifen) and 4-OH-N-desmethyltamoxifen (endoxifen). A series of studies carried out to characterize endoxifen pharmacology have demonstrated that it has equivalent potency in vitro to 4-hydroxytamoxifen in ER-α and -beta (ER-β) binding,[50] for the suppression of ER-dependent human breast cancer cell line proliferation,[22,50] and in global ER-responsive gene expression.[51] A recent study suggests that endoxifen's effect on the ER may differ from 4-hydroxytamoxifen based on the observation of ER-α degradation.[52]

In women who receive tamoxifen at a dose of 20 mg per day, plasma endoxifen steady-state concentrations are generally 6 to

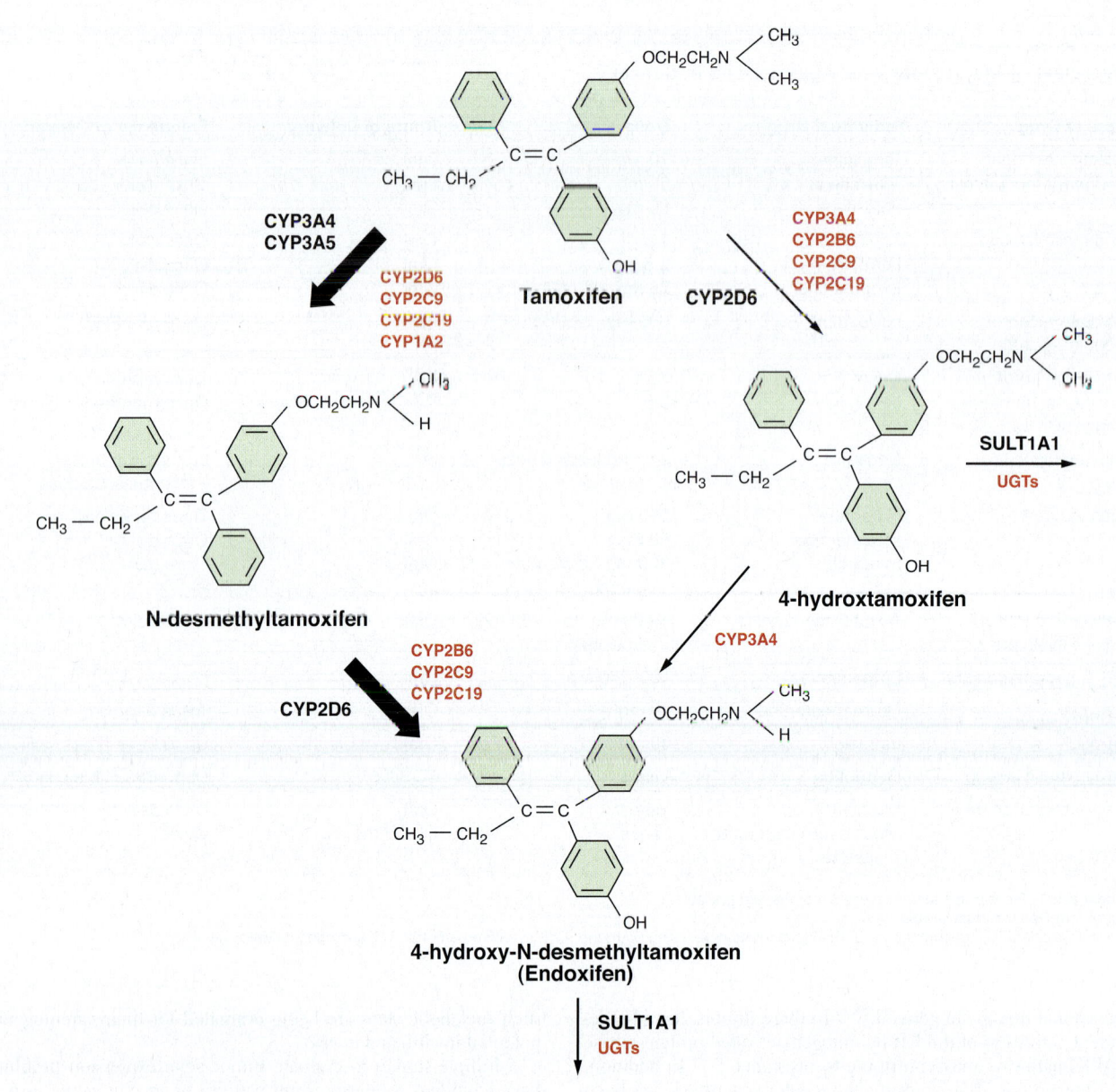

Figure 27.1 Metabolic pathway of tamoxifen biotransformation. (From Sideras K, Ingle JN, Ames MM, et al. Coprescription of tamoxifen and medications that inhibit CYP2D6. *J Clin Oncol* 2010;28:2768–2776.)

10 times higher than 4-hydroxytamoxifen.[53] Although the metabolism of tamoxifen to 4-OH-tamoxifen is catalyzed by multiple enzymes, endoxifen is formed predominantly by the CYP2D6-mediated oxidation of N-desmethyltamoxifen, the most abundant tamoxifen metabolite (see Fig. 27.1).[54] Multiple clinical studies have demonstrated that common *CYP2D6* genetic variation (leading to low or absent CYP2D6 activity) or the drug-induced inhibition of CYP2D6 significantly lowers endoxifen concentrations.[53,55] The *CYP2D6* gene is highly polymorphic, with more than 70 major alleles with four well-defined phenotypes: poor metabolizers (PM), intermediate metabolizers (IM), extensive metabolizers (EM), and ultrarapid metabolizers (UM).

The clinical studies to evaluate the association between *CYP2D6* polymorphisms and tamoxifen outcomes have yielded conflicting results. Initial[56] and follow-up data[57,58] demonstrated that CYP2D6 PM had an approximately two- to threefold higher risk of breast cancer recurrence (compared to CYP2D6 EM) and these data led an FDA special emphasis panel to recommend a tamoxifen label change to incorporate data that the *CYP2D6* genotype was an important biomarker associated with tamoxifen efficacy.[5] However, this label change has been delayed, in part because of conflicting data from secondary analyses of 5-year tamoxifen prospective trials (ATAC,[59] BIG 1-98,[60] and ABCSG8[61]) as well as meta-analyses,[62] which demonstrate that the *CYP2D6* genotype is associated with tamoxifen efficacy when tamoxifen is administered as monotherapy for the adjuvant treatment of postmenopausal, ER-positive breast cancer. Additional support for the importance of endoxifen concentrations came from a secondary analysis of a prospective study, which demonstrated a higher risk of recurrence for women with low endoxifen concentrations.[13]

Many drugs are known to inhibit CYP2D6 activity. In tamoxifen-treated women, the coadministration of potent CYP2D6 inhibitors, such as paroxetine, converts a patient with normal CYP2D6 metabolism to a phenotypic PM.[63] Many other clinically important drugs have been reported to inhibit the CYP2D6 enzyme system, but their effects on tamoxifen metabolism have not been prospectively studied. As with the data regarding *CYP2D6* genotype, the data regarding CYP2D6 inhibitors has additionally been controversial, including two studies that reported opposite findings with regard to CYP2D6 inhibitor use and breast cancer recurrence or death.[64,65] Although the *CYP2D6* data remain controversial, we conclude that until results from prospective adjuvant studies are available, women should be counseled regarding the potential impact of the *CYP2D6* genotype on the effectiveness of adjuvant tamoxifen, and potent CYP2D6 inhibitors should be avoided. Additional caution should be used with drugs that induce CYP3A, such as rifampicin, as a these drugs have been demonstrated to substantially reduce (up to 86%) the concentrations of tamoxifen and its metabolites.[66]

Strategies to overcome low endoxifen concentrations include dose escalation of tamoxifen to 40 mg per day, which has been demonstrated to significantly increase endoxifen concentrations,[67,68] as well as the direct administration of endoxifen itself. The latter strategy is ongoing in multiple different clinical trials, and early reports suggest clinical activity in aromatase inhibitors (AI)-resistant breast cancer.[69]

Following the metabolic activation of tamoxifen, the hydroxylated metabolites undergo both glucuronidation and sulfation. Peak plasma levels of tamoxifen (maximum concentration [Cmax]) are seen 3 to 7 hours after oral administration. Assuming an oral bioavailability of 30%, the volume of distribution has been calculated to be 20 L/kg, and plasma clearance ranges from 1.2 to 5.1 L per hour.[70] The terminal half-life of tamoxifen has been reported to range between 4 and 11 days.[71,72] The elimination half-life of tamoxifen increases with successive doses, which is consistent with saturable kinetics.[71,73] The drug's distribution in tissues is extensive. Levels of the parent drug and metabolites have been reported to be higher in tissue than in plasma in animal studies.[74,75] Reports of tamoxifen concentrations 10- to 60-fold higher than plasma concentrations in the liver, lungs, brain, pancreas, skin, and bones are reported.[76,77] Elevated levels of tamoxifen with biliary obstruction have been reported.[78]

Tamoxifen has been reported to interact with warfarin,[73,79–81] digitoxin, phenytoin,[82] and medroxyprogesterone.[73] Tamoxifen-induced activation of human transcription factor pregnane X receptor (hPXR), resulting in the induction of CYP3A4, may increase the elimination of concomitantly administered CYP3A substrates,[83] such as anastrozole.[84]

Toremifene

Toremifene is an agent similar to tamoxifen. It is available in the United States for the treatment of patients with metastatic breast cancer, and is approved in other countries for the adjuvant treatment of ER-positive breast cancer. Clinical trials have demonstrated no difference in either disease-free or overall survival when toremifene was compared with tamoxifen for the treatment of ER-positive breast cancer,[85,86] and evidence exists for major cross-resistance between tamoxifen and toremifene.[87,88]

Pharmacology

Toremifene is an antiestrogen with a chemical structure that differs from that of tamoxifen by the substitution of a chlorine for a hydrogen atom that is retained when toremifene undergoes metabolism.[89] Like tamoxifen, toremifene is metabolized by CYP3A,[90] with a secondary metabolism to form hydroxylated metabolites that appear to have similar binding affinities to 4-OH tamoxifen.[89,91] The importance of these metabolites or the role of metabolism to the hydroxylated metabolites is unknown, but may play a role given the structural similarity of toremifene to tamoxifen. Although the oral bioavailability has not been defined, toremifene's oral absorption appears to be good. The time to peak plasma concentrations after oral administration ranges from 1.5 to 6.0 hours,[92] with the terminal half-lives for toremifene and one metabolite, 4-hydroxytoremifene, being 5 to 6 days.[93,94] The apparent clearance is 5.1 L per hour. The terminal half-life for the major metabolite, N-desmethyltoremifene, is 21 days.[95] The time to reach plasma steady-state concentrations is 1 to 5 weeks. Plasma protein binding is more than 99%. As with tamoxifen, toremifene is present at higher concentrations in tissues compared to plasma with a high apparent volume of distribution (958 L). Seventy percent of the drug is excreted in feces as metabolites. Studies in patients with impaired liver function or those on anticonvulsants known to induce CYP3A have demonstrated that hepatic dysfunction decreases the clearance of toremifene and N-desmethyltoremifene,[95] whereas those patients on anticonvulsants had an increased clearance. Although toremifene appeared to be less carcinogenic than tamoxifen in preclinical models,[43,96,97] of the rates of endometrial cancer in the adjuvant studies have been similar to tamoxifen.[85]

Raloxifene

Raloxifene is an estrogen agonist and antagonist originally developed to treat osteoporosis. Large placebo-controlled randomized trials demonstrated reduced rates of osteoporosis and a reduction in new breast cancers in treated women, leading to the development of a second-generation breast cancer chemoprevention trial (National Surgical Adjuvant Breast and Bowel Project, NSAPB P2) in which raloxifene was compared with tamoxifen in high-risk postmenopausal women. In this study, tamoxifen was superior to raloxifene in terms of both invasive and noninvasive cancer events, but was associated with a higher risk of thromboembolic events and endometrial cancer.[98]

Pharmacology

Raloxifene is partially estrogenic in bone[99] and lowers cholesterol.[100] It is antiestrogenic in mammary tissue[101,102] and uterine tissue.[103]

The pharmacokinetics of raloxifene have been studied principally in postmenopausal women.[104–106] Pharmacokinetic parameters of raloxifene show considerable interindividual variation. Limited information is available on the pharmacokinetics of raloxifene in individuals with hepatic impairment, renal impairment, or both.

Raloxifene is rapidly absorbed from the gastrointestinal tract. Because raloxifene undergoes extensive first-pass glucuronidation, oral bioavailability of unchanged drug is low. Although approximately 60% of an oral dose is absorbed, the absolute bioavailability as unchanged raloxifene is only 2%. However, systemic availability of raloxifene may be greater than that indicated in bioavailability studies, because circulating glucuronide conjugates are converted back to the parent drug in various tissues.

After the oral administration of a single 120- or 150-mg dose of raloxifene hydrochloride, peak plasma concentrations of raloxifene and its glucuronide conjugates are achieved at 6 hours and 1 hour, respectively. After the oral administration of radiolabeled raloxifene, less than 1% of total circulating radiolabeled material in plasma represents the parent drug.

Results of a single-dose study in patients with liver dysfunction indicate that plasma raloxifene concentrations correlate with serum bilirubin concentrations and are 2.5 times higher than individuals with normal hepatic function. In postmenopausal women who received raloxifene in clinical trials, plasma concentrations of raloxifene and the glucuronide conjugates in those with renal impairment (i.e., estimated creatinine clearance values as low as 23 mL per minute) were similar to values in women with normal renal function.

Raloxifene and its monoglucuronide conjugates are more than 95% bound to plasma proteins. Raloxifene binds to albumin and α$_1$-acid glycoprotein. Raloxifene undergoes extensive first-pass metabolism to the glucuronide conjugates raloxifene 4′-glucuronide, 6-glucuronide, and 6,4′-diglucuronide. UGT1A1 and -1A8 have been found to catalyze the formation of both the 6-β-and 4′-β-glucuronides, whereas UGT1A10 formed only the 4′-β-glucuronide.[107] The metabolism of raloxifene does not appear to be mediated by CYP enzymes (such as CYP2D6), because metabolites other than glucuronide conjugates have not been identified.

The plasma elimination half-life of raloxifene at steady state averages 32.5 hours (range, 15.8 to 86.6 hours). Raloxifene is excreted principally in feces as an unabsorbed drug and via biliary elimination as glucuronide conjugates, which, subsequently, are metabolized by bacteria in the gastrointestinal tract to the parent drug. After oral administration, less than 0.2% of a raloxifene dose is excreted as the parent compound and less than 6% as glucuronide conjugates in urine.

Fulvestrant

Fulvestrant is an ER antagonist that has no known agonist activity and results in ER downregulation.[108–111] Like tamoxifen, fulvestrant competitively binds to the ER but with a higher affinity—approximately 100 times greater than that of tamoxifen,[108,112–114]—thus preventing endogenous estrogen from exerting its effect in target cells.

Results from two phase III clinical trials using the 250 mg per month dose demonstrated fulvestrant to be as effective as anastrozole in the treatment of postmenopausal women with advanced hormone receptor–positive breast cancer previously treated with antiestrogen therapy (mainly tamoxifen).[112–116] In the setting of first-line hormone-responsive metastatic breast cancer, a randomized phase III clinical trial to compare tamoxifen to fulvestrant (250 mg per month) demonstrated no differences in response or time to progression.[117] Because of pharmacology data (discussed in the following paragraphs), the 500 mg per day dose was developed. A randomized trial comparing the 250 mg per month with 500 mg per month dose demonstrated a 4-month improvement in median overall survival advantage for the higher dose.[118] For this reason, the higher dose is now the standard recommended dose.

Fulvestrant is well tolerated. The most common drug-related events (greater than 10% incidence) from the randomized phase III studies were injection-site reactions and hot flashes. Common events (1% to 10% incidence) included asthenia, headache, and gastrointestinal disturbances such as nausea, vomiting, and diarrhea, with minor gastrointestinal disturbances being the most commonly described adverse event.

Pharmacology

Fulvestrant is a steroidal molecule derived from E_2 with an alkylsulphonyl side chain in the 7-α position (Fig. 27.2). Because fulvestrant is poorly soluble and has low and unpredictable oral bioavailability, a parenteral formulation of fulvestrant was developed in an attempt to maximize delivery of the drug.[111] The intramuscular formulation provides prolonged release of the drug over several weeks. The pharmacokinetics of three different single doses of fulvestrant (50, 125, and 250 mg) have been published.[111] In this phase I/II multicenter study, postmenopausal women with primary breast cancer who were awaiting curative surgery received either fulvestrant, tamoxifen, or placebo. After single intramuscular injections of fulvestrant, the time of maximal concentration (t_{max}) ranged from 2 to 19 days, with the median being 7 days for each dose group. At the interval of 28 days, Cmin values were two- to fivefold lower than the Cmax values. For most patients in the 125- and 250-mg dose groups, significant levels of fulvestrant were still measurable 84 days after administration. Pharmacokinetic modeling of the pooled data from the 250-mg cohort was best described by a two-compartment model in which a longer terminal phase began approximately 3 weeks after administration. Because of the long time needed to reach a steady state, the 500-mg loading dose regimen was prospectively studied and determined to be superior to the 250 mg per month dose, both in terms of steady state concentrations achieved within 1 month[119] as well as progression-free and overall survival.[118]

AROMATASE INHIBITORS

At menopause, the synthesis of ovarian hormones ceases. However, estrogen continues to be converted from androgens (produced by the adrenal glands) by aromatase, an enzyme of the CYP superfamily. Aromatase is the enzyme complex responsible for the final step in estrogen synthesis via the conversion of androgens, androstenedione and testosterone, to estrogens, estrone (E_1) and E_2. This biologic pathway served as the basis for the development of the antiaromatase class of compounds. Alterations in aromatase expression have been implicated in the pathogenesis of estrogen-dependent disease, including breast cancer, endometrial cancer, and endometriosis. The importance of this enzyme is also highlighted by the fact that selective aromatase inhibitors are commonly used as first-line therapy for the treatment of postmenopausal women with estrogen-responsive breast cancer. Aminoglutethimide was the first clinically used aromatase inhibitor. When it became available, it was used to cause a *medical adrenalectomy*. Because of the lack of selectivity for aromatase and the resultant suppression of aldosterone and cortisol, aminoglutethimide is no longer recommended for treating metastatic breast cancer. Aminoglutethimide is also occasionally used to try to reverse excess hormone production by adrenocortical cancers.[120]

Aromatase (cytochrome P-450 19 [CYP19]) is encoded by the *CYP19* gene, which is highly polymorphic. Some of these variants are functionally important[121] and may have clinical significance.[122,123]

Aromatase inhibitors have been classified in a number of different ways, including first, second, and third generation; steroidal and nonsteroidal; and reversible (ionic binding) and irreversible (suicide inhibitor, covalent binding).[124] The nonsteroidal aromatase inhibitors include aminoglutethimide (first generation), rogletimide and fadrozole (second generation), and anastrozole, letrozole, and vorozole (third generation). The steroidal aromatase inhibitors include formestane (second generation) and exemestane (third generation).

Steroidal and nonsteroidal aromatase inhibitors differ in their modes of interaction with, and their inactivation of, the aromatase enzyme. Steroidal inhibitors compete with the endogenous

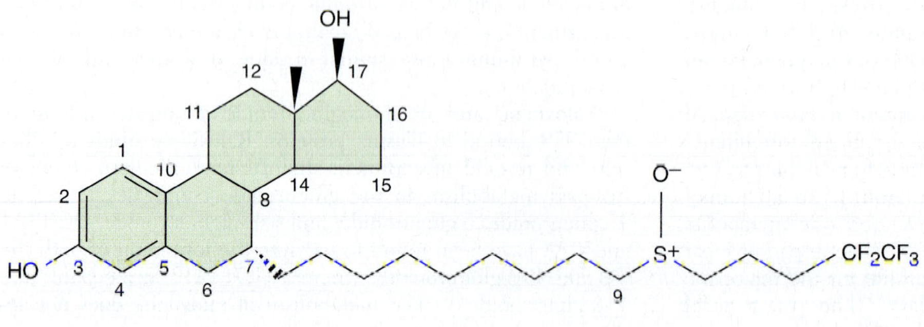

Figure 27.2 Structure of fulvestrant.

substrates, androstenedione and testosterone, for the active site of the enzyme and are processed into intermediates that bind irreversibly to the active site, causing irreversible enzyme inhibition.[19] Nonsteroidal inhibitors also compete with the endogenous substrates for access to the active site, where they then form a reversible bond to the heme iron atom so that enzyme activity can recover if the inhibitor is removed; however, inhibition is sustained whenever the inhibitor is present.[19]

Letrozole and Anastrozole

Both letrozole and anastrozole have been extensively studied in the metastatic and adjuvant settings. When compared to tamoxifen, both letrozole and anastrozole have demonstrated superior response rates and progression-free survival in the metastatic setting.[124,125] In the adjuvant setting, two trials have been performed and demonstrated superiority in terms of relapse-free survivals of both anastrozole (ATAC)[126] and letrozole (BIG 1-98).[127] Additionally, anastrozole has been studied in a sequential approach, and the sequence of tamoxifen followed by anastrozole is superior to 5 years of tamoxifen alone.[128] Anastrozole has recently been compared to placebo in women at an increased risk of developing breast cancer and was demonstrated to significantly reduce the incidence of invasive breast cancer.[129]

The side effects of both anastrozole and letrozole are similar and include arthralgias and myalgias in up to 50% of patients. Both letrozole and anastrozole are associated with a higher rate of bone fracture, compared with the tamoxifen.[130] At the present time, minimal long-term (longer than 5 years) clinical data regarding the effect of aromatase inhibitors on bones are available. When offering anastrozole for extended periods of time to patients with early breast cancer, attention to bone health is paramount, and bone density should be monitored in all patients. Prospective studies have demonstrated that bisphosphonates prevent aromatase-inhibitor–induced bone loss and a meta-analysis presented at the 2013 San Antonio Breast Cancer Symposium demonstrated that bisphosphonates reduce bone recurrences and prolong overall survival. Therefore, bisphosphonates should be considered in AI-treated patients, both in those with and without an increased risk of bone fractures.

A meta-analysis of toxicities comparing aromatase inhibitors with tamoxifen has demonstrated a 30% increase in grade 3 and 4 cardiac events with aromatase inhibitors.[131] However, prospective data demonstrate no differences in myocardial events comparing anastrozole with placebo, although an increase in hypertension was observed.[129]

No impact has been seen with anastrozole on adrenal steroidogenesis at up to 10 times the clinically recommended dose.[132] Although letrozole may decrease basal and adrenocorticotropic hormone–stimulated cortisol synthesis,[133,134] the clinical effect appears to be minimal. Aromatase inhibitors appear to have differential effects on lipids. In a study of over 900 patients with metastatic disease, anastrozole showed no marked effect on lipid profiles compared with baseline.[135] Conversely, the administration of letrozole in women with advanced breast cancer resulted in significant increases in total cholesterol and low-density lipoprotein, from baseline, after 8 and 16 weeks of therapy.[136] In the Breast International Group 1-98 trial, more women who received letrozole experienced grade 1 hypercholesterolemia compared to women who received tamoxifen.[127]

Letrozole is a nonsteroidal aromatase inhibitor with a high specificity for the inhibition of estrogen production (Fig. 27.3). Letrozole is 180 times more potent than aminoglutethimide as an inhibitor of aromatase in vitro. Aldosterone production in vitro is inhibited by concentrations 10,000 times higher than those required for inhibition of estrogen synthesis.[137,138] In a normal male volunteer study, letrozole was shown to decrease E_2 and serum E_1 levels to 10% of baseline with a single 3-mg dose. In phase I studies, letrozole caused a significant decline in plasma E_1 and E_2 within 24 hours of a single oral dose of 0.1 mg.[139,140] After 2 weeks of treatment, the blood levels of E_2, E_1, and estrone sulfate were suppressed 95% or more from baseline. This continued over the 12 weeks of therapy. There was no apparent alteration in plasma levels of cortisol and aldosterone with letrozole or after corticotropin stimulation.[139] In postmenopausal women with advanced breast cancer, the drug did not have any effect on follicle-stimulating hormone (FSH), luteinizing hormone (LH), thyrotropin (previously thyroid-stimulating hormone), cortisol, 17-α-hydroxyprogesterone, androstenedione, or aldosterone blood concentrations.[141,142]

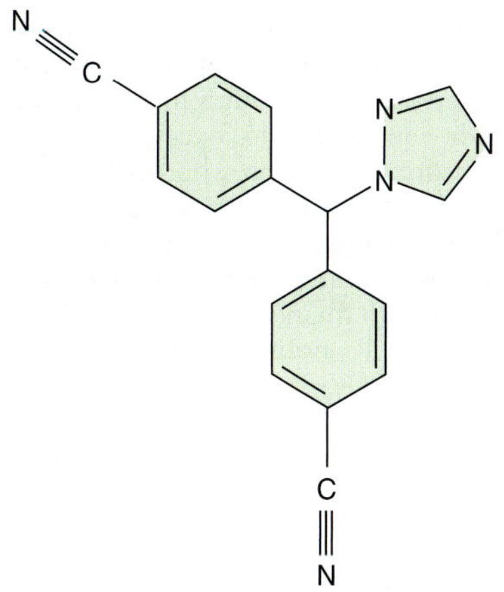

Figure 27.3 Structure of letrozole.

Anastrozole is a nonsteroidal aromatase inhibitor that is 200-fold more potent than aminoglutethimide.[143] No effect on the adrenal glands has been detected. In human studies, the t_{max} is 2 to 3 hours after oral ingestion.[144] Elimination is primarily via hepatic metabolism, with 85% excreted by that route and only 10% excreted unchanged in urine. The main circulating metabolite is triazole after cleavage of the two rings in anastrozole by N-dealkylation. Linear pharmacokinetics have been observed in the dose range of 1 to 20 mg and do not change with repeat dosing. The terminal half-life is approximately 50 hours, and steady-state concentrations are achieved in approximately 10 days with once-a-day dosing and are three to four times higher than peak concentrations after a single dose. Plasma protein binding is approximately 40%.[145] In one study, anastrozole 1 mg and 10 mg daily, inhibited in vivo aromatization by 96.7% and 98.1%, respectively, and plasma E_1 and E_2 levels were suppressed 86.5% and 83.5%, respectively, regardless of dose.[146] Thus, 1 mg of anastrozole achieves near maximal aromatase inhibition and plasma estrogen suppression in breast cancer patients.

A recent prospective study to evaluate the pharmacokinetics of anastrozole (1 mg per day) demonstrated large interindividual variations in plasma anastrozole and anastrozole metabolite concentrations, as well as pretreatment and postdrug plasma E_1, E_2, and E_1 conjugate and estrogen precursor (androstenedione and testosterone) concentrations.[147] Further research is needed to determine the basis for the wide variability in the pharmacokinetics of anastrozole and whether these findings are clinically relevant.

Exemestane

Exemestane has a steroidal structure and is classified as a type 1 aromatase inhibitor, also known as an *aromatase inactivator*, because it irreversibly binds with and permanently inactivates the enzyme.[134] Exemestane has been compared to tamoxifen in both the metastatic and adjuvant settings. In the setting of tamoxifen-refractory metastatic breast cancer, exemestane is superior to megestrol acetate, as demonstrated in a phase III trial in which improvements in both median time to tumor progression and median survival were observed.[148] In the adjuvant setting, the international exemestane study compared 2 to 3 years of tamoxifen with 2 to 3 years of exemestane in women who had previously competed 2 to 3 years of adjuvant tamoxifen. In this trial, a switch to exemestane resulted in superior disease-free and overall survival in the hormone receptor–positive subtype. Furthermore, exemestane has been compared with the nonsteroidal agent anastrozole in the adjuvant treatment of ER-positive breast cancer, and there were no differences in disease-free or overall survival.[149] Finally, exemestane has been compared to placebo in patients at increased risk of breast cancer, and a significant reduction in the risk of developing invasive breast cancer was observed.[150]

Side Effects of Exemestane

Although preclinical studies have suggested that exemestane prevented bone loss in ovariectomized rats,[151] the Intergroup Exemestane adjuvant trial still demonstrated a higher rate of bone fracture for patients randomized to the exemestane arm and there were no differences in fracture rates comparing anastrozole with exemestane.[149] Side effects, including arthralgias and myalgias, appear to be similar to the other AIs. With regard to steroidogenesis, no impact on either cortisol or aldosterone levels was seen in a small study after the administration of exemestane for 7 days.[152] Finally, exemestane has weak androgenic properties, and its use at higher doses has been associated with steroidal-like side effects, such as weight gain and acne.[153,154] However, these side effects have not been observed with the FDA-approved dose (25 mg per day).[155]

Pharmacology

Exemestane is administered once daily by mouth, with the recommended daily dose being 25 mg. The time needed to reach maximal E_2 suppression is 7 days,[156] and its half-life is 27 hours.[157] At daily doses of 10 to 25 mg, exemestane suppresses estrogen concentrations to 6% to 15% of pretreatment levels. This activity is more pronounced than that produced by formestane and comparable to that produced by the nonsteroidal AIs, anastrozole and letrozole.[158–160] Exemestane does not appear to affect cortisol or aldosterone levels when evaluated after 7 days of treatment based on dose-ranging studies, including doses from 0.5 to 800 mg.[152] Exemestane is metabolized by CYP3A4.[134] Although drug–drug interactions have not been formally reported for exemestane, there is the potential for interactions with drugs that affect CYP3A4.[134]

GONADOTROPIN-RELEASING HORMONE ANALOGS

Gonadotropin-releasing hormone (GnRH) analogs result in a *medical orchiectomy* in men and are used as a means of providing androgen ablation for hormone-sensitive and castration refractory metastatic prostate cancer.[161] Because the initial agonist activity of GnRH analogs can cause a *tumor flare* from temporarily increased androgen levels, concomitant use of the antiandrogen flutamide or bicalutamide has been used to prevent this effect. GnRH analogs can also cause tumor regressions in hormonally responsive breast cancers[162] and have received FDA approval for the treatment of metastatic breast cancer in premenopausal women. Data suggest that these drugs may be useful as adjuvant therapy of premenopausal women with resected breast cancer.[163] The use of these drugs in combination with tamoxifen or exemestane in premenopausal women with primary breast cancer is the subject of large, ongoing, international clinical trials. The primary toxicities of GnRH analogs are secondary to the ablation of sex steroid concentrations and include hot flashes, sweating, and nausea.[164] These symptoms can be reversed with low doses of progesterone analogs.[5] In males treated with GnRH analogs for prostate cancer, an alternate strategy of intermittent schedule of GnRH administration may result in improved tolerability and quality of life, with comparable efficacy compared with continuous GnRH analog administration in well-selected advanced prostate cancer patient cohorts.[165] However, in a recent trial comparing intermittent with continuous androgen ablation in newly diagnosed metastatic hormone sensitive prostate cancer patients, a greater risk for death from an intermittent strategy could not be conclusively ruled out although intermittent therapy resulted in small improvements in quality of life.[166]

GnRH analogs available for clinical use include goserelin[167,168] and leuprolide.[169] Both are available in depot intramuscular preparations to be given at monthly intervals. The recommended monthly dose of leuprolide is 7.5 mg and of goserelin is 3.6 mg. There are also longer acting depot preparations to be administered every 3, 4, 6, and 12 months.

Pharmacology

Analogs of the decapeptide GnRH[167,169,170] have been synthesized by modifications of position 6 in which the l-glycine has been exchanged for a d-amino acid and the C-terminal amino acid has been either replaced by an ethylamide or substituted for a modified amino acid. These changes increase the affinity of the analog for the GnRH receptor and decrease the susceptibility to enzymatic degradation. There is an amino acid structure of GnRH with the substitutions for leuprolide and goserelin. Initial administration of these compounds results in stimulation of gonadotropin release. However, prolonged administration has led to profound inhibition of the pituitary–gonadal axis.[170] Plasma E_2 and progesterone are consistently suppressed to postmenopausal or castrate levels after 2 to 4 weeks of treatment with goserelin or leuprolide.[164,171] These drugs are administered intramuscularly or subcutaneously in a parenteral sustained-release microcapsule preparation, because parenteral administration of the parent drug is otherwise associated with rapid clearance. The GnRH analogs are metabolized in the liver, kidney, hypothalamus, and pituitary gland by neutral peptidase cleavage of the peptide bond between the tyrosine in the 5 position and the amino acid in position 6 and by a postproline-cleaving enzyme that cleaves the peptide bond between proline in the 9 position and the glycine-NH_2 in the 10 position. Substitutions at the glycine 6 position and modification of the C-terminal make these analogs more resistant to this enzymatic cleavage.

Leuprolide is approximately 80 to 100 times more potent than endogenous GnRH. It induces castrate levels of testosterone in men with prostate cancer within 3 to 4 weeks of drug administration after an initial sharp increase in LH and FSH. The mechanisms of action include pituitary desensitization after a reduction in pituitary GnRH receptor binding sites and possibly a direct antitumor effect in ER-positive human breast cancer cells.[169] The depot form results in a dose rate of 210 μg per day of leuprolide. Peak concentrations of the depot form, achieved approximately 3 hours after drug administration, have been reported to range between 13.1 and 54.5 μg/L. There appears to be a linear increase in the area under the curve (AUC) for doses of 3.75, 7.5, and 15.0 mg in the depot form. The parenteral bioavailability of subcutaneously injected leuprolide is 94%. The volume of distribution ranges from 27.4 to 37.1 L. In human studies, leuprolide urinary excretion as a metabolite was the primary route of clearance.

Goserelin is approximately 100 times more potent than the naturally occurring GnRH. Like leuprolide, it causes the stimulation of LH and FSH acutely, and with subsequent administration, GnRH receptor numbers decrease, and the pituitary becomes desensitized with decreasing LH and FSH levels. Castrate levels of testosterone are achieved within 1 month. In women, goserelin inhibits ovarian androgen production, but serum levels of dehydroepiandrosterone sulfate and, to a lesser extent, androstenedione, are preserved. In vitro, goserelin has demonstrated antitumor activity in estrogen-dependent MCF7 human breast cancer cells and LNCaP2 prostate cancer cells. The drug is released at a continuous mean rate of 120 μg per day in the depot form, with peak concentrations in the range of 2 to 3 μg/L achieved. The mean volume of distribution in six patients has been reported to be 13.7 L,[172] which is consistent with extracellular fluid volume. Goserelin is principally excreted in the urine, with a mean total body clearance of 8 L per hour in patients with normal renal function. The total body clearance is reduced by approximately 75%, with renal dysfunction and the elimination half-life increased two- or threefold. However, dose adjustment for renal insufficiency does not appear to be necessary. The 5 to 10 hexapeptide and the 4 to 10 hexapeptide were detected in urine in animal studies.[173] The terminal half-life of goserelin is approximately 5 hours after subcutaneous injection. Protein binding is low, and no known drug interactions have been documented.

GONADOTROPIN-RELEASING HORMONE ANTAGONISTS

Modification to the structure of GnRH has resulted in the development of GnRH antagonist compounds that are currently being used in the treatment of prostate cancer. Abarelix was initially approved by the FDA in 2003 as the first depot-injectable GnRH antagonist, but was subsequently withdrawn in 2005. Degarelix is a synthetically modified compound with GnRH antagonist activity that was approved for use by the FDA in 2008 for the management of prostate cancer.[174] Its effect in prostate cancer treatment is to block the GnRH receptor, and thereby prevent the trigger for the production of LH, which mediates androgen synthesis. In contrast to GnRH analogs, degarelix does not cause *tumor flare* symptoms secondary to temporary increased androgen production. A large randomized clinical trial demonstrated that degarelix was associated with a rapid and sustained reduction in serum testosterone, prostate-specific antigen (PSA), FSH, and LH levels, with a loading dose of 240 mg subcutaneously, followed by a monthly maintenance dose of 80 mg[175] with comparable efficacy to leuprolide.[176] The most common side effects (greater than 10%) were hot flashes and pain at the injection site[176] when patients were provided degarelix for a 12-month period. It is unknown if degarelix will have a similar chronic side effect profile known to be associated with long-term GnRH analog use.

Pharmacology

The recommended loading dose of degarelix is 240 mg, administered as two injections of 120 mg each subcutaneously. Monthly maintenance doses of 80 mg as a 20 mg/mL solution is started 28 days after the loading dose. In an analysis of pharmacokinetic/pharmacodynamic (PK/PD) properties of degarelix in 60 healthy males, after a single subcutaneous dose, a terminal half life of 47 days was observed.[177] PK properties of degarelix have been evaluated when administered as a subcutaneous depot of drug as a gel in six different doses to 48 healthy males and when administered intravenously. Using data from several clinical trials, the rate of drug diffusion from subcutaneous administration results in detectable drug up to 60 days after a single dose compared to less than 4 days when the drug is injected intravenously.

ANTIANDROGENS

Flutamide

The antiandrogen flutamide is used in men with metastatic prostate cancer either as initial therapy, combined with GnRH analog administration, or when the metastatic prostate cancer is unresponsive, despite androgen ablation therapy. The recommended dose is 250 mg by mouth three times a day. In patients whose prostate cancer is growing despite flutamide use, stopping flutamide can sometimes cause a flutamide-withdrawal response.

The most common toxicity seen with flutamide is diarrhea, with or without abdominal discomfort. Gynecomastia, which can be tender, frequently occurs in men who are not receiving concomitant androgen ablation therapy.[178] Flutamide can rarely cause hepatotoxicity, a condition that is reversible if detected early, but this toxicity can also be fatal.[179] There is no accepted, clinically recommended testing schedule to screen for flutamide-induced hepatotoxicity other than being aware of this phenomenon and testing for liver function if hepatic symptoms develop.

Pharmacology

Flutamide is a pure antiandrogen with no intrinsic steroidal activity.[180] Flutamide's mechanism of action is as an androgen-receptor antagonist. This binding prevents dihydrotestosterone binding and subsequent translocation of the androgen-receptor complex into the nuclei of cells. Because it is a pure antiandrogen, it acts only at the cellular level. The administration of flutamide alone leads to increased LH and FSH production and a concomitant increase in plasma testosterone and E_2 levels. Plasma protein binding ranges between 94% and 96% for flutamide and between 92% and 94% for 2-hydroxyflutamide, its major metabolite. When the drug is administered three times a day, steady state levels are achieved by day 6. The elimination half-life at steady state is 7.8 hours, and 2-hydroxyflutamide achieves concentrations 50 times higher than the parent drug at steady state and has equal or greater potency than that of flutamide.[180] The elimination half-life for the metabolite is 9.6 hours. The high plasma concentrations of 2-hydroxyflutamide, as compared with flutamide, suggest that the therapeutic benefits of flutamide are mediated primarily through its active metabolite.[181]

Bicalutamide

Bicalutamide is another nonsteroidal antiandrogen that has been approved by the FDA for use in the United States. The recommended dose is one 50-mg tablet per day. One randomized trial reported that bicalutamide compared favorably with flutamide in patients with advanced prostate cancer.[182] Bicalutamide appears to be relatively well tolerated and is associated with a lower incidence of diarrhea than is flutamide.

Pharmacology

Bicalutamide has a binding affinity to the androgen receptor in the rat prostate that is four times greater than that of 2-hydroxyflutamide.[183,184] In vivo, bicalutamide caused a marked inhibition of growth of accessory sex organs in rats, with a potency 5 to 10 times greater than that of flutamide. Unlike flutamide, bicalutamide did not cause a significant increase in LH or testosterone in rats. In humans, the drug has a long plasma half-life of 5 to 7 days, so it may be administered on a weekly schedule. Pharmacokinetics of the drug showed a dose-dependent increase in mean peak plasma concentrations, and the AUC increased linearly with the dose. The half-life of bicalutamide in humans was approximately 6 days, and the drug clearance was not saturable at plasma concentrations up to 1,000 ng/mL. Daily dosing of the drug led to an approximately tenfold accumulation after 12 weeks of administration. In contrast to results in rats, serum concentrations of testosterone and LH increased significantly from baseline at all dose levels tested in humans. Whereas serum FSH concentrations remained essentially unchanged, the median serum E_2 concentrations increased significantly.[185]

Nilutamide

Nilutamide represents the third variation of an antiandrogen available for use in patients with prostate cancer. The observation of unique toxicities, night blindness, and pulmonary toxicity has limited its use.

NOVEL ANTIANDROGENS

Although testosterone depletion remains an unchallenged standard for advanced stage hormone-sensitive disease, evidence has emerged that *castration-recurrent* prostate cancer remains androgen receptor (AR) dependent and is neither *hormone refractory* nor *androgen independent*, which were commonly used terms to define the progression of advanced stage disease following androgen deprivation therapy. Recognition of AR functioning despite the paucity of circulating androgens is evidenced by the elevation of AR messenger RNA in castration-recurrent tumor tissue relative to androgen-dependent tumors and reexpression of some androgen-regulated genes during clinical castration resistance. Recently, the AR axis has been the focus of therapeutic targeting.

Abiraterone Acetate

After the failure of initial androgen manipulation with GnRH analogs and peripheral antiandrogens, prostate cancer continues to respond to a variety of second and third line hormonal interventions. Based on this observation, CYP17, a key enzyme in androgen and estrogen synthesis, was targeted using ketoconazole, which is a weak, reversible, and nonspecific inhibitor of CYP17 resulting in modest antitumor activity of short durability. More recently, abiraterone, a more potent (i.e., 20 times more than ketoconazole), selective, and irreversible inhibitor of CYP17, has been investigated in castration-recurrent prostate cancer, and significant objective responses have been observed.[186] Chemically, it is a 3-pyridyl steroid pregnenolone–derived compound available in an oral prodrug form of abiraterone acetate. Its main toxicity is from symptoms of mineralocorticoid excess (including hypokalemia, hypertension, and fluid overload), because continuous CYP17 blockade results in raising adrenocorticotrophic hormone (ACTH) levels that increase steroid levels upstream of CYP17, including corticosterone and deoxycorticosterone. These adverse effects are best avoided by the coadministration of steroids.

The established dose of abiraterone is 1,000 mg a day (four 250 mg tablets). Following oral administration of abiraterone acetate, the median time to maximum plasma abiraterone concentrations is 2 hours. At the dose of 1,000 mg daily, steady state values (mean ± standard deviation [SD]) of Cmax were 226 ± 178 ng/mL and of AUC were 1173 ± 690 ng.hr/mL. Abiraterone is highly bound (>99%) to the human plasma proteins, albumin and alpha-1 acid glycoprotein. The apparent steady state volume of distribution (mean ± SD) is 19,669 ± 13,358 L. No major deviation from dose proportionality was observed in the dose range of 250 mg to 1,000 mg. However, the exposure was not significantly increased when the dose was doubled from 1,000 to 2,000 mg (8% increase in mean AUC). The two main circulating metabolites of abiraterone in human plasma are abiraterone sulfate (inactive) and N-oxide abiraterone sulfate (inactive), which each account for about 43% of exposure. CYP3A4 and SULT2A1 are enzymes involved in the formation and conjugation of N-oxide abiraterone.

Enzalutamide

Enzalutamide is a new diarylthiohydantoin compound that binds AR with an affinity that is several-fold greater than the antiandrogens bicalutamide and flutamide. This class of novel AR inhibitor also disrupts the nuclear translocation of AR and impairs DNA binding to androgen response elements and the recruitment of coactivators.[187] In early clinical trials, promising results have been observed in castrate refractory and chemotherapy-resistant settings. The major metabolite of enzalutamide is N-desmethyl enzalutamide, and CYP2C8 is responsible for the formation of the active metabolite, N-desmethyl enzalutamide. Enzalutamide pharmacokinetics, in the studied dose range between 30 mg to 480 mg, exhibited a linear, two-compartment model with first-order kinetics. In patients with mCRPC, the mean (% coefficient of variation [CV]) predose Cmin values for enzalutamide and N-desmethyl enzalutamide were 11.4 (25.9%) μg/mL and 13.0 (29.9%) μg/mL, respectively. Enzalutamide is mainly metabolized by CYP2C8 and CYP3A4. Doses ranging from 30 to 600 mg daily have been evaluated, with dose-limiting toxicities including fatigue, seizure, asthenia, anemia, and arthralgia occurring at higher dose levels. At present, enzalutamide has been approved for treating advanced castrate-recurrent prostate cancer[188] after a failure of docetaxel chemotherapy at a dose of 160 mg (four, 40 mg oral capsules). Clinical trials are ongoing to evaluate the efficacy of enzalutamide in castrate-recurrent patients who are chemotherapy naïve.

Galeterone and Orteronel

Novel CYP17 inhibitors that are more selective for 17,20-lyase over 17 α-hydroxylase are currently being developed. Orteronel (TAK-700) is an example of a highly selective 17,20 lyase, which is currently undergoing phase III clinical trials in a pre- and post-chemotherapy castrate-recurrent setting after the failure of androgen deprivation therapy.[189] Other novel agents being developed include galeterone, which is an inhibitor of CYP 17 α-hydroxylase and C17,20 lyase. Survival mechanisms of prostate cancer cells targeted by galeterone include its binding to AR, competitive inhibition of testosterone binding, and a reduction in the quantity of AR protein within the prostate cancer cells. It can also enhance the degradation of constitutively active splice variants. Therefore, taken together, it diminishes the ability of the cells to respond to the low levels of androgenic growth signals. This agent is currently in early clinical safety and efficacy testing for advanced stage prostate cancer.

OTHER SEX STEROID THERAPIES

Fluoxymesterone

Fluoxymesterone is an androgen that has been used in women with metastatic breast cancer who have hormonally responsive cancers and who have progressed on other hormonal therapies such as tamoxifen, an aromatase inhibitor, or megestrol acetate. The usual dose is 10 mg given twice daily. Although the overall response rate is low for fluoxymesterone used in this clinical situation,[190] there are some patients who have substantial antitumor responses lasting for months or even years.

Toxicities associated with fluoxymesterone are those that would be expected with an androgen: hirsutism, male-pattern baldness, voice lowering (hoarseness), acne, enhanced libido, and erythrocytosis. Fluoxymesterone can also cause elevated liver function test results in some patients and, rarely, has been associated with hepatic neoplasms.

Pharmacology

Fluoxymesterone is a chlorinated synthetic analog of testosterone with potent androgenic and anabolic activity in humans. Limited pharmacologic information is available on this agent. Colburn,[191] using a radioimmunoassay, studied two patients after a single oral administration of a 50-mg dose. Peak serum concentrations were achieved between 1 and 3 hours after administration, with the average peak concentrations being 335 ng/mL. By 5 hours after drug administration, serum levels had declined to approximately 50% of the peak concentration. Urinary excretion of a 10-mg dose can be detected for 24 hours, and at least 6-hydroxy, 4-ene, 3-β, and 11-hydroxy metabolites of fluoxymesterone have been detected.[192]

Estrogens: Diethylstilbestrol and Estradiol

Diethylstilbestrol (DES) had been the primary hormonal therapy for postmenopausal metastatic breast cancer. Randomized comparative trials demonstrated it had a similar response rate to that of tamoxifen.[193,194] However, based on these trials, DES use was supplanted by tamoxifen, primarily because DES has more toxicity. DES is occasionally used in metastatic breast cancer patients who have hormonally sensitive cancers that have failed to respond to multiple other hormonal therapies. The usual dose in this situation is 15 mg per day, either as a single dose or as divided doses. DES was also used as androgen ablation therapy in men with metastatic prostate cancer.[195] Doses of approximately 3 mg per day result in testosterone levels that are seen in an anorchid state.

DES toxicities include nausea and vomiting, breast tenderness, and a darkening of the nipple–areolar complex. DES increases the risk of thromboembolic phenomenon, which may result in life-threatening complications. Although DES is not clinically available in the United States, similar antitumor effects and toxicities are seen with estradiol, with a target dose of 10 mg by mouth three times a day. The pharmacology of E_2 has been extensively described elsewhere.[196]

Medroxyprogesterone and Megestrol

Medroxyprogesterone and megestrol are 17-OH-progesterone derivatives differing in a double bond between C6 and C7 positions in megestrol. Historically, megestrol was used as a hormonal agent for patients with advanced breast cancer, usually at a total daily dose of 160 mg. Additionally, it is still used for the treatment of hormonally responsive metastatic endometrial cancer, at a dose of 320 mg per day. In addition, doses of 160 mg per day are occasionally used as a hormonal therapy for prostate cancer.[197] Megestrol has also been extensively evaluated for the treatment of anorexia/cachexia related to cancer or AIDS.[198–201] Various dosages ranging from 160 to 1,600 mg per day have been used. A prospective study has demonstrated a dose–response relationship with doses up to 800 mg per day.[202] Low dosages of megestrol (20 to 40 mg per day) have been shown to be an effective means of reducing hot flashes in women with breast cancer and in men who have undergone androgen ablation therapy.[5] Although megestrol had historically been commonly administered four times per day, the long terminal half-life supports once-per-day dosing.

Megestrol is a relatively well-tolerated medication, with its most prominent side effects being appetite stimulation and resultant weight gain. Although these may be beneficial effects in patients with anorexia/cachexia, they can be important problems in patients with breast or endometrial cancers. Another side effect of megestrol acetate is the marked suppression of adrenal steroid production by suppression of the pituitary–adrenal axis.[203] Although this appears to be asymptomatic in the majority of patients, reports suggest that this adrenal suppression can cause clinical problems in some patients.[204] This drug has been abruptly stopped for decades without the recognition of untoward sequelae in patients, and it seems reasonable to continue this practice. Nonetheless, if Addisonian signs or symptoms develop after drug discontinuation, corticosteroids should be administered.

Furthermore, if patients who receive megestrol have a significant infection, experience trauma, or undergo surgery, then corticosteroid coverage should be administered. There appears to be a slightly increased incidence of thromboembolic phenomena in patients receiving megestrol alone.[202] This risk appears to be higher if megestrol is administered with concomitant cytotoxic therapy.[205] There are conflicting reports regarding megestrol-causing edema.[206] If it does, the edema is generally minimal and easily handled with a mild diuretic. Megestrol may cause impotence in some men.[207] The incidence of this is controversial, although it is generally agreed that this is a reversible situation. Megestrol can cause menstrual irregularities, the most prominent of which is withdrawal menstrual bleeding within a few weeks of drug discontinuation.[5] Although nausea and vomiting have sometimes been attributed as a toxicity of this drug, there are data to demonstrate that this drug has antiemetic properties.[200,201,205] In terms of magnitude, megestrol appears to decrease both nausea and vomiting in advanced-stage cancer patients by approximately two thirds.

Medroxyprogesterone has many of the same properties, clinical uses, and toxicities as megestrol acetate. It has never been commonly used in the United States for the treatment of breast cancer but has been used more in Europe. Medroxyprogesterone is available in 2.5- and 10-mg tablets and in injectable formulations of 100 and 400 mg/L. Dosing for the treatment of metastatic breast or prostate cancer has commonly been 400 mg per week or more and 1,000 mg per week or more for metastatic endometrial cancer. Injectable or daily oral doses have been used for controlling hot flashes.

Pharmacology

The exact mechanism of antitumor effect of medroxyprogesterone and megestrol is unclear. These drugs have been reported to suppress adrenal steroid synthesis,[208] suppress ER levels,[209] alter tumor hormone metabolism,[210] enhance steroid metabolism,[211] and directly kill tumor cells.[212] In addition, progestins may influence some growth factors,[213] suppress plasma estrone sulfate formation, and, at high concentrations, inhibit P-glycoprotein.

The oral bioavailability of these progestational agents is unknown, although absorption appears to be poor for medroxyprogesterone relative to megestrol.

The terminal half-life for megestrol is approximately 14 hours,[214,215] with a t_{max} of 2 to 5 hours after oral ingestion.[216] The AUC for a single megestrol dose of 160 mg is between 2.5- and 8-fold higher than that for single-dose medroxyprogesterone at 1,000 mg with a radioactive dose of megestrol; 50% to 78% is found in the urine after oral administration, and 8% to 30% is found in the feces.

Metabolism and excretion of medroxyprogesterone have been incompletely characterized. In humans, 20% to 50% of a [^{3}H]medroxyprogesterone dose is excreted in the urine and 5% to 10% in the stool after intravenous administration.[217–219] Metabolism of medroxyprogesterone occurs via hydroxylation, reduction, demethylation, and combinations of these reactions.[220] The major urinary metabolite is a glucuronide. Less than 3% of the dose is excreted as unconjugated medroxyprogesterone in humans. Clearance of medroxyprogesterone has been reported to range between 27 and 70 L per hour.[219] The initial volume of distribution is between 4 and 8 L in humans. The mean terminal half-life is 60 hours. The t_{max} for medroxyprogesterone occurs 2 to 5 hours after oral administration. Medroxyprogesterone appears to be concentrated in the small intestine, the colon, and in adipose tissue in human autopsy studies.[221] Drug interactions of medroxyprogesterone have been reported with aminoglutethimide, which decreases plasma medroxyprogesterone levels.[222] Medroxyprogesterone may reduce the concentration of the N-desmethyltamoxifen metabolite concentration. Progestational agents also may increase plasma warfarin levels.[223] These reports are consistent with CYP3A being the site of interaction.

OTHER HORMONAL THERAPIES

Octreotide

Octreotide is a somatostatin analog that is administered for the treatment of carcinoid syndrome and other hormonal excess syndromes associated with some pancreatic islet cell cancers and acromegaly. Response rates (measured in terms of a reduction in diarrhea and flushing) are high and can last for several months to years. Occasionally, antitumor responses temporarily related to octreotide are seen with these tumors. Octreotide may be useful to alleviate 5-fluorouracil–associated diarrhea.[224–226]

Octreotide can be administered intravenously or subcutaneously. Initial doses of 50 µg are given two to three times on the first day. The dose is titrated upward, with a usual daily dose of 300 to 450 µg per day for most patients. A depot preparation is available, allowing doses to be administered at monthly intervals. Octreotide is generally well tolerated overall. It appears to cause more toxicity in acromegalic patients, with such problems as bradycardia, diarrhea, hypoglycemia, hyperglycemia, hypothyroidism, and cholelithiasis.

Pharmacology

Octreotide is an 8-amino acid synthetic analog of the 14-amino acid peptide somatostatin.[227] Octreotide has a similar high affinity for somatostatin receptors, as does its parent compound, with a concentration that inhibits the receptor by 50% in the subnanomolar range. Octreotide inhibits insulin, glucagon, pancreatic polypeptide, gastric inhibitory polypeptide, and gastrin secretion. It has a much longer duration of action than the parent compound because of its greater resistance to enzymatic degradation. Its absorption after subcutaneous administration is rapid, and bioavailability is 100% after subcutaneous injection. Peak concentrations of 4 µg/L after a 100-µg dose occur within 20 to 30 minutes of subcutaneous injection and are 20% to 40% of the corresponding intravenous injection. Both peak concentration and AUC for octreotide increase linearly with dose. The total body clearance in healthy volunteers is 9.6 L per hour. Hepatic metabolism of octreotide accounts for 30% to 40% of the drug's disposition, and 11% to 20% is excreted unchanged in the urine. The volume of distribution ranges between 18 and 30 L, and the terminal half-life is reported to be between 72 and 98 minutes. Sixty-five percent of the drug is protein bound primarily to the lipoprotein fraction.[227,228] Because of the short half-life, classic octreotide is administered subcutaneously two or three times per day.[229] A slow-release form of octreotide, designed for once-per-month administration, controls the symptoms of carcinoid syndrome at least as well as three-times-per-day octreotide.[230]

REFERENCES

1. Fisher B, Costantino JP, Wickerham DL, et al. Tamoxifen for the prevention of breast cancer: current status of the National Surgical Adjuvant Breast and Bowel Project P-1 study. *J Natl Cancer Inst* 2005;97:1652–1662.
2. Fisher B, Dignam J, Wolmark N, et al. Tamoxifen in treatment of intraductal breast cancer: National Surgical Adjuvant Breast and Bowel Project B-24 randomised controlled trial. *Lancet* 1999;353:1993–2000.
3. Colleoni M, Gelber S, Goldhirsch A, et al. Tamoxifen after adjuvant chemotherapy for premenopausal women with lymph node-positive breast cancer: International Breast Cancer Study Group Trial 13-93. *J Clin Oncol* 2006;24:1332–1341.
4. Davies C, Pan H, Godwin J, et al. Long-term effects of continuing adjuvant tamoxifen to 10 years versus stopping at 5 years after diagnosis of oestrogen receptor-positive breast cancer: ATLAS, a randomised trial. *Lancet* 2013;381:805–816.
5. Loprinzi CL, Michalak JC, Quella SK, et al. Megestrol acetate for the prevention of hot flashes. *N Engl J Med* 1994;331:347–352.
6. Loprinzi CL, Kugler JW, Sloan JA, et al. Venlafaxine in management of hot flashes in survivors of breast cancer: a randomised controlled trial. *Lancet* 2000;356:2059–2063.
7. Archer DF, Dupont CM, Constantine GD, et al. Desvenlafaxine for the treatment of vasomotor symptoms associated with menopause: a double-blind, randomized, placebo-controlled trial of efficacy and safety. *Am J Obstet Gynecol* 2009;200:238.e1–238e10.
8. Barton DL, LaVasseur BI, Sloan JA, et al. Phase III, placebo-controlled trial of three doses of citalopram for the treatment of hot flashes: NCCTG trial N05C9. *J Clin Oncol* 2010;28:3278–3283.
9. Freeman EW, Guthrie KA, Caan B, et al. Efficacy of escitalopram for hot flashes in healthy menopausal women: a randomized controlled trial. *JAMA* 2011;305:267–274.
10. Stearns V, Beebe KL, Iyengar M, et al. Paroxetine controlled release in the treatment of menopausal hot flashes: a randomized controlled trial. *JAMA* 2003;289:2827–2834.
11. Pandya KJ, Morrow GR, Roscoe JA, et al. Gabapentin for hot flashes in 420 women with breast cancer: a randomised double-blind placebo-controlled trial. *Lancet* 2005;366:818–824.
12. Loprinzi CL, Qin R, Balcueva EP, et al. Phase III, randomized, double-blind, placebo-controlled evaluation of pregabalin for alleviating hot flashes, N07C1. *J Clin Oncol* 2010;28:641–647.
13. Madlensky L, Natarajan L, Tchu S, et al. Tamoxifen metabolite concentrations, CYP2D6 genotype, and breast cancer outcomes. *Clin Pharmacol Ther* 2011;89:718–725.
14. Tamoxifen for early breast cancer: an overview of the randomised trials. Early Breast Cancer Trialists' Collaborative Group. *Lancet* 1998;351:1451–1467.
15. Wickerham DL, Fisher B, Wolmark N, et al. Association of tamoxifen and uterine sarcoma. *J Clin Oncol* 2002;20:2758–2760.
16. Dewar JA, Horobin JM, Preece PE, et al. Long term effects of tamoxifen on blood lipid values in breast cancer. *BMJ* 1992;305:225–226.
17. Love RR, Mazess RB, Barden HS, et al. Effects of tamoxifen on bone mineral density in postmenopausal women with breast cancer. *N Engl J Med* 1992;326:852–856.
18. Powles TJ, Hickish T, Kanis JA, et al. Effect of tamoxifen on bone mineral density measured by dual-energy x-ray absorptiometry in healthy premenopausal and postmenopausal women. *J Clin Oncol* 1996;14:78–84.
19. Buzdar A, Howell A, Cuzick J, et al. Comprehensive side-effect profile of anastrozole and tamoxifen as adjuvant treatment for early-stage breast cancer: long-term safety analysis of the ATAC trial. *Lancet Oncol* 2006;7:633–643.
20. Gorin MB, Day R, Costantino JP, et al. Long-term tamoxifen citrate use and potential ocular toxicity. *Am J Ophthalmol* 1998;125:493–501.
21. Tonetti DA, Jordan VC. Possible mechanisms in the emergence of tamoxifen-resistant breast cancer. *Anticancer Drugs* 1995;6:498–507.
22. Lim YC, Desta Z, Flockhart DA, et al. Endoxifen (4-hydroxy-N-desmethyl-tamoxifen) has anti-estrogenic effects in breast cancer cells with potency similar to 4-hydroxy-tamoxifen. *Cancer Chemother Pharmacol* 2005;55:471–478.
23. Benz CC, Scott GK, Sarup JC, et al. Estrogen-dependent, tamoxifen-resistant tumorigenic growth of MCF-7 cells transfected with HER2/neu. *Breast Cancer Res Treat* 1993;24:85–95.
24. Borg A, Baldetorp B, Ferno M, et al. ERBB2 amplification is associated with tamoxifen resistance in steroid-receptor positive breast cancer. *Cancer Lett* 1994;81:137–144.
25. Houston SJ, Plunkett TA, Barnes DM, et al. Overexpression of c-erbB2 is an independent marker of resistance to endocrine therapy in advanced breast cancer. *Br J Cancer* 1999;79:1220–1226.
26. Lipton A, Ali SM, Leitzel K, et al. Serum HER-2/neu and response to the aromatase inhibitor letrozole versus tamoxifen. *J Clin Oncol* 2003;21:1967–1972.
27. Bunone G, Briand PA, Miksicek RJ, et al. Activation of the unliganded estrogen receptor by EGF involves the MAP kinase pathway and direct phosphorylation. *Embo J* 1996;15:2174–2183.
28. Kato S, Endoh H, Masuhiro Y, et al. Activation of the estrogen receptor through phosphorylation by mitogen-activated protein kinase. *Science* 1995;270:1491–1494.
29. Pietras RJ, Arboleda J, Reese DM, et al. HER-2 tyrosine kinase pathway targets estrogen receptor and promotes hormone-independent growth in human breast cancer cells. *Oncogene* 1995;10:2435–2446.
30. Osborne CK, Bardou V, Hopp TA, et al. Role of the estrogen receptor coactivator AIB1 (SRC-3) and HER-2/neu in tamoxifen resistance in breast cancer. *J Natl Cancer Inst* 2003;95:353–361.
31. Encarnacion CA, Ciocca DR, McGuire WL, et al. Measurement of steroid hormone receptors in breast cancer patients on tamoxifen. *Breast Cancer Res Treat* 1993;26:237–246.
32. Watts CK, Handel ML, King RJ, et al. Oestrogen receptor gene structure and function in breast cancer. *J Steroid Biochem Mol Biol* 1992;41:529–536.
33. Zhang QX, Borg A, Wolf DM, et al. An estrogen receptor mutant with strong hormone-independent activity from a metastatic breast cancer. *Cancer Res* 1997;57:1244–1249.
34. Toy W, Shen Y, Won H, et al. ESR1 ligand-binding domain mutations in hormone-resistant breast cancer. *Nat Genet* 2013;45:1439–1445.
35. Robinson DR, Wu YM, Vats P, et al. Activating ESR1 mutations in hormone-resistant metastatic breast cancer. *Nat Genet* 2013;45:1446–1451.

36. Merenbakh-Lamin K, Ben-Baruch N, Yeheskel A, et al. D538G mutation in estrogen receptor-alpha: a novel mechanism for acquired endocrine resistance in breast cancer. *Cancer Res* 2013;73:6856–6864.
37. Fendl KC, Zimniski SJ. Role of tamoxifen in the induction of hormone-independent rat mammary tumors. *Cancer Res* 1992;52:235–237.
38. Williams GM. Tamoxifen experimental carcinogenicity studies: implications for human effects. *Proc Soc Exp Biol Med* 1995;208:141–143.
39. Williams GM, Iatropoulos MJ, Djordjevic MV, et al. The triphenylethylene drug tamoxifen is a strong liver carcinogen in the rat. *Carcinogenesis* 1993;14:315–317.
40. Rutqvist LE, Johansson H, Signomklao T, et al. Adjuvant tamoxifen therapy for early stage breast cancer and second primary malignancies. Stockholm Breast Cancer Study Group. *J Natl Cancer Inst* 1995;87:645–651.
41. Mani C, Kupfer D. Cytochrome P-450-mediated activation and irreversible binding of the antiestrogen tamoxifen to proteins in rat and human liver: possible involvement of flavin-containing monooxygenases in tamoxifen activation. *Cancer Res* 1991;51:6052–6058.
42. Mani C, Pearce R, Parkinson A, et al. Involvement of cytochrome P4503A in catalysis of tamoxifen activation and covalent binding to rat and human liver microsomes. *Carcinogenesis* 1994;15:2715–2720.
43. Styles JA, Davies A, Lim CK, et al. Genotoxicity of tamoxifen, tamoxifen epoxide and toremifene in human lymphoblastoid cells containing human cytochrome P450s. *Carcinogenesis* 1994;15:5–9.
44. Han XL, Liehr JG. Induction of covalent DNA adducts in rodents by tamoxifen. *Cancer Res* 1992;52:1360–1363.
45. Mani C, Hodgson E, Kupfer D. Metabolism of the antimammary cancer antiestrogenic agent tamoxifen. II. Flavin-containing monooxygenase-mediated N-oxidation. *Drug Metab Dispos* 1993;21:657–661.
46. Mani C, Gelboin HV, Park SS, et al. Metabolism of the antimammary cancer antiestrogenic agent tamoxifen. I. Cytochrome P-450-catalyzed N-demethylation and 4-hydroxylation. *Drug Metab Dispos* 1993;21:645–656.
47. Albain KS, Barlow WE, Shak S, et al. Prognostic and predictive value of the 21-gene recurrence score assay in postmenopausal women with node-positive, oestrogen-receptor-positive breast cancer on chemotherapy: a retrospective analysis of a randomised trial. *Lancet Oncol* 2010;11:55–65.
48. Dowsett M, Cuzick J, Wale C, et al. Prediction of risk of distant recurrence using the 21-gene recurrence score in node-negative and node-positive postmenopausal patients with breast cancer treated with anastrozole or tamoxifen: a TransATAC study. *J Clin Oncol* 2010;28:1829–1834.
49. Paik S, Shak S, Tang G, et al. A multigene assay to predict recurrence of tamoxifen-treated, node-negative breast cancer. *N Engl J Med* 2004;351:2817–2826.
50. Johnson MD, Zuo H, Lee KH, et al. Pharmacological characterization of 4-hydroxy-N-desmethyl tamoxifen, a novel active metabolite of tamoxifen. *Breast Cancer Res Treat* 2004;85:151–159.
51. Lim YC, Li L, Desta Z, et al. Endoxifen, a secondary metabolite of tamoxifen, and 4-OH-tamoxifen induce similar changes in global gene expression patterns in MCF-7 breast cancer cells. *J Pharmacol Exp Ther* 2006;318:503–512.
52. Wu X, Hawse JR, Subramaniam M, et al. The tamoxifen metabolite, endoxifen, is a potent antiestrogen that targets estrogen receptor alpha for degradation in breast cancer cells. *Cancer Res* 2009;69:1722–1727.
53. Jin Y, Desta Z, Stearns V, et al. CYP2D6 genotype, antidepressant use, and tamoxifen metabolism during adjuvant breast cancer treatment. *J Natl Cancer Inst* 2005;97:30–39.
54. Desta Z, Ward BA, Soukhova NV, et al. Comprehensive evaluation of tamoxifen sequential biotransformation by the human cytochrome P450 system in vitro: prominent roles for CYP3A and CYP2D6. *J Pharmacol Exp Ther* 2004;310:1062–1075.
55. Stearns V, Johnson MD, Rae JM, et al. Active tamoxifen metabolite plasma concentrations after coadministration of tamoxifen and the selective serotonin reuptake inhibitor paroxetine. *J Natl Cancer Inst* 2003;95:1758–1764.
56. Goetz MP, Rae JM, Suman VJ, et al. Pharmacogenetics of tamoxifen biotransformation is associated with clinical outcomes of efficacy and hot flashes. *J Clin Oncol* 2005;23:9312–9318.
57. Schroth W, Antoniadou L, Fritz P, et al. Breast cancer treatment outcome with adjuvant tamoxifen relative to patient CYP2D6 and CYP2C19 genotypes. *J Clin Oncol* 2007;25:5187–5193.
58. Schroth W, Goetz MP, Hamann U, et al. Association between CYP2D6 polymorphisms and outcomes among women with early stage breast cancer treated with tamoxifen. *JAMA* 2009;302:1429–1436.
59. Rae JM, Drury S, Hayes DF, et al. CYP2D6 and UGT2B7 genotype and risk of recurrence in tamoxifen-treated breast cancer patients. *J Natl Cancer Inst* 2012;104:452–460.
60. Regan MM, Leyland-Jones B, Bouzyk M, et al. CYP2D6 genotype and tamoxifen response in postmenopausal women with endocrine-responsive breast cancer: the breast international group 1-98 trial. *J Natl Cancer Inst* 2012;104:441–451.
61. Goetz MP, Suman VJ, Hoskin TL, et al. CYP2D6 metabolism and patient outcome in the Austrian Breast and Colorectal Cancer Study Group trial (ABCSG) 8. *Clin Cancer Res* 2013;19:500–507.
62. Province MA, Goetz MP, Brauch H, et al. CYP2D6 Genotype and adjuvant tamoxifen: meta-analysis of heterogeneous study populations. *Clin Pharmacol Ther* 2014;95:216–227.
63. Borges S, Desta Z, Li L, et al. Quantitative effect of CYP2D6 genotype and inhibitors on tamoxifen metabolism: implication for optimization of breast cancer treatment. *Clin Pharmacol Ther* 2006;80:61–74.
64. Dezentje VO, van Blijderveen NJ, Gelderblom H, et al. Effect of concomitant CYP2D6 inhibitor use and tamoxifen adherence on breast cancer recurrence in early-stage breast cancer. *J Clin Oncol* 2010;28:2423–2429.
65. Kelly CM, Juurlink DN, Gomes T, et al. Selective serotonin reuptake inhibitors and breast cancer mortality in women receiving tamoxifen: a population based cohort study. *BMJ* 2010;340:c693.
66. Binkhorst L, van Gelder T, Loos WJ, et al. Effects of CYP induction by rifampicin on tamoxifen exposure. *Clin Pharmacol Ther* 2012;92:62–67.
67. Irvin WJ Jr., Walko CM, Weck KE, et al. Genotype-guided tamoxifen dosing increases active metabolite exposure in women with reduced CYP2D6 metabolism: a multicenter study. *J Clin Oncol* 2011;29:3232–3239.
68. Kiyotani K, Mushiroda T, Imamura CK, et al. Dose-adjustment study of tamoxifen based on CYP2D6 genotypes in Japanese breast cancer patients. *Breast Cancer Res Treat* 2012;131:137–145.
69. Goetz MP, Suman VA, Reid JR, et al. A first-in-human phase I study of the tamoxifen (TAM) metabolite, Z-endoxifen hydrochloride (Z-Endx) in women with aromatase inhibitor (AI) refractory metastatic breast cancer (MBC) (NCT01327781). *Cancer Res* 2013;73(24 Suppl): Abstract nr PD3-4.
70. Lien EA, Anker G, Lonning PE, et al. Decreased serum concentrations of tamoxifen and its metabolites induced by aminoglutethimide. *Cancer Res* 1990;50:5851–5857.
71. Adam HK, Patterson JS, Kemp JV. Studies on the metabolism and pharmacokinetics of tamoxifen in normal volunteers. *Cancer Treat Rep* 1980;64:761–764.
72. Patterson JS, Settatree RS, Adam HK, et al. Serum concentrations of tamoxifen and major metabolite during long-term nolvadex therapy, correlated with clinical response. *Eur J Cancer Suppl* 1980;1:89–92.
73. Camaggi CM, Strocchi E, Canova N, et al. Medroxyprogesterone acetate (MAP) and tamoxifen (TMX) plasma levels after simultaneous treatment with 'low' TMX and 'high' MAP doses. *Cancer Chemother Pharmacol* 1985;14:229–231.
74. Lien EA, Solheim E, Lea OA, et al. Distribution of 4-hydroxy-N-desmethyl-tamoxifen and other tamoxifen metabolites in human biological fluids during tamoxifen treatment. *Cancer Res* 1989;49:2175–2183.
75. Lien EA, Solheim E, Ueland PM. Distribution of tamoxifen and its metabolites in rat and human tissues during steady-state treatment. *Cancer Res* 1991;51:4837–4844.
76. Daniel P, Gaskell SJ, Bishop H, et al. Determination of tamoxifen and biologically active metabolites in human breast tumours and plasma. *Eur J Cancer Clin Oncol* 1981;17:1183–1189.
77. Robinson SP, Langan-Fahey SM, Johnson DA, et al. Metabolites, pharmacodynamics, and pharmacokinetics of tamoxifen in rats and mice compared to the breast cancer patient. *Drug Metab Dispos* 1991;19:36–43.
78. DeGregorio MW, Wiebe VJ, Venook AP, et al. Elevated plasma tamoxifen levels in a patient with liver obstruction. *Cancer Chemother Pharmacol* 1989;23:194–195.
79. Lodwick R, McConkey B, Brown AM. Life threatening interaction between tamoxifen and warfarin. *Br Med J (Clin Res Ed)* 1987;295:1141.
80. Ritchie LD, Grant SM. Tamoxifen-warfarin interaction: the Aberdeen hospitals drug file. *BMJ* 1989;298:1253.
81. Tenni P, Lalich DL, Byrne MJ. Life threatening interaction between tamoxifen and warfarin. *BMJ* 1989;298:93.
82. Rabinowicz AL, Hinton DR, Dyck P, et al. High-dose tamoxifen in treatment of brain tumors: interaction with antiepileptic drugs. *Epilepsia* 1995;36:513–515.
83. Desai PB, Nallani SC, Sane RS, et al. Induction of cytochrome P450 3A4 in primary human hepatocytes and activation of the human pregnane X receptor by tamoxifen and 4-hydroxytamoxifen. *Drug Metab Dispos* 2002;30:608–612.
84. Dowsett M, Cuzick J, Howell A, et al. Pharmacokinetics of anastrozole and tamoxifen alone, and in combination, during adjuvant endocrine therapy for early breast cancer in postmenopausal women: a sub-protocol of the 'Arimidex and tamoxifen alone or in combination' (ATAC) trial. *Br J Cancer* 2001;85:317–324.
85. Pagani O, Gelber S, Price K, et al. Toremifene and tamoxifen are equally effective for early-stage breast cancer: first results of International Breast Cancer Study Group Trials 12-93 and 14-93. *Ann Oncol* 2004;15:1749–1759.
86. Hayes DF, Van Zyl JA, Hacking A, et al. Randomized comparison of tamoxifen and two separate doses of toremifene in postmenopausal patients with metastatic breast cancer. *J Clin Oncol* 1995;13:2556–2566.
87. Stenbygaard LE, Herrstedt J, Thomsen JF, et al. Toremifene and tamoxifen in advanced breast cancer—a double-blind cross-over trial. *Breast Cancer Res Treat* 1993;25:57–63.
88. Vogel CL, Shemano I, Schoenfelder J, et al. Multicenter phase II efficacy trial of toremifene in tamoxifen-refractory patients with advanced breast cancer. *J Clin Oncol* 1993;11:345–350.
89. Kangas L. Review of the pharmacological properties of toremifene. *J Steroid Biochem* 1990;36:191–195.
90. Berthou F, Dreano Y, Belloc C, et al. Involvement of cytochrome P450 3A enzyme family in the major metabolic pathways of toremifene in human liver microsomes. *Biochem Pharmacol* 1994;47:1883–1895.
91. Simberg NH, Murai JT, Siiteri PK. In vitro and in vivo binding of toremifene and its metabolites in rat uterus. *J Steroid Biochem* 1990;36:197–202.
92. Kohler PC, Hamm JT, Wiebe VJ, et al. Phase I study of the tolerance and pharmacokinetics of toremifene in patients with cancer. *Breast Cancer Res Treat* 1990;16 Suppl:S19–S26.
93. Tominaga T, Abe O, Izuo M. A phase I study of toremifene. *Breast Cancer Res Treat* 1990;16 (Suppl):27.
94. Wiebe VJ, Benz CC, Shemano I, et al. Pharmacokinetics of toremifene and its metabolites in patients with advanced breast cancer. *Cancer Chemother Pharmacol* 1990;25:247–251.

95. Anttila M, Laakso S, Nylanden P, et al. Pharmacokinetics of the novel antiestrogenic agent toremifene in subjects with altered liver and kidney function. Clin Pharmacol Ther 1995;57:628–635.
96. Hard GC, Iatropoulos MJ, Jordan K, et al. Major difference in the hepatocarcinogenicity and DNA adduct forming ability between toremifene and tamoxifen in female Crl:CD(BR) rats. Cancer Res 1993;53:4534–4541.
97. Montandon F, Williams GM. Comparison of DNA reactivity of the polyphenylethylene hormonal agents diethylstilbestrol, tamoxifen and toremifene in rat and hamster liver. Arch Toxicol 1994;68:272–275.
98. Vogel VG, Costantino JP, Wickerham DL, et al. Update of the National Surgical Adjuvant Breast and Bowel Project Study of Tamoxifen and Raloxifene (STAR) P-2 Trial: Preventing Breast Cancer. Cancer Prev Res (Phila) 2010;3:696–706.
99. Delmas PD, Balena R, Confravreux E, et al. Bisphosphonate risedronate prevents bone loss in women with artificial menopause due to chemotherapy of breast cancer: a double-blind, placebo-controlled study. J Clin Oncol 1997;15:955–962.
100. Draper MW, Flowers DE, Huster WJ, et al. A controlled trial of raloxifene (LY139481) HCl: impact on bone turnover and serum lipid profile in healthy postmenopausal women. J Bone Miner Res 1996;11:835–842.
101. Anzano MA, Peer CW, Smith JM, et al. Chemoprevention of mammary carcinogenesis in the rat: combined use of raloxifene and 9-cis-retinoic acid. J Natl Cancer Inst 1996;88:123–125.
102. Gottardis MM, Jordan VC. Antitumor actions of keoxifene and tamoxifen in the N-nitrosomethylurea-induced rat mammary carcinoma model. Cancer Res 1987;47:4020–4024.
103. Black LJ, Jones CD, Falcone JF. Antagonism of estrogen action with a new benzothiophene derived antiestrogen. Life Sci 1983;32:1031–1036.
104. Allerheiligen S, Geiser J, Knadler M. Raloxifene (RAL) pharmacokinetics and the associated endocrine effects in premenopausal women treated during the follicular, ovulatory, and luteal phases of the menstrual cycle. Pharmaceut Res 1996;13:S430.
105. Forgue ST, Rudy AC, Knadler MP. Raloxifene pharmacokinetics in healthy postmenopausal women. Pharmaceut Res 1996;13:S430.
106. Ni L, Allerheiligen S, Basson R. Pharacokinetics of raloxifene in men and postmenopausal women volunteers. Pharmaceut Res 1996;13:S430.
107. Kemp DC, Fan PW, Stevens JC. Characterization of raloxifene glucuronidation in vitro: contribution of intestinal metabolism to presystemic clearance. Drug Metab Dispos 2002;30:694–700.
108. [illegible] anti proliferative and anti estrogenic effects of ICI 164,384 and ICI 182,780 in 4 OH tamoxifen resistant human breast cancer cells. Int J Cancer 1994;56:295–300.
109. Howell A, DeFriend DJ, Robertson JF, et al. Pharmacokinetics, pharmacological and anti-tumour effects of the specific anti-oestrogen ICI 182780 in women with advanced breast cancer. Br J Cancer 1996;74:300–308.
110. Howell A, Osborne CK, Morris C, et al. ICI 182,780 (Faslodex): development of a novel, "pure" antiestrogen. Cancer 2000;89:817–825.
111. Robertson JF, Odling-Smee W, Holcombe C, et al. Pharmacokinetics of a single dose of fulvestrant prolonged-release intramuscular injection in postmenopausal women awaiting surgery for primary breast cancer. Clin Ther 2003;25:1440–1452.
112. Piccart M, Parker LM, Pritchard KI. Oestrogen receptor downregulation: an opportunity for extending the window of endocrine therapy in advanced breast cancer. Ann Oncol 2003;14:1017–1025.
113. Wakeling AE, Bowler J. Steroidal pure antioestrogens. J Endocrinol 1987;112:R7–R10.
114. Wakeling AE, Dukes M, Bowler J. A potent specific pure antiestrogen with clinical potential. Cancer Res 1991;51:3867–3873.
115. Howell A, Robertson JF, Quaresma Albano J, et al. Fulvestrant, formerly ICI 182,780, is as effective as anastrozole in postmenopausal women with advanced breast cancer progressing after prior endocrine treatment. J Clin Oncol 2002;20:3396–3403.
116. Osborne CK, Pippen J, Jones SE, et al. Double-blind, randomized trial comparing the efficacy and tolerability of fulvestrant versus anastrozole in postmenopausal women with advanced breast cancer progressing on prior endocrine therapy: results of a North American trial. J Clin Oncol 2002;20:3386–3395.
117. Howell A, Robertson JF, Abram P, et al. Comparison of fulvestrant versus tamoxifen for the treatment of advanced breast cancer in postmenopausal women previously untreated with endocrine therapy: a multinational, double-blind, randomized trial. J Clin Oncol 2004;22:1605–1613.
118. Leo AD, Jerusalem G, Petruzelka L, et al. Final overall survival: fulvestrant 500 mg vs 250 mg in the randomized CONFIRM trial. J Natl Cancer Inst 2014;106:djt337.
119. McCormack P, Sapunar F. Pharmacokinetic profile of the fulvestrant loading dose regimen in postmenopausal women with hormone receptor-positive advanced breast cancer. Clin Breast Cancer 2008;8:347–351.
120. Schteingart DE, Cash R, Conn JW. Amino-glutethimide and metastatic adrenal cancer. Maintained reversal (six months) of Cushing's syndrome. JAMA 1996;198:1007–1010.
121. Ma CX, Adjei AA, Salavaggione OE, et al. Human aromatase: gene resequencing and functional genomics. Cancer Res 2005;65:11071–11082.
122. Colomer R, Monzo M, Tusquets I, et al. A single-nucleotide polymorphism in the aromatase gene is associated with the efficacy of the aromatase inhibitor letrozole in advanced breast carcinoma. Clin Cancer Res 2008;14:811–816.
123. Wang L, Ellsworth KA, Moon I, et al. Functional genetic polymorphisms in the aromatase gene CYP19 vary the response of breast cancer patients to neoadjuvant therapy with aromatase inhibitors. Cancer Res 2010;70:319–328.
124. Goss PE, Ingle JN, Martino S, et al. A randomized trial of letrozole in postmenopausal women after five years of tamoxifen therapy for early-stage breast cancer. N Engl J Med 2003;349:1793–1802.
125. Mouridsen H, Gershanovich M, Sun Y, et al. Phase III study of letrozole versus tamoxifen as first-line therapy of advanced breast cancer in postmenopausal women: analysis of survival and update of efficacy from the International Letrozole Breast Cancer Group. J Clin Oncol 2003;21:2101–2109.
126. Howell A, Cuzick J, Baum M, et al. Results of the ATAC (Arimidex, Tamoxifen, Alone or in Combination) trial after completion of 5 years' adjuvant treatment for breast cancer. Lancet 2005;365:60–62.
127. Thurlimann B, Keshaviah A, Coates AS, et al. A comparison of letrozole and tamoxifen in postmenopausal women with early breast cancer. N Engl J Med 2005;353:2747–2757.
128. Jakesz R, Jonat W, Gnant M, et al. Switching of postmenopausal women with endocrine-responsive early breast cancer to anastrozole after 2 years' adjuvant tamoxifen: combined results of ABCSG trial 8 and ARNO 95 trial. Lancet 2005;366:455–462.
129. Cuzick J, Sestak I, Forbes JF, et al. Anastrozole for prevention of breast cancer in high-risk postmenopausal women (IBIS-II): an international, double-blind, randomised placebo-controlled trial. Lancet 2014;383:1041–1048.
130. Baum M, Budzar AU, Cuzick J, et al. Anastrozole alone or in combination with tamoxifen versus tamoxifen alone for adjuvant treatment of postmenopausal women with early breast cancer: first results of the ATAC randomised trial. Lancet 2002;359:2131–2139.
131. Amir E, Seruga B, Nira S, et al. Toxicity of adjuvant endocrine therapy in postmenopausal breast cancer patients: a systematic review and meta-analysis. J Natl Cancer Inst 2011;103:1299–1309.
132. Plourde PV, Dyroff M, Dukes M. Arimidex: a potent and selective fourth-generation aromatase inhibitor. Breast Cancer Res Treat 1994;30:103–111.
133. Bisagni G, Cocconi G, Scaglione F, et al. Letrozole, a new oral non-steroidal aromatase inhibitor in treating postmenopausal patients with advanced breast cancer. A pilot study. Ann Oncol 1996;7:99–102.
134. Buzdar AU. Pharmacology and pharmacokinetics of the newer generation aromatase inhibitors. Clin Cancer Res 2003;9:468S–472S.
135. Dewar JA, Nabholtz JM, Bonneterre J, et al. The effect of anastrozole (Arimidex) on serum lipids: data from a randomized comparison of anastrozole (AN) versus tamoxifen (TAM) in postmenopausal (PM) women with advanced breast cancer (ABC). Breast Cancer Res Treat 2000;64:51.
136. Elisaf MS, Bairaktari ET, Nicolaides C, et al. Effect of letrozole on the lipid profile in postmenopausal women with breast cancer. Eur J Cancer 2001;37:1510–1513.
137. Bhatnagar AS, Hausler A, Schieweck K. Inhibition of aromatase in vitro and in vivo by aromatase inhibitors. J Enzyme Inhib 1990;4:179–186.
138. Bhatnagar AS, Hausler A, Schieweck K, et al. Highly selective inhibition of estrogen biosynthesis by CGS 20267, a new non-steroidal aromatase inhibitor. J Steroid Biochem Mol Biol 1990;37:1021–1027.
139. Demers LM. Effects of Fadrozole (CGS 16949A) and Letrozole (CGS 20267) on the inhibition of aromatase activity in breast cancer patients. Breast Cancer Res Treat 1994;30:95–102.
140. Lipton A, Demers LM, Harvey HA, et al. Letrozole (CGS 20267). A phase I study of a new potent oral aromatase inhibitor of breast cancer. Cancer 1995;75:2132–2138.
141. Iveson TJ, Smith IE, Ahern J, et al. Phase I study of the oral nonsteroidal aromatase inhibitor CGS 20267 in postmenopausal patients with advanced breast cancer. Cancer Res 1993;53:266–270.
142. Trunet PF, Muller PH, Bhatnagar A. Phase I study in healthy male volunteers with the non-steroidal aromatase inhibitor GCS 20267. Eur J Cancer 1990;26:173.
143. Dukes M, Edwards PN, Large M, et al. The preclinical pharmacology of "Arimidex" (anastrozole; ZD1033)—a potent, selective aromatase inhibitor. J Steroid Biochem Mol Biol 1996;58:439–445.
144. Yates RA, Dowsett M, Fisher GV, et al. Arimidex (ZD1033): a selective, potent inhibitor of aromatase in postmenopausal female volunteers. Br J Cancer 1996;73:543–548.
145. Lonning PE, Geisler J, Dowsett M. Pharmacological and clinical profile of anastrozole. Breast Cancer Res Treat 1998;49:S53–S57.
146. Geisler J, King N, Dowsett M, et al. Influence of anastrozole (Arimidex), a selective, non-steroidal aromatase inhibitor, on in vivo aromatisation and plasma oestrogen levels in postmenopausal women with breast cancer. Br J Cancer 1996;74:1286–1291.
147. Ingle JN, Buzdar AU, Schaid DJ, et al. Variation in anastrozole metabolism and pharmacodynamics in women with early breast cancer. Cancer Res 2010;70:3278–3286.
148. Kaufmann M, Bajetta E, Dirix LY, et al. Exemestane is superior to megestrol acetate after tamoxifen failure in postmenopausal women with advanced breast cancer: results of a phase III randomized double-blind trial. The Exemestane Study Group. J Clin Oncol 2000;18:1399–1411.
149. Goss PE, Ingle JN, Pritchard KI, et al. Exemestane versus anastrozole in postmenopausal women with early breast cancer: NCIC CTG MA.27—a randomized controlled phase III trial. J Clin Oncol 2013;31:1398–1404.
150. Goss PE, Ingle JN, Ales-Martinez JE, et al. Exemestane for breast-cancer prevention in postmenopausal women. N Engl J Med 2011;364:2381–2391.
151. Goss PE, Grynpas M, Qi S, et al. The effects of exemestane on bone and lipids in the ovariectomized rat. Breast Cancer Res Treat 2001;69:224.
152. Evans TR, Di Salle E, Ornati G, et al. Phase I and endocrine study of exemestane (FCE 24304), a new aromatase inhibitor, in postmenopausal women. Cancer Res 1992;52:5933–5939.

153. Bajetta E, Zilembo N, Noberasco C, et al. The minimal effective exemestane dose for endocrine activity in advanced breast cancer. *Eur J Cancer* 1997;33:587–591.
154. Michaud LB, Buzdar AU. Risks and benefits of aromatase inhibitors in postmenopausal breast cancer. *Drug Saf* 1999;21:297–309.
155. Coombes RC, Hall E, Gibson LJ, et al. A randomized trial of exemestane after two to three years of tamoxifen therapy in postmenopausal women with primary breast cancer. *N Engl J Med* 2004;350:1081–1092.
156. Demers LM, Lipton A, Harvey HA, et al. The efficacy of CGS 20267 in suppressing estrogen biosynthesis in patients with advanced stage breast cancer. *J Steroid Biochem Mol Biol* 1993;44:687–691.
157. Spinelli R, Jannuzzo MG, Poggesi I, et al. Pharmacokinetics (PK) of Aromasin (Exemestane, EXE) after single and repeated doses in healthy postmenopausal volunteers (HPV). *Eur J Cancer* 1999;35:S295.
158. Buzdar A, Howell A. Advances in aromatase inhibition: clinical efficacy and tolerability in the treatment of breast cancer. *Clin Cancer Res* 2001;7:2620–2635.
159. Johannessen DC, Engan T, Di Salle E, et al. Endocrine and clinical effects of exemestane (PNU 155971), a novel steroidal aromatase inhibitor, in postmenopausal breast cancer patients: a phase I study. *Clin Cancer Res* 1997;3:1101–1108.
160. Jones S, Vogel C, Arkhipov A, et al. Multicenter, phase II trial of exemestane as third-line hormonal therapy of postmenopausal women with metastatic breast cancer. Aromasin Study Group. *J Clin Oncol* 1999;17:3418–3425.
161. Ahmann FR, Citrin DL, deHaan HA, et al. Zoladex: a sustained-release, monthly luteinizing hormone-releasing hormone analogue for the treatment of advanced prostate cancer. *J Clin Oncol* 1987;5:912–917.
162. Corbin A. From contraception to cancer: a review of the therapeutic applications of LHRH analogues as antitumor agents. *Yale J Biol Med* 1982;55:27–47.
163. Kaufmann M, Jonat W, Blamey R, et al. Survival analyses from the ZEBRA study. Goserelin (Zoladex) versus CMF in premenopausal women with node-positive breast cancer. *Eur J Cancer* 2003;39:1711–1717.
164. Harvey HA, Lipton A, Max DT, et al. Medical castration produced by the GnRH analogue leuprolide to treat metastatic breast cancer. *J Clin Oncol* 1985;3:1068–1072.
165. Abrahamsson PA. Potential benefits of intermittent androgen suppression therapy in the treatment of prostate cancer: a systematic review of the literature. *Eur Urol* 2010;57:49–59.
166. Hussain M, Tangen CM, Berry DL, et al. Intermittent versus continuous androgen deprivation in prostate cancer. *N Engl J Med* 2013;368:1314–1325.
167. Brogden RN, Faulds D. Goserelin. A review of its pharmacodynamic and pharmacokinetic properties and therapeutic efficacy in prostate cancer. *Drugs Aging* 1995;6:324–343.
168. Vogelzang NJ, Chodak GW, Soloway MS, et al. Goserelin versus orchiectomy in the treatment of advanced prostate cancer: final results of a randomized trial. Zoladex Prostate Study Group. *Urology* 1995;46:220–226.
169. Plosker GL, Brogden RN. Leuprorelin. A review of its pharmacology and therapeutic use in prostatic cancer, endometriosis and other sex hormone-related disorders. *Drugs* 1994;48:930–967.
170. Nillius SJ. *The Therapeutic Uses of Gonadotropin-Releasing Hormone and Its Analogues*. London: Butterworth; 1981.
171. Klijn JG, DeJong FH, Blankenstein MA. Anti-tumor and endocrine effects of chronic LHRH agonist treatment (buserelin) with or without tamoxifen in premenopausal metastatic breast cancer. *Breast Cancer Res Treat* 1984;4:209.
172. Clayton RN, Bailey LC, Cottam J, et al. A radioimmunoassay for GnRH agonist analogue in serum of patients with prostate cancer treated with D-Ser (tBu)6 AZA Gly10 GnRH. *Clin Endocrinol (Oxf)* 1985;22:453–462.
173. Chrisp P, Goa KL. Goserelin. A review of its pharmacodynamic and pharmacokinetic properties, and clinical use in sex hormone-related conditions. *Drugs* 1991;41:254–288.
174. Samant MP, Hong DJ, Croston G, et al. Novel gonadotropin-releasing hormone antagonists with substitutions at position 5. *Biopolymers* 2005;80:386–391.
175. Van Poppel H, Tombal B, de la Rosette JJ, et al. Degarelix: a novel gonadotropin-releasing hormone (GnRH) receptor blocker—results from a 1-yr, multicentre, randomised, phase 3 dosage-finding study in the treatment of prostate cancer. *Eur Urol* 2008;54:805–813.
176. Klotz L, Boccon-Gibod L, Shore ND, et al. The efficacy and safety of degarelix: a 12-month, comparative, randomized, open-label, parallel-group phase III study in patients with prostate cancer. *BJU Int* 2008;102:1531–1538.
177. Steinberg M. Degarelix: a gonadotropin-releasing hormone antagonist for the management of prostate cancer. *Clin Ther* 2009;31:2312–2331.
178. Brogden RN, Clissold SP. Flutamide. A preliminary review of its pharmacodynamic and pharmacokinetic properties, and therapeutic efficacy in advanced prostatic cancer. *Drugs* 1989;38:185–203.
179. Wysowski DK, Freiman JP, Tourtelot JB, et al. Fatal and nonfatal hepatotoxicity associated with flutamide. *Ann Intern Med* 1993;118:860–864.
180. Brogden RN, Chrisp P. Flutamide. A review of its pharmacodynamic and pharmacokinetic properties, and therapeutic use in advanced prostatic cancer. *Drugs Aging* 1991;1:104–115.
181. Radwanski E, Perentesis G, Symchowicz S, et al. Single and multiple dose pharmacokinetic evaluation of flutamide in normal geriatric volunteers. *J Clin Pharmacol* 1989;29:554–558.
182. Schellhammer PF, Sharifi R, Block NL, et al. A controlled trial of bicalutamide versus flutamide, each in combination with luteinizing hormone-releasing hormone analogue therapy, in patients with advanced prostatic carcinoma. Analysis of time to progression. CASODEX Combination Study Group. *Cancer* 1996;78:2164–2169.
183. Furr BJ. Casodex (ICI 176,334)—a new, pure, peripherally-selective anti-androgen: preclinical studies. *Horm Res* 1989;32:69.
184. Furr BJ. Casodex: preclinical studies. *Eur Urol* 1990;18:2.
185. Kennealey GT, Furr BJ. Use of the nonsteroidal anti-androgen Casodex in advanced prostatic carcinoma. *Urol Clin North Am* 1991;18:99–110.
186. Attard G, Reid AH, A'Hern R, et al. Selective inhibition of CYP17 with abiraterone acetate is highly active in the treatment of castration-resistant prostate cancer. *J Clin Oncol* 2009;27:3742–3748.
187. Tran C, Ouk S, Clegg NJ, et al. Development of a second-generation antiandrogen for treatment of advanced prostate cancer. *Science* 2009;324:787–790.
188. Scher HI, Fizazi K, Saad F, et al. Increased survival with enzalutamide in prostate cancer after chemotherapy. *N Engl J Med* 2012;367:1187–1197.
189. Zhu H, Garcia JA. Targeting the adrenal gland in castration-resistant prostate cancer: a case for orteronel, a selective CYP-17 17,20-lyase inhibitor. *Curr Oncol Rep* 2013;15:105–112.
190. Kennedy BJ. Hormonal therapies in breast cancer. *Semin Oncol* 1974;1:119–130.
191. Colburn WA. Radioimmunoassay for fluoxymesterone (Halotestin). *Steroids* 1975;25:43–52.
192. Kammerer RC, Merdink JL, Jagels M, et al. Testing for fluoxymesterone (Halotestin) administration to man: identification of urinary metabolites by gas chromatography-mass spectrometry. *J Steroid Biochem* 1990;36:659–666.
193. Ingle JN, Ahmann DL, Green SJ, et al. Randomized clinical trial of diethylstilbestrol versus tamoxifen in postmenopausal women with advanced breast cancer. *N Engl J Med* 1981;304:16–21.
194. Stewart HJ, Forrest AP, Gunn JM, et al. The tamoxifen trial - a double-blind comparison with stilboestrol in postmenopausal women with advanced breast cancer. *Eur J Cancer* 1980;Suppl 1:83–88.
195. Byar DP. Proceedings: The Veterans Administration Cooperative Urological Research Group's studies of cancer of the prostate. *Cancer* 1973;32:1126–1130.
196. Loose-Mitchell DS, Stancel GM. *Estrogens and Progestins*. 10 ed. New York: McGraw-Hill; 2001.
197. Bonomi P, Pessis D, Bunting N, et al. Megestrol acetate used as primary hormonal therapy in stage D prostatic cancer. *Semin Oncol* 1985;12:36–39.
198. Bruera E, Macmillan K, Kuehn N, et al. A controlled trial of megestrol acetate on appetite, caloric intake, nutritional status, and other symptoms in patients with advanced cancer. *Cancer* 1990;66:1279–1282.
199. Feliu J, Gonzalez-Baron M, Berrocal A, et al. Usefulness of megestrol acetate in cancer cachexia and anorexia. A placebo-controlled study. *Am J Clin Oncol* 1992;15:436–440.
200. Loprinzi CL, Ellison NM, Schaid DJ, et al. Controlled trial of megestrol acetate for the treatment of cancer anorexia and cachexia. *J Natl Cancer Inst* 1990;82:1127–1132.
201. Tchekmedyian NS, Hickman M, Siau J, et al. Megestrol acetate in cancer anorexia and weight loss. *Cancer* 1992;69:1268–1274.
202. Loprinzi CL, Michalak JC, Schaid DJ, et al. Phase III evaluation of four doses of megestrol acetate as therapy for patients with cancer anorexia and/or cachexia. *J Clin Oncol* 1993;11:762–767.
203. Loprinzi CL, Jensen MD, Jiang NS, et al. Effect of megestrol acetate on the human pituitary-adrenal axis. *Mayo Clin Proc* 1992;67:1160–1162.
204. Leinung MC, Liporace R, Miller CH. Induction of adrenal suppression by megestrol acetate in patients with AIDS. *Ann Intern Med* 1995;122:843–845.
205. Rowland KM Jr., Loprinzi CL, Shaw EG, et al. Randomized double-blind placebo-controlled trial of cisplatin and etoposide plus megestrol acetate/placebo in extensive-stage small-cell lung cancer: a North Central Cancer Treatment Group study. *J Clin Oncol* 1996;14:135–141.
206. Loprinzi CL, Johnson PA, Jensen M. Megestrol acetate for anorexia and cachexia. *Oncology* 1992;49:46–49.
207. Von Roenn JH, Armstrong D, Kotler DP, et al. Megestrol acetate in patients with AIDS-related cachexia. *Ann Intern Med* 1994;121:393–399.
208. Alexieva-Figusch J, Blankenstein MA, Hop WC, et al. Treatment of metastatic breast cancer patients with different dosages of megestrol acetate; dose relations, metabolic and endocrine effects. *Eur J Cancer Clin Oncol* 1984;20:33–40.
209. Tseng L, Gurpide E. Effects of progestins on estradiol receptor levels in human endometrium. *J Clin Endocrinol Metab* 1975;41:402–404.
210. Gurpide E, Tseng L, Gusberg SB. Estrogen metabolism in normal and neoplastic endometrium. *Am J Obstet Gynecol* 1977;129:809–816.
211. Gordon GG, Altman K, Southren AL, et al. Human hepatic testosterone A-ring reductase activity: effect of medroxyprogesterone acetate. *J Clin Endocrinol Metab* 1971;32:457–461.
212. Allegra JC, Kiefer SM. Mechanisms of action of progestational agents. *Semin Oncol* 1985;12:3–5.
213. Ewing TM, Murphy LJ, Ng ML, et al. Regulation of epidermal growth factor receptor by progestins and glucocorticoids in human breast cancer cell lines. *Int J Cancer* 1989;44:744–752.
214. Adlercreutz H, Eriksen PB, Christensen MS. Plasma concentration of megestrol acetate and medroxyprogesterone acetate after single oral administration to healthy subjects. *J Pharm Biomed Anal* 1983;1:153.
215. Martin F, Adlercreutz H, eds. *Aspects of Megestrol Acetate and Medroxyprogesterone Acetate Metabolism*. New York: Raven Press; 1977.
216. Gaver RC, Pittman KA, Reilly CM, et al. Bioequivalence evaluation of new megestrol acetate formulations in humans. *Semin Oncol* 1985;12:17–19.
217. Fotherby K, Kamyab S, Littleton P. Metabolism of synthetic progestational compounds in humans. *J Reprod Fertil* 1968;5:51–61.

218. Fukushima DK, Ievin J, Liang JS, et al. Isolation and partial synthesis of a new metabolite of medroxyrogesterone acetate. *Steroids* 1979;34: 57–72.
219. Utaaker E, Lundgren S, Kvinnsland S, et al. Pharmacokinetics and metabolism of medroxyprogesterone acetate in patients with advanced breast cancer. *J Steroid Biochem* 1988;31:437–441.
220. Sturm G, Haberlein H, Bauer T, et al. Mass spectrometric and high-performance liquid chromatographic studies of medroxyprogesterone acetate metabolites in human plasma. *J Chromatogr* 1991;562:351–362.
221. Pannuti F, Camaggi CM, Strocchi E, eds. *Medroxyprogesterone Acetate Pharmacokinetics.* New York. Raven Press, 1984.
222. Lundgren S, Lonning PE, Aakvaag A, et al. Influence of aminoglutethimide on the metabolism of medroxyprogesterone acetate and megestrol acetate in postmenopausal patients with advanced breast cancer. *Cancer Chemother Pharmacol* 1990;27:101–105.
223. Lundgren S, Kvinnsland S, Utaaker E, et al. Effect of oral high-dose progestins on the disposition of antipyrine, digitoxin, and warfarin in patients with advanced breast cancer. *Cancer Chemother Pharmacol* 1986;18:270–275.
224. Cascinu S, Fedeli A, Fedeli SL, et al. Control of chemotherapy-induced diarrhoea with octreotide in patients receiving 5-fluorouracil. *Eur J Cancer* 1992;28:182–183.
225. Cascinu S, Fedeli A, Fedeli SL, et al. Octreotide versus loperamide in the treatment of fluorouracil-induced diarrhea: a randomized trial. *J Clin Oncol* 1993;11:148–151.
226. Gebbia V, Carreca I, Testa A, et al. Subcutaneous octreotide versus oral loperamide in the treatment of diarrhea following chemotherapy. *Anticancer Drugs* 1993;4:443–445.
227. Harris AG. Somatostatin and somatostatin analogues: pharmacokinetics and pharmacodynamic effects. *Gut* 1994;35:S1–S4.
228. Chanson P, Timsit J, Harris AG. Clinical pharmacokinetics of octreotide. Therapeutic applications in patients with pituitary tumours. *Clin Pharmacokinet* 1993;25:375–391.
229. Marbach P, Briner U, Lemaire M. From somatostatin to Sandostatin: pharmacodynamics and pharmacokinetics. *Digestion* 1993;54:9–13.
230. Rubin J, Ajani J, Schirmer W, et al. Octreotide acetate long-acting formulation versus open-label subcutaneous octreotide acetate in malignant carcinoid syndrome. *J Clin Oncol* 1999;17:600–606.

28 Antiangiogenesis Agents

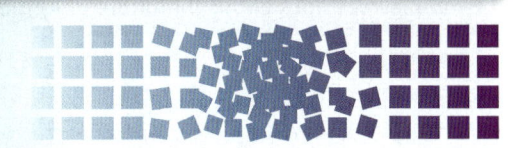

Cindy H. Chau and William Douglas Figg, Sr.

INTRODUCTION

Blood vessels are indispensable for tumor growth and metastasis, and the formation of a new network of blood vessels from the existing vasculature, termed *angiogenesis*, is one of the essential hallmarks of cancer development.[1] Indeed, it was over 70 years ago that the existence of tumor-derived factors responsible for promoting new vessel growth was postulated,[2] and that tumor growth is essentially dependent on vascular induction and the development of a neovascular supply.[3] By the late 1960s, Dr. Judah Folkman and colleagues[4] had begun the search for a tumor angiogenesis factor. In the 1971 landmark report, Folkman[5] proposed that inhibition of angiogenesis by means of holding tumors in a nonvascularized dormant state would be an effective strategy to treat human cancer, and hence laid the groundwork for the concept behind the development of *antiangiogenesis* agents. This fostered the search for angiogenic factors, regulators of angiogenesis, and antiangiogenic molecules over the next few decades and shed light on angiogenesis as an important therapeutic target for the treatment of cancer and other diseases.

A decade has passed since the regulatory approval of the first antiangiogenic drug bevacizumab, and while initial results were regarded as highly promising, clinical evidence indicated that antiangiogenic therapy also had limitations. Successful development and clinical translation of this novel class of agents depends on the complete understanding of the biology of angiogenesis and the regulatory proteins that govern this angiogenic process, topics that have been covered in greater detail in another section of this textbook. This chapter will briefly review the mechanisms underlying tumor angiogenesis followed by an in-depth discussion of antiangiogenic therapy, the modes of action of angiogenesis inhibitors, and the successes and challenges of this treatment modality.

UNDERSTANDING THE ANGIOGENIC PROCESS

Angiogenic Switch and Regulatory Proteins

Tumor development and progression depend on angiogenesis. Recruitment of new blood vessels to the tumor site is required for the delivery of nutrients and oxygen to the cancerous growths and for the removal of waste products.[6] Cancer cells promote angiogenesis at an early stage of tumorigenesis, beginning with the release of molecules that send signals to the surrounding normal host tissue and stimulate the migration of microvascular endothelial cells (EC) in the direction of the angiogenic stimulus. These angiogenic factors not only mediate EC migration, but also EC proliferation and microvessel formation in tumors undergoing the switch to the angiogenic phenotype.[7] Experimental evidence for this *angiogenic switch* was observed when hyperplastic islets in transgenic mice (RIP-Tag model) switch from small (<1 mm), white microscopic dormant tumors to red, rapidly growing tumors.[7] Dormant tumors have been discovered during autopsies of individuals who died of causes other than cancer.[8] These autopsy studies suggest that the vast majority of microscopic in situ cancers never switch to the angiogenic phenotype during a normal lifetime. Such incipient tumors are usually not neovascularized and can remain harmless to the host for long periods of time as microscopic lesions that are in a state of dormancy.[9,10] These nonangiogenic tumors cannot expand beyond the initial microscopic size and cannot become clinically detectable, lethal tumors until they have switched to the angiogenic phenotype[11–13] through neovascularization and/or blood vessel cooption.[14] Depending on the tumor type and the environment, this switch can occur at different stages of the tumor progression pathway and ultimately depends on a net balance of positive and negative regulators. Thus, the angiogenic phenotype may result from the production of growth factors by tumor cells and/or the downregulation of negative modulators.

Changes in this angiogenic balance affecting the levels of activator and inhibitor molecules dictate whether an EC will be in a quiescent or an angiogenic state. Normally, the inhibitors predominate, thereby blocking growth. Once the balance shifts in favor of the angiogenic state, proangiogenic factors prompts the activation, growth, and division of vascular ECs, resulting in the formation of new blood vessels. Activated ECs produce and release matrix metalloproteinases (MMP) into the surrounding tissue to break down the extracellular matrix to allow the ECs to migrate and organize themselves into hollow tubes that eventually evolve into a mature network of blood vessels. Proangiogenic factors or positive regulators of angiogenesis include vascular endothelial growth factor (VEGF), basic fibroblast growth factor (PlGF), platelet-derived growth factor (PDGF), placental growth factor, transforming growth factor-β, pleiotrophins, and others.[15] Activation of the hypoxia-inducible factor 1 (HIF-1) via tumor-associated hypoxic conditions is also involved in the upregulation of several angiogenic factors.[16] The angiogenic switch also involves the downregulation of angiogenesis suppressor proteins, which include endostatin, angiostatin, thrombospondin, and others.[17,18] Most notably, however, is the link between many oncogenes and angiogenesis and the significant role oncogenes play in driving the angiogenic switch.[19,20] These proangiogenic oncogenes not only induce the expression of stimulators, but may also downregulate inhibitors of angiogenesis.[21]

Endogenous Inhibitors of Angiogenesis

The infrequency of microscopic in situ tumors that actually undergo the angiogenic switch (<1%) suggests that naturally occurring endogenous inhibitors exist in the body to defend against the angiogenic switch in pathologic conditions and to limit physiologic angiogenesis.[9] These circulating endogenous inhibitors could also prevent microscopic metastases from growing into visible tumors. Early studies by Langer et al.[22,23] demonstrated the possible existence of such inhibitors through the extraction of a functional inhibitor from cartilage, a tissue that is poorly vascularized. Since then, dozens of endogenous angiogenesis inhibitors have been identified, some of which are listed in Table 28.1.[17,18,24] Many of the endogenous inhibitors of angiogenesis that have been discovered to date are proteolytically cleaved fragments of larger proteins that are members of either the clotting/coagulation system

TABLE 28.1

Examples of Endogenous Inhibitors of Angiogenesis

Alphastatin
Angiostatin
Antithrombin III (cleaved)
Arrestin
Canstatin
Endostatin
Interferon alpha/beta (IFN-α/β)
2-Methoxyestradiol (2-ME)
Pigment epithelial-derived factor (PEDF)
Platelet factor 4 (PF-4)
Tetrahydrocortisol-S
Thrombospondin 1
Tissue inhibitor of metalloproteinase 2 (TIMP-2)
Tumstatin
Vasohibin

or members of the extracellular matrix family of glycoproteins. Endostatin is the most well-studied endogenous angiogenesis inhibitor.[25,26] Other potent endogenous angiogenesis inhibitors include thrombospondin 1[27] and tumstatin.[28] The discovery of vasohibin, an endogenous inhibitor that is selectively induced in ECs by proangiogenic stimulatory growth factors such as VEGF, demonstrated the existence of an intrinsic and EC-specific feedback inhibitor control mechanism,[29,30] whereas most endogenous inhibitors of angiogenesis are extrinsic to ECs. More recently, a second endothelium-produced negative regulator of angiogenesis has been discovered, the Dll4-Notch signaling system.[31,32] Both intrinsic factors have since been shown to control tumor angiogenesis by an autoregulatory or negative-feedback mechanism. The Dll4-Notch axis has emerged as a critical regulator of tumor angiogenesis, and inhibitors of this pathway (e.g., demcizumab, the anti-Dll4 monoclonal antibody) are currently being investigated in early phase trials of solid tumors.[33]

Perhaps the most compelling genetic evidence that endogenous inhibitors suppress pathologic angiogenesis was observed in studies using mice deficient in tumstatin, endostatin, or thrombospondin 1 (TSP-1).[34] These experiments demonstrate that normal physiologic levels of the inhibitors can retard the tumor growth and that their absence leads to enhanced angiogenesis and increased tumor growth by two- to threefold, strongly suggesting that endogenous inhibitors of angiogenesis can act as endothelium-specific tumor suppressors. The connection between a tumor suppressor protein and angiogenesis is best illustrated by the classic tumor suppressor p53. p53 inhibits angiogenesis by increasing the expression of TSP-1[35] by repressing VEGF[36] and basic fibroblast growth factor–binding protein,[37] and by degrading HIF-1,[38] which blocks the downstream induction of VEGF expression. New evidence suggests that p53 also indirectly downregulates VEGF expression via the retinoblastoma pathway in a p21-dependent manner during sustained hypoxia.[39] Furthermore, p53-mediated inhibition of angiogenesis may also occur in part via the antiangiogenic activity of endostatin and tumstatin.[40] This landmark finding clearly demonstrates that p53 not only controls cell proliferation, but can also repress tumor angiogenesis through enzymatic mobilization of these endogenous angiogenesis inhibitor proteins to prevent ECs from being recruited into the dormant, microscopic tumors, thereby preventing the switch to the angiogenic phenotype.[41] The discovery that these endogenous angiogenesis inhibitors can suppress the growth of primary tumors raises the possibility that such inhibitors might also be able to slow tumor metastasis. Indeed, the inhibition of angiogenesis by angiostatin significantly reduced the rate of metastatic spread.

DRUG DEVELOPMENT OF ANGIOGENESIS INHIBITORS

The first angiogenesis inhibitor was reported in 1980 and involved the low-dose administration of interferon α (IFN-α).[42–44] Over the next decade, several compounds were discovered to have potent antiangiogenic activity, including protamine and platelet factor 4,[45] trahydrocortisol,[46] and the fumagillin analog TNP-470.[17] The proof of concept that targeting angiogenesis is an effective strategy for treating cancer came with the approval of the first angiogenesis inhibitor, bevacizumab, by the U.S. Food and Drug Administration (FDA). Since then, several antiangiogenic agents have received FDA approval for cancer treatment (Table 28.2), and three additional agents (pegaptanib, ranibizumab, and aflibercept) are approved for the treatment of wet age-related macular degeneration.

Rationale for Antiangiogenic Therapy

Antiangiogenic therapy stems from the fundamental concept that tumor growth, invasion, and metastasis are angiogenesis dependent; thus, blocking blood vessel recruitment to starve primary and metastatic tumors is a rational approach. The microvascular EC recruited by a tumor has become an important second target in cancer therapy. Unlike the cancer cell (the primary target of cytotoxic chemotherapy), which is genetically unstable with unpredictable mutations, the genetic stability of ECs may make them less susceptible to acquired drug resistance.[48] Moreover, ECs in the microvascular bed of a tumor may support 50 to 100 tumor cells. Coupling this amplification potential together with the lower toxicity of most angiogenesis inhibitors results in the use of antiangiogenic therapy, which should be significantly less toxic than conventional chemotherapy. However, the variable responses of antiangiogenic therapy observed in different tumor types and the fact that angiogenesis inhibitors have not delivered the benefits initially envisaged suggest that the precise mechanism of action of angiogenesis inhibitors is complex and remains incompletely understood.

Modes of Action of Antiangiogenic Agents

Various strategies for the development of antiangiogenic drugs have been investigated over the years, with these agents being classified into several different categories depending on their modes of action. Some inhibit ECs directly, whereas others inhibit the angiogenesis signaling cascade or block the ability of ECs to break down the extracellular matrix. Inhibitors may block one main angiogenic protein, two or three angiogenic proteins, or have a broad-spectrum effect by blocking a range of angiogenic regulators that can be located in both the tumor and ECs.[49] In some cases, the antiangiogenic activity is discovered as a secondary function after the drug has received regulatory approval for a different primary function. For example, bortezomib is a proteasome inhibitor that is approved for multiple myeloma and was later found to possess antiangiogenic activity via inhibiting VEGF. Some small-molecule drugs may display their antiangiogenic activity through inducing the expression of endogenous angiogenesis inhibitors such as celecoxib, a cyclooxygenase-2 (COX-2) inhibitor, which inhibits angiogenesis by increasing levels of endostatin.[25]

Some drugs possess antiangiogenic properties but with mechanisms that are not completely understood, such as thalidomide and its analogs, lenalidomide and pomalidomide, referred to as immunomodulatory drugs. Thalidomide was originally shown to inhibit angiogenesis by D'Amato et al,[50] in 1994 and this was subsequently confirmed in several different in vitro and ex vivo

TABLE 28.2
Antiangiogenic Agents that Have Received U.S. Food and Drug Administration Approval for Cancer Treatment

Drug	Class	Mechanism (Cellular Targets)	Year of Approval	Indications	Dosages
Bevacizumab (Avastin)	Anti-VEGF mAB	VEGF	2004	First- and second-line metastatic CRC	5 mg/kg IV q2wk + bolus IFL; 10 mg/kg IV q2wk + FOLFOX4
			2006	First-line NSCLC	15 mg/kg IV q3wk + carboplatin/paclitaxel
			2009	Second-line GBM	10 mg/kg IV q2wk
			2009	Metastatic RCC	10 mg/kg IV q2wk + IFN
			2013	Second-line metastatic CRC (after prior bevacizumab-containing regimen)	5 mg/kg IV q2wk or 7.5 mg/kg IV q3wk + fluoropyrimidine–irinotecan or fluoropyrimidine–oxaliplatin–based regimen
Ziv-aflibercept (Zaltrap, VEGF Trap)	Anti-VEGF mAB	VEGFA, VEGFB, PIGF1, PIGF2	2012	Metastatic CRC (after prior oxaliplatin-containing regimen)	4 mg/kg IV q2wk (1-hr infusion)
Sorafenib (Nexavar, BAY439006)	Small-molecule TKI	VEGFR2, VEGFR3, PDGFR, FLT3, c-Kit	2005	Advanced RCC	400 mg PO bid (w/o food)
			2007	Unresectable HCC	400 mg PO bid (w/o food)
			2013	RAI-refractory DTC	400 mg PO bid (w/o food)
Sunitinib (Sutent, SU11248)	Small-molecule TKI	VEGFR1, VEGFR2, VEGFR3, PDGFR, FLT3, c-Kit, RET	2006	Imatinib-resistant or -intolerant GIST	50 mg PO qd, 4 wk on/2 wk off
			2006	Advanced RCC	50 mg PO qd, 4 wk on/2 wk off
			2011	Advanced pNET	37.5 mg PO qd
Pazopanib (Votrient)	Small-molecule TKI	VEGFR1, VEGFR2, VEGFR3, PDGFR, Itk, Lck, c-Fms	2009	Advanced RCC	800 mg PO qd (w/o food)
			2012	Advanced soft tissue sarcoma	800 mg PO qd (w/o food)
Vandetanib (Caprelsa)	Small molecule TKI	RET, VEGFR, EGFR, BRK, TIE2	2011	Advanced MTC	300 mg PO qd
Axitinib (Inlyta)	Small molecule TKI	VEGFR1, VEGFR2, VEGFR3	2012	Advanced RCC (after failure of prior therapy)	5 mg PO bid
Cabozantinib (XL184, Cometriq)	Small molecule TKI	MET, VEGFR2, RET, KIT, AXL, FLT3	2012	Progressive, metastatic MTC	140 mg PO qd (w/o food)
Regorafenib (Stivarga)	Small molecule TKI	RET, VEGFR1, VEGFR2, VEGFR3, TIE2, KIT, PDGFR	2012	Previously treated metastatic CRC	160 mg PO qd × 21 days (q28-day cycle)
			2013	GIST	160 mg PO qd × days 1–21 (q28-day cycle)
Temsirolimus (Torisel)	mTOR inhibitor	mTOR	2007	Advanced RCC	25 mg IV qwk (infused over 30–60 min)
Everolimus (Afinitor, RAD-001)[a]	mTOR inhibitor	mTOR	2009	Second-line advanced RCC (after VEGFR TKI failure)	10 mg PO qd
			2010	SEGA associated w/TSC	4.5 mg/m^2 PO qd
			2011	pNET	10 mg PO qd
			2012	Advanced HR+, HER2- breast cancer	10 mg PO qd
			2012	AML associated w/TSC	10 mg PO qd

[a] Afinitor Disperz (everolimus tablets for oral suspension) was approved in 2012 for children aged 1 and older who have SEGA + TSC.

mAB, monoclonal antibody; CRC, colorectal cancer; IV, intravenous; IFL, irinotecan, 5-fluorouracil, and leucovorin; FOLFOX4, 5-flourouracil, leucovorin, and oxaliplatin; NSCLC, non–small-cell lung cancer; GBM, glioblastoma multiforme; RCC, renal cell carcinoma; VEGFA, vascular endothelial growth factor A; PIGF, placental growth factor; TKI, tyrosine–kinase inhibitor; VEGFR, VEGF receptor; PDGFR, platelet-derived growth factor receptor; FLT, Fms-like tyrosine kinase; c-Kit, stem cell factor receptor; HCC, hepatocellular carcinoma; RAI, radioactive iodine; DTC, differentiated thyroid carcinoma; PO, orally; RET, glial cell line-derived neurotrophic factor receptor; pNET, pancreatic neuroendocrine tumor; GIST, gastrointestinal stromal tumor; qd, every day; Itk, interleukin-2 receptor inducible T-cell kinase; Lck, leukocyte-specific protein tyrosine kinase; c-Fms, transmembrane glycoprotein receptor tyrosine kinase; bid, twice daily; EGFR, epidermal growth factor receptor; BRK, protein tyrosine kinase 6; MTC, medullary thyroid cancer; mTOR, mammalian target of rapamycin; SEGA, subependymal giant cell astrocytoma; TSC, tuberous sclerosis complex; HR, hormone receptor; HER2, human epidermal growth factor receptor 2; AML, angiomyolipoma.

assays.[51–54] Interestingly, unlike other mechanisms of action, the antiangiogenic activity of thalidomide is believed to require enzymatic activation. The extent to which the antiangiogenic properties of thalidomide and its analogs play a role in its antimyeloma activity is not clearly understood. Several mechanisms have been proposed that involve the downregulation of cytokines in EC, the inhibition of EC proliferation, the decrease in the level of circulating ECs, or the modulation of adhesion molecules between the multiple myeloma cells and the endogenous bone marrow stromal cells, thereby decreasing the production of VEGF and interleukin 6 (IL-6).[55–59] The immunomodulatory agents are discussed in greater detail in another section of this textbook. Examples of the various types of angiogenesis inhibitors are highlighted in Table 28.3.

Drugs with antiangiogenic activity may be classified as either direct or indirect angiogenesis inhibitors. A direct angiogenesis inhibitor blocks vascular ECs from proliferating, migrating, or increasing their survival in response to proangiogenic proteins. They target the activated endothelium directly and inhibit multiple angiogenic proteins. Examples of direct angiogenesis inhibitors include many of the endogenous inhibitors of angiogenesis, such as endostatin, angiostatin, and TSP-1. Indirect angiogenesis inhibitors decrease or block expression of a tumor cell product, neutralize the tumor product itself, or block its receptor on ECs. The limitation to indirect inhibitors is that, over time, tumor cells may acquire mutations that lead to increased expression of other proangiogenic proteins that are not blocked by the indirect inhibitor. This may give the appearance of drug resistance and warrants the addition of a second antiangiogenic agent, one that would target the expression of these upregulated proangiogenic proteins. Examples of drugs that interfere with the angiogenesis-signaling pathway include the anti-VEGF monoclonal antibodies and small-molecule tyrosine kinase inhibitors. These drugs target the major signaling pathways in tumor angiogenesis: VEGF, PDGF, and their respective receptors, as well as other growth factors and/or signaling pathways.

VEGF (also known as vascular permeability factor) is a potent proangiogenic growth factor and its expression is upregulated by most cancer cell types. It stimulates EC proliferation, migration, and survival as well as induces increased vascular permeability. The different forms of VEGF bind to transmembrane receptor tyrosine kinases (RTK) on ECs: VEGFR1 (Flt-1), VEGFR2 (KDR/Flk-1 or kinase insert domain receptor/fetal liver kinase 1), or VEGFR3 (Flt-4).[60] This results in receptor dimerization, activation, and autophosphorylation of the tyrosine–kinase domain, thereby triggering downstream signaling pathways. Other signaling molecules that may represent attractive therapeutic targets include PDGF and the angiopoietins (Ang1, Ang2). PDGF-B/PDGF receptor (R)-β plays an important role in the recruitment of pericytes and maturation of the microvasculature.[61] Ang2, which binds the Tie-2 receptor, is mostly expressed in tumor-induced neovasculature, whereby its selective inhibition results in reduced EC proliferation.[62] The angiopoietins are also involved in lymphangiogenesis, the formation of new lymphatic vessels, which plays a key role in tumor metastasis. An increased Ang2/Ang1 ratio correlates with tumor angiogenesis and poor prognosis in many cancers, thus making the angiopoietins an attractive therapeutic target. Angiopoietin inhibitors are currently under investigation in the preclinical and clinical setting.

Other strategies for targeting angiogenesis involve the tumor microenvironment. Breakdown of the extracellular matrix is required to allow ECs to migrate into surrounding tissues and proliferate into new blood vessels; thus, drugs that target MMPs, enzymes that catalyze the breakdown of the matrix, can also inhibit angiogenesis. However, clinical development of MMP inhibitors (MMPI) has yielded disappointing results.[63–66]

Integrins are cell surface adhesion molecules that play an essential role in cell–cell and cell–matrix adhesion as well as in transmitting signals important for cell migration, invasion, proliferation, and survival. The involvement of integrin in tumor angiogenesis was demonstrated in studies that show the β-4 subunit of integrin promoting endothelial migration and invasion.[67] Agents that target integrins (inhibitors of $\alpha_v\beta_3$ and $\alpha_v\beta_5$) have been evaluated as potential therapeutic options and include etaracizumab, cilengitide, and intetumumab. However, all three integrin inhibitors have proven to be largely ineffective in various early and late stage cancer trials.[68–73] In summary, the downstream effects of antiangiogenic agents, in addition to blocking angiogenesis, may involve inducing vessel regression, promoting sensitization to radiotherapy and chemotherapy by depriving ECs of VEGF's prosurvival signals, and inhibiting the recruitment of proangiogenic bone marrow–derived cells as well as reducing the self-renewal capability of cancer stem cells.[74]

CLINICAL UTILITY OF APPROVED ANTIANGIOGENIC AGENTS IN CANCER THERAPY

The following section reviews the current FDA-approved angiogenesis inhibitors (Table 28.2). These agents include: (1) the monoclonal anti-VEGF antibodies (bevacizumab and ziv-aflibercept); (2) small-molecule tyrosine kinase inhibitors (TKI) (sorafenib, sunitinib, pazopanib, vandetanib, axitinib, cabozantinib, and regorafenib); and (3) the mammalian target of rapamycin (mTOR) inhibitors (temsirolimus and everolimus), as examples of drugs that possess antiangiogenic activity. Other approved drugs that also inhibit angiogenesis as a secondary function, such as thalidomide, are discussed in greater detail in another section of this textbook and are presented in Table 28.3.

Anti-VEGF Therapy

Bevacizumab

Bevacizumab is a recombinant humanized anti–VEGF-A monoclonal antibody that received FDA approval in February 2004 for use in combination therapy with fluorouracil-based regimens for

TABLE 28.3
Examples of Drugs that Possess Antiangiogenic Activity or Inhibit Angiogenesis as a Secondary Function

Drug	Class
Cetuximab Panitumumab Trastuzumab	EGFR/HER monoclonal antibodies
Gefitinib Erlotinib	EGFR small-molecule tyrosine–kinase receptor inhibitors
Everolimus Temsirolimus	mTOR inhibitors
Thalidomide Lenalidomide Pomalidomide	Immunomodulatory agents
Belinostat (PXD101) LBH589 Vorinostat (SAHA)	HDAC inhibitors
Celecoxib	COX-2 inhibitors
Bortezomib	Proteasome inhibitors
Zoledronic acid	Bisphosphonates
Rosiglitazone	PPAR-γ agonists
Doxycycline	Antibiotic

EGFR, epidermal growth factor receptor; mTOR, mammalian target of rapamycin HDAC, histone deacetylase; COX-2, cyclooxygenase-2; PPAR, peroxisome proliferator–activated receptor.

metastatic colorectal cancer. Bevacizumab binds VEGF and prevents the interaction of VEGF to its receptors (Flt-1 and KDR) on the surface of ECs. It is the first antiangiogenic agent clinically proven to extend survival following a large, randomized, double-blind, phase III study in which bevacizumab was administered in combination with bolus irinotecan, 5-fluorouracil, and leucovorin (IFL) as first-line therapy for metastatic colorectal cancer (CRC).[75] In 2006, its approval extended to first- or second-line treatment of patients with metastatic carcinoma of the colon or rectum. This recommendation is based on the demonstration of a statistically significant improvement in overall survival (OS) in patients receiving bevacizumab plus FOLFOX4 (5-flourouracil, leucovorin, and oxaliplatin) when compared to those receiving FOLFOX4 alone. In January 2013, it was further approved to treat mCRC for second-line treatment when used with fluoropyrimidine-based (combined with irinotecan or oxaliplatin) chemotherapy after disease progression following a first-line treatment with a bevacizumab-containing regimen based on clinical benefits observed in the randomized phase III study (ML18147).[76] Despite the benefit in the metastatic setting, the addition of bevacizumab did not improve clinical outcomes in the adjuvant setting in CRC.[77,78] In 2006, bevacizumab received an additional approval for use in combination with carboplatin and paclitaxel, and is indicated for first-line treatment of patients with unresectable, locally advanced, recurrent, or metastatic nonsquamous, non–small-cell lung cancer (NSCLC) based on the demonstration of a statistically significant improvement in OS in patients in the bevacizumab arm compared to those receiving chemotherapy alone.[79] In February 2008, the FDA granted a conditional, accelerated approval for bevacizumab to be used in combination with paclitaxel for the treatment of patients who have not received chemotherapy for metastatic human epidermal growth factor receptor 2 (HER2)-negative breast cancer. However, additional clinical trials were conducted and the new data showed only a small effect on progression free survival (PFS) without evidence of an improvement in OS or a clinical benefit to patients sufficient to outweigh the risks; thus, the FDA rescinded its approval and removed the breast cancer indication from the drug's label in November 2011.[80–82] This controversial decision continues to be debated with ongoing subgroup analyses to identify patients who would likely benefit from bevacizumab.

Bevacizumab received another accelerated approval as a single agent for patients with glioblastoma multiforme (GBM) with progressive disease following therapy in May 2009. The approval was based on the demonstration of durable objective response rates observed in two single-arm trials, AVF3708g and NCI 06-C-0064E.[83] Currently, no data have shown whether bevacizumab improves disease-related symptoms or survival in people previously treated for GBM. Moreover, phase III trials of bevacizumab in newly diagnosed GBM (RTOG 8025 and AVAglio) have shown a 3- to 4-month improvement of PFS, but no OS advantage over the standard of care.[84] The AVAglio trial improved patients' quality of life, whereas the RTOG 0825 did not and instead increased the burden of symptoms with a negative impact on cognition. Although these two studies showed that bevacizumab had a modest benefit as the initial therapy for GBM, it remained effective to treat recurrences where treatment options are limited. In July 2009, bevacizumab was approved for use in combination with IFN-α for the treatment of patients with metastatic renal cell carcinoma (RCC). Results from the AVOREN trial demonstrated a 5-month improvement in median PFS in patients treated with bevacizumab plus IFN-α-2a versus IFN-α-2a plus placebo.[85] Another phase III trial (CALGB 90206) of bevacizumab plus IFN-α versus IFN-α monotherapy was conducted in patients with previously untreated, metastatic clear cell RCC. Median PFS was 8.4 months versus 4.9 months in favor of the bevacizumab arm.[86] Both studies did not demonstrate a statistically significant advantage in OS.[87,88]

Clinical studies of bevacizumab in combination with oxaliplatin-containing and 5-fluorouracil–based regimens have shown that combination therapy is well tolerated with toxicity not being substantially greater than that of the chemotherapy alone.[89] Side effects included grade 3 hypertension, grade 1 or 2 proteinuria, a slight increase (less than two percentage points) in grade 3 or 4 bleeding, and impaired surgical wound healing in patients who underwent surgery during treatment with bevacizumab. However, potentially life-threatening events (e.g., arterial and venous thromboembolic events, gastrointestinal perforation, hemoptysis, risk of ovarian failure) have occurred in some patients, thus requiring close patient monitoring in individuals who are at greater risk of adverse events.[90] In a recent meta-analysis of RCTs, bevacizumab in combination with chemotherapy or biologic therapy, compared with chemotherapy alone, was associated with increased treatment-related mortality.[91]

Although four phase III randomized studies have demonstrated improvements in PFS for ovarian cancer (OC)—two first-line trials (GOG 218 and ICON7) and two in recurrent OC [platinum-resistant (AURELIA Trial) or platinum-sensitive (OCEANS Trial)]—the role of bevacizumab in OC remains controversial. Bevacizumab is approved for use in combination with chemotherapy in the first- and second-line treatment of advanced OC in Europe, but it is not currently licensed in the United States for this indication. Mature OS data and predictive biomarkers are key to defining the subsets of patients who will most like benefit from this therapy. More recently, a randomized, phase III trial (GOG240) has demonstrated for the first time that bevacizumab can prolong OS and PFS for women with advanced, recurrent, or persistent cervical cancer that was not curable with standard chemotherapy. At the time of writing, there are currently over 400 actively recruiting, ongoing trials investigating the clinical benefits of bevacizumab in combination with chemotherapeutic regimens or as adjuvant therapy in various stages and types of cancer (http://clinicaltrial.gov).

Ziv-aflibercept

Ziv-aflibercept (previously known as aflibercept or VEGFTrap) is a recombinant humanized fusion protein of the extracellular domains of VEGF receptor 1 (VEGFR1) and VEGFR2 with the constant region (Fc) of human immunoglobulin (Ig)G1 that binds to VEGF-A, VEGF-B, PlGF1, and PlGF2, thereby preventing these ligands from binding to and activating their cognate receptors.[92] Ziv-aflibercept has a higher VEGF-A binding affinity and more potent blockade of VEGFR1 or VEGFR2 activation than bevacizumab.[93] In tumor models, ziv-aflibercept exerts its antiangiogenic effects through regressing tumor vasculature and size, remodeling or normalizing surviving vasculature, and inhibiting ascites formation.[94] In August 2012, ziv-aflibercept received regulatory approval for use in combination with 5-fluorouracil, leucovorin, and irinotecan (FOLFIRI) for the treatment of patients with metastatic CRC that is resistant to or that has progressed following treatment with an oxaliplatin-containing regimen. Results from the pivotal phase III VELOUR trial showed that ziv-aflibercept plus FOLFIRI statistically and significantly improved PFS (median PFS, 6.90 versus 4.67 months, respectively), OS (median OS, 13.50 versus 12.06 months, respectively), and overall response rates (19% versus 11.1%, respectively) relative to placebo plus FOLFIRI.[95] Toxicities related to ziv-aflibercept were consistent with those expected from the anti-VEGF drug class. The frequency of vascular-related adverse events appeared to be higher with ziv-aflibercept than bevacizumab treatment when compared across trials. Current clinical data are insufficient to directly compare ziv-aflibercept and bevacizumab in the first- or second-line setting for metastatic CRC.

Tyrosine–Kinase Inhibitor Therapy

Sorafenib

Sorafenib is a small-molecule Raf kinase and VEGF receptor kinase (VEGFR2 and VEGFR3) inhibitor. It has been shown to exhibit broad-spectrum effects on multiple targets (PDGF receptor (PDGFR), stem cell factor (c-KIT) receptor, p38) that affect the maintenance of the tumor vasculature and angiogenesis.[96] In December 2005, the FDA granted approval for sorafenib, which is considered the first multikinase inhibitor, for the treatment of patients with advanced RCC. Safety and efficacy of sorafenib was proven in the largest randomized phase III study conducted in advanced RCC that showed prolong PFS in favor of sorafenib.[97,98] In November 2007, sorafenib was approved for the treatment of patients with unresectable hepatocellular carcinoma (HCC) based on the study results in patients with advanced HCC who had not received previous systemic treatment. Median survival and the time to radiologic progression were nearly 3 months longer for patients treated with sorafenib than for those given placebo.[99] In November 2013, sorafenib received a new indication under the FDA's priority review program for the treatment of locally recurrent or metastatic, progressive differentiated thyroid carcinoma (DTC) refractory to radioactive iodine (RAI) treatment based on positive results from the phase III DECISION trial. Treatment with sorafenib improved PFS (the primary endpoint of the trial) by 41% compared with placebo (10.8 versus 5.8 months, respectively; hazard ratio [HR], 0.587, 95% confidence interval [CI] [0.454 to 0.758]; p <0.0001).[100] The overall response rates were 12% for patients who received sorafenib versus 1% for the placebo arm. Although only about 5% to 15% of thyroid cancer patients become refractory to RAI, no standard treatments are available and, thus, sorafenib is the first agent specifically approved for RAI-resistant DTC. Sorafenib was generally well tolerated with a predictable safety profile. Common adverse events include diarrhea, rash/desquamation, fatigue, hand-foot skin reaction, alopecia, and nausea/vomiting. Grade 3/4 adverse events were 38% for sorafenib versus 28% for placebo. Sorafenib-induced hypertension occurred in patients with metastatic RCC. The treatment-related hypertension was noted to be a class effect observed not only with VEGFR inhibitors, but also with the VEGF monoclonal antibody as well.[90] No significant relationship between previously described mediators of blood pressure and the magnitude of increase was found in a study evaluating the mechanism of sorafenib-induced hypertension in patients.[101]

Sunitinib

Sunitinib (SU11248) is a small-molecule, multitargeted TKI that exhibits potent antitumor and antiangiogenic activity and inhibits VEGFR-1, -2, -3, c-KIT, PDGFR; FLT-3; colony-stimulating factor receptor type 1 receptor; and the glial cell line–derived neurotrophic factor receptor. It was rationally designed and chosen for its high bioavailability and its nanomolar-range potency against the antiangiogenic RTKs. Sunitinib received its first U.S. regulatory approval in 2006 for the treatment of gastrointestinal stromal tumor (GIST) after disease progression on, or intolerance to, imatinib and accelerated approval for the treatment of advanced RCC.[102] Sunitinib demonstrated significant efficacy (prolonged median time to progression) in imatinib-resistant or -intolerant GIST in a randomized phase III trial.[103] The accelerated approval for RCC was based on durable partial responses, with a response rate of 26% to 37%, and a median duration of response of 54 weeks from two phase II, single-arm trials of patients with cytokine-refractory RCC.[104] The accelerated approval was converted to regular approval in 2007 following confirmation of an improvement in PFS and OS in a phase III trial of sunitinib for first-line treatment of patients with treatment-naïve, metastatic RCC.[105,106] In May 2011, the drug received a new indication for the treatment of progressive, well-differentiated pancreatic neuroendocrine tumors (pNET) in patients with unresectable, locally advanced, or metastatic disease. The randomized phase III trial was discontinued early after the independent data monitoring committee observed more serious adverse events and deaths in the placebo group as well as a difference in PFS favoring sunitinib. The median PFS for patients treated with sunitinib was 10.2 months, compared with 5.4 months for patients treated with placebo (HR, 0.427, 95% CI, 0.271 to 0.673], p <0.001).[107] Common adverse effects, including diarrhea, mucositis, asthenia, skin abnormalities, and altered taste, were more common in patients receiving sunitinib. In addition, a decrease in left ventricular ejection fraction and severe hypertension were also more commonly reported in the sunitinib arm. Grade 3 or 4 treatment-emergent adverse events were reported in 56% versus 51% of patients on sunitinib versus placebo, respectively.

Pazopanib

Pazopanib is a second-generation, multitargeted TKI that binds to VEGFR-1, -2, -3, PDGFR-α and -β, c-KIT, and several other key proteins responsible for angiogenesis, tumor growth, and cell survival. Pazopanib exhibited in vivo and in vitro activity against tumor growth, and early clinical trials demonstrated potent antitumor and antiangiogenic activity.[108] A phase III clinical trial in treatment-naïve and cytokine-pretreated patients with advanced and/or metastatic RCC showed a significant improvement in PFS and tumor response compared with placebo,[109] leading to the approval of pazopanib in the United States in October 2009. A recent, randomized phase III trial (COMPARZ) compared the efficacy and safety of pazopanib and sunitinib as first-line therapy involving patients with metastatic RCC and demonstrated that both pazopanib and sunitinib have similar efficacy, but the safety and quality-of-life profiles favor pazopanib.[110] In April 2012, pazopanib was approved for the treatment of patients with metastatic nonadipocytic soft tissue sarcoma who have received prior chemotherapy following a phase III trial that demonstrated a statistically significant improvement in PFS. The median PFS was 4.6 months for patients receiving pazopanib versus 1.6 months for the placebo arm.[111] The drug is generally well tolerated, with the most common adverse events being diarrhea, fatigue, anorexia, hypertension, and hair depigmentation, as well as laboratory abnormalities in elevated aspartate aminotransferase and alanine aminotransferase. Pazopanib has shown clinical activity in a variety of tumors, including breast cancer, thyroid cancer, HCC, and cervical cancer.[112] Ongoing phase II and III trials are further evaluating pazopanib in these malignancies.

Vandetanib

Vandetanib is an oral, small-molecule TKI that inhibits the activity of RET kinase, VEGFR, epidermal growth factor receptor (EGFR), protein tyrosine kinase 6 (BRK), TIE2, members of the ephrin (EPH) receptors kinase family, and members of the Src family of tyrosine kinases.[113] Vandetanib reduced endothelial cell migration, proliferation, survival, and angiogenesis in vitro, and it decreased tumor vessel permeability and inhibited tumor growth and metastasis in vivo. In April 2011, vandetanib received U.S. regulatory approval for the treatment of symptomatic or progressive medullary thyroid cancer (MTC) in patients with unresectable, locally advanced, or metastatic disease. Until the approval of vandetanib, no systemic therapy was approved for the treatment of unresectable MTC, making it the first molecularly targeted agent approved for this disease. Results of a randomized phase III trial of patients with unresectable, locally advanced, or metastatic MTC demonstrated statistically significant and clinically meaningful improvements in PFS for vandetanib compared with placebo (HR, 0.46; 95% CI, 0.31 to 0.69; p <0.001).[114] Common grade 3 and 4 toxicities (>5%) were diarrhea and/or colitis, hypertension and hypertensive crisis, fatigue, hypocalcemia, rash, and corrected QT interval (QTc) prolongation. Given the toxicity profile, which includes QTc prolongation and sudden death, vandetanib is only available through a restricted distribution program. Vandetanib is also the first targeted drug to show evidence of efficacy in a randomized phase II trial in patients with locally advanced or metastatic differentiated thyroid carcinoma,[115] and a phase III trial is currently underway. Early phase studies are also being conducted in solid tumors, including GIST and kidney and pancreatic cancers.

Axitinib

Axitinib is a potent and selective second-generation inhibitor of VEGFR-1, -2, and -3. The in vitro half-maximal inhibitory concentration (IC50) of axitinib is 10-fold lower for the VEGF family of receptors than for other TKIs such as pazopanib, sunitinib, or sorafenib.[116] In January 2012, axitinib received approval for the treatment of advanced RCC after the failure of one prior systemic therapy based on a phase III trial (AXIS) comparing the efficacy and safety of axitinib versus sorafenib as a second-line treatment for metastatic RCC.[117,118] The median PFS was 6.7 months with axitinib compared to 4.7 months with sorafenib (HR, 0.67; 95% CI, 0.54, 0.81; one-sided p <0.0001). This improvement in PFS was greater in the cytokine-pretreated subgroup in comparison with the sunitinib-pretreated subgroup. The most frequent adverse events with axitinib were diarrhea (all grade), hypertension (all grade), fatigue, decreased appetite, nausea, and dysphonia. Moreover, hypertension, nausea, dysphonia, and hypothyroidism were more common with axitinib, whereas palmar–plantar erythrodysesthesia, alopecia, and rash were more frequent with sorafenib. A phase III trial (AGILE) comparing axitinib with sorafenib as first-line therapy in patients with treatment-naïve metastatic RCC demonstrated no significant difference in median PFS between patients treated with axitinib or sorafenib.[119] Additionally, axitinib is being studied as a single agent as well as in combination with chemotherapy across several tumor types including HCC, NSCLC, and pancreatic and thyroid cancers.

Cabozantinib

Cabozantinib (XL184) is a small-molecule TKI with potent activity toward the MET receptor and VEGFR2, as well as a number of other receptor tyrosine kinases, including RET, KIT, AXL, and FLT-3. MET is the only known receptor for hepatocyte growth factor (HGF), and its signaling activity plays a key role in tumorigenic growth, metastasis, and therapeutic resistance. The dysregulated expression and/or activation of MET and HGF have been implicated in the development of numerous human cancers including glioma; melanoma; and hepatocellular, renal, gastric, pancreatic, prostate, ovarian, breast, and lung cancers, and is often correlated with poor prognosis.[120] Recent studies have determined that the MET pathway plays an important role in the development of resistance to VEGF pathway inhibition and that the use of VEGFR inhibitors, such as sunitinib, sorafenib, or a VEGFR2-targeting antibody, can result in the development of an aggressive tumor phenotype characterized by increased invasiveness and metastasis.[121–123] Thus, there is an advantage to targeting both the MET and VEGF pathways to disrupt angiogenesis, tumorigenesis, and cancer progression. In November 2012, cabozantinib received U.S. regulatory approval for progressive metastatic MTC based on the phase III trial that demonstrated a statistically significant PFS prolongation for the cabozantinib-treatment arm.[124] The estimated median PFS was 11.2 months for cabozantinib versus 4.0 months for placebo (HR, 0.28; 95% CI, 0.19 to 0.40; p <0.001). Manageable toxicities included diarrhea, palmar–plantar erythrodysesthesia, decreased weight and appetite, nausea, and fatigue. Cabozantinib has been effective against several solid cancers, including MTC, breast, NSCLC, melanoma, and liver cancer, and is currently being studied in clinical trials in a number of tumor types, with the most significant results observed in the reduction of bone metastatic lesions in castration-resistant prostate cancer.[125]

Regorafenib

Regorafenib is a small-molecule TKI of multiple membrane-bound and intracellular kinases including RET, VEGFR1, VEGFR2, VEGFR3, KIT, PDGFR-α, PDGFR-β, FGFR1, FGFR2, TIE2, DDR2, TrkA, Eph2A, RAF-1, BRAF, BRAFV600E, SAPK2, PTK5, and Abl pathways.[126] Regorafenib is structurally related to sorafenib and differs from the latter by the presence of a fluorine atom in the center phenyl ring, resulting in higher inhibitory potency against various proangiogenic receptors than sorafenib, including VEGFR2 and FGFR1. In September 2012, regorafenib was approved for the treatment of patients with mCRC who have been previously treated with fluoropyrimidine-, oxaliplatin-, and irinotecan-based chemotherapy, with an anti-VEGF therapy, and if KRAS wild type, with an anti-EGFR therapy. The phase III CORRECT trial that resulted in approval of the drug demonstrated a median OS of 6.4 months in the regorafenib group versus 5.0 months in the placebo group (HR, 0.77; 95% CI, 0.64 to 0.94; one-sided p = 0.0052).[127] Regorafenib is the first TKI with survival benefits in mCRC that has progressed after all standard therapies. In February 2013, it received another indication for the treatment of patients with locally advanced, unresectable, or metastatic GIST who have been previously treated with imatinib and sunitinib. This was based on positive findings of the phase III GRID trial that demonstrated a median PFS of 4.8 months for regorafenib and 0.9 months for placebo (HR, 0.27, 95% CI, 0.19 to 0.39; p <0.0001).[128] In both studies, regorafenib provided significant improvements in PFS to highly refractory patient populations who have progressed on standard treatments. The most common adverse events that were grade 3 or higher and related to regorafenib were hand–foot skin reaction, fatigue, diarrhea, hypertension, and rash or desquamation. Its clinical development as a single agent or in combination with standard chemotherapeutic agents in various malignant tumors is ongoing and includes a phase III trial in patients with HCC whose disease has progressed after treatment with sorafenib.

mTOR Inhibitors

The mTOR pathway is a central component of the PI3K/Akt signaling pathway and a regulator of many biologic processes that are essential for angiogenesis, cell proliferation, and metabolism.[129] Inhibition of the mTOR kinase prevents downstream signaling via the Akt pathway, resulting in inhibition of protein translation and cell growth. mTOR plays a key role in angiogenesis and specifically regulates the expression of HIF-1, which is upregulated by the loss of the von Hippel–Lindau gene in RCC. In May 2007, temsirolimus was approved for the treatment of advanced RCC. Efficacy and safety were demonstrated in a phase III study in previously untreated patients (n = 626) with poor risk features of metastatic RCC assigned to one of three treatment arms: IFN-α alone, temsirolimus 25 mg alone, or the combination of temsirolimus (15 mg) and IFN-α.[130] Single-agent temsirolimus was associated with a statistically significant improvement in OS when compared with IFN; the addition of temsirolimus to IFN did not improve OS. The results of the phase III INTORSECT trial compared the efficacy of temsirolimus and sorafenib in the second-line treatment of metastatic RCC after disease progression on sunitinib demonstrated that temsirolimus did not improve survival over sorafenib in the second-line setting.[131] The significant OS difference in favor of sorafenib (stratified HR, 1.31; 95% CI, 1.05 to 1.63; two-sided p = 0.01) suggested that VEGFR inhibition may be a better option than mTOR inhibitors for patients progressing on sunitinib. The most common adverse reactions that occurred were rash, asthenia, mucositis, nausea, edema, and anorexia. Rare, but serious adverse reactions associated with temsirolimus included interstitial lung disease, bowel perforation, and acute renal failure.

Everolimus (RAD001) was approved in March 2009 for patients with advanced RCC whose disease had progressed on VEGFR-targeted therapy (sunitinib or sorafenib). Efficacy was demonstrated in a phase 3 trial that study met its primary endpoint with a median PFS of 4.9 and 1.9 months in the everolimus and placebo arms, respectively (HR, 0.33; p <0.0001).[132] Everolimus is also indicated for subependymal giant cell astrocytoma (SEGA) associated with tuberous sclerosis complex (TSC), renal angiomyolipoma with TSC, progressive neuroendocrine tumors of pancreatic origin, and advanced hormone receptor-positive, HER2-negative breast cancer in combination with exemestane.[133] The most common adverse reactions were stomatitis, infections, asthenia, fatigue, cough, and diarrhea. The most common grade 3/4 adverse reactions were infections, dyspnea, fatigue, stomatitis, dehydration, pneumonitis, abdominal pain, and asthenia. Both temsirolimus and everolimus are currently being evaluated in phase I through III studies of various cancer types. By downregulating HIF-1 in the tumor cell, mTOR inhibitors may complement the effects of TKIs at the level of the EC; thus, the combination of mTOR inhibitors with other targeted agents such as bevacizumab or sorafenib/sunitinib are also being investigated.

On the Horizon: Anti-VEGFR2 Monoclonal Antibody

Ramucirumab (IMC-1121B) is a fully human IgG1 monoclonal antibody that binds with high affinity to the extracellular VEGF-binding domain of VEGFR-2. In a phase III trial (REGARD), ramucirumab monotherapy conferred a statistically significant benefit in OS and PFS compared to placebo in patients with advanced gastric or gastroesophageal junction adenocarcinoma in the second-line setting with an acceptable safety profile.[134] The survival advantage is the first to be elicited by a single-agent biologic treatment in this setting and, based on these findings, the FDA has assigned a priority review designation for ramucirumab. An ongoing phase III trial (RAINBOW) of ramucirumab in combination with chemotherapy as second-line treatment for patients with advanced gastric cancer is currently underway, and preliminary results demonstrated the trial met both its primary (OS) and secondary (PFS) endpoints. In April 2014, the U.S. FDA approved ramucirumab for use as a single agent for the treatment of patients with advanced or metastatic, gastric or gastroesophageal junction adenocarcinoma with disease progression on or after prior treatment with fluoropyrimidine- or platinum-containing chemotherapy. The recommended ramucirumab dose and schedule is 8 mg/kg administered as a 60-minute intravenous infusion every 2 weeks. The drug also marginally improved survival in the second-line treatment of NSCLC in an ongoing phase III (REVEL) trial.

COMBINATION THERAPIES

Tumor angiogenesis is a highly complex process involving multiple growth factors and their receptor signaling pathways. Based on current evidence, with a few exceptions, effective therapy will probably rely on a combinatorial approach that involves targeting multiple pathways simultaneously. However, a recent study has demonstrated that simultaneous inhibition of the VEGF and EGF pathways in combination with chemotherapy shortens rather than prolongs PFS as compared to inhibition of the VEGF pathway alone in combination with chemotherapy.[135] Whether other targeted agents exhibit beneficial effects when combined with VEGF inhibitors remains to be investigated. Moreover, a number of studies have shown that antiangiogenic agents in combination with chemotherapy or radiotherapy result in additive or synergistic effects. Several models have been proposed to explain the mechanism responsible for this potentiation, keying in on the chemosensitizing effects of antiangiogenic therapy.[136] One hypothesis is that antiangiogenic therapy may normalize the tumor vasculature, thus resulting in improved oxygenation, better blood perfusion, and consequently, improved delivery of chemotherapeutic drugs.[137] A second model suggests that chemotherapy delivered at low doses and at close, regular intervals with no extended drug-free break periods preferentially damages ECs in the tumor neovasculature,[138,139] and suppresses circulating endothelial progenitor cells.[140,141] This regimen, also called metronomic chemotherapy, sustains antiangiogenic activity and reduces acute toxicity.[142] Thus, the efficacy of metronomic chemotherapy may increase when administered in combination with specific antiangiogenic drugs. Another model addresses the use of antiangiogenic drugs to slow down tumor cell repopulation between successive cycles of cytotoxic chemotherapy.[143] This model underscores the importance of timing and sequence in achieving the maximal therapeutic benefit from combination therapies. In fact, a preclinical study in murine tumor models demonstrated that the administration of sunitinib markedly reduced chemotherapy-induced bone marrow toxicity, suggesting that the sequential treatment regimen (delivery of antiangiogenics followed by chemotherapy) showed superior survival benefits compared with the simultaneous administration of two drugs.[144] Finally, other mechanisms that might also contribute to the synergism include angiogenesis inhibitor–induced tumor blood vessel regression, the prevention of tumor coopting of vessels from surrounding healthy tissues, and the formation of abnormal vessels in the tumor microenvironment.[145] Nevertheless, it remains a challenge to determine why bevacizumab has proved largely ineffective as a single agent, whereas VEGF RTK inhibitors have repeatedly failed in randomized phase III trials when used in combination with chemotherapy. Furthermore, an additional challenge is to determine the optimal dose and duration of antiangiogenic drugs as well as the impact of drug sequencing in combination regimens. Studies are warranted to delineate the discrepancy of bevacizumab's efficacy in the macrometastatic versus micrometastatic disease settings.[146,147]

BIOMARKERS OF ANTIANGIOGENIC THERAPY

Antiangiogenic therapy has created a need to develop effective biomarkers to assess the activity of these inhibitors. Biomarkers of tumor angiogenesis activity are important to guide clinical development of these agents and to select patients most likely to benefit from this approach. Although there are currently no validated biomarkers for clinically assessing the efficacy of or selecting patients who will respond to antiangiogenic therapies, a number of candidate markers, including tissue, imaging, and circulating biomarkers, are emerging that need to be prospectively validated.[148,149] Several avenues are currently being investigated and include tumor biopsy analysis, microvessel density, noninvasive vascular imaging modalities (positron-emission tomography, dynamic contrast-enhanced magnetic resonance imaging), and measuring circulating biomarkers (levels of angiogenic factors in serum, plasma, urine, or circulating ECs and their precursors).[150–152] Recent research efforts have focused on identifying genetic and toxicity biomarkers to predict which patients will benefit from anti-VEGF/VEGFR therapy and identify patients at risk of adverse events. The existence of VEGF single-nucleotide polymorphisms (SNP) and their association with clinical outcomes may be predictive of patient response to bevacizumab. A recent study identified a locus in VEGFR1 that correlated with increased VEGFR1 expression and poor bevacizumab treatment outcomes.[153] Moreover, a breast cancer study (E2100) reported the VEGF-2578 AA and VEGF-1154 AA genotypes predicted an improved median OS, whereas the VEGF-634 CC and VEGF-1498 TT genotypes predicted protection from grade 3/4 hypertension in the combination-treatment arm.[154] The degree of hypertension can serve as a predictive biomarker of survival in patients after bevacizumab or TKI treatment. Although an association between hypertension and anti-VEGF therapy has been described, the clinical implications of this association and the predictive value of hypertension remains to be validated prospectively. A retrospective analysis of hypertension and efficacy outcomes was conducted in seven large phase III trials (n = 6,486 patients) and, in six of seven studies, early treatment-related blood pressure increase was neither predictive of clinical benefit from bevacizumab nor prognostic for the course of the disease.[155] However, one study (AVF2107g) showed early increased blood pressure was associated with longer PFS and OS. Because genetics play a significant role in modifying the risk of hypertension,[156] it remains to be determined whether polymorphisms in the VEGF/VEGFR pathway may function as potential biomarkers to predict the association between treatment-related hypertension and response to anti-VEGF therapy, as previously implicated in the E2100 trial.[154] Other biomarkers of response include elevated VEGF and placental growth factor levels,[148,152] whereas biomarkers of resistance, including circulating basic fibroblast growth factor, stromal cell-derived factor 1α, and viable circulating endothelial cells, increased when tumors escaped treatment.[157] A first prospective biomarker study (MERiDiAN) in metastatic breast cancer is currently underway to evaluate the impact of bevacizumab in patients stratified for plasma short VEGF-A isoforms. If validated, these findings could help identify which subgroup of patients should receive antiangiogenic therapy and could lead the way to possible future tailoring of individualized antiangiogenic therapy.

RESISTANCE TO ANTIANGIOGENIC THERAPY

Despite a decade of trials with angiogenesis inhibitors, clinical experience reveals that VEGF-targeted therapy often prolongs the survival of cancer patients by only months because tumors elicit evasive resistance.[145,158] Resistance to VEGF inhibitors may be observed in late-stage tumors when tumors regrow during treatment after an initial period of growth suppression from these antiangiogenic agents. This resistance involves the reactivation of tumor angiogenesis and increased expression of other proangiogenic factors. As the disease progresses, it is possible that redundant pathways might be implicated, with VEGF being replaced by other angiogenic pathways, warranting the addition of a second angiogenesis inhibitor that would target these secondary growth factors and/or their activated receptor pathways, or the use of a multitargeted TKI antiangiogenic drug (e.g., sunitinib, sorafenib).

However, resistance to these drugs eventually occurs, implicating the existence of additional pathways mediating resistance to antiangiogenic therapies. Moreover, tumor cells bearing genetic alterations of the $p53$ gene may display a lower apoptosis rate under hypoxic conditions, which might reduce their reliance on vascular supply and, therefore, their responsiveness to antiangiogenic therapy.[159] The selection and overgrowth of tumor-variant cells that are hypoxia resistant and, thus, less dependent[159] on angiogenesis and vasculature remodeling, resulting in vessel stabilization,[160] could also explain the resistance to antiangiogenic drugs. Other possible mechanisms for acquired resistance include tumor vessels becoming less sensitive to antiangiogenic agents, tumor regrowth via rebound revascularization, and vessel cooption.[161-166] Perhaps one of the most intriguing findings is that, although ECs are assumed to be genetically stable, they may under some circumstances harbor genetic abnormalities and thus acquire resistance as well.[167,168]

Recent studies report that VEGF-targeted therapies not only induce primary tumor shrinkage and inhibit tumor progression, but can also initiate mechanisms that increase malignancy to promote tumor invasiveness and metastasis.[122,123,169] These mechanisms of resistance to antiangiogenic therapy involve tumor- and host-mediated pathways and may allow for differential efficacy in different stages of disease progression.[163] Specifically, antiangiogenic drug–resistance mechanisms involve pathways mediated by the tumor, whether intrinsic or acquired in response to therapy or by the host, which is either responding directly to therapy or indirectly to tumoral cues. Taken together, antiangiogenic therapy can enhance tumor invasiveness and metastasis to facilitate and/or accelerate disease in microscopic tumors and, hence, reduce OS benefit. Understanding the mechanisms of resistance, whether intrinsic or acquired, after exposure to antiangiogenic drug treatment is essential for developing strategies that will allow for optimal exploitation of VEGF inhibitors. It is equally important to identify biomarkers of drug resistance and factors mediating this resistance because the development of reliable biomarkers can be invaluable to monitor the development of evasive resistance to angiogenesis inhibitors.

REFERENCES

1. Hanahan D, Weinberg RA. Hallmarks of cancer: the next generation. *Cell* 2011;144:646–674.
2. Ide AG, Baker NH, Warren SL. Vascularization of the Brown Pearce rabbit epithelioma transplant as seen in the transparent ear chamger. *Am J Roentgenol* 1939;42:891–899.
3. Algire GH, Chalkley HW, Legallais FY, et al. Vascular reactions of normal and malignant tissues in vivo. I. Vascular reactions of mice to wounds and to normal and neoplastic transplants. *J Natl Cancer Inst* 1945;6:73–85.
4. Folkman J, Merler E, Abernathy C, et al. Isolation of a tumor factor responsible for angiogenesis. *J Exp Med* 1971;133:275–288.
5. Folkman J. Tumor angiogenesis: therapeutic implications. *N Engl J Med* 1971;285:1182–1186.
6. Papetti M, Herman IM. Mechanisms of normal and tumor-derived angiogenesis. *Am J Physiol Cell Physiol* 2002;282:C947–C970.
7. Hanahan D, Folkman J. Patterns and emerging mechanisms of the angiogenic switch during tumorigenesis. *Cell* 1996;86:353–364.
8. Black WC, Welch HG. Advances in diagnostic imaging and overestimations of disease prevalence and the benefits of therapy. *N Engl J Med* 1993;328:1237–1243.
9. Folkman J, Kalluri R. Cancer without disease. *Nature* 2004;427:787.
10. Weidner N, Semple JP, Welch WR, et al. Tumor angiogenesis and metastasis—correlation in invasive breast carcinoma. *N Engl J Med* 1991;324:1–8.
11. Holmgren L, O'Reilly MS, Folkman J. Dormancy of micrometastases: balanced proliferation and apoptosis in the presence of angiogenesis suppression. *Nat Med* 1995;1:149–153.
12. Naumov GN, Bender E, Zurakowski D, et al. A model of human tumor dormancy: an angiogenic switch from the nonangiogenic phenotype. *J Natl Cancer Inst* 2006;98:316–325.
13. Udagawa T, Fernandez A, Achilles EG, et al. Persistence of microscopic human cancers in mice: alterations in the angiogenic balance accompanies loss of tumor dormancy. *Faseb J* 2002;16:1361–1370.
14. Holash J, Maisonpierre PC, Compton D, et al. Vessel cooption, regression, and growth in tumors mediated by angiopoietins and VEGF. *Science* 1999;284:1994–1998.
15. Relf M, LeJeune S, Scott PA, et al. Expression of the angiogenic factors vascular endothelial cell growth factor, acidic and basic fibroblast growth factor, tumor growth factor beta-1, platelet-derived endothelial cell growth factor, placenta growth factor, and pleiotrophin in human primary breast cancer and its relation to angiogenesis. *Cancer Res* 1997;57:963–969.
16. Carmeliet P, Dor Y, Herbert JM, et al. Role of HIF-1alpha in hypoxia-mediated apoptosis, cell proliferation and tumour angiogenesis. *Nature* 1998;394:485–490.
17. Folkman J. Endogenous angiogenesis inhibitors. *Apmis* 2004;112:496–507.
18. Nyberg P, Xie L, Kalluri R. Endogenous inhibitors of angiogenesis. *Cancer Res* 2005;65:3967–3979.
19. Rak J, Yu JL. Oncogenes and tumor angiogenesis: the question of vascular "supply" and vascular "demand". *Semin Cancer Biol* 2004;14:93–104.
20. Bottos A, Bardelli A. Oncogenes and angiogenesis: a way to personalize antiangiogenic therapy? *Cell Mol Life Sci* 2013;70:4131–4140.
21. Rak J, Yu JL, Klement G, et al. Oncogenes and angiogenesis: signaling three-dimensional tumor growth. *J Investig Dermatol Symp Proc* 2000;5:24–33.
22. Langer R, Brem H, Falterman K, et al. Isolations of a cartilage factor that inhibits tumor neovascularization. *Science* 1976;193:70–72.
23. Langer R, Conn H, Vacanti J, et al. Control of tumor growth in animals by infusion of an angiogenesis inhibitor. *Proc Natl Acad Sci U S A* 1980;77:4331–4335.
24. Ribatti D. Endogenous inhibitors of angiogenesis: a historical review. *Leuk Res* 2009;33:638–644.
25. Folkman J. Antiangiogenesis in cancer therapy—endostatin and its mechanisms of action. *Exp Cell Res* 2006;312:594–607.
26. Karamouzis MV, Moschos SJ. The use of endostatin in the treatment of solid tumors. *Expert Opin Biol Ther* 2009;9:641–648.
27. Lawler J. Thrombospondin-1 as an endogenous inhibitor of angiogenesis and tumor growth. *J Cell Mol Med* 2002;6:1–12.
28. Maeshima Y, Manfredi M, Reimer C, et al. Identification of the anti-angiogenic site within vascular basement membrane-derived tumstatin. *J Biol Chem* 2001;276:15240–15248.
29. Kerbel RS. Vasohibin: the feedback on a new inhibitor of angiogenesis. *J Clin Invest* 2004;114:884–886.
30. Sato Y. The vasohibin family: a novel family for angiogenesis regulation. *J Biochem* 2013;153:5–11.

31. Noguera-Troise I, Daly C, Papadopoulos NJ, et al. Blockade of Dll4 inhibits tumour growth by promoting non-productive angiogenesis. *Nature* 2006;444:1032–1037.
32. Ridgway J, Zhang G, Wu Y, et al. Inhibition of Dll4 signalling inhibits tumour growth by deregulating angiogenesis. *Nature* 2006;444:1083–1087.
33. Kuhnert F, Kirshner JR, Thurston G. Dll4-Notch signaling as a therapeutic target in tumor angiogenesis. *Vasc Cell* 2011;3:20.
34. Sund M, Hamano Y, Sugimoto H, et al. Function of endogenous inhibitors of angiogenesis as endothelium-specific tumor suppressors. *Proc Natl Acad Sci U S A* 2005;102:2934–2939.
35. Dameron KM, Volpert OV, Tainsky MA, et al. Control of angiogenesis in fibroblasts by p53 regulation of thrombospondin-1. *Science* 1994;265:1582–1584.
36. Zhang L, Yu D, Hu M, et al. Wild-type p53 suppresses angiogenesis in human leiomyosarcoma and synovial sarcoma by transcriptional suppression of vascular endothelial growth factor expression. *Cancer Res* 2000;60:3655–3661.
37. Sherif ZA, Nakai S, Pirollo KF, et al. Downmodulation of bFGF-binding protein expression following restoration of p53 function. *Cancer Gene Ther* 2001;8:771–782.
38. Ravi R, Mookerjee B, Bhujwalla ZM, et al. Regulation of tumor angiogenesis by p53 induced degradation of hypoxia inducible factor 1alpha. *Genes Dev* 2000;14:34–44.
39. Farhang Ghahremani M, Goossens S, Nittner D, et al. p53 promotes VEGF expression and angiogenesis in the absence of an intact p21-Rb pathway. *Cell Death Differ* 2013;20:888–897.
40. Teodoro JG, Parker AE, Zhu X, et al. p53-mediated inhibition of angiogenesis through up-regulation of a collagen prolyl hydroxylase. *Science* 2006;313:968–971.
41. Folkman J. Tumor suppression by p53 is mediated in part by the antiangiogenic activity of endostatin and tumstatin. *Sci STKE* 2006;2006:pe35.
42. Brouty-Boye D, Zetter BR. Inhibition of cell motility by interferon. *Science* 1980;208:516–518.
43. Dvorak HF, Gresser I. Microvascular injury in pathogenesis of interferon-induced necrosis of subcutaneous tumors in mice. *J Natl Cancer Inst* 1989;81:497–502.
44. Sidky YA, Borden EC. Inhibition of angiogenesis by interferons: effects on tumor- and lymphocyte-induced vascular responses. *Cancer Res* 1987;47:5155–5161.
45. Taylor S, Folkman J. Protamine is an inhibitor of angiogenesis. *Nature* 1982;297:307–312.
46. Crum R, Szabo S, Folkman J. A new class of steroids inhibits angiogenesis in the presence of heparin or a heparin fragment. *Science* 1985;230:1375–1378.
47. Ingber D, Fujita T, Kishimoto S, et al. Synthetic analogues of fumagillin that inhibit angiogenesis and suppress tumour growth. *Nature* 1990;348:555–557.
48. Kerbel RS. Inhibition of tumor angiogenesis as a strategy to circumvent acquired resistance to anti-cancer therapeutic agents. *Bioessays* 1991;13:31–36.
49. Folkman J. Angiogenesis: an organizing principle for drug discovery? *Nat Rev Drug Discov* 2007;6:273–286.
50. D'Amato RJ, Loughnan MS, Flynn E, et al. Thalidomide is an inhibitor of angiogenesis. *Proc Natl Acad Sci U S A* 1994;91:4082–4085.
51. Bauer KS, Dixon SC, Figg WD. Inhibition of angiogenesis by thalidomide requires metabolic activation, which is species-dependent. *Biochem Pharmacol* 1998;55:1827–1834.
52. Figg WD. The 2005 Leon I. Goldberg Young Investigator Award Lecture: development of thalidomide as an angiogenesis inhibitor for the treatment of androgen-independent prostate cancer. *Clin Pharmacol Ther* 2006;79:1–8.
53. Kenyon BM, Browne F, D'Amato RJ. Effects of thalidomide and related metabolites in a mouse corneal model of neovascularization. *Exp Eye Res* 1997;64:971–978.
54. Price DK, Ando Y, Kruger EA, et al. 5'-OH-thalidomide, a metabolite of thalidomide, inhibits angiogenesis. *Ther Drug Monit* 2002;24:104–110.
55. Dredge K, Marriott JB, Macdonald CD, et al. Novel thalidomide analogues display anti-angiogenic activity independently of immunomodulatory effects. *Br J Cancer* 2002;87:1166–1172.
56. Gupta D, Treon SP, Shima Y, et al. Adherence of multiple myeloma cells to bone marrow stromal cells upregulates vascular endothelial growth factor secretion: therapeutic applications. *Leukemia* 2001;15:1950–1961.
57. Ng SS, Gutschow M, Weiss M, et al. Antiangiogenic activity of N-substituted and tetrafluorinated thalidomide analogues. *Cancer Res* 2003;63:3189–3194.
58. Zhang H, Vakil V, Braunstein M, et al. Circulating endothelial progenitor cells in multiple myeloma: implications and significance. *Blood* 2005;105:3286–3294.
59. De Sanctis JB, Mijares M, Suarez A, et al. Pharmacological properties of thalidomide and its analogues. *Recent Pat Inflamm Allergy Drug Discov* 2010;4:144–148.
60. Ferrara N, Gerber HP, LeCouter J. The biology of VEGF and its receptors. *Nat Med* 2003;9:669–676.
61. Lindahl P, Johansson BR, Leveen P, et al. Pericyte loss and microaneurysm formation in PDGF-B-deficient mice. *Science* 1997;277:242–245.
62. Oliner J, Min H, Leal J, et al. Suppression of angiogenesis and tumor growth by selective inhibition of angiopoietin-2. *Cancer Cell* 2004;6:507–516.
63. Fingleton B. MMPs as therapeutic targets—still a viable option? *Semin Cell Dev Biol* 2008;19:61–68.
64. Roy R, Yang J, Moses MA. Matrix metalloproteinases as novel biomarkers and potential therapeutic targets in human cancer. *J Clin Oncol* 2009;27:5287–5297.
65. Shi ZG, Li JP, Shi LL, et al. An updated patent therapeutic agents targeting MMPs. *Recent Pat Anticancer Drug Discov* 2012;7:74–101.
66. Gialeli C, Theocharis AD, Karamanos NK. Roles of matrix metalloproteinases in cancer progression and their pharmacological targeting. *FEBS J* 2011;278:16–27.

67. Nikolopoulos SN, Blaikie P, Yoshioka T, et al. Integrin beta4 signaling promotes tumor angiogenesis. *Cancer Cell* 2004;6:471–483.
68. Bradley DA, Daignault S, Ryan CJ, et al. Cilengitide (EMD 121974, NSC 707544) in asymptomatic metastatic castration resistant prostate cancer patients: a randomized phase II trial by the prostate cancer clinical trials consortium. *Invest New Drugs* 2011;29:1432–1440.
69. Desgrosellier JS, Cheresh DA. Integrins in cancer: biological implications and therapeutic opportunities. *Nat Rev Cancer* 2010;10:9–22.
70. Hersey P, Sosman J, O'Day S, et al. A randomized phase 2 study of etaracizumab, a monoclonal antibody against integrin alpha(v)beta(3), + or − dacarbazine in patients with stage IV metastatic melanoma. *Cancer* 2010;116:1526–1534.
71. Heidenreich A, Rawal SK, Szkarlat K, et al. A randomized, double-blind, multicenter, phase 2 study of a human monoclonal antibody to human alphanu Integrins (intetumumab) in combination with docetaxel and prednisone for the first-line treatment of patients with metastatic castration-resistant prostate cancer. *Ann Oncol* 2013;24:329–336.
72. O'Day S, Pavlick A, Loquai C, et al. A randomised, phase II study of intetumumab, an anti-alphav-integrin mAb, alone and with dacarbazine in stage IV melanoma. *Br J Cancer* 2011;105:346–352.
73. Stupp R, Hegi M, Gorlia T, et al. Standard chemoradiotherapy ± cilengitide in newly diagnosed glioblastoma (GBM): updated results and subgroup analyses of the international randomized phase III CENTRIC trial (EORTC trial #26071-22072/Canadian Brain Tumor Consortium). Program and abstracts presented at: 2013 European Cancer Congress; 2013; Amsterdam.
74. Ellis LM, Hicklin DJ. VEGF-targeted therapy: mechanisms of anti-tumour activity. *Nat Rev Cancer* 2008;8:579–591.
75. Hurwitz H, Fehrenbacher L, Novotny W, et al. Bevacizumab plus irinotecan, fluorouracil, and leucovorin for metastatic colorectal cancer. *N Engl J Med* 2004;350:2335–2342.
76. Bennouna J, Sastre J, Arnold D, et al. Continuation of bevacizumab after first progression in metastatic colorectal cancer (ML18147): a randomised phase 3 trial. *Lancet Oncol* 2013;14:29–37.
77. Allegra CJ, Yothers G, O'Connell MJ, et al. Phase III trial assessing bevacizumab in stages II and III carcinoma of the colon: results of NSABP protocol C-08. *J Clin Oncol* 2011;29:11–16.
78. de Gramont A, Van Cutsem E, Schmoll HJ, et al. Bevacizumab plus oxaliplatin-based chemotherapy as adjuvant treatment for colon cancer (AVANT): a phase 3 randomised controlled trial. *Lancet Oncol* 2012;13:1225–1233.
79. Sandler A, Gray R, Perry MC, et al. Paclitaxel-carboplatin alone or with bevacizumab for non-small-cell lung cancer. *N Engl J Med* 2006;355:2542–2550.
80. Miles DW, Chan A, Dirix LY, et al. Phase III study of bevacizumab plus docetaxel compared with placebo plus docetaxel for the first-line treatment of human epidermal growth factor receptor 2-negative metastatic breast cancer. *J Clin Oncol* 2010;28:3239–3247.
81. Robert NJ, Dieras V, Glaspy J, et al. RIBBON-1: randomized, double-blind, placebo-controlled, phase III trial of chemotherapy with or without bevacizumab for first-line treatment of human epidermal growth factor receptor 2-negative, locally recurrent or metastatic breast cancer. *J Clin Oncol* 2011;29:1252–1260.
82. Brufsky AM, Hurvitz S, Perez E, et al. RIBBON-2: a randomized, double-blind, placebo-controlled, phase III trial evaluating the efficacy and safety of bevacizumab in combination with chemotherapy for second-line treatment of human epidermal growth factor receptor 2-negative metastatic breast cancer. *J Clin Oncol* 2011;29:4286–4293.
83. Cohen MH, Shen YL, Keegan P, et al. FDA drug approval summary: bevacizumab (Avastin) as treatment of recurrent glioblastoma multiforme. *Oncologist* 2009;14:1131–1138.
84. Soffietti R, Trevisan E, Ruda R. What have we learned from trials on antiangiogenic agents in glioblastoma? *Expert Rev Neurother* 2014;14:1–3.
85. Escudier B, Pluzanska A, Koralewski P, et al. Bevacizumab plus interferon alfa-2a for treatment of metastatic renal cell carcinoma: a randomised, double-blind phase III trial. *Lancet* 2007;370:2103–2111.
86. Rini BI, Halabi S, Rosenberg JE, et al. Bevacizumab plus interferon alfa compared with interferon alfa monotherapy in patients with metastatic renal cell carcinoma: CALGB 90206. *J Clin Oncol* 2008;26:5422–5428.
87. Escudier B, Bellmunt J, Negrier S, et al. Phase III trial of bevacizumab plus interferon alfa-2a in patients with metastatic renal cell carcinoma (AVOREN): final analysis of overall survival. *J Clin Oncol* 2010;28:2144–2150.
88. Rini BI, Halabi S, Rosenberg JE, et al. Phase III trial of bevacizumab plus interferon alfa versus interferon alfa monotherapy in patients with metastatic renal cell carcinoma: final results of CALGB 90206. *J Clin Oncol* 2010;28:2137–2143.
89. Hurwitz H, Saini S. Bevacizumab in the treatment of metastatic colorectal cancer: safety profile and management of adverse events. *Semin Oncol* 2006;33:S26–S34.
90. Chen HX, Cleck JN. Adverse effects of anticancer agents that target the VEGF pathway. *Nat Rev Clin Oncol* 2009;6:465–477.
91. Ranpura V, Hapani S, Wu S. Treatment-related mortality with bevacizumab in cancer patients: a meta analysis. *JAMA* 2011;305:487–494.
92. Holash J, Davis S, Papadopoulos N, et al. VEGF-Trap: a VEGF blocker with potent antitumor effects. *Proc Natl Acad Sci U S A* 2002;99:11393–11398.
93. Papadopoulos N, Martin J, Ruan Q, et al. Binding and neutralization of vascular endothelial growth factor (VEGF) and related ligands by VEGF Trap, ranibizumab and bevacizumab. *Angiogenesis* 2012;15:171–185.
94. Gaya A, Tse V. A preclinical and clinical review of aflibercept for the management of cancer. *Cancer Treat Rev* 2012;38:484–493.

95. Van Cutsem E, Tabernero J, Lakomy R, et al. Addition of aflibercept to fluorouracil, leucovorin, and irinotecan improves survival in a phase III randomized trial in patients with metastatic colorectal cancer previously treated with an oxaliplatin-based regimen. *J Clin Oncol* 2012;30:3499–3506.
96. Wilhelm SM, Carter C, Tang L, et al. BAY 43-9006 exhibits broad spectrum oral antitumor activity and targets the RAF/MEK/ERK pathway and receptor tyrosine kinases involved in tumor progression and angiogenesis. *Cancer Res* 2004;64:7099–7109.
97. Escudier B, Eisen T, Stadler WM, et al. Sorafenib in advanced clear-cell renal-cell carcinoma. *N Engl J Med* 2007;356:125–134.
98. Escudier B, Eisen T, Stadler WM, et al. Sorafenib for treatment of renal cell carcinoma: Final efficacy and safety results of the phase III treatment approaches in renal cancer global evaluation trial. *J Clin Oncol* 2009;27:3312–3318.
99. Llovet JM, Ricci S, Mazzaferro V, et al. Sorafenib in advanced hepatocellular carcinoma. *N Engl J Med* 2008;359:378–390.
100. Brose MS, Nutting C, Jarzab B, et al. Sorafenib in locally advanced or metastatic patients with radioactive iodine refractory differentiated thyroid cancer: the phase III DECISION trial. *J Clin Oncol* 2013;31.
101. Veronese ML, Mosenkis A, Flaherty KT, et al. Mechanisms of hypertension associated with BAY 43-9006. *J Clin Oncol* 2006;24:1363–1369.
102. Goodman VL, Rock EP, Dagher R, et al. Approval summary: sunitinib for the treatment of imatinib refractory or intolerant gastrointestinal stromal tumors and advanced renal cell carcinoma. *Clin Cancer Res* 2007;13:1367–1373.
103. Demetri GD, van Oosterom AT, Garrett CR, et al. Efficacy and safety of sunitinib in patients with advanced gastrointestinal stromal tumour after failure of imatinib: a randomised controlled trial. *Lancet* 2006;368:1329–1338.
104. Motzer RJ, Michaelson MD, Redman BG, et al. Activity of SU11248, a multitargeted inhibitor of vascular endothelial growth factor receptor and platelet-derived growth factor receptor, in patients with metastatic renal cell carcinoma. *J Clin Oncol* 2006;24:16–24.
105. Motzer RJ, Hutson TE, Tomczak P, et al. Sunitinib versus interferon alfa in metastatic renal-cell carcinoma. *N Engl J Med* 2007;356:115–124.
106. Motzer RJ, Hutson TE, Tomczak P, et al. Overall survival and updated results for sunitinib compared with interferon alfa in patients with metastatic renal cell carcinoma. *J Clin Oncol* 2009;27:3584–3590.
107. Raymond E, Dahan L, Raoul JL, et al. Sunitinib malate for the treatment of pancreatic neuroendocrine tumors. *N Engl J Med* 2011;364:501–513.
108. Kumar R, Knick VB, Rudolph SK, et al. Pharmacokinetic-pharmacodynamic correlation from mouse to human with pazopanib, a multikinase angiogenesis inhibitor with potent antitumor and antiangiogenic activity. *Mol Cancer Ther* 2007;6:2012–2021.
109. Sternberg CN, Davis ID, Mardiak J, et al. Pazopanib in locally advanced or metastatic renal cell carcinoma: results of a randomized phase III trial. *J Clin Oncol* 2010;28:1061–1068.
110. Motzer RJ, Hutson TE, Cella D, et al. Pazopanib versus sunitinib in metastatic renal-cell carcinoma. *N Engl J Med* 2013;369:722–731.
111. van der Graaf WT, Blay JY, Chawla SP, et al. Pazopanib for metastatic soft-tissue sarcoma (PALETTE): a randomised, double-blind, placebo-controlled phase 3 trial. *Lancet* 2012;379:1879–1886.
112. Schutz FA, Choueiri TK, Sternberg CN. Pazopanib: Clinical development of a potent anti-angiogenic drug. *Crit Rev Oncol Hematol* 2011;77:163–171.
113. Thornton K, Kim G, Maher VE, et al. Vandetanib for the treatment of symptomatic or progressive medullary thyroid cancer in patients with unresectable locally advanced or metastatic disease: U.S. Food and Drug Administration drug approval summary. *Clin Cancer Res* 2012;18:3722–3730.
114. Wells SA, Jr., Robinson BG, Gagel RF, et al. Vandetanib in patients with locally advanced or metastatic medullary thyroid cancer: a randomized, double-blind phase III trial. *J Clin Oncol* 2012;30:134–141.
115. Leboulleux S, Bastholt L, Krause T, et al. Vandetanib in locally advanced or metastatic differentiated thyroid cancer: a randomised, double-blind, phase 2 trial. *Lancet Oncol* 2012;13:897–905.
116. Gross-Goupil M, Francois L, Quivy A, et al. Axitinib: a review of its safety and efficacy in the treatment of adults with advanced renal cell carcinoma. *Clin Med Insights Oncol* 2013;7:269–277.
117. Rini BI, Escudier B, Tomczak P, et al. Comparative effectiveness of axitinib versus sorafenib in advanced renal cell carcinoma (AXIS): a randomised phase 3 trial. *Lancet* 2011;378:1931–1939.
118. Motzer RJ, Escudier B, Tomczak P, et al. Axitinib versus sorafenib as second-line treatment for advanced renal cell carcinoma: overall survival analysis and updated results from a randomised phase 3 trial. *Lancet Oncol* 2013;14:552–562.
119. Hutson TE, Lesovoy V, Al-Shukri S, et al. Axitinib versus sorafenib as first-line therapy in patients with metastatic renal-cell carcinoma: a randomised open-label phase 3 trial. *Lancet Oncol* 2013;14:1287–1294.
120. Graveel CR, Tolbert D, Vande Woude GF. MET: a critical player in tumorigenesis and therapeutic target. *Cold Spring Harb Perspect Biol* 2013;5.
121. Shojaei F, Lee JH, Simmons BH, et al. HGF/c-Met acts as an alternative angiogenic pathway in sunitinib-resistant tumors. *Cancer Res* 2010;70:10090–10100.
122. Ebos JM, Lee CR, Cruz-Munoz W, et al. Accelerated metastasis after short-term treatment with a potent inhibitor of tumor angiogenesis. *Cancer Cell* 2009;15:232–239.
123. Paez-Ribes M, Allen E, Hudock J, et al. Antiangiogenic therapy elicits malignant progression of tumors to increased local invasion and distant metastasis. *Cancer Cell* 2009;15:220–231.
124. Elisei R, Schlumberger MJ, Muller SP, et al. Cabozantinib in progressive medullary thyroid cancer. *J Clin Oncol* 2013;31:3639–3646.
125. Smith DC, Smith MR, Sweeney C, et al. Cabozantinib in patients with advanced prostate cancer: results of a phase II randomized discontinuation trial. *J Clin Oncol* 2013;31:412–429.
126. Strumberg D, Schultheis B. Regorafenib for cancer. *Expert Opin Investig Drugs* 2012;21:879–889.
127. Grothey A, Van Cutsem E, Sobrero A, et al. Regorafenib monotherapy for previously treated metastatic colorectal cancer (CORRECT): an international, multicentre, randomised, placebo-controlled, phase 3 trial. *Lancet* 2013;381:303–312.
128. Demetri GD, Reichardt P, Kang YK, et al. Efficacy and safety of regorafenib for advanced gastrointestinal stromal tumours after failure of imatinib and sunitinib (GRID): an international, multicentre, randomised, placebo-controlled, phase 3 trial. *Lancet* 2013;381:295–302.
129. Gibbons JJ, Abraham RT, Yu K. Mammalian target of rapamycin: discovery of rapamycin reveals a signaling pathway important for normal and cancer cell growth. *Semin Oncol* 2009;36 Suppl 3:S3–S17.
130. Hudes G, Carducci M, Tomczak P, et al. Temsirolimus, interferon alfa, or both for advanced renal-cell carcinoma. *N Engl J Med* 2007;356:2271–2281.
131. Hutson TE, Escudier B, Esteban E, et al. Randomized phase III trial of temsirolimus versus sorafenib as second-line therapy after sunitinib in patients with metastatic renal cell carcinoma. *J Clin Oncol* 2014;32:760–767.
132. Motzer RJ, Escudier B, Oudard S, et al. Efficacy of everolimus in advanced renal cell carcinoma: a double-blind, randomised, placebo-controlled phase III trial. *Lancet* 2008;372:449–456.
133. Lebwohl D, Anak O, Sahmoud T, et al. Development of everolimus, a novel oral mTOR inhibitor, across a spectrum of diseases. *Ann N Y Acad Sci* 2013;1291:14–32.
134. Fuchs CS, Tomasek J, Yong CJ, et al. Ramucirumab monotherapy for previously treated advanced gastric or gastro-oesophageal junction adenocarcinoma (REGARD): an international, randomised, multicentre, placebo-controlled, phase 3 trial. *Lancet* 2014;383:31–39.
135. Tol J, Koopman M, Cats A, et al. Chemotherapy, bevacizumab, and cetuximab in metastatic colorectal cancer. *N Engl J Med* 2009;360:563–572.
136. Kerbel RS. Antiangiogenic therapy: a universal chemosensitization strategy for cancer? *Science* 2006;312:1171–1175.
137. Jain RK. Normalization of tumor vasculature: an emerging concept in antiangiogenic therapy. *Science* 2005;307:58–62.
138. Browder T, Butterfield CE, Kraling BM, et al. Antiangiogenic scheduling of chemotherapy improves efficacy against experimental drug-resistant cancer. *Cancer Res* 2000;60:1878–1886.
139. Klement G, Baruchel S, Rak J, et al. Continuous low-dose therapy with vinblastine and VEGF receptor-2 antibody induces sustained tumor regression without overt toxicity. *J Clin Invest* 2000;105:R15–R24.
140. Bertolini F, Paul S, Mancuso P, et al. Maximum tolerable dose and low-dose metronomic chemotherapy have opposite effects on the mobilization and viability of circulating endothelial progenitor cells. *Cancer Res* 2003;63:4342–4346.
141. Mancuso P, Colleoni M, Calleri A, et al. Circulating endothelial-cell kinetics and viability predict survival in breast cancer patients receiving metronomic chemotherapy. *Blood* 2006;108:452–459.
142. Kerbel RS, Kamen BA. The anti-angiogenesis basis of metronomic chemotherapy. *Nat Rev Cancer* 2004;4:423–436.
143. Hudis CA. Clinical implications of antiangiogenic therapies. *Oncology (Williston Park)* 2005;19:26–31.
144. Zhang D, Hedlund EM, Lim S, et al. Antiangiogenic agents significantly improve survival in tumor-bearing mice by increasing tolerance to chemotherapy-induced toxicity. *Proc Natl Acad Sci U S A* 2011;108:4117–4122.
145. Kerbel RS. Tumor angiogenesis. *N Engl J Med* 2008;358:2039–2049.
146. Mountzios G, Pentheroudakis G, Carmeliet P. Bevacizumab and micrometastases: Revisiting the preclinical and clinical rollercoaster. *Pharmacol Ther* 2014;141:117–124.
147. Ebos JM, Kerbel RS. Antiangiogenic therapy: impact on invasion, disease progression, and metastasis. *Nat Rev Clin Oncol* 2011;8:210–221.
148. Jain RK, Duda DG, Willett CG, et al. Biomarkers of response and resistance to antiangiogenic therapy. *Nat Rev Clin Oncol* 2009;6:327–338.
149. Murukesh N, Dive C, Jayson GC. Biomarkers of angiogenesis and their role in the development of VEGF inhibitors. *Br J Cancer* 2010;102:8–18.
150. Davis DW, McConkey DJ, Abbruzzese JL, et al. Surrogate markers in antiangiogenesis clinical trials. *Br J Cancer* 2003;89:8–14.
151. Wehland M, Bauer J, Magnusson NE, et al. Biomarkers for anti-angiogenic therapy in cancer. *Int J Mol Sci* 2013;14:9338–9364.
152. Lambrechts D, Lenz HJ, de Haas S, et al. Markers of response for the antiangiogenic agent bevacizumab. *J Clin Oncol* 2013;31:1219–1230.
153. Lambrechts D, Claes B, Delmar P, et al. VEGF pathway genetic variants as biomarkers of treatment outcome with bevacizumab: an analysis of data from the AViTA and AVOREN randomised trials. *Lancet Oncol* 2012;13:724–733.
154. Schneider BP, Wang M, Radovich M, et al. Association of vascular endothelial growth factor and vascular endothelial growth factor receptor-2 genetic polymorphisms with outcome in a trial of paclitaxel compared with paclitaxel plus bevacizumab in advanced breast cancer: ECOG 2100. *J Clin Oncol* 2008;26:4672–4678.
155. Hurwitz HI, Douglas PS, Middleton JP, et al. Analysis of early hypertension and clinical outcome with bevacizumab: results from seven phase III studies. *Oncologist* 2013;18:273–280.
156. Levy D, Ehret GB, Rice K, et al. Genome-wide association study of blood pressure and hypertension. *Nat Genet* 2009;41:677–687.

157. Batchelor TT, Sorensen AG, di Tomaso E, et al. AZD2171, a pan-VEGF receptor tyrosine kinase inhibitor, normalizes tumor vasculature and alleviates edema in glioblastoma patients. *Cancer Cell* 2007;11:83–95.
158. Sennino B, McDonald DM. Controlling escape from angiogenesis inhibitors. *Nat Rev Cancer* 2012;12:699–709.
159. Yu JL, Rak JW, Coomber BL, et al. Effect of p53 status on tumor response to antiangiogenic therapy. *Science* 2002;295:1526–1528.
160. Glade Bender J, Cooney EM, Kandel JJ, et al. Vascular remodeling and clinical resistance to antiangiogenic cancer therapy. *Drug Resist Updat* 2004;7:289–300.
161. Bergers G, Hanahan D. Modes of resistance to anti-angiogenic therapy. *Nat Rev Cancer* 2008;8:592–603.
162. Crawford Y, Ferrara N. Tumor and stromal pathways mediating refractoriness/resistance to anti-angiogenic therapies. *Trends Pharmacol Sci* 2009;30:624–630.
163. Ebos JM, Lee CR, Kerbel RS. Tumor and host-mediated pathways of resistance and disease progression in response to antiangiogenic therapy. *Clin Cancer Res* 2009;15:5020–5025.
164. Kerbel RS, Yu J, Tran J, et al. Possible mechanisms of acquired resistance to anti-angiogenic drugs: implications for the use of combination therapy approaches. *Cancer Metastasis Rev* 2001;20:79–86.
165. Shojaei F, Ferrara N. Role of the microenvironment in tumor growth and in refractoriness/resistance to anti-angiogenic therapies. *Drug Resist Updat* 2008;11:219–230.
166. Sweeney CJ, Miller KD, Sledge GW Jr. Resistance in the anti-angiogenic era: nay-saying or a word of caution? *Trends Mol Med* 2003;9:24–29.
167. Hida K, Hida Y, Amin DN, et al. Tumor-associated endothelial cells with cytogenetic abnormalities. *Cancer Res* 2004;64:8249–8255.
168. Streubel B, Chott A, Huber D, et al. Lymphoma-specific genetic aberrations in microvascular endothelial cells in B-cell lymphomas. *N Engl J Med* 2004;351:250–259.
169. Loges S, Mazzone M, Hohensinner P, et al. Silencing or fueling metastasis with VEGF inhibitors: antiangiogenesis revisited. *Cancer Cell* 2009;15:167–170.

29 Monoclonal Antibodies

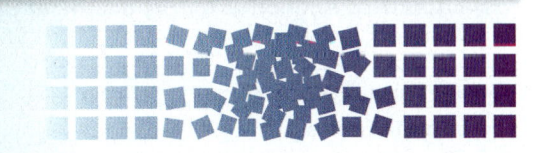

Hossein Borghaei, Matthew K. Robinson, Gregory P. Adams, and Louis M. Weiner

INTRODUCTION

Antibody-based therapeutics are important components of the cancer therapeutic armamentarium. Early antibody therapy studies attempted to explicitly target cancers based on the structural and biologic properties that distinguish neoplastic cells from their normal counterparts. The immunogenicity and inefficient effector functions of the first-generation murine monoclonal antibodies (MAb) that were evaluated in clinical trials limited their effectiveness.[1–3] Patients developed human antimouse antibody (HAMA) responses against the therapeutic agents that rapidly cleared it from the body and limited the number of times the therapy could be administered. The development of engineered chimeric, humanized, and fully human MAbs has identified a number of important and useful applications for antibody-based cancer therapy. Currently, the U.S. Food and Drug Administration (FDA) has approved 14 MAbs and MAb-conjugates for the treatment of cancer (Table 29.1) and many more are under evaluation in late-stage clinical trials.[4] Antibodies provide an important means by which to exploit the immune system by specifically recognizing and directing antitumor responses.

Antibodies are produced by B cells and arise in response to exposures to a variety of structures, termed antigens, as a result of a series of recombinations of V, D, and J germline genes. Immunoglobulin-G (IgG) molecules are most commonly employed as the working backbones of current therapeutic monoclonal antibodies, although various other isotypes of antibodies have specialized functions (e.g., IgA molecules play important roles in mucosal immunity, IgE molecules are involved in anaphylaxis). The advent of hybridoma technology by Kohler and Milstein[5] made it possible to produce large quantities of antibodies with high purity and monospecificity for a single binding region (epitope) on an antigen.

The mechanisms that antibody-based therapeutics employ to elicit antitumor effects include focusing components of the patient's immune system to attack tumor cells[6,7] and methods to alter signal transduction pathways that drive tumor progression.[8,9] Antibody-based conjugates employ the targeting specificity of antibodies to deliver toxic compounds, such as chemotherapeutics, specifically to the tumor sites.

IMMUNOGLOBULIN STRUCTURE

Structural and Functional Domains

An IgG molecule is typically divided into three domains consisting of two identical antigen-binding (Fab) domains connected to an effector or Fc domain by a flexible hinge sequence. Figure 29.1 shows the structure of an IgG molecule. IgG antibodies are comprised of two identical light chains and two identical heavy chains, with the chains joined by disulfide bonds, resulting in a bilaterally symmetrical complex. The Fab domains mediate the binding of IgG molecules to their cognate antigens and are composed of an intact light chain and half of a heavy chain. Each chain in the Fab domain is further divided into variable and constant regions, with the variable region containing hypervariable, or complementarity determining regions (CDR) in which the antigen-contact residues reside. The light and heavy chain variable regions each contain three CDRs (CDR1, CDR2, and CDR3). All six CDRs form the antigen-binding pocket and are collectively defined in immunologic terms as the idiotype of the antibody. In the majority of cases, the variable heavy chain CDR3 plays a dominant role in binding.[10]

The different isotypes of immunoglobulins are defined by the structure and function of their Fc domains. The Fc domain, composed of the CH2 and CH3 regions of the antibody's heavy chains, is the critical determinant of how an antibody mediates effector functions, transports across cellular barriers, and persists in circulation.[7,11]

MODIFIED ANTIBODY-BASED MOLECULES

Advances in antibody engineering and molecular biology have facilitated the development of many novel antibody-based structures with unique physical and pharmacokinetic properties (see Fig. 29.1). These include chimeric human-murine antibodies with human-constant regions and murine-variable regions,[12] humanized antibodies in which murine CDR sequences have been grafted into human IgG molecules, and entirely human antibodies derived from human hybridomas and, more recently, from transgenic mice expressing human immunoglobulin genes.[13] An accepted naming scheme based on "stems" was developed by the World Health Organization's International Nonproprietary Names (INN) for pharmaceuticals and is employed in the United States (Table 29.2). Engineering has also facilitated the development of antibody-based fragments. In addition to the classic, enzymatically derived Fab and F(ab')$_2$ molecules, a plethora of promising IgG-derivatives have been developed that retain antigen-binding properties of intact antibodies (see Fig. 29.1; for review see Robinson et al.[14]). The basic building block for these molecules is the 25 kDa, monovalent single-chain Fv (scFv) that is comprised of the variable domains (V$_H$ and V$_L$) of an antibody fused together with a short peptide linker. Novel, bispecific antibody-based structures can facilitate binding to two tumor antigens or bridge tumor cells with immune effector cells to focus antibody-dependent cell-mediated cytotoxicity (ADCC) or killing by T cells. An example of the former is MM-111, a bispecific gene-fused molecule composed of an anti-HER2 scFv connected to an anti-HER3 scFv via a modified form of human serum albumin.[15] Examples of the latter mechanism include small scFv-based bispecific T-cell engagers (BiTE) such as the anti-CD3/anti-CD19 molecule blinatumomab[16] and larger MAb-based antibodies such as catumaxomab, a rat/mouse anti-CD3/EpCAM bispecific MAb produced via quadroma technology.[17] Both classes of bispecifics endow selectivity and targeting properties that are not obtainable with natural antibody formats.

TABLE 29.1
FDA Approved Antibodies for the Treatment of Cancer

Generic Name (Trade Name)	Origin	Isotype (Conjugate)	Indication	Target	Initial Approval
Unconjugated MAbs					
Rituximab (Rituxan)	Chimeric	IgG1	NHL	CD20	1997
Trastuzumab (Herceptin)	Humanized	IgG1	BrCa	HER2	1998
Alemtuzumab (Campath 1H)	Humanized	IgG1	CLL	CD52	2001
Cetuximab (Erbitux)	Chimeric	IgG1	CRC, SCCHN	EGFR	2004
Bevacizumab (Avastin)	Humanized	IgG1	CRC, NSCLC, RCC, GBM	VEGF	2004
Panitumumab (Vectibix)	Human (XenoMouse)	IgG2	CRC	EGFR	2006
Ofatumumab (Arzerra)	Human (XenoMouse)	IgG1	CLL	CD20	2009
Denosumab (Prolia/Xgeva)	Human	IgG2	Metastasis-related SREs, ADT/AI-associated osteoporosis, GCT	RANKL	2010
Pertuzumab (Perjeta)	Humanized	IgG1	BrCa	HER2	2012
Immunoconjugates					
Gemtuzumab ozogamicin (Mylotarg)	Humanized	IgG4 (calicheamicin)	AML	CD33	2000[a]
Ibritumomab tiuxetan (Zevalin)	Murine	IgG1 (^{90}Y)	NHL	CD20	2002
Tositumomab (Bexxar)	Murine	IgG2A (^{131}I)	NHL	CD20	2003
Brentuximab vedotin (Adcetris)	Chimeric	IgG1 (MMAE)	HL, sALCL	CD30	2011
Ado-trastuzumab emtansine (Kadcyla)	Humanized	IgG1 (DM1)	BrCa	HER2	2013

[a] Withdrawn from the US market in June 2010.

NHL, non-Hodgkin lymphoma; BrCa, breast cancer; CLL, chronic lymphocytic leukemia; CRC, colorectal cancer; SCCHN, squamous cell carcinoma of head and neck; EGFR, epidermal growth factor receptor; NSCLC, non–small-cell lung cancer; RCC, renal cell carcinoma; GBM, glioblastoma multiforme; VEGF, vascular endothelial growth factor; SREs, skeletal-related events; ADT, androgen deprivation therapy; AI, aromatase inhibitor; GCT, giant cell tumor; RANKL, RANK ligand; AML, acute myelogenous leukemia; ^{90}Y, yttrium-90; ^{131}I, iodine-131; MMAE, Monomethyl auristatin E; HL, Hodgkin lymphoma; sALCL, systemic anaplastic large-cell lymphoma.

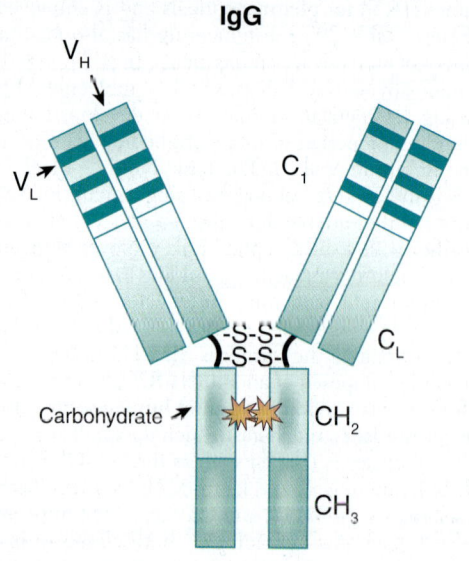

Figure 29.1 Structure of an IgG. C, constant; V, variable; H, heavy chain; L, light chain.

TABLE 29.2
Rules for Naming MAb for the Treatment of Cancer

The International Nonproprietary Names (INN) for monoclonal antibodies (MAbs) are composed of "stems" that indicate their origin, specificity, and modifications. The names include a random prefix to provide distinction from other names, a substem indicating the target specificity (-t[u]- for tumor), a substem indicating the species of origin (see the following) and a suffix (-mab), which indicates the presence of an immunoglobulin variable domain.

Substem Indication of the Species on Which the Immunoglobulin Sequence Is Based	
-o-	mouse
-xi-	chimeric
-zu-	humanized
-xizu-	chimeric/humanized
u	human

FACTORS REGULATING ANTIBODY-BASED TUMOR TARGETING

Antibody Size

Nonuniform distribution of systemically administered antibody is generally observed in biopsied specimens of solid tumors. Heterogeneous tumor blood supply limits uniform antibody delivery to tumors, and elevated interstitial pressures in the center of tumors oppose inward diffusion.[18] This high interstitial pressure slows the diffusion of molecules from their vascular extravasation site in a size-dependent manner.[19,20] The relatively large transport distances in the tumor interstitium also substantially increase the time required for large IgG macromolecules to reach target cells.[21]

Tumor Antigens

Access to the target antigen is undoubtedly a critical determinant of therapeutic effect of antibody-based applications. Such access is regulated by the heterogeneity of antigen expression by tumor cells. Shed antigen in the serum, tumor microenvironment, or both may saturate the antibody's binding sites and prevent binding to the cell surface. Alternatively, a rapid internalization of an antibody/antigen complex, although critical for antibody–drug conjugates (ADC), may deplete the quantity of cell surface MAb capable of initiating ADCC or cytotoxic signal transduction events. Finally, target antigens are normally *tumor associated* rather than *tumor specific*. Tumor-specific antigens are both highly desirable and rare. Typically, such antigens arise as a result of unique tumor-based genetic recombinations, such as clonal immunoglobulin idiotypes expressed on the surface of B-cell lymphomas.[22]

Antibody affinity for its target antigen has complex effects on tumor targeting. The *binding-site barrier* hypothesis postulates that antibodies with extremely high affinity for target antigen would bind irreversibly to the first antigen encountered upon entering the tumor, which would limit the diffusion of the antibody into the tumor and accumulate instead in regions surrounding the tumor vasculature.[23,24] Similarly, in tumor spheroids, the in vitro penetration of engineered antibodies is primarily limited by internalization and degradation.[25] The valence of an antibody molecule can increase the functional affinity of the antibody through an avidity effect.[26–28]

Half-Life/Clearance Rate

The concentration of intact IgG in mammalian serum is maintained at constant levels with half-lives of IgGs measured in days. This homeostasis is regulated in part by the major histocompatibility complex (MHC)-class I–related Fc receptor, FcRn (n = neonatal), a saturable, pH-dependent salvage mechanism that regulates quality and quantity of IgG in serum. This mechanism can be exploited via mutations in the Fc portion of an IgG to modulate IgGs pharmacokinetics.[29,30] Indeed, multiple strategies have been developed to increase the serum persistence of antibody-based fragments and other classes of protein therapeutics.[14,31]

Glycosylation

IgGs undergo N-linked glycosylation at the conserved Asn residue at position 297 within the C_H2 domain of the constant region. Glycosylation status of the residue has long been known to impact the ability of IgGs to bind effector ligands such as FcγR and C1q, which, in turn, affects their ability to participate in Fc-mediated functions such as ADCC and complement-dependent cytotoxicity (CDC).[32–34] The glycosylation of MAbs can be altered to increase ADCC by producing them in a cell line engineered to express β(1,4)-N-acetylglucosaminyltransferase III (GnTIII), the enzyme required to add the bisecting GlcNAc residues.[33] Defucosylation of antibody Fc domains is also associated with enhanced ADCC, and in a recently completed multicenter phase II trial of a defucosylated anti CC chemokine receptor 4 (CCR4), MAb was associated with meaningful antitumor activity, including complete responses and enhanced progression-free survival (PFS).[35]

UNCONJUGATED ANTIBODIES

The majority of monoclonal antibodies approved for clinical use display intrinsic antitumor effects that are mediated by one or more of the following mechanisms.

Cell-Mediated Cytotoxicity

As components of the immune system, effector cells such as natural killer (NK) cells and monocytes/macrophages represent natural lines of defense against oncologically transformed cells. These effector cells express Fcγ receptors (FcγR) on their cell surfaces, which interact with the Fc domain of IgG molecules. This family is comprised of three classes (type I, II, and III) that are further divided into subclasses (IIa/IIb and IIIa/IIIb).[36] Recognition of transformed cells by immune effector cells leads to cell-mediated killing through processes such as ADCC and phagocytosis, as shown in Figure 29.2, and can be mediated by FcγRI (CD64), a high affinity receptor capable of binding to monomeric IgG, or FcγRII (CD32) and FcγRIII (CD16), which are low affinity receptors that preferentially bind multimeric complexes of IgG. Signaling through type I, IIa, and IIIa receptors results in the activation of effector cells due to associated immunoreceptor tyrosine-based activation motifs (ITAM), whereas the engagement of type IIb receptors inhibits cell activation through associated immunoreceptor tyrosine-based inhibitory motifs (ITIM).[36] Clinical results support the idea that ADCC can play a role in the efficacy of antibody-based therapies. Naturally occurring polymorphisms in FcγRs alter their affinity for human IgG1 and have been linked to clinical response.[37,38] A polymorphism in the FCGR3A gene results in either a valine or phenylalanine at position 158 of FcγRIIIa. Human IgG1 binds more strongly to FcγRIIIa-158V than FcγRIIIa-158F, and likewise to NK cells from individuals that are either homozygous for 158F or heterozygous for this polymorphism.[39] The FcγRIIIa-158v was a predictor of early response and was associated with improved PFS.

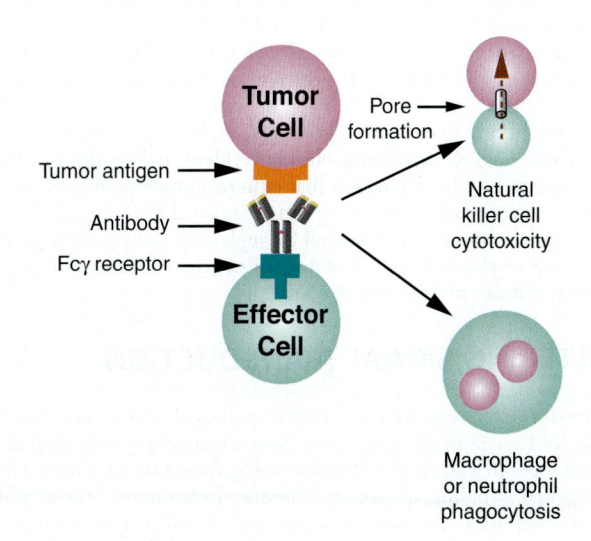

Figure 29.2 Antibody-dependent cellular cytotoxicity. The antibody engages the tumor antigen and the Fc domain binds to cellular Fc receptors to bridge effector and target cells. This bridging induces effector cell activation, resulting in natural killer cell cytotoxicity or phagocytosis by neutrophils, monocytes, or macrophages.

A second polymorphism, FcγRIIa-131H/R, did not predict early response but was an independent predictor of time to progression (TTP).[38] Taken together, these data suggest that modulating the affinity of MAbs for FcγRIIIa, FcγRIIa, or both may increase the efficacy of therapeutic MAbs.

Each class of FcγR exhibits a characteristic specificity for IgG subclasses.[40] Many groups have focused on modifying the Fc domain of IgGs to optimize the engagement of subclasses of FcγR and the induction of ADCC, based on the findings of Shields et al.,[29] who performed a series of mutagenesis experiments to map the residues required for IgG1-FcγR interaction. Antibodies such as ocrelizumab, a humanized version of rituximab, have increased binding to low affinity FcγRIIIa variants and are now in clinical trials.

An alternative to modifying the Fc region of MAbs is to create bispecific antibodies (bsAbs) that recognize both a tumor-associated antigen and a *trigger antigen* present on the surface of an immune effector cell.[43] Simultaneous engagement of both antigens can redirect the cytotoxic potential of the effector cell against the tumor.[41–43] Such antibodies are capable of eliciting effector function against tumor cell lines in vitro and in animal models. Two HER-2 directed bispecific antibodies, 2B1 and MDX-H210, have been tested in phase I clinical trials.[44,45]

Bispecific antibodies have a number of distinctive properties, including flexible choices of cytotoxic trigger molecules,[46] recruitment of effector function in the presence of excess IgG,[42] and custom tailoring of the affinity of the bsAb to match effector cell characteristics. These advantages have been facilitated by improved methods of bsAb production.[47] BiTE antibodies represent a novel class of bispecific, single chain Fv antibodies.[48] Promising results have been seen in early phase clinical trials with at least two BiTE antibodies, one of which, blinatumomab, targets CD19/CD3.[49] Promising phase I results have also been reported in an interim analysis of an anti-EpCAM/anti-CD3 MT110 BiTE in the setting of advanced lung and gastrointestinal tumors.[50]

Complement-Dependent Cytotoxicity

In addition to cell-mediated killing (see previous), MAbs can recruit the complement cascade to kill cells via CDC. Although IgM is the most effective isotype for complement activation, it is not widely used in clinical oncology. Similar to ADCC, the human IgG subclass used to construct a therapeutic MAb dictates its ability to elicit CDC; IgG1 is extremely efficient at fixing complement, in contrast to IgG2 and IgG4.[51] Antibodies activate complement through the classical pathway, by engaging multiple C1q to trigger activation of a cascade of serum proteases, which kill the antibody-bound cells.[52,53] The anti-CD20 MAb rituximab has been found to depend in part on CDC for its *in vivo* efficacy.[54] Antibody engineering approaches have identified residues in the C_H2 domain of the Fc region that either suppress or enhance the ability of rituximab to bind C1q and activate CDC.[55] The ability to manipulate complement fixation through engineering approaches warrants *in vivo* testing to determine the impact of these changes on the efficacy and toxicity of MAbs.

ALTERING SIGNAL TRANSDUCTION

Growth factor receptors represent a well-established class of targets for therapeutic intervention. Normal signaling through these receptors often leads to mitogenic and prosurvival responses. Unregulated signaling, as seen in a number of common cancers due to receptor overexpression, promotes tumor cell growth and insensitivity to chemotherapeutic agents. Clinically relevant MAbs can modulate signaling through their target receptors to normalize cell growth rates and sensitize tumor cells to cytotoxic agents. The binding of cetuximab or panitumumab to the epidermal growth factor receptor (EGFR) physically blocks ligand binding[56] and prevents the receptor from assuming the extended conformation required for dimerization.[57] Pertuzumab binds to the dimerization domain of HER-2, thereby sterically inhibiting subsequent receptor heterodimerization with other ligand-bound family members.[58] Alternatively, signaling through growth factor receptors can be indirectly modified by MAbs that bind to activating ligands, as is seen with the anti–vascular endothelial growth factor (VEGF) MAb, bevacizumab.[59]

IMMUNOCONJUGATES

MAbs that are not capable of directly eliciting antitumor effects, either by altering signal transduction or directing immune system cells, can still be effective against tumors by delivering cytotoxic payloads. MAbs have been employed to deliver a wide variety of agents, including chemotherapy, toxins, radioisotopes, and cytokines (for review see Adams and Weiner[60]). In theory, the appropriate combination of toxic agents and MAbs could lead to a synergistic effect. For example, delivery of a therapeutic radioisotope by a MAb would be significantly enhanced if, by binding to its target antigen, the MAb also activated a signaling event that increased the target cell's sensitivity to ionizing radiation.

Catalytic toxins derived from plants catalytic toxins derived from plants (e.g., ricin) and microorganisms (e.g., Pseudomonas) represent two classes of cytotoxic agent that have been investigated for their utility in immunoconjugate strategies.[61] Although there are promising preclinical studies,[62] few successful clinical trials have been reported using this approach. In a phase I clinical trial in hairy cell leukemia patients who were resistant to cladribine, 11 of 16 patients exhibited complete remissions with minimal side effects with an anti-CD22 immunotoxin with a truncated form of *Pseudomonas exotoxin*.[63] Clinical trials with other immunotoxins have been associated with unacceptable neurotoxicity[64] and life-threatening vascular leak syndrome.[65]

Immunocytokine fusions have also been investigated as an approach to direct the patient's immune response to his or her own tumor.[66] A number of cytokines have been incorporated into antibody-based constructs, including interleukin-2 (IL-2),[67,68] interferon γ (IFN-γ),[69] tumor necrosis factor α (TFN-α),[69] VEGF,[70] and IL-12.[71]

Antibody–Drug Conjugates

The first ADC, gemtuzumab ozogamicin (Mylotarg), was approved by the FDA in 2000 for the treatment of patients with relapsed CD33-positive acute myeloid leukemia, but was voluntarily withdrawn from the US market by its manufacturer in 2010 after a confirmatory phase III trial (SWOG S0106) recommended, based on results of a planned interim analysis, that Mylotarg randomizations be terminated due to a lack of efficacy in the presence of enhanced toxicity.[72] Although two additional randomized trials[73,74] suggested that some patient populations may benefit from Mylotarg therapy, the drug remains off the market in the United States.

The majority of ADCs under development employ potent cytotoxic agents that block the polymerization of tubulin (e.g., auristatins or maytansines) or damage DNA (e.g., calicheamicins or pyrrolobenzodiazepines) by employing a variety of linkers and conjugation strategies.[75]

A variety of ADCs specific for a wide range of oncology targets are currently in clinical evaluation, with the majority of the more advanced agents being tested in the setting of diffuse malignancies.[76] The majority of these employ auristatins or maytansines as their payloads. Early observations suggest that cumulative, dose-related peripheral sensory neuropathy can result when auristatins are conjugated to an antibody via a cleavable linker, and dose limiting thrombocytopenia can result when auristatins and maytansinoids are conjugated to the antibody via an uncleavable linker.[76,77]

Two ADCs are now approved for use in clinical practice. Ado-trastuzumab emtansine (T-DM1, Kadcyla), an ADC composed of the anti-HER2 MAb trastuzumab linked to DM1,[78] is now approved for the treatment of patients with refractory HER2/neu expressing breast cancers. The other, brentuximab vedotin (SGN-35, Adcetris), is an ADC consisting of the anti-CD30 chimeric MAb cAC10 that is linked to three to five molecules of the microtubule-disrupting agent Monomethyl auristatin E. At this point, this drug is approved for use in patients with recurrent systemic anaplastic large cell lymphoma. The clinical data associated with both of these ADCs will be discussed in subsequent sections of this chapter.

Antibodies also can be used to target liposome encapsulated drugs[79] and other cytotoxic agents, such as antisense RNA[80] or radionuclides to tumors.

Radioimmunoconjugates

Two anti-CD20 radioimmunoconjugates have been FDA approved for radioimmunotherapy (RIT) of non-Hodgkin lymphoma (NHL). Ibritumomab (Zevalin) and tositumomab (Bexxar) are murine MAbs labeled with yttrium-90 (^{90}Y) and iodine-131 (^{131}I), respectively. Both are associated with impressive clinical efficacy.[81,82] Although these radioimmunoconjugates are effective therapeutics, cumbersome logistics surrounding their administration have significantly limited their use. Despite significant preclinical evidence supporting the use of RIT for solid malignancies, clinical results have not demonstrated consistent antitumor activity.[60]

ANTIBODIES APPROVED FOR USE IN SOLID TUMORS

Trastuzumab

Trastuzumab (Herceptin) is a humanized IgG1[83] that targets domain IV of the HER2/ErbB2 member of the EGFR/ErbB family of receptor tyrosine kinases. Gene amplification as judged by fluorescence in situ hybridization (FISH) with concomitant overexpression of HER2 protein measured by immunohistochemistry (IHC) is seen in approximately 25% of breast cancers.[84,85] HER2 amplification and overexpression is now recognized to also be a critical driver in a subset (7% to 34%) of gastric cancers.[86] Trastuzumab inhibits tumor cell growth by binding to HER2 and blocking the unregulated HER2 signaling that is associated with its high level overexpression.

Trastuzumab became the first FDA-approved monoclonal antibody for the treatment of solid tumors based on a series of studies carried out in the setting of HER2-positive metastatic breast cancer.[87,88] A subsequent phase III trial investigating trastuzumab in combination with cytotoxic chemotherapy demonstrated an improved response rate compared to chemotherapy alone, from 25.0% to 57.3% with a taxane regimen.[89]

Trastuzumab is also approved for use in the adjuvant setting based on an approximately 50% reduction in recurrence after 1 year in multiple phase III trials.[90–92] Myocardial dysfunction, seen with anthracycline therapy, was observed with increased frequency in patients receiving antibody alone[93] or with doxorubicin or epirubicin.

Recognition of HER2 as a driver in a subset of gastric cancers led to an open-label, randomized, phase III trial (ToGA) that investigated the addition of trastuzumab to standard of care chemotherapy,[94] and showed increased median overall survival with higher levels of HER2 expression. A study by Gomez-Martin et al.[95] in 99 patients with metastatic gastric cancer being treated with first-line trastuzumab plus chemotherapy identified a mean HER2/CEP17 ratio of 4.7 to be an optimal cut-off to discriminate between trastuzumab-sensitive and refractory patients.

Pertuzumab

Pertuzumab (Perjeta) is a humanized IgG1 MAb that binds to domain II of HER2 and blocks ligand-dependent dimerization of HER2 with other members of the EGFR family.[96] Pertuzumab, in combination with trastuzumab and docetaxel, is approved for use as first-line therapy in HER2-positive metastatic breast cancer patients. Use of the combination is also approved for the treatment of HER2-positive, locally advanced, inflammatory, or high-risk early breast cancer (>2 cm node negative or node positive) in the neoadjuvant setting.

FDA-approval of pertuzumab was based on results of a phase III trial (CLEOPATRA) of 808 patients with locally recurrent, unresectable, or metastatic breast cancer randomized to receive trastuzumab plus docetaxel with or without the addition of pertuzumab. Inclusion of pertuzumab increased the independently assessed PFS by 6.1 months from 12.4 to 18.5 (hazard ratio [HR], 0.62 [95% confidence interval [CI], 0.51, 0.75], p <0.0001), with a trend toward improved overall survival[97] that reached statistical significance (p = 0.0008) after an additional year of follow-up.[98] The addition of pertuzumab did increase rates of grade 3 adverse events (AE), but it did not adversely affect cardiac function. Accelerated approval was granted for use of pertuzumab in combination with trastuzumab and docetaxel for the neoadjuvant treatment of high-risk early-stage breast cancer. This approval was based on results from a four-arm, open-label phase II study of 417 patients randomized to receive trastuzumab plus docetaxel, pertuzumab plus docetaxel, pertuzumab plus trastuzumab, or the triple combination. The triple combination improved the pathologic complete response (pCR) rate by 17.8% over the trastuzumab plus docetaxel arm (39.3% versus 21.5%) in the pertuzumab arm.[99] Follow-up studies to confirm a correlation between pCR and long-term clinical benefit are ongoing.

Cetuximab

Cetuximab (Erbitux) targets the EGFR. This chimeric IgG1 binds to domain III of the EGFR, with roughly a tenfold higher affinity than either EGF or transforming growth factor α (TGF-α) ligands and thereby inhibits ligand-induced activation of this tyrosine kinase receptor. Cetuximab may also function to downregulate EGFR-dependent signaling by stimulating EGFR internalization.[100] Cetuximab is approved for the treatment of colorectal cancer (CRC) and, more recently, for the treatment of squamous cell cancer of the head and neck (SCCHN).

The efficacy and safety of cetuximab against CRC was demonstrated alone and in combination with irinotecan in a phase II, multicenter, randomized, and controlled trial of 329 patients.[101] The combination of irinotecan plus cetuximab increased both the overall response and the median duration of response as compared to cetuximab alone. Additionally, patients with irinotecan refractory disease responded to treatment with the combination regimen. Recent studies in patients with colorectal cancers have indicated that patients with KRAS mutations in codon 12 or 13 should not receive anti-EGFR therapy.[101,102]

An international, multicenter, phase III trial comparing definitive radiotherapy to radiotherapy plus cetuximab in SCCHN demonstrated that EGFR blockade with radiotherapy significantly reduced the risk of locoregional failure by 32% and the risk of death by 26%. In advanced stage non–small-cell lung cancer (NSCLC) expressing EGFR, the combination of cetuximab and standard doublet chemotherapy (cisplatin plus vinorelbine) was studied in a prospective randomized phase III trial.[103] The addition of cetuximab was associated with a slight, but statistically significant, benefit in overall survival over chemotherapy alone (median overall survival 10.1 versus 11.3 months). A similar study using the carboplatin plus paclitaxel backbone in combination with cetuximab did not meet its primary endpoint of improved PFS, although cetuximab-treated patients exhibited higher objective response rates.[104] Therefore, the benefit of adding cetuximab to standard chemotherapy for patients with advanced NSCLC is unclear.

Panitumumab

Panitumumab (Vectibix) is a fully human IgG2 monoclonal antibody that binds to EGFR. Similar to cetuximab, panitumumab inhibits EGFR activation by blocking the binding of EGF and TGF-α. However, it does so by binding to EGFR with a higher affinity than cetuximab (5×10^{-11} M versus 1×10^{-10} M). As previously mentioned, the IgG2 class of antibodies does not induce activation of the immune system cell via the Fc-receptor mechanism, so panitumumab's primary action appears to be interference with EGFR–ligand interactions.

A phase III trial of 463 patients with metastatic colorectal cancer compared panitumumab plus best supportive care (BSC) to BSC alone.[105] A partial-response rate of 8% and a stable-disease rate of 28% were reported for the panitumumab arm compared with a 10% stable-disease rate in the best supportive care arm of the study. As with cetuximab, patients with metastatic colorectal cancers who have KRAS mutations in codons 12 or 13 are not routinely offered therapy with panitumumab.[106]

Bevacizumab

Bevacizumab (Avastin or rhuMAb VEGF) is a humanized monoclonal antibody targeting VEGF. VEGF is a critical determinant of tumor angiogenesis, a process that is a necessary component of tumor invasion, growth, and metastasis. VEGF expression by invasive tumors has been shown to correlate with vascularity and cellular proliferation and is prognostic for several human cancers.[107–109] Interestingly, the inhibition of VEGF signaling via bevacizumab treatment may normalize tumor vasculature, promoting a more effective delivery of chemotherapy agents.[110] Bevacizumab is approved for use as a first-line therapy for metastatic colorectal cancer and NSCLC when given in combination with appropriate cytotoxic chemotherapy regimens. Phase III clinical trials leading to the approval of bevacizumab for the treatment of colorectal cancer demonstrated improved response rates from 35% to 45% compared to fluorouracil (5-FU)–based chemotherapy alone. Enhanced response durations and improved patient survival were seen in patients treated with chemotherapy plus bevacizumab as compared to patients receiving chemotherapy alone.[111] A survival benefit was also seen in the setting of NSCLC. A randomized phase III trial (ECOG 4599) of paclitaxel and carboplatin with or without bevacizumab in patients with advanced nonsquamous NSCLC led to a significant improvement in median survival (12.5 months versus 10.2 months; p = 0.0075) for patients in the bevacizumab arm,[112] with significantly higher response rates. A higher incidence of bleeding was associated with bevacizumab (4.5% versus 0.7%). Five of 10 treatment-related deaths occurred as a result of hemoptysis, all in the bevacizumab arm.

A phase III trial randomized 722 patients with metastatic breast cancer with no prior chemotherapy for advanced disease to either paclitaxel or paclitaxel and bevacizumab.[113] PFS was significantly better in the paclitaxel plus bevacizumab arm (median, 11.8 versus 5.9 months; HR for progression, 0.60; p <0.001) with an increased response rate (36.9% versus 21.2%, p <0.001). Overall survival, however, was similar.

In contrast,[114] in a randomized phase III trial, capecitabine/bevacizumab increased response rates compared with capecitabine alone in 462 anthracycline and taxane pretreated metastatic breast cancer patients but did not meet its primary endpoint of improved PFS. Overall survival and time to deterioration in quality of life were comparable in both treatment groups.

Bevacizumab has not demonstrated activity in the adjuvant colorectal and breast cancer settings.[115,116] There was no improvement in overall survival between the two groups and the rate of invasive disease-free survival was also not significantly different between the treatment groups.

Bevacizumab is also approved for the management of recurrent glioblastomas based on results of phase II studies.[117]

Ado-Trastuzumab Emtansine

Ado-trastuzumab emtansine (T-DM1, Kadcyla) is an ADC composed of the anti-HER2 MAb trastuzumab linked to DM1, a highly potent derivative of maytansine, through a stable thioether linker.[78]

Based on two single-agent phase II trials of T-DM1[118,119] that demonstrated single-agent activity in the setting of metastatic breast cancer, two separate phase III studies were conducted. The 991 patient EMILIA trial demonstrated that T-DM1 significantly prolongs both PFS and overall survival as compared to a regimen of lapatinib plus capecitabine when used in the setting of metastatic breast cancer that had progressed after treatment with trastuzumab plus a taxane.[120] Grade 3 and worse AEs were lower in the T-DM1 arm (200, 40.8%) as compared to the lapatinib plus capecitabine arm (278, 57%). Results are still awaited from the ongoing MARIANNE trial that is assessing first-line efficacy and safety of T-DM1 alone and T-DM1 plus pertuzumab versus trastuzumab plus taxane (NCT01120184).

Denosumab

Denosumab (Xgeva) is a fully human IgG2 RANK ligand (RANKL) neutralizing antibody. Denosumab is FDA-approved for use in adults and skeletally mature adolescents who have either surgically unsalvageable giant cell tumors of the bone (GCTB) or where resection is anticipated to result in severe morbidity. Approval was based in part on two open-label, phase II trials examining subcutaneous administration of 120 mg q4 week with additional loading doses on days 8 and 15 of the first cycle.[121,122] Serious adverse events were seen in 9% of patients (n = 25). Of 187 patients, 47 (25%) exhibited partial objective responses based on modified Response Evaluation Criteria in Solid Tumors (RECIST) criteria.

Denosumab is also approved in for use in two supportive care settings based on three randomized, double-blind, placebo-controlled phase III trials evaluating its efficacy versus zoledronic acid[123–125] to reduce bone metastasis-related skeletal-related events (SRE). Based on data from two phase III trials, a second formulation and dosing schedule of denosumab is approved to increase bone mass in prostate cancer[126] and breast cancer[127] patients at high risk for bone fracture due to hormone-ablation therapies.

ANTIBODIES USED IN HEMATOLOGIC MALIGNANCIES

Rituximab

Rituximab (Rituxan) is a chimeric anti-CD20 monoclonal antibody that was the first MAb to be approved by the FDA for use in human malignancy.[128,129] Studies have shown that multiple doses can be safely administered, and *in vitro* studies have demonstrated multiple mechanisms by which anti-CD20 antibodies can lead to cell death.[130] Efficacy of rituximab monotherapy is well established.[131]

Rituximab has been tested in conjunction with chemotherapy based on supportive preclinical data.[132,133] The combination of rituximab with cyclophosphamide, doxorubicin, vincristine, and prednisolone (CHOP) resulted in a 95% overall response rate (55% complete response, 40% partial response) among 40 patients with low-grade or follicular B-cell non-Hodgkin lymphoma, with molecular complete remissions observed.[134] A long term study of elderly patients with previously untreated diffuse large-cell lymphoma randomized to either CHOP chemotherapy plus rituximab (R-CHOP) or CHOP alone demonstrated a significant improvement in event-free survival, PFS, disease-free survival, and overall survival for the combination arm.[135] No significant differences in long-term toxicity were noted.

Low-grade B-cell lymphoma patients possessing the 158V/V polymorphism in FcγRIII experience superior response rates and outcomes when treated with rituximab.[37,38] These findings signify that antibody Fc domain::Fc receptor interactions underlie at least some of the clinical benefit of rituximab, and indicate a possible role for ADCC that depends on such interactions.

A combination of active agents (such as lenalidomide and thalidomide) that are also immune modulating may be additive with rituximab,[136] and perhaps synergize by increasing ADCC.[137] Cytokines such as interleukin-2 (IL-2), IL-12, or IL-15 and myeloid growth factors may also enhance therapeutic antibody activity as suggested by preclinical data demonstrating that IL-2 can promote NK cell proliferation and activation and can enhance rituximab activity[138] and clinical efficacy.[139,140] Myeloid growth factors, in combination with rituximab, may also activate ADCC.[141] Alternative approaches to induce effector cell activity by combining Toll-like receptors (TLR) agonists, such as CpG oligonucleotides, have been investigated.[142] Altering the balance of proapoptotic and antiapoptotic signals could generate more rituximab-induced cytotoxicity. BCL-2 downregulation by antisense oligonucleotides was found to enhance rituximab efficacy in preclinical testing.[143,144] However, small molecules that bind to the BH-3 domain common to many members of the BCL-2 family of proteins may be better therapeutic agents.[145-147]

Ofatumumab

The anti-CD20 ofatumumab[148] is a fully human antibody that binds an epitope on CD20 distinct from that bound by rituximab and is engineered for better complement activation, although it induces less ADCC. Ofatumumab has received regulatory approval for the treatment of patients with fludarabine-refractory chronic lymphocytic leukemia (CLL). In a recently reported, planned interim analysis that included 138 CLL patients with treatment-refractory disease or bulky (>5 cm) lymphadenopathy, treatment with ofatumumab led to an overall response rate (primary endpoint) of 47% in patients with bulky disease and 5% in patients refractory to both alemtuzumab and fludarabine.[149]

Additional humanized anti-CD20 antibodies (veltuzumab[150] and ocrelizumab) are under development.

Alemtuzumab

Alemtuzumab (Campath-1H) targets the CD52 glycopeptide, which is highly expressed on T and B lymphocytes. It has been tested as a therapeutic agent for CLL and promyelocytic leukemias, as well as other non–Hodgkin lymphomas.

Brentuximab Vedotin

Brentuximab vedotin (SGN-35, Adcetris) is an ADC consisting of the anti-CD30 chimeric MAb cAC10 that is linked to three to five molecules of the microtubule-disrupting agent Monomethyl auristatin E (MMAE). MMAE is a highly potent derivative of dolastatin. Linkage of MMAE to cAC10 occurs through a protease-cleavable linker.[151] Brentuximab vedotin is approved for treating systemic, chemotherapy-refractory anaplastic large-cell lymphomas (sALCL). It is also approved to treat patients with Hodgkin lymphoma who have progressed after an autologous stem cell transplant (ASCT). Patients ineligible for ASCT must have failed two prior multidrug chemotherapy regimens.

Brentuximab vedotin received accelerated approval in 2011 based in part on the results of two phase II trials. In a multicenter trial conducted by Pro et al.,[152] 58 patients with relapsed or refractory sALCL received brentuximab vedotin (1.8 mg per kilogram per week), and 86% of patients achieved objective response. Complete responses occurred in 57% of patients, with a median duration of 13.2 months. An additional 17 patients (29%) had partial responses. Median overall response was 12.6 months. Most common grade 3 and 4 adverse events (AE) were neutropenia (21%), thrombocytopenia (14%), and peripheral sensory neuropathy (12%). A similar trial, in Hodgkin lymphoma, was reported by Younes et al.[153] Patients (n = 102) that had failed ASCT received brentuximab vedotin on the same schedule as listed previously and were assessed for the objective response rate. In this setting, 75% of patients had objective responses, with 34% being complete remissions. The median duration of complete responses was 20.5 months, and 31 patients were progression free after a median follow-up of 1.5 years. Phase III trials to assess the known risk of neuropathy (AETHERA) and to confirm overall clinical benefit seen in the phase II trials (ECHELON-2, or ClinicalTrials.gov Identifier NCT01712490) are ongoing.

CONCLUSION

In the 35 years since Kohler and Milstein first developed the hybridoma technology that enabled antibody-based therapeutics, the field has made remarkable progress. Numerous antibody-based molecules are currently in clinical trials and many more are in development. Multiple therapeutic antibodies have a proven clinical benefit and have been licensed by the FDA. The thoughtful application of advances in cancer biology and antibody engineering suggest that this progress will continue.

REFERENCES

1. Badger CC, Anasetti C, Davis J, et al. Treatment of malignancy with unmodified antibody. *Pathol Immunopathol Res* 1987;6:419–434.
2. Khazaeli MB, Conry RM, Lobuglio AF. Human immune-response to monoclonal-antibodies. *J Immunother Emphasis Tumor Immunol* 1994;15:42–52.
3. Lee J, Fenton BM, Koch CJ, et al. Interleukin 2 expression by tumor cells alters both the immune response and the tumor microenvironment. *Cancer Res* 1998;58:1478–1485.
4. Reichert JM, Dhimolea E. The future of antibodies as cancer drugs. *Drug Discov Today* 2012;17:954–963.
5. Kohler G, Milstein C. Continuous cultures of fused cells secreting antibody of predefined specificity. *Nature* 1975;256:495–497.
6. Houghton AN, Mintzer D, Cordon-Cardo C, et al. Mouse monoclonal IgG3 antibody detecting GD3 ganglioside: a phase I trial in patients with malignant melanoma. *Proc Natl Acad Sci U S A* 1985;82:1242–1246.
7. Steplewski Z, Lubeck MD, Koprowski H. Human macrophages armed with murine immunoglobulin G2a antibodies to tumors destroy human cancer cells. *Science* 1983;221:865–867.
8. Trauth BC, Klas C, Peters AM, et al. Monoclonal antibody-mediated tumor regression by induction of apoptosis. *Science* 1989;245:301–305.
9. Yang XD, Jia XC, Corvalan JR, et al. Eradication of established tumors by a fully human monoclonal antibody to the epidermal growth factor receptor without concomitant chemotherapy. *Cancer Res* 1999;59:1236–1243.
10. Komissarov AA, Calcutt MJ, Marchbank MT, et al. Equilibrium binding studies of recombinant anti-single-stranded DNA Fab. Role of heavy chain complementarity-determining regions. *J Biol Chem* 1996;271:12241–12246.
11. Ghetie V, Popov S, Borvak J, et al. Increasing the serum persistence of an IgG fragment by random mutagenesis. *Nat Biotechnol* 1997;15:637–640.
12. LoBuglio AF, Wheeler RH, Trang J, et al. Mouse/human chimeric monoclonal antibody in man: kinetics and immune response. *Proc Natl Acad Sci U S A* 1989;86:4220–4224.
13. Kudo T, Saeki H, Tachibana T. A simple and improved method to generate human hybridomas. *J Immunol Methods* 1991;145:119–125.
14. Robinson MK, Weiner LM, Adams GP. Improving monoclonal antibodies for cancer therapy. *Drug Dev Res* 2004;61:172–187.
15. Denlinger CS, Beeram M, Tolcher AW, et al. A phase I/II and pharmacologic study of MM-111 in patients with advanced, refractory HER2-positive (HER2+) cancers. *J Clin Oncol* 2010;28:15s.
16. Nagorsen D, Bargou R, Ruttinger D, et al. Immunotherapy of lymphoma and leukemia with T-cell engaging BiTE antibody blinatumomab. *Leuk Lymphoma* 2009;50:886–891.
17. Goere D, Flament C, Rusakiewicz S, et al. Potent immunomodulatory effects of the trifunctional antibody catumaxomab. *Cancer Res* 2013;73:4663–4673.
18. Jain RK. Transport of molecules in the tumor interstitium: a review. *Cancer Res* 1987;47:3039–3051.

19. Jain RK. Physiological barriers to delivery of monoclonal antibodies and other macromolecules in tumors. *Cancer Res* 1990;50:814s–819s.
20. Jain RK, Baxter LT. Mechanisms of heterogeneous distribution of monoclonal antibodies and other macromolecules in tumors: significance of elevated interstitial pressure. *Cancer Res* 1988;48:7022–7032.
21. Jain RK. Transport of molecules across tumor vasculature. *Cancer Metastasis Rev* 1987;6:559–593.
22. Miller RA, Maloney DG, Warnke R, et al. Treatment of B-cell lymphoma with monoclonal anti-idiotype antibody. *N Engl J Med* 1982;306:517–522.
23. Fujimori K, Covell DG, Fletcher JE, et al. A modeling analysis of monoclonal antibody percolation through tumors: a binding site barrier. *J Nucl Med* 1990;31:1191–1198.
24. Rudnick SI, Lou J, Shaller CC, et al. Influence of affinity and antigen internalization on the uptake and penetration of Anti-HER2 antibodies in solid tumors. *Cancer Res* 2011;71:2250–2259.
25. Thurber GM, Wittrup KD. Quantitative spatiotemporal analysis of antibody fragment diffusion and endocytic consumption in tumor spheroids. *Cancer Res* 2008;68:3334–3341.
26. Adams GP, Tai MS, McCartney JE, et al. Avidity-mediated enhancement of in vivo tumor targeting by single-chain Fv dimers. *Clin Cancer Res* 2006;12:1599–1605.
27. Wolff EA, Schreiber GJ, Cosand WL, et al. Monoclonal antibody homodimers: enhanced antitumor activity in nude mice. *Cancer Res* 1993;53:2560–2565.
28. Werlen RC, Lankinen M, Offord RE, et al. Preparation of a trivalent antigen-binding construct using polyoxime chemistry: improved biodistribution and potential for therapeutic application. *Cancer Res* 1996;56:809–815.
29. Shields RL, Namenuk AK, Hong K, et al. High resolution mapping of the binding site on human IgG1 for Fc gamma RI, Fc gamma RII, Fc gamma RIII, and FcRn and design of IgG1 variants with improved binding to the Fc gamma R. *J Biol Chem* 2001;276:6591–6604.
30. Kenanova V, Olafsen T, Crow DM, et al. Tailoring the pharmacokinetics and positron emission tomography imaging properties of anti-carcinoembryonic antigen single-chain Fv-Fc antibody fragments. *Cancer Res* 2005;65:622–631.
31. McDonagh CF, Huhalov A, Harms BD, et al. Antitumor activity of a novel bispecific antibody that targets the ErbB2/ErbB3 oncogenic unit and inhibits heregulin-induced activation of ErbB3. *Mol Cancer Ther* 2012;11:582–593.
32. Lund J, Takahashi N, Pound JD, et al. Multiple interactions of IgG with its core oligosaccharide can modulate recognition by complement and human Fc gamma receptor I and influence the synthesis of its oligosaccharide chains. *J Immunol* 1996;157:4963–4969.
33. Umana P, Jean-Mairet J, Moudry R, et al. Engineered glycoforms of an antineuroblastoma IgG1 with optimized antibody-dependent cellular cytotoxic activity. *Nat Biotechnol* 1999;17:176–180.
34. Wright A, Morrison SL. Effect of glycosylation on antibody function: implications for genetic engineering. *Trends Biotechnol* 1997;15:26–32.
35. Ishida T, Joh T, Uike N, et al. Defucosylated anti-CCR4 monoclonal antibody (KW-0761) for relapsed adult T-cell leukemia-lymphoma: a multicenter phase II study. *J Clin Oncol* 2012;30:837–842.
36. Raghavan M, Bjorkman PJ. Fc receptors and their interactions with immunoglobulins. *Annu Rev Cell Dev Biol* 1996;12:181–220.
37. Cartron G, Dacheux L, Salles G, et al. Therapeutic activity of humanized anti-CD20 monoclonal antibody and polymorphism in IgG Fc receptor FcgammaRIIIa gene. *Blood* 2002;99:754–758.
38. Weng WK, Levy R. Two immunoglobulin G fragment C receptor polymorphisms independently predict response to rituximab in patients with follicular lymphoma. *J Clin Oncol* 2003;21:3940–3947.
39. Koene HR, Kleijer M, Algra J, et al. Fc gammaRIIIa-158V/F polymorphism influences the binding of IgG by natural killer cell Fc gammaRIIIa, independently of the Fc gammaRIIIa-48L/R/H phenotype. *Blood* 1997;90:1109–1114.
40. Gessner JE, Heiken H, Tamm A, et al. The IgG Fc receptor family. *Ann Hematol* 1998;76:231–248.
41. Keler T, Graziano RF, Mandal A, et al. Bispecific antibody-dependent cellular cytotoxicity of HER2/neu-overexpressing tumor cells by Fcgamma receptor type I-expressing effector cells. *Cancer Res* 1997;57:4008–4014.
42. Weiner LM, Holmes M, Richeson A, et al. Binding and cytotoxicity characteristics of the bispecific murine monoclonal antibody 2B1. *J Immunol* 1993;151:2877–2886.
43. Shalaby MR, Shepard HM, Presta L, et al. Development of humanized bispecific antibodies reactive with cytotoxic lymphocytes and tumor cells overexpressing the HER2 protooncogene. *J Exp Med* 1992;175:217–225.
44. Valone FH, Kaufman PA, Guyre PM, et al. Phase Ia/Ib trial of bispecific antibody MDX-210 in patients with advanced breast or ovarian cancer that overexpresses the proto-oncogene HER-2/neu. *J Clin Oncol* 1995;13:2281–2292.
45. Weiner LM, Clark JI, Davey M, et al. Phase I trial of 2B1, a bispecific monoclonal antibody targeting c-erbB-2 and FcgammaRIII. *Cancer Res* 1995;55:4586–4593.
46. Liu MA, Kranz DM, Kurnick JT, et al. Heteroantibody duplexes target cells for lysis by cytotoxic T lymphocytes. *Proc Natl Acad Sci U S A* 1985;82:8648–8652.
47. Carter P. Bispecific human IgG by design. *J Immunol Methods* 2001;248:7–15.
48. Mack M, Riethmuller G, Kufer P. A small bispecific antibody construct expressed as a functional single-chain molecule with high tumor cell cytotoxicity. *Proc Natl Acad Sci U S A* 1995;92:7021–7025.
49. Bargou R, Leo E, Zugmaier G, et al. Tumor regression in cancer patients by very low doses of a T cell-engaging antibody. *Science* 2008;321:974–977.
50. Fiedler W, Hönemann D, Ritter B, et al. Safety and pharmacology of the EpCAM/CD3-bispecific BiTE antibody MT110 in patients with metastatic colorectal, gastric, and lung cancer. *Eur J Cancer* 2009;7:136–137.
51. Presta LG. Engineering antibodies for therapy. *Curr Pharm Biotechnol* 2002;3:237–256.
52. Makrides SC. Therapeutic inhibition of the complement system. *Pharmacol Rev* 1998;50:59–87.
53. Walport MJ. Complement, First of two parts. *N Engl J Med* 2001;344:1058–1066.
54. Di Gaetano N, Cittera E, Nota R, et al. Complement activation determines the therapeutic activity of rituximab in vivo. *J Immunol* 2003;171:1581–1587.
55. Idusogie EE, Presta LG, Gazzano-Santoro H, et al. Mapping of the C1q binding site on Rituxan, a chimeric antibody with a human IgG1 Fc. *J Immunol* 2000;164:4178–4184.
56. Sunada H, Magun BE, Mendelsohn J, et al. Monoclonal antibody against epidermal growth factor receptor is internalized without stimulating receptor phosphorylation. *Proc Natl Acad Sci U S A* 1986;83:3825–3829.
57. Li S, Schmitz KR, Jeffrey PD, et al. Structural basis for inhibition of the epidermal growth factor receptor by cetuximab. *Cancer Cell* 2005;7:301–311.
58. Franklin MC, Carey KD, Vajdos FF, et al. Insights into ErbB signaling from the structure of the ErbB2-pertuzumab complex. *Cancer Cell* 2004;5:317–328.
59. Presta LG, Chen H, O'Connor SJ, et al. Humanization of an anti-vascular endothelial growth factor monoclonal antibody for the therapy of solid tumors and other disorders. *Cancer Res* 1997;57:4593–4599.
60. Adams GP, Weiner LM. Monoclonal antibody therapy of cancer. *Nat Biotechnol* 2005;23:1147–1157.
61. Reiter Y, Pastan I. Recombinant Fv immunotoxins and Fv fragments as novel agents for cancer therapy and diagnosis. *Trends Biotechnol* 1998;16:513–520.
62. Kreitman RJ, Wang QC, FitzGerald DJ, et al. Complete regression of human B-cell lymphoma xenografts in mice treated with recombinant anti-CD22 immunotoxin RFB4(dsFv)-PE38 at doses tolerated by cynomolgus monkeys. *Int J Cancer* 1999;81:148–155.
63. Kreitman RJ, Wilson WH, Bergeron K, et al. Efficacy of the anti-CD22 recombinant immunotoxin BL22 in chemotherapy-resistant hairy-cell leukemia. *N Engl J Med* 2001;345:241–247.
64. Pai LH, Bookman MA, Ozols RF, et al. Clinical evaluation of intraperitoneal Pseudomonas exotoxin immunoconjugate OVB3-PE in patients with ovarian cancer. *J Clin Oncol* 1991;9:1105–1105.
65. Baluna R, Vitetta ES. Vascular leak syndrome: a side effect of immunotherapy. *Immunopharmacology* 1997;37:117–132.
66. Lode HN, Xiang R, Becker JC, et al. Immunocytokines: a promising approach to cancer immunotherapy. *Pharmacol Ther* 1998;80:277–292.
67. Hornick JL, Khawli LA, Hu P, et al. Pretreatment with a monoclonal antibody/interleukin-2 fusion protein directed against DNA enhances the delivery of therapeutic molecules to solid tumors. *Clin Cancer Res* 1999;5:51–60.
68. Lode HN, Xiang R, Duncan SR, et al. Tumor-targeted IL-2 amplifies T cell-mediated immune response induced by gene therapy with single-chain IL-12. *Proc Natl Acad Sci U S A* 1999;96:8591–8596.
69. Sharifi J, Khawli LA, Hu P, et al. Generation of human interferon gamma and tumor necrosis factor alpha chimeric TNT-3 fusion proteins. *Hybrid Hybridomics* 2002;21:421–432.
70. Halin C, Niesner U, Villani ME, et al. Tumor-targeting properties of antibody-vascular endothelial growth factor fusion proteins. *Int J Cancer* 2002;102:109–116.
71. Halin C, Rondini S, Nilsson F, et al. Enhancement of the antitumor activity of interleukin-12 by targeted delivery to neovasculature. *Nature Biotechnol* 2002;20:264–269.
72. Petersdorf SH, Kopecky KJ, Slovak M, et al. A phase 3 study of gemtuzumab ozogamicin during induction and postconsolidation therapy in younger patients with acute myeloid leukemia. *Blood* 2013;121:4854–4860.
73. Burnett AK, Hills RK, Milligan D, et al. Identification of patients with acute myeloblastic leukemia who benefit from the addition of gemtuzumab ozogamicin: results of the MRC AML15 trial. *J Clin Oncol* 2011;29:369–377.
74. Castaigne S, Pautas C, Terre C, et al. Effect of gemtuzumab ozogamicin on survival of adult patients with de-novo acute myeloid leukaemia (ALFA-0701): a randomised, open-label, phase 3 study. *Lancet* 2012;379:1508–1516.
75. Ducry L, Stump B. Antibody-drug conjugates: linking cytotoxic payloads to monoclonal antibodies. *Bioconjug Chem* 2010;21:5–13.
76. Lambert JM. Drug-conjugated antibodies for the treatment of cancer. *Br J Clin Pharmacol* 2013;76:248–262.
77. van de Donk NW, Dhimolea E. Brentuximab vedotin. *MAbs* 2012;4:458–465.
78. LoRusso PM, Weiss D, Guardino E, et al. Trastuzumab emtansine: a unique antibody-drug conjugate in development for human epidermal growth factor receptor 2-positive cancer. *Clin Cancer Res* 2011;17:6437–6447.
79. Park JW, Hong K, Kirpotin DB, et al. Anti-HER2 immunoliposomes: enhanced efficacy attributable to targeted delivery. *Clin Cancer Res* 2002;8:1172–1181.
80. Rodriguez M, Coma S, Noe V, et al. Development and effects of immunoliposomes carrying an antisense oligonucleotide against DHFR RNA and directed toward human breast cancer cells overexpressing HER2. *Antisense Nucleic Acid Drug Dev* 2002;12:311–325.
81. Juweid ME. Radioimmunotherapy of B-cell non-Hodgkin's lymphoma: from clinical trials to clinical practice. *J Nucl Med* 2002;43:1507–1529.
82. Witzig TE, White CA, Wiseman GA, et al. Phase I/II trial of IDEC-Y2B8 radioimmunotherapy for treatment of relapsed or refractory CD20(+) B-cell non-Hodgkin's lymphoma. *J Clin Oncol* 1999;17:3793–3803.

83. Carter P, Presta L, Gorman CM, et al. Humanization of an anti-p185HER2 antibody for human cancer therapy. *Proc Natl Acad Sci U S A* 1992;89:4285–4289.
84. Slamon DJ, Clark GM, Wong SG, et al. Human breast cancer: correlation of relapse and survival with amplification of the HER-2/neu oncogene. *Science* 1987;235:177–182.
85. Dawood S, Broglio K, Buzdar AU, et al. Prognosis of women with metastatic breast cancer by HER2 status and trastuzumab treatment: an institutional-based review. *J Clin Oncol* 2010;28:92–98.
86. Tanner M, Hollmen M, Junttila TT, et al. Amplification of HER-2 in gastric carcinoma: association with Topoisomerase IIalpha gene amplification, intestinal type, poor prognosis and sensitivity to trastuzumab. *Ann Oncol* 2005;16:273–278.
87. Baselga J, Tripathy D, Mendelsohn J, et al. Phase II study of weekly intravenous recombinant humanized anti-p185HER2 monoclonal antibody in patients with HER2/neu-overexpressing metastatic breast cancer. *J Clin Oncol* 1996;14:737–744.
88. Cobleigh MA, Vogel CL, Tripathy D, et al. Multinational study of the efficacy and safety of humanized anti-HER2 monoclonal antibody in women who have HER2-overexpressing metastatic breast cancer that has progressed after chemotherapy for metastatic disease. *J Clin Oncol* 1999;17:2639–2648.
89. Slamon DJ, Leyland-Jones B, Shak S, et al. Addition of Herceptin™ (humanized anti-HER2 antibody) to first line chemotherapy for HER2 overexpressing metastatic breast cancer (HER2/MBC) markedly increases anticancer activity: a randomized multinational controlled phase III trial. *Proc Am Soc Clin Oncol* 1998;17:A377.
90. Piccart-Gebhart MJ, Procter M, Leyland-Jones B, et al. Trastuzumab after adjuvant chemotherapy in HER2-positive breast cancer. *N Engl J Med* 2005;353:1659–1672.
91. Romond EH, Perez EA, Bryant J, et al. Trastuzumab plus adjuvant chemotherapy for operable HER2-positive breast cancer. *N Engl J Med* 2005;353:1673–1684.
92. Smith I, Procter M, Gelber RD, et al. 2-year follow-up of trastuzumab after adjuvant chemotherapy in HER2-positive breast cancer: a randomised controlled trial. *Lancet* 2007;369:29–36.
93. Ewer MS, Gibbs HR, Swafford J, et al. Cardiotoxicity in patients receiving transtuzumab (Herceptin): primary toxicity, synergistic or sequential stress, or surveillance artifact? *Semin Oncol* 1999;26:96–101.
94. Bang YJ, Van Cutsem E, Feyereislova A, et al. Trastuzumab in combination with chemotherapy versus chemotherapy alone for treatment of HER2-positive advanced gastric or gastro-oesophageal junction cancer (ToGA): a phase 3, open-label, randomised controlled trial. *Lancet* 2010;376:687–697.
95. Gomez-Martin C, Plaza JC, Pazo-Cid R, et al. Level of HER2 gene amplification predicts response and overall survival in HER2-positive advanced gastric cancer treated with trastuzumab. *J Clin Oncol* 2013;10:4445–4452.
96. Agus DB, Akita RW, Fox WD, et al. Targeting ligand-activated ErbB2 signaling inhibits breast and prostate tumor growth. *Cancer Cell* 2002;2:127–137.
97. Baselga J, Cortes J, Kim SB, et al. Pertuzumab plus trastuzumab plus docetaxel for metastatic breast cancer. *N Engl J Med* 2012;366:109–119.
98. Swain SM, Kim SB, Cortes J, et al. Pertuzumab, trastuzumab, and docetaxel for HER2-positive metastatic breast cancer (CLEOPATRA study): overall survival results from a randomised, double-blind, placebo-controlled, phase 3 study. *Lancet Oncol* 2013;14:461–471.
99. Gianni L, Pienkowski T, Im YH, et al. Efficacy and safety of neoadjuvant pertuzumab and trastuzumab in women with locally advanced, inflammatory, or early HER2-positive breast cancer (NeoSphere): a randomised multicentre, open-label, phase 2 trial. *Lancet Oncol* 2012;13:25–32.
100. Waksal HW. Role of an anti-epidermal growth factor receptor in treating cancer. *Cancer Metastasis Rev* 1999;18:427–436.
101. Van Cutsem ELI, D'haens G. KRAS status and efficacy in the first-line treatment of patients with metastatic colorectal cancer (metastatic CRC) treated with FOLFIRI with or without cetuximab: The CRYSTAL experience. Abstract 2. *J Clin Oncol* 2008;26:5s.
102. Bokemeyer CBI, Hartmann JT. KRAS status and efficacy of first-line treatment of patients with metastatic colorectal (metastatic CRC) with FOLFOX with or without cetuximab: The OPUS experience. Abstract 4000. *J Clin Oncol* 2008;26:178s.
103. Pirker R, Pereira JR, Szczesna A, et al. Cetuximab plus chemotherapy in patients with advanced non-small-cell lung cancer (FLEX): an open-label randomised phase III trial. *Lancet* 2009;373:1525–1531.
104. Lynch TJ, Patel T, Dreisbach L, et al. Cetuximab and first-line taxane/carboplatin chemotherapy in advanced non-small-cell lung cancer: results of the randomized multicenter phase III trial BMS099. *J Clin Oncol* 2010;28:911–917.
105. Gibson TB, Ranganathan A, Grothey A. Randomized phase III trial of panitumumab, a fully human anti-epidermal growth factor receptor monoclonal antibody, in metastatic colorectal cancer. *Clin Colorectal Cancer* 2006;6:29–31.
106. Amado RG, Wolf M, Peeters M, et al. Wild-type KRAS is required for panitumumab efficacy in patients with metastatic colorectal cancer. *J Clin Oncol* 2008;26:1626–1634.
107. Brown LF, Berse B, Jackman RW, et al. Expression of vascular permeability factor (vascular endothelial growth factor) and its receptors in breast cancer. *Hum Pathol* 1995;26:86–91.
108. Obermair A, Kohlberger P, Bancher-Todesca D, et al. Influence of microvessel density and vascular permeability factor/vascular endothelial growth factor expression on prognosis in vulvar cancer. *Gynecol Oncol* 1996;63:204–209.
109. Takahashi Y, Tucker SL, Kitadai Y, et al. Vessel counts and expression of vascular endothelial growth factor as prognostic factors in node-negative colon cancer. *Arch Surg* 1997;132:541–546.
110. Jain RK. Normalization of tumor vasculature: an emerging concept in antiangiogenic therapy. *Science* 2005;307:58–62.
111. Hurwitz H, Fehrenbacher L, Novotny W, et al. Bevacizumab plus irinotecan, fluorouracil, and leucovorin for metastatic colorectal cancer. *N Engl J Med* 2004;350:2335–2342.
112. Sandler A, Gray R, Perry MC, et al. Paclitaxel-carboplatin alone or with bevacizumab for non-small-cell lung cancer. *N Engl J Med* 2006;355:2542–2550.
113. Miller K, Wang M, Gralow J, et al. Paclitaxel plus bevacizumab versus paclitaxel alone for metastatic breast cancer. *N Engl J Med* 2007;357:2666.
114. Miller KD, Chap LI, Holmes FA, et al. Randomized phase III trial of capecitabine compared with bevacizumab plus capecitabine in patients with previously treated metastatic breast cancer. *J Clin Oncol* 2005;23:792–799.
115. Allegra CJ, Yothers G, O'Connell MJ, et al. Initial safety report of NSABP C-08: A randomized phase III study of modified FOLFOX6 with or without bevacizumab for the adjuvant treatment of patients with stage II or III colon cancer. *J Clin Oncol* 2009;27:3385–3390.
116. Cameron D, Brown J, Dent R, et al. Adjuvant bevacizumab-containing therapy in triple-negative breast cancer (BEATRICE): primary results of a randomised, phase 3 trial. *Lancet Oncol* 2013;14:933–942.
117. Kreisl TN, Kim L, Moore K, et al. Phase II trial of single-agent bevacizumab followed by bevacizumab plus irinotecan at tumor progression in recurrent glioblastoma. *J Clin Oncol* 2009;27:740–745.
118. Burris HA 3rd, Rugo HS, Vukelja SJ, et al. Phase II study of the antibody drug conjugate trastuzumab-DM1 for the treatment of human epidermal growth factor receptor 2 (HER2)-positive breast cancer after prior HER2-directed therapy. *J Clin Oncol* 2011;29:398–405.
119. Krop IE, LoRusso P, Miller KD, et al. A phase II study of trastuzumab emtansine in patients with human epidermal growth factor receptor 2-positive metastatic breast cancer who were previously treated with trastuzumab, lapatinib, an anthracycline, a taxane, and capecitabine. *J Clin Oncol* 2012;30:3234–3241.
120. Verma S, Miles D, Gianni L, et al. Trastuzumab emtansine for HER2-positive advanced breast cancer. *N Engl J Med* 2012;367:1783–1791.
121. Thomas D, Carriere P, Jacobs I. Safety of denosumab in giant-cell tumour of bone. *Lancet Oncol* 2012;11:815.
122. Chawla S, Henshaw R, Seeger L, et al. Safety and efficacy of denosumab for adults and skeletally mature adolescents with giant cell tumour of bone: interim analysis of an open-label, parallel-group, phase 2 study. *Lancet Oncol* 2013;14:901–908.
123. Fizazi K, Carducci M, Smith M, et al. Denosumab versus zoledronic acid for treatment of bone metastases in men with castration-resistant prostate cancer: a randomised, double-blind study. *Lancet* 2011;377:813–822.
124. Henry DH, Costa L, Goldwasser F, et al. Randomized, double-blind study of denosumab versus zoledronic acid in the treatment of bone metastases in patients with advanced cancer (excluding breast and prostate cancer) or multiple myeloma. *J Clin Oncol* 2011;29:1125–1132.
125. Stopeck AT, Lipton A, Body JJ, et al. Denosumab compared with zoledronic acid for the treatment of bone metastases in patients with advanced breast cancer: a randomized, double-blind study. *J Clin Oncol* 2010;28:5132–5139.
126. Smith MR, Egerdie B, Hernandez Toriz N, et al. Denosumab in men receiving androgen-deprivation therapy for prostate cancer. *N Engl J Med* 2009;361:745–755.
127. Ellis GK, Bone HG, Chlebowski R, et al. Randomized trial of denosumab in patients receiving adjuvant aromatase inhibitors for nonmetastatic breast cancer. *J Clin Oncol* 2008;26:4875–4882.
128. Maloney D, Grillo-López A, Bodkin D, et al. IDEC-C2B8: results of a phase I multiple-dose trial in patients with relapsed non-Hodgkin's lymphoma. *J Clin Oncol* 1997;15:3266–3274.
129. Maloney D, Grillo-López A, White C, et al. IDEC-C2B8 (Rituximab) anti-CD20 monoclonal antibody therapy in patients with relapsed low-grade non-Hodgkin's lymphoma. *Blood* 1997;90:2188–2195.
130. Shan D, Ledbetter J, Press O. Signaling events involved in anti-CD20-induced apoptosis of malignant human B cells. *Cancer Immunol Immunother* 2000;48:673–683.
131. Coiffier B, Haioun C, Ketterer N, et al. Rituximab (anti-CD20 monoclonal antibody) for the treatment of patients with relapsing or refractory aggressive lymphoma: a multicenter phase II study. *Blood* 1998;92:1927–1932.
132. Czuczman MS, Grillo-López AJ, White CA, et al. Treatment of patients with low-grade B-cell lymphoma with the combination of chimeric anti-CD20 monoclonal antibody and CHOP chemotherapy. *J Clin Oncol* 1999;17:268–276.
133. Demidem A, Lam T, Alas S, et al. Chimeric anti-CD20 (IDEC-C2B8) monoclonal antibody sensitizes a B cell lymphoma cell line to cell killing by cytotoxic drugs. *Cancer Biother Radiopharm* 1997;12:177–186.
134. Gribben JG, Freedman A, Woo SD, et al. All advanced stage non-Hodgkin's lymphomas with a polymerase chain reaction amplifiable breakpoint of bcl-2 have residual cells containing the rearrangement at evaluation and after treatment. *Blood* 1991;78:3275–3280.
135. Feugier P, Van Hoof A, Sebban C, et al. Long-term results of the R-CHOP study in the treatment of elderly patients with diffuse large B-cell lymphoma: a study by the Groupe d'Etude des Lymphomes de l'Adulte. *J Clin Oncol* 2005;23:4117–4126.

136. Kaufmann H, Raderer M, Wohrer S, et al. Antitumor activity of rituximab plus thalidomide in patients with relapsed/refractory mantle cell lymphoma. *Blood* 2004;104:2269–2271.
137. Reddy N, Hernandez-Ilizaliturri FJ, Deeb G, et al. Immunomodulatory drugs stimulate natural killer-cell function, alter cytokine production by dendritic cells, and inhibit angiogenesis enhancing the anti-tumour activity of rituximab in vivo. *Br J Haematol* 2008;140:36–45.
138. Hooijberg E, Sein JJ, van den Berk PC, et al. Eradication of large human B cell tumors in nude mice with unconjugated CD20 monoclonal antibodies and interleukin 2. *Cancer Res* 1995;55:2627–2634.
139. Friedberg JW, Neuberg D, Gribben JG, et al. Combination immunotherapy with rituximab and interleukin 2 in patients with relapsed or refractory follicular non-Hodgkin's lymphoma. *Br J Haematol* 2002;117:828–834.
140. Khan KD, Emmanouilides C, Benson DM Jr., et al. A phase 2 study of rituximab in combination with recombinant interleukin-2 for rituximab-refractory indolent non-Hodgkin's lymphoma. *Clin Cancer Res* 2006;12:7046–7053.
141. van der Kolk LE, Grillo-López AJ, Baars JW, et al. Treatment of relapsed B-cell non-Hodgkin's lymphoma with a combination of chimeric anti-CD20 monoclonal antibodies (rituximab) and G-CSF: final report on safety and efficacy. *Leukemia* 2003;17:1658–1664.
142. Warren TL, Dahle CE, Weiner GJ. CpG oligodeoxynucleotides enhance monoclonal antibody therapy of a murine lymphoma. *Clin Lymphoma* 2000;1:57–61.
143. Smith MR, Jin F, Joshi I. Enhanced efficacy of therapy with antisense BCL-2 oligonucleotides plus anti-CD20 monoclonal antibody in scid mouse/human lymphoma xenografts. *Mol Cancer Ther* 2004;3:1693–1699.
144. Ramanarayanan J, Hernandez-Ilizaliturri FJ, Chanan-Khan A, et al. Pro-apoptotic therapy with the oligonucleotide Genasense (oblimersen sodium) targeting Bcl-2 protein expression enhances the biological anti-tumour activity of rituximab. *Br J Haematol* 2004;127:519–530.
145. van Delft MF, Wei AH, Mason KD, et al. The BH3 mimetic ABT-737 targets selective Bcl-2 proteins and efficiently induces apoptosis via Bak/Bax if Mcl-1 is neutralized. *Cancer Cell* 2006;10:389–399.
146. Paoluzzi L, Gonen M, Gardner JR, et al. Targeting Bcl-2 family members with the BH3 mimetic AT-101 markedly enhances the therapeutic effects of chemotherapeutic agents in in vitro and in vivo models of B-cell lymphoma. *Blood* 2008;111:5350–5358.
147. Nguyen M, Marcellus RC, Roulston A, et al. Small molecule obatoclax (GX15-070) antagonizes MCL-1 and overcomes MCL-1-mediated resistance to apoptosis. *Proc Natl Acad Sci U S A* 2007;104:19512–19517.
148. Coiffier B, Lepretre S, Pedersen LM, et al. Safety and efficacy of ofatumumab, a fully human monoclonal anti-CD20 antibody, in patients with relapsed or refractory B-cell chronic lymphocytic leukemia: a phase 1-2 study. *Blood* 2008;111:1094–1100.
149. Wierda WG, Kipps TJ, Mayer J, et al. Ofatumumab as single-agent CD20 immunotherapy in fludarabine-refractory chronic lymphocytic leukemia. *J Clin Oncol* 2010;28:1749–1755.
150. Stein R, Qu Z, Chen S, et al. Characterization of a new humanized anti-CD20 monoclonal antibody, IMMU-106, and its use in combination with the humanized anti-CD22 antibody, epratuzumab, for the therapy of non-Hodgkin's lymphoma. *Clin Cancer Res* 2004;10:2868–2878.
151. Senter PD, Sievers EL. The discovery and development of brentuximab vedotin for use in relapsed Hodgkin lymphoma and systemic anaplastic large cell lymphoma. *Nat Biotechnol* 2012;30:631–637.
152. Pro B, Advani R, Brice P, et al. Brentuximab vedotin (SGN-35) in patients with relapsed or refractory systemic anaplastic large-cell lymphoma: results of a phase II study. *J Clin Oncol* 2012;30:2190–2196.
153. Younes A, Gopal AK, Smith SE, et al. Results of a pivotal phase II study of brentuximab vedotin for patients with relapsed or refractory Hodgkin's lymphoma. *J Clin Oncol* 2012;30:2183–2189.

30 Assessment of Clinical Response

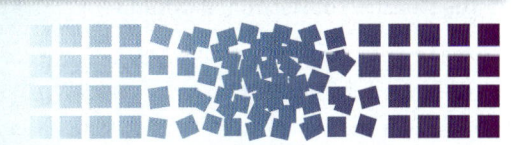

Antonio Tito Fojo and Susan E. Bates

INTRODUCTION

Approaches to response assessments have become increasingly important over the past decade as the drug development pipeline has steadily increased in volume. In 2012, an estimated 981 medicines were in development for cancer, and the number is certainly higher today.[1] The challenge is, first, how to measure the activity of an agent in the research setting, and, second, how to measure activity in the standard of care setting.

The "modern era" of drug development began in 1976 when 16 experienced oncologists treating lymphoma gathered to decide what would be considered a reliable measure of response to a therapy.[2] Each oncologist measured 12 *simulated tumor masses* employing *usual clinical methods* (i.e., calipers or rulers). A principal goal was to identify the amount of shrinkage that *could not* be ascribed to operator error and that *would not* be found if a *placebo* was administered. Moertel and Hanley recommended that *to avoid error, a 50% reduction in the product of perpendicular diameters be employed as the criterion for efficacy*.[2] It was from this beginning that our current methodologies of response assessment evolved. The important point to note is that the decision to use a 50% reduction in the product of perpendicular diameters as a measure of efficacy was made so as to reduce error and *not because it represented a value that conferred clinical benefit*.

From Calipers and Rulers in Lymphoma to the Bidimensional World Health Organization Criteria

In 1981, five years after the Moertel and Hanley report,[2] a World Health Organization (WHO) initiative developed standardized approaches for the "reporting of response, recurrence and disease-free interval."[3] The WHO criteria, like Moertel and Hanley, recommended that malignant disease be measured in two dimensions. Complete response (CR) was defined as the disappearance of all known disease, and a partial response (PR) was scored if there occurred a "50% decrease in the sum of the products of the perpendicular diameters of the multiple lesions." Thus, the 50% reduction initially chosen as an operationally optimal value became institutionalized as the threshold for declaring efficacy in the majority of cancers. This measure of efficacy was perpetuated in 2000 with the now widely used Response Evaluation Criteria in Solid Tumors (RECIST), but shifting to one dimension.[4] The authors noted "the definition of a partial response, in particular, is an arbitrary convention—there is no inherent meaning for an individual patient of a 50% decrease in overall tumor load." Nevertheless, the threshold chosen—a 30% reduction in one dimension—was comparable in volume to the 50% decrease in the sum of the products of the perpendicular diameters and thus perpetuated the 1976 standard. In spite of its arbitrary origins, the 50% reduction has held up over time. But the major impact of the WHO criteria was that it marked the beginning of a common language of response. These criteria have been revisited and refined over time, as technology and medicine advanced. Table 30.1 compares the WHO criteria with those of RECIST 1.0 and RECIST 1.1 and three modifications of RECIST, whereas Figure 30.1 provides a visual presentation of the RECIST threshold required to qualify as response or progression.[3-9]

ASSESSING RESPONSE

RECIST 1.1

The RECIST 1.0 guidelines were updated as RECIST 1.1 in 2009, with a number of differences between the two response criteria highlighted. RECIST 1.1 preserves the same categories of response found in RECIST 1.0:

- Complete response: Complete disappearance of all disease
- Partial response: ≥30% reduction in the sum of the longest diameter of target lesions
- Stable disease: Change not meeting criteria for response or progression
- Progression: ≥20% increase in the sum of the longest diameter of target lesions

However, a decade of experience with RECIST identified several problems with the criteria, some of which could be corrected. In RECIST 1.0, minimum size varied between 1 and 2 cm depending on technique; in RECIST 1.1, a 1-cm lesion is the minimum measurable. In RECIST 1.0, 10 lesions were to be measured, 5 per organ; RECIST 1.1 reduced that to 5 lesions, 2 per organ. Response criteria in RECIST 1.0 did not address lymph nodes; in RECIST 1.1, lymph nodes decreasing to <1 cm in their short axis could constitute a complete response. Disease progression in nontarget disease was further defined to indicate that in addition to a 20% increase in target lesions over the smallest sum on study, there must be an absolute increase of 5 mm, and that an increase of a single nontarget lesion should not trump an overall disease status assessment based on target lesions.

Variations of the RECIST Criteria

The RECIST criteria have been widely used for standardizing the reporting of clinical trial results and have improved reproducibility. However, the increasing precision and codification of RECIST has led to recognition of its limitations. For example, there are unique challenges in central nervous system (CNS) disease, relating response to tumor size measurements based on contrast enhancement. Pseudoprogression refers to an increase in contrast enhancement due to a transient increase in vascular permeability after irradiation, whereas pseudoresponse is a decrease in contrast enhancement that may occur due to a reduction in vascular permeability following corticosteroids or an antiangiogenic agent such as bevacizumab.[10-12] The McDonald criteria, traditionally used in determining glioma response based

TABLE 30.1
Key Features of Response Criteria

	WHO[3]	RECIST 1.0[4]	RECIST 1.1[5]	CNS RANO Criteria[7]	RECIST Mesothelioma[8]	RECIST Immunotherapy[9]
Dimension	Uni- and bidimensional	Unidimensional	Unidimensional	Bidimensional	Unidimensional	Bidimensional
Measurable Lesion	Not defined	Longest diameter, ≥20 mm with most modalities; ≥10 mm with spiral CT	Longest diameter ≥10 mm on CT or on skin if using calipers; ≥20 mm if using CXR	Two perpendicular diameters of contrast enhancing lesions ≥10 mm	Tumor thickness perpendicular to chest wall or mediastinum, measured in two positions at three levels on transverse cuts of CT scan	Longest perpendicular diameters
Measurable Lymph Nodes	Not defined	Not defined	≥15 mm short axis	—	—	—
Disease Burden to be Assessed at Baseline	All (not specified)	Measurable target lesions up to 10 total (5 per organ); other lesions nontarget	Measurable target lesions up to 5 total (2 per organ); other lesions nontarget	Two to five lesions in patients with several lesions	Pleural disease in perpendicular diameter; nodal, subcutaneous, and other bidimensional lesions measured unidimensionally as per the RECIST criteria	5 lesions per organ, up to 10 visceral lesions and five cutaneous lesions
Sum	Sum of the products of bidimensional diameters or sum of linear unidimensional diameters	Sum of longest diameters of all measurable lesions	Sum of the longest diameters of target lesions with only exception use of short axis for lymph nodes	Sum of the products of perpendicular diameters of all measurable enhancing target lesions	Sum of the six measurements defines a pleural unidimensional measure	SPD with new lesions incorporated into baseline; tumor burden = SPD$_{index\ lesions}$ + SPD$_{new\ lesions}$
Complete Response	Disappearance all known disease	Disappearance all known disease	Disappearance all known disease; lymph nodes <10 mm	—	Disappearance all target lesions with no evidence of tumor elsewhere	Disappearance all lesions in two consecutive observations
Partial Response	≥50% decrease	≥30% decrease; all other no evidence of progression	≥30% decrease; all other disease, no evidence of progression	≥50% reduction; stable or decreased steroid use compared to baseline	≥30% reduction in total tumor measurement	≥50% decrease compared with baseline in two observations
Response Confirmation?	≥4 weeks apart	≥4 weeks apart	≥4 weeks apart (if response primary end point); no, if secondary endpoint	≥4 weeks apart	Repeat on two occasions ≥4 weeks apart	≥4 weeks apart

(continued)

TABLE 30.1
Key Features of Response Criteria (continued)

	WHO[3]	RECIST 1.0[4]	RECIST 1.1[5]	CNS RANO Criteria[7]	RECIST Mesothelioma[8]	RECIST Immunotherapy[9]
Progressive Disease	≥25% increase in size of one or more measurable lesions or appearance of new lesions	≥20% increase, taking as reference smallest sum in study; or appearance of new lesions	≥20% increase, with absolute increase ≥5 mm, taking as reference smallest sum in study; or appearance of new lesions	≥25%, or any new lesions	≥20% increase in the total tumor measurement over the nadir measurement, or the appearance of one or more new lesions	≥25% increase compared with nadir confirmed ≥4 weeks apart; up to five new lesions (≥5 × 5 mm) per organ incorporated into tumor burden
	Nonmeasurable disease: Estimated increase of ≥25%	Nonmeasurable disease: unequivocal progression	Nonmeasurable disease: unequivocal progression	Nonmeasurable disease: >5 mm increase in maximal diameter; ≥25% increase in SPD; or significant increase in nonenhancing lesions on same or lower dose of corticosteroids	—	New, nonmeasurable lesions (i.e., <5 × 5 mm) do not define progression
Stable Disease	Stable disease or non-PR and non-PD ≥4 weeks	Non-PR, non-PD; minimum time defined by protocol	Non-PR, non-PD; minimum time defined by protocol	—	Non-PR, non-PD	Non-irPR, non-irPD

CXR, Chest X-ray; SPD, sum of products of two largest perpendicular diameters; PD, progressive disease; irPR, immune-related partial response; irPD, immune-related progressive disease.

on two-dimensional measurements, have been recently updated as part of the Response Assessment in Neuro-Oncology (RANO) response criteria and extended to include a response assessment for metastatic CNS disease.[7,13]

Other examples where RECIST is limited include mesothelioma, gastrointestinal stromal tumors (GIST), hepatocellular cancers, among others. The pleural disease of mesothelioma increases in depth while following the pleural surface. GIST tumors may remain unchanged in size after treatment, whereas the center of the tumor mass undergoes necrosis, and progression may occur in the remaining rim.[14] Hepatocellular cancers are often treated with local–regional therapy in which the goal is tumor necrosis and treatment failure occurs in surviving viable tumor.[15] Different strategies have emerged to quantify these diseases, including modifications of RECIST, quantifying positron-emission tomography (PET) imaging, and biomarker criteria, as will be discussed. The RECIST adaptation for mesothelioma, growing along the pleural surface, is to measure the diameter perpendicular to the chest wall or mediastinum, and to measure at three levels.[8] The adaptation for hepatocellular cancer following local therapy is measurement of the longest diameter of the tumor that shows enhancement on the arterial phase of the scan, bypassing the dense, homogeneous Lipiodol-containing necrotic area.[15]

Investigators have also observed that following immunotherapy, tumor lesions may increase in size due to the increased infiltration of T cells, even meeting criteria for RECIST-defined progressive

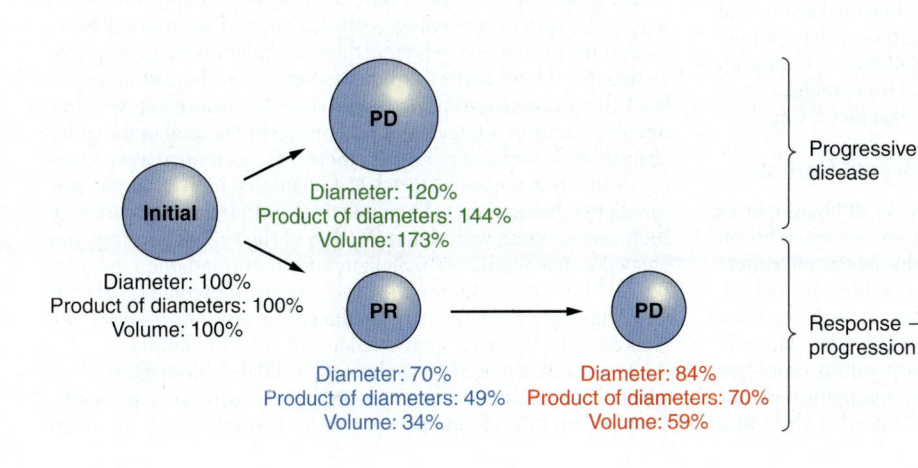

Figure 30.1 RECIST thresholds in three parameters: diameter, product of diameters, and volume. In the figure, spheres meeting RECIST criteria for progressive disease (PD) and for PR are shown with the percentage relative to the baseline calculated for each parameter. To meet the threshold for PD, the longest diameter must increase to 120%, which is equivalent to a 144% increase in the product of the perpendicular diameters and a 173% increase in the volume of a sphere. Although PR definitions are almost identical to those employed with WHO, RECIST has a higher threshold to meet PD.[6]

disease (PD). Previously radiographically undetectable lesions may appear. Departing from conventional RECIST, which defines any new lesion as PD, the immune response criteria allow the appearance of new lesions, adding them to the total tumor burden.[9] An increase in total tumor burden of >25% relative to baseline or nadir is required to define PD.

International Working Group Criteria for Lymphoma

Revised guidelines for lymphoma assessment were promulgated by the International Working Group (IWG) in 2007.[16] These guidelines incorporated 18F-fluorodeoxyglucose (FDG)-PET assessments in metabolically active lymphomas.[16] Although a CR requires the complete disappearance of detectable disease, a post-treatment residual mass is permitted if it is negative on FDG-PET and was positive at baseline. For lymphomas that are not consistently FDG avid, or if FDG avidity is unknown, a CR requires that nodes >1.5 cm before therapy regress to <1.5 cm, and nodes that were 1.1 to 1.5 cm in long axis and >1.0 cm in the short axis shrink to ≤1.0 cm in short axis. The definition of PR resembles the WHO criteria, in that a ≥50% decrease in the sum of the product of the diameters in up to six nodal masses or in hepatic or splenic nodules must be documented. Although RECIST 1.1 now includes lymph node assessment, the IWG criteria remain the assessment method typically used in lymphoma clinical trials.

ALTERNATE RESPONSE CRITERIA

The previous examples represent attempts to more accurately measure tumor burden. Evolving imaging technology enabling volumetric measurements of tumor masses may eventually resolve some of these problems, but effective therapeutic agents are required to enable validation and utilization of response assessment tools. The lack of an agent that can mediate substantial tumor shrinkage underlies the concept of *clinical benefit response* (CBR) as an endpoint in pancreatic cancer. Clinical benefit was defined as a combination of improvement in pain, performance status, and weight; the assessment of CBR supported the U.S. Food and Drug Administration (FDA) approval of gemcitabine in pancreatic cancer.[17,18] Better therapies for pancreatic cancer that result in tumor shrinkage or eradication should include and then eclipse clinical benefit.

Response criteria may be specific to a particular disease or clinical setting. Some diseases by their nature require specific strategies for response assessment.

Severity-Weighted Assessment Tool Score in Cutaneous T-Cell Lymphoma

Cutaneous T-cell lymphoma (CTCL) is a disease that can involve the entire epidermis, or comprise individual skin lesions varying widely in severity rather than size. The severity-weighted assessment tool (SWAT) assigns a factor for skin lesion severity—patch, plaque, or tumor—multiplies this factor by the percent of skin involved with each lesion type and then adds these together. This complex system formed the basis of the FDA approval of vorinostat for CTCL.[19]

Pathologic Complete Response in Breast Cancer

One unique response endpoint is the assessment of breast cancer treated in the neoadjuvant setting. The purpose of neoadjuvant therapy is to improve survival, render locally advanced cancer amenable to surgery, or to aid in breast conservation. In that setting, the absence of cancer cells in resected breast tissue has been used to define a pathologic complete response (pCR). The rate of pCR has been proposed as a surrogate endpoint for event-free survival (EFS) or overall survival (OS) to support approval of new agents or combinations of agents tested in clinical trials.[20] In a pooled analysis of 11,955 patients enrolled on 12 neoadjuvant trials, individual patients with pCR had improved EFS and OS.[21] However, at the trial level, pCR rates did not correlate with EFS or OS, a problem likely due to heterogeneity of breast cancer subtypes among the trials. Despite this, pCR rates were recently used to support the approval of pertuzumab and trastuzumab in the neoadjuvant setting.[21,22]

Computed Tomography-Based Tumor Density

One approach, often called the Choi criteria, advocates assessing tumor response in GIST, renal cell cancer, or hepatocellular cancer based on density on computed tomography (CT) scans (Table 30.2). This variation was prompted by the evident response to treatment with imatinib but with minimal tumor shrinkage.[23] The Choi criteria are still considered exploratory in GIST,[24,25] and it is too soon to know of benefits in other histologies.[26,27] Further study should determine its utility, although it will likely be confined to specific tumor types with specific drugs.

FDG-PET

Although widely used in clinical practice, FDG-PET has become part of standardized response criteria for clinical trials only in lymphoma (see Table 30.2). In solid tumors, FDG-PET can aid in the detection of new or recurrent sites of disease, and can be used as an adjunct during assessments for disease progression when using RECIST criteria.[5] Although FDG uptake is a powerful diagnostic tool and its uptake reflects a tumor's metabolic activity, it has some limitations. Some tumors have variable FDG avidity; differences can occur due to variations in patient activity, carbohydrate intake, blood glucose, and timing; and there are several benign sources of uptake, including inflammatory and postsurgical sites. Multiple methods of quantitating FDG-PET and assessing response have been proposed, but to date there is no consensus, particularly regarding the definition of a metabolic response.[28–33]

The two most widely used response criteria—the European Organisation for the Research and Treatment of Cancer (EORTC) criteria and PET Response Criteria in Solid Tumors (PERCIST) (see Table 30.2)—have been evaluated in specific disease types, but unifying FDG-PET response criteria remains a challenge in anticancer drug development.[28,30] We would note that, as shown in Figure 30.1, a 30% reduction in the diameter of a sphere—the magnitude of change required to score a response according to RECIST—represents a 65% decrease in volume. If an standardized uptake value (SUV) decrease is directly equated to a volume decrease, a reduction of 25% translates to a 10% reduction in diameter, a value that likely constitutes an insufficient response.

Serum Biomarkers of Response

The ideal response assessment method is an assay that could measure tumor quantity by a simple blood test (see Table 30.2). Circulating protein biomarkers have been identified and studied for several decades for screening, early detection of recurrent disease, determining prognosis, selecting therapy, and monitoring response to therapy. These serum tumor markers are to be distinguished from the assays determining the presence of an overexpressed or mutated molecular target. With the successful launch of therapies against such molecular targets, there has been increased interest in the assays needed to select therapy for individual patients (predictive biomarkers). The analytical and clinical validation of such assays, along with determination of their clinical utility, has created a new regulatory paradigm known as *companion diagnostics*.[34,35] This investment in the development of predictive markers for companion diagnostics has reduced the focus on protein biomarkers of treatment response relative to older literature.

As a result, there are few clinically validated biomarkers of response.[36] In addition to issues regarding sensitivity and specificity, their use and development has also been hindered by the often

TABLE 30.2
Alternate Response Criteria: Biomarkers

Criterion	Baseline	Response	Progression
CA-125 in ovarian cancer (GCIG criteria)[43]	CA 125 >2× ULN	CA 125 decline ≥50% confirmed at 28 days	2× nadir OR 2× ULN if normalized on therapy on two occasions 1 wk apart
PSA in prostate cancer (PSA WG1)[45,a]	PSA ≥5 ng/mL and documentation of two consecutive increases in PSA 1 wk apart	PSA decline of 50% from baseline (measured twice 3–4 wks apart)	After decrease from baseline, a 50% increase AND an increase ≥5 ng/mL, or back to baseline, whichever is lower
PSA in prostate cancer (PCWG2)[46,a]	PSA ≥2.0 ng/mL; estimate pretreatment PSA-DT: Need ≥3 values ≥4 wks apart	Report percent change from baseline (rise or fall) at 12 weeks, and separately, the maximal change (rise or fall) at any time using a waterfall plot	PSA increase ≥25% and absolute increase by ≥2 ng/mL above the nadir, confirmed by a second value ≥3 wks later (i.e., confirmed rising trend) OR PSA increase ≥25% and ≥2 ng/mL above baseline >12 wks
hCG and AFP in testicular cancer[50–51]		Decrease consistent with marker half-life: 2–3 d for hCG, 5–7 d for AFP	Rising levels usually indicate need to change therapy
Choi Criteria for CT Imaging			
Choi criteria[24–27]		≥10% decrease in tumor size OR ≥15% reduction in tumor density	An increase in tumor size ≥10% and does not meet criteria of PR by tumor attenuation on CT
FDG-PET Criteria			
EORTC criteria[29–31]	ROI should be drawn, SUV calculated	**CMR:** Complete resolution of uptake **PMR:** SUV reduction ≥25% **SMD:** SUV increase <25% and decrease <15%	**PMD:** SUV increase >25% in regions defined on baseline, or appearance of new FDG-avid lesions
PERCIST criteria[29]	SUL peak >1.5× normal liver	**CMR:** Complete resolution of uptake **PMR:** SUL reduction ≥30%	**PMD:** SUL increase >30% in regions defined on baseline, or appearance of new FDG avid lesions

[a] Guidelines for PSA assessment have evolved from those of the PSAWG1, where responses were dichotomized based on the percent decline, to those in the PCWG2 where PSA response is considered a continuous variable. Recently, emphasis has shifted to assessing PSA doubling time.

CA-125, cancer antigen 125; GCIG, Gynecologic Cancer InterGroup; ULN, upper limit of normal; PSA, prostate-specific antigen; PSAWG1, PSA Working Group 1; PCWG2, Prostate Cancer Working Group 2; PSA-DT, PSA-doubling time; hCG, human chorionic gonatropin; AFP, alpha-fetoprotein; EORTC, European Organisation for the Research and Treatment of Cancer; ROI, regions of interest; SUV, standardized uptake value; CMR, complete metabolic response; PMR, partial metabolic response; SMD, stable metabolic disease; PMD, progressive metabolic disease; PERCIST, PET response criteria in solid tumors; SUL, SUV normalized to lean body mass.

---

limited efficacy of therapies; response biomarkers are of little value without highly effective primary and salvage therapies. For example, a recent clinical trial indicates that in *asymptomatic patients with ovarian cancer whose only evidence of disease progression is an isolated rising CA-125*, nothing is gained by instituting treatment before there is other evidence of progression.[37,38]

- **Cancer Antigen 125 (CA-125):** Despite recognized limitations, CA-125 is widely used. For example, the Gynecologic Cancer InterGroup (GCIG) criteria have evolved to help determine whether a patient's tumor has responded to therapy.[39–41] Response is defined as a 50% decline from an elevated baseline value, whereas progression is defined as a doubling over the nadir or the upper limit of normal.[42] In clinical practice, CA-125 levels are followed as part of standard management, but making clinical decisions on marker changes alone is not recommended.[43]
- **Prostate-Specific Antigen (PSA):** Similar issues have confronted investigators caring for patients with prostate cancer. The PSA Working Group 1 (PCWG1) guidelines, first published in 1999, established PSA criteria, particularly for use in patients with disease that was difficult to quantify.[44] There followed a second working group (PCWG2) that recommended plotting the percent PSA change for each patient in a waterfall plot so as to avoid creating a dichotomous variable from the changes in PSA.[45] PCWG2 also recommended keeping patients on trial until evidence of a change in clinical status—either symptomatic or radiographic progression. The latter addressed concerns with patients in whom PSA changes did not reflect clinical status, particularly those with transient increases in the first 12 weeks of a new therapy.
- **Human Chorionic Gonadotropin (hCG) and alpha fetoprotein (AFP):** Because testicular cancer is a highly curable disease with validated biomarkers, outcome assessment has focused on the rapid detection of patients whose tumors have a poor response to therapy. Because both markers have relatively short half-lives—2 to 3 days for hCG and 5 to 7 days for serum AFP—the rate of decline can be determined. Various methods have demonstrated that a rapid decline or early normalization of marker levels is indicative of a good

outcome, without any one method achieving widespread acceptance.[46-48] Nonetheless, the 2010 American Society of Clinical Oncology (ASCO) guidelines on serum tumor markers concluded there was still insufficient evidence to recommend changing therapy solely on the basis of a slow marker decline.[49] Rising levels after two cycles of therapy (outside the first week of treatment when rises can be due to tumor lysis) can be considered an indication to change the treatment plan.[49,50]

Circulating Tumor Cells and Circulating Tumor DNA

Two response endpoints under recent investigation show a potential to detect the impact of therapy. One is the measurement of circulating tumor cells (CTC) in the bloodstream, enriched by one or more capture strategies, including one that has received FDA approval.[51] The number of CTCs in the blood has been shown to be prognostic, with higher levels conferring a poor prognosis, and to correlate with a response to therapy. A second approach is the determination of levels of circulating tumor DNA (ctDNA) in the blood. This is detected by quantitating the number of DNA molecules carrying a given mutation or gene rearrangement in the blood, typically detected through targeted sequencing of common mutations, or of a previously identified *mutation signature* or gene rearrangement. The amount of ctDNA appears to correlate with tumor burden, increases with stage, and in one study, was deemed more sensitive than CTC detection.[52-54] Whether these tests will ultimately prove to be more sensitive and accurate than the serum biomarkers discussed previously remains to be determined. Because targeted sequencing can be very sensitive, one concern is that false-positive ctDNA detection may occur after treatment, or intermittently in the setting of enlarging tumor masses. At the least, detection of CTCs and ctDNA is advancing our understanding of cancer biology, as studies reveal evidence of metastatic heterogeneity, clonal heterogeneity, and emergence of resistance mutations in clinical samples.

DETERMINING OUTCOME

The response measures described previously represent different approaches to quantitate tumor burden. What happens after those data are obtained varies depending on the clinical setting. In the community, less emphasis is placed on strict criteria. In the setting of a clinical trial, tumor size is measured and the response categorized. For FDA submission, these are but factors in the risk-benefit equation needed for drug approvals. The FDA conveys full approval to new agents based on true *clinical benefit* (i.e., an improvement in a *survival* endpoint or symptom relief).[55] Surrogates for clinical benefit, such as response rate, may support either regular approval or accelerated approval, depending on the setting.

Overall Response Rate, Duration of Response, and Stable Disease

Overall response rate (ORR) is the proportion of patients with a tumor size reduction of a predefined amount for a minimum time period. The FDA has generally defined ORR as the sum of PRs and CRs. Although OS remains the gold standard, ORR is often used both in drug development and in clinical practice to indicate antitumor efficacy of a given therapy. Table 30.3 summarizes the attributes and drawbacks of using ORR as a method of assessment. Using standardized definitions of response, it has been shown that ORR often correlates with OS, although ORR usually explains only a fraction of the variability of the survival benefits.[56-58] Equally important, however, is the duration of response, a value that is measured from the time of initial response until documented tumor progression, and which assumes added importance when ORR is the endpoint for regulatory approval.

Unlike PR and CR, the FDA has generally not been willing to include *stable disease (SD)*, defined as shrinkage that qualifies as neither response nor progression, as part of the ORR, feeling it is often indicative of the underlying disease biology rather than a drug's therapeutic effect.[55,59] Nevertheless, in reporting data, investigators are increasingly using the term CBR, which includes CR + PR + SD and which is a misuse of the term *clinical benefit* because neither CR, PR, or SD are objective tumor findings that address the true *clinical benefit* of a therapy.[58,60] In the absence of standardized definitions for SD that are shown to effect meaningful changes in a clinical outcome, SD should not be used as a response endpoint. A better approach is to use nondichotomized response assessments, such as the waterfall plot or one of the kinetic analyses, discussed later.

Progression-Free Survival, Time to Progression, and Time to Treatment Failure

In cancer drug development, one usually finds ORR assessed as an indicator of activity in phase II trials, whereas randomized phase III trials rely on other endpoints such as progression-free survival (PFS) and time to progression (TTP) (see Table 30.3). Although PFS and TTP attempt to assess efficacy in close proximity to a therapy, they score outcomes differently and are not interchangeable. TTP is defined as the time from randomization to *the time of disease progression*.[55] In TTP analyses, deaths are censored either at the time of death or at an earlier visit. In contrast, PFS is defined from the time of randomization to the time of *disease progression or death*. Although patients who discontinue trial participation for adverse events might be censored in both analyses, patients who die while on study are censored only in the TTP analysis. Those who favor TTP argue that if a patient dies without their tumor meeting criteria for progression, one cannot accurately estimate when progression might have occurred, so the data should be censored. However, those who favor PFS argue that, in some cases, death might be an adverse effect of the therapy. High-dose therapies represent an example of why PFS might be a preferable (regulatory) endpoint. If in a given tumor there is evidence of a dose-response relationship for an active drug, then high doses may have a greater response. However, such high doses may also be responsible for a greater number of deaths. Assessing only those who survive the high dose therapy and ignoring those who die (i.e., TTP) may lead to the conclusion that the high-dose therapy is more effective. The balance sheet that includes death (i.e., PFS) would clearly demonstrate this efficacy came at too great a price.

Although many have argued that PFS and TTP should be acceptable endpoints for cancer clinical trials, in the majority of tumors there is no convincing evidence PFS is a surrogate for OS, and in those where there is some evidence, its value is arguable.[61] Table 30.3 presents the attributes and drawbacks of PFS and TTP. Note that the definition of progression is often difficult, particularly in some tumor types, and that investigator bias can influence PFS and TTP. Problems with ascertainment bias and censoring, depicted in Figure 30.2, can also impact outcomes.

Alternate endpoints include time to treatment failure (TTF), defined as a composite endpoint measuring time from randomization to discontinuation of treatment for any reason, including disease progression, treatment toxicity, and death. The FDA has not recommended TTF as a regulatory endpoint for drug approval. However, the high rates of censoring due to toxicity seen in phase III clinical trials may lead to a reassessment of this position given that most can agree that not only is efficacy important, but so too is tolerability, and TTF can capture both of these attributes.

TABLE 30.3

A Comparison of Important Cancer Approval Endpoints

Regulatory Evidence	Endpoints	Advantages	Disadvantages
Clinical benefit used for regular approvals	Overall survival (OS)	■ Universally accepted direct measure of clinical benefit ■ Easily measured ■ Includes treatment-related mortality that can obscure benefit in a subset ■ Precisely measured; unambiguous ■ Not dependent on assessment intervals	■ May involve larger studies ■ May require long follow-up ■ May be affected by crossover and/or sequential therapies ■ Includes noncancer deaths
	Symptom endpoints (patient-reported outcomes)	■ Patient perspective of direct clinical benefit	■ Blinding is often difficult ■ Data are frequently missing or incomplete ■ Clinical significance of small changes is unknown ■ Multiple analyses ■ Lack of validated instruments
Surrogates used for accelerated approvals or regular approvals	Disease-free survival (DFS)	■ Smaller sample size and shorter follow-up necessary compared with survival studies	■ Not statistically validated as surrogate for survival in all settings ■ Not precisely measured; subject to assessment bias, particularly in open-label studies ■ Definitions vary among studies
	Objective response rate (ORR)	■ Can be assessed in single-arm studies ■ Assessed earlier and in smaller studies compared with survival studies ■ Effect attributable to drug, not natural history	■ Not a direct measure of benefit ■ Not a comprehensive measure of drug activity ■ Only a subset of patients who benefit
	Complete response (CR)	■ Can be assessed in single-arm studies ■ Durable complete responses can represent clinical benefit ■ Assessed earlier and in smaller studies compared with survival studies ■ Definition of progressive disease (PD) identifies uniform time to end treatment and data capture	■ Not a direct measure of benefit in all cases ■ Not a comprehensive measure of drug activity ■ Small subset of patients with benefit ■ Requires prospective, consistent definition. Meaningful response durations not standardized ■ Definition of PD is arbitrary without evidence it actually represents end of benefit period
	Progression-free survival (PFS) or time to progression (TTP)[a]	■ Smaller sample size and shorter follow-up necessary compared with survival studies ■ Measurement of stable disease included ■ Not confounded by crossover or subsequent therapies ■ Generally based on objective and quantitative assessment	■ Statistically validated as surrogate for survival only in some settings ■ Not precisely measured; subject to assessment bias particularly in open-label studies ■ Definitions vary among studies; little agreement on magnitude of difference that constitutes clinical benefit ■ Requires frequent and consistent radiological or other assessments ■ Involves balanced timing of assessments among treatment arms

[a] Progression-free survival includes all deaths; time to progression censors deaths that occur before progression.
Adapted from U.S. Department of Health and Human Services, Food and Drug Administration, Center for Drug Evaluation and Research (CDER), Center for Biologics Evaluation and Research (CBER). *Guidance from Industry. Clinical Trial Endpoints for the Approval of Cancer Drugs and Biologics.* 2007. http://www.fda.gov/downloads/Drugs/.../Guidances/ucm071590.pdf.

Prespecified evaluation interval
Ideally, disease progression is reported at a prespecified evaluation interval

Ascertainment (evaluation) bias
An earlier evaluation leads to earlier scoring of progression (e.g., concern for symptoms prompt earlier evaluation)

Ascertainment (evaluation) bias
A later evaluation leads to delay in scoring progression (e.g., evaluation delayed by toxicity or treatment delays)

Censoring bias
Patient whose disease would have progressed quickly is censored early. Here censoring is "beneficial."

Censoring bias
Patient whose disease would have progressed late is censored early. Here censoring is "detrimental."

Informative censoring
Central review cannot score progression with available data. Although progression had been scored, the data is instead censored centrally. This is usually "beneficial."

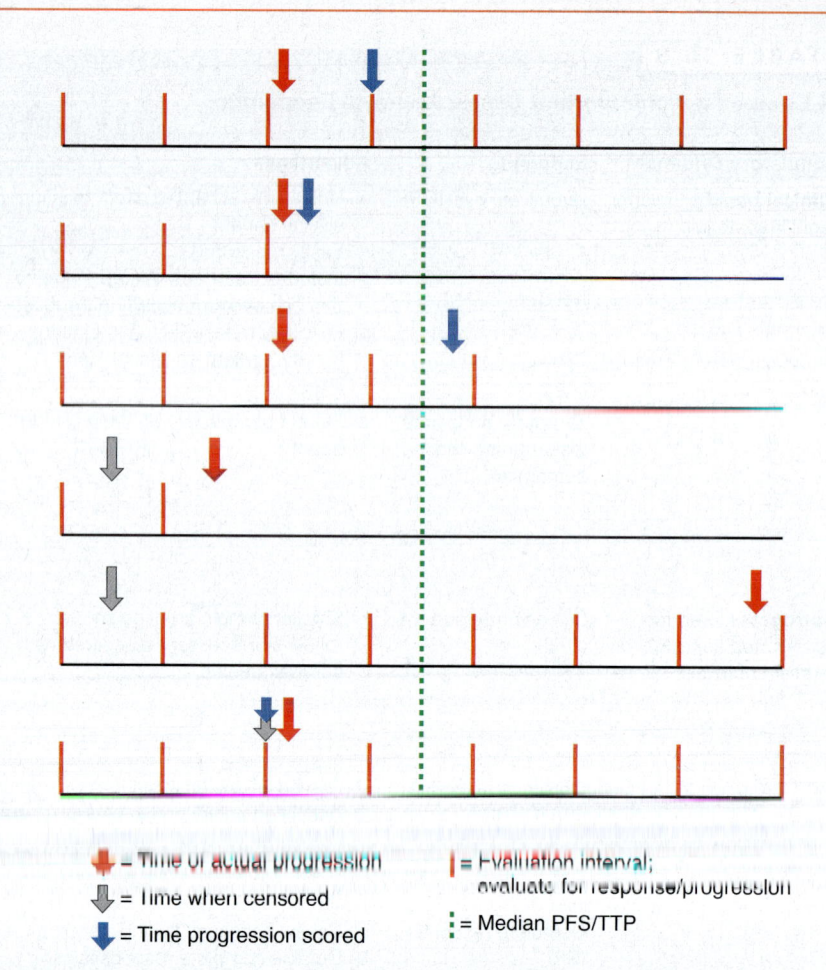

↓ = Time of actual progression
↓ = Time when censored
↓ = Time progression scored
| = Evaluation interval; evaluate for response/progression
┊ = Median PFS/TTP

Figure 30.2 The potential problems encountered when PFS is used as an endpoint. Ideally, as depicted at the *top*, response assessment will be conducted at a prespecified time. However, the date at which progression is scored may suffer from either ascertainment or censoring bias. Ascertainment bias can occur if either an evaluation occurs before the prespecified date or if it is delayed. For example, a clinician concerned about a patient who is not experiencing side effects and has likely been randomized to placebo may be more inclined to investigate symptoms early and document progression before the prespecified time, while delaying the evaluation of a patient randomized to the experimental arm who experiences some toxicity. Similarly, censoring—an increasing problem in randomized trials—may impact the outcome of a given study arm by either censoring patients who would experience early progression (beneficial impact) or censoring those who would have remained progression free for a long time (detrimental impact). Finally, informative censoring can occur when independent radiologic review cannot concur with an investigator's assessment of progression and censors the patient. This outcome is usually beneficial, because a patient who is very close to experiencing progression is censored. (Adapted from Villaruz LC, Socinski MA. The clinical viewpoint: definitions, limitations of RECIST, practical considerations of measurement. *Clin Cancer Res* 2013;19:2629–2636.)

Overall Survival

Defined as the time from randomization to death, OS has been considered the gold standard of clinical trial endpoints (see Table 30.3). In part, this is so because it is unambiguous and does not suffer from interpretation bias. An additional advantage of the survival endpoint is that it can balance the effect of therapies with high treatment-related mortality even if tumor control is substantially better with the new treatment. However, some worry that because patients may receive multiple lines of therapy following the clinical trial, the results may be confounded by those subsequent therapies. The latter concern is often cited as the reason why an advantage in PFS/TTP *disappears* when one looks to OS. But as a review of clinical trials confirms,[62] the magnitude of the difference does not disappear, only the statistical validity (Fig. 30.3).[63,64]

When evaluating a randomized controlled trial, it is important that the OS as well as the PFS analyses are always by intention to treat (ITT). In an ITT analysis, often described as *once randomized, always analyzed*, all patients assigned to a group at the time of randomization are analyzed regardless of what occurred subsequently.[65] An ITT analysis avoids the bias introduced by omitting dropouts and noncompliant patients that can negate randomization and overestimate clinical effectiveness.

Kaplan–Meier Plots

In a typical clinical trial, data are often presented as a Kaplan–Meier plots. In discrete time intervals, the number of patients in each group who are progression free and alive (PFS analysis) or alive (OS analysis) at the end of the interval are counted and divided by the total number of patients in that group at the beginning of the time interval. One excludes from this calculation patients censored for a reason other than progressive disease or death during the same interval. This has the advantage that it allows one to include censored patients in estimates of the probability of PFS or OS up to the point when they were censored (i.e., they are excluded only beyond the point of censoring). In most clinical trials, a fraction of patients are typically censored.

In constructing the Kaplan–Meier plot, probabilities are calculated for each interval of time. The probability of surviving

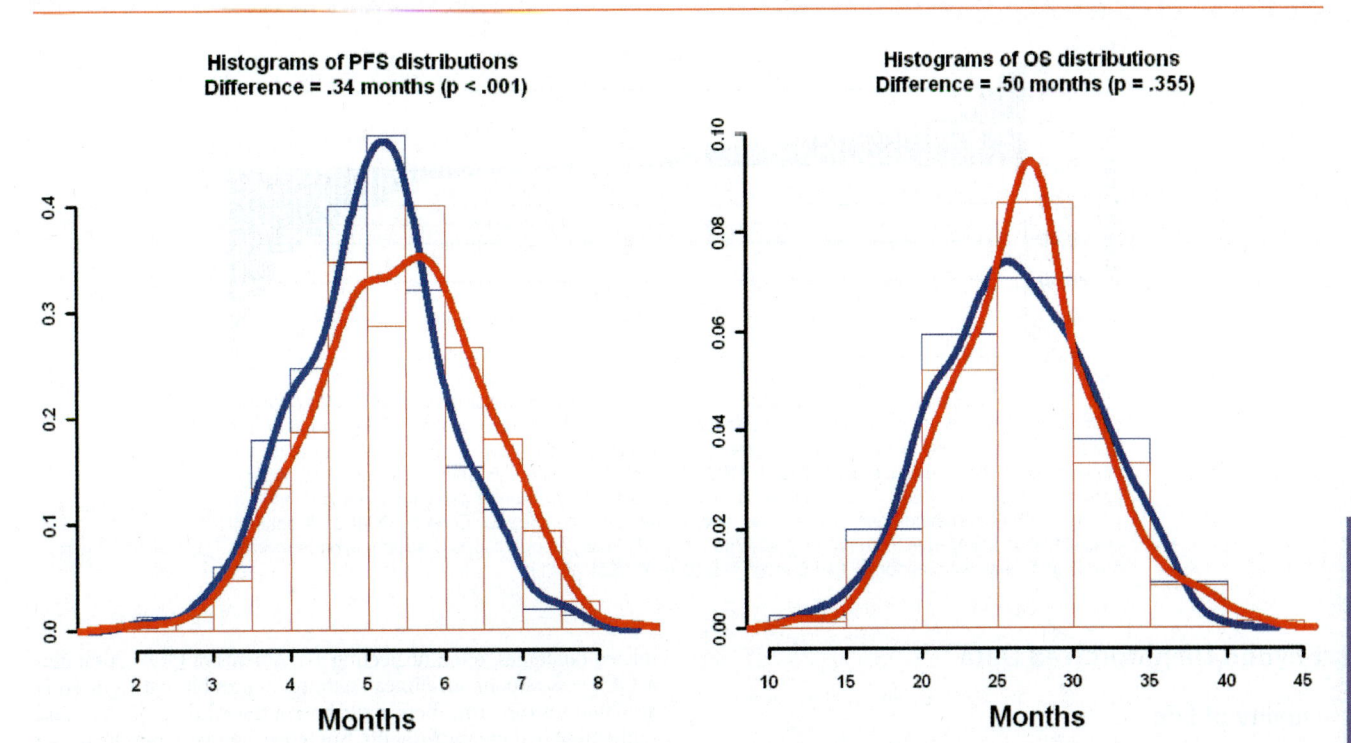

Figure 30.3 Hypothetical distribution of PFS and OS data demonstrating the *disappearance of PFS benefit*. Because chemotherapy does not exert a lasting effect on the underlying tumor biology and because PFS is a shorter interval (measured in increments, not daily as is OS) PFS differences often disappear. The *hypothetical example* shown illustrates this phenomenon. The *left panel* shows a histogram of PFS distributions with a difference of 0.34 months that nevertheless achieves statistical significance over the short interval when PFS is measured. The *right panel* depicts similar histograms for OS captured over a longer time period. Despite a larger absolute difference of 0.5 months, the OS difference does not reach statistical significance. For these hypothetical curves, random number generated data sets (with normal distribution), histograms and density plots were generated using R version 2.11.1 (2010-05-31).[76] The differences were deliberately chosen to be small, but a similar disappearance can also occur with larger differences. As can be seen, what disappears is not the absolute benefit, but the statistical validity.

progression free or being counted as a survivor to the end of any interval of assessment is the product of the probabilities of surviving in all the preceding assessment intervals multiplied by the probability for the interval of interest. One might ask to what extent the two curves in each study differ. One measure that is of value is the median PFS or OS—a value calculated in most studies from a Kaplan–Meier plot.

Hazard Ratios

Increasingly, however, hazard ratios are cited in preference to the more traditional measures of efficacy such as the median PFS and median OS. *However, because a hazard ratio is a value that has no dimensions, it has very limited value, informing the reader only with regard to the reliability and uniformity of the data.* It does not quantify the magnitude of the benefit. A physician and, especially, a patient want to know the magnitude of the benefit (i.e., the extent to which a life will be prolonged), not what a dimensionless hazard ratio is. By definition, the *hazard ratio* is a ratio of the *hazard rates*. The hazard rate quantifies the likelihood that a patient will experience a *hazardous event* or a hazard during a defined interval of observation, and this is expressed as a rate or percent. For example, if during a given period of observation 20 of 100 patients receiving a reference or control therapy experience progression or death, their hazard rate during this interval is 0.2 (20/100). If during this same interval, only 10 of the 100 patients receiving the experimental therapy experience progression or death, their hazard rate is 0.1 (10/100). In this simple example, the hazard ratio for the interval, calculated as *the ratio of the hazard rates* is 0.5 (0.1/0.2) and indicates the likelihood of experiencing a hazardous event is reduced by 50% in the experimental arm. As commonly presented, and as this simple example illustrates, the lower the hazard ratio, the better the experimental therapy. To determine whether the hazard ratio has statistical significance, one can (1) use a log-rank test to show that the null hypothesis that the two treatments lead to the same survival probabilities is wrong, or (2) use a parametric approach writing a regression model and fitting the data to the model so that one can establish the hazard ratio for the whole trial and its statistical significance. In many cases, the Cox proportional hazard model is used. Although the ideal hazard ratio would capture the differential benefit throughout the period of study, in practice, the extremes depicted in a Kaplan–Meier plot may not be analyzed.

Forest Plots

Interest in determining whether there is heterogeneity in a treatment effect, such that better outcomes occur in some subgroups, has led to the use of Forest plots to display treatment effects across subgroups. Although simple in concept, these plots are subject to error because subgroups are composed of smaller numbers and the confidence intervals are therefore wider than those for the entire group. The most common presentation includes a vertical line at the *no effect point* (e.g., a hazard ratio of 1.0), with symbols of varying size representing the subgroups, each with its confidence interval depicted by a line that stretches from the symbol to both sides (the symbol size is usually proportional to the size of the subgroup). If the confidence interval for a subgroup crosses the no effect point, this is commonly interpreted (not necessarily correctly) as a lack of effect in the subgroup. *The information one seeks from a Forest plot is whether the effect size for different subgroups varies significantly from the main effect, which is determined by a test for heterogeneity.*[66]

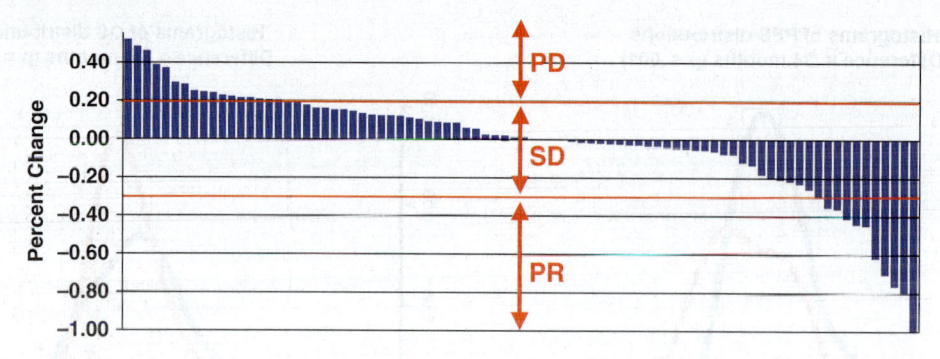

Figure 30.4 Example of a waterfall plot demonstrating for each patient the maximum benefit obtained with the study therapy. Those to the *left* represent patients whose tumors increased, and those on the *right* represent patients whose tumors regressed. The *vertical red lines* at +20% and −30% define the boundaries of stable disease according to RECIST. Ideally, all responses should be confirmed after a period of at least 4 weeks. The example shown is of patients with renal cell carcinoma treated with the microtubule targeting agent ixabepilone. (From Huang H, Menefee M, Edgerly M, et al. A phase II clinical trial of ixabepilone [Ixempra; BMS-247550; NSC 710428], an epothilone B analog, in patients with metastatic renal cell carcinoma. *Clin Cancer Res* 2010;16:1634–1641.)

Beyond Dichotomized Data

Quality of Life

The assessment of cancer patients enrolled on a clinical trial can be said to consist of two sets of endpoints: cancer outcomes and patient outcomes. Cancer outcomes measure the response of the tumor to treatment, the duration of the response, the symptom free period, and the early recognition of relapse. In contrast, patient outcomes assess the benefit achieved with a given therapy by measuring the increase in survival and the quality of life (QOL) before and after therapy. Unfortunately, physicians tend to concentrate on cancer-related outcomes, often neglecting assessments of QOL. Although a QOL assessment in clinical settings is possible with currently available instruments, there must be continued development and refinement of these instruments. Such development must focus not only on extracting valuable information in an unbiased manner, but also and equally important, developing an instrument that is user friendly and will be completed in a high percentage of encounters.

Waterfall Plots

The arbitrary nature of the 50% cutoff set by Moertel and Hanley and its evolution to the current RECIST threshold of 30%

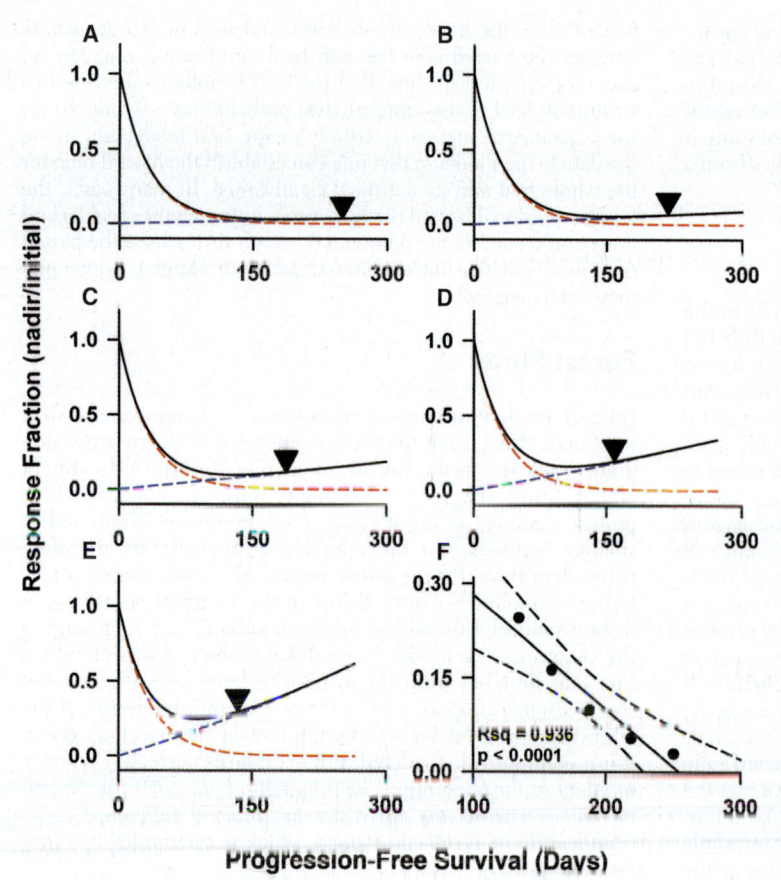

Figure 30.5 The effect of the growth rate constant, *g*, on two commonly reported clinical values: maximum tumor shrinkage and PFS. Tumor measurements obtained in patients can be analyzed mathematically. **(A–E)** The *black line* depicts idealized clinical data using tumor quantities measured as patients received chemotherapy. Actually, clinical measurements comprise concurrent tumor regression (*dashed red line*) and growth (*dashed blue line*) that can be described by a rate constant and a first order kinetic equation, $f(t) = \exp^{(-d \cdot t)} + \exp^{(g \cdot t)} - 1$, where exp is the base of the natural logarithm, $e = 2.7182...$, and *f* is the percent change in tumor measurement at time *t*, normalized to the value when treatment began. The rate constant *d* accounts for exponential decrease, whereas the rate constant *g* accounts for exponential growth occurring during treatment.[68,69] To demonstrate the correlation between the growth rate, tumor shrinkage and PFS, the *same* regression rate (*d*) has been modeled in panels A through E, whereas the growth rate constant, *g*, increases in each successive panel. The *black triangles* depict the point at which tumor size is 20% above the nadir (RECIST definition of PD). As the growth rate increases (i.e., faster tumor growth) from **A** to **E**, the nadir is reached sooner, and the depth of the nadir is less. **(F)** The correlation between PFS and maximum tumor shrinkage (nadir) is shown, plotting the correlation between PFS and response fraction, which is defined as the ratio of nadir to initial value.[68,69] Although idealized plots are given, the curves are based firmly on data obtained from patients enrolled on clinical trials.

reduction in the size of the maximum diameter raises valid queries as to why 30% is valuable and not 29% or 25%. On this background, waterfall plots such as the one shown in Figure 30.4 have become increasingly popular because they depict the benefit or lack thereof in all patients as a continuum of response, rather than a dichotomized response rate.[67] Waterfall plots can be generated from any quantitative assessment. If ctDNA or tumor cells prove to be as quantitative as hoped, the maximum decline could be plotted as a waterfall plot.

Growth Kinetics

Efforts to quantify tumor kinetic parameters from clinical data have been investigated in recent years. Different equations have been applied to describe the two-phase curve based on tumor size as observed in most solid tumor trials, where there is first shrinkage followed by regrowth (Fig. 30.5). These models show exponential tumor shrinkage after treatment, followed by tumor regrowth that is either exponential or linear and have been shown to correlate with OS and to discriminate effective therapies as well as individual patients within trials.[68–73] A major advantage is that more of the data are used, relative to dichotomized response assessment, and regression or growth rates can be determined even in patients who are censored in a Kaplan–Meier analysis. Equations that model both regression and growth rates confirm the clinical intuition that resistant disease is emerging even as overall tumor volume is reduced. Further, "the strategy of studying tumor growth kinetics circumvents one weakness of 'progression criteria,' which is that they inherently dichotomize a complex biological process that may be better characterized using a continuous function."[74] As shown in Figure 30.5, the response of a tumor to a therapy is exemplified by the nadir, the time to the nadir, and the time to progression or PFS, and these are all are all dependent on the growth rate.

REFERENCES

1. America's Biopharmaceutical Research Companies. *Medicines in Development for Cancer*. PhRMA Web site. http://www.phrma.org/sites/default/files/pdf/phrmamedicinesindevelopmentcancer2012.pdf.
2. Moertel CG, Hanley JA. The effect of measuring error on the results of therapeutic trials in advanced cancer. *Cancer* 1976;38:388–394.
3. Miller AB, Hoogstraten B, Staquet M, et al. Reporting results of cancer treatment. *Cancer* 1981;47:207–214.
4. Therasse P, Arbuck SG, Eisenhauer EA, et al. New guidelines to evaluate the response to treatment in solid tumors. European Organization for Research and Treatment of Cancer, National Cancer Institute of the United States, National Cancer Institute of Canada. *J Natl Cancer Inst* 2000;92:205–216.
5. Eisenhauer EA, Therasse P, Bogaerts J, et al. New response evaluation criteria in solid tumours: revised RECIST guideline (version 1.1). *Eur J Cancer* 2009;45:228–247.
6. Mazumdar M, Smith A, Schwartz LH. A statistical simulation study finds discordance between WHO criteria and RECIST guideline. *J Clin Epidemiol* 2004;57:358–365.
7. Wen PY, Macdonald DR, Reardon DA, et al. Updated response assessment criteria for high-grade gliomas: response assessment in neuro-oncology working group. *J Clin Oncol* 2010;28:1963–1972.
8. Byrne MJ, Nowak AK. Modified RECIST criteria for assessment of response in malignant pleural mesothelioma. *Ann Oncol* 2004;15:257–260.
9. Wolchok JD, Hoos A, O'Day S, et al. Guidelines for the evaluation of immune therapy activity in solid tumors: immune-related response criteria. *Clin Cancer Res* 2009;15:7412–7420.
10. Quant EC, Wen PY. Response assessment in neuro-oncology. *Curr Oncol Rep* 2011;13:50–56.
11. Hawkins-Daarud A, Rockne RC, Anderson AR, et al. Modeling tumor-associated edema in gliomas during anti-angiogenic therapy and its impact on imageable tumor. *Front Oncol* 2013;3:66.
12. Fink J, Born D, Chamberlain MC. Pseudoprogression: relevance with respect to treatment of high-grade gliomas. *Curr Treat Options Oncol* 2011;12:240–252.
13. Lin NU, Lee EQ, Aoyama H, et al. Challenges relating to solid tumour brain metastases in clinical trials, part 1: patient population, response, and progression. A report from the RANO group. *Lancet Oncol* 2013;14:e396–e406.
14. Mabille M, Vanel D, Albiter M, et al. Follow-up of hepatic and peritoneal metastases of gastrointestinal tumors (GIST) under Imatinib therapy requires different criteria of radiological evaluation (size is not everything!!!). *Eur J Radiol* 2009;69:204–208.
15. Liu L, Wang W, Chen H, et al. EASL- and mRECIST-evaluated responses to combination therapy of sorafenib with transarterial chemoembolization predict survival in patients with hepatocellular carcinoma. *Clin Cancer Res* 2014;20:1623–1631.
16. Cheson BD, Pfistner B, Juweid ME, et al. Revised response criteria for malignant lymphoma. *J Clin Oncol* 2007;25:579–586.
17. Bernhard J, Dietrich D, Scheithauer W, et al. Clinical benefit and quality of life in patients with advanced pancreatic cancer receiving gemcitabine plus capecitabine versus gemcitabine alone: a randomized multicenter phase III clinical trial—SAKK 44/00-CECOG/PAN.1.3.001. *J Clin Oncol* 2008;26:3695–3701.
18. Burris HA, Moore MJ, Andersen J, et al. Improvements in survival and clinical benefit with gemcitabine as first-line therapy for patients with advanced pancreas cancer: a randomized trial. *J Clin Oncol* 1997;15:2403–2413.
19. Mann BS, Johnson JR, He K, et al. Vorinostat for treatment of cutaneous manifestations of advanced primary cutaneous T-cell lymphoma. *Clin Cancer Res* 2007;13:2318–2322.
20. von Minckwitz G, Untch M, Blohmer JU, et al. Definition and impact of pathologic complete response on prognosis after neoadjuvant chemotherapy in various intrinsic breast cancer subtypes. *J Clin Oncol* 2012;30:1796–1804.
21. Cortazar P, Zhang L, Untch M, et al. Pathological complete response and long-term clinical benefit in breast cancer: the CTNeoBC pooled analysis. *Lancet* 2014 [Epub ahead of print].
22. Bardia A, Baselga J. Neoadjuvant therapy as a platform for drug development and approval in breast cancer. *Clin Cancer Res* 2013;19:6360–6370.
23. Choi H, Charnsangavej C, Faria SC, et al. Correlation of computed tomography and positron emission tomography in patients with metastatic gastrointestinal stromal tumor treated at a single institution with imatinib mesylate: proposal of new computed tomography response criteria. *J Clin Oncol* 2007;25:1753–1759.
24. Schramm N, Englhart E, Schlemmer M, et al. Tumor response and clinical outcome in metastatic gastrointestinal stromal tumors under sunitinib therapy: comparison of RECIST, Choi and volumetric criteria. *Eur J Radiol* 2013;82:951–958.
25. Dudeck O, Zeile M, Reichardt P, et al. Comparison of RECIST and Choi criteria for computed tomographic response evaluation in patients with advanced gastrointestinal stromal tumor treated with sunitinib. *Ann Oncol* 2011;22:1828–1833.
26. Ronot M, Bouattour M, Wassermann J, et al. Alternative response criteria (Choi, European Association for the Study of the Liver, and Modified Response Evaluation Criteria in Solid Tumors [RECIST]) versus RECIST 1.1 in patients with advanced hepatocellular carcinoma treated with sorafenib. *Oncologist* 2014. http://prostatecancer.theoncologist.com/article/alternative-response-criteria-choi-european-association-study-liver-and-modified-response.
27. van der Veldt AA, Meijerink MR, van den Eertwegh AJ, et al. Choi response criteria for early prediction of clinical outcome in patients with metastatic renal cell cancer treated with sunitinib. *Br J Cancer* 2010;102:803–809.
28. Wahl RL, Jacene H, Kasamon Y, et al. From RECIST to PERCIST: evolving considerations for PET response criteria in solid tumors. *J Nucl Med* 2009;50:122S–150S.
29. Shankar LK, Hoffman JM, Bacharach S, et al. Consensus recommendations for the use of 18F-FDG PET as an indicator of therapeutic response in patients in National Cancer Institute Trials. *J Nucl Med* 2006;47:1059–1066.
30. Young H, Baum R, Cremerius U, et al. Measurement of clinical and subclinical tumour response using [18F]-fluorodeoxyglucose and positron emission tomography: review and 1999 EORTC recommendations. European Organization for Research and Treatment of Cancer (EORTC) PET Study Group. *Eur J Cancer* 1999;35:1773–1782.
31. Kramer-Marek G, Capala J. Can PET imaging facilitate optimization of cancer therapies? *Curr Pharm Des* 2012;18:2657–2669.
32. Niederkohr RD, Greenspan BS, Prior JO, et al. Reporting guidance for oncologic 18F-FDG PET/CT imaging. *J Nucl Med* 2013;54:756–761.
33. Liu Y, Litière S, de Vries EG, et al. The role of response evaluation criteria in solid tumour in anticancer treatment evaluation: results of a survey in the oncology community. *Eur J Cancer* 2014;50:260–266.
34. Rubin EH, Allen JD, Nowak JA, et al. Developing precision medicine in a global world. *Clin Cancer Res* 2014;20:1419–1427.
35. Parkinson DR, McCormack RT, Keating SM. Evidence of clinical utility: an unmet need in molecular diagnostics for cancer patients. *Clin Cancer Res* 2014;20:1428–1444.
36. Buyse M, Sargent DJ, Grothey A, et al. Biomarkers and surrogate end points—the challenge of statistical validation. *Nat Rev Clin Oncol* 2010;7:309–317.
37. Karam AK, Karlan BY. Ovarian cancer: the duplicity of CA125 measurement. *Nat Rev Clin Oncol* 2010;7:335–339.

38. Rustin GJ, van der Burg ME, Griffin CL, et al. Early versus delayed treatment of relapsed ovarian cancer (MRC OV05/EORTC 55955): a randomised trial. Lancet 2010;376:1155–1163.
39. Vergote I, Rustin GJ, Eisenhauer EA, et al. Re: new guidelines to evaluate the response to treatment in solid tumors [ovarian cancer]. Gynecologic Cancer Intergroup. J Natl Cancer Inst 2000;92:1534–1535.
40. Guppy AE, Rustin GJ. CA125 response: can it replace the traditional response criteria in ovarian cancer? Oncologist 2002;7:437–443.
41. Rustin GJ, Quinn M, Thigpen T, et al. Re: New guidelines to evaluate the response to treatment in solid tumors (ovarian cancer). J Natl Cancer Inst 2004;96:487–488.
42. Rustin GJ, Vergote I, Eisenhauer E, et al. Definitions for response and progression in ovarian cancer clinical trials incorporating RECIST 1.1 and CA 125 agreed by the Gynecological Cancer Intergroup (GCIG). Int J Gynecol Cancer 2011;21:419–423.
43. Eisenhauer EA. Optimal assessment of response in ovarian cancer. Ann Oncol 2011;22:viii49–viii51.
44. Bubley GJ, Carducci M, Dahut W, et al. Eligibility and response guidelines for phase II clinical trials in androgen-independent prostate cancer: recommendations from the Prostate-Specific Antigen Working Group. J Clin Oncol 1999;17:3461–3467.
45. Scher HI, Halabi S, Tannock I, et al. Design and end points of clinical trials for patients with progressive prostate cancer and castrate levels of testosterone: recommendations of the Prostate Cancer Clinical Trials Working Group. J Clin Oncol 2008;26:1148–1159.
46. Mazumdar M, Bajorin DF, Bacik J, et al. Predicting outcome to chemotherapy in patients with germ cell tumors: the value of the rate of decline of human chorionic gonadotrophin and alpha-fetoprotein during therapy. J Clin Oncol 2001;19:2534–2541.
47. Fizazi K, Culine S, Kramar A, et al. Early predicted time to normalization of tumor markers predicts outcome in poor-prognosis nonseminomatous germ cell tumors. J Clin Oncol 2004;22:3868–3876.
48. Toner GC. Early identification of therapeutic failure in nonseminomatous germ cell tumors by assessing serum tumor marker decline during chemotherapy: still not ready for routine clinical use. J Clin Oncol 2004;22:3842–3845.
49. Gilligan TD, Seidenfeld J, Basch EM, et al. American Society of Clinical Oncology Clinical Practice Guideline on uses of serum tumor markers in adult males with germ cell tumors. J Clin Oncol 2010;28:3388–3404.
50. Albers P, Albrecht W, Algaba F, et al. EAU guidelines on testicular cancer: 2011 update. Eur Urol 2011;60:304–319.
51. Yap T, Lorente D, Omlin A, et al. Circulating tumor cells: a multifunctional biomarker. Clin Cancer Res 2014;20:2553–2568.
52. Dawson SJ, Tsui DW, Murtaza M, et al. Analysis of circulating tumor DNA to monitor metastatic breast cancer. N Engl J Med 2013;368:1199–1209.
53. Punnoose EA, Atwal S, Liu W, et al. Evaluation of circulating tumor cells and circulating tumor DNA in non-small cell lung cancer: association with clinical endpoints in a phase II clinical trial of pertuzumab and erlotinib. Clin Cancer Res 2012;18:2391–2401.
54. Bettegowda C, Sausen M, Leary RJ, et al. Detection of circulating tumor DNA in early- and late-stage human malignancies. Sci Transl Med 2014;6:224ra24.
55. Pazdur R. Endpoints for assessing drug activity in clinical trials. Oncologist 2008;13:19–21.
56. Buyse M, Thirion P, Carlson RW, et al. Relation between tumour response to first-line chemotherapy and survival in advanced colorectal cancer: a meta-analysis. Meta-Analysis Group in Cancer. Lancet 2000;356:373–378.
57. Bruzzi P, Del Mastro L, Sormani MP, et al. Objective response to chemotherapy as a potential surrogate end point of survival in metastatic breast cancer patients. J Clin Oncol 2005;23:5117–5125.
58. Vidaurre T, Wilkerson J, Simon R, et al. Stable disease is not preferentially observed with targeted therapies and as currently defined has limited value in drug development. Cancer J 2009;15:366–373.
59. McKee AE, Farrell AT, Pazdur R, et al. The role of the U.S. Food and Drug Administration review process: clinical trial endpoints in oncology. Oncologist 2010;15:13–18.
60. Ohorodnyk P, Eisenhauer EA, Booth CM. Clinical benefit in oncology trials: is this a patient-centred or tumour-centred end-point? Eur J Cancer 2009;45:2249–2252.
61. Buyse M. Use of meta-analysis for the validation of surrogate endpoints and biomarkers in cancer trials. Cancer J 2009;15:421–425.
62. Wilkerson J, Fojo T. Progression-free survival is simply a measure of a drug's effect while administered and is not a surrogate for overall survival. Cancer J 2009;15:379–385.
63. Reck M, von Pawel J, Zatloukal P, et al. Overall survival with cisplatin-gemcitabine and bevacizumab or placebo as first-line therapy for nonsquamous non-small-cell lung cancer: results from a randomised phase III trial (AVAiL). Ann Oncol 2010;21:1804–1809.
64. Hortobagyi GN, Gomez HL, Li RK, et al. Analysis of overall survival from a phase III study of ixabepilone plus capecitabine versus capecitabine in patients with MBC resistant to anthracyclines and taxanes. Breast Cancer Res Treat 2010;122:409–418.
65. Hennekens C, Buring J. Epidemiology in Medicine. 1st ed. Boston: Little, Brown and Co.; 1987.
66. Cuzick J. Forest plots and the interpretation of subgroups. Lancet 2005;365:1308.
67. Huang H, Menefee M, Edgerly M, et al. A phase II clinical trial of ixabepilone (Ixempra; BMS-247550; NSC 710428), an epothilone B analog, in patients with metastatic renal cell carcinoma. Clin Cancer Res 2010;16:1634–1641.
68. Stein WD, Gulley JL, Schlom J, et al. Tumor regression and growth rates determined in five intramural NCI prostate cancer trials: the growth rate constant as an indicator of therapeutic efficacy. Clin Cancer Res 2011;17:907–917.
69. Stein WD, Wilkerson J, Kim ST, et al. Analyzing the pivotal trial that compared sunitinib and IFN-α in renal cell carcinoma, using a method that assesses tumor regression and growth. Clin Cancer Res 2012;18:2374–2381.
70. Maitland ML, Wu K, Sharma MR, et al. Estimation of renal cell carcinoma treatment effects from disease progression modeling. Clin Pharmacol Ther 2013;93:345–351.
71. Claret L, Girard P, Hoff PM, et al. Model-based prediction of phase III overall survival in colorectal cancer on the basis of phase II tumor dynamics. J Clin Oncol 2009;27:4103–4108.
72. Claret L, Gupta M, Han K, et al. Evaluation of tumor-size response metrics to predict overall survival in Western and Chinese patients with first-line metastatic colorectal cancer. J Clin Oncol 2013;31:2110–2114.
73. Wang Y, Sung C, Dartois C, et al. Elucidation of relationship between tumor size and survival in non-small-cell lung cancer patients can aid early decision making in clinical drug development. Clin Pharmacol Ther 2009;86:167–174.
74. Oxnard GR, Morris MJ, Hodi FS, et al. When progressive disease does not mean treatment failure: reconsidering the criteria for progression. J Natl Cancer Inst 2012;104:1534–1541.
75. Team RDC. R: A language and environment for statistical computing. R Foundation for Statistical Computing. Vienna, Austria: R Foundation for Statistical Computing, 2010. http://www.r-project.org.

PART IV

Cancer Prevention and Screening

31 Tobacco Use and the Cancer Patient

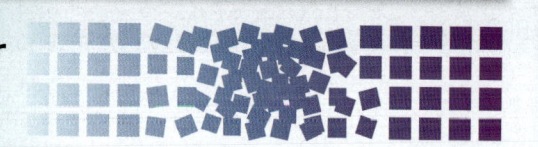

Graham W. Warren, Benjamin A. Toll, Irene M. Tamí-Maury, and Ellen R. Gritz

INTRODUCTION

Tobacco is commonly described as the largest preventable cause of cancer. Over 50 years ago, tobacco was increasingly recognized as the primary cause of lung cancer, with definitive recognition for tobacco use as a causative factor in the seminal 1964 U.S. Surgeon General's Report (SGR) on Smoking and Health.[1] Recent editions of the SGR have described the widespread adverse health effects of tobacco on a spectrum of diseases, including as a causative agent for a spectrum of cancers.[2,3] Tobacco use is an addiction usually initiated in youth prior to the age of 18 and is driven by the highly addictive drug, nicotine.[4] As related to the cancer patient, considerable work has been conducted to associate tobacco use with the risk of developing cancer and how tobacco cessation can substantially reduce cancer risks. However, there is a relative paucity of effort that has been put forth to identify the effects of smoking on outcomes for cancer patients or to establish methods to help cancer patients quit smoking. Fortunately, in recent years, the importance of tobacco use by the cancer patient has been increasingly recognized as an important health behavior, including a National Cancer Institute (NCI)–sponsored conference on tobacco use in 2010, a joint sponsored NCI–American Association of Cancer Research (AACR)–sponsored workshop at the Institute of Medicine in 2012, and recent recommendations by the AACR and the American Society of Clinical Oncology (ASCO) to address tobacco use in cancer patients.[5,6] The recently released 2014 SGR now provides substantial evidence behind the effects of smoking by cancer patients with the following conclusions[7]:

1. In cancer patients and survivors, the evidence is sufficient to infer a causal relationship between cigarette smoking and adverse health outcomes. Quitting smoking improves the prognosis of cancer patients.
2. In cancer patients and survivors, the evidence is sufficient to infer a causal relationship between cigarette smoking and increased all-cause mortality and cancer-specific mortality.
3. In cancer patients and survivors, the evidence is sufficient to infer a causal relationship between cigarette smoking and increased risk for second primary cancers known to be caused by cigarette smoking, such as lung cancer.
4. In cancer patients and survivors, the evidence is suggestive but not sufficient to infer a causal relationship between cigarette smoking and the risk of recurrence, poorer response to treatment, and increased treatment-related toxicity.

The overall objective of this chapter is to discuss tobacco use by cancer patients, the clinical effects of smoking in cancer patients, methods to address tobacco use by cancer patients, and areas of needed research.

NEUROBIOLOGY OF TOBACCO DEPENDENCE

Nicotine is the primary addictive component of tobacco that increases extracellular concentrations of dopamine in the nucleus accumbens and stimulates the mesolimbic dopaminergic system,[8,9] resulting in nicotine's rewarding effect experienced by tobacco users.[10–12] Dopaminergic neurotransmission may also be involved in the assignment of incentive salience, or stimulus for a pleasure based reward, to tobacco use–related environmental cues[13,14] that may become conditioned reinforcers of tobacco use behaviors. For example, an individual who smokes while drinking their morning coffee may associate coffee, or even holding a coffee cup in their hand, with the reward from smoking. Thus, cigarette smoking is directly linked to external nontobacco-based behavioral stimuli. Activation of the nucleus accumbens has further been implicated in drug reinstatement or relapse.[15,16] Individuals who have quit tobacco use for years have restarted a tobacco habit simply by sitting next to a smoker and being exposed to secondhand smoke. Substantial work has been conducted on the addictive nature of tobacco and nicotine, and readers are referred to several comprehensive reviews on this topic.[9,12,17]

TOBACCO USE PREVALENCE AND THE EVOLUTION OF TOBACCO PRODUCTS

Much of the discussion on tobacco use epidemiology and carcinogenesis is presented in Chapter 4. In brief, the prevalence of cigarette smoking among adults in the United States decreased to 19.0% as compared with 22.8% in 2001, but it did not meet the *Healthy People 2010* objective to reduce smoking prevalence to 12%.[18,19] There have been substantial changes in the landscape of tobacco use over time as a direct consequence of cigarette-centered policies and regulations aiming to reduce the harmful effects and number of deaths caused by smoking.[20–22] Under this new landscape, novel and reemergent noncigarette tobacco products such as cigars, cigarillos, snuff, chewing tobacco, water pipes (hookahs), and other forms of tobacco consumption have been growing in demand as a consequence of aggressive and sophisticated marketing by the tobacco industry.[23] Consumption patterns have also changed due to efforts by the tobacco industry to make cigarettes appear safer, such as low tar or filtered cigarettes, and the inclusion of flavoring (menthol, vanilla, fruits, etc.).[24] Although these efforts may have changed consumption patterns, they have not reduced cancer risk. Large patient cohorts demonstrate that the introduction of low tar and filtered cigarettes actually increased risk by promoting deeper inhalation and higher rates of addiction with no reductions in cancer risk,[24,25] resulting in subsequent changes in lung cancer from centrally located squamous cell cancers to peripherally located nonsquamous cell cancers.

The relatively recent introduction of electronic cigarettes (i.e., e-cigarettes, e-cigs, nicotine vaporizers, or electronic nicotine delivery systems [ENDS]) is noteworthy. These electronic or battery-powered devices activate a heating element that vaporizes a liquid solution contained in a cartridge, and then the user inhales this vapor. Levels of nicotine as well as other chemical additives and flavors in the cartridge are uncertain and vary according to the brand.[26] Although there are no research studies that have evaluated the potential harmful effects of the use of e-cigarettes for cancer patients,[27] organizations such as the World Health Organization have already expressed concerns about the safety of these increasingly popular products.[28,29] To date, e-cigarettes have not been approved by the U.S. Food and Drug Administration (FDA) as therapeutic devices to aid in quitting smoking.[26] Readers are referred to a recent editorial on the use of e-cigarettes by cancer patients[27]; however, it will likely be several years before evidence-based health information is available.

TOBACCO USE BY THE CANCER PATIENT

The prevalence of current smoking among long-term adult cancer survivors appears to have declined in the past decade,[30] but data suggest higher rates of smoking among cancer survivors than in the general population.[30–32] These data are often biased by the fact that assessments in cancer patients may not include cancer patients who were current smokers at the time of death. As a result, estimates of smoking rates in cancer survivors may be misleading and may underestimate true tobacco use patterns for cancer patients. Furthermore, alternative tobacco products are often not assessed in cancer patients. Data from the Childhood Cancer Survivor Study and the 2009 Behavioral Risk Factor Surveillance System indicate that approximately 3% to 8% of cancer survivors use smokeless tobacco products.[33,34] Patients may be attracted to these alternative products due to less social stigma and the nonevidence-based perception that these products are healthier alternatives compared to cigarette smoking.

Continued tobacco use by cancer patients often represents a combined failure by the patient to recognize the need to stop smoking even after a cancer diagnosis and the effort by health-care providers to address tobacco use with evidence-based assessments and tobacco cessation support. Approximately 30% of all cancer patients use tobacco at the time of cancer diagnosis with higher rates in traditionally tobacco-related disease sites, such as head and neck or lung cancers, and lower rates in traditionally nontobacco-related disease sites, such as breast or prostate cancers.[35–44] However, findings from several studies indicate that cancer patients are receptive to smoking cessation interventions even as they continue to smoke.[35,38,45–50]

A cancer diagnosis can be used as a window of opportunity, or *teachable moment*, to intervene and provide assistance in the quitting process.[51] A recent study in 12,000 cancer patients, including 2,700 patients who smoked, capitalized on the teachable moment and demonstrated that less than 3% of patients who were contacted by the cessation program rejected tobacco cessation assistance.[45] However, only 1.2% of patients who received a mailed invitation participated in the program. This highlights the idea that patients may be interested in quitting, but methods such as mailed tobacco cessation information may not yield effective participation by cancer patients. Once enrolled, patients and clinicians must realize that although relapses in the general population usually occur within 1 week of cessation, relapses in cancer patients may be delayed due to cancer treatment–related variables such as surgical or other posttreatment healing.[52] Consequently, it is important to continue offering tobacco assessments and cessation support for cancer survivorship efforts.

Defining Tobacco Use by the Cancer Patient

In dealing with tobacco use by cancer patients, it is important to note that virtually all of the evidence associating tobacco with cancer treatment outcomes deals with smoking. Few studies report associations between other forms of tobacco use (e.g., smokeless, cigars, cigarillos) and outcomes in cancer patients. Furthermore, the definition of smoking across published studies varies substantially.[53] In studies of cancer patients, smoking has been defined as current (e.g., smoking after diagnosis, at diagnosis, in the weeks before diagnosis, within the 12 months prior to diagnosis, after diagnosis, within the past 10 years), former (e.g., recent, intermediate-, or long-term quit for 1 month, 3 month, 6 month, 12 month, 2 years, 5 years, 10 years), never, quitting after diagnosis, and according to exposure (e.g., multiple pack year cutoffs, Brinkman index, years of smoking, years of smoking within a predefined period of time such as 5 years prior to diagnosis). Though the nonstandard method of addressing tobacco use in cancer patients has been observed in several reports,[54–57] there are no current standard recommendations for the definition of tobacco use by any national organization. There are four primary categories for smoking status:

1. **Never smoking** is typically defined as having smoked less than 100 cigarettes in a person's lifetime and no current cigarette use. These patients are generally considered as a reference group in many studies. Categories 2 through 4 require that a person has smoked at least 100 cigarettes in their lifetime.
2. **Former smoking** is typically defined as no current cigarette use, usually within the past year.
3. **Recent smoking** (or recent quit) is generally defined as having stopped smoking within the recent past, typically for a period of 1 week to 1 year.
4. **Current smoking** is typically defined as smoking one or more cigarettes per day every day or some days.

Ever smoking is a combination of categories 2 through 4 (i.e., former, recent, and current smokers) that has been used to report negative associations between smoking and cancer outcomes in a number of studies.[58–70] Defining smoking according to *ever* smoking status limits the ability to interpret the effects of current smoking on a clinical outcome, and nothing can be done to address a prior tobacco use history. However, defining exposure according to *current* smoking status allows for the analysis of potentially reversible effects as well as for the potential implementation of smoking cessation to prevent the adverse outcomes of smoking on cancer patients. The primary focus for the remainder of this chapter will be on *current* smoking and will include a discussion of methods to address tobacco use with the cancer patient through accurate assessments and structured tobacco cessation support.

THE CLINICAL EFFECTS OF SMOKING ON THE CANCER PATIENT

Cancer treatment is generally defined according to disease site, stage, treatment type (e.g., surgery, chemotherapy [CT], radiotherapy [RT], or biologic therapy), and primary treatment objective, such as cure or palliation. A comprehensive discussion of the effects of smoking on cancer patients is beyond the scope of a single chapter, but the 2014 SGR provides an excellent evidence base, concluding that "the evidence is sufficient to infer a causal relationship between cigarette smoking and adverse health outcomes."[7] Overall, approximately 75% to 80% of studies in the SGR demonstrated a negative association between smoking and outcome, with approximately 65% to 70% of studies demonstrating statistically significant negative associations. This chapter will provide an illustrative review of studies that demonstrate the adverse effects of tobacco across disease sites and treatment modalities (e.g., surgery, CT, RT), and effects will be discussed across the categories of *mortality, recurrence and cancer-related mortality, toxicity,* and *risk of a second primary cancer*. Evidence for the benefits of smoking cessation will also be presented within each section.

The Effect of Smoking on Overall Mortality

Substantial evidence demonstrates that current smoking by cancer patients increases the risk of overall mortality across virtually all cancer disease sites and for all treatment modalities. Currently smoking significantly increased the risk of overall mortality by between 17% to 38% as compared with never, former, and recent quit smokers in a large cohort of patients across 13 disease sites.[71] Similar but larger observations were noted in elderly current smokers from a separate cohort (hazard ratio [HR], 1.72, 95% confidence interval [CI], 1.23 to 2.42).[72] A large analysis of over 20,000 patients treated with surgery demonstrated that current smoking increased mortality by 62% in gastrointestinal cancer patients and by 50% in thoracic cancer patients with a nonsignificant trend in urologic cancer patients.[73] Several larger studies with at least 500 patients demonstrated that current smoking increases mortality in head and neck cancer,[74–77] breast cancer,[78–81] gastrointestinal cancers,[82,83] prostate cancer,[84–87] renal cancer,[88] gynecologic cancers,[89,90] and lung cancer.[91–102] Smaller studies demonstrate similar effects for hematolymphoid cancers such as leukemia and lymphoma.[103,104] Studies suggest that the effects of current smoking on mortality may be dose and time dependent, with higher risks in heavier smokers[105,106] and lesser risks in patients whose time since quitting was longer.[105]

Whereas many reports rely on retrospective chart reviews, several prospective studies demonstrate that current smoking increases mortality.[71] Browman et al.[107] was one of the first prospective studies to demonstrate that current smoking increased mortality by 2.3-fold in patients who continued to smoke during RT as compared with nonsmokers. Results from Radiation Therapy Oncology Group (RTOG) 9003 and 0129 cooperative group trials demonstrated that current smoking increased mortality in advanced head and neck cancer patients treated with RT or concurrent chemoradiotherapy (CRT),[108] with a similar effect noted in 165 cervical cancer patients treated with CRT.[109] In the randomized retinoid chemoprevention trial of 1,190 early stage head and neck cancer patients, current smoking increased mortality by 2.5-fold.[110]

Numerous studies have demonstrated that current smoking increases overall mortality as compared with former and never smokers combined.[72,75,76,101,102,107,108] The adverse effects of smoking compared with former and never smokers not only reflect the negative effects of smoking on mortality as a whole, but also demonstrate that the effects of smoking are reversible. Current smoking increased mortality risk as compared with patients who quit within the year[71] or 1 to 3 months prior to diagnosis.[111,112] Furthermore, in 284 limited-stage small-cell lung cancer patients, patients who quit smoking at or following a cancer diagnosis had a 45% reduction in mortality as compared with current smokers.[113] These studies suggest that the effects of smoking on mortality are reversible.

Collectively, these studies provide significant data associating current smoking with increased overall mortality across most disease sites, tumor stages, treatment modalities, and in both traditionally tobacco-related as well as nontobacco-related cancers. The potential significance of smoking is perhaps best exemplified by Bittner et al.,[114] who analyzed causes of death in prostate cancer patients and demonstrated that more than 90% died of causes other than prostate cancer, but that current smoking increased the risks of non–prostate cancer deaths between 3- and 5.5-fold. As a result, tobacco use and cessation may be of paramount importance to cancers with high cure rates, such as prostate cancer or breast cancer, simply because patients may be at the most risk of death from noncancer-related causes such as heart disease, pulmonary disease, or other diseases related to smoking and tobacco use.

The Effect of Smoking on Cancer Recurrence and Cancer-Related Mortality

The primary objective of cancer therapy is to cure cancer and prevent recurrence. However, smoking has been shown to increase cancer recurrence and cancer-related mortality. Across a broad spectrum of cancer patients, current smoking increased cancer mortality as compared with former and never smokers.[71] Current smoking has been shown to increase cancer mortality in patients with head and neck cancer,[106,115–118] breast cancer,[76,119] gastrointestinal cancers,[82,120,121] prostate cancer,[41,84,122] gynecologic cancers,[89,90,106,123–125] and lung cancer.[126] Cancer recurrence, whether local or metastatic, is a key driver behind cancer-related mortality. Several studies demonstrate that current smoking increases the risk of recurrence and decreases response across multiple disease sites.[76,84,107,127,128] The effects of smoking on increasing recurrence or cancer-related mortality have also been reported in several relatively rare cancers.[120,129] In a remarkable report of patients with recurrent head and neck cancers treated with salvage surgery, continued smoking after salvage treatment continued to increase the risk of yet another recurrence by 42%.[130] The striking nature of this last study highlights the continued risks even in recurrent cancer patients and the resilience with which some cancer patients will continue to smoke.

The effects of smoking are also noted in premalignant lesions. In patients with high-grade vulvar intraepithelial neoplasia, current smoking increased the risk of persistent disease after therapy by 30-fold.[131] In a prospective trial of progesterone to treat cervical intraepithelial neoplasia (CIN), current smoking increased the risk of progression as compared with former and never smokers combined.[132] A prospective trial of 516 low-grade cervical intraepithelial neoplasia patients demonstrated that current smoking decreased response by 36%, although a similar effect was also noted in former smokers.[133]

As noted with overall mortality, several studies demonstrated that the effects of current smoking are worse than the effects of former smoking[76,86,89,109,127,134–136,137] and that the effects of smoking may be acutely reversible. Several studies also demonstrate that current smoking increases recurrence or cancer mortality, whereas former smoking has no significant effect.[41,78,82,84,85,119,127,174,138] The acutely reversible effects of smoking were shown by Browman et al.[114] who demonstrated that continued smoking increased the risk of cancer-related mortality by 23% as compared with patients who quit within 12 weeks of starting RT. In 284 colorectal cancer patients, smoking at the first postoperative visit increased the risk of cancer mortality by 2.5-fold as compared with all other patients suggesting that smoking after treatment significantly predict for adverse outcome.[121] In a notable study of over 1,400 prostate cancer patients treated with surgery, continued smoking 1 year after treatment increased the risk of recurrence 2.3-fold, but quitting smoking 1 year after treatment did not confer an increased risk of recurrence.[128] Chen et al.[138] demonstrate that patients who continue to smoke before and following a bladder cancer diagnosis have an increased risk of recurrence as compared with patients who quit in the year prior to diagnosis or within the first 3 months after diagnosis. The reversible effects of smoking on recurrence and mortality are consistent with observations on overall mortality and continue to emphasize the benefit of tobacco cessation for cancer patients who smoke at diagnosis.

The Effect of Smoking on Cancer Treatment Toxicity

Discussion of the effects of smoking on cancer treatment toxicity is highly dependent upon disease site, treatment modality (e.g., surgery, CT, RT), and timing of toxicity. Across disease sites and treatments, current smoking has been shown to increase complications from surgery,[140–149] pulmonary complications,[150,151] toxicity from RT,[117,152–156] mucositis,[157] hospitalization,[158] and vasomotor symptoms.[159] One of the largest recent studies in over 20,000 gastrointestinal, pulmonary, and urologic patients demonstrates that former or current smoking increased the risk of surgical site infection, pulmonary complications, or 30-day mortality in a site-specific manner.[73] The effects of current smoking were most significant for pulmonary complications where former smoking had a lesser or nonsignificant effect. In 13,469 lung cancer patients treated with surgery, current smoking increased the risk of postoperative death with no increased risk in former smokers.[160] Current smoking increased the risk of complications, morbidity, or reoperation following esophagectomy, pancreatectomy, or colorectal surgery.[161-163] A study of 836 prostate cancer patients treated with RT demonstrated that current smoking increased abdominal cramps, rectal urgency, diarrhea, incomplete emptying, and sudden emptying between two- and nine-fold,[164] with similar effects noted in 3,489 cervical cancer patients who smoked more than 1 pack per day (PPD).[156]

Several studies have demonstrated that the effects of smoking on cancer treatment toxicity are reversible. Stopping smoking within 3 weeks of surgery reduced wound healing complications in esophageal cancer patients treated with surgery and reconstruction.[165] In 393 T1 laryngeal cancer patients treated with RT, quitting smoking after diagnosis reduced laryngeal complications as compared with continued smoking.[152] In a large study of 7,990 lung cancer patients from the Society of Thoracic Surgeons Database, current smoking increased the risk of pulmonary complications by 80% and hospital mortality 3.5-fold.[151] However, smoking cessation for 2 weeks eliminated the risks for pulmonary complications, and cessation for 1 month eliminated risks for hospital mortality. Vaporciyan et al.[166] also showed that current smoking increased the risk of pulmonary complications 2.7-fold as compared with smoking cessation for at least 1 month prior to surgery. In a striking example of the potentially reversible effects of smoking in 205 head and neck cancer patients treated with RT,[167] 43% of smoking patients treated in the morning experienced Grade 3+ mucositis compared with 72% of smokers treated in the afternoon (p = 0.04). These data suggest that reducing smoking overnight may yield a clinical benefit in reduced toxicity. Whereas all toxicity may not be acutely reversed, these encouraging data show that patients can make clinically meaningful improvements in their health and/or cancer treatment within a short time frame by quitting smoking.

The Effect of Smoking on Risk of Second Primary Cancer

Several studies have reported the effects of smoking on the risk of developing a second primary cancer. Park et al.[168] reported on over 14,000 male cancer patients and demonstrated that current smoking increased the risk of developing a second tobacco-related primary cancer twofold, with no increased risk in former smokers. A higher risk was observed in in head and neck cancer patients who smoked more than 10 cigarettes per day, with no increased risk in lighter smokers.[169] Kinoshita et al.[170] showed an 82% increased risk of developing a second primary in gastric cancer patients who are current smokers with no increased risk in former smokers. In the phase III randomized trial of isotretinoin for the prevention of a second primary tumor in 1,190 head and neck cancer patients, current smoking increased the risk of a second primary by 2.2-fold with a nonsignificant trend of 1.6-fold in former smokers.[110] Notably, 39% of patients who reported quitting within the previous year were biochemically confirmed smokers.[171] As a result, these data collectively suggest that some of the increased risk may be biased by continued smoking in patients who deny smoking by self-report.

The effects of smoking on the risk of a second primary cancer are also noted in nontobacco-related cancers and in long-term survivors. In 835 breast cancer patients, smoking increased the risk for the development of lung metastases after breast cancer by more than threefold.[172] Ford et al.[173] demonstrated that breast cancer patients who were former smokers had a threefold increased risk of developing lung cancer, but that current smokers had a 13-fold increased risk. In nearly 1,100 estrogen receptor (ER)-positive breast cancer patients, current smokers had a 1.8-fold increased risk of developing a second contralateral breast cancer, and current smokers at most recent follow-up had a 2.2-fold increased risk, but former smoking at the diagnosis or most recent follow-up had no increased risk.[174] In 2,700 5-year survivors of testicular cancer, current smokers had a 1.8-fold increased risk of developing a second primary as compared with all other survivors.[175]

There are some studies suggesting that smoking, combined with cytotoxic therapy, may have an additive or synergistic effect on the risk of developing a second primary cancer. In 9,780 prostate cancer patients from the Cancer of the Prostate Strategic Urologic Research Endeavor (CaPSURE) study, RT increased the risk of bladder cancer by 1.6-fold, smoking increased the risk by 2.1-fold, and smoking combined with RT increased risk by 3.7-fold.[176] In ER-positive breast cancer patients, treatment with RT had no significant effect on the risk of developing a contralateral breast cancer, but RT combined with current smoking increased the risk of contralateral cancer by ninefold.[173] In a detailed analysis of Hodgkin lymphoma patients, nonheavy smokers (defined as never, former, and less than one PPD) had a second primary relative risk of between fourfold and sevenfold when treated with CT or RT as compared with patients who received no RT or CT.[177] However, heavy smokers had a sixfold increased risk in the absence of RT and CT and a 17- to 49-fold increased risk when combined with RT and/or CT. These observations suggest that smoking combined with cytotoxic cancer therapy may complement the risk of developing a second primary cancer perhaps through the promotion of mutations induced by CT and/or RT in the presence of tobacco smoke. The potential mechanisms of this effect have not been tested or defined at this time, but the mechanism of tobacco-induced carcinogenesis in prior reports[3] supports these observations.

Human Papilloma Virus, Epidermal Growth Factor Receptor, Anaplastic Lymphoma Kinase, Programmed Cell Death Protein 1, and Smoking

Data over the past decade has shown that head and neck cancers that are human papilloma virus (HPV) positive are known to have an improved prognosis as compared with HPV-negative tumors.[178] Patients who have HPV-positive tumors typically have increased p16 expression and often respond better to conventional cancer therapy, including RT and CT. Many HPV-positive patients are never smokers or have a lighter smoking history. However, smoking was an independent adverse risk factor for both overall and cancer-related mortality with a 1% increase in risk per pack-year smoked.[178] Current smoking increased cancer mortality approximately fivefold even in p16-positive patients treated with surgery.[115] Smoking also increased the risk of developing second primary cancer in both HPV-positive and HPV-negative patients.[179] As a consequence, the presence of HPV does not appear to negate the adverse effects of smoking.

A similar effect is noted in lung cancer patients with epidermal growth factor receptor (EGFR)-mutated or anaplastic lymphoma kinase (ALK)-mutated tumors. As with HPV-positive head and neck cancer patients, lung cancer patients who are light or never smokers have a higher rate of EGFR-positive tumors that may respond to biologic therapy using EGFR tyrosine–kinase inhibitors. At this time, most information regarding EGFR-based therapy for lung cancer reports on the effects of ever smoking demonstrating that ever smokers have a decreased response to EGFR therapy. Early, large, randomized trials demonstrate that Tarceva (erlotinib) and Iressa (gefitinib) provide survival and tumor control benefits specifically in never smokers.[180,181] A very similar pattern is noted for ALK-positive patients with a much higher incidence in never smokers and high response rate to the ALK kinase inhibitor crizotinib.[182] Paik et al.[183] have described the importance of driver mutations in EGFR, ALK, and KRAS demonstrating that smokers have a higher preponderance for K-ras drivers, whereas nonsmokers tend to have EGFR or ALK driver mutations. In general, patients who are smokers may be best served with conventional cancer treatments rather than these biologic therapies, but randomized controlled trials confirming this suggestion are lacking at this time.

Although there are essentially no biologic therapies that have shown to have a better response in smokers, there are exciting data presented at the 2013 European CanCer Organization (ECCO) annual conference, suggesting that anti–programmed cell death protein 1 (PD-1)–based therapies may have a better response rate in smokers.[184] These very preliminary data have yet to be replicated or expanded into randomized trials, but if expanded trials prove effective, they may represent one of the only cancer treatments that may specifically benefit smokers.

Summarizing the Clinical Effects of Smoking on the Cancer Patient

Smoking by cancer patients increases mortality, toxicity, recurrence, and the risk of a second primary cancer. There are four important conclusions, and a fifth implied conclusion, to the evidence previously presented:

1. One or more adverse effects of smoking affect all cancer disease sites.
2. One or more adverse effects of smoking affect all treatment modalities.
3. The effects of current smoking are distinct from an ever or former smoking history.
4. Several lines of evidence demonstrate that many of the effects of smoking are reversible.

Although substantial data demonstrate that smoking by cancer patients increases the risk for one or more outcomes, the largest limitations are the lack of standard tobacco use definitions, the lack of assessing tobacco use in cancer patients at follow-up, and the lack of structured tobacco cessation for cancer patients. Importantly, patients may further misrepresent tobacco use. Several studies suggest that approximately 30% of cancer patients who smoke deny tobacco use.[171,185,186] Marin et al.[187] exemplify the importance of an accurate assessment, demonstrating that patients who self-reported smoking had no significant risk associated with surgical complications; however, biochemical confirmation of smoking significantly increased the risk of surgical wound complications. This highlights the potential discrepancy between the effects of smoking based on subjective versus biochemically confirmed assessments. Due to this discrepancy, the *fifth implied conclusion* is that the adverse effects of smoking and the benefits of cessation may be more pronounced than currently reported in the literature.

ADDRESSING TOBACCO USE BY THE CANCER PATIENT

National Oncology Association Statements and Clinical Practice Guidelines

Professional societies are taking leadership roles in recognizing the need to assess patients' tobacco use and to examine the effects of tobacco use in medical treatment, including the important role of tobacco cessation. The American Medical Association (AMA) passed a resolution supporting documentation of smoking behavior in clinical trials, from trial registration through treatment, follow-up, and to end of the study or death.[188] The Oncology Nursing Society (ONS) has also advocated for assessment and cessation.[189,190] Both the AACR[5,191] and ASCO[6,192] have issued policy statements specifically addressing tobacco use in cancer patients, detailing that clinicians have a responsibility to address tobacco use, that all patients should be screened, that all patients who use tobacco should receive evidence-based tobacco cessation support, and that tobacco use should be included in clinical practice and research. These provide strong counsel to address tobacco use in the general population as well as in cancer patients.

Smoking Cessation Guidelines

Overall, the approach to tobacco cessation for the cancer patient is very similar to the approach for the general population. However, there are a few specific details that are important to consider when approaching the cancer patient who smokes. It is important to recognize that virtually all newly diagnosed cancer patients are faced with a life-changing diagnosis that will require intensive treatment approaches. Treatments, toxicity, and outcomes differ according to disease site and treatment modality. Whereas some cancer patients may have a curable cancer, others may have incurable cancer. Smoking in cancer patients is also often associated with comorbid psychiatric diseases, such as depression, that may affect dependence.[193] The urgency of cessation is also important to consider. If smoking decreases the efficacy of cancer treatment, then every effort should be made to stop tobacco use as soon as possible rather than choosing a quit date several weeks or months after a cancer diagnosis. Patients may also be burdened with a "stigma" associated with certain tobacco-related cancers,[193–197] where they may be viewed by others, or themselves, as causing their cancer due to tobacco use. As a result, the rationale and motivation for quitting tobacco use likely differs among cancer patients, but there is a consistent theme that exists. (1) All patients should be asked about tobacco use with structured assessments; (2) all patients who use tobacco or are at risk for relapse should be offered evidence-based cessation support; and 3) tobacco assessment and cessation support should occur at the time of diagnosis, during treatment, and during follow up for all cancer patients.

Empiric treatment of tobacco use by cancer patients is fundamentally supported by Public Health Service (PHS) Guidelines that are based on evidence from tobacco cessation efforts in non-cancer patients. Originally issued in 1996 and renewed in 2008, *The Clinical Practice Guideline: Treating Tobacco Use and Dependence* is a PHS-sponsored, evidence-based guideline designed to assist health-care providers in delivering and supporting effective smoking cessation treatment.[198,199] The basic recommendation states that clinicians should consistently identify, document, and treat every tobacco user seen in a health-care setting. Details of cessation support range from brief to intensive intervention, but emphasize that consistent repeated cessation support and even brief counseling are effective methods to assist patients with stopping tobacco use. It is important to note that physician-delivered interventions significantly increase long-term abstinence rates.[199] Included are newer effective medication options and strong support for counseling and the use of quit lines as effective intervention strategies. As described in the PHS Guidelines, the principal steps in conducting effective smoking cessation interventions are referred to as The 5 A's:

1. *Ask* about tobacco use for every patient.
2. *Advise* every tobacco user to quit.
3. *Assess* the willingness of patients to quit.
4. *Assist* patients with quitting through counseling and pharmacotherapy.
5. *Arrange* follow-up cessation support, preferably within the first week after the quit date.

There is a strong evidence base for these interventions as documented in the clinical practice guideline.[199]

Implementing Smoking Cessation Into Clinical Practice

An algorithm is provided to guide clinicians in implementing the five A's into clinical cancer care (Fig. 31.1).[5,45,194,199] Included in the algorithm are suggested questions that are useful to accurately assess tobacco use by cancer patients where patients can generally be divided into *current*, *former*, or *never* smokers. The first step (ASK) is to inquire about and document tobacco use behaviors for every

ASK:

Baseline tobacco assessment questions to determine smoking/tobacco use status:
1. Have you smoked at least 100 cigarettes in you life?
   A. Yes
   B. No
2. Do you now smoke every day, some days, or not at all?
   A. Every day
   B. Some days
   C. Not at all
3. Do you use other forms of tobacco every day, some days, or not at all?
   A. Every day
   B. Some days
   C. Not at all

CURRENT = Answers 2A, 2B, 3A or 3B
FORMER = Answers 1A and 2C and 3C
NEVER = Answers 1B and 2C and 3C

For CURRENT smokers:
4. On average, how many cigarettes per day did you smoke in the past 7 days?
5. How soon after waking do you smoke your first cigarette?
   A. <30 min (higher nicotine dependence)
   B. >30 min (lower nicotine dependence)

For CURRENT and FORMER smokers:
6. At what age did you start smoking regularly?
7. At what age did you stop smoking regularly?
8. When you smoke regularly, how many cigarettes per day did you smoke on average?
9. How long has it been since you smoked even a single puff?
   A. <1 day
   B. 1–7 days
   C. 8–30 days
   E. 4–6 months
   F. 6–12 months
   G. More than 1 year

All CURRENT smokers and patients who smoked within the past 30 days

ADVISE patients to stop smoking with clear strong personalized advice

ASSESS willingness to quit immediately or set quit date as soon as possible

ASSIST patients with behavioral counseling and pharmacotherapy

ARRANGE follow-up, ideally within 1–2 weeks or in preparation for cancer treatment

Maintain abstinence, prevent relapse

All FORMER smokers

All CURRENT smokers and patients who smoked within the past 30 days

REASSESS current tobacco use at follow-up

Standard cancer care and follow-up

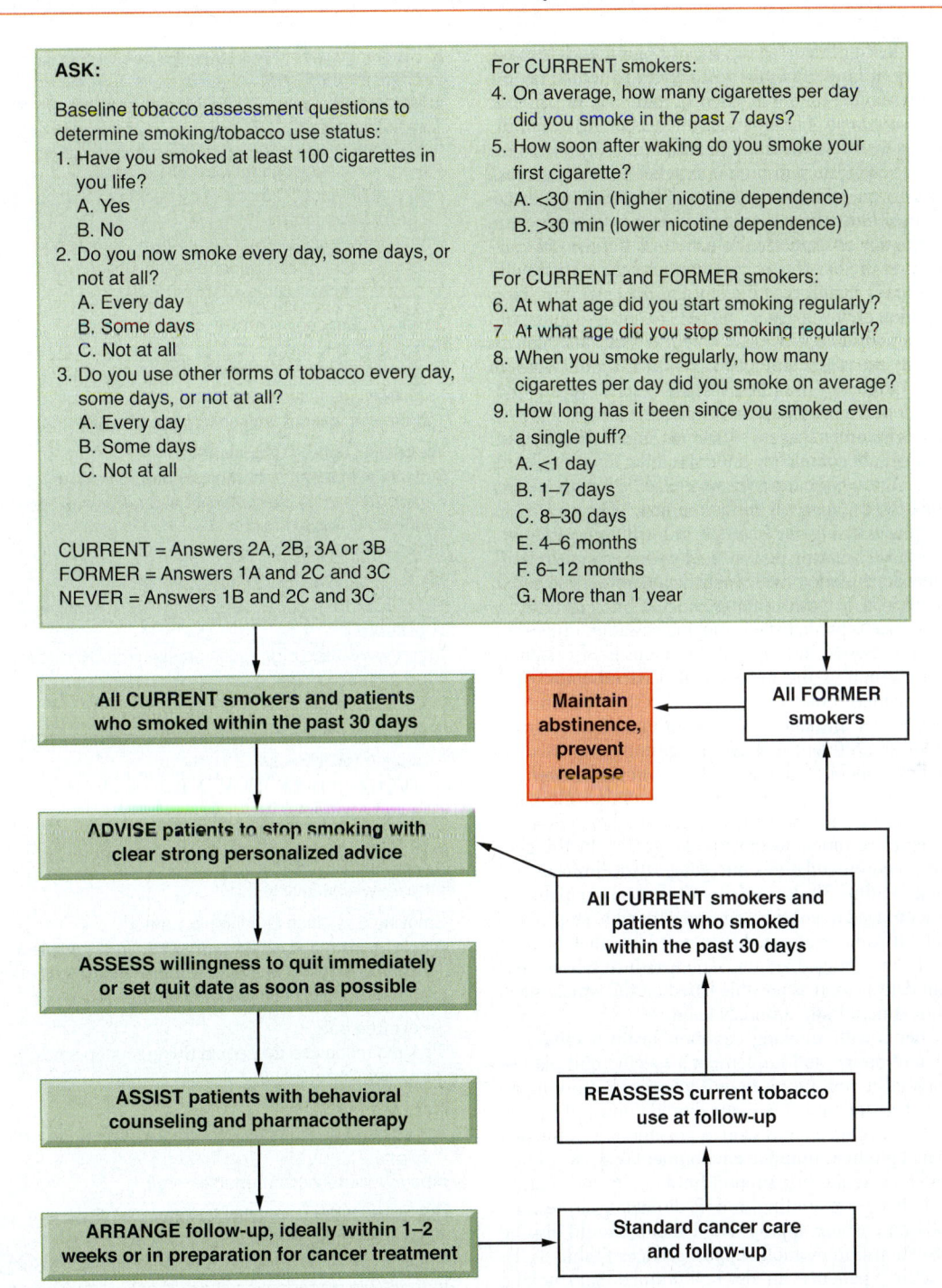

Figure 31.1 This 5 A's screening and smoking cessation treatment schema for cancer patients may be integrated into clinical oncology practice.

patient at every visit including follow-up visits. Whereas a more comprehensive evaluation is necessary at the first consult, only updates to current tobacco use are needed at follow-up. Including smoking status assessments as a "vital sign" for all patients significantly increases the identification and treatment for patients.[200] Tobacco-use status stickers on paper charts or an automated reminder system for electronic records can increase compliance with tobacco assessments.[45] With the recent Meaningful Use standards that were implemented in 2011, hospitals using an electronic medical record (EMR) are essentially required to document tobacco use.[201] A recent report utilized the EMR to implement mandatory tobacco assessments in cancer patients demonstrating that just a few questions at the initial evaluation and at follow-up could yield high referral. Less than 1% of referrals were delayed when assessments were repeated on a monthly basis rather than at every clinic visit.[45] These findings reduce the clinical burden and patient fatigue associated with repeated assessments as frequently as every day such as in patients who are treated with daily RT or CT.

At the time of this chapter release, there were no national guidelines for implementation of specific questions to assess tobacco use in cancer patients. However, Figure 31.1 provides effective questions for assessing tobacco use in cancer patients based on advice from published reports.[5,45,194,199] Current, former, and never smokers are identified in a structured manner. Patients who use tobacco within the past 30 days should have structured support to quit tobacco use, maintain abstinence, and prevent relapse.

Although not explicitly stated by any specific guidelines, asking about tobacco use in family members of cancer patients may be important because family members often support cancer patients during and following treatment, but continued smoking by family members can make quitting much more difficult.[202–204]

Advising is the second step in promoting effective tobacco cessation that involves giving clear, strong, and personalized advice to stop tobacco use. This advice should include the importance of quitting smoking, such as explicit information on the risks of continued smoking and the benefits of cessation for cancer treatment outcomes and overall health regardless of cancer diagnosis. This includes a discussion of how it is not "too late" to quit and that quitting will in fact benefit their cancer treatment efficacy and cancer outcome.[5] Patients can also consider the cost savings of stopping a smoking habit. Clinicians must be particularly sensitive to avoid contributing to any perceived blame for the patient's illness.[195–197,205] Clinicians must remember that most patients started smoking in adolescence and did not completely understand the risks associated with tobacco use. At the same time, the severe addiction associated with chronic tobacco use makes it difficult to stop.

The next step is *assessing* dependence and willingness to quit. Asking "How soon after waking do you smoke your first cigarette?" assesses nicotine dependence, with high dependence associated with a shorter interval between waking and the first cigarette.[206] Nicotine dependence is predictive of smoking cessation outcomes and can be used as a good indicator of the intensity of cessation treatment needed, such as the need for pharmacotherapy.[207,208] Determining the patient's motivation and interest in quitting are critical parameters that influence the types of intervention strategies to be employed. Different strategies for quitting are based on the transtheoretical model of change and motivational interviewing stance, which recognizes that unique intervention messages and strategies are needed to optimally promote smoking cessation based on a patient's readiness to quit smoking.[209,210] In the general population, recommendations encourage that clinicians set a target quit date within 30 days. However, for cancer patients, the reader is encouraged to consider an urgent need to stop smoking immediately. If patients are unable to quit immediately, then patients should be encouraged to immediately reduce tobacco use and to set a quit date as soon as possible based on the typical need to start cancer treatment in the immediate future.

Assisting patients with smoking cessation involves clinicians helping the patient design and implement a specific quit plan or broadly enhancing the motivation to quit tobacco. Promoting an effective quit strategy for cancer patients should consist of (1) setting a quit date (immediately or as soon as possible), (2) removing all tobacco-related products from the environment (e.g., cigarettes, ashtrays, lighters), (3) requesting support from family and friends, (4) discussing challenges to quitting, and (5) discussing or prescribing pharmacotherapy where appropriate. Patients should also be provided information on cessation support services (Table 31.1). In the cancer setting, patients can also be informed that smoking cessation is a critical component of cancer care over which they have complete control, thereby conferring some personal control over their cancer care.

Patients who are unwilling to quit should continue to receive repeated assessments and counseling to help motivate patients to quit smoking. These patients should be encouraged to make immediate reductions in tobacco use and work toward abstinence as soon as possible. Clinician education, reassurance, and gentle encouragement can help them to consider changing their smoking behaviors. Specific strategies include discussing the personal relevance of smoking and benefits to cessation, providing support and acknowledging the difficulty of quitting, educating patients about the positive consequences of quitting smoking, and discussing available pharmacologic methods to assist with quitting.[211] The emphasis should be placed on patient autonomy to quit. Motivational strategies for patients unwilling to quit can be employed (e.g., asking open-ended questions, providing affirmations, reflective listening, summarizing).[198,210,212,213] Table 31.2 provides suggested methods to help clinicians promote tobacco cessation.

The final step in a clinician-delivered smoking cessation intervention involves *arranging* a follow-up contact with the patient. Ideally, cancer patients will follow an immediate quit strategy and follow-up should occur preferably within 1 to 2 weeks. However, a short-term follow-up may also benefit patients who are reluctant to quit smoking. The clinician must remember that a new cancer diagnosis is stressful and patients may rely on continued smoking to

TABLE 31.1

Additional Tobacco Cessation Resources for Patients and Clinicians[a]

American Association for Cancer Research
Information about the adverse effects of tobacco and advocacy for tobacco control
(http://www.aacr.org/home/public--media/science-policy--government-affairs/science-policy--government-affairs-committee/tobacco-and-cancer.aspx)

American Cancer Society
A national cancer organization providing brochures and fact sheets on the health effects of tobacco and resources for smoking cessation
(http://www.cancer.org/cancer/cancercauses/tobaccocancer/)

American Legacy Foundation
A national independent public health foundation offering programs to help people quit and resources about the health effects of tobacco use
(http://www.legacyforhealth.org/)

American Society of Clinical Oncology
Resources for tobacco cessation with an emphasis on cancer patients
(http://www.asco.org/practice-research/tobacco-cessation-and-control-resources)

Centers for Disease Control and Prevention
A collection of online resources, information, and materials about quitting tobacco use
(http://www.cdc.gov/tobacco/)

North American Quitline Consortium
Information on local and national cessation quitlines, 1-800-QUIT-NOW
(http://www.naquitline.org/)

Smoking Cessation Leadership Center
A collaborative dedicated to disseminating knowledge about the health effects of tobacco and assistance in cessation
(http://smokingcessationleadership.ucsf.edu/)

Smokefree.gov
Tips and resources for people trying to stop smoking
(http://smokefree.gov/)

Tobacco Free Nurses
An organization aimed at engaging nurses in tobacco cessation efforts
(http://www.tobaccofreenurses.org/)

U.S. Department of Health & Human Services, Surgeon General.gov
Tobacco use and cessation information from the Surgeon General
(http://www.surgeongeneral.gov/initiatives/tobacco/index.html)

World Health Organization
An international organization tasked with implementing and monitoring public health with a focus on tobacco control
(http://www.who.int/topics/tobacco/en/)

[a] Current as of December 2013.

TABLE 31.2 Select Treatment Strategies Used for Tobacco Cessation Treatments

- Provide and monitor the use of nicotine replacement or other pharmacotherapy.
- Provide education regarding the health effects of tobacco use and its addictive and relapsing nature.
- Identify and change environmental and psychological cues for tobacco use.
- Generate alternative behaviors for tobacco use.
- Assist in optimization of social support for cessation efforts and address tobacco use in family members.
- Prevent relapse including the identification of future high-risk situations and plans for specific behaviors in those situations.
- Provide motivational interventions as needed throughout treatment.
- Identify relaxation techniques such as guided imagery and progressive muscle relaxation.
- Provide behavioral strategies to address depressed mood (e.g., increasing pleasurable activities).
- Provide crisis intervention including appropriate referrals and emergency intervention if indicated.
- Recognize and congratulate patients on success with reducing and/or quitting smoking.

relieve stress, but after absorbing the psychological effects of a new cancer diagnosis, patients may be more receptive to smoking cessation. During follow-up, clinicians should congratulate patients on successful cessation efforts, discuss accomplishments and setbacks, and assess pharmacotherapy use and problems. Patients should not be criticized for returning to smoking; rather, it is critical to create a supportive environment for patients to communicate progress, failure, and personal needs. Framing relapses as a learning experience can be helpful, and patients should be encouraged to set another quit date. Referrals to a psychologist or professionally trained smoking cessation counselor should be considered for patients with numerous unsuccessful quit attempts, comorbid depression, anxiety, additional substance abuse disorders, or inadequate social support.

Clinicians who are not well versed in tobacco cessation should realize that smoking is an extremely difficult addiction to overcome and should recognize the clinical pattern associated with cessation. As patients stop smoking, many will experience symptoms of withdrawal, including dry or sore throat, constipation, cravings to smoke, irritability, anxiety, trouble concentrating, restlessness, increased appetite, depression, and insomnia. In the first few weeks, patients may also report an increase in mucous secretions from the airways, a cough, and other upper respiratory tract symptoms. Patients and clinicians should realize that tobacco cessation requires a concerted effort, may require repeated attempts, and symptoms will not resolve immediately. Clinicians should counsel patients on a repeated basis, recognize success, and provide repeated assistance if patients relapse.

Pharmacologic Treatment for Smoking Cessation

The principles of pharmacotherapy to help patients quit smoking are fundamentally based on reducing the craving associated with nicotine withdrawal. Nicotine replacement therapy (NRT), in the form of patches, lozenges, inhalers, sprays, and gum, varenicline (Chantix), and bupropion (Zyban) are the three principal first-line pharmacotherapies recommended for use either alone or in combination according to PHS Guidelines.[199] Table 31.3 presents information on these first-line agents. Nicotine is the primary addictive substance in tobacco and NRT facilitates smoking cessation by reducing craving and withdrawal that smokers experience during abstinence. NRT also weans smokers off nicotine by providing a lower level and, in some cases, slower infusion of nicotine than smoking.[214] Strong evidence from over 100 randomized clinical trials support the use of NRT to increase the odds of quitting approximately twofold as compared with placebo.[215] Pooled analyses demonstrate that 17% of smokers receiving NRT were able to quit versus 10% with placebo after at least 6 months. Recent evidence further shows that combination therapy, or dual NRT (such as a nicotine patch and lozenge), is a very effective smoking cessation therapy that produces high quit rates.[216,217] Data suggest that activation of the nicotinic acetylcholine receptor (nAChR) may promote tumor development,[218] but evidence suggests that the negative aspects of smoking outweigh these concerns.[219,220] Furthermore, there are no clinical trials reporting negative outcomes for NRT in cancer patients as related to mortality or recurrence. Studies also demonstrate that NRT is not associated with an increased risk of carcinogenesis in the general population.[221,222] As a result, NRT should be used as a clinically proven method to help cancer patients stop smoking.

Antidepressants have been studied as non-nicotine–based pharmacotherapy in part due to depression and psychiatric disease being comorbid conditions in smokers.[223] Bupropion (Zyban) is currently the only FDA-approved antidepressant for the treatment of tobacco dependence.[199] Bupropion inhibits the reuptake of both dopamine and norepinephrine, thereby increasing dopamine and norepinephrine concentrations in the mesolimbic systems.[12,224] Bupropion also antagonizes the nAChR, thereby lowering the rewarding effects of nicotine.[225] Should an abstinent smoker relapse, bupropion may function to reduce the pleasure of cigarette smoking experienced by the smoker[226] and help to prevent further relapse. A meta-analysis found that smokers who received bupropion were twice as likely as those who received placebo to have achieved long-term abstinence at either a 6- or 12-month follow-up.[227]

Varenicline (Chantix) is a α4β2 nAChR partial agonist that produces sustained dopamine release in the mesolimbic system that received FDA approval for treating tobacco dependence in 2006. Sustained dopamine release maintains a normal systemic level of the neurotransmitter, which helps to reduce craving and withdrawal during abstinence.[228] Varenicline also antagonizes the rewarding effects of nicotine. Because varenicline attenuates the pleasure smokers experience from smoking, it may decrease motivation to smoke and protect them from relapse. One of the initially reported randomized clinical trials that compared varenicline (2 mg), bupropion (300 mg), and placebo showed that varenicline was superior to bupropion and placebo, with overall continuous abstinence rates between 10% to 23%.[229] A meta-analysis demonstrated that the 1-mg daily dose approximately doubled, whereas the 2-mg daily dose approximately tripled the likelihood of long-term abstinence at 6 months as compared to placebo.[199] As a result, the 1-mg daily dose can be considered as an alternative should the patient experience significant dose-related side effects. Several meta-analyses have shown that varenicline is superior to bupropion and placebo in the general population.[230–233]

In July 2009, the FDA issued a warning after reports that some patients attempting to quit smoking while using varenicline or bupropion experienced unusual changes in behavior, depressed mood, worsening of depression, or had thoughts of suicide. This has prompted recommendations that health-care providers elicit information about a patient's psychiatric history prior to prescribing varenicline or bupropion to closely monitor changes in mood and behavior during the course of treatment. However,

TABLE 31.3
First-Line Pharmacotherapy Agents for the Treatment of Nicotine Depedence

Agent	Dose	Mechanism	Use
Nicotine Replacement			
Transdermal (patches)	16 h or 24 h 7, 14, or 21 mg 1 patch/d	Steady state NRT to reduce craving and withdrawal	6–10 CPD: 14 mg daily × 8 wks then 7 mg daily × 2 wks >10 CPD: 21 mg daily × 6 wks, then 14 mg × 2 wks, then 7 mg × 2 wks
Gum	2 or 4 mg Max: 24 pieces/d	Short-term NRT to reduce craving and withdrawal	First cigarette >30 min after waking: 2 mg PO q1–2 hr First cigarette <30 min after waking: 4 mg PO q1–2 hr
Lozenge	2 or 4 mg Max: 20 lozenges/d	Short-term NRT to reduce craving and withdrawal	1st cigarette >30 min after waking: 2 mg PO q1–2 hr 1st cigarette <30 min after waking: 4 mg PO q1–2 hr
Nasal spray	0.5 mg/spray Max: 10 sprays/hr or 80 sprays/d	Short-term NRT to reduce craving and withdrawal	1 spray/nostril q1–5 hr
Inhaler	4 mg/cartridge Max: 16 cartridges/d	Short-term NRT to reduce craving and withdrawal	1 cartridge inhaled over 20 min q1.5–6 hr
Bupropion (Zyban)	150 mg	Block nicotinic receptors and reduces reward	1 tablet daily × 3 d, then 1 tablet twice daily for 7–12 wks
Varenicline (Chantix)	0.5 or 1 mg	Dopaminergic reward and partial nicotinic receptor antagonist	0.5 mg daily × 3 d, then 0.5 mg twice daily × 3 d, then 1 mg twice daily

CPD, cigarettes per day; PO, by mouth; NRT, nicotine replacement therapy.

updated recent safety studies examining very large databases (one database of N = 119,546, one database of N = 35,800) regarding safety have shown no difference in neuropsychiatric side effects between varenicline or bupropion as compared to NRT and no increased risk of depression.[234,235] Another prospective study showed no adverse events when treating participants with current or past major depression and also showed higher abstinence rates for the varenicline group as compared to placebo at weeks 9 to 52 (20.3% versus 10.4%, p <0.001).[236] Varenicline should be considered a viable cessation pharmacotherapy for cancer patients.

The clinical practice guideline also identifies two non-nicotine–based medications—clonidine and nortriptyline—as second-line pharmacotherapies for tobacco dependence. A second-line agent is used when a smoker cannot use first-line medications due to either contraindications or lack of effectiveness. Both clonidine, an antihypertensive, and nortriptyline, a tricyclic antidepressant, have been shown to effectively assist smokers achieve abstinence.[227,237] Unfortunately, many patients who quit will eventually relapse, and rates of long-term abstinence remain low. Because smoking poses enormous health risks to individuals and their families, even a modest reduction in smoking may translate into a significant impact on public health. Clinicians should continue to encourage recalcitrant smokers to stop tobacco use and use pharmacotherapy where appropriate with repeated quit attempts.

Empirically Tested Cessation Interventions with Cancer Patients

The overwhelming majority of cessation research has been performed in the general population, but there are several studies that have been performed in cancer patients. Gritz et al.[238] conducted the first physician- or dentist-delivered randomized cessation intervention comparison in 186 newly diagnosed head and neck cancer patients. Patients were treated with either minimal advice or an enhanced intervention with trained clinicians consisting of strong personalized advice to stop smoking, a contracted quit date, tailored written materials, and booster advice sessions. No significant differences were found between treatments, but a 70.2% continuous abstinence rate was found at 12-month follow-up regardless of treatment condition, suggesting that many cancer patients can benefit from brief physician-delivered advice. A later study by Schnoll et al.,[239] comparing cognitive behavioral treatment with standardized health education advice, also failed to find significant differences in quit rates. All patients received NRT, and quit rates in both groups approached 50% at 1-month follow-up and 40% at 3-month follow-up.

Additional studies, ranging from 15 to 80 patients, examined nurse-delivered cessation interventions for a variety of cancer patients. The lowest cessation rates were found with a single session intervention: a 21% cessation rate in the intervention group versus 14% in the usual care group 6 weeks' postintervention.[240] Higher cessation rates were associated with a more intensive intervention consisting of three inpatient visits, supplementary materials, and five postdischarge follow-up contacts. Additional studies demonstrate higher cessation rates with more intensive intervention (40% to 75%) as compared with usual care (43% to 50%), suggesting more intensive interventions may yield higher cessation rates.[241–243] In general, more intense interventions appear to be more efficacious, but even brief advice is important to achieve tobacco cessation.

In a randomized trial of 432 cancer patients coordinated by the Eastern Cooperative Oncology Group (ECOG) with a physician-delivered intervention (comprised of cessation advice, optional NRT, and written materials) or usual care (unstructured advice from physicians), there were no significant intervention effects and generally low abstinence rates (12% to 15%

at 6 to 12 months).[244] However, patients with head and neck or lung cancer were significantly more likely to have quit smoking compared to patients with tumors that were not smoking related. Analyses of outcomes from the Mayo Clinic Nicotine Dependence Center found that although lung cancer patients were more likely to achieve 6-month tobacco abstinence than controls (22% versus 14%), no significant differences were observed after adjusting for covariates.[245] Garces et al.[246] also found no significant differences in abstinence rates between head and neck cancer patients and controls (33% versus 26%). However, higher abstinence rates were found for both head and neck and lung cancer patients treated within 3 months of diagnosis compared to those treated for more than 3 months after the diagnosis, emphasizing the potential importance of the *teachable moment* at the time of the cancer diagnosis.

The potential importance of addressing smoking combined with considering comorbid disease has been noted in a few studies. In a randomized head and neck cancer patients of usual care versus 9 to 11 sessions of a nurse-administered intervention consisting of cognitive-behavioral therapy and medications, targeting comorbid smoking, drinking, and depression significantly increased quit rates at 6-month follow-up for the intervention group compared to the usual control group (47% versus 31%, p <0.05).[247] In a randomized trial of 246 cancer patients treated with 9 weeks of NRT with or without bupropion, there was no significant difference with the addition of bupropion to NRT, but in patients with depressive symptoms, bupropion increased abstinence rates, lowered withdrawal, and improved quality of life.[248] Patients without depression symptoms did equally well when treated with bupropion versus transdermal nicotine and counseling alone.

Patient recruitment has been a problem noted by some studies, including 5.5 years to accrue 246 patients with telephone screening of over 7,500 potential patients.[249] A pilot trial of varenicline in thoracic oncology patients required screening 1,130 patients to accrue 49 participants randomized to a 12-week course of either varenicline or placebo paired with a behavioral counseling platform of seven sessions.[250] A randomized trial of 185 smoking cancer patients comparing the efficacy of a hospital-based standard care smoking cessation model versus standard care augmented by a behavioral tapering regimen via a handheld device before inpatient hospitalization for cancer surgery demonstrated no difference in quit rates (both 32%).[251] However, over 29,000 patients were screened to conduct a randomized clinical trial with a smoking cancer patient population. These studies highlight the potential difficulty recruiting participants who smoke, including considerations for the importance of medical comorbidity in guiding smoking cessation treatment, patient mix (multiple tumor sites), treatment status (awaiting treatment to completed treatment), variation in stage of disease, and considering how psychiatric conditions such as depression reflect the difficulty of conducting research in the oncology setting and the importance of these variables in future studies.

Although accruing patients to intervention trials may seem discouraging, several studies demonstrate the benefit of counseling over self-help. Emmons et al.[252] conducted a randomized controlled trial in 796 young adult survivors of pediatric cancer that included six calls, tailored and targeted written materials, and optional NRT as compared with self-help. Significantly higher quit rates were found in the counseling group compared to the self-help group at all reported follow-up time points, including 12 months (15% versus 9%; p <0.01). A randomized trial of a motivational interviewing-based smoking cessation intervention in a south Australian hospital was delivered over a 3-month period, consisted of multiple contacts with a trained counselor, and provided supplementary material tailored to cancer patients with NRT.[253] The control group received brief advice to quit and generic supplementary material. Quit rates did not differ by treatment group (5% to 6% at 3-month follow-up), but the intervention group was significantly more likely to report attempts to quit smoking.

Current Tobacco Assessment and Cessation Support by Oncologists

Access to cessation support is critical to address tobacco use by cancer patients. A recent survey of 58 NCI-designated cancer centers indicated that about 80% reported a tobacco use program available to their patients and about 60% routinely offered educational materials, but less than 50% had a designated individual who provided services.[254] A recent survey of over 1,500 members of the International Association for the Study of Lung Cancer (IASLC)[255] and a parallel study of 1,197 ASCO members[256] observed that approximately 90% of physicians believe that tobacco affects outcomes, tobacco cessation should be a standard part of cancer care, and approximately 80% regularly advise patients to stop using tobacco, but only approximately 40% discuss medications or assist with quitting. Dominant perceived barriers to cessation support were patient resistance to treatment, an inability to get patients to quit, a lack of cessation resources, and a lack of clinician education. These data showed that even motivated clinicians are not regularly providing tobacco cessation support. A recent survey of 155 actively accruing cooperative group clinical trials further demonstrated that only 29% of active trials collected any tobacco use information, 4.5% collected any tobacco use information at follow-up, and none addressed tobacco cessation.[55] Few oncology meetings offer educational workshops or talks, and they are often poorly attended when they are offered.[257] Collectively, these data demonstrate that oncologists are not regularly providing cessation support and that we are not capturing tobacco use information that may be critical to understanding the effects of tobacco on cancer treatment outcomes.

More in-person talks as well as written and Web-based training should be made available, as well as new approaches that move from the traditional 5 A's model delivered by a single professional to referral systems that efficiently connect tobacco users to multiple resources for tobacco cessation.[258–260] The ASCO *Prevention Curriculum* has a chapter devoted to educating oncology healthcare professionals on the evaluation and treatment of tobacco use.[213] Innovative curricula, such as the Texas Tobacco Outreach Education Program (TOEP), are available and can facilitate program development in other states.[261] However, specialty programs in tobacco cessation treatment that are based in cancer centers and other medical centers are valuable resources that need to be further developed.

Addressing tobacco use in cancer patients may be approached in a systematic and efficient manner. A recent report highlighted the potential utility of automated tobacco assessment and smoking cessation using structured assessments in the EMR where all patients were automatically referred to a dedicated cessation program consisting of phone-based cessation support.[45] In 2,700 patients referred for cessation support, half received only a mailing and only 1% contacted the cessation program. However, in the arm with at least five phone call attempts made by the cessation service, 81% of patients were successfully contacted and only 3% refused cessation support. Furthermore, assessments implemented every 4 weeks, rather than more frequent assessments every 2 weeks, resulted in delayed cessation referrals in less than 1% of smokers. This is the first report to try and identify clinically efficient mechanisms of addressing tobacco use that may be useful in clinical practice or research that may be an effective method of increasing patient participation in cessation support, but substantial work is needed to assess who may benefit from low versus high intensity support in such a program.

Examples of Model Tobacco Treatment Programs

Several dedicated tobacco treatment programs at cancer centers have been developed. Table 31.4 contrasts the core elements of

TABLE 31.4
Attributes of Prototypical Tobacco Treatment Programs

Attribute	MDACC	RPCI	Yale	MSKCC
Tobacco assessment of all patients (EMR)	Yes	Yes	Yes	Yes
Automatic referral of all patients	Yes	Yes	No	Yes
In-person counseling	Yes	No	Yes	Yes
Telephone counseling	Yes	Yes	No	Yes
Medications prescribed	Yes	No	Yes	Yes
Biochemical confirmation (CO) testing	Yes	No	Yes	No
Free to patient	Yes	Yes	No	Yes
Third-party payment	No	No	Yes	Yes
Research studies of new treatments	Yes	Yes	Yes	Yes

MDACC, M.D. Anderson Cancer Center, Houston, TX; RPCI, Roswell Park Cancer Institute, Buffalo, NY; Yale, Yale University Hospital, Smilow Cancer Center, New Haven, CT; MSKCC, Memorial Sloan Kettering Cancer Center, New York, NY.

four active model programs at the end of 2013 (University of Texas M.D. Anderson Cancer Center, Roswell Park Cancer Institute, Yale Cancer Center, and Memorial Sloan Kettering Cancer Center), each of which employ different methods to help cancer patients quit smoking. All programs follow the evidence-based 5 A's model described previously from PHS Guidelines.[199] All programs were made available to patients at their respective medical centers and are now designed to evaluate and treat all patients who self-report current tobacco use. Importantly, not all cancer centers can treat smoking cessation in the same manner. Financing of a cessation program is critical and may include institutional funds, state funds, research funds, and third-party billing. Notably, given the broad spectrum of adverse health effects associated with smoking, cancer centers should carefully consider the potential health benefits and cost savings associated with tobacco cessation due to reductions in treatment complications and recurrence associated with smoking by cancer patients. There is no one "correct" way to create and sustain a tobacco treatment program at a cancer center, but at the very least and consistent with evidence, rigorous behavioral counseling should be provided and, if possible, medication management as well.

FUTURE CONSIDERATIONS

Research Considerations

The past several years have shown a surge in activities identifying the effects of tobacco in cancer patients and increasing awareness is being developed for cessation support at cancer centers as well as through several national organizations. There are three fundamental areas of research that need to be expanded:

1. *Evaluating the effects of tobacco use and cessation on clinical cancer outcomes.* The 2014 SGR concluded that smoking caused adverse outcomes in cancer patients,[7] but several limitations remain. Tobacco-use definitions should be standardized and implemented at diagnosis, during treatment, and follow-up. Biochemical confirmation with cotinine or exhaled carbon monoxide may improve the accuracy of tobacco assessment in at-risk groups such as current smokers who are trying to quit or patients who reported quitting in the past year.[171,185,186,262] Although smoking is the predominant form of tobacco consumption, all tobacco products should be considered. A further understanding of the effects of tobacco on the efficacy and toxicity of cancer treatment, tumor response, quality of life, survival, recurrence, compliance, second primary, and noncancer-related comorbidity is needed. All cancer disease sites and stages are important to consider.
2. *Understanding the effects of tobacco and cessation on cancer biology.* Although not a primary focus of this chapter, tobacco and tobacco-related products increase tumor growth, angiogenesis, migration, invasion and metastasis and decrease response to conventional cancer treatments such as CT and RT. These and other areas are important to consider, including the potential effects on immune-related therapy and vaccine development. *In vivo* models of exposure and cancer response are not well developed, yet are critical to this research area. Work is also needed to assess the effect of emerging tobacco-related products such as e-cigarettes.
3. *Advance understanding of models to increase access to cessation support and increase efficacy of tobacco cessation methods for cancer patients.* This diverse area includes assessing the timing of intervention, intensity, duration, follow-up, and the potential effects of harm-reduction strategies. Cessation pharmacology requires additional consideration in combination with unique approaches to motivational and behavioral counseling in cancer patients. Significant work is needed to disseminate evidence-based cessation support and to assess the cost-effectiveness of different cessation strategies, particularly with regard to improving the cost of cancer care as a whole. Preventing relapse and evaluating the safety of transition to alternative products such as e-cigarettes is equally important and increasingly complex with the addition of new tobacco-related products. Identifying and addressing barriers to effective cessation support is also needed. As related to the cancer patient, clinicians and cessation specialists should consider how their research relates to cancer care. Taking advantage of new integrated medical management systems presents a significant opportunity to improve cessation support access as well as to develop a more effective tracking of patient outcomes.

Policy Implications and Systematic Issues

Several national and international organizations have emphasized the importance of tobacco assessments and cessation for the general population and for cancer patients that include tools to evaluate tobacco use at diagnosis, during treatment, and follow-up appointments, as well as routine support for smoking cessation.[5,6,188–191] In 2012, ASCO, with the contribution of the American Legacy Foundation, published a Tobacco Cessation Toolkit for the oncology setting.[263] This evidence-based guideline intends to help oncology providers integrate tobacco cessation strategies into their patient care. Utilization of the EMR and standardized, automated systems for more efficacious and efficient access to tobacco cessation support has also been suggested,[45] but requires participation by clinicians, institutions, insurers, and health departments. Not only should providers be aware of the need for tobacco cessation and available interventions, but health-care institutions must also build such treatment into their overall system of care. Thus, the identification of patients who smoke or use any alternative tobacco product, referral or direct treatment by providers, billing and reimbursement for treatment provided, and consistent efforts from professional oncology organizations are critically important.[257] The tremendous public health burden from tobacco-related disability and death has not been countered by a proportional level of funding in tobacco control, cancer treatment research, or public advocacy. Researchers, clinicians, and advocates must come together to persuade policy makers to increase funding in tobacco-related research, treatment, and policy initiatives on behalf of healthy individuals and patients. A united front is critically needed in support of a common agenda that includes both increased tobacco-control efforts and additional funding for disease-related research and treatment. With clinical rationale, guidelines, and advocacy in place, the final steps in effective tobacco control and improving health outcomes are to implement these recommendations into practice.

REFERENCES

1. U.S. Department of Health, Education, and Welfare. *Smoking and Health: Report of the Advisory Committee to the Surgeon General of the Public Health Service.* PHS Publication No. 1103. Washington, D.C.: U.S. Department of Health, Education, and Welfare, Public Health Service, Center for Disease Control; 1964.
2. Office of the Surgeon General, Office on Smoking and Health. *The Health Consequences of Smoking. A Report of the Surgeon General.* Atlanta: Centers for Disease Control and Prevention; 2004.
3. Centers for Disease Control and Prevention, National Center for Chronic Disease Prevention and Health Promotion, Office on Smoking and Health. *How Tobacco Smoke Causes Disease: The Biology and Behavioral Basis for Smoking-Attributable Disease: A Report of the Surgeon General.* Atlanta: Centers for Disease Control and Prevention; 2010.
4. U.S. Department of Health and Human Services. *The Health Consequences of Smoking: Nicotine Addiction. A Report of the Surgeon General.* DHHS Publication No. (CDC) 88-8406. Atlanta: U.S. Department of Health and Human Services, Public Health Service, Centers for Disease Control, National Center for Chronic Disease Prevention and Health Promotion, Office on Smoking and Health; 1988.
5. Toll BA, Brandon TH, Gritz ER, et al. Assessing tobacco use by cancer patients and facilitating cessation: an American Association for Cancer Research policy statement. *Clin Cancer Res* 2013;19:1941–1948.
6. Hanna N, Mulshine J, Wollins DS, et al. Tobacco cessation and control a decade later: American society of clinical oncology policy statement update. *J Clin Oncol* 2013;31:3147–3157.
7. U.S. Department of Health and Human Services. *The Health Consequences of Smoking—50 Years of Progress: A Report of the Surgeon General.* Atlanta: U.S. Department of Health and Human Services, Centers for Disease Control and Prevention, National Center for Chronic Disease Prevention and Health Promotion, Office on Smoking and Health; 2014.
8. Brunzell DH. Preclinical evidence that activation of mesolimbic alpha 6 subunit containing nicotinic acetylcholine receptors supports nicotine addiction phenotype. *Nicotine Tob Res* 2012;14:1258–1269.
9. Benowitz NL. Nicotine addiction. *N Engl J Med.* 2010;362:2295–2303.
10. Nestler EJ. Is there a common molecular pathway for addiction? *Nat Neurosci* 2005;8:1445–1449.
11. Dani JA, De Biasi M. Cellular mechanisms of nicotine addiction. *Pharmacol Biochem Behav* 2001;70:439–446.
12. Balfour DJ. The neurobiology of tobacco dependence: a preclinical perspective on the role of the dopamine projections to the nucleus accumbens. *Nicotine Tob Res* 2004;6:899–912.
13. Berridge KC, Robinson TE. What is the role of dopamine in reward: hedonic impact, reward learning, or incentive salience? *Brain Res Brain Res Rev* 1998;28:309–369.
14. Schultz W. Multiple dopamine functions at different time courses. *Annu Rev Neurosci* 2007;30:259–288.
15. Kalivas PW, McFarland K. Brain circuitry and the reinstatement of cocaine-seeking behavior. *Psychopharmacology* 2003;168:44–56.
16. Dani JA, Balfour DJK. Historical and current perspective on tobacco use and nicotine addiction. *Trends Neurosci* 2011;34:383–439.
17. Di Chiara G. Role of dopamine in the behavioural actions of nicotine related to addiction. *Eur J Pharmacol* 2000;393:295–314.
18. Centers for Disease Control and Prevention. Current cigarette smoking among adults—United States, 2011. *MMWR Morb Mortal Wkly Rep* 2012;61:889–894.
19. Centers for Disease Control and Prevention. Cigarette smoking among adults—United States, 2001. *MMWR Morb Mortal Wkly Rep* 2003;52:953–956.
20. Smokefree Laws and Policies. American Lung Association Web site. http://www.lungusa2.org/slati/smokefree_laws.php. Accessed November 25, 2013.
21. Tobacco Policy Project/State Legislated Actions on Tobacco Issues (SLATI). American Lung Association Web site. http://www.lungusa2.org/slati. Accessed November 25, 2013.
22. Tobacco Taxes. American Lung Association Web site. http://www.lungusa2.org/slati/tobacco_taxes.php. Accessed November 25, 2013.
23. Tobacco Situation and Outlook Report, U.S. Department of Agriculture, U.S. Census 1880-2005.
24. Warren GW, Cummings KM. Tobacco and lung cancer: risks, trends, and outcomes in patients with cancer. In: *American Society of Clinical Oncology 2013 Educational Book.* 201; 359–364. ASCO University Web site. http://meetinglibrary.asco.org//content/200-132. Accessed November 25, 2013.
25. Thun MJ, Carter BD, Feskanich D, et al. 50-year trends in smoking-related mortality in the United States. *N Engl J Med.* 2013;368:351–364.
26. U.S. Food and Drug Administration. Summary of Results: Laboratory Analysis of Electronic Cigarettes Conducted by FDA. U.S. Food and Drug Administration Web site. http://www.fda.gov/NewsEvents/PublicHealthFocus/ucm173146.htm. Accessed November 25, 2013.
27. Cummings KM, Dresler CM, Field JK, et al. E-cigarettes and cancer patients. *J Thorac Oncol* 2014;9:438–441.
28. Kuschner WG, Reddy S, Mehrotra N, et al. Electronic cigarettes and thirdhand tobacco smoke: two emerging health care challenges for the primary care provider. *Int J Gen Med* 2011;4:115–120.
29. WHO Study Group on Tobacco Product Regulation. WHO Study Group on Tobacco Product Regulation. Report on the scientific basis of tobacco product regulation: third report of a WHO study group. *World Health Organ Tech Rep Ser* 2009;(955).1–41.
30. National Cancer Institute. Cancer Trends Progress Report – 2011/2012 Update. Nation Cancer Institute Web site. http://progressreport.cancer.gov. Published August 2012. Accessed November 25, 2013.
31. Bellizzi KM, Rowland JH, Jeffery DD, et al. Health behaviors of cancer survivors: examining opportunities for cancer control intervention. *J Clin Oncol* 2005;23:8884–8893.
32. Coups EJ, Ostroff JS. A population-based estimate of the prevalence of behavioral risk factors among adult cancer survivors and noncancer controls. *Prev Med* 2005;40:702–711.
33. Klosky JL, Hum AM, Zhang N, et al. Smokeless and dual tobacco use among males surviving childhood cancer: a report from the Childhood Cancer Survivor Study. *Cancer Epidemiol Biomarkers Prev* 2013;22:1025–1029.
34. Underwood JM, Townsend JS, Tai E, et al. Persistent cigarette smoking and other tobacco use after a tobacco-related cancer diagnosis. *J Cancer Surviv* 2012;6:333–344.
35. Walker MS, Vidrine DJ, Gritz ER, et al. Smoking relapse during the first year after treatment for early-stage non-small-cell lung cancer. *Cancer Epidemiol Biomarkers Prev* 2006;15:2370–2377.
36. Gritz ER. Smoking and smoking cessation in cancer patients. *Br J Addict* 1991;86:549–554.
37. Lippman SM, Lee JJ, Karp DD, et al. Randomized phase III intergroup trial of isotretinoin to prevent second primary tumors in stage I non-small-cell lung cancer. *J Natl Cancer Inst* 2001;93:605–618.
38. Ostroff JS, Jacobsen PB, Moadel AB, et al. Prevalence and predictors of continued tobacco use after treatment of patients with head and neck cancer. *Cancer* 1995;75:569–576.
39. Hickey K, Do KA, Green A. Smoking and prostate cancer. *Epidemiol Rev* 2001;23:115–125.
40. Plaskon LA, Penson DF, Vaughan TL, et al. Cigarette smoking and risk of prostate cancer in middle-aged men. *Cancer Epidemiol Biomarkers Prev* 2003;12:604–609.
41. Watters JL, Park Y, Hollenbeck A, et al. Cigarette smoking and prostate cancer in a prospective US cohort study. *Cancer Epidemiol Biomarkers Prev* 2009;18:2427–2435.
42. Alberg AJ, Singh S, May JW, et al. Epidemiology, prevention, and early detection of breast cancer. *Curr Opin Oncol* 2000;12:515–520.
43. Johnson KC, Miller AB, Collishaw NE, et al. Active smoking and secondhand smoke increase breast cancer risk: the report of the Canadian Expert Panel on Tobacco Smoke and Breast Cancer Risk (2009). *Tob Control* 2011;20:e2.
44. Breast Cancer Family Registry; Kathleen Cuningham Consortium for Research into Familial Breast Cancer (Australasia); Ontario Cancer Genetics Network (Canada). Smoking and risk of breast cancer in carriers of mutations in BRCA1 or BRCA2 aged less than 50 years. *Breast Cancer Res Treat* 2008;109:67–75.
45. Warren GW, Marshall JR, Cummings KM, et al. Automated tobacco assessment and cessation support for cancer patients. *Cancer* 2014;120:562–569.
46. Centers for Disease Control and Prevention. Cigarette smoking among adults—United States, 2004. *MMWR Morb Mortal Wkly Rep* 2005;54:1121–1124.

47. Centers for Disease Control and Prevention. Tobacco use among adults—United States, 2005. *MMWR Morb Mortal Wkly Rep* 2006;55:1145–1148.
48. Gritz ER, Nisenbaum R, Elashoff RE, et al. Smoking behavior following diagnosis in patients with stage I non-small cell lung cancer. *Cancer Causes Control* 1991;2:105–112.
49. Chen AM, Vazquez E, Courquin J, et al. Tobacco use among long-term survivors of head and neck cancer treated with radiation therapy. *Psychooncology* 2014;23:190–194.
50. Ostroff J, Garland J, Moadel A, et al. Cigarette smoking patterns in patients after treatment of bladder cancer. *J Cancer Educ* 2000;15:86–90.
51. McBride CM, Emmons KM, Lipkus IM. Understanding the potential of teachable moments: the case of smoking cessation. *Health Educ Res* 2003;18:156–170.
52. Gritz ER, Schacherer C, Koehly L, et al. Smoking withdrawal and relapse in head and neck cancer patients. *Head Neck* 1999;21:420–427.
53. Warren GW, Marshall JR, Cummings KM. Smoking, cancer treatment, and design of clinical trials. *Proc AACR* 2013:54:594.
54. Parsons A, Daley A, Begh R, et al. Influence of smoking cessation after diagnosis of early stage lung cancer on prognosis: systematic review of observational studies with meta-analysis. *BMJ* 2010;340:b5569.
55. Peters EN, Torres E, Toll BA, et al. Tobacco assessment in actively accruing National Cancer Institute Cooperative Group Program Clinical Trials. *J Clin Oncol* 2012;30:2869–2875.
56. Land SR. Methodologic barriers to addressing critical questions about tobacco and cancer prognosis. *J Clin Oncol* 2012;30:2030–2032.
57. Gritz ER, Dresler C, Sarna L. Smoking, the missing drug interaction in clinical trials: ignoring the obvious. *Cancer Epidemiol Biomarkers Prev* 2005;14:2287–2293.
58. Yu GP, Ostroff JS, Zhang ZF, et al. Smoking history and cancer patient survival: a hospital cancer registry study. *Cancer Detect Prev* 1997;21:497–509.
59. Dahlstrom KR, Calzada G, Hanby JD, et al. An evolution in demographics, treatment, and outcomes of oropharyngeal cancer at a major cancer center: a staging system in need of repair. *Cancer* 2012;119:81–89.
60. Molina MA, Cheung MC, Perez EA, et al. African American and poor patients have a dramatically worse prognosis for head and neck cancer: an examination of 20,915 patients. *Cancer* 2008;113:2797–2806.
61. Dragun AE, Huang B, Tucker TC, et al. Disparities in the application of adjuvant radiotherapy after breast-conserving surgery for early stage breast cancer: impact on overall survival. *Cancer* 2011;117:2590–2598.
62. Bostrom PJ, Alkhateeb S, Trotter G, et al. Sex differences in bladder cancer outcomes among smokers with advanced bladder cancer. *BJU Int* 2011;109:70–76.
63. Kroeger N, Klatte T, Birkhäuser FD, et al. Smoking negatively impacts renal cell carcinoma overall and cancer-specific survival. *Cancer* 2011;118:1795–1802.
64. Marks DI, Ballen K, Logan BR, et al. The effect of smoking on allogeneic transplant outcomes. *Biol Blood Marrow Transplant* 2009;15:1277–1287.
65. Gridelli C, Ciardiello F, Gallo C, et al. First-line erlotinib followed by second-line cisplatin-gemcitabine chemotherapy in advanced non-small-cell lung cancer: the TORCH randomized trial. *J Clin Oncol* 2012;30:3002–3011.
66. Maeda R, Yoshida J, Ishii G, et al. Influence of cigarette smoking on survival and tumor invasiveness in clinical stage IA lung adenocarcinoma. *Ann Thorac Surg* 2012;93:1626–1632.
67. Maeda R, Yoshida J, Ishii G, et al. The prognostic impact of cigarette smoking on patients with non-small cell lung cancer. *J Thorac Oncol* 2011;6:735–742.
68. Janjigian YY, McDonnell K, Kris MG, et al. Pack-years of cigarette smoking as a prognostic factor in patients with stage IIIB/IV nonsmall cell lung cancer. *Cancer* 2010;116:670–675.
69. Toyooka S, Takano T, Kosaka T, et al. Epidermal growth factor receptor mutation, but not sex and smoking, is independently associated with favorable prognosis of gefitinib-treated patients with lung adenocarcinoma. *Cancer Sci* 2008;99:303–308.
70. Kawai H, Tada A, Kawahara M, et al. Smoking history before surgery and prognosis in patients with stage IA non-small-cell lung cancer—a multicenter study. *Lung Cancer* 2005;49:63–70.
71. Warren GW, Kasza K, Reid M, et al. Smoking at diagnosis and survival in cancer patients. *Int J Cancer* 2013;132:401–410.
72. Kvale E, Ekundayo OJ, Zhang Y, et al. History of cancer and mortality in community-dwelling older adults. *Cancer Epidemiol* 2011;35:30–36.
73. Gajdos C, Hawn MT, Campagna EJ, et al. Adverse effects of smoking on postoperative outcomes in cancer patients. *Ann Surg Oncol* 2012;19:1430–1438.
74. Duffy SA, Ronis DL, McLean S, et al. Pretreatment health behaviors predict survival among patients with head and neck squamous cell carcinoma. *J Clin Oncol* 2009;27:1969–1975.
75. Farshadpour F, Kranenborg H, Calkoen EV, et al. Survival analysis of head and neck squamous cell carcinoma: influence of smoking and drinking. *Head Neck* 2011;33:817–823.
76. Meyer F, Bairati I, Fortin A, et al. Interaction between antioxidant vitamin supplementation and cigarette smoking during radiation therapy in relation to long-term effects on recurrence and mortality: a randomized trial among head and neck cancer patients. *Int J Cancer* 2008;122:1679–1683.
77. Shen GP, Xu FH, He F, et al. Pretreatment lifestyle behaviors as survival predictors for patients with nasopharyngeal carcinoma. *PLoS One* 2012;7:e36515.
78. Dal Maso L, Zucchetto A, Talamini R, et al. Effect of obesity and other lifestyle factors on mortality in women with breast cancer. *Int J Cancer* 2008;123:2188–2194.
79. Hellmann SS, Thygesen LC, Tolstrup JS, et al. Modifiable risk factors and survival in women diagnosed with primary breast cancer: results from a prospective cohort study. *Eur J Cancer Prev* 2010;19:366–673.
80. Holmes MD, Murin S, Chen WY, et al. Smoking and survival after breast cancer diagnosis. *Int J Cancer* 2007;120:2672–2677.
81. Sagiv SK, Gaudet MM, Eng SM, et al. Active and passive cigarette smoke and breast cancer survival. *Ann Epidemiol* 2007;17:385–393.
82. Phipps AI, Baron J, Newcomb PA. Prediagnostic smoking history, alcohol consumption, and colorectal cancer survival: the Seattle Colon Cancer Family Registry. *Cancer* 2011;117:4948–4957.
83. Huang XE, Tajima K, Hamajima N, et al. Effects of dietary, drinking, and smoking habits on the prognosis of gastric cancer. *Nutr Cancer* 2000;38:30–36.
84. Kenfield SA, Stampfer MJ, Chan JM, et al. Smoking and prostate cancer survival and recurrence. *JAMA* 2011;305:2548–2555.
85. Merrick GS, Butler WM, Wallner KE, et al. Androgen-deprivation therapy does not impact cause-specific or overall survival after permanent prostate brachytherapy. *Int J Radiat Oncol Biol Phys* 2006;65:669–677.
86. Pickles T, Liu M, Berthelet E, et al. The effect of smoking on outcome following external radiation for localized prostate cancer. *J Urol* 2004;171:1543–1546.
87. Taira AV, Merrick GS, Butler WM, et al. Long-term outcome for clinically localized prostate cancer treated with permanent interstitial brachytherapy. *Int J Radiat Oncol Biol Phys* 2011;79:1336–1342.
88. Sweeney C, Farrow DC. Differential survival related to smoking among patients with renal cell carcinoma. *Epidemiology* 2000;11:344–346.
89. Coker AL, DeSimone CP, Eggleston KS, et al. Smoking and survival among Kentucky women diagnosed with invasive cervical cancer: 1995–2005. *Gynecol Oncol* 2009;112:365–369.
90. Modesitt SC, Huang B, Shelton BJ, et al. Endometrial cancer in Kentucky: the impact of age, smoking status, and rural residence. *Gynecol Oncol* 2006;103:300–306.
91. Poullis M, McShane J, Shaw M, et al. Smoking status at diagnosis and histology type as determinants of long-term outcomes of lung cancer patients. *Eur J Cardiothorac Surg* 2012;43:919–924.
92. Kawaguchi T, Tamiya A, Tamura A, et al. Chemotherapy is beneficial for elderly patients with advanced non-small-cell lung cancer: analysis of patients aged 70–74, 75–79, and 80 or older in Japan. *Clin Lung Cancer* 2012;13:447–447.
93. Pirker R, Pereira JR, Szczesna A, et al. Prognostic factors in patients with advanced non-small cell lung cancer: data from the phase III FLEX study. *Lung Cancer* 2012;77:376–382.
94. Ferketich AK, Niland JC, Mamet R, et al. Smoking status and survival in the national comprehensive cancer network non-small cell lung cancer cohort. *Cancer* 2013;119:847–853.
95. Chansky K, Sculier JP, Crowley JJ, et al. The International Association for the Study of Lung Cancer Staging Project: prognostic factors and pathologic TNM stage in surgically managed non-small cell lung cancer. *J Thorac Oncol* 2009;4:792–801.
96. Myrdal G, Lamberg K, Lambe M, et al. Regional differences in treatment and outcome in non-small cell lung cancer: a population-based study (Sweden). *Lung Cancer* 2009;63:16–22.
97. Saito-Nakaya K, Nakaya N, Akechi T, et al. Marital status and non-small cell lung cancer survival: the Lung Cancer Database Project in Japan. *Psychooncology* 2008;17:869–876.
98. Zhou W, Heist RS, Liu G, et al. Smoking cessation before diagnosis and survival in early stage non-small cell lung cancer patients. *Lung Cancer* 2006;53:375–380.
99. Tsao AS, Liu D, Lee JJ, et al. Smoking affects treatment outcome in patients with advanced nonsmall cell lung cancer. *Cancer* 2006;106:2428–2436.
100. Ebbert JO, Williams BA, Sun Z, et al. Duration of smoking abstinence as a predictor for non-small-cell lung cancer survival in women. *Lung Cancer* 2005;47:165–172.
101. Tammemagi CM, Neslund-Dudas C, Simoff M, et al. Smoking and lung cancer survival: the role of comorbidity and treatment. *Chest* 2004;125:27–37.
102. Nordquist LT, Simon GR, Cantor A, et al. Improved survival in never-smokers vs current smokers with primary adenocarcinoma of the lung. *Chest* 2004;126:347–351.
103. Ehlers SL, Gastineau DA, Patten CA, et al. The impact of smoking on outcomes among patients undergoing hematopoietic SCT for the treatment of acute leukemia. *Bone Marrow Transplant* 2011;46:285–290.
104. Geyer SM, Morton LM, Habermann TM, et al. Smoking, alcohol use, obesity, and overall survival from non-Hodgkin lymphoma: a population-based study. *Cancer* 2010;116:2993–3000.
105. Deleyiannis FW, Thomas DB, Vaughan TL, et al. Alcoholism: independent predictor of survival in patients with head and neck cancer. *J Natl Cancer Inst* 1996;88:542–549.
106. Ngô C, Alran S, Plancher C, et al. Outcome in early cervical cancer following pre-operative low dose rate brachytherapy: a ten-year follow up of 257 patients treated at a single institution. *Gynecol Oncol* 2011;123:248–252.
107. Browman GP, Wong G, Hodson I, et al. Influence of cigarette smoking on the efficacy of radiation therapy in head and neck cancer. *N Engl J Med* 1993;328:159–163.
108. Gillison ML, Zhang Q, Jordan R, et al. Tobacco smoking and increased risk of death and progression for patients with p16-positive and p16-negative oropharyngeal cancer. *J Clin Oncol* 2012;30:2102–2111.
109. Waggoner SE, Darcy KM, Fuhrman B, et al. Association between cigarette smoking and prognosis in locally advanced cervical carcinoma treated with chemoradiation: a Gynecologic Oncology Group study. *Gynecol Oncol* 2006;103:853–858.

110. Khuri FR, Lee JJ, Lippman SM, et al. Randomized phase III trial of low-dose isotretinoin for prevention of second primary tumors in stage I and II head and neck cancer patients. *J Natl Cancer Inst* 2006;98:441–450.
111. Karvonen-Gutierrez CA, Ronis DL, Fowler KE, et al. Quality of life scores predict survival among patients with head and neck cancer. *J Clin Oncol* 2008;26:2754–2760.
112. Sardari Nia P, Weyler J, Colpaert C, et al. Prognostic value of smoking status in operated non-small cell lung cancer. *Lung Cancer* 2005;47:351–359.
113. Chen J, Jiang R, Garces YI, et al. Prognostic factors for limited-stage small cell lung cancer: a study of 284 patients. *Lung Cancer* 2010;67:221–226.
114. Bittner N, Merrick GS, Galbreath RW, et al. Primary causes of death after permanent prostate brachytherapy. *Int J Radiat Oncol Biol Phys* 2008;72:433–440.
115. Haughey BH, Sinha P. Prognostic factors and survival unique to surgically treated p16+ oropharyngeal cancer. *Laryngoscope* 2012;122:S13–S33.
116. Kawakita D, Hosono S, Ito H, et al. Impact of smoking status on clinical outcome in oral cavity cancer patients. *Oral Oncol* 2012;48:186–191.
117. Chen AM, Chen LM, Vaughan A, et al. Tobacco smoking during radiation therapy for head-and-neck cancer is associated with unfavorable outcome. *Int J Radiat Oncol Biol Phys* 2011;79:414–419.
118. Junor E, Kerr G, Oniscu A, et al. Benefit of chemotherapy as part of treatment for HPV DNA-positive but p16-negative squamous cell carcinoma of the oropharynx. *Br J Cancer* 2012;106:358–365.
119. Manjer J, Andersson I, Berglund G, et al. Survival of women with breast cancer in relation to smoking. *Eur J Surg* 2000;166:852–858.
120. Kountourakis P, Correa AM, Hofstetter WL, et al. Combined modality therapy of cT2N0M0 esophageal cancer: the University of Texas M. D. Anderson Cancer Center experience. *Cancer* 2011;117:925–930.
121. Munro AJ, Bentley AH, Ackland C, et al. Smoking compromises cause-specific survival in patients with operable colorectal cancer. *Clin Oncol (R Coll Radiol)* 2006;18:436–440.
122. Gong Z, Agalliu I, Lin DW, et al. Cigarette smoking and prostate cancer-specific mortality following diagnosis in middle-aged men. *Cancer Causes Control* 2008;19:25–31.
123. Kjaerbye-Thygesen A, Frederiksen K, Hogdall EV, et al. Smoking and overweight: negative prognostic factors in stage III epithelial ovarian cancer. *Cancer Epidemiol Biomarkers Prev* 2006;15:798–803.
124. Nagle CM, Bain CJ, Webb PM. Cigarette smoking and survival after ovarian cancer diagnosis. *Cancer Epidemiol Biomarkers Prev* 2006;15:2557–2560.
125. Wright JD, Li J, Gerhard DS, et al. Human papillomavirus type and tobacco use as predictors of survival in early stage cervical carcinoma. *Gynecol Oncol* 2005;98:84–91.
126. Sardari Nia P, Van Marck E, Weyler J, et al. Prognostic value of a biologic classification of non-small-cell lung cancer into the growth patterns along with other clinical, pathological and immunohistochemical factors. *Eur J Cardiothorac Surg* 2010;38:628–636.
127. Hoff CM, Grau C, Overgaard J. Effect of smoking on oxygen delivery and outcome in patients treated with radiotherapy for head and neck squamous cell carcinoma—a prospective study. *Radiother Oncol* 2012;103:38–44.
128. Joshu CE, Mondul AM, Meinhold CL, et al. Cigarette smoking and prostate cancer recurrence after prostatectomy. *J Natl Cancer Inst* 2011;103:835–838.
129. Mai SK, Welzel G, Haegele V, et al. The influence of smoking and other risk factors on the outcome after radiochemotherapy for anal cancer. *Radiat Oncol* 2007;2:30.
130. Kim AJ, Suh JD, Sercarz JA, et al. Salvage surgery with free flap reconstruction: factors affecting outcome after treatment of recurrent head and neck squamous carcinoma. *Laryngoscope* 2007;117:1019–1023.
131. Khan AM, Freeman-Wang T, Pisal N, et al. Smoking and multicentric vulval intraepithelial neoplasia. *J Obstet Gynaecol* 2009;29:123–125.
132. Hefler L, Grimm C, Tempfer C, et al. Treatment with vaginal progesterone in women with low-grade cervical dysplasia: a phase II trial. *Anticancer Res* 2010;30:1257–1261.
133. Matsumoto K, Oki A, Furuta R, et al. Tobacco smoking and regression of low-grade cervical abnormalities. *Cancer Sci* 2010;101:2065–2073.
134. Fleshner N, Garland J, Moadel A, et al. Influence of smoking status on the disease-related outcomes of patients with tobacco-associated superficial transitional cell carcinoma of the bladder. *Cancer* 1999;86:2337–2345.
135. Ioffe YJ, Elmore RG, Karlan BY, et al. Effect of cigarette smoking on epithelial ovarian cancer survival. *J Reprod Med* 2010;55:346–350.
136. Schlumbrecht MP, Sun CC, Wong KN, et al. Clinicodemographic factors influencing outcomes in patients with low-grade serous ovarian carcinoma. *Cancer* 2011;117:3741–3749.
137. Fortin A, Wang CS, Vigneault E. Influence of smoking and alcohol drinking behaviors on treatment outcomes of patients with squamous cell carcinomas of the head and neck. *Int J Radiat Oncol Biol Phys* 2009;74:1062–1069.
138. Chen CH, Shun CT, Huang KH, et al. Stopping smoking might reduce tumour recurrence in nonmuscle-invasive bladder cancer. *BJU Int* 2007;100:281–286.
139. Browman GP, Mohide EA, Willan A, et al. Association between smoking during radiotherapy and prognosis in head and neck cancer: a follow-up study. *Head Neck* 2002;24:1031–1037.
140. Clark JR, McCluskey SA, Hall F, et al. Predictors of morbidity following free flap reconstruction for cancer of the head and neck. *Head Neck* 2007;29:1090–1101.
141. Little SC, Hughley BB, Park SS. Complications with forehead flaps in nasal reconstruction. *Laryngoscope* 2009;119:1093–1099.
142. Patel RS, McCluskey SA, Goldstein DP, et al. Clinicopathologic and therapeutic risk factors for perioperative complications and prolonged hospital stay in free flap reconstruction of the head and neck. *Head Neck* 2010;32:1345–1353.
143. Baumann DP, Lin HY, Chevray PM. Perforator number predicts fat necrosis in a prospective analysis of breast reconstruction with free TRAM, DIEP, and SIEA flaps. *Plast Reconstr Surg* 2010;125:1335–1341.
144. Goodwin SJ, McCarthy CM, Pusic AL, et al. Complications in smokers after postmastectomy tissue expander/implant breast reconstruction. *Ann Plast Surg* 2005;55:16–19.
145. Bertelsen CA, Andreasen AH, Jorgensen T, et al. Anastomotic leakage after anterior resection for rectal cancer: risk factors. *Colorectal Dis* 2010;12:37–43.
146. Cooke DT, Lin GC, Lau CL, et al. Analysis of cervical esophagogastric anastomotic leaks after transhiatal esophagectomy: risk factors, presentation, and detection. *Ann Thorac Surg* 2009;88:177–184.
147. Richards CH, Platt JJ, Anderson JH, et al. The impact of perioperative risk, tumor pathology and surgical complications on disease recurrence following potentially curative resection of colorectal cancer. *Ann Surg* 2011;254:83–89.
148. Nickelsen TN, Jorgensen T, Kronborg O. Lifestyle and 30-day complications to surgery for colorectal cancer. *Acta Oncol* 2005;44:218–223.
149. Begum FD, Hogdall E, Christensen IJ, et al. Serum tetranectin as a preoperative indicator for postoperative complications in Danish ovarian cancer patients. *Gynecol Oncol* 2010;117:116–150.
150. Joo YH, Sun DI, Cho JH, et al. Factors that predict postoperative pulmonary complications after supracricoid partial laryngectomy. *Arch Otolaryngol Head Neck Surg* 2009;135:1154–1157.
151. Mason DP, Subramanian S, Nowicki ER, et al. Impact of smoking cessation before resection of lung cancer: a Society of Thoracic Surgeons General Thoracic Surgery Database study. *Ann Thorac Surg* 2009;88:362–370.
152. van der Voet JC, Keus RB, Hart AA, et al. The impact of treatment time and smoking on local control and complications in T1 glottic cancer. *Int J Radiat Oncol Biol Phys* 1998;42:247–255.
153. Wedlake LJ, Thomas K, Lalji A, et al. Predicting late effects of pelvic radiotherapy: is there a better approach? *Int J Radiat Oncol Biol Phys* 2010;78:1163–1170.
154. Hocevar-Boltezar I, Zargi M, Strojan P. Risk factors for voice quality after radiotherapy for early glottic cancer. *Radiother Oncol* 2009;93:524–529.
155. Lilla C, Ambrosone CB, Kropp S, et al. Predictive factors for late normal tissue complications following radiotherapy for breast cancer. *Breast Cancer Res Treat* 2007;106:143–150.
156. Eifel PJ, Jhingran A, Bodurka DC, et al. Correlation of smoking history and other patient characteristics with major complications of pelvic radiation therapy for cervical cancer. *J Clin Oncol* 2002;20:3651–3657.
157. Wuketich S, Hienz SA, Marosi C. Prevalence of clinically relevant oral mucositis in outpatients receiving myelosuppressive chemotherapy for solid tumors. *Support Care Cancer* 2012;20:175–183.
158. Zevallos JP, Mallen MJ, Lam CY, et al. Complications of radiotherapy in laryngopharyngeal cancer: effects of a prospective smoking cessation program. *Cancer* 2009;115:4636–4644.
159. Gold EB, Flatt SW, Pierce JP, et al. Dietary factors and vasomotor symptoms in breast cancer survivors: the WHEL Study. *Menopause* 2006;13:423–433.
160. Cheung MC, Hamilton K, Sherman R, et al. Impact of teaching facility status and high-volume centers on outcomes for lung cancer resection: an examination of 13,469 surgical patients. *Ann Surg Oncol* 2009;16:3–13.
161. Zingg U, Smithers BM, Gotley DC, et al. Factors associated with postoperative pulmonary morbidity after esophagectomy for cancer. *Ann Surg Oncol* 2011;18:1460–1468.
162. Kelly KJ, Greenblatt DY, Wan Y, et al. Risk stratification for distal pancreatectomy utilizing ACS-NSQIP: preoperative factors predict morbidity and mortality. *J Gastrointest Surg* 2011;15:250–259.
163. Merkow RP, Bilimoria KY, Cohen ME, et al. Variability in reoperation rates at 182 hospitals: a potential target for quality improvement. *J Am Coll Surg* 2009;209:557–564.
164. Alsadius D, Hedelin M, Johansson KA, et al. Tobacco smoking and long-lasting symptoms from the bowel and the anal-sphincter region after radiotherapy for prostate cancer. *Radiother Oncol* 2011;101:495–501.
165. Kuri M, Nakagawa M, Tanaka H, et al. Determination of the duration of preoperative smoking cessation to improve wound healing after head and neck surgery. *Anesthesiology* 2005;102:892–896.
166. Vaporciyan AA, Merriman KW, Ece F, et al. Incidence of major pulmonary morbidity after pneumonectomy: association with timing of smoking cessation. *Ann Thorac Surg* 2002;73:420–425.
167. Bjarnason GA, Mackenzie RG, Nabid A, et al. Comparison of toxicity associated with early morning versus late afternoon radiotherapy in patients with head-and-neck cancer: a prospective randomized trial of the National Cancer Institute of Canada Clinical Trials Group (HN3). *Int J Radiat Oncol Biol Phys* 2009;73:166–172.
168. Park SM, Lim MK, Jung KW, et al. Prediagnosis smoking, obesity, insulin resistance, and second primary cancer risk in male cancer survivors: National Health Insurance Corporation Study. *J Clin Oncol* 2007;25:4835–4843.
169. Leon X, del Prado Venegas M, Orus C, et al. Influence of the persistence of tobacco and alcohol use in the appearance of second neoplasm in patients with a head and neck cancer. A case-control study. *Cancer Causes Control* 2009;20:645–652.
170. Kinoshita Y, Tsukuma H, Ajiki W, et al. The risk for second primaries in gastric cancer patients: adjuvant therapy and habitual smoking and drinking. *J Epidemiol* 2000;10:300–304.
171. Khuri FR, Kim ES, Lee JJ, et al. The impact of smoking status, disease stage, and index tumor site on second primary tumor incidence and tumor recurrence in the head and neck retinoid chemoprevention trial. *Cancer Epidemiol Biomarkers Prev* 2001;10:823–829.

172. Scanlon EF, Suh O, Murthy SM, et al. Influence of smoking on the development of lung metastases from breast cancer. *Cancer* 1995;75:2693–2699.
173. Ford MB, Sigurdson AJ, Petrulis ES, et al. Effects of smoking and radiotherapy on lung carcinoma in breast carcinoma survivors. *Cancer* 2003;98:1457–1464.
174. Li CI, Daling JR, Porter PL, et al. Relationship between potentially modifiable lifestyle factors and risk of second primary contralateral breast cancer among women diagnosed with estrogen receptor-positive invasive breast cancer. *J Clin Oncol* 2009;27:5312–5318.
175. van den Belt-Dusebout AW, de Wit R, Gietema JA, et al. Treatment-specific risks of second malignancies and cardiovascular disease in 5-year survivors of testicular cancer. *J Clin Oncol* 2007;25:4370–4378.
176. Boorjian S, Cowan JE, Konety BR, et al. Cancer of the Prostate Strategic Urologic Research Endeavor Investigators. Bladder cancer incidence and risk factors in men with prostate cancer: results from Cancer of the Prostate Strategic Urologic Research Endeavor. *J Urol* 2007;177:883–887.
177. Travis LB, Gospodarowicz M, Curtis RE, et al. Lung cancer following chemotherapy and radiotherapy for Hodgkin's disease. *J Natl Cancer Inst* 2002;94:182–192.
178. Ang KK, Harris J, Wheeler R, et al. Human papillomavirus and survival of patients with oropharyngeal cancer. *N Engl J Med* 2010;363:24–35.
179. Peck BW, Dahlstrom KR, Gan SJ, et al. Low risk of second primary malignancies among never smokers with human papillomavirus-associated index oropharyngeal cancers. *Head Neck* 2012;35:794–799.
180. Herbst RS, Prager D, Hermann R, et al. TRIBUTE: a phase III trial of erlotinib hydrochloride (OSI-774) combined with carboplatin and paclitaxel chemotherapy in advanced non-small-cell lung cancer. *J Clin Oncol* 2005;23:5892–5899.
181. Thatcher N, Chang A, Parikh P, et al. Gefitinib plus best supportive care in previously treated patients with refractory advanced non-small-cell lung cancer: results from a randomised, placebo-controlled, multicentre study (Iressa Survival Evaluation in Lung Cancer). *Lancet* 2005;366:1527–1537.
182. Kwak EL, Bang YJ, Camidge DR, et al. Anaplastic lymphoma kinase inhibition in non-small-cell lung cancer. *N Engl J Med* 2010;363:1693–1703.
183. Paik PK, Johnson ML, D'Angelo SP, et al. Driver mutations determine survival in smokers and never-smokers with stage IIIB/IV lung adenocarcinomas. *Cancer* 2012;118:5840–5847.
184. Soria JC, Cruz C, Bahleda R, et al. Clinical activity, safety and biomarkers of PD-L1 blockade in non-small cell lung cancer (NSCLC): additional analyses from a clinical study of the engineered antibody MPDL3280A (anti-PDL1). Presented at: 2013 European Cancer Congress 2013-2015. Amsterdam.
185. Morales N, Romano M, Cummings KM, et al. Accuracy of self-reported tobacco use in newly diagnosed cancer patients. *Cancer Causes Control* 2013;24:1223–1230.
186. Warren GW, Arnold SM, Valentino JP, et al. Accuracy of self-reported tobacco assessments in a head and neck cancer treatment population. *Radiother Oncol* 2012;103:45–48.
187. Marin VP, Pytynia KB, Langstein HN, et al. Serum cotinine concentration and wound complications in head and neck reconstruction. *Plast Reconstr Surg* 2008;121:451–457.
188. American Medical Association. Tobacco use or exposure as a variable in clinical research (Resolution 424, A-06).www.ama-assn.org.ama1/pub/upload/mm/475/bot479i406.pdf.
189. Sarna L, Bialous SA. Nursing and tobacco cessation: setting a research agenda. Reports from a national conference. In: *Nursing Research*. Philadelphia: Lippincott Williams & Wilkins; 2006: 4S.
190. Sarna L, Bialous SA, Chan S, et al. International symposia: global perspectives on nursing involvement in tobacco control. Presented in: Oncology Nursing Society, 28th Annual Congress Syllabus, May 1-4, 2003, Denver, Colorado, Denver: Oncology Nursing Society; 2003: 112.
191. Viswanath K, Herbst RS, Land SR, et al. Tobacco and cancer: an American Association for Cancer research policy statement. *Cancer Res* 2010;70(17):3419–3430.
192. American Society of Clinical Oncology. American Society of Clinical Oncology policy statement update: tobacco control—Reducing cancer incidence and saving lives. 2003. *J Clin Oncol* 2003;21:2777–2786.
193. Gritz ER, Fingeret MC, Vidrine DJ, et al. Successes and failures of the teachable moment: smoking cessation in cancer patients. *Cancer* 2006;106:17–27.
194. Gritz ER, Dresler C, Sarna L. Smoking, the missing drug interaction in clinical trials: ignoring the obvious. *Cancer Epidemiol Biomarkers Prev* 2005;14:2287–2293.
195. Chapple A, Ziebland S, McPherson A. Stigma, shame, and blame experienced by patients with lung cancer: qualitative study. *BMJ* 2004;328:1470.
196. LoConte NK, Else-Quest NM, Eickhoff J, et al. Assessment of guilt and shame in patients with non-small cell lung cancer compared with patients with breast and prostate cancer. *Clin Lung Cancer* 2008;9:171–178.
197. Wassenaar TR, Eickhoff JC, Jarzemsky DR, et al. Differences in primary care clinicians' approach to non-small cell lung cancer patients compared with breast cancer. *J Thorac Oncol* 2007;2:722–728.
198. Fiore MC, Bailey WC, Cohen SJ, et al. *Quick Reference Guide for Clinicians. Treating Tobacco Use and Dependence*. Rockville, MD: U.S. Department of Health and Human Services, Public Health Services; 2000. http://health.state.tn.us/Downloads/TQL_Quick%20Reference.pdf. Accessed November 25, 2013.
199. Fiore MC, Jaén CR, Baker TB, et al. *Treating Tobacco Use and Dependence: 2008 Update*. Rockville, MD: U.S. Department of Health and Human Services; 2008. http://www.ncbi.nlm.nih.gov/books/NBK63952/. Accessed November 25, 2013.
200. Fiore MC, Jorenby DE, Schensky AE, et al. Smoking status as the new vital sign: effect on assessment and intervention in patients who smoke. *Mayo Clin Proc* 1995;70:209–213.

201. Blumenthal D, Tavenner M. The "meaningful use" regulation for electronic health records. *N Engl J Med* 2010;363:501–504.
202. Couple approaches to smoking cessation. In: Schmaling KB, Sher TG, eds. *The Psychology of Couples and Illness: Theory, Research, & Practice*. Washington, D.C.: American Psychological Association; 2000: 311–336.
203. Homish GG, Leonard KE. Spousal influence on smoking behaviors in a US community sample of newly married couples. *Soc Sci Med* 2005;61:2557–2567.
204. Hemsing N, Greaves L, O'Leary R, et al. Partner support for smoking cessation during pregnancy: a systematic review. *Nicotine Tob Res* 2012;14:767–776.
205. Tod AM, Joanne R. Overcoming delay in the diagnosis of lung cancer: a qualitative study. *Nurs Stan* 2010;24:35–43.
206. Fagerstrom KO, Schneider NG. Measuring nicotine dependence: a review of the Fagerstrom Tolerance Questionnaire. *J Behav Med* 1989;12:159–182.
207. Baker TB, Piper ME, Bolt DM, et al. Time to first cigarette in the morning smoking as an index of ability to quit smoking: implications for nicotine dependence. *Nicotine Tob Res* 2007;9:S555–S570.
208. Ferguson JA, Patten CA, Schroeder DR, et al. Predictors of 6-month tobacco abstinence among 1224 cigarette smokers treated for nicotine dependence. *Addict Behav* 2003;28:1203–1218.
209. Prochaska JO, DiClemente CC. Stages and processes of self-change of smoking: toward an integrative model of change. *J Consult Clin Psychol* 1983;51:390–395.
210. Prokhorov AV, Hudmon KS, Gritz ER. Promoting smoking cessation among cancer patients: a behavioral model. *Oncology (Williston Park)* 1997;11:1807–1813.
211. Toll BA, Rojewski AM, Duncan L, et al. "Quitting smoking will benefit your health": the evolution of clinician messaging to encourage tobacco cessation. *Clin Cancer Res* 2014;20:301–309.
212. Miller WR, Rose GS. Toward a theory of motivational interviewing. *Am Psychol* 2009;64:527–537.
213. Gritz ER, Fingeret MC, Vidrine DJ. Tobacco control in the oncology setting. In: Brawley OW, Khuri FR, Rock CL, eds. *ASCO Cancer Prevention Curriculum*. Alexandria, VA: American Society of Clinical Oncology; 2007.
214. Henningfield JE, Keenan RM. Nicotine delivery kinetics and abuse liability. *J Consult Clin Psychol* 1993;61:743–750.
215. Silagy C, Lancaster T, Stead L, et al. Nicotine replacement therapy for smoking cessation. *Cochrane Database Syst Rev* 2004;(3):CD000146.
216. Piper M, Smith S, Schlam T, et al. A randomized placebo-controlled clinical trial of 5 smoking cessation pharmacotherapies. *Arch Gen Psychiatry* 2009;66:1253–1262.
217. Smith S, McCarthy D, Japuntich S, et al. Comparative effectiveness of 5 smoking cessation pharmacotherapies in primary care clinics. *Arch Intern Med* 2009;169:2148–2155.
218. Warren GW, Singh AK. Nicotine and lung cancer. *J Carcinog* 2013;12:1–8.
219. Myles PS, Iacono GA, Hunt JO, et al. Risk of respiratory complications and wound infection in patients undergoing ambulatory surgery: smokers versus nonsmokers. *Anesthesiology* 2002;97:842–847.
220. Sørensen L, Hørby J, Friis E, et al. Smoking as a risk factor for wound healing and infection in breast cancer surgery. *Eur J Surg Oncol* 2002;28:815–820.
221. Jorgensen ED, Zhao H, Traganos F, et al. DNA damage response induced by exposure of human lung adenocarcinoma cells to smoke from tobacco- and nicotine-free cigarettes. *Cell Cycle* 2010;9:2170–2176.
222. Murray RP, Connett JE, Zapawa LM. Does nicotine replacement therapy cause cancer? Evidence from the Lung Health Study. *Nicotine Tob Res* 2009;11:1076–1082.
223. Hughes JR, Stead LF, Lancaster T. Nortriptyline for smoking cessation: a review. *Nicotine Tob Res* 2005;7:491–499.
224. Ascher JA, Cole JO, Colin JN, et al. Bupropion: a review of its mechanism of antidepressant activity. *J Clin Psychiatry* 1995;56:395–401.
225. Fryer JD, Lukas RJ. Noncompetitive functional inhibition at diverse, human nicotinic acetylcholine receptor subtypes by bupropion, phencyclidine, and ibogaine. *J Pharmacol Exp Ther* 1999;288:88–92.
226. Cryan JF, Bruijnzeel AW, Skjei KL, et al. Bupropion enhances brain reward function and reverses the affective and somatic aspects of nicotine withdrawal in the rat. *Psychopharmacology* 2003;168:347–358.
227. Hughes JR, Stead LF, Lancaster T. Antidepressants for smoking cessation. *Cochrane Database Syst Rev* 2003;(2):CD000031.
228. Coe JW, Brooks PR, Vetelino MG, et al. Varenicline: an alpha4beta2 nicotinic receptor partial agonist for smoking cessation. *J Med Chem* 2005;48:3474–3477.
229. Jorenby DE, Hays JT, Rigotti NA, et al. Efficacy of varenicline, an alpha4beta2 nicotinic acetylcholine receptor partial agonist, vs placebo or sustained-release bupropion for smoking cessation: a randomized controlled trial. *JAMA* 2006;296:56–63.
230. Cahill K, Stead LF, Lancaster T. Nicotine receptor partial agonists for smoking cessation. *Cochrane Database Syst Rev* 2012;4:CD006103.
231. Hoogendoorn M, Welsing P, Rutten-van Mölken MP. Cost-effectiveness of varenicline compared with bupropion, NRT, and nortriptyline for smoking cessation in the Netherlands. *Curr Med Res Opin* 2008;24:51–61.
232. Linden K, Jormanainen V, Linna M, et al. Cost effectiveness of varenicline versus bupropion and unaided cessation for smoking cessation in a cohort of Finnish adult smokers. *Curr Med Res Opin* 2010;26:549–560.
233. Zimovetz EA, Wilson K, Samuel M, et al. A review of cost-effectiveness of varenicline and comparison of cost-effectiveness of treatments for major smoking-related morbidities. *J Eval Clin Pract* 2011;17:288–297.
234. Gibbons RD, Mann JJ. Varenicline, smoking cessation, and neuropsychiatric adverse events. *Am J of Psychiatry* 2013;170:1460–1467.

235. Thomas KH, Martin RM, Davies NM, et al. Smoking cessation treatment and risk of depression, suicide, and self harm in the Clinical Practice Research Datalink: prospective cohort study. *BMJ* 2013;347:f5704.
236. Anthenelli RM, Morris C, Ramey TS, et al. Effects of varenicline on smoking cessation in adults with stably treated current or past major depression: a randomized trial. *Ann Intern Med* 2013;159:390–400.
237. Gourlay SG, Stead LF, Benowitz NL. Clonidine for smoking cessation. *Cochrane Database Syst Rev* 2004;(3):CD000058.
238. Gritz ER, Carr CR, Rapkin D, et al. Predictors of long-term smoking cessation in head and neck cancer patients. *Cancer Epidemiol Biomarkers Prev* 1993;2:261–270.
239. Schnoll RA, Rothman RL, Wielt DB, et al. A randomized pilot study of cognitive-behavioral therapy versus basic health education for smoking cessation among cancer patients. *Ann Behav Med* 2005;30:1–11.
240. Griebel B, Wewers ME, Baker CA. The effectiveness of a nurse-managed minimal smoking-cessation intervention among hospitalized patients with cancer. *Oncol Nurs Forum* 1998;25:897–902.
241. Wewers ME, Bowen JM, Stanislaw AE, et al. A nurse-delivered smoking cessation intervention among hospitalized postoperative patients—influence of a smoking-related diagnosis: a pilot study. *Heart Lung* 1994;23:151–156.
242. Wewers ME, Jenkins L, Mignery T. A nurse-managed smoking cessation intervention during diagnostic testing for lung cancer. *Oncol Nurs Forum* 1997;24:1419–1422.
243. Stanislaw AE, Wewers ME. A smoking cessation intervention with hospitalized surgical cancer patients: a pilot study. *Cancer Nurs* 1994;17:81–86.
244. Schnoll RA, Zhang B, Rue M, et al. Brief physician-initiated quit-smoking strategies for clinical oncology settings: a trial coordinated by the Eastern Cooperative Oncology Group. *J Clin Oncol* 2003;21:355–365.
245. Sanderson Cox L, Patten CA, Ebbert JO, et al. Tobacco use outcomes among patients with lung cancer treated for nicotine dependence. *J Clin Oncol* 2002;20:3461–3469.
246. Garces YI, Schroeder DR, Nirelli LM, et al. Tobacco use outcomes among patients with head and neck carcinoma treated for nicotine dependence: a matched-pair analysis. *Cancer* 2004;101:116–124.
247. Duffy SA, Ronis DL, Valenstein M, et al. A tailored smoking, alcohol, and depression intervention for head and neck cancer patients. *Cancer Epidemiol Biomarkers Prev* 2006;15:2203–2208.
248. Schnoll RA, Martinez E, Tatum KL, et al. A bupropion smoking cessation clinical trial for cancer patients. *Cancer Causes Control* 2010;21:811–820.
249. Martinez E, Tatum KL, Weber DM, et al. Issues related to implementing a smoking cessation clinical trial for cancer patients. *Cancer Causes Control* 2009;20:97–104.
250. Park ER, Japuntich S, Temel J, et al. A smoking cessation intervention for thoracic surgery and oncology clinics: a pilot trial. *J Thorac Oncol* 2011;6:1059–1065.
251. Ostroff JS, Burkhalter JE, Cinciripini PM, et al. Randomized trial of a presurgical scheduled reduced smoking intervention for patients newly diagnosed with cancer. *Health Psychol* 2013 [Epub ahead of print].
252. Emmons KM, Puleo E, Park E, et al. Peer-delivered smoking counseling for childhood cancer survivors increases rate of cessation: the partnership for health study. *J Clin Oncol* 2005;23:6516–6523.
253. Wakefield M, Olver I, Whitford H, et al. Motivational interviewing as a smoking cessation intervention for patients with cancer: randomized controlled trial. *Nurs Res* 2004;53:396–406.
254. Goldstein AO, Ripley-Moffitt CE, Pathman DE, et al. Tobacco use treatment at the U.S. National Cancer Institute's designated Cancer Centers. *Nicotine Tob Res* 2013;15:52–58.
255. Warren GW, Marshall JR, Cummings KM, et al. Practice patterns and perceptions of thoracic oncology providers on tobacco use and cessation in cancer patients. *J Thorac Oncol* 2013;8:543–548.
256. Warren GW, Marshall JR, Cummings KM, et al. Addressing tobacco use in cancer patients: a survey of American Society of Clinical Oncology (ASCO) members. *J Oncol Pract* 2013;9:258–262.
257. Gritz ER, Sarna L, Dresler C, et al. Building a united front: aligning the agendas for tobacco control, lung cancer research, and policy. *Cancer Epidemiol Biomarkers Prev* 2007;16:859–863.
258. Vidrine JI, Shete S, Cao Y, et al. Ask-Advise-Connect: a new approach to smoking treatment delivery in health care settings. *JAMA Intern Med* 2013;173:458–464.
259. Bernstein SL, Jearld S, Prasad D, et al. Rapid implementation of a smokers' quitline fax referral service in an urban area. *J Health Care Poor Underserved* 2009;20:55–63.
260. Sarna L, Bialous SA, Ong MK, et al. Increasing nursing referral to telephone quitlines for smoking cessation using a web-based program. *Nurs Res* 2012;61:433–440.
261. Stancic N, Mullen PD, Prokhorov AV, et al. Continuing medical education: what delivery format do physicians prefer? *J Contin Educ Health Prof* 2003;23:162–167.
262. Society for Research on Nicotine and Tobacco Committee on Biochemical Verification. Biochemical verification of tobacco use and cessation. *Nicotine Tob Res* 2002;4:149–159.
263. American Society of Clinical Oncology. Tobacco Cessation Guide for Oncology Providers. ASCO Web site. http://www.asco.org/sites/default/files/tobacco_cessation_guide.pdf. Accessed November 25, 2013.

32 Role of Surgery in Cancer Prevention

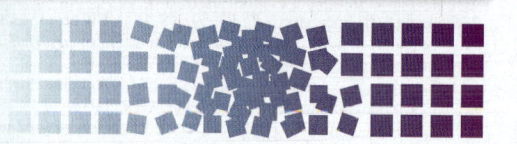

José G. Guillem, Andrew Berchuck, Jeffrey F. Moley, Jeffrey A. Norton, Sheryl G. A. Gabram-Mendola, and Vanessa W. Hui

INTRODUCTION

Since the heritable component of some cancer predispositions has been linked to mutations in specific genes, clinical interventions have been formulated for mutation carriers within affected families. The primary interventions for mutation carriers for highly penetrant syndromes, such as multiple endocrine neoplasia (MEN), familial adenomatous polyposis (FAP), hereditary nonpolyposis colorectal cancer (CRC), and hereditary breast and ovarian cancer syndromes, are primarily surgical. This chapter is divided into five sections addressing breast (S.G.A.G.), gastric (J.N.), ovarian and endometrial (A.B.), and MENs (J.F.M.) and colorectal (J.G.G., V.W.H.). For each, the clinical and genetic indications and timing of prophylactic surgery and its efficacy, when known, are provided.

Prophylactic surgery in hereditary cancer is a complex process, requiring a clear understanding of the natural history of the disease and variance of penetrance, a realistic appreciation of the potential benefit and consequence of a risk reducing procedure in an otherwise potentially healthy individual, and the long-term sequelae of such surgical intervention, as well as the individual patient's and family's perception of surgical risk and anticipated benefit.

PATIENTS AT HIGH RISK FOR BREAST CANCER

Identification of Patients at Risk

A detailed family history is the most important tool for identifying individuals at increased risk for hereditary cancers. The US Preventive Services Task Force updated their recommendation for risk assessment, genetic counseling, and genetic testing for asymptomatic women who have not been diagnosed with a *BRCA*-related cancer. In this update, the use of a risk screening tool is highly recommended to identify appropriate patients for referral for genetic counseling.[1] The American Society of Clinical Oncology has also updated the policy on genetic and genomic testing for cancer susceptibility, and this update includes information on genetic tests of uncertain clinical utility and direct-to-consumer marketing, both of which impact the practice of oncology and preventive medicine.[2] Historically, genetic counseling and testing were offered by health-care providers. However, with the advent of direct-to-consumer marketing, individuals may obtain tests and receive results directly from a company. The American Society of Clinical Oncology still endorses pre- and posttest counseling for thorough disclosure of the impact of testing. Before any woman considers risk-reduction surgery such as bilateral mastectomy or salpingo-oophorectomy, referral to a high-risk or genetic screening program is desirable, as women often overestimate their actual breast cancer risk.[3]

The most common cancer syndromes that place women at risk for breast cancer are *BRCA1*[4] and *BRCA2*[5] gene mutations. Other less common syndromes are listed in Table 32.1.[6,7]

Following referral for genetic assessment, three groups of patients emerge.[8] The first consists of those women who have undergone genetic testing and have been found to harbor a mutated gene associated with high penetrance for breast cancer. Given that the possibility of developing breast cancer in this group may be as high as 90%, there is a role for enhanced surveillance or risk-reduction surgery. The American Cancer Society has published guidelines for magnetic resonance imaging (MRI) screening as a method for enhanced surveillance.[9] Women in this first group qualify for such screening, which can be offered annually but scheduled at 6-month intervals with screening mammography to increase the rate of identifying interval cancers. Alternatively, simultaneous screening with MRI and mammography to compare one modality with the other on an annual basis may also be offered. Another choice for this group of women is to pursue bilateral risk-reduction mastectomy with an option for immediate reconstruction. Bilateral salpingo-oophorectomy for *BRCA1* and *BRCA2* mutation carriers may also be considered, as this procedure has been shown to reduce breast cancer risk by almost 50%.[8,10] This is especially true for *BRCA2* mutation carriers, who tend to develop hormone receptor–positive breast cancers.

The second group consists of women with strong family histories suggestive of hereditary breast cancer who test negative for both the *BRCA1* and *BRCA2* mutations as well as the other described syndromes. In this group, there may not have been a family member with cancer who was tested for the mutation. Therefore, a negative test does not necessarily indicate that a woman's risk is equivalent to that of the general population.[7] There may also be an undetected mutation in such a family, indicating the possibility of higher-than-average risk for that particular woman. These women may or may not qualify for enhanced surveillance with MRI screening,[9] and accurate assessment of their risk may require the use of other risk prediction tools,[3] in addition to evaluating for the presence of lobular carcinoma in situ, atypical lobular hyperplasia, or atypical ductal hyperplasia, and determining if a more intensive surveillance regimen is necessary based on heterogeneously or extremely dense breast tissue on mammography.

The third group consists of women with a strong family history of breast cancer, who for various reasons, have chosen not to pursue genetic testing. These individuals may have other health-related problems, psychological concerns, cost issues, or they may fear perceived medical insurance discrimination. Women in all groups can be educated that with passage of the Genetic Information Nondiscrimination Act in 2008, significant advances have occurred that protect patients from discrimination by employers and health insurers.[11]

Women in the second and third groups may still qualify for bilateral risk-reduction mastectomy and immediate reconstruction. Often, women who elect this path are influenced by their family history or by witnessing breast and/or ovarian cancer deaths in close family members, giving them a significant fear of a breast or ovarian cancer diagnosis. For women in all three groups, the decision of whether to pursue risk-reducing surgery is difficult. Often, the expertise of a cancer clinical psychologist or psychiatrist

TABLE 32.1 Hereditary Carcinoma Syndromes Including Breast Cancer

Syndrome	Chromosome/Gene	Primary Carcinoma	Secondary Carcinoma	Breast Cancer Penetrance
Familial breast cancer/ovarian cancer syndrome	17q21; BRCA1 Autosomal dominant	Breast cancer, ovarian cancer	Colon, prostate	60%–80%
Familial breast cancer/ovarian cancer syndrome	13q12; BRCA2 Autosomal dominant	Breast cancer, ovarian cancer	Male breast cancer, endometrial, prostate, oropharyngeal, pancreatic	60%–80%
Li-Fraumeni syndrome	17p13.1 and 22q12.1; TP53 and CHEK2 Autosomal dominant	Soft tissue cancers (including breast)	Soft tissue sarcoma, leukemia, osteosarcoma, melanoma, colon, pancreas, adrenal syndrome, cortex, and brain tumors	50%–85% (for all types of cancers in this syndrome)
PTEN hamartoma syndrome (Cowden's)	10q23.31; PTEN mutation Autosomal dominant	Breast cancer	Thyroid (follicular) and endometrial carcinoma	25%–50%
Peutz-Jeghers syndrome	19p13.3; STK11 Autosomal dominant	Gastrointestinal cancers	Esophagus, stomach, small intestine, large bowel, pancreas, lung, ovary, endometrial	29%
Diffuse gastric cancer	16q22.1; CDH1 Autosomal dominant	Diffuse gastric cancer	Colorectal, lobular breast cancer	39% (lobular breast cancer)
Louis-Bar syndrome	11q22.3; ATM Autosomal recessive	Leukemia and lymphoma	Ovarian, breast, gastric, melanoma, leiomyomas, sarcomas	38% (for all types of cancers in the syndrome)

PTEN, phosphatase and tensin homolog.
Data from Lux MR, Fasching PA, Beckmann MW. Hereditary breast and ovarian cancer: review and future perspectives. J Mol Med 2006;84:16–28, and Shannon KM, Chittenden A. Genetic testing by cancer site: breast. Cancer J 2012;18:310–319.

is enlisted, as risk-reduction mastectomy involves an irreversible procedure with body image and sexual implications.[8]

Updated in 2007, the Society of Surgical Oncology published a position statement on the role of prophylactic mastectomy for patients at high risk for breast cancer, as well as those patients recently diagnosed with breast cancer who are considering contralateral prophylactic breast surgery.[12] For women at high risk, indications fall into three broad categories: presence of a mutation in BRCA or other susceptible genes, strong family history with no demonstrable mutation, and histologic risk factors (biopsy-proven atypical ductal hyperplasia, atypical lobular hyperplasia, or lobular carcinoma in situ especially in patients with a strong family history of breast cancer). Recommendations for patients with recently diagnosed breast cancer are similar in that they include the indications for high-risk individuals previously noted, as well as future surveillance challenges for the opposite breast (clinically and mammographically dense breast tissue or diffuse, indeterminate microcalcifications in the contralateral breast). Another important consideration is the need for symmetry in patients with large, ptotic, or disproportionately sized contralateral breasts.

Surgical Issues and Technique

In a single institution's 33-year experience,[13] the risk for breast cancer in both moderate- and high-risk groups of women based on family history was reduced by at least 89% for women who underwent bilateral prophylactic mastectomy. From a technical perspective, in this study, women either had a subcutaneous mastectomy (removal of the majority of breast tissue with sparing of the nipple–areola complex) or total mastectomy (removal of the entire breast through the nipple–areola complex). Most of the recurrences occurred in women undergoing a subcutaneous mastectomy. However, this was the most frequent procedure performed at that time and thus may have contributed to the number of increased recurrences.

Another surgical option for high-risk women is bilateral salpingo-oophorectomy. Among a cohort of women with BRCA1 and BRCA2 mutations, this procedure has been associated with a lower risk of mortality from both breast and ovarian cancer.[10] As an additional benefit, this procedure also decreases the risk of breast cancer in this patient population, likely through the mechanism of decreasing hormonal exposure at a younger age.

Contemporary surgical procedures for risk-reducing bilateral mastectomy include total mastectomy, skin-sparing mastectomy (preservation of the skin envelope by removal of the entire breast through a circumareolar incision around the nipple–areola complex), subcutaneous mastectomy, areola-sparing mastectomy (removal of the nipple while sparing the areola), and nipple-sparing mastectomy (removal of entire breast and nipple core tissue but preservation of nipple–areolar skin).[14] Given advances in reconstructive nipple–areolar techniques, it appears that total mastectomy with or without skin-sparing methods reduces the risk of breast cancer to the greatest extent with reasonable cosmesis. More limited and long-term follow-up data are available on areola- and nipple-sparing techniques. The potential limitations of these procedures are distortion of the nipple–areola complex and lack of sensitivity after breast tissue has been completely removed.[8]

Immediate reconstruction is offered to patients and performed in the vast majority undergoing bilateral risk-reduction mastectomy. Choices of reconstruction include a bilateral pedicled or free tissue transverse rectus abdominis muscle flap, a free bilateral deep inferior epigastric perforator flap or superficial inferior epigastric artery flap, bilateral latissimus flaps with or without implant or expanders, or bilateral implant or expander placement alone.[14] Although tissue flap transfer gives a more natural appearance and texture to the reconstructed site, individual body contour drives the ultimate plan for reconstruction. The decision about the type of reconstruction should be made by the plastic surgeon with input from the surgical oncologist, especially for the group of women with breast cancer desiring bilateral mastectomies who may require adjuvant radiation for treatment.

Although the risk reduction is dramatic for bilateral mastectomy, residual breast tissue may be left behind, especially with skin-sparing procedures. Patients should be educated that careful chest wall surveillance is recommended after such a procedure. Local recurrences after bilateral implant reconstruction are reliably detected by clinical examination. Recurrences after reconstruction with autologous tissue present most commonly on the skin 50% to 72% of the time and are detectable by physician examination.[15] Nonpalpable deeper recurrences in this setting are less common, and use of mammography image surveillance may be indicated, especially if significant breast tissue was left behind unintentionally during the bilateral mastectomy procedure. At times, an initial "screening" mammogram may be performed, if significant residual breast tissue is suspected; this should occur well after all healing has taken place to delineate the amount of visible breast tissue on imaging. This drives future decisions of whether to follow a patient with imaging. Finally, all patients should be instructed to return for clinical breast examination with the health provider if any change is noted on the reconstructed breasts, regardless of imaging plan.

Although risk-reduction bilateral mastectomy may be exceedingly beneficial for high-risk women, especially for those testing positive for *BRCA1*, *BRCA2*, or other deleterious mutations, or belonging to a family afflicted with a cancer syndrome, they are never emergent procedures. Along with risk-reduction bilateral salpingo-oophorectomy, risk-reduction bilateral mastectomy resides at the far end of the spectrum of an individual's choices.[16] These procedures should be offered only after appropriate genetic counseling and accurate assessment of a woman's actual risk for breast and ovarian cancer. An in-depth consultation with the patient and her family members is necessary prior to proceeding with an operative plan.

HEREDITARY DIFFUSE GASTRIC CANCER

Gastric cancer is the fourth most common cause of cancer worldwide and is the second leading cause of cancer mortality.[17] Although environmental agents, including *Helicobacter pylori* and diet, are the primary risk factors for this disease, approximately 10% of gastric cancers are a result of familial clustering.[18,19] Histologically, gastric cancers may be classified as either intestinal or diffuse types. The intestinal type histopathology is linked to environmental factors and advanced age. The diffuse type occurs in younger patients and is associated with a familial predisposition. Because of a decrease in intestinal-type gastric cancers, the overall incidence of gastric cancer has declined significantly in the past 50 years. However, the incidence of diffuse gastric cancer (DGC), which is also called signet ring cell or linitis plastica, has remained stable and, by some reports, may be increasing.

Hereditary DGC (HDGC) is a genetic cancer susceptibility syndrome defined by one of the following: (1) two or more documented cases of DGC in first- or second-degree relatives, with at least one diagnosed before the age of 50; or (2) three or more cases of documented DGC in first- or second-degree relatives, independent of age of onset. The average age of onset of HDGC is 38, and the pattern of inheritance is autosomal dominant.[20] Figure 32.1 shows a pedigree with HDGC.

In 1998, inactivating germline mutations in the E-cadherin gene *CDH1* were identified in three Maori families, each with multiple cases of poorly differentiated DGC.[21] The *CDH1* mutations in these families were inherited in an autosomal dominant pattern, with incomplete but high penetrance. Onset of clinically apparent cancer was early, with the youngest affected individual dying of DGC at the age of 14.[21] Since then, germline mutations of *CDH1* have been identified in 30% to 50% of all patients with HDGC.[19,22] More than 50 mutations have been recognized across diverse ethnic backgrounds, including European, African American, Pakistani, Japanese, Korean, and others.[19] In addition to gastric cancers, germline *CDH1* mutations are associated with increased risk of lobular carcinoma of the breast, and this was the first manifestation of a *CDH1* mutation in one series.[23] *CDH1* is, to date, the only gene implicated in HDGC. Penetrance of DGC in patients carrying a *CDH1* mutation is estimated at 70% to 80%, but may be higher. The need for a systematic study of specimens is supported by recent work by Gaya et al.[24] in which initial total gastrectomy specimens were reported as negative, but detailed sectioning and analysis showed invasive carcinoma.

CDH1 is localized on chromosome 16q22.1 and encodes the calcium-dependent cell adhesion glycoprotein E-cadherin. Functionally, E-cadherin impacts maintenance of normal tissue morphology and cellular differentiation. It is hypothesized that *CDH1* acts as a tumor suppressor gene in HDGC, with loss of function leading to loss of cell adhesion and subsequently to proliferation, invasion, and metastases. Figure 32.2 shows the *CDH1* mutation for the pedigree depicted in Figure 32.1.

The germline *CDH1* mutation is most frequently a truncating mutation. Germline missense mutations are causative in a few HDGC kindreds, but are more often clinically insignificant. In vitro assays for cellular invasion and aggregation may predict the functional impact of missense mutations to aid in this distinction.[22] Within the gastric mucosa, the "second hit" leading to complete loss of E-cadherin function results from *CDH1* promoter methylation, as has been described in sporadic gastric cancer.[25]

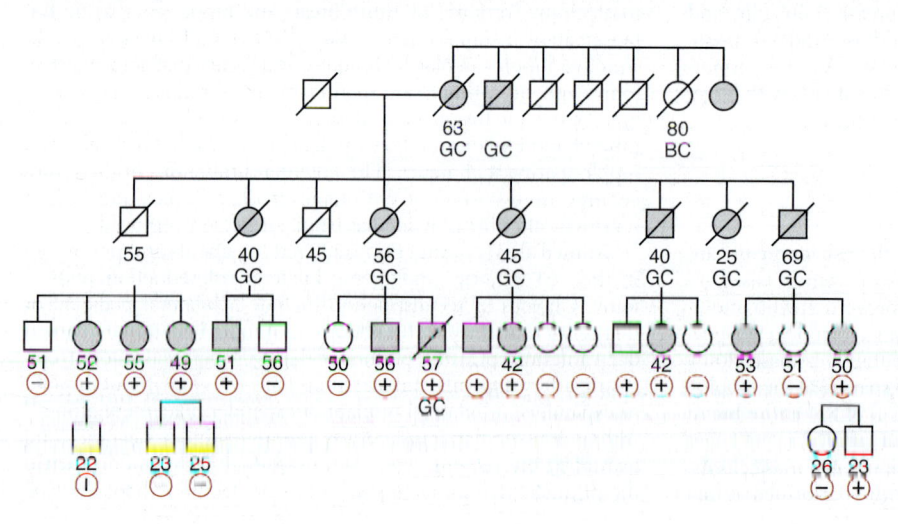

Figure 32.1 A family pedigree showing autosomal dominant inheritance of gastric cancer. Individual mutation testing results for the codon 1003 CDH1 mutation are indicated by + or −. Individuals affected with gastric cancer are shaded. (From Norton JA, Ham CM, Van Dam J, et al. CDH1 truncating mutations in the E-cadherin gene: an indication for total gastrectomy to treat hereditary diffuse gastric cancer. *Ann Surg* 2007;245:873.)

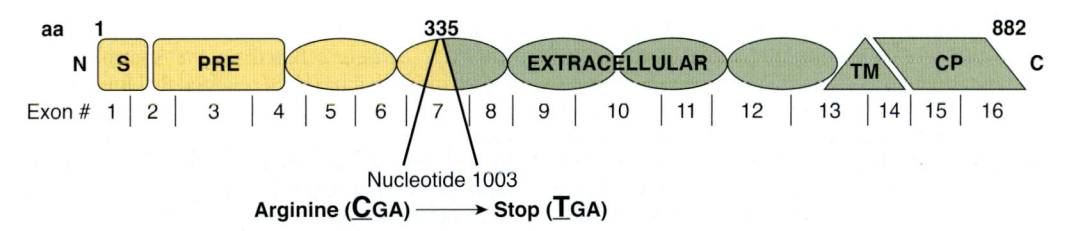

Figure 32.2 The mutation in this kindred is located in the central region of the E-cadherin gene that codes for the extracellular cadherin domains of the protein containing calcium-binding motifs important in the adhesion process. The C → T transition in exon 7 of nucleotide 1003 results in a premature stop codon (R335X), producing truncated peptides that lack the transmembrane and cytoplasmic β-catenin–binding domains essential for tight cell-cell adhesion. Black area indicates truncated portion of peptide. N, N-terminus; C, C-terminus; S, signal peptide; PRE, precursor sequence; TM, transmembrane domain; CP, cytoplasmic domain. (From Norton JA, Ham CM, Van Dam J, et al. CDH1 truncating mutations in the E-cadherin gene: an indication for total gastrectomy to treat hereditary diffuse gastric cancer. *Ann Surg* 2007;245:873.)

It remains unclear whether specific *CDH1* mutations are associated with distinctive phenotypic characteristics or rates of penetrance, although this may become apparent as more recurrent mutations are recognized. To date, most mutations identified have been novel and distributed throughout *CDH1*. Recognition of recurrent mutations has usually resulted from independent events; however, there is evidence for the role of founder effects in certain kindreds.[22] At present, it is also unclear whether patients with HDGC without detectable *CDH1* mutations have mutation of a different gene or merely a *CDH1* mutation that has gone unrecognized.

New recommended screening criteria for *CDH1* mutations are as follows:

1. Families with one or more cases of DGC
2. Individuals with DGC before the age of 40 years without a family history
3. Families or individuals with cases of DGC (one case below the age of 50 years) and lobular breast cancer
4. Cases where pathologists detect in situ signet ring cells or pagetoid spread of signet ring cells adjacent to diffuse type gastric cancer[18,26]

As in other familial cancer syndromes, genetic counseling should take place prior to genetic testing so that the family understands the potential impact of the results. After obtaining informed consent, a team comprising a geneticist, gastroenterologist, surgeon, and oncologist should discuss the possible outcomes of testing and the management options associated with each. Genetic testing should first be performed on a family member with HDGC or on a tissue sample if no affected relative is living. In addition to direct sequencing, multiplex ligation-dependent probe amplification is recommended to test for large genomic rearrangements. If a *CDH1* mutation is identified, asymptomatic family members may proceed with genetic testing, preferably by the age of 20.[19] If no mutation is identified in the family member with DGC, the value of testing asymptomatic relatives is low.

Among individuals found to carry a germline *CDH1* mutation, clinical screening is problematic. Histologically, DGC is characterized by multiple infiltrates of malignant signet ring cells, which may underlie normal mucosa.[27] Because these malignant foci are small in size and widely distributed, they are difficult to identify via random endoscopic biopsy. Chromoendoscopy and positron emission tomography have reportedly been used, but the clinical utility of these tools in early detection remains unproven. Lack of a sensitive screening test for HDGC makes early diagnosis extremely challenging. By the time patients are symptomatic and present for treatment, many have diffuse involvement of the stomach or linitis plastica, and rates of mortality are high. Published case reports describe patients who have presented with extensive DGC despite recent normal endoscopy and negative biopsies.[28] The 5-year survival rate for individuals who develop clinically apparent DGC is only 10%, with the majority dying before age 40.

Because of high cancer penetrance, poor outcome, and inadequacy of clinical screening tools for HDGC, prophylactic total gastrectomy is recommended as a management option for asymptomatic carriers of *CDH1* mutations.[18] Although total gastrectomy is performed with prophylactic intent in these cases, most specimens have been found to contain foci of diffuse signet ring cell cancer.[19,28,29] Foci of DGC have been identified even in patients who have undergone extensive negative screening, including high-resolution computed tomography, positron emission tomography scan, chromoendoscopy-guided biopsies, and endoscopic ultrasonography.[19] However, HGDC in asymptomatic *CDH1* carriers is usually completely resected by prophylactic gastrectomy, as pathologic analyses of resected specimens have shown only T1N0 disease.

Because these signet ring cell cancers are multifocal and distributed throughout the entire stomach, especially in the cardia,[30] prophylactic gastrectomy should include the entire stomach, and the surgeon must transect the esophagus and not the proximal stomach. Furthermore, it should be performed by a surgeon experienced in the technical aspects of the procedure and familiar with HDGC. In asymptomatic patients, lymph node metastases have not been observed; therefore, D2 lymph node resection is not necessary. The optimal timing of prophylactic gastrectomy in individuals with *CDH1* mutations is unknown, but recent consensus recommendations indicate that age 20 is reasonable.[18]

Although it is a potentially lifesaving procedure, prophylactic gastrectomy for *CDH1* mutation carries significant risks that must be considered. Overall mortality for total gastrectomy is estimated to be as high as 2% to 4%, although it is estimated to be 1% when performed prophylactically. Patients must also be aware that there is a nearly 100% risk of long-term morbidity associated with this procedure, including diarrhea, dumping, weight loss, and difficulty eating.[19] A recent study of the effects of prophylactic gastrectomy for *CDH1* mutation demonstrated that physical and mental function were normal at 12 months, but specific digestive issues were recognized. Overall, 70% had diarrhea, 63% fatigue, 81% eating discomfort, 63% reflux, 45% eating restrictions, and 44% had altered body image, suggesting that this operation impacted negatively on quality of life.[31] Because of these complications and the fact that lymph node spread has not been observed, some recommend vagus-preserving gastrectomy done either open or laparoscopically. In addition, because the penetrance of *CDH1* mutations is incomplete, some patients who undergo prophylactic gastrectomy would never have gone on to develop clinically significant gastric cancer. Prophylactic gastrectomy has, in fact, been performed on several patients reported to show no evidence of gastric cancer on pathology.[29]

Some individuals with *CDH1* mutations choose not to pursue prophylactic gastrectomy. These individuals should undergo careful surveillance, including biannual chromoendoscopy with biopsies, beginning when they are at least 10 years younger than the youngest family member with DGC was at time of diagnosis. It is recommended that any endoscopically visible lesion is targeted and that six random biopsies are taken from the following regions: antrum, transitional zone, body, fundus, and cardia. Careful white-light examination with targeted and random biopsies combined with detailed histopathology can identify early lesions and help to inform decision making with regard to gastrectomy.[32] Additionally, because women with *CDH1* mutations have a nearly 40% lifetime risk of developing lobular breast carcinoma, they should be carefully screened with annual mammography and breast MRI starting at age 35.[23] They should also do monthly self-examinations and have a breast examination by a physician every 6 months. The same surveillance recommendations are probably appropriate for HDGC families without identifiable *CDH1* mutations, although no current guidelines for this exist.

The emergence of gene-directed gastrectomy as a treatment strategy for patients with HDGC represents the culmination of a successful collaboration between molecular biologists, geneticists, oncologists, gastroenterologists, and surgeons. It is anticipated that the recognition of similar molecular markers in other familial cancer syndromes will transform the approach to the early diagnosis and treatment of a variety of tumors.

SURGICAL PROPHYLAXIS OF HEREDITARY OVARIAN AND ENDOMETRIAL CANCER

Hereditary Ovarian Cancer (*BRCA1, BRCA2*)

Inherited mutations in *BRCA1* and *BRCA2* strongly predispose women to breast cancer and to high-grade serous cancers of the ovary, fallopian tube, and peritoneum.[33,34] About two-thirds are due to *BRCA1* mutations and one-third *BRCA2* mutations, and these account for about 15% to 20% of high-grade serous cases. The lifetime risk of these gynecologic cancers increases from a baseline of 1.5% to about 15% to 25% in *BRCA2* carriers and 30% to 60% in *BRCA1* carriers.[33,34] *BRCA1/2* mutations are rare in most populations (<1 in 500 individuals); one notable exception is the Ashkenazi Jewish population, in which the carrier frequency is 1 in 40.[35] *BRCA1*-associated cases peak in the 50s and *BRCA2*-associated cancers in the 60s.[36] In addition to *BRCA1/2* mutations, germline mutations in a number of other genes in the homologous recombination DNA repair pathway confer high penetrance susceptibility to ovarian cancer (e.g., *RAD51C, RAD51D, BRIP1, PALB2*).[37] This has led to the development of more comprehensive cancer genetic testing panels that are increasingly being used to identify women who are candidates for risk-reducing salpingo-oophorectomy (RRSO).

Genetic testing for inherited high-penetrance mutations in *BRCA1/2* and other genes should be discussed with women who have a significant family history of early onset breast cancer and/or cancers of the ovary, fallopian tube, or peritoneum. Involvement of a genetic counselor prior to testing is helpful, as they have expertise in managing the inherent clinical and social issues. Most *BRCA1/2* mutations involve base deletions or insertions in the coding sequence or splice sites that encode truncated protein products that are clearly dysfunctional. Less frequently, disease-causing mutations may occur that alter a single amino acid, though most of these missense variants represent innocent polymorphisms. The clinical significance of missense mutations can sometimes be elucidated by determining whether they segregate with cancer in other family members. In addition, genomic rearrangements may occur that inactivate *BRCA1* or *BRCA2*, and identification of such alterations requires molecular testing beyond sequencing.

Penetrance of ovarian cancer is not 100% in those with clearly deleterious *BRCA1/2* mutations, but presently it is not possible to provide more precise personalized risk estimates to guide the use of RRSO. However, common variants have been discovered in other genes that appear to affect the risk of ovarian cancer in *BRCA1/2* carriers.[38] Based on the known ovarian cancer risk–modifying loci, it has been reported that the 5% of *BRCA1* carriers at lowest risk have a lifetime risk of ≤28% of developing ovarian cancer, whereas the 5% at highest risk have a ≥63% lifetime risk. In the future, when modifier loci are more completely catalogued, more precise estimates of cancer risk may be provided to individual patients who are considering RRSO.

As about 20% of women with high-grade serous ovarian cancers have *BRCA1/2* mutations, it has been suggested that all of these women undergo genetic testing regardless of family history.[39] Mutational analysis in women with these cancers may increasingly become standard practice as the cost of genetic testing declines. Testing may also be driven by the availability of poly(ADP-ribose) polymerase inhibitor therapy for women whose cancers have germline or sporadic mutations in genes such as *BRCA1/2* and others that are involved in homologous recombination DNA repair.

RRSO is strongly recommended in women who carry *BRCA1/2* mutations because of the high mortality rate of ovarian cancer and the lack of effective screening and prevention approaches. Although screening with pelvic ultrasound and serum CA125 is generally recommended for *BRCA1/2* carriers during their 20s and 30s, it is not proven to reduce ovarian cancer mortality because even early stage high-grade cancers have a very high mortality. Oral contraceptives reduce the risk of ovarian cancer in the general population and appear to have a similar effect in *BRCA1/2* carriers, but this must be balanced against concerns regarding increased breast cancer risks.

The past practice of performing RRSO based solely on family history has been replaced by reliance on genetic testing. Clinical management of women with a strong family history in whom a deleterious germline mutation is not found, or those with variants of uncertain significance, should be resolved on a case-by-case basis. RRSO may be deemed appropriate in some cases, despite the absence of a clearly deleterious mutation. Fortunately, the risk of hereditary ovarian cancer does not rise dramatically until the mid-30s in women with *BRCA1* mutations and the 40s for women with *BRCA2* mutations.[36] As a result, most women are able to complete childbearing prior to undergoing RRSO. It is advisable for *BRCA1* carriers to undergo RRSO around age 35, as there is a 4% risk of ovarian cancer being discovered clinically or at the time of RRSO by age 40.[10] *BRCA2* carriers may choose to delay surgery into their 40s due to their lower risk of ovarian cancer, but this could diminish the protection against breast cancer that is afforded by RRSO. If a mutation carrier, particularly a *BRCA1* carrier, chooses to pursue fertility into her 40s, then she should be counseled that she is at considerable risk of developing a life-threatening cancer that is largely preventable.

Several studies have provided evidence of the efficacy of RRSO. In one early study of *BRCA1/2* carriers, RRSO reduced the rate of breast and ovarian cancer by 75% over several years of follow-up.[40] A separate study in 2002 examined outcome in 551 *BRCA1/2* carriers from various registries.[41] Among 259 women who had undergone RRSO, 6 (2.3%) were found to have stage I ovarian cancer at the time of the procedure and 2 (0.8%) subsequently developed serous peritoneal carcinoma. Among the controls, 58 (20%) women developed ovarian cancer after a mean follow-up of 8.8 years. With the exclusion of the six women whose cancers were diagnosed at surgery, RRSO reduced ovarian cancer risk by 96%. More recently, in 2014, an international registry study of over 5,783 subjects with median follow-up of 5.6 years found that RRSO reduced ovarian, tubal, and peritoneal cancer risk by 80%.[36] There was an estimated lifetime risk of primary peritoneal cancer after RRSO of about 4% for *BRCA1* carriers and 2% for *BRCA2* carriers.[36] The risk of death from all causes was reduced by 77%. A prospective cohort study noted that RRSO was associated with reduction in breast cancer–specific (hazard ratio [HR] = 0.44; 95% confidence interval [CI] = 0.26 to 0.76), ovarian cancer–specific (HR = 0.21; 95% CI = 0.06 to 0.80), and all-cause mortality (HR = 0.40; 95% CI = 0.26 to 0.61).[10]

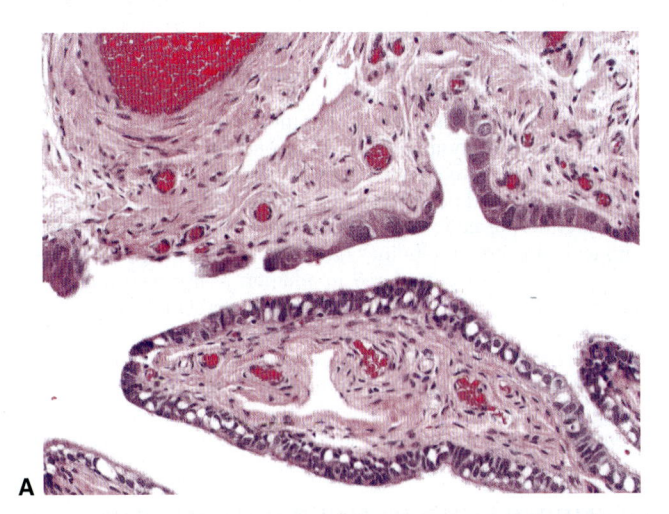

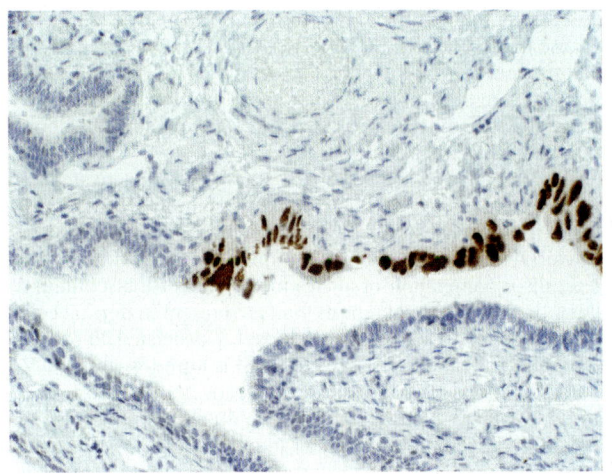

Figure 32.3 Hematoxylin and eosin (A) and immunohistochemical staining (B) demonstrating overexpression of mutant *TP53* in serous carcinoma in situ of the fallopian tube from a *BRCA1* mutation carrier who underwent risk-reducing bilateral salpingo-oophorectomy.

Removal of the ovaries, as internal organs, usually has little effect on body image and self-esteem, and most *BRCA1/2* mutation carriers elect to undergo RRSO. Insurance payers will almost always pay for RRSO in proven mutation carriers.

RRSO can be performed laparoscopically in most women, with discharge to home the same day. If a laparoscopic approach is problematic due to obesity or adhesions, the surgery can be performed through a small lower abdominal incision. Morbidity including bleeding, infection, and damage to the urinary or gastrointestinal tracts can occur, but the incidence of serious complications is very low. As the fallopian tubes and ovaries are small discrete organs, they are relatively easy to remove completely. Attention should be paid to transecting the ovarian artery and vein proximal to the ovary and tube so that remnants are not left behind. This involves opening the pelvic sidewall peritoneum, visualizing the ureter, and then isolating the ovarian blood supply. If there are adhesions between the adnexa and adjacent structures, careful dissection should be performed to ensure complete removal of the ovaries and fallopian tubes. If the uterus is not removed, care should be taken to remove the entire fallopian tube. A small portion of the tube inevitably will be left in the cornu of the uterus, but the risk of fallopian tube cancer developing in such remnants appears to be negligible.

Though there is not strong evidence that *BRCA1/2* mutations increase uterine cancer risk, many women elect to have the uterus removed as part of the surgical procedure because they have completed their family or have other gynecologic indications. Although the addition of a hysterectomy may increase operative time, blood loss, surgical complications, and hospital stay, it usually can be performed laparoscopically and serious adverse outcomes are infrequent. Furthermore, the likelihood of future exposure to tamoxifen in the context of breast cancer prevention or treatment, which increases endometrial cancer risk two- to three-fold, also argues for concomitant hysterectomy. Women who receive hormone replacement therapy after surgery will require a progestin along with estrogen to protect against the development of endometrial cancer if the uterus is not removed.

In younger women, surgical menopause after RRSO is associated with vasomotor symptoms, vaginal atrophy, decreased libido, and an accelerated onset and incidence of osteoporosis and cardiovascular disease. In premenopausal women who do not have a personal history of breast cancer, estrogen replacement can be administered to ameliorate many of the deleterious effects of premature menopause. Systemic estrogen levels are lower in oophorectomized premenopausal women taking hormone replacement than if the ovaries had been left in place. The therapeutic benefit of oophorectomy in women with breast cancer has long been appreciated, and more recent studies support the contention that RRSO reduces the risk of breast cancer by about half in *BRCA1/2* carriers.[42] However, a meta-analysis showed that while RRSO was strongly protective against estrogen receptor–positive breast cancer (HR = 0.22), there was no protection against estrogen receptor–negative breast cancer.[42] Many cancers are identified after developing early onset breast cancer, and this group represents the most difficult in which to balance the potential risks and benefits of estrogen replacement therapy.

Early stage high-grade serous cancers and in situ lesions with *TP53* mutations have been identified in the fallopian tubes of some RRSO specimens (Fig. 32.3). This has led to a paradigm shift in which it is now thought that most high-grade serous cancers found in the ovary, fallopian tube, and peritoneum are derived from cells that originate in the tubal fimbria.[43] The frequency of occult malignancies has varied between reports, but appears to be about 3%.[43] In view of this, the pelvis and peritoneal cavity should be examined carefully. Malignant cells also have been found in peritoneal cytologic specimens, and washings of the pelvis should be obtained when performing RRSO. The pathologist should be informed of the indication for surgery and serial sections of the fallopian tubes should be performed to look for the presence of early lesions. Patients found to have occult invasive high-grade serous cancers should be treated with chemotherapy after surgery. Those with in situ lesions appear to have a good outcome without chemotherapy.[44]

Cases of peritoneal serous carcinoma indistinguishable from ovarian cancer have been observed years after RRSO, but the origin of these cancers is unclear. Some may represent recurrences of occult ovarian or tubal cancers. In this regard, retrospective examination of the ovaries and fallopian tubes sometimes has revealed primary cancers that were not originally recognized. In contrast, some of these cancers likely arise directly from fallopian tube cells that have implanted in the peritoneum and subsequently become malignant. Patients who undergo RRSO should be made aware of their residual risk of peritoneal cancer, but there is no evidence that continued surveillance using CA125 and/or ultrasound is beneficial.

HEREDITARY ENDOMETRIAL CANCER (LYNCH SYNDROME)

Although Lynch syndrome (LS, also known as hereditary nonpolyposis CRC syndrome) typically manifests as familial clustering of early onset CRC, there is also an increased incidence of several other types of cancers—most notably endometrial cancer in women.[45] About 3% of endometrial cancers are attributable to inherited mutations in the DNA mismatch repair (MMR) genes that cause LS. Most often, *MSH2* and *MLH1* are implicated, but mutations in *MSH6* and *PMS2* also occur.[45] The risk of ovarian cancer is also significantly increased in LS, but to a lesser degree than in *BRCA1/2* mutation carriers, and accounts for only about 1% of all ovarian cancers.

Cells in which one of the LS genes have been inactivated exhibit a phenomenon called microsatellite instability (MSI).[46] This occurs as DNA mismatches cause shortening or lengthening of repetitive DNA sequences and these mismatches go unrepaired. This results in generation of alleles in the cancer that contain a greater or lesser number of repeats than are present in normal cells from that individual. MSI occurs in most LS-associated colorectal and endometrial cancers.[46] However, MSI is found in about 20% of sporadic cancers that arise in these organs, and in most cases is caused by silencing of the *MLH1* gene due to promoter hypermethylation. Screening strategies for identification of MMR gene alterations in families with LS-associated cancers include analysis of tumor tissue for MSI and/or loss of DNA MMR gene expression using immunohistochemistry (IHC).[46] In cancers with MSI or loss of expression of one of the MMR genes, or in families with pedigrees suggestive of LS, these genes can be sequenced to identify disease-causing mutations, most of which cause truncated protein products.[47] Although it has been suggested that it may be cost-effective to do these tests on all endometrial cancers, this approach has not been widely adopted.[47]

The risk of a woman who carries a LS mutation developing endometrial cancer ranges from 20% to 60% in various reports.[45,48] The risk of ovarian cancer is increased to about 5% to 12%. Whereas the mean age of women with sporadic endometrial cancers is in the early 60s, cancers that arise in association with LS are often diagnosed before menopause, with the average age in the 40s. The clinical features of these endometrial cancers are similar to those of most sporadic cases (well-differentiated, endometrioid histology, early stage), and survival is about 90%. The mean age of onset of ovarian cancer in LS is in the early 40s, and the clinical features of these cancers are generally more favorable than in sporadic cases. They usually are identified at an early stage, are well- or moderately differentiated, have favorable survival, and some occur in the setting of a synchronous endometrial cancer.

Recommendations for screening and risk-reducing surgery in LS are better established for CRC than for extracolonic malignancies.[49] Transvaginal ultrasound has been proposed as a screening test for endometrial cancer (and ovarian cancer), but its efficacy is unproven.[50] Endometrial biopsy is the most sensitive means of diagnosing endometrial cancer, and it has been suggested that this should be employed periodically beginning around age 30 to 35. However, there are no published studies demonstrating that this approach prevents endometrial cancer deaths compared to simply performing a biopsy if abnormal uterine bleeding occurs.

Most experts believe that risk-reducing hysterectomy has a role in the management of some women with LS because of the high incidence of endometrial cancer. The risk of endometrial cancer is low during the prime reproductive years, and the uterus does not serve a vital function once childbearing has been completed. In view of the increased risk of ovarian cancer in LS, concomitant bilateral salpingo-oophorectomy should also be considered. One study demonstrated that there were no cases of endometrial or ovarian cancer in 61 LS carriers who underwent risk-reducing hysterectomy and bilateral salpingo-oophorectomy, while endometrial cancer occurred in 33% and ovarian cancer in 5% who retained their uterus and ovaries.[51] Despite the low risk of death from gynecologic cancers in LS, cost-effectiveness analyses of various approaches suggest that risk-reducing hysterectomy and salpingo-oophorectomy leads to both the lowest cost and the greatest increase in quality-adjusted life-years.[52] Estrogen replacement after removal of the ovaries in premenopausal women with LS is not contraindicated, as there is no evidence that this adversely affects the incidence of other cancers.

Many women with LS elect to undergo risk-reducing colectomy, which provides an opportunity to perform concomitant hysterectomy. Hysterectomy in concert with colectomy, either via laparoscopy or laparotomy, does not greatly increase operative time or surgical complications. If an endometrial biopsy has not been performed preoperatively, an intraoperative inspection of the uterine cavity and possibly frozen section should be performed to exclude the presence of cancer. If cancer is found in the uterus, surgical staging—including sampling of the regional lymph nodes—should be considered in addition to hysterectomy.[53] It is also appropriate to discuss risk-reducing hysterectomy with LS carriers who do not elect to undergo prophylactic colectomy. The operative approach (vaginal versus laparotomy versus laparoscopy) can be determined based on the presence or absence of uterine pathology (e.g., myomas), whether the patient has had prior abdominal surgery, and whether the ovaries are also to be removed.

GYNECOLOGIC CANCER RISK IN VERY RARE HEREDITARY CANCER SYNDROMES

Several very rare hereditary cancer syndromes also increase the risk of gynecologic cancers, and some of these women could potentially benefit from risk-reducing surgery to remove the ovaries and/or uterus. Peutz-Jeghers syndrome is characterized by intestinal polyps and an increased risk of colorectal and breast cancers. This rare syndrome is due to inherited mutations in the *STK11* gene. Affected women also have an increased risk of ovarian sex cord-stromal tumors with annular tubules and adenoma malignum of the cervix. Li-Fraumeni syndrome is caused by inherited mutations in the *TP53* gene, and carriers are predisposed to a number of types of cancers including sarcomas and breast cancer. The risk of ovarian cancer is increased as well, but is not a major cause of cancer in these families. Cowden syndrome is due to germline *PTEN* mutations and increases the risk of several malignancies including breast, thyroid, mucocutaneous, and endometrial cancers. Finally, small cell carcinoma of the ovary, hypercalcemic type, is due to mutations in the *SMARCA4* gene. These highly lethal ovarian cancers occur at a very young age (median 24 years) and present difficult challenges related to timing of RRSO. There are no well-accepted evidence-based guidelines for early detection and prevention of gynecologic cancers in these very rare hereditary cancer syndromes. An awareness of the risk and natural history of gynecologic cancers in these families provides a basis for counseling individual patients.

MULTIPLE ENDOCRINE NEOPLASIA TYPE 2

Gene Carriers

The MEN type 2 syndromes include MEN 2A, MEN 2B, and familial (non-MEN) medullary thyroid carcinoma (FMTC).[54–56] These are autosomal dominant inherited syndromes caused by germline mutations in the *RET* proto-oncogene. Their hallmark is the development of multifocal bilateral medullary thyroid carcinoma (MTC) associated with C-cell hyperplasia. MTCs arise from the thyroid C-cells, also called parafollicular cells. C-cells secrete the hormone calcitonin, a specific tumor marker for MTC. A slow-growing tumor in most cases, MTC causes significant morbidity and death in patients with uncontrolled local or metastatic spread. Large tumor burden is associated with diarrhea and flushing. In the MEN 2 syndromes, there is almost complete penetrance of MTC. Other features are variably expressed, with incomplete penetrance (summarized in Table 32.2).

In MEN 2A, all patients develop MTC. Approximately 42% of affected patients also develop pheochromocytomas, associated with adrenal medullary hyperplasia. Hyperparathyroidism develops in

TABLE 32.2

Clinical Features of Sporadic Medullary Thyroid Carcinoma, Multiple Endocrine Neoplasia 2A, Multiple Endocrine Neoplasia 2B, and Familial Medullary Thyroid Carcinoma

Clinical Setting	Features of MTC	Inheritance Pattern	Associated Abnormalities	Genetic Defect
Sporadic MTC	Unifocal	None	None	Somatic RET mutations in >20% of tumors
MEN 2A	Multifocal, bilateral	Autosomal dominant	Pheochromocytomas, hyperparathyroidism, cutaneous lichen amyloidosis, Hirshprung's disease	Germline missense mutations in extracellular cysteine codons of RET
MEN 2B	Multifocal, bilateral	Autosomal dominant	Pheochromocytomas, mucosal neuromas, megacolon, skeletal abnormalities	Germline missense mutation in tyrosine kinase domain of RET
FMTC	Multifocal, bilateral	Autosomal dominant	None	Germline missense mutations in extracellular or intracellular cysteine codons of RET

MTC, medullary thyroid carcinoma; MEN, multiple endocrine neoplasia; FMTC, familial medullary thyroid carcinoma.

10% to 35%. Cutaneous lichen amyloidosis and Hirschsprung's disease are infrequently associated with MEN 2A.[57–60]

MEN 2B appears to be the most aggressive form of hereditary MTC. In MEN 2B, MTC develops in all patients at a very young age (infancy). All affected individuals develop neural gangliomas particularly in the mucosa of the digestive tract, conjunctiva, lips, and tongue; 40% to 50% develop pheochromocytomas. Patients with MEN 2B may also have megacolon, skeletal abnormalities, and markedly enlarged peripheral nerves. They do not develop hyperparathyroidism.

FMTC is characterized by development of MTC in the absence of any other endocrinopathies. MTC in these patients has a more indolent clinical course. Some individuals with FMTC may never manifest clinical evidence (i.e., symptoms or a lump in the neck), although biochemical testing and histologic evaluation of the thyroid demonstrates MTC.[55,56]

RET Genotype-Phenotype Correlations

Mutations in the RET proto-oncogene are responsible for MEN 2A, MEN 2B, and FMTC.[61–64] This gene encodes a transmembrane tyrosine kinase protein.[57,65] The mutations that cause the MEN 2 syndromes are activating gain-of-function mutations affecting constitutive activation of the protein. This is unusual among hereditary cancer syndromes, which are usually caused by loss-of-function mutations in the predisposition gene (e.g., familial polyposis, BRCA1 and 2, von Hippel-Lindau, and MEN 1). More than 30 missense mutations have been described in patients affected by the MEN 2 syndromes (Fig. 32.4).

There is a relationship between the type of inherited RET mutation and presentation of MTC. The most virulent form is seen in patients with MEN 2B. These patients most commonly have a germline mutation in codon 918 of RET (ATG->ACG), although other mutations have been described (codon 883 and 922). As noted previously, MTC in MEN 2B has an extremely early age of onset (infancy). Despite its distinctive clinical appearance and associated gastrointestinal difficulties, the disease is often not detected until the patient develops a neck mass. Metastatic spread is usually present at the time of initial treatment, and calcitonin levels often remain elevated postoperatively.

MTC has a variable course in patients with MEN 2A, similar to that of sporadic MTC. Codon 634 and 618 mutations are the most common RET mutations associated with MEN 2A, although mutations at other codons are also observed (see Fig. 32.4). Some patients do extremely well for many years, even with distant metastases, while others develop inanition, symptomatic liver, lung or skeletal metastases, as well as disabling diarrhea. Recurrence in the central neck, with invasion of the airway or great vessels, may cause death.

In patients with FMTC, MTC is usually indolent. These individuals most commonly have mutations of codons 609, 611, 618, 620, 768, 804, or 891, although mutations of other codons have been identified (see Fig. 32.4). Many patients with FMTC are cured by thyroidectomy alone, and even those with persistent elevation of calcitonin levels do well for many years. Occasionally, patients with FMTC survive into the seventh or eighth decade without clinical signs of disease, although pathologic examination of the thyroid will reveal MTC or C-cell hyperplasia.[66]

Risk-Reducing Thyroidectomy in RET Mutation Carriers

Genetic counseling and informed consent should be obtained prior to genetic testing. Specific issues that should be covered in genetic counseling sessions include explaining the patterns of heritability, likelihood of expression of different tumors, their prevention and treatment, insurability, nonpaternity, survivor guilt, and others.

It has been shown that RET mutation carriers may harbor foci of MTC in the thyroid gland, even when calcitonin levels are normal.[67] While the age of onset and rate of disease progression may differ, the lifetime penetrance of MTC is near 100% in carriers of RET mutations associated with MEN 2 syndromes. At-risk individuals who are found to have inherited a RET gene mutation are therefore candidates for thyroidectomy, regardless of their plasma calcitonin levels.

The best option for prevention of MTC in RET mutation carriers is complete surgical resection prior to malignant transformation. Prophylactic thyroidectomy prior to the development of MTC is the goal in these patients. A number of studies have demonstrated improved biochemical cure rates and/or decreased recurrence rates from early thyroidectomy, performed after positive screening by calcitonin testing or RET mutation testing.[68–70]

MEN 2B mutations are the highest risk level, designated level III (see Fig. 32.4).[55,71] Patients with MEN 2B have the most aggressive form of MTC, with invasive disease reported in patients <1 year of age. These patients should have preventative surgery

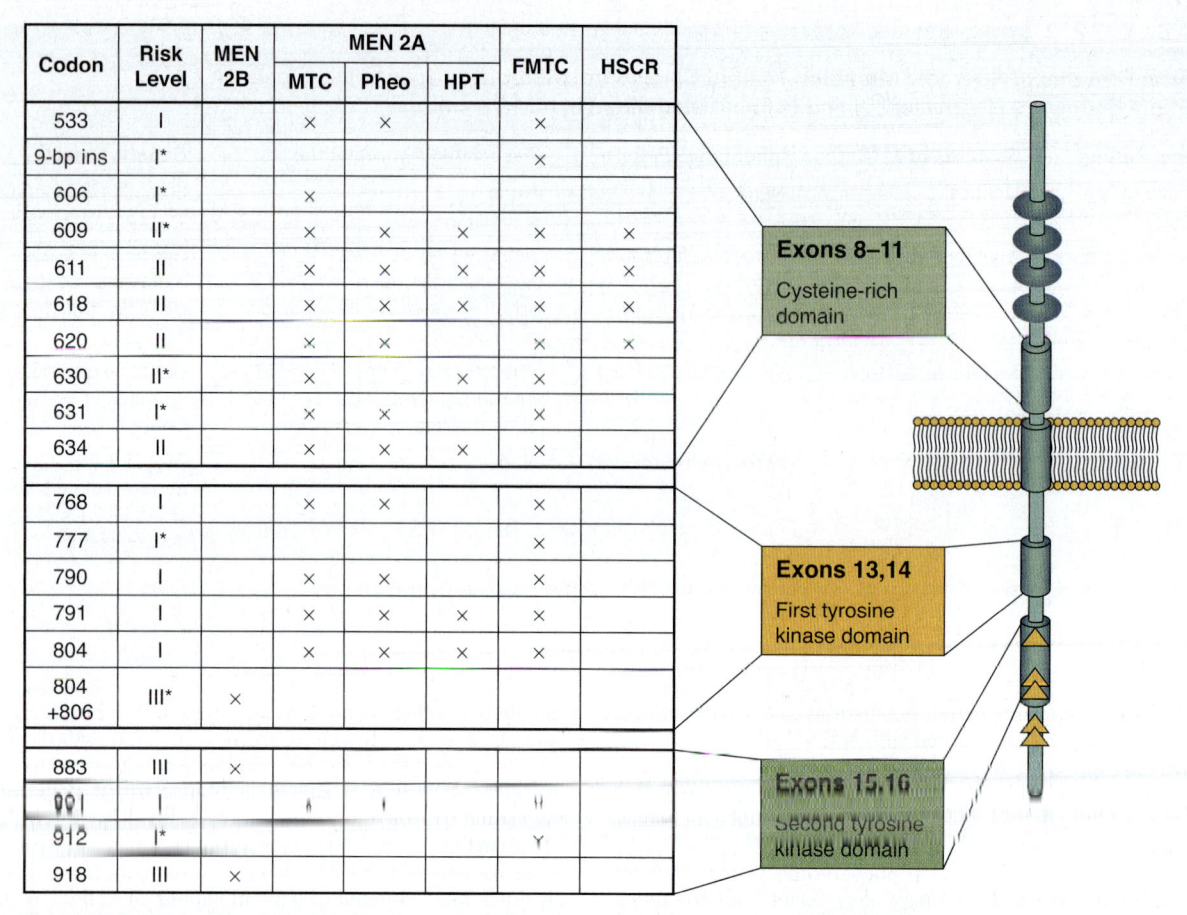

Codon	Risk Level	MEN 2B	MEN 2A MTC	MEN 2A Pheo	MEN 2A HPT	FMTC	HSCR
533	I		×	×		×	
9-bp ins	I*					×	
606	I*		×				
609	II*		×	×	×	×	×
611	II		×	×	×	×	×
618	II		×	×	×	×	×
620	II		×	×		×	×
630	II*		×		×	×	
631	I*		×	×		×	
634	II		×	×	×	×	
768	I		×			×	
777	I*					×	
790	I		×	×		×	
791	I		×	×	×	×	
804	I		×	×	×	×	
804 +806	III*	×					
883	III	×					
891	I		×			×	
912	I*					×	
918	III	×					

Figure 32.4 *RET* mutation sites associated with multiple endocrine neoplasia (MEN) 2 syndromes. Codons previously reported in association with MEN-2 syndromes are listed by structural domain within the RET protein. Risk level is based on consensus guidelines or more recent clinical reports. Previously reported phenotypes for each codon are shown. MTC, medullary thyroid carcinoma; Pheo, pheochromocytoma; HPT, hyperparathyroidism; FMTC, familial medullary thyroid carcinoma; HSCR, Hirschsprung's disease. *Asterisk* indicates risk level based on recent clinical reports not available at publication of the consensus guidelines. (From Traugott AL, Moley JF. The RET protooncogene. *Cancer Treat Res* 2010;153:303–319.)

Exons 8–11: Cysteine-rich domain

Exons 13,14: First tyrosine kinase domain

Exons 15,16: Second tyrosine kinase domain

early in the first year of life, if possible. Identification and preservation of parathyroid glands can be extremely difficult in these infants, due to their small size, translucent appearance, and the presence of exuberant thymic and perithyroidal nodal tissue. These procedures should be performed by surgeons experienced in parathyroid and/or pediatric thyroid operations.

Patients with MEN 2A with mutations in codons 634, 620, 618, and 611 are also considered high risk (level II).[55,71] Patients with level II mutations should undergo a total thyroidectomy at 5 to 6 years of age. There is evidence that the risk of lymph node metastasis is very low in patients with MEN 2A under the age of 8, with normal calcitonin levels. Central lymph node dissection is associated with higher risk of hypoparathyroidism, and recurrent laryngeal nerve injury and should be reserved for patients with elevated calcitonin levels.

A larger subset of *RET* mutations, associated with MEN 2A and/or FMTC, is considered the lowest risk (level I).[55,71] These include mutations at codons 768, 790, 791, 804, and 891. For patients with low-risk level I mutations, total thyroidectomy is recommended before age 5 to 10 years. This decision, however, regarding ideal age at preventative thyroidectomy in low-risk mutation carriers, is currently being reviewed, and may be driven by additional clinical data such as the basal or stimulated serum calcitonin level.[72,73] There are no guidelines at present that address the issue of timing of surgery based on calcitonin level, and at present, pentagastrin (the primary calcitonin secretagogue used in testing) is not available in the United States. It is anticipated that within a decade, there will

be enough published data to direct timing of interventions based upon this information. As with the level II mutations, the need for central lymph node dissection should be guided by calcitonin levels and clinical features of the patient and kindred.

Until recently, some groups recommended total thyroidectomy with central neck lymph node dissection and total parathyroidectomy with autotransplantation for all *RET* mutation carriers. Recent studies and personal experience, however, have demonstrated an extremely low likelihood of nodal metastases in patients with MEN 2A or FMTC younger than 8 years of age, and in patients with a normal calcitonin level.[70] Our current strategy is to leave the parathyroid in situ in these patients, if possible.[74] Often, however, the desired complete removal of thyroid tissue results in compromise of parathyroid blood supply. In these situations, autotransplantation of devascularized parathyroid is required. We routinely remove and autotransplant the parathyroid if a central node dissection is done. In parathyroid autotransplantation, parathyroid glands are sliced into 1 mm × 3 mm fragments and autotransplanted into individual muscle pockets in the muscle of the nondominant forearm in patients with MEN 2A, or in the sternocleidomastoid muscle in patients with FMTC or MEN 2B. Patients are maintained on calcium and vitamin D supplementation for 4 to 6 weeks postoperatively.

In a recent series of thyroidectomies performed in 50 individuals with MEN 2A (identified by genetic screening), total thyroidectomy and central node dissection with parathyroidectomy and parathyroid autografting were performed in all patients (Fig. 32.5).[70]

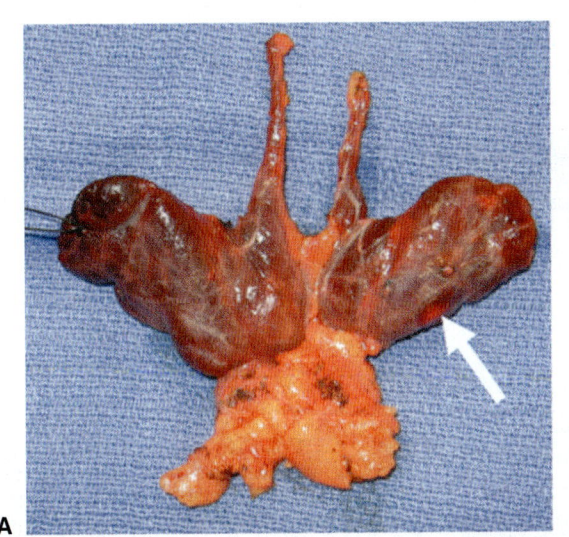

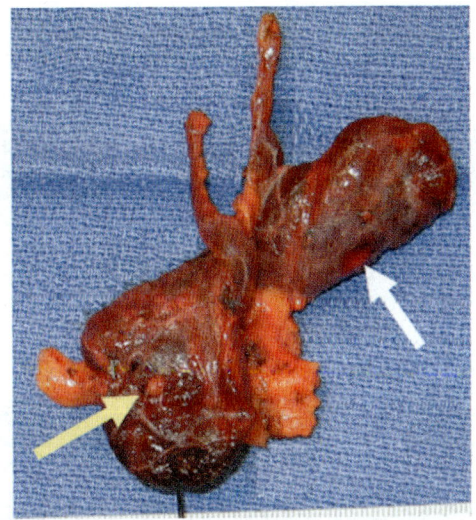

Figure 32.5 Total thyroidectomy specimen with attached central nodes from a patient with germline *RET* mutation and elevated calcitonin levels. Note small visible foci of medullary thyroid carcinoma (*arrows*).

All autografts functioned, but three patients required supplemental calcium. The percentage of individuals requiring calcium supplementation following parathyroidectomy with parathyroid autografting reportedly ranges from 0% to 18%. Parathyroidectomy should be performed in all patients showing gross parathyroid enlargement or biochemical evidence of parathyroid disease at time of surgery. The operating surgeon should have expertise in preservation of parathyroid function. It is important that the surgeon performing an operative procedure for MTC be familiar with the techniques described here. If not, the patient should be referred to a center where these procedures are routinely performed.

Some patients with MEN 2 will be found to have elevated calcitonin levels prior to thyroidectomy. This is usually associated with medullary thyroid carcinoma or C-cell hyperplasia in the gland, and may be associated with lymph node metastases. Much has been written about the correlation between preoperative calcitonin levels and extent of nodal involvement. It has been suggested that preoperative calcitonin level may guide the extent of node dissection. In a study of 300 European patients with MTC, node metastases were not identified when the preoperative basal calcitonin level was <20 pg/ml.[75] Involvement of nodal groups was correlated with basal calcitonin level as follows: ipsilateral central and lateral neck nodes (basal calcitonin >20 pg/ml), contralateral central nodes (basal calcitonin >50 pg/ml), contralateral lateral neck nodes (basal calcitonin >200 pg/ml), and mediastinal nodes (basal calcitonin >500 pg/ml). Based upon these findings, this group (who also wrote the European guidelines) recommends thyroidectomy only if basal calcitonin is <20 pg/ml, ipsilateral central and lateral neck dissection if the calcitonin is 20 to 50 pg/ml, and contralateral central neck dissection if the basal calcitonin is 50 to 200 pg/ml, with the addition of contralateral lateral neck dissection if the calcitonin is 200 to 500 pg/ml. Most experts agree that sternotomy with mediastinal neck dissection should be reserved for patients with image evidence of mediastinal disease. In contrast, most North American surgeons rely heavily upon preoperative ultrasound imaging to map the extent of nodal involvement and determine extent of surgery based upon calcitonin and imaging results.[55,74,76]

Follow-up

Following thyroidectomy, thyroid hormone replacement is required for life. Patients may need several weeks of oral calcium and vitamin D until parathyroid function recovers. Intermittent calcitonin testing may be done to monitor for persistent or recurrent MTC. The importance of regular monitoring of patients' compliance with thyroid medication following thyroidectomy should not be underestimated. Children and teenagers are frequently noncompliant, and this can be determined by routine measurement of thyroid-stimulating hormone levels. Continued noncompliance can result in growth problems. Occasionally, local human services agencies may need to be involved in particularly difficult cases.

The term "biochemical cure" is used to refer to patients with normal calcitonin levels after surgery for MTC. Complete postoperative normalization of calcitonin has been associated with decreased long-term risk of MTC recurrence, though the evidence is less clear for a survival benefit. A persistent or recurrent elevation in calcitonin indicates residual or recurrent MTC and warrants additional investigation by imaging. However, as most MTC has a fairly indolent course, patients with biochemical evidence of recurrent disease may not have corollary imaging findings for some time.

Conclusions

Identification of *RET* gene mutations in individuals at risk for developing hereditary forms of MTC has simplified management, expanding the scope of indications for surgical intervention. Patients who carry this mutation can be offered operative treatment at a very young age, hopefully before the cancer has developed or spread, and those identified as not having the mutation are spared further genetic and biochemical screening. This achievement marks a new paradigm in surgery: the indication that an operation be performed based on the results of a genetic test. As in the decision to perform any surgical procedure, meticulous preparation and detailed discussion with patient and family must precede the final recommendation. It is also important that the patient and family be involved in preoperative discussions with genetic counselors. Postoperative follow-up for compliance with thyroid medication is important, especially in children and teenagers who are still growing and developing into adults.

FAMILIAL ADENOMATOUS POLYPOSIS, *MYH*-ASSOCIATED POLUPOSIS, AND LYNCH SYNDROME

Inherited CRC syndromes with multiple adenomatous polyps include FAP, *MYH*-associated polyposis (MAP), and LS. In some cases, the diagnosis is suspected because of a striking family history

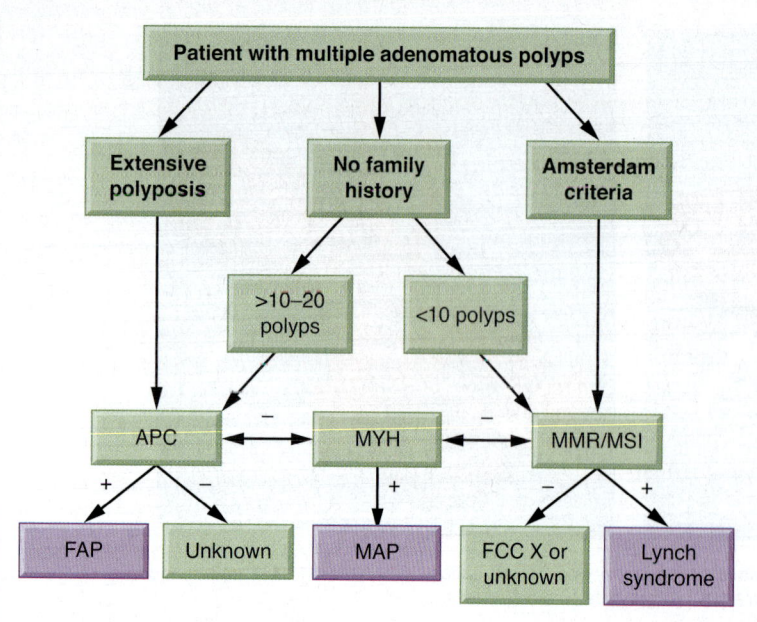

Figure 32.6 Schematic demonstrating the potential genetic workup for a patient with multiple adenomatous colorectal polyps and suspected of having an inherited colorectal cancer syndrome. APC, adenomatous polyposis coli; MMR, mismatch repair; MSI, microsatellite instability; FAP, familial adenomatous polyposis; MAP, MYH-associated polyposis; FCC X, familial colorectal cancer syndrome X.

of CRC, while in others, suspicion arises from a very young onset of CRC or florid polyposis.

Although adenomatous polyp burden and family history may suggest one syndrome over another, an initial negative genetic test result should be followed by further evaluation for other syndromes. For example, in clinical practice, a negative adenomatous polyposis coli (APC) gene test in a patient with a suspected CRC syndrome is followed by reflex testing for MAP and LS, as shown in Figure 32.6.

FAP is an autosomal dominant syndrome that accounts for <1% of the annual CRC burden, is caused by mutations in the tumor-suppressor APC gene. It is characterized by the presence of ≥100 adenomatous polyps in the colorectum, nearly 100% penetrance, and an inevitable risk of CRC if prophylactic colectomy is not performed.[8,77] Patients with a less severe form known as attenuated FAP (AFAP) usually present with <100 colorectal adenomas that tend to be proximally located. MAP is an autosomal recessive syndrome that often presents phenotypically as attenuated polyposis. While an estimated 2% of the general population are monoallelic carriers of a mutated base-excision-repair MUTYH (MYH) gene, biallelic germline mutations may account for 9% to 18% of patients with FAP or AFAP phenotypes who have no demonstrable APC mutation.[78–80]

LS accounts for 1% to 4% of all newly diagnosed CRC and is attributable to a germline mutation in one of the DNA MMR genes (MLH1, MSH2, MSH6, and PMS2).[81–83] Epigenetic silencing of the MSH2 gene via a 3′-end deletion in EPCAM (TACSTD1), a neighbor of MSH2 that plays a role in cell adhesion, also accounts for 20% to 25% of all suspected MSH2 cases and 1% to 6% of LS cases overall.[84–86] LS is characterized by early age-of-onset CRC, predominance of lesions proximal to the splenic flexure, an increased rate of metachronous CRC, and a unique spectrum of benign and malignant extracolonic tumors. Lifetime risk of CRC in patients with LS may be as high as 80%.[83,87] MSI reflects a deficiency in DNA repair secondary to MMR gene mutation and is a hallmark feature of LS-associated tumors.

Variability in penetrance, phenotypic expression, and certainty of disease development mandate distinctly different surgical approaches in these three syndromes, including the type and timing of risk-reducing colon and rectal surgery.[88]

Familial Adenomatous Polyposis

Surveillance of at-risk family members should begin around age 10 to 15 years with an annual colonoscopy or flexible sigmoidoscopy.[89] At-risk individuals who belong to families with an AFAP phenotype should undergo colonoscopic screening every 2 to 3 years starting in their late teens. Informative genetic testing is possible in families with a demonstrated APC mutation, and mutations are detected in most pedigrees. However, approximately 25% of patients with FAP will have a de novo APC mutation.[8] Severity of polyposis should be established during colonoscopy, as the timing of surgery and the risk of developing colorectal is dependent on the extent of polyp burden. Patients with mild polyposis and a correspondingly lower CRC risk can undergo surgery in their late teens. Patients with severe polyposis, a high degree of dysplasia, multiple adenomas >5 mm in size, and symptoms (bleeding, persistent diarrhea, anemia, failure to thrive, psychosocial stress, etc.) should undergo risk-reducing colorectal surgery as soon as is practical after diagnosis.[90,91] However, in carefully selected, fully asymptomatic patients who have small adenomas but a strong family history of aggressive abdominal desmoid disease, consideration can be given to delaying prophylactic colectomy, as the risk of desmoid-related complication may be greater than the risk of CRC development.

The three current surgical options for patients with FAP are total proctocolectomy (TPC) with permanent ileostomy, total colectomy with ileorectal anastomosis (IRA), and proctocolectomy with ileal pouch-anal anastomosis (IPAA). IPAA can be a double-stapled, end-of-pouch-to-anus anastomosis, which may leave behind approximately 1 cm of anal transition zone. An alternative approach, which is preferred when there is carpeting of the anal transition zone with adenomas, is to perform a mucosal stripping of the anal transition zone down to the dentate line followed by a hand-sewn per anal anastomosis of pouch to the dentate line. Selection of the optimal procedure for an individual patient is based on several factors, including characteristics of the FAP syndrome within the patient and family, differences in likely postoperative functional outcome, preoperative anal sphincter status, and patient preference.[8]

TPC with permanent ileostomy, although rarely chosen as a primary procedure, is used in patients with invasive cancer involving the sphincters or levator complex, or patients for whom an IPAA is not technically feasible (secondary to desmoid disease and foreshortening of the small bowel mesentery, making it surgically impossible to bring the ileal pouch to the anus) nor likely to lead to good function such as massive obesity or weak anal sphincters. However, TPC is occasionally chosen as a primary procedure by patients who perceive that their lifestyle would be compromised by the frequent bowel movements (five to six per day) sometimes associated with the IPAA procedure.

In addition to these issues, the key in deciding between an IPAA and an IRA is based primarily on the risk of rectal cancer development if the rectum is left in situ. The risk of rectal cancer following IRA may range from 3% to 10% at 10 years, while the risk for a secondary proctectomy for uncontrolled rectal polyposis ranges from 10% to 61% at 20 years following initial colectomy with IRA.[92–94] The magnitude of risk in an individual patient is, however, related to the overall extent of colorectal polyposis. IRA may be considered for patients with <1,000 colorectal polyps (including those with attenuated FAP) and <20 rectal adenomas, as these individuals have a relatively low risk of developing rectal cancer.[88,93] Patients with severe rectal (>20 adenomas) or colonic (>1,000 adenomas) polyposis, an adenoma >3 cm, or an adenoma with severe dysplasia should ideally undergo a risk reducing procedure that will include a proctectomy.[90,91,93]

The risk of secondary rectal excision, due to uncontrollable rectal polyposis or rectal cancer, may be estimated by identifying the specific location of the causative *APC* mutation. Patients with mutations located between codons 1250 and 1464 have been shown to have a six-fold increased risk of developing rectal cancer, compared to those with mutations prior to codon 1250 or after codon 1464 (mean number of rectal polyps 42 versus 22, respectively).[8,92] Although the use of the genotype-phenotype relationship to guide patient management may be appealing,[92] it is important to recognize the variability of phenotypic expression that exists even among members of the same family. This suggests that at the current time, the choice between an IRA and an IPAA should be based primarily on clinical (rather than genetic) grounds.[90]

The risk of polyp and cancer development following primary surgery is not limited to patients undergoing IRA. In patients undergoing IPAA, neoplasia may occur at the site of ileal pouch anastomosis; the frequency appears to be greater after stapled anastomosis (28% to 31%) than after mucosectomy and hand-sewn anastomosis (10% to 14%).[95] In the case of neoplasia developing at the anal transition zone after a stapled anastomosis, transanal mucosectomy may be performed, followed by advancement of the pouch to the dentate line. Of additional concern is the development of adenomatous polyps in the ileal pouch, which occurs in approximately 45% of patients by 10-year follow-up.[96] Consequently, depending on polyp burden, lifetime endoscopic surveillance of the rectal remnant (after IRA) every 6 to 12 months or the ileal pouch (after IPAA) every 1 to 3 years is required following either procedure.[89]

Another important consideration in choosing between IPAA and IRA is postoperative bowel function and quality of life. Some studies have associated IPAA with higher frequency of both daytime and nocturnal bowel movements, higher incidence of passive incontinence and incidental soiling, and greater postoperative morbidity.[97] However, long-term follow-up demonstrates a comparable quality of life following IPAA for FAP relative to the patient's preoperative baseline.[98] Therefore, although the choice of procedure must be carefully individualized, because of the risk of rectal cancer associated with IRA, the authors favor IPAA for most patients with FAP whenever feasible. However, an IRA should be considered in specific circumstances, such as when there is mild rectal polyposis (as in AFAP), or a young patient with rectal sparing who is not interested in undergoing the multiple procedures that accompany an IPAA and diverting loop ileostomy, or a young woman interested in having children and trying to avoid the decreased fecundity associated with an IPAA procedure.[99] The use of minimally invasive techniques such as laparoscopy may reduce the risk of infertility associated with IPAA.[100,101] Though a diverting loop ileostomy should be performed in all IPAA procedures, it is not always feasible due to a number of anatomic factors such as body habitus.

Endoscopic surveillance of the rectal segment at 6- to 12-month intervals after the index surgery is recommended, with subsequent surveillance frequencies dependent on the number and size of adenomas observed.[89] Although small (<5 mm) scattered adenomas can be safely observed or removed with biopsy forceps, polyps >5 mm should be removed by snare. However, repeated fulguration and polypectomy over many years can lead to difficulty with subsequent polypectomy, reduced rectal compliance, and difficulty identifying flat cancers in the background of scar tissue. The development of severe dysplasia and/or villous adenomas not amenable to endoscopic removal is indication for proctectomy.

Long-Term Considerations from Extracolonic Manifestations

Despite the reduced risk of CRC-related death following prophylactic colectomy, patients with FAP are still at increased risk of mortality from both rectal cancer and other causes relative to the general population. The three main causes of death following IRA are progression of desmoid disease, stomach and duodenal cancer, and perioperative mortality. Additional FAP-related extraintestinal manifestations include epidermoid cysts, supernumerary teeth, osteomas of the jaw and/or skull, congenital hypertrophy of the retinal pigment epithelium, cancers of the hepatopancreatobiliary tract and genitourinary tract, and thyroid cancer.[102–104]

Desmoids

Desmoids may occur in 10% to 25% of patients with FAP.[105,106] Unlike those found in the general population, FAP-associated desmoids tend to be intra-abdominal and arise following abdominal surgery.[106,107] Although conflicting reports exist, it appears that female patients, those with extracolonic manifestations of FAP, a positive family history of desmoids, and *APC* mutations located at 3' of codon 1440 are at increased risk of developing desmoids.[106,108,109] These tumors often involve the small bowel mesentery as well as the retroperitoneum and are often life-threatening due to invasion or compression of adjacent viscera. Further, recurrence and morbidity rates are high following attempted resection, with recurrent disease often more aggressive than the initial desmoid. Estimated 5-year overall survival for patients with intra-abdominal desmoids causing severe symptoms such as significant pain and septic fistula/abscess, diameter >20 cm or rapidly growing, and/or need for parenteral nutrition is only 53%.[107] Therefore, desmoid resection is evaluated on an individualized case-by-case basis with surgery reserved for highly select cases.

Desmoids that involve the small bowel mesentery may preclude the formation of an IPAA secondary to foreshortening of the small bowel mesentery, especially in patients undergoing proctectomy after an initial IRA.[110] Surgery for intra-abdominal and abdominal wall desmoids should be reserved for limited disease where the likelihood of clear margins is high.

In symptomatic cases where resection of an intra-abdominal desmoid may not be feasible, intestinal bypass or ureteral stenting may be necessary to alleviate bowel or urinary obstruction secondary to mass effect. In addition to surgical intervention, several medical options with variable efficacy are available for the management of desmoid disease and include nonsteroidal anti-inflammatory drugs (e.g., sulindac), selective estrogen receptor modulators (e.g., tamoxifen), immunomodulators (e.g., imatinib, sorafenib, interferon), doxorubin-based cytotoxic chemotherapy, and radiation.

MYH-Associated Polyposis

MAP should be suspected in patients with >10 colorectal adenomas, a weak history of CRC, and no family history of FAP. The diagnosis is confirmed by *MUTYH* (*MYH*) gene testing.[80,88]

Depending on the polyp burden, the management of the colon and rectum of a patient with a biallelic *MYH* mutation can be endoscopic or surgical. If the polyp burden is limited and an endoscopic approach is pursued, colonoscopy should be performed every 1 to 3 years.[87,89] If the polyp burden is not amenable to an endoscopic approach at the time of diagnosis, then a resection is indicated. In most cases in which surgery is deemed necessary, an IRA is sufficient. However, if rectal polyposis is severe, an IPAA may be indicated. Indications for surgery following an endoscopic surveillance program include increasing polyp size or number, or worsening histology.

Extracolonic manifestations of MAP are similar to FAP and include osteomas, desmoids, congenital hypertrophy of the retinal pigment epithelium, as well as cancers of the thyroid, ovary, bladder, sebaceous gland, and breast. In addition, patients with MAP are also at a 4% lifetime risk of developing duodenal cancer and require upper endoscopies every 1 to 3 years beginning as early as ages 18 to 20 years and starting no later than ages 30 to 35 years.[87,89,111]

Lynch Syndrome

Due to the discordance associated with the term hereditary nonpolyposis colorectal cancer, the use of this term has largely been abandoned with reversion back to the eponym LS, which refers to individuals with a predisposition to CRC and other malignancies as a result of a germline MMR mutation.[112] Overall, CRC occurs in up to 80% of patients with LS by their mid-40s.[8,82] Endometrial cancer occurs in 40% to 60%, gastric cancer in 11% to 19%, urinary tract cancer in 5% to 18%, and ovarian cancer in 9% to 15% of affected individuals.[8,82,87]

The Amsterdam criteria and revised Bethesda guidelines[113] (Table 32.3) are used in clinical practice to identify patients at risk for LS who require further genetic evaluation. The Amsterdam criteria, which led to the identification of the LS-causing MMR gene mutations require that there be:

- Three relatives (one a first-degree relative of the other two) with colorectal, endometrial, stomach, ovary, small bowel, ureteral/renal pelvis, brain, hepatobiliary, and/or sebaceous cancer;
- In two or more successive generations;
- With at least one case of cancer diagnosed before the age of 50;
- And that FAP as a diagnosis is excluded.[114]

Though the Amsterdam criteria can be used clinically to identify potential patients with LS, using it alone will result in identification of only 42% of LS mutation carriers.[115] Families meeting Amsterdam criteria but lacking an MMR mutation are referred to as having "familial colorectal cancer type X" and appear to have a lower incidence of colorectal and extracolonic cancers than those with a LS germline MMR mutation (see Fig. 32.6). Of note, they have an increased incidence of left-sided and nonmucinous microsatellite stable tumors.[77,88]

Patients with CRC who belong to pedigrees suspicious for LS should be offered screening by IHC for loss of MMR protein expression or by MSI analysis. As the sensitivity of IHC testing for loss of MMR protein expression is comparable to MSI testing, either approach can be pursued.[112] However, IHC testing is less expensive and can also identify a specific MMR protein loss, which can help target subsequent germline testing. Routine IHC testing for loss of MMR protein in individuals younger than 50 years at the time of CRC diagnosis is feasible and has led to the identification of patients with LS who might otherwise have been missed.[116,117] Patients with MSI-high tumors should undergo testing for germline MMR mutations in *MSH2*, *MLH1*, *MSH6*, and *PMS2*. Reflex IHC and/or MSI testing on all newly diagnosed CRC has been advocated by some expert groups and has been successfully implemented at some institutions.[83,112,118] However, a majority of cancer programs nationwide currently do not have a protocol for reflex testing for LS, citing lack of institutional protocols as well as fear of nonreimbursement.[119] As such, a unified move toward universal testing remains some time away. In families for which tumor tissue is not available, initial germline testing may be considered though the financial burden is not insignificant, with the cost of finding a single LS carrier measuring approximately $58,000 (compared to the $5,000 spent in finding a single LS carrier using IHC screening).[120] As in FAP, a mutation in an affected individual must be established for testing in at-risk individuals to be conclusive.

In lieu of universal testing, several predictive models such as the MMRpredict, MMRpro, and PREMM$_{1,2,6}$ have been devised in order to assess an individual's likelihood of harboring LS.[115,121,122] These models quantify an individual's risk for carrying an *MLH1*, *MSH2*, or *MSH6* germline mutation by using clinical characteristics such as age at onset of CRC and/or other LS-associated cancers, location of CRC, family history, history of synchronous or metachronous CRC, among others. A study of these predictive models demonstrated that they all performed better than the revised Bethesda guidelines in terms of identifying patients with germline mutations for LS.[123] The MMRpredict model appeared to have to be the best predictor, with a sensitivity and specificity for LS of 94% and 91%, respectively. Other validation studies, however, have not demonstrated the superiority of MMRpredict compared to the other aforementioned models.[124,125] It appears that the use of clinical characteristics in combination with MSI or MMR protein expression status in predictive models may potentially improve our ability to establish LS diagnoses in patients with CRC. However, the practicality and applicability of these tools in a clinical setting requires further assessment.

Although development of CRC in LS is not a certainty, the 80% lifetime risk, the 16% to 30% risk of metachronous CRC, and the possibly accelerated adenoma-to-carcinoma sequence mandate consideration of prophylactic surgical options.[82,87,126–129] Patients with LS who have a CRC or more than one advanced adenoma should be offered the options of prophylactic total colectomy with IRA or segmental colectomy with annual postoperative surveillance colonoscopy. Careful surveillance is also necessary after total colectomy and IRA, as the risk of high-risk adenomas and cancer in the retained rectum at a median of 104 months are 11% and 8%, respectively.[126] Although there has been no study demonstrating an improved survival for patients with LS undergoing total colectomy and IRA versus segmental colectomy, mathematical models suggest a slight survival benefit for total colectomy and IRA, especially for individuals under the age of 30.[130,131] In addition, because of increased rates of metachronous CRC development and the risk of multiple abdominal surgeries

TABLE 32.3

The Revised Bethesda Guidelines for Testing Colorectal Tumors for Microsatellite Instability

Tumors from individuals should be tested for MSI in the following situations:

1. Colorectal cancer diagnosed in a patient who is <50 y of age
2. Presence of synchronous, metachronous colorectal, or other HNPCC-associated tumors,[a] regardless of age.
3. Colorectal cancer with the MSI-H[b] histology[c] diagnosed in a patient who is <60 y of age.[d]
4. Colorectal cancer diagnosed in one or more first-degree relatives with an HNPCC-related tumor, with one of the cancers being diagnosed under age 50 years.
5. Colorectal cancer diagnosed in two or more first- or second-degree relatives with HNPCC-related tumors, regardless of age.

MSI, microsatellite instability; HNPCC, hereditary nonpolyposis colorectal cancer; MSI-H, microsatellite instability–high.
[a] HNPCC-related tumors include colorectal, endometrial, stomach, ovarian, pancreas, ureter and renal pelvis, biliary tract, and brain (usually glioblastoma as seen in Turcot syndrome) tumors, sebaceous gland adenomas and keratoacanthomas in Muir-Torre syndrome, and carcinoma of the small bowel.
[b] MSI-H in tumors refers to changes in two or more of the five National Cancer Institute–recommended panels of microsatellite markers.
[c] Presence of tumor-infiltrating lymphocytes, Crohn's-like lymphocytic reaction, mucinous/signet ring differentiation, or medullary growth pattern.
[d] There was no consensus among the workshop participants on whether to include the age criteria in guideline 3; participants voted to keep <60 years of age in the guidelines.
From Umar A, Boland CR, Terdiman JP, et al. Revised Bethesda Guidelines for hereditary nonpolyposis colorectal cancer (Lynch syndrome) and microsatellite instability. *J Natl Cancer Inst* 2004;96:261–268.

in those undergoing a segmental resection, a total colectomy and IRA has emerged as the procedure of choice for the index cancer, with consideration for TPC in cases where a high risk of metachronous rectal cancer can be predicted.[126–128] Targeted genetic testing approaches—such as the single amplicon MSH2 A636P mutation test in Ashkenazi Jewish patients with CRC—have demonstrated how a rapid and inexpensive preoperative genetic test can help direct the extent of colon resection.[132]

LS mutation carriers with a normal colon and without a history of CRC may also be offered prophylactic colectomy in highly select situations. One rationale for this approach is the similarity of lifetime cancer risk between patients with APC and MMR gene mutations, and the fact that total abdominal colectomy with IRA produces less functional disturbance than the prophylactic procedure recommended for FAP (TPC with IPAA). However, an alternate strategy for these individuals is surveillance by colonoscopy, which is cost-effective and greatly reduces the rate of CRC development and overall mortality.[133] There is a risk of CRC development in the interval between colonoscopies, though most interval cancers tend to be early stage.[134,135] As such, given that metachronous CRC may develop in as short a duration as a median of 11.3 months,[136] the recommended interval for surveillance colonoscopies is now every 1 to 2 years.[89] While prophylactic colectomy is not routinely recommended, it may be indicated in highly select patients for whom colonoscopic surveillance is not technically possible or in those who refuse to undergo regular surveillance. A decision analysis model suggests that prophylactic subtotal colectomy at age 25 may offer a survival benefit of 1.8 years, compared with surveillance colonoscopy. The benefit of prophylactic colectomy decreases when surgery is delayed until later in life and is negligible when performed at the time of cancer development.[137] Thus, the decision between prophylactic surgery and surveillance for a gene-positive mutation individual is based on many factors including penetrance of disease in the family, early age-of-onset in affected family members, functional and quality-of-life considerations, and likelihood of compliance with surveillance. Table 32.4 lists some of the pros and cons of a prophylactic colectomy for germline mutation carriers for LS without a history of CRC. Patients with LS and an index rectal cancer should be offered the options of TPC with IPAA or anterior proctosigmoidectomy with primary reconstruction.[128,138] The rationale for TPC is the 10% to 15% associated risk of metachronous colon cancer in the remaining colon following the index rectal cancer. Choosing between the two procedures depends, in part, on the patient's willingness to undergo intensive surveillance in the remnant proximal colon, as well as issues regarding quality of life and bowel function.

TABLE 32.4
Prophylactic Total Abdominal Colectomy and Ileorectal Anastomosis for Lynch Syndrome Patients without Cancer

Pros
- Elimination of colon cancer risk
- Elimination of need for surveillance colonoscopy
- Alleviating patient anxiety over the prospect of colon cancer development

Cons
- Persistence of risk of rectal cancer development
- Rectum still requires flexible endoscopic surveillance
- Patient anxiety of prospect of rectal cancer persists
- Possible altered bowel function
- Risk of surgery and possible associated complications

REFERENCES

1. Moyer VA, US Preventive Services Task Force. Risk Assessment, Genetic Counseling, and Genetic Testing for BRCA-Related Cancer in Women: U.S. Preventive Services Task Force Recommendation Statement. *Ann Intern Med* 2014;160.
2. Robson ME, Storm CD, Weitzel J, et al. American Society of Clinical Oncology policy statement update: genetic and genomic testing for cancer susceptibility. *J Clin Oncol* 2010;28:893–901.
3. Amir E, Freedman OC, Seruga B, et al. Assessing women at high risk of breast cancer: a review of risk assessment models. *J Natl Cancer Inst* 2010;102:680–691.
4. Miki Y, Swensen J, Shattuck-Eidens D, et al. A strong candidate for the breast and ovarian cancer susceptibility gene BRCA1. *Science* 1994;266:66–71.
5. Wooster R, Neuhausen SL, Mangion J, et al. Localization of a breast cancer susceptibility gene, BRCA2, to chromosome 13q12-13. *Science* 1994;265:2088–2090.
6. Lux MP, Fasching PA, Beckmann MW. Hereditary breast and ovarian cancer: review and future perspectives. *J Mol Med* 2006;84:16–28.
7. Shannon KM, Chittenden A. Genetic testing by cancer site: breast. *Cancer J* 2012;18:310–319.
8. Guillem JG, Wood WC, Moley JF, et al. ASCO/SSO review of current role of risk-reducing surgery in common hereditary cancer syndromes. *J Clin Oncol* 2006;24:4642–4660.
9. Saslow D, Boetes C, Burke W, et al. American Cancer Society guidelines for breast screening with MRI as an adjunct to mammography. *CA Cancer J Clin* 2007;57:75–89.
10. Domchek SM, Friebel TM, Singer CF, et al. Association of risk-reducing surgery in BRCA1 or BRCA2 mutation carriers with cancer risk and mortality. *JAMA* 2010;304:967–975.
11. US Equal Employment Opportunity Commission. Genetic information discrimination. http://www.eeoc.gov/laws/types/genetic.cfm. Accessed January 2, 2014.
12. Society of Surgical Oncology. Position statement on prophylactic mastectomy. http://www.surgonc.org/practice-policy/practice-management/consensus-statements/position-statement-on-prophylactic-mastectomy. Accessed February 1, 2014.
13. Hartmann LC, Schaid DJ, Woods JE, et al. Efficacy of bilateral prophylactic mastectomy in women with a family history of breast cancer. *N Engl J Med* 1999;340:77–84.
14. Eldor L, Spiegel A. Breast reconstruction after bilateral prophylactic mastectomy in women at high risk for breast cancer. *Breast J* 2009;15:S81–S89.
15. Zakhireh J, Fowble B, Esserman LJ. Application of screening principles to the reconstructed breast. *J Clin Oncol* 2010;28:173–180.
16. Gabram SG, Dougherty T, Albain KS, et al. Assessing breast cancer risk and providing treatment recommendations: immediate impact of an educational session. *Breast J* 2009;15:S39–S45.
17. Nadauld LD, Ford JM. Molecular profiling of gastric cancer: toward personalized cancer medicine. *J Clin Oncol* 2013;31:838–839.
18. Bardram L, Hansen TV, Gerdes AM, et al. Prophylactic total gastrectomy in hereditary diffuse gastric cancer: identification of two novel CDH1 gene mutations-a clinical observational study. *Fam Cancer* 2014;13:231–242.
19. Norton JA, Ham CM, Van Dam J, et al. CDH1 truncating mutations in the E-cadherin gene: an indication for total gastrectomy to treat hereditary diffuse gastric cancer. *Ann Surg* 2007;245:873–879.
20. Lynch HT, Grady W, Suriano G, et al. Gastric cancer: new genetic developments. *J Surg Oncol* 2005;90:114–133, discussion 133.
21. Guilford P, Hopkins J, Harraway J, et al. E-cadherin germline mutations in familial gastric cancer. *Nature* 1998;392:402–405.
22. Kaurah P, MacMillan A, Boyd N, et al. Founder and recurrent CDH1 mutations in families with hereditary diffuse gastric cancer. *JAMA* 2007;297:2360–2372.
23. Benusiglio PR, Malka D, Rouleau E, et al. CDH1 germline mutations and the hereditary diffuse gastric and lobular breast cancer syndrome: a multicentre study. *J Med Genet* 2013;50:486–489.
24. Gaya DR, Stuart RC, Going JJ, et al. Hereditary diffuse gastric cancer associated with E-cadherin mutation: penetrance after all. *Eur J Gastroenterol Hepatol* 2008;20:1249–1251.
25. Lee KH, Hwang D, Kang KY, et al. Frequent promoter methylation of CDH1 in non-neoplastic mucosa of sporadic diffuse gastric cancer. *Anticancer Res* 2013;33:3765–3774.
26. Oliveira C, Sousa S, Pinheiro H, et al. Quantification of epigenetic and genetic 2nd hits in CDH1 during hereditary diffuse gastric cancer syndrome progression. *Gastroenterology* 2009;136:2137–2148.
27. Carneiro F, Huntsman DG, Smyrk TC, et al. Model of the early development of diffuse gastric cancer in E-cadherin mutation carriers and its implications for patient screening. *J Pathol* 2004;203:681–687.
28. Huntsman DG, Carneiro F, Lewis FR, et al. Early gastric cancer in young, asymptomatic carriers of germ-line E-cadherin mutations. *N Engl J Med* 2001;344:1904–1909.
29. Suriano G, Yew S, Ferreira P, et al. Characterization of a recurrent germ line mutation of the E-cadherin gene: implications for genetic testing and clinical management. *Clin Cancer Res* 2005;11:5401–5409.

30. Rogers WM, Dobo E, Norton JA, et al. Risk-reducing total gastrectomy for germline mutations in E-cadherin (CDH1): pathologic findings with clinical implications. Am J Surg Pathol 2008;32:799–809.
31. Worster E, Liu X, Richardson S, et al. The impact of prophylactic total gastrectomy on health-related quality of life: a prospective cohort study. Ann Surg 2014;260:87–93.
32. Lim YC, di Pietro M, O'Donovan M, et al. Prospective cohort study assessing outcomes of patients from families fulfilling criteria for hereditary diffuse gastric cancer undergoing endoscopic surveillance. Gastrointest Endosc 2014;80:78–87.
33. Mavaddat N, Peock S, Frost D, et al. Cancer risks for BRCA1 and BRCA2 mutation carriers: results from prospective analysis of EMBRACE. J Natl Cancer Inst 2013;105:812–822.
34. Risch HA, McLaughlin JR, Cole DE, et al. Prevalence and penetrance of germline BRCA1 and BRCA2 mutations in a population series of 649 women with ovarian cancer. Am J Hum Genet 2001;68:700–710.
35. Struewing JP, Hartge P, Wacholder S, et al. The risk of cancer associated with specific mutations of BRCA1 and BRCA2 among Ashkenazi Jews. N Engl J Med 1997;336:1401–1408.
36. Finch AP, Lubinski J, Moller P, et al. Impact of oophorectomy on cancer incidence and mortality in women with a BRCA1 or BRCA2 mutation. J Clin Oncol 2014;32:1547–1553.
37. Walsh T, Casadei S, Lee MK, et al. Mutations in 12 genes for inherited ovarian, fallopian tube, and peritoneal carcinoma identified by massively parallel sequencing. Proc Natl Acad Sci U S A 2011;108:18032–18037.
38. Couch FJ, Wang X, McGuffog L, et al. Genome-wide association study in BRCA1 mutation carriers identifies novel loci associated with breast and ovarian cancer risk. PLoS Genet 2013;9:e1003212.
39. Schrader KA, Hurlburt J, Kalloger SE, et al. Germline BRCA1 and BRCA2 mutations in ovarian cancer: utility of a histology-based referral strategy. Obstet Gynecol 2012;120:235–240.
40. Kauff ND, Satagopan JM, Robson ME, et al. Risk-reducing salpingo-oophorectomy in women with a BRCA1 or BRCA2 mutation. N Engl J Med 2002;346:1609–1615.
41. Rebbeck TR, Lynch HT, Neuhausen SL, et al. Prophylactic oophorectomy in carriers of BRCA1 or BRCA2 mutations. N Engl J Med 2002;346:1616–1622.
42. Kauff ND, Domchek SM, Friebel TM, et al. Risk-reducing salpingo-oophorectomy for the prevention of BRCA1- and BRCA2-associated breast and gynecologic cancer: a multicenter, prospective study. J Clin Oncol 2008;26:1331–1337.
43. Folkins AK, Jarboe EA, Roh MH, et al. Precursors to pelvic serous carcinoma and their clinical implications. Gynecol Oncol 2009;113:391–396.
44. Wethington SL, Park KJ, Soslow RA, et al. Clinical outcome of isolated serous tubal intraepithelial carcinomas (STIC). Int J Gynecol Cancer 2013;23:1603–1611.
45. Bonadona V, Bonaiti B, Olschwang S, et al. Cancer risks associated with germline mutations in MLH1, MSH2, and MSH6 genes in Lynch syndrome. JAMA 2011;305:2304–2310.
46. Leenen CH, van Lier MG, van Doorn HC, et al. Prospective evaluation of molecular screening for Lynch syndrome in patients with endometrial cancer ≤70 years. Gynecol Oncol 2012;125:414–420.
47. Resnick K, Straughn JM Jr, Backes F, et al. Lynch syndrome screening strategies among newly diagnosed endometrial cancer patients. Obstet Gynecol 2009;114:530–536.
48. Watson P, Vasen HF, Mecklin JP, et al. The risk of endometrial cancer in hereditary nonpolyposis colorectal cancer. Am J Med 1994;96:516–520.
49. Koornstra JJ, Mourits MJ, Sijmons RH, et al. Management of extracolonic tumours in patients with Lynch syndrome. Lancet Oncol 2009;10:400–408.
50. Dove-Edwin I, Boks D, Goff S, et al. The outcome of endometrial carcinoma surveillance by ultrasound scan in women at risk of hereditary nonpolyposis colorectal carcinoma and familial colorectal carcinoma. Cancer 2002;94:1708–1712.
51. Schmeler KM, Lynch HT, Chen LM, et al. Prophylactic surgery to reduce the risk of gynecologic cancers in the Lynch syndrome. N Engl J Med 2006;354:261–269.
52. Yang KY, Caughey AB, Little SE, et al. A cost-effectiveness analysis of prophylactic surgery versus gynecologic surveillance for women from hereditary nonpolyposis colorectal cancer (HNPCC) Families. Fam Cancer 2011;10:535–543.
53. Pistorius S, Kruger S, Hohl R, et al. Occult endometrial cancer and decision making for prophylactic hysterectomy in hereditary nonpolyposis colorectal cancer patients. Gynecol Oncol 2006;102:189–194.
54. Traugott AL, Moley JF. Multiple endocrine neoplasia type 2: clinical manifestations and management. Cancer Treat Res 2009;153:321–337.
55. American Thyroid Association Guidelines Task Force, Kloos RT, Eng C, et al. Medullary thyroid cancer: management guidelines of the American Thyroid Association. Thyroid 2009;19:565–612.
56. Wells SA Jr, Pacini F, Robinson BG, et al. Multiple endocrine neoplasia type 2 and familial medullary thyroid carcinoma: an update. J Clin Endocrinol Metab 2013;98:3149–3164.
57. Eng C, Clayton D, Schuffenecker I, et al. The relationship between specific RET proto-oncogene mutations and disease phenotype in multiple endocrine neoplasia type 2. International RET mutation consortium analysis. JAMA 1996;276:1575–1579.
58. Howe JR, Norton JA, Wells SA Jr. Prevalence of pheochromocytoma and hyperparathyroidism in multiple endocrine neoplasia type 2A: results of long-term follow-up. Surgery 1993;114:1070–1077.
59. Machens A, Niccoli-Sire P, Hoergel J, et al. Early malignant progression of hereditary medullary thyroid cancer. N Engl J Med 2003;349:1517–1525.
60. Gagel RF, Levy ML, Donovan DT, et al. Multiple endocrine neoplasia type 2A associated with cutaneous lichen amyloidosis. Ann Intern Med 1989;111:802–806.
61. Santoro M, Carlomagno F, Romano A, et al. Activation of RET as a dominant transforming gene by germline mutations of MEN2A and MEN2B. Science 1995;267:381–383.
62. Mulligan LM, Ponder BA. Genetic basis of endocrine disease: multiple endocrine neoplasia type 2. J Clin Endocrinol Metab 1995;80:1989–1995.
63. Mulligan L, Kwok J, Healy C. Germ-line mutations of the RET protooncogene in multiple endocrine neoplasia type 2A (MEN 2A). Nature 1993;363:458–460.
64. Donis-Keller H, Dou S, Chi D, et al. Mutations in the RET proto-oncogene are associated with MEN 2A and FMTC. Hum Mol Genet 1993;2:851–856.
65. Traugott AL, Moley JF. The RET Protooncogene. Cancer Treat Res 2010;153:303–319.
66. Quayle FJ, Benveniste R, DeBenedetti MK, et al. Hereditary medullary thyroid carcinoma in patients greater than 50 years old. Surgery 2004;136:1116–1121.
67. Lips CJ, Landsvater RM, Hoppener JW, et al. Clinical screening as compared with DNA analysis in families with multiple endocrine neoplasia type 2A. N Engl J Med 1994;331:828–835.
68. Niccoli-Sire P, Murat A, Baudin E, et al. Early or prophylactic thyroidectomy in MEN 2/FMTC gene carriers: results in 71 thyroidectomized patients. The French Calcitonin Tumours Study Group (GETC). Eur J Endocrinol 1999;141:468–474.
69. Rodriguez GJ, Balsalobre MD, Pomares F, et al. Prophylactic thyroidectomy in MEN 2A syndrome: experience in a single center. J Am Coll Surg 2002;195:159–166.
70. Skinner MA, Moley JA, Dilley WG, et al. Prophylactic thyroidectomy in multiple endocrine neoplasia type 2A. N Engl J Med 2005;353:1105–1113.
71. Brandi ML, Gagel RF, Angeli A, et al. Guidelines for diagnosis and therapy of MEN type 1 and type 2. J Clin Endocrinol Metab 2001;86:5658–5671.
72. Elisei R, Romei C, Renzini G, et al. The timing of total thyroidectomy in RET gene mutation carriers could be personalized and safely planned on the basis of serum calcitonin: 18 years experience at one single center. J Clin Endocrinol Metab 2012;97:426–435.
73. Waguespack SG, Rich TA, Perrier ND, et al. Management of medullary thyroid carcinoma and MEN2 syndromes in childhood. Nat Rev Endocrinol 2011;7:596–607.
74. Moley JF. Medullary thyroid carcinoma: management of lymph node metastases. J Natl Compr Canc Netw 2010;8:549–556.
75. Machens A, Dralle H. Biomarker-based risk stratification for previously untreated medullary thyroid cancer. J Clin Endocrinol Metab 2010;95:2655–2663.
76. Solorzano CC, Evans DB. Same-day ultrasound guidance in reoperations for locally recurrent papillary thyroid cancer. Surgery 2007;142:973–975.
77. Patel SG, Ahnen DJ. Familial colon cancer syndromes: an update of a rapidly evolving field. Curr Gastroenterol Rep 2012;14:428–438.
78. Aretz S, Uhlhaas S, Goergens H, et al. MUTYH-associated polyposis: 70 of 71 patients with biallelic mutations present with an attenuated or atypical phenotype. Int J Cancer 2006;119:807–814.
79. Russell AM, Zhang J, Luz J, et al. Prevalence of MYH germline mutations in Swiss APC mutation-negative polyposis patients. Int J Cancer 2006;118:1937–1940.
80. Jasperson KW. Genetic testing by cancer site: colon (polyposis syndromes). Cancer J 2012;18:328–333.
81. Hampel H, Frankel WL, Martin E, et al. Screening for the Lynch syndrome (hereditary nonpolyposis colorectal cancer). N Engl J Med 2005;352:1851–1860.
82. Lynch HT, Lynch PM, Lanspa SJ, et al. Review of the Lynch syndrome: history, molecular genetics, screening, differential diagnosis, and medicolegal ramifications. Clin Genet 2009;76:1–18.
83. Vasen HF, Blanco I, Aktan-Collan K, et al. Revised guidelines for the clinical management of Lynch syndrome (HNPCC): recommendations by a group of European experts. Gut 2013;62:812–823.
84. Niessen RC, Hofstra RM, Westers H, et al. Germline hypermethylation of MLH1 and EPCAM deletions are a frequent cause of Lynch syndrome. Genes Chromosomes Cancer 2009;48:737–744.
85. Kuiper RP, Vissers LE, Venkatachalam R, et al. Recurrence and variability of germline EPCAM deletions in Lynch syndrome. Hum Mutat 2011;32:407–414.
86. Rumilla K, Schowalter KV, Lindor NM, et al. Frequency of deletions of EPCAM (TACSTD1) in MSH2-associated Lynch syndrome cases. J Mol Diagn 2011;13:93–99.
87. Jasperson KW, Tuohy TM, Neklason DW, et al. Hereditary and familial colon cancer. Gastroenterology 2010;138:2044–2058.
88. Steinhagen E, Markowitz AJ, Guillem JG. How to manage a patient with multiple adenomatous polyps. Surg Oncol Clin N Am 2010;19:711–723.
89. National Comprehensive Cancer Network. NCCN Clinical Practice Guidelines in Oncology: Colorectal Cancer Screening. http://www.nccn.org/professionals/physician_gls/pdf/colorectal_screening.pdf. Accessed February 19, 2014.
90. Vasen HF, Moslein G, Alonso A, et al. Guidelines for the clinical management of familial adenomatous polyposis (FAP). Gut 2008;57:704–713.
91. Church J. Familial adenomatous polyposis. Surg Oncol Clin N Am 2009;18:585–598.
92. Nieuwenhuis MH, Bulow S, Bjork J, et al. Genotype predicting phenotype in familial adenomatous polyposis: a practical application to the choice of surgery. Dis Colon Rectum 2009;52:1259–1263.

93. Sinha A, Tekkis PP, Rashid S, et al. Risk factors for secondary proctectomy in patients with familial adenomatous polyposis. Br J Surg 2010;97: 1710–1715.
94. Koskenvuo L, Renkonen-Sinisalo L, Jarvinen HJ, et al. Risk of cancer and secondary proctectomy after colectomy and ileorectal anastomosis in familial adenomatous polyposis. Int J Colorectal Dis 2014;29:225–230.
95. Remzi FH, Church JM, Bast J, et al. Mucosectomy vs. stapled ileal pouch-anal anastomosis in patients with familial adenomatous polyposis: functional outcome and neoplasia control. Dis Colon Rectum 2001;44:1590–1596.
96. Friederich P, de Jong AE, Mathus-Vliegen LM, et al. Risk of developing adenomas and carcinomas in the ileal pouch in patients with familial adenomatous polyposis. Clin Gastroenterol Hepatol 2008;6:1237–1242.
97. Aziz O, Athanasiou T, Fazio VW, et al. Meta-analysis of observational studies of ileorectal versus ileal pouch-anal anastomosis for familial adenomatous polyposis. Br J Surg 2006;93:407–417.
98. Fazio VW, Kiran RP, Remzi FH, et al. Ileal pouch anal anastomosis: analysis of outcome and quality of life in 3707 patients. Ann Surg 2013;257: 679–685.
99. Rajaratnam SG, Eglinton TW, Hider P, et al. Impact of ileal pouch-anal anastomosis on female fertility: meta-analysis and systematic review. Int J Colorectal Dis 2011;26:1365–1374.
100. Bartels SA, D'Hoore A, Cuesta MA, et al. Significantly increased pregnancy rates after laparoscopic restorative proctocolectomy: a cross-sectional study. Ann Surg 2012;256:1045–1048.
101. Beyer-Berjot L, Maggiori L, Birnbaum D, et al. A total laparoscopic approach reduces the infertility rate after ileal pouch-anal anastomosis: a 2-center study. Ann Surg 2013;258:275–282.
102. Steinhagen E, Guillem JG, Chang G, et al. The prevalence of thyroid cancer and benign thyroid disease in patients with familial adenomatous polyposis may be higher than previously recognized. Clin Colorectal Cancer 2012;11: 304–308.
103. Steinhagen E, Hui VW, Levy RA, et al. Results of a prospective thyroid ultrasound screening program in adenomatous polyposis patients. Am J Surg [ePub ahead of print].
104. Jarrar AM, Milas M, Mitchell J, et al. Screening for thyroid cancer in patients with familial adenomatous polyposis. Ann Surg 2011;253:515–521.
105. Giardiello FM, Burt RW, Jarvinen H, et al. Familial adenomatous polyposis. In: Bosman FT, Carneiro F, Hruban RH, et al, eds. Classification of Tumours of the Digestive System. Lyon: IARC Press; 2010:147–151
106. Nieuwenhuis MH, Lefevre JH, Bulow S, et al. Family history, surgery, and APC mutation are risk factors for desmoid tumors in familial adenomatous polyposis: an international cohort study. Dis Colon Rectum 2011;54: 1229–1234.
107. Quintini C, Ward G, Shatnawei A, et al. Mortality of intra-abdominal desmoid tumors in patients with familial adenomatous polyposis: a single center review of 154 patients. Ann Surg 2012;255:511–516.
108. Sinha A, Gibbons DC, Phillips RK, et al. Surgical prophylaxis in familial adenomatous polyposis: do pre-existing desmoids outside the abdominal cavity matter? Fam Cancer 2010;9:407–411.
109. Schiessling S, Kihm M, Ganschow P, et al. Desmoid tumour biology in patients with familial adenomatous polyposis coli. Br J Surg 2013;100:694–703.
110. von Roon AC, Tekkis PP, Lovegrove RE, et al. Comparison of outcomes of ileal pouch-anal anastomosis for familial adenomatous polyposis with and without previous ileorectal anastomosis. Br J Surg 2008;95:494–498.
111. Nieuwenhuis MH, Vogt S, Jones N, et al. Evidence for accelerated colorectal adenoma–carcinoma progression in MUTYH-associated polyposis? Gut 2012;61:734–738.
112. Palomaki GE, McClain MR, Melillo S, et al. EGAPP supplementary evidence review: DNA testing strategies aimed at reducing morbidity and mortality from Lynch syndrome. Genet Med 2009;11:42–65.
113. Umar A, Boland CR, Terdiman JP, et al. Revised Bethesda Guidelines for hereditary nonpolyposis colorectal cancer (Lynch syndrome) and microsatellite instability. J Natl Cancer Inst 2004;96:261–268.
114. Vasen HF, Watson P, Mecklin JP, et al. New clinical criteria for hereditary nonpolyposis colorectal cancer (HNPCC, Lynch syndrome) proposed by the International Collaborative group on HNPCC. Gastroenterology 1999; 116:1453–1456.
115. Barnetson RA, Tenesa A, Farrington SM, et al. Identification and survival of carriers of mutations in DNA mismatch-repair genes in colon cancer. N Engl J Med 2006;354:2751–2763.
116. Lee-Kong SA, Markowitz AJ, Glogowski E, et al. Prospective immunohistochemical analysis of primary colorectal cancers for loss of mismatch repair protein expression. Clin Colorectal Cancer 2010;9:255–259.
117. Steinhagen E, Shia J, Markowitz AJ, et al. Systematic immunohistochemistry screening for Lynch syndrome in early age-of-onset colorectal cancer patients undergoing surgical resection. J Am Coll Surg 2012;214:61–67.
118. Heald B, Plesec T, Liu X, et al. Implementation of universal microsatellite instability and immunohistochemistry screening for diagnosing lynch syndrome in a large academic medical center. J Clin Oncol 2013;31:1336–1340.
119. Beamer LC, Grant ML, Espenschied CR, et al. Reflex immunohistochemistry and microsatellite instability testing of colorectal tumors for Lynch syndrome among US cancer programs and follow-up of abnormal results. J Clin Oncol 2012;30:1058–1063.
120. Mvundura M, Grosse SD, Hampel H, et al. The cost-effectiveness of genetic testing strategies for Lynch syndrome among newly diagnosed patients with colorectal cancer. Genet Med 2010;12:93–104.
121. Chen S, Wang W, Lee S, et al. Prediction of germline mutations and cancer risk in the Lynch syndrome. JAMA 2006;296:1479–1487.
122. Kastrinos F, Steyerberg EW, Mercado R, et al. The PREMM(1,2,6) model predicts risk of MLH1, MSH2, and MSH6 germline mutations based on cancer history. Gastroenterology 2011;140:73–81.
123. Green RC, Parfrey PS, Woods MO, et al. Prediction of Lynch syndrome in consecutive patients with colorectal cancer. J Natl Cancer Inst 2009;101:331–340.
124. Khan O, Blanco A, Conrad P, et al. Performance of Lynch syndrome predictive models in a multi-center US referral population. Am J Gastroenterol 2011;106:1822–1827, quiz 1828.
125. Tresallet C, Brouquet A, Julie C, et al. Evaluation of predictive models in daily practice for the identification of patients with Lynch syndrome. Int J Cancer 2012;130:1367–1377.
126. Kalady MF, McGannon E, Vogel JD, et al. Risk of colorectal adenoma and carcinoma after colectomy for colorectal cancer in patients meeting Amsterdam criteria. Ann Surg 2010;252:507–511, discussion 511–513.
127. Parry S, Win AK, Parry B, et al. Metachronous colorectal cancer risk for mismatch repair gene mutation carriers: the advantage of more extensive colon surgery. Gut 2011;60:950–957.
128. Kalady MF, Lipman J, McGannon E, et al. Risk of colonic neoplasia after proctectomy for rectal cancer in hereditary nonpolyposis colorectal cancer. Ann Surg 2012;255:1121–1125.
129. Cirillo L, Urso ED, Parrinello G, et al. High risk of rectal cancer and of metachronous colorectal cancer in probands of families fulfilling the Amsterdam criteria. Ann Surg 2013;257:900–901.
130. Stupart DA, Goldberg PA, Baigrie RJ, et al. Surgery for colonic cancer in HNPCC: total vs segmental colectomy. Colorectal Dis 2011;13: 1395–1399.
131. Maeda T, Cannom RR, Beart RW Jr, et al. Decision model of segmental compared with total abdominal colectomy for colon cancer in hereditary nonpolyposis colorectal cancer. J Clin Oncol 2010;28:1175–1180.
132. Guillem JG, Glogowski E, Moore HG, et al. Single-amplicon MSH2 A636P mutation testing in Ashkenazi Jewish patients with colorectal cancer: role in presurgical management. Ann Surg 2007;245:560–565.
133. Barrow P, Khan M, Lalloo F, et al. Systematic review of the impact of registration and screening on colorectal cancer incidence and mortality in familial adenomatous polyposis and Lynch syndrome. Br J Surg 2013;100: 1719–1731.
134. Vasen HF, Abdirahman M, Brohet R, et al. One to 2-year surveillance intervals reduce risk of colorectal cancer in families with Lynch syndrome. Gastroenterology 2010;138:2300–2306.
135. Stuckless S, Green JS, Morgenstern M, et al. Impact of colonoscopic screening in male and female Lynch syndrome carriers with an MSH2 mutation. Clin Genet 2012;82:439–445.
136. Engel C, Rahner N, Schulmann K, et al. Efficacy of annual colonoscopic surveillance in individuals with hereditary nonpolyposis colorectal cancer. Clin Gastroenterol Hepatol 2010;8:174–182.
137. Syngal S, Weeks JC, Schrag D, et al. Benefits of colonoscopic surveillance and prophylactic colectomy in patients with hereditary nonpolyposis colorectal cancer mutations. Ann Intern Med 1998;129:787–796.
138. Giardiello FM, Allen JI, Axilbund JE, et al. Guidelines on genetic evaluation and management of Lynch syndrome: a consensus statement by the US Multi-Society Task Force on Colorectal Cancer. Dis Colon Rectum 2014; 57(8):1025–1048.

33 Cancer Risk–Reducing Agents

Dean E. Brenner, Scott M. Lippman, and Susan T. Mayne

WHY CANCER PREVENTION AS A CLINICAL ONCOLOGY DISCIPLINE

Until recently, clinical oncology has been defined as a medical specialty that attempts to intervene in order to slow or reverse the final stage of the cancer process—the clonally derived, genomically damaged, invasive cell mass. Cancer is a long process, a stepwise carcinogenic progression that encompasses critical molecular events that culminate in the loss of key cellular control homeostatic functions (e.g., control of proliferation, apoptosis, invasion, angiogenesis).[1] These events occur prior to and during the morphologic changes that have historically defined neoplasia. Morphologic changes, such as subtle increases in cellular proliferation that progress to early and late precancerous lesions containing dysplastic cells, characterize the carcinogenesis process (Fig. 33.1).[1-3] Opportunities for intervention in this process can include diverse, nonpharmacologic approaches (e.g., obesity management via diet/lifestyle interventions) or pharmacologic interventions (e.g., drugs or nutrients/nonnutrient substances used as drugs) aimed at delaying or reversing the carcinogenesis process prior to or following the appearance of early morphologic changes. Cancer screening and early detection strategies (e.g., surveillance endoscopy, fecal occult blood testing, mammography) identify not only those individuals with early stage, curable malignant transformations, but also those individuals with noninvasive neoplasias who are at risk for progression to transformed invasive malignancies.

Recognizing that cancer is a continuum, oncologists are increasingly expected to be knowledgeable about a diverse array of cancer-related topics including lifestyle behaviors such as diet and exercise, risk assessment, screening, other preventive interventions, in addition to current treatments for advanced malignancy. The understanding, use, and management of interventions designed to delay or reverse the carcinogenesis process have become integral components of the this role.[4]

DEFINING CANCER RISK–REDUCING AGENTS (CHEMOPREVENTION)

Cancer risk reduction, commonly referred to as chemoprevention, is the use of a range of interventions from drugs to isolated dietary components to whole-diet modulation to block, reverse, or prevent the development of invasive cancer.[5,6] Human cancer risk reduction asserts that one can intervene at many steps in the carcinogenic process, which occurs over many years. This prolonged latency provides opportunities to intervene at many time points and at multiple events in the carcinogenic process. Successful deployment of cancer risk–reducing agent interventions requires evidence of reduced cancer-associated incidence and/or mortality.

The concept of field carcinogenesis was first described in the early 1950s as *field cancerization* in squamous cell carcinomas of the head and neck, and subsequently ascribed to many epithelial sites. The field carcinogenesis concept is that patients have a wide surface area of precancerous or cancerous tissue change that can be detected at the gross (oral premalignant lesions, polyps), microscopic (metaplasia, dysplasia), and/or molecular (gene loss or amplification) levels. Recent molecular studies detecting profound genetic alterations in histologically normal tissue from high-risk individuals have provided strong support for the field carcinogenesis concept. The implication of the field effect is that multifocal, genetically distinct, and clonally related premalignant lesions can progress over a broad tissue region.[1] The essence of cancer risk reduction, then, is intervention within the multistep carcinogenic process and throughout a wide field.

IDENTIFYING POTENTIAL CANCER RISK–REDUCING AGENTS

Cancer risk–reducing agent identification results from the synthesis of data from population, basic, translational, and clinical sciences. Findings from all of these disciplines are combined to contribute to the identification of agents with the potential to delay or reverse the carcinogenesis process (see Fig. 33.1).

The Hanahan and Weinberg hallmarks of malignant transformation—self-sufficiency in growth signals, insensitivity to growth-inhibitory signals, evasion of apoptosis, limitless replication potential, sustained angiogenesis, and tissue invasion and metastasis[7]—reflect the loss of cellular signaling control. The molecular damage that results in transformation is triggered by a large array of genetic and environmental stressors such as chronic inflammation, oxidation, inherited genetic mutations, and exogenous environmental exposures. Many such signaling intermediates have common functions in multiple organ sites (see Fig. 33.1). The complexity and overlap of signal transduction pathways suggests that single molecular therapeutic/preventive targets may have limited effectiveness. Interventions aimed at preventing the occurrence of or overcoming the effects of molecular defects in multiple pathways or targets may be required to arrest or reverse carcinogenesis. Using the Hanahan and Weinberg hallmarks, examples of possible targets are shown in Table 33.1.

PRECLINICAL DEVELOPMENT OF CANCER RISK–REDUCING AGENTS

Similar to the development of therapeutic interventions, the assessment of efficacy and toxicity of single chemically synthesized entities, agents designed *in silico*, botanicals, nutrients/nonnutrient substances used as drugs for cancer risk–reducing agent efficacy proceeds through a translational paradigm that identifies efficacy in cell culture models, in live animal models, and in humans. Preclinical models that simulate the carcinogenesis process in target epithelia identify molecular biomarkers for modulation by interventions. These models can be used to identify potential toxicity of interventions and to assess the effect of interventions on the development and progression of preneoplasia/neoplasia.[8]

The U.S. National Cancer Institute's (NCI) PREVENT Cancer Preclinical Drug Development Program is a prime example of a

Molecular Biomarkers of Carcinogenesis

Dysplasia = Intraepithelial Neoplasia (IEN)

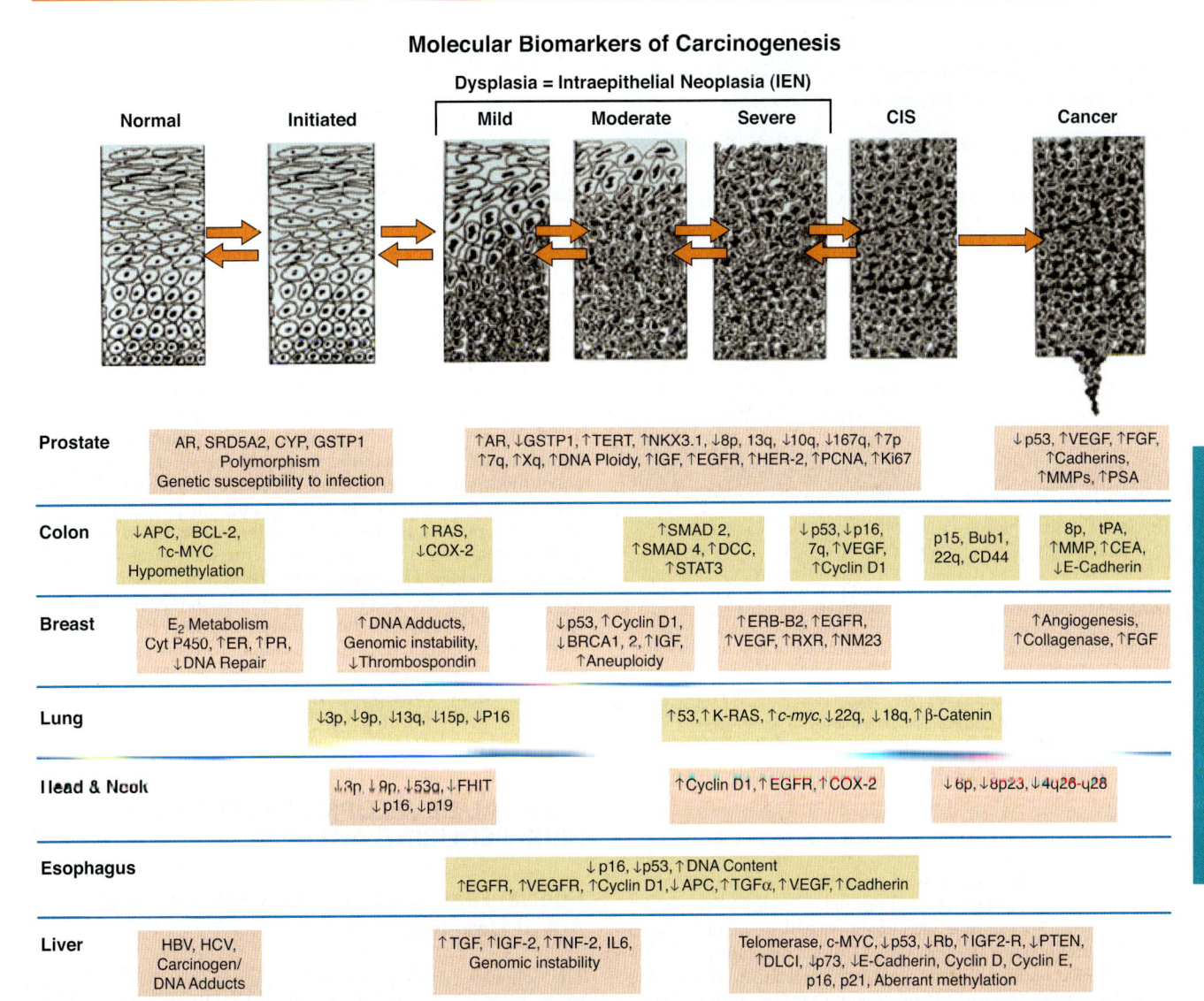

	Normal	Initiated	Mild	Moderate	Severe	CIS	Cancer
Prostate	AR, SRD5A2, CYP, GSTP1 Polymorphism Genetic susceptibility to infection		↑AR, ↓GSTP1, ↑TERT, ↑NKX3.1, ↓8p, 13q, ↓10q, ↓167q, ↑7p ↑7q, ↑Xq, ↑DNA Ploidy, ↑IGF, ↑EGFR, ↑HER-2, ↑PCNA, ↑Ki67				↓p53, ↑VEGF, ↑FGF, ↑Cadherins, ↑MMPs, ↑PSA
Colon	↓APC, BCL-2, ↑c-MYC Hypomethylation		↑RAS, ↓COX-2	↑SMAD 2, ↑SMAD 4, ↑DCC, ↑STAT3	↓p53, ↓p16, 7q, ↑VEGF, ↑Cyclin D1	p15, Bub1, 22q, CD44	8p, tPA, ↑MMP, ↑CEA, ↓E-Cadherin
Breast	E₂ Metabolism Cyt P450, ↑ER, ↑PR, ↓DNA Repair		↑DNA Adducts, Genomic instability, ↓Thrombospondin	↓p53, ↑Cyclin D1, ↓BRCA1, 2, ↑IGF, ↑Aneuploidy	↑ERB-B2, ↑EGFR, ↑VEGF, ↑RXR, ↑NM23		↑Angiogenesis, ↑Collagenase, ↑FGF
Lung			↓3p, ↓9p, ↓13q, ↓15p, ↓P16		↑53, ↑K-RAS, ↑c-myc, ↓22q, ↓18q, ↑β-Catenin		
Head & Neck			↓3p, ↓9p, ↓53q, ↓FHIT ↓p16, ↓p19		↑Cyclin D1, ↑EGFR, ↑COX-2	↓6p, ↓8p23, ↓4q26-q28	
Esophagus			↓p16, ↓p53, ↑DNA Content ↑EGFR, ↑VEGFR, ↑Cyclin D1, ↓APC, ↑TGFα, ↑VEGF, ↑Cadherin				
Liver	HBV, HCV, Carcinogen/ DNA Adducts		↑TGF, ↑IGF-2, ↑TNF-2, IL6, Genomic instability		Telomerase, c-MYC, ↓p53, ↓Rb, ↑IGF2-R, ↓PTEN, ↑DLCI, ↓p73, ↓E-Cadherin, Cyclin D, Cyclin E, p16, p21, Aberrant methylation		

Figure 33.1 Genetic progression in major cancers. Carcinogenesis is driven by genetic progression. This progression is marked by the appearance of molecular biomarkers in distinctive patterns representing accumulating changes in gene expression and correlating with changes in histologic phenotype as cells move from normal through the early stages of clonal expansion to dysplasia and finally to early invasive, locally advanced, and metastatic cancer. The figure[257] shows candidate molecular biomarkers of genetic progression in seven target organs: the prostate,[300-302] the colon,[2] the breast,[303,304] the lung,[305-307] the head and neck,[308-311] the esophagus,[312,313] and the liver.[314] CIS, carcinoma in situ; AR, androgen receptor; CYP, cytochrome P-450; GSTP1, glutathione S transferase P1; TERT, telomerase reverse transcriptase; NKX3.1, NK 3 transcription factor related, locus 1 (prostate specific, androgen regulated); IGF, insulin-like growth factor; EGFR, epidermal growth factor receptor; HER-2, human epidermal growth factor receptor-2; PCNA, proliferating cell nuclear antigen; VEGF, vascular endothelial growth factor; FGF, fibroblast growth factor; MMP, matrix metalloproteinase; PSA, prostate-specific antigen; APC, adenomatous polyposis coli; BCL-2, B-cell lymphoma 2 gene, apoptosis control; c-MYC, v-myc avian myelocytomatosis viral oncogene homolog; COX-2, cyclooxygenase-2; SMAD, homolog of mothers against decapentaplegic + *C. Elegans* SMA protein; DCC, deleted in colon cancer gene; CEA, carcinoembryonic antigen; ER, estrogen receptor; PR, progesterone receptor; ERB-B2, Receptor tyrosine-protein kinase erbB-2, same as HER-2; RXR, retinoid X receptor; NM23, Nucleoside disphosphate kinase A; K-RAS, Kirsten rat sarcoma viral oncogene homolog; FHIT, fragile histidine triad protein; TGFα, tumor growth factor alpha; HBV, hepatitis B virus; HCV, hepatitis C virus; TNF-2, tumor necrosis factor 2; IL6, interleukin 6; PTEN, phosphatase and tensin homolog. (Figure and revised caption from Kelloff GJ, Lippman SM, Dannenberg AJ, et al. Progress in chemoprevention drug development: the promise of molecular biomarkers for prevention of intraepithelial neoplasia and cancer—a plan to move forward. *Clin Cancer Res* 2006;12:3661–3697, published with permission from the American Association for Cancer Research.)

rational strategy to select promising agents for clinical trials through a stepwise approach of preclinical in vitro testing followed by *in vivo* screening.[8-10] This system involves several phases: biochemical prescreening assays, in vitro efficacy models, in vivo short-term screening, animal efficacy testing, and preclinical toxicology testing.

Biochemical Prescreening Assays

Prescreening assays are a series of short-term, mechanistic assays developed to evaluate the ability of a test compound to modulate biochemical events presumed to be mechanistically linked to carcinogenesis.[8] These in vitro assays are rapidly completed for potential cancer risk–reducing agents. Examples of such assays include carcinogen-DNA binding, prostaglandin synthesis inhibition, glutathione–S-transferase inhibition, and ornithine decarboxylase inhibition.

In Vitro Efficacy Models

In vitro assays test the cancer risk–reducing activity of a screened compound in four epithelial cell systems (primary rat tracheal epithelial cells, human lung tumor [A427] cells, mouse mammary organ cultures [MMOC], and human foreskin epithelial cells).

TABLE 33.1
Molecular Mechanisms Common to Transforming Cells and Potential Preventive Interventions

Characteristics of Neoplasia	Possible Molecular Targets
■ Self-sufficiency in cell growth	EGFR, platelet-derived growth factor, MAPK, PI3K
■ Insensitivity to antigrowth signals	SMADs, pRb, cyclin-dependent kinases, MYC
■ Limitless replicative potential	hTERT, pRb, p53
■ Evading apoptosis	Bcl-2, BAX, caspases, Fas, tumor necrosis factor receptor, insulin growth factor/PI3K/Akt, mTOR, p53, NF-κB, PTEN, RAS
■ Sustained angiogenesis	VEGF, basic fibroblast growth factor, integrins ($\alpha_v\beta_3$), thrombospondin-1, HIF-1α
■ Tissue invasion and metastases	MMPs, MAPK, E-cadherin

EGFR, epidermal growth factor receptor; MAPK, mitogen-activated protein kinase; PI3K, phosphoinositide 3-kinase; SMAD, drosophila protein, mothers against decapentaplegic gene and the *Elegans* protein SMA; pRb, phosphorylated Rb protein; hTERT, human telomerase reverse transcriptase; mTOR, mammalian target of rapamycin; NF-κB, nuclear factor kappa B; PTEN, phosphatase and tensin homolog, VEGF, vascular endothelial growth factor; HIF-1α, hypoxia inducible factor-1α; MMP, Matrix metalloproteinases. Adapted from Kelloff GJ, Lippman SM, Dannenberg AJ, et al. Progress in chemoprevention drug development: the promise of molecular biomarkers for prevention of intraepithelial neoplasia and cancer—a plan to move forward. *Clin Cancer Res* 2006;12:3661–3697 and derived from Hanahan D, Weinberg RA. The hallmarks of cancer. *Cell* 2000;100:57–70.

The assays measure the ability of potential cancer risk–reducing agents to reverse transformation in normal epithelial cells exposed to carcinogens. For example, after treatment with a carcinogen such as 7,12-demethylbenz(a)anthracene, MMOCs develop lesions similar to alveolar nodules that are considered precancerous in mouse mammary glands in vivo.[11] Pretreatment of organ cultures before carcinogen exposure measures the effect of cancer risk–reducing agents in the initiation stage of carcinogenesis, whereas treatment after carcinogen exposure measures activity during tumor promotion. Three of these assays (using rat tracheal epithelial, A427, and MMOC cells) have shown predictive values of 76% to 83% for cancer risk–reducing agent efficacy in in vivo models.[8]

Preclinical In Vivo Models for Cancer Risk–Reducing Agent Efficacy Testing

Animal models remain a crucial link in the efficacy assessment of cancer risk–reducing agents for epithelial cancer. Chemical carcinogenesis models provide the reproducible development of tumors in animals following the administration of a known chemical initiator or combination initiator/promoter and have been the primary in vivo screening tool for cancer risk–reducing agents (Table 33.2A).[12,13] Carcinogenesis models employing genetically engineered mice permit the interrogation of targeted pathways and the corresponding efficacy of cancer risk–reducing agents. Although useful for mechanistic studies, knockout or genetic mutational models create accelerated neoplastic progression that does not accurately recapitulate the more complex, stepwise, human carcinogenesis process. Recombinant alleles can be driven by the addition of drug-sensitive regulatory elements, such as tetracycline or tamoxifen analogs. The drug-sensitive regulatory elements achieve temporal control over a gene promoter through the administration of the drug that binds to the regulatory element. Such a system permits the inhibition or overexpression of the organ-specific gene using Cre recombinase, a site specific DNA recombinase that targets DNA regions flanked by loxP sequences. Tables 33.2A and 2B list in pictorial form higher updated chemical and transgenic mouse models that may be used for cancer risk-reducing agent testing.

CLINICAL DEVELOPMENT OF CANCER RISK–REDUCING AGENTS

Special Features of Cancer Risk–Reducing Agent Development

The clinical efficacy assessment of cancer risk–reducing agents employs phased testing (phase I to III) models used for development of drugs[14] but with crucial differences in study design and end points. Special features for the clinical development of

TABLE 33.2A
Chemical Carcinogenesis Models Used for Screening of Cancer Risk–Reducing Agents for Common Epithelial Neoplasms in Animals

Organ Site	Species	Carcinogen	End Point
Colon	Rat, mouse	Azoxymethane (AOM)	Aberrant crypts, adenomas, adenocarcinomas
Lung	Mouse	N—butyl-N-(4-hydroxybutyl)nitrosamine (NNK); benzo[a]pyrene; cigarette smoke	Adenomas, adenocarcinomas
	Hamster	Methylnitrosourea (MNU)	Squamous cell carcinomas
	Mouse	N-nitroso-tris-chloroethylurea	Squamous cell carcinomas
Breast	Rat	Dimethylbenz[a]anthracene (DMBA); MNU	Adenocarcinomas, adenomas
Prostate	Rat	MNU + testosterone	Adenocarcinomas
Bladder	Rat, mouse	N-butyl-N-(4-hydroxybutyl)nitrosamine (OH-BBN)	Transitional cell carcinoma
Pancreas	Hamster	N-nitrobis-(2-oxopropyl)amine (BOP)	Ductal carcinomas
Head and neck	Rat	4-nitroquinoline-1-oxide (4-NQO)	Tongue squamous cell carcinomas
	Mouse	DMBA	Squamous cell carcinomas
Esophagus	Rat	Dimethylbenz[a]anthracene	Squamous cell carcinomas
	Rat	Esophagogastroduodenal anastomosis + iron	Adenocarcinomas

Adapted from Steele VE, Lubet RA. The use of animal models for cancer chemoprevention drug development. *Semin Oncol* 2010;37:327–338.

TABLE 33.2B

Selected Transgenic Animal Models for Carcinogenesis Evaluation

Organ Site	Genes Targeted	End Point	References
Colon	*Apc, Lrig1, gp130, Stat3, Smad3, Wnt-β-catenin, villin, TGFBR2, Kras, Ink4a*	Adenomas and adenocarcinomas	(258, 259)
Lung	*KrasG12D, KrasG12Vgeo, PTEN, BrafV600E, cRaf, Egfr* L858R±T790M, *PIK3CA*, EMLA4-ALK fusion *Rb, P53*	Adenomas and adenocarcinomas Small cell	(260)
Breast	Mouse mammary tumor virus long terminal repeat promoter (MMTV) driven *BRCA1, p53, ERα, aromatase, TGFα, Her2/neu, wnt, PELP-1, AIB-1*	DCIS, adenocarcinomas	(261)
Prostate	Probasin promotor driving SV40 large T antigen (*TRAMP/LADY*), *c-Myc, TMPRSS-ERG, Akt, Wnt-β-catenin*, androgen receptor *Nkx3.1, FGFR1, TGF, PTEN*	Prostate intraepithelial neoplasia, neuroendocrine tumors (TRAMP); adenocarcinomas (*c-Myc, TMPRESS-ERG, Akt, Wnt*, androgen receptor) Adenocarcinomas	(262)
Pancreas	*KrasG12D* alone, *LSL-Kras, PDX-1, R26Notch, Tif1γ* Combined *PDX-1, LSL-Kras, LSL-Trp53*; combined *PDX-1, Brca2, LSL-Kras Trp53; KrasG12D* on *Mist1* locus; *PDX-1, KrasG12D+ Ink4a/Arf* or *Smad4*; *Ptf1a, KrasG12D, TGFBR2*	Pancreatic intraepithelial neoplasia Pancreatic adenocarcinoma	(263)

Note: Most models are mouse models. Such models will permit efficacy testing of specific pathway targets using single agent interventions, combinations, or multimechanism-based natural products.

---

cancer risk–reducing agents create the following challenges to be overcome: (1) the need for large therapeutic index (doses associated with potential toxicity of an intervention need to substantially exceed doses aimed at delaying or reversing transformation) for use in individuals who are asymptomatic yet may benefit from an extended (years) treatment course; (2) the long latency to malignant transformation (an assessment of effectiveness based on the reduction in cancer incidence requires studies lasting for years and involving thousands of participants); (3) adherence (once-daily dosing regimens using interventions that have sufficiently long half-lives may minimize the impact of a missed dose yet maintain the biologic impact on the physiologic target; minimal toxicity and strong psychological commitment to preventive goals also enhance adherence[15]); and (4) complex risk assessment for cancer (individuals with highly penetrant but infrequent, germ-line genetic susceptibility to breast and colon cancers[16,17] are excellent candidates for cancer risk–reducing agents and are likely to accept some toxicity for reduced cancer risk). For individuals at more modestly increased risk (e.g., long-term, current smokers; persons with a family history of cancer; women with mammographically dense breasts), quantitative risk assessment algorithms may be useful in the future to identify optimal cancer risk–reducing agents. The refinement of cancer risk calculators for breast,[18] colon,[19] and prostate cancer[20] promises to appropriately select high-risk individuals for cancer risk–reducing agents such that anticipated benefits exceed potential risks.

Biomarkers as Cancer Risk–Reducing Agent Targets and Efficacy End Points

A biomarker is a characteristic that is measured and evaluated as an indicator of normal biologic processes, pathogenic processes, or pharmacologic responses to therapeutic interventions.[21] A surrogate end point for cancer prevention assumes that a measured biologic feature will predict the presence or future development of a cancer outcome.[22] Biomarkers enable a reduction in the size and duration of an intervention trial by replacing a rare or distal end point with a more frequent, proximate end point.[23] Intraepithelial neoplasia has served and continues to serve as a biomarker for invasive malignancy (Table 33.3). Although many advocate the use of intraepithelial neoplasia based biomarkers as regulatory surrogate end points, others caution that intraepithelial neoplasias may not serve as sufficiently robust surrogate biomarkers for cancer incidence or mortality.[24]

In order to be useful as end points for cancer risk–reducing agent efficacy testing as regulatory end points, any biomarker must have statistical accuracy, precision, and effectiveness of results[24] that demonstrate prediction of a *hard* disease end point—cancer incidence or mortality. An independent validation data set must address defined standards of validation that minimize bias in the study design and the populations studied.[25] The biomarker must be generalizable to the specific clinical or screening population (Table 33.4).

Phases of Cancer Risk–Reducing Agent Development

Phase I cancer risk–reducing agent trials define an optimal cancer risk–reducing agent dose. An optimal cancer risk–reducing agent dose is one that is usually nontoxic, scheduled once daily, and modulates a tissue, cellular, or serum biomarker of drug activity (e.g., the dose of aspirin that inhibits prostaglandin production in a target tissue site). The definition of a maximum tolerated dose is not an essential end point of a phase I cancer risk–reducing agent trial. Higher, yet nontoxic doses may lower cancer risk–reducing agent efficacy. For example, β-carotene at high doses has pro-oxidant activity and may enhance the carcinogenesis process, whereas at low doses, it is a potent antioxidant and differentiating agent.[26]

Phase II cancer risk–reducing agent trials begin to define cancer risk–reduction efficacy. These short-term (6 months to 1 year) treatment periods gather evidence of risk reduction by assessing drug effects on tissue, cellular, or blood surrogate markers of carcinogenesis. Phase IIa trials are nonrandomized, biomarker modulation trials. Phase IIb trials are randomized, placebo-controlled trials of several hundred subjects testing, for example, whether a risk-reducing agent reduces recurrence of a previously resected intraepithelial neoplastic lesion as the primary end point. Cellular dynamic

TABLE 33.3
Common Intraepithelial Neoplasias

Epithelium	Intraepithelial Neoplasia	References
Colon and rectum	Adenoma	(264)
Lower esophagus	Barrett esophagus	(265)
Upper esophagus	Squamous dysplasia	(266, 267)
Skin: Squamous/basal cell	Actinic keratosis	(268)
Skin: Pigmented	Dysplastic nevus	(269)
Cervix	Cervical intraepithelial neoplasia	(270)
Head and neck	Leukoplakia/oral epithelial dysplasia	(271)
Prostate	Prostate intraepithelial neoplasia (PIN), intraductal carcinoma of the prostate	(272)
Lung	Bronchial dysplasia	(273)
Pancreas	Pancreatic intraepithelial neoplasia	(274)

(e.g., proliferation, apoptotic index), biochemical, or molecular (e.g., p53, cyclin D) end points may be used as secondary end points. Preoperative or window of opportunity trials enroll subjects for brief study periods prior to obtaining tissue by a planned resection of an invasive neoplasm. Such designs permit the exploration of biomarker modulation in the invasive neoplasm and in contiguous epithelial fields proximal and distal to the invasive neoplasm.[27]

Phase III cancer risk–reducing agent trials define reduction in a hard cancer end point such as cancer incidence or mortality. Such trials, using large, higher risk populations in a randomized, double-blinded intervention, are designed to identify a standard of preventive care for a given risk population. For example, trials of tamoxifen for the reduction of breast cancer incidence,[28,29] finasteride for the reduction of prostate cancer incidence,[30] and β-carotene for the reduction of lung cancer incidence[31] serve as examples of well-conducted, definitive phase III cancer risk–reducing agent clinical trials.

Some investigators consider randomized, controlled clinical trials with an end point sufficient for regulatory review as phase III.

TABLE 33.4
Characteristics of Biomarkers for Use as End Points in Cancer Risk–Reducing Agent Efficacy Assessment

- Variability of expression between phases of the carcinogenesis process
- Detected early in the carcinogenesis process
- Genetic progression or protein pathway based
- Target of modulation by preventive interventions
- Changes in biomarker linked to reduction in incident cancer of epithelial target
- Changes in biomarker linked to clinical benefit
- Can be quantified directly or via closely related activity such as a downstream target or upstream kinase
- Measurable in an accessible biosample (preferably urine, serum, saliva, stool, or breath)
- High throughput, technically feasible, analytical procedure with strong quality assurance/quality control procedures
- Cost-effective

Using such a definition, a clinical trial with an end point of reduction in adenoma recurrence is considered a phase III trial. Other investigators define phase III cancer risk–reducing agent trials as randomized, controlled clinical trials with a cancer incidence or mortality end point. This controversy causes confusion in the literature. For the purpose of clarity in this textbook, the latter definition of phase III trial is used—a prospective, randomized, controlled clinical trial with a cancer incidence or mortality end point. Randomized, controlled clinical trials with a surrogate biomarker end point such as an intraepithelial neoplasia (e.g., adenoma) are defined as phase IIb cancer risk–reducing agent trials.

MICRONUTRIENTS

Definition

Micronutrients comprise a large, diverse group of molecules typically ingested as part of the diet that play roles in normal human biology. This group of compounds has been investigated extensively as cancer risk–reducing agents in purified forms (i.e., supplements), as components of multiagent cocktails, and occasionally, as components of food extracts/other mixtures. Although retinoids are not micronutrients per se, they are related to retinol (vitamin A) and share certain properties with carotenoids, which are diet derived and, therefore, included along with micronutrients.

Retinoids, Carotenoids, and Antioxidant Nutrients

Overview and Mechanisms

Retinoids are the natural derivatives and synthetic analogs of vitamin A.[32] Cancer risk–reduction intervention studies have evaluated the parent compound (retinol, typically given as retinyl acetate or palmitate), naturally occurring retinoids such as all-trans–retinoic acid (ATRA) and 13-cis-retinoic acid (13cRA), and also synthetic retinoids such as etretinate and fenretinide (4-hydroxy[phenyl]retinamide [4HPR]). These agents have been of interest for cancer risk reduction for decades. Mechanistically, retinoids have been shown to modulate cellular growth and differentiation, as well as apoptosis.[32] A large body of research indicates that retinoids have activity in the promotion and progression phases of carcinogenesis, including extensive evidence of efficacy in the setting of premalignant lesions, leading to their evaluation in human Phase III trials. Nuclear retinoic acid receptors mediate many of the retinoid-signaling effects; however, retinoids interact with other signaling pathways, such as estrogen signaling in breast cancer.[33]

Carotenoids are a group of naturally occurring plant pigments, only some of which are found in appreciable levels in the human diet and human tissues, including beta-carotene, alpha-carotene, lycopene, lutein, and β-cryptoxanthin.[34] Of these, the most widely studied carotenoids for cancer risk reduction are beta-carotene and lycopene. Beta-carotene has the highest pro–vitamin A activity of the carotenoids, but alpha-carotene and β-cryptoxanthin also possess pro–vitamin A activity. Other carotenoids, such as lycopene, do not possess vitamin A activity but are known to have potent antioxidant activity, particularly with regard to singlet oxygen quenching.[35] Furthermore, eccentric cleavage products of beta-carotene,[36] as well as other non-pro–vitamin A carotenoids such as lycopene (e.g., apocarotenals, apocarotenoic acids) appear to be biologically active and may also act via retinoid-signaling pathways.[37]

Because of the known antioxidant function of carotenoids, they are often studied for risk-reducing efficacy in combination with other antioxidant nutrients, especially vitamins E and C and selenium (sometimes as a cocktail, versus placebo). Thus, we will consider this group of nutrients first, followed by other micronutrients that are thought to act via different mechanisms and/or pathways.

Epidemiology

A large body of literature indicates that people who consume greater amounts of carotenoids from foods (primarily fruits and vegetables) and people with higher serum or plasma levels of various carotenoids have a lower risk for various cancers.[38] In particular, according to the systematic review of the literature conducted by the World Cancer Research Fund/American Institute for Cancer Research,[38] foods containing carotenoids are "probably" associated with lower risks of cancers of the mouth/pharynx/larynx and lung; foods containing beta-carotene are "probably" associated with lower risks of cancers of the esophagus; and foods containing lycopene are "probably" associated with lower risks of prostate cancer. Preformed retinol intake is inconsistently associated with risks of various cancers but that, in part, likely reflects confounding, because dietary sources of preformed retinol primarily include foods of animal origin (e.g., liver, eggs, milk). Vitamin C in the diet comes primarily from the consumption of fruits and vegetables; therefore, vitamin C and carotenoids often trend together in epidemiologic findings. Vitamin E, in contrast, is found in different foods, especially nuts, seeds, and vegetable oils; intake and blood concentrations are somewhat inconsistently associated with cancer risk.[39] Selenium, being a trace mineral, is difficult to measure in the diet, but higher selenium status has been associated with a lower risk of certain cancers, although the results are not entirely consistent.[39]

Preclinical In Vivo Models

In preclinical models, retinoids induce differentiation as well as arrest proliferation[33] of various cancers, making them attractive agents for cancer risk reduction.[40] The International Agency for Research on Cancer reviewed the preclinical research involving beta-carotene, concluding that there was sufficient evidence of cancer preventive activity, particularly involving mouse skin tumor models and the hamster buccal pouch model.[41] Notably, there was inconsistent evidence of efficacy in respiratory tract models. Lycopene has been evaluated in numerous cell culture systems and in a variety of models of prostate carcinogenesis, including chemically induced, orthotopic implantation, transgenic, and xenotransplantation, with mixed evidence of efficacy.[42] Evidence, primarily from cell culture studies, suggests that lycopene metabolites may be at least partially responsible for anticarcinogenic activity.[37]

Clinical Trials: Retinoids, Carotenoids, and Antioxidant Nutrients

Retinoids, carotenoids, and antioxidant nutrients have been evaluated in the setting of preneoplasia/neoplasia in many different organ sites, as will be discussed. Of the many clinical trials of retinoids and carotenoids/other antioxidant nutrients, key trials with cancer incidence/recurrence as primary outcomes are tabulated (see Tables 33.5 and 33.6) and reviewed.

Clinical Efficacy in the Upper Airway

Many trials of cancer risk–reducing agents have been done in the setting of squamous cell carcinomas of the head and neck, in large part because of the substantial clinical problem of relatively high rates of recurrences and second primary tumors in curatively treated cancer patients. Early work demonstrated that high-dose 13cRA (50 to 100 mg/m² per day) produced no significant differences in disease recurrence (local, regional, or distant) but significantly lowered the rate of second primary invasive neoplasms,[43] with the benefits persisting for at least 5 years.[44] Substantial retinoid toxicity, however, including skin dryness and peeling, cheilitis, conjunctivitis, and hypertriglyceridemia, was evident in a large proportion of patients. Subsequent trials thus used lower doses of retinoids (13cRA or a synthetic retinoid, etretinate), but failed to show efficacy in reducing second primary tumor formation (Table 33.5).[45,46]

Supplemental beta-carotene has also been studied as a single agent and in combination with other agents for the prevention of second primary cancers of the mouth and throat (Table 33.6). One trial of beta-carotene alone observed no harm or benefit[47]; another observed nonsignificantly fewer second head and neck cancers but more lung cancers[48]; and a third gave beta-carotene with α-tocopherol (400 IU per day).[49] In the third trial, beta-carotene was discontinued early due to adverse findings from lung cancer prevention trials (see the following); however, after a median follow-up of 6.5 years, all-cause mortality was increased, which the authors attributed to the supplemental α-tocopherol. As will be discussed later, adverse effects of antioxidant nutrients are not limited to head and neck cancer patients; potential mechanisms for adverse effects are discussed further.

Clinical Efficacy in the Lung (Lower Airway)

Reversal of Metaplasia or Dysplasia. Active smokers and recent quitters have multiple preinvasive metaplastic and dysplastic lesions in the pulmonary tree. Most of these lesions resolve upon smoking cessation, but some remain and progress to invasive neoplasms. Unfortunately, micronutrient or retinoid interventions have not demonstrated preventive efficacy in most rigorous trials in patients with early lesions. For example, a US trial randomized 755 asbestos workers to receive beta-carotene (50 mg per day) and retinol (25,000 IU every other day) versus placebo; sputum atypia was not reduced after 5 years.[50] As another example, eligible smokers with lung metaplasia or dysplasia were randomized to 6 months of 13cRA or placebo. The extent of metaplasia decreased similarly (in approximately 50% of subjects) in both study arms.[51] Only smoking cessation was associated with a significant reduction in the metaplasia index during the 6-month intervention.

Prevention of Invasive Neoplasms. Large, phase III efficacy trials of beta-carotene plus other micronutrients for primary prevention of lung cancer have been completed, as summarized in Table 33.6. The Alpha-Tocopherol, Beta-carotene (ATBC) Trial involved 29,133 men from Finland who were heavy cigarette smokers at entry.[52] In a two-by-two factorial design, participants were randomized to receive either supplemental α-tocopherol, beta-carotene, the combination, or placebo. Unexpectedly, participants receiving beta-carotene (alone or in combination with α-tocopherol) had a statistically significant 18% increase in lung cancer incidence and an 8% increase in total mortality relative to participants receiving placebo. α-Tocopherol had no effect.

The finding of an increased incidence of lung cancer in the beta-carotene–supplemented smokers was replicated in the Carotene and Retinol Efficacy Trial (CARET), a large randomized trial of supplemental beta-carotene plus retinol versus placebo in asbestos workers and smokers.[53] This trial was terminated early, but, at the time of termination, overall lung cancer incidence was increased by 28% in the supplemented subjects and total mortality was also increased by 17%. In contrast, the Physicians' Health Study (PHS) of supplemental beta-carotene versus placebo in 22,071 male US physicians reported no significant effect—positive or negative—of 12 years of supplementation of beta-carotene on total cancer, lung cancer, or cardiovascular disease (see Table 33.6).[54] Two other trials involving supplemental beta-carotene alone (the Women's Health Study[55]) or with other antioxidant nutrients (the Medical Research Council/British Heart Foundation Heart Protection Study[56]) on overall cancer incidence also failed to observe efficacy.

Prevention of Second Primary Invasive Neoplasms. EUROSCAN was a multicenter trial employing a two-by-two factorial design to test retinyl palmitate and N-acetylcysteine (also a compound with known antioxidant activity) in preventing second primary invasive neoplasms in patients with early stage cancers

TABLE 33.5

Larger, Randomized Trials of Retinoids in Human Cancer Risk Reduction with Cancer Outcomes[a,b]

Population	Drug (Dose)	End Point	Outcomes	References
United States, prior HNSCC	13cRA (50–100 mg/m²/d)	Second primary tumor	Significant reduction in second primary tumors at 32 and 55 mos; however, substantial toxicity	(43, 44)
France, prior HNSCC	Etretinate (50/25 mg/d)	Second primary tumor	No difference	(46)
United States, prior HNSCC	13cRA (30 mg/d)	Second primary tumor	No difference	(45)
Europe, prior HNSCC, NSCLC	Vitamin A (300,000/150,000 IU/d) +/− N-acetylcysteine	Second primary tumor	No difference	(57)
United States, Prior NSCLC	13cRA (30 mg/d)	Second primary tumor	No difference, but second primary tumors were lower in nonsmokers on drug but higher in smokers on drug	(58)
Italy, prior breast cancer	4HPR (200 mg/d) No treatment	Contralateral breast cancer	Nonsignificant reduction; premenopausal women did better but opposite in postmenopausal women	(60)
United States, prior BCC	13cRA (10 mg/d)	Second basal cell carcinoma	No difference	(65)
United States, prior actinic keratosis	Retinol (25,000 IU/d)	Skin cancer incidence	Reduction in squamous cell carcinomas but not basal cell carcinomas	(67)
United States, prior BCC/SCC of the skin	13cRA (5–10 mg/d) Retinol (25,000 IU/d)	Second skin cancer	No significant difference for either agent	(66)
Netherlands, renal transplant patients	Acitretin (30 mg/d)	Skin cancer	Significant reduction	(64)
United States, aggressive SCC of the skin	13cRA (1 mg/kg/d) + interferon alpha	Second primary tumors and tumor recurrences	No effect	(275)
United States, prior bladder TCC	Megadose vitamins (40,000 IU retinol/d) versus RDA vitamins	Recurrence	Significant reduction in recurrence	(73)
United States, prior bladder TCC	4HPR (200 mg/d)	Recurrence	No difference	(72)

[a]Trials of retinoids that also included beta-carotene are listed under Table 33.2 only.
[b]Versus placebo unless otherwise indicated.
HNSCC, head and neck squamous cell carcinoma; NSLC, non–small-cell lung cancer; BCC, basal cell carcinoma; TCC, transitional cell carcinoma; RDA, recommended dietary allowance.

of the head and neck or lung. None of the interventions reduced second airway primary invasive neoplasms.[57] The Lung Intergroup Trial randomized patients with surgically resected lung cancer to 13cRA versus placebo and found no significant differences between the two arms in second primary tumors.[58] Notably, smoking status modified the effect of the 13cRA intervention, which was harmful in current smokers yet beneficial in former smokers.

Thus, phase III trials of both carotenoids/antioxidants and retinoids indicate that these agents overall do not reduce the risk of developing invasive lung cancers, nor do they prevent the development of second primary invasive neoplasms. However, the finding that former smokers seemed to benefit from both 13cRA[58] and beta-carotene[53] is intriguing. Mechanistic work suggests this interaction is real rather than chance (see the following), suggesting that (1) risk-reduction in smokers is especially challenging,[59] and (2) trials in former smokers may merit consideration.

Clinical Efficacy in the Breast

Moon et al[40] first showed that fenretinide was a promising cancer risk–reducing agent for the breast, having a high therapeutic index and synergistic interaction with tamoxifen in mammary carcinogenesis model studies. This laboratory work led to a large-scale randomized trial of fenretinide (versus no treatment) for 5 years to prevent contralateral breast cancer in women aged 30 to 70 years with a history of resected early breast cancer and no prior adjuvant therapy.[60] The intervention produced no significant overall effect, although fenretinide reduced contralateral and ipsilateral breast cancer rates in premenopausal women, with an opposite (adverse) trend observed in postmenopausal women. The reduced incidence of second breast cancer in premenopausal patients persisted with longer follow-up.[61]

Retinoid X receptor (RXR)–selective retinoids are also being evaluated in preclinical and clinical studies. Ongoing work suggests that combination treatment may represent a promising new strategy to suppress both estrogen receptor–negative and estrogen receptor–positive breast tumors, and the combination of retinoids with antiestrogens may be particularly effective.[62]

Clinical Efficacy in the Skin

Retinoids have been widely studied for cancer risk–reducing efficacy in skin. Early work was done in patients who have substantial skin cancer risk either due to xeroderma pigmentosum or medication-induced immunosuppression for transplants. For example, 13cRA reduced skin cancer by 63% in patients with

TABLE 33.6
Randomized Trials of Antioxidant Nutrients in Human Cancer Risk Reduction with Cancer Outcomes[a]

Population	Drug (Dose)	End Point	Outcomes	References
United States, prior head/neck cancer	Beta-carotene (50 mg/d)	Second primary head and neck cancers	Nonsignificant reduction in second head and neck cancer, increase in lung cancer	(48)
Italy, prior head/neck cancer	Beta-carotene (75 mg/d) for 3 mos with 1 mo off	Second primary head and neck cancers	No effect on second primary tumors, nonsignificant decrease in death	(47)
Canada, prior head/neck cancer	30 mg beta-carotene/d + 400 IU vitamin E/d	Deaths	Beta-carotene discontinued, mortality increased at end of trial	(49)
Finland, male smokers	20 mg beta-carotene/d +/− 50 mg vitamin E/d	Lung cancer	Lung cancer increased with beta-carotene, no effect vitamin E	(52)
United States, smokers and asbestos workers	Beta-carotene (30 mg/d) + retinol (25,000 IU/d)	Lung cancer	Lung cancer increased with beta-carotene + vitamin A	(53)
United States, resected stage I non–small-cell lung cancer	Selenized yeast, 200 µg/d versus placebo	Second primary cancer	No effect	(276)
United States, male physicians	Beta-carotene (50 mg every other day)	Total cancer	No effect	(54)
United States, female health professionals	Beta-carotene (50 mg/ every other day)	All cancers	No effect	(55)
United Kingdom, adults at risk for coronary heart disease	20 mg beta-carotene/d + 600 mg vitamin E/d + 250 mg vitamin C/d	Total cancers	No effect	(56)
United States, prior skin cancer	50 mg beta-carotene/d	Second skin cancer	No effect	(68)
Australia	Beta-carotene (30 mg/d)	Incident squamous cell skin cancer incident basal cell skin cancer	No effect	(69)
United States, prior skin cancer	200 µg selenium/d	Second skin cancer	No effect, with longer follow-up became adverse	(70)
Linxian County, China, general population	15 mg beta-carotene/d + 30 mg vitamin E/d + 50 µg selenium/d	Stomach cancer death Esophageal cancer death	Significant decrease in stomach cancer death; no effect on esophageal cancer death	(75)
Linxian County, China, esophageal dysplasia	Multivitamin/multimineral + 15 mg beta-carotene/d	Stomach cancer death Esophageal cancer death	No effect	(78)
United States, males	200 µg selenium/d +/− 400 IU vitamin E/d	Prostate cancer incidence	No effect; with longer follow-up vitamin E became adverse	(84)
United States, male physicians II	500 mg vitamin C/d + 400 IU vitamin E every other day	Prostate cancer incidence, total cancer incidence	No effect	(86)

[a] All versus placebo.

---

xeroderma pigmentosum; however, severe, acute mucocutaneous toxicity with the 13cRA occurred.[63] Also, the preventive effect of the retinoid was lost after stopping retinoid therapy. In renal transplant patients, acitretin (30 mg per day) reduced the numbers of premalignant lesions, the number of patients with skin cancer, and the cumulative number of skin cancers.[64]

In lower risk populations, low-dose 13cRA (10 mg per day)[65] and retinol or 13cRA alone did not reduce the recurrence of basal or squamous cell skin cancers,[66] although retinol alone reduced squamous but not basal cell carcinomas in patients with prior actinic keratoses.[67]

Beta-carotene (50 mg per day), in a randomized trial did not reduce the recurrence of nonmelanoma skin cancers.[68] Consistent with findings in the lung, the risk was increased by 44% in current smokers randomized to beta-carotene but not in never smokers randomized to beta-carotene as compared with placebo.

Supplemental beta-carotene (30 mg per day) also did not prevent basal cell carcinoma or squamous cell carcinoma of the skin in an Australian trial.[69]

Clark et al.[70] randomized patients with a history of nonmelanoma skin cancer to 200 µg per day selenium or placebo.[70] Selenium did not reduce the incidence of second skin cancers; a further report of this trial with longer follow-up[71] indicated that there was instead a significant increase in total nonmelanoma skin cancer (hazard ratio [HR] = 1.17; 95% confidence interval [CI], 1.02 to 1.34) and squamous cell skin cancer (HR = 1.25; 95% CI, 1.03 to 1.51).

Clinical Efficacy in the Bladder

A trial of fenretinide (200 mg per day orally for 12 months) versus placebo was conducted for preventing tumor recurrence in patients with nonmuscle-invasive bladder transitional cell carcinoma after transurethral resection with or without adjuvant intravesical bacillus Calmette-Guérin; recurrence rates were similar in both groups.[72] Another trial randomized 65 patients with biopsy-confirmed transitional cell carcinoma of the bladder to a multivitamin (recommended dietary allowance [RDA] levels) alone or supplemented with 40,000 IU retinol, 100 mg pyridoxine, 2,000 mg ascorbic acid, 400 U of α-tocopherol, and 90 mg zinc.[73] The 5-year estimate of tumor recurrence was 91% in the RDA arm versus 41% in the higher-dose nutrient arm ($p = 0.0014$).

Clinical Efficacy in the Cervix

Randomized trials include four with beta-carotene (alone or with other antioxidant nutrients), and five with retinoids. Only one of these trials, involving ATRA,[74] found a significant treatment effect. This trial administered a 0.372% ATRA solution by collagen sponge in a cervical cap delivery system. There was a higher complete response rate in the ATRA group (43%) than the placebo group (27%; $p = 0.041$) among the 141 patients with moderate dysplasia; no significant differences in dysplasia regression rates between the two study arms were detected in patients with severe dysplasia. The investigators experienced substantial losses to follow-up in this patient population.

Clinical Efficacy in the Esophagus and Stomach

Certain regions of China (Huixian and Linxian) have strikingly high incidence rates of esophageal and gastric cancers. Two trials were done in Linxian County; one was a general population trial that tested the efficacy of four different nutrient combinations at inhibiting the development of esophageal and gastric cancers.[75] Those who were given the combination of beta-carotene, vitamin E, and selenium had a 13% reduction in total cancer deaths, a 4% reduction in esophageal cancer deaths, and a 21% reduction in gastric cancer deaths (see Table 33.6). None of the other nutrient combinations reduced gastric or esophageal cancer deaths significantly in this trial. The treatment benefit has been shown to persist for 10 years postintervention, with greater efficacy seen in participants under age 55 years.[76] This finding stands in contrast to most other antioxidant nutrient supplement intervention trials, suggesting that the applicability of these results for populations with adequate nutritional status and for other tumor sites may be limited.[77]

The other Linxian trial evaluated a multivitamin/multimineral preparation plus beta-carotene (15 mg per day) in residents with esophageal dysplasia.[78] There was no clear evidence of efficacy, although confidence intervals were wide.

Clinical Efficacy in the Colon/Rectum

Of the randomized trials aimed at the prevention of recurrent colorectal adenomas with micronutrients that have been completed, some used beta-carotene alone[79] or with other nonmicronutrient interventions.[80] Others evaluated beta-carotene with and without supplemental vitamins C and E.[81] None of the trials observed benefit with supplementation. A subsequent report from one trial noted that alcohol intake and cigarette smoking modified the efficacy of beta-carotene.[82] Among nonsmokers and nondrinkers, beta-carotene was associated with a significant decrease in the risk of one or more recurrent adenomas (relative risk [RR] = 0.56). Among persons who smoked and also drank more than one alcoholic drink per day, beta-carotene significantly increased the risk of recurrent adenoma (RR = 2.07).

Clinical Efficacy in the Prostate

Because oxidative stress may play a role in the etiology of prostate cancer, several antioxidant nutrients, including vitamin E, selenium, and lycopene, have been of interest for preventing prostate cancer. The largest trial to date of these nutrients is the Selenium and Vitamin E Cancer Prevention Trial (SELECT), which tested selenium and vitamin E in a two-by-two factorial design for the primary prevention of prostate cancer. Despite preliminary indications of prostate cancer risk–reducing efficacy for selenium (from a trial of selenium for skin cancer[70]) and vitamin E (from a trial of vitamin E to prevent lung cancer[83]), there was no evidence of efficacy.[84] With extended follow-up, the nonsignificant adverse effect of vitamin E became significantly adverse.[85] Negative/neutral findings also were reported for vitamins E and C and prostate and total cancer in the PHS II randomized controlled trial.[86]

The carotenoid lycopene has generated much interest with regard to prostate cancer risk, and several intervention trials have been conducted based on lycopene supplements. These studies have been small, short term, based on intermediate end points, and often lack adequate control groups. The use of a tomato sauce–based intervention is arguably a better approach to evaluate, based on animal data indicating that tomato powder (which includes lycopene along with other phytochemicals), but not lycopene alone, was effective at inhibiting prostate carcinogenesis.[87]

Mechanisms for Ineffective Retinoid and Carotenoid Cancer Risk–Reducing Activity

There are now a number of trials demonstrating that supplemental beta-carotene/retinoids given to current smokers can produce increases rather than reductions in cancer incidence. In tobacco users, beta-carotene and other carotenoids may produce oxidative carotenoid breakdown products that alter retinoid metabolism and signaling pathways, along with pro-oxidation.[88] For retinoids such as 13cRA, smoking may induce genetic and epigenetic changes in the lung that affect retinoid activity; for example, tobacco smoking can affect RAR-β expression.[58] The adverse effects of supplemental nutrients are not limited to smokers; α-tocopherol increased rather than reduced prostate cancer in SELECT (which had relatively few smokers) and selenium increased prostate cancer among men without a baseline selenium deficiency.[89] This may be a consequence of the relatively high doses used in SELECT,[77] but certainly calls into question the notion that reducing oxidative stress is a pivotal cancer risk–reduction strategy, even in nonsmokers.

It has become clear that reactive oxygen species (ROS), such as hydrogen peroxide, can act as important physiologic regulators of intracellular signaling pathways.[90,91] Data in mouse models have shown that vitamin E accelerates lung tumor growth by disrupting the ROS–p53 axis, potentially by removing oxidative damage to DNA, which can serve as a potent stimulus for p53 activation.[92] Although some of the large cancer risk–reducing trials may have failed in their primary objective, they may indirectly contribute to a clearer understanding of cancer biology, leading to the recognition that the role of oxidative stress and ROS in human disease is much more nuanced than originally hypothesized.[93]

As for the retinoids, these agents are generally too toxic to be used as single agents for risk-reducing efficacy; however, a major area of ongoing research is examining retinoids (low doses) given in combination with other agents, especially those that regulate the epigenome, such histone deacetylase (HDAC) inhibitors.[33]

Folic Acid and Other B Vitamins

Overview and Mechanisms. Folate is a water-soluble B vitamin found in foods, whereas folic acid is the synthetic form found in supplements and fortified foods. Adequate folate is critical for DNA methylation, repair, and synthesis.[94,95] The methylation status of genes can play a key role in gene silencing and gene expression, lending plausibility to the idea that folate could be a key nutrient in regulating cell growth and proliferation.

Epidemiology. Epidemiologic studies have linked low folate intake with higher risk of several cancers, most notably colorectal cancer.[96] Long-term use of multivitamin supplements, which are a major source of folate and other B vitamins, has been associated with a reduction in the risk of colon cancer in some studies, including recent (postfortification) findings.[97–99] Supporting an anticancer role of folate is that genotypes for methylene tetrahydrofolate reductase, an enzyme known to be involved in folate metabolism, predict the risk of colon cancer dependent on folate intake or status.[100] Vitamin B_6 has been less studied in relation to cancer than folate, but some epidemiologic studies suggest that vitamin B_6 may be important for colorectal cancer.[101,102] A higher risk of cancer related to deficiencies of these vitamins has been suggested for alcohol drinkers.[103]

Clinical Trials: Folic Acid and B Vitamins. Risk-reducing efficacy for supplemental folic acid has been primarily evaluated in the setting of prevention of recurrent colorectal adenomas (i.e., in patients with prior adenomas). Of six randomized trials of folic acid, two small trials reported suggestions of benefit of folic acid supplementation.[104,105] However, benefits were not observed in two much larger trials, the Aspirin/Folate Polyp Prevention Study (AFPPS) (dose: 1 mg of folic acid daily)[106] and the United Kingdom Colorectal Adenoma Prevention (ukCAP) trial (dose: 500 μg of folic acid daily).[107] AFPPS found indications of an increased risk for advanced lesions and multiple adenomas with prolonged treatment and follow-up. A third large trial, the Nurses Health Study/Health Professionals Follow-up Study (NHS/HPFS) folic acid polyp prevention trial, showed no overall risk reduction.[108] The most recent trial, done in a Chinese population >50 years of age,[109] reported that 1 mg folic acid per day reduced sporadic colorectal adenomas when compared to no intervention (not a placebo-controlled study). One possible explanation for the discrepancy of the Chinese trial versus North American and European trials is the baseline plasma folate status. In the Chinese trial, the mean baseline folate concentration of 5 ng/mL[109] was half of the reported 10 ng/mL in a United States trial,[106] where folate fortification of the food supply occurs.

Calcium and Vitamin D

Overview and Mechanisms. There are two major forms of vitamin D: ergocalciferol (D_2) and cholecalciferol (D_3). Vitamin D_2 is absorbed through dietary sources such as fortified milk products, and D_3 is synthesized via ultraviolet (UV) B light isomerization of 7-dehydrocholesterol in the epidermis.[110] Vitamin D_3 is converted to calcitriol (1, 25-$[OH]_2$ D_3) in a two-step process requiring both hepatic and renal hydroxylation. Calcitriol binds to the vitamin D receptor, which translocates to the nucleus and binds to multiple gene promoter sites. Through this mechanism, vitamin D regulates cytoplasmic signaling pathways that impact cellular differentiation and growth through proteins such as Ras and mitogen-activated protein kinase (MAPK), protein lipase A, prostaglandins, cyclic adenosine monophosphate (AMP), protein kinase A, and phosphatidyl inositol 3 kinase.[110] 1,25$(OH)_2D_3$ regulates cellular proliferation and apoptosis. For example, 1,25$(OH)_2D_3$ can induce cleavage of caspase 3, poly (ADP-ribose) polymerase (PARP), and MAPK, leading to apoptosis. 1,25$(OH)_2D_3$ inhibits the expression and phosphorylation of Akt, a key regulator of cellular proliferation. The differentiation properties of 1,25$(OH)_2D_3$ are mediated through transcriptional activation of the CDK inhibitor p21. The effects of vitamin D on multiple signal transduction pathways operational in cancer cells are reviewed by Deeb et al.[111]

Epidemiology. Observational epidemiologic studies have shown a relatively consistent inverse association between low calcium intake, including that from supplements, and increased colorectal and colon cancer risk.[112,113] Vitamin D exposure is typically assessed by measuring 25(OH)vitamin D in plasma, but also exposure is derived not only from diet and supplements, but also from cutaneous synthesis following dermal exposure to UV radiation. A large number of observational studies have evaluated the association between vitamin D status and cancer risk, as systematically reviewed by the Agency for Healthcare Research and Quality (AHRQ).[114] The evidence is inconsistent for most cancer sites, with the exception of studies showing that individuals with lower blood vitamin D levels have a higher risk of colorectal cancer or adenoma. Although some observational studies have reported that higher serum vitamin D is associated with lower breast cancer risk, the association is inconsistent.[114,115] Also, there are some studies suggesting high serum vitamin D is associated with increases in certain cancers, particularly pancreatic cancer.[116]

Clinical Trials: Calcium and Vitamin D

Clinical Efficacy in the Colon. Baron et al.[117] randomized subjects with a recent history of colorectal adenomas to either calcium carbonate (1,200 mg per day of elemental calcium) or placebo. Results showed significant benefit for the calcium arm (adjusted RR = 0.81; 95% CI, 0.67 to 0.99; $p = 0.04$). In a smaller, similar study of calcium gluconolactate and carbonate (2 g elemental calcium daily), the adjusted odds ratio (OR) for adenoma recurrence was 0.66 (95% CI, 0.38 to 1.17; $p = 0.16$) for calcium treatment,[118] and while not statistically significant, it was similar to the data of Baron et al.[117]

In the largest trial of calcium and vitamin D with primary cancer end points (e.g., colon, breast), the US Women's Health Initiative (WHI) evaluated the combination of 400 IU of vitamin D per day plus 1,000 mg of calcium per day in 36,282 postmenopausal women. For colon cancer, there was no benefit observed,[119] although the mean baseline intake of calcium was already very high (more than 1,151 mg per day). With regard to vitamin D as a single agent, there was also no suggestion of benefit for colon cancer incidence in a 5-year British trial of vitamin D (100,000 IU every 4 months) that reported colon cancer incidence,[120] although this was not a primary end point.

Clinical Efficacy in the Breast. Vitamin D has received considerable attention for a possible role in the prevention of breast cancer,[121] although no trials have yet investigated vitamin D as a single agent for breast cancer risk reduction. The large WHI trial gave a combination of calcium and vitamin D, as noted previously, and there was no significant effect of this combination on breast cancer risk (HR, 0.96; 95% CI, 0.85 to 1.09).[122] Lappe et al.[123] conducted a trial that examined the relation between calcium plus vitamin D (1,100 IU per day) supplementation (versus calcium alone or placebo) in 1,179 healthy postmenopausal women in Nebraska.[123] Although fracture was the primary outcome of the trial, total cancer incidence was reportedly lower in the calcium plus vitamin D group, although the number of end points was very small (n = 50 total cancers observed during the follow-up). An ongoing randomized trial of vitamin D and omega-3 fatty acids (the VITamin D and OmegA-3 TriaL [VITAL]) among 20,000 participants is expected to provide more definitive data on a possible role of vitamin D in the prevention of breast and other cancers.[124]

Summary and Conclusion: Micronutrients

Certain agents, including the retinoids, beta-carotene, folic acid, calcium plus vitamin D, vitamin E, and selenium, have received substantial attention for a possible role in reducing the risk of cancer in humans. As reviewed herein, some of the trials have observed statistically significant reductions in the risk of the primary end point (e.g., retinoids in skin carcinogenesis models, calcium in colorectal adenomas, antioxidant nutrients in Linxian, China, for gastric cancer prevention), whereas others have observed statistically significant increases in the risk of the primary end points (beta-carotene and retinoid lung cancer prevention trials in smokers, vitamin E and prostate cancer, selenium and nonmelanoma skin cancer). Considering the completed trials, there is clear evidence against the general use of nutrient *supplements* for cancer prevention, which is the conclusion also reached by the World Cancer Research Fund/American Institute for Cancer Research.[38] Note that there is no evidence that food sources of these nutrients increase risk.

Having noted that, there are other key themes emerging from this growing body of research. One such theme is that nutrient supplementation may be of benefit to some but not all. One such population that may benefit includes persons who are low in the nutrient of interest at baseline.[77] This was initially suggested in the Linxian County trial (done in a micronutrient-deficient population), with growing support from subgroup analyses of several completed trials.[77] However, the hypothesis that nutrient supplementation can reduce cancer risk in subgroups selected based on inadequate nutritional status has, to date, not been formally evaluated in intervention trials.

Another consistent theme is that lifestyle factors (e.g., smoking) and genetics (polymorphisms) may determine who is most likely to benefit from supplementation. Trial data will likely be increasingly mined to identify genetic profiles associated with both better outcomes (risk prediction) and response to intervention.[125,126] Ultimately, a more personalized approach to cancer risk reduction may emerge, consistent with the movement toward a more personalized approach for cancer treatment.

Finally, nearly all of these trials initiate intervention with older adults (who are more likely to develop cancer end points during the follow-up); but, animal models suggest that the timing of exposure may likely be quite relevant. For example, folic acid may protect against initiation, but may also promote the proliferation of existing neoplasms.[127] Thus, the dose, form (food versus supplement), timing, and nutritional and lifestyle characteristics may all be relevant in affecting the efficacy of risk-reducing interventions involving nutrients and related substances. Further research, drawing upon newer tools now available through the field of nutritional genomics, will be needed to gain greater clarity on the heterogeneous biologic effects observed in nutrient-based risk reduction.

ANTI-INFLAMMATORY DRUGS

Mechanism

Nonsteroidal anti-inflammatory drugs (NSAIDs) represent a class of drugs that reduce cellular inflammation through multiple mechanisms, the most prominent of them being the modulation of eicosanoid metabolism.[128] Eicosanoids are metabolites of dietary fatty acids, primarily linoleic acid. Linoleic acid is metabolized to arachidonic acid, which is stored in the lipid membrane and, once mobilized from the membrane, further metabolized by prostaglandin-H synthases (PGHS) 1 and 2 to PGD_2, PGE_2, $PGF_{2\alpha}$, PGI_2, or thromboxane A_2 (TxA_2) by specific syntheses. Leukotriene pathways involve the conversion of arachidonic acid to leukotriene A_4 by 5-lipoxygenase and subsequent hydrolysis of leukotriene A_4 to other downstream leukotrienes. Newly formed prostaglandins function primarily through binding to prostaglandin receptors (EP receptors), releasing coupled G-proteins to elicit responses in the same or neighboring cells.[129]

Prostaglandins (PG) play crucial roles in controlling cellular proliferation, apoptosis, cellular invasiveness, and angiogenesis and in modulating immunosuppression.[129] Because PGE_2 is the most abundant PG in tumors, reducing local concentrations of PGE_2 may be a pivotal cancer preventive strategy.[129]

PGHS-independent mechanisms of NSAID action may, at least in part, explain NSAID preventive efficacy.[130] A diverse group of NSAIDs inhibit apoptosis via multiple mechanisms. Among the more prominent of these mechanisms is the inhibition of cyclic guanosine monophosphate (cGMP) phosphodiesterase activity, attenuation of beta-catenin mRNA through suppressing transcription of the CTNNB1 gene, and activation of c-Jun N-terminal kinase 1.[130] NSAIDs activate peroxisome proliferator–activated receptor (PPAR)γ, leading to increased E-cadherin expression and reduced colony formation in vitro, while reducing PPARδ, leading to reduced resistance to apoptosis.[130] Selective cyclooxygenase 2 (COX-2) inhibitors inhibit Akt signaling and induce apoptosis of human colorectal and prostate cancer cells in vitro in a COX-2–independent manner via the inhibition of phosphoinositide-dependent kinase-1 (PDK-1). NSAIDs inhibit nuclear factor kappa B (NF-κB) at pharmacologic concentrations and key cellular proliferation signaling intermediates such as activator protein 1 (AP-1) and other intermediates of the MAPK pathway.[130] The impact of NSAIDs on carcinogenic events driven by these upstream pathways in humans as opposed to preliminary in vitro or in vivo models remains unclear.

Epidemiology

Pooled analyses of 34 controlled trials of aspirin 75 mg to 100 mg daily (69,224 participants), conducted primarily for cardiovascular disease reduction, observed reduced cancer deaths (OR, 0.63; 95% CI, 0.49 to 0.82). Most of the benefit occurred after 5 years follow-up.[131] In a pooled analysis of 150 case control and 45 cohort studies, in addition to a reduced risk of death from colorectal cancer (OR, 0.58; 95% CI, 0.44 to 0.78), chronic and frequent (once daily or more) use of aspirin also reduced the risk of death from esophageal (OR, 0.58; 95% CI, 0.44 to 0.76), gastric (OR, 0.61; 95% CI, 0.40 to 0.93), and breast (OR, 0.81; 95% CI, 0.72 to 0.93) cancers.[132] An analysis of 662,624 men and women enrolled in the American Cancer Society's Cancer Prevention Study II found that aspirin taken at least 16 times per month over a 6-year period conferred a 40% reduced risk of colorectal cancer mortality.[133] Both the 46,363 male patients of the Health Professional Study[134] and the 82,911 patients of the Nurse's Health Study[135] suggest that prolonged use (>10 years) of 325 mg of aspirin twice weekly or more reduces colorectal cancer risk (RR, 0.77; 95% CI, 0.67 to 0.88, from the Nurse's Health Study). Daily NSAID intake is associated with a 40% reduction (OR, 0.56; 95% CI, 0.43 to 0.73) in the risk of esophageal adenocarcinoma.[136]

Evidence in Preclinical In Vivo Carcinogenesis Models

NSAIDs, including aspirin, indomethacin, piroxicam, sulindac, ibuprofen, and ketoprofen, suppress colonic tumorigenesis induced chemically (1,2-dimethylhydrazine or its metabolites) or transgenically (Min+).[137,138] The selective COX-2 inhibitors were the most efficacious colon tumorigenesis inhibitors in both chemical and transgenic rodent models.[139,140] In preclinical models, NSAIDs affect the onset and progression of cancers in the stomach, skin, breast, lung, prostate, and urinary bladder, although the evidence is more limited than for colon cancers.[141]

Clinical Trials

Key clinical trials of NSAIDs for the prevention of colorectal cancer are summarized in Table 33.7. Sulindac reduced the size and number of preexisting adenomas in patients with familial adenomatous polyposis but did not suppress the development of new adenomas,[142] whereas the selective COX-2 inhibitor, celecoxib, suppressed the development of new adenomatous polyps in patients with familial adenomatous polyposis.[143] Although these results are promising, reports of invasive neoplasms developing in familial adenomatous polyposis patients being treated with sulindac[144] raise the question of whether NSAIDs preferentially alter the formation or regression of those adenomas less likely to progress to invasive adenocarcinomas, as compared to those more likely to progress.

Randomized, double-blinded placebo controlled trials of NSAIDs as cancer risk reducing agents for colorectal adenocarcinoma (see Table 33.7) have confirmed that aspirin suppresses

TABLE 33.7
Summary of Clinical Trials of Nonsteroidal Anti-Inflammatory Drugs as Colorectal Cancer Risk–Reducing Agents

Population	Drug (Dose), Duration	Phase	Endpoint	Outcome	References
Gene Associated					
Familial adenomatous polyposis (FAP)	Sulindac (300–400 mg/d, divided doses)	IIb	Polyp regression	Colorectal and duodenal polyps regressed in ~50%	(277, 278) (279)
Hereditary nonpolyposis colon cancer (Lynch syndrome)	Aspirin 600 mg/d, resistant starch	III	Cancer	≥2 yr, hazard ratio (HR) colon cancer 0.41; 95% CI, 0.19–0.86; all cancers incidence rate ratio 0.37, 95% CI, 0.18–0.78; no effect of starch	(280, 281)
Sporadic Risk					
Previous adenomatous polyps, healthy subjects	Aspirin (40, 81, 325, 650 mg once per day)	I, IIa	Dose-biomarker	Aspirin dose of 81 mg daily sufficient to suppress colorectal mucosal prostaglandin E_2	(282–284)
Previous adenomatous polyps	Sulindac (300 mg), 4 mos	IIb	Polyp regression	Sulindac did not significantly decrease the number or size of polyps	(146)
Previous adenomatous polyps	Piroxicam (7.5 mg), 2 yr	IIb	Polyp recurrence	Colorectal mucosal PGE_2 reduced in piroxicam treated arm, unacceptable toxicity	(145)
Prior colorectal cancer	Aspirin (325 mg once per day), 3 yr	IIb	Polyp recurrence	Aspirin use associated with delayed development of adenomatous polyps	(285)
Previous adenomatous polyps	Aspirin (81 mg once per day or 325 mg once per day) and/or folate, 3 yr	IIb	Polyp recurrence	Low-dose aspirin reduced the recurrence of adenomatous polyps	(286)
Previous adenomatous polyps	Celecoxib and rofecoxib	IIb	Polyp recurrence	Celecoxib and rofecoxib reduced the recurrence of adenomatous polyps, unacceptable toxicity	(148–150)

adenoma recurrence in patients previously treated for adenomas or for cancer. Neither sulindac nor piroxicam alone suppressed adenoma formation in high-risk, sporadic populations at tolerable doses.[145,146] Sulindac, in combination with difluoromethylornithine, has potent colorectal anticarcinogenesis effects.[147] Selective COX-2 inhibitors (celecoxib, rofecoxib) reduce the recurrence of adenomas by one-third in all patients previously treated for adenomas and by one-half in patients with previously resected large (≥1 cm) adenomas,[148–150] but they are too toxic as cancer risk–reducing agents due to their cardiovascular toxicity.[151,152] Although most NSAIDs (piroxicam, indomethacin) have sufficient gastrointestinal (GI) toxicity to reduce their acceptability as cancer risk–reducing agents,[153,154] the long-term administration of low-dose aspirin in vascular prevention trials demonstrates acceptable GI toxicity.[155]

Up to 40% of individuals screened for colorectal neoplasms will have an adenomatous polyp detected and removed, yet only 10% of these lesions will progress to invasive neoplasms. To date, prospective NSAID trials of only 2 to 3 years cannot substitute for cancer incidence or mortality end points. Given the 10-year latency between adenoma formation and a cancer event, prospective trials sufficiently powered to detect colorectal cancer incidence end points are unlikely in the future.[156] Alternatively, a follow-up of patients randomized on trials of aspirin in the prevention of vascular events in the 1980s and 1990s offers secondary analysis opportunities. In a pooled analysis of three prospective vascular end point cohort studies, 20-year low-dose aspirin treatments reduced cancer deaths from all solid tumors (OR, 0.69; CI, 0.54 to 0.88) and from lung and esophageal adenocarcinomas (OR, 0.66; CI, 0.56 to 0.77).[155] Despite this, the U.S. Preventive Services Task Force (USPSTF) does not recommend the use of aspirin or NSAIDs as cancer risk–reducing agents for normal risk populations, preferring adherence to colorectal cancer screening recommendations (fecal occult blood testing and endoscopy).[153,154,157]

Minimal prospective cancer risk reduction data are available at other epithelial organ sites. Ketorolac, given as a 1% rinse solution, did not reduce the size or histology of leukoplakia lesions.[158] Celecoxib reduces the Ki67 labeling index and increases the expression of nuclear survivin without significantly changing the cytoplasmic survivin in bronchial biopsies of smokers.[159] Cancer prevention trials of aspirin as interventions for delaying progression from intraepithelial neoplasias in other epithelial sites remain ongoing for the lower esophagus.[136] No prospective, randomized trials or data are available for breast, prostate, or gynecologic cancer prevention.

EPIGENETIC TARGETING AGENTS (SELECTIVE ESTROGEN RECEPTOR MODULATORS, 5α-STEROID REDUCTASE INHIBITORS, POLYAMINE INHIBITORS)

Posttranslational pathway targets remain a fertile source of chemopreventive strategies. Phase III data support cancer risk–reduction agent efficacy of selective estrogen receptor modulators (SERM) and 5α-steroid reductase inhibitors for breast and prostate cancer prevention, respectively. Inhibitors of the polyamine pathway may be useful preventives for colorectal cancer.

Selective Estrogen Receptor Modulators

Mechanism

SERMs function as estrogen receptor (ER) agonists and antagonists depending on the SERM structure and target tissue. Predominant ERα receptors occur in the human uterus, cortical bone, and the liver; whereas predominant ERβ receptors occur in blood vessels, cancellous bone, the whole brain, and immune cells.[160,161] During carcinogenesis, the amount of ERα increases while the amount of ERβ decreases in breast tissues.[162] Ideally, a desirable SERM for cancer prevention will function as an antiestrogen in the breast and uterus, but a partial estrogen agonist in skeletal, cardiovascular, central nervous system (CNS), GI tract, and vaginal tissues. In addition, an ideal SERM will not have procoagulant effects and will not cause perimenopausal symptoms such as hot flashes.[162]

Tamoxifen. Tamoxifen is a triphenylethylene compound developed for the treatment of ER-positive breast cancer in the 1960s and 1970s.[163,164] Tamoxifen inhibits the initiation and promotion phases of breast carcinogenesis in the dimethylbenzanthracene chemical carcinogenesis model.[164,165] When tamoxifen binds to ERβ, which then binds to an AP-1 type gene promoter, it functions as an estrogen agonist. When bound to ERα, which binds to an estrogen response element (ERE) target gene promoter, tamoxifen functions as an estrogen antagonist.[162,166] Tamoxifen has estrogen antagonist effects in the human breast; partial estrogen agonist effects in bone, the cardiovascular system, and CNS; and predominant estrogen agonist effects in the uterus, liver, and vagina. The estrogen agonist effects in the liver and uterus result in tamoxifen's toxicities of thromboembolism and endometrial cancer, respectively. The clinical finding that tamoxifen reduces the incidence of contralateral second primary breast cancers during adjuvant treatment regimens catalyzed the push for its development as a cancer risk–reduction agent.[167,168]

Raloxifene. The benzothiophene structure of raloxifene confers a different tissue-specific ER-binding profile than the triphenylethylene tamoxifen. Raloxifene has greater estrogen agonist activity in bone but reduced estrogen agonist activity in the uterus. Raloxifene was studied for the treatment and prevention of osteoporosis in a large, pivotal trial (the Multiple Outcomes of Raloxifene Evaluation [MORE]) and was found to reduce the rate of vertebral fracture as compared to placebo in postmenopausal women.[169]

Lasofoxifene and Arzoxifene. Lasofoxifene and arzoxifene are third-generation SERMs developed as more potent blockers of bone resorption with the goal of reducing the risk of fractures, breast cancer, and heart disease while minimizing the SERM-induced risk of endometrial hyperplasia in postmenopausal women. Both agents proved potent in vitro and in preliminary clinical trials for bone fracture prevention.[170–173]

Selective Estrogen Receptor Modulators as Risk-Reducing Agents for Breast Cancer Prevention

Efficacy. Table 33.8 summarizes the phase III data for SERM-based breast cancer–risk reduction. In a systematic review of MEDLINE and Cochrane databases through December, 2012, the USPSTF identified seven trials of tamoxifen or raloxifene that showed a reduced incidence of invasive breast cancer by 7 to 9 cases in 1,000 women over 5 years compared to placebo.[174] Tamoxifen is more effective than raloxifene; it reduces breast cancer incidence more than raloxifene by 5 cases in 1,000 women. Both drugs reduce the incidence of ER-positive breast cancer, but neither reduces the risk of ER-negative breast cancer. Neither drug reduced breast cancer–specific or all cause mortality rates. Based on benefit–risk models, women with estimated 5-year risks of breast cancer of 3% or greater are likely to benefit from treatment.[175] Using similar

TABLE 33.8

Phase III, Randomized, Controlled Clinical Trials of SERMs for the Prevention of Breast Cancer

Study	Drug and Daily Dose	N =	Treatment Duration (Years)	Entry Criteria	Overall Outcome HR (95% CI)	References
NSABP P-1	Tamoxifen 20 mg Placebo	13,388	5	Gail model: 5 yr predicted risk of ≥1.66%	0.52 (0.42–0.64)	(28,287)
IBIS-I	Tamoxifen 20 mg Placebo	7,139	5	>Twofold relative risk	0.72 (0.58–0.90)	(288)
Marsden	Tamoxifen 20 mg Placebo	2,471	8	Family history	0.87 (0.63–1.21)	(289)
Italian	Tamoxifen 20 mg Placebo	5,408	5	Normal risk, hysterectomy	0.67 (0.59–0.76)	(290)
NSABP P-2 (STAR)	Raloxifene 60 mg Tamoxifen 20 mg	19,747	5	Gail model: 5 yr predicted risk of ≥1.66%	RR Raloxifene versus tamoxifen 1.02 (0.81–1.28)	(29)
MORE/CORE	Raloxifene 60 mg Placebo Raloxifene 120 mg Placebo	7,705 6,511	5	Normal risk, postmenopausal with osteoporosis	0.42 (0.29–0.60)	(291,292)
RUTH	Raloxifene 60 mg Placebo	10,101	5	Normal risk, postmenopausal with risk of coronary heart disease	0.67 (0.47–0.96)	(179)
PEARL	Lasofoxifene 0.5 mg Lasofoxifene 0.25 mg Placebo	8,856	5	Normal risk, postmenopausal, with osteoporosis	0.25 mg: 0.82 (0.45–1.49) 0.5 mg: 0.21 (0.08–0.55)	(170)
GENERATIONS	Arzoxifene 20 mg Placebo	9,354	4	Normal risk, postmenopausal, with osteoporosis	0.42 (0.26–0.68)	(172)

Table and data adapted from Cuzick J, Sestak I, Bonanni B, et al. Selective oestrogen receptor modulators in prevention of breast cancer: an updated meta-analysis of individual participant data. *Lancet* 2013;381:1827–1834.

analysis methods as the USPSTF, the American Society of Clinical Oncology recommends the use of tamoxifen (20 mg per day orally for 5 years) or raloxifene (60 mg per day orally for 5 years) "in premenopausal women who are age ≥35 years with a 5-year projected absolute breast cancer risk ≥1.66% according to the NCI Breast Cancer Risk Assessment Tool (or equivalent measures), or with lobular carcinoma in situ."[176] Tamoxifen reduces the risk of in situ (preinvasive) breast neoplasms (lobular carcinoma in situ, ductal carcinoma in situ) by 50%.[177,178] The reduction during treatment persists for at least 5 years after treatment.[177,178] Raloxifene does not reduce the risk of in situ breast neoplasms.

Data from two trials designed to evaluate the safety and efficacy of lasofoxifene (PEARL)[170,171] and arzoxifene (GENERATIONS)[172,173] as bone fracture preventives have been analyzed for breast cancer–risk reduction. Their effect at reducing breast cancer incidence was captured in secondary analyses (see Table 33.8). Neither lasofoxifene nor arzoxifene have been evaluated in phase III randomized controlled breast cancer prevention trials. Arzoxifene development has been discontinued in the United States.

Toxicity Profiles. Tamoxifen causes a twofold increase in the risk of endometrial adenocarcinoma (RR, 2.13; 95% CI, 1.36 to 3.32) and is related to more benign gynecologic conditions, uterine bleeding, and surgical procedures than the placebo controls, whereas raloxifene did not increase the risk for endometrial cancer or uterine bleeding.[174] Tamoxifen causes a twofold increase in thrombotic embolic events (RR, 1.93; 95% CI, 1.41 to 2.64), whereas raloxifene causes a 60% increase in risk of venous thromboembolism (RR, 1.60; 95% CI, 1.15 to 2.23).[174] Raloxifene does not differ from tamoxifen in risk of fractures, other cancers, or cardiovascular events.[177] Raloxifene's lower risk of endometrial adenocarcinomas compared to tamoxifen needs to be weighed against the increased risk of stroke seen in in the MORE/CORE trials (see Table 33.8).[179] Raloxifene's effectiveness in the community may also be compromised by its poor bioavailability (2%) due to rapid phase II enzyme metabolism in the gut and liver,[180] whereas tamoxifen is more bioavailable and has active metabolites that permit a prolonged drug effect. Missed raloxifene doses may potentially compromise efficacy and prevention outcomes in widespread, community use.

Aromatase Inhibitors. In adjuvant clinical trials for breast cancer, aromatase inhibitors (anastrozole, exemestane, letrozole) given after 5 years of tamoxifen enhance the reduction of breast cancer recurrence in the contralateral breast compared to tamoxifen alone.[181] In a phase I cancer risk–reducing agent trial, letrozole reduced the Ki-67 proliferation index of breast epithelial cells aspirated from high-risk women.[182] Exemestane reduced the overall risk of ER-positive invasive breast cancer (Table 33.9). It did not reduce the risk of noninvasive breast neoplasms or ER-negative breast cancer.[183] Exemestane has no increased risk of venous thromboembolism, endometrial cancer, fracture, or cataract,[183] but losses in bone mineral density and cortical thickness of the distal tibia and radius occurred after 2 years of treatment despite calcium and vitamin D supplementation.[184] The results of the International Breast Cancer Intervention Study II (IBIS-II), comparing anastrozole with placebo, are similar to those reported for exemestane.[185] Compared to exemestane, anastrozole decreases the incidence of ductal carcinoma in situ (DCIS), whereas exemestane does not. Neither aromatase inhibitor increased survival compared to placebo controls. The American Society of Clinical Oncology recommends exemestane for breast cancer prevention in addition to tamoxifen and raloxifene.

Use Counseling. Despite the widespread evidence of breast cancer preventive efficacy for tamoxifen and raloxifene, only 3% to 20% of eligible high-risk women agree to take tamoxifen for primary prevention.[186] The low willingness of eligible women to take tamoxifen for 5 years demonstrates the issue of risk benefit for cancer risk–reducing agents. Women with high short-term risk (5 year Gail risk of >3%)—for example, those with ER-positive atypical hyperplasia, lobular carcinoma in situ, and the majority of non–high-grade ductal carcinoma in situ lesions—have an acceptable risk to benefit ratio and are the most likely to benefit from a 5-year cancer risk–reducing agent intervention with a SERM.[175,176] The toxicity profile of aromatase inhibitors differs from SERMs. Although aromatase inhibitors may have a more favorable risk to benefit profile than SERMs, long-term outcomes and toxicity experience for aromatase inhibitor risk-reducing agent intervention are not available to date. In the National Surgical Adjuvant Breast and Bowel Project, tamoxifen-treated women with a *BRCA2* mutation but not a *BRCA1* mutation had reduced cancer incidence,[187] but subsequent data from another group have found reduced cancer risk in women with both BRCA mutations.[188] Data remain insufficient to recommend the use of SERMs for risk reduction in women with BRCA mutations.

5α-Steroid Reductase Inhibitors

Mechanism

Prostate cancers require androgens to proliferate and evade apoptosis. The primary nuclear androgen responsible for the maintenance of epithelial function is dihydrotestosterone. The testes and adrenal gland synthesize dihydrotestosterone by the conversion of testosterone by 5α-steroid reductase types 1 and 2 isozymes. Dihydrotestosterone binds to intracellular androgen receptors to form a complex that binds to DNA hormone response elements controlling cellular proliferation and apoptosis. Finasteride, a selective, competitive inhibitor of type 2 5α-steroid reductase,[189] inhibits proliferation in the transformed prostate cell. In the 3,2′-dimethyl-4-aminobiphenyl (DMAB), methylnitrosourea (MNU), and testosterone chemical carcinogenesis models in rats, finasteride reduces prostate tumor incidence by close to six-fold. Finasteride appears to be more effective in the promotion phase of prostate carcinogenesis.[190] Dutasteride inhibits both 5α-steroid reductase inhibitor[190] types 1 and 2 isoforms and has similar anticarcinogenesis activity in preclinical models to finasteride.

TABLE 33.9

Phase III, Randomized, Controlled Clinical Trials of Aromatase Inhibitors for the Prevention of Breast Cancer

Study	Drug and Daily Dose	N =	Treatment Duration (Years)	Entry Criteria	Overall Outcome HR (95% CI)	References
MAP.3	Exemestane 25 mg Placebo	4,560	5	Gail model 5 yr predicted risk of ≥2.3%	0.35 (0.18–0.70)	(183)
IBIS-II	Anastrozole 1 mg Placebo	3,851	5	RR twofold higher than general population or Tyrer-Cuzick 10-yr risk >5%	0.47 (0.32–0.68)	(185)

TABLE 33.10
Phase III, Randomized, Controlled Clinical Trials of 5α-Steroid Reductase Inhibitors for the Prevention of Prostate Cancer

Study	Drug and Daily Dose	N =	Treatment Duration (Years)	Entry Criteria	Overall Outcome HR (95% CI)	References
PCPT	Finasteride 5 mg Placebo	18,880	7	Age ≥55 y, PSA ≤3 ng/mL	0.70 (0.65–0.76)	(30, 193)
REDUCE	Dutaseride 0.5 mg Placebo	6,729	4	Age 50–75 y, PSA 2.5–10.0 ng/mL, core biopsies within 6 mos	RR = 0.77 (0.70–0.85)	(192)

PSA, prostate specific antigen.

Cancer Risk–Reducing Agent Activity

Randomized, placebo-controlled cancer incidence end point risk-reducing agent clinical trials demonstrated that finasteride and dutasteride reduced the incidence of prostate cancer by approximately 22% (Table 33.10).[30,191,192] Patients who are treated with either drug yet progress to transformed neoplasms develop more tumors of a high Gleason grade (7 to 10) compared to the placebo arm (22%). After 18 years of follow-up, no significant differences in overall survival or survival after prostate cancer diagnosis were found in the finasteride-treated group compared to the placebo-treated group.[193] Sexual function side effects (e.g., erectile dysfunction, loss of libido, gynecomastia) were more common in the finasteride- or dutasteride-treated groups.[30,192]

The 5α-steroid reductase inhibitors, finasteride and dutasteride, prevent or delay carcinogenesis progression in the prostate, yet progression of high-grade lesions is unaffected. Use of finasteride for a period of 7 years reduced the incidence of prostate cancer but did not significantly affect mortality.[193] Increasing the diagnosis of low-grade prostate cancer through prostate-specific antigen (PSA) testing or intervention with a drug with a minimal toxicity profile without reducing mortality is of no benefit and "all forms of therapy cause considerable burden to the patient and to society."[193]

SIGNAL TRANSDUCTION MODIFIERS

Both cancer therapy and cancer prevention have investigated drugs that modify specific targets in signal transduction pathways. Although the emphasis in drug development has focused on cancer treatment, interventions aimed at modulating signal transduction pathways promise new approaches to interventions in the carcinogenic process. Because of the complexity of signaling systems, the inhibition of single targets may not be effective or may cause unacceptable toxicity.

Difluoromethylornithine

Mechanism

Polyamines (spermidine, spermine, and the diamine, putrescine) are required to maintain cellular growth and function.[194] In mammalian cells, polyamine inhibition by genetic mutation or pharmaceutical agents is associated with virtual cessation in cellular growth. Difluoromethylornithine (DFMO) is an enzyme-activated irreversible inhibitor of ornithine decarboxylase (which is transactivated by the c-MYC oncogene and cooperates with the RAS oncogene in malignant transformation).[195]

Evidence in Preclinical In Vivo Carcinogenesis Models

Extensive preclinical data has found that DFMO prevents tumor promotion in a variety of systems, including skin, mammary, colon, cervical, and bladder carcinogenesis models.[194] Synergistic or additive activity with retinoids, butylated hydroxyanisole, tamoxifen, piroxicam, and fish oil has been demonstrated with low concentrations of DFMO.[194]

Clinical Trials

In phase I prevention trials, DFMO at a dose of 0.5 mg/m² per day reduced tissue polyamines in the colon and skin[196,197] and causes regression of cervical intraepithelial neoplasia when used topically,[198] but does not reduce tissue polyamines or other biomarkers of cellular proliferation in the human breast.[199] As a single agent, DFMO has anticarcinogenic activity for nonmelanoma skin cancers, primarily basal cell carcinoma. In combination with an NSAID (sulindac), DFMO reduced adenoma recurrences, suggesting a synergistic reduction of colorectal cancer risk (Table 33.11). Preliminary data suggest some cancer risk–reducing agent activity for the lower esophagus and the prostate (see Table 33.11).[200]

Statins

Mechanism

Statins are hydroxyl-3-methylglutaryl coenzyme A (HMG-CoA) reductase inhibitors that inhibit the conversion of HMG-CoA to mevalonate, a cholesterol precursor. The statins are a class of medications with similar structures but with variable moieties that can result in hydrophilic forms (e.g., pravastatin, rosuvastatin) and lipophilic forms (e.g., lovastatin, simvastatin, fluvastatin, atorvastatin).[201] Statins decrease the risk of cancer in preclinical studies by inhibiting RAS- and RHO-mediated cell proliferation, upregulating cell cycle inhibitors (e.g., p21 and p27), and inducing apoptosis of transformed cells and the inhibition of angiogenesis.[202]

Evidence in Preclinical In Vivo Carcinogenesis Models

Lipophilic statins delay progression of pancreatic intraepithelial neoplasias and the growth of pancreatic carcinoma xenografts. Atorvastatin alone and in combination with NSAIDs reduced colonic adenoma and adenocarcinoma incidence and multiplicity by half in rodent transgenic and chemical carcinogenesis models. Lovastatin reduced lung adenoma multiplicity but not incidence.[201]

Clinical Trials

Although several large trials of pravastatin or simvastatin on cardiovascular disease risk with cancer as secondary end points have shown no benefit for reducing cancer risk with follow-ups between 18 months to 4 years, these trials were not adequately powered to examine cancer end points.[201] Several case control studies evaluating statin effects have shown a significant association with lower risk of colorectal adenocarcinoma with odds ratios ranging from 0.53 to 0.91 for arroxifene. A secondary analysis of a celecoxib prevention trial demonstrated no statin protection against colorectal

TABLE 33.11
Summary of Clinical Trials of Difluoromethylornithine as a Cancer Risk–Reducing Agent

Population	Dose per Day, Duration	Phase	Endpoint	Outcome	References
Low risk bladder cancer (Ta. T1. Grades 1 or 2)	1 gm versus placebo × 1 year	III	Bladder cancer recurrence	Did not prevent or delay recurrence	(293)
Prostate risk: men with family history prostate cancer, age 35–70 yr	500 mg versus placebo × 1 yr	IIb	Prostate volume, polyamines, PSA	10-fold reduction of prostate size increase over 1 yr compared to placebo, PSA reduction not significant	(294)
Nonmelanoma skin cancer	500 mg/m² versus placebo × 4–5 y	III	New nonmelanoma skin cancers	Lower rate of basal cell carcinomas per year (0.28 versus 0.40); persistent reduction in nonmelanoma skin cancers, not statistically significant	(295, 296)
Colon adenomas	DFMO: 500 mg Sulindac: 150 mg versus placebo × 3 y	IIb	Adenoma recurrence	RR for adenoma recurrence for DFMO/sulindac treatment 5 0.30 (0.18–0.49)	(147)

PSA, prostate specific antigen.

neoplasms.[203] The Women's Health Initiative (prospective longitudinal cohort of 159,319 women) found that lovastatin was associated with a lower risk of developing colorectal cancer (HR = 0.62; 95% CI, 0.39 to 0.99).[204] Prospective longitudinal studies have shown mixed results. The PHS reported statin use was inversely associated with prostate cancer (adjusted RR, 0.51),[205] whereas the Nurse's Health Study showed no association with risk of breast cancer.[206] Interventional trials to determine statin preventive efficacy for colon and breast cancer are ongoing.[201] Statins may be effective risk-reducing agents in individuals with the A/A variant of the predominant T/T genotype of rs12654264 of the HMG-CoA reductase gene.[207]

Bisphosphonates

Mechanism

Bisphosphonates are pyrophosphate analogs with a central phosphorus-carbon-phosphorus bond that resists bone degradation preventing bone loss and fractures. Second- and third-generation amino bisphosphonates (pamidronic, alendronic, risedronic, ibandronic, and zoledronic acids) inhibit farnesyl diphosphate synthase downstream of HMG-CoA reductase, leading to decreased posttranslational prenylation of GTP-binding proteins such as RAS and Rho. Amino bisphosphonates inhibit cell proliferation, angiogenesis, and cell cycle arrest while inducing apoptosis.[201]

Evidence in In Vivo Preclinical and Clinical Models

HER2-transgenic mice treated with zoledronic acid had increased tumor-free survival and overall survival. Zoledronic acid suppressed bone, lung, and liver metastases when treated prior to an injection of breast cancer cells.[201] The short-term use of bisphosphonates is associated with reduced breast cancer incidence in case control studies[208,209] and prospective cohort studies (HR = 0.68; 95% CI, 0.52 to 0.88 in a prospective cohort study).[210] Randomized trials of amino-bisphosphonates in postmenopausal women with breast cancer treated for 1 year have found a reduction of breast cancer risk in the contralateral breast (HR = 0.39; 95% CI, 0.18 to 0.88).[211] Case control data suggesting a bisphosphonate-associated reduction in colorectal cancer risk have not been confirmed by prospective cohort studies (i.e., Women's Health Initiative, Nurse's Health Study).[201]

Metformin

Mechanism

Metformin, an oral antidiabetic drug in the biguanide class, is the first-line drug of choice for the treatment of type 2 diabetes.[212] Cancers are more common in diabetics and obese individuals than their normal weight and normoglycemic counterparts, leading to the hypothesis that elevated serum insulin concentrations promote cancer risk.[213,214] Insulin and insulin-like growth factors (IGF1 and 2) stimulate cellular DNA synthesis, proliferation, and tumor growth through phosphoinositide-3 kinase (PI3K), mammalian target of rapamycin (mTOR), and the RAS-MAPK signaling pathways.[213] Metformin activates the adenosine monophosphate-activated protein kinase (AMPK) via LKB1, a protein-threonine kinase that has tumor-suppressor activity.[201] Metformin anticarcinogenesis activity appears to be broad and includes downregulation of erbB-2 and epidermal growth factor receptor (EGFR) expression, inhibiting the phosphorylation of erbB family members, IGF1R, Akt, mTOR, and STAT3 in vivo. Low doses of metformin inhibit the self-renewal/proliferation of cancer stem cells in breast, colon, and pancreatic models.[215,216]

Evidence in Preclinical In Vivo Carcinogenesis Models

Metformin reduces tobacco carcinogen–induced tumors in mice, and pancreatic premalignant and malignant tumors in hamsters.[201] However, metformin's anticarcinogenic activity appears dependent on the dose and the induced carcinogenesis process. Metformin promoted carcinogenesis in MNU-induced rat breast cancers, MMTV-Neu ER-negative breast cancers, OH-BBN induced bladder cancer, and Min+ mouse intestinal tumors using nonobese rodents.[217] Metformin cancer risk–reducing agent effects may be limited to obesity- and diabetes-associated carcinogenesis mechanisms.

Clinical Trials

Two large retrospective cohort studies have shown that metformin therapy is associated with a reduced risk of solid tumors by 25% to 30%.[201] The Women's Health Initiative observed a lower incidence of invasive breast cancer in metformin-treated women with type 2 diabetes mellitus.[218] Phase II window of opportunity randomized trials have shown reduced proliferation and increased apoptosis in resected tissue of breast cancer patients.[201]

Diet-Derived Natural Products

Mechanism

Polyphenolic phytochemicals, such as curcumin, resveratrol, epigallocatechin gallate (EGCG), genistein, and ginger, are attractive as cancer risk–reducing agents for their low toxicity and multimechanism anticarcinogenic properties. They have anti-inflammatory activity, in part through scavenging of ROS, modulation of protein kinase signal transduction pathways (e.g., STAT-3, HER2/neu, MAPK, and Akt), and downstream inhibition of eicosanoid synthesis potentially due to upstream inhibition of NF-κB and PPAR or direct blockade or inhibition of eicosanoid-metabolizing enzymes.[219–221] Curcumin, and presumably other polyphenolics, downregulate stem cell driver signaling systems Wnt, Hedgehog, and Notch with subsequent reductions of breast, pancreatic, and colonic stem cell self-renewal.[222,223]

Omega-3 fatty acids (derived from marine products) compete with omega-6 fatty acid substrates for eicosanoid-metabolizing enzymes with subsequent tissue reduction of these inflammatory mediators.[224,225] These fatty acids have other diverse anticarcinogenic mechanisms (e.g., G-protein inhibition, changes in membrane physical characteristics that alter transmembrane signaling protein dynamics) that make them attractive as cancer risk–reducing agents.[226,227]

Whole berries, black raspberries, and strawberries contain mixtures of multiple anticarcinogenic compounds such as ellagic acid, anthocyanins, and tocopherols.[228] Research-grade berries are grown in a standardized cultivation environment and assayed for key components to ensure year-to-year reproducibility despite yearly climatologic variation. Berries have potent stabilization of methylation properties in addition to the expected anti-inflammatory and antioxidative properties associated with the prominent components.[229,230]

Preclinical and Clinical Anticarcinogenesis Efficacy. Diverse diet-derived natural products have moderate-to-strong anticarcinogenic effects in both chemical and transgenic rodent carcinogenesis models (Table 33.12). Phase I clinical trials of curcumin detected little parent compound in plasma or tissues, raising the possibility of biologically active conjugates or deconjugation at the target site.[231] Resveratrol's plasma bioavailability exceeds that of curcumin and ginger, and partitions into human colon tissue at 10-fold concentrations compared to plasma.[219,234,235] No natural products have been studied in large prospective, cancer incidence risk–reduction trials. Using intraepithelial biomarker end points in human phase II trials, berry formulations reduce esophageal dysplasia and oral leukoplakia.[236,237] Curcumin reduces the number of colon aberrant crypt foci in human smokers.[238]

ANTI-INFECTIVES

Many infectious agents are known causes of human cancers, including the human hepatitis viruses, hepatitis B virus (HBV) and hepatitis C virus (HCV) for hepatocellular carcinoma[239]; Helicobacter pylori for gastric adenocarcinoma[240]; human papilloma viruses (HPV) for cervical, anal, vulva, penis, and oral cavity and pharynx carcinomas[241]; herpes virus-8 for Kaposi sarcoma[242]; Epstein-Barr virus for Burkitt and other lymphomas[243]; liver flukes for cholangiocarcinoma[244]; and schistosomes for bladder carcinoma.[245] The success of the HPV vaccine at reducing the incidence of intraepithelial neoplasia of the cervix is one example that demonstrates the potential of immunochemoprevention for epithelial targets for which an etiologic agent can be identified.

Helicobacter pylori

Intestinal-type gastric adenocarcinoma arises through a multistep process that begins with chronic gastritis initiated by H. pylori, progressing through gastric mucosal atrophy, intestinal metaplasia to dysplasia, and ultimately, to adenocarcinoma.[246] H. pylori infects 50% of the world's population.[240] Infection occurs early in life, remains quiescent, and may be associated with chronic gastritis of variable intensity but with minimal symptoms. Although the majority of H. pylori organisms remain in the gastric mucous layer, 10% adhere to the gastric mucosa through adhesion BabA, an outer membrane protein that binds to the Lewis-B histo-blood group antigen.[240] Progression to atrophic gastritis and peptic ulcer disease (occurs in 10% to 15% of infected individuals) requires other bacterial and host cofactors.[245,246] Infection with H. pylori is associated with an OR of 2.7 to 6.0 for gastric cancer; CagA increases this risk by 20- to 40-fold. The risk of developing gastric adenocarcinoma with an H. pylori infection is estimated to be 1% to 3%.[245,246]

The eradication of H. pylori with antibiotics and anti-inflammatory agents—for example, amoxicillin, metronidazole, and bismuth subsalicylate—increases the rate of regression of nonmetaplastic gastric atrophy and intestinal metaplasia in geographically diverse regions.[247,248] A combination of a 2-week course of a proton pump inhibitor (omeprazole) and an antibiotic (amoxicillin) reduced the risk of gastric cancer in a high-risk population in China (OR = 0.61; 95% CI, 0.36 to 0.96) for 14.7 years after the treatment.[249] The sequence of giving proton pump inhibitors and antibiotic therapy does not alter the treatment outcome. In addition to contributing to gastric cancer risk, H. pylori infections may also contribute to pancreatic cancer risk.[250] Because H. pylori infections are so widespread, mass eradication campaigns in high-risk regions are being considered.[251] However, complicating this is that H. pylori infections have also been associated with a reduced risk of both esophageal adenocarcinoma and gastric cardia carcinoma.[252]

MULTIAGENT APPROACHES TO CANCER RISK REDUCTION

In the transition to molecularly targeted interventions, combinations of targets that logically address critical carcinogenic pathways may have greater efficacy than single agents. For example, previously demonstrated interactive signaling of EGFRs and COX-2 experiments in Min+ mice[253] demonstrates cancer preventive synergism. Combining atorvastatin with selective or nonselective COX inhibitors enhanced the inhibition of azoxymethane-induced colon carcinogenesis in F344 rats and reduced the dose of the combined drugs required to achieve a reduction of colon carcinogenesis.[254]

DFMO plus sulindac inhibited adenoma formation in a phase IIb trial of 375 patients with a prior history of adenomas followed for 36 months (see Table 33.11).[147] Cardiovascular-adverse outcomes were higher in DFMO/sulindac-treated patients who had preexisting high baseline cardiovascular risk; however, the cardiovascular-adverse events were similar to placebo in moderate or low cardiovascular risk patients.[255] Using IGF-1 as a biomarker, Guerrieri-Gonzaga et al.[256] showed that the combination of low-dose tamoxifen with low-dose fenretinide is safe but not synergistic. As more data accumulate from in vivo models, combined drugs aimed at specific targets in coordinated signaling pathways will enter clinical biomarker-based trials. Optimal doses, toxicity, and biomarker modulation data will select those combinations useful for risk reduction trials and, ultimately, generalized use in at-risk populations.

TABLE 33.12

Selected Diet-Derived Natural Products with Cancer Risk–Reducing Activity

Nutritional Extract	Source	Mechanisms	In Vivo Anticarcinogenesis Efficacy	Human Trials	References
Curcumin ([1E,6E]-1,7-bis-[4-hydroxy-3-methoxyphenyl]-1,6-heptadiene-3,5-dione/diferuloylmethane)	Turmeric, rhizome of *Curcuma longa*	Inhibits: PGE$_2$ synthesis via direct binding to COX-2 and through inhibition of NF-κB, angiogenesis. ErbB2 transduction; PI3K-Akt transduction; Inhibits stem cell self renewal Agonist: vitamin D receptor	Colon, breast, skin	Phase I: Poor bioavailability due to biotransformation in gut, enterohepatic cycling of metabolites; Phase IIa: reduced aberrant crypt foci	(219, 238)
Resveratrol (3,5,4′-trihydroxy-trans-stilbene)	Grapes, mulberries, peanuts, and *Cassia quinquangulata* plants	Inhibits: Carcinogen activation via inhibition of phase I isozyme, eicosanoids via direct binding; NF-κB; Nrf2. Acts as a caloric restriction mimetic, activates the histone deacetylase SIRT1 and AMPK	Colorectal, breast, pancreas, skin, and prostate	Phase I: 1 g dose generated peak concentration ~2 μM, conjugates 10-fold higher; resveratrol tissue concentrations 10-fold higher than plasma; Phase IIa: Small reduction in IGF-1 and IGFBP-1	(220, 234)
Ginger (gingerols, paradols, shagaols)	Rhizome of *Zingiber officinale*	Induces apoptosis via caspase-3 mechanisms; Inhibits NF-κB activation and downstream COX-2 expression; reduces iNOS expression and ornithine decarboxylase activity	Colon, breast, skin, oral cavity, liver	Phase I: 2 g dose nontoxic; Phase IIa: Small reductions in PGE$_2$, increased Bax in upper colon crypt	(235, 297, 298)
Green tea (epigallocatechin gallate, other catechins)	Green tea extract	Inhibits: PI3K-Akt transduction, IGF-1, IGFBP-3; NK-κB; catenin reduces methylation via inhibition of DNA methyltransferase 1	Lung, prostate, skin, colorectal	Phase IIa: 500–1,000 mg/m^2 × 12 wk reduced oral premalignant lesions in 50%; Phase IIb: 2.5 g × 1 yr reduced colorectal adenoma recurrence by 50%	(221)
Omega-3 fatty acids (eicosapentaenoic acid; docosahexaenoic acid)	Fish oil	Reduction of inflammation via eicosanoid reduction; direct binding to G receptor proteins; PPAR activation; induction of anti-inflammatory lipid mediators (resolvins, protectins, maresins)	Colon, breast, prostate	Phase II: 4–7 mg/d reduced colon adenomas in familial adenomatous polyposis; ongoing trials for sporadic; extensive case control studies	(226, 299)
Berries	Black raspberries, strawberries	Reduction of methylation via inhibition of methyltransferases, re-regulated Wnt; inhibits NF-κB; inhibits cyclooxygenases; inhibits proliferation	Esophageal squamous cell, colon, skin	Phase IIb: Freeze dried strawberries reduced esophageal dysplasia; Phase IIa: Blackberry gel reduced leukoplakia	(228, 229, 236, 237)

IGFBP-1, insulin growth factor binding protein-1; iNOS, inducible isoform of nitric oxide synthase.

REFERENCES

1. Vogelstein B, Papadopoulos N, Velculescu VE, et al. Cancer genome landscapes. *Science* 2013;339:1546–1558.
2. Fearon ER, Vogelstein B. A genetic model for colorectal tumorigenesis. *Cell* 1990;61:759–767.
3. Sidransky D. Emerging molecular markers of cancer. *Nat Rev Cancer* 2002;2:210–219.
4. Lippman SM, Levin B, Brenner DE, et al. Cancer prevention and the American Society of Clinical Oncology. *J Clin Oncol* 2004;22:3848–3851.
5. Wattenberg L. Chemoprevention of cancer. *Cancer Res* 1985;45:1–8.
6. Greenwald P, Kelloff G. The role of chemoprevention in cancer control. *IARC Scientific Publications (Lyon)* 1996;139:13–22.
7. Hanahan D, Weinberg RA. The hallmarks of cancer. *Cell* 2000;100:57–70.
8. Steele VE, Boone CW, Lubet RA, et al. Preclinical drug development paradigms for chemopreventives. *Hematol Oncol Clin North Am* 1998;12:943–961.
9. Perloff M, Steele VE. Early-phase development of cancer prevention agents: challenges and opportunities. *Cancer Prev Res (Phila)* 2013;6:379–383.
10. National Cancer Institute. PREVENT Cancer Preclinical Drug Development Program. National Cancer Institute Web site. http://prevention.cancer.gov/programs-resources/programs/prevent. Accessed December 7, 2013.
11. Mehta RG, Naithani R, Huma L, et al. Efficacy of chemopreventive agents in mouse mammary gland organ culture (MMOC) model: a comprehensive review. *Curr Med Chem.* 2008;15:2785–2825.
12. Hoenerhoff MJ, Hong HH, Ton TV, et al. A review of the molecular mechanisms of chemically induced neoplasia in rat and mouse models in National Toxicology Program bioassays and their relevance to human cancer. *Toxicol Pathol* 2009;37:835–848.
13. Steele VE, Lubet RA. The use of animal models for cancer chemoprevention drug development. *Semin Oncol* 2010;37:327–338.
14. Shureiqi I, Reddy P, Brenner DE. Chemoprevention: general perspective. *Crit Rev Oncol Hematol* 2000;33:157–167.
15. Becker M. Adherence to prescribed therapies. *Med Care* 1985;23:539–554.
16. Miki Y, Swensen J, Shattuck-Eidens D, et al. A strong candidate for the breast and ovarian cancer susceptibility gene BRCA1. *Science* 1994;266:66–71.
17. Powell SM, Petersen GM, Krush AJ, et al. Molecular diagnosis of familial adenomatous polyposis. *N Engl J Med* 1993;329:1982–1987.
18. Meads C, Ahmed I, Riley RD. A systematic review of breast cancer incidence risk prediction models with meta analysis of their performance. *Breast Cancer Res Treat* 2012;132:365–377.
19. Kastrinos F, Steyerberg EW, Balmana J, et al. Comparison of the clinical prediction model PREMM(1,2,6) and molecular testing for the systematic identification of Lynch syndrome in colorectal cancer. *Gut* 2013;62:272–279.
20. Ankerst DP, Boeck A, Freedland SJ, et al. Evaluating the PCPT risk calculator in ten international biopsy cohorts: results from the Prostate Biopsy Collaborative Group. *World J Urol* 2012;30:181–187.
21. National Institutes of Health, U.S. Food and Drug Administration. *Biomarkers and Surrogate Endpoints: Advancing Clinical Research and Applications.* Bethesda, MD: National Insitutes of Health; 1999.
22. Schatzkin A, Freedman LS, Schiffman MH, et al. Validation of intermediate end points in cancer research. *J Natl Cancer Inst* 1990;82:1746–1752.
23. Prentice R. Surrogate endpoints in clinical trials: definition and operational criteria. *Statistics Med* 1989;8:431–440.
24. Ransohoff DF. Rules of evidence for cancer molecular-marker discovery and validation. *Nat Rev Cancer* 2004;4:309–314.
25. Pepe MS, Feng Z, Janes H, et al. Pivotal evaluation of the accuracy of a biomarker used for classification or prediction: standards for study design. *J Natl Cancer Inst* 2008;100:1432–1438.
26. Pryor WA, Stahl W, Rock CL. Beta carotene: from biochemistry to clinical trials. *Nutr Rev* 2000;58:39–53.
27. Brenner DE, Hawk E. Trials and tribulations of interrogating biomarkers to define efficacy of cancer risk reductive interventions. *Cancer Prev Res (Phila)* 2013;6:71–73.
28. Fisher B, Costantino J, Wickerham D, et al. Tamoxifen for prevention of breast cancer: report of the National Surgical Adjuvant Breast and Bowel Project P-1 study. *J Natl Cancer Inst* 1998;90:1371–1388.
29. Vogel VG, Costantino JP, Wickerham DL, et al. Update of the National Surgical Adjuvant Breast and Bowel Project Study of Tamoxifen and Raloxifene (STAR) P-2 Trial: Preventing breast cancer. *Cancer Prev Res (Phila)* 2010;3:696–706.
30. Thompson IM, Goodman PJ, Tangen CM, et al. The influence of finasteride on the development of prostate cancer. *N Engl J Med* 2003;349:215–224.
31. Omenn G, Goodman G, Thornquist M, et al. Effects of a combination of beta carotene and vitamin A on lung cancer and cardiovascular disease. *N Engl J Med* 1996;334:1150–1155.
32. Lotan R. Retinoids in cancer chemoprevention. *Faseb J* 1996;10:1031–1039.
33. Tang X-H, Gudas LJ. Retinoids, retinoic acid receptors, and cancer. *Annu Rev Pathol* 2011;6:345–364.
34. Khachik F, Beecher G, Smith JC Jr. Lutein, lycopene, and their oxidative metabolites in chemoprevention of cancer. *J Cell Biochem* 1995;22:236–246.
35. Di Mascio P, Kaiser S, Sies H. Lycopene as the most efficient biological carotenoid singlet oxygen quencher. *Arch Biochem Biophys* 1989;274:532–538.
36. Eroglu A, Hruszkewycz DP, dela Sena C, et al. Naturally occurring eccentric cleavage products of provitamin A β-carotene function as antagonists of retinoic acid receptors. *J Biol Chem* 2012;287:15886–15895.
37. Ford NA, Erdman JW Jr. Are lycopene metabolites metabolically active? *Acta Biochim Pol* 2012;59:1–4.
38. World Cancer Research Fund, American Institute for Cancer Research. *Food, Nutrition, Physical Activity, and the Prevention of Cancer: A Global Perspective.* Washington, DC: AICR; 2007.
39. Panel on Dietary Antioxidants and Related Compounds, Subcommittees on Upper Reference Levels of Nutrients and Interpretation and Uses of DRIs, Standing Committee on the Scientific Evaluation of Dietary Reference Intakes, Food and Nutrition Board, Institute of Medicine. *Dietary Reference Intakes for Vitamin C, Vitamin E, Selenium, and Carotenoids.* Washington, DC: National Academy Press; 2000.
40. Moon RC, Mehta RG, Rao KVN. Retinoids and cancer in experimental animals. In: Sporn MB, Roberts AB, Goodman DS, eds., *The Retinoids.* 2nd ed. New York: Raven Press; 1994: 573–595.
41. International Agency for Research on Cancer World Health Organization. *Carotenoids.* Lyon: International Agency for Research on Cancer; 1998.
42. Holzapfel NP, Holzapfel BM, Champ S, et al. The potential role of lycopene for the prevention and therapy of prostate cancer: from molecular mechanisms to clinical evidence. *Int J Mol Sci* 2013;14:14620–14646.
43. Hong WK, Lippman SM, Itri LM, et al. Prevention of second primary tumors with 13cRA in squamous-cell carcinoma of the head and neck. *N Engl J Med* 1990;323:795–801.
44. Benner SE, Pajak TF, Lippman SM, et al. Prevention of second primary tumors with isotretinoin in patients with squamous cell carcinoma of the head and neck: long term follow-up. *J Natl Cancer Inst* 1994;86:140–141.
45. Khuri FR, Lee JJ, Lippman SM, et al. Randomized phase III trial of low-dose isotretinoin for prevention of second primary tumors in stage I and II head and neck cancer patients. *J Natl Cancer Inst* 2006;98:441–450.
46. Bolla M, Lefur R, Ton Van J, et al. Prevention of second primary tumours with etretinate in squamous cell carcinoma of the oral cavity and oropharynx. Results of a multicentric double-blind randomised study. *Eur J Cancer* 1994;30A:767–772.
47. Toma S, Bonelli L, Sartoris A, et al. beta-carotene supplementation in patients radically treated for stage I–II head and neck cancer: results of a randomized trial. *Oncol Rep* 2003;10:1895–1901.
48. Mayne ST, Cartmel B, Baum M, et al. Randomized trial of supplemental beta-carotene to prevent second head and neck cancer. *Cancer Res* 2001;61:1457–1463.
49. Bairati I, Meyer F, Jobin E, et al. Antioxidant vitamins supplementation and mortality: a randomized trial in head and neck cancer patients. *Int J Cancer* 2006;119:2221–2224.
50. McLarty JW, Holiday DB, Girard WM, et al. Beta-carotene, vitamin A and lung cancer chemoprevention: results of an intermediate endpoint study. *Am J Clin Nutr* 1995;62:1431S–1438S.
51. Lee JS, Lippman SM, Benner SE, et al. Randomized placebo-controlled trial of isotretinoin in chemoprevention of bronchial squamous metaplasia. *J Clin Oncol* 1994;12:937–945.
52. The Alpha-Tocopherol Beta Carotene Cancer Prevention Study Group. The effect of vitamin E and beta carotene on the incidence of lung cancer and other cancers in male smokers. *N Engl J Med* 1994;330:1029–1035.
53. Omenn GS, Goodman G, Thornquist M, et al. Chemoprevention of lung cancer: the beta-Carotene and Retinol Efficacy Trial (CARET) in high-risk smokers and asbestos-exposed workers. *IARC Sci Publ* 1996;67–85.
54. Hennekens CH, Buring JE, Manson JE, et al. Lack of effect of long-term supplementation with beta carotene on the incidence of malignant neoplasms and cardiovascular disease. *N Engl J Med* 1996;334:1145–1149.
55. Lee IM, Cook NR, Manson JE, et al. Beta-carotene supplementation and incidence of cancer and cardiovascular disease: the Women's Health Study. *J Natl Cancer Inst* 1999;91:2102–2106.
56. Heart Protection Study Collaborative Group. MRC/BHF Heart Protection Study of antioxidant vitamin supplementation in 20,536 high-risk individuals: a randomised placebo-controlled trial. *Lancet* 2002;360:23–33.
57. van Zandwijk N, Dalesio O, Pastorino U, et al. EUROSCAN, a randomized trial of vitamin A and N-acetylcysteine in patients with head and neck cancer or lung cancer. For the European Organization for Research and Treatment of Cancer Head and Neck and Lung Cancer Cooperative Groups. *J Natl Cancer Inst* 2000;92:977–986.
58. Lippman SM, Lee JJ, Karp DD, et al. Randomized phase III intergroup trial of isotretinoin to prevent second primary tumors in stage I non-small-cell lung cancer. *J Natl Cancer Inst* 2001;93:605–618.
59. Mayne ST, Lippman SM. Cigarettes: a smoking gun in cancer chemoprevention. *J Natl Cancer Inst* 2005;97:1319–1321.
60. Veronesi U, De Palo G, Marubini E, et al. Randomized trial of fenretinide to prevent second breast malignancy in women with early breast cancer. *J Natl Cancer Inst* 1999;91:1847–1856.
61. De Palo G, Mariani L, Camerini T, et al. Effect of fenretinide on ovarian carcinoma occurrence. *Gynecol Oncol* 2002;86:24–27.
62. Gray JP, Brown PH. Chemoprevention of hormone receptor-negative breast cancer: new approaches needed. *Recent Results Cancer Res* 2011;188:147–162.
63. Kraemer KH, DiGiovanna JJ, Moshell AN, et al. Prevention of skin cancer in xeroderma pigmentosum with the use of oral isotretinoin. *N Engl J Med* 1988;318:1633–1637.
64. Bouwes Bavinck JN, Tieben LM, Van Der Woude FJ, et al. Prevention of skin cancer and reduction of keratotic skin lesions during acitretin therapy in renal

transplant recipients: a double-blind, placebo-controlled study. *J Clin Oncol* 1995;13:1933–1938.
65. Tangrea JA, Edwards BK, Taylor PR, et al. Long-term therapy with low-dose isotretinoin for prevention of basal cell carcinoma: a multicenter clinical trial Isotretinoin-Basal Cell Carcinoma Study Group. *J Natl Cancer Inst* 1992;84:328–332.
66. Levine N, Moon TE, Cartmel B, et al. Trial of retinol and isotretinoin in skin cancer prevention: a randomized, double-blind, controlled trial. Southwest Skin Cancer Prevention Study Group. *Cancer Epidemiol Biomarkers Prev* 1997;6:957–961.
67. Moon TE, Levine N, Cartmel B, et al. Effect of retinol in preventing squamous cell skin cancer in moderate-risk subjects: a randomized, double-blind, controlled trial. Southwest Skin Cancer Prevention Study Group. *Cancer Epidemiol Biomarkers Prev* 1997;6:949–956.
68. Greenberg ER, Baron JA, Stukel TA, et al. A clinical trial of beta carotene to prevent basal-cell and squamous-cell cancers of the skin. The Skin Cancer Prevention Study Group. *N Engl J Med* 1990;323:789–795.
69. Green A, Williams G, Neale R, et al. Daily sunscreen application and beta-carotene supplementation in prevention of basal-cell and squamous-cell carcinomas of the skin: a randomised controlled trial. *Lancet* 1999;354:723–729.
70. Clark LC, Combs GF Jr, Turnbull BW, et al. Effects of selenium supplementation for cancer prevention in patients with carcinoma of the skin. A randomized controlled trial. Nutritional Prevention of Cancer Study Group. *JAMA* 1996;276:1957–1963.
71. Duffield-Lillico AJ, Slate EH, Reid ME, et al. Nutritional Prevention of Cancer Study Group. Selenium supplementation and secondary prevention of nonmelanoma skin cancer in a randomized trial. *J Natl Cancer Inst* 2003;95:1477–1481.
72. Sabichi AL, Lerner SP, Atkinson EN, et al. Phase III prevention trial of fenretinide in patients with resected non-muscle-invasive bladder cancer. *Clin Cancer Res* 2008;14:224–229.
73. Lamm DL, Riggs DR, Shriver JS, et al. Megadose vitamins in bladder cancer: a double-blind clinical trial. *J Urol* 1994;151:21–26.
74. Meyskens FL Jr, Surwit E, Moon TE, et al. Enhancement of regression of cervical intraepithelial neoplasia II (moderate dysplasia) with topically applied all-trans-retinoic acid: a randomized trial. *J Natl Cancer Inst* 1994;86:539–543.
75. Blot WJ, Li JY, Taylor PR, et al. Nutrition intervention trials in Linxian, China: supplementation with specific vitamin/mineral combinations, cancer incidence, and disease-specific mortality in the general population. *J Natl Cancer Inst* 1993;85:1483–1492.
76. Qiao YL, Dawsey SM, Kamangar F, et al. Total and cancer mortality after supplementation with vitamins and minerals: follow-up of the Linxian General Population Nutrition Intervention Trial. *J Natl Cancer Inst* 2009;101:507–518.
77. Mayne ST, Ferrucci LM, Cartmel B. Lessons learned from randomized clinical trials of micronutrient supplementation for cancer prevention. *Annu Rev Nutr* 2012;32:369–390.
78. Li JY, Taylor PR, Li B, et al. Nutrition intervention trials in Linxian, China: multiple vitamin/mineral supplementation, cancer incidence, and disease-specific mortality among adults with esophageal dysplasia. *J Natl Cancer Inst* 1993;85:1492–1498.
79. Kikendall JW, Mobarhan S, Nelson R, et al. Oral beta carotene does not reduce the recurrence of colorectal adenomas [Abstract]. *Am J Gastroenterol* 1991;36:1356.
80. MacLennan R, Macrae F, Bain C, et al. Randomized trial of intake of fat, fiber, and beta carotene to prevent colorectal adenomas. *J Natl Cancer Inst* 1995;87:1760–1766.
81. Greenberg ER, Baron JA, Tosteson TD, et al. A clinical trial of antioxidant vitamins to prevent colorectal adenoma. Polyp Prevention Study Group. *N Engl J Med* 1994;331:141–147.
82. Baron JA, Cole BF, Mott L, et al. Neoplastic and antineoplastic effects of beta-carotene on colorectal adenoma recurrence: results of a randomized trial. *J Natl Cancer Inst* 2003;95:717–722.
83. Heinonen OP, Albanes D, Virtamo J, et al. Prostate cancer and supplementation with alpha-tocopherol and beta-carotene: incidence and mortality in a controlled trial. *J Natl Cancer Inst* 1998;90:440–446.
84. Lippman SM, Klein EA, Goodman PJ, et al. Effect of selenium and vitamin E on risk of prostate cancer and other cancers: the Selenium and Vitamin E Cancer Prevention Trial (SELECT). *JAMA* 2009;301:39–51.
85. Klein EA, Thompson IM Jr, Tangen CM, et al. Vitamin E and the risk of prostate cancer: the Selenium and Vitamin E Cancer Prevention Trial (SELECT). *JAMA* 2011;306:1549–1556.
86. Gaziano JM, Glynn RJ, Christen WG, et al. Vitamins E and C in the prevention of prostate and total cancer in men: the Physicians' Health Study II randomized controlled trial. *JAMA* 2009;301:52–62.
87. Boileau TW, Liao Z, Kim S, et al. Prostate carcinogenesis in N-methyl-N-nitrosourea (NMU)-testosterone-treated rats fed tomato powder, lycopene, or energy-restricted diets. *J Natl Cancer Inst* 2003;95:1578–1586.
88. Goralczyk R. Beta-carotene and lung cancer in smokers: review of hypotheses and status of research. *Nutr Cancer* 2009;61:767–774.
89. Kristal AR, Darke AK, Morris JS, et al. Baseline Selenium Status and Effects of Selenium and Vitamin E Supplementation on Prostate Cancer Risk. *J Natl Cancer Inst* 2014;106:djt456.
90. Stone JR, Yang S. Hydrogen peroxide: a signaling messenger. *Antioxid Redox Signal* 2006;8:243–270.
91. Finkel T. Signal transduction by reactive oxygen species. *J Cell Biol* 2011;194:7–15.
92. Sayin V, Ibrahim M, Larsson E, et al. Antioxidants accelerate lung cancer progression in mice. *Sci Transl Med* 2014;6:ra15.
93. Mayne ST. Oxidative stress, dietary antioxidant supplements, and health: is the glass half full or half empty? *Cancer Epidemiol Biomarkers Prev* 2013;22:2145–2147.
94. Duthie SJ, Narayanan S, Blum S, et al. Folate deficiency in vitro induces uracil misincorporation and DNA hypomethylation and inhibits DNA excision repair in immortalized normal human colon epithelial cells. *Nutr Cancer* 2000;37:245–251.
95. Blount BC, Mack MM, Wehr CM, et al. Folate deficiency causes uracil misincorporation into human DNA and chromosome breakage: implications for cancer and neuronal damage. *Proc Natl Acad Sci U S A* 1997;94:3290–3295.
96. Giovannucci E. Epidemiologic studies of folate and colorectal neoplasia: a review. *J Nutr* 2002;132:2350S–2355S.
97. White E, Shannon JS, Patterson RE. Relationship between vitamin and calcium supplement use and colon cancer. *Cancer Epidemiol Biomarkers Prev* 1997;6:769–774.
98. Jacobs EJ, Connell CJ, Patel AV, et al. Multivitamin use and colon cancer mortality in the Cancer Prevention Study II cohort (United States). *Cancer Causes Control* 2001;12:927–934.
99. Gibson TM, Weinstein SJ, Pfeiffer RM, et al. Pre- and postfortification intake of folate and risk of colorectal cancer in a large prospective cohort study in the United States. *Am J Clin Nutr* 2011;94:1053–1062.
100. Chen J, Giovannucci E, Kelsey K, et al. A methylenetetrahydrofolate reductase polymorphism and the risk of colorectal cancer. *Cancer Res* 1996;56:4862–4864.
101. Larsson S, Giovannucci, E, Wolk A. Vitamin B6 intake, alcohol consumption, and colorectal cancer: a longitudinal population-based cohort of women. *Gastroenterology* 2005;128:1830–1837.
102. Wei E, Giovannucci E, Selhub J, et al. Plasma vitamin B6 and the risk of colorectal cancer and adenoma in women. *J Natl Cancer Inst* 2005;97:684–692.
103. Giovannucci E, Rimm EB, Ascherio A, et al. Alcohol, low-methionine-low-folate diets, and risk of colon cancer in men. *J Natl Cancer Inst* 1995;87:265–273.
104. Jaszewski R, Misra S, Tobi M, et al. Folic acid supplementation inhibits recurrence of colorectal adenomas: a randomized chemoprevention trial. *World J Gastroenterol* 2008;14:4492–4498.
105. Paspatis GA, Karamanolis DG. Folate supplementation and adenomatous colonic polyps. *Dis Colon Rectum* 1994;37:1340–1341.
106. Cole BF, Baron JA, Sandler RS, et al. Folic acid for the prevention of colorectal adenomas: a randomized clinical trial. *JAMA* 2007;297:2351–2359.
107. Logan RF, Grainge MJ, Shepherd VC, et al. Aspirin and folic acid for the prevention of recurrent colorectal adenomas. *Gastroenterology* 2008;134:29–38.
108. Wu K, Platz EA, Willett WC, et al. A randomized trial on folic acid supplementation and risk of recurrent colorectal adenoma. *Am J Clin Nutr* 2009;90:1623–1631.
109. Gao Q-Y, Chen H-M, Chen Y-X, et al. Folic acid prevents the initial occurrence of sporadic colorectal adenoma in Chinese older than 50 years of age: a randomized clinical trial. *Cancer prevention research (Phila)* 2013;6:744–752.
110. Ramnath N, Kim S, Christensen PJ. Vitamin D and lung cancer. *Expert Rev Respir Med* 2011;5:305–309.
111. Deeb KK, Trump DL, Johnson CS. Vitamin D signalling pathways in cancer: potential for anticancer therapeutics. *Nat Rev Cancer* 2007;7:684–700.
112. McCullough M, Robertson AS, Rodriguez C, et al. Calcium, vitamin D, dairy products, and risk of colorectal cancer in the cancer prevention study II nutrition cohort (United States). *Cancer Causes Control* 2003;14:1–12.
113. Wu K, Willett WC, Fuchs CS, et al. Calcium intake and risk of colon cancer in women and men. *J Natl Cancer Inst* 2002;94:437–446.
114. Chung M, Balk EM, Brendel M, et al. *Vitamin D and Calcium: A Systematic Review of Health Outcomes.* Evidence Report No. 183 (Prepared by the Tufts Evidence-based Practice Center). Rockville, MD: Agency for Healthcare Research and Quality; 2009.
115. World Health Organization, International Agency for Research on Cancer. Vitamin D and Cancer. Working Group Reports, Volume 5. Lyon, France: IARC; 2008.
116. Stolzenberg-Solomon RZ, Jacobs EJ, Arslan AA, et al. Circulating 25-hydroxyvitamin D and risk of pancreatic cancer: Cohort Consortium Vitamin D Pooling Project of Rarer Cancers. *Am J Epidemiol* 2010;172:81–93.
117. Baron J, Beach M, Mandel JS, et al. Calcium supplements for the prevention of colorectal adenomas. The Calcium Polyp Prevention Study Group. *N Engl J Med* 1999;340:101–107.
118. Bonithon-Kopp C, Kronborg O, Giacosa A, et al. Calcium and fibre supplementation in prevention of colorectal adenoma recurrence: a randomized intervention trial. *Lancet* 2000;356:1300–1306.
119. Wactawski-Wende J, Kotchen JM, Anderson GL, et al. Calcium plus vitamin D supplementation and the risk of colorectal cancer. *N Engl J Med* 2006;354:684–696.
120. Trivedi DP, Doll R, Khaw KT. Effect of four monthly oral vitamin D3 (cholecalciferol) supplementation on fractures and mortality in men and women living in the community: randomised double blind controlled trial. *BMJ* 2003;326:469.
121. Cui Y, Rohan TE. Vitamin D, calcium, and breast cancer risk: a review. *Cancer Epidemiol Biomarkers Prev* 2006;15:1427–1437.
122. Chlebowski RT, Johnson KC, Kooperberg C, et al. Calcium plus vitamin D supplementation and the risk of breast cancer. *J Natl Cancer Inst* 2008;100:1581–1591.
123. Lappe JM, Travers-Gustafson D, Davies KM, et al. Vitamin D and calcium supplementation reduces cancer risk: results of a randomized trial. *Am J Clin Nutr* 2007;85:1586–1591.

124. Manson JE, Bassuk SS, Lee IM, et al. The VITamin D and OmegA-3 TriaL (VITAL): rationale and design of a large randomized controlled trial of vitamin D and marine omega-3 fatty acid supplements for the primary prevention of cancer and cardiovascular disease. *Contemp Clin Trials* 2012;33:159–171.
125. Wu X, Spitz MR, Lee JJ, et al. Novel susceptibility loci for second primary tumors/recurrence in head and neck cancer patients: large-scale evaluation of genetic variants. *Cancer Prev Res (Phila)* 2009;2:617–624.
126. Platz EA. Is prostate cancer prevention with selenium all in the genes? *Cancer Prev Res (Phila)* 2010;3:576–578.
127. Miller JW, Ulrich CM. Folic acid and cancer—where are we today? *Lancet* 2013;381:974–976.
128. Thun MJ, Henley SJ, Patrono C. Nonsteroidal anti-inflammatory drugs as anticancer agents: mechanistic, pharmacologic, and clinical issues. *J Natl Cancer Inst* 2002;94:252–266.
129. Wang D, Mann JR, DuBois RN. The role of prostaglandins and other eicosanoids in the gastrointestinal tract. *Gastroenterology* 2005;128:1445–1461.
130. Gurpinar E, Grizzle WE, Piazza GA. COX-Independent Mechanisms of Cancer Chemoprevention by Anti-Inflammatory Drugs. *Front Oncol* 2013;3:181.
131. Rothwell PM, Wilson M, Price JF, et al. Effect of daily aspirin on risk of cancer metastasis: a study of incident cancers during randomised controlled trials. *Lancet* 2012;379:1591–1601.
132. Rothwell PM, Price JF, Fowkes FG, et al. Short-term effects of daily aspirin on cancer incidence, mortality, and non-vascular death: analysis of the time course of risks and benefits in 51 randomised controlled trials. *Lancet* 2012;379:1602–1612.
133. Thun MJ, Namboodiri MM, Heath C Jr. Aspirin use and reduced risk of fatal colon cancer. *N Engl J Med* 1991;325:1593–1596.
134. Chan AT, Giovannucci EL, Meyerhardt JA, et al. Aspirin dose and duration of use and risk of colorectal cancer in men. *Gastroenterology* 2008;134:21–28.
135. Chan AT, Giovannucci EL, Meyerhardt JA, et al. Long-term use of aspirin and nonsteroidal anti-inflammatory drugs and risk of colorectal cancer. *JAMA* 2005;294:914–923.
136. Liao LM, Vaughan TL, Corley DA, et al. Nonsteroidal anti-inflammatory drug use reduces risk of adenocarcinomas of the esophagus and esophagogastric junction in a pooled analysis. *Gastroenterology* 2012;142:442–452.
137. DuBois M, Lucker PH. Effect of indomethacin on intestinal tumor induced in rats by the acetate derivative of dimethylnitrosamine. *Cancer* 1981;44:558–559.
138. Jacoby RF, Marshall DJ, Newton MA, et al. Chemoprevention of spontaneous intestinal adenomas in the Apc Min mouse model by the nonsteroidal anti-inflammatory drug piroxicam. *Cancer Res* 1996;56:710–714.
139. Kawamori T, Rao C, Seibert K, et al. Chemopreventive effect of celecoxib, a specific cyclooxygenase-2 inhibitor on colon carcinogenesis. *Cancer Res* 1998;58:409–412.
140. Oshima M, Dinchuk JE, Kargman SL. Suppression of intestinal polyposis in Apc delta 716 knockout ice by inhibition of cyclooxygenase 2 (COX-2). *Cell* 1996;87:803–809.
141. Anderson WF, Umar A, Viner JL, et al. The role of cyclooxygenase inhibitors in cancer prevention. *Curr Pharm Des* 2002;8:1035–1062.
142. Giardiello FM, Yang VW, Hylind LM, et al. Primary chemoprevention of familial adenomatous polyposis with sulindac. *N Engl J Med* 2002;346:1054–1059.
143. Steinbach G, Lynch PM, Phillips RK. The effect of celecoxib, a cyclooxygenase-2 inhibitor, in familial adenomatous polyposis. *N Engl J Med* 2000;342:1946–1952.
144. Thorson AG, Lynch HT, Smyrk TC. Rectal cancer in FAP patient after sulindac. *Lancet* 1994;343:180.
145. Calaluce R, Earnest DL, Heddens D, et al. Effects of piroxicam on prostaglandin E2 levels in rectal mucosa of adenomatous polyp patients: a randomized phase IIb trial. *Cancer Epidemiol Biomarkers Prev* 2000;9:1287–1292.
146. Ladenheim J, Garcia G, Titzer D, et al. Effects of sulindac on sporadic colonic polyps. *Gastroenterology* 1995;108:1083–1087.
147. Meyskens FL Jr, McLaren CE, Pelot D, et al. Difluoromethylornithine plus sulindac for the prevention of sporadic colorectal adenomas: a randomized placebo-controlled, double-blind trial. *Cancer Prev Res (Phila)* 2008;1:32–38.
148. Arber N, Eagle CJ, Spicak J, et al. Celecoxib for the prevention of colorectal adenomatous polyps. *N Engl J Med* 2006;355:885–895.
149. Bertagnolli MM, Eagle CJ, Zauber AG, et al. Celecoxib for the prevention of sporadic colorectal adenomas. *N Engl J Med* 2006;355:873–884.
150. Baron JA, Sandler RS, Bresalier RS, et al. A randomized trial of rofecoxib for the chemoprevention of colorectal adenomas. *Gastroenterology* 2006;131:1674–1682.
151. Bresalier RS, Sandler RS, Quan H, et al. Cardiovascular events associated with rofecoxib in a colorectal adenoma chemoprevention trial. *N Engl J Med* 2005;352:1092–1102.
152. Solomon SD, McMurray JJ, Pfeffer MA, et al. Cardiovascular risk associated with celecoxib in a clinical trial for colorectal adenoma prevention. *N Engl J Med* 2005;352:1071–1080.
153. Rostom A, Dube C, Lewin G, et al. Nonsteroidal anti-inflammatory drugs and cyclooxygenase-2 inhibitors for primary prevention of colorectal cancer: a systematic review prepared for the U.S. Preventive Services Task Force. *Ann Intern Med* 2007;146:376–389.
154. Dube C, Rostom A, Lewin G, et al. The use of aspirin for primary prevention of colorectal cancer: a systematic review prepared for the U.S. Preventive Services Task Force. *Ann Intern Med* 2007;146:365–375.
155. Rothwell PM, Fowkes FG, Belch JF, et al. Effect of daily aspirin on long-term risk of death due to cancer: analysis of individual patient data from randomised trials. *Lancet* 2011;377:31–41.
156. Rothwell PM. Aspirin in prevention of sporadic colorectal cancer: current clinical evidence and overall balance of risks and benefits. *Recent Results Cancer Res* 2013;191:121–142.
157. U.S. Preventive Services Task Force. Routine aspirin or nonsteroidal anti-inflammatory drugs for the primary prevention of colorectal cancer: U.S. Preventive Services Task Force recommendation statement. *Ann Intern Med* 2007;146:361–364.
158. Mulshine JL, Atkinson JC, Greer RO, et al. Randomized, double-blind, placebo-controlled phase IIb trial of the cyclooxygenase inhibitor ketorolac as an oral rinse in oropharyngeal leukoplakia. *Clin Cancer Res* 2004;10:1565–1573.
159. Mao JT, Fishbein MC, Adams B, et al. Celecoxib decreases Ki-67 proliferative index in active smokers. *Clin Cancer Res* 2006;12:314–320.
160. Bord S, Horner A, Beavan S, et al. Estrogen receptors alpha and beta are differentially expressed in developing human bone. *J Clin Endocrinol Metab* 2001;86:2309–2314.
161. Kuiper GG, Carlsson B, Grandien K, et al. Comparison of the ligand binding specificity and transcript tissue distribution of estrogen receptors alpha and beta. *Endocrinology* 1997;138:863–870.
162. Fabian CJ, Kimler BF. Selective estrogen-receptor modulators for primary prevention of breast cancer. *J Clin Oncol* 2005;23:1644–1655.
163. Jordan VC. SERMs: meeting the promise of multifunctional medicines. *J Natl Cancer Inst* 2007;99:350–356.
164. Jordan VC. Tamoxifen (ICI46,474) as a targeted therapy to treat and prevent breast cancer. *Br J Pharmacol* 2006;147:S269–S276.
165. Jordan VC. Effect of tamoxifen (ICI 46,474) on initiation and growth of DMBA-induced rat mammary carcinomata. *Eur J Cancer* 1976;12:419–424.
166. Jordan VC. Chemoprevention of breast cancer with selective oestrogen-receptor modulators. *Nat Rev Cancer* 2007;7:46–53.
167. Cuzick J, Baum M. Tamoxifen and contralateral breast cancer. *Lancet* 1985;2:282.
168. Fisher B, Redmond C. New perspective on cancer of the contralateral breast: a marker for assessing tamoxifen as a preventive agent. *J Natl Cancer Inst* 1991;83:1278–1280.
169. Ettinger B, Black DM, Mitlak BH, et al. Reduction of vertebral fracture risk in postmenopausal women with osteoporosis treated with raloxifene: results from a 3-year randomized clinical trial. Multiple Outcomes of Raloxifene Evaluation (MORE) Investigators. *JAMA* 1999;282:637–645.
170. LaCroix AZ, Powles T, Osborne CK, et al. Breast cancer incidence in the randomized PEARL trial of lasofoxifene in postmenopausal osteoporotic women. *J Natl Cancer Inst* 2010;102:1706–1715.
171. Cummings SR, Ensrud K, Delmas PD, et al. Lasofoxifene in postmenopausal women with osteoporosis. *N Engl J Med* 2010;362:686–696.
172. Cummings SR, McClung M, Reginster JY, et al. Arzoxifene for prevention of fractures and invasive breast cancer in postmenopausal women. *J Bone Miner Res* 2011;26:397–404.
173. Powles TJ, Diem SJ, Fabian CJ, et al. Breast cancer incidence in postmenopausal women with osteoporosis or low bone mass using arzoxifene. *Breast Cancer Res Treat* 2012;134:299–306.
174. Nelson HD, Smith ME, Griffin JC, et al. Use of medications to reduce risk for primary breast cancer: a systematic review for the U.S. Preventive Services Task Force. *Ann Intern Med* 2013;158:604–614.
175. Moyer VA. Medications for risk reduction of primary breast cancer in women: U.S. Preventive Services Task Force recommendation statement. *Ann Intern Med* 2013;159:698-708.
176. Visvanathan K, Hurley P, Bantug E, et al. Use of pharmacologic interventions for breast cancer risk reduction: American Society of Clinical Oncology clinical practice guideline. *J Clin Oncol* 2013;31:2942–2962.
177. Vogel VG, Costantino JP, Wickerham DL, et al. Carcinoma in situ outcomes in National Surgical Adjuvant Breast and Bowel Project Breast Cancer Chemoprevention Trials. *J Natl Cancer Inst Monogr* 2010;2010:181–186.
178. Cuzick J, Sestak I, Bonanni B, et al. Selective oestrogen receptor modulators in prevention of breast cancer: an updated meta-analysis of individual participant data. *Lancet* 2013;381:1827–1834.
179. Barrett-Connor E, Mosca L, Collins P, et al. Effects of raloxifene on cardiovascular events and breast cancer in postmenopausal women. *N Engl J Med* 2006;355:125–137.
180. Snyder KR, Sparano N, Malinowski JM. Raloxifene hydrochloride. *Am J Health Syst Pharm* 2000;57:1669–1675.
181. Goss PE, Ingle JN, Martino S, et al. A randomized trial of letrozole in postmenopausal women after five years of tamoxifen therapy for early-stage breast cancer. *N Engl J Med* 2003;349:1793–1802.
182. Fabian CJ, Kimler BF, Zalles CM, et al. Reduction in proliferation with six months of letrozole in women on hormone replacement therapy. *Breast Cancer Res Treat* 2007;106:75–84.
183. Goss PE, Ingle JN, Ales-Martinez JE, et al. Exemestane for breast-cancer prevention in postmenopausal women. *N Engl J Med* 2011;364:2381–2391.
184. Cheung AM, Tile L, Cardew S, et al. Bone density and structure in healthy postmenopausal women treated with exemestane for the primary prevention of breast cancer: a nested substudy of the MAP.3 randomised controlled trial. *Lancet Oncol* 2012;13:275–284.
185. Cuzick J, Sestak I, Forbes JF, et al. Anastrozole for prevention of breast cancer in high-risk postmenopausal women (IBIS-II): an international, double blind, randomised placebo-controlled trial. *Lancet* 2014;383:1041–1048.
186. Waters EA, McNeel TS, Stevens WM, et al. Use of tamoxifen and raloxifene for breast cancer chemoprevention in 2010. *Breast Cancer Res Treat* 2012;134:875–880.

187. King MC, Wicand S, Hale K, et al. Tamoxifen and breast cancer incidence among women with inherited mutations in BRCA1 and BRCA2: National Surgical Adjuvant Breast and Bowel Project (NSABP-P1) Breast Cancer Prevention Trial. *JAMA* 2001;286:2251–2256.
188. Gronwald J, Tung N, Foulkes WD, et al. Tamoxifen and contralateral breast cancer in BRCA1 and BRCA2 carriers: an update. *Int J Cancer* 2006; 118:2281–2284.
189. Hess-Wilson JK, Knudsen KE. Endocrine disrupting compounds and prostate cancer. *Cancer Lett* 2006;241:1–12.
190. Andriole G, Bostwick D, Civantos F, et al. The effects of 5alpha-reductase inhibitors on the natural history, detection and grading of prostate cancer: current state of knowledge. *J Urol* 2005;174:2098–2104.
191. Thompson IM, Tangen CM, Goodman PJ, et al. Chemoprevention of prostate cancer. *J Urol* 2009;182:499–507.
192. Andriole GL, Bostwick DG, Brawley OW, et al. Effect of dutasteride on the risk of prostate cancer. *N Engl J Med* 2010;362:1192–1202.
193. Thompson IM Jr, Goodman PJ, Tangen CM, et al. Long-term survival of participants in the prostate cancer prevention trial. *N Engl J Med* 2013;369:603–610.
194. Gerner EW, Meyskens FL Jr. Polyamines and cancer: old molecules, new understanding. *Nat Rev Cancer* 2004;4:781–792.
195. Meyskens FL Jr, Gerner EW. Development of difluoromethylornithine (DFMO) as a chemoprevention agent. *Clin Cancer Res* 1999;5:945–951.
196. Love R, Carbone P, Verma A, et al. Randomized phase I chemoprevention dose seeking study of alpha-difluoromethylornithine. *J Natl Cancer Inst* 1993;85:732–737.
197. Alberts DS, Dorr RT, Einspahr JG, et al. Chemoprevention of human actinic keratoses by topical 2-(difluoromethyl)-dl-ornithine. *Cancer Epidemiol Biomarkers Prev* 2000;9:1281–1286.
198. Meyskens FL Jr, Surwit E, Moon TE, et al. Enhancement of regression of cervical intraepithelial neoplasia II (moderate dysplasia) with topically applied all-trans-retinoic acid: randomized trial. *J Natl Cancer Inst* 1994;86:539–543.
199. Fabian CJ, Kimler BF, Brady DA, et al. A phase II breast cancer chemoprevention trial of oral alpha-difluoromethylornithine: breast tissue, imaging, and serum and urine biomarkers. *Clin Cancer Res* 2002;8:3105–3117.
200. Jeter JM, Alberts DS. Difluoromethylornithine: the proof is in the polyamines. *Cancer Prev Res (Phila)* 2012;5:1341–1344.
201. Gronich N, Rennert G. Beyond aspirin-cancer prevention with statins, metformin and bisphosphonates. *Nat Rev Clin Oncol* 2013;10:625–642.
202. Moyad MA. Why a statin and/or another proven heart healthy agent should be utilized in the next major cancer chemoprevention trial: part II. *Urologic Oncol* 2004;22:472–477.
203. Bertagnolli MM, Hsu M, Hawk ET, et al. Statin use and colorectal adenoma risk: results from the adenoma prevention with celecoxib trial. *Cancer Prev Res (Phila)* 2010;3:588–596.
204. Simon MS, Rosenberg CA, Rodabough RJ, et al. Prospective analysis of association between use of statins or other lipid-lowering agents and colorectal cancer risk. *Ann Epidemiol* 2012;22:17–27.
205. Platz EA, Leitzmann MF, Visvanathan K, et al. Statin drugs and risk of advanced prostate cancer. *J Natl Cancer Inst* 2006;98:1819–1825.
206. Eliassen AH, Colditz GA, Rosner B, et al. Serum lipids, lipid-lowering drugs, and the risk of breast cancer. *Arch Intern Med* 2005;165:2264–2271.
207. Lipkin SM, Chao EC, Moreno V, et al. Genetic variation in 3-hydroxy-3-methylglutaryl CoA reductase modifies the chemopreventive activity of statins for colorectal cancer. *Cancer Prev Res (Phila)* 2010;3:597–603.
208. Rennert G. Bisphosphonates: beyond prevention of bone metastases. *J Natl Cancer Inst* 2011;103:1728–1729.
209. Rennert G, Pinchev M, Rennert HS. Use of bisphosphonates and risk of postmenopausal breast cancer. *J Clin Oncol* 2010;28:3577–3581.
210. Chlebowski RT, Chen Z, Cauley JA, et al. Oral bisphosphonate use and breast cancer incidence in postmenopausal women. *J Clin Oncol* 2010;28:3582–3590.
211. Monsees GM, Malone KE, Tang MT, et al. Bisphosphonate use after estrogen receptor-positive breast cancer and risk of contralateral breast cancer. *J Natl Cancer Inst* 2011;103:1752–1760.
212. Kirpichnikov D, McFarlane SI, Sowers JR. Metformin: an update. *Ann Intern Med* 2002;137:25–33.
213. Pollack MN. Insulin, insulin-like growth factors, insulin resistance, and neoplasia. *Am J Clin Nutr* 2007;86:s820–s822.
214. Evans JM, Donnelly LA, Emslie-Smith AM, et al. Metformin and reduced risk of cancer in diabetic patients. *BMJ* 2005;330:1304–1305.
215. Zhu P, Davis M, Blackwelder A, et al. Metformin selectively targets tumor initiating cells in erbB-2 overexpressing breast cancer models. *Cancer Prev Res (Phila)* 2014;7:199–210.
216. Lonardo E, Cioffi M, Sancho P, et al. Metformin targets the metabolic achilles heel of human pancreatic cancer stem cells. *PLoS One* 2013;8:e76518.
217. Grubbs C, Clapper M, Reid J, et al. *Metformin Promotes Tumorigenesis in Animal Models of Cancer Prevention.* Washington, DC: American Association for Cancer Research; 2013.
218. Chlebowski RT, McTiernan A, Wactawski-Wende J, et al. Diabetes, metformin, and breast cancer in postmenopausal women. *J Clin Oncol* 2012;30:2844–2852.
219. Heger M, van Golen RF, Broekgaarden M, et al. The molecular basis for the pharmacokinetics and pharmacodynamics of curcumin and its metabolites in relation to cancer. *Pharmacol Rev* 2014;66:222–307.
220. Whitlock NC, Baek SJ. The anticancer effects of resveratrol: modulation of transcription factors. *Nutr Cancer* 2012;64:493–502.
221. Lambert JD. Does tea prevent cancer? Evidence from laboratory and human intervention studies. *Am J Clin Nutr* 2013;98:1667S–1675S.
222. Kakarala M, Brenner DE, Korkaya H, et al. Targeting breast stem cells with the cancer preventive compounds curcumin and piperine. *Breast Cancer Res Treat* 2010;122:777–785.
223. Norris L, Karmokar A, Howells L, et al. The role of cancer stem cells in the anti-carcinogenicity of curcumin. *Mol Nutr Food Res* 2013;57:1630–1637.
224. Zou H, Yuan C, Dong L, et al. Human cyclooxygenase-1 activity and its responses to COX inhibitors are allosterically regulated by nonsubstrate fatty acids. *J Lipid Res* 2012;53:1336–1347.
225. Wada M, Delong CJ, Hong YH, et al. Enzymes and receptors of prostaglandin pathways with arachidonic acid- vs. eicosapentaenoic acid derived substrates and products. *J Biol Chem* 2007;282:22254–22266.
226. Laviano A, Rianda S, Molfino A, et al. Omega-3 fatty acids in cancer. *Curr Opin Clin Nutr Metab Care* 2013;16:156–161.
227. Cockbain AJ, Toogood GJ, Hull MA. Omega-3 polyunsaturated fatty acids for the treatment and prevention of colorectal cancer. *Gut* 2012;61:135–149.
228. Stoner GD, Wang LS, Casto BC. Laboratory and clinical studies of cancer chemoprevention by antioxidants in berries. *Carcinogenesis* 2008;29:1665–1674.
229. Wang LS, Dombkowski AA, Seguin C, et al. Mechanistic basis for the chemopreventive effects of black raspberries at a late stage of rat esophageal carcinogenesis. *Mol Carcinog* 2011;50:291–300.
230. Wang LS, Kuo CT, Stoner K, et al. Dietary black raspberries modulate DNA methylation in dextran sodium sulfate (DSS)-induced ulcerative colitis. *Carcinogenesis* 2013;34:2842–2850.
231. Ireson C, Orr S, Jones DJ, et al. Characterization of metabolites of the chemopreventive agent curcumin in human and rat hepatocytes and in the rat in vivo, and evaluation of their ability to inhibit phorbol ester-induced prostaglandin E2 production. *Cancer Res* 2001;61:1058–1064.
232. Ireson CR, Jones DJ, Orr S, et al. Metabolism of the cancer chemopreventive agent curcumin in human and rat intestine. *Cancer Epidemiol Biomarkers Prev* 2002;11:105–111.
233. Vareed SK, Kakarala M, Ruffin MT, et al. Pharmacokinetics of curcumin conjugate metabolites in healthy human subjects. *Cancer Epidemiol Biomarkers Prev* 2008;17:1411–1417.
234. Gescher A, Steward WP, Brown K. Resveratrol in the management of human cancer: how strong is the clinical evidence? *Ann N Y Acad Sci* 2013;1290:12–20.
235. Stoner GD. Ginger: Is it ready for prime time? *Cancer Prev Res (Phila)* 2013;6:257–262.
236. Stoner GD, Wang LS. Chemoprevention of esophageal squamous cell carcinoma with berries. *Top Curr Chem* 2013;329:1–20.
237. Mallery SR, Zwick JC, Pei P, et al. Topical application of a bioadhesive black raspberry gel modulates gene expression and reduces cyclooxygenase 2 protein in human premalignant oral lesions. *Cancer Res* 2008;68:4945–4957.
238. Carroll RE, Benya RV, Turgeon DK, et al. Phase IIa clinical trial of curcumin for the prevention of colorectal neoplasia. *Cancer Prev Res (Phila)* 2011;4:354–364.
239. Seeff LB, Hoofnagle JH. Epidemiology of hepatocellular carcinoma in areas of low hepatitis B and hepatitis C endemicity. *Oncogene* 2006;25:3771–3777.
240. Fox JG, Wang TC. Inflammation, atrophy, and gastric cancer. *J Clin Invest* 2007;117:60–69.
241. Saslow D, Castle PE, Cox JT, et al. American Cancer Society Guideline for human papillomavirus (HPV) vaccine use to prevent cervical cancer and its precursors. *CA Cancer J Clin* 2007;57:7–28.
242. Mohanna S, Maco V, Bravo F, et al. Epidemiology and clinical characteristics of classic Kaposi's sarcoma, seroprevalence, and variants of human herpesvirus 8 in South America: a critical review of an old disease. *Int J Infect Dis* 2005;9:239–250.
243. Castillo JJ, Reagan JL, Bishop KD, et al. Viral lymphomagenesis: from pathophysiology to the rationale for novel therapies. *Br J Haematol* 2014;165:300–315.
244. Al-Bahrani R, Abuetabh Y, Zeitouni N, et al. Cholangiocarcinoma: risk factors, environmental influences and oncogenesis. *Ann Clin Lab Sci* 2013;43:195–210.
245. Mostafa MH, Sheweita SA, O'Connor PJ. Relationship between schistosomiasis and bladder cancer. *Clin Microbiol Rev* 1999;12:97–111.
246. Zivny J, Wang TC, Yantiss R, et al. Role of therapy or monitoring in preventing progression to gastric cancer. *J Clin Gastroenterol* 2003;36:S50–S60.
247. Correa P, Fontham ET, Bravo JC, et al. Chemoprevention of gastric dysplasia: randomized trial of antioxidant supplements and anti-helicobacter pylori therapy. *J Natl Cancer Inst* 2000;92:1881–1888.
248. Wong BC, Zhang L, Ma JL, et al. Effects of selective COX-2 inhibitor and Helicobacter pylori eradication on precancerous gastric lesions. *Gut* 2012;61:812–818.
249. Ma JL, Zhang L, Brown LM, et al. Fifteen-year effects of Helicobacter pylori, garlic, and vitamin treatments on gastric cancer incidence and mortality. *J Natl Cancer Inst* 2012;104:488–492.
250. Risch HA, Lu L, Kidd MS, et al. Helicobacter pylori seropositivities and risk of pancreatic carcinoma. *Cancer Epidemiol Biomarkers Prev* 2014;23:172–178.
251. Mazzoleni LE, Francesconi CF, Sander GB. Mass eradication of *Helicobacter pylori*: feasible and advisable? *Lancet* 2011;378:462–464.
252. Whiteman DC, Parmar P, Fahey P, et al. Association of Helicobacter pylori infection with reduced risk for esophageal cancer is independent of environmental and genetic modifiers. *Gastroenterology* 2010;139:73–83.

253. Torrance CJ, Jackson PE, Montgomery E, et al. Combinatorial chemoprevention of intestinal neoplasia. *Nat Med* 2000;6:1024–1028.
254. Reddy BS, Wang CX, Kong AN, et al. Prevention of azoxymethane-induced colon cancer by combination of low doses of atorvastatin, aspirin, and celecoxib in F 344 rats. *Cancer Res* 2006;66:4542–4546.
255. Zell JA, Pelot D, Chen WP, et al. Risk of cardiovascular events in a randomized placebo-controlled, double-blind trial of difluoromethylornithine plus sulindac for the prevention of sporadic colorectal adenomas. *Cancer Prev Res (Phila)* 2009;2:209–212.
256. Guerrieri-Gonzaga A, Robertson C, Bonanni B, et al. Preliminary results on safety and activity of a randomized, double-blind, 2 x 2 trial of low-dose tamoxifen and fenretinide for breast cancer prevention in premenopausal women. *J Clin Oncol* 2006;24:129–135.
257. Kelloff GJ, Lippman SM, Dannenberg AJ, et al. Progress in chemoprevention drug development: the promise of molecular biomarkers for prevention of intraepithelial neoplasia and cancer—a plan to move forward. *Clin Cancer Res* 2006;12:3661–3697.
258. Washington MK, Powell AE, Sullivan R, et al. Pathology of rodent models of intestinal cancer: progress report and recommendations. *Gastroenterology* 2013;144:705–717.
259. Nandan MO, Yang VW. Genetic and chemical models of colorectal cancer in mice. *Curr Colorectal Cancer Rep* 2010;6:51–59.
260. Kwon MC, Berns A. Mouse models for lung cancer. *Mol Oncol* 2013;7:165–177.
261. Kirma NB, Tekmal RR. Transgenic mouse models of hormonal mammary carcinogenesis: advantages and limitations. *J Steroid Biochem Mol Biol* 2012;131:76–82.
262. Irshad S, Abate-Shen C. Modeling prostate cancer in mice: something old, something new, something premalignant, something metastatic. *Cancer Metastasis Rev* 2013;32:109–122.
263. Herreros-Villanueva M, Hijona E, Cosme A, et al. Mouse models of pancreatic cancer. *World J Gastroenterol* 2012;18:1286–1294.
264. Winawer SJ, Zauber AG, Ho MN, et al. Prevention of colorectal cancer by colonoscopic polypectomy. The National Polyp Study Workgroup. *N Engl J Med* 1993;329:1977–1981.
265. Spechler S. Barrett's esophagus. *Semin Oncol* 1994;21:431–437.
266. Shen Q, Liu S, Dawsey S, et al. Cytology screening for esophageal cancer from a high risk population in China. *Int J Cancer* 1993;54:185–188.
267. Taylor P, Li B, Dawsey S, et al. Prevention of esophageal cancer: the nutrition intervention trials in Linxian, China. Linxian Nutrition Intervention Trials Study Group. *Cancer Res* 1994;54:2029s–2031s.
268. Sober A, Burstein J. Precursors to skin cancer. *Cancer* 1995;75:645–650.
269. Tucker M, Halpern A, Holly E, et al. Clinically recognized dysplastic nevi. A central risk factor for cutaneous melanoma. *JAMA* 1997;277:1439–1444.
270. Gustafsson L, Adami H-O. Natural history of cervical neoplasia: consistent results obtained by an identification technique. *Br J Cancer* 1989;60:132–137.
271. Cawson R. Premalignant lesions in the mouth. *Br Med Bull* 1975;31:164–180.
272. Zhou M. Intraductal carcinoma of the prostate: the whole story. *Pathology* 2013;45:533–539.
273. Saccomanno G, Archer VE, Auerbach O, et al. Development of carcinoma of the lung as reflected in exfoliated cells. *Cancer* 1974;33:256–270.
274. Cooper CL, O'Toole SA, Kench JG. Classification, morphology and molecular pathology of premalignant lesions of the pancreas. *Pathology* 2013;45:286–304.
275. Brewster AM, Lee JJ, Clayman GL, et al. Randomized trial of adjuvant 13-cis-retinoic acid and interferon alfa for patients with aggressive skin squamous cell carcinoma. *J Clin Oncol* 2007;25:1974–1978.
276. Karp DD, Lee SJ, Keller SM, et al. Randomized, double-blind, placebo-controlled, phase III chemoprevention trial of selenium supplementation in patients with resected stage I non-small-cell lung cancer: ECOG 5597. *J Clin Oncol* 2013;31:4179–4187.
277. Labayle D, Fischer D, Vielh P. Sulindac causes regression of rectal polyps in familial adenomatous polyposis. *Gastroenterology* 1991;101:635–639.
278. Giardiello FM, Hamilton SR, Krush AJ, et al. Treatment of colonic and rectal adenomas with sulindac in familial adenomatous polyposis. *N Engl J Med* 1993;328:1313–1316.
279. Nugent KP, Farmer KC, Sipgelman AD, et al. Randomized controlled trial of the effect of sulindac on duodenal and rectal polyposis and cell proliferation in patients with familial adenomatous polyposis. *Br J Surg* 1993;80:1618–1619.
280. Mathers JC, Movahedi M, Macrae F, et al. Long-term effect of resistant starch on cancer risk in carriers of hereditary colorectal cancer: an analysis from the CAPP2 randomised controlled trial. *Lancet Oncol* 2012;13:1242–1249.
281. Burn J, Gerdes AM, Macrae F, et al. Long-term effect of aspirin on cancer risk in carriers of hereditary colorectal cancer: an analysis from the CAPP2 randomised controlled trial. *Lancet* 2011;378:2081–2087.
282. Ruffin MT, Krishnan K, Rock CL, et al. Suppression of human colorectal mucosal prostaglandins: determining the lowest effective aspirin dose. *J Natl Cancer Inst* 1997;89:1152–1160.
283. Krishnan K, Ruffin MT, Normolle D, et al. Colonic mucosal prostaglandin E2 and cyclooxygenase expression before and after low aspirin doses in subjects at high risk or at normal risk for colorectal cancer. *Cancer Epidemiol Biomarkers Prev* 2001;10:447–453.
284. Sample D, Wargovich M, Fischer SM, et al. A dose-finding study of aspirin for chemoprevention utilizing rectal mucosal prostaglandin E(2) levels as a biomarker. *Cancer Epidemiol Biomarkers Prev* 2002;11:275–279.

285. Sandler RS, Halabi S, Baron JA, et al. A randomized trial of aspirin to prevent colorectal adenomas in patients with previous colorectal cancer. *N Engl J Med* 2003;348:883–890.
286. Baron JA, Cole BF, Sandler RS, et al. A randomized trial of aspirin to prevent colorectal adenomas. *N Engl J Med* 2003;348:891–899.
287. Fisher B, Costantino JP, Wickerham DL, et al. Tamoxifen for the prevention of breast cancer: current status of the National Surgical Adjuvant Breast and Bowel Project P-1 study. *J Natl Cancer Inst* 2005;97:1652–1662.
288. Cuzick J, Forbes JF, Sestak I, et al. Long-term results of tamoxifen prophylaxis for breast cancer—96-month follow-up of the randomized IBIS-I trial. *J Natl Cancer Inst* 2007;99:272–282.
289. Powles TJ, Ashley S, Tidy A, et al. Twenty-year follow-up of the Royal Marsden randomized, double-blinded tamoxifen breast cancer prevention trial. *J Natl Cancer Inst* 2007;99:283–290.
290. Veronesi U, Maisonneuve P, Rotmensz N, et al. Tamoxifen for the prevention of breast cancer: Late results of the Italian randomzied tamoxifen prevention trial among women with hysterectomy. *J Natl Cancer Inst* 2007;99:727–737.
291. Cauley JA, Norton L, Lippman ME, et al. Continued breast cancer risk reduction in postmenopausal women treated with raloxifene: 4-year results from the MORE trial. Multiple outcomes of raloxifene evaluation. *Breast Cancer Res Treat* 2001;65:125–134.
292. Martino S, Cauley JA, Barrett-Connor E, et al. Continuing outcomes relevant to Evista: breast cancer incidence in postmenopausal osteoporotic women in a randomized trial of raloxifene. *J Natl Cancer Inst* 2004;96:1751–1761.
293. Messing E, Kim KM, Sharkey F, et al. Randomized prospective phase III trial of difluoromethylornithine vs placebo in preventing recurrence of completely resected low risk superficial bladder cancer. *J Urol* 2006;176:500–504.
294. Simoneau AR, Gerner EW, Nagle R, et al. The effect of difluoromethylornithine on decreasing prostate size and polyamines in men: results of a yearlong phase IIb randomized placebo-controlled chemoprevention trial. *Cancer Epidemiol Biomarkers Prev* 2008;17:292–299.
295. Bailey HH, Kim K, Verma AK, et al. A randomized, double-blind, placebo-controlled phase 3 skin cancer prevention study of (alpha)-difluoromethylornithine in subjects with previous history of skin cancer. *Cancer Prev Res (Phila)* 2010;3:35–47.
296. Kreul SM, Havighurst T, Kim K, et al. A phase III skin cancer chemoprevention study of DFMO: long-term follow-up of skin cancer events and toxicity. *Cancer Prev Res (Phila)* 2012;5:1368–1374.
297. Zick SM, Ruffin MT, Djuric Z, et al. Quantitation of 6-, 8- and 10-gingerols and 6-shogaol in human plasma by high-performance liquid chromatography with electrochemical detection. *Int J Biomed Sci* 2010;6:233–240.
298. Zick SM, Turgeon DK, Vareed SK, et al. Phase II study of the effects of ginger root extract on eicosanoids in colon mucosa in people at normal risk for colorectal cancer. *Cancer Prev Res (Phila)* 2011;4:1929–1937.
299. Hull MA. Nutritional agents with anti-inflammatory properties in chemoprevention of colorectal neoplasia. *Recent Results Cancer Res* 2013;191:143–156.
300. Nelson WG, De Marzo AM, Isaacs WB. Prostate cancer. *N Engl J Med* 2003;349:366–381.
301. von Knobloch R, Konrad L, Barth PJ, et al. Genetic pathways and new progression markers for prostate cancer suggested by microsatellite allelotyping. *Clin Cancer Res* 2004;10:1064–1073.
302. Palapattu GS, Sutcliffe S, Bastian PJ, et al. Prostate carcinogenesis and inflammation: emerging insights. *Carcinogenesis* 2005;26:1170–1181.
303. Dontu G, Liu S, Wicha MS. Stem cells in mammary development and carcinogenesis: implications for prevention and treatment. *Stem Cell Rev* 2005;1:207–213.
304. Liu S, Dontu G, Mantle ID, et al. Hedgehog signaling and Bmi-1 regulate self-renewal of normal and malignant human mammary stem cells. *Cancer Res* 2006;66:6063–6071.
305. Wistuba II, Lam S, Behrens C, et al. Molecular damage in the bronchial epithelium of current and former smokers. *J Natl Cancer Inst* 1997;89:1366–1373.
306. Massion PP, Carbone DP. The molecular basis of lung cancer: molecular abnormalities and therapeutic implications. *Respir Res* 2003;4:12.
307. Mao C, Koutsky LA, Ault KA, et al. Efficacy of human papillomavirus-16 vaccine to prevent cervical intraepithelial neoplasia: a randomized controlled trial. *Obstet Gynecol* 2006;107:18–27.
308. Califano J, van der Riet P, Westra W, et al. Genetic progression model for head and neck cancer: implications for field cancerization. *Cancer Res* 1996;56:2488–2492.
309. Califano J, Westra WH, Meininger G, et al. Genetic progression and clonal relationship of recurrent premalignant head and neck lesions. *Clin Cancer Res* 2000;6:347–352.
310. Braakhuis BJ, Tabor MP, Kummer JA, et al. A genetic explanation of Slaughter's concept of field cancerization: evidence and clinical implications. *Cancer Res* 2003;63:1727–1730.
311. Ha PK, Benoit NE, Yochem R, et al. A transcriptional progression model for head and neck cancer. *Clin Cancer Res* 2003;9:3058–3064.
312. Barrett MT, Sanchez CA, Prevo LJ, et al. Evolution of neoplastic cell lineages in Barrett oesophagus. *Nat Genet* 1999;22:106–109.
313. Reid BJ, Levine DS, Longton G, et al. Predictors of progression to cancer in Barrett's esophagus: baseline histology and flow cytometry identify low- and high-risk patient subsets. *Am J Gastroenterol* 2000;95:1669–1676.
314. Thorgeirsson SS, Grisham JW. Molecular pathogenesis of human hepatocellular carcinoma. *Nat Genet* 2002;31:339–346.

34 Cancer Screening

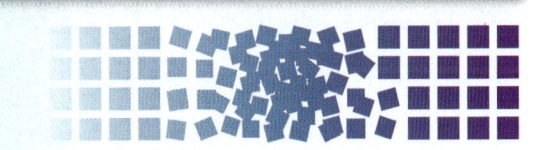

Otis W. Brawley and Howard L. Parnes

INTRODUCTION

Cancer screening refers to a test or examination performed on an asymptomatic individual. The goal is not simply to find cancer at an early stage, nor is it to diagnose as many patients with cancer as possible. The goal of cancer screening is to prevent death and suffering from the disease in question through early therapeutic intervention.

The assumption that early detection improves outcomes can be traced back to the concept that cancer inexorably progresses from a small, localized, primary tumor to local–regional spread, to distant metastases and death. This linear model of disease progression predicts that early intervention would reduce cancer mortality.

Cancer screening was an element of the "periodic physical examination," as espoused by the American Medical Association in the 1920s.[1] It consisted of palpation to find a mass or enlarged lymph nodes and auscultation to find a rub or abnormal sound. Today, screening has grown to include radiologic testing, the measurement of serum markers of disease, and even molecular testing. A positive screening test leads to further diagnostic testing, which might lead to a cancer diagnosis.

The intuitive appeal of early detection accounts for the emphasis that has long been placed on screening. However, it is not widely understood that screening tests are always associated with some harm (e.g., anxiety, financial costs) and may actually cause substantial harm (e.g., invasive follow-up diagnostic or therapeutic procedures). Because screening is, by definition, done in healthy people, all early detection tests should be carefully studied and their risk–benefit ratio determined before they are adopted for widespread usage.

Screening is a public health intervention. However, some draw a distinction between screening an individual within the doctor–patient relationship and mass screening, a program aimed at screening a large population. The latter may involve advertising campaigns to encourage people to be screened for a particular cancer at a shopping mall or at a community event, such as state fair.

Screening may be either *opportunistic* (i.e., a patient sees a health-care provider who chooses to screen or not to screen) or *programmatic*. Programmatic refers to a standardized approach with algorithms for screening and follow-up as well as recall of patients for regular routine screening with quality control measures. Programmatic screening is usually more effective.

PERFORMANCE CHARACTERISTICS

The degree to which a screening test can discriminate between individuals with and without a particular disease is described by its performance characteristics. These include the a test's sensitivity, specificity, positive predictive value (PPV), and negative predictive value (NPV) (Table 34.1). It should be noted that these measures relate to the accuracy of a screening test; they do not provide any information regarding a test's efficacy or effectiveness.

- Sensitivity is the proportion of persons designated positive by the screening test among all individuals who have the disease: true positive (TP)/(TP + false negative [FN]).
- Specificity is the proportion of persons designated negative by the screening test among all individuals who do not have the disease: true negative TN/(TN + false positive [FP]).
- Positive predictive value is the proportion of individuals with a positive screening test who have the disease: (TP)/(TP + FP).
- Negative predictive value is the proportion of individuals with a negative screening test who do not have the disease: (TN)/(TN + false negative [FN]).[2]

For a given screening test, sensitivity and specificity are inversely related. For example, as one lowers the threshold for considering a serum prostate-specific antigen (PSA) level to represent a *positive* screen, the sensitivity of the test increases and more cancers will be detected. This increased sensitivity comes at the cost of decreased specificity (i.e., more men without cancer will have *positive* screenings tests and, therefore, will be subjected to unnecessary diagnostic procedures).

Some screening tests, such as mammograms, are more subjective and operator dependent than others. For this reason, the sensitivity and specificity of screening mammography varies among radiologists. For a given radiologist, the lower his or her threshold for considering a mammogram to be suspicious, the higher the sensitivity and lower the specificity will be for them. However, mammography can have both a higher sensitivity and higher specificity in the hands of a more experienced versus a less experienced radiologist.

As opposed to sensitivity and specificity, the PPV and NPV of a screening test are dependent on disease prevalence. PPV is also highly responsive to small increases in specificity. As shown in Table 34.2, given a disease prevalence of 5 cases per 1,000 (0.005), the PPV of a hypothetical screening test increases dramatically as specificity goes from 95% to 99.9%, but only marginally as sensitivity goes from 80% to 95%. Given a disease prevalence of only 1 per 10,000 (0.0001), the PPV of the same test is poor even at high sensitivity and specificity. The positive association between breast cancer prevalence and age is the major reason why screening mammography is a better test (higher PPV) for women aged 50 to 59 than for women 40 to 49 years of age.

ASSESSING SCREENING TESTS AND OUTCOMES

Screening Test Results

Lead time bias occurs whenever screening results in an earlier diagnosis than would have occurred in the absence of screening.

TABLE 34.1

Performance Characteristics of a Screening Test

Sensitivity is the proportion designated positive by the screening test among all individuals who have the disease.

$$\frac{TP}{TP + FN}$$

Specificity is the proportion designated negative by the screening test among all those who do not have the disease.

$$\frac{TN}{TN + FP}$$

Positive predictive value is the proportion of individuals with a positive test who have the disease.

$$\frac{TP}{TP + FP}$$

Negative predictive value is the proportion of individuals with a negative test negative who do not have the disease.

$$\frac{TN}{TN + FN}$$

TP, true positive, the condition present and the test is positive; FN, false negative, the condition is present and the test is negative; FP, false positive, the condition is absent and the test is positive; TN, true negative, the condition is absent and test is negative.

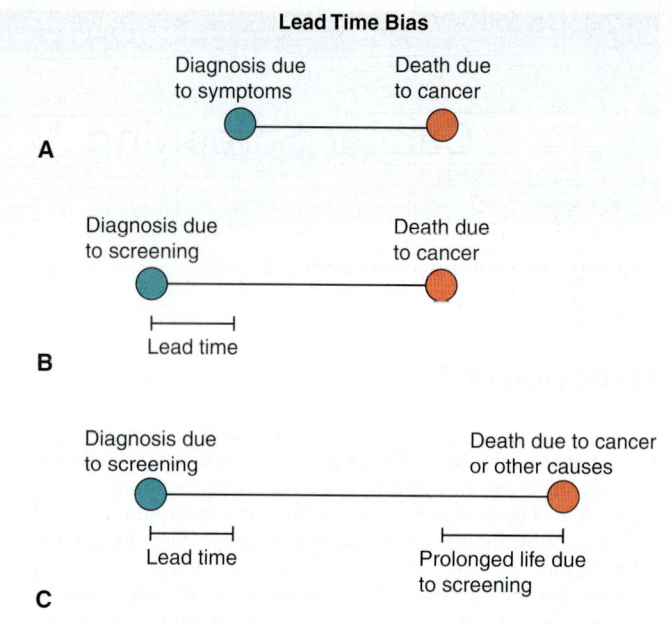

Figure 34.1 Survival is the time from cancer diagnosis to death. **(A)** Lead time bias occurs when screening results in an earlier diagnosis. Without screening, a patient is diagnosed with cancer due to symptoms. **(B)** With screening, the patient is often diagnosed earlier. When screening and treatment do not prolong life, the screened patient can have a longer survival solely due to the earlier diagnosis. The survival increase is pure lead time bias. **(C)** When screening and treatment are beneficial, the patient is diagnosed before the onset of symptoms and the patient lives beyond the point in which death would have occurred without screening.

Because survival is measured *from the time of diagnosis*, an earlier diagnosis, by definition, increases survival. Unless an effective intervention is available, lead time bias has no impact on the natural history of a disease and death will occur at the same time it would have in the absence of early detection (Fig. 34.1).

Length bias is a function of the biologic behavior of a cancer. Slower growing, less aggressive cancers are more likely to be detected by a screening test than faster growing cancers, which are more likely to be diagnosed due to the onset of symptoms between scheduled screenings (interval cancers). Length bias has an even greater effect on survival statistics than lead time bias (Fig. 34.2).

Overdiagnosis is an extreme form of length bias and represents pure harm. It refers to the detection of tumors, often through highly sensitive modern imaging modalities and other diagnostic tests, that fulfill the histologic criteria for malignancy but are not biologically destined to harm the patient (see Fig. 34.2).

There are two categories of overdiagnosis: the detection of histologically defined *cancers* not destined to metastasize or harm the patient, and the detection of cancers not destined to metastasize or cause harm *in the life span of the specific patient*. The importance of this second category is illustrated by the widespread practice in the United States of screening elderly patients with limited life expectancies, who are thus unlikely to benefit from early cancer diagnosis.

Overdiagnosis occurs with many malignancies, including lung, breast, prostate, renal cell, melanoma, and thyroid cancers.[3] Neuroblastoma provides one of the most striking examples of overdiagnosis.[4] Urine vanillylmandelic acid (VMA) testing is a highly sensitive screening test for the detection of this pediatric disease. After screening programs in Germany, Japan, and Canada showed marked increases in the incidence of this disease without a concomitant decline in mortality, it was noticed that nearby areas that did not screen had similar death rates with lower incidence.[4,5] It is now appreciated that screen-detected neuroblastomas have a very good prognosis with minimal or no treatment. Many actually regress spontaneously.

Stage shift—i.e., a cancer diagnosis at an earlier stage than would have occurred in the absence of screening—is necessary, but not sufficient, for a screening test to be effective in terms of reducing mortality. Both lead time bias and length bias contribute to this phenomenon. Although it is tempting to speculate that diagnosis at an earlier stage must confer benefit, this is not necessarily the case. For example, a substantial proportion of men treated with radical prostatectomy for what appears to be a localized prostate cancer relapse after undergoing surgery. Conversely, some men who are treated with definitive therapy would never have gone on to develop metastatic disease in the absence of treatment.

TABLE 34.2

Positive Predictive Value Given Varying Sensitivity and Specificity and Prevalence

Prevalence 0.005		Sensitivity %		
		80	90	95
Specificity %	95	7	8	9
	99	29	31	32
	99.9	80	82	83

Prevalence 0.0001		Sensitivity %		
		80	90	95
Specificity %	95	0.2	0.2	2.0
	99	0.8	0.9	0.9
	99.9	0.7	8.0	0.0

PPV improves dramatically in response to small changes in specificity. Changes in specificity influence PPV much more than changes in sensitivity. Note the influence of prevalence on PPV. Screening tests do not perform as well in populations with a low prevalence of disease.

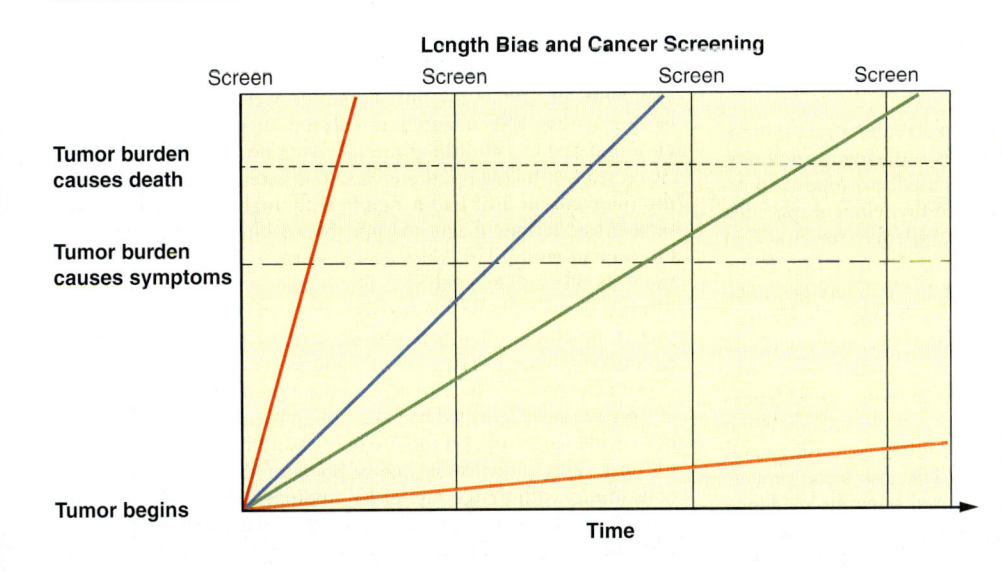

Figure 34.2 Length bias and cancer screening. The *red line* is indicative of a fast-growing tumor that is not amenable to regular screening. The *blue line* is indicative of a fast-growing tumor that can be diagnosed by screening or later by symptoms; death may possibly be prevented by treatment. The *green line* is a slower growing but potentially deadly cancer that can be detected by symptoms or several screenings and treated, possibly preventing death. The *orange line* is indicative of a very slow growing tumor that would never cause death and would never need treatment despite being screen detected. This is classic overdiagnosis.

Selection bias occurs when enrollees in a clinical study differ from the general population. In fact, people who voluntarily participate in clinical trials tend to be healthier than the general population, perhaps due to a greater interest in health and healthcare research. Screening studies tend to enroll individuals healthier than the general population. This so-called *healthy volunteer effect*[6,7] can introduce a powerful bias if not adequately controlled for by randomization procedures.

Assessing Screening Outcomes

The usual primary goal of cancer screening is to reduce mortality from the disease in question (a reduction in disease-specific mortality). Screening studies generally do not have sufficient statistical power to assess the impact of screening for a specific malignancy on overall mortality. (Lung cancer screening provides an exception to this rule; see the following.) As discussed previously, the fact that a screening test increases the percentage of people diagnosed with early stage cancer and decreases that of late stage cancer (stage shift) is not equivalent to proof of mortality reduction. Further, due to the healthy volunteer effect, case control and cohort studies cannot provide definitive evidence of mortality benefit. Prospective, randomized clinical trials are required to address this issue. In such trials, volunteers are randomized to be screened or not and are then followed longitudinally to determine if there is a difference in disease-specific or overall mortality.

A reduction in mortality rates or in the risk of death is often stated in terms of relative risk. However, this method of reporting may be misleading. It is preferable to report both the relative and absolute reduction in mortality. For example, the European Randomized Study of Screening for Prostate Cancer (ERSPC) showed that screening reduced the risk of prostate cancer death by 20%. However, this translates into only 1 prostate cancer death averted per 1,000 men screened (5 prostate cancer deaths per 1,000 men not screened versus 4 prostate cancer deaths per 1,000 men screened) and a relatively modest lifetime reduction in the absolute risk of prostate cancer death of only 0.6%, from 3.0% to 2.4%.[8]

PROBLEMS WITH RANDOMIZED TRIALS

It is important to acknowledge that even prospective, randomized trials can have serious methodologic shortcomings. For example, imbalances caused by flaws in the randomization scheme can prejudice the outcome of a trial. Other flaws include so-called *drop-in* or *contamination*, in which some participants on the control arm get the intervention. Patients on the intervention arm may also *drop out* of the study. Both drop-ins and drop-outs reduce the statistical power of a clinical trial.

In the United States, it is now considered standard to obtain informed consent before randomization takes place. However, there have been several published studies that randomized participants from rosters of eligible subjects such as census lists. In these trials, informed consent was obtained after randomization and only among those randomized to the screening arm of the study. Those randomized to the control arm were not contacted, and indeed, did not know they were in a clinical trial. They were followed through national death registries. Although the study was analyzed on an intent-to-screen basis, this method can still introduce biases. For example, only patients on the intervention arm had access to the screening facility and staff for counseling and treatment if diagnosed; those in the control group were more likely to be treated in the community as opposed to high-volume centers of excellence and were less likely to be treated with surgery and more likely to be treated with hormones alone than those on the screened arm. The study arms would also tend to differ in their knowledge of the disease, which may contribute to an overestimate of the benefits of a screening test.[9]

Virtually every screening test is a balance between known harms and potential benefits. The most important risk of screening is the detection and subsequent treatment of a cancer that would never have come to clinical detection or harmed the patient in the absence of screening (i.e., overdiagnosis and overtreatment). Treatment can cause emotional and physical morbidity and even death.[10] Even when screening has a net mortality benefit, there can be considerable harm. For example, in the recent randomized trial of spiral lung computed tomography (CT) scan, approximately 27,000 current smokers and former smokers were given three annual low-dose CT scans. More than 20% had a *positive* screening CT scan, necessitating further testing. About 1,000 subsequently underwent invasive diagnostic procedures and 16 deaths were reported within 60 days of the procedure.[11] It is not known how many of these deaths were directly related to the screening.

It can be dangerous to extrapolate estimates of benefit from one population to another. In particular, studies showing that a radiographic test is beneficial to average risk individuals may not mean that it is beneficial to a population at high risk, and vice versa. For example, women at high risk for breast cancer due to an inherited mutation of a DNA repair gene may be at higher risk for radiation-induced cancer from mammographies compared to the general population; a screening test (e.g., spiral lung CT scan), shown to be efficacious in a high-risk population of heavy smokers may result in net harm if applied to a low or average risk population.

SCREENING GUIDELINES AND RECOMMENDATIONS

A number of organizations develop cancer screening recommendations or guidelines. These organizations use varying methods. The Institute of Medicine (IOM) has released two reports to establish standards for developing trustworthy clinical practice guidelines and conducting systematic evidence reviews that serve as their basis.[12,13] The U.S. Preventive Services Task Force (USPSTF) and the American Cancer Society (ACS) are two organizations that issue respected and widely used cancer guidelines (Table 34.3). Both have changed their methods to comply with the IOM standards.

The USPSTF is a panel of experts in prevention and evidence-based medicine.[14] They are primary care providers specializing in internal medicine, pediatrics, family practice, gynecology and obstetrics, nursing, and health behavior. The task force process begins by conducting an extensive structured scientific evidence review. The task force then develops recommendations for primary care clinicians and health-care systems. They adhere to some of the highest standards for recommending a screening test. They are very much concerned with the question, "Does the evidence supporting a screening test demonstrate that the benefits outweigh its harms?"

The ACS guidelines date back to the 1970s. The current process for making guidelines involves commissioning academics to do an independent systematic evidence review. A single generalist group digests the evidence review, listens to public input, and writes the guidelines. The ACS panel tries to clearly articulate the benefits, limitations, and harms associated with a screening test.[15]

BREAST CANCER

Mammographies, clinical breast examinations (CBE) by a healthcare provider, and breast self-examinations (BSE) have long been advocated[16] for the early detection of breast cancer. In recent years, ultrasound, magnetic resonance imaging (MRI), and other technologies have been added to the list of proposed screening modalities.

Mammographic screening was first advocated in the 1950s. The Health Insurance Plan (HIP) Study was the first prospective, randomized clinical trial to formally assess its value in reducing death from breast cancer. In this study, started in 1963, about 61,000 women were randomized to three annual mammograms with clinical breast examination versus no screening, which was the standard practice at that time. HIP first reported that mammography reduced breast cancer mortality by 30% at about 10 years after study entry. With 18 years of follow-up, those in the screening arm had a 25% lower breast cancer mortality rate.[16]

Nine additional prospective randomized studies have been published. These studies provide the basis for the current consensus that screening women 40 to 75 years of age does reduce the relative risk of breast cancer death by 10% to 25%. The 10 studies demonstrate that the risk–benefit ratio is more favorable for women over 50 years of age. Mammography has also been shown to be operator dependent, with better performance characteristics (higher sensitivity and specificity and lower FP rates) reported by high-volume centers (Table 34.4).

It is important to note that every one of these studies has some flaws and limitations. They vary in the questions asked and their findings. The Canadian screening trial suggests mammographies and clinical breast examinations do not decrease risk of death for women aged 40 to 49 and that mammographies add nothing to CBEs for women age 50 to 59 years.[17] On the other extreme, the Kopparberg, Sweden study suggests that mammographies are associated with a 32% reduction in the risk of death for women aged 40 to 74 years.[18]

To date, no study has shown that BSEs decrease mortality. BSEs have been studied in two large randomized trials. In one, approximately 266,000 Chinese women were randomized to receive intensive BSE instruction with reinforcements and reminders compared to a control group receiving no instruction on BSE. At 10 years of follow-up, there was no difference in mortality, but the intervention arm had a significantly higher incidence of benign breast lesions diagnosed and breast biopsies preformed. In the second study, 124,000 Russian women were randomized to monthly BSEs versus no BSEs. There was no difference in mortality rates, despite the BSE group having a higher proportion of early stage tumors and a significant increase in the proportion of cancer patients surviving 15 years after diagnosis.

Ultrasonography is primarily used in the diagnostic evaluation of a breast mass identified by palpation or mammography. There is little evidence to support the use of ultrasound as an initial screening test. This modality is highly operator dependent and time consuming, with a high rate of FP findings.[19] An MRI is used for screening women at elevated breast cancer risk due to BRCA1 and BRCA2 mutations, Li-Fraumeni syndrome, Cowden disease, or a very strong family history. MRI is more sensitive but less specific than mammography, leading to a high FP rate and more unnecessary biopsies, especially among young women.[20] The impact of MRI breast screening on breast cancer mortality has not yet been determined.

Thermography, an infrared imaging technology, has some advocates as a breast cancer screening modality despite a lack of evidence from several small cohort studies.[21] Nipple aspirate cytology and ductal lavage have also been suggested as possible screening methods. Both should be considered experimental at this time.[22]

Effectiveness of Breast Cancer Screening

Breast cancer screening has been associated with a dramatic rise in breast cancer incidence. At the same time, there has been a dramatic decrease in breast cancer mortality rates. However, in the United States and Europe, incidence-by-stage data show a dramatic increase in the proportion of early stage cancers without a concomitant decrease in the incidence of regional and metastatic cancers.[23] These findings are at odds with the clinical trials data and raise questions regarding the extent to which early diagnosis is responsible for declining breast cancer mortality rates.

From 1976 to 2008, the incidence of early-stage breast cancer for American women aged 40 and older increased from 112 to 234 per 100,000. This is a rise of 122 cases per 100,000, whereas the absolute decrease in late-stage cancers was only 8 cases per 100,000 (from 102 to 94 cases per 100,000). These data raise questions regarding the magnitude of benefit, as well as the potential risks, of breast cancer screening. The discrepancy between the magnitude of the increase of early disease and the decrease of late-stage cancer and cancer mortality suggests that a proportion of invasive breast cancers diagnosed by screening represents overdiagnosis. These data suggest that overdiagnosis accounts for up to 31% of all breast cancers diagnosed by screening.[24] Others have estimated that up to 50% of breast cancers detected by screening mammography are overdiagnosed cancers. In an exhaustive review of the screening literature, a panel of experts concluded that overdiagnosis does exist and estimated it to be 11% to 19% of breast cancers diagnosed by screening.[25]

A confounding factor with regard to the mortality benefits of breast cancer screening is the improvement that has occurred in breast cancer treatment over this period of time. The effects of the advances in therapy are supported by cancer modeling studies. Indeed, the Cancer Intervention and Surveillance Modeling Network (CISNET), supported by the U.S. National Cancer Institute (NCI), has estimated that two-thirds of the observed breast cancer mortality reduction is attributable to modern therapy, rather than to screening.[26]

TABLE 34.3
Screening Recommendations for Normal-Risk Asymptomatic Subjects

Cancer Type	Test or Procedure	American Cancer Society	U.S. Preventive Services Task Force
Breast	Self-examination	Women ≥20 years: Breast self-exam is an option	"D"
	Clinical examination	Women 20–39 years: Perform every 3 years Women ≥40 years: Perform annually	Women ≥40 years: "I" (as a stand alone without mammography)
	Mammography	Women ≥40 years: Screen annually for as long as the woman is in good health	Women 40–49 years: The decision should be an individual one, and take patient context/values into account ("C") Women 50–74 years: Every 2 years ("B") Women ≥75 years: "I"
	MRI	Women >20% lifetime risk of breast cancer: Screen with MRI plus mammography annually Women 15%–20% lifetime risk of breast cancer: Discuss option of MRI plus mammography annually Women <15% lifetime risk of breast cancer: Do not screen annually with MRI	"I"
Cervical	Pap test (cytology)	Women ages 21–29 years: Screen every 3 years Women 30–65 years: Acceptable approach to screen with cytology every 3 years (see HPV test) Women <21 years: No screening Women >65 years: No screening following adequate negative prior screening Women after total hysterectomy for noncancerous causes: Do not screen	Women ages 21–65 years: Screen every 3 years ("A") Women <21 years: "D" Women >65 years, with adequate, normal prior Pap screenings: "D" Women after total hysterectomy for noncancerous causes: "D"
	HPV test	Women <30 years: Do not use HPV testing Women ages 30–65 years: Preferred approach to screen with HPV and cytology cotesting every 5 years (see Pap test) Women >65 years: No screening following adequate negative prior screening Women after total hysterectomy for noncancerous causes: Do not screen	Women ages 30–65 years: Screen in combination with cytology every 5 years if woman desires to lengthen the screening interval (see Pap test) ("A") Women <30 years: "D" Women >65 years, with adequate, normal prior Pap screenings: "D" Women after total hysterectomy for noncancerous causes: "D"
Colorectal	Sigmoidoscopy	Adults ≥50 years: Screen every 5 years Note: For all CRC screening tests, stop screening when benefits are unlikely due to life-limiting comorbidity.	Adults 50–75 years: Every 5 years in combination with high-sensitivity fecal occult blood testing (FOBT) every 3 years ("A")[a] Adults 76–85 years: "C" Adults ≥85 years: "D"
	Fecal occult blood testing (FOBT)	Adults ≥50 years: Screen every year with high sensitivity guaiac based FOBT or fecal immunochemical test (FIT) only	Adults 50–75 years: Annually, for high-sensitivity FOBT ("A") Adults 76–85 years: "C" Adults ≥85 years: "D"
	Colonoscopy	Adults ≥50 years: Screen every 10 years	Adults 50–75 years: every 10 years ("A") Adults 76–85 years: "C" Adults ≥85 years: "D"
	Fecal DNA testing	Adults ≥50 years: Screen, but interval uncertain	"I"
	Fecal immunochemical testing (FIT)	Adults ≥50 years: Screen every year	"I"
	CT colonography	Adults ≥50 years: Screen every 5 years	"I"
Lung	Complete skin examination by clinician or patient	Men and women, 55–74 years, with ≥30 pack-year smoking history, still smoking or have quit within past 15 years: Discuss benefits, limitations, and potential harms of screening. Only perform screening in facilities with the right type of CT scanner and with high expertise/specialists.	"I" ("B" draft recommendation issued for public comment in July 2013)

(continued)

TABLE 34.3

Screening Recommendations for Normal-Risk Asymptomatic Subjects *(continued)*

Cancer Type	Test or Procedure	American Cancer Society	U.S. Preventive Services Task Force
Ovary	CA-125 Transvaginal ultrasound	There is no sufficiently accurate test proven effective in the early detection of ovarian cancer. For women at high risk of ovarian cancer and/or who have unexplained, persistent symptoms, the combination of CA-125 and transvaginal ultrasound with pelvic exam may be offered.	"D" "D"
Prostate	Prostate-specific antigen (PSA)	Starting at age 50, men should talk to a doctor about the pros and cons of testing so they can decide if testing is the right choice for them. If African American or have a father or brother who had prostate cancer before age 65, men should have this talk starting at age 45. How often they are tested will depend on their PSA level. As for PSA; if men decide to be tested, they should have the PSA blood test with or without a rectal exam.	Men, all ages: "D"
	Digital rectal examination (DRE)		No individual recommendation
Skin	Complete skin examination by clinician or patient	Self-examination monthly; clinical exam as part of routine cancer-related checkup	"I"

Note: Summary of the screening procedures recommended for the general population by the American Cancer Society and the U.S. Preventive Services Task Force. These recommendations refer to asymptomatic persons who have no risk factors for the cancer, other than age or gender.

[a] USPSTF lettered recommendations are defined as follows:
"A": The USPSTF recommends the service, because there is high certainty that the net benefit is substantial.
"B": The USPSTF recommends the service, because there is high certainty that the net benefit is moderate or moderate certainty that the net benefit is moderate to substantial.
"C": The USPSTF recommends selectively offering or providing this service to individual patients based on professional judgment and patient preferences. There is at least moderate certainty that the net benefit is small.
"D": The USPSTF recommends against the service, because there is moderate or high certainty that the service has no net benefit or that the harms outweigh the benefits.
"I": The USPSTF concludes that the current evidence is insufficient to assess the balance of benefits and harms of the service.

Questions have also been raised regarding the quality of the randomized screening trials that demonstrated the mortality benefits of mammography and clinical breast examination because these trials suffered from a variety of design flaws. In some, randomization methods were suboptimal, others reported varying numbers of participants over the years, and still others had substantial contamination (drop-ins). Perhaps more importantly, most trials were started and concluded before the widespread use of more advanced mammographic technology, before the modern era of adjuvant therapy, and before the advent of targeted therapy.

Although randomized control trials (RCT) remain the gold standard for assessing the benefits of a clinical intervention, they cannot take into account improvements in both treatment and patient awareness that occurred over time. For this reason, observational and modeling studies can provide important, complementary information.

One systematic review of 17 published population-based and cohort studies compared breast cancer mortality in groups of women aged 50 to 69 years who started breast cancer screening at different times. Although these studies are subject to methodologic limitations, only four suggested that breast cancer screening reduced the relative risk of breast cancer mortality by 33% or more and five suggested no benefit from screening. The review concluded that breast cancer screening likely reduces the risk of breast cancer death by no more than 10%.[27]

Even with these limitations, a systematic review of the data sponsored by the USPSTF concluded that regular mammography reduces breast cancer mortality in women aged 40 to 74 years.[28] The task force also concluded that the benefits of mammography are most significant in women aged 50 to 74 years.

Screening Women Age 40 to 49

Experts disagree about the utility of screening women in their forties. In the HIP Randomized Control Trial, women who entered at age 40 to 49 years had a mortality benefit at 18 years of follow-up. However, to a large extent, the mortality benefit among those aged 45 to 49 years at entry was driven by breast cancers diagnosed after they reached age 50 years.[16]

Mammography, like all screening tests, is more efficient (higher PPV) for the detection of disease in populations with higher disease prevalence (see Table 34.2). Mammography is, therefore, a better test in women age 50 to 59 years than it is among women age 40 to 49 years because the risk of breast cancer increases with age. Mammography is also less optimal in women age 40 to 49 years compared to women 50 to 59 years of age for the following reasons:

- A larger proportion have increased breast density, which can obscure lesions (lower sensitivity).
- Younger women are more likely to develop aggressive, fast-growing breast cancers that are diagnosed between regular screening visits. By definition, these *interval cancers* are not screen detected.[29]

The USPSTF meta-analysis of eight large randomized trials suggested a 15% relative reduction in mortality (relative risk [RR], 0.85; 95% confidence interval [CI], 0.75 to 0.96) from mammography screening for women aged 40 to 49 years after 11 to 20 years of follow-up. This is equivalent to a needing to invite 1,904 women to screenings over 10 years to prevent one breast cancer death. Studies, however, show that more than half of women aged 40 to 49 years screened annually over a 10-year period will have an FP mammogram necessitating further evaluation, often including biopsy. In addition, estimates of overdiagnosis in this group range from 10% to 40% of diagnosed invasive cancers.[30]

In an effort to decrease FP rates, some have suggested screening every 2 years rather than yearly. Comparing biennial with annual screening, the USPSTF model demonstrated that biennial screening of women ages 40 to 70 only marginally decreases the number of lives saved while halving the false positive rate.[31] Notably, the Swedish two-county trial, which had a planned 24-month screening interval (the actual interval was 33 months) reported one

TABLE 34.4
Randomized Controlled Trials

Study	Randomization	Sample Size	Intervention and Age at Entry	Follow-up	Finding
Health Insurance Plan, United States 1963[a,b]	Individual	60,565–60,857	MMG and CBE for 3 years Age 40–64 years	18 years	RR 0.77 (95% CI: 0.61–0.97)
Malmo, Sweden 1976[c,d]	Individual	42,283	Two-view MMG every 18–24 months × 5 Age 45–69 years	12 years	RR 0.81 (95% CI: 0.62–1.07)
Ostergotland (County E of Two-County Trial) Sweden 1977[e-g]	Geographic cluster	38,405–39,034 study 37,145–37,936 control	Three single-view MMG every 2 years women, Age 40–50 years Every 33 months women, Age 50–74	12 years	RR 0.82 (95% CI: 0.64–1.05)
Kopparberg (County W of Two-County Trial) Sweden 1977[e-g]	Geographic cluster	38,562–39,051 intervention 18,478–18,846 control	Three single-view MMG every 2 years women, Age 40–50 years Every 33 months women, Age 50–74 years	12 years	RR 0.68 (95% CI: 0.52–0.89)
Edinburgh, United Kingdom[h]	Cluster by physician practice	23,266 study 21,904 control	Initially, two-view MMG and CBE Then annual CBE with single-view MMG years 3, 5, and 7, Age 45–64 years	10 years	RR 0.84 (95% CI: 0.63–1.12)
NBSS-1, Canada 1980[i,j]	Individual	25,214 study (100% screened after entry CBE) 25,216 control	Annual two-view MMG and CBE for 4–5 years, Age 40–49 years	13 years	RR 0.97 (95% CI: 0.74–1.27)
NBSS-2, Canada 1980[i,j]	Individual	19,711 study (100% screened after entry CBE) 19,694 control	Annual two-view MMG and CBE versus CBE, Age 50–59 years	11–16 years (mean 13 years)	RR 1.02 (95% CI: 0.78–1.33)
Stockholm, Sweden 1981[k]	Cluster by birth date	40,318–38,525 intervention group 19,943–20,978 control group	Single view MMG every 28 months × 2 Age 40–64 years	8 years	RR 0.80 (95%) CI: 0.53–1.22)
Gothenberg, Sweden 1982[d]	Complex	21,650 invited 29,961 control	Initial two-view MMG, then single-view MMG every 18 months × 4 Single read first three rounds, then double-read, Age 39–59 years	12–14 years	RR 0.79 (95% CI 0.58–1.08) In the evaluation phase RR 0.77 (95% CI 0.60–1.00) In follow-up phase
Age Trial[l]	Individual	160,921 (53,884 invited; 106,956 not invited)	Invited group aged 48 and younger offered annual screening by MMG (double-view first screen, then single mediolateral oblique view thereafter); 68% accepted screening on the first screen an 69% and 70% were reinvited (81% attended at least one screen) Age 39–41 years	10.7 years	RR 0.83 (95% CI: 0.66–1.04)

[a] Shapiro S, Venet W, Strax P, et al. Ten- to fourteen-year effect of screening on breast cancer mortality. *J Natl Cancer Inst* 1982;69:349–355.
[b] Shapiro S. Periodic screening for breast cancer: the HIP Randomized Controlled Trial. Health Insurance Plan. *J Natl Cancer Inst Monogr* 1997:27–30.
[c] Andersson I, Aspegren K, Janzon L, et al. Mammographic screening and mortality from breast cancer: the Malmo mammographic screening trial. *BMJ* 1988;297:943–948.
[d] Nystrom L, Rutqvist LE, Wall S, et al. Breast cancer screening with mammography: overview of Swedish randomised trials. *Lancet* 1993;341:973–978.
[e] Tabar L, Fagerberg CJ, Gad A, et al. Reduction in mortality from breast cancer after mass screening with mammography. Randomised trial from the Breast Cancer Screening Working Group of the Swedish National Board of Health and Welfare. *Lancet* 1985;1:829–832.
[f] Tabar L, Fagerberg G, Duffy SW, Day NE. The Swedish two county trial of mammographic screening for breast cancer: recent results and calculation of benefit. *J Epidemiol Community Health* 1989;43:107–114.
[g] Tabar L, Fagerberg G, Duffy SW, et al. Update of the Swedish two-county program of mammographic screening for breast cancer. *Radiol Clin North Am* 1992;30:187–210.
[h] Roberts MM, Alexander FE, Anderson TJ, et al. Edinburgh trial of screening for breast cancer: mortality at seven years. *Lancet* 1990;335:241–246.
[i] Miller AB, To T, Baines CJ, Wall C. The Canadian National Breast Screening Study-1: breast cancer mortality after 11 to 16 years of follow-up. A randomized screening trial of mammography in women age 40 to 49 years. *Ann Intern Med* 2002;137:305–312.
[j] Miller AB, Wall C, Baines CJ, et al. Twenty five year follow-up for breast cancer incidence and mortality of the Canadian National Breast Screening Study: randomised screening trial. *BMJ* 2014;348–366.
[k] Frisell J, Eklund G, Hellstrom L, et al. Randomized study of mammography screening—preliminary report on mortality in the Stockholm trial. *Breast Cancer Res Treat* 1991;18:49–56.
[l] Moss SM, Cuckle H, Evans A, et al. Effect of mammographic screening from age 40 years on breast cancer mortality at 10 years' follow-up: a randomised controlled trial. *Lancet* 2006;368:2053–2060.

of the greatest reductions in breast cancer mortality among the RCTs conducted to date.

Screening Women at High Risk

There is interest in creating risk profiles as a way of reducing the inconveniences and harms of screening. It might be possible to identify women who are at greater risk of breast cancer and refocus screening efforts on those most likely to benefit.

Risk factors for breast cancer include the following:

- Extremely dense breasts on mammography or a first-degree relative with breast cancer are each associated with at least a twofold increase in breast cancer risk
- Prior benign breast biopsy, second-degree relatives with breast cancer, or heterogeneously dense breasts each increase risk 1.5- to twofold
- Current oral contraceptive use, nulliparity, and age at first birth 30 years and older increase risk 1- to 1.5-fold.[31]

Importantly, these are risk factors for breast cancer diagnosis, not breast cancer mortality. Few studies have assessed the association between these factors and death from breast cancer; however, reproductive factors and breast density have been shown to have limited influence on breast cancer mortality.[32,33]

Genetic testing for BRCA1 and BRCA2 mutations and other markers of breast cancer risk has identified a group of women at high risk for breast cancer. Unfortunately, when to begin and the optimal frequency of screening have not been defined. Mammography is less sensitive at detecting lesions in women carrying BRCA1 and BRCA2 mutations, possibly because such cancers occur in younger women in whom mammography is known to be less sensitive.

MRI screening may be more sensitive than mammography in women at high risk, but specificity is lower. MRIs are associated with both an increase in FP and an increase in the detection of smaller cancers, which are more likely to be biologically indolent. The impact of MRIs on breast cancer mortality with or without concomitant use of mammographies has not been evaluated in a randomized controlled trial.

Breast Density

It is well established that mammogram sensitivity is lower in women with heterogeneously dense or very dense breasts.[29,32] However, at this time, there are no clear guidelines regarding whether or how screening algorithms should take breast density into account.

In the American College of Radiology's Imaging Network (ACRIN)/NCI 666 Trial, breast ultrasound was offered to women with increased mammographic breast density and, if either test was positive, they were referred for a breast biopsy.[34] The radiologists performing the ultrasounds were not aware of the mammographic findings. Mammography detected 7.6 cancers per 1,000 women screened; ultrasound increased the cancer detection rate to 11.8 per 1,000. However, the PPV for mammography alone was 22.6%, whereas the PPV for mammography with ultrasound was only 11.2%.

It has yet to be determined whether supplemental imaging reduces breast cancer mortality in women with increased breast density. Although it continues to be strongly advocated by some, systematic reviews have concluded that the evidence is currently insufficient to recommend for or against this approach.[35] There are also a number of barriers to supplemental imaging, including inconsistent insurance coverage, lack of availability in many communities, concerns about cost-effectiveness (particularly with regard to MRI), and the increased FP rate associated with supplemental imaging leading to unnecessary biopsies.[36]

Newer technologies may improve screening accuracy for women with dense breasts. Compared to conventional mammography, full-field digital mammography (FFDM) appears to have less FPs. This could reduce the number of women needing supplemental imaging and biopsies.[37] Digital breast tomosynthesis (DBT) uses x-rays and a digital detector to generate cross-sectional images of the breasts. Data are limited, but compared to mammograms, DBT appears to offer increased sensitivity and a reduction in the recall rates.[38] Another potential supplementary imaging modality currently under investigation is three-dimensional (3-D) automated breast ultrasound, and having screening ultrasounds performed by technologists rather than radiologists.

Ductal Carcinoma In Situ

The incidence of noninvasive ductal carcinoma in situ (DCIS) has increased more than fivefold since 1970 as a direct consequence of widespread screening mammographies.[39] DCIS is a heterogeneous condition with low- and intermediate-grade lesions taking a decade or more to progress. Nevertheless, women with this diagnosis are uniformly subjected to treatment. A better understanding of this entity and an increased ability to predict its biologic behavior may enable more judicious, personalized treatment of DCIS.

There is little evidence that the early detection and aggressive treatment of low- and intermediate-grade DCIS reduces breast cancer mortality. The standard of care for all grades of DCIS is lumpectomy with radiation or mastectomy, followed by tamoxifen for 5 years. Interestingly, patterns of care studies indicate that mastectomy rates are increasing,[40] and that women are more often choosing double mastectomies for the treatment of DCIS.[41] Genomic characterization will hopefully lead to the identification of a subset of noninvasive cancers that can be treated less aggressively or even observed.

Harms

The harms and disadvantages of mammography screening include overdiagnosis, FP tests, FN tests, and the possibility of radiation-induced breast cancer.

The fact that mammography screening has increased the incidence of localized disease without a significant change in metastatic disease at the time of diagnosis suggests that there is some degree of overdiagnosis. The risk of overdiagnosis is greatest at the first screening[3] and varies with patient age, tumor type, and grade of disease.

FP screening tests lead to substantial inconvenience and anxiety in addition to unnecessary invasive biopsies with their attendant complications. In the United States, about 10% of all women screened for breast cancer are called back for additional testing, and less than half of them will be diagnosed with breast cancer. The risk of a FP mammogram is greater for women under the age of 50.[37]

FN tests delay diagnosis and provide false reassurance. They are more common in younger women and in women with dense breasts.[42,43] Certain histologic subtypes are also more difficult to see on mammogram. Mucinous and lobular tumors and rapidly growing tumors tend to blend in with normal breast architecture.[44]

A typical screening mammogram provides approximately 4 mSv of radiation. It has been estimated that annual mammographies will cause up to 1 case of breast cancer per 1,000 women screened from age 40 to age 80 years. Radiation exposure at younger ages causes a greater risk of breast cancer.[45] There is also concern that ionizing radiation from mammographies might disproportionately increase the breast cancer risk for women with certain BRCA1 or BRCA2 mutations, because these genes are related to DNA repair.[46]

Recommendations

Women at Average Risk

The ACS and most other medical groups recommend that average risk women undergo a CBE every 3 years starting at age 20 and that women 40 years of age and over should undergo CBEs and screening mammograms annually. Women should be informed of the benefits, limitations, and harms associated with breast cancer screening. A mammography will not detect all breast cancers, and some breast cancers detected with mammographies may still have a poor prognosis. The harms associated with breast cancer screening also include the potential for FP results, causing substantial anxiety. When abnormal findings cannot be resolved with additional imaging, a biopsy is required to rule out the possibility of breast cancer. A majority of biopsies are benign. Finally, some breast cancers detected by a mammography may be biologically indolent, meaning they would not have caused a problem or have been detected in a woman's lifetime had she not undergone a mammography.

The USPSTF, the American College of Physicians, and the Canadian Task Force on the Periodic Health Examination recommend routine screening beginning at age 50 years.[30,47,48] For women aged 40 to 49 years of age, these groups advise physicians to enter into a discussion with the patient. The physician and patient should take into account individual risks and concerns before deciding to screen.[47]

An Advisory Committee on Cancer Prevention in the European Union recommends that women between the ages of 50 and 69 years be offered mammogram screening in an organized screening program with quality assurance.[49] This committee says women aged 40 to 49 years should be advised of the potential harms of screening and, if mammographic screening is offered, it should be performed with strict quality standards and double reading.

Women at High Risk

The ACS has issued guidelines for women who are known to likely carriers of a BRCA mutation and other rarer high-risk genetic syndromes, or at high risk for other reasons.[50] Annual screening mammographies and MRIs starting at age 30 is recommended for women:

- With a known *BRCA* mutation
- Who are untested but have a first-degree relative with a *BRCA* mutation
- Who had been treated with radiation to the chest for Hodgkin disease
- Who have an approximately 20% to 25% or greater lifetime risk of breast cancer based on specialized breast cancer risk estimation models.

COLON CANCER SCREENING

Colorectal cancer screening with the rigid sigmoidoscope dates back to the late 1960s. The desire to examine the entire colon led to the use of a barium enema and the development of fecal occult blood tests. With the development of fiber optics, flexible sigmoidoscopies and, later, colonoscopies were employed. Today, fecal occult blood testing (FOBT), stool DNA testing, flexible sigmoidoscopies, colonoscopies, and CT colonographies and, occasionally, barium enemas are all used in colorectal cancer screening. MRI colonoscopy is in development.

Screening examinations of the colon and rectum can find cancer early, but also find precancerous polyps. Randomized trials have demonstrated that endoscopic polypectomies reduce the incidence of colorectal cancer by about 20%.[51–53]

FOBT was the first colorectal screening test studied in a prospective randomized clinical trial. The Minnesota Colon Cancer Control Study randomized 46,551 adults to one of three arms: annual FOBTs, biennial screening, or usual care. A rehydrated guaiac test was used. With 13 years of follow-up, the annual screened arm had a 33% relative reduction in colorectal cancer mortality compared to the usual care group.[54] At 18 years of follow-up, the biennially screened group had a 21% reduction in colorectal cancer mortality.[55] This study would subsequently show that stool blood testing was associated with a 20% reduction in colon cancer incidence.[51] These results were confirmed by two other randomized trials.[56,57] A reduction in colon cancer-specific mortality persisted in the Minnesota trial through 30 years of follow-up. Overall mortality was not affected.

Rehydration increases the sensitivity of FOBT at the expense of lowering specificity.[58] Indeed, rehydrated specimens have a very high FP rate. Overall, 1% to 5% of FOBTs are positive, but only 2% to 10% of those with a positive FOBT have cancer.

Fecal immunochemical tests (FIT) are stool tests that do not react to hemoglobin in dietary products. They appear to have higher sensitivity and specificity for colorectal cancer when compared to nonrehydrated FOBT tests.[59]

Fecal DNA testing is an emerging modality. These tests look for DNA sequences specific to colorectal polyps and colorectal cancer. They may have increased sensitivity and specificity compared to FOBT. Although fecal DNA tests appear to find cancer, the body of evidence on their ability to reduce colorectal cancer mortality is limited due to a lack of study. This test has been intermittently available.

Flexible sigmoidoscopies are, of course, limited to an examination of the rectum and sigmoid colon. A prospective randomized trial of once-only flexible sigmoidoscopies demonstrated a 23% reduction in colorectal cancer incidence and a 31% reduction in colorectal cancer mortality after a median 11.2 years of follow-up.[60] In the NCI's Prostate, Lung, Colorectal, and Ovarian Cancer Screening Trial (PLCO), there was a 21% reduction in colorectal cancer incidence and a 26% reduction in colorectal cancer mortality with two sigmoidoscopies done 3 to 5 years apart compared with the usual care group after a median followup of 11.9 years.[53] In both studies, there was no effect on proximal lesions (i.e., right and transverse colon) due to the limited reach of the scope. It is estimated that flexible sigmoidoscopies can find 60% to 80% of cancers and polyps found by colonoscopies.[61]

In two meta-analyses of five randomized controlled trials of sigmoidoscopies, there was an 18% relative reduction in colorectal cancer incidence and a 28% relative reduction in colorectal cancer mortality.[62,63] Participants ranged in age from 50 to 74 years. Follow-up ranged from 6 to 13 years.

The *colonoscopy* has become the preferred screening method of many, although there have been no prospective, randomized trials of colonoscopy screening. A positive FOBT, FIT, fecal DNA test, or sigmoidoscopy warrants a follow-up diagnostic colonoscopy. Perhaps the best support for colonoscopy screening is indirect evidence from the Minnesota Colon Cancer Control Study, which required that all participants with a positive stool blood test have diagnostic imaging of the entire colon. In the Minnesota study, more than 40% of those screened annually eventually received a colonoscopy. One can also make the argument that the sigmoidoscopy studies indirectly support the efficacy of colonoscopy screening, although it can be argued that embryologic and epidemiologic evidence indicate that the right and left colon are biologically distinct and, therefore, the mortality benefits from sigmoidoscopies do not constitute proof that a colonoscopy would similarly reduce mortality from proximal colon lesions.

In studies involving repeat colonoscopies by a second physician, 21% of all adenomas were missed, including 26% of 1 to 5 mm adenomas and 2% of adenomas 10 mm or more in length.[64] Other limitations of colonoscopies include the inconvenience of the bowel preparation and the risk of bowel perforation (about 3 out of 1,000 procedures, overall, with nearly all of the risk among patients who undergo colonoscopic polypectomies). The cost of the procedure and the limited number of physicians who can do the procedure are also of concern.

A *CT colonography* or *virtual* colonoscopy allows a physician to visually reproduce the endoscopic examination on a computer screen. A CT colonography involves the same prep as a colonoscopy, but is less invasive. It might have a higher compliance rate.

In experienced hands, the sensitivity of a CT colonography for the detection of polyps ≥6 mm appears to be comparable to that of a colonoscopy. In a meta-analysis of 30 studies, 2-D and 3-D CT colonographies performed equally well.[65]

The disadvantages of a CT colonography include the fact that it requires a colonic prep and a finding on CT requires a follow-up diagnostic colonoscopy. The rate of extracolonic findings of uncertain significance is high (~15% to 30%), and each one must be evaluated, thereby contributing to additional expense and potential morbidity. The long-term, cumulative radiation risk of repeated colonography screenings is also a concern.

Current Recommendations

The ACS, the American College of Gastroenterology, the American Gastroenterological Association, the American Society for Gastrointestinal Endoscopy, and the American College of Radiology have issued joint colorectal cancer guidelines. These groups consider FOBT, FIT, rigid and flexible sigmoidoscopies, colonoscopies, and CT colonographies to all be reasonable screening methodologies.

They recommend the following: (1) Screening modalities be chosen based on personal preference and access, and (2) average risk adults should begin colorectal cancer screening at age 50 years with one of the following options:

1. Annual high sensitivity FOBT or FIT
2. A flexible sigmoidoscopy every 5 years
3. A colonoscopy every 10 years
4. A double contrast barium enema every 5 years
5. A CT colonography every 5 years

No test is of unequivocal superiority. Patient preferences should be incorporated into screening in order to increase compliance. The guidelines also stress that a single screening examination is far from optimal and that patients should be in a program of regular screening.

Although some colorectal cancers are diagnosed in persons under the age of 50 years, screening persons age 40 to 49 years has low yield.[66] The guidelines also state that patients with less than a 10-year life expectancy should not be screened.

The USPSTF issued colorectal cancer screening guidelines in 2008.[67] The guidelines were based on a systematic literature review and decision models. The task force concluded that three screening strategies appear to be equivalent for adults age 50 to 75 years:

1. An annual FOBT with a sensitive test
2. A flexible sigmoidoscopy every 5 years, with a sensitive FOBT every 3 years
3. A colonoscopy every 10 years

The task force recommends that patients age 76 to 85 years be evaluated individually for screening. They found "insufficient evidence" to recommend CT colonographies or fecal DNA testing.

Patients at Increased Risk of Colorectal Cancer

Patients can have higher than average risk of colorectal cancer due to familial or hereditary factors and clinical conditions such as inflammatory bowel disease. These patients technically undergo surveillance and not screening. Nevertheless, there are few clinical studies to guide recommendations. Guidelines have been created based on professional opinion and an understanding of the biology of colorectal cancer (Table 34.5).[68]

OTHER CANCERS OF THE GASTROINTESTINAL TRACT

There are no widely accepted screening guidelines for cancers of the esophagus, stomach, pancreas, and liver. However, surveillance is advocated for some patients at high risk.

Esophageal Cancer Screening

Esophageal cancer screening has centered on endoscopic examinations for those at high risk due to chronic, severe gastroesophageal reflux disease.[69] Some physicians advocate routine endoscopic surveillance of patients with Barrett esophagus. At this time, there is no evidence that such surveillance is effective at reducing cancer mortality.

TABLE 34.5

Colon Cancer Screening Recommendations for People with Familial or Inherited Risk

Familial Risk Category	Screening Recommendation
First-degree relative[a] affected with colorectal cancer or an adenomatous polyp at age ≥60 years, or two second-degree relatives[b] affected with colorectal cancer	Same as average risk but starting at age 40 years
Two or more first-degree relatives with colon cancer, or a single first-degree relative with colon cancer or adenomatous polyps diagnosed at an age <60 years	Colonoscopy every 5 years, beginning at age 40 years or 10 years younger than the earliest diagnosis in the family, whichever comes first
One second-degree or any third-degree relative[b,c] with colorectal cancer	Same as average risk
Gene carrier or at risk for familial adenomatous polyposis[d]	Sigmoidoscopy annually, beginning at age 10–12 years[e]
Gene carrier or at risk for HNPCC	Colonoscopy, every 1–2 years, beginning at age 20–25 years or 10 years younger than the earliest case in the family, whichever comes first

[a] First-degree relatives include patients, siblings, and children.
[b] Second-degree relatives include grandparents, aunts, and uncles.
[c] Third-degree relatives include great-grandparents and cousins.
[d] Includes the subcategories of familial adenomatous polyposis, Gardner syndrome, some Turcot syndrome families, and attenuated adenomatous polyposis coli (AAPC).
[e] In AAPC, colonoscopy should be used instead of sigmoidoscopy because of the preponderance of proximal colonic adenomas. Colonoscopy screening in AAPC should probably begin in the late teens or early 20s.
HNPCC, hereditary nonpolyposis colon cancer.
From Winawer S, Fletcher R, Rex D, et al. Colorectal cancer screening and surveillance: clinical guidelines and rationale: update based on new evidence. Gastroenterology 2003;124:544–560, with permission.

Gastric Cancer Screening

Barium-meal photofluorography, serum pepsinogen, and gastric endoscopy have been proposed as screening methods for the early detection of gastric cancer. There are no randomized trials evaluating the impact of these modalities on gastric cancer mortality. Indeed, screening with barium-meal photofluorography has been studied in high-risk populations for more than 40 years without clear evidence of benefit.

Time-trend analysis and case control studies of gastric endoscopy have suggested a decrease in gastric cancer mortality among those at high risk in screened versus unscreened individuals; however, a large observational study in a high-risk population failed to demonstrate a benefit.[70,71]

Although widespread gastric screenings cannot be advocated, there may be justification for endoscopic screenings of high-risk populations. Candidates for screening might include elderly individuals with atrophic gastritis or pernicious anemia, patients who have had partial gastrectomy,[72] those with a history of sporadic adenomas, and patients with familial adenomatous polyposis or hereditary nonpolyposis colon cancer.

Pancreatic Cancer Screening

At this time, there are no data from prospective clinical trials to support a role for pancreatic cancer screening. Some patients with an extensive family history have undergone periodic CT scanning of the abdomen, but this approach has not been shown to reduce pancreatic cancer mortality. There is an ongoing search for screening biomarkers. There is a need to follow large cohorts prospectively after collecting and storing biologic samples to identify biomarkers of risk.[73]

Liver Cancer Screening

Screening for liver cancer or hepatocellular carcinoma (HCC) has focused on very high-risk individuals, such as those with cirrhosis.[54] To date, trial results are unreliable due to small study sizes and a lack of randomization.

Serum alpha-fetoprotein (AFP), a fetal-specific glycoprotein antigen, is an HCC tumor marker used in screening. It is not specific to HCC because it may be elevated in hepatitis, pregnancy, and some germ cell tumors. AFP has variable sensitivity and has not been tested in any randomized clinical trial with a mortality end point.

In one prospective, 16-year, population-based observational study, screening was done on 1,487 Alaska natives with chronic hepatis B virus (HBV) infection. The survival of those with screen-detected HCC was compared with a historical group of clinically diagnosed HCC patients.[74] With a target of AFP determination every 6 months, there was a 97% sensitivity and 95% specificity for HCC. Such high sensitivity and specificity have not been found in other studies. It is not known if AFP screening decreases HCC mortality.[75]

Hepatic ultrasound has been used as an additional method for detection of HCC. This procedure is operator dependent with variable sensitivity and specificity. Ultrasound screening is commonly used in patients with hepatitis and cirrhosis.[76,77]

Interest in CT scanning has grown due to the limitations of AFP and ultrasound. CT scans may be a more sensitive test for HCC than ultrasound or AFP.[75]

GYNECOLOGIC CANCER

Cervical Cancer Screening

Dr. George Papanicolaou first introduced the Pap smear or Pap test in the early 1940s. The test was widely adopted based on its ability to identify squamous premalignancies and malignancies (from the ectodermal cervix) and glandular dysplasia and adenocarcinomas (from the endocervix). It is, however, more sensitive at detecting squamous lesions.

The Pap test was introduced before the advent of the prospective, randomized clinical trial and, therefore, has never been so tested. However, a number of observational studies over the past 60 years support the effectiveness of this screening test.[78,79] Multiple ecologic studies have shown an inverse correlation between the introduction of Pap testing in a given country and reductions in both cervical cancer incidence and mortality.[80] Importantly, mortality reductions in these studies have been proportional to the intensity of screening. In one series, more than half of women diagnosed with cervical cancer either had never had a Pap test or had not been screened within 5 years of diagnosis.[80]

Cervical cytology has evolved over the years. The original Pap smear used an ectocervical spatula to apply a specimen ("smear") to glass slides. It later included an endocervical brush. The smear was fixed, stained, and manually examined under a microscope. That method is still used today, but a liquid-based/thin-layer system capable of being analyzed by computer is gaining in popularity.[81]

Human papillomavirus (HPV) 16 and 18 are the cause of more than 70% of cervical cancers. Thirteen other HPV subtypes are known to be associated with cervical cancer. With increasing understanding of the role of HPV in cervical disease, interest in developing tests to determine the presence of HPV DNA and RNA has grown. HPV screening can be used along with cytology (*cotesting*), in response to an abnormal cytologic test (*reflexive testing*), or as a stand-alone test. One advantage of the liquid-based/thin-layer tests over the older smears is that it makes reflexive testing easier to perform. An abnormal cytology screen can be objectively verified by testing for the presence of the HPV virus without calling the patient back.

HPV testing is especially useful because of its negative predictive value. Although a positive test for HPV infection is not diagnostic of cervical disease, a negative HPV test strongly suggests that the abnormal Pap does not represent a premalignant condition.

The utility of the HPV test is limited in younger women because one-third or more of women in their 20s have active cervical infections at any given time. The overwhelming majority of these infections and resultant dysplasia will regress and resolve within 8 to 24 months. For women over the age of 30, screening for the presence of HPV DNA or RNA appears to be superior to cytology in identifying women at risk for cervical dysplasia and cancer.[82] An HPV infection in women over the age of 30 is more likely to be persistent and clinically significant.[83] The risk of cervical cancer also increases with age, and most cervical cancer deaths occur in women over 50 years of age.

Cytologic Terminology

The terminology of the Pap smear has changed over time. The traditional cytologic categories were mild, moderate, and severe dysplasia and carcinoma in situ. *Mild* correlated with cervical intraepithelial neoplasia (CIN)1 histology on biopsy; *moderate* usually indicated CIN2; and *severe* dysplasia indicated CIN3 or carcinoma in situ.

There was some subjectivity and some overlap, especially in the area of mild and moderate dysplasia. The NCI sponsored the development of the Bethesda system in 1988. This system provides an assessment of the adequacy of the cervical specimen and a way of categorizing and describing the Pap smear findings. It more effectively and uniformly communicates cytology results from the laboratory to the patient caregiver. The Bethesda system was modified in 1991 and again in 2001.[84] Today, more than 40 international professional societies have endorsed the Bethesda system.

The Bethesda system recognizes both squamous and glandular cytologic abnormalities.

Squamous cell abnormalities include:

- Atypical squamous cells (ASC), which are categorized as either:
  - Of undetermined significance (ASC-US)
  - Cannot exclude high-grade squamous intraepithelial lesions (ASC-H)
- Low-grade squamous intraepithelial lesion (LSIL), which correlates with histologic CIN1
- High-grade squamous intraepithelial lesion (HSIL), which correlates with histologic CIN2, CIN3, and carcinoma in situ

Glandular cell abnormalities (features suggestive of adenocarcinoma) include:

- Atypical glandular cells (AGC): endocervical, endometrial, or not otherwise specified
- AGCs, favor neoplastic
- Endocervical or not otherwise specified
- Endocervical adenocarcinoma in situ (AIS)
- Adenocarcinoma

ASCs differ from normal cells but do not meet criteria for LSIL or HSIL. A small proportion of ASC-US smears are from CIN1 lesions; a smaller proportion are from CIN2 or 3. LSILs are usually due to a transient HPV infection. HSILs are more likely to be due to a persistent HPV infection and are more likely to progress to cervical cancer than LSILs.

The Lower Anogenital Squamous Terminology (LAST) project of the College of American Pathology and the American Society for Colposcopy and Cervical Pathology has proposed that histologic cervical findings be described using the same terminology as cytologic findings.[85]

Women under the age of 30 who have not received the HPV vaccine have a high incidence of HPV infection[86] and the highest prevalence of CIN. However, the overwhelming majority of these HPV infections and associated CIN will spontaneously regress.[87,88] Due to the high regression rates, cervical screening and treatment in women aged 20 to 24 years appear to have little or no impact on the incidence of invasive cervical cancer. It is estimated that about 6% of CIN1 lesions progress to CIN3, and 10% to 20% of CIN3 lesions progress to invasive cancer.[89]

The Atypical Squamous Cells of Undetermined Significance (ASCUS)-LSIL Triage Study (ALTS) evaluated women with abnormal Pap smears.[90] The investigators concluded that women with ASC-US should be tested for HPV. Those who are HPV positive should receive a colposcopy. In addition, because most women with LSIL or HSIL had an HPV infection, an immediate colposcopy and a biopsy of lesions was recommended.[91] HPV DNA testing is very sensitive for identifying CIN2 or worse pathology. Among women 30 to 69 years of age, the sensitivity of the Pap test with HPV testing was 95% compared with 55% for the Pap test alone.[92]

Performance Characteristics of Cervical Cytology

The sensitivity of cytology varies and is a function of the adequacy of the cervical specimen. It is also affected by the age of the woman and the experience of the cytologist. The addition of HPV testing increases the number of women referred for a colposcopy. Not surprisingly, sensitivity is improved by serial examinations over time versus a single screen.

Screening Recommendations

Cervical screening, like other screening tests, is associated with some degree of overdiagnosis as evidenced by the phenomenon of spontaneous regression (see previous) and, therefore, potential harm from overtreatment, such as cervical incompetence, which may reduce fertility and the ability to carry a pregnancy to term. Because dysplasia takes years to progress to cervical cancer, increasing the screening interval can reduce overdiagnosis and excessive treatment without decreasing screening efficacy.

In 2012, the ACS, the American Society for Colposcopy and Cervical Pathology (ASCCP), and the American Society for Clinical Pathology (ASCP) issued joint screening guidelines.[93] These guidelines recommend different surveillance strategies and options based on a woman's age, screening history, risk factors, and choice of screening tests. The following are the recommendations for a woman at average risk.

- Screening for cervical cancer should begin at 21 years of age. Women aged 21 to 29 years should receive cytology screening (with either conventional cervical cytology smears or liquid-based cytology) every 3 years. HPV testing should not be performed in this age group (although it can be used to follow-up a diagnosis of ASC-US). Women under 21 years of age should not be screened regardless of their age of sexual initiation.
- For women aged 30 to 65 years, the preferred approach is to be screened every 5 years with both HPV testing and cytology (cotesting). It is also acceptable to continue screening every 3 years with cytology alone.
- Women should discontinue screening after age 65 years if they have had three consecutive negative cytology tests or two consecutive negative HPV test results within the 10-year period before ceasing screening, with the most recent test occurring within the last 5 years.
- Women who have undergone a hysterectomy for noncancerous conditions do not need to undergo cervical cancer screening
- Women, regardless of age, should NOT be screened annually by any screening method.
- Women who have received HPV vaccinations should still be screened according to the previously listed schedule.

Screening in Low Resource Countries

Cytology and HPV testing is not widely available in much of the world. Cervical cancer remains a leading cause of death in many of these areas. Visual inspection of the cervix is a low-tech method of screening that is now recognized as having the potential to save thousands of lives per year. A clustered, randomized trial in India compared one-time cervical visual inspection and immediate colposcopy, biopsy, and/or cryotherapy (where indicated) versus counseling on cervical cancer deaths in women aged 30 to 59 years. After 7 years of follow-up, the age-standardized rate of death due to cervical cancer was 76.6 per 100,000 person-years in the intervention group versus 56.7 per 100,000 person-years in unscreened controls.[94,95] This was the first prospective randomized clinical trial to evaluate cervical cancer screening.

Ovarian Cancer Screening

Modalities proposed for ovarian cancer screening include the bimanual pelvic examination, serum CA-125 antigen measurement, and transvaginal ultrasound (TVU). The bimanual pelvic examination is subjective and not very reproducible, but serum CA-125 can be objectively measured. Unfortunately, CA-125 is neither sensitive nor specific. It is elevated in only about half of women with ovarian cancer and may be elevated in a number of nonmalignant diseases (e.g., diverticulosis, endometriosis, cirrhosis, normal menstruation, pregnancy, uterine fibroids).[96–98] TVU has shown poor performance in the detection of ovarian cancer in average and high risk women.[99] There is interest in the analysis of serum proteomic patterns, but this should be considered experimental.[100,101]

The combination of CA-125 and TVU has been assessed in two large, prospective trials. The U.S. trial, the Prostate Lung Colorectal and Ovarian trial (PLCO), enrolled

78,216 women of average risk age 55 to 74 years.[102,103] Participants were randomized to receive annual examinations with CA-125 (at entry and then annually for 5 years) and TVU (at entry and then annually for 3 years) (n = 39,105), or usual care (n = 39,111). Participants were followed for a maximum of 13 years, with mortality from ovarian cancer as the main study outcome. At the conclusion of the study, the number of deaths from ovarian cancer was similar in each group. There were 3.1 ovarian cancer deaths per 10,000 women years in the screened group versus 2.6 deaths per 10,000 women years in the control group (RR = 1.18; 95% CI, 0.82 to 1.71).[103]

The U.K. Collaborative Trial of Ovarian Cancer Screening (UKCTOCS) is a randomized trial assessing the efficacy of CA-125 and TVU in more than 200,000 postmenopausal women. In this trial, CA-125 is being used as a first-line test and TVU as a follow-up test using a risk of ovarian cancer algorithm (ROCA).[104] The ROCA measures changes in CA-125 over time rather than using a predefined cut point.[105] ROCA is believed to improve sensitivity for smaller tumors without measurably increasing the FP rate. A mortality assessment is expected in 2015.[106]

No organization currently recommends screening average risk women for ovarian cancer. In 2012, the USPSTF recommended against screening for ovarian cancer, concluding that there was "adequate evidence" that (1) annual screening with TVU and CA-125 does not reduce ovarian cancer mortality and (2) screening for ovarian cancer can lead to important harms, mainly surgical interventions in women without ovarian cancer.[107]

Women at High Risk for Ovarian Cancer

Although no study has shown a mortality benefit for ovarian cancer screening of high-risk individuals, a National Institutes of Health (NIH) consensus panel concluded that it was prudent for women with a known hereditary ovarian cancer syndrome, such as BRCA1/2 mutations or HNPCC, to have annual rectovaginal pelvic examinations, CA-125 determinations, and TVU until childbearing is completed or at least until age 35 years, at which time a prophylactic bilateral oophorectomy is recommended.[108]

Endometrial Cancer Screening

There is insufficient evidence to recommend endometrial cancer screening either for women at average risk or for those at increased risk due to a history of unopposed estrogen therapy, tamoxifen therapy, late menopause, nulliparity, infertility or failure to ovulate, obesity, diabetes, or hypertension.[109] The ACS recommends that women be informed about the symptoms of endometrial cancer—in particular, vaginal bleeding and spotting—after the onset of menopause. Women should be encouraged to immediately report these symptoms to their physician.

Women at High Risk for Endometrial Cancer

Women with a suspected autosomal-dominant predisposition to colon cancer (e.g. Lynch syndrome), should consider undergoing an annual endometrial biopsy to evaluate endometrial histology, beginning at age 35 years.[110,111] This is based only on *expert opinion*, given the paucity of clinical trial data. Women should be informed about the potential benefits, harms, and limitations of testing for early endometrial cancer.

LUNG CANCER SCREENING

Lung cancer screening programs using chest radiographs (CXR) and sputum cytology began in the late 1940s.[112] An evaluation of these programs showed that screening led to the diagnosis of an increased number of cancers, an increased proportion of early stage cancers, and a larger proportion of screen-diagnosed patients surviving more than 5 years.

These findings led many to advocate for mass lung cancer screening, whereas others called for a prospective, randomized trial with a lung cancer mortality endpoint.[113] The Mayo Lung Project (MLP), which began in 1971, was such a trial. More than 9,200 male smokers were enrolled and randomized to either have sputum cytology collected and CXRs done every 4 months for 6 years or to have these same tests performed annually.

At 13 years of follow-up, there were more early stage cancers in the intensively screened arm (n = 99) than in the control arm (n = 51), but the number of advanced tumors was nearly identical (107 versus 109, respectively).[114] Despite an increase in 5-year survival (35% versus 15%) intensive screening was not associated with a reduction in lung cancer mortality (3.2 versus 3.0 deaths per 1,000 person-years, respectively).[115]

The impact of screening on cancer incidence persisted through nearly 20 years of follow-up. There were 585 lung cancers diagnosed on the intensive screening arm versus 500 on the control arm (p = 0.009) and intensive screening continued to be associated with a significant increase in disease-specific survival. However, a concomitant decrease in lung-cancer mortality did not emerge with long-term follow-up (4.4 lung cancer deaths per 1,000 person-years in the intensively screened arm versus 3.9 per 1,000 person-years in the control arm).[116] This suggests that some lung cancers diagnosed by screening would not have resulted in death had they not been detected (i.e., overdiagnosis).[116]

Two other large, randomized studies of CXR and sputum cytology were conducted in the United States during the same time period. All three studies evaluated different screening schedules rather than screening versus no screening. Paradoxically, a meta-analysis of the three studies found that more frequent screening was associated with an increase (albeit not statistically significant), rather than a decrease, in lung cancer mortality when compared with less frequent screening.[117] A study conducted in Czechoslovakia in the 1980s also failed to show a reduction in lung cancer mortality with CXR screening.[118]

More recently, the NCI conducted the PLCO trial at 10 sites across the United States. This was a prospective, randomized trial of nearly 155,000 men and women, aged 55 to 74 years. Participants were randomized to receive annual, single-view, posteroanterior CXRs for 4 years versus routine care. With 13 years of follow-up, no significant difference in lung cancer mortality was observed. A total of 1,213 lung cancer deaths occurred on the intervention arm versus 1,230 in the control group (RR, 0.99; 95% CI, 0.87 to 1.22).[119]

Low-dose computerized tomography (LDCT) is an appealing technology for lung cancer screening. It uses an average of 1.5 mSv of radiation to perform a lung scan in 15 seconds. A conventional CT scan uses 8 mSv of radiation and takes several minutes. The LDCT image is not as sharp as the conventional image, but sensitivity and specificity for the detection of lung lesions are similar.

As in the early chest radiograph trials, a number of single-arm LDCT studies reported a substantial increase in the number of early stage lung cancers diagnosed. These studies also demonstrated that 5-year survival rates were increased in screened compared to unscreened populations.

These findings led to the conduct of several randomized trials of LDCT for the early detection of lung cancer. The largest, longest, and first to report a mortality end point is the National Lung Screening Trial (NLST). In this trial, approximately 53,000 persons were randomized to receive three annual LDCT scans or single-view posteroanterior CXRs. Eligible participants were current and former smokers between 55 and 74 years of age at the time of randomization with at least a 30 pack-year smoking history; former smokers were eligible if they had quit smoking within the previous 15 years.

With a median follow-up of 6.5 years, 13% more lung cancers were diagnosed and a 20% (95% CI, 6.8 to 26.7; p = 0.004) relative reduction in lung cancer mortality was observed in the LDCT arm compared to the CXR arm.[11] This corresponds to rates of death from lung cancer of 247 and 309 per 100,000 person-years, respectively.[11] Another important finding from the NLST was a 6.7% (95% CI, 1.2 to 13.6; p = 0.02) decrease in death from any cause in the LDCT group.

NLST participants were at high risk for developing lung cancer based on their smoking history. Indeed, 25% of all participant deaths were due to lung cancer. A further analysis of the NLST shows that screening prevented the greatest number of lung cancer deaths among participants who were at the highest risk but prevented very few deaths among those at the lowest risk. These findings provide empirical support for risk-based screening.[120]

LDCT screening is clearly promising, but there are some notable caveats. The risk of a FP finding in the first screen was 21%. Overall, after three CT scans, 39.1% of participants had at least one positive screening result. Of those who screened positive, the FP rate was 96.4% in the LDCT group.[11] Positive results require additional workup, which can include conventional CT scans, a needle biopsy, bronchoscopy, mediastinoscopy, or thoracotomy. These diagnostic procedures are associated with anxiety, expense, and complications (e.g., pneumo- or hemothorax after a lung biopsy). In the LDCT study arm, there were 16 deaths within 60 days of an invasive diagnostic procedure. Of the 16 deaths, 6 ultimately did not have cancer. Although it is not known whether these deaths were directly caused by the invasive procedure, such findings do give pause. Although the radiation dose from LDCT is low, the possibility that this screening test could cause radiation-induced cancers is at least a theoretical concern. The possibility of this long-term phenomenon will have to be assessed in future analyses.

The CXR lung screening studies suggested that there is a reservoir of biologically indolent lung cancer and that a percentage of screen-detected lung cancers represent overdiagnosis. The estimated rate of overdiagnosis in the long-term follow-up of the Mayo Lung Study and the other CXR studies was 17 to 18.5%.[121] Similarly, it is estimated that 18.5% of the cancers diagnosed on the LDCT arm of the NLST represented overdiagnosis.[122]

There are estimates that widespread, high-quality screening has the potential to prevent 12,000 lung cancer deaths per year in the United States.[123] However, the NLST was performed at 33 centers specifically chosen for their expertise in the screening, diagnosis, and treatment of lung cancer. It is not known whether the widespread adoption of LDCT lung cancer screening will result in higher complication rates and a less favorable risk–benefit ratio.

Although LDCT lung cancer screening should clearly be considered for those at high risk of the disease, those at lower risk are equally likely to suffer the harms associated with screening but less likely to reap the benefits.

Following the announcement of the NLST results, the ACS, the American College of Chest Physicians (AACP), the American Society of Clinical Oncology (ASCO), and the National Comprehensive Cancer Network (NCCN) recommended that clinicians should initiate a discussion about lung cancer screening with patients who would have qualified for the trial. That is:

- Age 55 to 74 years
- At least a 30 pack-year smoking history
- Currently smoke or have quit within the past 15 years
- Relatively good health

Core elements of this discussion should include the benefits, uncertainties, and harms associated with screening for lung cancer with LDCT. Adults who choose to be screened should enter an organized screening program at an institution with expertise in LDCT screening, with access to a multidisciplinary team skilled in the evaluation, diagnosis, and treatment of abnormal lung lesions. If such a program is not available, the risks of harm due to screening may be greater than the benefits.[124,125] The guidelines recommend an annual LDCT screening with the caveat that participants in NLST had only three annual screens.

The USPSTF guidelines give LDCT a grade B recommendation, concluding that there is moderate certainty that annual screening for lung cancer with LDCT is of moderate net benefit in asymptomatic persons at high risk for lung cancer based on age, total cumulative exposure to tobacco smoke, and years since quitting.

PROSTATE CANCER SCREENING

Hugh Hampton Young first advocated the early detection of prostate cancer with a careful digital rectal examination (DRE) in 1903. Screening for prostate cancer with the DRE and serum PSA was first advocated in the mid 1980s and became commonplace by 1992. PSA screening is directly responsible for prostate cancer becoming the most common nonskin cancer in American men.

PSA is a glycoprotein produced almost exclusively by the epithelial component of the prostate gland. This protein was discovered in the late 1970s, and a serum test to measure circulating levels was developed in the early 1980s. Although PSA is prostate specific, it is not prostate cancer specific and may be elevated in a variety of conditions (e.g., benign prostatic hyperplasia, inflammation and following trauma to the gland, the presence of prostate cancer).

The PSA test has been widely advocated for prostate cancer screening because it is objective, easily measured, reproducible, noninvasive, and inexpensive. Although PSA screening increases the detection of potentially curable disease, there is substantial debate about the overall utility of the test. This is because PSA screening introduces substantial lead time and length bias as well as being associated with a high FN and FP rates and having a low positive predictive value. The prostate cancer conundrum was best summarized by the distinguished urologist, Willet Whitmore when he said, "Is cure necessary for those in whom it is possible? Is cure possible for those in whom it is necessary?"[126]

Observational studies suggest that the problem of prostate cancer overdiagnosis precedes the PSA era. In a landmark analysis with 20-year follow-up, only a small proportion of 767 men, diagnosed with localized prostate cancer in the 1970s and early 1980s and followed expectantly, died from prostate cancer: 4% to 7% of those with Gleason 2 to 4 tumors, 6% to 11% of those with Gleason 5 disease, and 18% to 30% of men with Gleason 6 cancer.[127]

Although obviously present in the pre-PSA era, overdiagnosis increased substantially after the introduction of PSA screening. This is illustrated by an examination of the prostate cancer incidence and mortality rates in Washington state and Connecticut. Due to the earlier uptake of PSA screening, the incidence of prostate cancer in Washington increased to twice that of Connecticut during the 1990s. However, mortality rates remained similar throughout the decade and, in fact, have remained similar to this day. The Surveillance, Epidemiology, and End Results (SEER) cancer registries show that, over the last 2 decades, a larger proportion of men living in western Washington have been diagnosed with prostate cancer and definitively treated, without a concomitant reduction in prostate cancer mortality compared to that of men living in Connecticut.[128]

Additional evidence of the potential for overdiagnosis comes from the unexpectedly large number of men diagnosed with prostate cancer in the Prostate Cancer Prevention Trial (PCPT). The PCPT was a prospective, randomized, placebo-controlled trial of finasteride for prostate cancer prevention. Men were screened annually during this trial, and those who had not been diagnosed with prostate cancer after 7 years on-study were asked to undergo an end-of-study prostate biopsy. Of 4,692 men on the placebo arm whose prostate cancer status had been determined by biopsy or transurethral resection (TURP), 24.4% were diagnosed with prostate cancer. Given that the lifetime risk of prostate cancer mortality in the United States is less than 3%, it is clear that many men harbor indolent prostate cancer and, therefore, are at risk of being overdiagnosed.

The unexpectedly high rate of positive end-of-study biopsies in men with PSA levels less than or equal to 4.0 ng/mL provided a more accurate assessment of disease prevalence and thus a more accurate assessment of PSA sensitivity than was previously possible. Of the 2,950 men on the placebo arm of the PCPT with PSA levels consistently less than or equal to 4 ng/mL who underwent end-of-study biopsies, 449 (15.2%) were diagnosed with prostate cancer. Accordingly, a PSA level <4.0 ng/mL is more likely to be a *false* negative. Because Sensitivity = True Positives / (True Positives + False Negatives), a higher FN rate means a lower sensitivity at any given PSA threshold. This has prompted some to advocate using a lower PSA threshold for recommending biopsies. However, although lowering the PSA threshold from 4.0 to 2.5 ng/mL increases the sensitivity from 24% to 42.8%, it reduces specificity from 92.7% to an unacceptably low 80%.[129]

In the PCPT, cancer was found on end-of-study biopsies at all PSA levels (e.g., including 10% of biopsies in men with PSA levels between 0.6 and 1.0 ng/mL and 6% of biopsies in men with PSA levels between 0 and 0.6 were positive), suggesting a continuum of prostate cancer risk and no cut point with simultaneously high sensitivity and high specificity. High-grade disease was also documented at all PSA levels, albeit at an overall frequency of only 2.3% of men with PSAs <4 ng/mL.[130,131]

Does Prostate Cancer Treatment Prevent Deaths?

In order for screening to work, treatment has to work. The first prospective, randomized studies showing that any prostate cancer treatment saves lives were published in the mid-1990s. These studies demonstrated an overall survival benefit for the addition of long-term androgen deprivation to radiation therapy in men with locally advanced, high-risk prostate cancer.[132]

The value of surgery for localized disease was assessed by the Scandinavian Prostate Cancer Group 4 study (SPCG-4). In this trial, 695 men with clinically localized prostate cancer were prospectively randomized to receive radical prostatectomy (RP) or watchful waiting (WW). In the expectant management group, hormonal therapy was given at the time of symptomatic metastases. About 60% of those enrolled had low-grade, 23% had moderate-grade, 5% had high-grade tumors, and 12% had tumors of unknown grade. At a median follow-up of 12.8 years, the RP group had significantly lower overall (RR 0.75; p = 0.007) and prostate cancer–specific mortality (RR 0.62; p = 0.01), with 14.6% of the PR group and 20.7% of the WW group having died of prostate cancer. The number needed to treat or prevent one prostate cancer death was 15. The survival benefit associated with RP was similar before and after 9 years of follow-up and for men with low and high-risk disease. However, a subset analysis suggested that the mortality benefit of surgery was limited to men less than 65 years of age. An important limitation of this trial is that 75% of the study participants had palpable disease, only 12% had nonpalpable disease, and only 5% of the cancers had been screen detected. It is, therefore, difficult to apply these data to the US prostate cancer population, which is dominated by nonpalpable, screen-detected disease.[133]

In contrast to the SPCG-4, the Prostate Intervention versus Observation Trial (PIVOT) was conducted in the United States during the early PSA era. In this study, 731 men with screen-detected prostate cancer were randomized to receive RP or WW. Of the participants, 50% had nonpalpable disease and, using established criteria for PSA levels, grade, and tumor stage, 43% of men had low-risk, 36% had intermediate-risk, and 21% had high-risk prostate cancer. With a median follow-up of 12 years, during which time 48.4% (354 of 731) of the study participants had died, RP was associated with statistically insignificant 2.9% and 2.6% absolute reductions in overall and prostate cancer specific mortality, respectively. Subgroup analyses suggested mortality benefits for men with PSA values greater than 10 ng/mL and for those with intermediate- and high-risk disease.[154]

The Prospective Randomized Screening Trials

The PLCO Cancer Screening Trial was a multicenter, phase III trial conducted in the United States by the NCI. In this trial, nearly 77,000 men age 55 to 74 years were randomized to receive annual PSA testing for 6 years or usual care. At 13 years of follow-up, a nonsignificant increase in cumulative prostate cancer mortality was observed among men randomized to annual screening (RR, 1.09; 95% CI, 0.87 to 1.36).[135] The most important limitation of this trial was the high rate of PSA testing among men randomized to the control arm. This *drop-in* or *contamination* served to reduce the statistical power of the study to detect differences in outcome between the two arms. It has also been argued that, due to the high rate of PSA screening on the control arm, PLCO effectively compared regular prostate cancer screening to opportunistic screening rather than comparing screening to no screening.

The ERSPC is a multicenter trial initiated in 1991 in the Netherlands and Belgium; five additional European countries joined between 1994 and 1998.[136,137] The frequency of PSA testing was every 4 years in all countries except Sweden, in which it was every 2 years. The study results were initially reported in 2009 and updated in 2012.[136,137] Although the overall analysis of 182,160 men, aged 50 to 74, did not show a reduction in prostate cancer–specific mortality, screening was associated with a significant decrease in prostate cancer mortality in the prespecified core age group, 55 to 69 years, which included 162,243 men. After a median follow-up of 11 years, a 21% relative reduction of prostate cancer death (RR, 0.79; 95% CI, 0.68 to 0.91) was observed in this group. In absolute terms, prostate cancer mortality was reduced from 5 to 4 men per 1,000 screened and 37 men had to be diagnosed to avert one prostate cancer death. It remains to be seen whether the benefits of screening will increase with continued follow-up.

The recruitment and randomization procedures of the ERSPC differed among countries. Notably, potential participants in Finland, Sweden, and Italy were identified from population registries and underwent randomization *before* written informed consent was obtained. In some trials, men on the control arm were not aware they were in the study. Therefore, men on the intervention arm in these countries were more likely to be cared for at high-volume referral centers. This may have contributed to the higher proportion of men on the screening arm, with clinically localized cancer being treated with RPs.[138]

In a separate report on 20,000 men randomized to screening or a control group in Göteborg, Sweden, there was a 40% (95% CI, 1.50 to 1.80) risk reduction at 14 years of follow-up.[139] They reported 293 (95% CI, 177 to 799) needed to be screened and 12 needed to be diagnosed in order to prevent one prostate cancer death. Three-fourths of the men in this report and 89% of the prostate cancer deaths were included in the published ERSPC analysis. Given this, these data do not constitute independent evidence of the efficacy of prostate cancer screening.

The other site to report separately was in Finland. A total of 80,144 men were randomized to a screening or usual care arm. At 12 years after randomization, there was no statistical difference in risk of prostate cancer death (hazard ratio [HR] = 0.85; 95% CI, 0.69 to 1.04).[140] Possible explanations as to why Sweden and Finland would have such different outcomes include differences in the frequency of screening (every 2 years versus every 4 years, respectively) and the higher background rate of death from prostate cancer in the control group in the Goteborg cohort. Given that the mortality data from these two cohorts have been largely included in the ERSPC analyses, they do not provide independent evidence of the efficacy of prostate cancer screening.

The decline in prostate cancer mortality in the United States since the introduction of PSA screening 2 decades ago is often offered as evidence supporting a mortality benefit for prostate cancer screening. However, prostate cancer mortality rates have also declined in many countries that have not widely adopted screening.[141] Thus, it is likely that improvements in treatment have contributed, at least in part, to the observed decline in prostate cancer mortality. Another possible contributing factor may be the World Health Organization (WHO) algorithm for adjudicating cause of death. A change occurred just as mortality rates began to go up in the late 1970s, and WHO changed back to the older algorithm in 1991 when prostate cancer mortality began declining in many countries.[142] All of these factors, including a beneficial effect from screening, may be contributing to the declining prostate cancer mortality rates in the United States.

Screening Recommendations

The topic of prostate cancer screening tends to evoke strong emotional reactions. Although the intuitive appeal of early detection is undeniable and screening may save some lives, the magnitude of the mortality reduction is relatively small, whereas the harms associated with screening can be substantial. Whether the potential benefits outweigh the known harms is a question that each man must answer for himself based on his individual preferences.

Several professional organizations in the United States, Europe, and Canada have recently reviewed the screening data and issued screening guidelines. All acknowledge that legitimate concerns remain regarding the risk–benefit ratio of prostate cancer screening. There is also general agreement that prostate cancer screening should only be done in the context of fully informed consent and that men should know that experts do not agree as to whether the benefits of screening for this disease outweigh the harms. Most recommend against mass screening in public meeting places, malls, churches, etc.

In 2009, the American Urological Association (AUA) PSA Best Practice Statement was published, which stated, "Given the uncertainty that PSA testing results in more benefit than harm, a thoughtful and broad approach to PSA is critical. Patients need to be informed of the risks and the benefits of testing before it is undertaken. The risks of over-detection and over-treatment should be included in this discussion."[143]

In 2010, the ACS updated their guidelines, stating that the balance of benefits and harms related to prostate cancer early detection are uncertain and the existing evidence is insufficient to support a recommendation for or against the routine use of PSA screening.[144] The ACS called for discussion and shared decision making within the physician–patient relationship.

The most recent 2012 USPSTF guidelines recommend against the use of PSA screening on the basis that there is moderate certainty that the harms of PSA testing outweigh the benefits and, on that basis, recommended against PSA-based screening for all men.[14] The task force did acknowledge that some men will continue to request screening and some physicians will continue to offer it. Like the ACS and AUA, they state that screening under such circumstances should respect patient preferences.

In 2013, the AUA conducted a systematic review of over 300 studies. They recommended against screening men younger than 40 years of age, and against screening average-risk men age 40 to 54 years, most men over 70 years of age, and men with a life expectancy of less than 10 to 15 years. They recommend that screening decisions be individualized for higher risk men ages 40 to 54 years and men over 70 years of age who are in excellent health. They placed primacy on shared decision making versus physician judgments about the balance of benefits and harms at the population level.[145] Even for men aged 55 to 69 years, the AUA concluded that the quality of evidence for benefits associated with screening was moderate, whereas the quality of the evidence for harm was high. They recommended shared decision making for this group, in whom they have concluded the benefits may outweigh the harm.

SKIN CANCER SCREENING

Assessments of skin cancer screening have focused on melanoma end points with very little attention to screening for nonmelanoma skin cancer. A systematic review of skin cancer screening studies examining the available evidence through mid 2005 concluded that direct evidence of improved health outcomes associated with skin cancer screening is lacking.[146]

No randomized, clinical trial of skin cancer screening has been attempted. However, several observational studies have suggested that melanoma screening might reduce mortality. For example, a decrease in melanoma mortality did occur after a Scottish campaign to promote awareness of the signs of suspicious skin lesions and encourage early self-referral. However, uncontrolled, ecologic studies such as this provide a relatively low level of evidence, because it is not possible to determine whether the observed mortality reduction was due to screening or other factors.

More recently, the Skin Cancer Research to Provide Evidence for Effectiveness of Screening project, or SCREEN project, compared a region of Germany in which intensive skin cancer screening was performed to areas of Germany without intensive screening. Approximately 360,000 residents of the Schleswig-Holstein region aged 20 years and older participated. They chose either to be screened by a nondermatologist physician trained in skin examinations or by a dermatologist. Almost 16,000 biopsies were performed and 585 melanomas were diagnosed. Overall, 1 in 23 participants had an excisional skin biopsy and 620 persons needed to be screened to detect one melanoma. This screening effort led to a 16% and 38% increase in melanoma incidence among men and women, respectively, compared to 2 years earlier. The melanoma incidence rate returned to preprogram levels after the program ended. Of the screen-detected melanomas, 90% were less than 1 mm thick. Screening was performed in 2003 to 2004, and melanoma mortality in this region subsequently declined. In 2008, it was nearly 50% lower in both men and women compared to the rest of Germany.[147,148]

Recommendations of Experts

Skin cancer screening recommendations are based on *expert opinion*, given the absence of a randomized clinical trial data and limited observational studies. The ACS recommends monthly skin self-examinations and a yearly clinical skin examination as part of a routine cancer-related checkup.[149] The USPSTF finds insufficient evidence to recommend for or against either routine skin cancer screening of the general population by primary care providers or counseling patients to perform periodic skin self-examinations. The task force does recommend that clinicians "remain alert" for skin lesions with malignant features when performing a physical examination for other purposes, particularly in high-risk individuals. The American Academy of Dermatology recommends that persons at highest risk (i.e., those with a strong family history of melanoma and multiple atypical nevi), perform frequent self-examination and seek a professional evaluation of the skin at least once per year.[150]

High-risk individuals are persons with multiple nevi or atypical moles. There is consensus they should be educated about the need for frequent surveillance by a trained health-care provider beginning at an early age. In the United States, Australia, and Western Europe, Caucasian men age 50 years and over account for nearly half of all melanoma cases. There is some discussion that melanoma early detection efforts should be focused on this population.

REFERENCES

1. Collen MF, Dales LG, Friedman GD, et al. Multiphasic checkup evaluation study. 4. Preliminary cost benefit analysis for middle-aged men. *Prev Med* 1973;2:236–246.
2. Prorok PC, Kramer BS, Gohagan JK. Screening theory and study design: the basics. In: Kramer B, Prorok P, eds. *Cancer Screening*. New York: Marcel Dekker; 1999:29–53.
3. Welch HG, Black WC. Overdiagnosis in cancer. *J Natl Cancer Inst* 2010;102:605–613.
4. Yamamoto K, Hayashi Y, Hanada R, et al. Mass screening and age-specific incidence of neuroblastoma in Saitama Prefecture, Japan. *J Clin Oncol* 1995;13:2033–2038.
5. Woods WG, Gao RN, Shuster JJ, et al. Screening of infants and mortality due to neuroblastoma. *N Engl J Med* 2002;346:1041–1046.
6. Friedman GD, Collen MF, Fireman BH. Multiphasic Health Checkup Evaluation: a 16-year follow-up. *J Chronic Dis* 1986;39:453–463.
7. Pinsky PF, Miller A, Kramer BS, et al. Evidence of a healthy volunteer effect in the prostate, lung, colorectal, and ovarian cancer screening trial. *Am J Epidemiol* 2007;165:874–881.
8. Boyle P, Brawley OW. Prostate cancer: current evidence weighs against population screening. *CA Cancer J Clin* 2009;59:220–224.
9. Autier P, Boyle P, Buyse M, et al. Is FOB screening really the answer for lowering mortality in colorectal cancer? *Recent Results Cancer Res* 2003;163:254–263.
10. de Boer AG, Taskila T, Ojajarvi A, et al. Cancer survivors and unemployment: a meta-analysis and meta-regression. *JAMA* 2009;301:753–762.
11. Aberle DR, Adams AM, Berg CD, et al. Reduced lung-cancer mortality with low-dose computed tomographic screening. *N Engl J Med* 2011;365:395–409.
12. Eden J, Levit L, Berg A, et al., eds. *Finding What Works in Health Care: Standards for Systematic Reviews*. Washington, DC: The National Academies Press; 2011.
13. Graham R, Mancher M, Wolman DM, et al. *Medicine CoSfDTCPCIo*. Washington, DC: The National Academies; 2011.
14. Moyer VA. Screening for prostate cancer: U.S. Preventive Services Task Force recommendation statement. *Ann Intern Med* 2012;157:120–134.
15. Brawley O, Byers T, Chen A, et al. New American Cancer Society process for creating trustworthy cancer screening guidelines. *JAMA* 2011;306:2495–2499.
16. Shapiro S. Periodic screening for breast cancer: the HIP Randomized Controlled Trial. Health Insurance Plan. *J Natl Cancer Inst Monogr* 1997:27–30.
17. Miller AB, Wall C, Baines CJ, et al. Twenty five year follow-up for breast cancer incidence and mortality of the Canadian National Breast Screening Study: randomised screening trial. *BMJ* 2014;348:g366.
18. Tabar L, Fagerberg G, Duffy SW, et al. Update of the Swedish two-county program of mammographic screening for breast cancer. *Radiol Clin North Am* 1992;30:187–210.
19. Moy L, Slanetz PJ, Moore R, et al. Specificity of mammography and US in the evaluation of a palpable abnormality: retrospective review. *Radiology* 2002;225:176–181.
20. Lord SJ, Lei W, Craft P, et al. A systematic review of the effectiveness of magnetic resonance imaging (MRI) as an addition to mammography and ultrasound in screening young women at high risk of breast cancer. *Eur J Cancer* 2007;43:1905–1917.
21. Wishart GC, Campisi M, Boswell M, et al. The accuracy of digital infrared imaging for breast cancer detection in women undergoing breast biopsy. *Eur J Surg Oncol* 2010;36:535–540.
22. Dooley WC, Ljung BM, Veronesi U, et al. Ductal lavage for detection of cellular atypia in women at high risk for breast cancer. *J Natl Cancer Inst* 2001;93:1624–1632.
23. Autier P, Boniol M, Middleton R, et al. Advanced breast cancer incidence following population-based mammographic screening. *Ann Oncol* 2011;22:1726–1735.
24. Bleyer A, Welch HG. Effect of three decades of screening mammography on breast-cancer incidence. *N Engl J Med* 2012;367:1998–2005.
25. Marmot MG, Altman DC, Cameron DA, et al. The benefits and harms of breast cancer screening: an independent review. *Br J Cancer* 2013;108:2205–2240.
26. Berry DA, Cronin KA, Plevritis SK, et al. Effect of screening and adjuvant therapy on mortality from breast cancer. *N Engl J Med* 2005;353:1784–1792.
27. Harris R, Yeatts J, Kinsinger L. Breast cancer screening for women ages 50 to 69 years a systematic review of observational evidence. *Prev Med* 2011;53:108–114.
28. Nelson HD, Tyne K, Naik A, et al. Screening for breast cancer: an update for the U.S. Preventive Services Task Force. *Ann Intern Med* 2009;151:727–737.
29. Mandelblatt JS, Cronin KA, Bailey S, et al. Effects of mammography screening under different screening schedules: model estimates of potential benefits and harms. *Ann Intern Med* 2009;151:738–747.
30. U.S. Preventive Services Task Force. Screening for breast cancer: U.S. Preventive Services Task Force recommendation statement. *Ann Intern Med* 2009;151:716–726.
31. Nelson HD, Zakher B, Cantor A, et al. Risk factors for breast cancer for women aged 40 to 49 years: a systematic review and meta-analysis. *Ann Intern Med* 2012;156:635–648.
32. Barnett GC, Shah M, Redman K, et al. Risk factors for the incidence of breast cancer: do they affect survival from the disease? *J Clin Oncol* 2008;26:3310–3316.
33. Gierach GL, Ichikawa L, Kerlikowske K, et al. Relationship between mammographic density and breast cancer death in the Breast Cancer Surveillance Consortium. *J Natl Cancer Inst* 2012;104:1218–1227.
34. Berg WA, Blume JD, Cormack JB, et al. Combined screening with ultrasound and mammography vs mammography alone in women at elevated risk of breast cancer. *JAMA* 2008;299:2151–2163.
35. Gartlehner G, Thaler K, Chapman A, et al. Mammography in combination with breast ultrasonography versus mammography for breast cancer screening in women at average risk. *Cochrane Database Syst Rev* 2013;4:CD009632.
36. Tice JA, O'Meara ES, Weaver DL, et al. Benign breast disease, mammographic breast density, and the risk of breast cancer. *J Natl Cancer Inst* 2013;105:1043–1049.
37. Kerlikowske K, Hubbard RA, Miglioretti DL, et al. Comparative effectiveness of digital versus film-screen mammography in community practice in the United States: a cohort study. *Ann Intern Med* 2011;155:493–502.
38. Haas BM, Kalra V, Geisel J, et al. Comparison of tomosynthesis plus digital mammography and digital mammography alone for breast cancer screening. *Radiology* 2013;269:694–700.
39. Rosenberg RD, Yankaskas BC, Abraham LA, et al. Performance benchmarks for screening mammography. *Radiology* 2006;241:55–66.
40. Gomez SL, Lichtensztajn D, Kurian AW, et al. Increasing mastectomy rates for early-stage breast cancer? Population-based trends from California. *J Clin Oncol* 2010;28:e155–e157.
41. Tuttle TM, Jarosek S, Habermann EB, et al. Increasing rates of contralateral prophylactic mastectomy among patients with ductal carcinoma in situ. *J Clin Oncol* 2009;27:1362–1367.
42. Rosenberg RD, Hunt WC, Williamson MR, et al. Effects of age, breast density, ethnicity, and estrogen replacement therapy on screening mammographic sensitivity and cancer stage at diagnosis: review of 183,134 screening mammograms in Albuquerque, New Mexico. *Radiology* 1998;209:511–518.
43. Kerlikowske K, Grady D, Barclay J, et al. Effect of age, breast density, and family history on the sensitivity of first screening mammography. *JAMA* 1996;276:33–38.
44. Porter PL, El-Bastawissi AY, Mandelson MT, et al. Breast tumor characteristics as predictors of mammographic detection: comparison of interval- and screen-detected cancers. *J Natl Cancer Inst* 1999;91:2020–2028.
45. Ronckers CM, Erdmann CA, Land CE. Radiation and breast cancer: a review of current evidence. *Breast Cancer Res* 2005;7:21–32.
46. Pijpe A, Andrieu N, Easton DF, et al. Exposure to diagnostic radiation and risk of breast cancer among carriers of BRCA1/2 mutations: retrospective cohort study (GENE-RAD-RISK). *BMJ* 2012;345:e5660.
47. Qaseem A, Snow V, Sherif K, et al. Screening mammography for women 40 to 49 years of age: a clinical practice guideline from the American College of Physicians. *Ann Intern Med* 2007;146:511–515.
48. Tonelli M, Connor Gorber S, Joffres M, et al. Recommendations on screening for breast cancer in average-risk women aged 40-74 years. *CMAJ* 2011;183:1991–2001.
49. Recommendations on cancer screening in the European Union. Advisory Committee on Cancer Prevention. *Eur J Cancer* 2000;36:1473–1478.
50. Saslow D, Boetes C, Burke W, et al. American Cancer Society guidelines for breast screening with MRI as an adjunct to mammography. *CA Cancer J Clin* 2007;57:75–89.
51. Mandel JS, Church TR, Bond JH, et al. The effect of fecal occult-blood screening on the incidence of colorectal cancer. *N Engl J Med* 2000;343:1603–1607.
52. Nishihara R, Wu K, Lochhead P, et al. Long-term colorectal-cancer incidence and mortality after lower endoscopy. *N Engl J Med* 2013;369:1095–1105.
53. Schoen RE, Pinsky PF, Weissfeld JL, et al. Colorectal-cancer incidence and mortality with screening flexible sigmoidoscopy. *N Engl J Med* 2012;366:2345–2357.
54. Mandel JS, Bond JH, Church TR, et al. Reducing mortality from colorectal cancer by screening for fecal occult blood. Minnesota Colon Cancer Control Study. *N Engl J Med* 1993;328:1365–1371.
55. Mandel JS, Church TR, Ederer F, et al. Colorectal cancer mortality: effectiveness of biennial screening for fecal occult blood. *J Natl Cancer Inst* 1999;91:434–437.
56. Hardcastle JD, Chamberlain JO, Robinson MH, et al. Randomised controlled trial of faecal-occult-blood screening for colorectal cancer. *Lancet* 1996;348:1472–1477.
57. Kronborg O, Fenger C, Olsen J, et al. Randomised study of screening for colorectal cancer with faecal-occult-blood test. *Lancet* 1996;348:1467–1471.
58. Ahlquist DA, Wieand HS, Moertel CG, et al. Accuracy of fecal occult blood screening for colorectal neoplasia. A prospective study using Hemoccult and HemoQuant tests. *JAMA* 1993;269:1262–1267.
59. Levin B, Brooks D, Smith RA, et al. Emerging technologies in screening for colorectal cancer: CT colonography, immunochemical fecal occult blood tests, and stool screening using molecular markers. *CA Cancer J Clin* 2003;53:44–55.
60. Atkin WS, Edwards R, Kralj-Hans I, et al. Once-only flexible sigmoidoscopy screening in prevention of colorectal cancer: a multicentre randomised controlled trial. *Lancet* 2010;375:1624–1633.
61. Levin TR. Flexible sigmoidoscopy for colorectal cancer screening: valid approach or short-sighted? *Gastroenterol Clin North Am* 2002;31:1015–1029.

62. Littlejohn C, Hilton S, Macfarlane GJ, et al. Systematic review and meta-analysis of the evidence for flexible sigmoidoscopy as a screening method for the prevention of colorectal cancer. Br J Surg 2012;99:1488–1500.
63. Elmunzer BJ, Hayward RA, Schoenfeld PS, et al. Effect of flexible sigmoidoscopy-based screening on incidence and mortality of colorectal cancer: a systematic review and meta-analysis of randomized controlled trials. PLoS Med 2012;9:e1001352.
64. van Rijn JC, Reitsma JB, Stoker J, et al. Polyp miss rate determined by tandem colonoscopy: a systematic review. Am J Gastroenterol 2006;101:343–350.
65. Rosman AS, Korsten MA. Meta-analysis comparing CT colonography, air contrast barium enema, and colonoscopy. Am J Med 2007;120:203–210.
66. Imperiale TF, Wagner DR, Lin CY, et al. Using risk for advanced proximal colonic neoplasia to tailor endoscopic screening for colorectal cancer. Ann Intern Med 2003;139:959–965.
67. U.S. Preventive Services Task Force. Screening for colorectal cancer: U.S. Preventive Services Task Force recommendation statement. Ann Intern Med 2008;149:627–637.
68. Winawer S, Fletcher R, Rex D, et al. Colorectal cancer screening and surveillance: clinical guidelines and rationale-Update based on new evidence. Gastroenterology 2003;124:544–560.
69. Quintero E, Castells A, Bujanda L, et al. Colonoscopy versus fecal immunochemical testing in colorectal-cancer screening. N Engl J Med 2012;366:697–706.
70. Murakami R, Tsukuma H, Ubukata T, et al. Estimation of validity of mass screening program for gastric cancer in Osaka, Japan. Cancer 1990;65:1255–1260.
71. Kampschoer GH, Fujii A, Masuda Y. Gastric cancer detected by mass survey. Comparison between mass survey and outpatient detection. Scand J Gastroenterol 1989;24:813–817.
72. Stael von Holstein C, Eriksson S, Huldt B, et al. Endoscopic screening during 17 years for gastric stump carcinoma. A prospective clinical trial. Scand J Gastroenterol 1991;26:1020–1026.
73. Shaukat A, Mongin SJ, Geisser MS, et al. Long-term mortality after screening for colorectal cancer. N Engl J Med 2013;369:1106–1114.
74. McMahon BJ, Bulkow L, Harpster A, et al. Screening for hepatocellular carcinoma in Alaska natives infected with chronic hepatitis B: a 16-year population-based study. Hepatology 2000;32:842–846.
75. Ghalasani N, Horlander JC Sr, Said A, et al. Screening for hepatocellular carcinoma in patients with advanced cirrhosis. Am J Gastroenterol 1999;94:2988–2993.
76. Sherman M, Peltekian KM, Lee C. Screening for hepatocellular carcinoma in chronic carriers of hepatitis B virus: incidence and prevalence of hepatocellular carcinoma in a North American urban population. Hepatology 1995;22:432–438.
77. Dodd GD 3rd, Miller WJ, Baron RL, et al. Detection of malignant tumors in end-stage cirrhotic livers: efficacy of sonography as a screening technique. AJR Am J Roentgenol 1992;159:727–733.
78. Laara E, Day NE, Hakama M. Trends in mortality from cervical cancer in the Nordic countries: association with organised screening programmes. Lancet 1987;1:1247–1249.
79. Christopherson WM, Lundin FE Jr, Mendez WM, et al. Cervical cancer control: a study of morbidity and mortality trends over a twenty-one-year period. Cancer 1976;38:1357–1366.
80. Janerich DT, Hadjimichael O, Schwartz PE, et al. The screening histories of women with invasive cervical cancer, Connecticut. Am J Public Health 1995;85:791–794.
81. Sawaya GF, McConnell KJ, Kulasingam SL, et al. Risk of cervical cancer associated with extending the interval between cervical-cancer screenings. N Engl J Med 2003;349:1501–1509.
82. Sankaranarayanan R, Nene BM, Shastri SS, et al. HPV screening for cervical cancer in rural India. N Engl J Med 2009;360:1385–1394.
83. Vesco KK, Whitlock EP, Eder M, et al. In: Screening for Cervical Cancer: A Systematic Evidence Review for the US Preventive Services Task Force. Rockville, MD: Agency for Healthcare Research and Quality; 2011.
84. Solomon D, Davey D, Kurman R, et al. The 2001 Bethesda System: terminology for reporting results of cervical cytology. JAMA 2002;287:2114–2119.
85. Darragh TM, Colgan TJ, Thomas Cox J, et al. The Lower Anogenital Squamous Terminology Standardization project for HPV-associated lesions: background and consensus recommendations from the College of American Pathologists and the American Society for Colposcopy and Cervical Pathology. Int J Gynecol Pathol 2013;32:76–115.
86. Ho GY, Bierman R, Beardsley L, et al. Natural history of cervicovaginal papillomavirus infection in young women. N Engl J Med 1998;338:423–428.
87. Holowaty P, Miller AB, Rohan T, et al. Natural history of dysplasia of the uterine cervix. J Natl Cancer Inst 1999;91:252–258.
88. Richardson H, Kelsall G, Tellier P, et al. The natural history of type-specific human papillomavirus infections in female university students. Cancer Epidemiol Biomarkers Prev 2003;12:485–490.
89. Melnikow J, Nuovo J, Willan AR, et al. Natural history of cervical squamous intraepithelial lesions: a meta-analysis. Obstet Gynecol 1998;92:727–735.
90. Cox JT, Schiffman M, Solomon D. Prospective follow-up suggests similar risk of subsequent cervical intraepithelial neoplasia grade 2 or 3 among women with cervical intraepithelial neoplasia grade 1 or negative colposcopy and directed biopsy. Am J Obstet Gynecol 2003;188:1406–1412.
91. Guido R, Schiffman M, Solomon D, et al. Postcolposcopy management strategies for women referred with low-grade squamous intraepithelial lesions or human papillomavirus DNA positive atypical squamous cells of undetermined significance: a two-year prospective study. Am J Obstet Gynecol 2003;188:1401–1405.

92. Mayrand MH, Duarte-Franco E, Rodrigues I, et al. Human papillomavirus DNA versus Papanicolaou screening tests for cervical cancer. N Engl J Med 2007;357:1579–1588.
93. Saslow D, Solomon D, Lawson HW, et al. American Cancer Society, American Society for Colposcopy and Cervical Pathology, and American Society for Clinical Pathology screening guidelines for the prevention and early detection of cervical cancer. CA Cancer J Clin 2012;62:147–172.
94. Sankaranarayanan R, Esmy PO, Rajkumar R, et al. Effect of visual screening on cervical cancer incidence and mortality in Tamil Nadu, India: a cluster-randomised trial. Lancet 2007;370:398–406.
95. Szarewski A. Cervical screening by visual inspection with acetic acid. Lancet 2007;370:365–366.
96. Johnson CC, Kessel B, Riley TL, et al. The epidemiology of CA-125 in women without evidence of ovarian cancer in the Prostate, Lung, Colorectal and Ovarian Cancer (PLCO) Screening Trial. Gynecol Oncol 2008;110:383–389.
97. Duffy MJ, Bonfrer JM, Kulpa J, et al. CA125 in ovarian cancer: European Group on Tumor Markers guidelines for clinical use. Int J Gynecol Cancer 2005;15:679–691.
98. Moss EL, Hollingworth J, Reynolds TM. The role of CA125 in clinical practice. J Clin Pathol 2005;58:308–312.
99. Fishman DA, Cohen L, Blank SV, et al. The role of ultrasound evaluation in the detection of early-stage epithelial ovarian cancer. Am J Obstet Gynecol 2005;192:1214–1221.
100. Kobayashi E, Ueda Y, Matsuzaki S, et al. Biomarkers for screening, diagnosis, and monitoring of ovarian cancer. Cancer Epidemiol Biomarkers Prev 2012;21:1902–1912.
101. Ren J, Cai H, Li Y, et al. Tumor markers for early detection of ovarian cancer. Expert Rev Mol Diagn 2010;10:787–798.
102. Prorok PC, Andriole GL, Bresalier RS, et al. Design of the Prostate, Lung, Colorectal and Ovarian (PLCO) Cancer Screening Trial. Control Clin Trials 2000;21:273S–309S.
103. Buys SS, Partridge E, Black A, et al. Effect of screening on ovarian cancer mortality: the Prostate, Lung, Colorectal and Ovarian (PLCO) Cancer Screening Randomized Controlled Trial. JAMA 2011;305:2295–2303.
104. Menon U, Gentry-Maharaj A, Hallett R, et al. Sensitivity and specificity of multimodal and ultrasound screening for ovarian cancer, and stage distribution of detected cancers: results of the prevalence screen of the UK Collaborative Trial of Ovarian Cancer Screening (UKCTOCS). Lancet Oncol 2009;10:327–340.
105. Drescher CW, Shah C, Thorpe J, et al. Longitudinal screening algorithm that incorporates change over time in CA125 levels identifies ovarian cancer earlier than a single-threshold rule. J Clin Oncol 2013;31:387–392.
106. Sharma A, Apostolidou S, Burnell M, et al. Risk of epithelial ovarian cancer in asymptomatic women with ultrasound-detected ovarian masses: a prospective cohort study within the UK collaborative trial of ovarian cancer screening (UKCTOCS). Ultrasound Obstet Gynecol 2012;40:338–344.
107. Moyer VA. Screening for ovarian cancer: U.S. Preventive Services Task Force reaffirmation recommendation statement. Ann Intern Med 2012;157:900–904.
108. NIH consensus conference. Ovarian cancer. Screening, treatment, and follow-up. NIH Consensus Development Panel on Ovarian Cancer. JAMA 1995;273:491–497.
109. Smith RA, von Eschenbach AC, Wender R, et al. American Cancer Society guidelines for the early detection of cancer: update of early detection guidelines for prostate, colorectal, and endometrial cancers. Also: update 2001—testing for early lung cancer detection. CA Cancer J Clin 2001;51:38–75.
110. Burke W, Petersen G, Lynch P, et al. Recommendations for follow-up care of individuals with an inherited predisposition to cancer. I. Hereditary nonpolyposis colon cancer. Cancer Genetics Studies Consortium. JAMA 1997;277:915–919.
111. Gull B, Karlsson B, Milsom I, et al. Can ultrasound replace dilation and curettage? A longitudinal evaluation of postmenopausal bleeding and transvaginal sonographic measurement of the endometrium as predictors of endometrial cancer. Am J Obstet Gynecol 2003;188:401–408.
112. Scamman CL. Follow-up study of lung cancer suspects in a mass chest X-ray survey. N Engl J Med 1951;244:541–544.
113. Croswell JM, Ransohoff DF, Kramer BS. Principles of cancer screening: lessons from history and study design issues. Semin Oncol 2010;37:202–215.
114. Fontana RS, Sanderson DR, Taylor WF, et al. Early lung cancer detection: results of the initial (prevalence) radiologic and cytologic screening in the Mayo Clinic study. Am Rev Respir Dis 1984;130:561–565.
115. Fontana RS, Sanderson DR, Woolner LB, et al. Screening for lung cancer. A critique of the Mayo Lung Project. Cancer 1991;67:1155–1164.
116. Marcus PM, Bergstralh EJ, Zweig MH, et al. Extended lung cancer incidence follow-up in the Mayo Lung Project and overdiagnosis. J Natl Cancer Inst 2006;98:748–756.
117. Manser R, Wright G, Hart D, et al. Surgery for early stage non-small cell lung cancer. Cochrane Database Syst Rev 2005:CD004699.
118. Kubik A, Parkin DM, Khlat M, et al. Lack of benefit from semi-annual screening for cancer of the lung: follow-up report of a randomized controlled trial on a population of high-risk males in Czechoslovakia. Int J Cancer 1990;45:26–33.
119. Oken MM, Hocking WG, Kvale PA, et al. Screening by chest radiograph and lung cancer mortality: the Prostate, Lung, Colorectal, and Ovarian (PLCO) randomized trial. JAMA 2011;306:1865–1873.
120. Kovalchik SA, Tammemagi M, Berg CD, et al. Targeting of low-dose CT screening according to the risk of lung-cancer death. N Engl J Med 2013;369:245–254.

121. Kubik AK, Parkin DM, Zatloukal P. Czech Study on Lung Cancer Screening: post-trial follow-up of lung cancer deaths up to year 15 since enrollment. *Cancer* 2000;89:2363–2368.
122. Patz EF Jr, Pinsky P, Gatsonis C, et al. Overdiagnosis in low dose computed tomography screening for lung cancer. *JAMA Intern Med* 2014;174:269–274.
123. Ma J, Ward EM, Smith R, et al. Annual number of lung cancer deaths potentially avertable by screening in the United States. *Cancer* 2013;119:1381–1385.
124. Wender R, Fontham ET, Barrera E Jr, et al. American Cancer Society lung cancer screening guidelines. *CA Cancer J Clin* 2013;63:107–117.
125. Bach PB, Mirkin JN, Oliver TK, et al. Benefits and harms of CT screening for lung cancer: a systematic review. *JAMA* 2012;307:2418–2429.
126. Montie JE, Smith JA. Whitmoreisms: memorable quotes from Willet F. Whitmore, Jr, M.D. *Urology* 2004;63:207–209.
127. Albertsen PC, Hanley JA, Fine J. 20-year outcomes following conservative management of clinically localized prostate cancer. *JAMA* 2005;293:2095–2101.
128. Lu-Yao G, Albertsen PC, Stanford JL, et al. Screening, treatment, and prostate cancer mortality in the Seattle area and Connecticut: fifteen-year follow up. *J Gen Intern Med* 2008;23:1809–1814.
129. Thompson IM, Chi C, Ankerst DP, et al. Effect of finasteride on the sensitivity of PSA for detecting prostate cancer. *J Natl Cancer Inst* 2006;98:1128–1133.
130. Thompson IM, Pauler DK, Goodman PJ, et al. Prevalence of prostate cancer among men with a prostate-specific antigen level < or =4.0 ng per milliliter. *N Engl J Med* 2004;350:2239–2246.
131. Thompson IM, Ankerst DP, Chi C, et al. Operating characteristics of prostate-specific antigen in men with an initial PSA level of 3.0 ng/ml or lower. *JAMA* 2005;294:66–70.
132. Widmark A, Klepp O, Solberg A, et al. Endocrine treatment, with or without radiotherapy, in locally advanced prostate cancer (SPCG-7/SFUO-3): an open randomised phase III trial. *Lancet* 2009;373:301–308.
133. Bill-Axelson A, Holmberg L, Ruutu M, et al. Radical prostatectomy versus watchful waiting in early prostate cancer. *N Engl J Med* 2011;364:1708–1717.
134. Wilt TJ, Brawer MK, Jones KM, et al. Radical prostatectomy versus observation for localized prostate cancer. *N Engl J Med* 2012;367:203–213.
135. Andriole GL, Crawford ED, Grubb RL 3rd, et al. Prostate cancer screening in the randomized Prostate, Lung, Colorectal, and Ovarian Cancer Screening Trial: mortality results after 13 years of follow-up. *J Natl Cancer Inst* 2012;104:125–132.
136. Schroder FH, Hugosson J, Roobol MJ, et al. Screening and prostate-cancer mortality in a randomized European study. *N Engl J Med* 2009;360:1320–1328.
137. Schroder FH, Hugosson J, Roobol MJ, et al. Prostate-cancer mortality at 11 years of follow-up. *N Engl J Med* 2012;366:981–990.
138. Wolters T, Roobol MJ, Steyerberg EW, et al. The effect of study arm on prostate cancer treatment in the large screening trial ERSPC. *Int J Cancer* 2010;126:2387–2393.
139. Hugosson J, Carlsson S, Aus G, et al. Mortality results from the Goteborg randomised population-based prostate-cancer screening trial. *Lancet Oncol* 2010;11:725–732.
140. Kilpelainen TP, Tammela TL, Malila N, et al. Prostate cancer mortality in the Finnish randomized screening trial. *J Natl Cancer Inst* 2013;105:719–725.
141. Center MM, Jemal A, Lortet-Tieulent J, et al. International variation in prostate cancer incidence and mortality rates. *Eur Urol* 2012;61:1079–1092.
142. Boyle P. Screening for prostate cancer: have you had your cholesterol measured? *BJU Int* 2003;92:191–199.
143. Greene KL, Albertsen PC, Babaian RJ, et al. Prostate specific antigen best practice statement: 2009 update. *J Urol* 2009;182:2232–2241.
144. Wolf AM, Wender RC, Etzioni RB, et al. American Cancer Society guideline for the early detection of prostate cancer: update 2010. *CA Cancer J Clin* 2010;60:70–98.
145. Carter HB. American Urological Association (AUA) guideline on prostate cancer detection: process and rationale. *BJU Int* 2013;112:543–547.
146. Wolff T, Tai E, Miller T. Screening for skin cancer: an update of the evidence for the U.S. Preventive Services Task Force. *Ann Intern Med* 2009;150:194–198.
147. Katalinic A, Waldmann A, Weinstock MA, et al. Does skin cancer screening save lives?: an observational study comparing trends in melanoma mortality in regions with and without screening. *Cancer* 2012;118:5395–5402.
148. Breitbart EW, Waldmann A, Nolte S, et al. Systematic skin cancer screening in Northern Germany. *J Am Acad Dermatol* 2012;66:201–211.
149. Smith RA, Brooks D, Cokkinides V, et al. Cancer screening in the United States, 2013: a review of current American Cancer Society guidelines, current issues in cancer screening, and new guidance on cervical cancer screening and lung cancer screening. *CA Cancer J Clin* 2013;63:88–105.
150. U.S. Preventive Services Task Force. Screening for skin cancer: U.S. Preventive Services Task Force recommendation statement. *Ann Intern Med* 2009;150:188–193.

35 Genetic Counseling

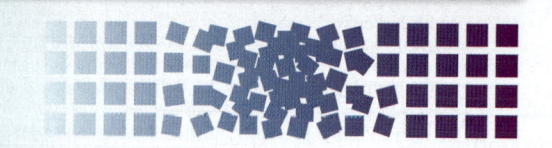

Ellen T. Matloff and Danielle C. Bonadies

INTRODUCTION

Clinically based genetic testing has evolved from an uncommon analysis ordered for the rare hereditary cancer family to a widely available tool ordered on a routine basis to assist in surgical and radiation decision making, chemoprevention, and surveillance of the patient with cancer, as well as management of the entire family. The evolution of this field has created a need for accurate cancer genetic counseling and risk assessment. Extensive coverage of this topic by the media, including Angelina Jolie's public disclosure of her *BRCA1+* status in May 2013, and widespread advertising by commercial testing laboratories have further fueled the demand for counseling and testing.

Cancer genetic counseling is a communication process between a health care professional and an individual concerning cancer occurrence and risk in his or her family.[1] The process, which may include the entire family through a blend of genetic, medical, and psychosocial assessments and interventions, has been described as a bridge between the fields of traditional oncology and genetic counseling.[1]

The goals of this process include providing the client with an assessment of individual cancer risk, while offering the emotional support needed to understand and cope with this information. It also involves deciphering whether the cancers in a family are likely to be caused by a mutation in a cancer gene and, if so, *which one*. There are >30 hereditary cancer syndromes, many of which can be caused by mutations in different genes. Therefore, testing for these syndromes can be complicated. Advertisements by genetic testing companies bill genetic testing as a simple process that can be carried out by health-care professionals with no training in this area; however, there are many genes involved in cancer, the interpretation of the test results is often complicated, the risk of result misinterpretation is great and associated with potential liability, and the emotional and psychological ramifications for the patient and family can be powerful.[2,3] A few hours of training by a company generating a profit from the sale of these tests does not adequately prepare providers to offer their own genetic counseling and testing services.[4] Furthermore, the delegation of genetic testing responsibilities to office staff and, recently, mammography technicians, is alarming and likely presents a huge liability for these ordering physicians, their practices, and their institutions.[5,6] *Providers should proceed with caution before taking on the role of primary genetic counselor for their patients.*

Counseling about hereditary cancers differs from *traditional* genetic counseling in several ways. Clients seeking cancer genetic counseling are rarely concerned with reproductive decisions, which are often the primary focus in traditional genetic counseling, but are instead seeking information about their own and other relatives' chances of developing cancer.[1] Additionally, the risks given are not absolute but change over time as the family and personal history changes and the patient ages. The risk reduction options available are often radical (e.g., chemoprevention or prophylactic surgery), and are not appropriate for every patient at every age. The surveillance and management plan must be tailored to the patient's age, childbearing status, menopausal status, risk category, ease of screening, and personal preferences and will likely change over time with the patient. The ultimate goal of cancer genetic counseling is to help the patient reach the decision best suited to her personal situation, needs, and circumstances.

There are now a significant number of referral centers across the country specializing in cancer genetic counseling, and the numbers are growing. However, some experts insist that the only way to keep up with the overwhelming demand for counseling will be to educate more physicians and nurses in cancer genetics. The feasibility of adding another specialized and time-consuming task to the clinical burden of these professionals is questionable, particularly with average patient encounters of 19.5 and 21.6 minutes for general practitioners and gynecologists, respectively.[7,8] A more practical goal is to better educate clinicians in the area of risk assessment so that they can screen their patient populations for individuals at high risk for hereditary cancer and refer them on to comprehensive counseling and testing programs. Access to genetic counseling is no longer an issue because there are now internet, phone, and satellite-based telemedicine services available (Table 35.1), with most major health insurance companies now covering these services[9–11] and several requiring them.[12]

WHO IS A CANDIDATE FOR CANCER GENETIC COUNSELING?

Only 5% to 10% of most cancer is thought to be caused by single mutations within autosomal-dominant inherited cancer susceptibility genes.[13] The key for clinicians is to determine which patients are at greatest risk to carry a hereditary mutation. There are seven critical risk factors in hereditary cancer (Table 35.2). The first is *early age of cancer onset*. This risk factor, *even in the absence of a family history*, has been shown to be associated with an increased frequency of germline mutations in many types of cancers.[14] The second risk factor is the presence of the same cancer in multiple affected relatives on the same side of the pedigree. These cancers do not need to be of similar histologic type in order to be caused by a single mutation. The third risk factor is the clustering of cancers known to be caused by a single gene mutation in one family (e.g., breast/ovarian/pancreatic cancer or colon/uterine/ovarian cancers). The fourth risk factor is the occurrence of multiple primary cancers in one individual. This includes multiple primary breast or colon cancers as well as a single individual with separate cancers known to be caused by a single gene mutation (e.g., breast and ovarian cancer in a single individual). Ethnicity also plays a role in determining who is at greatest risk to carry a hereditary cancer mutation. Individuals of Jewish ancestry are at increased risk to carry three specific *BRCA1/2* mutations.[15] The presence of a cancer that presents unusually—in this case, breast cancer in a male—represents a sixth risk factor and is important even when it is the only risk factor present. Finally, the last risk factor is pathology. Certain types of cancer are overrepresented in hereditary cancer families. For example, medullary and triple negative breast

TABLE 35.1
How to Find a Genetic Counselor for Your Patient

American Board of Genetic Counselors
https://abgcmember.goamp.com/Net/ABGCWcm/Find_Counselor/ABGCWcm/PublicDir.aspx?hkey=0ad511c0-d9e9-4714-bd4b-0d73a59ee175
http://bit.ly/1kzTbk9
Directory of board-certified genetic counselors

InformedDNA
www.informeddna.com
(800) 975-4819
A nationwide network of independent genetic counselors that use telephone and internet technology to bring genetic counseling to patients and providers. Covered by many insurance companies.

National Society of Genetic Counselors
www.nsgc.org (click "Find a Counselor" button)
(312) 321-6834
For a listing of genetic counselors in your area who specialize in cancer.

National Cancer Institute Cancer Genetics Services Directory
www.cancer.gov/cancertopics/genetics/directory
(800) 4-CANCER
A free service designed to locate providers of cancer risk counseling and testing services.

---

cancers (where the estrogen, progesterone and Her2 receptors are all negative, often abbreviated ER/PR/Her2) are overrepresented in BRCA1 families,[16,17] and the National Comprehensive Cancer Network (NCCN) BRCA testing guidelines now include individuals diagnosed with a triple negative breast cancer <age 60 years.[18] However, breast cancer patients without these pathologic findings are *not* necessarily at lower risk to carry a mutation. In contrast, patients with a borderline or mucinous ovarian carcinoma are at lower risk to carry a *BRCA1* or *BRCA2* mutation[19] and may instead carry a mutation in a different gene. It is already well-established that medullary thyroid carcinoma, sebaceous adenoma or carcinoma, adrenocortical carcinoma before the age of 25 years, and multiple adenomatous, hamartomatous, or juvenile colon polyps are indicative of other rare hereditary cancer syndromes.[11,20] These risk factors should be viewed in the context of the entire family history, and must be weighed in proportion to the number of individuals who have not developed cancer. The risk assessment is often limited in families that are small or have few female relatives; in such families, a single risk factor may carry more weight.

A less common, but extremely important, finding is the presence of unusual physical findings or birth defects that are known to be associated with rare hereditary cancer syndromes. Examples include benign skin findings, autism, large head circumference,[20,21] and thyroid disorders in Cowden syndrome, odontogenic keratocysts in Gorlin syndrome,[22] and desmoid tumors or dental abnormalities in familial adenomatous polyposis (FAP).[23] These and other findings should prompt further investigation of the patient's family history and consideration of a referral to genetic counseling.

In this chapter, the breast/ovarian cancer counseling session with a female patient will serve as a paradigm by which all other sessions may follow broadly.

COMPONENTS OF THE CANCER GENETIC COUNSELING SESSION

Precounseling Information

Before coming in for genetic counseling, the counselee should be informed about what to expect at each visit, and what information he/she should collect ahead of time. The counselor can then begin to collect medical and family history information and pathology reports that will be essential for the genetic counseling session.

Family History

An accurate family history is undoubtedly one of the most essential components of the cancer genetic counseling session. Optimally, a family history should include at least three generations; however, patients do not always have this information. For each individual affected with cancer, it is important to document the exact diagnosis, age at diagnosis, treatment strategies, and environmental exposures (i.e., occupational exposures, cigarettes, other agents).[24] The current age of the individual, laterality, and occurrence of any other cancers must also be documented. Cancer diagnoses should be confirmed with pathology reports whenever possible. A study by Love et al.[25] revealed that individuals accurately reported the primary site of cancer only 83% of the time in their first degree relatives with cancer, and 67% and 60% of the time in second and third degree relatives, respectively. It is common for patients to report a uterine cancer as an ovarian cancer, or a colon polyp as an invasive colorectal cancer. These differences, although seemingly subtle to the patient, can make a tremendous difference in risk assessment. Individuals should be asked if there are any consanguineous (inbred) relationships in the family, if any relatives were born with birth defects or mental retardation, and whether other genetic diseases run in the family (e.g., Fanconi anemia, Cowden syndrome), because these pieces of information could prove to be important in reaching a diagnosis.

The most common misconception in family history taking is that somehow a maternal family history of breast, ovarian, or uterine cancer is more significant than a paternal history. Conversely, many still believe that a paternal history of prostate cancer is more significant than a maternal history. Few cancer genes discovered thus far are located on the sex chromosomes and, therefore, both maternal and paternal history are significant and must be explored thoroughly. It has also become necessary to elicit the spouse's personal and family history of cancer. This has bearing on

---

TABLE 35.2
Risk Factors that Warrant Genetic Counseling for Hereditary Cancer Syndromes

1. Early age of onset (e.g., <50 years for breast, colon, and uterine cancer)
2. Multiple family members on the same side of the pedigree with the same cancer
3. Clustering of cancers in the family known to be caused by a single gene mutation (e.g., breast/ovarian/pancreatic; colon/uterine/ovarian; colon cancer/polyps/desmoid tumors/osteomas)
4. Multiple primary cancers in one individual (e.g., breast/ovarian cancer; colon/uterine; synchronous/metachronous colon cancers; <15 gastrointestinal polyps; <5 hamartomatous or juvenile polyps)
5. Ethnicity (e.g., Jewish ancestry for breast/ovarian cancer syndrome)
6. Unusual presentation of cancer/tumor (e.g., breast cancer in a male; medullary thyroid cancer; retinoblastoma; even one sebaceous carcinoma or adenoma)
7. Pathology (e.g., triple negative [ER/PR/Her-2] breast cancer <60; medullary breast cancers are overrepresented in women with hereditary breast and ovarian cancer; a colon tumor with an abnormal microsatellite instability (MSI) or immunohistochemistry (IHC) result increases the risk for a hereditary colon cancer syndrome)

the cancer status of common children, but may also determine if children are at increased risk for a serious recessive genetic disease such as Fanconi anemia.[26] Children who inherit two copies of a *BRCA2* mutation (one from each parent) are now known to have this serious disorder characterized by defective DNA repair and high rates of birth defects, aplastic anemia, leukemia, and solid tumors.[26] Patients should be encouraged to report changes in their family history over time (e.g., new cancer diagnoses, genetic testing results in relatives), because this may change their risk assessment and counseling.

A detailed family history should also include genetic diseases, birth defects, mental retardation, multiple miscarriages, and infant deaths. A history of certain recessive genetic diseases (e.g., ataxia telangiectasia, Fanconi anemia) can indicate that healthy family members who carry just one copy of the genetic mutation may be at increased risk to develop cancer.[26,27] Other genetic disorders, such as hereditary hemorrhagic telangiectasia, can be associated with a hereditary cancer syndrome caused by a mutation in the same gene—in this case, juvenile polyposis.[28]

Dysmorphology Screening

Congenital anomalies, benign tumors, and unusual dermatologic features occur in a large number of hereditary cancer predisposition syndromes. Examples include osteomas of the jaw in FAP, palmar pits in Gorlin syndrome, and papillomas of the lips and mucous membranes in Cowden syndrome. Obtaining an accurate past medical history of benign lesions and birth defects, and screening for such dysmorphology can greatly impact diagnosis, counseling, and testing. For example, *BRCA1/2* testing is inappropriate in a patient with breast cancer who has a family history of thyroid cancer and the orocutaneous manifestations of Cowden syndrome.

Risk Assessment

Risk assessment is one of the most complicated components of the genetic counseling session. It is crucial to remember that risk assessment changes over time as the person ages and as the health statuses of their family members change. Risk assessment can be broken down into three separate components.

- What is the chance that the counselee will develop the cancer observed in his/her family (or a genetically related cancer such as ovarian cancer due to a family history of breast cancer)?
- What is the chance that the cancers in this family are caused by a single gene mutation?
- What is the chance that we can identify the gene mutation in this family with our current knowledge and laboratory techniques?

Cancer clustering in a family may be due to genetic and/or environmental factors, or may be coincidental because some cancers are very common in the general population.[29] Although inherited factors may be the primary cause of cancers in some families, in others, cancer may develop because an inherited factor increases the individual's susceptibility to environmental carcinogens. It is also possible that members of the same family may be exposed to similar environmental exposures due to shared geography or patterns in behavior and diet that may increase the risk of cancer.[30] Therefore, it is important to distinguish the difference between a familial pattern of cancer (due to environmental factors or chance) and a hereditary pattern of cancer (due to a shared genetic mutation). Emerging research is also evaluating the role and clinical utility of more common low-penetrance susceptibility genes and single nucleotide polymorphisms (SNP) that may account for a proportion of familial cancers.[31]

Several models are available to calculate the chance that a woman will develop breast cancer, including the Gail and Claus models.[32,33] Computer-based models are also available to help determine the chance that a *BRCA* mutation will be found in a family.[34] At first glance, many of these models appear simple and easy to use, and it may be tempting to exclusively rely on these models to assess cancer risk. However, each model has its strengths and weaknesses, and the counselor needs to understand the limitations well and know which are validated, which are considered problematic, when a model will not work on a particular patient, or when another genetic syndrome should be considered. For example, none of the existing models are able to factor in other risks that may be essential in hereditary risk calculation (e.g., a sister who was diagnosed with breast cancer after radiation treatment for Hodgkin disease).

The risk of a detectable mutation will also vary based on cancer history and the degree of relationship to an affected family member. For example, family members with early-onset breast cancer have a higher likelihood of testing positive than unaffected family members. Therefore, the risk assessment process should include a discussion of which family member is the best candidate for testing.

DNA Testing

DNA testing is now available for a variety of hereditary cancer syndromes. However, despite misrepresentation by the media, testing is feasible for only a small percentage of individuals with cancer. DNA testing offers the important advantage of presenting clients with *actual risks* instead of the empiric risks derived from risk calculation models. DNA testing can be very expensive; full sequencing and rearrangement testing of the *BRCA1/2* genes currently averages $3,500, and full panel testing costs up to $7,000 per patient. Importantly, testing should begin in an affected family member whenever possible to maximize scientific accuracy. Most insurance companies now cover cancer genetic testing in families where the test is medically indicated.

One of the most crucial aspects of DNA testing is accurate result ordering and interpretation. Unfortunately, errors in ordering and interpretation are the greatest risk of genetic testing and are very common.[35] Emerging data reveal that between 30% to 50% of genetic tests are ordered inappropriately, which is problematic for patients, clinicians, and insurers.[36–38] Recent data demonstrate that many medical providers have difficulty interpreting even basic pedigrees and genetic test results.[33–35] Additional studies have demonstrated that an inaccurate interpretation of genetic testing has been shown to result in inappropriate medical management recommendations, unnecessary prophylactic surgeries, a massive waste of health-care dollars, psychosocial distress, and false reassurance for patients.[2,3]

Interpretations are becoming increasingly complicated as more tests and gene panels become available. For example, one study demonstrated that approximately 25% of high-risk families that were *BRCA1* and *BRCA2* negative by commercially available sequencing were found to carry a deletion or duplication in one of these genes, or a mutation in another gene.[39]

This is particularly concerning in an era in which testing companies are canvassing physicians, and now mammography technicians, and encouraging them to perform their own counseling and testing. The potential impact of test results on the patient and his/her family is great and, therefore, accurate interpretation of the results is paramount. Professional groups have recognized this and have adopted standards encouraging clinicians to refer patients to genetics experts to ensure proper ordering and interpretation of genetic tests. The U.S. Preventive Services Task Force recommends that women whose family history is suggestive of a *BRCA* mutation be referred for genetic counseling before being offered genetic testing.[40] The American College of Surgeons' Commission on Cancer standards include "cancer risk assessment, genetic counseling and testing services provided to patients either on site or by referral, by a qualified genetics professional."[4] In an effort to reduce errors, some insurance companies are requiring genetic counseling by a certified genetic counselor before testing for hereditary breast or colon cancer syndromes.[12]

Results can fall into a few broad categories. It is important to note that a negative test result can actually be interpreted in three different ways, detailed in #2, #3, and #4, which follows.

1. <u>Deleterious mutation "positive."</u> When a deleterious mutation in a well-known cancer gene is discovered, the cancer risks for the patient and her family are relatively straightforward. However, with the development of multigene panels and the inclusion of many lesser known genes, the risks of detecting a mutation within a gene whose cancer risks are ill defined and medical management options unknown is much greater. Even for well-known genes, the risks are not precise and should be presented to patients as a risk range.[41,42] When a true mutation is found, it is critical to test both parents (whenever possible) to determine from which side of the family the mutation is originating, even when the answer appears obvious.

2. <u>True negative.</u> An individual does not carry the deleterious mutation found in her family, which ideally, has been proven to segregate with the cancer family history. In this case, the patient's cancer risks are usually reduced to the population risks.

3. <u>Negative.</u> A mutation was not detected, and the cancers in the family are not likely to be hereditary based on the personal and family history assessment. For example, a patient is diagnosed with breast cancer at age 38 years and comes from a large family with no other cancer diagnoses and relatives who died at old ages of other causes.

4. <u>Uninformative.</u> A mutation cannot be found in affected family members of a family in which the cancer pattern appears to be hereditary; there is likely an undetectable mutation within the gene, or the family carries a mutation in a different gene. If, for example, the patient developed breast cancer at age 38 years, has a father with breast cancer, and has a paternal aunt who developed breast and ovarian cancers before age 50 years, a negative test result would be almost meaningless. It would simply mean that the family has a mutation that could not be identified with our current testing methods or a mutation in another cancer gene. The entire family would be followed as high risk.

5. <u>Variant of uncertain significance.</u> A genetic change is identified, the significance of which is unknown. It is possible that this change is deleterious or completely benign. It may be helpful to test other *affected* family members to see if the mutation segregates with disease in the family. If it does not segregate, the variant is less likely to be significant. If it does, the variant is more likely to be significant. Other tools, including a splice site predictor, in conjunction with data on species conservation and amino acid difference scores, can also be helpful in determining the likelihood that a variant is significant. It is rarely helpful (and can be detrimental) to test *unaffected* family members for such variants. The rates of variants of uncertain significance vary greatly depending on the reporting protocols of the lab and the genes analyzed. Creation of open databases through a nationwide movement called Free the Data will likely improve variant reporting for all laboratories.

In order to pinpoint the mutation in a family, an affected individual most likely to carry the mutation should be tested first whenever possible. This is most often a person affected with the cancer in question at the earliest age. Test subjects should be selected with care, because it is possible for a person to develop sporadic cancer in a hereditary cancer family. For example, in an early-onset breast cancer family, it would not be ideal to first test a woman diagnosed with breast cancer at age 65 years because she may represent a sporadic case.

If a mutation is detected in an affected relative, other family members can be tested for the same mutation with a great degree of accuracy. Family members who do not carry the mutation found in their family are deemed true negative. Those who are found to carry the mutation in their family will have more definitive information about their risks to develop cancer. This information can be crucial in assisting patients in decision making regarding surveillance and risk reduction.

If a mutation is not identified in the affected relative, it usually means that either the cancers in the family are (1) not hereditary, or (2) caused by an undetectable mutation or a mutation in a different gene. A careful review of the family history and the risk factors will help to decipher whether interpretation 1 or 2 is more likely. Additional genetic testing may need to be ordered at this point. In cases in which the cancers appear hereditary and no mutation is found, DNA banking should be offered to the proband for a time in the future when improved testing may become available. A letter indicating exactly who in the family has access to the DNA should accompany the banked sample.

The genetic counseling result disclosure session should also include a detailed discussion of which other family members would benefit from genetic counseling and testing and referral information. This can apply not only to families who have been found to carry a deleterious mutation, but may also prove useful in other families (e.g., test a higher risk relative or determine segregation of a variant within a family).

The penetrance of mutations in cancer susceptibility genes is also difficult to interpret. Initial estimates derived from high-risk families provided very high cancer risks for *BRCA1* and *BRCA2* mutation carriers.[43] More recent studies done on populations that were not selected for family history have revealed lower penetrances.[44] Because exact penetrance rates cannot be determined for individual families at this time, and because precise genotype/phenotype correlations remain unclear, it is prudent to provide patients with a range of cancer risk and to explain that their risk probably falls somewhere within this spectrum. This can prove challenging for genes that lack published long-term data on cancer associations and risks.

Female carriers of *BRCA1* and *BRCA2* mutations have a 50% to 85% lifetime risk to develop breast cancer and between a 15% to 60% lifetime risk to develop ovarian cancer.[15,42,43] It is important to note that the classification "ovarian cancer" also includes cancer of the fallopian tubes and primary peritoneal carcinoma.[44,45] *BRCA2* carriers also have an increased lifetime risk of male breast cancer, pancreatic cancer, and possibly, melanoma.[46,47]

Options for Surveillance, Risk Reduction, and Tailored Treatment

The cancer risk counseling session is a forum to provide counselees with information, support, options, and hope. Mutation carriers can be offered: earlier and more aggressive surveillance, chemoprevention, and/or prophylactic surgery. Detailed management options for *BRCA* carriers are discussed in this chapter.

Surveillance recommendations are evolving with newer techniques and additional data. At this time, it is recommended that individuals at increased risk for breast cancer, particularly those who carry a *BRCA* mutation, have annual mammograms beginning at age 25 years, with a clinical breast exam by a breast specialist, a yearly breast magnetic resonance imaging (MRI) with a clinical breast exam by a breast specialist, and a yearly clinical breast exam by a gynecologist.[48,49] It is suggested that the mammogram and MRI be spaced out around the calendar year so that some intervention is planned every 6 months. Recent data suggest that MRI may be safer and more effective in *BRCA* carriers <40 years of age and may someday replace mammograms in this population.[50]

BRCA carriers may take a selective estrogen-receptor modulator (SERM) or aromatase inhibitor in hopes of reducing their risks of developing breast cancer. These medications have been proven effective in women at increased risk due to a positive family history of breast cancer.[51-53] There are limited data on the effectiveness of such medications in unaffected BRCA carriers[54-56]; however, there are some data to suggest that BRCA carriers taking tamoxifen as treatment for a breast cancer reduce their risk of a contralateral breast cancer.[57] Additionally, the majority of BRCA2 carriers who develop breast cancer develop an estrogen-positive form of the disease,[58] and it is hoped that this population will respond especially well to chemoprevention. Further studies in this area are necessary before drawing conclusions about the efficacy of chemoprevention in this population. Prophylactic bilateral mastectomy reduces the risk of breast cancer by >90% in women at high-risk for the disease.[59] Before genetic testing was available, it was not uncommon for entire generations of cancer families to have at-risk tissues removed without knowing if they were *personally* at increased risk for their familial cancer. Fifty percent of unaffected individuals in hereditary cancer families will *not* carry the inherited predisposition gene and can be spared prophylactic surgery or invasive high-risk surveillance regimens. Therefore, it is clearly not appropriate to offer prophylactic surgery until a patient is referred for genetic counseling and, if possible, testing.[60]

Women who carry BRCA1/2 mutations are also at increased risk to develop second contralateral and ipsilateral primaries of the breast.[61] These data bring into question the option of breast conserving surgery in women at high risk to develop a second primary within the same breast. For this reason, the BRCA1/2 carrier status can have a profound impact on surgical decision making,[62] and many patients have genetic counseling and testing immediately after diagnosis and before surgery or radiation therapy. Those patients who test positive and opt for prophylactic mastectomy can often be spared radiation and the resulting side effects that can complicate reconstruction. Approximately 30% to 80% of previously irradiated patients who later opt for mastectomy with reconstruction report significant complications or unfavorable cosmetic results.[62,63]

Women who carry BRCA1/2 mutations are also at increased risk to develop ovarian, fallopian tube, and primary peritoneal cancer, even if no one in their family has developed these cancers. Surveillance for ovarian cancer includes transvaginal ultrasounds and CA-125 testing; however, the effectiveness of such surveillance in detecting ovarian cancers at early, more treatable stages has not been proven in any population. Oral contraceptives reduce the risk of ovarian cancer in all women, including BRCA carriers.[64] Recent data indicate that the impact of this intervention on increasing breast cancer risk, if any, is low.[56,65] Given the difficulties in screening and in the treatment of ovarian cancer, the risk/benefit analysis likely favors the use of oral contraceptives in young carriers of BRCA1/2 mutations who are not yet ready to have their ovaries removed. Prophylactic bilateral salpingo-oophorectomy (BSO) is currently the most effective means to reduce the risk of ovarian cancer and is recommended to BRCA1/2 carriers by the age of 35 to 40 or when childbearing is complete.[66] Specific operative and pathologic protocols have been developed for this prophylactic surgery.[67] In BRCA1/2 carriers whose pathologies come back normal, this surgery is highly effective at reducing the subsequent risk of ovarian cancer.[68] A decision analysis, comparing various surveillance and risk-reducing options available to BRCA carriers, has shown an increase in life expectancy if BSO is pursued by age 40.[69] Emerging data indicate that most ovarian cancers begin in the fallopian tube, and that salpingectomy may someday be sufficient in reducing ovarian cancer risk in young women; however, more data are needed before this option is offered to patients outside of clinical trials.[70] A relatively small percentage of women who pursue BSO may develop primary peritoneal carcinoma.[44,71] There has been some debate about whether BRCA1/2 carriers should also opt for total abdominal hysterectomy (TAH) due to the fact that small stumps of the fallopian tubes remain after BSO alone. The question of whether BRCA carriers are at increased risk for uterine serous papillary carcinoma (USPC) has also been raised.[72-74] If a relationship does exist between BRCA mutations and uterine cancer, the risk appears to be low and not elevated over that of the general population.[75] Removing the uterus may make it possible for a BRCA carrier to take unopposed estrogen or tamoxifen in the future without the risk of uterine cancer, but this surgery is associated with a longer recovery time and has more side effects than does BSO alone. Each patient should be counseled about the pros and cons of each procedure and the risks associated with premature menopause before having surgery.[76]

A secondary, but important, reason for female BRCA carriers to consider prophylactic oophorectomy is that it also significantly reduces the risk of a subsequent breast cancer, particularly if they have this surgery before menopause.[77,78] The reduction in breast cancer risk remains even if a healthy premenopausal carrier elects to take low-dose hormone-replacement therapy (HRT) after this surgery[79]. Early data suggest that tamoxifen, in addition to premenopausal oophorectomy, in BRCA carriers may have little additional benefit in terms of breast cancer risk reduction.[80] Research is needed in balancing quality of life issues secondary to estrogen deprivation with cancer risk reduction in these young female BRCA1/2 carriers.

New developments are also emerging in the treatment and, possibly, the prevention of BRCA-related cancers. Early data revealed that breast and ovarian cancers in BRCA carriers were particularly sensitive to treatment with poly adenosine diphosphate (ADP)-ribose polymerases (PARP) inhibitors in combination with chemotherapy.[81,82] New trials are focusing on which chemotherapeutic regimens are most effective in mutation carriers. More data are needed on larger cohorts of patients and are currently being studies in multiple clinical trials.

Genetic counseling and testing is also available for dozens of cancer syndromes, including Lynch syndrome, von Hippel Lindau syndrome, multiple endocrine neoplasias, and familial adenomatous polyposis. Surveillance and risk reduction for patients who are known mutation carriers for such conditions may decrease the associated morbidity and mortality of these syndromes.

Follow-up

A follow-up letter to the patient is a concrete means of documenting the information conveyed in the sessions so that the patient and his/her family members can review it over time. This letter should be sent to the patient and health-care professionals to whom the patient has granted access to this information. A follow-up phone call and/or counseling session may also be helpful, particularly in the case of a positive test result. Some programs provide patients with an annual or biannual newsletter updating them on new information in the field of cancer genetics or patient support groups. It is now recommended that patients return for follow-up counseling sessions months, or even years, after their initial consult to discuss advances in genetic testing and changes in surveillance and risk reduction options. This can be beneficial for individuals who have been found to carry a hereditary predisposition, for those in whom a syndrome/mutation is suspected but yet unidentified, and for those who are ready to move forward with genetic testing. Follow-up counseling is also recommended for patients whose life circumstances have changed (e.g., preconception, after childbearing is complete), who are preparing for prophylactic surgery, or who are ready to discuss the family genetics with their children.

ISSUES IN CANCER GENETIC COUNSELING

Psychosocial Issues

The psychosocial impact of cancer genetic counseling cannot be underestimated. Just the process of scheduling a cancer risk counseling session may be quite difficult for some individuals with a family history who are not only frightened about their own cancer risk, but also are reliving painful experiences associated with the cancer of their loved ones.[13] Counselees may be faced with an onslaught of emotions, including anger, fear of developing cancer, fear of disfigurement and dying, grief, lack of control, negative body image, and a sense of isolation.[24] Some counselees wrestle with the fear that insurance companies, employers, family members, and even future partners will react negatively to their cancer risks. For many, it is a double-edged sword as they balance their fears and apprehensions about dredging up these issues with the possibility of obtaining reassuring news and much needed information.

A person's perceived cancer risk is often dependent on many "nonmedical" variables. They may estimate that their risk is higher if they look like an affected individual, or share some of their personality traits.[24] Their perceived risks will vary depending on if their relatives were cancer survivors or died painful deaths from the disease. Many people wonder not *if* they are going to get cancer, but *when*.

The counseling session is an opportunity for individuals to express why they believe they have developed cancer, or why their family members have cancer. Some explanations may revolve around family folklore, and it is important to listen to and address these explanations rather than dismiss them.[24] In doing this, the counselor will allow the clients to alleviate their greatest fears and to give more credibility to the medical theory. Understanding a patient's perceived cancer risk is important, because that fear may *decrease* surveillance and preventive health-care behaviors.[83] For patients and families who are moving forward with DNA testing, a referral to a mental health-care professional is often very helpful. Genetic testing has an impact not only on the patient, but also on his/her children, siblings, parents, and extended relatives. This can be overwhelming for an individual and the family, and should be discussed in detail prior to testing.

To date, studies conducted in the setting of pre- and post-genetic counseling have revealed that, at least in the short term, most patients do not experience adverse psychological outcomes after receiving their test results.[84,85] In fact, preliminary data have revealed that individuals in families with known mutations who seek testing seem to fare better psychologically at 6 months than those who avoid testing.[84] Among individuals who learn they are *BRCA* mutation carriers, anxiety and distress levels appear to increase slightly after receiving their test results but returned to pre-test levels in several weeks.[86] Although these data are reassuring, it is important to recognize that genetic testing is an individual decision and will not be right for every patient or every family.

Presymptomatic Testing in Children

Presymptomatic testing in children has been widely discussed, and most concur that it is appropriate only when the onset of the condition regularly occurs in childhood or if there are useful interventions that can be applied.[87] For example, genetic testing for mutations in the *BRCA* genes and other adult-onset diseases is generally limited to individuals who are >18 years of age. The American College of Medical Genetics states that if the "medical or psychosocial benefits of a genetic test will not accrue until adulthood . . . genetic testing generally should be deferred."[88] In contrast, the DNA-based diagnosis of children and young adults at risk for hereditary medullary thyroid carcinoma (MTC) is appropriate and has improved the management of these patients.[89] DNA-based testing for MTC is virtually 100% accurate and allows at-risk family members to make informed decisions about prophylactic thyroidectomy. FAP is a disorder that occurs in childhood and in which mortality can be reduced if detection is presymptomatic.[90] Testing is clearly indicated in these instances.

Questions have been raised about the parents' right to demand testing for adult-onset diseases, and this is now happening regularly with direct-to-consumer tests and whole exome testing of children.[91] The risks of such testing to the child, and the child's right *not* to be tested must be considered. Whenever childhood testing is not medically indicated, it is preferable that testing decisions are postponed until the children are adults and can decide for themselves whether to be tested.

Confidentiality

The level of confidentiality surrounding cancer genetic testing is paramount due to concerns of genetic discrimination. Careful consideration should be given to the confidentially of family history information, pedigrees, genetic test results, pathology reports, and the carrier status of other family members as most hospitals and clinicians transition to electronic medical records systems. The goal of electronic records is to share information about the patient with his/her entire health-care team. However, genetics is a unique specialty that involves the whole family. Patient's charts often contain Health Insurance Portability and Accountability Act (HIPAA)–protected health information and genetic test results for many other family members. This information may not be appropriate to enter into an electronic record. The unique issues of genetics services need to be considered when designing electronic medical record standards.

Confidentiality of test results *within* a family can also be of issue, because genetic counseling and testing often reveals the risk statuses of family members other than the patient. Under confidentiality codes, the patient needs to grant permission before at-risk family members can be contacted. For this reason, many programs have built in a "share information with family members" clause to their informed consent documents. It has been questioned whether or not a family member could sue a health-care professional for negligence if they were identified at high risk yet not informed.[92] Most recommendations have stated that the burden of confidentiality lies between the provider and the patient. However, more recent recommendations state that confidentiality *should* be violated if the potential harm of not notifying other family members outweighs the harm of breaking a confidence to the patient.[93] There is no patent solution for this difficult dilemma, and situations must be considered on a case-by-case basis with the assistance of the in-house legal department and ethics committee.

Insurance and Discrimination Issues

When genetic testing for cancer predisposition first became widely available, the fear of health insurance discrimination by both patients and providers was one of the most common concerns.[94,95] It appears that the risks of health insurance discrimination were overstated and that almost no discrimination by health insurers has been reported.[96] HIPAA banned the use of genetic information as a preexisting condition.[97,98] In May of 2008, Congress passed the Genetic Information Nondiscrimination Act (GINA, HR 493), which provides broad protection of an individual's genetic information against health insurance and employment discrimination.[99] In addition, the Heath Care and Education Reconciliation Act of 2010 (HR 4872) prohibits group health plans from denying insurance based on preexisting conditions and from increasing premiums based on health status.[100] Health-care providers can now more confidently reassure their patients that genetic counseling and testing will not put them at risk of losing group or individual health insurance.

More and more patients are choosing to submit their genetic counseling and/or testing charges to their health insurance companies. In the past few years, more insurance companies have agreed to pay for counseling and/or testing,[101] perhaps in light of data that show these services reduce errors related to ordering and interpreting genetic testing and that decision analyses have revealed subsequent prophylactic surgeries to be cost effective.[102] The risk of life or disability insurance discrimination, however, is more realistic. Patients should be counseled about such risks before they pursue genetic testing.

Reproductive Issues

Reproductive technology in the form of preimplantation genetic diagnosis, prenatal testing, or sperm sorting are options[103] for men and women with a hereditary cancer syndrome, but are requested by few patients for adult-onset conditions in which there are viable options for surveillance and risk reduction. Importantly, if a BRCA2 carrier is considering having a child, it is important to assess the spouse's risk of also carrying a BRCA2 mutation. If the spouse is of Jewish ancestry or has a personal or family history of breast, ovarian, or pancreatic cancer, BRCA testing should be considered and a discussion of the risk of Fanconi anemia in a child with two BRCA2 mutations should take place.[104]

RECENT ADVANCES AND FUTURE DIRECTIONS

Cancer genetic counseling and testing were thrust into the national spotlight in the spring of 2013 when Hollywood icon Angelina Jolie publically disclosed that she was a BRCA1 carrier. One month later the Supreme Court unanimously ruled against gene patents. Referrals for genetic testing spiked across the country and have not returned to baseline levels at most centers. Within hours of the ruling, other labs began offering less expensive and more comprehensive BRCA testing, dramatically changing the marketplace of genetic testing for hereditary breast cancer.

All laboratories that have entered the BRCA marketplace have done so by including BRCA1 and BRCA2 in gene panels. These panels simultaneously analyze groups of genes that contribute to increased risk for breast, colon, ovarian, uterine, and other cancers. The cost of this technology continues to decrease with some multi-gene panels costing just a few hundred dollars *less* than traditional BRCA testing (~$4,000). Some panels include only well-known genes (e.g., *p53, APC, MLH1*), although many include lesser known genes (e.g., *BRIP1, NBN, MRE11A*) for which cancer risks are ill defined and medical management options are unknown. Because testing for these genes is new to the clinical setting, it is expected to take several years to compile accurate cancer risk estimates and appropriate recommendations for surveillance and risk reduction. Furthermore, the rate of *variants of uncertain significance* will likely be more common in the lesser known genes. These changes have increased the complexity of genetic testing exponentially. In response, several state and one national insurance company have mandated genetic counseling by certified providers before they will cover cancer genetic testing. In a surprising response, the American Society of Clinical Oncology (ASCO) opposed this insurer's decision, despite more than a decade's worth of data demonstrating that the majority of physicians do not have the time or expertise to offer genetic counseling and testing[38,105-108]. The AMA will decide whether to back the ASCO resolution in June 2014.

Some companies are now offering direct-to-consumer (DTC) genetic testing via websites. The accuracy of some of these DTC genetic tests are in question, and the leading company, 23andMe, has recently come under fire by the U.S. Food and Drug Administration.[105]

Maintaining high standards for thorough genetic counseling, informed consent, and accurate result interpretation will be paramount in reducing potential risks and maximizing the benefits of genetic technology in the next century.

REFERENCES

1. Peters J. Breast cancer genetics: relevance to oncology practice. *Cancer Control* 1995;2:195–208.
2. Brierley KL, Campfield D, Ducaine W, et al. Errors in delivery of cancer genetics services: implications for practice. *Conn Med* 2010;74:413–423.
3. Brierley KL, Blouch E, Cogswell W, et al. Adverse events in cancer genetic testing: medical, ethical, legal, andt financial implications. *Cancer J* 2012;18:303–309.
4. American College of Surgeons, Commission on Cancer: Cancer Program Standards 2012: Ensuring Patient-Centered Care. http://www.facs.org/cancer/coc/programstandards2012.html Accessed on December 3, 2012.
5. Yale Cancer Genetic Counseling Program. Mammography techs ordering their own genetic testing? It appears our suspicion was correct. yalecancergeneticcounseling.blogspot.com October 2, 2013. http://yalecancergeneticcounseling.blogspot.com/2013/10/mammography-techs-ordering-their-own.html
6. Lubin IM, Caggana M, Constantin C, et al. Ordering molecular genetic tests and reporting results: practices in laboratory and clinical settings. *J Mol Diagn* 2008;10:459–468.
7. Weeks WB, Wallace AE. Time and money: a retrospective evaluation of the inputs, outputs, efficiency, and incomes of physicians. *Arch Intern Med* 2003;163(8):944–948.
8. Doksum T, Bernhardt BA, Holtzman NA. Does knowledge about the genetics of breast cancer differ between nongeneticist physicians who do or do not discuss or order BRCA testing? *Genet Med* 2003;5:99–105.
9. Rosenthal ET. Shortage of genetics counselors may be anecdotal, but need is real. *Oncology Times* 2007;29:34–36.
10. Informed Medical Decisions. Adult Genetics: Genetic counseling for your health concerns. Available at: http://www.informeddna.com/index.php/patients/adult-genetics.html. Accessed August 24, 2009.
11. Informed Medical Decisions. News: Aetna Press Release: Aetna to offer access to confidential telephonic cancer genetic counseling to health plan members. Available at: http://www.informeddna.com/images/stories/news_articles/news%20press%20release%20Aetna.pdf. Accessed August 24, 2009.
12. Schneider, ME. Cigna to require counseling for some genetic tests. Internal Medicine News Digital Network. July 26, 2013. http://www.internalmedicinenews.com/single-view/cigna-to-require-counseling-for-some-genetic-tests/efd4f471df8b46ba2208da423adf198d.html
13. Claus E, Schildkraut J, Thompson W, et al. The genetic attributable risks of breast and ovarian cancer. *Cancer* 1996;77:2318–2324.
14. Loman N, Johannsson O, Kristoffersson U. Family history of breast and ovarian cancers and BRCA1 and BRCA2 mutations in a population-based series of early-onset breast cancer. *J Natl Cancer Inst* 2001;93:1215.
15. Struewing J, Hartge P, Wacholder S. The risk of cancer associated with specific mutations of BRCA1 and BRCA2 among Ashkenazi Jews. *N Engl J Med* 1997;336:1401–1408.
16. Eisinger F, Jacquemier J, Charpin C, et al. Mutations at BRCA1: the medullary breast carcinoma revisited. *Cancer Res* 1998;58:1588–1592.
17. Kandel M, Stadler Z, Masciari S, et al. Prevalence of BRCA1 mutations in triple negative breast cancer. Paper presented at: 2006 42nd Annual ASCO Meeting; 2006; Atlanta, GA.
18. National Comprehensive Cancer Network Clinical Guidelines in Oncology: Genetics/Familial High-Risk Assessment - Breast and Ovarian Cancer. http://www.nccn.org/professionals/physician_gls/f_guidelines.asp#detection Accessed November 2, 2012.
19. Risch H, McLaughlin J, Cole D, et al. Population BRCA1 and BRCA2 mutation frequencies and cancer penetrances: a kin-cohort study in Ontario, Canada. *JNCI* 2006;98:1694–706.
20. Matloff E, Brierley K, Chimera C. A clinician's guide to hereditary colon cancer. *Cancer J* 2004;10(5):280–287.
21. Pilarski R. Cowden syndrome: a critical review of the clinical literature. *J Genet Couns* 2009 Feb;18:13–27.
22. Varga EA, Pastore M, Prior T, et al. The prevalence of PTEN mutations in a clinical pediatric cohort with autism spectrum disorders, developmental delay, and macrocephaly. *Genet Med* 2009;11:111–117.
23. Gorlin R. Nevoid basal-cell carcinoma syndrome. *Medicine* 1987;66(2):98–113.
24. Schneider K. *Counseling About Cancer: Strategies for Genetic Counseling*. 2nd ed. Wiley-Liss; 2001.
25. Love R, Evan A, Josten D. The accuracy of patient reports of a family history. *J Chronic Dis* 1985;38(4):289–293.
26. Alter B, Rosenberg P, Brody L. Clinical and molecular features associated with biallelic mutations in FANCD1/BRCA2. *J Med Genet* 2007;44:1–9.
27. Thompson D, Duedal S, Kirner J, et al. Cancer risks and mortality in heterozygous ATM mutation carriers. *J Natl Cancer Inst* 2005;97:813–822.
28. Korzenik J, Chung D, Digumarthy S, et al. Case 33-2005: a 43-year-old man with lower gastrointestinal bleeding. *N Engl J Med* 2005;353:1836–1844.
29. American Cancer Society. *Cancer Facts and Figures 2009*. Atlanta, GA: American Cancer Society; 2009.

30. Olopade O, Weber B. Breast cancer genetics: toward molecular characterization of individuals at increased risk for breast cancer. Part II. PPO Updates 1998;12:1–8.
31. Stratton MR, Rahman N. The emerging landscape of breast cancer susceptibility. Nat Genet 2008;40:17–22.
32. Gail M, Brinton L, Byar D. Projecting individualized probabilities of developing breast cancer for white females who are being examined annually. J Natl Cancer Inst 1989;81:1879–1886.
33. Claus E, Risch N, Thompson W. Autosomal dominant inheritance of early-onset breast cancer. Cancer 1994;73:643.
34. Parmigiani G, Berry D, Agilar O. Determining carrier probabilities for breast cancer susceptibility genes BRCA1 and BRCA2. Am J Hum Genet 1998;62:145–158.
35. Friedman S. Thoughts from FORCE: Comments Submitted to the Secretary's Advisory Committee on Genetics Health and Society. http://facingourrisk.wordpress.com/2008/12/03/comments-submitted-to-the-secretarys-advisory-committee-on-genetics-health-and-society/. Accessed April 6, 2010.
36. UnitedHealth. Personalized Medicine: Trends and Prospects for the New Science of Genetic Testing and Molecular Diagnostics. Working Paper 7. Minnetonka, MN: UnitedHealth Center for Health Reform & Modernization; March 2012.
37. ARUP Laboratories. Value of Genetic Counselors in the Laboratory. Salt Lake City: ARUP Laboratories; March 2011.
38. Plon SE, Cooper HP, Parks B, et al. Genetic testing and cancer risk management recommendations by physicians for at-risk relatives. Genet Med 2011;13:148–154.
39. Walsh T. More Than 25% of Breast Cancer Families with Wild-Type Results from Commercial Genetic Testing of BRCA1 and BRCA2 Are Resolved by BROCA Sequencing of All Known Breast Cancer Genes. Paper presented at: 2013 American Society of Human Genetics Meeting Session #19; 2013; Boston, MA.
40. U.S. Preventive Services Task Force. Genetic Risk Assessment and BRCA Mutation Testing for Breast and Ovarian Cancer Susceptibility. Rockville, MD: Agency for Healthcare Research and Quality; 2013. http://www.uspreventiveservicestaskforce.org/uspstf12/breastcnxr/breastfinalrs.htm. Accessed June 2, 2014.
41. King MC, Marks JH, Mandell JB, et al. Breast and ovarian cancer risks due to inherited mutations in BRCA1 and BRCA2. Science 2003;302:643–646.
42. Antoniou A, Pharoah PD, Narod S, et al. Average risks of breast and ovarian cancer associated with BRCA1 or BRCA2 mutations detected in case Series unselected for family history: a combined analysis of 22 studies. Am J Hum Genet 2003;72:1117–1130.
43. Ford D, Easton D, Bishop D, et al. Risks of cancer in BRCA1 mutation carriers. Lancet 1994;343:692–695.
44. Piver M, Jishi M, Tsukada Y. Primary peritoneal carcinoma after prophylactic ooophorectomy in women with a family history of ovarian cancer. Cancer 1993;71:2751–2755.
45. Aziz S, Kuperstein G, Rosen B. A genetic epidemiological study of carcinoma of the fallopian tube. Gynecol Oncol 2001;80:341–345.
46. van Asperen C, Brohet R, Meijers-Heijboer A, et al. Cancer risks in BRCA2 families: estimates for sites other than breast and ovary. J Med Genet 2005;42:711–719.
47. Breast Cancer Linkage Consortium. Cancer risks in BRCA2 mutation carriers. J Natl Cancer Inst 1999;91:1310–1316.
48. Warner E, Plewes D, Hill K, et al. Surveillance of BRCA1 and BRCA2 mutation carriers with magnetic resonance imaging, ultrasound, mammography, and clinical breast examination. JAMA 2004;202:1317–1325.
49. Kriege M, Brekelmans CT, Boetes C, et al. Efficacy of MRI and mammography for breast-cancer screening in women with a familial or genetic predisposition. N Engl J Med 2004;29:351:427–437.
50. Kuhl C, Weigel S, Schrading S, et al. Prospective multicenter cohort study to refine management recommendations for women at elevated familial risk of breast cancer: the EVA Trial. J Clin Oncol 2010:1450–1457.
51. Powles T, Ashley S, Tidy A, et al. Twenty-year follow-up of the Royal Marsden randomized, double-blinded tamoxifen breast cancer prevention trial. J Natl Cancer Inst 2007;99:283–290.
52. Cuzick J, Forbes J, Sestak I, et al. Long-term results of tamoxifen prophylaxis for breast cancer: 96 month follow-up of the randomized IBIS-I trial. J Natl Cancer Inst 2007;99:272–282.
53. Goss PE, Ingle JN, Alés-Martínez JE, et al. Exemestane for breast-cancer prevention in postmenopausal women. N Engl J Med 2011;364:2381.
54. Fisher B, Constantino J, Wickerman D. Tamoxifen for the prevention of breast cancer: report of the National Surgical Adjuvant Breast and Bowel Project P-1 Study. J Natl Cancer Inst 1998;90:1371–1388.
55. King M, Wieand S, Hale K. Tamoxifen and breast cancer incidence among women with inherited mutations in BRCA1 and BRCA2. JAMA 2001;286:2251–2256.
56. Narod S, Brunet J, Ghadirian P. Tamoxifen and risk of contralateral breast cancer in BRCA1 and BRCA2 mutation carriers: a case-control study. Lancet 2000;356:1876–1881.
57. Phillips KA, Milne RL, Rookus MA, et al. Tamoxifen and risk of contralateral breast cancer for BRCA1 and BRCA2 mutation carriers. J Clin Oncol 2013;31:3091–3099.
58. Lakhani S, van de Vijver M, Jacquemier J, et al. The pathology of familial breast cancer: predictive value of immunohistochemical markers estrogen receptor, progesterone receptor, HER-2, and p53 in patients with mutations in BRCA1 and BRCA2. J Clin Oncol 2002;20:2310–2318.
59. Hartmann L, Schaid D, Woods J. Efficacy of bilateral prophylactic mastectomy in women with a family history of breast cancer. N Engl J Med 1999;340:77–84.
60. Matloff E. The breast surgeon's role in BRCA1 and BRCA2 testing. Am J Surg 2000;180:294–298.
61. Turner B, Harold E, Matloff E, et al. BRCA1/BRCA2 germline mutations in locally recurrent breast cancer patients after lumpectomy and radiation therapy: Implications for breast-conserving management in patients with BRCA1/BRCA2 mutations. J Clin Oncol 1999;17:3017–3024.
62. Contant CM, et al. Clinical experience of prophylactic mastectomy followed by immediate breast reconstruction in women at hereditary risk of breast cancer (HBOC) or a proven BRCA1 or BRCA2 germ-line mutation. Eur J Surg Oncol 2002;28:627–632.
63. Forman DL, Chiu J, Restifo RJ, et al. Breast reconstruction in previously irradiated patients using tissue expanders and implants: a potentially unfavorable result. Ann Plast Surg 1998;40:360–363.
64. McLaughlin J, Risch H, Lubinski J, et al. Reproductive risk factors for ovarian cancer in carriers of BRCA1 or BRCA2 mutations: a case-control study. Lancet 2007;8:26–34.
65. Milne R, Knight J, John E, et al. Oral contraceptive use and risk of early-onset breast cancer in carriers and noncarriers of BRCA1 and BRCA2 mutations. Cancer Epidemiol Biomarkers Prev 2005;14:350–356.
66. Domchek S, Friebel T, Neuhausen S, et al. Mortality reduction after risk-reducing bilateral salpingo-oophorectomy in a prospective cohort of BRCA1 and BRCA2 mutation carriers. Lancet Oncol 2006;7:223–229.
67. Powel CB, Kenley E, Chen LM, et al. Risk-reducing salpingo-oophorectomy in BRCA mutation carriers: role of serial sectioning in the detection of occult malignancy. J Clin Oncol 2005;23:127–132.
68. Finch A, Beiner M, Lubinski J, et al. Salpingo-oophorectomy and the risk of ovarian, fallopian tube, and peritoneal cancers in women with a BRCA1 or BRCA2 mutation. JAMA 2006;296:185–192.
69. Kurian AW, Sigal BM, Plevritis SK. Survival analysis of cancer risk reduction strategies for BRCA1/2 mutation carriers. J Clin Oncol 2010;10;28:222–231.
70. Kwon JS, Tinker A, Pansegrau G, et al. Prophylactic salpingectomy and delayed oophorectomy as an alternative for BRCA mutation carriers. Obstet Gynecol 2013;121:14–24.
71. American College of Obstetricians and Gynecologists. ACOG committee opinion. Breast-ovarian cancer screening. Number 176, October 1996. Committee on Genetics. The American College of Obstetricians and Gynecologists. Int J Gynaecol Obstet 1997;56:82–83.
72. Hornreich G, Beller U, Lavie O. Is uterine serous papillary carcinoma a BRCA1 related disease? Case report and review of the literature. Gynecol Oncol 1999;75(2):300–304.
73. Levine D, Lin P, Barakat R. Risk of endometrial carcinoma associated with BRCA mutation. Gynecol Oncol 2001;80(3):395–398.
74. Goshen R, Chu W, Elit L. Is uterine papillary serous adenocarcinoma a manifestation of the hereditary breast-ovarian cancer syndrome? Gynecol Oncol 2000;79(3):477–481.
75. Boyd J. The breast, ovarian, and other cancer genes. Gynecol Oncol 2001;80(3):337–340.
76. Campfield Bonadies D, Moyer A, Matloff ET. What I wish I'd known before surgery: BRCA carriers' perspectives after bilateral salpingo-oophorectomy. Fam Cancer 2011;10:79–85.
77. Rebbeck T, Lynch H, Neuhausen S, et al. Prophylactic oophorectomy in carriers of BRCA1 or BRCA2 mutations. N Engl J Med 2002;346:1616–1622.
78. Kauff N, Satagopan J, Robson M, et al. Risk-reducing salpingo-oophorectomy in women with a BRCA1 or BRCA2 mutation. N Engl J Med 2002;346:1609–1615.
79. Rebbeck T, Friebel T, Wagner T, et al. Effect of short-term hormone replacement therapy on breast cancer risk reduction after bilateral prophylactic oophorectomy in BRCA1 and BRCA2 mutation carriers: the PROSE study group. J Clin Oncol 2005;23:7804–7810.
80. Gronwald J, Tung N, Foulkes W, et al. Tamoxifen and contralateral breast cancer in BRCA1 and BRCA2 carriers: an update. Int J Cancer 2006;118:2281–2284.
81. Fong PC, Boss DS, Yap TA, et al. Inhibition of Poly (ADPRibose) Polymerase in Tumors from BRCA Mutation Carriers. N Engl J Med 2009;361:1–12.
82. Inglhart JD, Silver DP. Synthetic lethality – a new direction in cancer-drug development. N Engl J Med 2009;361:1–3.
83. Kash K, Holland J, Halper M, et al. Psychological distress and surveillance behaviors of women with a family history of breast cancer. J Natl Cancer Inst 1992;84:24–30.
84. Lerman C, Hughes C, Lemon S. What you don't know can hurt you: adverse psychologic effects in members of BRCA1-linked and BRCA2-linked families who decline genetic testing. J Clin Oncol 1998;16:1650–1654.
85. Croyle R, Smith K, Botkin J. Psychological responses to BRCA1 mutation testing: preliminary findings. Health Psychol 1997;16:63–72.
86. Hamilton JG, Lobel M, Moyer A. Emotional distress following genetic testing for hereditary breast and ovarian cancer: a meta-analytic review. Health Psychol 2009;28:510–518.
87. Clayton E. Removing the shadow of the law from the debate about genetic testing of children. Am J Med Genet 1995;57:630–634.
88. ASHG/ACMG. Points to consider: ethical, legal, and psychosocial implications of genetic testing in children and adolescents. American Society of Human Genetics Board of Directors, American College of Medical Genetics Board of Directors. Am J Hum Genet 1995;57:1233–1241.
89. Ledger G, Khosia S, Lindor N, et al. Genetic testing in the diagnosis and management of multiple endocrine neoplasia type II. Ann Intern Med 1995;122:118–124.

90. Rhodes M, Bradburn D. Overview of screening and management of familial adenomatous polyposis. *Br J Surg* 1992;33:125–123.
91. Howard HC, Avard D, Borry P. Are the kids really all right? Direct-to-consumer genetic testing in children: are company policies clashing with professional norms? *Eur J Hum Genet* 2011;19:1122–1126.
92. Tsoucalas C. Legal aspects of cancer genetics - screening, counseling, and registers. In: Lynch H, Kullander S, eds. *Cancer Genetics in Women*. Vol I. Boca Raton, FL: CRC Press, Inc.; 1987:9.
93. American Society of Human Genetics. ASHG Statement: professional disclosure of familial genetic information. *Am J Hum Genet* 1998;62:474–483.
94. Bluman L, Rimer B, Berry D. Attitudes, knowledge, and risk perceptions of women with breast and/or ovarian cancer considering testing for BRCA1 and BRCA2. *J Clin Oncol* 1999; 17:1040–1046.
95. Matloff E, Shappell H, Brierley K, et al. What would you do? Specialists' perspectives on cancer genetic testing, prophylactic surgery and insurance discrimination. *J Clin Oncol* 2000;18:2484–2492.
96. Hall MA, Rich SS. Patients' fear of genetic discrimination by health insurers: the impact of legal protections *Genet Med* 2000:2:214–221.
97. Leib JR, Hoodfar E, Larsen Haidle J, Nagy R. The new genetic privacy law. *Community Oncol* 2008;5:351–354.
98. Hudson KL, Holohan JD, Collins FS. Keeping pace with the times — the Genetic Information Nondiscrimination Act of 2008. *N Engl J Med* 2008;358:2661–2663.
99. The Genetic Information Nondiscrimination Act of 2008 (H.R. 493). Library of Congress Web site. http://beta.congress.gov/bill/110th-congress/house-bill/493. Accessed June 2, 2014.
100. The Health Care and Education Affordability Reconciliation Act of 2010 (H.R. 4872). Library of Congress Web site. http://beta.congress.gov/bill/111th-congress/house-bill/4872: Accessed June 2, 2014.
101. Manley S, Pennell R, Frank T. Insurance coverage of BRCA1 and BRCA2 sequence analysis. *J Genet Couns* 1998;7:A462.
102. Grann V, Whang W, Jabcobson J, et al. Benefits and costs of screening Ashkenazi Jewish women for BRCA1 and BRCA2. *J Clin Oncol* 1999;17: 494–500.
103. Offit K, Kohut K, Clagett B, et al. Cancer genetic testing and assisted reproduction. *J Clin Oncol* 2006;24:4775–4782.
104. Offit K, Levran O, Mullaney B, et al. Shared genetic susceptibility to breast cancer, brain tumors, and Fanconi anemia. *J Natl Cancer Inst* 2003;95(20): 1548–1551.
105. Greendale K, Pyeritz RE. Empowering primary care health professionals in medical genetics: How soon? How fast? How far? *Am J Med Genet* 2001;106:223–232.
106. Wilkins-Haug L, Hill LD, Power ML, et al. Gynecologists' training, knowledge, and experiences in genetics: a survey. *Obstet Gynecol* 2000;95:421–424.
107. Wood ME, Stockdale A, Flynn BS. Interviews with primary care physicians regarding taking and interpreting the cancer family history. *Fam Pract* 2008; 25:334–340.
108. Bellcross CA, Kolor K, Goddard K, et al. Awareness and utilization of BRCA1/2 testing among U.S. primary care physicians. *Am J Prev Med* 2011;40:61–66.
109. Pollack A. F.D.A. Orders genetic testing firm to stop selling DNA analysis service. *New York Times*. November 25, 2013. http://www.nytimes.com/2013/11/26/business/fda-demands-a-halt-to-a-dna-test-kits-marketing.html?_r=0

PART V

Lymphomas and Leukemias

Section 1 Leukemias and Lymphomas in Children

36 Leukemias and Lymphomas of Childhood

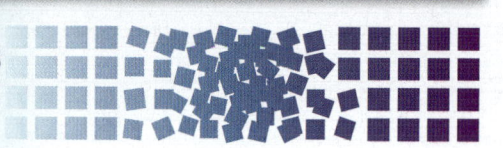

Karen R. Rabin, Judith F. Margolin, Kala Y. Kamdar, and David G. Poplack

INTRODUCTION

The cure rates seen in pediatric oncology are some of the best in modern oncology. These are largely related to the remarkable progress in the treatment of leukemias and lymphomas, where cure rates have improved from less than 10% to 80% to 95%.[1-4] Cure rates for pediatric myeloid leukemia are lower, in the 60% to 70% range.[5,6] The improvement in outcomes for all of pediatric cancer are the result of the successful implementation of cooperative group clinical trials at the national and even international level.[7] Currently, more than two-thirds of children with cancer in the United States are treated in clinical trials.[7] Although there are many similarities in treating children and adults with these diseases, there are also differences that pertain to development and growth, drug metabolism, and psychosocial issues.

LEUKEMIAS

Incidence, Histology, and General Outcomes

Acute lymphoblastic leukemia (ALL), the most common malignancy of childhood, accounts for 75% of leukemias and is curable in 80% to 95% of cases.[8] Figure 36.1 demonstrates the improvement in survival in pediatric ALL on successive cooperative group trials from 1968 to 2005.[1] Although there are variations with age, sex, and ethnicity, the majority of ALL cases have pre–B immunophenotype and FAB L1 histology (80% of cases); 20% are of T-cell origin. The peak incidence of pediatric ALL is between ages 2 and 5 years. ALL is slightly more common in American Caucasians than in African Americans, and there is a slightly increased incidence in male patients.[9] Approximately 5,000 children are diagnosed with ALL each year in the United States, with an incidence of 29.2 per million.[9] The Surveillance, Epidemiology, and End Results (SEER) program data show that the incidence of ALL has been climbing slowly. Controversy exists concerning whether and how incidence and outcomes differ between racial and ethnic groups. Studies from the 1990s suggest that Caucasians have slightly higher survival rates than those of African ancestry and Hispanics, although this is confounded in part by the fact that those of African ancestry and Hispanics more often develop high-risk forms of ALL.[10-12] Racial and ethnic disparities in access to care and adherence to treatment may also have an adverse impact on survival.[13,14]

Acute myeloid leukemia (AML) accounts for approximately 15% to 20% of childhood leukemias, chronic myelogenous leukemia (CML) accounts for 3% to 4%, and juvenile myelomonocytic leukemia (JMML) and other rarer histologies account for less than 1%. The incidence of AML is currently estimated to be 5 to 7 cases per million in the United States.[15] Myelodysplastic syndrome (MDS) is a relatively rare diagnosis in childhood, generally progresses to AML, and is treated with similar regimens (including bone marrow transplant) as AML.[16] AML incidence is slightly higher in African Americans and Hispanics in the United States, and survival is slightly lower.[17,18]

Because of intrinsic differences in drug sensitivity between ALL and AML cells, progress in treating AML has been less dramatic than that of ALL. Nevertheless, current cure rates in AML have risen to approximately 45% to 65% with the advent of more intensive conventional chemotherapy and bone marrow transplant (BMT) (Fig. 36.2).[19,20]

Etiology

Environmental Factors

There is extensive literature and a continued interest in exploring possible relationships between infectious or environmental exposures and increased risk of childhood leukemia. However, most studies show weak or no correlation of these factors with the incidence of leukemia.[21-23] Electromagnetic fields have not been found to be significant in pediatric malignancies.[24-26] There is an emerging body of evidence from population-based studies of polymorphisms of drug-metabolizing genes, such as *NQO1* and *GST* polymorphisms, that may be associated with an increase or decrease in an individual's risk for developing leukemia based on exposures to particular environmental toxins like benzene and other organic solvents, quinine-containing substances, and flavonoids.[27]

Genetics

There is significant evidence that genetic factors play a role in the etiology of pediatric leukemia. Within the leukemic blasts themselves, there are characteristic cytogenetic changes (Table 36.1), many of which have prognostic significance (see later discussion). Key genetic changes found in childhood leukemia (especially in younger patients) may occur in utero or very early in life.[28,29] Evidence includes the detection of cells bearing these changes in neonatal blood spots[30] and transmission of leukemia by twin–twin transfusion.[31] The *delayed infection* hypothesis holds that children in developed countries are spared the frequent early infections that are necessary for normal development of the immune system. An infection occurring at a later time is then hypothesized to elicit a pathologic, myelosuppressive response, providing a selective growth advantage to the pre-leukemic clone, leading to development of overt leukemia.[32]

In most cases, leukemia appears to result from a complex interplay between environmental and genetic factors. Recently, genome-wide association studies have identified several constitutional genetic variations with moderate but statistically significant effects on the relative risk of ALL.[33-36] Collectively, variants in *IKZF1*, *ARID5B*, *CEBPE*, and *CDKN2A* may account for up to 80% of the attributable risk of developing ALL in Europeans.[35] *ARID5B* and *GATA3* polymorphisms have been identified as associated with both ALL susceptibility and relapse hazard, and may contribute to racial disparities in outcome, because high-risk alleles occurred more frequently in subjects with a greater degree of Native American ancestry.[33]

In addition to somatic and germ-line genetic changes associated with leukemia, there are well-described cases of familial

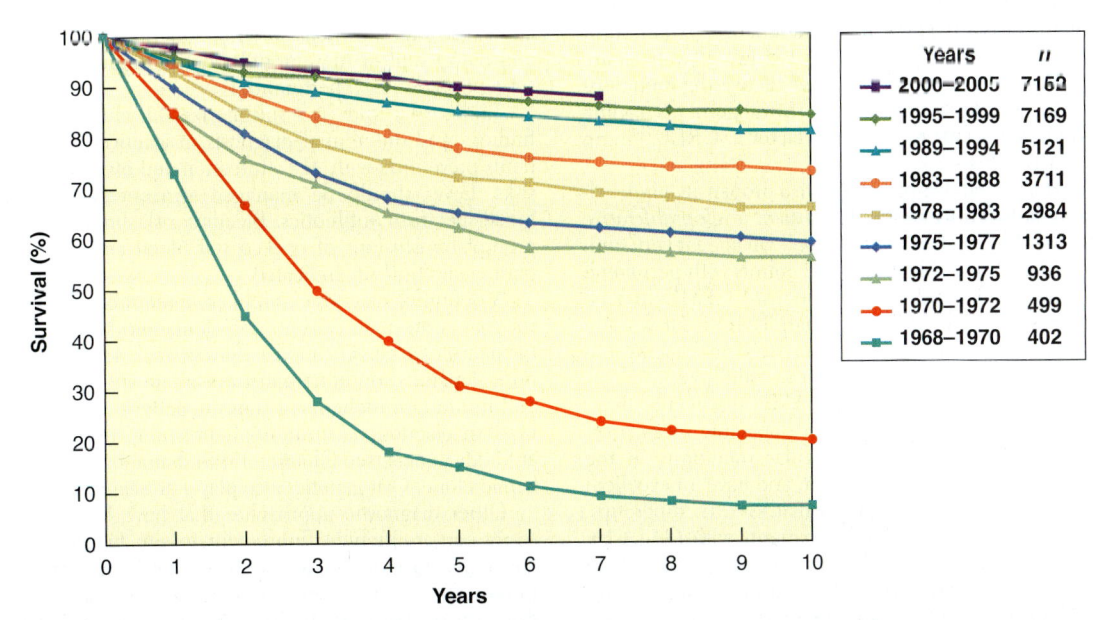

Figure 36.1 Improvement in survival of children with acute lymphoblastic leukemia. Overall survival probability by treatment era for 29,287 children with ALL who enrolled in trials from 1968 to 2005 conducted by the Children's Oncology Group (COG), the Pediatric Oncology Group (POG), and the Children's Cancer Group (CCG). The 2000 to 2005 curve includes CCG, POG, and COG. The 1995 to 1999 curve includes CCG and POG. All other curves are CCG. (Adapted from Hunger SP, Lu X, Devidas M, et al. Improved survival for children and adolescents with acute lymphoblastic leukemia between 1990 and 2005: a report from the children's oncology group. *J Clin Oncol* 2012;30:1663–1669.)

leukemia, including recently described mutations in the hematopoietic transcription factor PAX5,[38] as well as strong associations between leukemia risk and immunodeficiency and several somatic genetic disorders (e.g., Down syndrome [DS], Bloom syndrome, ataxia telangiectasia, Shwachman-Diamond syndrome, Noonan syndrome, neurofibromatosis).[8] Recently, a new association has been described between Li-Fraumeni syndrome, a well-known cancer predisposition syndrome, and hypodiploid ALL.[39]

Patients with DS have a 10- to 20-fold increased risk of developing leukemia.[40] The occurrence of leukemia in DS patients appears to be unrelated to the other congenital abnormalities and

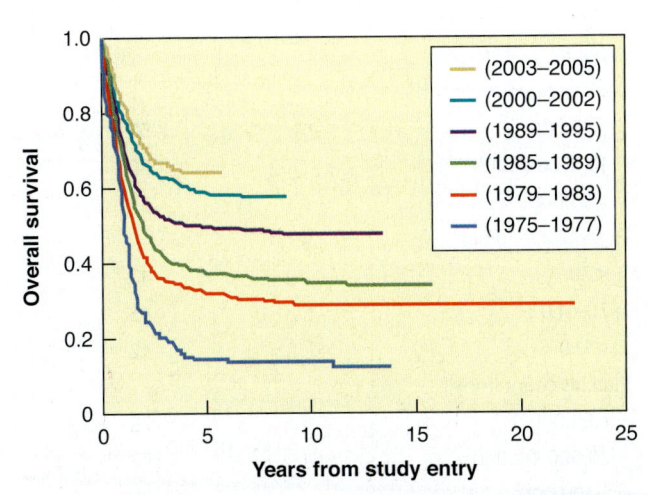

Figure 36.2 Improvement in survival of children with acute myeloid leukemia. Incremental improvements in overall survival in Children's Oncology Group and legacy trials in de novo childhood AML during the years indicated. (From Gamis AS, Alonzo TA, Perentesis JP, et al. Children's Oncology Group's 2013 blueprint for research: acute myeloid leukemia. *Pediatr Blood Cancer* 2013;60:964–971.)

TABLE 36.1 Acute Leukemia: Favorable and Unfavorable Prognostic Factors

Acute Lymphoblastic Leukemia

Favorable	Unfavorable
■ Age, 1–9 years	■ Age, <1 or ≥10 years
■ White blood cell count <50,000/mcL	■ White blood cell count ≥50,000/mcL
■ High hyperdiploidy (DNA index >1.16; and especially trisomies of chromosomes 4 and 10)	■ Hypodiploidy (DNA index <0.81 or <44 chromosomes)
■ Chromosomal translocation t(12;21) or ETV6-RUNX1	■ Chromosomal alterations ■ t(9;22) or BCR-ABL1 ■ MLL gene rearrangement ■ iAMP21 (intrachromosomal amplification of chromosome 21)
■ CNS-1	■ IKZF1 gene deletion or mutation
■ Rapid response to induction chemotherapy	■ Ph-like gene expression profile
	■ Extramedullary disease
	■ Slow response to induction chemotherapy

Acute Myeloid Leukemia

Favorable	Unfavorable
■ Core binding factor transcription complex, t(8;21) or inv(16)	■ Monosomy 5, 5q deletion
	■ Monosomy 7
■ Acute promyelocytic leukemia t(15;17)	■ FLT3 internal tandem duplication
■ Down syndrome	■ Secondary AML/myelodysplastic syndrome
■ Rapid response to induction chemotherapy	■ Slow response to induction chemotherapy

CNS, central nervous system.

medical problems of DS.[41] The cytogenetic changes common in ALL occur less frequently in DS-ALL,[42–45] but two alterations are markedly enriched: (1) Janus kinase 2 (*JAK2*) activating mutations in approximately 20% of DS-ALL, and (2) rearrangements leading to overexpression of cytokine receptor-like factor 2 (*CRLF2*) in up to 50% of DS-ALL.[46–48]

In the neonatal period, DS patients have a propensity for developing a nonneoplastic entity known as *transient myeloproliferative disease* (TMD) of DS, which at presentation, can appear very similar to AML (i.e., very high white blood cell counts with peripheral myeloblasts), but usually resolves spontaneously.[49] TMD may be difficult to distinguish from AML. Although TMD itself is not a form of malignancy or leukemia, approximately 30% of the DS patients with TMD will develop AML later in childhood.[49]

When patients with DS do develop AML (especially those younger than age 2 years), they tend to develop acute megakaryoblastic leukemia (AMKL), display particular mutations in the *GATA-1* hematopoietic transcription factor, and have an excellent prognosis compared to other adult and pediatric AML subgroups. The disease-free survival (DFS) for DS patients with *GATA-1*+ AMKL is over 90%, with regimens significantly less intensive than those required for other AML cases.[50] The reasons behind the increased risk of leukemia in DS remain unknown.

Clonal Nature of Lymphoid Cancers

Lymphoid malignancies appear to have derived from an original abnormal progenitor that lost the ability to fully differentiate and formed a *clone* of leukemic blast cells. ALL blasts are characterized by early cytoplasmic and surface lymphoid antigens (detectable by flow cytometry) as well as incomplete immunoglobulin (Ig) and T cell receptor (TCR) gene rearrangements, suggesting they arise from a precursor T- or B-lymphoid progenitor. AML may arise from a multipotent or committed myeloid progenitor. Persistence of subclinical amounts of leukemia during or after therapy is called minimal residual disease (MRD).[51] MRD may be detected by flow cytometry or polymerase chain reaction (PCR)-based detection of Ig/TCR rearrangements or chromosomal translocations.[52] Use of high-throughput sequencing technologies for MRD detection is being undertaken on a research basis and may hold promise as a future clinical test with even higher sensitivity and precision.[53]

Diagnosis

The presenting signs and symptoms of a child with leukemia reflect the impact of bone marrow infiltration, the extent of extramedullary disease spread, and problems arising from changes in blood viscosity and chemistry related to the size, number, and breakdown products of leukemic blasts (tumor lysis).[12] Leukostasis from high white blood cell (WBC) counts may cause signs and symptoms ranging from mild respiratory symptoms and pulmonary infiltrates, to stroke, cranial or peripheral neuropathies, hematuria, renal failure, and ocular findings.[8] AML blasts are larger, less flexible, and contain granules that can cause inflammation and clotting. Thus, AML has a higher risk of serious systemic problems then ALL for a given high WBC (e.g., >100,000/mm³). Gingival infiltration and orbital and periorbital soft tissue masses (chloromas) are often seen in AML.[54] AML FAB subtypes 4 and 5 have a tendency to present with chloromas.

Central nervous system (CNS) involvement is more common in ALL but is also possible with AML.[55,56] CNS involvement is most often meningeal involvement, but may manifest as cranial nerve involvement, and occasionally, frank leukemic infiltrates in the parenchyma of the brain. CNS involvement may be asymptomatic or manifest as cranial nerve palsies, seizures, or focal neurologic findings. Testicular involvement generally manifests as a painless, palpable mass. Hepatosplenomegaly is common in both ALL and AML, and may compromise respiration in small children. Lymphomatous involvement of nodes or extranodal tissue can cause superior mediastinal or superior vena cava syndromes, and bowel wall or mesenteric node infiltrations can cause intussusception or bowel perforation.

Tables 36.2 and 36.3 summarize the clinical and laboratory findings and differential diagnosis, respectively, for pediatric patients presenting with ALL. Infection and bleeding are significant risks. Fever should be managed aggressively with intravenous broad-spectrum antibiotics. Bleeding risk should be addressed by prompt transfusions of packed red blood cells, platelets, and/or plasma, as clinically indicated.

A definitive diagnosis of leukemia requires that the bone marrow has more than 20% to 25% leukemic blasts (depending on the pathologic classification system used).[57] Traditionally, the diagnosis depended on bone marrow aspirate and biopsy morphology and immunohistochemical staining patterns. The cornerstone of modern diagnosis is immunophenotyping, using flow cytometry antibody panels (see Chapter 43) to define the lineage of the leukemic clone. Cytogenetics also play a critical role.

Other diagnostic approaches that have become standard in many centers include fluorescent in situ hybridization (FISH), and PCR (to identify specific fusion proteins arising from chromosomal rearrangements). Finally, several techniques are used primarily on a research basis, such as RNA expression arrays, DNA copy number and single-nucleotide polymorphism (SNP) arrays, and whole-genome and whole-exome sequencing.[58–61] These techniques will be used increasingly for clinical decision making as well, such as to identify cryptic, actionable mutations[62] or to predict susceptibility to targeted therapy.[63,64]

TABLE 36.2

Clinical and Laboratory Features at Diagnosis in Children with Acute Lymphoblastic Leukemia

Clinical and Laboratory Features	Percentage of Patients
Symptoms and Physical Findings	
Fever	61
Bleeding (e.g., petechiae or purpura)	48
Bone pain	23
Lymphadenopathy	50
Splenomegaly	63
Hepatosplenomegaly	68
Laboratory Features	
Leukocyte count (mm³)	
<10,000	53
10,000–49,000	30
>50,000	17
Hemoglobin (g/dL)	
<7.0	43
7.0–11.0	45
>11.0	12
Platelet count (mm³)	
<20,000	28
20,000–99,000	47
≥100,000	25
Lymphoblast morphology	
L1	84
L2	15
L3	1

TABLE 36.3
Differential Diagnosis in Childhood Acute Lymphoblastic Leukemia

- Nonmalignant conditions
  - Juvenile rheumatoid arthritis
  - Infectious mononucleosis
  - Idiopathic thrombocytopenic purpura
  - Pertussis; parapertussis
  - Aplastic anemia
  - Acute infectious lymphocytosis
- Malignancies
  - Neuroblastoma
  - Retinoblastoma
  - Rhabdomyosarcoma
- Unusual presentations
  - Hypereosinophilic syndrome

TABLE 36.4
Definitions of Central Nervous System Disease Status at Diagnosis of Acute Lymphoblastic Leukemia Based on Cerebrospinal Fluid Findings[65]

Status	Cerebrospinal Fluid Findings
CNS-1	No lymphoblasts
CNS-2	<5 WBCs/mcL with definable blasts on cytocentrifuge examination
CNS-3	≥5 WBCs/mcL with blast cells (or cranial nerve palsy)

Management

Prognostic Factors in Management of Pediatric Acute Lymphoblastic Leukemia

As outcomes with modern therapy in pediatric ALL have improved, many factors previously shown to be important for predicting a prognosis have lost statistical significance. Five factors have retained prognostic significance and constitute the basis on which patients are stratified in most treatment protocols. These factors are (1) age at presentation, (2) WBC at presentation, (3) specific cytogenetic abnormalities, (4) presence or absence of CNS involvement (Table 36.4), and (5) rapidity of initial response to chemotherapy.[8] The 1996 National Cancer Institute (NCI) consensus criteria standardized definitions of age, initial WBC, and CNS involvement to facilitate a comparison of clinical trial results between groups.[65] Cooperative groups differ in incorporation of cytogenetics and response to therapy. General principles of modern ALL protocols include treatment of low-risk disease with less-intensive chemotherapy to minimize toxicity while maintaining excellent overall survival (OS) (90% to 95%), whereas high-risk disease (OS, 40% to 85%) is treated with more intensive therapy.[8]

The age-determined risk groups are less than 1 year (infant ALL), 1.0 to 9.99 years (standard risk ALL), and ≥10 years (high-risk ALL). Infants constitute a very high-risk group. MLL (11q23) rearrangements are frequent, especially t(4;11)(q21;q23), and are associated with hyperleukocytosis, extramedullary disease, and common acute lymphoblastic leukemia antigen (CALLA) (CD10) negativity.[66,67] Cure rates on current infant protocols have improved modestly to approximately 50%.[68,69] Results are poorest in infants under 3 months of age with MLL rearrangement. Unlike for some other high-risk ALL subgroups, current evidence does not suggest a benefit of stem cell transplant.[69]

Adolescents and young adults have also traditionally demonstrated lower cure rates, although survival has improved significantly with early intensive postinduction therapy.[17,70] In B-lineage ALL, presenting with a WBC count more than 50,000/mcL, and particularly over 100,000/mcL, is associated with a high risk of relapse.

Blast cell cytogenetics and ploidy have a significant prognostic impact in ALL (Fig. 36.3). High hyperdiploidy (≥50 chromosomes or DNA index >1.16) is associated with good prognosis, particularly with trisomies of chromosomes 4 and 10.[71-73] Hypodiploidy (<45 chromosomes) and especially haploidy

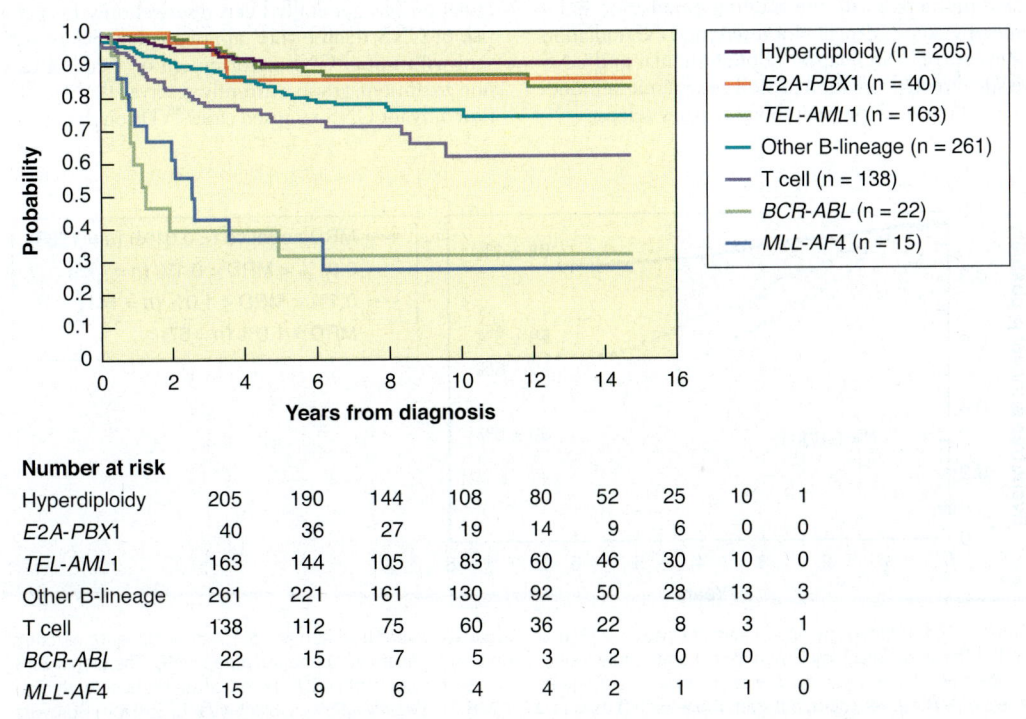

Figure 36.3 Kaplan-Meier analysis of event-free survival according to biologic subtype of leukemia. (From Pui CH, Robison LL, Look AT. Acute lymphoblastic leukaemia. *Lancet* 2008;371:1030–1043.)

Number at risk								
Hyperdiploidy	205	190	144	108	80	52	25	10	1
E2A-PBX1	40	36	27	19	14	9	6	0	0
TEL-AML1	163	144	105	83	60	46	30	10	0
Other B-lineage	261	221	161	130	92	50	28	13	3
T cell	138	112	75	60	36	22	8	3	1
BCR-ABL	22	15	7	5	3	2	0	0	0
MLL-AF4	15	9	6	4	4	2	1	1	0

Curves shown:
- Hyperdiploidy (n = 205)
- E2A-PBX1 (n = 40)
- TEL-AML1 (n = 163)
- Other B-lineage (n = 261)
- T cell (n = 138)
- BCR-ABL (n = 22)
- MLL-AF4 (n = 15)

(23 chromosomes) are associated with a poor prognosis.[72,74] Two other recently identified unfavorable abnormalities are *IKZF1* alterations[75] and intrachromosomal amplification of chromosome 21 (iAMP21).[76] *CRLF2* overexpression has been found to have an independent adverse prognostic impact in some studies, but not others.[77,78]

The most common translocation in pediatric ALL is t(12;21)(p12;q22), forming the *ETV6-RUNX1* (also known as *TEL-AML1*) fusion. This cryptic translocation occurs in 25% of US pediatric ALL cases, less frequently in other geographic and ethnically defined populations, and is associated with a favorable prognosis.[79,80] The Philadelphia chromosome (Ph+) refers to the t(9;22)(9q34;q11) translocation, forming the *BCR-ABL1* fusion. Ph+ ALL is less prevalent in children than adults and was historically associated with a dismal prognosis. Treatment of Ph+ ALL and CML were revolutionized by imatinib mesylate, a selective tyrosine kinase inhibitor active against the *BCR-ABL1* fusion. The addition of imatinib to conventional chemotherapy has improved survival from approximately 30% to 40% to 80%, and hematopoietic stem cell transplant (HSCT) in first remission is no longer considered as the standard of care.[81–83] Ongoing studies are investigating the efficacy of later generation tyrosine kinase inhibitors such as dasatinib.[84]

Numerous translocations occur in T-lineage ALL, but they are not generally associated with a prognosis. Activating *NOTCH1* mutations occur in over 50% of T-ALL cases, and are associated with a favorable prognosis.[85,86] Because mutated *NOTCH1* activity depends on γ-secretase activity, γ-secretase inhibitors are being investigated as a novel therapeutic approach. Early T-cell precursor (ETP) is a very unfavorable prognostic subgroup identified based on a distinctive immunophenotype, constituting approximately 10% of T-lineage ALL, which bears a gene expression signature and mutational profile similar to myeloid leukemia.[61,87]

CNS and testicular involvement are unfavorable prognostic signs, for which therapy is intensified.[56] The CNS is considered a sanctuary site because many systemic treatments do not adequately penetrate the blood–brain barrier, so CNS preventive therapy is required in all patients to prevent eventual CNS relapse. CNS prophylaxis is usually achieved through systemic and intrathecal chemotherapy. Although CNS involvement at diagnosis has generally been treated in the past with the addition of radiation to intensive chemotherapy, some advocate for reserving CNS radiation for use only in the case of CNS relapse.[88] Both testicular and CNS relapses require site-directed radiation as well as systemic reinduction due to increased risk of subsequent bone marrow relapse.[12,89]

All modern pediatric ALL treatment protocols use the prognostic factors outlined here, in varying ways, to stratify patients into different risk groups that receive treatment of different intensity. The first phase of treatment (*induction*) lasts 4 to 6 weeks and includes a glucocorticoid, vincristine (VCR), asparaginase, and for high-risk patients, an anthracycline (usually daunomycin).[12] The Berlin-Frankfurt-Munster group begins induction with a *steroid window*, and the degree of cytoreduction during this window is used in risk assessments.[90] Some groups intensify induction with additional medications. Rapid response to induction is an important prognostic variable (Fig. 36.4).[8,73] Induction failure (≥25% marrow blasts at the end of induction) is rare (2% to 5% of cases) and generally associated with a poor prognosis, although a recent large retrospective analysis reported an unexpected heterogeneity in survival, ranging from 10% to 70%, depending on age, cytogenetics, and B- versus T-lineage disease.[91]

Induction is usually followed by a *consolidation phase* to reinforce the bone marrow remission and to administer CNS prophylaxis. Subsequent intensive phases may be termed *intensification*, *delayed intensification*, or *reinduction/reconsolidation*, with the intensity depending on the risk group.[12,92,93] These intensive courses are generally delivered within the first 6 to 12 months of treatment, followed by a *maintenance* or *continuation* phase lasting 2 to 3 years, which consists of antimetabolite treatment (usually consisting of methotrexate weekly and 6-mercaptopurine daily), periodic intrathecal (IT) treatments, and periodic *pulses* of VCR and oral glucocorticoids with the frequency of these pulses varying by protocol and treatment group. To minimize and avoid treatment-related toxicities, strict supportive care guidelines are employed. Therapy-related mortality on frontline pediatric ALL protocols is generally under 2% to 3%. Overall treatment duration is usually between 2 and 3.5 years. On current Children's Oncology Group regimens, boys receive an additional year of maintenance, but many other cooperative study groups treat both genders for approximately 2 years.

CNS-directed therapy is usually present in all phases, but is most intensive during the first several months. CNS therapy uses intrathecal chemotherapy, high-dose systemic chemotherapy (principally, higher dose methotrexate or cytarabine), and/or cranial radiation.[56,94] Because it is often associated with neurocognitive deficits, endocrine, and growth abnormalities, cranial radiation has generally been reserved only for patients at highest risk of CNS relapse (i.e., approximately 5% of patients who present with initial CNS involvement or T-cell disease), but at least one treatment group currently reserves the use of cranial irradiation only for CNS-relapsed cases.[88] Through the years, the doses of

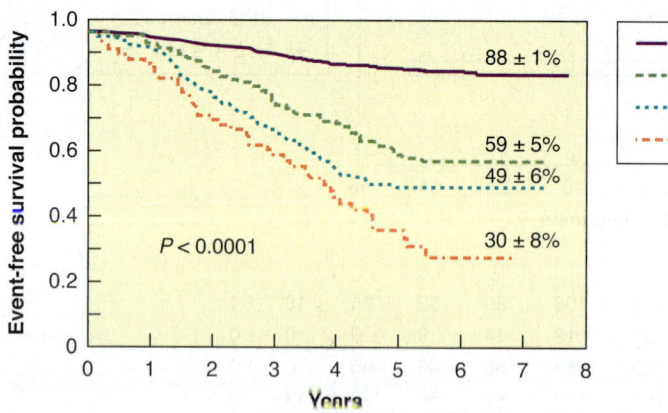

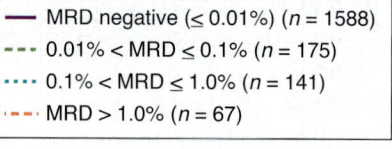

Figure 36.4 Effect of minimal residual disease (MRD) on prognosis. Event-free survival (EFS) of all patients enrolled on the Pediatric Oncology Group 9900 series therapeutic studies with satisfactory end-induction MRD. The 5 year EFS values plus or minus standard error are shown for patients with varying levels of MRD. The outcome of those with high levels of MRD is very poor, but even those with 0.01% to 0.1% MRD have only a 59% ± 5% 5-year EFS. (From Borowitz MJ, Devidas M, Hunger SP, et al. Clinical significance of minimal residual disease in childhood acute lymphoblastic leukemia and its relationship to other prognostic factors: a Children's Oncology Group study. *Blood* 2008;111:5477–5485.)

cranial radiation have decreased from the 24- to 36-Gy range that was used on early protocols to 18 Gy for treatment and 12 Gy on some CNS preventive therapy regimens.[56]

Therapy for relapsed ALL depends on the location of relapse (isolated extramedullary, bone marrow, or combined) and the duration of initial remission. Extramedullary relapse generally has a better prognosis than bone marrow relapse, but requires localized in addition to systemic chemotherapy.[12] For testicular relapse, local therapy involves orchiectomy, followed by irradiation of the remaining testicle and scrotal area.[12,95] Fertility will be compromised (so postpubertal males should be offered sperm banking), and hormonal supplements should be offered as needed. Prognosis after a testicular relapse remains quite good. For CNS relapse, local therapy involves intensified intrathecal therapy, varying regimens of high-dose systemic therapy, and the addition of cranial and/or craniospinal radiation.

All relapse types have a worse prognosis if they occur during therapy or within 6 months of completing therapy.[96] Interestingly, a recent study indicated that postrelapse survival does not differ according to the intensity of chemotherapy received prior to relapse.[97] Multiple medications and regimens are being tested for induction in relapsed and refractory leukemia. A common approach is to administer several intensive blocks of conventional chemotherapy agents, with or without a concomitant novel investigational agent.[98] Promising results have been recently obtained with clofarabine and clofarabine-containing regimens.[99–101] Blinatumomab, a CD19/CD3-bispecific T-cell engaging (BiTE) antibody, has shown promising response rates and prolonged survival in relapsed B-lineage ALL in adults, and is currently in a phase II international trial in pediatrics.[102,103] Promising recent results have been obtained using chimeric antigen receptor-modified T cells with specificity for CD19, termed CTL019 cells.[104] The most recent update on this trial reported that among 20 patients (including 16 pediatric) with treatment refractory CD19+ ALL, 14 patients (82%) achieved complete remission, with robust in vivo expansion of CTL019 cells, and 11 of 17 evaluable patients maintained an ongoing CR during median follow-up of 2.6 months.[105]

The decision between chemotherapy and HSCT for second complete remission has been controversial. HSCT is usually used for relapse within 6 months of the completion of initial treatment (CR1 <30 months), but the decision also depends on suitable donor availability, the difficulty (number and intensity of induction attempts needed to achieve CR2), and the overall health of the recipient.[106] Prior to HSCT, patients with relapsed ALL typically receive induction and consolidative chemotherapy, because the chances of success with HSCT are extremely low in the setting of continued active disease. Autologous BMT in ALL is no longer recommended.

Prognostic Factors and Management of Pediatric Acute Myeloid Leukemia

In contrast with ALL, there are fewer standard clinical or laboratory-based factors in AML that consistently relate to prognosis. Table 36.1 reviews prognostic factors in pediatric ALL and AML. Poor prognostic factors that predict lower remission rates and/or decreased event-free survival (EFS) include blast cytogenetics with monosomy 5 or 7, 5q deletion, FLT3/ITD, and secondary AML/MDS.[19,107–109] Adolescents and young adults have an increased risk of treatment-related mortality, but no significant difference in OS.[110] A swift response to induction chemotherapy (i.e., remission after one cycle of chemotherapy), favorable cytogenetics, and DS (with FAB M7) are predictive of better outcomes.[108] Favorable cytogenetics in AML include core binding factor alterations (the t[8;21] AML1/ETO fusion and inv[16]), and the t(15;17) PML/RARα fusion seen in acute promyelocytic leukemia (APL) (see Chapter 43). Two other recently identified favorable cytogenetic alterations (CCAAT) are mutations in NPM1[111] and CCAAT/enhancer-binding protein alpha (CEBP).[112] In addition to genetic alterations, MRD is being integrated into current AML studies as an important prognostic marker.[113] Although many findings in AML are similar between adults and children, important biologic and therapeutic differences are emerging. An example of this is that mutations of the KIT receptor tyrosine kinase have a similar frequency in pediatric core binding factor AML as those found in adult AML, but lack the poor prognosis seen in adults.[109]

There have been incremental improvements in AML outcomes over recent decades, with current overall survival in the 60% to 70% range (see Fig. 36.2). These improvements have come through increased intensity of therapy and improved supportive care.[114,115] The inherent drug resistance of AML cells poses challenges because the intensification of therapy required is associated with significant treatment-related toxicity, particularly infections.[19]

With the exception of DS patients with FAB M7 AML and patients with APL, most pediatric AML induction therapies include two cycles of ara-C and daunomycin, with or without thioguanine and/or etoposide. Studies have shown that the intensity of induction therapy is important for OS.[19] In the Children's Cancer Group 2891 protocol, intensively timed induction (starting the second cycle on day 14 regardless of count recovery) did not change the induction (CR1) rate, but it did have a profound effect on eventual cure rate.[116] Although fewer than 5% of pediatric AML patients present with CNS disease, as many as 20% will suffer an isolated CNS relapse.[55] Intrathecal chemotherapy (usually ara-C) has been found by several groups to effectively reduce the risk of CNS relapse.[19]

Conventional postinduction consolidative chemotherapy in pediatric AML usually involves two to three cycles of high-dose ara-C based combinations, to which anthracycline, etoposide, or ifosfamide/cyclophosphamide may be added. There is no proven benefit to maintenance chemotherapy, so conventional treatment is rarely more than four to eight cycles.[110,111]

Gemtuzumab ozogamicin (GO), a newer agent consisting of an antibody to CD33 coupled to calicheamicin (a toxic antitumor antibiotic), has shown some promise in relapsed AML and was recently tested in a randomized, prospective trial for frontline disease by the Children's Oncology Group.[118] GO was significantly associated with improved EFS, but not OS. Other adult and pediatric trials of GO in AML have yielded mixed results, and at present, it has been voluntarily withdrawn from the commercial market and its role in AML therapy remains to be determined. Two promising novel biologic agents, the proteasome inhibitor bortezomib[119] and the kinase inhibitor sorafenib (which inhibits FLT3)[120] are currently being tested for efficacy in combination with frontline conventional chemotherapy. The indications for HSCT in pediatric AML, preparative regimens, timing (CR1 or later), and type of donor are the focus of intensive ongoing controversy and research.[116,121,122]

Pediatric APL has among the highest cure rates in pediatric AML. These patients should receive all-*trans*-retinoic acid (ATRA), which directly binds to the t(15;17) translocation, which forms a fusion protein combining the promyelocytic leukemia (PML) gene with the retinoic acid receptor alpha (RARα) gene, which is causative for this form of AML.[123] They should also receive conventional chemotherapy during both induction and consolidation phases. Patients who respond to this therapy have an 80% to 85% survival rate and should not be subjected to HSCT.[124] Similar to adult therapies for APL (see Chapter 43), arsenic trioxide, found to be useful for salvage in patients who became resistant to ATRA, is currently being tested in upfront pediatric APL regimens (both alone and in combination with ATRA and conventional chemotherapy) in an effort to improve DFS in CR1.[125] Rapid initiation of therapy is particularly important in APL due to the risk of severe bleeding complications in untreated disease. Early deaths from bleeding are often not captured on clinical trials, but population-based studies indicate that they are a significant cause of mortality.[126] Despite the remarkable successes with ATRA and arsenic trioxide with and without conventional chemotherapy, there remain patients with APL with relapsed and refractory disease, and many of these can still be cured with HSCT.[127]

DS patients with AMKL (see earlier discussion) do well with lower dose ara-C regimens and standard timing of their induction cycles. Current results in DS AMKL are the best of any AML subgroup outside of APL, with 70% to 85% EFS, with patients under 2 years showing the best results, and thus not requiring intensive chemotherapy or HSCT.[128–130]

The prognosis for pediatric patients who relapse after either conventional or HSCT therapy for AML is poor. A second CR can be obtained using similar ara-C and anthracycline-containing regimens in 20% to 70% of patients, but the likelihood of obtaining a cure is approximately half the rate for de novo AML.[131] Clofarabine alone and in combination (see ALL relapse discussion) with other chemotherapeutic agents also shows some efficacy.[100,101] HSCT in early relapse or CR2 for AML patients who were previously transplanted in CR1 is a strategy that has had some success.[131–133] Other novel therapies, including FLT3 inhibitors and hypomethylating agents, are currently being studied.[134]

Rarer Forms of Leukemia in Children

Chronic leukemias, with the exception of CML, do not occur in children. Ph+ CML is rare in childhood (<1% to 2% of all pediatric leukemia cases).[135] When it does occur, it typically presents in adolescents and is in the chronic phase. Therapy is similar to that recommended in adults, with imatinib (along with hydroxyurea if the initial counts are high, and/or the patient presents with a high degree of hepatosplenomegaly) as the mainstay of induction and maintenance therapy. The use of alternative tyrosine kinase inhibitors such as dasatinib and nilotinib are being investigated in children as well as adults.[136] Because there is no clear end point for when or whether any of these tyrosine kinase inhibitors can be safely discontinued, many pediatric oncologists continue to consider hematopoietic stem cell transplantation in remission.

JMML, a myeloproliferative disorder unique to childhood, is characterized by extreme monocytosis, hepatosplenomegaly, thrombocytopenia, and increased fetal hemoglobin.[137] Bone marrow morphology is often consistent with myelodysplasia as well as myeloproliferation, and cytogenetics frequently reveals a monosomy 7 clone. Mutations in *PTN11*, *CBL*, and other *RAS* pathway genes have also been noted.[138,139] Although the clinical course can be indolent (requiring only intermittent blood product and antibiotic support), JMML patients often progress to frank marrow failure. Neither aggressive AML-type chemotherapy nor splenectomy has been shown to significantly prolong survival, so these approaches are starting to be reserved for those patients who are symptomatic. The most definitive therapy in JMML is an allogeneic BMT.[140] Overall DFS with BMT in JMML has been in the 40% to 55% range, with relapse the major reason for failure. Novel therapies targeting the rat sarcoma (*RAS*), rapidly accelerated fibrosarcoma (*RAF*), mitogen activated protein kinase (*MEK*), mammalian target of rapamycin (mTOR), signal transducer and activator of transcription 5 (*STAT5*), and other signaling pathways are currently under investigation.[137]

Mixed phenotype acute leukemia (MPAL) is a new designation established by the World Health Organization (WHO) 2008 classification, replacing the prior diagnosis of biphenotypic acute leukemia, which was based on the European Group for the Immunological Classification of Leukemias (EGIL) and the WHO 2001 classification.[141] MPALs constitute only approximately 0.5% to 1% of acute leukemias, with combined lineage differentiation that is most often B- and myeloid, followed by T- and myeloid, and rarely B- and T- or trilineage. The WHO classification recognizes two specific subgroups, characterized by a *BCR-ABL* rearrangement and *MLL* rearrangement, as well as a subgroup for the remainder of cases, which have other nonspecific chromosomal abnormalities. There are little systematic data about this rare form of leukemia, but outcomes are generally poor. Some data suggest that ALL-directed therapy may be more effective than AML-directed therapy. Allogeneic stem cell transplant is frequently employed.

LYMPHOMAS

Lymphomas constitute approximately 10% of cancer in children, and are the third most common pediatric malignancy (behind leukemias and brain tumors).[142] Two-thirds of lymphomas in children are a heterogeneous group of lymphomas categorized as non-Hodgkin lymphomas (NHL), and the remainder are Hodgkin lymphomas (HL). Table 36.5 compares the differences in presenting and staging features between pediatric NHL and HL. The histology, biology, and management of lymphoma differs in children compared to adults. For example, the indolent, low-grade lymphomas seen in adults are rarely seen in children. Additionally, radiation and certain types of chemotherapy are minimized when possible to reduce detrimental effects on growth and development and other late effects of therapy such as second malignancies.

Non-Hodgkin Lymphoma

The Revised European–American Classification of Lymphoid Neoplasms (REAL) classification, which has served as the basis for the WHO classification of hematopoietic and lymphoid tumors, categorizes lymphomas according to phenotype and differentiation.[143]

TABLE 36.5

Comparison of Hodgkin Lymphoma and Non-Hodgkin Lymphoma in Pediatric Patients

Feature	Hodgkin Lymphoma	Non-Hodgkin Lymphoma
Age	Mostly >10 y	Any age in children
Stage at diagnosis	Mostly localized	Commonly widespread
Constitutional symptoms	Alter prognosis	Do not affect prognosis
CNS involvement	Rare	Occurrence increases with AIDS
Mediastinal involvement	Most common with nodular sclerosing Hodgkin lymphoma	Most common with lymphoblastic lymphoma
Gastrointestinal involvement	Rare	Occurs
Abdominal nodal involvement	Can be small or large, mesenteric rare	Usually enlarged, mesenteric common
Bone involvement	Rare	Occurs
Marrow involvement	Rare	Common

Adapted from Rademaker, J. Hodgkin's and non-Hodgkin's lymphomas. *Radiol Clin North Am* 2007;45:69–83.

Pediatric NHLs appear in four major categories: (1) precursor T- and, less commonly, precursor B-lymphoblastic lymphoma (30% of pediatric NHLs), (2) Burkitt and Burkitt-like lymphoma (40% to 50%), (3) diffuse large B-cell lymphoma (15%), and (4) anaplastic large cell lymphoma (10%).[142] These subtypes are high-grade, acute diseases and, rarely, truly localized diseases. Major improvement in the survival of children with NHL has occurred during the past 20 years, correlating with the advent of systemic multiagent chemotherapy regimens, as opposed to a reliance on localized therapies such as surgery and radiation.

The Cotswold revision of the Ann Arbor NHL staging and classification system used in adult NHLs has mostly been replaced in pediatrics by the St. Jude's Research Hospital staging system outlined in Table 36.6, which incorporates common presentations of pediatric NHL including increased extranodal involvement, bone marrow and CNS involvement, and on contiguous spread of disease.[144] Surgical/pathologic staging is no longer carried out in either pediatric NHL or HL cases. Diagnosis generally relies on biopsy and radiologic scans, usually a combination of computed tomography (CT) and nuclear medicine scans and, occasionally, magnetic resonance imaging.[145] The current 5-year EFS rates for early low-stage disease are in the 90% to 95% range and from 70% to 90% for the higher stage presentations.[4,142]

Unlike ALL or HL, there is no sharp age peak for the occurrence of NHL in children. There is a marked imbalance in the male to female incidence, which approaches a 3:1 ratio.[142,146] With the exception of children with rare, inherited, or acquired immunodeficiency syndromes (e.g., Wiskott-Aldrich syndrome, common variable immune deficiency, ataxia telangiectasia, X-linked lymphoproliferative syndrome, HIV/AIDS, or exposure to immunosuppressive drugs after solid organ or bone marrow transplants), most children who develop NHL have a history of normal health and no known risk factors. The main exception to this concerns the possible etiologic role of the Epstein-Barr virus (EBV). EBV is strongly associated with lymphomas in HIV patients, lymphoproliferative diseases found in posttransplant patients, and endemic Burkitt lymphoma, and it is found in many cases of HL (see later discussion) in otherwise healthy children.[147,148]

Lymphoblastic lymphomas share many molecular, biologic, cytogenetic, and therapeutic characteristics with ALL, and are now treated with similar chemotherapy protocols.[12,146] The distinction between ALL and lymphoblastic lymphoma is somewhat arbitrary because those patients with more than 25% lymphoblasts in their bone marrow at diagnosis (despite the existence of a large lymphomatous mass elsewhere in the body) are designated as having ALL. Morphologically, the cells are indistinguishable, and the immunophenotypes generally overlap.[146,149] In contrast to ALL however, precursor T-lymphoblastic lymphoma is more common than precursor B-lymphoblastic lymphoma, with more than 75% of lymphoblastic lymphoma cases demonstrating precursor T-cell immunophenotype.

The typical presentation of children with lymphoblastic lymphoma is that of a patient with rapidly enlarging neck and mediastinal lymphadenopathy. Particular attention needs to be paid to hydration status, kidney function, and whether the kidneys are directly involved with the disease. CT and positron-emission tomography (PET) are helpful for assessing the degree of organ involvement, but care must be taken in requiring children with mediastinal masses to lie supine (which can compress both central blood vessels and airways) or undergo sedation (which causes vasodilation and decreased blood return to the heart).[150] A histologic diagnosis should be sought in the least invasive way possible. Prebiopsy steroids or *postage stamp irradiation* (use of a small radiation field to emergently relieve airway compression) can be done, but the steroids may jeopardize obtaining the histologic diagnosis or accurate staging. CNS status should be assessed prior to systemic chemotherapy, and prophylactic intrathecal chemotherapy should be administered early.[146] Prognostic factors include the level of bone marrow involvement at diagnosis and CNS involvement at diagnosis.

Primary therapy for lymphoblastic lymphoma (of either B- or T-cell histology) consists of multiagent chemotherapy with or without radiation. Stage I lymphoblastic cases do very well with short treatments (three to five cycles) of cyclophosphamide, doxorubicin, vincristine, and prednisone (CHOP regimen or similar), and a relatively short (24 weeks versus 2 to 3 years with ALL) maintenance phase of antimetabolite (6-mercaptopurine daily and weekly oral methotrexate).[142,146] Higher stage (stages II, III, and IV) lymphoblastic cases require more intensive regimens and a prolonged maintenance phase such as that used for ALL. The benefit of high-dose methotrexate and cranial radiation remain controversial in lymphoblastic lymphoma.[151-153] Nelarabine is a novel nucleoside analog with preferential cytotoxicity in T-lineage lymphoid malignancies that is being studied in current protocols.[154] Because activating NOTCH1 mutations are found in the majority of T-cell

TABLE 36.6

St. Jude Children's Research Hospital Staging System for Pediatric Non-Hodgkin Lymphoma

Stage	Description
I	A single tumor (extranodal) or single anatomic area (nodal), with the exclusion of mediastinum or abdomen
II	A single tumor (extranodal) with regional node involvement Two or more nodal areas on the same side of the diaphragm Two single (extranodal) tumors with or without regional node involvement on the same side of the diaphragm A primary gastrointestinal tract tumor, usually in the ileocecal area, with or without involvement of associated mesenteric nodes only[a]
III	Two single tumors (extranodal) on opposite sides of the diaphragm Two or more nodal areas above and below the diaphragm All the primary intrathoracic tumors (mediastinal, pleural, thymic) All extensive primary intra-abdominal disease[a] All paraspinal or epidural tumors, regardless of other tumor sites
IV	Any of the previous with initial central nervous system or bone marrow involvement[b]

[a] Stage II abdominal disease typically is limited to a segment (usually distal ileum) of the gut plus or minus the associated mesenteric nodes only, and the primary tumor can be completely removed grossly by segmental excision. Stage III abdominal disease typically exhibits spread to para-aortic and retroperitoneal areas by implants and plaques in mesentery or peritoneum, or by direct infiltration of structures adjacent to the primary tumor. Ascites may be present, and the complete resection of all gross tumor is not possible.
[b] If bone marrow involvement is present at diagnosis, the percentage of blasts or abnormal cells must be 25% or less to be classified as stage IV non-Hodgkin lymphoma. If there are more than 25% blasts, the patient is classified as having acute leukemia (either precursor B- or T-acute lymphoblastic leukemia or L3 acute lymphoblastic leukemia).

leukemias, gamma-secretase inhibitors that block Notch 1 signaling are another class of agents whose role in treatment regimens is being assessed.[155,156] Relapse in lymphoblastic lymphoma is, fortunately, an uncommon problem, but when it does occur it happens either during or shortly after completion of therapy. Relapse of low-stage disease can frequently be salvaged using the more intensive chemotherapy designed for high-stage disease.[157] Lymphoblastic lymphoma patients who relapse after higher stage treatment have a poor prognosis and are candidates for nelarabine, phase I agents and/or BMT if response is obtained to salvage therapy.[157] Radiation to areas of bulk disease and total-body irradiation are incorporated into the transplant regimens, but, in general, radiation does not have a role in primary treatment or reinduction at relapse.

Burkitt and Burkitt-like lymphoma are mature B-cell lymphomas. Endemic Burkitt lymphoma (usually presenting with localized head and neck masses—most frequently, the jaw) in Africa is quite common (100 cases per million children), and 95% are associated with EBV. Sporadic Burkitt lymphoma, as seen in the United States, typically presents with an abdominal mass, occurs in 1 to 2 cases per million children, and only 15% are associated with EBV.[158] The most common presentation in the United States is of a boy age 5 to 10 years, with a right lower quadrant mass and/or acute abdomen secondary to an ileocecal intussusception. If the tumor is limited to the distal ileum or cecum, it should be completely excised along with its associated mesentery, and the bowel repaired with an end-to-end anastomosis.[159] These children have low-stage disease, require less chemotherapy, and have an excellent outcome. More frequently, the abdominal involvement is much more diffuse.

Burkitt lymphoma cells have a mature B-cell immunophenotype (expressing cell surface immunoglobulin, usually IgM) and are characterized morphologically by homogeneous round-to-oval nuclei, multiple nucleoli, and intensely basophilic cytoplasm with large vacuolated areas containing fat. Burkitt-like lymphoma shares pathologic and molecular features with diffuse large B-cell lymphoma and responds to similar chemotherapy as Burkitt lymphoma. The majority of Burkitt lymphoma cases display the t(8;14) (q24;q32) translocation in which *c-myc* from chromosome 8 is translocated to the Ig heavy-chain locus on chromosome 14. In this translocation and in two less common variants, t(2;8) (p12;q24) and t(8;22) (q24;q11), the *c-myc* oncogene is overexpressed because of the influence of Ig regulatory regions (enhancers).[160]

The diagnosis of Burkitt lymphoma must be done very expeditiously as these tumors grow swiftly and patients are at high risk of intestinal obstruction (from intussusception) and metabolic problems related to tumor lysis syndrome. Tumor lysis often begins even before chemotherapy. Special attention must be paid to serum electrolyte balance (including calcium/phosphate balance), and vigorous intravenous hydration and alkalinization to improve uric acid excretion is essential. Allopurinol or recombinant urate oxidase, rasburicase, is used to block uric acid production. Occasionally, the lysis syndrome can be severe enough to cause acute renal failure, and dialysis must be used to maintain fluid and reestablish electrolyte balance.

Children with low-stage, African-endemic Burkitt lymphoma have been successfully treated with single or multiple doses of cyclophosphamide. Therapies as brief as 4 weeks have been successfully employed.[161] These strategies result in lower cure rates, but they make it feasible to treat large numbers of children with lower toxic death and complication rates in resource-poor settings.[162] Higher stage Burkitt lymphoma (stages 3 and 4) requires significantly more intensive chemotherapy, involving much higher doses of cyclophosphamide, and the addition of an anthracycline, high-dose ara-C, methotrexate, and VP-16 to the CHOP schemas. Many current high-stage Burkitt lymphoma protocols use hematopoietic growth factor support to enhance bone marrow recovery in order to allow intensive cycles to be given approximately every 3 weeks. These protocols are intensive, but they are usually of a short (6- to 8-month) duration. There have been some efforts to reduce chemotherapy and to add biologic agents like rituximab (anti-CD20 antibody) to reduce toxicity of treatment in patients who have HIV or other medical problems.[163,164] Currently, the efficacy of the addition of rituximab to advanced stage Burkitt lymphoma protocols is being investigated.[165] The cure rate for pediatric patients with higher stage (stage III and IV) Burkitt lymphoma is now 80% to 90%.[166] The management of relapsed Burkitt lymphoma is problematic. Relapses usually occur during therapy or shortly after the cessation of therapy. Low-stage patients can sometimes be effectively treated using a high-stage primary protocol. Higher stage relapsed patients may try a salvage therapy such as R-ICE (rituximab, ifosfamide, carboplatin, etoposide) or phase I therapies, and BMT should be considered if a response is achieved.[167]

The workup and staging of large cell lymphomas are similar to that described for other forms of NHL. Diffuse large B cell lymphoma (DLBCL) tends to present with large mediastinal masses, but bone, lymph node, and abdominal presentations are also seen. Bone marrow and CNS involvement are not common. Combination chemotherapy is effective against DLBCL, and radiation does not have a role in therapy for most cases. DLBCL and anaplastic large cell lymphoma (ALCL) used to be treated similarly as large cell lymphomas, the mature B-cell lymphomas (DLBCL and Burkitt lymphoma) are now grouped together on contemporary treatment protocols. However, it is not clear that DLBCL requires as much CNS-directed therapy as Burkitt lymphoma because CNS involvement is less common for DLBCL. Primary mediastinal B-cell lymphoma (PMBL) is a subtype of DLBCL that often presents with sclerosis and has a less favorable prognosis. PMBL shares some biologic features with Hodgkin lymphoma, and alternate treatment regimens are being investigated for PMBL based on differences in biology and prognosis.[168]

ALCL tends to present with involvement of lymph nodes and extranodal sites including the skin, the lung, other soft tissues, and bone. Bone marrow and CNS involvement are uncommon. The majority of ALCL cases have T-cell immunophenotype. ALCL is also known for cytogenetically presenting with the t(2;5) (p23;q35) translocation, which fuses nucleophosmin with a transmembrane tyrosine-specific protein kinase known as anaplastic lymphoma kinase. Three to five cycles of CHOP or APO (adriamycin, prednisone, Oncovin/VCR) have been used, and more recently, Associazione Italiana Ematologia Oncologia Pediatrica (AIEOP) ALCL-99 with EFS that ranges from 70% to 85%.[169] Targeted therapy with crizotinib, an inhibitor of the anaplastic lymphoma kinase (ALK), a tyrosine kinase, has produced promising responses in early studies in relapsed ALK-positive ALCL.[170] Another targeted therapy demonstrating promising activity against both ALCL and Hodgkin lymphoma is brentuximab vedotin, an anti-CD30 directed monoclonal antibody conjugated to a microtubule-disrupting agent.[171]

Hodgkin Lymphoma

The natural history and outcome of treatment in HL is similar in young children and adults, but treatment decisions (and regimens) are different in children based on the need for attention to late effects of therapy. Risk-adapted therapy seeks to maintain excellent cure rates of 80% to 90%, whereas limiting radiation and certain types of chemotherapy that may cause long-term organ damage, growth problems, infertility, and second malignancies.[3,172] HL is rare below the age of 5 years, with the majority of pediatric cases presenting in children older than 11 years. Young patients (<10 years) have a 3:1 male to female ratio. This imbalance returns to the approximately equal male to female ratio seen in adult disease as the age of presentation climbs. The age of HL incidence in industrialized countries is bimodal, with the first peak in adults 20 to 30 years of age and the second peak occurring much later in adulthood.[173]

The etiology of HL is unknown, but EBV is found in up to 40% of cases.[174] There are also familial and geographic clusters that suggest an inherited, environmental, or infectious contribution to etiology.[174] Most children (90%) present with painless adenopathy in the neck, and 60% have involvement of anterior mediastinum, paratracheal, or hilar lymph nodes. The Cotswold modification of the Ann Arbor Staging System (described in Chapter 39) is used for all ages. B symptoms (defined as in adults) include unexplained fever (more than 38°C [100.4°F]), drenching night sweats, and more than 10% weight loss. B symptoms are present in approximately 30% of newly diagnosed pediatric HL cases.[175] The process of clinical staging includes both site of involvement and the presence of B symptoms and is described in detail for adult patients in Chapter 38. There is no longer any role for staging laparotomy, because localized radiation is no longer used as a sole treatment modality in pediatric HL. Increasingly, PET scans are being used to assess staging and early response and to guide further treatment, as opposed to exclusive reliance on CT.[176]

The malignant cells in HL constitute a minority (estimated at 0.1% to 10%) of the cell population of the discernible tumor.[177] Inflammatory cells (histiocytes, plasma cells, lymphocytes, eosinophils, and neutrophils) make up the bulk of the tumor. The malignant cells are actually malignant lymphocytes with specific, characterized immunophenotypes. The WHO classifies four subtypes of classic HL: (1) nodular sclerosing, (2) mixed cellularity, (3) lymphocyte rich, and (4) lymphocyte depleted. Nodular lymphocyte-predominant HL (NLPHL) is another important subtype of HL.

The most common presenting histology in pediatric HL is nodular sclerosing type, which accounts for more than 50% of the cases (40% of the younger patients but 70% of the adolescents).[173] It is characterized by bands of fibrosis and a thickened lymph node capsule that are discernible even in a gross pathologic section. These nodes and masses tend to form scars that can lead to residual masses, which appear as opacified lesions on radiologic studies for years after a full clinical response. Mixed cellularity is responsible for approximately 30% of pediatric cases. It is commonly seen in children less than 10 years of age and is highly associated with EBV positivity. The lymphocyte depleted form of HL is quite rare, except in children with HIV. The lymphocyte-rich variant is quite rare in children (approximately 5% of the cases), has a high incidence of mediastinal masses and stage III disease, but has an older average age of presentation (32 years).[173]

With the exception of NLPHL, treatment for all of the various HL histologies is the same and is based on staging. Risk-adapted therapy in pediatric HL is composed of three to six cycles of combination chemotherapy followed by involved field radiation therapy (IFRT) for higher risk patients. The composition of the chemotherapy regimens has varied during the years, but combinations of vinca alkaloids, alkylating agents (cyclophosphamide commonly used now), steroids, anthracyclines, and bleomycin have been used. Current therapies for low-risk HL attempt to reduce exposure to alkylators, anthracyclines, and bleomycin and IFRT to reduce the risk of late effects.

Therapy for higher risk HL (higher stage at presentation or slow response to therapy) currently involves additional cycles of higher dose combination chemotherapy and IFRT, with EFS rates still in the 80% to 90% range when risk-adapted therapy is given.[3] Targeted therapy such as brentuximab vedotin, discussed previously, will be studied in frontline therapy regimens. Treatment for relapsed or refractory pediatric HL is beyond the scope of this chapter, but the medications (e.g., ifosfamide and vinorelbine) and approaches (e.g., BMT) are usually similar to those used in adults (see Chapter 38). Novel therapies under investigation include antibodies targeting CD30 (brentuximab vedotin), CD25, and other antigens; the proteasome inhibitor bortezomib; and histone deacetylase inhibitors; as well as cytotoxic T-cell based therapies directed against both EBV-associated and EBV-negative lymphomas.[3]

NLPHL disease affects 10% to 15% of pediatric patients, is more common among male and younger patients, and is usually clinically localized (low stage). Stage I patients do well with surgical resection only (no chemotherapy or radiotherapy) and close follow-up.[178] For stage II/III, most would be treated with several cycles of relatively low-dose chemotherapy (i.e., avoiding the use of alkylators, topoisomerase inhibitors) and radiation therapy. Preliminary evidence suggests that this approach for NLPHL leads to an overall survival close to 100%, and should decrease the late effects of secondary malignancy and infertility.[179] Many current study protocols would forgo even low-dose IFRT for those young patients who achieve a complete response with low-dose chemotherapy, but this should still be considered an experimental approach because combination low-dose chemotherapy and IFRT has been the standard of care, and there are reports of relapse after chemotherapy-only treatments.

SUPPORTIVE CARE

There is no question that a large part of the success of modern leukemia and lymphoma treatment is related to the major improvements in supportive care that coincided with improvements in chemotherapy. These advances have included improved blood products, antibiotics, antifungals, and better intensive care unit support of critically ill pediatric patients. Erythropoietin has been used sparingly in pediatric oncology, and is not generally incorporated in frontline therapies for any of the lymphoid cancers. Leukocyte growth factors (granulocyte colony-stimulating factor, granulocyte-macrophage colony-stimulating factor, and PEGylated forms, such as pegfilgrastim) are used sparingly in pediatric leukemia and lymphoma therapies for multiple reasons, including (1) concerns (mostly not substantiated in the literature) that these factors may stimulate the growth of these diseases, (2) multiple studies that show no changes in overall outcome when these factors are used, (3) financial burden, and (4) the addition of needle sticks and/or the increased infection risk from entering central lines daily. Growth factors are, however, used routinely in many relapse and higher stage lymphoma protocols to enable a dose-intensive chemotherapy schedule and avoid long periods of profound neutropenia.

LONG-TERM, PALLIATIVE, AND HOSPICE CARE IN PEDIATRIC ONCOLOGY

The survivors of current lower risk (less intensively treated) forms of ALL, NHL, and HL in childhood can now expect prolonged DFS, intact fertility, lesser cognitive and social disruption, and an easier integration into standard medical and social environments than in the past. Survivors from higher doses and larger radiation fields used in the 1960s and 1970s, as well as from regimens involving higher cumulative doses of chemotherapy, continue to have an increased risk of important long-term toxicities, including endocrine, growth, fertility, and learning disabilities, along with cardiac, renal, liver, and other end-organ toxicities.[180] Second malignancies are another serious problem, arising from carcinogenic exposures to chemotherapy and radiotherapy, as well as possibly an innate propensity to develop cancer.[181] It has been estimated that pediatric cancer survivors will soon represent as many as 1 in 250 adult Americans in the 15- to 45-year-old population.[182] Reducing late effects of therapy while preserving cure rates is a crucial goal in improving outcomes in childhood leukemia and lymphoma.[183]

Even with cure rates that reach, in many categories of disease, into the over 90% region, a substantial number of children still die of leukemia and lymphoma. A small number die after failing their first regimens, but many succumb after alternately succeeding and then failing several attempts at cure. A discussion of hospice and palliative care for these children and support for their families is beyond the scope of this chapter, but this is an area of active interest and involvement in most pediatric oncology programs. Hospice and palliative care treatments in pediatrics share some of the same concerns, goals, and methods as programs for adults. However, the unique requirements of psychosocial support in children, and the impact of a possible death of a child on a family, lead most experts to guide these patients to pediatric centers.

REFERENCES

1. Hunger SP, Lu X, Devidas M, et al. Improved survival for children and adolescents with acute lymphoblastic leukemia between 1990 and 2005: a report from the Children's Oncology Group. J Clin Oncol 2012;30:1663–1669.
2. Inaba H, Greaves M, Mullighan CG. Acute lymphoblastic leukaemia. Lancet 2013;381:1943–1955.
3. Freed J, Kelly KM. Current approaches to the management of pediatric Hodgkin lymphoma. Paediatr Drugs 2010;12:85–98.
4. Reiter A. Non-Hodgkin lymphoma in children and adolescents. Klin Padiatr 2013;225:S87–S93.
5. Creutzig U, van den Heuvel-Eibrink MM, Gibson B, et al. Diagnosis and management of acute myeloid leukemia in children and adolescents: recommendations from an international expert panel. Blood 2012;120:3187–3205.
6. Rubnitz JE, Gibson B, Smith FO. Acute myeloid leukemia. Hematol Oncol Clin North Am 2010;24:35–63.
7. Bleyer A, Morgan S, Barr R. Proceedings of a workshop: bridging the gap in care and addressing participation in clinical trials. Cancer 2006;107:1656–1658.
8. Pui CH, Robison LL, Look AT. Acute lymphoblastic leukaemia. Lancet 2008;371:1030–1043.
9. Jemal A, Siegel R, Ward E, et al. Cancer statistics, 2009. CA Cancer J Clin 2009;59:225–249.
10. Bhatia S, Sather HN, Heerema NA, et al. Racial and ethnic differences in survival of children with acute lymphoblastic leukemia. Blood 2002;100:1957–1964.
11. Kadan-Lottick NS, Ness KK, Bhatia S, et al. Survival variability by race and ethnicity in childhood acute lymphoblastic leukemia. JAMA 2003;290:2008–2014.
12. Pui CH, Evans WE. Treatment of acute lymphoblastic leukemia. N Engl J Med 2006;354:166–178.
13. Pui CH, Pei D, Pappo AS, et al. Treatment outcomes in black and white children with cancer: results from the SEER database and St Jude Children's Research Hospital, 1992 through 2007. J Clin Oncol 2012;30:2005–2012.
14. Bhatia S, Landier W, Shangguan M, et al. Nonadherence to oral mercaptopurine and risk of relapse in Hispanic and non-Hispanic white children with acute lymphoblastic leukemia: a report from the Children's Oncology Group. J Clin Oncol 2012;30:2094–2101.
15. Xie Y, Davies SM, Xiang Y, et al. Trends in leukemia incidence and survival in the United States (1973–1998). Cancer 2003;97:2229–2235.
16. Glaubach T, Robinson LJ, Corey SJ. Pediatric myelodysplastic syndromes: they do exist! J Pediatr Hematol Oncol 2014;36:1–7.
17. Bhatia S, Neglia JP. Epidemiology of childhood acute myelogenous leukemia. J Pediatr Hematol Oncol 1995;17:94–100.
18. Children's Oncology Group, Aplenc R, Alonzo TA, et al. Ethnicity and survival in childhood acute myeloid leukemia: a report from the Children's Oncology Group. Blood 2006;108:74–80.
19. Meshinchi S, Arceci RJ. Prognostic factors and risk-based therapy in pediatric acute myeloid leukemia. Oncologist 2007;12:341–355.
20. Hann IM, Webb DK, Gibson BE, et al. MRC trials in childhood acute myeloid leukaemia. Ann Hematol 2004;83:S108–S112.
21. Kim AS, Eastmond DA, Preston RJ. Childhood acute lymphocytic leukemia and perspectives on risk assessment of early-life stage exposures. Mutat Res 2006;613:138–160.
22. McNally RJ, Eden TO. An infectious aetiology for childhood acute leukaemia: a review of the evidence. Br J Haematol 2004;127:243–263.
23. Mallol-Mesnard N, Menegaux F, Auvrignon A, et al. Vaccination and the risk of childhood acute leukaemia: the ESCALE study (SFCE). Int J Epidemiol 2007;36:110–116.
24. Kleinerman RA, Kaune WT, Hatch EE, et al. Are children living near high-voltage power lines at increased risk of acute lymphoblastic leukemia? Am J Epidemiol 2000;151:512–515.
25. Kabuto M, Nitta H, Yamamoto S, et al. Childhood leukemia and magnetic fields in Japan: a case-control study of childhood leukemia and residential power-frequency magnetic fields in Japan. Int J Cancer 2006;119:643–650.
26. Svendsen AL, Weihkopf T, Kaatsch P, et al. Exposure to magnetic fields and survival after diagnosis of childhood leukemia: a German cohort study. Cancer Epidemiol Biomarkers Prev 2007;16:1167–1171.
27. Bolufer P, Collado M, Barragan E, et al. The potential effect of gender in combination with common genetic polymorphisms of drug-metabolizing enzymes on the risk of developing acute leukemia. Haematologica 2007;92:308–314.
28. Ford AM, Ridge SA, Cabrera ME, et al. In utero rearrangements in the trithorax-related oncogene in infant leukaemias. Nature 1993;363:358–360.
29. Bateman CM, Colman SM, Chaplin T, et al. Acquisition of genome-wide copy number alterations in monozygotic twins with acute lymphoblastic leukemia. Blood 2010;115:3553–3558.
30. Gale KB, Ford AM, Repp R, et al. Backtracking leukemia to birth: identification of clonotypic gene fusion sequences in neonatal blood spots. Proc Natl Acad Sci U S A 1997;94:13950–13954.
31. Greaves MF, Maia AT, Wiemels JL, et al. Leukemia in twins: lessons in natural history. Blood 2003;102:2321–2333.
32. Greaves M. Infection, immune responses and the aetiology of childhood leukaemia. Nat Rev Cancer 2006;6:193–203.
33. Trevino LR, Yang W, French D, et al. Germline genomic variants associated with childhood acute lymphoblastic leukemia. Nat Genet 2009;41:1001–1005.
34. Papaemmanuil E, Hosking FJ, Vijayakrishnan J, et al. Loci on 7p12.2, 10q21.2 and 14q11.2 are associated with risk of childhood acute lymphoblastic leukaemia. Nat Genet 2009;41:1006–1010.
35. Sherborne AL, Hosking FJ, Prasad RB, et al. Variation in CDKN2A at 9p21.3 influences childhood acute lymphoblastic leukemia risk. Nat Genet 2010;42:492–494.
36. Perez-Andreu V, Roberts KG, Harvey RC, et al. Inherited GATA3 variants are associated with Ph-like childhood acute lymphoblastic leukemia and risk of relapse. Nat Genet 2013;45:1494–1498.
37. Xu H, Cheng C, Devidas M, et al. ARID5B genetic polymorphisms contribute to racial disparities in the incidence and treatment outcome of childhood acute lymphoblastic leukemia. J Clin Oncol 2012;30:751–757.
38. Shah S, Schrader KA, Waanders E, et al. A recurrent germline PAX5 mutation confers susceptibility to pre-B cell acute lymphoblastic leukemia. Nat Genet 2013;45:1226–1231.
39. Holmfeldt L, Wei L, Diaz-Flores E, et al. The genomic landscape of hypodiploid acute lymphoblastic leukemia. Nat Genet 2013;45:242–252.
40. Zwaan MC, Reinhardt D, Hitzler J, et al. Acute leukemias in children with Down syndrome. Pediatr Clin North Am 2008;55:53–70.
41. Linabery AM, Blair CK, Gamis AS, et al. Congenital abnormalities and acute leukemia among children with Down syndrome: a Children's Oncology Group study. Cancer Epidemiol Biomarkers Prev 2008;17:2572–2577.
42. Rabin KR, Whitlock JA. Malignancy in children with trisomy 21. Oncologist 2009;14:164–173.
43. Arico M, Ziino O, Valsecchi MG, et al. Acute lymphoblastic leukemia and Down syndrome: presenting features and treatment outcome in the experience of the Italian Association of Pediatric Hematology and Oncology (AIEOP). Cancer 2008;113:515–521.
44. Forestier E, Izraeli S, Beverloo B, et al. Cytogenetic features of acute lymphoblastic and myeloid leukemias in pediatric patients with Down syndrome: an iBFM-SG study. Blood 2008;111:1575–1583.
45. Maloney KW, Carroll WL, Carroll AJ, et al. Down syndrome childhood acute lymphoblastic leukemia has a unique spectrum of sentinel cytogenetic lesions that influences treatment outcome: a report from the Children's Oncology Group. Blood 2010;116:1045–1050.
46. Bercovich D, Ganmore I, Scott LM, et al. Mutations of JAK2 in acute lymphoblastic leukaemias associated with Down's syndrome. Lancet 2008;372:1484–1492.
47. Russell LJ, Capasso M, Vater I, et al. Deregulated expression of cytokine receptor gene, CRLF2, is involved in lymphoid transformation in B cell precursor acute lymphoblastic leukemia. Blood 2009;114:2688–2698.
48. Mullighan CG, Collins-Underwood JR, Phillips LA, et al. Rearrangement of CRLF2 in B-progenitor- and Down syndrome-associated acute lymphoblastic leukemia. Nat Genet 2009;41:1243–1246.
49. Massey GV, Zipursky A, Chang MN, et al. A prospective study of the natural history of transient leukemia (TL) in neonates with Down syndrome (DS): Children's Oncology Group (COG) study POG-9481. Blood 2006;107:4606–4613.
50. Ge Y, Dombkowski AA, LaFiura KM, et al. Differential gene expression, GATA1 target genes, and the chemotherapy sensitivity of Down syndrome megakaryocytic leukemia. Blood 2006;107:1570–1581.
51. Pui CH, Campana D. New definition of remission in childhood acute lymphoblastic leukemia. Leukemia 2000;14:783–785.
52. Campana D. Minimal residual disease in acute lymphoblastic leukemia. Semin Hematol 2009;46:100–106.
53. Faham M, Zheng J, Moorhead M, et al. Deep-sequencing approach for minimal residual disease detection in acute lymphoblastic leukemia. Blood 2012;120:5173–5180.
54. Arceci RJ. Progress and controversies in the treatment of pediatric acute myelogenous leukemia. Curr Opin Hematol 2002;9:353–360.
55. Dusenbery KE, Howells WB, Arthur DC, et al. Extramedullary leukemia in children with newly diagnosed acute myeloid leukemia: a report from the Children's Cancer Group. J Pediatr Hematol Oncol 2003;25:760–768.
56. Pui CH, Howard SC. Current management and challenges of malignant disease in the CNS in paediatric leukaemia. Lancet Oncol 2008;9:257–268.
57. Swerdlow SH, Campo E, Harris NL. WHO Classification of Tumours of Haematopoietic and Lymphoid Tissues. Lyon, France: WHO: 2008.
58. Holleman A, Cheok MH, den Boer ML, et al. Gene-expression patterns in drug-resistant acute lymphoblastic leukemia cells and response to treatment. N Engl J Med 2004;351:533–542.
59. Lu XY, Harris CP, Cooley L, et al. The utility of spectral karyotyping in the cytogenetic analysis of newly diagnosed pediatric acute lymphoblastic leukemia. Leukemia 2002;16:2222–2227.
60. Mullighan CG, Goorha S, Radtke I, et al. Genome-wide analysis of genetic alterations in acute lymphoblastic leukaemia. Nature 2007;446:758–764.
61. Zhang J, Ding L, Holmfeldt L, et al. The genetic basis of early T-cell precursor acute lymphoblastic leukaemia. Nature 2012;481:157–163.
62. Welch JS, Westervelt P, Ding L, et al. Use of whole genome sequencing to diagnose a cryptic fusion oncogene. JAMA 2011;305:1577–1584.
63. Wei G, Twomey D, Lamb J, et al. Gene expression-based chemical genomics identifies rapamycin as a modulator of MCL1 and glucocorticoid resistance. Cancer Cell 2006;10:331–342.
64. Roberts KG, Morin RD, Zhang J, et al. Genetic alterations activating kinase and cytokine receptor signaling in high-risk acute lymphoblastic leukemia. Cancer Cell 2012;22:153–166.
65. Smith M, Arthur D, Camitta B, et al. Uniform approach to risk classification and treatment assignment for children with acute lymphoblastic leukemia. J Clin Oncol 1996;14:18–24.

66. Hilden JM, Dinndorf PA, Meerbaum SO, et al. Analysis of prognostic factors of acute lymphoblastic leukemia in infants: report on CCG 1953 from the Children's Oncology Group. Blood 2006;108:441–451.
67. Nagayama J, Tomizawa D, Koh K, et al. Infants with acute lymphoblastic leukemia and a germline MLL gene are highly curable with use of chemotherapy alone: results from the Japan Infant Leukemia Study Group. Blood 2006;107:4663–4665.
68. Pieters R, Schrappe M, De Lorenzo P, et al. A treatment protocol for infants younger than 1 year with acute lymphoblastic leukaemia (Interfant-99): an observational study and a multicentre randomised trial. Lancet 2007;370:240–250.
69. Dreyer ZE, Dinndorf PA, Camitta B, et al. Analysis of the role of hematopoietic stem-cell transplantation in infants with acute lymphoblastic leukemia in first remission and MLL gene rearrangements: a report from the Children's Oncology Group. J Clin Oncol 2011;29:214–222.
70. Nachman JB, La MK, Hunger SP, et al. 2009. Young adults with acute lymphoblastic leukemia have an excellent outcome with chemotherapy alone and benefit from intensive postinduction treatment: a report from the Children's Oncology Group. J Clin Oncol 27:5189–5194.
71. Trueworthy R, Shuster J, Look T, et al. Ploidy of lymphoblasts is the strongest predictor of treatment outcome in B-progenitor cell acute lymphoblastic leukemia of childhood: a Pediatric Oncology Group study. J Clin Oncol 1992;10:606–613.
72. Heerema NA, Raimondi SC, Anderson JR, et al. Specific extra chromosomes occur in a modal number dependent pattern in pediatric acute lymphoblastic leukemia. Genes Chromosomes Cancer 2007;46:684–693.
73. Borowitz MJ, Devidas M, Hunger SP, et al. Clinical significance of minimal residual disease in childhood acute lymphoblastic leukemia and its relationship to other prognostic factors: a Children's Oncology Group study. Blood 2008;111:5477–5485.
74. Nachman JB, Heerema NA, Sather H, et al. Outcome of treatment in children with hypodiploid acute lymphoblastic leukemia. Blood 2007;110:1112–1115.
75. Mullighan CG, Su X, Zhang J, et al. Deletion of IKZF1 and prognosis in acute lymphoblastic leukemia. N Engl J Med 2009;360:470–480.
76. Rand V, Parker H, Russell LJ, et al. Genomic characterization implicates IKZF1 as a likely primary genetic event in childhood B-cell precursor acute lymphoblastic leukemia. Blood 2011;117:6848–6855.
77. Chen IM, Harvey RC, Mullighan CG, et al. Outcome modeling with CRLF2, IKZF1, JAK, and minimal residual disease in pediatric acute lymphoblastic leukemia: a Children's Oncology Group study. Blood 2012;119:3512–3522.
78. van der Veer A, Waanders E, Pieters R, et al. Independent prognostic value of BCR-ABL1-like signature and IKZF1 deletion, but not high CRLF2 expression, in children with B-cell precursor ALL. Blood 2013;122:2622–2629.
79. Rubnitz JE, Wichlan D, Devidas M, et al. Prospective analysis of TEL gene rearrangements in childhood acute lymphoblastic leukemia: a Children's Oncology Group study. J Clin Oncol 2008;26:2186–2191.
80. Aldrich MC, Zhang L, Wiemels JL, et al. Cytogenetics of Hispanic and White children with acute lymphoblastic leukemia in California. Cancer Epidemiol Biomarkers Prev 2006;15:578–581.
81. Arico M, Valsecchi MG, Camitta B, et al. Outcome of treatment in children with Philadelphia chromosome-positive acute lymphoblastic leukemia. N Engl J Med 2000;342:998–1006.
82. Schultz KR, Carroll A, Heerema NA, et al. Long-term follow-up of imatinib in pediatric Philadelphia chromosome-positive acute lymphoblastic leukemia: Children's Oncology Group Study AALL0031. Leukemia 2014 Jul;28(7):1467–1471. Epub 2014 Jan 20.
83. Schultz KR, Bowman WP, Aledo A, et al. Improved early event-free survival with imatinib in Philadelphia chromosome-positive acute lymphoblastic leukemia: a Children's Oncology Group study. J Clin Oncol 2009;27:5175–5181.
84. Foa R, Vitale A, Vignetti M, et al. Dasatinib as first-line treatment for adult patients with Philadelphia chromosome-positive acute lymphoblastic leukemia. Blood 2011;118:6521–6528.
85. Breit S, Stanulla M, Flohr T, et al. Activating NOTCH1 mutations predict favorable early treatment response and long-term outcome in childhood precursor T-cell lymphoblastic leukemia. Blood 2006;108:1151–1157.
86. Weng AP, Ferrando AA, Lee W, et al. Activating mutations of NOTCH1 in human T cell acute lymphoblastic leukemia. Science 2004;306:269–271.
87. Coustan-Smith E, Mullighan CG, Onciu M, et al. Early T-cell precursor leukaemia: a subtype of very high-risk acute lymphoblastic leukaemia. Lancet Oncol 2009;10:147–156.
88. Pui CH, Campana D, Pei D, et al. Treating childhood acute lymphoblastic leukemia without cranial irradiation. N Engl J Med 2009;360:2730–2741.
89. Einsiedel HG, von Stackelberg A, Hartmann R, et al. Long-term outcome in children with relapsed ALL by risk-stratified salvage therapy: results of trial acute lymphoblastic leukemia-relapse study of the Berlin-Frankfurt-Munster Group 87. J Clin Oncol 2005;23:7942–7950.
90. Schrappe M, Reiter A, Riehm H. Cytoreduction and prognosis in childhood acute lymphoblastic leukemia. J Clin Oncol 1996;14:2403–2406.
91. Schrappe M, Hunger SP, Pui CH, et al. Outcomes after induction failure in childhood acute lymphoblastic leukemia. N Engl J Med 2012;366:1371–1381.
92. Schrappe M, Nachman J, Hunger S, et al. 'Educational symposium on long-term results of large prospective clinical trials for childhood acute lymphoblastic leukemia (1985–2000)'. Leukemia 2010;24:253–254.
93. Pui CH, Pei D, Sandlund JT, et al. Long-term results of St Jude Total Therapy Studies 11, 12, 13A, 13B, and 14 for childhood acute lymphoblastic leukemia. Leukemia 2010;24:371–382.
94. Tubergen DG, Gilchrist GS, O'Brien RT, et al. Prevention of CNS disease in intermediate-risk acute lymphoblastic leukemia: comparison of cranial radiation and intrathecal methotrexate and the importance of systemic therapy: a Childrens Cancer Group report. J Clin Oncol 1993;11:520–526.
95. Finklestein JZ, Miller DR, Feusner J, et al. Treatment of overt isolated testicular relapse in children on therapy for acute lymphoblastic leukemia. A report from the Children's Cancer Group. Cancer 1994;73:219–223.
96. Nguyen K, Devidas M, Cheng SC, et al. Factors influencing survival after relapse from acute lymphoblastic leukemia: a Children's Oncology Group study. Leukemia 2008;22:2142–2150.
97. Freyer DR, Devidas M, La M, et al. Postrelapse survival in childhood acute lymphoblastic leukemia is independent of initial treatment intensity: a report from the Children's Oncology Group. Blood 2011;117:3010–3015.
98. Raetz EA, Borowitz MJ, Devidas M, et al. Reinduction platform for children with first marrow relapse of acute lymphoblastic leukemia: a Children's Oncology Group Study [corrected]. J Clin Oncol 2008;26:3971–3978.
99. Jeha S. New therapeutic strategies in acute lymphoblastic leukemia. Semin Hematol 2009;46:76–88.
100. Jeha S, Gaynon PS, Razzouk BI, et al. Phase II study of clofarabine in pediatric patients with refractory or relapsed acute lymphoblastic leukemia. J Clin Oncol 2006;24:1917–1923.
101. Hijiya N, Gaynon P, Barry E, et al. A multi-center phase I study of clofarabine, etoposide and cyclophosphamide in combination in pediatric patients with refractory or relapsed acute leukemia. Leukemia 2009;23:2259–2264.
102. Topp MS, Kufer P, Gokbuget N, et al. Targeted therapy with the T-cell-engaging antibody blinatumomab of chemotherapy-refractory minimal residual disease in B-lineage acute lymphoblastic leukemia patients results in high response rate and prolonged leukemia-free survival. J Clin Oncol 2011;29:2493–2498.
103. Topp MS, Gokbuget N, Zugmaier G, et al. Long-term follow-up of hematologic relapse-free survival in a phase 2 study of blinatumomab in patients with MRD in B-lineage ALL. Blood 2012;120:5185–5187.
104. Grupp SA, Kalos M, Barrett D, et al. Chimeric antigen receptor-modified T cells for acute lymphoid leukemia. N Engl J Med 2013;368:1509–1518.
105. Grupp SA, Frey NV, Aplenc R T cells engineered with a chimeric antigen receptor (CAR) targeting CD19 (CTL019) produce significant in vivo proliferation, complete responses and long-term persistence without GVHD in children and adults with relapsed, refractory ALL. Blood 2013;122(abstract 67).
106. Mehta PA, Davies SM. Allogeneic transplantation for childhood ALL. Bone Marrow Transplant 2008;41:133–139.
107. Kaspers GJ, Creutzig U. Pediatric acute myeloid leukemia: towards high-quality cure of all patients. Haematologica 2007;92.1519–1532.
108. Kaspers GJ, Creutzig U. Pediatric acute myeloid leukemia: international progress and future directions. Leukemia 2005;19:2025–2029.
109. Pollard JA, Alonzo TA, Gerbing RB, et al. Prevalence and prognostic significance of KIT mutations in pediatric patients with core binding factor AML enrolled on serial pediatric cooperative trials for de novo AML. Blood 2010;115:2372–2379.
110. Canner J, Alonzo TA, Franklin J, et al. Differences in outcomes of newly diagnosed acute myeloid leukemia for adolescent/young adult and younger patients: a report from the Children's Oncology Group. Cancer 2013;119:4162–4169.
111. Hollink IH, Zwaan CM, Zimmermann M, et al. Favorable prognostic impact of NPM1 gene mutations in childhood acute myeloid leukemia, with emphasis on cytogenetically normal AML. Leukemia 2009;23:262–270.
112. Ho PA, Alonzo TA, Gerbing RB, et al. Prevalence and prognostic implications of CEBPA mutations in pediatric acute myeloid leukemia (AML): a report from the Children's Oncology Group. Blood 2009;113:6558–6566.
113. Buccisano F, Maurillo L, Del Principe MI, et al. Prognostic and therapeutic implications of minimal residual disease detection in acute myeloid leukemia. Blood 2012;119:332–341.
114. Woods WG. Curing childhood acute myeloid leukemia (AML) at the half-way point: promises to keep and miles to go before we sleep. Pediatr Blood Cancer 2006;46:565–569.
115. Gamis AS, Alonzo TA, Perentesis JP, et al. Children's Oncology Group's 2013 blueprint for research: acute myeloid leukemia. Pediatr Blood Cancer 2013;60:964–971.
116. Woods WG, Neudorf S, Gold S, et al. A comparison of allogeneic bone marrow transplantation, autologous bone marrow transplantation, and aggressive chemotherapy in children with acute myeloid leukemia in remission. Blood 2001;97:56–62.
117. Kardos G, Zwaan CM, Kaspers GJ, et al. Treatment strategy and results in children treated on three Dutch Childhood Oncology Group acute myeloid leukemia trials. Leukemia 2005;19:2063–2071.
118. Gamis A, Aplenc R, Alonzo T, et al. Gemtuzumab Ozogamicin (GO) in children with de novo acute myeloid leukemia (AML) improves event-free survival (EFS) by reducing relapse risk—results from the randomized phase III Children's Oncology Group (COG) trial, AAML0531. ASH Annual Meeting 2013;(abstract 355).
119. Horton TM, Pati D, Plon SE, et al. A phase 1 study of the proteasome inhibitor bortezomib in pediatric patients with refractory leukemia: a Children's Oncology Group study. Clin Cancer Res 2007;13:1516–1522.
120. Widemann BC, Kim A, Fox E, et al. A phase I trial and pharmacokinetic study of sorafenib in children with refractory solid tumors or leukemias: a Children's Oncology Group Phase I Consortium report. Clin Cancer Res 2012;18:6011–6022.
121. Bunin NJ, Davies SM, Aplenc R, et al. Unrelated donor bone marrow transplantation for children with acute myeloid leukemia beyond first remission or refractory to chemotherapy. J Clin Oncol 2008;26:4326–4332.

122. Horan JT, Alonzo TA, Lyman GH, et al. Impact of disease risk on efficacy of matched related bone marrow transplantation for pediatric acute myeloid leukemia: the Children's Oncology Group. J Clin Oncol 2008;26:5797–5801.
123. Biondi A, Rovelli A, Cantu-Rajnoldi A, et al. Acute promyelocytic leukemia in children: experience of the Italian Pediatric Hematology and Oncology Group (AIEOP). Leukemia 1994;8:S66–S70.
124. Ribeiro R. Update on the management of pediatric acute promyelocytic leukemia. Clin Adv Hematol Oncol 2006;4:263–265.
125. Zhou J, Zhang Y, Li J, et al. Single-agent arsenic trioxide in the treatment of children with newly diagnosed acute promyelocytic leukemia. Blood 2010;115:1697–1702.
126. Juliusson G, Lazarevic V, Horstedt AS, et al. Acute myeloid leukemia in the real world: why population-based registries are needed. Blood 2012;119:3890–3899.
127. Dvorak CC, Agarwal R, Dahl GV, et al. Hematopoietic stem cell transplant for pediatric acute promyelocytic leukemia. Biol Blood Marrow Transplant 2008;14:824–830.
128. Gamis AS, Woods WG, Alonzo TA, et al. Increased age at diagnosis has a significantly negative effect on outcome in children with Down syndrome and acute myeloid leukemia: a report from the Children's Cancer Group Study 2891. J Clin Oncol 2003;21:3415–3422.
129. Abildgaard L, Ellebaek E, Gustafsson G, et al. Optimal treatment intensity in children with Down syndrome and myeloid leukaemia: data from 56 children treated on NOPHO-AML protocols and a review of the literature. Ann Hematol 2006;85:275–280.
130. Rao A, Hills RK, Stiller C, et al. Treatment for myeloid leukaemia of Down syndrome: population-based experience in the UK and results from the Medical Research Council AML 10 and AML 12 trials. Br J Haematol 2006;132:576–583.
131. Aladjidi N, Auvrignon A, Leblanc T, et al. Outcome in children with relapsed acute myeloid leukemia after initial treatment with the French Leucemie Aique Myeloide Enfant (LAME) 89/91 protocol of the French Society of Pediatric Hematology and Immunology. J Clin Oncol 2003;21:4377–4385.
132. Oda M, Isoyama K, Ito E, et al. Survival after cord blood transplantation from unrelated donor as a second hematopoietic stem cell transplantation for recurrent pediatric acute myeloid leukemia. Int J Hematol 2009;89:374–382.
133. Meshinchi S, Leisenring WM, Carpenter PA, et al. Survival after second hematopoietic stem cell transplantation for recurrent pediatric acute myeloid leukemia. Biol Blood Marrow Transplant 2003;9:706–713.
134. Moore AS, Kearns PR, Knapper S, et al. Novel therapies for children with acute myeloid leukaemia. Leukemia 2013;27:1451–1460.
135. Millot F, Traore P, Guilhot J, et al. Clinical and biological features at diagnosis in 40 children with chronic myeloid leukemia. Pediatrics 2005;116:140–143.
136. Suttorp M, Eckardt L, Tauer JT, et al. Management of chronic myeloid leukemia in childhood. Curr Hematol Malig Rep 2012;7:116–124.
137. Loh ML. Recent advances in the pathogenesis and treatment of juvenile myelomonocytic leukaemia. Br J Haematol 2011;152:677–687.
138. Hasle H. Myelodysplastic and myeloproliferative disorders in children. Curr Opin Pediatr 2007;19:1–8.
139. Loh ML, Sakai DS, Flotho C, et al. Mutations in CBL occur frequently in juvenile myelomonocytic leukemia. Blood 2009;114:1859–1863.
140. Locatelli F, Nollke P, Zecca M, et al. Hematopoietic stem cell transplantation (HSCT) in children with juvenile myelomonocytic leukemia (JMML): results of the EWOG-MDS/EBMT trial. Blood 2005;105:410–419.
141. Matutes E, Pickl WF, Van't Veer M, et al. Mixed-phenotype acute leukemia: clinical and laboratory features and outcome in 100 patients defined according to the WHO 2008 classification. Blood 2011;117:3163–3171.
142. Shukla NN, Trippett TM. Non-Hodgkin's lymphoma in children and adolescents. Curr Oncol Rep 2006;8:387–394.
143. Swerdlow SH. Lymphoma classification and the tools of our trade: an introduction to the 2012 USCAP Long Course. Mod Pathol 2013;26:S1–S14.
144. Cairo MS, Perkins S. Non-Hodgkin's lymphoma in children. In: Bast RC, Bast RC Jr, Holland JF, eds. Holland-Frei Cancer Medicine. Ontario: Hamilton; 2000.
145. Miller E, Metser U, Avrahami G, et al. Role of 18F-FDG PET/CT in staging and follow-up of lymphoma in pediatric and young adult patients. J Comput Assist Tomogr 2006;30:689–694.
146. Pinkerton R. Continuing challenges in childhood non-Hodgkin's lymphoma. Br J Haematol 2005;130:480–488.
147. Saha A, Robertson ES. Epstein-Barr virus-associated B-cell lymphomas: pathogenesis and clinical outcomes. Clin Cancer Res 2011;17:3056–3063.
148. Rezk SA, Weiss LM. Epstein-Barr virus-associated lymphoproliferative disorders. Hum Pathol 2007;38:1293–1304.
149. Mann G, Attarbaschi A, Steiner M, et al. Early and reliable diagnosis of non-Hodgkin lymphoma in childhood and adolescence: contribution of cytomorphology and flow cytometric immunophenotyping. Pediatr Hematol Oncol 2006;23:167–176.
150. Perger L, Lee EY, Shamberger RC. Management of children and adolescents with a critical airway due to compression by an anterior mediastinal mass. J Pediatr Surg 2008;43:1990–1997.
151. Asselin BL, Devidas M, Wang C, et al. Effectiveness of high-dose methotrexate in T-cell lymphoblastic leukemia and advanced-stage lymphoblastic lymphoma: a randomized study by the Children's Oncology Group (POG 9404). Blood 2011;118:874–883.
152. Sandlund JT, Pui CH, Zhou Y, et al. Effective treatment of advanced-stage childhood lymphoblastic lymphoma without prophylactic cranial irradiation: results of St Jude NHL13 study. Leukemia 2009;23:1127–1130.
153. Burkhardt B, Woessmann W, Zimmermann M, et al. Impact of cranial radiotherapy on central nervous system prophylaxis in children and adolescents with central nervous system-negative stage III or IV lymphoblastic lymphoma. J Clin Oncol 2006;24:491–499.
154. DeAngelo DJ. Nelarabine for the treatment of patients with relapsed or refractory T-cell acute lymphoblastic leukemia or lymphoblastic lymphoma. Hematol Oncol Clin North Am 2009;23:1121–1135.
155. Ferrando AA. The role of NOTCH1 signaling in T-ALL. Hematology Am Soc Hematol Educ Program 2009:353–361.
156. Real PJ, Ferrando AA. NOTCH inhibition and glucocorticoid therapy in T-cell acute lymphoblastic leukemia. Leukemia 2009;23:1374–1377.
157. Attarbaschi A, Dworzak M, Steiner M, et al. Outcome of children with primary resistant or relapsed non-Hodgkin lymphoma and mature B-cell leukemia after intensive first-line treatment: a population-based analysis of the Austrian Cooperative Study Group. Pediatr Blood Cancer 2005;44:70–76.
158. Lombardi L, Newcomb EW, Dalla-Favera R. Pathogenesis of Burkitt lymphoma: expression of an activated c-myc oncogene causes the tumorigenic conversion of EBV-infected human B lymphoblasts. Cell 1987;49:161–170.
159. Fleming ID, Turk PS, Murphy SB, et al. Surgical implications of primary gastrointestinal lymphoma of childhood. Arch Surg 1990;125:252–256.
160. Molyneux EM, Rochford R, Griffin B, et al. Burkitt's lymphoma. Lancet 2012;379:1234–1244.
161. Hesseling P, Molyneux E, Kamiza S, et al. Endemic Burkitt lymphoma: a 28-day treatment schedule with cyclophosphamide and intrathecal methotrexate. Ann Trop Paediatr 2009;29:29–34.
162. Hesseling P, Broadhead R, Mansvelt E, et al. The 2000 Burkitt lymphoma trial in Malawi. Pediatr Blood Cancer 2005;44:245–250.
163. Patte C, Auperin A, Gerrard M, et al. Results of the randomized international FAB/LMB96 trial for intermediate risk B-cell non-Hodgkin lymphoma in children and adolescents: it is possible to reduce treatment for the early responding patients. Blood 2007;109:2773–2780.
164. Crosswell HE, Bergsagel DJ, Yost R, et al. Successful treatment with modified CHOP-rituximab in pediatric AIDS-related advanced stage Burkitt lymphoma. Pediatr Blood Cancer 2008;50:883–885.
165. Meinhardt A, Burkhardt B, Zimmermann M, et al. Phase II window study on rituximab in newly diagnosed pediatric mature B-cell non-Hodgkin's lymphoma and Burkitt leukemia. J Clin Oncol 2010;28:3115–3121.
166. Harris NL, Jaffe ES, Stein H, et al. A revised European-American classification of lymphoid neoplasms: a proposal from the International Lymphoma Study Group. Blood 1994;84:1361–1392.
167. Griffin TC, Weitzman S, Weinstein H, et al. A study of rituximab and ifosfamide, carboplatin, and etoposide chemotherapy in children with recurrent/refractory B-cell (CD20+) non-Hodgkin lymphoma and mature B-cell acute lymphoblastic leukemia: a report from the Children's Oncology Group. Pediatr Blood Cancer 2009;52:177–181.
168. Attias D, Hodgson D, Weitzman S. Primary mediastinal B-cell lymphoma in the pediatric patient: Can a rational approach to therapy be based on adult studies? Pediatr Blood Cancer 2009;52:566–570.
169. Grigg AP, Seymour JF. Graft versus Burkitt's lymphoma effect after allogeneic marrow transplantation. Leuk Lymphoma 2002;43:889–892.
170. Gambacorti-Passerini C, Messa C, Pogliani EM. Crizotinib in anaplastic large-cell lymphoma. N Engl J Med 2011;364:775–776.
171. Younes A, Gopal AK, Smith SE, et al. Results of a pivotal phase II study of brentuximab vedotin for patients with relapsed or refractory Hodgkin's lymphoma. J Clin Oncol 2012;30:2183–2189.
172. Sandlund JT, Hudson MM. Hematology: Treatment strategies for pediatric Hodgkin lymphoma. Nat Rev Clin Oncol 2010;7:243–244.
173. Rademaker J. Hodgkin's and non-Hodgkin's lymphomas. Radiol Clin North Am 2007;45:69–83.
174. Preciado MV, De Matteo E, Diez B, et al. Epstein-Barr virus (EBV) latent membrane protein (LMP) in tumor cells of Hodgkin's disease in pediatric patients. Med Pediatr Oncol 1995;24:1–5.
175. Schwartz CL. Prognostic factors in pediatric Hodgkin disease. Curr Oncol Rep 2003;5:498–504.
176. Furth C, Denecke T, Steffen I, et al. Correlative imaging strategies implementing CT, MRI, and PET for staging of childhood Hodgkin disease. J Pediatr Hematol Oncol 2006;28:501–512.
177. Stein H. Hodgkin lymphoma. In: Jaffe ES, Harris NL, Stein H, et al. eds. World Health Organization Classification of Tumors: Tumors of Hematopoietic and Lymphoid Tissues. Lyon: IARC Press; 2001:237.
178. Murphy SB, Morgan ER, Katzenstein HM, et al. Results of little or no treatment for lymphocyte-predominant Hodgkin disease in children and adolescents. J Pediatr Hematol Oncol 2003;25:684–687.
179. Pellegrino B, Terrier-Lacombe MJ, Oberlin O, et al. Lymphocyte-predominant Hodgkin's lymphoma in children: therapeutic abstention after initial lymph node resection—a Study of the French Society of Pediatric Oncology. J Clin Oncol 2003;21:2948–2952.
180. Fulbright JM, Raman S, McClellan WS, et al. Late effects of childhood leukemia therapy. Curr Hematol Malig Rep 2011;6:195–205.
181. Mody R, Li S, Dover DC, et al. Twenty-five-year follow-up among survivors of childhood acute lymphoblastic leukemia: a report from the Childhood Cancer Survivor Study. Blood 2008;111:5515–5523.
182. Bleyer WA. The impact of childhood cancer on the United States and the world. CA Cancer J Clin 1990;40:355–367.
183. Robison LL. Late effects of acute lymphoblastic leukemia therapy in patients diagnosed at 0-20 years of age. Hematology Am Soc Hematol Educ Program 2011:238–242.

Section 2 Lymphomas in Adults

37 Molecular Biology of Lymphomas

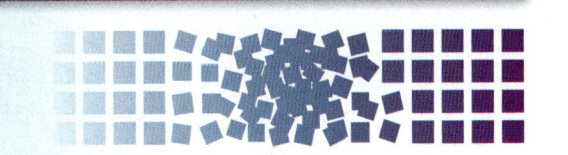

Laura Pasqualucci and Riccardo Dalla-Favera

INTRODUCTION

The term lymphoma identifies a heterogeneous group of biologically and clinically distinct neoplasms that originate from cells in the lymphoid organs and have been historically divided into two distinct categories: non-Hodgkin lymphoma (NHL) and Hodgkin lymphoma (HL).[1] During the past few decades, significant progress has been made in elucidating the molecular pathogenesis of lymphoid malignancies as a clonal expansion of B cells (in the majority of cases) or T cells. The molecular characterization of the most frequent genetic abnormalities associated with lymphoma has led to the identification of multiple proto-oncogenes and tumor suppressor genes, whose abnormal functioning contributes to lymphoma pathogenesis. Relatively less is known about the pathogenesis of T-cell NHL (T-NHL) and HL. This chapter will focus on the molecular pathogenesis of the most common and well-characterized types of lymphoma, including B-cell NHL (B-NHL), T-NHL, HL, and chronic lymphocytic leukemia (CLL), which also derives from mature B cells. Emphasis will be given to the mechanisms of genetic lesion and the nature of the involved genes in relationship to the normal biology of lymphocytes.

THE CELL OF ORIGIN OF LYMPHOMA

The number of B and T cells in the adult are not significantly different; however, 85% of lymphomas originate from mature B cells, whereas only 10% to 15% derive from the T-cell lineage. This bias may be explained in part by the unique DNA modification events that take place in normal B lymphocytes in order to enable the production of highly efficient neutralizing antibodies and that are mechanistically more complex than those utilized by T cells to encode T-cell receptors. The biology of these processes thus represents a key concept for the understanding of lymphomagenesis.

B-Cell Development and the Dynamics of the Germinal Center Reaction

B lymphocytes are generated from a common pluripotent stem cell in the bone marrow, where precursor B cells first assemble their immunoglobulin heavy chain locus (*IGH*) followed by the light chain loci (*IGL*) through a site-specific process of cleavage and rejoining, known as V(D)J recombination.[2] Cells that fail to express a functional (and nonautoreactive) antigen receptor are eliminated within the bone marrow, whereas B-cell precursors that have successfully rearranged their antibody genes are positively selected to migrate into peripheral lymphoid organs as mature, naïve B cells.[3] In most B cells, the subsequent maturation steps are linked to the histologic structure of the germinal center (GC), a specialized microenvironment that forms following the encounter of naïve B cells with a foreign antigen, in the context of signals delivered by CD4+ T cells and antigen-presenting cells (Fig. 37.1).[3-5]

GCs are highly dynamic structures in which B cells transit back and forth between two zones that are conserved across several species: the dark zone (DZ), which consists of rapidly proliferating centroblasts (CB) (doubling time: 6 to 12 hours), and the light zone (LZ), which consists of more quiescent cells termed centrocytes (CC), amidst a network of resident accessory cells (follicular dendritic cells [FDC] and human T follicular helper [TFH] cells).[6-9] According to currently accepted models, the DZ is the site where GC B cells modify the variable region of their IG genes (IgV) by the process of somatic hypermutation (SHM), which introduces mostly single nucleotide substitutions with few deletions and duplications in order to change their affinity for the antigen.[3,5,10-12] Conversely, the LZ is the site of selection based on affinity to the antigen. A critical regulator of the GC reaction is BCL6,[13,14] a transcriptional repressor[15] that negatively modulates the expression of a broad set of genes, including those involved in B-cell receptor (BCR) and CD40 signaling,[16,17] T-cell mediated B-cell activation,[16] induction of apoptosis,[16,18] response to DNA damage (by modulation of genes involved in the sensing and execution of DNA damage responses),[19-22] various cytokine and chemokine signaling pathways (e.g., those triggered by interferon and transforming growth factor beta [TGFβ]),[16,18] and plasma cell differentiation, via suppression of the PRDM1/BLIMP1 master regulator.[23-26] This transcriptional program suggests that BCL6 is critical to establish the proliferative status of CBs and to allow the execution of antigen-specific DNA modification processes (SHM and class-switch recombination) without eliciting responses to DNA damage; furthermore, BCL6 keeps in check a variety of signaling pathways that could lead to premature activation and differentiation prior to the selection for the survival of cells producing high affinity antibodies.

CBs are then believed to cease proliferation and shuttle to the LZ, where they are rechallenged by the antigen through the interaction with CD4+ T cells and FDCs.[3,4,7,8] CCs expressing a BCR with reduced affinity for the antigen will be eliminated by apoptosis, whereas a few cells with greater affinity will be selected for survival and differentiation into memory cells and plasma cells,[4] or reenter the DZ following stimulation by a variety of different signals.[9] Iterative rounds of mutations and selections lead to affinity maturation at the population level. In the GC, CCs also undergo class-switch recombination (CSR), a DNA remodeling event that confers distinct effector functions to antibodies with identical specificities.[27] SHM and CSR represent B-cell–specific functions that modify the genome of B cells via mechanisms involving single- or double-strand breaks and which depend on the activity of the activation-induced cytidine deaminase (AID) enzyme,[28-30] a notion that will become important in the understanding of the mechanisms generating genetic alterations in B-NHL.

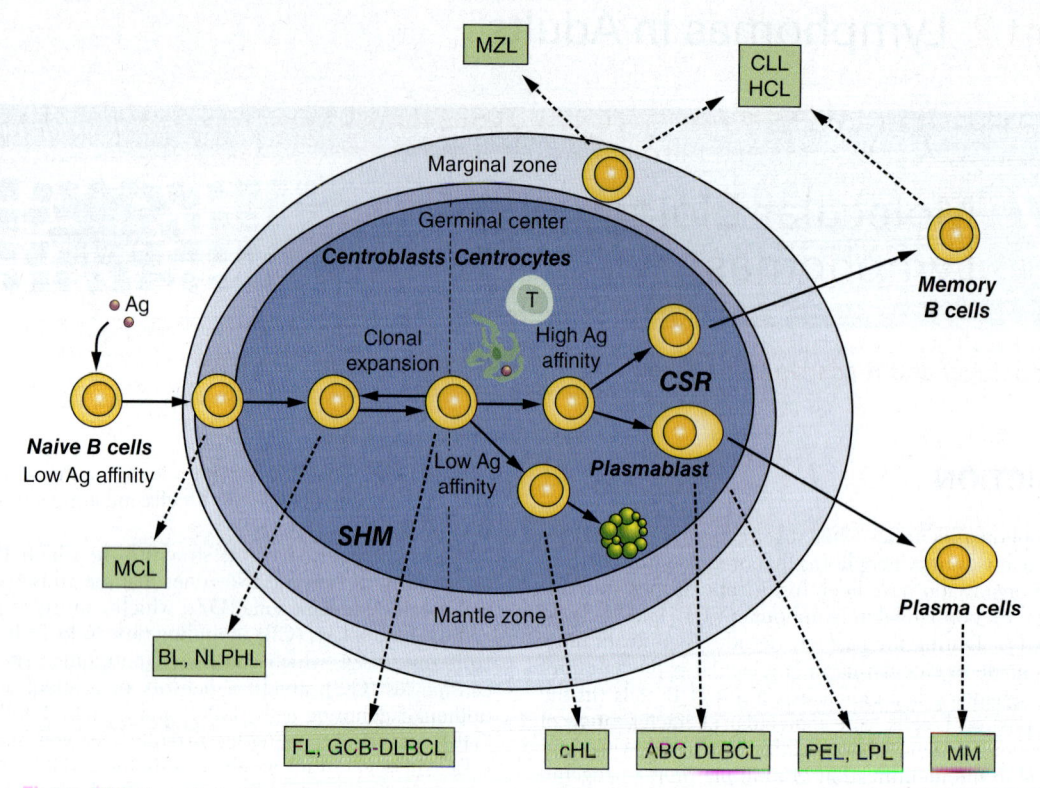

Figure 37.1 Normal B-cell development and lymphomagenesis. Schematic representation of a lymphoid follicle, constituted by the germinal center (GC), the mantle zone, and the surrounding marginal zone. B cells that have successfully rearranged their *IG* genes in the bone marrow move to peripheral lymphoid organs as naïve B cells. Upon encounter with a T-cell dependent antigen, B cells become proliferating centroblasts in the GC and eventually transition into centrocytes, which shuttle back and forth between the dark and light zone while undergoing iterative rounds of SHM and selection. Only GC B cells with high affinity for the antigen will be positively selected to exit the GC and further differentiate into plasma cells or memory B cells, whereas low-affinity clones are eliminated by apoptosis. *Dotted arrows* link various lymphoma types to their putative normal counterpart, identified based on the presence of somatically mutated IgV genes, as well as on distinctive phenotypic features. CSR, class-switch recombination; SHM, somatic hypermutation; MCL, mantle-cell lymphoma; FL, follicular lymphoma; BL, Burkitt lymphoma; GCB-DLBCL, germinal center B cell-like diffuse large B-cell lymphoma; ABC-DLBCL, activated B cell-like diffuse large B-cell lymphoma; PEL, primary effusion lymphoma; LPL, lymphoplasmacytic lymphoma; NLPHL, nodular lymphocyte predominance Hodgkin lymphoma; cHL, classical Hodgkin lymphoma; MZL, marginal zone lymphoma; HCL, hairy cell leukemia; CLL, chronic lymphocytic leukemia; MM, multiple myeloma.

Once these processes are completed, two critical signals for licensing GC exit are represented by engagement of the BCR by the antigen and activation of the CD40 receptor by the CD40 ligand present on CD4+ T cells. These signals induce the downregulation of BCL6 at the translational and transcriptional level, respectively, thus restoring DNA damage responses, as well as activation and differentiation capabilities.

Although oversimplified, this schematic description of the GC reaction is useful to introduce two basic concepts for the understanding of B-NHL pathogenesis. First, the activity of SHM, which introduces irreversible DNA changes in the genome, allowed for the conclusion that most B-NHL types, with the exception of most mantle-cell lymphoma (MCL), derive from GC-experienced B cells that underwent clonal expansion within the GC, because the malignant clones harbor hypermutated IgV sequences containing largely identical mutations, suggesting the derivation from a single founder cell.[31] Second, two common mechanisms of oncogenic lesions in B-NHL—namely, chromosomal translocations and aberrant somatic hypermutation (ASHM)—result from mistakes in the machinery that normally diversifies the Ig genes during B lymphocyte differentiation, further supporting the GC origin of most B-NHL (Fig. 37.2).[32] Finally, the definition of two distinct phases during GC development reflects different transient states within the same B-cell developmental step, which can be recognized in different B-NHL subtypes to some extent.

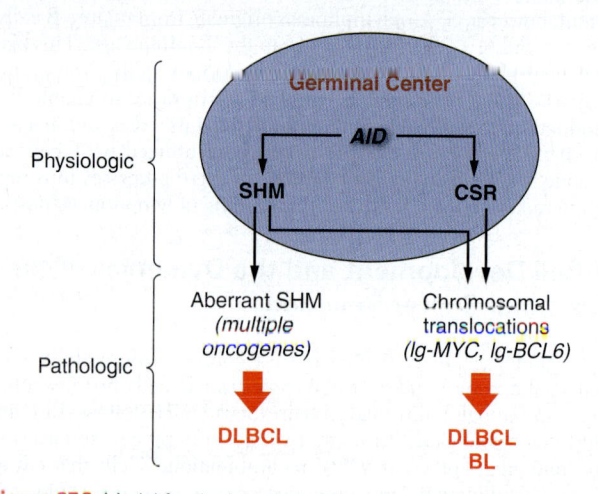

Figure 37.2 Model for the initiation of chromosomal translocations and ASHM during lymphomagenesis. B-NHL-associated genetic lesions are favored by mistakes occurring during the physiologic processes of SHM and CSR in the highly proliferative environment of the GC (top). These events lead to chromosomal translocations, which in most cases juxtapose the *IG* genes to one of several proto-oncogenes (e.g., *BCL2* or *MYC*), and ASHM of multiple target genes, thus contributing to the pathogenesis of lymphoma. DLBCL, diffuse large B-cell lymphoma; BL, Burkitt lymphoma.

T-Cell Development

The process of T-cell development proceeds through sequential stages defined according to the expression of the molecules CD4 and CD8. Committed lymphoid progenitors exit the bone marrow and migrate to the thymus as early T-cell progenitors or double negative 1 (DN1) cells, which lack the expression of both CD4 and CD8 and harbor unrearranged T-cell receptor (TCR) genes.[33] In the thymic cortex, T cells advance through the double negative stages DN2, DN3, and DN4, while undergoing specific rearrangements at the TCRβ locus in order to acquire expression of the pre-TCR.[33] Those thymocytes that have successfully recombined the pre-TCR will be selected to further differentiate into double positive cells (CD4+CD8+), which express a complete surface TCR and can then enter a process of positive and negative selection in the medulla, before exiting the thymus as single positive T cells.[33] The end result of this process is a pool of mature T cells that exhibit coordinated TCR and coreceptor specificities, as required for effective immune responses to foreign antigens. Most mature T-NHLs arise from postthymic T cells in the lymphoid organs.

GENERAL MECHANISMS OF GENETIC LESIONS IN LYMPHOMA

Analogous to other cancers, lymphoma represents a multistep process deriving from the accumulation of multiple genetic lesions affecting oncogenes and tumor suppressor genes, including chromosomal translocations, point mutations, genomic deletions, and copy number (CN) gains/amplifications.

Chromosomal Translocations

Although also found in nonlymphoid tumors, chromosomal translocations represent the genetic hallmark of malignancies derived from the hematopoietic system. These events are generated through the reciprocal and balanced recombination of two specific chromosomes and are often recurrently associated with a given tumor type, where they are clonally represented in each tumor case.

The precise molecular mechanisms underlying the generation of translocations remain partially unclear; however, significant advances have been made in our understanding of the events that are required for their initiation.[34] It has been documented that chromosomal translocations occur at least in part as a consequence of mistakes during Ig and TCR gene rearrangements in B and T cells, respectively, and, based on the characteristics of the chromosomal breakpoint, can be broadly divided into three groups: (1) translocations derived from mistakes of the recombination activating gene RAG-mediated V(D)J recombination process, as is the case for translocations involving IGH and CCND1 in MCL or IGH and BCL2 in follicular lymphoma (FL)[34–36]; (2) translocations mediated by errors in the AID dependent CSR process, such as those involving the Ig genes and MYC in sporadic Burkitt lymphoma (BL)[34]; (3) translocations occurring as by-products of the AID-mediated SHM mechanism, which also generates DNA breaks, such as those joining the Ig and MYC loci in endemic BL.[34] Conclusive experimental evidence for the involvement of antibody-associated remodeling events has been provided through in vivo studies performed in lymphoma-prone mouse models, where the removal of the AID enzyme was sufficient to abrogate the generation of MYC-IGH translocations in normal B cells undergoing CSR[37,38] and to prevent the development of GC-derived B-NHL.[39]

The common feature of all NHL-associated chromosomal translocations is the presence of a proto-oncogene in the proximity of the chromosomal recombination sites. In most lymphoma types, and in contrast with acute leukemias, the coding domain of the oncogene is not affected by the translocation, but its pattern of expression is altered as a consequence of the juxtaposition of heterologous regulatory sequences derived from the partner chromosome (proto-oncogene deregulation) (Fig. 37.3). This process of proto-oncogene deregulation is defined as homotopic if a proto-oncogene whose expression is tightly regulated in the normal tumor counterpart becomes constitutively expressed in the lymphoma cell, and heterotopic when the proto-oncogene is not expressed in the putative normal counterpart of the tumor cell and undergoes ectopic expression in the lymphoma. In most types of NHL-associated translocations, the heterologous regulatory sequences responsible for proto-oncogene deregulation are derived from antigen receptor loci, which are expressed at high levels in the target tissue.[34] However, in certain translocations, such as the ones involving BCL6 in diffuse large B-cell lymphoma (DLBCL), different promoter regions from distinct chromosomal sites can be found juxtaposed to the proto-oncogene in individual tumor cases, a concept known as promiscuous translocations.[40–47]

Less commonly, B-NHL associated chromosomal translocations juxtapose the coding regions of the two involved genes to form a chimeric unit that encodes for a novel fusion protein, an outcome typically observed in chromosomal translocation

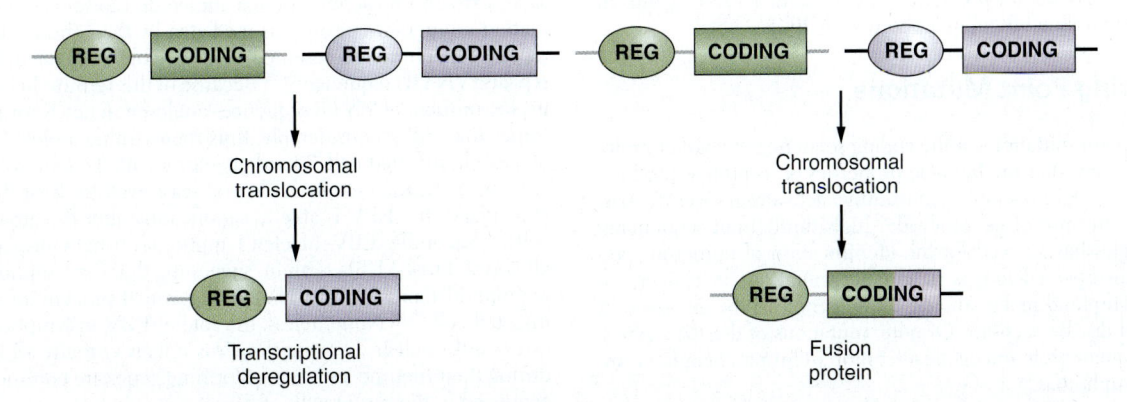

Figure 37.3 Molecular consequences of chromosomal translocations. *Top panel*: The two genes involved in prototypic chromosomal translocations are graphically represented, with their regulatory (REG) and coding sequences. Only one side of the balanced, reciprocal translocations is indicated in the figure. *Bottom panel*: Distinct outcomes of chromosomal translocations. In the case of transcriptional deregulation (*left scheme*), the normal regulatory sequences of the proto-oncogene are substituted with regulatory sequences derived from the partner chromosome, leading to deregulated expression of the proto-oncogene. In most B-NHLs, the heterologous regulatory regions derive from the IG loci. In the case of fusion proteins (*right scheme*), the coding sequences of the two involved genes are joined in frame into a chimeric transcriptional unit that encodes for a novel fusion protein, characterized by novel biochemical and functional properties.

associated with acute leukemia (see Fig. 37.3). Examples are the t(11;18) of mucosa-associated lymphoid tissue (MALT) lymphoma and the t(2;5) of anaplastic large-cell lymphoma (ALCL). The molecular cloning of the genetic loci involved in most recurrent translocations has led to the identification of a number of proto-oncogenes involved in lymphomagenesis.

Aberrant Somatic Hypermutation

The term aberrant somatic hypermutation defines a mechanism of genetic lesion that appears to derive from a malfunction in the physiologic SHM process, leading to the mutation of multiple non-Ig genes.[48] This phenomenon is uniquely associated with B-NHL and particularly with DLBCL, where over 10% of actively transcribed genes have been found mutated as a consequence of ASHM.

In GC B cells, SHM is tightly regulated both spatially and temporally to introduce mutations only in the rearranged IgV genes[49] as well as in the 5' region of a few other genes, including BCL6 and the CD79 components of the B-cell receptor,[50-53] although the functional role of mutations found in these other genes remains obscure. On the contrary, multiple mutational events were found to affect numerous loci have been found mutated in over half of DLBCL cases and, at lower frequencies, in few other lymphoma types.[54-58] The identified target loci include several well known proto-oncogenes such as PIM1, PAX5, and MYC, one of the most frequently altered human oncogenes.[48] These mutations are typically distributed within ~2 kb from the transcription initiation site (i.e., the hypermutable domain in the Ig locus)[59] and, depending on the genomic configuration of the target gene, may affect nontranslated as well as coding regions, thus holding the potential of altering the response to factors that normally regulate their expression or changing key structural and functional properties.[48] This is the case of MYC, where a significant number of amino acid substitutions have proven functional consequences in activating its oncogenic potential. Nonetheless, a comprehensive characterization of the potentially extensive genetic damage caused by ASHM is still lacking, and the mechanism involved in this malfunction has not been elucidated.

Copy Number Gains and Amplifications

In addition to chromosomal translocations and ASHM, the structure of proto-oncogenes and their pattern of expression can be altered by CN gains and amplifications, leading to overexpression of an intact protein. Compared to epithelial cancer, only a few genes have been identified so far as specific targets of amplification in B-NHL, as exemplified by REL and BCL2 in DLBCL[60-63] and by the genes encoding for programmed cell death 1 PD-1 ligands in primary mediastinal B-cell lymphoma (PMBCL).[64,65]

Activating Point Mutations

Somatic point mutations in the coding sequence of a target proto-oncogene may alter the biologic properties of its protein product, leading to its stabilization or constitutive activation. Over the past few years, the use of genomewide, high throughput sequencing technologies has allowed for the identification of numerous previously unsuspected targets of somatic mutations in cancer, including lymphoid malignancies. These genes will be discussed in individual disease sections. Of note, mutations of the RAS genes, a very frequent proto-oncogene alteration in human neoplasia, are rare in lymphomas.[66]

Inactivating Mutations and Deletions

Until recently, the TP53 gene, possibly the most common target of genetic alteration in human cancer,[67] remained one of few bona fide tumor suppressor genes involved in the pathogenesis of NHL, although at generally low frequencies and restricted to specific disease subtypes, such as BL and DLBCL derived from the transformation of FL or CLL.[68,69] The mechanism of TP53 inactivation in NHL is analogous to the one observed in human neoplasia in general, entailing a point mutation of one allele and a chromosomal deletion or mutation of the second allele. However, recent efforts taking advantage of genomewide technologies revealed several additional candidate tumor suppressor genes that are lost in B-NHL through specific chromosomal deletions and/or deleterious mutations. Two such genes lie on the long arm of chromosome 6 (6q), a region long known to be deleted in a large percentage of aggressive lymphomas associated with poor prognoses.[70,71] The PRDM1/BLIMP1 gene on 6q21 is biallelically inactivated in ~25% of ABC-DLBCL cases,[72-74] and the gene encoding for the negative nuclear factor kappa B (NF-κB) regulator A20 on chromosome 6q23 is commonly lost in ABC-DLBCL, PMBCL, and subtypes of marginal zone lymphoma and HL.[75-78] Monoallelic inactivating mutations and deletions were found to affect the acetyltransferase genes CREBBP and EP300 in a significant proportion of DLBCL and FL, suggesting a role as haploinsufficient tumor suppressors.[79] These two lymphoma types also harbor truncating mutations of MLL2,[80] which is emerging as one of the most commonly mutated genes in cancer. Among the tumor suppressors preferentially inactivated by CN losses, it is important to mention the DLEU2/miR15-a/16.1 cluster on chromosome 13q14.3, the most frequent alteration in CLL (>50% of cases),[81] and CDKN2A/B (p16/INK4a), which is inactivated by focal homozygous deletions in transformed FL (tFL), Richter syndrome (RS), and ABC-DLBCL,[82-84] and less frequently, by epigenetic transcriptional silencing in various B-NHL.[85]

Infectious Agents

Viral and bacterial infections have both been implicated in the pathogenesis of lymphoma. At least three viruses are associated with specific NHL subtypes: the Epstein-Barr virus (EBV), the human herpesvirus-8/Kaposi sarcoma–associated herpesvirus (HHV-8/KSHV), and the human T-lymphotropic virus type 1 (HTLV-1). Other infectious agents, including HIV, hepatitis C virus (HCV), Helicobacter pylori, and Chlamydophila psittaci have an indirect role in NHL pathogenesis by either impairing the immune system and/or providing chronic antigenic stimulation.

EBV was initially identified in cases of endemic African BL,[86,87] and was subsequently also detected in a fraction of sporadic BL, HIV-related lymphomas, and primary effusion lymphomas (PEL).[88-92] Upon infection, the EBV genome is transported into the nucleus of the B lymphocyte, where it exists predominantly as an extrachromosomal circular molecule (episome).[93] The formation of circular episomes is mediated by the cohesive terminal repeats, which are represented by a variable number of tandem repeats (VNTR) sequence.[93,94] Because of this termini heterogeneity, the number of VNTR sequences enclosed in newly formed episomes may differ considerably, thus representing a clonal marker of a single infected cell.[94] Evidence for a pathogenetic role of the virus in NHL infected by EBV is at least twofold. First, it is well recognized that EBV is able to significantly alter the growth of B cells.[95] Secondly, EBV-infected lymphomas usually display a single form of fused EBV termini, suggesting that the lymphoma cell population represents the clonally expanded progeny of a single infected cell.[88,89] Nonetheless, the role of EBV in lymphomagenesis is still unclear, because the virus infects virtually all humans during their lifetime and its transforming genes are commonly not expressed in the tumor cells of BL.

HHV-8 is a gammaherpesvirus initially identified in tissues of HIV-related Kaposi sarcoma[96] and subsequently found to infect PEL cells as well as a substantial fraction of multicentric Castleman disease.[96-98] Phylogenetic analysis has shown that the closest relative of HHV-8 is herpesvirus saimiri (HVS), a gamma-2 herpesvirus of primates associated with T-cell lymphoproliferative disorders.[99] Like other gammaherpesviruses, HHV-8 is also lymphotropic, and infect lymphocytes both in vitro and in vivo.[95,97,98] Lymphoma cells naturally infected by HHV-8 harbor the viral genome in its episomal configuration and display a marked restriction of viral gene expression, suggesting a pattern of latent infection.[99]

The HTLV-1 RNA retrovirus was first isolated from a cell line established from an adult T-cell leukemia/lymphoma (ATLL) patient.[100] Unlike acutely transforming retroviruses, the HTLV-1 genome does not encode a viral oncogene nor does it transform T cells by cis-activation of an adjacent cellular proto-oncogene, because the provirus appears to integrate randomly within the host genome.[101–103] The pathogenetic effect of HTLV-1 was initially attributed to the viral production of a trans-regulatory protein (HTLV-1 tax) that can activate the transcription of several host genes.[104–110] However, Tax expression is suppressed in vivo, most likely to allow for an immune escape of the infected cells, questioning its role in transformation. More recently, a viral factor has been identified, which is thought to be involved in cell proliferation and viral replication and which may be responsible for HTLV-1–mediated lymphomagenesis.

An association between B-NHL and infection by HCV, a single stranded RNA virus of the Flaviviridae family, has been proposed based on the increased risk of developing lymphoproliferative disorders observed among HCV-positive patients[111] and also on the results of interventional studies demonstrating that eradication of HCV with antiviral treatment could directly induce lymphoma regression in seropositive patients affected by indolent NHL.[112] Although the underlying mechanisms remain unclear, current models suggest that chronic B-cell stimulation by antigens associated with HCV infection may induce nonmalignant B-cell expansion, which subsequently evolves into B-NHL by accumulating additional genetic lesions.

The causative link between antigen stimulation by *H. pylori* and MALT lymphoma originating in the stomach is documented by the observation that *H. pylori* can be found in the vast majority of the lymphoma specimens,[113–115] and eradication of infection with antibiotics leads to long-term complete regression in 70% of cases.[116] However, cases with t(11;18)(q21;21) respond poorly to antibiotic eradication,[117] suggesting additional players.

C. psittaci, an obligate intracellular bacterium, was recently linked to the development of ocular adnexal marginal zone B-cell lymphoma (MZL), although variations in prevalence among different geographical areas remain a major investigational issue.[118,119] In this indolent lymphoma, *C. psittaci* causes both local and systemic persistent infection, and presumably contributes to lymphomagenesis through its mitogenic activity and its ability to promote polyclonal cell proliferation and resistance to apoptosis in the infected cells in vivo. Notably, bacterial eradication with antibiotic therapy is often followed by lymphoma regression.[120]

MOLECULAR PATHOGENESIS OF B-NHL

The following section will focus on well-characterized genetic lesions that are associated with the most common types of B-NHL, classified according to the World Health Organization (WHO) classification of lymphoid neoplasia.[1] The molecular pathogenesis of HIV-related NHL will also be addressed, whereas the pathogenesis of other B-cell NHLs remains far less understood. Lymphoblastic lymphoma, which is considered the same disease as T- and B-acute lymphoblastic leukemia, will not be covered in this chapter.

Mantle Cell Lymphoma

Cell of Origin

Mantle cell lymphoma is an aggressive disease representing ~5% of all NHL diagnoses and generally regarded as incurable.[1] Based on immunophenotype, gene expression profile, and molecular features, such as the presence of unmutated IgV genes in the vast majority of cases, MCL has been historically considered as derived from naïve, pre-GC peripheral B cells located in the inner mantle zone of secondary follicles (see Fig. 37.1).[171] More recently, the observation of BCR diversity, including *IGHV* hypermutation, in a subset of tumor cases (15% to 40%) has shifted this paradigm, suggesting the existence of distinct molecular subtypes, including one influenced by the CG environment.

Genetic Lesions

MCL is typically associated with the t(11;14)(q13;q32) translocation, that juxtaposes the *IGH* gene at 14q32 to a region containing the *CCND1* gene (also known as *BCL1*) on chromosome 11q13.[122–124] The translocation consistently leads to homotopic deregulation and overexpression of cyclin D1, a member of the D-type G1 cyclins that regulates the early phases of the cell cycle and is normally not expressed in resting B cells.[125–127] By deregulating cyclin D1, t(11;14) is thought to contribute to malignant transformation by perturbing the G1-S phase transition of the cell cycle.[121] Importantly, the frequency and specificity of this genetic lesion, together with the expression of cyclin D1 in the tumor cells, provides an excellent marker for MCL diagnosis.[1]

In addition to t(11;14), up to 10% of MCLs overexpress aberrant or shorter cyclin D1 transcripts, as a consequence of secondary rearrangements, microdeletions, or point mutations in the gene 3′ untranslated region.[128–130] These alterations lead to cyclin D1 overexpression through the removal of destabilizing sequences and the consequent increase in the mRNA half life, and are more commonly observed in cases characterized by high proliferative activity and a more aggressive clinical course. The pathogenic role of cyclin D1 deregulation in human neoplasia is suggested by the ability of the encoded protein to transform cells in vitro and to promote B-cell lymphomagenesis in transgenic mice, although only when combined to other oncogenic events[131,132]; however, an animal model that faithfully recapitulates the features of the human MCL is still lacking.

Other genetic alterations involved in MCL include biallelic inactivation of the *ATM* gene by genomic deletions and mutations,[133] loss of *TP53* (20% of patients, where it represents a marker of poor prognosis),[134] and inactivation of the *CDKN2A* gene by deletions, point mutations, or promoter hypermethylation (approximately half of the cases belonging to the MCL variant characterized by a blastoid cell morphology).[135] Also associated with aggressive tumors are mutations activating the Notch signaling pathway, including *NOTCH1* (12% of clinical samples) and *NOTCH2* (5% of samples); these lesions, which are mutually exclusive, mostly consist of truncating events that remove the PEST sequences required for NOTCH protein degradation and, thus, lead to protein stabilization.[136,137] Other recurrent mutations were reported in genes encoding the antiapoptotic protein BIRC3, the Toll-like receptor 2 (TLR2), the chromatin modifiers WHSC1 and MLL2, and the MEF2B transcription factor.[136] In a small number of cases, *BMI1* is amplified and/or overexpressed, possibly as an alternative mechanism to the loss of *CDKN2A*.[138,139]

Burkitt Lymphoma

Cell of Origin

BL is an aggressive lymphoma comprising three clinical variants, namely sporadic BL (sBL), endemic BL (eBL), and HIV-associated BL, often diagnosed as the initial manifestation of AIDS.[1] In all variants, the presence of highly mutated IgV sequences[140–143] and the expression of a distinct transcriptional signature[144,145] unequivocally confirm the derivation from a GC B cell.

Genetic Lesions

All BL cases, including the leukemic variants, share a virtually obligatory genetic lesion (i.e., chromosomal translocations involving the MYC gene on region 8q24 and one of the Ig loci on the partner chromosome).[146,147] In ~80% of cases, this is represented by the IGH locus, leading to t(8;14)(q24;q32), whereas in the remaining 20% of cases, either IGκ (2p12) or IGλ (22q11) are involved.[146–149] Although fairly homogeneous at the microscopic level, these translocations display a high degree of molecular heterogeneity, the breakpoints being located 5' and centromeric to MYC in t(8;14), but mapping 3' to MYC in t(2;8) and t(8;22).[146–150] Further molecular heterogeneity derives from the exact breakpoint sites observed on chromosomes 8 and 14 in t(8;14): Translocations of eBL tend to involve sequences at an undefined distance (>1,000 kb) 5' to MYC on chromosome 8 and sequences within or in proximity to the IGHJ region on chromosome 14.[151,152] In sBL, t(8;14) preferentially involves sequences within or immediately 5' to MYC (<3 kb) on chromosome 8 and within the IGH switch regions on chromosome 14.[151,152]

The common consequence of t(8;14), t(2;8) and t(8;22) is the ectopic and constitutive overexpression of the MYC proto-oncogene,[153–155] which is normally absent in the majority of proliferating GC B cells,[13] in part due to BCL6-mediated transcriptional repression.[156] Oncogenic activation of MYC in BL is mediated by at least three distinct mechanisms: (1) juxtaposition of the MYC coding sequences to heterologous enhancers derived from the Ig loci;[153–155] (2) structural alterations of the gene 5' regulatory sequences, which affect the responsiveness to cellular factors controlling its expression[157] — in particular, the MYC exon 1/intron 1 junction encompasses critical regulatory elements that are either decapitated by the translocation or mutated in the translocated alleles; and (3) amino acid substitutions within the gene exon 2, encoding for the protein transactivation domain.[158,159] These mutations can abolish the ability of p107, a nuclear protein related to RB1, to suppress MYC activity[160] or increase protein stability.[161,162]

MYC is a nuclear phosphoprotein that functions as a sequence-specific DNA-binding transcriptional regulator controlling proliferation, cell growth, differentiation, and apoptosis, all of which are implicated in carcinogenesis.[163] In addition, MYC controls DNA replication independent of its transcriptional activity, a property that may promote genomic instability by inducing replication stress.[164] Consistent with its involvement in multiple cellular processes, the MYC target gene network is estimated to include ~15% of all protein-coding genes as well as noncoding RNAs.[163,165] In vivo, MYC is found mainly in heterodimeric complexes with the related protein MAX, and such interaction is required for MYC-induced stimulation of transcription and cell proliferation.[166–172] In NHL carrying MYC translocations, constitutive expression of MYC induces the transcription of target genes with diverse roles in regulating cell growth by affecting DNA replication, energy metabolism, protein synthesis, and telomere elongation.[163,172,173] Furthermore, deregulated MYC expression is thought to cause genomic instability, and thus contributes to tumor progression by facilitating the occurrence of additional genetic lesions.[174] Dysregulation of MYC expression in a number of transgenic mouse models leads to the development of aggressive B-cell lymphomas with high penetrance and short latency.[162,175,176] These mouse models confirm the pathogenetic role of deregulated MYC in B cells, although the resulting tumors tend to be more immature than the human BL, most likely due to the early activation of the promoter sequences used for the expression of the MYC transgene.

More recently, the application of new genomics technologies revealed additional oncogenic mechanisms that cooperate with MYC in the development of this aggressive lymphoma. Mutations of the transcription factor 3 (TCF3) (10% to 25%) and its negative regulator ID3 (35% to 58%) are highly recurrent in all three subtypes of BL, where they promote tonic (antigen-independent) BCR signaling and sustain survival of the tumor cell by engaging the phosphoinositide 3-kinase (PI3K) pathway (Fig. 37.4).[177] In addition, TCF3 can promote cell-cycle progression by transactivating CCND3. Notably, CCND3 is itself a target of gain-of-function mutations in 38% of sBL, where these events affect conserved residues in the carboxyl terminus of this D-type cyclin, which are implicated in the control of protein stability, leading to higher expression levels. Interestingly, CCND3 mutations occur in only 2.6% of eBL, suggesting alternative oncogenic mechanisms in this subtype.[177] Other common genetic lesions include the loss of TP53 by mutation and/or deletion (35% of both sBL and eBL cases),[68] inactivation of CDKN2B by deletion or hypermethylation (17% of samples),[85] and deletions of 6q, detected in ~30% of cases, independent of the clinical variant.[70] Finally, one contributing factor to the development of BL is monoclonal EBV infection, present in virtually all cases of eBL and in ~30% of sBL.[86,88,178,179] The consistent expression of EBER, a class of small RNA molecules, has been proposed to mediate the transforming potential of EBV in BL.[180] However, EBV infection in BL displays a peculiar latent infection phenotype characterized by negativity of both EBV-transforming antigens LMP1 and EBNA2; thus, the precise pathogenetic role of this virus has remained elusive.[181]

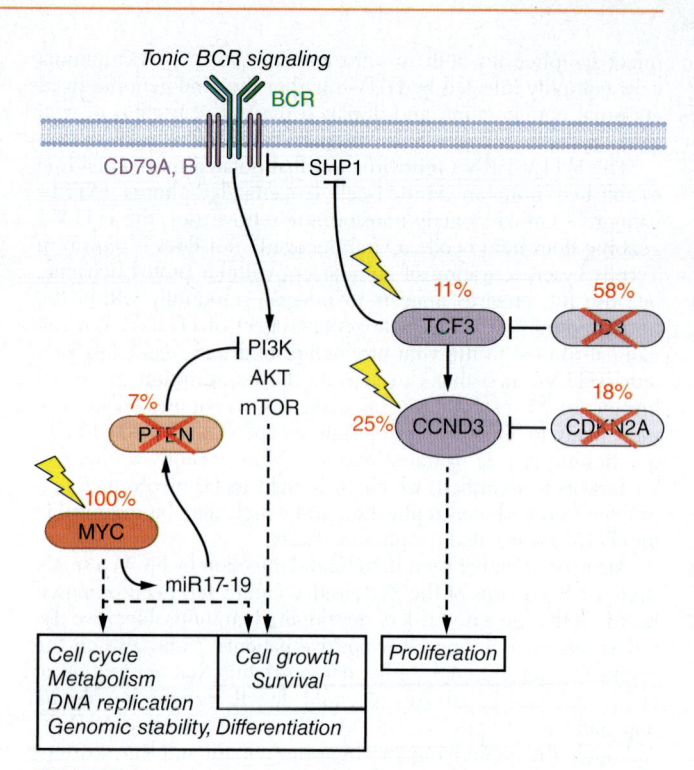

Figure 37.4 Most common genetic lesions identified in BL. *Lightning bolts* indicate activating mutations and *crosses* denote inactivating events. mTOR, mammalian target of rapamycin.

Follicular Lymphoma

FL represents the second most common type of B-NHL (~20% of diagnoses) and the most common low-grade B-NHL.[1] It is an indolent but largely incurable disease, characterized by a continuous pattern of progression and relapses that often culminates in its histologic transformation to an aggressive lymphoma with a diffuse large cell architecture and a dismal prognosis (20% to 30% of cases).[182,183]

Cell of Origin

The ontogeny of FL from a GC B cell is supported by the expression of specific GC B-cell markers such as BCL6 and CD10, together with the presence of somatically mutated Ig genes showing evidence of ongoing SHM activity.[1]

Genetic Lesions

The genetic hallmark of FL is represented by chromosomal translocations affecting the BCL2 gene on chromosome band 18q21, which are detected in 80% to 90% of cases independent of cytologic subtype, although less frequent in grade 3 FL.[184–187] These rearrangements join the 3' untranslated region of BCL2 to an IG J_H segment, resulting in the ectopic expression of BCL2 in GC B cells,[184,185,188–192] where its transcription is normally repressed by BCL6.[18,193] Approximately 70% of the breakpoints on chromosome 18 cluster within the major breakpoint region, whereas the remaining 5% to 25% map to the more distant minor cluster region, located ~20 kb downstream of the BCL2 gene.[184,185,188,189] Rearrangements involving the 5' flanking region of BCL2 have been described in a minority of cases.[194] The BCL2 gene encodes a 26-kd integral membrane protein that controls the cell apoptotic threshold by preventing programmed cell death and, thus, may contribute to lymphomagenesis by inducing apoptosis resistance in tumor cells independent of antigen selection. Nevertheless, additional genetic aberrations are required for malignant transformation. Most prominent among them are mutations in multiple epigenetic modifiers, including the methyltransferase MLL2 (80% to 90% of cases),[80] the polycomb-group oncogene EZH2 (7% of patients),[195] the acetyltransferases CREBBP and EP300 (40% of cases),[79,80] and multiple core histones,[196] which may all contribute to transformation by remodeling the epigenetic landscape of the precursor tumor cell. A major role is also played by chronic antigen stimulation.[197,198]

Whole-exome sequencing and CN analysis of sequential, clonally related FL and tFL biopsies has recently provided the ability to characterize the molecular events that are specifically acquired during histologic progression to DLBCL, and thus presumably play a major role in governing this process. tFL-specific lesions include inactivation of CDKN2A/B through deletion, mutation, and hypermethylation (one-third of patients),[84,136,199] rearrangements and amplifications of MYC,[84,200] TP53 mutations/deletions (25% to 30% of cases),[69,201–203] loss of chromosome 6 (20%),[70] ASHM, and although larger cohorts of patients will need to be studied, biallelic loss of the immune regulator B2M.[84] Chromosomal translocations of the BCL6 gene are detected in 6% to 14% of all FL cases, and were shown to have a significantly higher prevalence in the group of patients that undergo transformation into aggressive DLBCL.[204–207]

Diffuse Large B-Cell Lymphoma

DLBCL is the most common form of B-NHL, accounting for ~40% of all new diagnoses in adulthood and including cases that arise de novo, as well as cases that derive from the clinical evolution of various, less aggressive B-NHL types (i.e., FL and CLL).[1,208]

Cell of Origin

Based on gene expression profile analysis, at least three well-characterized molecular subtypes have been recognized within this diagnostic entity, which reflect the derivation from B cells at various developmental stages. Germinal center B-cell–like (GCB) DLBCL appears to derive from proliferating GC cells; ABC-DLBCL shows a transcriptional signature related to BCR-activated B cells or to B cells committed to plasmablastic differentiation; and PMBCL is postulated to arise from post-GC thymic B cells. The remaining 15% to 30% of cases remain unclassified.[209–212] Stratification according to gene expression profiles has prognostic value, because patients diagnosed with GCB-DLBCL display better overall survival compared to ABC-DLBCL,[63] but is imperfectly replicated by immunophenotyping or morphology and does not presently inform differential therapy[213,214]; thus, it is not officially incorporated into the WHO classification. A separate classification schema identified three discrete subsets defined by the expression of genes involved in oxidative phosphorylation, B-cell receptor/proliferation, and tumor microenvironment/host inflammatory response.[215]

Genetic Lesions

The heterogeneity of DLBCL is reflected in the catalog of genetic lesions that are associated with its pathogenesis, and include balanced reciprocal translocations, gene amplifications, chromosomal deletions, single point mutations, and relatively unique among all NHL, ASHM. During the past few years, the application of genomewide approaches such as whole-exome/transcriptome/genome sequencing and single nucleotide polymorphism (SNP) array analysis have provided a comprehensive picture of the DLBCL genomic landscape. One important finding of these studies is that, compared to other B-cell malignancies, DLBCL shows a significantly higher degree of genomic complexity, harboring on average 50 to more than 100 lesions per case, with great diversity across patients.[80,216,217] Although many of the identified lesions can be variably found in both molecular subtypes of the disease, consistent with a general role during transformation, others appear to be preferentially or exclusively associated with individual DLBCL subtypes, indicating that GCB and ABC-DLBCL utilize distinct oncogenic pathways (Fig. 37.5).

GCB and ABC Shared Lesions. The most prominent program disrupted in DLBCL, independent of subtype, is represented by epigenetic regulation of chromatin due to mutations in the CREBBP/EP300 acetyltransferase genes (35% of cases) and the MLL2 H3K4 trimethyltransferase (~30% of cases).[79,80,217] These lesions may favor tumor development by reprogramming the cancer epigenome and, in the case of CREBBP/EP300, by altering the balance between the activity of the BCL6 oncogene, which is typically inactivated by acetylation, and the tumor suppressor p53, which requires acetylation at specific residues for its function.[79]

Deregulated activity of the BCL6 oncoprotein due to a multitude of genetic lesions is also a major contributor to DLBCL pathogenesis, in both GCB and ABC-DLBCL. Chromosomal rearrangements of the BCL6 gene at band 3q27 are observed in up to 35% of cases,[71,205,218] although with a twofold higher frequency in the ABC-DLBCL subtype (see Fig. 37.4).[219] These rearrangements juxtapose the intact coding domain of BCL6 downstream and in the same transcriptional orientation to heterologous sequences derived from the partner chromosome, including IGH (14q23), IGκ (2p12), IGλ (22q11), and at least 20 other chromosomal sites unrelated to the IG loci.[40–47] The majority of these translocations result in a fusion transcript in which the promoter region and the first noncoding exon of BCL6 are replaced by sequences derived from the partner gene.[41,220] Because the common denominator of these promoters is a broader spectrum of activity throughout B-cell development, including expression in the post-GC differentiation stage, the translocation is thought to prevent the downregulation of BCL6 expression that is normally associated with differentiation into post-GC cells. Deregulated expression of an intact BCL6 gene product is also sustained by a variety of indirect mechanisms, including gain-of-function mutations in its positive regulator MEF2B (~11% of cases),[221] inactivating mutations/deletions of CREBBP/EP300,[79] and mutations/deletions of FBXO11 (~5%),[222] which encodes a ubiquitin ligase involved in the control of BCL6 protein degradation. These lesions play a critical role in lymphomagenesis by enforcing the proliferative phenotype typical of GC cells, while suppressing proper DNA damage responses; moreover, constitutive expression of BCL6 blocks terminal differentiation, as confirmed by a mouse model in which deregulated BCL6 expression causes DLBCL.[223]

DLBCL cells have also acquired the ability to escape both arms of immune surveillance, including cytotoxic T lympocytes (CTL)-mediated cytotoxicity (through genetic loss of the B2M/human leukocyte antigen class I [HLA-I] genes) and natural killer (NK) cell–mediated death (through genetic loss of the CD58 molecule).[224] Analogous effects may be achieved in PMBCL by disruption of the major histocompatibility complex class II

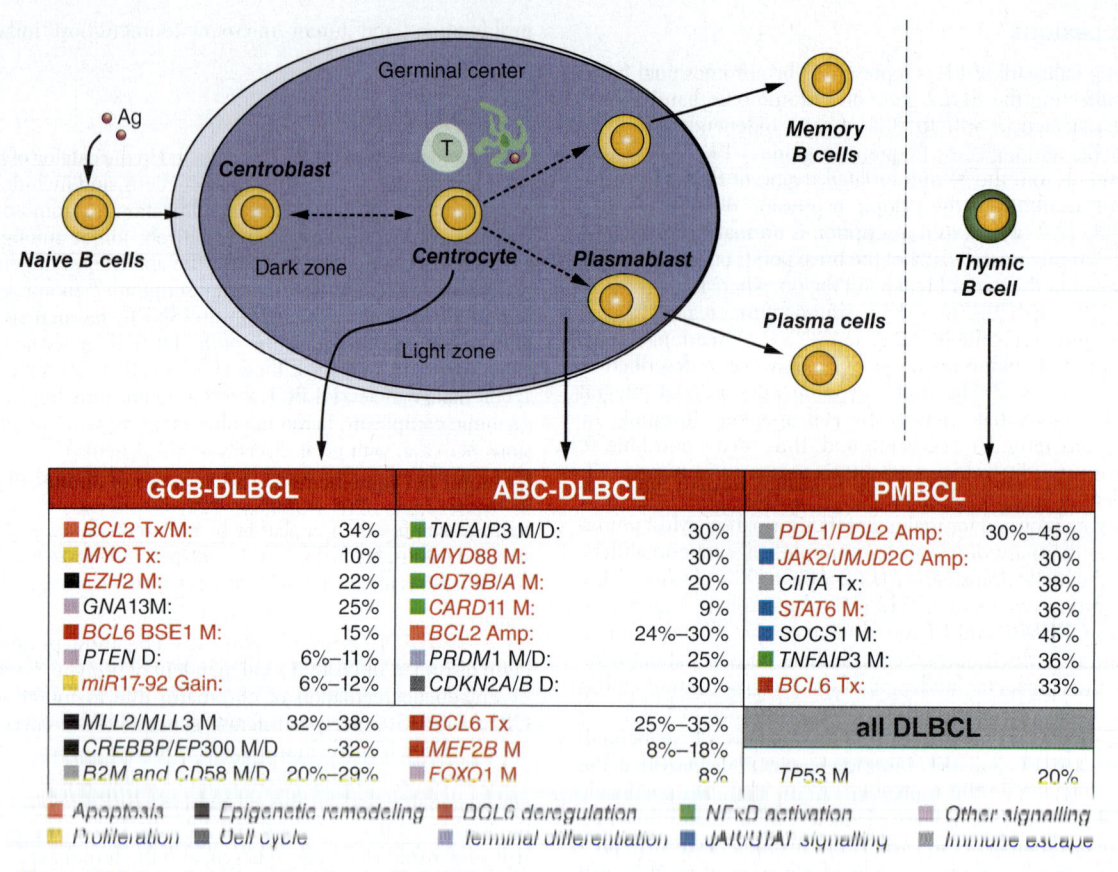

Figure 37.5 Genetic lesions associated with DLBCL. Most common genetic lesions identified in the three major DLBCL subtypes, including lesions that are shared between GCB- and ABC-DLBCL and lesions that are preferentially segregating with individual molecular subtypes. Loss-of-function alterations are in *black* and gain-of-function events are in *red*. Color-coded squares denote the biologic function/signaling pathway affected by the alteration.

(MHC-II) transactivator class II major histocompatibility complex transactivator (CIITA) and amplification of the genes encoding for the immunomodulatory proteins PDL1/PDL2.

Finally, approximately 50% of all DLBCL are associated with ASHM.[48] The number and identity of the genes that accumulate mutations in their coding and noncoding regions due to this mechanism varies in different cases and is still largely undefined. However, preferential targeting of individual genes has been observed in the two main DLBCL subtypes, with mutations of MYC and BCL2 being found at significantly higher frequencies in GCB-DLBCL, and mutations of PIM1 almost exclusively observed in ABC-DLBCL. ASHM may, therefore, contribute to the heterogeneity of DLBCL via the alteration of different cellular pathways in different cases. Mutations and deletions of the TP53 tumor suppressor gene are detectable in ~20% of cases, including those that originate from the transformation of FL, and are more often associated with chromosomal translocations involving BCL2.[69]

GCB-DLBCL. Genetic lesions specific to GCB-DLBCL include the t(14;18) and t(8;14) translocations, which deregulate the BCL2 and MYC oncogenes in 34% and 10% of cases, respectively.[63,193,225,226] Also exquisitely restricted to this subtype are mutations of the EZH2 gene,[195] which encodes a histone methyltransferase responsible for trimethylating Lys27 of histone H3 (H3K27), mutations of the S1PR2 adaptor protein GNA13, mutations affecting an autoregulatory domain within the BCL6 5' untranslated exon 1,[219,227,228] and deletions of the tumor suppressor PTEN.[83,229]

Somatic mutations of the BCL6 5' regulatory sequences are detected in up to 75% of DLBCL cases[52,230,231] and reflect the activity of the physiologic SHM mechanism that operates in normal GC B cells.[52,53] However, a functional analysis of numerous mutated BCL6 alleles uncovered a subset of mutations that are specifically associated with GCB-DLBCL and that are not observed in normal GC cells or in other B-cell malignancies.[227] These mutations deregulate BCL6 transcription by disrupting an autoregulatory circuit through which the BCL6 protein controls its own expression levels via binding to the promoter region of the gene[227,228] or by preventing CD40-induced BCL6 downregulation in post-GC B cells.[232] Because the full extent of mutations deregulating BCL6 expression has not been characterized, the fraction of DLBCL cases carrying abnormalities in BCL6 cannot be determined.

ABC-DLBCL. Several genetic abnormalities are observed almost exclusively in ABC-DLBCL, including amplifications of the BCL2 locus on 18q24[233,234]; mutations within the NF-κB (CARD11, TNFAIP3/A20),[75,235] B-cell receptor (CD79B),[236] and TLR (MYD88)[237] signaling pathways; inactivating mutations and deletions of BLIMP1[72–74]; chromosomal translocations deregulating the BCL6 oncogene; and deletion or lack of expression of the p16 tumor suppressor. Mutations of the ATM gene have been reported in a small subset of cases.[238]

A predominant feature of ABC-DLBCL is the constitutive activation of the NF-κB signaling pathway, initially evidenced by the selective expression of a signature enriched in NF-κB target genes, and by the requirement of NF-κB for proliferation and survival of ABC-DLBCL cell lines. This phenotype is sustained by a variety of alterations affecting positive and negative regulators of NF-κB, as well as other adaptor molecules converging on activation of NF-κB, specifically in this disease subtype. In up to 30% of cases, the TNFAIP3 gene, encoding for the negative regulator A20, is biallelically inactivated by mutations and/or deletions, thus preventing termination of NF-κB responses.[75,76] The tumor suppressor role of A20 was documented by the observation that reconstitution of A20 knockout cell lines with a wild-type protein induces apoptosis and blocks proliferation, in part due to suppression of NF-κB activity.[75,76] In an additional ~10% of ABC-DLBCL, the *CARD11* gene is targeted by oncogenic mutations clustering in the protein coiled-coil domain and enhancing its ability to transactivate NF-κB target genes.[235] Less commonly, mutations were found in a variety of other genes encoding for NF-κB components, overall accounting for over half of all ABC-DLBCL[75] and suggesting that yet unidentified lesions may be responsible for the NF-κB activity in the remaining fraction of cases.

In addition to constitutive NF-κB activity, ABC-DLBCLs display evidence of chronic active BCR signaling, which is associated with somatic mutations affecting the immunoreceptor tyrosine-based activation motif (ITAM) signaling modules of *CD79B* and *CD79A* in 10% of ABC-DLBCL biopsy samples, but rarely in other DLBCLs.[236] Moreover, silencing several BCR proximal and distal subunits is toxic to ABC-DLBCL. These findings provided genetic evidence in support of the development of therapies targeting BCR signaling,[236] and indeed, kinase inhibitors that interfere with this signaling pathway are emerging as a new treatment paradigm for ABC-DLBCL.

Approximately 30% of ABC-DLBCL patients harbor a recurrent change in the intracellular Toll/interleukin-1 receptor domain of the MYD88 adaptor molecule, which has the potential to activate NF-κB as well as JAK/STAT3 transcriptional responses.[237] Although the relationship between *MYD88* mutations and TLR signaling has not been studied, MYD88 was shown to be required for the survival of ABC-DLBCLs, indicating a pathogenic role for TLR in this disease type.

A second important program that is disrupted by genetic lesions in ABC-DLBCL includes terminal B-cell differentiation. In up to 25% of ABC-DLBCL cases, the *PRDM1* gene is inactivated by biallelic truncating or missense mutations and/or genomic deletions, as well as by transcriptional repression through constitutively active, translocated *BCL6* alleles.[72-74] The *PRDM1* gene encodes for a zinc finger transcriptional repressor that is expressed in a subset of GC B cells undergoing plasma cell differentiation and in all plasma cells,[239,240] and is an essential requirement for terminal B-cell differentiation.[241] Thus, BLIMP1 inactivation contributes to lymphomagenesis by blocking post-GC B-cell differentiation. Consistently, translocations deregulating the *BCL6* gene are exceedingly rare in *BLIMP1* mutated DLBCLs, suggesting that BCL6 deregulation and BLIMP1 inactivation represent alternative oncogenic mechanisms converging on the same pathway (Fig. 37.6).

PMBCL. PMBCL is a tumor observed most commonly in young female adults, which involves the mediastinum and displays a distinct gene expression profile, largely similar to HL.[211,212] A genetic hallmark of both PMBCL and HL is the amplification of chromosomal region 9q24, detected in nearly 50% of patients.[83,242] This relatively large interval encompasses multiple genes of possible pathogenetic significance, including the gene encoding for the JAK2 tyrosine kinase and the *PDL1/PDL2* genes, which encode for inhibitors of T-cell responses[64,83,242] and have been linked to impaired antitumor immune responses in several cancers. Other lesions affecting regulators of immune responses in PMBCL include genomic breakpoints and mutations of the MHC class II transactivator gene *CIITA*, which may reduce tumor cell immunogenicity by downregulating surface HLA class II expression.[64,65,243] The ability of the previously mentioned lesions to interfere with the interaction between the lymphoma cells and the microenvironment suggests a central role for escape from immuno-surveillance mechanisms. Besides contributing to lymphomagenesis, elevated expression levels of these genes may, in part, explain the unique features of these lymphoma types, which are characterized by a significant inflammatory infiltrate. PMBCL also shares with HL the presence of genetic lesions affecting the NF-κB pathway and

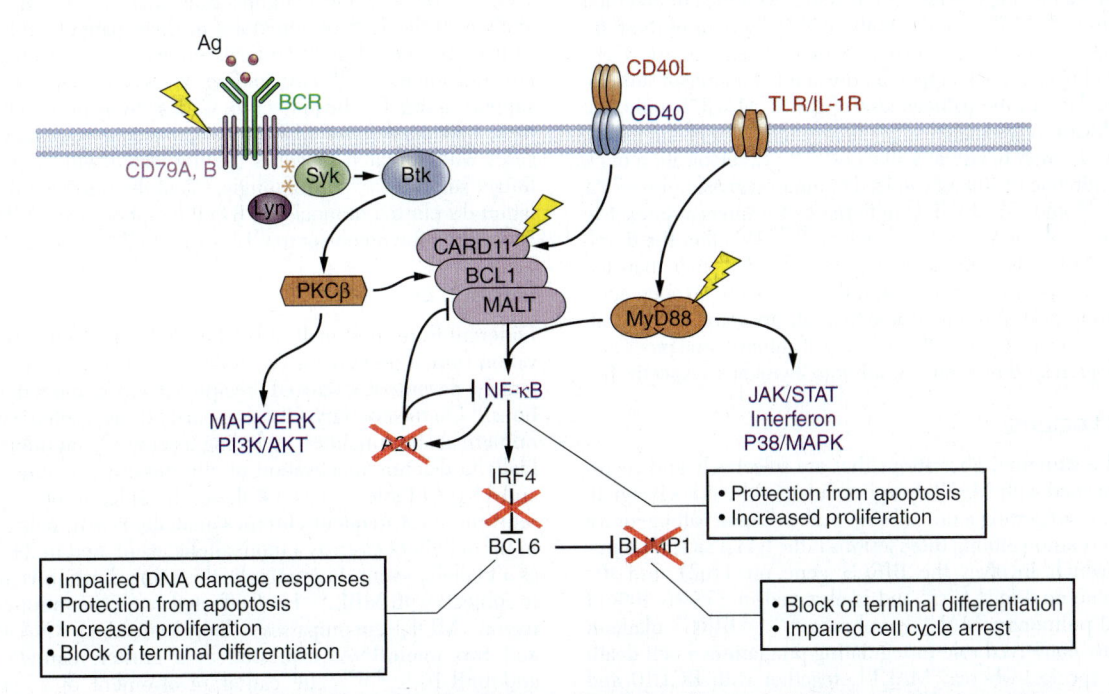

Figure 37.6 Pathway lesions in ABC-DLBCL. Schematic representation of a germinal center centrocyte, expressing a functional surface BCR, a CD40 receptor and a TLR. In normal B cells, engagement of the BCR by the antigen (spheres), interaction of the CD40 receptor with the CD40L presented by T-cells, and activation of the TLR converge on activation of the NF-κB pathway, including its targets IRF4 and A20 among others. IRF4, in turn, downregulates BCL6 expression, allowing the release of BLIMP1 expression, a master plasma cell regulator required for terminal differentiation. In ABC-DLBCL, multiple genetic lesions disrupt this pathway at multiple levels in different cases (percentages as indicated); these lesions contribute to lymphomagenesis by favoring the antiapoptotic and pro-proliferative function of NF-κB, as well as chronic active BCR and JAK/STAT3 signaling, while blocking terminal B-cell differentiation through mutually exclusive deregulation of BCL6 and inactivation of BLIMP1.

the deregulated expression of receptor tyrosine kinases.[78,244–246] In particular, mutations of the transcription factor *STAT6*, amplifications/overexpression of *JAK2* (which promote STAT6 activation via interleukin 3 (IL-3)/IL-4), and inactivating mutations of its negative regulator *SOCS1* are highly recurrent in PMBCL, pointing to the JAK/STAT signaling pathway as a major disease contributor.

DLBCL Derived from CLL and FL Transformation. Recently, exome sequencing studies examining sequential biopsies of CLL/RS or FL/tFL have provided insights onto the molecular mechanisms that drive the transformation process. These analyses extended the set of genetic lesions that are specifically acquired during transformation and include *CDKN2A/B* loss, *TP53* loss, and *MYC* translocations (in both conditions), along with ASHM and *B2M* inactivation in tFL, or *NOTCH1* mutations in RS.[82,84] They also allowed for reconstruction of the evolutionary history of the dominant tumor clone during transformation, revealing that FL and tFL derive from a common ancestor mutated clone through divergent evolution, as opposed to RS, which, analogous to CLL progression,[247] arises from the predominant CLL clone through a linear pattern. Finally, comparison with de novo DLBCL showed that, despite their morphologic resemblance, the genomic landscapes of RS and tFL are largely unique in that they are characterized by distinct combinations of alterations otherwise not commonly observed in de novo DLBCL/NOS.[82,84]

Extranodal Marginal Zone Lymphoma of Mucosa-Associated Lymphoid Tissue (MALT)

Cell of Origin

Mucosa-associated lymphoid tissue (MALT) lymphoma represents the third most common form of NHL,[1] and has steadily risen in incidence over the last 2 decades.[248] The presence of rearranged and somatically mutated IgV genes,[31,249] together with the architectural relationship with MALT,[1] indicate the post-GC origin of these tumors, possibly from a marginal zone memory B cell (see Fig. 37.1). A number of observations support a critical role for antigen stimulation, particularly in the pathogenesis of gastric MALT lymphoma: (1) This disease is associated with chronic infection of the gastric mucosa by *H. pylori* in virtually all cases[113–115]; (2) eradication of *H. pylori* by antibiotic treatment can lead to tumor regression in ~70% of cases[116,250]; and (3) MALT lymphoma cells express autoreactive BCR, in particular to rheumatoid factors.[251,252] Whether the development of MALT lymphoma arising in body sites other than the stomach also depends on antigen stimulation remains an open question. In this respect, it is remarkable that salivary gland and thyroid MALT lymphoma are generally a sequela of autoimmune processes, namely Sjögren syndrome and Hashimoto thyroiditis, respectively.

Genetic Lesions

Most of the structural aberrations that are selectively and recurrently associated with MALT lymphoma target the NF-κB signaling pathway, suggesting a critical role in the disease pathogenesis. The most common among these lesions is the t(11;18)(q21;q21) translocation, which involves the *BIRC3* gene on 11q21 and the *MALT1* gene on 18q21,[253,254] and is observed in 25% to 40% of gastric and pulmonary MALT lymphomas.[255–257] BIRC3 plays an evolutionary conserved role in regulating programmed cell death in diverse species, whereas MALT1, together with BCL10 and CARD11, is a component of the ternary complex that plays a central role in BCR and NF-κB signaling activation.[258] Notably, the wild-type proteins encoded by these two genes are incapable of activating NF-κB, in contrast to the BIRC3/MALT1 fusion protein, suggesting that the translocation confer a survival advantage to the tumor by leading to inhibition of apoptosis and constitutive NF-κB activation without the need for upstream signaling.[253,254,259] In an additional 15% to 20% of cases, *MALT1* is translocated to the IGH locus as a consequence of t(14;18)(q32;q21),[260,261] whereas ~5% of patients harbor abnormalities of chromosomal band 1p22, generally represented by t(1;14)(p22;q32); the latter deregulates the expression of *BCL10*, a cellular homolog of the equine herpesvirus-2 *E10* gene, which contains an amino-terminal caspase recruitment domain (CARD) homologous to that found in several apoptotic molecules.[262,263] BCL10, however, does not have proapoptotic activity in vivo, where it functions as a positive regulator of antigen-induced activation of NF-κB.[258,264,265] Thus, the translocation may provide both antiapoptotic and proliferative signals mediated via NF-κB transcriptional targets.

A more recently identified translocation associated, although not restricted to, MALT lymphoma is t(3;14)(p13;q32),[266,267] which leads to the deregulated expression of FOXP1, a member of the Forkhead box family of winged-helix transcription factors involved in the regulation of Rag1 and Rag2 and essential for B-cell development.[268] Finally, homozygous or hemizygous loss of *TNFAIP3* due to mutations and/or deletions has been reported in 20% of MALT lymphoma patients, typically in a mutually exclusive pattern with other alterations leading to NF-κB activation.[77] Other recurrent genetic lesions in this disease include trisomy 3,[269,270] *BCL6* alterations, and *TP53* mutations.[271–273]

Chronic Lymphocytic Leukemia

Cell of Origin

CLL is a malignancy of mature, resting B lymphocytes that originates from the oncogenic transformation of a common precursor resembling an antigen experienced B cell.[274] This notion was conclusively demonstrated when gene expression profile studies revealed that, although CLL can express somatically mutated or unmutated IgV genes at approximately equal percentages,[275,276] all cases share a homogeneous signature more related to that of CD27+ memory and marginal zone B cells.[277,278] Moreover, an analysis of the Ig gene repertoire in these patients indicates very similar, at times almost identical, antigen receptors among different individuals.[279–284] This finding, known as *stereotypy*, strongly supports a role for the antigen in CLL pathogenesis. The histogenetic heterogeneity of CLL carries prognostic relevance, because cases with mutated Ig genes are associated with a significantly longer survival.[285,286] Intriguingly, 6% of the normal elderly population develops a monoclonal B-cell lymphocytosis (MBL) that is considered the precursor to CLL in 1% to 2% of cases.[287]

Genetic Lesions

Different from most mature B-NHL and consistent with the derivation from a post-GC or GC-independent B cell, CLL cases are largely devoid of balanced, reciprocal chromosomal translocations.[81] On the contrary, CLL is recurrently associated with several numerical abnormalities, including trisomy 12 and monoallelic or biallelic deletion/inactivation of chromosomal regions 17p, 11q, and 13q14 (Table 37.1).[81] Of these, the deletion of 13q14 represents the most frequent chromosomal aberration, being observed in up to 76% of cases as a monoallelic event, and in 24% of cases as a biallelic event. Interestingly, this same deletion is also found in subjects with MBL.[287] In all affected cases, the minimal deleted region (MDR) encompasses a long noncoding RNA (*DLEU2*) and two microRNAs expressed as a cluster, namely miR-15a and miR-16-1.[288–290] The causal involvement of 13q14–MDR-encoded tumor suppressor genes in CLL pathogenesis was demonstrated in vivo in two animal models, which developed clonal lymphoproliferative diseases with features of MBL, CLL, and DLBCL at 75% to 40% penetrance.[291] Trisomy 12 is found in approximately 16% of patients evaluated by interphase fluorescent in situ hybridization and correlates with poor survival, but no specific gene(s) have been identified.[292–294] Deletions of chromosomal region 11q22-23 (18% of cases) almost invariably encompass the

TABLE 37.1 Most Common Genetic Lesions Associated with Non-Hodgkin Lymphoma

NHL Subtype	Genetic Abnormality	Cases Affected (%)	Involved Gene	Functional Consequences	Gene Function
Mantle cell lymphoma	t(11;14)(q13;q32)	95	CCND1	Transcriptional deregulation	Cell-cycle regulation
Burkitt lymphoma	t(8;14)(q24;q32)	80	MYC	Transcriptional deregulation	Control of proliferation and growth
	t(2;8)(p11;q24)	15	MYC	Transcriptional deregulation	
	t(8;22)(q24;q11)	5	MYC	Transcriptional deregulation	
Follicular lymphoma	t(14;18)(q32;q21)	90	BCL2	Transcriptional deregulation	Antiapoptosis
	t(2;18)(p11;q21)	Rare	BCL2	Transcriptional deregulation	
	t(18;22)(q21;q11)	Rare	BCL2	Transcriptional deregulation	
Diffuse large B-cell lymphoma (GCB)	t(8;14)(q24;q32)	10	MYC	Transcriptional deregulation	Proliferation and growth
	t(14;18)(q32;q21)	30	BCL2	Transcriptional deregulation	Antiapoptosis
	t(3;other)(q27;other)	15	BCL6	Transcriptional deregulation	Master regulator of GC responses
	EZH2 M	20	EZH2	Unknown	Chromatin remodeling
Diffuse large B-cell lymphoma (ABC)	t(3;other)(q27;other)	25	BCL6	Transcriptional deregulation	Master regulator of GC responses
	TNFAIP3 M/D	20	TNFAIP3	Loss of function	Negative NF-κB regulator
	PRDM1 M/D	20	PRDM1	Loss of function	Terminal B-cell differentiation
	CD79B M	18	CD79B	Gain of function	Activation of BCR signaling
	CARD11 M	9	CARD11	Gain of function	Positive NF-κB regulator
	18q21 amplification	30	BCL2	Increased gene dosage	Antiapoptosis
Primary mediastinal B-cell lymphoma	9p24.1 amplification	50	JAK2	Increased gene dosage	JAK/STAT pathway regulation
			PDL1, PDL2	Increased gene dosage	Immunomodulatory responses
Mucosa associated lymphoid tissue (MALT) lymphoma	t(11;18)(q21;q21)	30	API2-MALT1 MALT1	Fusion protein	Positive NF-κB regulator
	t(14;18)(q32;q21)	15–20	FOXP1	Transcriptional deregulation	Positive NF-κB regulator
	t(3;14)(p13;q32)	10	BCL10	Transcriptional deregulation	Transcription factor
	t(1;14)(p22;q32)	5		Transcriptional deregulation	Positive NF-κB regulator
Lymphoplasmacytic lymphoma	t(9;14)(p13;q32)	50	PAX5	Transcriptional deregulation	B-cell proliferation and differentiation
Anaplastic large cell lymphoma	t(2;5)(p23;q35)	60[a]	NPM/ALK	Fusion protein	Tyrosine kinase
Classic Hodgkin lymphoma	TNFAIP3 M/D	40[b]	TNFAIP3	Loss of function	Negative NF-κB regulator
	SOCS1 M/D	45	SOCS1	Loss of function	Inhibition of JAK-STAT pathway
	2p13 amplification	50	REL	Increased gene dosage	Positive NF-κB regulator
	9p24.1 amplification	50	JAK2	Increased gene dosage	Inhibition of JAK/STAT pathway
			PDL1, PDL2	Increased gene dosage	Immunomodulatory responses

GCB, germinal center B-cell–like; ABC, activated B-cell–like; M, mutation; D, deletion. See also Fig. 37.5 for a more complete list of the recurrent genetic lesions in DLBCL.
[a] In the adult population; 85% in childhood.
[b] Sixty percent in Epstein-Barr Virus-negative cases.

ATM gene and may thus promote genomic instability.[295–297] These lesions can be observed in the patient germ line, and may thus account, at least in part, for the familial form of the disease. Another important target within the 11q22-23 deleted region is the BIRC3 gene, encoding for a negative regulator of NF-κB.[298] The identification of inactivating mutations and the evidence of constitutive NF-κB activation in these cases suggests that NF-κB could serve as a therapeutic target in this poor prognostic category of patients. Deletions of 17p13, which include the TP53 tumor suppressor and which are frequently accompanied by a mutation of the second allele,[68,299] are observed in ~7% of CLL at diagnosis but are enriched in cases that underwent transformation to RS, a highly aggressive lymphoma with poor clinical outcome.[82] More recently, gain-of-function mutations of NOTCH1 and mutations of SF3B1 were discovered in 5% to 10% of diagnostic CLL samples,[300–303] where they seem to predict an adverse outcome, as supported by their preferential enrichment in RS (30% of cases) and fludarabine refractory cases (25%), respectively (Fig. 37.7).[82,300–304]

HIV-Related Non-Hodgkin Lymphoma

The association between an immunodeficiency state and the development of lymphoma has been recognized in several clinical conditions, including congenital (e.g., Wiskott-Aldrich syndrome), iatrogenic (e.g., treatment with immunosuppressive agents), and viral-induced (e.g., AIDS) immunodeficiencies. Detailed investigations have been conducted on the molecular pathophysiology of HIV-related NHL, which are primarily classified into three clinico-pathologic categories: BL, DLBCL, and PEL.[1,305,306] Based

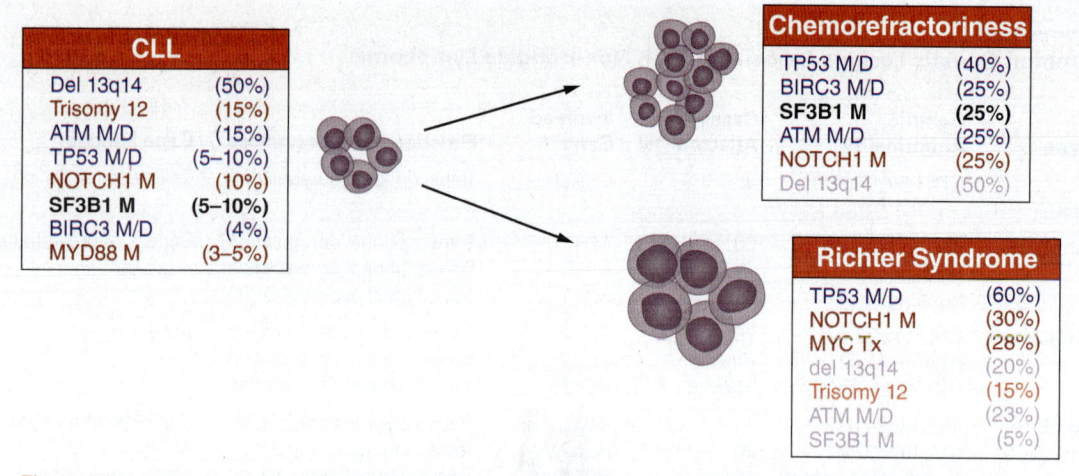

Figure 37.7 Genetic lesions associated with CLL. Frequency of common genetic alterations observed in unselected CLL cases at diagnosis, fludarabine-resistant CLL and RS. Blue, loss of function mutations; Red, gain-of-function mutations.

on the site of origin, HIV-related NHLs are generally grouped into systemic HIV-related NHL (i.e., DLBCL and BL) and HIV-related PCNSL, which is characterized by a uniform morphology consistent with a diffuse architecture of large cells.[1,305,306]

Cell of Origin

HIV-related NHLs invariably derive from B cells that have experienced the GC reaction, as indicated by the presence of somatic mutations in the *IG* and *BCL6* genes, as well as by several phenotypic and transcriptional features.[305–307] Based on the presence or absence of immunoblastic features and on the expression pattern of BCL6, CD138, and the EBV-encoded LMP1, both HIV-related DLBCL and PCNSL can be segregated into two distinct histogenetic categories. Cases displaying the BCL6+/CD138−/LMP1− phenotype closely resemble the phenotype of GC B cells, whereas BCL6−/CD138+/LMP1+ cases are morphologically consistent with immunoblastic lymphoma, plasmacytoid, and reflect a post-GC stage of B-cell differentiation.[305,306] PEL consistently derives from B cells, reflecting a preterminal stage of differentiation.[97,308–310]

Genetic Lesions. The three categories of HIV-related NHL associate with distinctive molecular pathways. HIV-related BLs consistently displays activation of MYC due to chromosomal translocations that are structurally similar to those found in sBL, whereas rearrangements of *BCL6* are always absent.[307] HIV related BLs also frequently harbor mutations in *TP53* (60%), *BCL6* 5′ noncoding sequences (60%), and, in 30% of cases, infection of the tumor clone by EBV, although the EBV-encoded antigens LMP1 and EBNA2 are not expressed.[311,312] Stimulation and selection by antigens, frequently represented by autoantigens, appear to be a prominent feature.[142,313]

Different from BL, the most frequent genetic alteration detected in HIV-related DLBCL is infection by EBV, which occurs in approximately 60% to 70% of cases and is frequently, although not always, associated with the expression of LMP1.[89,91,312] Moreover, HIV-related DLBCLs carry *BCL6* rearrangements in 20% of cases,[314] and mutations of the *BCL6* 5′ noncoding region in 70% of cases.[315]

All HIV-related PCNSLs show evidence of EBV infection.[316] However, only the subset with immunoblastic morphology expresses the LMP1 transforming protein.[317] These tumors display ASHM[57] and harbor oncogenic mutations in the *CARD11* gene (16% of cases),[318] which may explain, in part, the constitutive NF-κB activity previously recognized in this lymphoma subtype. Although some reports have suggested that HHV-8 may be related to PCNSL pathogenesis in immunocompromised patients, extensive analyses have unequivocally ruled out this hypothesis.[319,320]

The last type of HIV-related NHL that has been characterized at the molecular level is PEL, also known as body cavity–based lymphoma.[97,308,309] This entity is associated with HHV-8 infection in 100% of cases and clinically presents as effusions in the serosal cavities of the body (pleura, pericardium, peritoneum) in the absence of solid tumor masses.[97,308,309] In addition to HHV-8, PEL cases frequently show coinfection of the tumor clone by EBV.[90,92,97,308,309]

MOLECULAR PATHOGENESIS OF T-CELL NON-HODGKIN LYMPHOMA

Peripheral T-cell lymphoma (PTCL) encompasses a highly heterogeneous and relatively uncommon group of diseases representing 5% to 10% of all NHLs worldwide, with significant geographical variation in both incidence and relative prevalence.[1] PTCLs arise from mature post-thymic T cells and, according to the clinical presentation of the disease, are listed as leukemic or disseminated, predominantly extranodal, cutaneous, and predominantly nodal.[1] Although the study of T-cell neoplasms is hampered by the rarity of these diseases and the difficulty of collecting homogeneous sample series, significant advances were made over the past decades in our understanding of their biology, classification, and prognosis.

Adult T-Cell Lymphoma/Leukemia (HTLV-1 Positive)

Cell of Origin

The term ATLL identifies a spectrum of lymphoproliferative diseases associated with HTLV-I infection that is mainly restricted to southwestern Japan and the Caribbean basin.[1,321] The United States and Europe are considered low-risk areas, because less than 1% of the population are HTLV-I carriers[322] and only 2% to 4% of seropositive individuals eventually develop ATLL.[1,101,102] Clonal rearrangement of the TCR is evident in all cases, and clonal integration of the virus has been observed.[323,324]

Genetic Lesions

Compared to other mature T-cell tumors, the molecular pathogenesis of ATLL has been elucidated to a wider extent. Particularly, the role of HTLV-I has been linked to the production of a transregulatory protein (HTLV-1 tax), that markedly increases expression of all viral gene products and transcriptionally activates the expression of certain host genes, including IL-2, CD25, c-sis, c-fos, and granulocyte-macrophage colony-stimulating factor (GM-CSF).[104–106,107,108] Indeed, a property of ATLL cells is the constitutively high expression of the IL-2 receptor. The central role of these genes in normal T-cell activation and growth, together with the results of in vitro studies, support the notion that tax-mediated activation of these host genes represents an important mechanism by which HTLV-1 initiates T-cell transformation.[104] In addition, tax interferes with DNA damage repair functions and with mitotic checkpoints,[109,110,325] which is consistent with the fact that ATLL cells harbor a high frequency of karyotypic abnormalities.

The long period of clinical latency that precedes the development of ATLL (usually 10 to 30 years), the small percentage of infected patients that develop this malignancy, and the observation that leukemic cells from ATLL are monoclonal suggest that HTLV-1 is not sufficient to cause the full malignant phenotype.[101–103] A model for ATLL, therefore, implies an early period of tax-induced polyclonal T-cell proliferation that, in turn, would facilitate the occurrence of additional genetic events leading to the monoclonal outgrowth of a fully transformed cell. In this respect, a recurrent genetic lesion in ATLL is represented by mutations of the TP53 tumor suppressor gene, which is inactivated in 40% of cases.[326,327]

Peripheral T-Cell Lymphoma, Not Otherwise Specified

This category represents the largest and most heterogeneous group of PTCLs, and includes all cases that lack specific features allowing classification within another entity. The majority of these cases derive from αβ CD4+ T cells and show aberrant defective expression of one or several T-cell–associated antigens.[328] Based on gene expression profiling, peripheral T cell lymphoma/not otherwise specified (PTCL/NOS) as a group appears to be most closely related to activated T cells than to resting T cells and can be segregated according to similarities with the transcriptional signature of CD4+ and CD8+ T cells. However, no correlation is observed between gene expression profiles (GEP) and immunophenotype, likely reflecting the variable detection of T-cell antigens in the disease.

Genetic Lesions

Clonal numerical and structural aberrations are found in most PTCL/NOS by conventional cytogenetics and in all cases by more sensitive approaches such as array-based methods. For a few loci, the correlation between gene CN and expression has been confirmed, suggesting a pathogenetic role. Candidate genes include CDK6 on chromosome 7q, MYC on chromosome 8, and the NF-κB regulator CARD11 at 7p22, whereas losses of 9p21 are associated with a reduced expression of CDKN2A/B.[329] Chromosomal translocations involving the TCR loci have been reported in rare cases and remain poorly understood, because the identity of the translocation partner has not been identified, with few exceptions: the BCL3 gene, the poliovirus receptor-related 2 (PVRL2) gene found in the t(14;19)(q11;q13) translocation, and the IRF4 gene, which is cloned in two cases.[330–332] More recently, whole-exome sequencing studies revealed the presence of recurrent heterozygous mutations in the RHOA small GTPase gene (18% of patients), including a hot-spot Gly17Val substitution that was shown to have inhibitory effects in the Rho-signaling pathway, potentially via the sequestration of GEP proteins.[333,334] These mutations appear to segregate with a subset of Tfh-like PTCL/NOS, characterized by the expression of CD10 and PD-1, the proliferation of CD21+FDCs, and EBER positivity. In a smaller number of cases, mutations were also found in TET2, DNM3TA, IDH2, TET3, FYN, and B2M.[333,334]

Angioimmunoblastic T-Cell Lymphoma

Cell of Origin

Angioimmunoblastic T-cell lymphoma (AITL) is an aggressive disease of the elderly and accounts for about one-third of all PTCL cases in Western countries.[335] The tumor cells display a mature CD4+CD8- T-cell phenotype, with frequent aberrant loss of one or several T-cell markers and coexpression of BCL6 and CD10 in at least a fraction of cells. Gene expression profile studies have conclusively established the cellular derivation of AITL from follicular helper T cells,[336] as initially suspected based on the expression of single markers.[337]

Genetic Lesions

Until recently, the scarce number of genetic studies had failed to provide any significant clues regarding the oncogenic pathways involved in AITL. However, a major discovery emerged in 2013 from two whole-exome sequencing studies that identified highly recurrent mutations of RHOA in 67% of all AITL cases.[333,334] These mutations are analogous to those observed in PTCL/NOS, but are not found in other mature B- and T-cell neoplasms, strongly suggesting a role for the disruption of the RHO-signaling pathway in the pathogenesis of this disease. Additional clonal aberrations have been reported in up to 90% of AITL patients and include chromosomal imbalances as well as mutations in TET2, IDH2, and DNMT3A, which are common to various hematologic malignancies, whereas chromosomal translocations affecting the TCR loci are extremely rare.[329,333,334]

Cutaneous T-Cell Lymphoma

Genetic lesions are involved in a limited but significant fraction of primary CTCLs showing a molecular marker of clonality. Most notable among them are rearrangements of the NFKB2 gene at 10q24, leading to a chimeric protein that retains the rel effector domain and can bind κB sequences in vitro,[338,339] but that lacks the ankyrin regulatory domain required for regulating the physiologic nuclear/cytoplasm distribution. The translocation may thus contribute to lymphoma development by causing constitutive activation of the NF-κB pathway.

Anaplastic Large Cell Lymphoma

Cell of Origin

ALCL is a distinct subset of T-NHL (~12% of cases), whose normal cellular counterpart has not yet been established.[1,321] The tumor is composed of large pleomorphic cells that exhibit a unique phenotype characterized by positivity for the CD30 antigen and the loss of most T-cell markers.[1,340] Based on the expression of a chimeric protein containing the cytoplasmic portion of anaplastic lymphoma kinase (ALK) (see the following), ALCL may be subdivided in two groups, displaying distinct transcriptional signatures[341]: The most common and curable is ALK-positive ALCL, and the more aggressive is ALK-negative ALCL.[1,342–344] However, the identification of a common 30-genes predictor that can discriminate ALCL from other T-NHL, independent of ALK status, suggests that these two subgroups are closely related and may derive from a common precursor.[345]

Genetic Lesions

The genetic hallmark of ALK+ALCL is a chromosomal translocation involving band 2p23 and a variety of chromosomal partners, with t(2;5)(p23;q35) accounting for 70% to 80% of the cases.[1,346] Cloning of the translocation breakpoint in t(2;5) demonstrated the involvement of the ALK gene on 2p23 and the nucleophosmin (NPM1) gene on 5q35.[347] As a consequence, the aminoterminus of NPM is linked in frame to the catalytic domain of ALK, driving transformation through multiple molecular mechanisms[347]: (1) the ALK gene, which is not expressed in normal T-lymphocytes, becomes inappropriately expressed in lymphoma cells, conceivably because of its juxtaposition to the promoter sequences of NPM, which are physiologically expressed in T cells; and (2) all translocations involving ALK produce proteins with constitutive tyrosine activity, due in most cases to spontaneous dimerization induced by the various fusion partners.[346] Constitutive ALK activity, in turn, results in the activation of several downstream signaling cascades, with the JAK/STAT and PI3K/AKT pathways playing central roles.[348–351] The transforming ability of the chimeric NPM/ALK protein has been proven both in vitro and in vivo in transgenic mouse models.[352–354]

In a minority of cases, fusions other than NPM/ALK cause the abnormal subcellular localization of the corresponding chimeric ALK proteins and the constitutive activation of ALK. Among these alternative rearrangements, the most frequent involve TPM3/TPM4, TRK-fused genes,[355] ATIC,[356,357] CLTCL1, and MSN. The diversity of known ALK fusion partners was further expanded by the recent identification of a novel TRAF1/ALK fusion transcript leading to constitutive NF-κB expression.[358] No recurrent cytogenetic abnormality has been described in ALK-negative ALCL, leaving the molecular events responsible for this disease subtype largely unknown.

MOLECULAR PATHOGENESIS OF HODGKIN LYMPHOMA

HL is a B-lymphoid malignancy characterized by the presence of scattered large atypical cells—the mononucleated Hodgkin cells and the multinucleated Reed-Sternberg cells (HRS)—residing in a complex admixture of inflammatory cells.[1,359] Based on the morphology and phenotype of the neoplastic cells, as well as on the composition of the infiltrate, HL is segregated in two major subgroups: nodular lymphocyte-predominant HL (NLPHL) (~5% of cases) and classic HL (cHL), comprising the nodular sclerosis, mixed cellularity, lymphocyte-depleted, and lymphocyte-rich variants. Until recently, molecular studies of HL have been hampered by the paucity of the tumor cells in the biopsy (typically less than 1%, although occasional cases can present more than 10% HRS cells). However, the introduction of sophisticated laboratory techniques allowing for the isolation and enrichment of neoplastic cells has markedly improved our understanding of HL histogenesis.

Cell of Origin

Despite the fact that HRS of cHL cells have lost the expression of nearly all B-cell–specific genes,[360–362] both HL types represent clonal populations of B cells, as revealed by the presence of clonally rearranged and somatically mutated Ig genes.[363,364] In about 25% of cHL cases, nonsense mutations disrupt originally in-frame IGHV gene rearrangements (crippling mutations), thereby preventing antigen selection. These data suggest that HRS cells of cHL have escaped apoptosis through a mechanism not linked to antigen stimulation.[364]

Genetic Lesions

A number of structural alterations lead to the constitutive activation of NF-κB in cHL. Nearly half of the cases display amplification of REL, which is associated with increased protein expression levels[365,366]; gains or translocations of the positive NF-κB regulator BCL3 were also reported.[330] More recently, a number of inactivating mutations were found in genes coding for negative regulators of NF-κB, including NFKBIA (20% of cases), NFKBIE (15%), and TNFAIP3 (40%), among others.[78,367–369] Notably, TNFAIP3-mutated cases are invariably EBV negative, suggesting that EBV infection may substitute, in part, for the pathogenic function of its protein product A20 in causing NF-κB constitutive activation.[78,369] In the past few years, genetic aberrations that modulate the tumor microenvironment have been uncovered using massively parallel DNA sequencing techniques, including genomic gains of PD-L1 (CD274) and PD-L2 (CD273) and translocations of CIITA.[64,65,243] Amplification of JAK2, mutations of STAT6, and inactivating mutations of SOCS1, a negative regulator of the JAK/STAT signaling pathway, are often found in NLPHL[747,746]; in an additional large fraction of cases, constitutive JAK/STAT activity is sustained by autocrine and paracrine signals.[359] BCL6 translocations have been reported in the lymphocyte and histiocytic (L&H) cells of NLPHL, but only rarely in cHL,[370,371] and translocations of BCL2 or mutations in positive or negative regulators of apoptosis (e.g., TP53, FAS, BAD, and ATM) are virtually absent.[369] As mentioned, an important pathogenic cofactor in cHL, but not NLPHL, is represented by monoclonal EBV infection, which occurs in approximately 40% of cHLs and up to 90% of HIV-related HLs, suggesting that infection precedes clonal expansion.[359] Of the viral proteins encoded by the EBV genome, infected HRS cells most commonly express LMP1, LMP2, and EBNA1, but not EBNA2.[359]

REFERENCES

1. Swerdlow SH, Campo E, Harris NL, et al., eds. WHO Classification of Tumours of Haematopoietic and Lymphoid Tissues. Lyon: International Agency for Research on Cancer; 2008.
2. Jung D, Giallourakis C, Mostoslavsky R, et al. Mechanism and control of V(D)J recombination at the immunoglobulin heavy chain locus. Annu Rev Immunol 2006;24:541–570.
3. Rajewsky K. Clonal selection and learning in the antibody system. Nature 1996;381:751–758.
4. Klein U, Dalla-Favera R. Germinal centres: role in B-cell physiology and malignancy. Nat Rev Immunol 2008;8:22–33.
5. MacLennan IC. Germinal centers. Annu Rev Immunol 1994;12:117–139.
6. Green JA, Cyster JG. S1PR2 links germinal center confinement and growth regulation. Immunol Rev 2012;247:36–51.
7. Allen CD, Okada T, Tang HL, et al. Imaging of germinal center selection events during affinity maturation. Science 2007;315:528–531.
8. Schwickert TA, Lindquist RL, Shakhar G, et al. In vivo imaging of germinal centres reveals a dynamic open structure. Nature 2007;446:83–87.
9. Victora GD, Schqickert TA, Fooksman DR, et al. Germinal center dynamics revealed by multiphoton microscopy with a photoactivatable fluorescent reporter. Cell 2010;143:592–605.
10. Di Noia JM, Neuberger MS. Molecular mechanisms of antibody somatic hypermutation. Annu Rev Biochem 2007;76:1–22.
11. Goossens T, Klein U, Küppers R. Frequent occurrence of deletions and duplications during somatic hypermutation: implications for oncogene translocations and heavy chain disease. Proc Natl Acad Sci U S A 1998;95:2463–2468.
12. Kuppers R, Zhao M, Hansmann ML, et al. Tracing B cell development in human germinal centres by molecular analysis of single cells picked from histological sections. EMBO J 1993;12:4955–4967.
13. Klein U, Tu Y, Stolovitzky GA, et al. Transcriptional analysis of the B cell germinal center reaction. Proc Natl Acad Sci U S A 2003;100:2639–2644.
14. Cattoretti G, Chang CC, Cechova K, et al. BCL-6 protein is expressed in germinal center B cells. Blood 1995;86:45–53.
15. Chang CC, Ye BH, Chaganti RS, et al. BCL-6, a POZ/zinc-finger protein, is a sequence-specific transcriptional repressor. Proc Natl Acad Sci U S A 1996;93:6947–6952.
16. Basso K, Saito M, Sumazin P, et al. Integrated biochemical and computational approach identifies BCL6 direct target genes controlling multiple pathways in normal germinal center B cells. Blood 2010;115:975–984.
17. Niu H, Cattoretti G, Dalla-Favera R. BCL6 controls the expression of the B7-1/CD80 costimulatory receptor in germinal center B cells. J Exp Med 2003;198:211–221.
18. Ci W, Polo JM, Cerchietti L, et al. The BCL6 transcriptional program features repression of multiple oncogenes in primary B cells and is deregulated in DLBCL. Blood 2009;113:5536–5548.
19. Phan RT, Dalla-Favera R. The BCL6 proto-oncogene suppresses p53 expression in germinal-centre B cells. Nature 2004;432:635–639.
20. Phan RT, Saito M, Basso K, et al. BCL6 interacts with the transcription factor Miz-1 to suppress the cyclin-dependent kinase inhibitor p21 and cell cycle arrest in germinal center B cells. Nat Immunol 2005;6:1054–1060.
21. Ranuncolo SM, Polo JM, Dierov J, et al. Bcl-6 mediates the germinal center B cell phenotype and lymphomagenesis through transcriptional repression of the DNA-damage sensor ATR. Nat Immunol 2007;8:705–714.
22. Ranuncolo SM, Polo JM, Melnick A. BCL6 represses CHEK1 and suppresses DNA damage pathways in normal and malignant B-cells. Blood Cells Mol Dis 2008;41:95–99.
23. Keller AD, Maniatis T. Identification and characterization of a novel repressor of beta-interferon gene expression. Genes Dev 1991;5:868–879.
24. Turner CA Jr, Mack DH, Davis MM. Blimp-1, a novel zinc finger-containing protein that can drive the maturation of B lymphocytes into immunoglobulin-secreting cells. Cell 1994;77:297–306.

25. Shaffer AL, Yu X, He Y, et al. BCL-6 represses genes that function in lymphocyte differentiation, inflammation, and cell cycle control. *Immunity* 2000;13:199-212.
26. Tunyaplin C, Shaffer AL, Angelin-Duclos CD, et al. Direct repression of prdm1 by Bcl-6 inhibits plasmacytic differentiation. *J Immunol* 2004;173: 1158–1165.
27. Honjo T, Kinoshita K, Muramatsu M. Molecular mechanism of class switch recombination: linkage with somatic hypermutation. *Annu Rev Immunol* 2002; 20:165–196.
28. Longerich S, Basu U, Alt F, et al. AID in somatic hypermutation and class switch recombination. *Curr Opin Immunol* 2006;18:164–174.
29. Muramatsu M, Kinoshita K, Fagarasan S, et al. Class switch recombination and hypermutation require activation-induced cytidine deaminase (AID), a potential RNA editing enzyme. *Cell* 2000;102:553–563.
30. Revy P, Muto T, Levy Y, et al. Activation-induced cytidine deaminase (AID) deficiency causes the autosomal recessive form of the Hyper-IgM syndrome (HIGM2). *Cell* 2000;102:565–575.
31. Kuppers R, Klein U, Hansmann ML, et al. Cellular origin of human B-cell lymphomas. *N Engl J Med* 1999;341:1520–1529.
32. Nussenzweig A, Nussenzweig MC. Origin of chromosomal translocations in lymphoid cancer. *Cell* 2010;141:27–38.
33. von Boehmer H, Aifantis I, Gounari F, et al. Thymic selection revisited: how essential is it? *Immunol Rev* 2003;191:62–78.
34. Kuppers R, Dalla-Favera R. Mechanisms of chromosomal translocations in B cell lymphomas. *Oncogene* 2001;20:5580–5594.
35. Tsujimoto Y, Gorham J, Cossman J, et al. The t(14;18) chromosome translocations involved in B-cell neoplasms result from mistakes in VDJ joining. *Science* 1985;229:1390–1393.
36. Tsujimoto Y, Louie E, Bashir MM, et al. The reciprocal partners of both the t(14; 18) and the t(11; 14) translocations involved in B-cell neoplasms are rearranged by the same mechanism. *Oncogene* 1988;2:347–351.
37. Ramiro AR, Jankovic M, Eisenreich T, et al. AID is required for c-myc/IgH chromosome translocations in vivo. *Cell* 2004;118:431–438.
38. Robbiani DF, Bothmer A, Callen E, et al. AID is required for the chromosomal breaks in c-myc that lead to c-myc/IgH translocations. *Cell* 2008;135: 1028–1038.
39. Pasqualucci L, Bhagat G, Jankovic M, et al. AID is required for germinal center-derived lymphomagenesis. *Nat Genet* 2008;40:108–112.
40. Akasaka H, Akasaka T, Kurata M, et al. Molecular anatomy of BCL6 translocations revealed by long-distance polymerase chain reaction-based assays. *Cancer Res* 2000;60:2335–2341.
41. Chen W, Iida S, Louie DC, et al. Heterologous promoters fused to BCL6 by chromosomal translocations affecting band 3q27 cause its deregulated expression during B-cell differentiation. *Blood* 1998;91:603–607.
42. Ye BH, Lista F, Lo Coco F, et al. Alterations of a zinc finger-encoding gene, BCL-6, in diffuse large- cell lymphoma. *Science* 1993;262:747–750.
43. Ye BH, Rao PH, Chaganti RS, et al. Cloning of bcl-6, the locus involved in chromosome translocations affecting band 3q27 in B-cell lymphoma. *Cancer Res* 1993;53:2732–2735.
44. Yoshida S, Kaneita Y, Aoki Y, et al. Identification of heterologous translocation partner genes fused to the BCL6 gene in diffuse large B-cell lymphomas: 5'-RACE and LA - PCR analyses of biopsy samples. *Oncogene* 1999;18:7994–7999.
45. Baron BW, Nucifora G, McCabe N, et al. Identification of the gene associated with the recurring chromosomal translocations t(3;14)(q27;q32) and t(3;22)(q27;q11) in B-cell lymphomas. *Proc Natl Acad Sci U S A* 1993;90:5262–5266.
46. Kerckaert JP, Deweindt C, Tilly H, et al. LAZ3, a novel zinc-finger encoding gene, is disrupted by recurring chromosome 3q27 translocations in human lymphomas. *Nat Genet* 1993;5:66–70.
47. Miki T, Kawamata N, Aria A, et al. Molecular cloning of the breakpoint for 3q27 translocation in B-cell lymphomas and leukemias. *Blood* 1994;83: 217–222.
48. Pasqualucci L, Neumeister P, Goossens T, et al. Hypermutation of multiple proto-oncogenes in B-cell diffuse large-cell lymphomas. *Nature* 2001;412: 341–346.
49. Neuberger MS. Antibody diversification by somatic mutation: from Burnet onwards. *Immunol Cell Biol* 2008;86:124–132.
50. Gordon MS, Kanegai CM, Doerr JR, et al. Somatic hypermutation of the B cell receptor genes B29 (Igbeta, CD79b) and mb1 (Igalpha, CD79a). *Proc Natl Acad Sci U S A* 2003;100:4126–4131.
51. Müschen M, Re D, Jungnickel B, et al. Somatic mutation of the CD95 gene in human B cells as a side-effect of the germinal center reaction. *J Exp Med* 2000;192:1833–1840.
52. Pasqualucci L, Migliazza A, Fracchiolla N, et al. BCL-6 mutations in normal germinal center B cells: evidence of somatic hypermutation acting outside Ig loci. *Proc Natl Acad Sci U S A* 1998;95:11816–11821.
53. Shen HM, Peters A, Baron B, et al. Mutation of BCL-6 gene in normal B cells by the process of somatic hypermutation of Ig genes. *Science* 1998;280: 1750–1752.
54. Cerri M, Capello D, Muti G, et al. Aberrant somatic hypermutation in post-transplant lymphoproliferative disorders. *Br J Haematol* 2004;127:362–364.
55. Deutsch AJ, Aigelsreiter A, Staber PB, et al. MALT lymphoma and extranodal diffuse large B-cell lymphoma are targeted by aberrant somatic hypermutation. *Blood* 2007;109:3500–3504.
56. Gaidano G, Pasqualucci L, Capello D, et al. Aberrant somatic hypermutation in multiple subtypes of AIDS-associated non-Hodgkin lymphoma. *Blood* 2003;102:1833–1841.

57. Montesinos-Rongen M, Van Roost D, Schaller C, et al. Primary diffuse large B-cell lymphomas of the central nervous system are targeted by aberrant somatic hypermutation. *Blood* 2004;103:1869–1875.
58. Vakiani E, Basso K, Klein U, et al. Genetic and phenotypic analysis of B-cell post-transplant lymphoproliferative disorders provides insights into disease biology. *Hematol Oncol* 2008;26:199–211.
59. Storb U, Peters A, Klotz E, et al. Cis-acting sequences that affect somatic hypermutation of Ig genes. *Immunol Rev* 1998;162:153–160.
60. Houldsworth J, Mathew S, Rao PH, et al. REL proto-oncogene is frequently amplified in extranodal diffuse large cell lymphoma. *Blood* 1996;87:25–29.
61. Houldsworth J, Oishen AB, Cattoretti G, et al. Relationship between REL amplification, REL function, and clinical and biologic features in diffuse large B-cell lymphomas. *Blood* 2004;103:1862–1868.
62. Rao PH, Houldsworth J, Dyomina K, et al. Chromosomal and gene amplification in diffuse large B-cell lymphoma. *Blood* 1998;92:234–240.
63. Rosenwald A, Wright G, Chan WC, et al. The use of molecular profiling to predict survival after chemotherapy for diffuse large-B-cell lymphoma. *N Engl J Med* 2002;346:1937–1947.
64. Green MR, Monti S, Rodig SJ, et al. Integrative analysis reveals selective 9p24.1 amplification, increased PD-1 ligand expression, and further induction via JAK2 in nodular sclerosing Hodgkin lymphoma and primary mediastinal large B-cell lymphoma. *Blood* 2010;116:3268–3277.
65. Rui L, Emre NC, Kruhlak MJ, et al. Cooperative epigenetic modulation by cancer amplicon genes. *Cancer Cell* 2010;18:590–605.
66. Neri A, Knowles DM, Greco A, et al. Analysis of RAS oncogene mutations in human lymphoid malignancies. *Proc Natl Acad Sci U S A* 1988;85: 9268–9272.
67. Hollstein M, Sidransky D, Vogelstein B, et al. p53 mutations in human cancers. *Science* 1991;253:49–53.
68. Gaidano G, Ballerini P, Gong JZ, et al. p53 mutations in human lymphoid malignancies: association with Burkitt lymphoma and chronic lymphocytic leukemia. *Proc Natl Acad Sci U S A* 1991;88:5413–5417.
69. Lo Coco F, Gaidano G, Louie DC, et al. p53 mutations are associated with histologic transformation of follicular lymphoma. *Blood* 1993;82:2289–2295.
70. Gaidano G, Hauptschein RS, Parsa NZ, et al. Deletions involving two distinct regions of 6q in B-cell non-Hodgkin lymphoma. *Blood* 1992;80: 1781–1787.
71. Offit K, Wong G, Filippa DA, et al. Cytogenetic analysis of 434 consecutively ascertained specimens of non-Hodgkin's lymphoma: clinical correlations. *Blood* 1991;77:1508–1515.
72. Mandelbaum J, Bhagat G, Tang H, et al. BLIMP1 is a tumor suppressor gene frequently disrupted in activated B cell-like diffuse large B cell lymphoma. *Cancer Cell* 2010;18:568–579.
73. Pasqualucci L, Compagno M, Houldsworth J, et al. Inactivation of the PRDM1/BLIMP1 gene in diffuse large B cell lymphoma. *J Exp Med* 2006;203:311–317.
74. Tam W, Gomez M, Chadburn A, et al. Mutational analysis of PRDM1 indicates a tumor-suppressor role in diffuse large B-cell lymphomas. *Blood* 2006; 107:4090–4100.
75. Compagno M, Lim WK, Grunn A, et al. Mutations of multiple genes cause deregulation of NF-kappaB in diffuse large B-cell lymphoma. *Nature* 2009;459:717–721.
76. Kato M, Sanada M, Kato I, et al. Frequent inactivation of A20 in B-cell lymphomas. *Nature* 2009;459:712–716.
77. Novak U, Rinaldi A, Kwee I, et al. The NF-(kappa)B negative regulator TNFAIP3 (A20) is inactivated by somatic mutations and genomic deletions in marginal zone lymphomas. *Blood* 2009;113:4918–4921.
78. Schmitz R, Hansmann ML, Bohle V, et al. TNFAIP3 (A20) is a tumor suppressor gene in Hodgkin lymphoma and primary mediastinal B cell lymphoma. *J Exp Med* 2009;206:981–989.
79. Pasqualucci L, Dominguez-Sola D, Chiarenza A, et al. Inactivating mutations of acetyltransferase genes in B-cell lymphoma. *Nature* 2011;471: 189–195.
80. Morin RD, Mendez-Lago M, Mungall AJ, et al. Frequent mutation of histone-modifying genes in non-Hodgkin lymphoma. *Nature* 2011;476: 298–303.
81. Dohner H, Stilgenbauer S, Benner A, et al. Genomic aberrations and survival in chronic lymphocytic leukemia. *N Engl J Med* 2000;343:1910–1916.
82. Fabbri G, Khiabanian H, Holmes AB, et al. Genetic lesions associated with chronic lymphocytic leukemia transformation to Richter syndrome. *J Exp Med* 2013;210:2273–2288.
83. Lenz G, Wright GW, Emre NC, et al. Molecular subtypes of diffuse large B-cell lymphoma arise by distinct genetic pathways. *Proc Natl Acad Sci U S A* 2008;105:13520–13525.
84. Pasqualucci L, Khiabanian H, Fangazio M, et al. Genetics of follicular lymphoma transformation. *Cell Rep* 2014;6:130–140.
85. Martinez-Delgado B, Robledo M, Arranz E, et al. Hypermethylation of p15/ink4b/MTS2 gene is differentially implicated among non-Hodgkin's lymphomas. *Leukemia* 1998;12:937–941.
86. zur Hausen H, Schulte-Holthausen H, Klein G, et al. EBV DNA in biopsies of Burkitt tumours and anaplastic carcinomas of the nasopharynx. *Nature* 1970;228:1056–1058.
87. Magrath IT. African Burkitt's lymphoma. History, biology, clinical features, and treatment. *Am J Pediatr Hematol Oncol* 1991;13:222–246.
88. Neri A, Barriga F, Inghirami G, et al. Epstein-Barr virus infection precedes clonal expansion in Burkitt's and acquired immunodeficiency syndrome-associated lymphoma. *Blood* 1991;77:1092–1095.

89. Ballerini P, Gaidano G, Gong JZ, et al. Multiple genetic lesions in acquired immunodeficiency syndrome-related non-Hodgkin's lymphoma. Blood 1993; 81:166–176.
90. Horenstein MG, Nador RG, Chadburn A, et al. Epstein-Barr virus latent gene expression in primary effusion lymphomas containing Kaposi's sarcoma-associated herpesvirus/human herpesvirus-8. Blood 1997;90:1186–1191.
91. Cingolani A, Gastaldi R, Fassone L, et al. Epstein-Barr virus infection is predictive of CNS involvement in systemic AIDS-related non-Hodgkin's lymphomas. J Clin Oncol 2000;18:3325–3330.
92. Fassone L, Bhatia K, Gutierrez M, et al. Molecular profile of Epstein-Barr virus infection in HHV-8-positive primary effusion lymphoma. Leukemia 2000;14:271–277.
93. Kieff E, Leibowitz D. Oncogenesis by herpesvirus. In: Weinberg RA, ed. Oncogenes and the Molecular Origin of Cancer. Cold Spring Harbor, NY: Cold Spring Harbor Laboratory Press; 1989: 259.
94. Raab-Traub N, Flynn K. The structure of the termini of the Epstein-Barr virus as a marker of clonal cellular proliferation. Cell 1986;47:883–889.
95. Chang Y, Cesarman E, Pessin MS, et al. Identification of herpesvirus-like DNA sequences in AIDS-associated Kaposi's sarcoma. Science 1994;266: 1865–1869.
96. Soulier J, Grollet L, Oksenhendler E, et al. Kaposi's sarcoma-associated herpesvirus-like DNA sequences in multicentric Castleman's disease. Blood 1995;86:1276–1280.
97. Cesarman E, Chang Y, Moore PS, et al. Kaposi's sarcoma-associated herpesvirus-like DNA sequences in AIDS-related body-cavity-based lymphomas. N Engl J Med 1995;332:1186–1191.
98. Gaidano G, Pastore C, Gloghini A, et al. Distribution of human herpesvirus-8 sequences throughout the spectrum of AIDS-related neoplasia. Aids 1996; 10:941–949.
99. Moore PS, Gao SJ, Dominguez G, et al. Primary characterization of a herpesvirus agent associated with Kaposi's sarcomae. J Virol 1996;70:549–558.
100. Poiesz BJ, Ruscetti FW, Gazdar AF, et al. Detection and isolation of type C retrovirus particles from fresh and cultured lymphocytes of a patient with cutaneous T-cell lymphoma. Proc Natl Acad Sci U S A 1980;77:7415–7419.
101. Ferreira OC Jr, Planelles V, Rosenblatt JD. Human T-cell leukemia viruses: epidemiology, biology, and pathogenesis. Blood Rev 1997;11:91–104.
102. Uchiyama T. Human T-cell leukemia virus type I (HTLV-I) and human diseases. Annu Rev Immunol 1997;15:15–37.
103. Yoshida M. Howard Temin Memorial Lectureship. Molecular biology of HTLV-1: deregulation of host cell gene expression and cell cycle. Leukemia 1997;11:1–2.
104. Cross SL, Feinberg MB, Wolf JB, et al. Regulation of the human interleukin-2 receptor alpha chain promoter: activation of a nonfunctional promoter by the transactivator gene of HTLV-I. Cell 1987;49:47–56.
105. Fujii M, Sassone-Corsi P, Verma IM. c-fos promoter trans-activation by the tax1 protein of human T-cell leukemia virus type I. Proc Natl Acad Sci U S A 1988;85:8526–8530.
106. Inoue J, Seiki M, Taniguchi T, et al. Induction of interleukin 2 receptor gene expression by p40x encoded by human T-cell leukemia virus type 1. Embo J 1986;5:2883–2888.
107. Nimer SD, Gasson JC, Hu K, et al. Activation of the GM-CSF promoter by HTLV-I and -II tax proteins. Oncogene 1989;4:671–676.
108. Wano Y, Feinberg M, Hosking JB, et al. Stable expression of the tax gene of type I human T-cell leukemia virus in human T cells activates specific cellular genes involved in growth. Proc Natl Acad Sci U S A 1988;85:9733–9737.
109. Jeang KT, Widen SG, Semmes OJ 4th, et al. HTLV-I trans-activator protein, tax, is a trans-repressor of the human beta-polymerase gene. Science 1990;247:1082–1084.
110. Jin DY, Spencer F, Jeang KT. Human T cell leukemia virus type 1 oncoprotein Tax targets the human mitotic checkpoint protein MAD1. Cell 1998;93:81–91.
111. Marcucci F, Mele A. Hepatitis viruses and non-Hodgkin lymphoma: epidemiology, mechanisms of tumorigenesis, and therapeutic opportunities. Blood 2011;117:1792–1798.
112. Hermine O, Lefrere F, Bronowicki JP, et al. Regression of splenic lymphoma with villous lymphocytes after treatment of hepatitis C virus infection. N Engl J Med 2002;347:89–94.
113. Wotherspoon AC, Ortiz-Hidalgo C, Falzon MR, et al. Helicobacter pylori-associated gastritis and primary B-cell gastric lymphoma. Lancet 1991;338: 1175–1176.
114. Doglioni C, Wotherspoon AC, Moschini A, et al. High incidence of primary gastric lymphoma in northeastern Italy. Lancet 1992;339:834–835.
115. Parsonnet J, Hansen S, Rodriguez L, et al. Helicobacter pylori infection and gastric lymphoma. N Engl J Med 1994;330:1267–1271.
116. Wotherspoon AC, Doglioni C, Diss TC, et al. Regression of primary low-grade B-cell gastric lymphoma of mucosa-associated lymphoid tissue type after eradication of Helicobacter pylori. Lancet 1993;342:575–577.
117. Liu H, Ruskon-Fourmestraux A, Lavergne-Slove A, et al. Resistance of t(11;18) positive gastric mucosa-associated lymphoid tissue lymphoma to Helicobacter pylori eradication therapy. Lancet 2001;357:39–40.
118. Ferreri AJ, Dolcetti R, Magnino S, et al. Chlamydial infection: the link with ocular adnexal lymphomas. Nat Rev Clin Oncol 2009;6:658–669.
119. Stefanovic A, Lossos IS. Extranodal marginal zone lymphoma of the ocular adnexa. Blood 2009;114:501–510.
120. Ferreri AJ, Ponzoni M, Guidoboni M, et al. Regression of ocular adnexal lymphoma after Chlamydia psittaci-eradicating antibiotic therapy. J Clin Oncol 2005;23:5067–5073.
121. Jares P, Colomer D, Campo E. Genetic and molecular pathogenesis of mantle cell lymphoma: perspectives for new targeted therapeutics. Nat Rev Cancer 2007;7:750–762.
122. Tsujimoto Y, Jaffe E, Cossman J, et al. Clustering of breakpoints on chromosome 11 in human B-cell neoplasms with the t(11;14) chromosome translocation. Nature 1985;315:340–343.
123. Tsujimoto Y, Yunis J, Onorato-Showe L, et al. Molecular cloning of the chromosomal breakpoint of B-cell lymphomas and leukemias with the t(11;14) chromosome translocation. Science 1984;224:1403–1406.
124. Erikson J, Finan J, Tsujimoto Y, et al. The chromosome 14 breakpoint in neoplastic B cells with the t(11;14) translocation involves the immunoglobulin heavy chain locus. Proc Natl Acad Sci U S A 1984;81:4144–4148.
125. Motokura T, Bloom T, Kim HG, et al. A novel cyclin encoded by a bcl1-linked candidate oncogene. Nature 1991;350:512–515.
126. Rosenberg CL, Wong E, Petty EM, et al. PRAD1, a candidate BCL1 oncogene: mapping and expression in centrocytic lymphoma. Proc Natl Acad Sci U S A 1991;88:9638–9642.
127. Withers DA, Harvey RC, Faust JB, et al. Characterization of a candidate bcl-1 gene. Mol Cell Biol 1991;11:4846–4853.
128. Seto M, Yamamoto K, Iida S, et al. Gene rearrangement and overexpression of PRAD1 in lymphoid malignancy with t(11;14)(q13;q32) translocation. Oncogene 1992;7:1401–1406.
129. Komatsu H, Iida S, Yamamoto K, et al. A variant chromosome translocation at 11q13 identifying PRAD1/cyclin D1 as the BCL-1 gene. Blood 1994;84: 1226–1231.
130. Wiestner A, Tehrani M, Chiorazzi M, et al. Point mutations and genomic deletions in CCND1 create stable truncated cyclin D1 mRNAs that are associated with increased proliferation rate and shorter survival. Blood 2007;109:4599–4606.
131. Bodrug SE, Warner BJ, Bath ML, et al. Cyclin D1 transgene impedes lymphocyte maturation and collaborates in lymphomagenesis with the myc gene. Embo J 1994;13:2124–2130.
132. Lovec H, Grzeschiczek A, Kowalski MB, Moroy T. Cyclin D1/bcl-1 cooperates with myc genes in the generation of B-cell lymphoma in transgenic mice. Embo J 1994;13:3487–3495.
133. Schaffner C, Idler I, Stilgenbauer S, et al. Mantle cell lymphoma is characterized by inactivation of the ATM gene. Proc Natl Acad Sci U S A 2000;97: 2773–2778.
134. Louie DC, Offit K, Jaslow R, et al. p53 overexpression as a marker of poor prognosis in mantle cell lymphomas with t(11;14)(q13;q32). Blood 1995;86: 2892–2899.
135. Pinyol M, Hernandez L, Cazorla M, et al. Deletions and loss of expression of p16INK4a and p21Waf1 genes are associated with aggressive variants of mantle cell lymphomas. Blood 1997;89:272–280.
136. Bea S, Valdes-Mas R, Navarro A, et al. Landscape of somatic mutations and clonal evolution in mantle cell lymphoma. Proc Natl Acad Sci U S A 2013;110:18250–1825.
137. Kridel R, Meissner B, Rogic S, et al. Whole transcriptome sequencing reveals recurrent NOTCH1 mutations in mantle cell lymphoma. Blood 2012;119:1963–1971.
138. Bea S, Tort F, Pinyol M, et al. BMI-1 gene amplification and overexpression in hematological malignancies occur mainly in mantle cell lymphomas. Cancer Res 2001;61:2409–2412.
139. Bea S, Salaverria I, Armengol L, et al. Uniparental disomies, homozygous deletions, amplifications, and target genes in mantle cell lymphoma revealed by integrative high-resolution whole-genome profiling. Blood 2009;113:3059–3069.
140. Chapman CJ, Mockridge CI, Rowe M, et al. Analysis of VH genes used by neoplastic B cells in endemic Burkitt's lymphoma shows somatic hypermutation and intraclonal heterogeneity. Blood 1995;85:2176–2181.
141. Chapman CJ, Zhou JX, Gregory C, et al. VH and VL gene analysis in sporadic Burkitt's lymphoma shows somatic hypermutation, intraclonal heterogeneity, and a role for antigen selection. Blood 1996;88:3562–3568.
142. Jain R, Roncella S, Hashimoto S, et al. A potential role for antigen selection in the clonal evolution of Burkitt's lymphoma. J Immunol 1994;153:45–52.
143. Tamaru J, Hummel M, Marafioti T, et al. Burkitt's lymphomas express VH genes with a moderate number of antigen-selected somatic mutations. Am J Pathol 1995;147:1398–1407.
144. Dave SS, Fu K, Wright GW, et al. Molecular diagnosis of Burkitt's lymphoma. N Engl J Med 2006;354:2431–2442.
145. Hummel M, Bentink S, Berger H, et al. A biologic definition of Burkitt's lymphoma from transcriptional and genomic profiling. N Engl J Med 2006; 354:2419–2430.
146. Dalla-Favera R, Bregni M, Erikson J, et al. Human c-myc onc gene is located on the region of chromosome 8 that is translocated in Burkitt lymphoma cells. Proc Natl Acad Sci U S A 1982;79:7824–7827.
147. Dalla-Favera R, Martinotti S, Gallo RC, et al. Translocation and rearrangements of the c-myc oncogene locus in human undifferentiated B-cell lymphomas. Science 1983;219:963–967.
148. Dalla-Favera R. Chromosomal translocations involving the c-myc oncogene in lymphoid neoplasia. In: Kirsch IR, ed. The Causes and Consequences of Chromosomal Aberrations. Boca Raton, FL: CRC Press; 1993: 312.
149. Taub R, Kirsch I, Morton C, et al. Translocation of the c-myc gene into the immunoglobulin heavy chain locus in human Burkitt lymphoma and murine plasmacytoma cells. Proc Natl Acad Sci U S A 1982;79:7837–7841.
150. Davis M, Malcolm S, Rabbitts TH. Chromosome translocation can occur on either side of the c-myc oncogene in Burkitt lymphoma cells. Nature 1984;308:286–288.

151. Neri A, Barriga F, Knowles DM, et al. Different regions of the immunoglobulin heavy-chain locus are involved in chromosomal translocations in distinct pathogenetic forms of Burkitt lymphoma. *Proc Natl Acad Sci U S A* 1988;85:2748–2752.
152. Pelicci PG, Knowles DM 2nd, Magrath I, et al. Chromosomal breakpoints and structural alterations of the c-myc locus differ in endemic and sporadic forms of Burkitt lymphoma. *Proc Natl Acad Sci U S A* 1986;83:2984–2988.
153. ar-Rushdi A, Nishikura K, Erikson J, et al. Differential expression of the translocated and the untranslocated c-myc oncogene in Burkitt lymphoma. *Science* 1983;222:390–393.
154. Hayday AC, Gillies SD, Saito H, et al. Activation of a translocated human c-myc gene by an enhancer in the immunoglobulin heavy-chain locus. *Nature* 1984;307:334–340.
155. Rabbitts TH, Forster A, Baer R, et al. Transcription enhancer identified near the human C mu immunoglobulin heavy chain gene is unavailable to the translocated c-myc gene in a Burkitt lymphoma. *Nature* 1983;306:806–809.
156. Dominguez-Sola D, Victora GD, Ying CY, et al. The proto-oncogene MYC is required for selection in the germinal center and cyclic reentry. *Nat Immunol* 2012;13:1083–1091.
157. Cesarman E, Dalla-Favera R, Bentley D, et al. Mutations in the first exon are associated with altered transcription of c-myc in Burkitt lymphoma. *Science* 1987;238:1272–1275.
158. Bhatia K, Huppi K, Spangler G, et al. Point mutations in the c-Myc transactivation domain are common in Burkitt's lymphoma and mouse plasmacytomas. *Nat Genet* 1993;5:56–61.
159. Bhatia K, Spangler G, Gaiano G, et al. Mutations in the coding region of c-myc occur frequently in acquired immunodeficiency syndrome-associated lymphomas. *Blood* 1994;84:883–888.
160. Gu W, Bhatia K, Magrath IT, et al. Binding and suppression of the Myc transcriptional activation domain by p107. *Science* 1994;264:251–254.
161. Gregory MA, Hann SR. c-Myc proteolysis by the ubiquitin-proteasome pathway: stabilization of c-Myc in Burkitt's lymphoma cells. *Mol Cell Biol* 2000;20:2423–2435.
162. Hemann MT, Bric A, Teruya-Feldstein J, et al. Evasion of the p53 tumour surveillance network by tumour-derived MYC mutants. *Nature* 2005;436:807–811.
163. Meyer N, Penn LZ. Reflecting on 25 years with MYC. *Nat Rev Cancer* 2008;8:976–990.
164. Dominguez-Sola D, Ying CY, Grandori C, et al. Non-transcriptional control of DNA replication by c-Myc. *Nature* 2007;448:445–451.
165. Eilers M, Eisenman RN. Myc's broad reach. *Genes Dev* 2008;22:2755–2766.
166. Amati B, Brooks MW, Levy N, et al. Oncogenic activity of the c-Myc protein requires dimerization with Max. *Cell* 1993;72:233–245.
167. Amati B, Dalton S, Brooks MW, et al. Transcriptional activation by the human c-Myc oncoprotein in yeast requires interaction with Max. *Nature* 1992;359:423–426.
168. Blackwood EM, Eisenman RN. Max: a helix-loop-helix zipper protein that forms a sequence-specific DNA-binding complex with Myc. *Science* 1991;251:1211–1217.
169. Blackwood EM, Luscher B, Eisenman RN. Myc and Max associate in vivo. *Genes Dev* 1992;6:71–80.
170. Gu W, Cechova K, Tassi V, et al. Opposite regulation of gene transcription and cell proliferation by c-Myc and Max. *Proc Natl Acad Sci U S A* 1993;90:2935–2939.
171. Kretzner L, Blackwood EM, Eisenman RN. Myc and Max proteins possess distinct transcriptional activities. *Nature* 1992;359:426–429.
172. Grandori C, Cowley SM, James LP, et al. The Myc/Max/Mad network and the transcriptional control of cell behavior. *Annu Rev Cell Dev Biol* 2000;16:653–699.
173. Dang CV, O'Donnell KA, Zeller KI, et al. The c-Myc target gene network. *Semin Cancer Biol* 2006;16:253–264.
174. Felsher DW, Bishop JM. Transient excess of MYC activity can elicit genomic instability and tumorigenesis. *Proc Natl Acad Sci U S A* 1999;96:3940–3944.
175. Adams JM, Harris AW, Pinkert CA, et al. The c-myc oncogene driven by immunoglobulin enhancers induces lymphoid malignancy in transgenic mice. *Nature* 1985;318:533–538.
176. Kovalchuk AL, Qi CF, Torrey TA, et al. Burkitt lymphoma in the mouse. *J Exp Med* 2000;192:1183–1190.
177. Schmitz R, Young RM, Ceribelli M, et al. Burkitt lymphoma pathogenesis and therapeutic targets from structural and functional genomics. *Nature* 2012;490:116–120.
178. Lombardi L, Newcomb EW, Dalla-Favera R. Pathogenesis of Burkitt lymphoma: expression of an activated c-myc oncogene causes the tumorigenic conversion of EBV-infected human B lymphoblasts. *Cell* 1987;49:161–170.
179. Prevot S, Hamilton-Dutoit S, Audouin J, et al. Analysis of African Burkitt's and high-grade B cell non-Burkitt's lymphoma for Epstein-Barr virus genomes using in situ hybridization. *Br J Haematol* 1992;80:27–32.
180. Bornkamm GW. Epstein-Barr virus and its role in the pathogenesis of Burkitt's lymphoma: an unresolved issue. *Semin Cancer Biol* 2009;19:351–365.
181. Thorley-Lawson DA, Allday MJ. The curious case of the tumour virus: 50 years of Burkitt's lymphoma. *Nat Rev Microbiol* 2008;6:913–924.
182. Kridel R, Sehn LH, Gascoyne RD. Pathogenesis of follicular lymphoma. *J Clin Invest* 2012;122:3424–3431.
183. Montoto S, Fitzgibbon J. Transformation of indolent B-cell lymphomas. *J Clin Oncol* 2011;29:1827–1834.
184. Bakhshi A, Jensen JP, Goldman P, et al. Cloning the chromosomal breakpoint of t(14;18) human lymphomas: clustering around JH on chromosome 14 and near a transcriptional unit on 18. *Cell* 1985;41:899–906.
185. Cleary ML, Sklar J. Nucleotide sequence of a t(14;18) chromosomal breakpoint in follicular lymphoma and demonstration of a breakpoint-cluster region near a transcriptionally active locus on chromosome 18. *Proc Natl Acad Sci U S A* 1985;82:7439–7443.
186. Cleary ML, Smith SD, Sklar J. Cloning and structural analysis of cDNAs for bcl-2 and a hybrid bcl-2/immunoglobulin transcript resulting from the t(14;18) translocation. *Cell* 1986;47:19–28.
187. Ott G, Katzenberger T, Lohr A, et al. Cytomorphologic, immunohistochemical, and cytogenetic profiles of follicular lymphoma: 2 types of follicular lymphoma grade 3. *Blood* 2002;99:3806–3812.
188. Tsujimoto Y, Finger LR, Yunis J, et al. Cloning of the chromosome breakpoint of neoplastic B cells with the t(14;18) chromosome translocation. *Science* 1984;226:1097–1099.
189. Cleary ML, Galili N, Sklar, J. Detection of a second t(14;18) breakpoint cluster region in human follicular lymphomas. *J Exp Med* 1986;164:315–320.
190. Graninger WB, Seto M, Boutain B, et al. Expression of Bcl-2 and Bcl-2-Ig fusion transcripts in normal and neoplastic cells. *J Clin Invest* 1987;80:1512–1515.
191. Ngan BY, Chen-Levy Z, Weiss LM, et al. Expression in non-Hodgkin's lymphoma of the bcl-2 protein associated with the t(14;18) chromosomal translocation. *N Engl J Med* 1988;318:1638–1644.
192. Petrovic AS, Young RL, Hilgarth B, et al. The Ig heavy chain 3' end confers a posttranscriptional processing advantage to Bcl-2-IgH fusion RNA in t(14;18) lymphoma. *Blood* 1998;91:3952–3961.
193. Saito M, Novak U, Piovan E, et al. BCL6 suppression of BCL2 via Miz1 and its disruption in diffuse large B cell lymphoma. *Proc Natl Acad Sci U S A* 2009;106:11294–11299.
194. Buchonnet G, Jardin F, Jean N, et al. Distribution of BCL2 breakpoints in follicular lymphoma and correlation with clinical features: specific subtypes or same disease? *Leukemia* 2002;16:1852–1856.
195. Morin RD, Johnson NA, Severson TM, et al. Somatic mutations altering EZH2 (Tyr641) in follicular and diffuse large B-cell lymphomas of germinal-center origin. *Nat Genet* 2010;42:181–185.
196. Okosun J, Bodor C, Wang J, et al. Integrated genomic analysis identifies recurrent mutations and evolution patterns driving the initiation and progression of follicular lymphoma. *Nat Genet* 2014;46:176–181.
197. Cleary ML, Meeker TC, Levy S, et al. Clustering of extensive somatic mutations in the variable region of an immunoglobulin heavy chain gene from a human B cell lymphoma. *Cell* 1986;44:97–106.
198. Bahler DW, Levy R. Clonal evolution of a follicular lymphoma: evidence for antigen selection. *Proc Natl Acad Sci U S A* 1992;89:6770–6774.
199. Elenitoba-Johnson KS, Gascoyne RD, Lim MS, et al. Homozygous deletions at chromosome 9p21 involving p16 and p15 are associated with histologic progression in follicle center lymphoma. *Blood* 1998;91:4677–4685.
200. Yano T, Jaffe ES, Longo DL, et al. MYC rearrangements in histologically progressed follicular lymphomas. *Blood* 1992;80:758–767.
201. Ichikawa A, Hotta T, Takagi N, et al. Mutations of p53 gene and their relation to disease progression in B-cell lymphoma. *Blood* 1992;79:2701–2707.
202. O'Shea D, O'Riain C, Taylor C, et al. The presence of TP53 mutation at diagnosis of follicular lymphoma identifies a high-risk group of patients with shortened time to disease progression and poorer overall survival. *Blood* 2008;112:3126–3129.
203. Sander CA, Yano T, Clark HM, et al. p53 mutation is associated with progression in follicular lymphomas. *Blood* 1993;82:1994–2004.
204. Bastard C, Deweindt C, Kerckaert JP, et al. LAZ3 rearrangements in non-Hodgkin's lymphoma: correlation with histology, immunophenotype, karyotype, and clinical outcome in 217 patients. *Blood* 1994;83:2423–2427.
205. Lo Coco F, Ye BH, Lista F, et al. Rearrangements of the BCL6 gene in diffuse large cell non-Hodgkin's lymphoma. *Blood* 1994;83:1757–1759.
206. Otsuki T, Yano T, Clark HM, et al. Analysis of LAZ3 (BCL-6) status in B-cell non-Hodgkin's lymphomas: results of rearrangement and gene expression studies and a mutational analysis of coding region sequences. *Blood* 1995;85:2877–2884.
207. Akasaka T, Lossos IS, Levy R. BCL6 gene translocation in follicular lymphoma: a harbinger of eventual transformation to diffuse aggressive lymphoma. *Blood* 2003;102:1443–1448.
208. A clinical evaluation of the International Lymphoma Study Group classification of non-Hodgkin's lymphoma. The Non-Hodgkin's Lymphoma Classification Project. *Blood* 1997;89:3909–2918.
209. Alizadeh AA, Eisen MB, Davis RE, et al. Distinct types of diffuse B-cell lymphoma identified by gene expression profiling. *Nature* 2000;403:503–511.
210. Wright G, Tan B, Rosenwald A, et al. A gene expression-based method to diagnose clinically distinct subgroups of diffuse large B cell lymphoma. *Proc Natl Acad Sci U S A* 2003;100:9991–9996.
211. Savage KJ, Monti S, Kutok JL, et al. The molecular signature of mediastinal large B-cell lymphoma differs from that of other diffuse large B-cell lymphomas and shares features with classical Hodgkin lymphoma. *Blood* 2003;102:3871–3879.
212. Rosenwald A, Wright G, Leroy K, et al. Molecular diagnosis of primary mediastinal B cell lymphoma identifies a clinically favorable subgroup of diffuse large B cell lymphoma related to Hodgkin lymphoma. *J Exp Med* 2003;198:851–862.
213. Choi WW, Weisenburger DD, Greiner TC, et al. A new immunostain algorithm classifies diffuse large B-cell lymphoma into molecular subtypes with high accuracy. *Clin Cancer Res* 2009;15:5494–5502.
214. Hans CP, Weisenburger DD, Greiner TC, et al. Confirmation of the molecular classification of diffuse large B-cell lymphoma by immunohistochemistry using a tissue microarray. *Blood* 2004;103:275–282.

215. Monti S, Savage KJ, Kutok JL, et al. Molecular profiling of diffuse large B-cell lymphoma identifies robust subtypes including one characterized by host inflammatory response. *Blood* 2005;105:1851–1861.
216. Lohr JG, Stojanov P, Lawrence MS, et al. Discovery and prioritization of somatic mutations in diffuse large B-cell lymphoma (DLBCL) by whole-exome sequencing. *Proc Natl Acad Sci U S A* 2012;109:3879–3884.
217. Pasqualucci L, Trifonov V, Fabbri G, et al. Analysis of the coding genome of diffuse large B-cell lymphoma. *Nat Genet* 2011;43:830–837.
218. Offit K, Jhanwar S, Ebrahim SA, et al. t(3;22)(q27;q11): a novel translocation associated with diffuse non-Hodgkin's lymphoma. *Blood* 1989;74:1876–1879.
219. Iqbal J, Greiner TC, Patel K, et al. Distinctive patterns of BCL6 molecular alterations and their functional consequences in different subgroups of diffuse large B-cell lymphoma. *Leukemia* 2007;21:2332–2343.
220. Ye BH, Chaganti S, Chang CC, et al. Chromosomal translocations cause deregulated BCL6 expression by promoter substitution in B cell lymphoma. *Embo J* 1995;14:6209–6217.
221. Ying CY, Dominguez-Sola D, Fabi M, et al. MEF2B mutations lead to deregulated expression of the oncogene BCL6 in diffuse large B cell lymphoma. *Nat Immunol* 2013;14:1084–1092.
222. Duan S, Cermak L, Pagan JK, et al. FBXO11 targets BCL6 for degradation and is inactivated in diffuse large B-cell lymphomas. *Nature* 2012;481:90–93.
223. Cattoretti G, Pasqualucci L, Ballon G, et al. Deregulated BCL6 expression recapitulates the pathogenesis of human diffuse large B cell lymphomas in mice. *Cancer Cell* 2005;7:445–455.
224. Challa-Malladi M, Lieu YK, Califano O, et al. Combined genetic inactivation of β2-Microglobulin and CD58 reveals frequent escape from immune recognition in diffuse large B cell lymphoma. *Cancer Cell* 2011;20:728–740.
225. Iqbal J, Sanger WG, Horsman DE, et al. BCL2 translocation defines a unique tumor subset within the germinal center B-cell-like diffuse large B-cell lymphoma. *Am J Pathol* 2004;165:159–166.
226. Ladanyi M, Offit K, Jhanwar SC, et al. MYC rearrangement and translocations involving band 8q24 in diffuse large cell lymphomas. *Blood* 1991;77:1057–1063.
227. Pasqualucci L, Migliazza A, Basso K, et al. Mutations of the BCL6 proto-oncogene disrupt its negative autoregulation in diffuse large B-cell lymphoma. *Blood* 2003;101:2914–2923.
228. Wang X, Li Z, Naganuma A, et al. Negative autoregulation of BCL-6 is bypassed by genetic alterations in diffuse large B cell lymphomas. *Proc Natl Acad Sci U S A* 2002;99:15018–15023.
229. Ueda Y, Gao JJ, Lemmon EE, et al. PTEN loss defines a PI3K/AKT pathway-dependent germinal center subtype of diffuse large B-cell lymphoma. *Proc Natl Acad Sci U S A* 2013;110:12420–12425.
230. Capello D, Vitolo U, Pasqualucci L, et al. Distribution and pattern of BCL-6 mutations throughout the spectrum of B-cell neoplasia. *Blood* 2000;95:651–659.
231. Migliazza A, Martinotti S, Chen W, et al. Frequent somatic hypermutation of the 5' noncoding region of the BCL6 gene in B-cell lymphoma. *Proc Natl Acad Sci U S A* 1995;92:12520–12524.
232. Saito M, Gao J, Basso K, et al. A signaling pathway mediating downregulation of BCL6 in germinal center B cells is blocked by BCL6 gene alterations in B cell lymphoma. *Cancer Cell* 2007;12:280–292.
233. Iqbal J, Neppalli VT, Wright G, et al. BCL2 expression is a prognostic marker for the activated B-cell-like type of diffuse large B-cell lymphoma. *J Clin Oncol* 2006;24:961–968.
234. Monni O, Joensuu H, Franssila K, et al. BCL2 overexpression associated with chromosomal amplification in diffuse large B-cell lymphoma. *Blood* 1997;90:1168–1174.
235. Lenz G, Davis RE, Ngo VN, et al. Oncogenic CARD11 mutations in human diffuse large B cell lymphoma. *Science* 2008;319:1676–1679.
236. Davis RE, Ngo VN, Lenz G, et al. Chronic active B-cell-receptor signalling in diffuse large B-cell lymphoma. *Nature* 2010;463:88–92.
237. Ngo VN, Young RM, Schmitz R, et al. Oncogenically active MYD88 mutations in human lymphoma. *Nature* 2011;470:115–119.
238. Gronbaek K, Worm J, Ralkiaer E, et al. ATM mutations are associated with inactivation of the ARF-TP53 tumor suppressor pathway in diffuse large B-cell lymphoma. *Blood* 2002;100:1430–1437.
239. Angelin-Duclos C, Cattoretti G, Lin KI, et al. Commitment of B lymphocytes to a plasma cell fate is associated with Blimp-1 expression in vivo. *J Immunol* 2000;165:5462–5471.
240. Cattoretti G, Angelin-Duclos C, Shaknovich R, et al. PRDM1/Blimp-1 is expressed in human B-lymphocytes committed to the plasma cell lineage. *J Pathol* 2005;206:76–86.
241. Shapiro-Shelef M, Lin KI, McHeyzer-Williams LJ, et al. Blimp-1 is required for the formation of immunoglobulin secreting plasma cells and pre-plasma memory B cells. *Immunity* 2003;19:607–620.
242. Joos S, Kupper M, Ohl S, et al. Genomic imbalances including amplification of the tyrosine kinase gene JAK2 in CD30+ Hodgkin cells. *Cancer Res* 2000;60:549–552.
243. Steidl C, Shah SP, Woolcock BW, et al. MHC class II transactivator CIITA is a recurrent gene fusion partner in lymphoid cancers. *Nature* 2011;471:377–381.
244. Mestre C, Rubio-Moscardo F, Rosenwald A, et al. Homozygous deletion of SOCS1 in primary mediastinal B-cell lymphoma detected by CGH to BAC microarrays. *Leukemia* 2005;19:1082–1084.
245. Melzner I, Bucur AJ, Bruderlein S, et al. Biallelic mutation of SOCS-1 impairs JAK2 degradation and sustains phospho-JAK2 action in the MedB-1 mediastinal lymphoma line. *Blood* 2005;105:2535–2542.
246. Weniger MA, Melzner I, Menz CK, et al. Mutations of the tumor suppressor gene SOCS-1 in classical Hodgkin lymphoma are frequent and associated with nuclear phospho-STAT5 accumulation. *Oncogene* 2006;25:2679–2684.
247. Landau DA, Carter SL, Stojanov P, et al. Evolution and impact of subclonal mutations in chronic lymphocytic leukemia. *Cell* 2013;152:714–726.
248. Muller AM, Ihorst G, Mertelsmann R, et al. Epidemiology of non-Hodgkin's lymphoma (NHL): trends, geographic distribution, and etiology. *Ann Hematol* 2005;84:1–12.
249. Bertoni F, Cazzaniga G, Bosshard G, et al. Immunoglobulin heavy chain diversity genes rearrangement pattern indicates that MALT-type gastric lymphoma B cells have undergone an antigen selection process. *Br J Haematol* 1997;97:830–836.
250. Wotherspoon AC. Gastric lymphoma of mucosa-associated lymphoid tissue and Helicobacter pylori. *Annu Rev Med* 1998;49:289–299.
251. Bende RJ, Aarts WM, Riedl RG, et al. Among B cell non-Hodgkin's lymphomas, MALT lymphomas express a unique antibody repertoire with frequent rheumatoid factor reactivity. *J Exp Med* 2005;201:1229–1241.
252. Hussell T, Isaacson PG, Crabtree JE, et al. Immunoglobulin specificity of low grade B cell gastrointestinal lymphoma of mucosa-associated lymphoid tissue (MALT) type. *Am J Pathol* 1993;142:285–292.
253. Akagi T, Motegi M, Tamura A, et al. A novel gene, MALT1 at 18q21, is involved in t(11;18) (q21;q21) found in low-grade B-cell lymphoma of mucosa-associated lymphoid tissue. *Oncogene* 1999;18:5785–5794.
254. Dierlamm J, Baens M, Wlodarska I, et al. The apoptosis inhibitor gene API2 and a novel 18q gene, MLT, are recurrently rearranged in the t(11;18)(q21;q21) associated with mucosa-associated lymphoid tissue lymphomas. *Blood* 1999;93:3601–3609.
255. Remstein ED, James CD, Kurtin PJ. Incidence and subtype specificity of API2-MALT1 fusion translocations in extranodal, nodal, and splenic marginal zone lymphomas. *Am J Pathol* 2000;156:1183–1188.
256. Baens M, Maes B, Steyls A, et al. The product of the t(11;18), an API2-MLT fusion, marks nearly half of gastric MALT type lymphomas without large cell proliferation. *Am J Pathol* 2000;156:1433–1439.
257. Motegi M, Yonezumi M, Suzuki H, et al. API2-MALT1 chimeric transcripts involved in mucosa-associated lymphoid tissue type lymphoma predict heterogeneous products. *Am J Pathol* 2000;156:807–812.
258. Thome M. CARMA1, BCL-10 and MALT1 in lymphocyte development and activation. *Nat Rev Immunol* 2004;4:348–359.
259. Lucas PC, Kuffa P, Gu S, et al. A dual role for the API2 moiety in API2-MALT1-dependent NF-kappaB activation: heterotypic oligomerization and TRAF2 recruitment. *Oncogene* 2007;26:5643–5654.
260. Sanchez-Izquierdo D, Buchonnet G, Siebert R, et al. MALT1 is deregulated by both chromosomal translocation and amplification in B-cell non-Hodgkin lymphoma. *Blood* 2003;101:4539–4546.
261. Streubel B, Lamprecht A, Dierlamm J, et al. T(14;18)(q32;q21) involving IGH and MALT1 is a frequent chromosomal aberration in MALT lymphoma. *Blood* 2003;101:2335–2339.
262. Willis TG, Jadayel DM, Du MQ, et al. Bcl10 is involved in t(1;14)(p22;q32) of MALT B cell lymphoma and mutated in multiple tumor types. *Cell* 1999;96:35–45.
263. Zhang Q, Siebert R, Yan M, et al. Inactivating mutations and overexpression of BCL10, a caspase recruitment domain-containing gene, in MALT lymphoma with t(1;14)(p22;q32). *Nat Genet* 1999;22:63–68.
264. Ruland J, Duncan GS, Elia A, et al. Bcl10 is a positive regulator of antigen receptor-induced activation of NF-kappaB and neural tube closure. *Cell* 2001;104:33–42.
265. Xue L, Morris SW, Orihuela C, et al. Defective development and function of Bcl10-deficient follicular, marginal zone and B1 B cells. *Nat Immunol* 2003;4:857–865.
266. Wlodarska I, Veyt E, De Paepe P, et al. FOXP1, a gene highly expressed in a subset of diffuse large B-cell lymphoma, is recurrently targeted by genomic aberrations. *Leukemia* 2005;19:1299–1305.
267. Streubel B, Vinatzer U, Lamprecht A, et al. T(3;14)(p14.1;q32) involving IGH and FOXP1 is a novel recurrent chromosomal aberration in MALT lymphoma. *Leukemia* 2005;19:652–658.
268. Hu H, Wang B, Borde M, et al. Foxp1 is an essential transcriptional regulator of B cell development. *Nat Immunol* 2006;7:819–826.
269. Wotherspoon AC, Finn TM, Isaacson PG. Trisomy 3 in low-grade B-cell lymphomas of mucosa-associated lymphoid tissue. *Blood* 1995;85:2000–2004.
270. Ott G, Kalla J, Steinhoff A, et al. Trisomy 3 is not a common feature in malignant lymphomas of mucosa-associated lymphoid tissue type. *Am J Pathol* 1998;153:689–694.
271. Du M, Peng H, Singh N, et al. The accumulation of p53 abnormalities is associated with progression of mucosa-associated lymphoid tissue lymphoma. *Blood* 1995;86:4587–4593.
272. Gaidano G, Capello D, Gloghini A, et al. Frequent mutation of bcl-6 proto-oncogene in high grade, but not low grade, MALT lymphomas of the gastrointestinal tract. *Haematologica* 1999;84:582–588.
273. Gaidano G, Volpe G, Pastore C, et al. Detection of BCL-6 rearrangements and p53 mutations in Malt-lymphomas. *Am J Hematol* 1997;56:206–213.
274. Klein U, Dalla-Favera R. New insights into the pathogenesis of chronic lymphocytic leukemia. *Semin Cancer Biol* 2010;20:377–383.
275. Fais F, Ghiotto F, Hashimoto S, et al. Chronic lymphocytic leukemia B cells express restricted sets of mutated and unmutated antigen receptors. *J Clin Invest* 1998;102:1515–1525.
276. Oscier DG, Thompsett A, Zhu D, et al. Differential rates of somatic hypermutation in V(H) genes among subsets of chronic lymphocytic leukemia defined by chromosomal abnormalities. *Blood* 1997;89:4153–4160.
277. Klein U, Tu Y, Stolovitzky GA, et al. Gene expression profiling of B cell chronic lymphocytic leukemia reveals a homogeneous phenotype related to memory B cells. *J Exp Med* 2001;194:1625–1638.

278. Rosenwald A, Alizadeh AA, Widhopf G, et al. Relation of gene expression phenotype to immunoglobulin mutation genotype in B cell chronic lymphocytic leukemia. *J Exp Med* 2001;194:1639–1647.
279. Widhopf GF 2nd, Rassenti LZ, Toy TL, et al. Chronic lymphocytic leukemia B cells of more than 1% of patients express virtually identical immunoglobulins. *Blood* 2004;104:2499–2504.
280. Messmer BT, Albesiano E, Efremov DG, et al. Multiple distinct sets of stereotyped antigen receptors indicate a role for antigen in promoting chronic lymphocytic leukemia. *J Exp Med* 2004;200:519–525.
281. Tobin G, Thunberg U, Karlsson K, et al. Subsets with restricted immunoglobulin gene rearrangement features indicate a role for antigen selection in the development of chronic lymphocytic leukemia. *Blood* 2004;104:2879–2885.
282. Murray F, Darzentas N, Hadzidimitriou A, et al. Stereotyped patterns of somatic hypermutation in subsets of patients with chronic lymphocytic leukemia: implications for the role of antigen selection in leukemogenesis. *Blood* 2008;111:1524–1533.
283. Stamatopoulos K, Belessi C, Moreno C, et al. Over 20% of patients with chronic lymphocytic leukemia carry stereotyped receptors: Pathogenetic implications and clinical correlations. *Blood* 2007;109:259–270.
284. Tobin G, Thunberg U, Johnson A, et al. Chronic lymphocytic leukemias utilizing the VH3-21 gene display highly restricted Vlambda2-14 gene use and homologous CDR3s: implicating recognition of a common antigen epitope. *Blood* 2003;101:4952–4957.
285. Damle RN, Wasil T, Fais F, et al. Ig V gene mutation status and CD38 expression as novel prognostic indicators in chronic lymphocytic leukemia. *Blood* 1999;94:1840–1847.
286. Hamblin TJ, Davis Z, Gardiner A, et al. Unmutated Ig V(H) genes are associated with a more aggressive form of chronic lymphocytic leukemia. *Blood* 1999;94:1848–1854.
287. Rawstron AC, Bennett FL, O'Connor SJ, et al. Monoclonal B-cell lymphocytosis and chronic lymphocytic leukemia. *N Engl J Med* 2008;359:575–583.
288. Calin GA, Dumitru CD, Shimizu M, et al. Frequent deletions and down-regulation of micro-RNA genes miR15 and miR16 at 13q14 in chronic lymphocytic leukemia. *Proc Natl Acad Sci U S A* 2002;99:15524–15529.
289. Kalachikov S, Migliazza A, Cayanis E, et al. Cloning and gene mapping of the chromosome 13q14 region deleted in chronic lymphocytic leukemia. *Genomics* 1997;42:369–377.
290. Migliazza A, Bosch F, Komatsu H, et al. Nucleotide sequence, transcription map, and mutation analysis of the 13q14 chromosomal region deleted in B-cell chronic lymphocytic leukemia. *Blood* 2001;97:2098–2104.
291. Klein U, Lia M, Crespo M, et al. The DLEU2/miR-15a/16-1 cluster controls B cell proliferation and its deletion leads to chronic lymphocytic leukemia. *Cancer Cell* 2010;17:28–40.
292. Anastasi J, Le Beau MM, Vardiman JW, et al. Detection of trisomy 12 in chronic lymphocytic leukemia by fluorescence in situ hybridization to interphase cells: a simple and sensitive method. *Blood* 1992;79:796–1801.
293. Hjalmar V, Kimby E, Matutes E, et al. Trisomy 12 and lymphoplasmacytoid lymphocytes in chronic leukemic B-cell disorders. *Haematologica* 1998;83:602–609.
294. Juliusson G, Oscier DG, Fitchett M, et al. Prognostic subgroups in B-cell chronic lymphocytic leukemia defined by specific chromosomal abnormalities. *N Engl J Med* 1990;323:720–724.
295. Bullrich F, Rasio D, Kitada S, et al. ATM mutations in B-cell chronic lymphocytic leukemia. *Cancer Res* 1999;59:24–27.
296. Stankovic T, Weber P, Stewart G, et al. Inactivation of ataxia telangiectasia mutated gene in B-cell chronic lymphocytic leukaemia. *Lancet* 1999;353:26–29.
297. Starostik P, Manshouri T, O'Brien S, et al. Deficiency of the ATM protein expression defines an aggressive subgroup of B-cell chronic lymphocytic leukemia. *Cancer Res* 1998;58:4552–4557.
298. Rossi D, Fangazio M, Rasi S, et al. Disruption of BIRC3 associates with fludarabine chemorefractoriness in TP53 wild-type chronic lymphocytic leukemia. *Blood* 2012;119:2854–2862.
299. Gaidano G, Foa R, Dalla-Favera R. Molecular pathogenesis of chronic lymphocytic leukemia. *J Clin Invest* 2012;122:3432–3438.
300. Fabbri G, Rasi S, Rossi D, et al. Analysis of the chronic lymphocytic leukemia coding genome: role of NOTCH1 mutational activation. *J Exp Med* 2011;208:1389–1401.
301. Puente XS, Pinyol M, Quesada V, et al. Whole-genome sequencing identifies recurrent mutations in chronic lymphocytic leukaemia. *Nature* 2011;475:101–105.
302. Quesada V, Conde L, Villamor N, et al. Exome sequencing identifies recurrent mutations of the splicing factor SF3B1 gene in chronic lymphocytic leukemia. *Nat Genet* 2012;44:47–52.
303. Wang L, Lawrence MS, Wan Y, et al. SF3B1 and other novel cancer genes in chronic lymphocytic leukemia. *N Engl J Med* 2011;365:2497–2506.
304. Rossi D, Bruscaggin A, Spina V, et al. Mutations of the SF3B1 splicing factor in chronic lymphocytic leukemia: association with progression and fludarabine-refractoriness. *Blood* 2011;118:6904–6908.
305. Carbone A, Gloghini A. AIDS-related lymphomas: from pathogenesis to pathology. *Br J Haematol* 2005;130:662–670.
306. Knowles DM. Etiology and pathogenesis of AIDS-related non-Hodgkin's lymphoma. *Hematol Oncol Clin North Am* 2003;17:785–820.
307. Gaidano G, Capello D, Carbone A. The molecular basis of acquired immunodeficiency syndrome-related lymphomagenesis. *Semin Oncol* 2000;27:431–441.
308. Carbone A, Gaidano G. HHV-8-positive body-cavity-based lymphoma: a novel lymphoma entity. *Br J Haematol* 1997;97:515–522.
309. Gaidano G, Carbone A. Primary effusion lymphoma: a liquid phase lymphoma of fluid-filled body cavities. *Adv Cancer Res* 2001;80:115–146.
310. Gaidano G, Gloghini A, Gattei V, et al. Association of Kaposi's sarcoma-associated herpesvirus-positive primary effusion lymphoma with expression of the CD138/syndecan-1 antigen. *Blood* 1997;90:4894–4900.
311. Carbone A, Gaidano G, Gloghini A, et al. BCL-6 protein expression in AIDS-related non-Hodgkin's lymphomas: inverse relationship with Epstein-Barr virus-encoded latent membrane protein-1 expression. *Am J Pathol* 1997;150:155–165.
312. Carbone A, Gaidano G, Gloghini A, et al. Differential expression of BCL-6, CD138/syndecan-1, and Epstein-Barr virus-encoded latent membrane protein-1 identifies distinct histogenetic subsets of acquired immunodeficiency syndrome-related non-Hodgkin's lymphomas. *Blood* 1998;91:747–755.
313. Riboldi P, Gaidano G, Schettino EW, et al. Two acquired immunodeficiency syndrome-associated Burkitt's lymphomas produce specific anti-i IgM cold agglutinins using somatically mutated VH4-21 segments. *Blood* 1994;83:2952–2961.
314. Gaidano G, Lo Coco F, Ye BH, et al. Rearrangements of the BCL-6 gene in acquired immunodeficiency syndrome-associated non-Hodgkin's lymphoma: association with diffuse large-cell subtype. *Blood* 1994;84:397–402.
315. Gaidano G, Carbone A, Pastore C, et al. Frequent mutation of the 5' noncoding region of the BCL-6 gene in acquired immunodeficiency syndrome-related non-Hodgkin's lymphomas. *Blood* 1997;89:3755–3762.
316. MacMahon EM, Glass JD, Hayward SD, et al. Epstein-Barr virus in AIDS-related primary central nervous system lymphoma. *Lancet* 1991;338:969–973.
317. Larocca LM, Capello D, Rinelli A, et al. The molecular and phenotypic profile of primary central nervous system lymphoma identifies distinct categories of the disease and is consistent with histogenetic derivation from germinal center-related B cells. *Blood* 1998;92:1011–1019.
318. Montesinos-Rongen M, Godlewska E, Brunn A, et al. Mutations of CARD11 but not TNFAIP3 may activate the NF-kappaB pathway in primary CNS lymphoma. *Acta Neuropathol* 2010;120:529–535.
319. Antinori A, Larocca LM, Fassone L, et al. HHV-8/KSHV is not associated with AIDS-related primary central nervous system lymphoma. *Brain Pathol* 1999;9:199–208.
320. Gaidano G, Capello D, Pastore C, et al. Analysis of human herpesvirus type 8 infection in AIDS-related and AIDS-unrelated primary central nervous system lymphoma. *J Infect Dis* 1997;175:1193–1197.
321. de Leval L, Bisig B, Thielen C, et al. Molecular classification of T-cell lymphomas. *Crit Rev Oncol Hematol* 2009;72:125–143.
322. Taylor GP. The epidemiology of HTLV-I in Europe. *J Acquir Immune Defic Syndr Hum Retrovirol* 1996;13:S8–14.
323. Tsukasaki K, Tsushima H, Yamamura M, et al. Integration patterns of HTLV-I provirus in relation to the clinical course of ATL: frequent clonal change at crisis from indolent disease. *Blood* 1997;89:948–956.
324. Takatsuki K, Matsuoka M, Yamaguchi K. Adult T-cell leukemia in Japan. *J Acquir Immune Defic Syndr Hum Retrovirol* 1996;13:S15–S19.
325. Uittenbogaard MN, Giebler HA, Reisman D, et al. Transcriptional repression of p53 by human T-cell leukemia virus type I Tax protein. *J Biol Chem* 1995;270:28503–28506.
326. Cesarman E, Chadburn A, Inghirami G, et al. Structural and functional analysis of oncogenes and tumor suppressor genes in adult T-cell leukemia/lymphoma shows frequent p53 mutations. *Blood* 1992;80:3205–3216.
327. Sakashita A, Hattori T, Miller CW, et al. Mutations of the p53 gene in adult T-cell leukemia. *Blood* 1992;79:477–480.
328. Gaulard P, Bourquelot P, Kanavaros P, et al. Expression of the alpha/beta and gamma/delta T-cell receptors in 57 cases of peripheral T-cell lymphomas. Identification of a subset of gamma/delta T-cell lymphomas. *Am J Pathol* 1990;137:617–628.
329. de Leval L, Rickman DS, Thielen C, et al. The gene expression profile of nodal peripheral T-cell lymphoma demonstrates a molecular link between angioimmunoblastic T-cell lymphoma (AITL) and follicular helper T (TFH) cells. *Blood* 2007;109:4952–4963.
330. Martin-Subero JI, Wlodarska I, Bastard C, et al. Chromosomal rearrangements involving the BCL3 locus are recurrent in classical Hodgkin and peripheral T-cell lymphoma. *Blood* 2006;108:401–402.
331. Almire C, Bertrand P, Ruminy P, et al. PVRL2 is translocated to the TRA@ locus in t(14;19)(q11;q13)-positive peripheral T-cell lymphomas. *Genes Chromosomes Cancer* 2007;46:1011–1018.
332. Feldman AL, Law M, Remstein ED, et al. Recurrent translocations involving the IRF4 oncogene locus in peripheral T-cell lymphomas. *Leukemia* 2009;23:574–580.
333. Palomero T, Couronne L, Khiabanian H, et al. Recurrent mutations in epigenetic regulators, RHOA and FYN kinase in peripheral T cell lymphomas. *Nat Genet* 2014;46:166–170.
334. Sakata-Yanagimoto M, Enami T, Yoshida K, et al. Somatic RHOA mutation in angioimmunoblastic T cell lymphoma. *Nat Genet* 2014;46:171–175.
335. Panwalkar AW, Armitage JO. T-cell/NK-cell lymphomas: a review. *Cancer Lett* 2007;253:1–13.
336. Piccaluga PP, Agostinelli C, Califano A, et al. Gene expression analysis of angioimmunoblastic lymphoma indicates derivation from T follicular helper cells and vascular endothelial growth factor deregulation. *Cancer Res* 2007;67:10703–10710.
337. Grogg KL, Attygalle AD, Macon WR, et al. Angioimmunoblastic T-cell lymphoma: a neoplasm of germinal-center T-helper cells? *Blood* 2005;106:1501–1502.

338. Chang CC, Zhang J, Lombardi L, et al. Rearranged NFKB-2 genes in lymphoid neoplasms code for constitutively active nuclear transactivators. *Mol Cell Biol* 1995;15:5180–5187.
339. Neri A, Chang CC, Lombardi L, et al. B cell lymphoma-associated chromosomal translocation involves candidate oncogene lyt-10, homologous to NF-kappa B p50. *Cell* 1991;67:1075–1087.
340. Fornari A, Piva R, Chiarle R, et al. Anaplastic large cell lymphoma: one or more entities among T-cell lymphoma? *Hematol Oncol* 2009;27:161–170.
341. Lamant L, de Reynies A, Duplantier MM, et al. Gene-expression profiling of systemic anaplastic large-cell lymphoma reveals differences based on ALK status and two distinct morphologic ALK+ subtypes. *Blood* 2007;109:2156–2164.
342. Gascoyne RD, Aoun P, Wu D, et al. Prognostic significance of anaplastic lymphoma kinase (ALK) protein expression in adults with anaplastic large cell lymphoma. *Blood* 1999;93:3913–3921.
343. Savage KJ, Harris NL, Vose JM, et al. ALK- anaplastic large-cell lymphoma is clinically and immunophenotypically different from both ALK+ ALCL and peripheral T-cell lymphoma, not otherwise specified: report from the International Peripheral T-Cell Lymphoma Project. *Blood* 2008;111:5496–5504.
344. Shiota M, Nakamura S, Ichinohasama R, et al. Anaplastic large cell lymphomas expressing the novel chimeric protein p80NPM/ALK: a distinct clinicopathologic entity. *Blood* 1995;86:1954–1960.
345. Piva R, Agnelli L, Pellegrino E, et al. Gene expression profiling uncovers molecular classifiers for the recognition of anaplastic large-cell lymphoma within peripheral T-cell neoplasms. *J Clin Oncol* 2010;28:1583–1590.
346. Chiarle R, Voena C, Ambrogio C, et al. The anaplastic lymphoma kinase in the pathogenesis of cancer. *Nat Rev Cancer* 2008;8:11–23.
347. Morris SW, Kirstein MN, Valentine MB, et al. Fusion of a kinase gene, ALK, to a nucleolar protein gene, NPM, in non-Hodgkin's lymphoma. *Science* 1994;263:1281–1284.
348. Kasprzycka M, Marzec M, Liu X, et al. Nucleophosmin/anaplastic lymphoma kinase (NPM/ALK) oncoprotein induces the T regulatory cell phenotype by activating STAT3. *Proc Natl Acad Sci U S A* 2006;103:9964–9969.
349. Marzec M, Zhang Q, Goradia A, et al. Oncogenic kinase NPM/ALK induces through STAT3 expression of immunosuppressive protein CD274 (PD-L1, B7-H1). *Proc Natl Acad Sci U S A* 2008;105:20852–20857.
350. Zhang Q, Wang HY, Liu X, et al. STAT5A is epigenetically silenced by the tyrosine kinase NPM1-ALK and acts as a tumor suppressor by reciprocally inhibiting NPM1-ALK expression. *Nat Med* 2007;13:1341–1348.
351. Bai RY, Ouyang T, Miething C, et al. Nucleophosmin-anaplastic lymphoma kinase associated with anaplastic large-cell lymphoma activates the phosphatidylinositol 3-kinase/Akt antiapoptotic signaling pathway. *Blood* 2000;96:4319–4327.
352. Chiarle R, Gong JZ, Guasparri I, et al. NPM-ALK transgenic mice spontaneously develop T-cell lymphomas and plasma cell tumors. *Blood* 2003;101:1919–1927.
353. Kuefer MU, Look AT, Pulford K, et al. Retrovirus-mediated gene transfer of NPM-ALK causes lymphoid malignancy in mice. *Blood* 1997;90:2901–2910.
354. Lange K, Uckert W, Blankenstein T, et al. Overexpression of NPM-ALK induces different types of malignant lymphomas in IL-9 transgenic mice. *Oncogene* 2003;22:517–527.
355. Hernandez L, Bea S, Bellosillo B, et al. Diversity of genomic breakpoints in TFG-ALK translocations in anaplastic large cell lymphomas: identification of a new TFG-ALK(XL) chimeric gene with transforming activity. *Am J Pathol* 2002;160:1487–1494.
356. Colleoni GW, Bridge JA, Garicochea B, et al. ATIC-ALK: A novel variant ALK gene fusion in anaplastic large cell lymphoma resulting from the recurrent cryptic chromosomal inversion, inv(2)(p23q35). *Am J Pathol* 2000;156:781–789.
357. Ma Z, Cools J, Marynen P, et al. Inv(2)(p23q35) in anaplastic large-cell lymphoma induces constitutive anaplastic lymphoma kinase (ALK) tyrosine kinase activation by fusion to ATIC, an enzyme involved in purine nucleotide biosynthesis. *Blood* 2000;95:2144–2149.
358. Feldman AL, Vasmatzis G, Asmann YW, et al. Novel TRAF1-ALK fusion identified by deep RNA sequencing of anaplastic large cell lymphoma. *Genes Chromosomes Cancer* 2013;52:1097–1102.
359. Kuppers R. The biology of Hodgkin's lymphoma. *Nat Rev Cancer* 2009;9:15–27.
360. Schwering I, Brauninger A, Klein U, et al. Loss of the B-lineage-specific gene expression program in Hodgkin and Reed-Sternberg cells of Hodgkin lymphoma. *Blood* 2003;101:1505–1512.
361. Re D, Muschen M, Ahmadi T, et al. Oct-2 and Bob-1 deficiency in Hodgkin and Reed Sternberg cells. *Cancer Res* 2001;61:2080–2084.
362. Stein H, Marafioti T, Foss HD, et al. Down-regulation of BOB.1/OBF.1 and Oct2 in classical Hodgkin disease but not in lymphocyte predominant Hodgkin disease correlates with immunoglobulin transcription. *Blood* 2001;97:496–501.
363. Küppers R, Rajewsky K, Zhao M, et al. Hodgkin disease: Hodgkin and Reed-Sternberg cells picked from histological sections show clonal immunoglobulin gene rearrangements and appear to be derived from B cells at various stages of development. *Proc Natl Acad Sci U S A* 1994;91:10962–10966.
364. Kanzler H, Kuppers R, Hansmann ML, et al. Hodgkin and Reed-Sternberg cells in Hodgkin's disease represent the outgrowth of a dominant tumor clone derived from (crippled) germinal center B cells. *J Exp Med* 1996;184:1495–1505.
365. Martin-Subero JI, Gesk S, Harder L, et al. Recurrent involvement of the REL and BCL11A loci in classical Hodgkin lymphoma. *Blood* 2002;99:1474–1477.
366. Barth TF, Martin-Subero JI, Joos S, et al. Gains of 2p involving the REL locus correlate with nuclear c-Rel protein accumulation in neoplastic cells of classical Hodgkin lymphoma. *Blood* 2003;101:3681–3686.
367. Jungnickel B, Staratschek-Jox A, Brauninger A, et al. Clonal deleterious mutations in the IkappaBalpha gene in the malignant cells in Hodgkin's lymphoma. *J Exp Med* 2000;191:395–402.
368. Emmerich F, Meiser M, Hummel M, et al. Overexpression of I kappa B alpha without inhibition of NF-kappaB activity and mutations in the I kappa B alpha gene in Reed-Sternberg cells. *Blood* 1999;94:3129–3134.
369. Schmitz R, Stanelle J, Hansmann ML, et al. Pathogenesis of classical and lymphocyte-predominant Hodgkin lymphoma. *Annu Rev Pathol* 2009;4:151–174.
370. Wlodarska I, Nooyen P, Maes B, et al. Frequent occurrence of BCL6 rearrangements in nodular lymphocyte predominance Hodgkin lymphoma but not in classical Hodgkin lymphoma. *Blood* 2003;101:706–710.
371. Martin-Subero JI, Klapper W, Sotnikova A, et al. Chromosomal breakpoints affecting immunoglobulin loci are recurrent in Hodgkin and Reed-Sternberg cells of classical Hodgkin lymphoma. *Cancer Res* 2006;66:10332–10338.

38 Hodgkin's Lymphoma

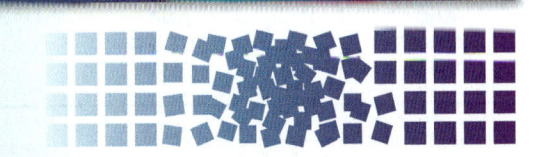

Anas Younes, Antonino Carbone, Peter Johnson, Bouthaina Dabaja, Stephen Ansell, and John Kuruvilla

INTRODUCTION

Although a relatively rare type of cancer, with an estimated 8,000 new cases per year in the United States, Hodgkin's lymphoma (HL) have fascinated scientists and clinicians for more than a century.[1,2] Remarkably, before the cell of origin and the biology of HL were elucidated, it became one of the earliest human cancers to be cured with multiagent chemotherapy.[1,3] Over the past 50 years, a significant progress has been made toward our understanding of HL biology, cell of origin, pathology, and treatment options. Therefore, many seminal observations that were made during the past few decades are now considered of historical value. For example, HL histologic classification evolved through multiple systems, starting from the initial histologic classification by Jackson and Parker in 1944, to the current system which is based on the World Health Organization (WHO) classification (Fig. 38.1).[4,5]

BIOLOGY OF HODGKIN'S LYMPHOMA

Cell of Origin

Molecular studies of isolated tumor cells have demonstrated that lymphocyte-predominant (LP) cells of nodular lymphocyte-predominant Hodgkin's lymphoma (NLPHL) are derived from antigen-selected germinal center (GC) B cells, whereas Reed-Sternberg (RS) cells in classic HL (cHL) appear to be derived from preapoptotic *crippled* GC B cells (Table 38.1).[6–9] Molecular features of LP cells include the presence of clonally rearranged and somatically mutated immunoglobulin (Ig)V gene cells, with signs of ongoing somatic hypermutation in a fraction of cases (see Table 38.1). These data linked the origin of LP cells in NLPHL to GC B cells. Another important feature supporting this linking was the immunohistochemical expression of BCL6 (a typical GC B-cell marker) in LP cells (Table 38.2).[10,11] Accordingly, LP cells can morphologically be observed in an environmental architecture resembling the structure of a secondary follicle, which contains a reactive GC. In fact, in the early phases of NLPHL, LP cells can be found in follicular structures in association with follicular dendritic cells (FDC) and GC type T-helper cells, in this regard resembling GC.[12]

The derivation of NLPHL from GCs is supported by the following features: (1) the expression of the BCL6 gene product and CD40 by LP cells[13,14]; (2) the occurrence of numerous CD4+/CD57+/PD1 T cells surrounding the LP cells, as seen in normal GCs and progressively transformed GCs (PTGC)[6]; (3) the presence of an FDC meshwork (CD21+/CD35+) within the tumor nodules[15]; and (4) the global gene expression profile.[16] Conversely, molecular features of RS cells in cHL demonstrate that they are probably derived from GC B cells that have acquired disadvantageous immunoglobulin variable chain gene mutations and normally would have undergone apoptosis.[6–8] In parallel to molecular investigations, biologic markers identifying distinct subsets of *mature* B cells have been used to study the cell of origin (see Table 38.2). According to the differential expression of these markers, LP and RS cells resemble *mature* B cells deriving from different stages of B-cell differentiation (i.e., GC and post-GC, respectively).

Reed-Sternberg Cells Lack Common B-Cell Markers

The loss of the B-cell phenotype in RS cells is unique among human lymphomas in the extent to which the lymphoma cells have undergone reprogramming of gene expression. As shown in gene expression profiling (GEP) studies, RS cells have lost the expression of most B-cell–typical genes and acquired expression of multiple genes that are typical for other types of cells in the immune system. Moreover, RS cell gene expression is most similar to that of Epstein-Barr virus (EBV)-transformed B cells, and cell lines derived from diffuse large-cell lymphomas showing features of in vitro activated B cells.[17]

The deregulated expression of inhibitors of B-cell molecules (inhibitor of differentiation and DNA binding 2 [ID2], activated B-cell factor 1 [ABF1], and notch 1), the downregulation of B-cell transcription factors (OCT2, BOB1, and PU.1), and the epigenetic silencing of B-cell genes (CD19 and immunoglobulin H [IgH]) all seem to be involved in the loss of the B-cell phenotype in RS cells.[17,18]

Multiple Signaling Pathways and Transcription Factors Have Deregulated Activity in Reed-Sternberg Cells

Very recently, biologic studies on HL cell lines using new technologies have shown that multiple signaling pathways and transcription factors have deregulated activity in RS cells. Involved pathways and transcription factors included nuclear factor kappa B (NF-κB), Janus kinase/signal transducers and activators of transcription (Jak-Stat), phosphoinositide 3-kinase (PI3K)–Akt, extracellular signal-regulated kinase (ERK), activating protein-1 (AP-1), notch 1, and receptor tyrosine kinases.[7,19] Functional studies have shown that in normal B GC cells, the activation of the CD40 receptor leads to NF-κB–mediated induction of the interferon regulatory factor 4/multiple myeloma oncogene 1 (IRF4/MUM1) transcription factor. CD40 engagement in HL cell lines by both soluble (s) CD40L and membrane-bound (mb) CD40L upregulates IRF4/MUM1 expression by HL cells.[20] CD40 engagement in HL cells by both sCD40L and mbCD40L enhances both clonogenic capacity and colony cell survival of HL cell lines, stimulates proliferation and rescue from apoptosis, mediates in vitro rosetting of activated CD4+ T cells to HL cells, and increases ERK phosphorylation and cell survival.[14,21]

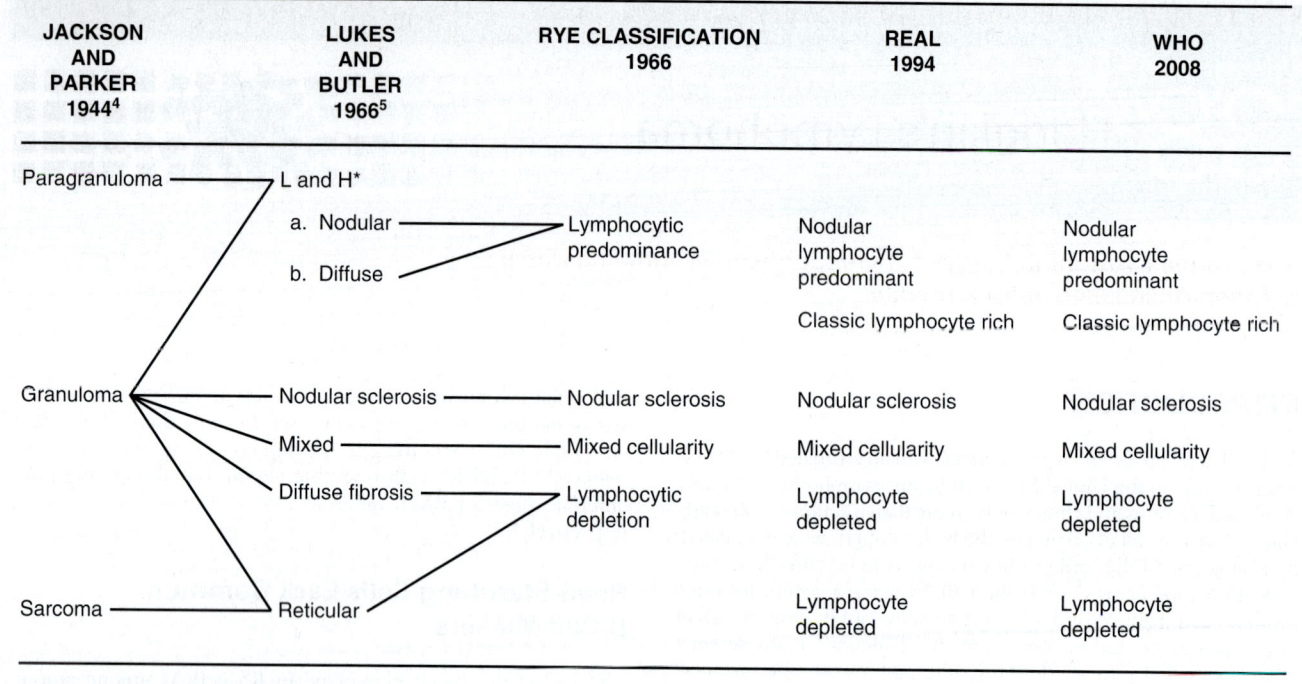

JACKSON AND PARKER 1944[4]	LUKES AND BUTLER 1966[5]	RYE CLASSIFICATION 1966	REAL 1994	WHO 2008
Paragranuloma	L and H* a. Nodular b. Diffuse	Lymphocytic predominance	Nodular lymphocyte predominant	Nodular lymphocyte predominant
			Classic lymphocyte rich	Classic lymphocyte rich
Granuloma	Nodular sclerosis	Nodular sclerosis	Nodular sclerosis	Nodular sclerosis
	Mixed	Mixed cellularity	Mixed cellularity	Mixed cellularity
	Diffuse fibrosis	Lymphocytic depletion	Lymphocyte depleted	Lymphocyte depleted
Sarcoma	Reticular		Lymphocyte depleted	Lymphocyte depleted

Figure 38.1 Comparison of classifications of Hodgkin's lymphoma. *Lymphocytic and histiocytic

PATHOLOGY OF HODGKIN'S LYMPHOMA

The REAL Classification and the WHO Proposal

The most recent contribution is provided by the Revised European American Lymphoma (REAL) classification[22] and the WHO proposal, which, on the basis of a combination of phenotypic and morphologic features, subdivided HL into two distinct pathologic and biologic entities: NLPHL and cHL. cHL includes four subtypes (see Table 38.2) (see the following). LP cells of NLPHL and RS cells of cHL have different morphology, different phenotype, and different infection pattern with the EBV. LP cells express CD20, CD45, and epithelial membrane antigen (EMA) antigens, whereas RS cells display CD15-positive, CD30-positive, and CD45-negative phenotypes. EBV infection is usually present only in the RS cells of cHL, which express EBV encoded latent membrane protein 1 (LMP1) (Table 38.3).[22,23]

Nodular Lymphocyte-Predominant Hodgkin's Lymphoma

Morphology

NLPHL is characterized by a nodular, or a nodular and diffuse, proliferation of RS cell variants known as LP cells. LP cells are large and usually have one large multilobated nucleus and scant cytoplasm. The nucleoli are usually multiple, basophilic, and smaller than those seen in classical RS cells.

TABLE 38.1
Cell of Origin and Cell Lineage of Hodgkin's Lymphoma

Feature[1-3]/Expression	RS Cells of cHL	LP Cells of NLPHL
Proposed cellular origin	Preapoptotic GC B cell	Ag-selected, mutating GC B cell
Ig gene (single-cell PCR)	Rearranged, clonal, mutated, "crippled"	Rearranged, clonal, mutated ongoing
Somatically mutated Ig VAR genes	Yes	Yes
Presence of destructive somatic mutation	Yes (25%)	No
BCR	No	Yes
B-cell specific transcription factors (OCT-2, BOB1, PU.1)	Very rarely	Yes
B-lineage commitment and maintenance factor PAX-5	Yes (low level)	Yes

PCR, polymerase chain reaction; Ig, immunoglobulin; VAR, variable; BCR, B-cell receptor.

TABLE 38.2
Expression of Molecular Markers in Hodgkin's Lymphoma

Expression[5,6]	RS Cells of cHL	LP Cells of NLPHL
B-cell markers (CD20, CD79)	Rarely	Yes
GC B-cell markers (BCL6, AID)	Rarely	Yes
Plasma cell markers (MUM1, CD138)	Often	No
Molecules involved in Ag presentation (MHC class II, CD40, CD80, CD86)	Yes	Yes
Markers for non–B cells (e.g., TARC, granzyme B, perforin)	Yes (variably)	No
T-cell markers	Yes (rarely)	No

AID, activation-induced cytidine deaminase; MUM1, multiple myeloma oncogene 1; Ag, antigen; MHC, major histocompatibility complex; TARC, thymus and activation-regulated chemokine.

TABLE 38.3

Morphologic, Phenotypic and Virologic Features of Reed-Sternberg Cells of Classic Hodgkin's Lymphoma, and Lymphocyte-Predominant Cells of Nodular Lymphocyte Predominant Hodgkin's Lymphoma[25]

Features/Expression	cHL/RS Cells	NLPHL LP Cells
Tumor cells	Diagnostic RS cells	LP or "popcorn" cells
Pattern	Diffuse, interfollicular, nodular	Nodular
Background	Lymphocytes, (T cells > B cells) histiocytes, eosinophils, plasma cells	Lymphocytes, (B cells > T cells) histiocytes
Fibrosis	Common	Rare
CD15	+	−
CD19	+ (20%–30%)	+
CD20	+ (20%–30%)	+
CD22	+ (20%–30%)	−
CD30	+	−
CD40	+	+
CD45	−	+
EMA	−	+
IRF4/MUM1	+	+
BCL6	+ (30%)	+
EBV infection	+ (30%–40%)	−

TABLE 38.4

Comparative Expression of Molecular Markers and Cell Microenvironment[10,11,15,26,27]

	NLPHL	THCRBCL
Expression		
CD15	−	−
CD30	Usually −	− or +
EMA	+	Usually +
CD20	+	+
CD79a	+	+
IRF4	+	− or +
EBV	−	Usually −
Cell population		
T cells	v or +	+
B cells/B and T cells	+	−
CD57 + rosetting T cells	+ or −	−
CD40L + rosetting T cells	−	−
IRF4/MUM1 + rosetting T cells	+	−
Histiocytes	− or +	+
DRCs meshworks	+	−

THCRBCL, T/histiocyte cell–rich B-cell lymphoma; DRCs, dendritic reticulum cells.

normal GC environment. Although LP cells are found to be even more similar to diffuse large B-cell lymphoma (including T-cell/histiocyte-rich large B-cell lymphoma) in terms of phenotypic and gene expression aspects, the environmental characteristics discriminate between these lymphomas (Table 38.4).

Phenotype

LP cells are positive for CD20, CD79a, CD75, BCL6, and CD45 and epithelial membrane antigen in nearly all cases (see Table 38.3).[11,19] CD75, formerly LN1, is superior to CD20 and CD79a in detecting LP cells. LP cells express CD75 strongly, whereas small reactive B cells in the background show weak cytoplasmic positivity in the Golgi area but no membranous staining, in accordance with their mantle cell phenotype. CD20 is expressed in LP cells equally or less than in the small reactive B cells in the background. CD79a is even worse than CD20 in detecting LP cells because preferentially stains of small reactive B cells. The OCT2, BOB1, PAX5, and PU.1 B-cell transcription factors and the activation-induced deaminase enzyme (which is involved in somatic hypermutation and class switch recombination mechanisms in Ig genes), are consistently coexpressed (see Table 38.1).[11,19]

Microenvironment

The LP cells reside within nodules consisting of spherical meshworks of FDCs that are filled with nonneoplastic inflammatory cells. Inflammatory cells include small B cells, T cells that specifically express CD3 and CD4, and histiocytes. Furthermore, the inflammatory cells of nodules of NLPHL are characterized by an increase in GC-derived CD57+, IRF4/MUM1+, and PD-1+ T cells (see Table 38.3). Tia1 and CD40L-positive CD3/CD4 positive T cells are absent. PD1 ringing is a feature commonly seen in NLPHL.[15,19,24,25]

In conclusion, LP cells of NLPHL clearly resemble GC B cells in many phenotypic and genetic aspects, and proliferate in association with a cellular microenvironment that retains key features of a

Microenvironment and Histologic Patterns

Well-recognized morphologic features of NLPHL include a nodular, or a nodular and diffuse, proliferation of scattered LP tumor cells, set against a background of reactive lymphocytes reminiscent of a primary follicle. Different patterns are recognizable in NLPHL on morphologic and immunohistologic grounds. Fan and colleagues[26] identified six distinct immunoarchitectural patterns (*classical* nodular, serpiginous/interconnected nodular, nodular with prominent extranodular LP cells, T-cell–rich nodular, diffuse with a T-cell–rich background, and diffuse, B-cell–rich pattern) and two variant patterns (presence of small GCs within the nodules and the presence of prominent sclerosis) (Fig. 38.2). In the nodular pattern originally described by Fan and colleagues[26] as pattern A, rare LP cells are seen outside of the nodule. In other patterns, however, increasing numbers of LP cells extend outside of the neoplastic nodules and infiltrate the perinodular space (see Fig. 38.2).[26]

A recent study recognized an additional nodular pattern of NLPHL in which LP cells reside in an environment reminiscent of lymphoid follicles and do not invade the extranodular space (Fig. 38.3).[12,27] The recognition of this pattern primarily relies on the identification within the nodules of BCL6+ and CD20+ LP cells, surrounded by rosetting PD1+ T cells. CD23 and CD21 immunostaining usually detects meshworks of FDCs, which entrap the LP cells and the surrounding T-cell rosettes. LP tumor cells are localized within an environment reminiscent of a secondary follicle or, more frequently, within neoplastic nodules reminiscent of a primary follicle without residual GCs (see Fig. 38.3).

Regarding the relationship of these histopathologic patterns to the clinical course of the disease, the pattern A of Fan and colleagues was usually seen in those patients presenting with earlier

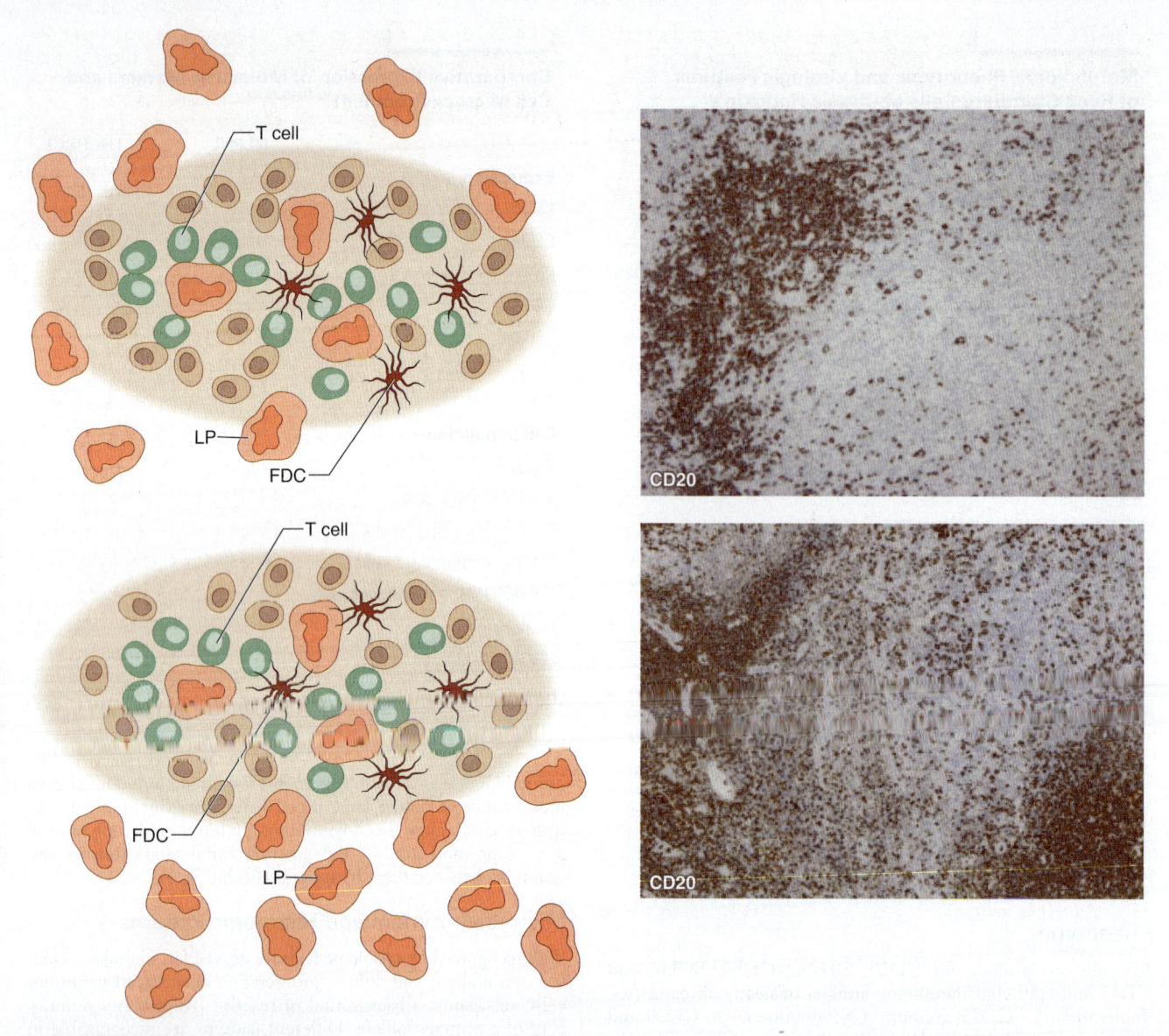

Figure 38.2 Major patterns on nodular lymphocyte predominate Hodgkin's lymphoma, as described by Fan and colleagues. Schematic representation *(to the left)*, microphotographs of CD20 immunostaining of LP cells *(to the right)*. *(Top)* Pattern A of Fan and colleagues.[26] *Classical* nodular pattern with rare extranodular LP cells. *(Top left)* In the *classical* nodular pattern, described by Fan and colleagues, the B cell rich nodules usually contain a prominent FDC meshwork that encompassed the LP cells. In these cases, the neoplastic LP cells are found to be located predominantly within the nodular structures, but rare LP cells extend outside of the nodule. *(Top right)* Classical nodular pattern. The pattern is characterized by scattered CD20+ LP cells within a nodular, reactive background dominated by small IgD+ B cells (not shown). The nodules contain a prominent CD23+ positive FDC meshwork that encompasses the LP cells (not shown). Rare LP cells can be found outside of the nodules. *(Bottom)* Pattern C of Fan and colleagues.[26] Nodular pattern with prominent extranodular LP cells. *(Bottom left)* During the progression of the disease, more LP cells extend outside of the nodules and infiltrate the perinodular space. Importantly, the presence of numerous LP cells outside the nodules may predict for progression to a diffuse pattern. The presence of many extranodular LP cells may characterize the pattern described by Fan and colleagues as "nodular with prominent extranodular LP cells". *(Bottom right)* Microphotograph of CD20 immunostaining of LP cells. This pattern shows more CD20+ LP cells *(at the center)* extending outside of the nodules. The extranodular LP cells are set in a background of reactive T cells and are not associated with FDC meshworks (not shown). Images were acquired with the Olympus dotSlide Virtual microscopy system using an Olympus BX51 microscopy equipped with PLAN APO 2×/0.08 and UPLAN SApo 40×/0.95 objectives.

clinical stage NLPHL. In general, the clinical impact of the different histopathologic patterns is still uncertain. Understanding this issue is difficult, because more than one pattern is frequently present at the same time.[28]

Classic Hodgkin's Lymphoma

Morphology

The so-called RS cell is the diagnostic key for this lymphoma because of its typical morphology: a giant cell with bi- or multinucleation and huge nucleoli. The typical morphology of binucleated and multinucleated RS cells and their mononuclear variant, the so-called Hodgkin's cell, are not specific to cHL, because they can also be observed in B-NHL (especially in diffuse large B-cell lymphoma [DLBCL] of the anaplastic variant), but they are pathognomonic for cHL in conjunction with an abundant cellular background composed of a varying spectrum of nonneoplastic inflammatory cells.[5]

Based on the characteristics of the reactive infiltrate, four histologic subtypes have been distinguished: lymphocyte-rich cHL (LRCHL), nodular sclerosis (NS) cHL, mixed cellularity (MC) cHL, and lymphocyte depletion (LD) cHL. LRCHL accounts for only a small fraction (3% to 5%) of all HLs. Most LRCHLs

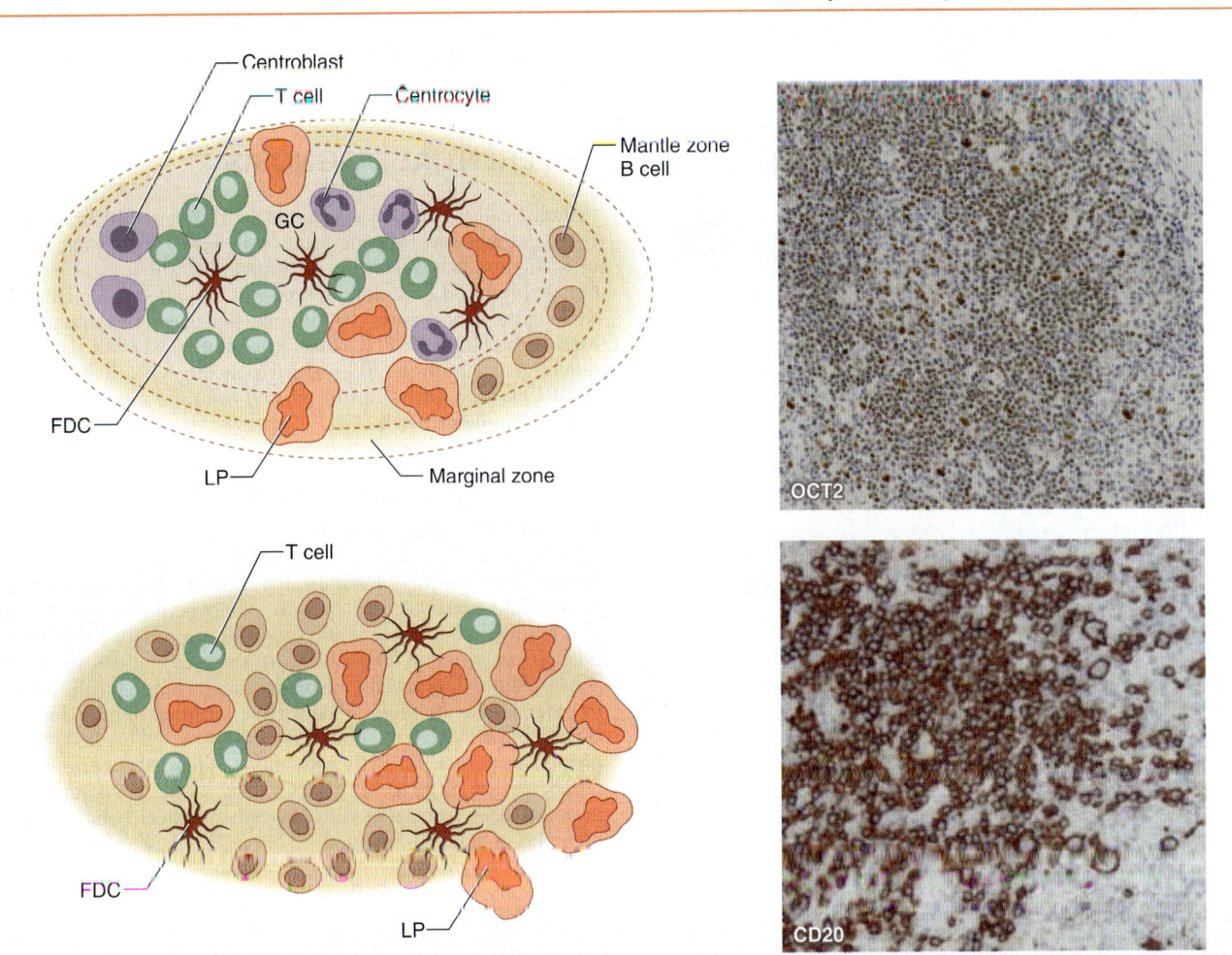

Figure 38.3 Nodular lymphocyte-predominant Hodgkin's lymphoma (NLPHL) may show a nodular pattern in which tumor cells do not invade the surrounding spaces. Schematic representation and microphotographs of OCT2, BCL6, and CD20 immunostaining of LP cells. OCT-2+, BCL6+, and CD20+ LP cells, surrounded by rosetting T cells (see schematic representation, *to the left*), are localized in an environment reminiscent of lymphoid follicles with (*Top*) or without (*Bottom*) a recognizable germinal center containing reactive B cells. In this pattern, LP cells do not extend outside of the nodules. *Top*: A schematic figure and microphotographs of OCT2 immunostaining of LP cells located in a follicle with recognizable germinal center. *Bottom*: A schematic figure and microphotograph of CD20 immunostainings of LP cells located in a nodule without a recognizable germinal center. Images were acquired with the Olympus dotSlide Virtual microscopy system using an Olympus BX51 microscopy equipped with PLAN APO 2×/0.08 and UPLAN SApo 40×/0.95 objectives.

have a better prognosis than do other cHLs and are characterized histologically by a small number of RS cells expressing a cHL immunophenotype. Based on these histologic and clinical features, there is no clear consensus on whether LRCHL represents a distinct disorder or just an early presentation of cHL. On the other hand, LRCHL cases display features intermediate between those of cHL and NLPHL.[11,19]

Phenotype

Phenotypically, RS cells of cHL are consistently positive for CD30, CD15, CD40, and IRF4/MUM1 (see Table 38.3).[23]

Microenvironment

cHL is a lymphoid neoplasm, derived from B cells, composed of mononuclear Hodgkin's cells and multinucleated RS cells residing in an abundant cellular microenvironment. In cHL, microenvironmental cell types include T- and B-reactive lymphocytes, eosinophils, mast cells, histiocytes/macrophages, plasma cells, and granulocytes (Fig. 38.4).[25,29–33] In addition, a great number of fibroblast-like cells and interdigitating reticulum cells are detectable, often in association with RS cells, within the collagen bands of NS cHL. Fibrosis—considered a common morphologic feature of HL lesions—is found more frequently in cHL subtypes than in NLPHL. An abnormal network of cytokines and chemokines and/or their receptors in RS cells is involved in the attraction of many of the microenvironmental cells into the lymphoma background (see Fig. 38.4).[8,34]

Nonmalignant inflammatory/immune cellular components of the HL microenvironment express molecules involved in cancer cell growth and survival, such as CD30L or CD40L, or in immune escape, such as programmed death 1 (PD-1). For example, CD30L+ eosinophils and mast cells, and proliferation-inducing ligand (APRIL)+ neutrophils, are consistently admixed to RS cells, whereas CD40L-expressing CD4+ T lymphocytes rosette RS cells. A considerable fraction of infiltrating CD4+ T cells are regulatory T (Treg) cells. Treg cells and PD-1+ T cells also interact with RS cells, which produce the Treg attractant galectin-1 and the PD-1 ligand (PDL-1).[7,25,29] The nonmalignant cells that compose most of the cellular background of cHL are recruited and/or induced to proliferate by tumor cells. They in turn produce soluble or membrane-bound molecules involved in tumor cell growth and survival. Numerous molecules are involved directly or indirectly in the recruitment and/or proliferation of cells constituting the cHL microenvironment. Normal cells may be recruited by cytokines/chemokines produced by RS cells or by T cells and

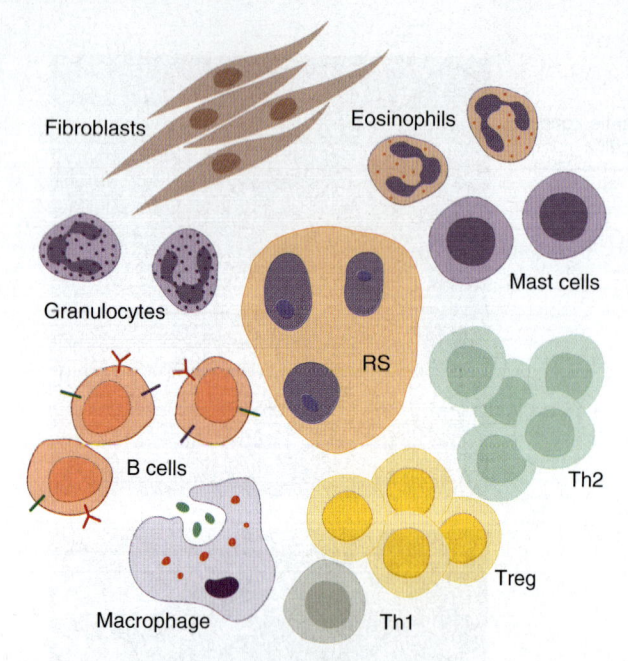

Figure 38.4 Reed-Sternberg (RS) cell and its microenvironment. An RS cell is shown within a rich, polymorphic cellular microenvironment that expresses members of the TNFR family protein and is embedded in a network of cytokines and chemokines. Treg, regulatory T cell; Th1, T helper cell type 1; Th2, T helper cell type 2.

fibroblasts activated by RS cells. RS cells produce molecules capable of inducing proliferation and/or differentiation of eosinophils, Treg cells, and fibroblasts.[29]

Epstein-Barr Virus Infection

Generally, in the different histologic subtypes of cHL, the immunophenotypic and genetic features of RS cells are identical, whereas their association with EBV shows differences. EBV is found in RS cells in about 40% of cHL cases in the Western world, mostly in cases of MC and LD HL, and less frequently in NS and LRCHL. Conversely, EBV is found in RS cells in nearly all cases of HL occurring in patients infected with HIV.[35] Independent studies have recently demonstrated that EBV can transform antigen receptor–deficient GC B cells, which enables their escape from apoptosis. The continued survival of the *rescued* preapoptotic B cells allows their proliferation. The EBV-encoded latent membrane protein (LMP) 2A is likely to function as the surrogate receptor through which B-cell signaling is triggered. This mechanism of EBV/LMP2A-induced the escape of antigen receptor-deficient GC B cells from apoptosis offers an intriguing model of lymphomagenesis. EBV infection might also affect the microenvironment composition by increasing the production of molecules involved in immune escape and T-cell recruitment, such as interleukin 10 (IL-10), CCL5, CCL20, and CXCL10.[36] LMP1 could have an interacting role with the microenvironment. Recent evidence indicates that EBV can manipulate the tumor microenvironment through the secretion of specific viral and cellular components into exosomes, small endocytically derived vesicles that are released from cells.[37,38] Exosomes produced by tumor cells from EBV-infected nasopharyngeal carcinoma contain LMP1, which can activate critical signaling pathways in uninfected neighboring cells, suggesting messenger functions of virus-modified exosomes.[37] Moreover, in B-cell lines, EBV-modified exosomes would activate cellular signaling mediated through integrins, actin, interferon, and NF-κB.[38] Further insights in these mechanisms are emerging from the understanding of the capability of EBV to modulate the (tumor-like) microenvironment.

DIFFERENTIAL DIAGNOSIS

Pathologically, HL subtypes should be distinguished from other B-cell lymphomas showing large and CD30 expressing tumor cells. Figure 38.5 shows B-cell lymphomas, which can be differentiated from NLPHL and cHL on immunophenotypic grounds. The figure also includes lymphomas that have overlapping features with cHL or NLPHL. Most importantly, NLPHL should be differentiated from T-cell/histiocyte-rich large B-cell lymphoma (THRLBCL), a DLBCL subtype, and from the rare cHL variant termed lymphocyte-rich cHL.[11,19]

Nodular Lymphocyte-Predominant Hodgkin's Lymphoma

According to current criteria, the detection of one nodule showing the typical features of NLPHL in an otherwise diffuse growth pattern is sufficient to exclude the diagnosis of primary THRLBCL. NLPHL may mimic THRLBCL in a subset of cases in which T cells, rather than B cells, are predominant. This typically occurs in older lesions in which T cells have infiltrated the nodules of B cells and disrupted the nodular architecture.[11] This finding was previously termed NLPHL with diffuse areas; the current preferred term is NLPHL, THRLBCL-like. These kinds of lesions have not been associated with aggressive clinical behavior. The presence of small B-cells and CD4+/CD57+ T cells points to a NLPHL diagnosis, whereas the absence of small B cells, and the presence of CD8+ cells and TIA1+ cells points to primary

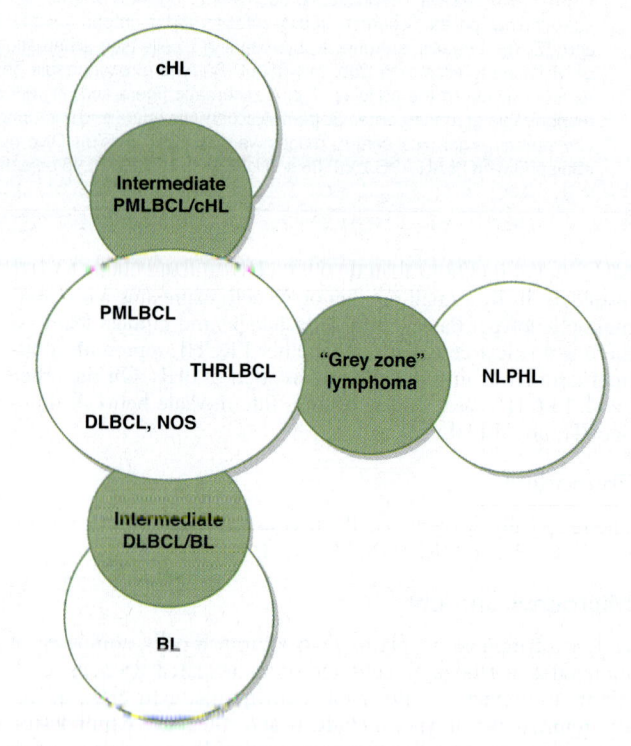

Figure 38.5 Provisional borderline categories for B cell lymphomas that do not clearly fit into one entity. They include the intermediate PMLBCL/cHL category and a "grey zone" lymphoma between THRLBCL and NLPHL. PMLBCL, primary mediastinal large B-cell lymphoma; THRLBCL, T-cell/histiocyte-rich large B-cell lymphoma; NOS, not otherwise specified.

THRLBCL (see Table 38.4). However, there may be a morphologic and phenotypic gray area between THRLBCL and NLPHL. CD4+/CD57+/TD1 small lymphocytes resetting around typical CD20+/BCL6+ LP cells are useful for the differential diagnosis with PTGC, LRCHL, and THRLBCL. In addition, staining for OCT2, PAX5, and PU1 should be considered as an important diagnostic tool. Interestingly, IgD identifies a subgroup of cases (10% to 20%) with peculiar phenotypical and clinical features.

LRCHL is the most difficult cHL subtype to differentiate from NLPHL, and misclassification has frequently been found in retrospective studies. RS cells in LRCHL can resemble LP cells morphologically; but, immunophenotypically RS cells in LRCHL are positive for CD30 and often express CD15. CD20 can be expressed but is typically weaker and less uniform than CD30 expression. NLPHL is PAX5+, OCT2+, and PU.1+, whereas cHL, including LRCHL, is PAX5+/−, OCT2−, and PU.1−. The distinction between NLPHL and LRCHL is essential, owing to therapeutic and prognostic differences.

cHL

cHL variants should be distinguished from DLBCL subtypes or DLBCL NOS variants that express CD30 (see Fig. 38.5), despite the fact that RS cells have lost much of the B-cell–specific markers. Most or all RS cells also lack the transcription factors OCT2, BOB.1, and PU.1. Instead, RS cells display, in varying frequency, molecules not normally expressed by B cells and B-NHL, such as CD30, CD15, CD70, thymus and activation-regulated chemokine (TARC), A20, fascin, and RANTES.

Finally, cHL cases rich in neoplastic cells may resemble, in particular, large B-cell lymphoma displaying anaplastic morphology and expressing CD30 or primary mediastinal large B-cell lymphoma (PMBCL). There is also a true morphologic and biologic overlap between PMBCL and cHL cases (see Fig. 38.5).

Overlapping Features of PMLBCL with cHL: The So-Called Mediastinal Gray Zone Lymphoma

Mediastinal B-cell lymphomas are mostly represented by NS cHL and PMLBCL. Although PMLBCL and NS cHL have several distinctive pathologic features (Table 38.5),[39–42] these entities exhibit strikingly similar clinical presentations (young women with an anterior mediastinal mass) and, in some cases, show overlap in pathologic, genetic, and molecular features (see Table 38.5). A provisional category, designated *B-cell lymphoma, unclassifiable, with features intermediate between DLBCL and cHL* has been introduced in the WHO proposal to encompass such cases. Table 38.5 shows the main morphologic, phenotypic, and genetic features that may be useful in distinguishing PMLBCL, cHL, and the provisional intermediate category PMLBCL/cHL.

Variant sharing features of DLBCL with anaplastic morphology and cHL may also occur. This shows an expression of CD30, CD15, surface markers, and transcription factors of B cells, commonly absent from RS cells (CD45RB, CD20, CD79, and OCT2).

Molecular Features

In accordance with overlapping phenotypes between cHL and B-cell lymphomas, these lymphomas have a gene expression profile that is intermediate between DLBCL and HL, but closely resembles PMLBCL. Activation of the NF-κB pathway, known to enhance the survival of RS cells, is also a feature of PMLBCL and may represent a survival pathway shared by both neoplasms, likely through the activation of antiapoptotic genes. Activation of the PI3K/AKT pathway were recently identified as a further shared pathogenic mechanism between PMLBCL and cHL. Taken together, molecular features that are common to both lymphoma

TABLE 38.5
Morphologic and Phenotypic Features that may be Useful in a Differential Diagnosis among Primary Mediastinal Large B-Cell Lymphoma, Classical Hodgkin's Lymphoma, and the Provisional Intermediate Category PMLBCL/cHL[23,43–48]

cHL	Typical RS cells (CD30+, CD15+)
	Background containing T cells, B cells, plasma cells, eosinophils, fibroblasts
	Abundant sclerosis
Intermediate	Large cells resembling RS cells (CD20+, B-cell transcription factors +)
PMLBCL/cHL	Admixed large cells with clear cytoplasm (CD20−, CD15−, B-cell transcription factors + weak)
	Large cells resembling centroblasts
	Background containing sparse inflammatory infiltrate with eosinophils, plasma cells, histiocytes, and T cells
	Sclerosis (variable)
	Necrosis (frequent)
PMLBCL	Large cells with clear cytoplasm, multilobated nuclei, large cells with RS-like morphology (CD30+, CD15−, CD20+, B-cell transcription factors +).
	Diminished background containing eosinophils, plasma cells, T cells
	Fine compartmentalizing sclerosis

entities include a decrease of BCR pathway signaling, constitutive NF-κB activation, activation of the cytokine–JAK-STAT pathway, and aberrant activation of the PI3K/AKT pathway. The identification of molecular links between PMLBCL and cHL supports the hypothesis that there may be some pathogenetic overlap between the two entities and that these diseases may in fact represent opposite ends of a continuum.[39–42]

HIV-Associated Hodgkin's Lymphoma

The Pre-Highly Active Antiretroviral Therapy Era

In the first years of the AIDS epidemic, HIV-associated HL displayed clinical, pathologic, and biologic peculiarities when compared with HL in people uninfected with HIV. First, HIV-associated HL exhibited unusually aggressive clinical behavior, which mandated the use of specific therapeutic strategies, and it was associated with a poor prognosis. Second, the pathologic spectrum of HIV-associated HL differed markedly from that of HL in people uninfected with HIV. In particular, the aggressive histologic subtypes of cHL, namely MC and LD, predominated among HIV-associated HL.[43] Tumor tissue was characterized by an unusually large proportion of RS cells infected by EBV. The fact that LMP1 was expressed in virtually all HIV-associated HL cases suggested that EBV plays an etiologic role in the pathogenesis of HIV-associated HL.

The Highly Active Antiretroviral Therapy Era

People with HIV/AIDS (PWHA) seem to be at increased risk of HL than in first years of the epidemic. HL is presently the most common non–AIDS-defining cancer. Patients infected with HIV, who are modestly immunocompromised due to the improvement in CD4 counts associated with this treatment, are more at risk for the development of the nodular sclerosis subtype.[44] In this regard, it has been postulated that with increasing CD4+ T cells resulting from highly active antiretroviral therapy (HAART), the appropriate cellular milieu of cHL, surrounding the RS cells, may again be available. In PWHA with improved immunity, CD4+ T cells provide adequate antiapoptotic pathways and mechanisms for immune escape by tumor cells allowing, in this way, the expansion and maintenance of full expression of the disease, as occurs in cHL among people without AIDS.[35,45-47] Alternatively, HL may arise as part of an immune reconstitution syndrome. Hypothetically, RS cell may already be present in severe immunosuppressed patients, and partial restoration may allow for the recruitment of surrounding immune cells and the manifestation of the tumor.[48,49] A recent study evaluating the effect of immune reconstitution on HL incidence among a cohort of male veterans infected with HIV ever receiving combination antiretroviral therapy (cART) highlighted that immunosuppression and poor viral control may increase HL risk, specifically during immune reconstitution in the interval post-cART initiation. These findings further suggested an immune reconstitution–type mechanism in HIV-related HL development.[50]

EARLY-STAGE HODGKIN'S LYMPHOMA

The management of early-stage Hodgkin's lymphoma exemplifies several important principles of oncology. These include the progressive improvement of cure rates through careful clinical research; the identification of prognostic features and new markers of optimal response; the refinement of treatment by the exploration of multimodality approaches; the vital importance of long-term follow-up; and a holistic analysis of the outcomes of treatment. Overall, this is one of the success stories of modern oncology, with modern treatment achieving high initial cure rates (up to 90% with the first-line of therapy) and good overall survival at around 95% after 5 years or more. Because it most often affects younger people in the 2nd to 4th decade of life, this has important implications for the goals of treatment, which must include not only the maximization of initial tumor control but also the avoidance of preventable long-term side effects.

Prognostic Features

The relatively orderly progression of cHL has long been recognized.[51] It generally develops through involvement of adjacent nodes in the same anatomical site, then in adjacent nodal areas, and it is extremely rare to find isolated deposits in two distant nodes. The same is not true for nodular lymphocyte-predominant disease, which, in this respect, more closely resembles a low-grade non-Hodgkin's lymphoma: It often presents with a single isolated node in the neck, but if it does progress, the dissemination is often to distant sites without intervening nodal involvement.

The predictable spread of cHL has allowed for the construction of a staging system based on anatomical extent, so that early-stage disease is defined by involvement of nodal groups on one side of the diaphragm only, more usually the thorax. Stage I disease is confined to a single anatomical nodal group (cervical, supraclavicular, axillary, anterior mediastinal, etc.), whereas a disease affecting more than one such group is stage II.

Beyond this division on the basis of nodal involvement, many studies have identified further prognostic features through retrospective analyses of large series of patients in clinical trials, mostly treated with extended field radiotherapy. This has allowed for the subdivision of early-stage disease into favorable and unfavorable categories. These do not represent biologically distinct processes, but act as a useful indicator of the severity of the illness and its optimum management, even though the current approaches to treatment are different to those in use when the factors were identified. Although a variety of stratification systems have been devised, common features include the presence of bulky disease (usually in the mediastinum), more advanced age (with a cutoff of 40 or 50 years of age), elevated erythrocyte sedimentation rate (ESR), systemic symptoms, and multiple or extranodal sites of involvement (Table 38.6).

Radiation Therapy

The effective treatment of HL by radiotherapy began with the work of Gilbert in the 1920s.[52] He introduced the rationale for treating both the evident sites of nodal involvement and adjacent but clinically uninvolved lymph nodes, on the basis that these were likely to contain microscopic disease. Peters[53] took the same approach at the Princess Margaret Hospital in the 1940s, publishing a landmark paper in the *American Journal of Roentgenology* in 1950, which described the cure of limited HL by high-dose, fractionated radiation. She reported 5- and 10-year survival rates of 88% and 79%, respectively, for patients with stage I disease, which transformed the outlook for an illness previously thought to have no long-term survivors.

In the early days, radiation therapy utilized fields that included the entire lymphatic system, total lymphoid irradiation (TLI), to

TABLE 38.6
Criteria Used to Stratify Early-Stage Hodgkin's Lymphoma

	EORTC	GHSG	NCIC/ECOG	NCCN 2010
Risk factors	a) Large mediastinal mass (>1/3) b) Age ≥50 years c) ESR ≥50 without B symptoms or ≥30 with B symptoms d) ≥4 nodal areas	a) Large mediastinal mass b) Extranodal disease c) ESR ≥50 without B symptoms or ≥30 with B symptoms d) ≥3 nodal areas	a) Histology other than LP/NS b) Age ≥40 years c) ESR ≥50 d) ≥4 nodal areas	a) Large mediastinal mass (>1/3) or >10 cm b) ESR ≥50 or any B symptoms c) ≥3 nodal areas d) >1 extranodal lesion
Favorable	CS I–II (supradiaphragmatic without risk factors	CS I–II without risk factors	CS I–II without risk factors	CS I–II without risk factors
Unfavorable	CS I–II (supradiaphragmatic with ≥1 risk factors	CS I or CS IIA with ≥1 risk factors CS IIB with c) or d) but without a) and b)	CS I–II with ≥1 risk factors	CS I–II with ≥1 risk factors (differentiating between bulky disease and other risk factors for treatment guidelines)

EORTC, European Organisation for Research and Treatment of Cancer; GHSG, German Hodgkin's Lymphoma Study Group; NCIC, National Cancer Institute of Canada; CS, Clinical stage.

relatively higher biologic radiation dosages compared to contemporary treatment. Extended field radiation therapy (EFRT) included all nodal sites using three radiation fields classically known as mantle, para-aortic–spleen, and inverted Y. A variation of EFRT was also used known as subtotal nodal irradiation (STNI).[54] This was effective, and in many cases curative, but was accompanied by important long-term toxicities, especially the induction of second malignancies and accelerated cardiovascular disease.[55–60] It remained the principal approach to treatment of early disease until clinical trials demonstrated that a combination strategy with chemotherapy could produce superior cure rates with much less irradiation, leading to a reduction of the irradiated field size to only the involved field (IF); the latter was based on a series of studies aimed at minimizing the toxicity of radiation therapy treatment. The German Hodgkin's Lymphoma Study Group (GHSG) HD8 showed in a randomized trial that reducing the treatment volume from EFRT to involved field radiation therapy (IFRT), when combined with chemotherapy, is equally effective. The European Organisation for Research and Treatment of Cancer (EORTC) H7 showed a similar outcome comparing IFRT to STNI.[61,62]

The developments in functional imaging, treatment planning, and image-guided radiation therapy have made it possible to better define and further decrease the radiation fields. Thus, IFRT, which is based on anatomic landmarks and encompassing adjacent uninvolved nodal stations, is no longer appropriate. Based on the fact that most recurrences occur in the original nodal sites, involved node irradiation therapy (INRT) was suggested; the field, in this case, is confined to the macroscopically involved nodes on imaging studies at diagnosis. Although this requires a significant margin around the node to allow and ensure adequate coverage, it can still result in significantly lower exposure to adjacent critical structures.[63] No formal comparison has been made to the results with IFRT, but multiple studies have shown no loss of efficacy with INRT (Fig. 38.6).[64,65]

Using INRT requires acquiring images at diagnosis in treatment positions and prior to the start of chemotherapy to minimize anatomic position variations between diagnostic and radiation treatment planning imaging. Because that is not practical in most cases, new guidelines defining involved site radiation therapy (ISRT) has been introduced by the International Lymphoma Radiation Oncology Group (ILROG). The new standard of care represents a significant reduction in the volume included in the previously used IFRT by using modern imaging and radiation planning techniques to limit the amount of normal tissue being irradiated.

Combined Modality Therapy

The recognition that HL is highly sensitive to cytotoxic chemotherapy led to the testing of systemic treatment in early stage disease. By administering limited doses of chemotherapy, it has been shown possible to reduce both the extent and dose of radiotherapy, while still maintaining high cure rates.[66–68] The success of this approach has depended on the different treatment of favorable and unfavorable disease, with results in favorable groups excellent even after low impact chemotherapy, such as two cycles of doxorubicin, bleomycin, vinblastine, and dacarbazine (ABVD) or the attenuated EBVP regimen. The EORTC H7-F study compared STNI to six cycles of EBVP followed by IFRT (36 to 40 Gy), with better results from the combined modality treatment: 10-year event-free survival was 88% versus 78%, and overall survival was 92% in both arms.[62] The GHSG HD10 study in favorable early disease compared results in a 2 × 2 randomization between two or four cycles of ABVD and 20 or 30 Gy of IFRT. All four groups had very high cure rates, with progression-free survival of 92% and overall survival of 97% at 5 years,[69] suggesting that two cycles of ABVD and 20 Gy of IFRT is sufficient treatment for carefully selected favorable disease.

A slightly different picture has emerged from studies of unfavorable early disease, where many patients present with bulky mediastinal nodes. Here, there is a threshold of treatment intensity below which the results become less favorable, with an apparent interaction between the efficacy of chemotherapy and the dose of irradiation used. Attenuated use of either modality can be compensated by the other, but if both elements are reduced too far, the freedom from treatment failure is lowered as the result of the excess of early recurrences. The EORTC H8-U trial showed the equivalence of either six or four cycles of MOPP-ABV when given before IFRT (36 to 40 Gy), or four cycles of MOPP-ABV before STNI, with 5-year event-free survivals of 84%, 88%, and 87%, respectively, and 10-year overall survival estimates of 88%, 85%, and 84%, respectively, indicating that treatment more intensive than four cycles of MOPP-ABV and IFRT was unnecessary, and that less toxic treatment might be possible.[70] More recently, the GHSG HD11 study has tested a 2 × 2 randomization between four cycles of ABVD and four cycles of the baseline bleomycin, etoposide, doxorubicin, cyclophosphamide, vincristine, procarbazine, and prednisone (BEACOPP) regimen before either 20 Gy or 30 Gy IFRT. The least intensive arm, four cycles of ABVD and 20 Gy, showed inferior 5-year progression-free survival at 82%, compared to 87%, although overall survival was unaffected, at 94.5%.[71] This suggests that for the unfavorable early-stage group, it may hazardous to reduce treatment below a threshold of four cycles of ABVD and 30 Gy IFRT, unless some means can be found to select those patients for whom further deintensification can be attempted, such as the use of functional imaging.

Chemotherapy Alone

Recognition of the long-term toxicity of extended field irradiation has led many investigators to test approaches by which radiotherapy may be omitted altogether from the treatment of early HL.[72,73] Two large randomized trials have been performed, in pediatric and adult patients, respectively, and both demonstrated that the omission of radiotherapy slightly reduced control of the disease,

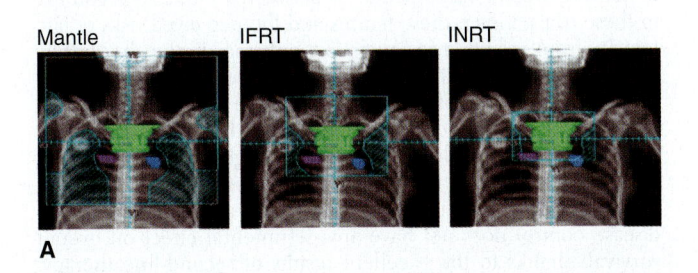

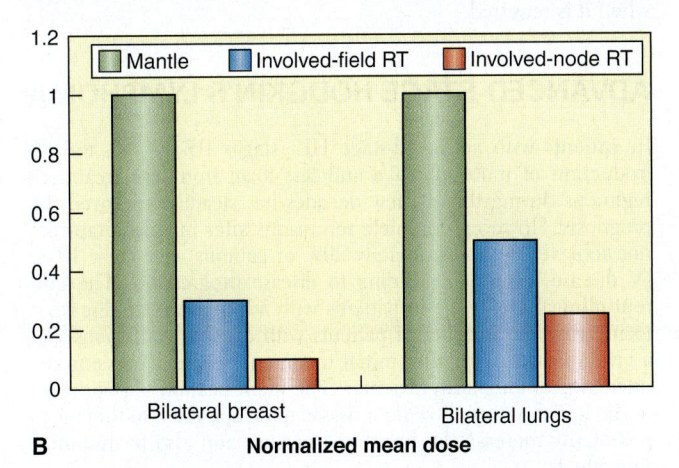

Figure 38.6 Differing radiation volumes in Hodgkin's lymphoma.

reflected in lower progression-free survival, but had no adverse impact on overall survival.

The North American Children's Oncology Group study CCG 5942, tested the omission of low-dose IFRT (21 Gy) for those in complete remission after four cycles of COPP-ABV chemotherapy. The study was closed prematurely when an interim analysis showed a difference in the progression rates in the two arms. With a median 7.7 years follow-up, the event-free survival favored the radiotherapy group (93% versus 83%; $p = 0.004$), with most recurrences in the chemotherapy-alone group seen at the sites of original disease. There was, however, no difference in overall survival, estimated at 97% at 10 years.[74]

In adults with early-stage nonbulky disease, the intergroup Eastern Oncology Cooperative Group (ECOG)/National Cancer Institute of Canada (NCIC) study tested treatment with ABVD alone to either 35 Gy STNI in favorable disease, or two cycles of ABVD followed by STNI in unfavorable cases. The first report of this study, with a median follow-up of 4.2 years, showed inferior freedom from progression in the chemotherapy-alone arms (87% versus 93%), with the unfavorable group particularly disadvantaged by the omission of radiotherapy.[75] The initial analysis showed no difference in overall survival, but with longer follow-up, a different picture emerged, with inferior 10-year survival among the patients who had received radiotherapy (87% versus 94%, respectively; $p = 0.04$). The risk of death from lymphoma was not different between the arms, but the risk of death from other causes was more than threefold higher among those treated with radiotherapy, and much of the excess was due to second cancers.[76] It is important to note, however, that this protocol involved much more extensive irradiation than is currently in use, making extrapolation of the results difficult.

In the absence of direct comparative trials between modern combined modality therapy and chemotherapy alone, a meta-analysis was performed using the intergroup study ABVD-alone group and the comparable patients from the GHSG HD10 and HD 11 studies who received ABVD and IFRT. This showed that the short-term disease control was inferior with ABVD alone, reflected in worse 8-year time to progression (93% versus 87%; hazard ratio [HR], 0.44; 95% confidence interval [CI], 0.24 to 0.78), but that overall survival was not adversely affected in these groups, with 95% alive in the long-term follow-up.[77] The impact of combined modality treatment was particularly apparent among patients who showed less than complete remission after chemotherapy, suggesting that some means of selecting those with chemosensitive disease for deescalation of therapy would be attractive, and might allow radiotherapy to be omitted without a loss of disease control.

Response-Adapted Treatment

Much interest has been generated in the possible use of functional imaging to give an early indication of chemosensitivity in HL. The technique most widely tested is 2-(18F)fluoro-2-deoxy-D-glucose positron emission tomography (FDG-PET), the application of which as an interim readout of efficacy has been enhanced by the development of a highly reproducible five-point scale for reporting the results (Table 38.7).[78] This approach appears to improve the sensitivity for the detection of residual active lymphoma when compared to conventional computed tomography,[79] but the data from prospective randomized studies using it as a guide to therapy are not yet mature enough for firm conclusions, and it is clear that there is a small but definite false-negative rate for FDG-PET, probably of the order of 5% to 10%.

Two studies have reported early results, with broadly similar outcomes (Table 38.8). The United Kingdom National Cancer Research Institute RAPID study randomized patients with nonbulky early stage disease who had an interim PET score of 1 or 2 after three cycles of ABVD to either 30 Gy IFRT or no further therapy, and found that the 3-year progression-free survival and overall survival

TABLE 38.7
Five-Point Scale for the Interpretation of Interim FDG-PET Scanning

Score	PET/CT Result
1	No uptake above background
2	Uptake ≤ mediastinum
3	Uptake > mediastinum but ≤ liver
4	Uptake moderately increased compared to the liver at any site
5	Uptake markedly increased compared to the liver at any site
X	New areas of uptake unlikely to be related to lymphoma

were not significantly different.[80] There was, however, a trend toward inferior disease control, which became significant when patients who did not receive the radiotherapy as allocated were excluded (97% versus 90.7%; HR, 2.39; $p = 0.003$). Similarly, the EORTC H10 study compared two strategies of therapy: standard treatment with ABVD and IFRT, stratified according to baseline prognostic factors, versus a nonradiotherapy approach, but using further chemotherapy, for those with negative FDG-PET scans after two cycles of ABVD.[81] The results with a short follow-up suggested inferior disease control in the experimental PET directed arms, although the number of progressions was small and a much longer follow-up will be required to determine whether there is any detrimental effect on survival.

Taken overall, the evidence suggests that for early HL, the use of combined modality treatment produces optimum results in terms of disease control, with a very high expectation of cure from the initial therapy. There is, however, a large proportion of patients (around 90%) who will be curable with chemotherapy alone, and the number needed to treat with radiation in order to achieve 1 extra cured patient is between 15 and 30 according to these trials. Given these figures and the perceived risks of late toxicity from radiotherapy, many patients may prefer the slightly higher risk of recurrent lymphoma to the potential for longer term morbidity. This will, of course, be subject to other variables such as their age, the sites of involvement (and thus the radiotherapy fields), and their baseline risk category. In general, the results of treatment from either approach are very good, and it is reassuring that in almost all the trials carried out, a small reduction in disease control does not have any detrimental effect on overall survival, thanks to the excellent results of second-line therapy, when it is required.

ADVANCED-STAGE HODGKIN'S LYMPHOMA

In patients with advanced-stage HL (stages IIB to IV), the introduction of more effective and less toxic front-line treatment regimens during the last few decades has steadily improved the prognosis. However, complete remissions after initial therapy are not achieved in approximately 20% of patients with stage III to IV disease, eventually leading to disease progression. The current clinical challenge in patients with advanced stage disease is to increase the number of patients with durable remissions and a favorable outcome after initial treatment, while decreasing the incidence of long-term toxicities. The identification of poor prognostic features may allow for a risk-adapted approach to therapy to potentially increase the likelihood of cure and also to minimize side effects.

TABLE 38.8
Response-Adapted Clinical Trials for Early-Stage Hodgkin's Lymphoma

Trial	Eligibility	Treatment Regimens	N	Outcome	Reference
RAPID	Nonbulky Stage I/II Favorable and Unfavorable	ABVD × 3 cycles PET positive: A: ABVD + IFRT 30 Gy PET negative: B: IFRT 30 Gy C: Observation	A: 145 B: 209 C: 211	A: OS at 3 years = 93.9% PFS at 3 years = 85.9% B: OS at 3 years = 97% PFS at 3 years = 93.8% C: OS at 3 years = 99.5% PFS at 3 years = 90.7%	80
EORTC H10	Favorable Stage I/II	ABVD × 3 + INRT 20 Gy A: PET positive B: PET negative ABVD × 2 C: PET positive: Esc BEACOPP × 2 + INRT 30 Gy D: PET negative: ABVD × 2	A: 33 B: 188 C: 27 D: 193	A: Data not available B: PFS at 1 year = 100% C: Data not available D: PFS at 1 year = 94.9%	81
EORTC H10	Unfavorable Stage I/II	ABVD × 4 + INRT 30 Gy A: PET positive B: PET negative ABVD × 2 C: PET positive: Esc BEACOPP × 2, INRT 30 Gy D: PET negative: ABVD × 4	A: 88 B: 251 C: 76 D: 268	A: Data not available B: PFS at 1 year = 97.3% C: Data not available D: PFS at 1 year = 94.7%	81

OS, Overall survival; PFS, Progression free survival.

In general, ABVD chemotherapy remains the most widely used treatment for newly diagnosed patients with advanced-stage HL in the United States. Dose-intense regimens such as escalated BEACOPP are more commonly used in Europe, but are also considered in North America in patients with multiple poor prognostic factors. The future management of advanced-stage HL patients, however, is being shaped by PET-directed approaches and the incorporation of novel agents into these standard combinations.

Prognostic Factors in Advanced Disease

The presence of adverse prognostic factors at diagnosis is one of the methods used to select therapy in HL and the International Prognostic Score (IPS) is an established risk stratification system for advanced disease patients (Table 38.9).[82] This prognostic model was constructed using seven factors associated with a poor outcome (serum albumin less than 4 g per deciliter, hemoglobin less than 10.5 g per deciliter, male sex, age 45 years or older, stage IV disease, leukocytosis of at least 15,000 per cubic millimeter, and lymphocytopenia of less than 600 per cubic millimeter or less than 8% of the white cell count). Although the IPS is highly predictive of freedom from disease progression, it does have limitations. The IPS does not adequately define the truly high-risk patients, because only 7% of the patients in the original study were in the high-risk group and their failure-free survival (FFS) at 5 years was still quite reasonable at 42%.[82] Furthermore, treatment strategies and supportive care have changed since the development of this prognostic model, and although the IPS is still clearly predictive of outcome, its performance may not be as good as originally described.[83–85]

Therefore, efforts have been made to improve the prognostication of the IPS by the incorporation of additional clinical prognostic factors,[86,87] the inclusion of biologic parameters,[88–99] or the addition of an early disease response assessment.[100,101] Biologic factors that have been studied include molecular profiling of the tumor and the RS cells[88,93–95]; the measurement of circulating cytokines or receptors including IL-10, CCL17, or soluble CD30[89–92,98]; and the enumeration of immune cells such as macrophages in the tumor microenvironment.[96,97,99] Although many of the biologic factors have prognostic significance independent of the IPS, they have not been adopted in everyday practice due to issues of reproducibility and a lack of prospective validation. On the other hand, an early response assessment as measured by an interim PET/computed tomography (PET/CT) scan has been shown to be a very powerful prognostic tool that is independent of clinical and biologic prognostic factors, including the IPS.[100–102] Interim PET/CT scanning has been introduced into standard

TABLE 38.9
International Prognostic Score (IPS)[82]

Adverse Prognostic Factors for Advanced Hodgkin's Lymphoma

≥45 years
Stage IV
Male
WBC ≥ 15,000 cells/μL
Lymphocytes < 600 cells/μL or <8% of WBC count, or both
Albumin < 4.0 g/dL
Hemoglobin < 10.5 g/dL

WBC, white blood cell count.

Choice of Initial Therapy

Combination chemotherapy forms the basis of treatment for patients with advanced-stage HL (Table 38.10). Initially, the MOPP regimen (nitrogen mustard, vincristine, procarbazine, and prednisone) was developed for previously untreated patients with very advanced HL, and a long-term follow-up of patients treated with the MOPP regime has confirmed that this combination can cure advanced HL. MOPP resulted in a freedom from progression rate of 54% and an overall survival of 48 % at 20 and now 40 years.[103] Although the MOPP regimen had a significant impact on the survival of patients who may previously have died of progressive disease, at least one-third of patients relapsed after MOPP chemotherapy and long-term complications were frequently seen in patients who received the combination.

To improve patient outcomes and decrease toxicity, other chemotherapy combinations such as ABVD were developed. An initial randomized trial compared alternating cycles of ABVD and MOPP chemotherapy to a dose and scheduled modified MOPP chemotherapy, and the alternating regimen was found to be superior in respect to the complete remission rate, freedom from progression, and overall survival.[104] Subsequently, a number of randomized trials were performed using ABVD in combination with MOPP chemotherapy or using ABVD alone. MOPP, ABVD, and MOPP alternating with ABVD were compared and the complete response rate and freedom from progression was initially found to be superior in patients receiving ABVD or the alternating program, but subsequent follow-up reports of the study show no difference in disease-free or overall survival when compared to a MOPP program also given at reduced doses.[105] Two further studies compared the MOPP/ABVD hybrid regimen to MOPP alternating with ABVD, and the regimens were found to be equivalent.[106,107] When the MOPP/ABV hybrid regimen was compared to ABVD, ABVD chemotherapy was found to be superior with less toxicity.[83] The results of these trials led to ABVD chemotherapy being regarded as a standard of care for patients with advanced HL based on the clinical efficacy of the combination, the ease of administration, and the acceptable toxicity profile.

As an alternative to ABVD, the Stanford V regimen was developed as a short duration regimen combined with radiation therapy.[108] The initial single institution results with the regimen showed excellent results with a 5-year freedom from progression of 89% and an overall survival of 96%. These promising results were confirmed in a multi-institutional study.[109] The Stanford V regimen has subsequently been compared to ABVD in a number of randomized trials. Initial studies suggested that ABVD might be superior to Stanford V with a 10-year failure-free survival that was superior in ABVD treated patients; however, it has been argued that the differences in outcome may be due to the fact that radiotherapy in the Stanford V arm was administered differently from what was originally described.[110] Two subsequent randomized trials comparing ABVD to Stanford V have found no difference in response rate, failure-free survival, or overall survival between the regimens.[111,112] Overall, ABVD is felt to be superior to Stanford V in patients with advanced disease.

The GHSG also developed new regimens for patients with advanced HL, particularly standard dose and dose-escalated BEACOPP.[113] A randomized trial comparing COPP (cyclophosphamide, vincristine, procarbazine, and prednisone) alternating with ABVD to escalated or standard BEACOPP showed that patients receiving escalated BEACOPP had improved disease control and overall survival.[114] The improvement in outcome for patients treated with escalated BEACOPP was sustained with long-term follow-up.[115] Although these results were encouraging, long-term complications including acute myeloid leukemia or myelodysplastic syndrome appeared to be more frequent in patients treated with escalated BEACOPP. A similar Italian study compared six cycles of ABVD to four cycles of escalated BEACOPP followed by two cycles of standard BEACOPP and to six cycles of a multidrug intensive regimen. When the results from the ABVD arm were compared the BEACOPP arm, there was an improved progression-free survival with BEACOPP, but the overall survival was not different. Although more toxicity was seen in the BEACOPP-treated patients, poor-risk patients tended to benefit most when treated with BEACOPP.[116]

Since these initial studies, a number of randomized studies have been performed to determine the optimal number of cycles of BEACOPP needed to maintain the clinical benefit but potentially decrease toxicity, and also to define the subgroup of patients most likely to benefit from a more intensive treatment approach. In a study restricted to those younger than 60 years of age, the GHSG found that six cycles of escalated BEACOPP followed by radiotherapy to PET-positive masses was more effective in terms of freedom from treatment failure and less toxic than eight cycles of the same regimen.[117] This led the GHSG to conclude that six cycles of escalated BEACOPP is their standard for advanced HL. To determine whether the high-risk group of patients are those who benefit most from escalated BEACOPP, the EORTC 20012 trial randomized advanced-stage Hodgkin patients with an IPS ≥3 to either eight cycles of ABVD or four cycles of escalated BEACOPP followed by four cycles of standard or baseline BEACOPP.[118] At a median follow-up of 3.9 years, event-free survival, which was the primary endpoint, was similar between treatment arms. Although more relapses were observed with ABVD treatment, early discontinuations were more common in BEACOPP-treated patients. In this high-risk group of patients, however, overall survival was not significantly improved with the use of BEACOPP.

Treating physicians who favor using escalated BEACOPP as initial therapy for advanced-stage HL have pointed to the high response rate and improved event-free survival as the reason to use this combination. In contrast, those who favor using ABVD as initial therapy have cited the complication rate with escalated BEACOPP, as well as the ability to salvage relapsing patients with stem cell transplantation, as reasons to use a less intensive treatment first. To compare these approaches, a randomized comparison of ABVD and escalated BEACOPP was reported, but the analysis included second-line therapy if administered.[119] Patients with residual or progressive disease after initial ABVD or escalated BEACOPP were treated with salvage therapy, including stem cell transplantation. The authors analyzed the outcome after initial therapy, but also analyzed the outcome after salvage therapy. The freedom from first progression significantly favored patients receiving escalated BEACOPP when compared to patients treated with ABVD (85% compared to 73%; $p = 0.004$). However, after completion of all planned therapy including salvage therapy for those with residual or progressive disease, the 7-year rate of freedom from second progression was not significantly different (88% in the escalated BEACOPP group and 82% in the ABVD group; $p = 0.12$) and the 7-year overall survival rate was 89% and 84%, respectively ($p = 0.39$). Severe adverse events were more commonly seen in patients receiving escalated BEACOPP. These results have led some to suggest that initial therapy may not need to be highly aggressive in all patients due to the fact that relapsing patients may be salvaged with subsequent intensive therapy.[120] Others have pointed out that overall survival was a secondary endpoint in this study and that the study was small compared to other similar trials.[121] In an attempt to clarify whether a survival difference exists, a meta-analysis was performed that suggested that six cycles of escalated BEACOPP may well improve overall survival when compared to ABVD.[122]

Overall, it is clear that escalated BEACOPP has greater efficacy than ABVD in patients up to 60 years of age, although escalated BEACOPP-treated patients experience more toxicity, particularly if they are in the upper segment of this age range. Acute and long-term toxicity may, however, be improved by the use of six

TABLE 38.10
Frontline Regimens Commonly Used for Newly Diagnosed Patients with Hodgkin's Lymphoma

Regimen/Drug	Dose	Route	Schedule (Day)	Cycle Length (Days)	Reference
ABVD				28	105
Doxorubicin (adriamycin)	25 mg/m²	IV	1, 15		
Bleomycin	10 units/m²	IV	1, 15		
Vinblastine	6 mg/m²	IV	1, 15		
Dacarbazine	375 mg/m²	IV	1, 15		
BEACOPP (baseline)				21	113
Etoposide	100 mg/m², 200 mg/m² if PO	IV	1–3, or PO days 2–3		
Doxorubicin	25 mg/m²	IV	1		
Cyclophosphamide	650 mg/m²	IV	1		
Vincristine	1.4 mg/m² (cap at 2 mg/m²)	IV	8		
Bleomycin	10 units/m²	IV	8		
Procarbazine	100 mg/m²	PO	1–7		
Prednisone	40 mg/m²	PO	1–14		
Escalated BEACOPP				21	243
Etoposide	200 mg/m²	IV	1–3		
Doxorubicin	35 mg/m²	IV	1		
Cyclophosphamide	1250 mg/m²	IV	1		
Vincristine	1.4 mg/m² (cap at 2 mg/m²)	IV	8		
Bleomycin	10 units/m²	IV	8		
Procarbazine	100 mg/m²	PO	1–7		
Prednisone	40 mg/m²	PO	1–14		
COPP				28	114
Cyclophosphamide	650 mg/m²	IV	1, 8		
Vincristine	1.4 mg/m² (cap at 2 mg/m²)	IV	1, 8		
Procarbazine	100 mg/m²	PO	1–14		
Prednisone	40 mg/m²	PO	1–14		
MOPP				28	105
Mechlorethamine	6 mg/m²	IV	1, 8		
Vincristine	1.4 mg/m² (cap at 2 mg/m²)	IV	1, 8		
Procarbazine	100 mg/m²	PO	1–14		
Prednisone	40 mg/m²	PO	1–14		
Stanford V				28	108
Mechlorethamine	6 mg/m²	IV	1		
Doxorubicin	25 mg/m²	IV	1, 15		
Vinblastine	6 mg/m²	IV	1, 15		
Vincristine	1.4 mg/m² (cap at 2 mg/m²)	IV	8, 22		
Bleomycin	5 units/m²	IV	8, 22		
Etoposide	60 mg/m²	IV	15		
Etoposide	120 mg/m² or 60 mg/m² IV	PO	16		
Prednisone	40 mg/m²	PO	Every other day Start taper day 10		
VEPEMB				28	244
Vinblastine	6 mg/m²	IV	1		
Cyclophosphamide	500 mg/m²	IV	1		
Procarbazine	100 mg/m²	PO	1–5		
Prednisone	30 mg/m²	PO	1–5		
Etoposide	60 mg/m²	PO	15–19		
Mitoxantrone	6 mg/m²	IV	15		
Bleomycin	10 mg/m²	IV	15		
VBM				21–28	245
Vinblastine	6 mg/m²	IV	1, 8		
Bleomycin	10 mg/m²	IV	1, 8		
Methotrexate	30 mg/m²	IV	1, 8		

IV, intravenous; PO, by mouth.

rather than eight cycles of escalated BEACOPP. It is also clear that approximately two-thirds of patients with advanced HL may not need intensive therapy such as escalated BEACOPP, because they will be cured with ABVD. Clinical risk factors, treatment burden and cost, fertility issues, the risk of long-term relapses, as well as potential short- and long-term complications should be considered as physicians and patients decide which regimen to use as initial treatment for advanced-stage HL.

Positron-Emission Tomography–Directed Approaches

A strategy to potentially optimize therapy for HL, by possibly increasing efficacy and decreasing toxicity, is to utilize PET scans during treatment. Because changes in glucose metabolism precede changes in tumor size, responses can be assessed earlier during treatment with PET scans than with CT. Early interim PET scan imaging after chemotherapy for HL has been shown to be a sensitive prognostic indicator of outcome in patients with advanced disease.[123] In prospective studies, interim PET scans after two cycles of ABVD chemotherapy was a significant predictor of progression-free or event-free survival in patients with advanced-stage disease.[101,102] Similar findings were reported for patients treated with Stanford V or escalated BEACOPP.[124,125] Current clinical trials are now testing whether patient outcomes can be improved by modifying treatment based on the interim PET scan results. In patients who have an inadequate response based on the interim PET scan, treatment is either intensified or salvage therapy is contemplated.

Initial studies testing whether deescalation to less intense or ablated therapy maintains efficacy in patients who have a complete response by the interim PET scan suggest that this approach is feasible. Avigdor et al.[126] treated advanced-stage HL patients with two cycles of escalated BEACOPP and deescalated to ABVD chemotherapy for four cycles if the PET scan after the initial two cycles was negative. Patients who did not achieve a negative scan were removed from the study and considered for salvage therapy followed by high-dose chemotherapy and autologous stem-cell transplantation. Seventy-two percent of patients had a negative scan, and deescalation to ABVD resulted in a 4-year progression-free survival of 87%.[126] In a similar fashion, the GHSG HD18 trial is testing whether the number of cycles of escalated BEACOPP can be reduced from six to four in patients with a negative interim PET scan.

An alternative approach is to intensify therapy in patients who do not have a negative interim PET scan. Initial studies have explored whether patients can start treatment with two cycles of ABVD and escalate to BEACOPP if the interim scan is positive.[127,128] Initial reports suggest that this strategy, with BEACOPP intensification only in interim PET-positive patients, showed better results than ABVD-treated historic controls, and spared BEACOPP toxicity in the majority of patients.[127] A similar strategy is being prospectively explored in the UK National Cancer Research Institute Response Adapted Therapy using FDG-PET imaging in the advanced HL (RATHL) trial. In this study, all patients receive two courses of ABVD chemotherapy, and PET-negative patients are randomized between ABVD and AVD, to test whether the omission of bleomycin reduces lung toxicity while achieving an equivalent outcome. Patients who remain PET positive undergo treatment escalation with BEACOPP, thereby attempting to improve remission rates. These studies are still in progress.

Consolidation Radiotherapy

An alternative strategy to modifying the initial treatment for advanced-stage HL is to attempt to consolidate the response following initial chemotherapy. Radiotherapy is commonly used as consolidation following primary chemotherapy, with the goal of improving responses or preventing progression in patients with residual masses.

The precise subgroup of patients with advanced-stage HL who benefit from consolidative radiotherapy has changed over time with the use of different chemotherapy regimens and the routine use of PET scans in clinical practice. For patients treated with standard anthracycline-based chemotherapy, those with only a partial response to treatment as determined by conventional restaging may convert to complete remissions after consolidation radiotherapy. Patients with a complete response to initial treatment, however, do not appear to benefit from consolidation radiotherapy.[129]

As more intensive regimens have been used, resulting in more complete responses, the need for consolidation radiotherapy has decreased. This may be particularly true when intensive approaches are coupled with a PET-based evaluation of residual masses to confirm a complete response. In three successive GHSG trials for advanced HL, the use of radiotherapy was reduced in each study as treatment was intensified and a PET scan analysis was included. In the HD9 trial, two-thirds of patients treated with COPP/ABVD or BEACOPP received radiotherapy. In contrast, in the HD15 trial where PET scans guided the decision, only 11% of patients were treated with radiotherapy after escalated BEACOPP without compromising patient outcome.[117] These studies suggest that the use of radiotherapy can possibly be restricted to patients with PET-positive residual masses after escalated BEACOPP treatment; however, the exact role of radiotherapy in ABVD-treated patients in the era of PET scans is not well defined.

Incorporating Novel Agents into Frontline Therapy

Previous strategies to improve the outcome of patients with advanced-stage HL have largely focused on the intensification of therapy. This has resulted in trials becoming focused on younger patients who are in good health and has also resulted in increased toxicity of therapy. However, not all newly diagnosed patients with HL are young with a good performance score. Also, patients and physicians are concerned about toxicity associated with treatment and want to minimize complications. New treatment approaches that benefit a greater proportion of patients and that are associated with less toxicity are, therefore, needed. The most promising strategy to achieve this may be to add novel agents to less intense chemotherapy regimens. Novel agents currently being used in combination with chemotherapy in the frontline setting include brentuximab vedotin, rituximab, and lenalidomide.

The use of brentuximab vedotin is currently attracting substantial interest, and this agent is being combined with modified forms of the ABVD and BEACOPP combinations. Brentuximab vedotin was initially combined with ABVD, and then substituted for bleomycin in a phase 1 study.[130] In this study, complete responses after the conclusion of front-line therapy were achieved in 95% of the 22 patients receiving ABVD plus brentuximab and in 96% of the 25 receiving AVD plus brentuximab. Significant pulmonary toxicity, however, was seen when brentuximab vedotin was given with the bleomycin-containing regimen, resulting in the concurrent use of bleomycin and brentuximab vedotin being contraindicated. Based on the very high response rate, and the fact that brentuximab vedotin when given with AVD was well tolerated, a randomized phase 3 trial comparing ABVD and AVD plus brentuximab vedotin (ECHELON-1 trial) has been initiated.

The GHSG is also exploring the use of brentuximab in combination with BEACOPP variants, namely a more conservative variant BrECAPP (brentuximab vedotin, etoposide, cyclophosphamide, doxorubicin, procarbazine, and prednisone) and a more aggressive variant BrECADD (brentuximab vedotin, etoposide, cyclophosphamide, doxorubicin, dacarbazine, and dexamethasone). The interim results of a randomized phase 2 trial suggest that use of these anti-CD30 targeted BEACOPP variants is feasible without compromising the efficacy associated with escalated BEACOPP.[131]

Two clinical trials have added rituximab to ABVD chemotherapy to deplete intratumoral B cells and that express CD20 and which may support the growth and survival of the malignant cells. Both studies demonstrated high complete response rates, and the event-free survival in both studies suggested promising activity of the combination. Furthermore, the combination was also effective in patients with high IPS scores. However, the efficacy of this combination will need to be confirmed in a randomized trial.[132,133]

A further strategy being evaluated by the GHSG is the addition of lenalidomide to moderate-dose chemotherapy for newly diagnosed advanced-stage patients. In a recent phase 1/2 study, the efficacy and safety of four to eight cycles of AVD chemotherapy plus lenalidomide at doses of 5 to 35 mg per day, followed by radiotherapy, was tested in elderly patients.[134] The regimen was well tolerated and the preliminary response results were encouraging, suggesting that adding new drugs to modified chemotherapy regimens holds significant promise for the future.

Complications of Treatment

The initial treatment of patients with HL with chemotherapy, often in combination with radiotherapy, results in a significant proportion of patients who are cured of their disease. The toxicity of treatment, however, is a significant limitation to its use. Although early toxicities of therapy are commonly manageable and of short duration, late toxicities are often irreversible and may result in life-threatening complications. The late effects of treatment determine the long-term morbidity, mortality, and quality of life of patients with HL. In the first 10 years after treatment, most deaths are due to disease progression or relapse, but beyond this time point, deaths due to late effects predominate.[135]

Acute hematologic toxicity, with possible infectious complications and treatment-related mortality, is associated with the intensity of the treatment combination, the age of the patient, and their comorbid conditions.[136,137] These toxicities are commonly managed by dose modifications and growth factor support. For patients receiving bleomycin, pulmonary toxicity is a concern. Bleomycin lung toxicity is a potentially life-threatening complication and may be more prevalent in patients receiving ABVD chemotherapy.[138]

A significant complication after treatment is the development of second malignancies. These can involve solid organs (most commonly lung, skin, breast, or gastrointestinal) or be hematologic (leukemia, myelodysplasia, or secondary lymphomas).[139] The risk of second malignancies is highest after treatment for childhood HL.[140,141] In those patients treated for HL before adulthood, the risk of developing a second malignant disease has been estimated to be almost 20 times greater than the general population, with a 30-year cumulative risk of 18% for male patients and 26% for female patients.[141] The most common second malignancy in female patients is breast cancer. Important risk factors for therapy-associated breast cancer are age of younger than 20 years at the time of treatment and treatment with extended field radiotherapy that includes the mediastinum.[142,143] The risk of breast cancer is estimated to be approximately 30% in patients who received 40 Gy to the mediastinum before 25 years of age.[144]

Chemotherapy drugs, especially alkylating agents, contribute to the risk of hematologic malignancies, particularly acute myeloid leukemia (AML) and myelodysplasia. The cumulative risk of developing AML is approximately 1.5% for patients treated for advanced stage Hodgkin lymphoma with chemotherapy regimens such as ABVD.[145] There may be an increase in the incidence of myelodysplasia and AML when more intensive regimens such as escalated BEACOPP are used. The overall rate of other second malignancies, however, appears similar when more intensive and less intensive chemotherapy regimens are compared.[115]

Other late effects include infertility, cardiac effects, endocrine dysfunction, peripheral neuropathy, and local effects from radiotherapy. Alkylating agents may induce male and female sterility, but this is far less frequent in patients treated with ABVD-like regimens than alkylating-containing regimens such as BEACOPP.[146–149] An increase in myocardial infarction, congestive cardiac failure, asymptomatic coronary disease, valvular dysfunction, and stroke have been recorded after treatment for HL, and the risk of cardiac mortality may persist for many years after completing therapy.[150]

SPECIAL CIRCUMSTANCES

Elderly Patients

Elderly patients with HL are a heterogeneous population, particularly when life expectancy, comorbidities, and functional status are considered. Patients older than 65 years constitute approximately 20% of the HL population, but less than 10% of patients included in clinical trials are >60 years. The results of clinical trials are, therefore, not broadly applicable to the elderly who often have difficulty tolerating aggressive treatment approaches. Elderly patients may even have difficulty tolerating ABVD chemotherapy, and response rates to ABVD in elderly patients are typically lower than those seen in younger patients. Older patients often have a poorer event-free survival after ABVD treatment when compared to younger patients.[151]

One reason for the relatively poor outcome in elderly patients is their susceptibility to the toxic effects of intensive therapy, and many have coexisting conditions that affect their ability to tolerate standard treatments. Although fit elderly patients can be treated with curative intent using the same therapeutic regimens as used in younger patients, toxicities and complications are more frequent.[151,152] For more frail elderly patients or those with significant comorbidities, alternative regimens such as VEPEMB (vinblastine, cyclophosphamide, procarbazine, prednisolone, etoposide, mitoxantrone, and bleomycin) or VBM (vinblastine, bleomycin, and methotrexate) could be considered.[153–155] New targeted agents such as brentuximab vedotin, alone or in combination with less toxic agents, are being studied in the treatment of elderly patients with HL.

Pregnancy

HL is one of the most common cancers in pregnant patients, with concurrent pregnancy reported in approximately 3% of all patients.[156,157] Overall, the prognosis and clinical course of HL diagnosed in pregnant women are similar to other patients.[158]

If possible, treatment of asymptomatic, early-stage, pregnant patients should be delayed until after the second trimester or until they complete their pregnancy. If treatment is required, it may be possible to control the disease with single-agent vinblastine to allow the pregnancy to go to term.[156,158,159] Patients who progress while receiving vinblastine can be treated with ABVD chemotherapy during the second or third trimester. Although radiotherapy should be generally avoided during pregnancy, advances in radiotherapy techniques have significantly reduced the risk of fetal complications and radiotherapy could be used if needed.[160] Treatment should not be delayed if the patient has symptomatic, advanced-stage, or progressive HL. If treatment is required and the patient does not want a therapeutic abortion, the successful completion of pregnancy without fetal malformation is possible with the use of ABVD or similar regimens.[161]

Salvage Chemotherapy and Stem Cell Transplantation

Salvage chemotherapy followed by autologous stem cell transplantation (ASCT) has become the treatment of choice in patients with relapsed HL or if the disease is refractory to initial chemotherapy.[162,163] Two randomized phase 3 clinical trials showed improved progression-free survival in patients receiving high-dose chemotherapy (HDCT), compared to those treated with standard-dose salvage chemotherapy, although there was no statistically significant difference in overall survival.[164,165]

Although these randomized controlled trials form the basis for the management of patients with relapsed or refractory HL (RR-HL), the challenge to clinicians remains how best to apply these data to patients as primary treatment strategies evolve. Improvements in the management of patients undergoing ASCT (the use of peripheral blood stem cells [PBSC] and modern supportive care) and allogeneic stem cell transplantation (alloSCT; the use of nonmyeloablative or reduced-intensity conditioning techniques and increased experience with matched unrelated and alternative donor stem cell sources) have led to improved safety, increasing age, and comorbidity cutoffs for transplant patients. These technical advances have granted further accessibility to stem cell transplant therapies. With the advent of active novel agents, the role of stem cell transplantation in the management of HL may need to be addressed again in randomized controlled trials.

Prognostic Factors in Relapsed/Refractory Hodgkin's Lymphoma

Multiple studies have identified prognostic factors in RR-HL who undergo salvage chemotherapy and ASCT. The largest studies of prognostic factors in patients not specifically selected for ASCT have been performed by the GHSG. Separate studies have examined prognostic factors in primary refractory HL (defined as progressing while on primary treatment or within 3 months of completion) and the second paper examined patients who relapsed beyond 3 months after completion of primary therapy. In the primary treatment setting, 206 patients were identified with the significant adverse prognostic factors identified from multivariate analysis being poor performance status (ECOG >0), age >50 years, and failure to obtain a temporary remission to initial therapy.[166] In the relapse setting, 422 patients were studied and the significant adverse prognostic factors for overall survival identified in multivariate analysis were anemia (hemoglobin <120 in males, <105 in females), advanced clinical stage (III or IV), and time to treatment failure of <12 months.[167]

In summary, other series and institutional reviews generally confirm that that time to relapse after initial therapy along with advanced stage and poor performance status at relapse are consistent predictors of poor outcome. Time to relapse is of clinical significance because the GHSG primary refractory series had a 5-year OS of 26% compared to 46% for early relapsers after chemotherapy (3 to 12 months) and 71% for late relapsers (after 12 months) in their series studying relapsers.[16,18] Prospective validation of the predictors of outcome identified by Josting et al.[16,18] have yet to be performed.

TREATMENT

Salvage Chemotherapy Prior to Autologous Stem Cell Transplantation and Peripheral Blood Stem Cell Mobilization

Despite a multitude of published phase 2 studies reporting results of salvage regimens for RR-HL,[168–178] Randomized control trial (RCTs) of second-line regimens have not been performed and, thus, there is no obvious *standard of care* regimen. The published RCTs of ASCT for RR-HL employed mini-BEAM or dexa-BEAM and the control arm of the most recent GHSG trial used dexamethasone, cytarabine, and cisplatin (DHAP), so these regimens can be considered as *standard* regimens in this setting.[164,165,179] Because the goal of salvage chemotherapy is to enable patients to proceed to ASCT, the ideal regimen should have a high response rate with minimal toxicity, and not impair the collection of peripheral blood stem cells for ASCT. Although the RCTs of ASCT support the use of multidrug regimens including carmustine (BCNU), etoposide, cytarabine, and melphalan (mini-BEAM), these regimens have significant hematologic toxicity, requiring frequent hospitalization for febrile neutropenia, and a high incidence of transfusion support (Table 38.11). Stem cell mobilization appears to be compromised following treatment with mini-BEAM.[180]

Given the multicenter experience with DHAP reported by the GHSG, a platinum-based regimen such as DHAP is a reasonable choice given comparable response rates and less toxicity.[179] When given prior to randomization in the HD-R2 study, DHAP lead to complete response (CR)/complete response unconfirmed (CRu) in 24%, PR in 46%, and SD in 20%. As the trial allowed patients to proceed to randomization as long as they did not have PD, 90% of patients proceeded toward transplant. Several published and widely used salvage chemotherapy regimens are summarized in Figure 38.1. These trials report similar response rates to DHAP, and there is no evidence to demonstrate that one is superior over others. Although the dexa-BEAM regimen had an overall response rate (ORR) of 81% in the GHSG/EBMT phase 3 ASCT trial, treatment related mortality (TRM) from salvage chemotherapy in that study was 5%. Other trials have reported a lower TRM between zero to 2%, a more acceptable level given the typically young age and lack of comorbidity typical of patients in this setting. Although the optimal number of cycles of salvage chemotherapy is unknown, two to three cycles of treatment are usually given by convention with a need to balance optimizing response and the risk of further toxicity.

The available institutional series reporting response rates to salvage chemotherapy often include a mixture of patients with primary refractory and relapsed disease with most series likely unable to demonstrate differences due to a lack of statistical power. Patients with primary refractory HL have an inferior response rate to second-line chemotherapy (51% versus 83%; p <0.0001),[181] which highlights the unique and inferior biology in this group of patients. The proportion of primary refractory patients in reported series along with other imbalances of prognostic factors and typically small sample sizes in these series likely explain any potential variation in reported response rates.[163,166,176,182–184]

Despite aggressive combination chemotherapy, between 10% to 40% of patients do not achieve a response to salvage chemotherapy and there are no RCT data supporting ASCT in nonresponders. Courses of alternative salvage chemotherapy have been given in an attempt to demonstrate chemosensitive disease prior to transplant. Studies have largely assessed responses using CT scan–based criteria. These series have largely reported selected patient populations and are characterized by small numbers, although the goal of achieving a response and proceeding to ASCT occurs in approximately half of the patients.[185–188]

An important issue related to salvage chemotherapy is the potential for second-line therapy to impair the ability to mobilize peripheral blood stem cells to support potentially curative high-dose chemotherapy. The efficacy of salvage chemotherapy for HL must be balanced by toxicity and the impact on subsequent PBSC mobilization. Success rates for PBSC mobilization have not been consistently reported in the RCTs or trials assessing the efficacy of salvage therapy. Some studies report that regimens containing melphalan, such as dexa-BEAM or mini-BEAM, may result in reduced stem cell mobilization.[189–191] Available results for commonly employed regimens demonstrate that at least 80% of patients undergoing PBSC mobilization reach a minimum threshold of 2.0×10^6 CD34 cells per kilogram.[180,192]

The Role of Functional Imaging in Response Assessment Prior to Autologous Stem Cell Transplantation

The use of FDG-PET in response assessment postsalvage chemotherapy and prior to ASCT is increasing despite a lack of large prospective data. Outside of response assessment, FDG-PET

TABLE 38.11
Salvage Regimens Commonly Used for the Treatment of Relapsed and Refractory Hodgkin's Lymphoma

Regimen/Drug	Dose	Route	Schedule (Day)	Cycle Length (Days)	Reference
GVD				21	246
Gemcitabine	1,000 mg/m²	IV	1, 8		
Vinorelbine	20 mg/m²	IV	1, 8		
Liposomal doxorubicin	15 mg/m²	IV	1, 8		
IGEV				21	247
Vinorelbine	20 mg/m²	IV	1		
Gemcitabine	800 mg/m²	IV	1, 4		
Ifosfamide	2,000 mg/m²	IV	1–4		
Prednisone	100 mg	PO	1–4		
MESNA	1,200 mg/m²	IV	1–4, 30 min prior then at 4 and 8 h		
DHAP				14–21	248
Cisplatin	100 mg/m²	IV	1		
Cytarabine	2,000 mg/m²	IV	Day 2, Q12 h × 2 doses		
Prednisone	40 mg	IV	1–4		
ICE				14	249
Ifosfamide	5,000 mg/m²	IV	2		
Carboplatin	AUC5	IV	2		
Etoposide	100 mg/m²	IV	1–3		
MESNA	5,000 mg/m²	IV	2		
Augmented ICE				14	195
Ifosfamide	5,000 mg/m²	IV	1, 2		
Carboplatin	AUC5	IV	3		
Etoposide	200 mg/m²	IV	Day 1, Q12 hours × 3 doses		
MESNA	5,000 mg/m²	IV	1, 2		
Brentuximab vedotin	1.8 mg/kg	IV	1	21	229
Dexa-BEAM				28	168, 250
Dexamethasone	8 mg	PO	Day 1–10, Q8 hour		
Carmustine	60 mg/m²	IV	2		
Etoposide	75–150 mg/m²	IV	4–7		
Cytarabine	100 mg/m²	IV	Day 4–7, Q12 hour × 8 doses		
Melphalan	20 mg/m²	IV	3		
Mini-BEAM				28	164, 169
Carmustine	60 mg/m²	IV	1		
Etoposide	75 mg/m²	IV	2–5		
Cytarabine	100 mg/m²	IV	Day 2–5, Q12 hour × 8 doses		
Melphalan	30 mg/m²	IV	6		
ASHAP				21	171
Doxorubicin	10 mg/m²	IV, continuous infusion	1–4		
Cisplatin	25 mg/m²	IV, continuous infusion	1–4		
Cytarabine	1,500 mg/m²	IV	5		
Methylprednisolone	500 mg	IV	1–5		
VIP				28	172
Etoposide	75 mg/m²	IV	1–5		
Ifosfamide	1,200 mg/m²	IV	1–5		
Cisplatin	20 mg/m²	IV	1–5		
GDP				21	174
Gemcitabine	1,000 mg/m²	IV	1, 8		
Dexamethasone	40 mg	PO	1–4		
Cisplatin	75 mg/m²	IV	1		

(continued)

TABLE 38.11
Salvage Regimens Commonly Used for the Treatment of Relapsed and Refractory Hodgkin's Lymphoma *(continued)*

Regimen/Drug	Dose	Route	Schedule (Day)	Cycle Length (Days)	Reference
GEM-P				28	175
Gemcitabine	1,000 mg/m²	IV	1, 8		
Methylprednisolone	1,000 mg	PO or IV	1–5		
Cisplatin	75 mg/m²	IV	15		
MINE				28	176
Mitoguazone	500 mg/m²	IV	1, 5		
Ifosfamide	1,500 mg/m²	IV	1–5		
Vinorelbine	15 mg/m²	IV	1, 5		
Etoposide	150 mg/m²	IV	1–3		
IVE				21	251
Epirubicin	50 mg/m²	IV	1		
Etoposide	200 mg/m²	IV	1–3		
Ifosfamide	3,000 mg/m²	IV	1–3		
MESNA	3,000 mg/m²	IV	1–3		

IV, intravenous; PO, by mouth.

scanning can also be viewed as a biomarker with a positive test after salvage therapy, suggesting a higher rate of relapse post-ASCT (whether this is due to tumor-related or other factors in the FDG-PET avid lesion remains to be elucidated). Retrospective institutional series suggest that abnormal functional imaging (FI; either gallium or FDG-PET scan) after salvage therapy and prior to ASCT are predictive of poor outcome (3-year OS of 35% versus 87% if negative FI). In particular, patients who had achieved a PR with CT imaging could be discriminated by FI; in those with negative FI, outcome was similar to patients in CR (3-year OS of 90% in CR, 80% in PR with negative functional imaging) but significantly inferior if positive (65%).[193] A large series studying FI after ifosfamide, carboplatin, etoposide (ICE) chemotherapy reported similar results with a 5-year event-free survival (EFS) of 31% for FI-positive disease compared to 75% if negative.[194]

The group at MSKCC has reported results of a prospective study that tested the strategy of attempting to achieve a negative FDG-PET scan prior to ASCT.[195] In patients that had a positive FDG-PET scan following ICE salvage chemotherapy, a non–cross-resistant chemotherapy regimen to ICE (GVD [gemcitabine, vinorelbine, and liposomal doxorubicin]) was given as a second-line salvage chemotherapy regimen. A positive FDG-PET scan was seen in 38% of cases post-ICE; 26 of 33 patients that received GVD achieved a response (CR, PR, or MR) and went onto transplant. Of these 33 patients, a negative FDG-PET scan was achieved in 52% and their outcome appeared similar to the patients who were FDG-PET negative after ICE. These data demonstrate that the goal of FDG-PET negativity prior to autograft is likely of value and that the use of a non–cross-resistant regimen can be successful in approximately half of patients. Unfortunately, the outcome of FDG-PET–avid patients that were transplanted remains poor with an EFS of 25% at a median follow-up beyond 4 years. Validation of this observation in other series and with other commonly used regimens would help to confirm this treatment approach.

Autologous Stem Cell Transplantation High-Dose Therapy Regimens and Strategies

The role of ASCT in HL has been defined by two published phase 3 RCTs.[164,165] The GHSG/EBMT assigned 161 patients with relapsed HL to receive two cycles of dexa-BEAM chemotherapy, and randomized responding patients to either two additional cycles of dexa-BEAM or high-dose therapy and ASCT. Freedom from treatment failure at 3 years was significantly improved in the ASCT group (55 versus 34%; p = 0.02), although there was no difference in overall survival.[165] These trials of ASCT did not include chemorefractory patients; only cohort and registry data address the benefit of ASCT in these patients.[162,163,166]

The role of ASCT in lymphoma overtly refractory to chemotherapy has not been well defined in the modern literature. The Seattle group reported the outcome of 64 chemoresistant (defined as less than a partial remission) HL patients who were transplanted on protocols conducted between 1986 and 2005. At a median follow-up of 4.2 years post-ASCT, 5-year PFS and OS were 17% and 31%, respectively, suggesting inferior outcomes when compared to ASCT in chemosensitive patients.

The two randomized trials of ASCT for RR-HL used BCNU, etoposide, Ara-C, melphalan (BEAM) HDCT. Other single institution studies report outcomes with diverse regimens.[50,196–200] The lack of randomized comparisons of HDCT regimens makes it difficult to conclude that there is an optimum regimen in terms of toxicity and efficacy. Late effects including second primary malignancies, cognitive deficits, and chronic fatigue are important considerations, but the impact of HDCT on these outcomes and if they vary between regimens remain unclear.

Further intensification of high-dose regimens has not been a successful strategy in RR-HL,[50] but single-arm studies augmented-dose mobilization regimens,[47] or additional therapy after stem cell collection[52] have been reported to improve outcomes. The Cologne high-dose sequential (HDS) protocol begins with an induction phase of two cycles of DHAP chemotherapy followed by response assessment. Responders proceed to HDS, which consists of 4g/m² of cyclophosphamide followed by G-CSF and subsequent PBSC collection, 8 g/m² of methotrexate with vincristine 1.4 mg/m², etoposide 2 g/m² with G-CSF and an optional second PBSC collection, and finally, BEAM HDCT and ASCT. Based on a multicenter phase 2 pilot trial showing HDS to be feasible with acceptable toxicity, the GHSG subsequently led an RCT.[201] The HD-R2 trial, a randomized comparison of HDS therapy followed by ASCT to standard DHAP and ASCT failed to show any benefit for the experimental HDS arm over the standard arm with no significant differences in freedom from treatment failure, progression-free, or overall survival were observed.[202]

An alternative intensification strategy that has been tested is the use of tandem autologous transplants.[203] This approach was prospectively tested in a large GELA cohort study. The multicenter

CELA-led H96 trial tested a risk-adapted approach in which patients were assigned to a single or tandem autograft based on the presence of risk factors at the initiation of salvage therapy. Patients with primary refractory disease or at least two poor risk factors (time to relapse <12 months, relapse in a prior radiation field, or stage III/IV disease at the time of relapse) were considered high risk and planned to receive tandem ASCT, whereas patients with standard risk received a single autograft.[204] With an acceptable TRM of 6% and a 5-year OS of 46% in the poor-risk group, this trial demonstrated feasibility, but it does not address the benefit of this strategy in a controlled trial.

Consolidation Strategies: Radiation Postautograft and Maintenance

Many transplant centers use radiation therapy (RT) peri- and post-ASCT in order to maximize treatment because autograft remains the last standard curative treatment option in RR-HL. Unfortunately, the role of radiation around ASCT has not been evaluated in prospective randomized trials. In the GHSG randomized study of ASCT versus dexa-BEAM, 11 of the randomized patients (approximately 10% of the patients on trial) received radiation (6 in the ASCT arm) for what was felt to be residual disease.[165] In the HD-R2 study, consolidative IFRT of 30 Gy was given per protocol in patients who had a >1.5 cm lesion on CT scan at day 100 post-BEAM HDCT and ASCT.[179] In total, 25 of 241 patients randomized (10%) received radiation for residual CT findings.

Outside of the RCT setting, institutional practice incorporating RT varies substantially. The transplant regimens used at MSKCC employ either subtotal or total lymphoid irradiation (STLI or TLI) to 18 Gy, accelerated involved field radiation (IFRT to 18-Gy total given as twice per day fractions for 5 days) or IFT with a total dose of 18-36 Gy in patients who have received prior radiation or had a contraindication to TLI. Thus, effectively all patients receive some radiation as part of their salvage therapy.[195] In contrast, patients at Princess Margaret would receive IFRT if they had a localized recurrence prior to salvage therapy or the presence of a lesion >5 cm if technically feasible. This policy led to the use of posttransplant radiation in 26% of patients.[205]

In contrast, maintenance therapy has been tested in two RCTs, although there are no data currently unavailable. The histone deacetylase inhibitor panobinostat was tested in patients post-ASCT with the trial terminated early and without meaningful numbers to report. The other study tested brentuximab vedotin (an antibody-drug conjugate targeting CD30) against placebo in a large RCT. Results are expected in 2014.

Allogeneic Stem Cell Transplants

AlloSCT continues to be emphasized as a treatment option in advanced HL due to the young age and lack of comorbidity in many patients. Historically, myeloablative alloSCT has been employed in advanced phases of the disease but with poor results because NRM often exceeded 50% and relapses were not uncommon.[206–209] The role of myeloablative alloSCT in HL appeared limited; although dose intensity can be delivered in the context of a myeloablative allograft and donor stem cells are free of tumor cell contamination, the presence of a clinically significant graft-versus-Hodgkin's lymphoma (GVHL) effect has not been clearly demonstrated.

More recently, reports have demonstrated signs of GVHL following donor lymphocyte infusion (DLI).[210–213] In addition to this antitumor effect, the safety of allogeneic transplantation has improved with the use of reduced intensity allogeneic stem cell transplantation (RIC-allo). These approaches have become increasingly popular due to decreased rates of early treatment-related mortality.[214–217] Despite early favorable outcomes, mature results of RIC-allo available in the literature consistently demonstrate a lack of long-term disease control with progression-free survival estimates of approximately 25% to 30% and overall survival estimates of 35% to 60% at least 2 years post-SCT.[212,214–217]

The Grupo Español de Linfomas/Trasplante Autólogo de Médula Ósea (GEL/TAMO) and EBMT have reported the results of a large prospective study of RIC-allo in RR-HL.[218] Although the trial was incompletely accrued over 7 years, 78 patients ultimately proceeded through a RIC-allo transplant with a preparative regimen consisting of fludarabine 150 mg/m^2, melphalan 140 mg/m^2, and Graft versus host disease (GVHD) prophylaxis of cyclosporine and short-course methotrexate. With a median follow-up of 38 months, 3-year outcomes included a relapse rate of 59%, PFS of 25%, and OS of 43%. Although post-SCT outcomes were similar in matched sibling and unrelated donors, patients with chemorefractory disease had an inferior PFS (25% versus 64% at 1 year). Chronic GVHD was associated with a reduced rate of relapse posttransplant. In patients with relapse after allo-SCT, DLI alone generate an overall response rate of 40%. These results suggest the presence of a GVHL effect in a prospective multicenter trial, but highlight the high relapse rate and not insignificant toxicity even with RIC-allo approaches.

Given the increasing usage of unrelated and alternative donors for allografts, it becomes critical to review disease-specific results in homogeneous patient populations because there are few prospective or multicenter trials. The M.D. Anderson Cancer Center has reported a prospective trial of RIC-allo in both sibling and matched unrelated donor (MUD) using fludarabine-based regimens with the majority accrued onto the fludarabine-melphalan 140 mg/m^2 arm.[219] The 2-year OS and PFS were reported at 64% and 32%, respectively, with no differences in OS, PFS, or relapse between related and MUD transplants. The study is limited by sample size, with 58 patients in total, although the majority (33) received MUD allografts. In a series from the United Kingdom, investigators reported the outcome of RIC-allo in 49 patients (31 related, 18 MUD) who underwent transplants using a regimen consisting of fludarabine-melphalan 140 mg/m^2 and alemtuzumab.[211] Although OS and PFS were not statistically significantly different, nonrelapse mortality was significantly inferior in MUD transplants (34.1% versus 7.2%). Four-year OS and PFS estimates were 55.7% and 39%, respectively.

Retrospective institutional and registry series have also been published. The Center for International Blood and Marrow Transplant Research (CIBMTR) reviewed 143 allografts from matched unrelated donors using reduced intensity or nonmyeloablative regimens reported between 1999 and 2004.[220] The results demonstrate feasibility with a 2-year TRM of 33% and 2-year OS and PFS of 37% and 20%, respectively. Reduced intensity and nonmyeloablative transplants did not differ significantly in outcome. Another large study reported the outcome of 90 nonmyeloablative transplants from related (n = 38), MUD (n = 24), or haploidentical (n = 28) donors at the Baltimore and Seattle programs.[215] A multivariate analysis did not demonstrate any differences in OS between the three donor sources; however, significantly improved PFS (HR, 0.3) was found in haploidentical transplants compared to related or unrelated transplants. Matched related and unrelated donors had similar PFS. NRM was also significantly lower for haploidentical recipients (HR, 0.14) compared to related recipients. An interpretation of this result is difficult given the patient inclusion from two centers and how biases may influence the prognostic factors in patients undergoing allograft from these varied donor sources.

Finally, the outcome of umbilical cord blood transplants (UCBT) has also been reported in RR-HL. The Minnesota group reported their results in lymphoma in which 23 patients received cord blood transplants for HL; the TRM was 13%, the cumulative relapse rate was 43%, PFS was 33%, and the OS at 3 years was 43%.

The age range for the entire lymphoma cohort was 6 to 68 years of age (median of 46 years of age), and 86% of patients received double cord transplants.[221] A slightly larger series of 29 UCBT patients older than 15 years was reported by Eurocord-Netcord with the Lymphoma Working Party of the EBMT. At 1-year posttransplant, PFS was 30%; OS, NRM, and relapse rates were not reported for the HL subgroup.[222]

In summary, the available data regarding allo-SCT in HL only confirms the feasibility of the procedure. In the datasets that present homogeneous patient populations, it appears that there are signs of reasonable efficacy, although the relapse rates remain troubling and few studies are being performed to address this issue. Given advances in the field of alternative donor transplantation, it is reasonable to consider MUD, haploidentical, and UCBT in the management of patients with RR-HL. Unfortunately, prospective trials have done little more than demonstrate a potential role for these procedures in the management of the disease; they have not established the optimal timing of RIC-allo, and these series include a heterogeneous patient population, including patients who have not received an autograft. Given the evidence and lack of toxicity with ASCT, it becomes difficult to justify the toxicity and mortality of an allograft from any donor source prior to an autograft regardless of the perceived risk of the disease without high quality data.

The role of allograft is best established in patients who have failed an autograft. There are many possible options for treatment in this setting, which include conventional cytotoxics, radiation therapy, and investigational agents. In the absence of randomized comparisons with standard therapy, RIC-allo transplant has been compared to retrospective cohorts by two groups.[223,224] Both the UK and Italian reports demonstrated an overall survival advantage favoring allografting. Unfortunately, both studies suffer from the standard issues surrounding retrospective cohort comparisons and relatively small sample sizes. These results can only remain hypothesis generating. Patient selection remains a potential confounding issue in all allo-SCT reports (particularly in retrospective institutional or registry reviews), and the benefit of RIC-allo to patients with RR-HL remains open to debate.

Second Autologous Stem Cell Transplants

A second autograft has been considered an option for patients who relapse after a prior ASCT. In such cases, stem cells must be available from the initial procedure or need to be collected a second time. There are limited institutional and registry data to support such a strategy and such cases are obviously highly selected. The CIBMTR reported a series that included 21 HL patients who underwent a second autograft.[225] With day 100 TRM of 11%, 5-year PFS and OS were 30% for the entire cohort, with no difference in outcome between NHL and HL cases. Outcomes were inferior in patients who were retransplanted within 1 year of the initial autograft (5-year PFS of zero versus 32%; p = 0.001).

The role of a second autograft remains unclear but can be considered in patients with a time to relapse of greater than 1 year after the initial transplant. Integrating the data regarding second autografts, allografts along with the increasing number of targeted therapies, conventional palliative systemic approaches, and radiation becomes more challenging as options continue to increase.

The challenge remains how best to manage patients who progress or relapse after ASCT given the variety of standard treatment options (single and multiagent chemotherapy, radiation therapy), intensive treatment strategies (second autografts, RIC-allo transplants) or drug development trials that are currently available. Because no comparative prospective data are available to inform this decision, clinicians and patients will have to make careful choices.

Management of Patients with Relapsed Hodgkin's Lymphoma After Stem Cell Transplant

Approximately 20% of patients with HL will not be cured with currently available first-line and second-line treatment modalities, and will require additional therapy. Patients with relapsed or refractory HL after receiving ASCT have unmet medical needs, and are considered candidates for drug development. The median survival following relapse from ASCT is estimated to be only 2.4 years, which is even shorter for those whose disease relapsed within 1 year from the transplant.[226] Because of the poor prognosis, several novel agents are being evaluated in this patient population, but brentuximab vedotin remains the only drug approved by the U.S. Food and Drug Administration (FDA) for this indication.

Brentuximab Vedotin

Since its initial identification as a possible Hodgkin's and Reed-Sternberg (HRS)-associated antigen, CD30 became a widely sought after target for novel therapy of patients with HL. In the following 3 decades, the expression and function of CD30 were further clarified by several independent groups. CD30 is a member of the tumor necrosis factor cell receptor superfamily. CD30 is highly expressed in HRS cells, but is also expressed by the malignant cells of anaplastic large cell lymphoma, peripheral T-cell lymphoma, primary mediastinal diffuse large B-cell lymphoma, and other uncommon solid tumors. Several attempts to develop naked anti-CD30 antibody therapy failed to produce meaningful clinical responses. In contrast, major clinical responses were achieved by conjugating the naked anti-CD30 antibody SGN30 to antitubulin monomethyl auristatin E (MMAE), to generate the antibody drug-conjugate (ADC) brentuximab vedotin.

Based on promising preclinical activity, a first-in-man phase 1 study of brentuximab vedotin was initiated to evaluate its safety. The study rapidly enrolled 45 patients with relapsed or refractory CD30-positive HL (93%) and anaplastic large cell lymphoma, of whom 73% received prior ASCT.[227] Escalating doses of brentuximab vedotin (from 0.1 mg per kg to 3.6 mg per kg) were administered intravenously every 3 weeks. Treatment was very well tolerated, but rare dose-limiting toxicities were observed, including grade 4 thrombocytopenia, grade 3 hyperglycemia, and febrile neutropenia. The recommended phase 2 dose was established as 1.8 mg per kg every 3 weeks. Although the study primary objective was to evaluate the safety of brentuximab vedotin, 86% of the patients had tumor reductions, and 17 patients achieved complete or partial remissions. A second phase 1 study investigated the safety and tolerability of brentuximab vedotin administered on a weekly schedule for 3 weeks, followed by 1 week of rest.[228] A total of 37 patients (31 had HL) were enrolled and treated, of whom 62% previously received an ASCT. The dose-limiting toxicities were grade 3 diarrhea and/or vomiting and grade 4 hyperglycemia. Complete and partial clinical remissions were observed in 46% of the patients. Collectively, these two phase 1 studies demonstrated the safety of brentuximab vedotin, and provided valuable information on the potential clinical efficacy in patients with relapsed and refractory HL.

In a follow-up pivotal phase 2 clinical trial, 102 patients with relapsed HL after receiving ASCT were treated with 1.8 mg per kilogram brentuximab vedotin given every 3 weeks.[229] Of 102 patients, 76 (75%) achieved partial or complete remissions (34% CRs). The median duration of response in patients who achieved complete remissions was approximately 2 years. The most common treatment-related side effects were peripheral neuropathy (42%), nausea (35%), and fatigue (34%). Grade 3 or higher neuropathy was seen in 8% of patients and was the most common reason for the discontinuation of brentuximab vedotin. Results of this study lead to the approval of brentuximab vedotin by the FDA in 2011.

Current strategies are aiming at incorporating brentuximab vedotin in front-line and second-line chemotherapy regimens. In the front-line setting, brentuximab vedotin was initially combined with standard ABVD in patients with advanced stage HL. In this phase 1 study, 51 patients with newly diagnosed patients with advanced stage HL were treated with brentuximab vedotin administered every 2 weeks on the same day of each ABVD therapy. The phase 2 recommended dose was established at 1.2 mg per kilogram of brentuximab vedotin given with standard dose and the schedule of ABVD. However, this combination was associated with an unexpected increase in pulmonary toxicity that was similar to bleomycin lung toxicity. Subsequently, an additional cohort of patients was treated without bleomycin (brentuximab vedotin + AVD), which resulted in a similar high response rate, but with no pulmonary toxicity. Of 22 patients, 21 (95%) patients given brentuximab vedotin and ABVD achieved complete remission, as did 24 (96%) of 25 patients given brentuximab vedotin and AVD. Based on these data, an international randomized study comparing standard ABVD with AVD plus brentuximab vedotin was initiated. In the second-line setting, a sequential therapy of brentuximab vedotin followed by ICE chemotherapy is currently being investigated in transplant-eligible patients with relapsed and refractory HL.

Investigational Agents

Histone Deacetylase Inhibitors

Histone deacetylase (HDAC) inhibitors are good candidates for HL therapy due to their unique mechanisms of action. HDAC inhibitors have been shown to have a direct antitumor effect by activating the intrinsic caspase pathway and downregulating antiapoptotic proteins, in addition to an indirect effect by disrupting the favorable microenvironment and activating the immune response.[230] For example, HDAC inhibitors can alter the phenotype and function of T cells in the HL microenvironment by decreasing the expression of the chemotaxis chemokine CCL17 (TARC).[230,231] Furthermore, HDAC inhibitors may restore antitumor immunity by upregulating OX40L.[232]

Several HDAC inhibitors have recently been evaluated for the treatment of relapsed HL with variable results. Vorinostat demonstrated the weakest clinical activity, with only 1 of 25 patients achieving a partial remission.[233] On the other hand, panobinostat and mocetinostat demonstrated higher response rates, but also more toxic effects. Mocetinostat (MGCD0103) is an oral non-hydroxamate HDAC inhibitor that preferentially inhibits HDAC class I and IV.[234,235] In a phase 2 study, 51 patients with relapsed or refractory HL were treated with 110 mg or 85 mg of mocetinostat three times a week.[236] Approximately 60% of patients had a reduction in their tumor measurements, with 24% achieving partial remissions. Toxicities include thrombocytopenia, fatigue, pneumonia, anemia, and pericardial effusion.[236] Panobinostat, a pan HDAC inhibitor, also demonstrated a promising clinical activity in patients with relapsed HL. In a phase 2 study, 129 patients were treated with 40 mg panobinostat and 27% achieved partial or complete remissions.[237]

PI3K/AKT/mTOR Pathway Inhibitors

The PI3K signaling pathway regulates a wide variety of essential cellular functions, including glucose metabolism, cell survival, and proliferation.[238–240] The PI3K signaling pathway is activated in many malignancies, including in Hodgkin's and non-Hodgkin's lymphomas, making it an appealing target for therapeutic intervention. There are four isoforms of PI3K (α, β, γ, and δ) that can be selectively inhibited by a variety of small molecules. Idelalisib (GS-1101 or CAL101) is an oral PI3K-δ–selective small molecule inhibitor that demonstrated promising clinical activity in a variety of B-cell malignancies, but it showed a limited clinical activity in patients with relapsed HL.[241] In a different study, the dual PI3K-δ/γ inhibitor IPI-145 produced a 33% response rate in an ongoing phase 1 clinical trial. Targeting the downstream mammalian target of rapamycin (mTOR) kinase also demonstrated promising clinical activity in patients with relapsed HL. For example, everolimus produced an overall response rate of 42% of patients.[242]

REFERENCES

1. Canellos GP, Rosenberg SA, Friedberg JW, et al. Treatment of Hodgkin lymphoma: a 50-year perspective. *J Clin Oncol* 2014;32:163–168.
2. Siegel R, Naishadham D, Jemal A. Cancer statistics, 2013. *CA Cancer J Clin* 2013;63:11–30.
3. Re D, Thomas RK, Behringer K, et al. From Hodgkin disease to Hodgkin lymphoma: biologic insights and therapeutic potential. *Blood* 2005;105:4553–4560.
4. Jackson H Jr, Parker F Jr. Hodgkin's disease. *N Engl J Med* 1944;230:1–8.
5. Lukes RJ, Butler JJ. The pathology and nomenclature of Hodgkin's disease. *Cancer Res* 1966;26:1063–1083.
6. Kuppers R, Rajewsky K. The origin of Hodgkin and Reed/Sternberg cells in Hodgkin's disease. *Annu Rev Immunol* 1998;16:471–493.
7. Kuppers R. The biology of Hodgkin's lymphoma. *Nat Rev Cancer* 2009;9:15–27.
8. Re D, Kuppers R, Diehl V. Molecular pathogenesis of Hodgkin's lymphoma. *J Clin Oncol* 2005;23:6379–6386.
9. Kuppers R, Rajewsky K, Zhao M, et al. Hodgkin disease: Hodgkin and Reed-Sternberg cells picked from histological sections show clonal immunoglobulin gene rearrangements and appear to be derived from B cells at various stages of development. *Proc Natl Acad Sci U S A* 1994;91:10962–10966.
10. Eberle FC, Mani H, Jaffe ES. Histopathology of Hodgkin's lymphoma. *Cancer J* 2009;15:129–137.
11. Smith LB. Nodular lymphocyte predominant Hodgkin lymphoma: diagnostic pearls and pitfalls. *Arch Pathol Lab Med* 2010;134:1434–1439.
12. Carbone A, Gloghini A. "Intrafollicular neoplasia" of nodular lymphocyte predominant Hodgkin lymphoma: description of a hypothetic early step of the disease. *Hum Pathol* 2012;43:619–628.
13. Falini B, Bigerna B, Pasqualucci L, et al. Distinctive expression pattern of the BCL-6 protein in nodular lymphocyte predominance Hodgkin's disease. *Blood* 1996;87:465–471.
14. Carbone A, Gloghini A, Gattei V, et al. Expression of functional CD40 antigen on Reed-Sternberg cells and Hodgkin's disease cell lines. *Blood* 1995;85:780–789.
15. Mason DY, Banks PM, Chan J, et al. Nodular lymphocyte predominance Hodgkin's disease. A distinct clinicopathological entity. *Am J Surg Pathol* 1994;18:526–530.
16. Brune V, Tiacci E, Pfeil I, et al. Origin and pathogenesis of nodular lymphocyte-predominant Hodgkin lymphoma as revealed by global gene expression analysis. *J Exp Med* 2008;205:2251–2268.
17. Schwering I, Brauninger A, Klein U, et al. Loss of the B-lineage-specific gene expression program in Hodgkin and Reed-Sternberg cells of Hodgkin lymphoma. *Blood* 2003;101:1505–1512.
18. Stein H, Marafioti T, Foss HD, et al. Down-regulation of BOB.1/OBF.1 and Oct2 in classical Hodgkin disease but not in lymphocyte predominant Hodgkin disease correlates with immunoglobulin transcription. *Blood* 2001;97:496–501.
19. Stein H, Bob R. Is Hodgkin lymphoma just another B-cell lymphoma? *Curr Hematol Malig Rep* 2009;4:125–128.
20. Aldinucci D, Rapana B, Olivo K, et al. IRF4 is modulated by CD40L and by apoptotic and anti-proliferative signals in Hodgkin lymphoma. *Br J Haematol* 2010;148:115–118.
21. Zheng B, Fiumara P, Li YV, et al. MEK/ERK pathway is aberrantly active in Hodgkin disease: a signaling pathway shared by CD30, CD40, and RANK that regulates cell proliferation and survival. *Blood* 2003;102:1019–1027.
22. Harris NL, Jaffe ES, Stein H, et al. A revised European-American classification of lymphoid neoplasms: a proposal from the International Lymphoma Study Group. *Blood* 1994;84:1361–1392.
23. Younes A, Carbone A. Clinicopathologic and molecular features of Hodgkin's lymphoma. *Cancer Biol Ther* 2003;2:500–507.
24. Carbone A, Gloghini A, Aldinucci D, et al. Expression pattern of MUM1/IRF4 in the spectrum of pathology of Hodgkin's disease. *Br J Haematol* 2002;117:366–372.
25. Carbone A, Gloghini A, Cabras A, et al. The Germinal centre-derived lymphomas seen through their cellular microenvironment. *Br J Haematol* 2009;145:468–480.

26. Fan Z, Natkunam Y, Bair E, et al. Characterization of variant patterns of nodular lymphocyte predominant hodgkin lymphoma with immunohistologic and clinical correlation. Am J Surg Pathol 2003;27:1346–1356.
27. Carbone A, Gloghini A. Nodular lymphocyte predominant Hodgkin lymphoma may show a nodular pattern in which tumour cells do not invade the surrounding spaces. Br J Haematol 2013;163:537–538.
28. Carbone A, Spina M, Gloghini A, et al. Nodular lymphocyte predominant Hodgkin lymphoma with non-invasive or early invasive growth pattern suggests an early step of the disease with a highly favorable outcome. Am J Hematol 2013;88:161–162.
29. Aldinucci D, Gloghini A, Pinto A, et al. The classical Hodgkin's lymphoma microenvironment and its role in promoting tumour growth and immune escape. J Pathol 2010;221:248–263.
30. Poppema S, van den Berg A. Interaction between host T cells and Reed-Sternberg cells in Hodgkin lymphomas. Semin Cancer Biol 2000;10:345–350.
31. Carbone A, Gloghini A, Gruss HJ, et al. CD40 ligand is constitutively expressed in a subset of T cell lymphomas and on the microenvironmental reactive T cells of follicular lymphomas and Hodgkin's disease. Am J Pathol 1995;147:912–922.
32. Steidl C, Lee T, Shah SP, et al. Tumor-associated macrophages and survival in classic Hodgkin's lymphoma. N Engl J Med 2010;362:875–885.
33. Ma Y, Visser L, Roelofsen H, et al. Proteomics analysis of Hodgkin lymphoma: identification of new players involved in the cross-talk between HRS cells and infiltrating lymphocytes. Blood 2008;111:2339–2346.
34. Skinnider BF, Mak TW. The role of cytokines in classical Hodgkin's lymphoma. Blood 2002;99:4283–4297.
35. Carbone A, Gloghini A, Serraino D, et al. HIV-associated Hodgkin lymphoma. Curr Opin HIV AIDS 2009;4:3–10.
36. Aldinucci D, Gloghini A, Pinto A, et al. The role of CD40/CD40L and interferon regulatory factor 4 in Hodgkin lymphoma microenvironment. Leuk Lymphoma 2012;53:195–201.
37. Meckes DG Jr, Shair KH, Marquitz AR, et al. Human tumor virus utilizes exosomes for intercellular communication. Proc Natl Acad Sci U S A 2010;107:20370–20375.
38. Meckes DG Jr, Gunawardena HP, Dekroon RM, et al. Modulation of B-cell exosome proteins by gamma herpesvirus infection. Proc Natl Acad Sci U S A 2013;110:E2925–2933.
39. Carbone A, Gloghini A, Aiello A, et al. B-cell lymphomas with features intermediate between distinct pathologic entities. From pathogenesis to pathology. Hum Pathol 2010;41:621–631.
40. Rosenwald A, Wright G, Leroy K, et al. Molecular diagnosis of primary mediastinal B cell lymphoma identifies a clinically favorable subgroup of diffuse large B cell lymphoma related to Hodgkin lymphoma. J Exp Med 2003;198:851–862.
41. Savage KJ, Monti S, Kutok JL, et al. The molecular signature of mediastinal large B-cell lymphoma differs from that of other diffuse large B-cell lymphomas and shares features with classical Hodgkin lymphoma. Blood 2003;102:3871–3879.
42. Gualco G, Natkunam Y, Bacchi CE. The spectrum of B-cell lymphoma, unclassifiable, with features intermediate between diffuse large B-cell lymphoma and classical Hodgkin lymphoma: a description of 10 cases. Mod Pathol 2012;25:661–674.
43. Tirelli U, Errante D, Dolcetti R, et al. Hodgkin's disease and human immunodeficiency virus infection: clinicopathologic and virologic features of 114 patients from the Italian Cooperative Group on AIDS and Tumors. J Clin Oncol 1995;13:1758–1767.
44. Biggar RJ, Jaffe ES, Goedert JJ, et al. Hodgkin lymphoma and immunodeficiency in persons with HIV/AIDS. Blood 2006;108:3786–3791.
45. Gloghini A, Carbone A. Why would the incidence of HIV-associated Hodgkin lymphoma increase in the setting of improved immunity? Int J Cancer 2007;120:2753–2754.
46. Deeken JF, Tjen ALA, Rudek MA, et al. The rising challenge of non-AIDS-defining cancers in HIV-infected patients. Clin Infect Dis 2012;55:1228–1235.
47. Engels EA. Non-AIDS-defining malignancies in HIV-infected persons: etiologic puzzles, epidemiologic perils, prevention opportunities. AIDS 2009;23:875–885.
48. Novak RM, Richardson JT, Buchacz K, et al. Immune reconstitution inflammatory syndrome: incidence and implications for mortality. AIDS 2012;26:721–730.
49. Rajasuriar R, Khoury G, Kamarulzaman A, et al. Persistent immune activation in chronic HIV infection. do any interventions work? AIDS 2013;27:1199–1208.
50. Kowalkowski MA, Mims MP, Amiran ES, et al. Effect of immune reconstitution on the incidence of HIV-related Hodgkin lymphoma. PLoS One 2013;8:e77409.
51. Rosenberg SA, Kaplan HS. Evidence for an orderly progression in the spread of Hodgkin's disease. Cancer Res 1966;26:1225–1231.
52. Gilbert R. Radiotherapy in Hodgkin's disease (malignant granulomatosis): anatomic and clinical foundations, governing principles, results. Am J Roentgenol Radium Ther 1939;41:198–241.
53. Peters MV. A study of survivals in Hodgkin's disease treated radiologically. Am J Roentgenol Radium Ther Nucl Med 1950;63:299–311.
54. Kaplan HS. Clinical evaluation and radiotherapeutic management of Hodgkin's disease and the malignant lymphomas. N Engl J Med 1968;278:892–899.
55. Bowers DC, McNeil DE, Liu Y, et al. Stroke as a late treatment effect of Hodgkin's Disease: a report from the Childhood Cancer Survivor Study. J Clin Oncol 2005;23:6508–6515.
56. Franklin J, Pluetschow A, Paus M, et al. Second malignancy risk associated with treatment of Hodgkin's lymphoma: meta-analysis of the randomised trials. Ann Oncol 2006;17:1749–1760.
57. Hancock SL, Tucker MA, Hoppe RT. Factors affecting late mortality from heart disease after treatment of Hodgkin's disease. JAMA 1993;270:1949–1955.
58. Mulrooney DA, Yeazel MW, Kawashima T, et al. Cardiac outcomes in a cohort of adult survivors of childhood and adolescent cancer: retrospective analysis of the Childhood Cancer Survivor Study cohort. BMJ 2009;339:b4606.
59. Travis LB, Hill D, Dores GM, et al. Cumulative absolute breast cancer risk for young women treated for Hodgkin lymphoma. J Natl Cancer Inst 2005;97:1428–1437.
60. Swerdlow AJ, Cooke R, Bates A, et al. Breast cancer risk after supradiaphragmatic radiotherapy for Hodgkin's lymphoma in England and Wales: a National Cohort Study. J Clin Oncol 2012;30:2745–2752.
61. Engert A, Schiller P, Josting A, et al. Involved-field radiotherapy is equally effective and less toxic compared with extended-field radiotherapy after four cycles of chemotherapy in patients with early-stage unfavorable Hodgkin's lymphoma: results of the HD8 trial of the German Hodgkin's Lymphoma Study Group. J Clin Oncol 2003;21:3601–3608.
62. Noordijk EM, Carde P, Dupouy N, et al. Combined-modality therapy for clinical stage I or II Hodgkin's lymphoma: long-term results of the European Organisation for Research and Treatment of Cancer H7 randomized controlled trials. J Clin Oncol 2006;24:3128–3135.
63. Girinsky T, Specht L, Ghalibafian M, et al. The conundrum of Hodgkin lymphoma nodes: to be or not to be included in the involved node radiation fields. The EORTC-GELA lymphoma group guidelines. Radiother Oncol 2008;88:202–210.
64. Campbell BA, Voss N, Pickles T, et al. Involved-nodal radiation therapy as a component of combination therapy for limited-stage Hodgkin's lymphoma: a question of field size. J Clin Oncol 2008;26:5170–5174.
65. Paumier A, Ghalibafian M, Beaudre A, et al. Involved-node radiotherapy and modern radiation treatment techniques in patients with Hodgkin lymphoma. Int J Radiat Oncol Biol Phys 2011;80:199–205.
66. Bonadonna G, Bonfante V, Viviani S, et al. ABVD plus subtotal nodal versus involved-field radiotherapy in early-stage Hodgkin's disease: long-term results. J Clin Oncol 2004;22:2835–2841.
67. Hoskin PJ, Smith P, Maughan TS, et al. Long term results of a randomised trial of involved field radiotherapy vs extended field radiotherapy in stage I and II Hodgkin lymphoma. Clin Oncol 2005;17:47–53.
68. Sasse S, Klimm B, Görgen H, et al. Comparing long-term toxicity and efficacy of combined modality treatment including extended- or involved-field radiotherapy in early-stage Hodgkin's lymphoma. Ann Oncol 2012;23:2953–2959.
69. Engert A, Plutschow A, Eich HT, et al. Reduced treatment intensity in patients with early-stage Hodgkin's lymphoma. N Engl J Med 2010;363:640–652.
70. Fermé C, Eghbali H, Meerwaldt JH, et al. Chemotherapy plus involved-field radiation in early-stage Hodgkin's disease. N Engl J Med. 2007;357(19):1916-1927.
71. Eich HT, Diehl V, Görgen H, et al. Intensified chemotherapy and dose-reduced involved-field radiotherapy in patients with early unfavorable Hodgkin's lymphoma: final analysis of the German Hodgkin Study Group HD11 trial. J Clin Oncol 2010;28:4199–4206.
72. Canellos GP, Abramson JS, Fisher DC, et al. Treatment of favorable, limited-stage Hodgkin's lymphoma with chemotherapy without consolidation by radiation therapy. J Clin Oncol 2010;28:1611–1615.
73. Straus DJ, Portlock CS, Qin J, et al. Results of a prospective randomized clinical trial of doxorubicin, bleomycin, vinblastine, and dacarbazine (ABVD) followed by radiation therapy (RT) versus ABVD alone for stages I, II, and IIIA nonbulky Hodgkin disease. Blood 2004;104:3483–3489.
74. Wolden SL, Chen L, Kelly KM, et al. Long-term results of CCG 5942: a randomized comparison of chemotherapy with and without radiotherapy for children with Hodgkin's lymphoma—a report from the Children's Oncology Group. J Clin Oncol 2012;30:3174–3180.
75. Meyer RM, Gospodarowicz MK, Connors JM, et al. Randomized comparison of ABVD chemotherapy with a strategy that includes radiation therapy in patients with limited-stage Hodgkin's lymphoma: National Cancer Institute of Canada Clinical Trials Group and the Eastern Cooperative Oncology Group. J Clin Oncol 2005;23:4634–4642.
76. Meyer RM, Gospodarowicz MK, Connors JM, et al. ABVD alone versus radiation-based therapy in limited-stage Hodgkin's lymphoma. N Engl J Med 2012;366:399–408.
77. Hay AE, Klimm B, Chen BE, et al. An individual patient-data comparison of combined modality therapy and ABVD alone for patients with limited-stage Hodgkin lymphoma. Ann Oncol 2013;24:3065–3069.
78. Barrington SF, Qian W, Somer EJ, et al. Concordance between four European centres of PET reporting criteria designed for use in multicentre trials in Hodgkin lymphoma. Eur J Nucl Med Mol Imaging 2010;37:1824–1833.
79. Hutchings M, Loft A, Hansen M, et al. FDG-PET after two cycles of chemotherapy predicts treatment failure and progression-free survival in Hodgkin lymphoma. Blood 2006;107:52–59.
80. Radford J, Barrington S, Counsell N, et al. Involved field radiotherapy versus no further treatment in patients with clinical stages IA and IIA Hodgkin lymphoma and a 'negative' PET scan after 3 cycles ABVD. Results of the UK NCRI RAPID Trial. ASH Annual Meeting Abstracts 2012;120:a547.
81. Andre M, Reman O, Federico M, et al. Interim analysis of the randomized EORTC/LYSA/FIL intergroup H10 trial on early PET-scan driven treatment adaptation in stage I/II Hodgkin lymphoma. ASH Annual Meeting Abstracts 2012;120:a549.

82. Hasenclever D, Diehl V. A prognostic score for advanced Hodgkin's disease. International Prognostic Factors Project on Advanced Hodgkin's Disease. N Engl J Med 1998;339:1506-1514.
83. Duggan DB, Petroni GR, Johnson JL, et al. Randomized comparison of ABVD and MOPP/ABV hybrid for the treatment of advanced Hodgkin's disease: report of an intergroup trial. J Clin Oncol 2003;21:607-614.
84. Guisado-Vasco P, Arranz-Saez R, Canales M, et al. Stage IV and age over 45 years are the only prognostic factors of the International Prognostic Score for the outcome of advanced Hodgkin lymphoma in the Spanish Hodgkin Lymphoma Study Group series. Leuk Lymphoma 2012;53:812-819.
85. Moccia AA, Donaldson J, Chhanabhai M, et al. International Prognostic Score in advanced-stage Hodgkin's lymphoma: altered utility in the modern era. J Clin Oncol 2012;30:3383-3388.
86. Gobbi PG, Ghirardelli ML, Solcia M, et al. Image-aided estimate of tumor burden in Hodgkin's disease: evidence of its primary prognostic importance. J Clin Oncol 2001;19:1388-1394.
87. Vassilakopoulos TP, Angelopoulou MK, Siakantaris MP, et al. Prognostic factors in advanced stage Hodgkin's lymphoma: the significance of the number of involved anatomic sites. Eur J Haematol 2001;67:279-288.
88. Scott DW, Chan FC, Hong F, et al. Gene expression-based model using formalin-fixed paraffin-embedded biopsies predicts overall survival in advanced-stage classical Hodgkin lymphoma. J Clin Oncol 2013;31:692-700.
89. Sarris AH, Kliche KO, Pethambaram P, et al. Interleukin-10 levels are often elevated in serum of adults with Hodgkin's disease and are associated with inferior failure-free survival. Ann Oncol 1999;10:433-440.
90. Vassilakopoulos TP, Nadali G, Angelopoulou MK, et al. Serum interleukin-10 levels are an independent prognostic factor for patients with Hodgkin's lymphoma. Haematologica 2001;86:274-281.
91. Visco C, Nadali G, Vassilakopoulos TP, et al. Very high levels of soluble CD30 recognize the patients with classical Hodgkin's lymphoma retaining a very poor prognosis. Eur J Haematol 2006;77:387-394.
92. Casasnovas RO, Mounier N, Brice P, et al. Plasma cytokine and soluble receptor signature predicts outcome of patients with classical Hodgkin's lymphoma: a study from the Groupe d'Etude des Lymphomes de l'Adulte. J Clin Oncol 2007;25:1732-1740.
93. Rassidakis GZ, Medeiros LJ, Vassilakopoulos TP, et al. BCL-2 expression in Hodgkin and Reed-Sternberg cells of classical Hodgkin disease predicts a poorer prognosis in patients treated with ABVD or equivalent regimens. Blood 2002;100.3935-3941.
94. Sanchez-Espiridion B, Montalban C, Lopez A, et al. A molecular risk score based on 4 functional pathways for advanced classical Hodgkin lymphoma. Blood 2010;116:e12-e17.
95. Chetaille B, Bertucci F, Finetti P, et al. Molecular profiling of classical Hodgkin lymphoma tissues uncovers variations in the tumor microenvironment and correlations with EBV infection and outcome. Blood 2009;113:2765-3775.
96. Steidl C, Lee T, Shah SP, et al. Tumor-associated macrophages and survival in classic Hodgkin's lymphoma. N Engl J Med 2010;362:875-885.
97. Steidl C, Connors JM, Gascoyne RD. Molecular pathogenesis of Hodgkin's lymphoma: increasing evidence of the importance of the microenvironment. J Clin Oncol 2011;29:1812-1826.
98. Sauer M, Plutschow A, Jachimowicz RD, et al. Baseline serum TARC levels predict therapy outcome in patients with Hodgkin lymphoma. Am J Hematol 2013;88:113-115.
99. His ED. Biologic features of Hodgkin lymphoma and the development of biologic prognostic factors in Hodgkin lymphoma: tumor and microenvironment. Leuk Lymphoma 2008;49:1668-1680.
100. Hutchings M, Loft A, Hansen M, et al. FDG-PET after two cycles of chemotherapy predicts treatment failure and progression-free survival in Hodgkin lymphoma. Blood 2006;107:52-59.
101. Gallamini A, Hutchings M, Rigacci L, et al. Early interim 2-[18F]fluoro-2-deoxy-D-glucose positron emission tomography is prognostically superior to international prognostic score in advanced-stage Hodgkin's lymphoma: a report from a joint Italian-Danish study. J Clin Oncol 2007;25:3746-3752.
102. Cerci JJ, Pracchia LF, Linardi CC, et al. 18F-FDG PET after 2 cycles of ABVD predicts event-free survival in early and advanced Hodgkin lymphoma. J Nucl Med 2010;51:1337-1343.
103. Longo DL, Young RC, Wesley M, et al. Twenty years of MOPP therapy for Hodgkin's disease. J Clin Oncol 1986;4:1295-1306.
104. Bonadonna G, Valagussa P, Santoro A. Alternating non-cross-resistant combination chemotherapy or MOPP in stage IV Hodgkin's disease. A report of 8-year results. Ann Intern Med 1986;104:739-746.
105. Canellos GP, Anderson JR, Propert KJ, et al. Chemotherapy of advanced Hodgkin's disease with MOPP, ABVD, or MOPP alternating with ABVD. N Engl J Med 1992;327:1478-1484.
106. Viviani S, Bonadonna G, Santoro A, et al. Alternating versus hybrid MOPP and ABVD combinations in advanced Hodgkin's disease: ten-year results. J Clin Oncol 1996;14:1421-1430.
107. Connors JM, Klimo P, Adams G, et al. Treatment of advanced Hodgkin's disease with chemotherapy—comparison of MOPP/ABV hybrid regimen with alternating courses of MOPP and ABVD: a report from the National Cancer Institute of Canada clinical trials group. J Clin Oncol 1997;15:1638-1645.
108. Bartlett NL, Rosenberg SA, Hoppe RT, et al. Brief chemotherapy, Stanford V, and adjuvant radiotherapy for bulky or advanced-stage Hodgkin's disease: a preliminary report. J Clin Oncol 1995;13:1080-1088.
109. Horning SJ, Williams J, Bartlett NL, et al. Assessment of the stanford V regimen and consolidative radiotherapy for bulky and advanced Hodgkin's disease: Eastern Cooperative Oncology Group pilot study E.1492. J Clin Oncol 2000;18:972-980.
110. Chisesi T, Bellei M, Luminari S, et al. Long-term follow-up analysis of HD9601 trial comparing ABVD versus Stanford V versus MOPP/EBV/CAD in patients with newly diagnosed advanced-stage Hodgkin's lymphoma: a study from the Intergruppo Italiano Linfomi. J Clin Oncol 2011;29:4227-4233.
111. Hoskin PJ, Lowry L, Horwich A, et al. Randomized comparison of the stanford V regimen and ABVD in the treatment of advanced Hodgkin's Lymphoma: United Kingdom National Cancer Research Institute Lymphoma Group Study ISRCTN 64141244. J Clin Oncol 2009;27:5390-5396.
112. Gordon LI, Hong F, Fisher RI, et al. Randomized phase III trial of ABVD versus Stanford V with or without radiation therapy in locally extensive and advanced-stage Hodgkin lymphoma: an intergroup study coordinated by the Eastern Cooperative Oncology Group (E2496). J Clin Oncol 2013;31:684-691.
113. Diehl V, Sieber M, Ruffer U, et al. BEACOPP: an intensified chemotherapy regimen in advanced Hodgkin's disease. The German Hodgkin's Lymphoma Study Group. Ann Oncol 1997;8:143-148
114. Diehl V, Franklin J, Pfreundschuh M, et al. Standard and increased-dose BEACOPP chemotherapy compared with COPP-ABVD for advanced Hodgkin's disease. N Engl J Med 2003;348:2386-2395.
115. Engert A, Diehl V, Franklin J, et al. Escalated-dose BEACOPP in the treatment of patients with advanced-stage Hodgkin's lymphoma: 10 years of follow-up of the GHSG HD9 study. J Clin Oncol 2009;27:4548-4554.
116. Federico M, Luminari S, Iannitto E, et al. ABVD compared with BEACOPP compared with CEC for the initial treatment of patients with advanced Hodgkin's lymphoma: results from the HD2000 Gruppo Italiano per lo Studio dei Linfomi Trial. J Clin Oncol 2009;27:805-811.
117. Engert A, Haverkamp H, Kobe C, et al. Reduced-intensity chemotherapy and PET-guided radiotherapy in patients with advanced stage Hodgkin's lymphoma (HD15): a randomised, open-label, phase 3 non-inferiority trial. Lancet 2012;379:1791-1799.
118. Carde PP, Karrasch M, Fortpied C, et al. ABVD (8 cycles) versus BEACOPP (4 escalated cycles => 4 baseline) in stage III-IV high-risk Hodgkin lymphoma (HL): First results of EORTC 20012 Intergroup randomized phase III clinical trial. ASCO Meeting Abstracts 2012;30:8002.
119. Viviani S, Zinzani PL, Rambaldi A, et al. ABVD versus BEACOPP for Hodgkin's lymphoma when high-dose salvage is planned. N Engl J Med 2011;365:203-212.
120. Connors JM. Hodgkin's lymphoma—the great teacher. N Engl J Med 2011;365:264-265.
121. Tam CS, Hersehtal A, Seymour JF. ABVD versus BEACOPP for Hodgkin's lymphoma. N Engl J Med 2011;365:1544-1545.
122. Skoetz N, Trelle S, Rancea M, et al. Effect of initial treatment strategy on survival of patients with advanced-stage Hodgkin's lymphoma: a systematic review and network meta-analysis. Lancet Oncol 2013;14:943-952.
123. Terasawa T, Lau J, Bardet S, et al. Fluorine-18-fluorodeoxyglucose positron emission tomography for interim response assessment of advanced-stage Hodgkin's lymphoma and diffuse large B-cell lymphoma: a systematic review. J Clin Oncol 2009;27:1906-1914.
124. Advani R, Maeda L, Lavori P, et al. Impact of positive positron emission tomography on prediction of freedom from progression after Stanford V chemotherapy in Hodgkin's disease. J Clin Oncol 2007;25:3902-3907.
125. Markova J, Kahraman D, Kobe C, et al. Role of [18F]-fluoro-2-deoxy-D-glucose positron emission tomography in early and late therapy assessment of patients with advanced Hodgkin lymphoma treated with bleomycin, etoposide, adriamycin, cyclophosphamide, vincristine, procarbazine and prednisone. Leuk Lymphoma 2012;53:64-70.
126. Avigdor A, Bulvik S, Levi I, et al. Two cycles of escalated BEACOPP followed by four cycles of ABVD utilizing early-interim PET/CT scan is an effective regimen for advanced high-risk Hodgkin's lymphoma. Ann Oncol 2010;21:126-132.
127. Gallamini A, Patti C, Viviani S, et al. Early chemotherapy intensification with BEACOPP in advanced-stage Hodgkin lymphoma patients with a interim-PET positive after two ABVD courses. Br J Haematol 2011;152:551-560.
128. Gallamini A, Rossi A, Patti C, et al. Early Treatment Intensification in Advanced-Stage High-Risk Hodgkin Lymphoma (HL) Patients, with a Positive FDG-PET Scan After Two ABVD Courses – First Interim Analysis of the GITIL/FIL HD0607 Clinical Trial. Blood 2012;120:550.
129. Aleman BM, Raemaekers JM, Tirelli U, et al. Involved-field radiotherapy for advanced Hodgkin's lymphoma. N Engl J Med 2003;348:2396-2406.
130. Younes A, Connors JM, Park SI, et al. Brentuximab vedotin combined with ABVD or AVD for patients with newly diagnosed Hodgkin's lymphoma: a phase 1, open-label, dose-escalation study. Lancet Oncol 2013;14:1348-1356.
131. Borchmann P, Eichenauer DA, Plütschow A, et al. Targeted beacopp variants in patients with newly diagnosed advanced stage classical hodgkin lymphoma: interim results of a randomized phase II study. Blood 2013;Abst# 4344.
132. Kasamon YL, Jacene HA, Gocke CD, et al. Phase 2 study of rituximab-ABVD in classical Hodgkin lymphoma. Blood 2012;119:4129-4132.
133. Younes A, Oki Y, McLaughlin P, et al. Phase 2 study of rituximab plus ABVD in patients with newly diagnosed classical Hodgkin lymphoma. Blood 2012;119:4123-4128.
134. Böll B, Plütschow A, Fuchs M, et al. German Hodgkin Study Group Phase I trial of doxorubicin, vinblastine, dacarbazine, and lenalidomide (AVD-Rev) for older Hodgkin lymphoma patients. Blood 2013;Abst# 3054.
135. Ng AK, Bernardo MP, Weller E, et al. Long-term survival and competing causes of death in patients with early-stage Hodgkin's disease treated at age 50 or younger. J Clin Oncol 2002;20:2101-2108.

136. Boll B, Gorgen H, Fuchs M, et al. ABVD in older patients with early-stage Hodgkin lymphoma treated within the German Hodgkin Study Group HD10 and HD11 trials. *J Clin Oncol* 2013;31:1522–1529.
137. Wongso D, Fuchs M, Plutschow A, et al. Treatment-related mortality in patients with advanced-stage Hodgkin lymphoma: an analysis of the German Hodgkin Study Group. *J Clin Oncol* 2013;31:2819–2824.
138. Martin WG, Ristow KM, Habermann TM, et al. Bleomycin pulmonary toxicity has a negative impact on the outcome of patients with Hodgkin's lymphoma. *J Clin Oncol* 2005;23:7614–7620.
139. Cote GM, Canellos GP. Can low-risk, early-stage patients with Hodgkin lymphoma be spared radiotherapy? *Curr Hematol Malig Rep* 2011;6:180–186.
140. Bhatia S, Yasui Y, Robison LL, et al. High risk of subsequent neoplasms continues with extended follow-up of childhood Hodgkin's disease: report from the Late Effects Study Group. *J Clin Oncol* 2003;21:4386–4394.
141. Hodgson DC, Gilbert ES, Dores GM, et al. Long-term solid cancer risk among 5-year survivors of Hodgkin's lymphoma. *J Clin Oncol* 2007;25:1489–1497.
142. Franklin J, Pluetschow A, Paus M, et al. Second malignancy risk associated with treatment of Hodgkin's lymphoma: meta-analysis of the randomised trials. *Ann Oncol* 2006;17:1749–1760.
143. Baxi SS, Matasar MJ. State-of-the-art issues in Hodgkin's lymphoma survivorship. *Curr Oncol Rep* 2010;12:366–373.
144. Travis LB, Hill D, Dores GM, et al. Cumulative absolute breast cancer risk for young women treated for Hodgkin lymphoma. *J Natl Cancer Inst* 2005;97:1428–1437.
145. Scholz M, Engert A, Franklin J, et al. Impact of first- and second-line treatment for Hodgkin's lymphoma on the incidence of AML/MDS and NHL—experience of the German Hodgkin's Lymphoma Study Group analyzed by a parametric model of carcinogenesis. *Ann Oncol* 2011;22:681–688.
146. Behringer K, Breuer K, Reineke T, et al. Secondary amenorrhea after Hodgkin's lymphoma is influenced by age at treatment, stage of disease, chemotherapy regimen, and the use of oral contraceptives during therapy: a report from the German Hodgkin's Lymphoma Study Group. *J Clin Oncol* 2005;23:7555–7564.
147. Sieniawski M, Reineke T, Josting A, et al. Assessment of male fertility in patients with Hodgkin's lymphoma treated in the German Hodgkin Study Group (GHSG) clinical trials. *Ann Oncol* 2008;19:1795–1801.
148. Hodgson DC, Pintilie M, Gitterman L, et al. Fertility among female hodgkin lymphoma survivors attempting pregnancy following ABVD chemotherapy. *Hematol Oncol* 2007;25:11–15.
149. Kulkarni SS, Sastry PS, Saikia TK, et al. Gonadal function following ABVD therapy for Hodgkin's disease. *Am J Clin Oncol* 1997;20:354–357.
150. Swerdlow AJ, Higgins CD, Smith P, et al. Myocardial infarction mortality risk after treatment for Hodgkin disease: a collaborative British cohort study. *J Natl Cancer Inst* 2007;99:206–214.
151. Evens AM, Hong F, Gordon LI, et al. The efficacy and tolerability of adriamycin, bleomycin, vinblastine, dacarbazine and Stanford V in older Hodgkin lymphoma patients: a comprehensive analysis from the North American intergroup trial E2496. *Br J Haematol* 2013;161:76–86.
152. Evens AM, Sweetenham JW, Horning SJ. Hodgkin lymphoma in older patients: an uncommon disease in need of study. *Oncology* 2008;22:1369–1379.
153. Gobbi PG, Federico M. What has happened to VBM (vinblastine, bleomycin, and methotrexate) chemotherapy for early-stage Hodgkin lymphoma? *Crit Rev Oncol Hematol* 2012;82:18–24.
154. Levis A, Anselmo AP, Ambrosetti A, et al. VEPEMB in elderly Hodgkin's lymphoma patients. Results from an Intergruppo Italiano Linfomi (IIL) study. *Ann Oncol* 2004;15:123–128.
155. Proctor SJ, Wilkinson J, Jones G, et al. Evaluation of treatment outcome in 175 patients with Hodgkin lymphoma aged 60 years or over: the SHIELD study. *Blood* 2012;119:6005–6015.
156. Pereg D, Koren G, Lishner M. The treatment of Hodgkin's and non-Hodgkin's lymphoma in pregnancy. *Haematologica* 2007;92:1230–1237.
157. Woo SY, Fuller LM, Cundiff JH, et al. Radiotherapy during pregnancy for clinical stages IA-IIA Hodgkin's disease. *Int J Radiat Oncol Biol Phys* 1992;23:407–412.
158. Yahalom J. Treatment options for Hodgkin's disease during pregnancy. *Leuk Lymphoma* 1990;2:151.
159. Connors JM. Challenging problems: coincident pregnancy, HIV infection, and older age. *Hematology Am Soc Hematol Educ Program* 2008:334–339.
160. Kal HB, Struikmans H. Radiotherapy during pregnancy: fact and fiction. *Lancet Oncol*. 2005;6:328–333.
161. Rizack T, Mega A, Legare R, et al. Management of hematological malignancies during pregnancy. *Am J Hematol* 2009;84:830–841.
162. Lazarus HM, Rowlings PA, Zhang MJ, et al. Autotransplants for Hodgkin's disease in patients never achieving remission: a report from the Autologous Blood and Marrow Transplant Registry. *J Clin Oncol* 1999;17:534–545.
163. André M, Henry-Amar M, Pico JL, et al. Comparison of high-dose therapy and autologous stem-cell transplantation with conventional therapy for Hodgkin's disease induction failure: a case-control study. *J Clin Oncol* 1999;17:222.
164. Linch DC, Winfield D, Goldstone AH, et al. Dose intensification with autologous bone-marrow transplantation in relapsed and resistant Hodgkin's disease: results of a BNLI randomised trial. *Lancet* 1993;341:1051–1054.
165. Schmitz N, Pfistner B, Sextro M, et al. Aggressive conventional chemotherapy compared with high-dose chemotherapy with autologous haemopoietic stem-cell transplantation for relapsed chemosensitive Hodgkin's disease: a randomised trial. *Lancet* 2002;359:2065–2071.
166. Josting A, Rueffer U, Franklin J, et al. Prognostic factors and treatment outcome in primary progressive Hodgkin lymphoma: a report from the German Hodgkin Lymphoma Study Group. *Blood* 2000;96:1280–1286.
167. Josting A, Franklin J, May M, et al. New prognostic score based on treatment outcome of patients with relapsed Hodgkin's lymphoma registered in the database of the German Hodgkin's lymphoma study group. *J Clin Oncol* 2002;20:221–230.
168. Pfreundschuh MG, Rueffer U, Lathan B, et al. Dexa-BEAM in patients with Hodgkin's disease refractory to multidrug chemotherapy regimens: a trial of the German Hodgkin's Disease Study Group. *J Clin Oncol* 1994;12:580–586.
169. Colwill R, Crump M, Couture F, et al. Mini-BEAM as salvage therapy for relapsed or refractory Hodgkin's disease before intensive therapy and autologous bone marrow transplantation. *J Clin Oncol* 1995;13:396–402.
170. Martin A, Fernandez-Jimenez MC, Caballero MD, et al. Long-term follow-up in patients treated with Mini-BEAM as salvage therapy for relapsed or refractory Hodgkin's disease. *Br J Haematol* 2001;113:161–171.
171. Rodriguez J, Rodriguez MA, Fayad L, et al. ASHAP: a regimen for cytoreduction of refractory or recurrent Hodgkin's disease. *Blood* 1999;93:3632–3636.
172. Ribrag V, Nasr F, Bouhris JH, et al. VIP (etoposide, ifosfamide and cisplatinum) as a salvage intensification program in relapsed or refractory Hodgkin's disease. *Bone Marrow Transplant* 1998;21:969–974.
173. Josting A, Rudolph C, Reiser M, et al. Time-intensified dexamethasone/cisplatin/cytarabine: an effective salvage therapy with low toxicity in patients with relapsed and refractory Hodgkin's disease. *Ann Oncol* 2002;13:1628–1635.
174. Baetz T, Belch A, Couban S, et al. Gemcitabine, dexamethasone and cisplatin is an active and non-toxic chemotherapy regimen in relapsed or refractory Hodgkin's disease: a phase II study by the National Cancer Institute of Canada Clinical Trials Group. *Ann Oncol* 2003;14:1762–1767.
175. Chau I, Harries M, Cunningham D, et al. Gemcitabine, cisplatin and methylprednisolone chemotherapy (GEM-P) is an effective regimen in patients with poor prognostic primary progressive or multiply relapsed Hodgkin's and non-Hodgkin's lymphoma. *Br J Haematol* 2003;120:970–977.
176. Ferme C, Mounier N, Divine M, et al. Intensive salvage therapy with high-dose chemotherapy for patients with advanced Hodgkin's disease in relapse or failure after initial chemotherapy: results of the Groupe d'Etudes des Lymphomes de l'Adulte H89 Trial. *J Clin Oncol* 2002;20:467–475.
177. Proctor SJ, Jackson GH, Lennard A, et al. Strategic approach to the management of Hodgkin's disease incorporating salvage therapy with high-dose ifosfamide, etoposide and epirubicin: a Northern Region Lymphoma Group study (UK). *Ann Oncol* 2003;14:147–150.
178. Bonfante V, Viviani S, Devizzi L, et al. High dose ifosfamide and vinorelbine as salvage therapy for relapsed or refractory Hodgkin's disease. *Eur J Haematol Suppl* 2001;64:51–55.
179. Josting A, Müller H, Borchmann P, et al. Dose intensity of chemotherapy in patients with relapsed Hodgkin's lymphoma. *J Clin Oncol* 2010;28:5074–5080.
180. Kuruvilla J, Nagy T, Pintilie M, et al. Similar response rates and superior early progression-free survival with gemcitabine, dexamethasone, and cisplatin salvage therapy compared with carmustine, etoposide, cytarabine, and melphalan salvage therapy prior to autologous stem cell transplantation for recurrent or refractory Hodgkin lymphoma. *Cancer* 2006;106:353–360.
181. Puig N, Pintilie M, Seshadri T, et al. Different response to salvage chemotherapy but similar post-transplant outcomes in patients with relapsed and refractory Hodgkin's lymphoma. *Haematologica* 2010;95:1496–1502.
182. Moskowitz CH, Kewalramani T, Nimer SD, et al. Effectiveness of high dose chemoradiotherapy and autologous stem cell transplantation for patients with biopsy-proven primary refractory Hodgkin's disease. *Br J Haematol* 2004;124:645–652.
183. Akhtar S, El Weshi A, Abdelsalam M, et al. Primary refractory Hodgkin's lymphoma: outcome after high-dose chemotherapy and autologous SCT and impact of various prognostic factors on overall and event free survival. A single institution result of 66 patients. *Bone Marrow Transplant* 2007;40:651–658.
184. Czyz J, Szydlo R, Knopinska-Posluszny W, et al. Treatment for primary refractory Hodgkin's disease: a comparison of high-dose chemotherapy followed by ASCT with conventional therapy. *Bone Marrow Transplant* 2004;33:1225–1229.
185. Brandwein JM, Callum J, Sutcliffe SB, et al. Evaluation of cytoreductive therapy prior to high dose treatment with autologous bone marrow transplantation in relapsed and refractory Hodgkin's disease. *Bone Marrow Transplant* 1990;5:99–103.
186. Stewart AK, Brandwein JM, Sutcliffe SB, et al. Mini-beam as Salvage Chemotherapy for Refractory Hodgkin's Disease and Non-Hodgkin's Lymphoma. *Leuk Lymphoma* 1991;5:111–115.
187. Ardeshna KM, Kakouros N, Qian W, et al. Conventional second-line salvage chemotherapy regimens are not warranted in patients with malignant lymphomas who have progressive disease after first-line salvage therapy regimens. *Br J Haematol* 2005;130:363–372.
188. Villa D, Seshadri T, Puig N, et al. Second-line salvage chemotherapy for transplant-eligible patients with Hodgkin's lymphoma resistant to platinum-containing first-line salvage chemotherapy. *Haematologica* 2012;97:751–757.
189. Dreger P, Kloss M, Petersen B, et al. Autologous progenitor cell transplantation: prior exposure to stem cell-toxic drugs determines yield and engraftment of peripheral blood progenitor cell but not of bone marrow grafts. *Blood* 1995;86:3970–3978.
190. Watts MJ, Sullivan AM, Jamieson E, et al. Progenitor-cell mobilization after low-dose cyclophosphamide and granulocyte colony-stimulating factor: an analysis of progenitor-cell quantity and quality and factors predicting for these parameters in 101 pretreated patients with malignant lymphoma. *J Clin Oncol* 1997;15:535–546.

191. Weaver CH, Zhen B, Buckner CD. Treatment of patients with malignant lymphoma with Mini-BEAM reduces the yield of CD34+ peripheral blood stem cells. *Bone Marrow Transplant* 1998;21:1169–1170.
192. Moskowitz CH, Nimer SD, Zelenetz AD, et al. A 2-step comprehensive high-dose chemoradiotherapy second-line program for relapsed and refractory Hodgkin disease: analysis by intent to treat and development of a prognostic model. *Blood* 2001;97:616–623.
193. Jabbour E, Hosing C, Ayers G, et al. Pretransplant positive positron emission tomography/gallium scans predict poor outcome in patients with recurrent/refractory Hodgkin lymphoma. *Cancer* 2007;109:2481–2489.
194. Moskowitz AJ, Yahalom J, Kewalramani T, et al. Pre-transplant functional imaging predicts outcome following autologous stem cell transplant for relapsed and refractory Hodgkin lymphoma. *Blood* 2010;116:4934–4937.
195. Moskowitz CH, Matasar MJ, Zelenetz AD, et al. Normalization of pre-ASCT, FDG-PET imaging with second-line, non cross resistant, chemotherapy programs improves event-free survival in patients with Hodgkin lymphoma. *Blood* 2012;119:1665–1670.
196. Crump M, Smith AM, Brandwein J, et al. High-dose etoposide and melphalan, and autologous bone marrow transplantation for patients with advanced Hodgkin's disease: importance of disease status at transplant. *J Clin Oncol* 1993;11:704–711.
197. Stewart DA, Guo D, Gluck S, et al. Double high-dose therapy for Hodgkin's disease with dose-intensive cyclophosphamide, etoposide, and cisplatin (DICEP) prior to high-dose melphalan and autologous stem cell transplantation. *Bone Marrow Transplant* 2000;26:383–388.
198. Stuart MJ, Chao NS, Horning SJ, et al. Efficacy and toxicity of a CCNU-containing high-dose chemotherapy regimen followed by autologous hematopoietic cell transplantation in relapsed or refractory Hodgkin's disease. *Biol Blood Marrow Transplant* 2001;7:552–560.
199. Evens A, Altman J, Mittal B, et al. Phase I/II trial of total lymphoid irradiation and high-dose chemotherapy with autologous stem-cell transplantation for relapsed and refractory Hodgkin's lymphoma. *Ann Oncol* 2007;18:679–688.
200. Bains T, Chen AI, Lemieux A, et al. Improved outcome with busulfan, melphalan and thiotepa conditioning in autologous hematopoietic stem cell transplant for relapsed/refractory Hodgkin lymphoma. *Leuk Lymphoma* 2014;55:583–587.
201. Josting A, Rudolph C, Mapara M, et al. Cologne high-dose sequential chemotherapy in relapsed and refractory Hodgkin lymphoma: results of a large multicenter study of the German Hodgkin Lymphoma Study Group (GHSG). *Ann Oncol* 2005;16:116–123.
202. Josting A, Muller H, Borchmann P, et al. Dose intensity of chemotherapy in patients with relapsed Hodgkin's lymphoma. *J Clin Oncol* 2010;28:5074–5080.
203. Fung HC, Stiff P, Schriber J, et al. Tandem autologous stem cell transplantation for patients with primary refractory or poor risk recurrent Hodgkin lymphoma. *Biol Blood Marrow Transplant* 2007;13:594–600.
204. Morschhauser F, Brice P, Ferme C, et al. Risk-adapted salvage treatment with single or tandem autologous stem-cell transplantation for first relapse/refractory Hodgkin's lymphoma: results of the prospective multicenter h96 trial by the GELA/SFGM study group. *J Clin Oncol* 2008; 26:5980–5987.
205. Puig N, Pintilie M, Seshadri T, et al. Different response to salvage chemotherapy but similar post-transplant outcomes in patients with relapsed and refractory Hodgkin's lymphoma. *Haematologica* 2010;95:1496–1502.
206. Gajewski JL, Phillips GL, Sobocinski KA, et al. Bone marrow transplants from HLA-identical siblings in advanced Hodgkin's disease. *J Clin Oncol* 1996;14:572–578.
207. Peniket AJ, Ruiz de Elvira MC, Taghipour G, et al. An EBMT registry matched study of allogeneic stem cell transplants for lymphoma: allogeneic transplantation is associated with a lower relapse rate but a higher procedure-related mortality rate than autologous transplantation. *Bone Marrow Transplant* 2003;31:667–678.
208. Anderson JE, Litzow MR, Appelbaum FR, et al. Allogeneic, syngeneic, and autologous marrow transplantation for Hodgkin's disease: the 21-year Seattle experience. *J Clin Oncol* 1993;11:2342–2350.
209. Akpek G, Ambinder RF, Piantadosi S, et al. Long-term results of blood and marrow transplantation for Hodgkin's lymphoma. *J Clin Oncol* 2001;19:4314–4321.
210. Anderlini P, Acholonu SA, Okoroji GJ, et al. Donor leukocyte infusions in relapsed Hodgkin's lymphoma following allogeneic stem cell transplantation: CD3+ cell dose, GVHD and disease response. *Bone Marrow Transplant* 2004;34:511–514.
211. Peggs KS, Hunter A, Chopra R, et al. Clinical evidence of a graft-versus-Hodgkin's-lymphoma effect after reduced-intensity allogeneic transplantation. *Lancet* 2005;365:1934–1941.
212. Peggs KS, Sureda A, Qian W, et al. Reduced-intensity conditioning for allogeneic haematopoietic stem cell transplantation in relapsed and refractory Hodgkin lymphoma: impact of alemtuzumab and donor lymphocyte infusions on long-term outcomes. *Br J Haematol* 2007;139:70–80.
213. Alvarez I, Sureda A, Caballero MD, et al. Nonmyeloablative stem cell transplantation is an effective therapy for refractory or relapsed hodgkin lymphoma: results of a Spanish prospective cooperative protocol. *Biol Blood Marrow Transplant* 2006;12:172–183.
214. Burroughs LM, O'Donnell PV, Sandmaier BM, et al. Fludarabine-melphalan as a preparative regimen for reduced-intensity conditioning allogeneic stem cell transplantation in relapsed and refractory Hodgkin lymphoma: the updated M.D. Anderson Cancer Center experience. *Haematologica* 2008;93:257–264.
215. Burroughs LM, O'Donnell PV, Sandmaier BM, et al. Comparison of outcomes of HLA-matched related, unrelated, or HLA-haploidentical related hematopoietic cell transplantation following nonmyeloablative conditioning for relapsed or refractory Hodgkin lymphoma. *Biol Blood Marrow Transplant* 2008;14:1279–1287.
216. Marcel PD, Parameswaran NH, Jeanette C, et al. Unrelated donor reduced-intensity allogeneic hematopoietic stem cell transplantation for relapsed and refractory Hodgkin lymphoma. *Biol Blood Marrow Transplant* 2009;15:109–117.
217. Sureda A, Robinson S, Canals C, et al. Reduced-intensity conditioning compared with conventional allogeneic stem-cell transplantation in relapsed or refractory Hodgkin's lymphoma: an analysis from the Lymphoma Working Party of the European Group for Blood and Marrow Transplantation. *J Clin Oncol* 2008;26:455–462.
218. Sureda A, Canals C, Arranz R, et al. Allogeneic stem cell transplantation after reduced intensity conditioning in patients with relapsed or refractory Hodgkin's lymphoma. Results of the HDR ALLO study - a prospective clinical trial by the Grupo Espanol de Linfomas/Trasplante de Medula Osea (GEL/TAMO) and the Lymphoma Working Party of the European Group for Blood and Marrow Transplantation. *Haematologica* 2012;97:310–317.
219. Anderlini P, Saliba R, Acholonu S, et al. Fludarabine-melphalan as a preparative regimen for reduced-intensity conditioning allogeneic stem cell transplantation in relapsed and refractory Hodgkin's lymphoma: the updated M.D. Anderson Cancer Center experience. *Haematologica* 2008;93:257–264.
220. Devetten MP, Hari PN, Carreras J, et al. Unrelated donor reduced-intensity allogeneic hematopoietic stem cell transplantation for relapsed and refractory Hodgkin lymphoma. *Biol Blood Marrow Transplant* 2009;15:109–117.
221. Brunstein CG, Cantero S, Cao Q, et al. Promising progression-free survival for patients low and intermediate grade lymphoid malignancies after nonmyeloablative umbilical cord blood transplantation. *Biol Blood Marrow Transplant* 2009;15:214–222.
222. Rodrigues CA, Sanz G, Brunstein CG, et al. Analysis of risk factors for outcomes after unrelated cord blood transplantation in adults with lymphoid malignancies: a study by the Eurocord-Netcord and lymphoma working party of the European group for blood and marrow transplantation. *J Clin Oncol* 2009;27:256–263.
223. Thomson KJ, Peggs KS, Smith P, et al. Improved outcome following reduced intensity allogeneic transplantation in Hodgkin's lymphoma relapsing post-autologous transplantation. *Blood* 2005;106:abstract 657.
224. Sarina B, Castagna L, Todisco E, et al. Allogeneic stem cell transplantation compared with chemotherapy for poor-risk Hodgkin lymphoma. *Biol Blood Marrow Transplant* 2009;15:432–438.
225. Smith SM, van Besien K, Carreras J, et al. Second autologous stem cell transplantation for relapsed lymphoma after a prior autologous transplant. *Biol Blood Marrow Transplant* 2008;14:904–912.
226. Arai S, Fanale M, Devos S, et al. Defining a Hodgkin lymphoma population for novel therapeutics after relapse from autologous hematopoietic cell transplantation. *Leuk Lymphoma* 2013;54:2531–2533.
227. Younes A, Bartlett NL, Leonard JP, et al. Brentuximab vedotin (SGN-35) for relapsed CD30-positive lymphomas. *N Engl J Med* 2010;363:1812–1821.
228. Fanale MA, Forero-Torres A, Rosenblatt JD, et al. A phase I weekly dosing study of brentuximab vedotin in patients with relapsed/refractory CD30-positive hematologic malignancies. *Clin Cancer Res* 2012;18:248–255.
229. Younes A, Gopal AK, Smith SE, et al. Results of a pivotal phase II study of brentuximab vedotin for patients with relapsed or refractory Hodgkin's lymphoma. *J Clin Oncol* 2012;30:2183–2189.
230. Buglio D, Georgakis GV, Hanabuchi S, et al. Vorinostat inhibits STAT6-mediated TH2 cytokine and TARC production and induces cell death in Hodgkin lymphoma cell lines. *Blood* 2008;112:1424–1433.
231. Buglio D, Mamidipudi V, Khaskhely NM, et al. The class-I HDAC inhibitor MGCD0103 induces apoptosis in Hodgkin lymphoma cell lines and synergizes with proteasome inhibitors by an HDAC6-independent mechanism. *Br J Haematol* 2010;151:387–396.
232. Sharpe AH, Wherry EJ, Ahmed R, et al. The function of programmed cell death 1 and its ligands in regulating autoimmunity and infection. *Nat Immunol* 2007;8:239–245.
233. Kirschbaum MH, Goldman BH, Zain JM, et al. A phase 2 study of vorinostat for treatment of relapsed or refractory Hodgkin lymphoma: Southwest Oncology Group Study S0517. *Leuk Lymphoma* 2012;53:259–262.
234. Zhou N, Moradei O, Raeppel S, et al. Discovery of N-(2-aminophenyl)-4-[(4-pyridin-3-ylpyrimidin-2-ylamino)methyl]benzamide (MGCD0103), an orally active histone deacetylase inhibitor. *J Med Chem* 2008;51:4072–4075.
235. Fournel M, Bonfils C, Hou Y, et al. MGCD0103, a novel isotype-selective histone deacetylase inhibitor, has broad spectrum antitumor activity in vitro and in vivo. *Mol Cancer Ther* 2008;7:759–768.
236. Younes A, Oki Y, Bociek RG, et al. Mocetinostat for relapsed classical Hodgkin's lymphoma: an open-label, single-arm, phase 2 trial. *Lancet Oncol* 2011;12:1222–1228.
237. Younes A, Sureda A, Ben-Yehuda D, et al. Panobinostat in patients with relapsed/refractory Hodgkin's lymphoma after autologous stem-cell transplantation: results of a phase II study. *J Clin Oncol* 2012;30:2197–2203.
238. Engelman JA. Targeting PI3K signalling in cancer: opportunities, challenges and limitations. *Nat Rev Cancer* 2009;9:550–562.
239. Yuan TL, Cantley LC. PI3K pathway alterations in cancer: variations on a theme. *Oncogene* 2008;27:5497–5510.
240. Hennessy BT, Smith DL, Ram PT, et al. Exploiting the PI3K/AKT pathway for cancer drug discovery. *Nat Rev Drug Discov* 2005;4:988–1004.

241. Meadows SA, Vega F, Kashishian A, et al. PI3Kdelta inhibitor, GS-1101 (CAL-101), attenuates pathway signaling, induces apoptosis, and overcomes signals from the microenvironment in cellular models of Hodgkin lymphoma. *Blood* 2012;119:1897–1900.
242. Johnston PB, Pinter-Brown L, Rogerio J, et al. Everolimus for relapsed/refractory classical Hodgkin lymphoma: multicenter, open-label, single-arm, phase 2 study. *54th ASH Annual Meeting* 2012;Abstract 2740.
243. von Tresckow B, Plütschow A, Fuchs M, et al. Dose-intensification in early unfavorable Hodgkin's lymphoma: final analysis of the German Hodgkin Study Group HD14 trial. *J Clin Oncol* 2012;30:907–913.
244. Levis A, Anselmo AP, Ambrosetti A, et al. VEPEMB in elderly Hodgkin's lymphoma patients. Results from an Intergruppo Italiano Linfomi (IIL) study. *Ann Oncol* 2004;15:123–128.
245. Gobbi PG, Federico M. What has happened to VBM (vinblastine, bleomycin, and methotrexate) chemotherapy for early-stage Hodgkin lymphoma? *Crit Rev Oncol Hematol* 2012;82:18–24.
246. Bartlett NL, Niedzwiecki D, Johnson JL, et al. Gemcitabine, vinorelbine, and pegylated liposomal doxorubicin (GVD), a salvage regimen in relapsed Hodgkin's lymphoma: CALGB 59804. *Ann Oncol* 2007;18:1071–1079.
247. Santoro A, Magagnoli M, Spina M, et al. Ifosfamide, gemcitabine, and vinorelbine: a new induction regimen for refractory and relapsed Hodgkin's lymphoma. *Haematologica* 2007;92:35–41.
248. Josting A, Rudolph C, Reiser M, et al. Time-intensified dexamethasone/cisplatin/cytarabine: an effective salvage therapy with low toxicity in patients with relapsed and refractory Hodgkin's disease. *Ann Oncol* 2002;13:1628–1635.
249. Moskowitz CH, Bertino JR, Glassman JR, et al. Ifosfamide, carboplatin, and etoposide: a highly effective cytoreduction and peripheral-blood progenitor-cell mobilization regimen for transplant-eligible patients with non-Hodgkin's lymphoma. *J Clin Oncol* 1999;17:3776–3785.
250. Schmitz N, Pfistner B, Sextro M, et al. Aggressive conventional chemotherapy compared with high-dose chemotherapy with autologous haemopoietic stem-cell transplantation for relapsed chemosensitive Hodgkin's disease: a randomised trial. *Lancet* 2002;359:2065–2071.
251. Proctor SJ, Jackson GH, Lennard A, et al. Strategic approach to the management of Hodgkin's disease incorporating salvage therapy with high-dose ifosfamide, etoposide and epirubicin: a Northern Region Lymphoma Group study (UK). *Ann Oncol* 2003;14:i47–i50.

39 Non-Hodgkin's Lymphoma

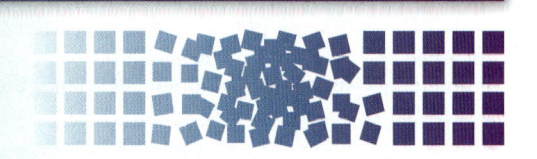

Arnold S. Freedman, Caron A. Jacobson, Peter Mauch, and Jon C. Aster

INTRODUCTION

Non-Hodgkin's lymphomas (NHL) are neoplastic transformations of mature B, T, and natural killer (NK) cells. Although NHLs and Hodgkin's lymphoma (HL) both infiltrate lymphohematopoietic tissues, their biologic and clinical behaviors are distinct. And although both are among the most sensitive malignancies to radiation and cytotoxic therapy, their cure rates differ. HLs are cured in about 80% of all patients employing both conventional and salvage treatment strategies, whereas NHLs are cured in less than 50% of patients.

EPIDEMIOLOGY AND ETIOLOGY

In 2011, there were an estimated 70,090 new cases of NHL in the United States, which constituted 4% of all new cancers in both males and females.[1] This is more than seven times the incidence of HL. There is a slight male-to-female predominance, and a higher incidence for Caucasians than for African Americans. The incidence rises steadily with age, especially after age 40. Lymphomas are among the most common malignancies in patients between the ages of 20 and 40 years. Moreover, the incidence of NHL nearly doubled between 1970 and 1995. Although the rate of increase has slowed since the mid 1990s the incidence has continued to rise by 1.5% to 2% each year. NHL ranks as the ninth most common cause of cancer-related death in men in the United States and eighth in women. In 2014, 18,990 deaths from NHL were predicted. The 5-year survival rates for NHL is 72% for Caucasians and 63% for African Americans.

There are striking differences in the age-dependent incidence of NHL by histologic subtype. In children, diffuse large B-cell lymphoma (DLBCL), Burkitt's lymphoma (BL), and lymphoblastic lymphoma are most common. Although DLBCL is also the most common histologic subtypes in adults, the indolent lymphomas (small lymphocytic and follicular lymphomas [FL]) are extremely rare in children.

Exposures and Diseases Associated with Non-Hodgkin's Lymphoma

Infectious agents are involved in the pathogenesis of some NHLs. Epstein-Barr virus (EBV) is most commonly associated with a variety of B-cell NHLs, including endemic, sporadic, and AIDS-associated BL, lymphomas that arise in the setting of immunosuppression, including after organ transplantation and treatment of autoimmune diseases, in the setting of HIV infection, and a subset of lymphomas that arise in otherwise normal elderly individuals (Table 39.1).[2] EBV infection is also implicated in extranodal NK cell and T-cell lymphomas that involve the upper aerodigestive tract as well as other extranodal sites, as well as a small number of other unusual and uncommon T-cell malignancies.[3] Infection with human T-lymphotropic virus type 1 (HTLV-1) has been implicated in adult T-cell leukemia-lymphoma (ATLL) seen in the Caribbean and Japan.[4] Human herpes virus 8 (HHV-8) infection is associated with primary effusion lymphoma, where the viral genome is found within tumor cells in virtually 100% of cases.[5] Chronic hepatitis B infection has also been associated with an increased risk of NHL.[6] The marginal zone lymphomas (MZL) have been linked to many infectious agents. The gastric extranodal MZLs are associated with *Helicobacter pylori* infection.[7] Splenic MZL has been associated with hepatitis C infections.[8] The ocular adnexal MZL has been linked with *Chlamydia psittaci* infections,[9] and immunoproliferative small intestinal disease (Mediterranean lymphoma, alpha heavy chain disease) has been associated with *Campylobacter jejuni*.[10] *Borrelia burgdorferi* infection has been associated with extranodal MZLs of the skin in cases from Europe.[11]

An increased risk of NHL has been associated with a number of environmental exposures and/or disease states (see Table 39.1).[12,13] There is controversial evidence that certain chemical exposures, specifically the herbicide phenoxyacetic acid, increase the risk of NHL.[14] Other potential environmental associations include exposure to arsenic, pesticides, fungicides, chlorophenols, or organic solvents, halomethane, lead, vinyl chloride, or asbestos.[15,16] Occupational exposures associated with an increased risk include agricultural work, welding, and work in the lumber industry.[17] NHL has been observed as a late complication of prior chemotherapy and/or radiation therapy. Specifically, patients with HL treated with radiation therapy and chemotherapy exhibit an increased risk of developing secondary DLBCL.[18]

Diseases of inherited and acquired immunodeficiency as well as autoimmune diseases are associated with an increased incidence of lymphoma (see Table 39.1). The association between immunosuppression and induction of NHLs is compelling because, if the immunosuppression can be reversed, a percentage of these lymphomas regress spontaneously.[19] The incidence of NHL is nearly 100-fold increased for patients undergoing organ transplantation necessitating chronic immunosuppression, and is greatest in the first year posttransplant. About 30% of these arise as a polyclonal B-cell proliferation that evolves into a clonal B-cell malignancy. The NHLs that occur in the context of immunosuppression or immunodeficiency, including human immunodeficiency virus 1 (HIV-1) infection, are frequently associated with EBV.[20] Histologically, DLBCLs are most frequently associated with immunosuppression and autoimmune diseases, although almost all histologies can be seen. The rare inherited immunodeficiency diseases (X-linked lymphoproliferative syndrome, Wiskott-Aldrich syndrome, Chédiak-Higashi syndrome, ataxia telangiectasia, and common variable immunodeficiency syndrome) are complicated by highly aggressive lymphomas. The elevated incidence of lymphoma in iatrogenic immunosuppression, AIDS, and autoimmune disease argues strongly for immune dysregulation contributing in the pathogenesis of some lymphomas.[21,22] An increased risk of NHL has been observed in first-degree relatives with NHL, HL, or chronic lymphocytic leukemia (CLL). In large databases studies, about 9% of patients with lymphoma or CLL have a first-degree relative with a lymphoproliferative disorder.[23,24]

TABLE 39.1
Conditions Associated with the Development of Lymphoma

Inherited Immunodeficiency States	Acquired Immunodeficiency States	Autoimmune and Inflammatory Disorders	Chemicals and Drugs	Infectious Agents (Other than HIV)
Klinefelter's syndrome	Acquired agammaglobulinemia	Rheumatoid arthritis	Phenytoin	Epstein-Barr virus
Chédiak-Higashi syndrome	HIV-1 infection	Autoimmune hemolytic anemia	Dioxin, agent orange, pesticides	HTLV-1
Ataxia telangiectasia	Iatrogenic	Systemic lupus erythematosus	Ionizing radiation	HHV-8
Wiskott-Aldrich syndrome	Multicentric Castleman's disease	Sjögren's syndrome	Chemotherapy, radiation therapy	*Helicobacter pylori*
Common variable immunodeficiency		Hashimoto's thyroiditis	Tumor necrosis factor agonists	*Campylobacter jejuni*
X-linked lymphoproliferative disease		Acquired angioedema	Hair dyes	*Chlamydia psittaci*
Autoimmune lymphoproliferative disease		Inflammatory bowel disease		*Borrelia afzelii*
Bloom syndrome		Celiac disease		HCV
				MTB

HIV-1, human immunodeficiency virus-1; HTLV-1, human T cell lymphotropic virus-1; HHV-8, human herpes virus-8; HCV, hepatitis C virus; MTB, *Mycobacterium tuberculosis*.

BIOLOGIC BACKGROUND FOR CLASSIFICATION OF LYMPHOID NEOPLASMS

Current lymphoma classification systems divide the lymphomas into different entities based, in part, on their perceived cell of origin (Fig. 39.1, Table 39.2). During embryogenesis, hematopoietic stem cells (HSC) from the liver and the placenta give rise to progenitor cells that migrate to the thymus and bone marrow where they undergo a program of antigen-independent differentiation into T- and B-cell lineage precursor cells, directed largely by the microenvironment.[25] Postnatally, all lymphoid cells are derived from bone marrow HSCs, which give rise to very early lymphoid progenitors with B, T, and NK lymphocyte potential. These cells, in turn, yield B-cell progenitors in the marrow, the site of early stages of B-cell differentiation, as well as other progenitors that migrate to the thymus and undergo T-cell differentiation.

B-Cell Development

The initial commitment to B-cell differentiation by lymphoid progenitors in the bone marrow requires the expression of the master B lineage transcription factor PAX5, which directly upregulates the expression of early B lineage markers such as CD19.[26] Subsequent precursor B cell development depends on a transcriptional program that is driven by PAX5 and downstream transcription factors and prosurvival signals produced by stepwise rearrangement of immunoglobulin (Ig) genes, which requires the lymphoid-specific recombination factors RAG1 and RAG2 and also involves the specialized DNA polymerase terminal deoxynucleotidyl transferase (TdT).[27] During development, pre-B cells pass through checkpoints that correspond to specific stages of Ig gene assembly, beginning with rearrangement of the Ig heavy chain locus (IgH).[28] Productive (in-frame) rearrangement of IgH leads to the expression of IgM heavy chain, which combines with a lambdalike polypeptide to enable the assembly of pre–B-cell receptors. The pre–B-cell receptor generates signals that prevent apoptosis, turns off further IgH gene rearrangement (contributing to allelic exclusion, the expression of only a single IgH in each B cell clone), and turns on rearrangements of the Ig light chain loci, first the kappa loci and, if these rearrangements are nonproductive, then the lambda light chain loci. During the period of Ig gene rearrangement, pre-B cells lack complete surface Ig and express CD19 and CD10, the common acute lymphoblastic leukemia antigen.[29] Precursor B cells that productively rearrange one or another light chain locus express the surface Ig receptor (sometimes referred to as the B-cell receptor [BCR]), which also transmits key survival signals that prevent apoptosis. Cells that express surface Ig upregulate additional B-cell markers such as CD79a, cytoplasmic and surface CD22, and CD20, as well as prosurvival factors such as BCL2, and downregulate CD10 and TdT emerging from the process as mature, immunologically naïve B cells.

In mice, two major types of naïve B cells have been defined. Roughly 90% of circulating and tissue-based B cells fall into the B2 class. B2 cells are widely distributed and largely respond to antigens in a T-cell–dependent fashion, a process that yields class-switched plasma cells expressing high-affinity Ig. B1 cells can be further subdivided into those that do or do not express the antigen CD5.[30] CD5+ B1a cells produce broadly reactive natural IgM, whereas CD5− B1b cells can generate T-independent, long-lasting memory-type IgM responses to some infectious pathogens. Whether B1 cells exist as a distinct B-cell lineage in humans has been (and remains) controversial, but it is notable that some human B-cell tumors, particularly CLL, is comprised of cells bearing some similarity to murine B1 cells.

From the marrow, naïve B cells migrate through the blood and extravasate into secondary lymphoid tissues, such as the spleen, the lymph nodes, and mucosa-associated lymphoid tissues in the gut. Homing of B cells to specific tissues appears to be controlled largely by chemokines that activate chemokine receptors expressed on B cells.[31] Upon encountering an antigen in peripheral tissues, B cells may either be induced to differentiate directly into short-lived IgM secreting plasma cells or may migrate to B-cell follicles. Antigen-mediated B-cell activation requires the transcription factor MYC and is accompanied by an increase in cell size and entry into cell cycle.[32,33] Once in follicles, the B cells downregulate MYC and BCL2 and upregulate the transcriptional repressor

Figure 39.1

B Cell	Precursor Cell	Disease
Bone marrow	Common Lymphocyte Progenitor	
	Pre-B Lymphoblast	Precursor B lymphoblastic lymphoma/leukemias
	Naïve B cell	Chronic lymphocytic leukemia/small lymphocytic lymphoma (CLL/SLL)
	Plasma cell	Multiple myeloma
Lymph node	Mantle B cell	Mantle cell lymphoma
	Germinal center B cell	Follicular lymphoma, Burkitt's lymphoma, diffuse large B-cell lymphoma (DLBCL)
	Marginal zone B cell	Marginal zone lymphoma, DLBCL, CLL/SLL
T cell		
Thymus	Double-negative T cell	Precursor T lymphoblastic lymphoma/leukemias
	Double-positive T cell	
	CD4-positive or CD8-positive T cell	
Lymph node	Peripheral T cell	Peripheral T-cell lymphomas

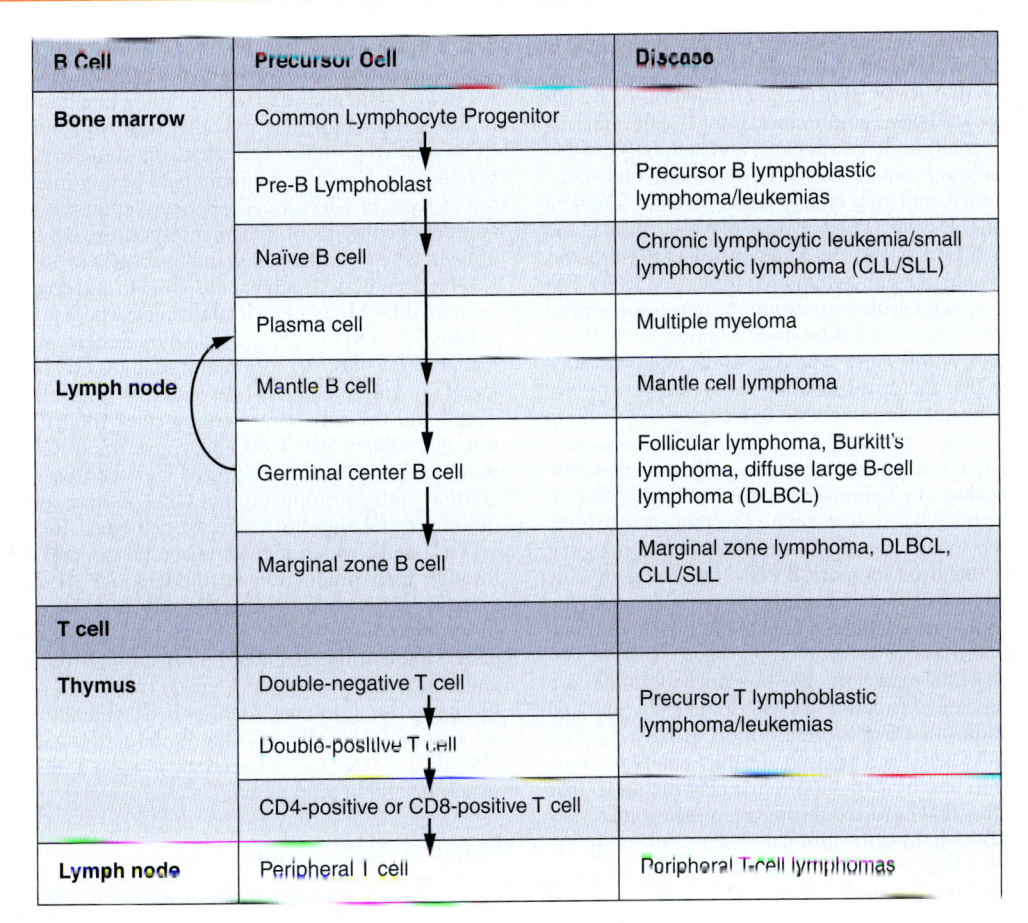

Figure 39.1 B- and T-cell development and cell of origin of lymphomas.

TABLE 39.2

Cluster Designations (CD) of Antigens Useful in Non-Hodgkin Lymphoma Classification

CD	Normal Lymphocyte Expression	Neoplastic Lymphocyte Expression
1a	Cortical thymocytes; Langerhans cells	Precursor T-lymphoblastic lymphoma/leukemia; Langerhans cell neoplasms
2	T and NK cells	T- and NK cell lymphomas
3	T (cytoplasmic and surface) and NK (cytoplasmic only) cells	T- and NK cell lymphomas
4	T and NK cells	T- and NK cell lymphomas
5	T cells, naïve B cells	Chronic lymphocytic leukemia/small lymphocytic lymphoma (CLL/SLL); mantle cell lymphoma; T-cell neoplasms
7	T and NK cells	T and NK cell lymphomas
8	T- and NK cell subsets	Some T and NK cell lymphomas
10	Precursor and germinal center B cells	Precursor B and T lymphoblastic lymphoma/leukemia; follicular lymphoma; Burkitt's lymphoma; diffuse large B cell lymphoma (DLBCL)
11c	B cell subset; CD8 T cells; NK cells	Hairy cell leukemia; splenic marginal zone lymphoma; CLL/SLL
16	NK cells	NK cell and some T-cell lymphomas
19	B cells	B-cell lymphomas
20	Mature B cells (except plasma cells)	Mature B-cell lymphomas
23	Activated B cells, follicular dendritic cells	CLL/SLL
25	Activated T and B cells	Hairy cell leukemia; adult T-cell leukemia/lymphoma
30	Activated lymphocytes (B, T, and NK cells)	Anaplastic large cell lymphoma (ALCL)
56	NK and activated T cells	NK and T-cell lymphomas; plasma cell neoplasms
57	NK and T-cell subsets	NK and T-cell lymphomas
103	Mucosal intraepithelial lymphocytes	Hairy cell leukemia; enteropathy-type T-cell lymphoma
138	Plasma cells	Plasma cell neoplasms; plasmablastic lymphoma

BCL6, which, like MYC, is essential for secondary B-cell follicle formation; secondary follicles are also known as germinal centers.[34] Downregulation of BCL2 may permit the elimination of B cells making low affinity antibodies, and in fact, most B cells entering into the germinal centers undergo apoptosis and are phagocytosed by resident macrophages (often referred to as tingible body macrophages because they contain a readily visible nuclear fragment derived from defunct B cells). The key roles of MYC, BCL2, and BCL6 in this process explain why the genes encoding these factors are commonly mutated in B-cell lymphomas (discussed later). Follicular B cells also upregulate the expression of activation-induced cytosine deaminase (AID), a gene product required for both somatic hypermutation and Ig class switching. Cells that by chance acquire mutations that increase Ig affinity for an antigen survive thanks to signals transmitted through the Ig receptor and go on to undergo class-switching, a process that is regulated by cytokines.[35] The germinal center reaction also requires follicular dendritic cells and a special class of CD4-positive follicular T cells that express the CD40 ligand.[36] B cells that survive this process may leave the germinal centers to take up residence in surrounding marginal zones to become long-lived memory B cells, or may terminally differentiate into plasma cells, which may take up residence in the medulla of the lymph nodes or the red pulp of the spleen, or home back to the bone marrow.

It is notable that the most common human lymphomas are B-cell tumors composed of lymphocytes with somatically mutated Ig genes, an alteration that marks these tumors as having arisen from cells that have experienced a germinal center reaction. Many of these same tumors also have mutations that bear the molecular hallmarks of mistakes that occurred during attempted somatic hypermutation or class-switching in germinal centers; indeed, mutations involving MYC, BCL2, and BCL6 identical to those found in lymphomas are also found at a low frequency in normal germinal center B cells obtained from both children and adults. Thus, the relatively high frequency of tumors derived from germinal center B cells likely reflects the error-prone nature of the molecular events that permit antibody class-switching and affinity maturation.

T-Cell Development

Progenitors from the bone marrow that travel to the thymus become committed to T-cell differentiation via interactions with thymic epithelial cells (TEC) (see Fig. 39.1). TECs express ligands for Notch receptors such as DLL4, leading to activation of the receptor NOTCH1, which is essential for early stages of T-cell development.[37] As during early B-cell development, early T-cell development is controlled by a transcriptional program induced by a master transcription factor (NOTCH1) and by survival signals mediated by complexes containing components of the T-cell receptor (TCR).[38] In most developing T cells, this begins with rearrangement of the TCRβ genes, which (as in B cells) requires RAG1 and RAG2 and involves the participation of TdT. Productive, in-frame rearrangement of the TCRβ gene permits expression of the TCRβ polypeptide, which pairs with pre-Tα polypeptides and assembles into the pre-T cell receptor. Prosurvival signals transmitted by pre-Tα allow cells to go on to rearrange the TCRα genes, and cells with productive TCRα rearrangements express TCRαβ receptors on their cell surfaces in complex with CD3 polypeptides. Surviving cells also upregulate the CD4 and CD8 coreceptors and proceed through both negative and positive antigenic selection, during which cells expressing autoreactive TCRs or TCRs that fail to recognize antigen in the context of major histocompatibility complex (MHC) antigens are eliminated by apoptosis.[39] Cells emerging from the thymus as naïve T cells express either CD4, a coreceptor for MHC class II antigens, or CD8, a coreceptor for MHC class I antigens. A much smaller subset of thymic T-cell progenitors productively rearrange their δ and γ TCR genes, and emerge from the thymus as naïve γδ-TCR–expressing T cells.

Like naïve B cells, naïve T cells home to peripheral tissues under the influence of chemokines, with most γδ T cells homing to gut and skin, and αβ T cells homing much more widely to secondary lymphoid tissues and other sites. γδ T cells are considered to be relative primitive cells that contribute to *natural* immunity, whereas αβ T cells can differentiate further into a number of different types of effector cells, depending on the dose, timing, and context of subsequent antigenic exposures. αβ T cells recognize antigen when it is presented in the context of an MHC molecule. CD4+ T cells, or T-helper cells, bind to and recognize an antigen presented by MHC class II molecules, whereas CD8+ T cells or cytotoxic T cells bind to and recognize antigen presented by MHC class I molecules. Activation also requires CD40 and CD40L interaction and CD28/CTLA4 and B7 interaction between the T cell and the antigen presenting cell (APC).[40] Antigen stimulation of CD8-positive T cells may give rise to CD8-positive effector cytotoxic cells or to long-lived CD8-positive memory cells. By contrast, antigen stimulation of CD4-positive cells can produce a number of CD4-positive effector cell types, including: T helper 1 (Th1) cells, which activate macrophages and cytotoxic T cells through their production of interleukin 2 (IL-2) and interferon gamma; T helper 2 (Th2) cells, which activate B cells through their production of IL-4, -5, -6, and -13[41,42]; T helper 17 (Th17) cells, which stimulate neutrophils through production of IL-17 and IL-22; and regulatory T cells (Treg), which produce immunosuppressive cytokines such as IL-10. Finally, follicular helper T cells are CD4+ T cells that home to the germinal center via CXCR5 and CXCL13 interactions and play a role in B cell Ig class switching and Ig production.[43]

Natural Killer Cells

There is a third class of lymphocytes that can kill targets without MHC restriction, namely NK cells, which are a component of the innate host immune system. NK cells recognize and kill cells that lack MHC class I molecules (including virally infected cells and malignant cells), as well as antibody-coated targets through interactions with Fc receptors on the NK cell surface. NK cells lack surface CD3 and do not have rearranged TCR genes. Morphologically, these cells are slightly larger than resting T and B cells and have paler cytoplasm that contains azurophilic granules, an appearance similar to that of activated cytotoxic T cells.

Immunophenotyping of Lymphoid Cells

As has been alluded to, lymphocytes at various stages in ontologic development can be defined and differentiated by the detection of certain antigens on the cell surface (see Table 39.2). This antigen footprint is referred to as the immunophenotype of the cell. It can be detected by a flow cytometric analysis of single cell suspensions from whole blood, bone marrow, body fluid, or disaggregated tissue using fluorescently labeled antibodies against these antigens or by immunohistochemistry, which involves the incubation of paraffin embedded tissue sections with enzyme-linked antibodies against these antigens followed by a colorimetric reaction. These techniques have become vital in diagnosing and monitoring lymphomas, and have provided insight into the normal counterparts of the malignant lymphocyte.

Chromosomal Translocations and Oncogene Rearrangements

Given the mechanism of Ig and TCR gene rearrangements in lymphoid cells—namely, the formation of DNA breaks with the joining of new pieces of DNA—it is not surprising that lymphomas are frequently found to have chromosomal translocations that involve the activation of an oncogene or inactivation of a tumor suppressor

TABLE 39.3 Genetic Features of B- and T-Cell Lymphomas

Genetic Feature	Genes	Lymphoma
t(8;14) t(2;8) t(8;22)	MYC/IgH MYC/Igκ MYC/Igλ	Burkitt's lymphoma
t(11;14)	BCL1 (CCND1)/IgH	Mantle cell lymphoma; multiple myeloma
t(14;18) t(3;14)	BCL2/IgH BCL6/IgH	Follicular lymphoma; diffuse large B-cell lymphoma (DLBCL)
t(11;18) t(1;14) t(14;18) t(3;14)	API2/MALT1 BCL10/IgH MALT1/IgH FOXP1/IgH	MALT lymphoma
Trisomy 3 7q21 deletion	Unknown CDK6	Splenic marginal zone lymphoma
11q23 deletion 13q14 deletion 17p13 deletion Trisomy 12	ATM Unknown TP53 Unknown	Chronic lymphocytic leukemia/small lymphocytic lymphoma (CLL/SLL); del(17p) and del(13q) also in multiple myeloma; del(11q) also in T-cell prolymphocytic leukemia (T-PLL)
t(9;14) 6q21 deletion	PAX5/IgH Unknown	Lymphoplasmacytic lymphoma
9p gain	JAK2, PDL1, PDL2	Mediastinal large B-cell lymphoma
inv(14) t(14;14)	TCRα/TCL1	Peripheral T-cell lymphoma, NOS; T-PLL
t(2;5) t(1;2) t(2;3) t(2;17) inv(2)	NPM1/ALK TPM3/ALK TFG/ALK CTLC/ALK ATIC/ALK	Anaplastic large cell lymphoma (ALCL)
Trisomy 3 Trisomy 5	Unknown Unknown	Angioimmunoblastic T-cell lymphoma
Isochromosome 7q	Unknown	Hepatosplenic T-cell lymphoma

MALT, mucosa-associated lymphoid tissue; CTLC, clathrin heavy chain 1.

gene (Table 39.3). The former is more common, whereby a proto-oncogene is brought under the control of a constitutively active promoter. The resulting overexpression of the involved gene (now called an oncogene) conveys oncogenic properties on the gene and its protein product, which is responsible for induction and/or maintenance of some aspect of the transformed phenotype. Examples of this type of event include the (8;14)(q24;q32) translocation in BL, involving the MYC proto-oncogene and the IgH gene; the (14;18)(q32;q32) translocation in follicular lymphoma, involving the BCL2 proto-oncogene and the IgH gene; and the (11;14)(q13;q32) translocation in mantle cell lymphoma, involving the gene encoding cyclin D1 (CCDN1) and the IgH gene. Less commonly, chromosomal translocations produce fusion genes that encode chimeric oncogenic proteins. Examples of this include the (2;5)(p23;q35) translocation involving the ALK and NPM1 genes in anaplastic large cell lymphoma (ALCL) and the t(11;18)(q21;q21) translocation involving the API2 and MLT genes in mucosa-associated lymphoid tissue (MALT) lymphoma. These translocations and rearrangements can be detected by polymerase chain reaction (PCR) using probes that span the chromosomal breakpoints, reverse transcriptase PCR (RT-PCR) to detect the RNA product of the fusion gene, or fluorescence in situ hybridization (FISH) using probes to specific chromosomal segments. In cases where the translocation results in the expression of a protein or portion of a protein that is never expressed in normal lymphocytes (e.g., anaplastic lymphoma kinase [ALK] kinase), immunohistochemistry can be used to detect the protein and infer the presence of a rearrangement involving the gene that encodes that protein.

LYMPHOMA CLASSIFICATION: THE PRINCIPLES OF THE WORLD HEALTH ORGANIZATION (WHO) CLASSIFICATION OF LYMPHOID NEOPLASMS

In 2001, the World Health Organization (WHO) published a new classification of tumors of the hematopoietic and lymphoid tissues (Table 39.4).[44] It was the end result of a project that began in 1995 with 10 committees of pathologists and a Clinical Advisory Committee of international experts to ensure the clinical utility of the classification system. It incorporated, with minor edits, the 1994 consensus by the International Lymphoma Study Group regarding a list of lymphoid neoplasms that were distinct and recognizable by pathologists called the Revised European and American Lymphoma (REAL) classification.[45] The principle behind the classification system is to use and integrate all of the relevant information, including morphology, immunophenotype, genetics, and clinical features, to define disease entities with the relative importance of each type of information varying from disease to disease. The WHO classification system was recently updated and diseases were

TABLE 39.4

World Health Organization Classification of Lymphoid Neoplasms 2008

Precursor B- and T-Cell Neoplasms
Precursor B-lymphoblastic leukemia/lymphoma
Precursor T-lymphoblastic leukemia/lymphoma

Mature B-Cell Neoplasms
Chronic lymphocytic leukemia/small lymphocytic lymphoma
B-cell prolymphocytic leukemia
Lymphoplasmacytic lymphoma
Splenic marginal zone lymphoma
Hairy cell leukemia
Splenic B-cell lymphoma, unclassifiable
    Splenic diffuse red pulp small B-cell lymphoma
    Hairy cell leukemia – variant
Plasma cell neoplasms
    Monoclonal gammopathy of undetermined significance (MGUS)
    Plasma cell myeloma
    Solitary plasmacytoma of bone
    Extraosseous plasmacytoma
    Monoclonal immunoglobulin deposition disease
Extranodal marginal zone lymphoma
Nodal marginal zone lymphoma
Follicular lymphoma
Primary cutaneous follicle center lymphoma
Mantle cell lymphoma
Diffuse large B-cell lymphoma (DLBCL)
    T cell/histiocyte-rich large B-cell lymphoma
    Primary DLBCL of the central nervous system
    Primary cutaneous DLBCL, leg type
    EBV-positive DLBCL of the elderly
DLBCL associated with chronic inflammation
Lymphomatoid granulomatosis
Primary mediastinal large B-cell lymphoma
Intravascular large B-cell lymphoma
ALK-positive large B-cell lymphoma
Plasmablastic lymphoma
Large B-cell lymphoma arising in HHV-8–associated multicentric
    Castleman's disease
Burkitt's lymphoma (BL)
B-cell lymphoma, unclassifiable, with features intermediate
    between DLBCL and BL
B-cell lymphoma, unclassifiable, with features intermediate
    between DLBCL and HL

Mature T- and NK Cell Neoplasms
T-cell prolymphocytic leukemia
T-cell large granular lymphocytic leukemia
Chronic lymphoproliferative disorder of NK cells
Aggressive NK cell leukemia
EBV-positive T-cell lymphoproliferative diseases of childhood
    Systemic EBV+ T-cell lymphoproliferative disease of childhood
    Hydroa vacciniforme-like lymphoma
Adult T-cell leukemia/lymphoma
Extranodal NK/T-cell lymphoma, nasal type
Enteropathy-type T-cell lymphoma
Hepatosplenic T-cell lymphoma
Subcutaneous panniculitis-like T-cell lymphoma
Mycosis fungoides
Sézary's syndrome
Primary cutaneous CD30+ T-cell lymphoproliferative disorders
    Primary cutaneous anaplastic large cell lymphoma
    Lymphomatoid papulosis
Primary cutaneous peripheral T-cell lymphomas, rare subtypes
    Primary cutaneous γ-δ T-cell lymphoma
    Primary cutaneous CD8+ aggressive epidermotropic cytotoxic
        T-cell lymphoma
    Primary cutaneous CD4+ small/medium T-cell lymphoma
Peripheral T-cell lymphoma, not otherwise specified
Angioimmunoblastic T-cell lymphoma
Anaplastic large cell lymphoma, ALK+
Anaplastic large cell lymphoma, ALK–

Immunodeficiency-Associated Lymphoproliferative Disorders
Lymphoproliferative diseases associated with primary immune
    disorders
Lymphomas associated with HIV infection
Posttransplant lymphoproliferative disorders (PTLD)
    Plasmacytic hyperplasia and infectious mononucleosis-like PTLD
    Polymorphic PTLD
    Monomorphic PTLD
    Classical HL-type PTLD
Other iatrogenic immunodeficiency-associated lymphoproliferative
    disorders

---

reclassified in 2008 based on new and evolving information with regard to each of these disease characteristics.

Categories of Lymphoid Neoplasms

There are five main categories of lymphoid neoplasms defined by the WHO: precursor B and T-cell neoplasms, mature B-cell neoplasms, mature T/NK cell neoplasms, HL, and immunodeficiency-associated lymphoproliferative disorders (see Table 39.4). Each category is a set of distinct diagnoses that are not further classified or grouped by grade, prognosis, or clinical behavior but instead are considered unique entities. In 2001, there were 48 such entities plus additional variants. In 2008, several additions were made, and several provisional diagnostic categories were created that reflect the additional information being gleaned from technology, such as gene expression profiling (GEP) and the consequent recognition of heterogeneity within existing disease entities. For example, within DLBCL, GEP can differentiate between two broad categories of disease, namely the germinal center B-cell type (GCB) and the activated B-cell type (ABC), with different prognoses.[46] These categories have not yet been adopted into the WHO because they are not yet relevant to differential treatment strategies, but new treatments are being developed with these GEPs in mind, and treatment effect is being stratified by DLBCL subtype in ongoing clinical trials, and this will likely become clinically relevant in the near future. Furthermore, disease location is being recognized as important in distinguishing one DLBCL from another, with DLBCL of certain locations like the central nervous system (CNS) or primary cutaneous DLBCL, leg type, having unique clinical presentations, clinical behavior, and GEPs compared with nodal DLBCL; these have been added as distinct entities to the 2008 WHO. The microenvironment is another important defining feature of some lymphomas and, as such, T-cell/histiocyte–rich large B-cell lymphoma was added to the updated classification. Finally, two provisional categories have been created to recognize lymphomas that have features intermediate between two types of lymphoma, the so-called gray zone lymphomas: B-cell lymphoma unclassifiable (BCLU) with features intermediate between BL and DLBCL (BCLU-BL/DLBCL) and BCLU with features intermediate between HL and DLBCL (BCLU-HL/DLBCL). These categories were created recognizing that they are likely a heterogenous group of disease, with some most closely resembling BL or HL, some most closely resembling DLBCL, and some belonging to distinct entities, helping to create a more systematic approach to their study and classification.

PRINCIPLES OF MANAGEMENT OF NON-HODGKIN'S LYMPHOMA

Differential Diagnosis and Sites of Disease at Presentation

More than two-thirds of patients with NHL present with persistent painless peripheral lymphadenopathy. At the time of presentation, a differential diagnosis of generalized lymphadenopathy necessitates the exclusion of infectious etiologies such as bacteria (including mycobacteria), viruses (e.g., infectious mononucleosis, cytomegalovirus, hepatitis B, HIV), and parasites (toxoplasmosis) as well as inflammatory and autoimmune diseases, and metastatic malignancies. It is generally agreed that a lymph node larger than 1.5 × 1.5 cm that is not associated with a documented infection and that persists longer than 4 weeks should be considered for a biopsy.[47] A biopsy should be performed immediately for patients with other findings suggesting malignancy (e.g., systemic complaints or B symptoms, such as fever, night sweats, weight loss). However, lymph nodes in several histopathologic subtypes of NHLs frequently wax and wane. In teenagers and young adults, infectious mononucleosis and HL should be placed high in the differential diagnosis. Involvement of Waldeyer's ring, epitrochlear, and mesenteric nodes are more frequently observed in patients with NHL than in patients with HL. About 10% of all patients with NHL present with systemic complaints. B symptoms are more common in patients with aggressive histologies approaching 50%. Less frequent presenting symptoms, occurring in less than 20% of patients, include fatigue, malaise, and pruritus.

NHLs also present with thoracic, abdominal, and/or extranodal symptoms. Although much less common than with HL, approximately 20% of patients with NHL have mediastinal adenopathy. These patients most frequently present with persistent cough, chest discomfort, or without clinical symptoms but have an abnormal chest radiograph. Occasionally, a superior vena cava syndrome accompanies presentation. A differential diagnosis of mediastinal presentation includes infections (e.g., histoplasmosis, tuberculosis, infectious mononucleosis), sarcoidosis, HL, as well as other malignancies. Involvement of retroperitoneal, mesenteric, and pelvic nodes is common in most histologic subtypes of NHL. Unless massive or leading to obstruction, nodal enlargement in these sites often does not produce symptoms. In contrast, patients with an abdominal mass, massive splenomegaly, or primary gastrointestinal (GI) lymphoma present with complaints similar to those caused by other space-occupying lesions. These complaints include chronic pain, abdominal fullness, and early satiety, symptoms associated with visceral obstruction or even acute perforation and GI hemorrhage. Rarely, patients present with symptoms of unexplained anemia. Those with aggressive NHLs can present with primary cutaneous lesions, testicular masses, acute spinal cord compression, solitary bone lesions, and rarely, lymphomatous meningitis. Symptoms of primary NHL of the CNS include headache, lethargy, focal neurologic symptoms, seizures, and paralysis.

When NHL involves an extranodal site, the differential diagnosis is more difficult. NHL uncommonly presents in the lungs as bronchovascular, lymphangitic, nodular, or alveolar patterns of involvement.[48] Between 25% and 50% of patients with NHLs present with hepatic infiltration, although relatively few present with large hepatic masses. Of the advanced-stage indolent lymphomas, nearly 75% of patients have microscopic hepatic infiltration at presentation. In contrast, primary hepatic lymphoma is rare and is nearly always an aggressive histology. Primary lymphoma of bone is another uncommon extranodal site, occurring in less than 5% of patients and often presenting as bone pain. Most frequently, lytic lesions are observed on standard radiographs. The most common sites of primary lymphoma of bone include the femur, the pelvis, and the vertebrae. Approximately 5% of NHLs are primary GI lymphomas. These tumors are often associated with hemorrhage, pain, or obstruction. The stomach is most frequently involved, followed by the small intestine, and the colon. Most GI lymphomas are of the diffuse aggressive histologies, specifically DLBCL, mantle cell lymphoma (MCL), and intestinal T-cell lymphoma. The most common site for extranodal MZLs is the stomach. A subset of MCLs presents as multiple intestinal polyposis, which may arise at any site in the GI tract. An uncommon presentation (2% to 14%) of NHL is renal infiltration, and even less common is localized presentation in the prostate, testis, or ovary. The typical histologic subtypes of these sites are DLBCL, BL, and gray zone tumors with features intermediate between DLBCL and BL. Rare sites of primary lymphoma include the orbit, heart, breast, salivary glands, the thyroid, and the adrenal gland.

Diagnosis and Initial Management

After the initial biopsy, a careful history and physical exam should be done to help assess the extent and pace of disease. Attention should be paid to the duration of symptoms and pace of symptomatic progression, whether symptoms associated with a poorer prognosis, such as fevers, night sweats, or unexplained weight loss are present, and to localizing symptoms that may point toward lymphomatous involvement of specific sites, such as the chest, abdomen, or CNS. Concurrent illness that may impact therapy or monitoring on therapy should be ascertained, including a history of diabetes or congestive heart failure. A physical exam should pay close attention to all the peripherally accessible sites of lymph nodes; the liver and spleen size; Waldeyer's ring; whether there is a pleural or pericardial effusion or abdominal ascites; whether there is an abdominal, testicular or breast mass; and whether there is cutaneous involvement because all of these findings may influence further evaluation and disease management.

Laboratory studies should be obtained, including complete blood count, routine chemistries, liver function tests, and serum protein electrophoresis to document the presence of circulating monoclonal paraproteins. The serum beta-2 microglobulin level and serum lactate dehydrogenase (LDH) are important independent prognostic factors in NHL. A bone marrow biopsy should be considered for staging and prognostic purposes depending on the disease histology and the results of other laboratory and staging studies. An evaluation of the cerebrospinal fluid (CSF) for lymphomatous involvement may be indicated in the setting of concerning neurologic signs or symptoms or a disease that has a high propensity to spread to the CNS. The latter includes a disease involving the paranasal sinuses, testes, and epidural space, as well as highly aggressive histologies like BL.

Imaging studies depend on the histology of the lymphoma as well as the clinical presentation. Chest, abdominal, and pelvic computed tomography (CT) scans are essential for accurate staging to assess lymphadenopathy for indolent lymphomas. Radionuclide scans have clinical utility as diagnostic and monitoring studies. ^{67}Gallium scanning, used based on the ability of this isotope to bind transferrin receptors on tumor cells, has been replaced by positron-emission tomography (PET) using ^{18}F-fluorodeoxyglucose (FDG). FDG-PET scanning is highly sensitive for detecting both nodal and extranodal sites involved by NHL. PET scanning is particularly useful for the histologically aggressive lymphomas, including BL, DLBCL, plasmablastic lymphoma, and the aggressive T-cell lymphomas, but is less reliable in lower grade histologies like MZLs.[49] The intensity of FDG avidity, or standardized uptake value (SUV), correlates with histologic aggressiveness.[50,51] PET scanning detects an actively metabolizing tumor in residual masses following or during chemotherapy, and persistent abnormal uptake predicts for early relapse and/or reduced survival.[52] It is more accurate than the detection of a residual mass on CT scans, which can often be a false positive. Consensus recommendations regarding PET scanning were published as a result of an International Harmonization Project. Among the recommendations are that PET only be used for DLBCL and HL, scanning during therapy be only part of clinical trials, and the scan after all therapy is completed should be done at least 3 but preferably 6 to 8 weeks after chemotherapy and 8 to 12 weeks after radiation or chemoradiotherapy. There is no evidence that a long-term follow up should include PET scanning.[53] Finally, magnetic resonance imaging (MRI) is useful in detecting bone, bone marrow, and CNS disease in the brain and spinal cord.

Staging and Prognostic Systems

The Ann Arbor staging system developed in 1971 for HL was adapted for staging NHLs (Table 39.5).[54] This staging system focuses on the number of tumor sites (nodal and extranodal), the location, and the presence or absence of systemic, or B, symptoms. Table 39.5 summarizes the essential features of the Ann Arbor system.

The concept of staging has less impact in NHL than in HL. Only a minority of patients with both indolent and aggressive NHL have localized disease at diagnosis, and there is little therapeutic benefit to distinguish between stage III and stage IV disease because the treatment options are identical. The prognosis is more dependent on histology and clinical parameters than the stage at presentation. Staging in NHLs, therefore, is done to identify the minority of patients who can be treated with local therapy or combined modality treatment and to stratify within histologic subtypes to determine the prognosis and to assess the impact of treatment.

Probably more important than staging is the International Prognostic Index (IPI), which provides risk stratification (Table 39.6).[55] The IPI was developed based on an analysis of over 2,000 patients with diffuse aggressive NHLs treated with an anthracycline-containing regimen. This analysis identified age (≤60 years versus >60 years); serum LDH (≤ normal versus > normal); performance status (0 or 1 versus 2 to 4); stage (I or II versus III or IV); and extranodal involvement (≤ one site versus > one site) to be independently prognostic for overall survival. Four risk groups were identified based on the number of risk factors: low risk (0 or 1); low intermediate (2); high intermediate (3); and high (4 to 5). The 5-year overall survival rates for patients with scores of 0 to 1, 2, 3, and 4 to 5 were 73%, 51%, 43%, and 26%, respectively. For the patients aged 60 years or less, only stage, LDH, and performance status were of prognostic significance. Patients ≤60 years with zero, one, two, or three risk factors had 5-year survival rates of 83%, 69%, 46%, and 32%, respectively. Survival rates for those age >60 years with the same scores were 56%, 44%, 37%, and 21%, respectively. The IPI has been adapted following treatment with cyclophosphamide, adriamycin, vincristine, and prednisone plus rituximab (CHOP-R) therapy for DLBCL. Within that model, the 4-year progression-free survival is 94%, 80%, and 53% for zero and one, two, or three or more risk factors, respectively.[56]

A similar predictive model has been developed for follicular lymphoma based on the analysis of over 4,000 patients with follicular NHL, known as the follicular lymphoma IPI or FLIPI (Table 39.7).[57] This study identified the following prognostic

TABLE 39.6

International Prognostic Index (IPI)

Age >60 years

LDH > upper limit normal

ECOG Performance Status ≥2

Ann Arbor Stage III or IV

Number of extranodal disease sites >1

# of Factors	Risk Group	3-year EFS (%)	3-year PFS (%)	3-year OS (%)
0–1	Low	81	87	91
2	Low Intermediate	69	75	81
3	High Intermediate	53	59	65
4–5	High	50	50	59

ECOG, Eastern Cooperative Oncology Group; EFS, event-free survival; PFS, progression-free survival; OS, overall survival.
Adapted from Ziepert M, Hasenclever D, Kuhnt E, et al. Standard International Prognostic Index remains a valid predictor of outcome for patients with aggressive CD20+ B-cell lymphoma in the rituximab era. *J Clin Oncol* 2010;28:2373–2380.

TABLE 39.5

Ann Arbor Staging for Lymphoma

Stage	Description
I	Involvement of a single lymph node region (I) or single extranodal site (IE)
II	Involvement of two or more lymph node regions or lymphatic structures on the same side of the diaphragm alone (II) or with involvement of limited, contiguous, extralymphatic organ or tissue (IIE)
III	Involvement of lymph node regions on both sides of the diaphragm (III), which may include the spleen (IIIS), or limited, contiguous, extralymphatic organ or tissue (IIIE), or both (IIIES)
IV	Diffuse or disseminated foci of involvement of one or more extralymphatic organs or tissues, with or without associated lymphatic involvement

Note. All stages are further subdivided according to the absence (A) or presence (B) of systemic B symptoms including fevers, night sweats, and/or weight loss (>10% of body weight over 6 months prior to diagnosis).

TABLE 39.7

Follicular Lymphoma International Prognostic Index (FL-IPI)

Age >60 years

LDH > upper limit normal

Hgb <12 g/dL

Ann Arbor Stage III or IV

Number of involved nodal areas >4

# of Factors	Risk Group	5-year OS (%)	10-year OS (%)
0–1	Low	91	71
2	Intermediate	78	51
3–5	High	52	36

LDH, lactate dehydrogenase; Hgb, hemoglobin; OS, overall survival.
Adapted from Solal-Celigny P, Roy P, Colombat P, et al. Follicular lymphoma international prognostic index. *Blood* 2004;104:1258.

factors: age >60 years, stage III/IV, more than four nodal sites, elevated serum LDH concentration, and hemoglobin less than 12. The 10-year survival rates for patients with zero to one (low risk), two (intermediate risk), or three or more (high risk) of these adverse factors averaged 71%, 51%, and 36%, respectively. Similar disease-specific IPIs have been developed for mantle cell lymphoma and peripheral T-cell lymphoma as well. These prognostic indices take into account the proliferative index and cell surface markers, respectively.[58,59]

More recently, as discussed in the section on the 2008 update to the WHO, GEP has been used to examine DLBCL to identify patients with different prognoses.[46] Based on gene expression, DLBCLs have been subclassified into GCB or ABC types. Patients with GCB-like DLBCL had significantly better overall survival than those with the ABC-like variant. Based on findings from GEP, immunohistochemical staining of a limited number of proteins has been proposed as an alternative method for subtyping of DLBCL and prognostication.[60] Germinal center and nongerminal center B-cell derivation can be determined by the expression of markers such as CD10, B cell lymphoma–6 protein (BCL-6), and multiple myeloma oncogene 1 (MUM1). Based on immunohistochemistry, it is estimated that approximately 40% of DLBCLs are of the GCB subtype, with the remainder falling into the non-GCB group.

Restaging after treatment is typically done 6 to 8 weeks following the completion of chemotherapy (or chemoimmunotherapy), or 8 to 12 weeks after the completion of radiotherapy or combination chemotherapy and radiotherapy, to assess for disease response to treatment. The most important prognostic factor is the achievement of a complete response to therapy. Restaging at the completion of treatment is often with the repetition of studies that were abnormal at diagnosis. It should be noted that patients with certain lymphomas or bulky disease may not have complete regression of their lymphadenopathy despite there not being any remaining active lymphoma. Nuclear studies, like PET/CT scans, and/or rebiopsy can be helpful in differentiating residual fibrotic tissue from active lymphoma.

SPECIFIC DISEASE ENTITIES

Precursor B-Cell and T-Cell Leukemia/Lymphoma

Lymphoblastic lymphoma and acute lymphoblastic leukemia appear to be different manifestations of the same disease entity (see Chapter 46). Cytologically, both are composed of blasts with a high nuclear-to-cytoplasmic ratio, scant cytoplasm, and nuclei with slightly coarse chromatin with multiple small nucleoli. The nuclei may be oval, but more often are folded or convoluted. The blasts are usually intermediate in size, but they may be large, or in unusual cases, so small that there may be confusion morphologically with CLL. When lymph nodes are involved, they are diffusely effaced by blasts. Mitotic figures are usually frequent, and (as with all high-grade lymphomas) some cases contain frequent tingible body macrophages, producing a starry-sky appearance that mimics BL.

Approximately 85% to 90% of lymphoblastic lymphomas are of the T-cell lineage, with the remainder being of the B-cell type. Both are comprised of tumor cells with immunophenotypes that correspond to stages of pre-T and pre-B–cell development, respectively. B-lymphoblastic tumors express CD19 and are variably positive for other B lineage markers and negative in most cases for surface immunoglobulin. T lymphoblastic tumors usually express cytoplasmic CD3 but may be surface CD3 negative, and show variable expression of other T-cell markers. Most lymphoblastic tumors are positive for TdT, a specific marker of immature lymphoid cells that can be detected by flow cytometry or immunohistochemistry.

Although lymphoblastic lymphomas represent a major subgroup of childhood NHLs, they are unusual in adults (2% of adult NHLs). Patients are usually adolescent or young adult males who present with lymphadenopathy in cervical, supraclavicular, and axillary regions (50%) or with a mediastinal mass (50% to 75%). These masses can be associated with superior vena cava syndrome, tracheal obstruction, and pericardial effusions. Less commonly, patients present with extranodal disease (skin, testicular, or bony involvement). More than 80% of patients present with stage III or stage IV disease, almost 50% have B symptoms, and the majority has an elevated LDH. Although the bone marrow can be uninvolved at presentation, virtually all patients develop bone marrow infiltration and a subsequent leukemic phase indistinguishable from T-cell acute lymphoblastic leukemia. Patients with bone marrow involvement have a very high incidence of CNS infiltration. B-cell lymphoblastic lymphoma is a very rare entity, with patients having a median age of 39 years.[61] B-cell lymphoblastic lymphomas present without a mediastinal mass but instead involve lymph nodes and extranodal sites.

The treatment of precursor B-cell and T-cell lymphoblastic leukemia/lymphoma is detailed in Chapter 46.

Follicular Lymphoma

Introduction

FL is the second most common lymphoma diagnosed in the United States and western Europe, making up approximately 20% of all NHLs, and 70% of indolent lymphomas.[62] The median age at diagnosis is 60 years, and there is a slight female predominance.[63,64] The incidence is increased among relatives of persons with FL.[65]

Pathology

FLs are malignant counterparts of normal germinal center B cells.[44] FL recapitulates the architecture of normal germinal centers (GC) of secondary lymphoid follicles.[44] The neoplastic cells consist of a mixture of centrocytes (small- to medium-sized cells with irregular or cleaved nuclei and scant cytoplasm) and centroblast (large cells with oval nuclei, several nucleoli, and moderate amounts of cytoplasm). The clinical aggressiveness of the tumor correlates with the number of centroblasts that are present. The WHO classification[44] adopted grading from 1 to 3 based on the number of centroblasts counted per high power field (hpf): Grade I, 0 to 5 centroblasts/hpf; Grade II, 6 to 15 centroblasts/hpf; Grade III, more than 15 centroblasts/hpf. Grade III has been subdivided into grade IIIa, in which centrocytes predominate, and grade IIIb, in which there are sheets of centroblasts.[66] Although the grading system remains in place, clinically, grade I and II and many cases of grade IIIa FLs are approached similarly. Akin to normal GCs, small numbers of T cells and follicular dendritic cells are present in the malignant follicles; however, tingible body macrophages, cells that have ingested apoptotic cells that are common in reactive GCs, are not observed. Involvement of the peripheral blood with malignant cells is commonly seen, and morphologically, these cells have notches and have been referred to as *buttock cells*. FL grade IIIb is an aggressive disease grouped with diffuse large B-cell lymphoma. Bone marrow involvement is exceedingly common in FL patients, usually taking the form of paratrabecular lymphoid aggregates.[44]

Immunophenotype and Genetics

FL cells express monoclonal immunoglobulin light chain, CD19, CD20, CD10, and BCL6 and are negative for CD5 and CD23. In virtually all cases, FL cells overexpress BCL-2. Clonal Ig gene rearrangements are present and, in most cases, the Ig loci have extensive somatic mutations, further supporting a GC origin. Approximately 85% of FLs have the t(14;18), which drives overexpression of BCL-2, a member of a family of proteins that blocks apoptosis. However, multiple genetic events are required for the development of FL, because the t(14;18) can be identified in a small fraction of normal B cells in most normal children and adults. Deep sequencing studies have established that the most common mutations in FL (90% of tumors) involve mixed-lineage leukemia 2 protein (MLL2), a gene encoding a histone H3 methylase.[67,68] Less common recurrent mutations involve other genes involving epigenetic modifying genes, such as EZH2, CREBBP, and EP300, indicating that genetically determined alterations in the epigenome contribute to FL in ways that remain to be defined. Other recent studies suggest that reactive cells within the malignant microenvironment also contribute to the pathobiology of FL, based on evidence that immune signatures of T cell and macrophage infiltration defined by gene expression profiling are predictive of outcome.[69]

Clinical Features

Patients with FL generally present with asymptomatic lymphadenopathy, which often waxes and wanes over the course of years. Bone marrow involvement is present in 70% of patients, whereas involvement of other nonlymphoid organs is uncommon. Less than 20% of patients present with B symptoms or an increased serum LDH. In a small subset of patients, the disease presents in the intestine; such patients usually have an early stage and a favorable prognosis.[70] Histologic transformation of FL to DLBCL occurs in 10% to 70% of patients over time, with a risk of about 2% to 3% per year[71–73] and is associated with the rapid progression of lymphadenopathy, extranodal disease (besides the marrow), B symptoms, elevated serum LDH, and calcium.

Prognosis

Measures of outcome include the FLIPI (see Table 39.7) and tumor grade.[74] A modified version of this score, the FLIPI2, evaluated five parameters, with some overlap of the FLIPI.[75] The utility of the FLIPI2 model remains uncertain. Since the incorporation of rituximab into the mainstream therapy of FL, the FLIPI has continued to be a useful prognostic model.[76]

FL tumors are graded from 1 to 3 and this grade has some prognostic utility. There has generally been suboptimal consensus of pathologists on grading FL. There is no evidence to support a different treatment approach between grade I and grade II FL. Differences in molecular genetics as well as clinical behavior suggest that FL grade IIIa is more commonly an indolent disease, whereas grade IIIb is an aggressive disease.[44,77]

The investigation of the cellular microenvironment of FL has provided interesting insights into prognosis.[78–87] It has been suggested that FL is an immunologically functional disease in which an interaction between the tumor cells and the microenvironment modulates clinical behavior. These studies, which have observed an impact on the prognosis of reactive macrophages and T cells, need additional study in larger data sets and a prospective design with uniformly treated patient populations.

Treatment of Early Stage Disease

Less than 10% of patients with FL have stage I/II disease.[88] Radiation therapy is the treatment of choice for limited stage FL and results in a 5-, 10-, and 15-year freedom from treatment failure of 72%, 46%, and 39%, and an overall 5-, 10-, and 15-year survival rates of 93%, 75%, and 62%, respectively, with a median survival of approximately 19 years.[89] A dose of 24 to 30 Gy appears to be highly effective, with no evidence of benefit for higher doses.[90] However, most patients with stage I disease treated in the United States do not receive radiation therapy.[88] This is surprising given a large study of over 6,000 patients with stage I or stage II FL diagnosed from 1973 to 2004, 34% of whom were initially treated with RT, where patients who received initial radiation therapy (RT) had higher rates of disease-specific survival at 5 years (90% versus 81%), 10 years (79% versus 66%), 15 years (68% versus 57%), and 20 years (63% versus 51%).[91]

In pre-rituximab era studies, adjuvant chemotherapy probably does not add additional benefit after local RT.[92] A recent retrospective analysis suggested an improved progression-free survival (PFS) outcome with chemoimmunotherapy or systemic therapy plus RT as compared to RT alone, with no impact on overall survival (OS).[93] This will require additional study. If significant morbidity is possible from RT based on the location of the disease area or if the patient chooses to not receive RT, observation may be a reasonable alternative, especially for stage II patients.[94] In this report, the median OS of selected untreated patients was 19 years. At a median follow-up of 7 years, 63% of patients had not required treatment.

Treatment of Advanced Stage Disease

The overwhelming majority of patients have advanced stage disease at diagnosis. Patients with asymptomatic FL do not require immediate treatment unless they have symptomatic nodal disease, compromised end organ function, B symptoms, symptomatic extranodal disease, or cytopenias. This approach is supported by randomized prospective trials of observation versus immediate treatment. One of the largest trials compared immediate treatment with chlorambucil to observation.[95] At a median follow-up of 16 years, no difference in OS and cause-specific survival was seen between the two approaches. Similar results have been noted in other prospective trials of initial treatment versus observation.[96]

A major question is whether rituximab might change this approach in early treatment in asymptomatic patients. A retrospective analysis of good risk patients who were either observed or received single-agent rituximab[97] found no negative impact of watchful waiting. A prospective study compared observation to rituximab alone or rituximab followed by maintenance in previously untreated FL. The median time to next treatment was 34 months in the watch and wait patient but was not reached in the rituximab-treatment arm. The 3-year PFS was 33%, 80%, and 90% of the observed, rituximab, or rituximab followed by maintenance patients, respectively, with 95% OS in all three groups. The important issues of time to second therapy, quality of life, impact on histologic transformation, cost, toxicity, and future responses to rituximab are not yet addressed.[98]

Rituximab has changed the paradigm of treating FL. The recent improvement in survival of patients with FL is largely due to the use of anti-CD20 monoclonal antibody-based therapy.[99] The benefit of adding rituximab to combination chemotherapy for the initial treatment has been demonstrated in multiple randomized trials of chemotherapy with or without rituximab (see Table 39.2).[100,101] All of these trials have demonstrated improved response rates and time to progression in the rituximab plus chemotherapy arms, as well as improvement in OS. FDG-PET scanning has been employed to evaluate responses to CHOP-R in previously untreated patients. PET scanning was predictive when performed after four cycles and at the end of therapy. The 2-year PFS was significantly higher for PET-negative than PET-positive patients when employed as an interim or end of therapy scan. The 2-year OS was also significantly higher for PET-negative than PET-positive patients. This will require further study but may change management in the future.[105]

Other chemotherapy drugs plus rituximab have also been used for the initial therapy of FL. Bendamustine plus rituximab (BR) has been compared to CHOP-R in a randomized phase III trial with bendamustine (90 mg/m^2 days 1 and 2) plus rituximab (375 mg/m^2 day 1) in 513 patients with advanced follicular, marginal zone, lymphoplasmacytic, and mantle cell lymphoma.[106] In this study, a superior median PFS in favor of BR versus CHOP-R was seen (69.5 versus 31.2 months) at 45 months. Moreover with BR, less toxicity, including lower rates of grade 3 and 4 neutropenia and leukopenia were observed. There was no difference in OS at a median follow-up of 45 months. Intensifying the schedule of CHOP-R from every 21 to every 14 days was also of no benefit.[107] Fludarabine plus rituximab[108] and fludarabine, mitoxantrone, dexamethasone, and rituximab[109] both showed response rates of over 90% in previously untreated patients. However, significant neutropenia and opportunistic infections were observed with these regimens. A randomized phase III trial compared three regimens in previously untreated stage II to IV FL patients: CHOP-R; cyclophosphamide, vincristine, prednisone, and rituximab (CVP-R); or rituximab, fludarabine, and mitoxantrone (R-FM). Both R-FM and CHOP-R were superior to CVP-R in 3-year PFS and time to treatment failure (TTF), but there was no difference in OS.[110] The current impact of this study is uncertain given the favorable results and lower toxicity seen with BR.

Rituximab alone has been used as the first therapy in patients with FL, with overall response rates of around 70% and complete response (CR) rates of over 30% reported.[111–113] The most favorable data of single-agent rituximab is the recent update of the swiss group for clinical cancer research (SAKK) trial.[114] Patients received four weekly doses, and then patients with stable disease or better were randomized to observation or four doses of maintenance therapy, one dose every 2 months. In this study, 202 patients with previously untreated or relapsed/refractory FL administered four weekly doses of single-agent rituximab has been reported. The 151 patients with responding or stable disease at week 12 were randomized to no further treatment or prolonged rituximab maintenance every 2 months for four doses. At a median follow-up of 35 months, patients who received the prolonged rituximab maintenance had a twofold increase in event-free-survival (23 months versus 12 months). With a longer follow-up, 45% of newly diagnosed patients in this study were in remission at 8 years with the addition of maintenance rituximab.

Maintenance rituximab has also been shown to benefit patients who received chemotherapy without rituximab as part of the initial treatment. A randomized trial of maintenance rituximab versus observation after CVP with the majority having FL, reported that patients who received maintenance rituximab had improved rates of 3-year PFS (68% versus 33%). Survival rates were similar between the two groups.[115] With the current paradigm of treating patients with concurrent chemotherapy plus rituximab, this study has less applicability.

The use of maintenance rituximab after chemoimmunotherapy in patients with FL has been examined in a large randomized trial.[116] Although maintenance rituximab appears to improve PFS rates, toxicities, albeit tolerable, are increased and the effect on OS is, to date, unclear. The Primary Rituximab and Maintenance (PRIMA) phase III intergroup trial randomly assigned 1,018 patients with previously untreated FL that responded to chemoimmunotherapy (CVP-R, CHOP-R, or fludarabine, cyclophosphamide, mitoxantrone, and rituximab [FCM-R]) maintenance with rituximab (375 mg/m^2 every 8 weeks for 24 months) or placebo.[116] At a median follow-up of 36 months from randomization, patients assigned to rituximab maintenance had a higher rate of PFS (75% versus 58%). A higher percentage of patients in complete response/complete response, unconfirmed (CRu) at 24 months (72% versus 52%) was also seen 2 years postrandomization in patients receiving maintenance rituximab. There was a significantly higher percentage of grade III/IV adverse events and infections in the rituximab maintenance group. At this time, OS is the same in both groups.

Radioimmunotherapy alone has been used as the initial treatment in a limited number of patients with FL. ^{131}I-tositumomab was given to 76 previously untreated patients with FL leading to overall and complete response rates of 95% and 75%, respectively, and, at 5-years, OS and PFS rates of 89% and 59%, respectively.[117] [131]I tositumomab is no longer commercially available. [90]Yttrium ([90]Yi)-ibritumomab tiuxetan has also been studied as sole initial therapy with excellent results with limited follow-up.[118]

Radioimmunotherapy has also been used as consolidation following conventional chemotherapy induction in patients with FL. Both [90]Yi-ibritumomab tiuxetan and ^{131}I-tositumomab have been studied. This approach has been associated with very high response rates, conversions of partial response (PR) to CR, and well-maintained responses.[119–121] A phase III trial compared [90]Yi-ibritumomab tiuxetan to observation following a CR or PR to induction chemotherapy for treatment-naïve patients with FL.[122] Of note, the majority of patients did not receive rituximab along with the induction chemotherapy. At 8 years, both the PR and CR patients who received [90]Yi-ibritumomab tiuxetan had significantly longer median PFS with improvement of about 36 months. In contrast to this study, a randomized trial of CHOP plus rituximab to CHOP followed by ^{131}I-tositumomab did not see any differences in PFS between the two arms.[123]

High-dose therapy and autologous stem cell transplantation (ASCT) has been used to consolidate first remission for patients with FL. These studies generally preceded the widespread use of rituximab. With ASCT in first remission, about 50% of patients are disease free at 10 years and beyond following ASCT, but an increased risk of second malignancies, including myelodysplastic syndrome (MDS), acute myelogenous leukemia (AML), and solid tumors, has been observed with long follow ups of these patients. Several randomized trials have examined the role of ASCT in previously untreated patients with FL following an induction therapy.[124–129] The majority of these studies have demonstrated a significant improvement in PFS, but no impact on OS.[130] One reason for the lack of impact on OS has been the excess number of second malignancies.

Although allogeneic stem cell transplantation (alloSCT) can potentially lead to a cure for patients with FL due to the significant treatment related mortality, this is largely reserved for patients with relapsed and more refractory disease.

Treatment of Relapsed FL

When patients with relapsed FL require treatment, there are many options, ranging from rituximab alone to combination chemotherapy plus rituximab, radioimmunotherapy, and for selected patients, stem cell transplantation.

A recent update of single-agent rituximab therapy in patients with relapsed FL is from the randomized SAKK trial.[114] With a long follow-up, 35% of responders remain in remission at 8 years. However, in the context of current induction therapy that includes chemotherapy and rituximab in the majority of patients, it is uncertain if the response data to single-agent rituximab is as high or durable as in patients who received chemotherapy without rituximab as induction therapy. There is a evidence, however, that retreatment with rituximab in patients with relapsed, largely FL, who had previously responded to rituximab had a response rate of 40% with a median time to progression of 18 months following retreatment.[131]

The combination of chemotherapy and rituximab has enhanced the efficacy of treatment of relapsed FL. Probably the largest study treated selected patients with relapsed FL who were previously not treated with an anthracycline- or rituximab-containing regimen.[132] Patients were randomized to CHOP or CHOP-R and responding patients were randomized to 2 years of maintenance rituximab or observation. The overall and CR rates were significantly improved in the CHOP-R group, and the median PFS was improved by approximately 12 months. An update of this study with a median follow-up of 6 years reported that maintenance rituximab also improved median PFS by 2.4 years. The OS at 5 years following maintenance was 74% versus 64% with observation alone. Given the current paradigm of chemoimmunotherapy and maintenance, the applicability of these data to presently treated patients is uncertain.

Another regimen in which a benefit for the addition of rituximab was seen for relapsed disease in a randomized trial employing FCM.[133] A number of phase 2 trials of other agents plus rituximab associated with quite high response rates included BR with 90% response rate (RR) and median PFS of 2 years.[134–136] Single-agent bendamustine has an overall RR of 77% with a median response duration of 6.7 months.[134] With more widespread use of BR as initial therapy, BR will be employed less for recurrent disease. The regimen FCR has a similarly high response rate but with significant myelosuppression.[137] Phase 2 studies employing bortezomib and rituximab and bortezomib, rituximab, and bendamustine have reported RRs of approximately 50% and 93%, respectively.[138,139]

The anti-CD20 radioimmunotherapy agents have been employed for treatment of patients with relapsed and refractory FL.[140] The RRs in this patient population are similar with both agents, with 60% to 80% of patients responding. The median PFS is about 12 months, although the approximately 20% to 37% of patients who achieve a CR have a median time to progression of approximately 4 years.[141,142] A randomized trial compared single-agent rituximab to [90]Yi-ibritumomab in patients with relapsed indolent (predominantly FL).[143] The overall and CR rates were significantly higher with radioimmunotherapy (RIT), but no difference in time to progression or OS was observed. Retreatment with these agents remains controversial, with uncertainty of delivery of full dose and concerns of second malignancies.[144]

FL is extremely responsive to RT; low-dose RT (e.g., total dose of 4 Gy, given as two consecutive daily 2-Gy fractions) can be used for the palliation of patients who have symptoms related to a single disease site, with CR rates of 57% and overall RRs of 82%.[145] Patients who go into CR have long, durable local control rates. There are no significant side effects of treatment, even in the head and neck region where higher doses would cause xerostomia and mucositis.

The use of either ASCT or alloSCT in FL is controversial and the subject of numerous clinical trials.[146] A large number of phase 2 studies prior to the availability of rituximab, involving high-dose therapy and autologous hematopoietic stem cell transplantation (HCT) have shown that approximately 40% of patients with good performance status and chemosensitive relapsed disease may experience prolonged PFS and OS.[147–151] Prior to the widespread use of rituximab for in vivo purging, many strategies were taken to render the autologous stem cell collections free of lymphoma cells. Although single institution studies suggested that reinfusion of tumor-free stem cells led to a decreased relapse rate, it remains controversial as to whether there is a benefit, particularly now with rituximab treatment. The only phase 3 randomized trial (the chemotherapy, unpurged stem cell transplantation, purged stem cell transplantation [CUP] trial) comparing ASCT to conventional chemotherapy in relapsed FL patients demonstrated a higher PFS and OS for ASCT, and no benefit for purging the stem cell graft.[152] A retrospective analysis of patients undergoing ASCT following rituximab-based salvage therapy did not suggest a benefit of ASCT as compared to conventional therapy. Unfortunately, as has been seen in ASCT in first remission, second malignancies—both solid tumors and MDS and AML—are reported following ASCT.

Phase 2 studies have looked at the use of in vivo purging pre-ASCT and maintenance therapy with rituximab following ASCT in patients with relapsed FL. These suggest an improvement in PFS, similar to what has been seen following conventional chemotherapy and chemoimmunotherapy. A phase 3 trial in patients with relapsed FL has investigated the inclusion of rituximab for in vivo purging pre-ASCT and 2 years of maintenance post-ASCT.[153] There was an improvement in PFS for patients receiving rituximab for in vivo purging, maintenance, and the combination of both as compared to no rituximab, but no OS benefit.

AlloSCT has been investigated in patients with relapsed FL. Both myeloablative and reduced intensity conditioning (RIC) approaches have been employed. Unfortunately, myeloablative conditioning has a treatment related mortality of up to 40%; however, the relapse rate is less than 20%.[154] There is enthusiasm for RIC alloSCT because it has lower treatment-related mortality,[155–157] but some reports suggest that the relapse rate may be higher than conventional myeloablative conditioning. The role of alloSCT versus ASCT for FL remains uncertain. A recent National Comprehensive Cancer Network (NCCN) database retrospective analysis found significantly higher 3-year OS for ASCT versus alloSCT (87% versus 61%).[158] Certainly, for younger patients with more resistant disease, alloSCT remains a potentially curative option for relapsed FL.

Histologic Transformation

Part of the natural history of any indolent B-cell NHLs is progression to a higher grade histologic subtype, most commonly DLBCL, but much less commonly, BL or even HL can be seen.[71,159] Histologic transformation (HT) is most commonly seen in FL, but is also seen in patients with MZL, lymphoplasmacytic lymphoma, and small lymphocytic lymphoma/CLL (where this is referred to as a Richter transformation), and a biopsy is critical in order to demonstrate transformation. HT occurs at a rate of approximately 2% to 3% per year.[72] The clinical presentation of HT includes rapid growing masses, extranodal disease, B symptoms, hypercalcemia, and elevated serum LDH. *TP53* mutations and translocations or amplifications of *MYC* are the most common genetic abnormalities seen in HT.

Historically, HT to DLBCL has been associated with a very poor prognosis. In a series from Stanford, previously untreated patients and patients with limited disease and no prior therapy at transformation had improved prognoses.[160] Although the median survival for all patients with transformation was only 22 months, those who achieved a CR to combination chemotherapy had an actuarial survival of 75% at 5 years. More recent studies suggest that CHOP-R may improve OS for patients with transformed disease. Patients who have not previously received an anthracycline-containing regimen should be treated with CHOP-R and, assuming a CR is obtained, monitored. For previously treated patients, high-dose therapy and ASCT should be considered assuming the patient has chemosensitive disease. Patients with histologic transformation can have later relapses with indolent lymphoma.

Newer Agents

There are a multitude of new approaches that have been studied in patients with FL. This includes monoclonal antibodies, idiotype vaccines, immunomodulatory agents, and novel drugs such as kinase inhibitors.

Monoclonal antibodies directed against other B-cell–associated antigens as well as new anti-CD20 monoclonal antibodies (mAb) are being investigated in FL. These have included anti-CD80,[161,162] anti-CD22 mAbs,[163,164] and anti-CD40.[165] Several new anti-CD20 monoclonal antibodies are being evaluated in patients with FL who are refractory to rituximab. These include several humanized antibodies that are designed to have less infusion toxicity and a better antibody-dependent cell-mediated cytotoxicity effector function.[166–168] The other mAb of interest is obinutuzumab, the first type II, glycoengineered, and humanized monoclonal anti-CD20 antibody.[169] In rituximab-refractory patients in the high-dose cohort, the RR was 55% with a median PFS of 11.9 months. Studies of obinutuzumab in combination with chemotherapy have shown 93% to 98% RRs in relapsed and refractory FL patients.[170]

A number of immunostimulatory agents have been studied to enhance the activity of rituximab. These include cytokines such as IL-2 and immunostimulatory DNA sequences known as CpGs.[171] To date, although having immunomodulatory effects, the impact on enhancing the therapeutic effect of rituximab has been limited. A phase 2 study of lenalidomide plus rituximab has reported high RRS, but a phase 3 study will be needed to demonstrate superiority over rituximab alone.[172]

The other area of interest has been in active immunization, focusing largely on the idiotype protein as the antigen. To date, there have been three randomized studies employing idiotype proteins coupled to a protein called keyhole limpet hemocyanin (KLH) following the induction of remission in patients with FL. The Favrille trial used rituximab for induction therapy. The median time to progression (TTP) was 9 months for the idiotype-KLH (Id-KLH) vaccinated patients and 12.6 months in the control group (p = 0.019).[173] However, this difference was attributed to more patients with high-risk FLIPI scores in the Id-KLH arm. The Biovax study reported showing a 14-month improvement in PFS for the Id-KLH vaccinated patients as compared to control; however, the induction chemotherapy was intense and remissions had to be sustained for 12 months prior to the initiation of vaccination.[174] The trial using the MyVax Id-KLH conjugate following CVP chemotherapy failed to show any PFS advantage. Based on these studies, it is unlikely at the present time that idiotype vaccinations will be pursued in FL.

B-cell kinases are logical targets for therapy in FL. To date, three kinase inhibitors, idelalisib, ibrutinib, and fostamatinib, which target the phosphoinositide 3-kinase (PI3k) p110δ, Bruton's tyrosine kinase (BTK), and spleen tyrosine kinase (SYK), respectively, have been tested. In relapsed and refractory FL patients, the response rates to idelalisib,[175] ibrutinib,[176] and fostamatinib[177] were 62% (including other indolent NHLs besides FL), 27%, and 10%, respectively. These agents are undergoing additional study, in combination with chemotherapy and as maintenance following remission induction, to better define their role.

Follicular Lymphoma Grade III

FL grade III has been historically referred to as follicular large cell lymphoma. It is histologically defined by the presence of more than 15 centroblasts per hpf. It is further subdivided into grade IIIa, where centrocytes are present, and grade IIIb, where there are sheets of centroblasts. These are further differentiated by the presence of BCL6 rearrangements in a high fraction of grade IIIb cases. Because many studies likely include both grade IIIa and IIIB, this heterogeneity may affect an interpretation of the outcomes. Although the follicular architecture is intact, the clinical presentation, behavior, and outcome with treatment in many patients with FL grade IIIb more closely approximates that of DLBCL.[178–180] In contrast to DLBCL, the relapse rate of FL grade IIIb is higher in some series, but survival is longer.[181] A recent series suggested similar outcomes of grade IIIa and IIIB cases and no benefit for the inclusion of anthracyclines in the treatment regimen.[182]

Small Lymphocytic Lymphoma/B-Cell Chronic Lymphocytic Leukemia

Introduction

Small lymphocytic lymphoma (SLL) is a mature (peripheral) B-cell malignancy. It is synonymous with CLL. The malignant cells in SLL and CLL are morphologically, immunophenotypically, and genetically identical. The difference between these two diagnoses is the clinical presentation, with a nonleukemic presentation in SLL. The diagnosis is made by an examination of involved tissue, such as the lymph node or bone marrow.

SLL represents less than 5% of all NHLs. CLL/SLL comprises 90% of chronic lymphocytic leukemias in Western countries. Less than 10% of patients present with only nodal involvement (i.e., SLL). However, most patients with SLL at presentation ultimately develop bone marrow and blood infiltration. The median age at diagnosis is 65 years.[63] At least 80% have stage IV disease due to bone marrow involvement at diagnosis.

Pathology

The cells within lymphoid tissues in CLL/SLL are small lymphocytes with condensed chromatin, round nuclei, and occasionally, a small nucleolus.[44] Larger lymphoid cells with prominent nucleoli and dispersed chromatin are also seen. These larger lymphoid cells are usually clustered together in so-called proliferation centers, which are pathognomonic. Roughly 60% of SLL/CLLs have Ig genes that show evidence of *significant* somatic mutation, defined as a rearranged Ig heavy-chain gene with a sequence that differs from germ-line position at 2% or more of the Ig V region nucleotides, which is taken as evidence of origin from an antigen-stimulated B cell.[183]

Immunophenotype and Genetics

SLL/CLL cells express low-level monoclonal surface Ig, usually IgM or IgM and IgD. They also express human leukocyte antigen-DR (HLA-DR) and the B-cell antigens CD19, CD20, and CD23, and are characteristically CD5 positive. About 40% of cases express CD38. Expression of the tyrosine kinase ZAP70 is also observed in a subset of cases and correlates with a more aggressive clinical course.[184]

Immunoglobulin genes are clonally rearranged, with IgV region somatic mutations in up to 60% of patients. Cytogenetic abnormalities include trisomy 12, which is present in about 40% of cases, as well as 13q deletions (45% to 55% of cases), 11q deletions (17% to 20% of cases), and 17p deletions (7% to 10% of cases). Cases with 13q deletions have the most favorable prognosis, whereas those with del(11q) or del(17p) have an unfavorable prognosis.[185] The t(11;14) involving the cyclin D1 (CCDN1) gene has been described, but many of these cases are believed to be leukemic variants of mantle cell lymphoma. Deep sequencing studies of CLL have revealed a number of recurrent mutations, the most common of which involve the NOTCH1, MYD88, and SF3B1 genes.[186]

Clinical Presentation

Most patients with SLL present with painless generalized lymphadenopathy, which has frequently been present for several years. B symptoms are rare. Hepatosplenomegaly is present in less than 50% of patients. The peripheral blood in patients with SLL may be normal or reveal only a mild lymphocytosis; by definition, patients with SLL have an absolute lymphocyte count of $<5,000/\mu L$ at the time of diagnosis. A serum paraprotein is found in about 20% of cases, and hypogammaglobulinemia is present in about 40%. Both CLL and SLL patients may develop autoimmune hemolytic anemia, pure red cell aplasia, and autoimmune thrombocytopenia. Elevated serum LDH is uncommon, whereas increased levels of serum beta-2 microglobulin are more frequently seen and can be a marker of disease burden. SLL/CLL can transform to DLBCL (Richter syndrome), an event that is associated with a short survival.[187] These patients present with rapidly growing masses, elevated serum LDH, and B symptoms. Rarely, transformation can be to B-cell prolymphocytic leukemia (B-PLL), which is characterized by high white cell counts and splenomegaly. It also has a poor prognosis.

Treatment of Small Lymphocytic Lymphoma

Patients with stage I SLL should be treated with involved field radiation, and not combined modality therapy or chemotherapy alone. In one limited series of 14 patients with stage I or II disease treated with 40 to 44 Gy, the 10-year freedom from relapse rates were 80% and 62% for stage I and stage II disease, respectively. Generally, patients with stage II or more advanced SLL are treated with chemotherapy regimens used for CLL (see Chapter 46). For patients with advanced stage disease who do not need systemic therapy but have one site causing symptoms, low-dose radiation (200 cGy for two fractions) can provide reasonable palliation, although the local control rates are not as high as seen with FL.[145]

Lymphoplasmacytic Lymphoma

Lymphoplasmacytic lymphoma represents about 1% of all NHLs. In some cases, patients present with mixed cryoglobulinemia, possibly related to concurrent hepatitis C virus infection.[188,189]

Pathology

Lymphoplasmacytic lymphoma is an indolent lymphoma composed of a diffuse proliferation comprised of a mixture of small lymphocytes, lymphoplasmacytic cells, and plasma cells.[190] Immunoglobulin inclusions in the cytoplasm (Russell bodies) or invaginating into the nucleus (Dutcher bodies) are commonly seen. Unlike multiple myeloma, amyloidosis is rare. Occasional cases may also contain frequent larger immunoblast-like cells.

Immunophenotype and Genetics

Monoclonal cytoplasmic immunoglobulin is seen within the plasmacytoid cells and plasma cells by immunohistochemistry. The admixed lymphoid cells express B-cell antigens CD19, CD20, and surface IgM, and in general, do not express CD10 or CD23. A minor subset of cases is positive for CD5. Waldenström macroglobulinemia is an entity caused by high levels of monoclonal IgM that is generally associated with lymphoplasmacytic lymphoma (LPL). Deletions of 6q21 have been identified in 40% to 60% of patients with Waldenström macroglobulinemia. Activating mutations in MYD88, an adaptor protein that appears to function in signaling pathways downstream of the Ig receptor that lead to activation of the transcription factor nuclear factor kappa B (NF-κB) activation, are highly associated with LPL, being present in close to 100% of cases. However, mutations of MYD88 are not specific for LPL, because they are also seen less commonly in DLBCL and other low-grade B-cell NHLs.

Clinical Presentation

Clinically, this disease is similar to small lymphocytic lymphoma. The median age is early 60s, and nearly all patients have stage IV disease by virtue of bone marrow involvement. B symptoms and elevated serum LDH are uncommon. Lymph node and splenic involvement are common. In the WHO clinical study, 5-year OS (58%) and failure-free survival (25%) were similar to SLL.

Treatment

At least 25% of patients with LPL/waldenstrom's macroglobulinemia (WM) have no indications for therapy at initial presentation. The indications for treatment include constitutional symptoms, cytopenias, or less commonly, symptomatic lymphadenopathy or splenomegaly. Other reasons for treatment are hyperviscosity related to the elevated serum IgM and paraneoplastic neuropathy.

Analogous to other indolent B-cell NHLs, rituximab plays a significant role in the therapy of LPL. Single-agent rituximab is indicated for minimally symptomatic patients. Approximately half of patients will have a partial response to single-agent rituximab.[191] One can see transient increases in serum IgM levels after rituximab that can cause or exacerbate hyperviscosity.

Chemoimmunotherapy has largely replaced single agents for the treatment of LPL. Commonly used regimens include: dexamethasone, rituximab, cyclophosphamide (DRC)[192]; bortezomib plus rituximab with or without dexamethasone (BRD)[193]; or thalidomide plus rituximab.[194] The latter two have limitations due to neuropathy. For DRC, the overall and complete response rates were 83% and 7%, respectively, and 2-year OS and PFS rates were 81% and 67%, respectively. Bortezomib and rituximab and thalidomide-rituximab have similar response rates. Alkylating agents, including chlorambucil and bendamustine, have RRs in excess of 80%. Purine analogs are active agents; however, stem cell toxicity can be an issue with purine analogs as well as chlorambucil.[195] For recurrent disease, one can often utilize agents that were previously used. For patients with more refractory LPL, the mammalian target of rapamycin (mTOR) inhibitor everolimus, anti-CD52 mAb, and the oral Bruton's tyrosine-kinase inhibitor, ibrutinib, are active. Selected patients with relapsed disease are considered for high-dose therapy with ASCT or alloSCT. The results seen are similar to that of other indolent lymphomas.

There are rare patients who have stage IE disease with this histology (i.e., renal involvement). In this case, modest dose RT (12 to 18 Gy) within the organ tolerance can provide long-term control and, occasionally, a cure.

Marginal Zone Lymphomas

MZLs are indolent NHLs that include three diseases arising from post-GC marginal zone B cells: splenic marginal zone B-cell lymphoma (± villous lymphocytes), extranodal marginal zone B-cell lymphoma of mucosa-associated lymphoid tissue (MALT) type (MALT-type lymphoma, or MALT lymphoma); and nodal marginal zone B-cell lymphoma.[196,197]

Nodal MZL

Nodal MZLs constitute less than 1% of all NHLs. These lymphomas are primarily nodal diseases without evidence of extranodal involvement.

Pathology

Within lymph nodes, there are collections of B cells in a parafollicular, perivascular, and perisinusoidal distribution that often bear a monocytoid appearance, having folded nuclear contours and moderate abundant pale cytoplasm. These cells may surround reactive-appearing GCs and mantle zones. A subset of cases is also associated with variable degrees of plasmacytoid differentiation.

Immunophenotype and Genetics

Cells express monoclonal surface immunoglobulin (IgM > IgG > IgA) as well as CD19, CD20, CD79a, and are negative for CD10 and CD23. A minor subset of cases may be CD5 positive. Cases with plasmacytoid differentiation may show monoclonal expression of cytoplasmic kappa or lambda light chain by immunohistochemistry. Such cases may be associated with small monoclonal immunoglobulin spikes, but these are generally under 0.5 g/dL and are not associated with hyperviscosity. A subset of cases expresses surface IgD, analogous to splenic MZL. Immunoglobulin genes are rearranged with evidence of somatic mutation, implying a post-GC origin. There are no known chromosomal abnormalities specific to nodal MZL.

Clinical Features

Over 70% of patients present with stage III/IV disease, and the majority are asymptomatic. Bone marrow involvement is less common (45%) than in most indolent lymphomas. The 5-year survival for patients with nodal MZL is 55% to 79%. Similar to other indolent lymphomas, histologic transformation can occur with nodal MZL.

Treatment

The optimal therapy for patients with nodal MZL is not known. Patients are frequently treated with chemoimmunotherapy, typically either alkylating agents or purine analogs plus rituximab, which produce RRs in excess of 80%. A recent phase III study comparing CHOP-R to BR included 67 patients with MZL not otherwise specified.[106] There was no difference (p < 0.32) in median PFS between CHOP-R (47 months) and BR (57 months). For now, patients should be offered either clinical trials or treated with regimens used for FL.

Splenic Marginal Zone Lymphoma (± Villous Lymphocytes)

Splenic MZL (± villous lymphocytes) constitutes less than 1% of all NHLs, with a median age of 65 to 70 years and uncommon before the age of 50 years.[63] It is more common in Caucasians, with no gender predominance. Splenic MZL has been associated with viral infections, specifically hepatitis C and Kaposi's sarcoma–associated herpesvirus (KSHV). In one study, treatment of hepatitis C induced regression of the lymphoma.

Pathology

In splenic MZL, there is an expansion of marginal zones in the spleen. Plasma cell differentiation may be seen in a subset of cases, but as in nodal MZL, monoclonal spikes, if present, are less than 0.5 mg/dL. Bone marrow, lymph nodes, and peripheral blood involvement (referred to as splenic lymphoma with villous or nonvillous lymphocytes) can also be present. Generally, cells have small nuclei, but in the peripheral blood, they typically have abundant cytoplasm with "shaggy" or villous projections.

Immunophenotype and Genetics

Splenic MZL cells express monoclonal surface IgM, IgD, CD19, and CD20. The tumor cells generally lack CD5 and CD10, helping to distinguish this tumor from SLL/CLL, MCL, and FL. They also typically are negative for CD25, CD103, and annexin A1, which helps to distinguish splenic MZL from hairy cell leukemia. Ig genes have evidence for somatic hypermutation in about half the cases. In splenic MZL, trisomy 3 is present in 39% of cases, which is found in other MZLs. Abnormalities of chromosome 7q are also frequently seen. Deep sequencing identified recurrent somatic mutations in genes involved in the NOTCH, NF-κB, and B-cell receptor pathways, as well as mutations in TP53.[198] NOTCH2 mutations have been reported in 21% to 25% of cases, and were associated with a poor prognosis.

Clinical Features

Patients typically present with splenomegaly, lymphocytosis, and cytopenias, with lymphadenopathy being a much less common feature. B symptoms and elevated LDH are uncommon. Because of marrow and peripheral blood involvement, over 90% of cases have stage IV disease at diagnosis. IgM monoclonal gammopathies and mixed cryoglobulinemia can be seen, especially with a hepatitis C infection. Acquired C1 esterase deficiency seen in many B-cell lymphoproliferative disorders and can be a feature of splenic MZL.[199] The survival of patients is in excess of 70% at 10 years. A prognostic model based on three risk factors—hemoglobin less than 12 g/dL, LDH level greater than normal, and albumin level less than 3.5 g/dL—could identify patients with 5-year cause-specific survivals of 88% for patients with zero risk factors, 73% for patients with one factor, and 50% for patients with two or three factors.[200]

Therapy

Similar to other indolent NHLs, many patients with splenic MZL do not require immediate therapy. Asymptomatic patients without splenomegaly or cytopenias can be observed. Patients with symptomatic splenomegaly and or significant cytopenias merit treatment. Those uncommon patients who also have hepatitis C may benefit from treatment of the infection, suggesting that tumor growth and survival is promoted by factors or signals elaborated in response to hepatitis C antigens. Splenectomy is reasonable for selected patients with excellent relief of symptoms and cytopenias. Splenectomy was associated with an overall response rate of 85% and an estimated PFS and OS at 5 years of 58% and 77%, respectively. For patients who are not surgical candidates, splenic radiation has some utility. In general, 150 cGy is given to the entire spleen three times per week. The total dose must remain under renal tolerance because the left kidney is almost always in the field. Single-agent rituximab can improve splenomegaly and cytopenias in over 90% of patients.[201] In a study of induction with weekly rituximab followed by maintenance, the RR was 95%, with OS and PFS at 5 years of 92% and 73%, respectively.[202] Other options for therapy at relapse are similar to those used for FL, and include retreatment with rituximab, alkylating agents, and purine analogs in combination with rituximab.

Extranodal Marginal Zone Lymphoma

MALT lymphoma is a subtype of MZL involving extranodal tissues. The most common site is the stomach, but MALT lymphoma has been described in a number of different organs and tissues including the skin, salivary glands, the lung, the small bowel, ocular adnexa, the breasts, the bladder, the thyroid, the dura, and the synovium. It has been associated with a variety of chronic inflammatory and infectious conditions, including autoimmune diseases such as Sjögren's syndrome and Hashimoto's thyroiditis, and infections with Helicobacter pylori (H. pylori), Borrelia burgdorferi (B. burgdorferi), Chlamydophila psittaci (C. psittaci), Campylobacter jejuni (C. jejuni), and hepatitis C virus (HCV).[203–206] MALT lymphoma behaves indolently and is principally observed until symptoms related to organ impairment become evident; however, in many cases, early stage disease treatment with radiation therapy or antibiotic therapy appears to be curative. There are few dedicated studies of MALT lymphoma outside of early stage disease and much of the management of advanced stage disease is extrapolated from the FL literature, which often includes a small number of MZL patients.

Epidemiology

MALT lymphomas account for approximately 5% to 8% of all NHLs, but represent 50% to 70% of all MZLs.[63,207] It is the third most common subtype of NHL after DLBCL and FL. The median age at diagnosis is 60 years, with incidence nearly equal in men and women. Two-thirds of patients present with stage I/II disease, with a minority of patients having more advanced disease at diagnosis. B symptoms and bone marrow involvement are rare. MALT lymphomas can transform into a more aggressive lymphoma, but this occurs rarely. The most common transformation is into an activated B-cell–like DLBCL.[208] Nearly half of all MALT lymphomas involve the gastric mucosa, where over 60% are associated with an H. pylori infection.

Pathology

MALT lymphomas are malignancies of antigen-stimulated B cells, which normally reside in lymph nodes within the marginal zone that is found outside the mantle zones of B-cell follicles.[197] Histologically, they are characterized by a monoclonal infiltrate of small- to medium-sized cells with abundant cytoplasm and irregular nuclear contours. Variable numbers of larger centroblast-like cells may also be present, and a subset of cases exhibit plasmacytic differentiation. An essential pathologic feature is the presence of lymphoepithelial lesions created by the invasion of mucosal glands and crypts by aggregates of lymphoma cells, producing an appearance that resembles the lymphocyte M-cell structures found in normal Peyer patches.

Immunophenotype and Genetics

MALT lymphomas are surface Ig positive, and are also positive for B-cell markers (CD19, CD20, CD79a, and CD22), and negative for CD5, CD10, CD23, and cyclin D1.[44] Uncommonly, MALT lymphomas are CD5 positive and this is associated with a worse prognosis; these lymphomas may have cytogenetic changes such as trisomy 3 and del7q.[209] Distinguishing MALT lymphomas from benign reactive lymphoid infiltrates may be difficult; in this circumstance, light chain restriction by flow cytometry or immunoglobulin heavy chain gene rearrangement studies by PCR can be helpful.

Other cytogenetic abnormalities that have been reported in MALT lymphomas include t(11;18), t(14;18), t(1;14), t(3;14), and trisomy 8. The t(11;18) is the most common; it occurs in 18% to 53% of MALT lymphomas of any site and is associated with a low-grade histology.[210,211] It produces the fusion of the apoptosis inhibitor 2 (API2) gene and the MALT1 gene. The resulting fusion gene encodes a chimeric protein that stimulates the activation of NF-κB, a transcription factor that turns on a number of genes that promote proliferation and inhibit apoptosis.[212] The t(11;18) translocation predicts for a poor response to H. pylori–directed therapies in gastric MALT lymphoma.[213] A substantial proportion of malignant B cells in MALT lymphomas express B-cell receptors with strong homology to rheumatoid factors, and this appears to be mutually exclusive with the presence of the t(11;18) translocation.[214] This suggests that t(11;18)-negative MALT lymphomas are driven by the stimulation of high-affinity B-cell receptors by antibody–antigen immune complexes and activated T cells, whereas t(11;18)-positive MALT lymphomas are not dependent on B-cell receptor signaling, but instead are driven by constitutive activation of NF-κB. The t(14;18), which pairs the MALT1 gene with the IgH gene and drives overexpression of MALT1 protein, is more common in nongastric MALT lymphomas.[215] The t(1;14), which results in the overexpression of BCL10, is rarer overall but more frequent in gastric and pulmonary MALT lymphomas. The t(3;14) translocation is present in 10% of thyroid, ocular adnexal, and cutaneous MALT lymphomas.[216] This translocation involves the IgH and FOXP1 genes and drives overexpression of the FOXP1 transcription factor. Of note, overexpression of MALT1, BCL10, and FOXP1 are all believed to result in NF-κB hyperactivation, making this a common feature of genetically diverse MALT lymphomas. MALT lymphomas are also more often associated with gains at chromosomes 3p, 6p, and 18p, and del(6q23) than the other subtypes of MZL.[217]

Clinical Presentation

The clinical presentation of MALT lymphoma depends in large part on the site of disease. Gastric and intestinal MALT lymphomas may present with symptoms of dyspepsia and abdominal pain, sometimes with signs and symptoms of bowel obstruction, but rarely with bleeding. These lymphomas are diagnosed on endoscopy with biopsies from multiple areas of endoscopically abnormal tissue as well as random sampling of macroscopically uninvolved mucosa. Involvement of the salivary and lacrimal glands, on the other hand, can result in Sjögren's-like syndromes of dry eyes and mouth. MALT lymphomas involving the ocular adnexa typically present with painless conjunctival injection and photophobia, resembling allergic conjunctivitis. Patients with bronchus-associated lymphoid tissue (BALT) lymphomas typically are older men and can have symptoms including cough, fever, and/or weight loss.[218] Other sites of disease often present with an obstructing mass. Some patients are diagnosed incidentally, either because of imaging studies or an exam of the eye or GI track done for another reason or as part of an evaluation for a monoclonal gammopathy, which is present in approximately 25% to 35% of MALT lymphoma patients; this feature is generally associated with plasmacytoid differentiation.[219] B symptoms are rare in this disease.[63] Bone marrow involvement is present in a minority of patients; therefore, cytopenias are rare, as is disease in the peripheral blood.

In addition to the blood tests that are standard for patients with NHL at diagnosis, patients with MALT lymphomas should have a few additional tests. HCV testing should be performed given its association with MALT lymphoma; an HIV virus test is advised. Additional laboratory studies to consider include a β2-microglobulin, serum protein electrophoresis and immunofixation, and serum light chains. Staging is done with CT scans of the chest, abdomen, and pelvis, as well as imaging of the neck, including the parotids and salivary glands, and orbits with CT or MRI. A bone marrow biopsy should be considered for patients with multifocal disease, and an evaluation of the gastric mucosa is reasonable for all patients with nongastric MALT lymphoma given the documented high rate of gastric involvement in these patients.[220]

Treatment

Management of MALT lymphoma depends both on stage and site of disease. As an indolent lymphoma with a long OS, close observation at diagnosis until the development of signs, symptoms, or organ function impairment as a result of the disease is appropriate for patients with advanced stage disease. An exception is patients with advanced stage MALT lymphoma and concomitant HCV infection; a trial of anti-HCV antiviral therapy in these patients may result in regression of their lymphoma. For patients with early stage and localized disease, however, treatment with radiation therapy or treatment with antibiotics, such as for H. pylori–positive gastric MALT lymphoma, has been associated with high RRs and durable responses, many of which may represent cures.

Treatment of symptomatic or organ impairing relapsed, refractory, or advanced stage disease is similar to approaches used in FL with chemotherapy, immunotherapy, or chemoimmunotherapy.

Gastric MALT lymphoma represents a paradigm for treating early stage, localized MALT lymphomas. For those associated with an H. pylori infection that do not harbor a t(11;18) translocation, eradication of H. pylori is effective treatment and results in good long-term disease control and OS.[221–223] In patients with H. pylori–negative lymphomas, MALT lymphomas with a t(11;18) translocation, or lymphomas that fail to respond to H. pylori therapy, RT is the preferred treatment modality.[224] Chemotherapy, immunotherapy, or chemoimmunotherapy is active in this disease but is generally reserved for patients with relapsed or refractory disease to antibiotic therapy or RT, or patients with more advanced stage or aggressive disease.[225,226] Similarly, MALT lymphoma of the ocular adnexa is primarily treated with RT.[227] However, given the association described by some groups between C. psittaci infection and MALT lymphoma in this area, antibiotic therapy with doxycycline has been studied.[228] The RR of single-agent doxycycline for MALT lymphoma of the ocular adnexa was 83%, with two-thirds of patients having partial responses. The 2-year PFS was 55%.

For relapsed or refractory disease or disease that is more extensive at presentation, agents that have been used and reported include single-agent therapy with alkylating agents such as chlorambucil or cyclophosphamide, purine analogs such as cladribine, bortezomib, and rituximab, and occasionally, multiagent anthracycline-based chemotherapy for younger patients with more aggressive disease. The use of single-agent, continuous, low-dose oral chlorambucil or cyclophosphamide in patients with early or advanced stage disease yielded CR rates of 75% and a relapse rate of 21% during the 11-year follow-up.[229] Single-agent rituximab in patients with stage I through IV MALT lymphoma (15 gastric, 10 nongastric) who were either chemotherapy naïve or who had progressed following chemotherapy resulted in an overall response rate of 73% and was better for chemotherapy-naïve patients than for previously treated patients (87% versus 45%).[225] Duration of response was short, however, with 36% of responders progressing at a median of 10.5 months. Combination chemoimmunotherapy with rituximab and fludarabine results in response rates of 85% to 100% and 2- to 3-year PFS of 80% to 100% at the expense, however, of significantly greater toxicity.[230] MALT lymphoma is extremely sensitive to radiation therapy, and this modality has a role in the palliation of patients with advanced disease.

Mantle Cell Lymphoma

MCL is a malignancy of monomorphous small- to medium-sized B cells with the characteristic t(11;14) leading to overexpression of the cyclin D1 cell cycle regulator in the majority of cases.

Pathology

MCLs are neoplastic counterparts of naïve "mantle zone" B cells. Morphologically, MCL can have either diffuse architecture, or a vaguely nodular appearance, occasionally growing predominantly in expanded mantle zones around reactive CCs. Cytologically, in most cases, the neoplastic cells are small- to medium-sized and have irregular nuclei and scant cytoplasm. Some cases of MCL have a predominance of intermediate-size cells with more open "blastic" chromatin; such blastic variants are associated with a high mitotic rate. Other cases are comprised of a spectrum of cells, including large cells (pleomorphic variant).

Immunophenotype and Genetics

MCLs express B-cell antigens, surface IgM (usually together with surface IgD), CD5, and CD43 and usually lack CD10 and CD23. Overexpression of cyclin D1 further distinguishes these tumors from most other entities. IgH variable gene segments lack a somatic mutation in 84% of cases (pre-GC), with the remainder being mutated.[231] By FISH, greater than 90% of MCLs have the t(11;14) associated with the rearrangement of the cyclin D1 gene (*CCDN1*). The remaining cases do not overexpress cyclin D1, but instead usually overexpress cyclin D2, cyclin D3, or cyclin E due to the presence of translocations involving these genes and the IgH locus.[232] Cyclin D1–negative cases are similar clinically to cyclin D1–positive cases[233] and have a similar gene expression profile. Deep sequencing[234] has identified *NOTCH1* mutations in a minority of cases, which may be associated with a poor prognosis. SOX11 overexpression is also associated with a worse prognosis.[232,235]

Clinical Features. MCL constitutes about 7% of all NHLs. About 75% of patients are males, with a median age of 63 years. Approximately 70% of patients have stage IV disease, and B symptoms are observed in approximately one-third of patients. Typical sites of involvement are the lymph nodes, the spleen, the liver, Waldeyer's ring, and bone marrow. Peripheral blood involvement is present in 25% to 50% of patients at presentation. MCL can involve any region of the GI tract (88% lower tract, 43% upper tract by endoscopy), occasionally presenting as multiple intestinal polyposis.[236] CNS involvement is rare and is usually associated with a leukemic phase.

The median survival of patients with MCL is 4 to 5 years and improving. Approximately 10% to 15% of patients have a disease with a more indolent disease, with minimal lymphadenopathy, mild splenomegaly, and a proliferation index measured by Ki 67 staining of around 10%.[237] These patients have a disease that behaves more like an indolent NHL, where a *watchful waiting* approach does not compromise response to therapy or survival. In contrast, patients with the blastic variant at diagnosis have a median survival of 18 months. Blastic transformation occurs in 35% of patients, with a risk of 42% at 4 years, and once occurring, the median survival is 3.8 months.[238]

Prognostic models have been employed for patients with MCL. The IPI developed for diffuse aggressive NHLs provides stratification of patients. Attempts to improve on the IPI include the mantle cell lymphoma International Prognostic Index (MIPI), which includes age, performance status (PS), LDH, and white blood cell count (WBC)[58] as prognostic factors, and several reports show that the MIPI is better than the IPI at stratifying patients.[239] The proliferation index alone and also when incorporated into the MIPI provides additional predictive power.[240] Gene expression profiling has been examined in MCL patients. In those studies, the proliferation signature and high expression of cyclin D1 were associated with an unfavorable prognosis.[241] Mutations and deletions of p53 are also associated with a worse prognosis.[242]

Treatment. The majority of patients with MCL have a disseminated disease requiring treatment. An indolent behaving disease is seen in 10% to 15% of patients, where a delay of initiation of treatment was not deleterious.[241] The treatment of MCL historically involved single alkylating agents as well as combination chemotherapy (CVP, CHOP) to which 30% to 50% of patients had a CR, with a median duration of 1 to 3 years.[243] In a meta-analysis, single alkylating agents offered results similar to combination chemotherapy.[244] A small number of patients with MCL will present with stage I to II disease. These patients are potentially curable with combined chemotherapy and involved field radiation (30 Gy). Chemoimmunotherapy has shown a significant impact in the treatment of MCL. A meta analysis of 638 patients with MCL showed that rituximab-containing regimens significantly increased median survival (37 versus 27 months)[245] as compared to chemotherapy alone. One of the mainstays of chemoimmunotherapy for the initial treatment of MCL is CHOP-R. However, results of a randomized trial comparing CHOP-R to BR reported superior PFS with BR with less toxicity.[106] In patients with a median age of 70 years, the median PFS for BR was 35 months, compared to 22 months with CHOP-R. One other randomized study compared CHOP-R to the fludarabine, cyclophosphamide, rituximab (FCR) regimen. In that study, for patients over age 60 years, CHOP-R and FCR had similar CR rates, but CHOP-R had less toxicity, and the OS at 4 years was 62% versus 47% in favor of CHOP-R.[246] This study included a second randomization of maintenance with interferon-α or rituximab until progression. For the patients who received CHOP-R, a significant survival benefit from maintenance rituximab was observed, with an estimated 4-year OS rate of 87% versus 63%.

More aggressive approaches for the initial treatment of MCL have been the rituximab, hyperfractionated cyclophosphamide, vincristine, doxorubicin, dexamethasone (R-HyperCVAD) regimen or the consolidation of first remission following chemoimmunotherapy with high-dose therapy and ASCT. The most recent update from the M.D. Anderson Cancer Center of R-HyperCVAD reported a median OS not reached at 8 years, and a median time to failure of 4.6 years.[247] A multi-institution SWOG phase 2 trial of R-HyperCVAD reported median PFS and OS of 4.8 and 6.8 years, respectively. However, 39% of patients were unable to complete the planned treatment.[248] A similar issue was found in a report from academic centers in Italy, where, despite excellent disease control with R-HyperCVAD, with OS and FFS of 86% and 61%, respectively, 63% of patients were unable to complete the planned treatment course with the most common reason being treatment-related toxicity.[249] There has been only one randomized trial comparing ASCT to conventional therapy, and this was in the pre-rituximab era. Autologous transplant for patients younger than 65 years, in first CR or PR, demonstrated improvements in PFS as compared to interferon-α maintenance, but a nonstatistically significant improvement in OS.[250] Many phase 2 studies have intensified the induction therapy prior to ASCT in an attempt to improve outcomes. The Nordic regimen (CHOP-R + high-dose cytarabine [HiDAC] and ASCT for mantle cell lymphoma)[251] has yielded excellent results, with median OS and response duration longer than 10 years, and a median event-free survival (EFS) of 7.4 years. An analysis of outcome by MIPI score found that, at 10 years, 70% of patients with low-intermediate MIPI-B were alive, but only 23% of the patients were still alive with high MIPI-B.

The majority of patients with MCL relapse from primary therapy. Three agents are U.S. Food and Drug Administration (FDA) approved for relapsed MCL: bortezomib, lenalidomide, and ibrutinib. Bortezomib has a 29% overall RR, and a 5% CR/Cru with a median duration of 7 months.[252] Lenalidomide is FDA approved for bortezomib failures, with a 26% RR (CR, 7%), and a median duration of response of 17 months.[253,254] Ibrutinib has a 68% RR, with a 21% CR, and a median duration of 17.5 months.[255] Another oral kinase inhibitor targeting CDK4/6 is under investigation for relapsed patients.[256] Conventional chemotherapy agents, including purine analogs and bendamustine, are active in relapsed patients.[135] For patients with localized progression, local RT can provide reasonable palliation.[257] MCL is one of the most sensitive tumors to RT, and modest doses of radiation (20 Gy) can shrink even large masses and, therefore, should be considered in chemorefractory patients.

SCT for relapsed MCL patients has been of limited benefit. With long follow-ups, patients undergoing ASCT have a high relapse rate.[258] There is interest in nonmyeloablative alloSCT for select patients with relapsed disease. The 3-year PFS and OS are 30% and 40%, respectively.[259] Given the poor prognosis for patients with relapsed MCL, clinical trials should be explored for these patients.

Diffuse Large B-Cell Lymphoma

DLBCL constitutes 31% of all NHLs, and is the most common histologic subtype. Although, in the past, DLBCL was considered one disease, in the 2008 WHO classification, DLBCL is recognized to encompass many entities (see Table 39.4). Caucasian Americans have a higher incidence of DLBCL than African Americans, Asian Americans, and Native or Alaskan Native Americans. There is a slight male predominance, and the median age is 64 years. There is a familial component in some cases, with about a 3.5-fold increased risk in relatives of probands with DLBCL. Patients with congenital or acquired immunodeficiency, patients on immunosuppression, and patients with autoimmune disorders have a higher risk of developing DLBCL, often EBV related. This implicated immune dysfunction is a risk factor for the disease. DLBCL can arise as a histologic transformation from any indolent B-cell NHL or CLL.

Pathology

DLBCLs consist of a diffuse proliferation of large cells that have a high mitotic rate. The only unifying feature is the large size of the tumor cells, which may have centroblastic, immunoblastic, plasmablastic, or anaplastic morphologies. In a subset of cases, classified as T-cell/histiocyte-rich large B-cell lymphoma, there are only scattered large tumor cells in a background of abundant small T cells and epithelioid histiocytes.[260]

Immunophenotype and Genetics

The normal cellular counterparts for DLBCL are GC and post-GC activated B cells. Tumor cells generally express B-cell antigens (CD19, CD20, CD79a), monoclonal sIgM, and occasionally, other heavy chain isotypes. CD5-positive cases are uncommon and may have a worse prognosis.[261] CD10 and BCL6 expression typifies tumors of GC origin (GCB), whereas expression of MUM1 favors a non-GC activated B cell type (ABC). In DLBCL, 1% to 10% are reported to express BCL2, whereas approximately 70% express BCL6, and CD30 positivity (11% of cases) is associated with better survival.[263]

Several chromosomal abnormalities have been observed in DLBCL. Rearrangements of BCL6 are found in a small proportion of FLs (6% to 13%), but occur in about 30% of DLBCLs.[264] Many different BCL6 translocations have been described, all of which replace the BCL6 promoter with the promoter of another gene that is highly expressed in GC B cells, thus driving the overexpression of BCL6. Other tumors have point mutations in the BCL6 promoter that prevent BCL6 (a transcriptional repressor) from negatively regulating its own expression.[265] BCL6 overexpression leads to increased proliferation and survival of GC B cells, and also blocks differentiation into plasma cells by interfering with the activity of the transcription factor PRDM1 (also known as BLIMP1).[266] Another 20% to 30% of DLBCLs are associated with the t(14,18). Surprisingly, the t(14;18) is not always associated with BCL2 protein overexpression by immunohistochemistry.[267] Ig genes consistently show somatic mutations in the Ig variable region genes.[268] By GEP, the GCB type is often associated with the t(14;18) and amplifications of the REL oncogene on chromosome 2. In contrast, the ABC type is associated with a loss of 6q21 and trisomy 3, gains of 3q and 18q21-22, and mutations of EZH2.[269,270] The involved area on 6q includes PRDM1 (BLIMP1), reinforcing the idea that PRDM1, a master regulator of plasma cell differentiation, functions as a tumor suppressor in B cells.[271] ABC cases also have a high level activation of NF-κB, a transcription factor implicated in the B-cell receptor signaling pathway that supports B-cell proliferation and survival.[272] Recently, there has been great interest in the clinical implications of MYC rearrangements and overexpression in DLBCL. MYC is rearranged in 10% of DLBCLs, with the partner gene being one of the Ig genes in 60% of cases and some other gene in 40% of cases. Approximately 20% of MYC rearranged cases have concurrent BCL2 or BCL6 rearrangements, a combination referred to as double hit lymphoma.[273] Amplification and/or overexpression of MYC independent of rearrangements or amplification has also been described and is also associated with a poor prognosis.[274,275] Deep sequencing of DLBCL samples have found extensive mutations, especially in the same histone-modifying genes implicated in FL—the histone acetyltransferases EP300 and CREBP and the histone methyltransferase MLL2. Thus, like FL, epigenetic changes are likely to have a central pathogenic role in DLBCL.[276]

Clinical Features

Patients have a median of age 64 years, although younger in African Americans versus Caucasians.[277] Patients present with rapidly enlarging masses, either nodal enlargement or extranodal disease. DLBCL presents as stage I or IE disease approximately 20% of the time. The disease is confined to one side of the diaphragm (stage I or II) in approximately 30% to 40% of patients. Stage IV disease is seen in approximately 40% of patients. B symptoms occur in 30% of patients, and serum LDH is elevated in over half the patients. Extranodal sites are common, occurring in 40% of cases, including the GI tract, the testis,[278] the bone, the thyroid, the skin, the CNS, and bone marrow. DLBCL is highly invasive, with local compression of blood vessels, airways, involvement of peripheral nerves, and destruction of bone. Bone marrow involvement initially is found in only 10% to 20% of patients and has a strong correlation with the risk of spread to the CNS.[279] Other sites of extranodal disease, specifically testicular, paranasal sinus, epidural, and the presence of multiple extranodal sites, are other risks for CNS dissemination.

Therapy of Early Stage Diffuse Large B-Cell Lymphoma

Less than 20% of patients with DLBCL have localized disease. The recommended treatment for localized disease outside of clinical trials is abbreviated combination chemoimmunotherapy plus involved field radiotherapy, or combination chemoimmunotherapy alone. The benefit of adding radiotherapy to 6 to 8 cycles of chemotherapy remains unclear. The SWOG randomized trial from the pre-rituximab era in patients with localized diffuse aggressive lymphoma compared eight cycles of CHOP to three cycles of CHOP plus involved field radiotherapy.[280] Patients treated with three cycles of CHOP plus radiotherapy had a significantly better 5-year PFS and OS than patients treated with eight cycles of CHOP (77% versus 64% for PFS, 82% versus 72% for OS). Overall life-threatening toxicity and cardiac toxicity were significantly higher in the patients receiving CHOP alone. The benefit of attenuated chemotherapy was largely found in patients over the age of 60 years. Although there is no analogous randomized trial that includes rituximab, there is a phase II trial of patients with early stage DLBCL employing three cycles of CHOP-R followed by involved field RT.[281] Patients had at least one adverse risk factor for early stage disease specifically: age >60 years, increased serum LDH, stage II disease, or performance status ≥1. The PFS and OS at 2 and 4 years was 93% and 88%, and 95% and 92%, respectively.

In the pre-rituximab era, another randomized trial compared eight courses of CHOP with or without involved field radiotherapy in patients with previously untreated bulky or extranodal stage I or stage II diffuse aggressive NHL. The disease-free survival was greater for CR patients who received radiotherapy (73% versus 56%), although 10-year OS was similar in the two treatment arms (68% versus 65%).[282] The role of RT remains uncertain in patients with stage I or II disease. In patients aged 60 years or younger with low-risk disease, an aggressive regimen (rituximab, doxorubicin, cyclophosphamide, vindesine, bleomycin, and prednisone [ACVBP]) was superior to CHOP plus radiation.[283] Similarly, in patients over age 60 years, the addition of RT did not improve DFS or OS for patients who received four cycles of CHOP alone.[284] A phase III study in patients age 60 years or under with IPI score of 0 or 1 compared six cycles of CHOP to CHOP-R, with all patients with bulk disease (masses greater than 7.5 cm) or extranodal sites receiving involved field radiation. If one looks at the patients with an IPI score of 0 with no bulk, which includes early stage patients, the 5-year EFS is approximately 90% with CHOP-R alone. This supports the notion that chemoimmunotherapy alone is a reasonable option for early stage disease. However, in patients with bulk disease often defined as masses greater than 7.5 cm, the outcome is worse than for patients without bulk. In the randomized MabThera International Trial (MInT) trial of CHOP versus CHOP-R, all patients (IPI 0 or IPI 1) with masses >7.5 cm received 30 to 40 Gy of involved field radiation to those sites. Those patients with IPI of 0 and bulk disease had a 10% to 15% lower PFS than patients without bulk.[285] A randomized trial of a similar patient population is examining whether involved field radiation impacts outcomes for patients with bulk disease or extranodal disease (the UNFOLDER trial). Early data in this trial suggests a benefit for RT after chemotherapy. Presently, the most appropriate management of patients with early stage DLBCL with bulk disease remains controversial.

Therapy of Advanced Stage Diffuse Large B-Cell Lymphoma

If a clinical trial is not available, the current recommendation for the treatment of advanced stage DLBCL is combination chemotherapy with CHOP-R for patients both under age 60 years as well as over age 60 years. Questions that have been addressed in trials has been the number of cycles, the interval for those cycles, and whether more intensive therapy including high-dose therapy and stem cell support has a significant impact on outcome.

In patients with DLBCL ages 60 to 80 years, the Groupe d'Etude des Lymphomes de l'Adulte (GELA) group reported that eight cycles of CHOP-R was superior to CHOP alone in terms of PFS, disease free survival (DFS) and OS with no added toxicity.[286,287] A U.S. Intergroup study compared in a similar population administering CHOP or CHOP-R given on a different schedule.[288] Responding patients were randomly assigned to receive either rituximab maintenance therapy or no maintenance. A beneficial impact of rituximab added to CHOP chemotherapy on EFS and OS was observed; however, no benefit was seen for maintenance rituximab following CHOP-R induction. Similarly, in patients less than 60 years of age, with an IPI of 0 and 1, the addition of rituximab to CHOP improved time to treatment failure and OS compared to CHOP alone.[285]

The number of cycles of therapy has been examined in the rituximab with CHOP over age 60 years (RICOVER-60) trial, in patients over age 60 years. This study compared six to eight cycles of CHOP or CHOP-R administered every 14 days (CHOP-R 14). CHOP-R was superior to CHOP given for six or eight cycles (70% versus 57%), and there was no benefit of eight cycles of CHOP-R over six cycles (with two additional doses of rituximab).[289] In another study, CHOP-R given every 21 days (CHOP-R 21) for eight cycles was compared to six cycles of CHOP-R 14.[290] More grade III/IV neutropenia was seen in the CHOP-R 21 (57%/31%) treated patients, whereas more thrombocytopenia occurred in the CHOP-R 14–treated patients. With a median follow-up of 40 months, there was no difference in PFS or OS. Another study from the GELA trial did not find an improvement in outcome with CHOP-R 14. This supports the notion that CHOP-R 21 for six to eight cycles is the standard of care.

Attempts to intensify therapy have included alternative regimens and ASCT. The GELA group treated patients under age 60 years with IPI of 1 with the more aggressive regimen R-ACVBP followed by consolidation with methotrexate and leucovorin.[291] When compared to CHOP-R plus intrathecal methotrexate, R-ACVBP plus methotrexate and leucovorin led to higher PFS and OS. Several studies have examined the role of high-dose therapy and ASCT in first CR/PR for patients with aggressive NHL prior to the addition of rituximab to combination chemotherapy. In the pre-rituximab era, the overall benefit of ASCT in first remission for patients with DLBCL remains uncertain despite many randomized trials. A meta-analysis of 3,079 patients treated on 15 randomized trials with either conventional therapy or ASCT in first CR, showed no difference in EFS, OS, or treatment-related mortality.[292] Two recent studies in the rituximab era have not resolved this issue of ASCT in first CR. R-CHOEP (rituximab, cyclophosphamide, adriamycin, vincristine, etoposide, and prednisone) was compared to R-MegaCHOEP, sequential high-dose therapy with stem cell support, for high-intermediate or high-risk age adjusted IPI score patients. There was more hematologic toxicity with R-MegaCHOEP. With a median follow-up of 42 months, no statistical difference was seen in 3-year EFS (70% versus 61%) or OS (74% versus 70%).[293] More recently, a US intergroup trial treated patients with age-adjusted high-intermediate and high-risk IPI scores with at least a PR after five cycles of CHOP-based therapy (CHOP or CHOP-R), to a total of six cycles of CHOP-based therapy followed by ASCT versus a total of eight cycles of CHOP-based therapy alone.[294] Patients who relapsed after chemotherapy alone could undergo ASCT as salvage therapy. After a median follow-up of 6.3 years, ASCT was associated with a higher PFS at 2 years (69 versus 55%; hazard ratio [HR] 1.72; 95% confidence interval [CI], 0.82 to 1.94) but no difference in OS (74 versus 71%; HR 1.26; 95% CI, 0.82 to 1.94). To date, the data do not support ASCT as a consolidation for first remission.

Treatment of Relapsed or Refractory Diffuse Large B-Cell Lymphoma

The majority of relapses from CHOP-R therapy are seen within the first 2 years after the completion of treatment. However, 18% of relapses occur greater than 5 years after the initial treatment.[295] The failure of primary therapy to induce a CR or early relapse within the first few months of completing treatment is associated with a particularly poor prognosis. We generally recommend that patients who relapse after a CR be rebiopsied, because a subset will have FL.

Once relapse or refractory disease has been determined, the next issue to resolve is whether the goal is potential curative therapy or palliation. For patients with poor performance status, particularly elderly patients, the goal is often palliation. Local radiation can provide transient palliation. Other chemotherapy agents, including single agents such as cytarabine[296] or bendamustine,[297] are associated with overall RRs of 50% to 63%, a CR rate of 37%, and a median PFS of approximately 6 months.[298] The all oral-agent regimen PEPC (prednisone, etoposide, cyclophosphamide, and procarbazine) can induce remission in over 50% of patients.[299] Clinical trials may be an option for some of these patients depending on eligibility criteria.

The majority of patients with relapsed and refractory DLBCL receive combination chemotherapy, often with rituximab. Various combinations of drugs, including ifosfamide, carboplatin, etoposide, cytarabine, gemcitabine, and cisplatin, have been utilized for relapsed disease. The goal is to identify patients with chemosensitive disease who have the greatest likelihood of benefiting from high-dose therapy and ASCT, which leads to a higher long-term DFS and OS for relapsed DLBCL. A major question has been whether one second-line regimen is superior. The collaborative trial in relapsed aggressive lymphoma (CORAL) study compared R-ICE (rituximab, ifosfamide, carboplatin, and etoposide) to R-DHAP (rituximab, dexamethasone, high-dose cytarabine, and cisplatin), followed by ASCT.[300,301] No difference in overall RR, EFS, or OS was seen between the two regimens, with approximately 60% of patients responding. A subset analysis suggested that patients with a GCB DLBCL may have a better treatment outcome with R-DHAP versus R-ICE. The ultimate goal of salvage therapy is to achieve disease control to proceed to ASCT. It has been known since 1987 that disease sensitivity is the best determinant of outcome with high-dose therapy and ASCT. Three patient groups were identified based on the response to most recent treatment. Patients with chemosensitive disease have 30% to 50% long-terms DFS, those with chemorefractory disease have 10% to 15% long-term DFS and those with primary refractory disease have essentially no benefit from ASCT.[302] A major question was whether patients with chemosensitive disease benefit from ASCT or simply continuing salvage chemotherapy. The Parma study addressed this question, where 109 patients who had relapsed after having achieved a CR and responded to two cycles of DHAP were randomized to high-dose therapy and ASCT or four additional cycles of DHAP. ASCT was associated with a superior failure-free survival (51% versus 12% at 5 years) and OS (53% versus 32% at 5 years).[303] In the rituximab era, the long-term results of ASCT are less favorable than reported in the Parma trial, with about 30% long-term survivors in remission. Investigators have, to date, failed to improve on these results with the addition of maintenance therapy posttransplant with rituximab,[304] an anti-CD19 immunotoxin, or the oral kinase inhibitor enzastaurin, or adding radioimmunotherapy to the conditioning regimen. For patients with relapsed or refractory DLBCL, high-dose therapy and ASCT remain the treatments of choice for patients with chemosensitive disease. If the recurrence is localized, adjuvant RT either before or after high-dose therapy and ASCT may be beneficial. For patients with chemorefractory disease, clinical trials or palliative therapy should be considered. Several new agents have shown some promise in patients with relapsed DLBCL, including ibrutinib, particularly in the ABC cell of origin subtype, lenalidomide[253] and everolimus.[305]

Allogeneic bone marrow transplantation is generally not the favored approach for relapsed DLBCL patients. Although highly selected patients can have prolonged remission, this is at the expense of a high treatment-related mortality. Overall, there is no advantage for alloSCT. Patients with recurrent disease following ASCT who have good performance status and chemosensitive disease are now considered for alloSCT usually with reduced intensity conditioning, rather than ablative alloSCT where morbidity and mortality are exceedingly high. Studies have reported a 40% to 60% year PFS with this approach, but with a treatment-related mortality of 20% for RIC alloSCT and up to 40% for myeloablative transplants.[306,307]

Chimeric antigen receptor T (CAR-T) cells are another investigational immunotherapy approach to treating malignancies that have had some early success in CLL and B-cell acute lymphoblastic leukemia.[308–310] This strategy uses T cells collected from a patient that are genetically modified to express a receptor that will bind to a surface antigen expressed on the patient's own tumor cells. In the case of B-cell malignancies, this antigen has been CD19. After infusion, autologous CAR-T cells home to sites of disease and also persist over time. The CARs consist of an extracellular antigen recognition domain (typically a single chain Fv variable fragment from a monoclonal antibody) linked via a transmembrane domain to an intracellular signaling domain (usually the CD3ζ endodomain), resulting in the redirection of T-cell specificity toward target antigen-positive cells, and one or more costimulatory domains including CD28, 4-1BB, or OX40 to enhance cytokine secretion and effector cell expansion, and prevent activation-induced apoptosis and immune suppression by tumor-related metabolites.[311] Eight patients with DLBCL and/or primary mediastinal large B-cell lymphoma (PMLBCL) who have been treated with anti-CD19 CAR-T cells have been reported.[312] Five of these patients had a CR (2) or PR (3) that persisted for up to 19 months following therapy.

Other Large B-Cell Lymphomas

Intravascular Large B-Cell Lymphoma

Intravascular large B-cell lymphoma (ILCL) is a rare subtype in which lymphoma cells proliferate within small blood vessels without producing a tumor mass or detectable circulating tumor cells.[313–315] The tumor cells resemble centroblasts or immunoblasts, express B-cell–associated antigens, and are usually CD10 negative and MUM1 positive. Patients present with a variety of symptoms caused by the occlusion of small vessels. These include B symptoms, rapidly progressive neurologic signs (dementia, cerebral vascular accident, and/or peripheral neuropathy), and skin lesions imitating an inflammatory rash. Western and Asian subtypes have been identified, with less frequent CNS and skin involvement in the former. Laboratory abnormalities include elevated serum LDH and anemia. The diagnosis is made by demonstrating large lymphoma cells within small to medium blood vessels. The diagnosis can be difficult, but if the disease is suspected, a *blind* biopsy of normal-appearing skin can be diagnostic. If this is not informative, a biopsy of other sites of suspected involvement may necessary. The treatment of patients with ILBL includes both systemic chemoimmunotherapy and therapy for the CNS. Prior to rituximab, the prognosis for these patients was poor, with less than 10% long-term survivors. With an earlier diagnosis and therapy with CHOP-R, the 2-year PFS and OS have been reported to be 56% and 66%, respectively. CNS prophylaxis with either intrathecal or high-dose systemic methotrexate is recommended. Patients with secondary involvement of the brain or spinal cord at diagnosis, depending on the clinical situation, may need intrathecal chemotherapy, systemic high-dose methotrexate, and/or radiation to the sites of involvement.

T-Cell Histiocyte-Rich Large B-Cell Lymphoma

In this uncommon subtype of DLBCL, the majority of the tumor cell mass is comprised of nonneoplastic T cells and/or histiocytes, with malignant B cells making up less than 10% of the cellularity.[316] The lymphoma cells express CD20 but lack CD5, CD10, and CD138. An IPI of 2 or greater was reported in one series in a majority (77%) of patients, often with spleen, liver, and marrow involvement. The outcome of treatment is controversial, with one large series showing a less favorable prognosis, and a second suggesting a similar outcome to other forms of DLBCL when matched for risk factors.

EBV-Positive DLBCL of the Elderly.
EBV-positive DLBCL of the elderly is a provisional entity in the 2008 WHO classification. It is seen in patients greater than age 50 years, without known immunodeficiency or prior lymphoma. In Asian countries, this accounts for 8% to 10% of DLBCL in patients without a known immunodeficiency.[317,318] It is less common in Western countries. Patients often present with extranodal disease in addition to lymph nodes. Due to older age, frequent extranodal disease, and poor performance status, these patients often have a poor prognosis.

ALK-Positive Large B-Cell Lymphoma.
These are rare variants of large B-cell lymphomas that expresses CD30 and ALK kinase, usually due to a t(2;17) that fuses *ALK* to the clathrin heavy chain 1 gene (*CTLC*). These tumors often have a plasmablastic appearance and have been reported to have a poor prognosis.[319]

Special Situations

Testicular Diffuse Large B-Cell Lymphoma

DLBCL presenting in the testis is the most common malignant tumor in that site in men over 60 years of age, and constitute 1% of all lymphomas.[278,320] Other less common histologies include BL in children and, rarely, FL. Historically, the long-term results of treatment are worse for these patients than predicted by the IPI. Despite therapy, patients are at risk for relapse systemically, in the CNS, and in the contralateral testis. Therefore, following orchiectomy, patients require systemic therapy, and strong consideration should be given to CNS prophylaxis with either systemic or intrathecal methotrexate, as well as prophylactic radiation to the contralateral testis. Much of the data for treating this condition is from small series without randomized trials to address management issues. A recent international prospective trial of 53 patients with untreated stage I or II primary testicular lymphoma treated with six to eight cycles of CHOP-R 21, four weekly doses of intrathecal methotrexate (12 mg), and RT to the contralateral testis (30 Gy) for all patients and (30 to 36 Gy) to regional nodes for patients with stage II disease.[278] With a median follow-up of 65 months, the OS and

PFS at 5 years was 85% and 71%, respectively. Only three relapses were seen in the CNS. This study defines the current standard of care with chemoimmunotherapy, CNS prophylaxis, and radiation to the contralateral testis.

Treatment of the Aggressive Non-Hodgkin's Lymphoma in the Elderly

Lymphoma occurs at a higher incidence with increasing age.[321–323] Patients over age 60 years as shown in the IPI have a lower CR rate, PFS, and OS than patients 60 years of age or less. The reasons are probably a combination of increased treatment-related mortality and comorbidities. Biologically, the disease may also be different in older individuals, which may account, in part, for the higher IPI scores that have been reported in elderly patients. Dose reductions in these patients may also explain the less favorable outcome. The SWOG reported a CR rate of 37% in patients 65 years of age and older who received initial 50% dose reductions of cyclophosphamide and doxorubicin. Complete remission rates were 52%, a rate similar to those of younger patients, when full-dose chemotherapy was used.

Randomized trials have clearly demonstrated a significant survival benefit for the addition of rituximab to combination chemotherapy for DLBCL in patients over age 60 years.[289,321–323,324] In light of the concerns of increased toxicity of treatment in elderly patients, several regimens have been reported with this in mind. A recent report of 149 patients age 80 years or older, employed reduced doses of cyclophosphamide, adriamycin, and vincristine at about 50% of standard dosing of CHOP-R (R-mini CHOP).[325] Grade 3/4 neutropenia and thrombocytopenia was seen in 39% and 7% of patients, respectively, and 12 toxic deaths were seen. The 2-year OS and PFS were 59% and 47%, respectively. For patients who are not considered candidates for combination or reduced-dose chemoimmunotherapy, regimens such as PEPC or BR[326] can be useful for palliation in elderly patients, with over 50% RRs and a median PFS of over 6 months.

The approach toward elderly patients with aggressive lymphoma should be similar to patients age 60 years or younger, with curative intent. Supportive care measures with hematopoietic growth factors can be considered, albeit controversially, as well as prophylactic antibiotics. Analogous to younger patients, elderly patients should be considered for clinical trials if eligible and feasible.

Primary Mediastinal Large B-Cell Lymphoma

Within the category of DLBCL is a distinct clinical entity known as PMLBCL, representing 2.4% of all NHLs and 7% of all cases of DLBCL.[327]

Pathology

Histologically, the large tumor cells often have finer nuclear membranes and smaller nucleoli than other subtypes of DLBCL, sometimes making it difficult to distinguish the tumor cells from reactive macrophages in small biopsies. Not infrequently, a few multinucleated cells reminiscent of Reed-Sternberg variants may be admixed with more typical tumor cells. The tumor cells diffusely infiltrate the mediastinum and often elicit dense fibrosis, another feature that may render biopsies difficult to interpret.

Immunophenotype and Genetics

PMLBCLs express B-cell antigens CD19, CD20, CD22, TRAF1, and c-Rel, but lack sIg and CD5.[323] Unlike other DLBCLs, a low level expression of CD30 is seen in most cases, and a high fraction of tumors expresses TRAF1 and have nuclear REL. *BCL2* and *BCL6* rearrangements are absent. Translocations of the *CIITA* (major histocompatibility complex class II transactivator) gene are noted in about 40% of cases. Copy number gains in the region on chromosome 9p containing the genes for janus kinase 2 (*JAK2*) and programmed cell death ligand 1 and 2 (*PDL1* and *PDL2*) are common. PDL1 and PDL2 are ligands for the programmed cell death receptor 1 (PD-1), which has a role in suppressing T cell function.[209] PMLBCL resembles classical Hodgkin's disease (HD) by GEP,[329] because one-third of the most highly expressed genes in PMLBCLs are also expressed in the Reed-Sternberg cells of HL.

Clinical Features

PMLBCLs have a female predominance, with median age of 40 years. Over 70% of these patients present with stage I/II bulky disease involving the mediastinum, with pleural and pericardial effusions in about 50% of the patients. Superior vena cava syndrome is frequently seen in these patients. An elevated LDH (77%) and B symptoms (47%) are common. Relapses occur locally or in extranodal sites, including the liver, the GI tract, the kidneys, the ovaries, and the CNS.

Treatment

The general approach toward patients with PMLBCL has been similar to patients with localized DLBCL, with the majority of patients receiving combined modality therapy. The most recent results with chemoimmunotherapy demonstrate a 3-year OS of 89% with CHOP-R therapy. In the MInT trial, 87 patients with PMLBCL[330] received six cycles of CHOP-R, 75% of whom also received RT; only 7% of patients who received radiation subsequently progressed or relapsed. A recent study of 51 patients treated with dose-adjusted etoposide, prednisone, vincristine, cyclophosphamide, doxorubicin (EPOCH) plus rituximab (DA-EPOCH-R), and no radiotherapy, reported an outstanding PFS (93%) and OS (100%). The two failures received radiation and were rendered disease free.[331] These studies suggest that six cycles of CHOP-R followed by RT, or six to eight cycles of DA-EPOCH-R and no RT gives excellent results in PMBCL.

Grey Zone Lymphoma

In 2008, the WHO created provisional diagnoses to capture B-cell lymphomas with features between two established diagnoses: BL and DLBCL, and classical Hodgkin's lymphoma (cHL) and DLBCL.[332] These lymphomas constitute the grey zone lymphomas.

B-Cell Lymphoma, Unclassifiable, with Features Intermediate Between B-Cell Lymphoma and Diffuse Large B-Cell Lymphoma

These lymphomas differ morphologically from DLBCL in that the neoplastic cells often range from intermediate to large in size, may have a very high Ki-67 index, and are uniformly CD10 positive. They differ from BL in that the cells are more variable in size, are often BCL2 positive, may be BCL6 negative, and may have a Ki-67 index lower than 100%. Although defined by morphologic features, GEP has, likewise, identified a group of lymphomas with a GEP between that of BL and DLBCL.[333] This group is not synonymous with B-cell lymphoma, unclassifiable (B-UNC)/BL/DLBCL but the two overlap, suggesting B-UNC/BL/DLBCL is not a unique entity but rather a group of distinct lymphomas, including true BL, DLBCL, and unclassifiable lymphomas, which require further characterization.

Although potentially heterogeneous, these lymphomas carry a poor prognosis and are associated with high IPIs and frequent extranodal sites; this trend may be driven by inclusion of a subset of tumors with a particularly poor prognosis.[334,335] Although the IPI remains the most powerful prognostic tool we have for DLBCL, certain genetic events are being recognized as indicators of particularly high-risk disease. Most notably, the presence of multiple concurrent chromosomal translocations, commonly involving *MYC* and *BCL2*, defines a group with an extraordinarily poor prognosis.[273] This was first noted in Burkitt-like lymphoma, many of which were B-UNC/BL/DLBCL. No patients with these *double-hit* lymphomas were alive at 1 year. In DLBCL, dual translocations are present in 12% to 14% of cases and are similarly associated with a poor prognosis.[336] B-UNC/BL/DLBCL is enriched for these *double-hit* lymphomas, with 30% to 45% harboring both *MYC* and *BCL2* translocations. Although the majority of double-hit lymphomas fall into this diagnostic category, not all B-UNC/BL/DLBCLs are double-hit lymphomas. Double-hit lymphomas with this histology, however, appear to have a particularly poor prognosis, with a median OS of 4 months compared to 3 years in double-hit DLBCL with typical morphologic features.[337]

Although the prognosis for this group as a whole is poor, there has been no systematic investigation of the treatment of B-UNC/BL/DLBCL, and thus, no prospective evidence supporting the intensification of therapy over CHOP-R. However, three groups have retrospectively looked at the impact of intensified chemotherapy on outcomes for B-UNC/BL/DLBCL.[343,338] These analyses are limited in that they are retrospective, small, and likely included patients without B-UNC/BL/DLBCL. However, each showed that intensive regimens such as a modified Magrath regimen with cyclophosphamide, vincristine, doxorubicine, methotrexate/ifosphamide, etoposide, cytarabine (CODox-M/IVAC), HyperCVAD, and DA-EPOCH-R had better outcomes over CHOP-R (overall response rate [ORR] 86% versus 57%, 4-year PFS approximately 50% to 65% versus 0% to 30%). Another group retrospectively examined the outcomes following intensive therapy compared with CHOP-R in 53 patients with aggressive B-cell lymphoma with high-grade features with or without an *MYC* translocation.[335] Notably, patients in this study had a lower risk than is typical for B-UNC/BL/DLBCL. Amongst all patients, there was no improvement in OS with intensive regimens (4-year OS of 50% to 60%); this relatively good OS is widely different from previous reports and perhaps reflects the good risk profile of this cohort. However, among patients with an *MYC* translocation, intensive regimens resulted in a significantly longer PFS and a trend toward longer OS over CHOP-R, and, for double-hit lymphomas in this category, there was a nonsignificant trend toward a shorter PFS and OS compared with patients with an isolated MYC translocation. This suggests that perhaps it is the double-hit lymphomas within the category of B-UNC/BL/DLBCL that drives their poor prognosis, and these are patients that might benefit from intensive chemotherapy like modified Magrath or DA-EPOCH-R. Data from patients with MYC translocation-positive DLBCL treated with DA-EPOCH-R by the National Cancer Institute phase 2 studies are promising; nine patients (8%) harbored an *MYC* translocation and had a 4-year EFS of 83%.[339] This regimen is currently being explored further in BL and MYC translocation-positive DLBCL in a multicenter trial.

At the present time, there is not sufficient evidence to suggest that all patients with B-UNC/BL/DLBCL should be treated with regimens more intense than CHOP-R. This is a heterogenous group of patients with varied prognoses and natural histories, some of whom may do well with standard CHOP-R. However, for double-hit lymphomas, many of which are B-UNC/BL/DLBCL, CHOP-R is insufficient. These patients should be encouraged to participate in clinical trials. In the absence of a trial, intensified regimens of DA-EPOCH-R or modified Magrath, with or without an ASCT or alloSCT, can be considered. Agents that target BCL2 and an MYC-driven protein, aurora A kinase, are currently in development and may prove useful in these lymphomas; these patients should be considered for clinical trials when available.

B-Cell Lymphoma, Unclassifiable, with Features Intermediate Between DLBCL and Classical Hodgkin's Lymphoma

An overlap between the clinical and pathologic features of PMLBCL and cHL has been recognized for some time. Both typically occur in younger female patients, involve contiguous nodal stations, and on biopsy, demonstrate a variable number of malignant B cells within a fibrotic inflammatory infiltrate. In 2003, two groups explored GEPs of newly diagnosed PMLBCL, DLBCL, and cHL and found that the GEP of PMLBCL more closely resembled cHL than DLBCL.[329,340] Specifically, PMLBCL had a low expression of genes involved in B-cell receptor signaling but a high expression of genes involved in IL-13 receptor signaling as well as immunomodulatory genes such as *PDL1* and *PDL2*. In addition, both cHL and PMLBCL are associated with amplification of 9p24.1, which contains the genes for *JAK2* and *PDL1*, and this correlated with increased PD-L1 expression.[341] The recognition of some lymphomas with features intermediate between PMLBCL and cHL, or B-UNC/cHL/DLBCL, further supports the pathologic relationship between these two malignancies.

Among patients with B-UNC/cHL/DLBCL, the majority are men, with presentations in the mediastinum. Histopathologically, one sees pleomorphic tumor cells resembling both the Hodgkin Reed-Sternberg (HRS) cell of cHL and the large, atypical B cell of DLBCL or PMLBCL. These cells appear in sheets, separated by fibrotic stroma with an associated inflammatory infiltrate. Immunohistochemical profiles of the malignant cells demonstrate frequent positivity for CD45, CD20, CD79a, and CD30, but are often CD15 negative; other B-cell markers like PAX5, organic cation transporter 2 (OCT-2), and BOB1 are often positive. Methylation profiling reveals a profile intermediate between that of PMLBCL and cHL, corroborating that it is distinct, perhaps on a continuum between the two.[342] Interestingly, patients can have composite lymphomas in which DLBCL and cHL present sequentially; whether these lymphomas relate to B-UNC/cHL/DLBCL is unknown. However, the methylation profiles of both components of a single case of a composite lymphoma were most similar to that of B-UNC/cHL/DLBCL, suggesting that they are related.

The prognosis is notably poorer in B-UNC/cHL/DLBCL than in cHL or PMLBCL.[343] This is partly due to differences in pathobiology, but may also result from not knowing whether to treat with an NHL or a cHL regimen. There are no large prospective studies, but consensus has favored treating like NHL. There are single-arm studies demonstrating good activity of CHOP in HL, making CHOP-R an acceptable first-line therapy.[344,345] More recently, 16 patients with B-UNC/cHL/DLBCL were treated with DA-EPOCH-R, and 4-year EFS and OS was only 45% and 75%, respectively.[339] This regimen, however, was more effective in PMLBCL, where the 5-year EFS and OS were 93% and 97%, respectively.[331] Following combination chemotherapy, the role of involved field radiation therapy (IFRT) in both cHL and PMLBCL is debated. Despite frequently presenting with bulky mediastinal disease, patients with PMLBCL enjoy a favorable prognosis, with a 5-year OS >80% following CHOP-R and 97% following DA-EPOCH-R. Whether to radiate patients who achieve a complete metabolic response following CHOP-R is uncertain, but radiation was omitted in such cases in the DA-EPOCH-R series. The only published randomized trial of radiotherapy for this disease was stopped early due to increased relapses in the nonradiated group at the interim analysis; all patients on this study had a complete response to CHOP-R.[346] A large randomized clinical trial is ongoing in Europe to decidedly answer this question. Despite the lack of evidence supporting RT in patients who have a complete response to chemotherapy with B-UNC/cHL/DLBCL, many are referred for radiation given their worse prognosis.

Burkitt's Lymphoma

Burkitt's lymphoma is a rare disease in adults, comprising less than 1% of adult NHLs, whereas BL constitutes 30% of nonendemic pediatric lymphomas.[347]

Pathology

BL cells resemble the small noncleaved cells within normal GCs of secondary lymphoid follicles. The mitotic rate is high, and analogous to normal GCs, frequent tingible body macrophages are seen, producing the classical *starry sky* appearance. The fraction of Ki-67 positive (proliferating cells) in BL is typically 99% or greater.[64]

Immunophenotype and Genetics

BL is a tumor of B-lineage derivation identified by the expression of CD19, CD20, sIgM, CD10, and BCL6, but not BCL2.[348] Endemic BLs are EBV positive, whereas the majority of non-endemic BLs are EBV negative. BL is associated with a translocation involving MYC on chromosome 8q24 in over 95% of the cases. The most common partners are chromosomes 14, 2, or 22, rearrangements that produce fusions of MYC with either the IgH (80%), kappa (15%), or lambda (5%) light chain genes. The breakpoints in MYC and IgH differ in endemic versus sporadic BL. MYC translocation is absent in <5% of cases, so-called atypical BL.[44] These cases are otherwise typical of BL, and share a characteristic GEP with cases of BL that are associated with MYC rearrangements.[333,349,350]

Clinical Features

BL is, in general, a pediatric tumor that has three major clinical presentations. The endemic (African) form presents as a jaw or facial bone tumor that spreads to extranodal sites, including the ovary, the testis, the kidney, the breast, and especially to the bone marrow and meninges. The nonendemic form has an abdominal presentation with massive disease, ascites, and renal, testis, and/or ovarian involvement, and, like the endemic form, also spreads to the bone marrow and CNS. Immunodeficiency-related cases more often involve lymph nodes and may present as acute leukemia. BL has a male predominance and is typically seen in patients less than 35 years of age.

Treatment

BL in adults has been similarly treated with regimens designed for pediatric populations. CHOP with intrathecal methotrexate should be considered insufficient treatment. Short, intensive therapy with CNS prophylaxis is the standard approach.[338,351] The original Magrath regimen (CODOX-M/IVAC) had a 92% 2-year OS.[352] Other, more recent series with this regimen in older patients have reported a 2-year OS of 82% for low-risk patients and 70% for high-risk patients.[353,354] Similar results have been seen with HyperCVAD rituximab-methotrexate-cytarabine.[355] A recent study of DA-EPOCH-R for six to eight cycles (two cycles past complete response) reported outstanding results with freedom from progression (FFP) of 95% and OS of 100% at a median follow-up of 86 months.[356] There is presently no evidence that first remission autologous transplant is indicated for adult BL.[357] The outcome for relapsed patients is dismal, with adults rarely cured with ASCT.[358]

MATURE T-CELL AND NATURAL KILLER CELL NEOPLASMS

Mycosis Fungoides

For a discussion of mycosis fungoides, see Chapter 40.

Peripheral T-Cell Lymphomas, Not Otherwise Specified

Peripheral T-cell lymphomas (PTCL) includes a number of entities, which constitute 15% of all NHLs in adults.[359] PTCL, not otherwise specified (NOS), comprising 6% of all NHLs, is the term used for cases that are not other entities defined in the WHO classification (e.g., ALCL).

Pathology

Features of PTCL, NOS vary widely and lack findings typical of other specific subtypes of PTCL. Lymph nodes are diffusely effaced by atypical lymphoid cells, which may include a spectrum of cell sizes or may be comprised mainly of large cells. The tumor cells may induce some degree of vascular proliferation and may be associated with varied stromal and host cell responses, sometimes including prominent infiltrates composed of eosinophils and/or macrophages. Mitoses, apoptosis, and geographic necrosis may also be seen.

Immunophenotype and Genetics

In contrast to B-cell lymphomas, the pattern of expression of T-cell surface antigens is variable. The normal cellular counterparts of PTCL NOS are mature peripheral T cells. T-cell-associated antigens are expressed (CD3+/−, CD2+/−).[360] CD4 is more often more expressed than CD8 and tumors may be CD4−/CD8−. In most cases, one or more "mature" T-cell antigens are lost, such as CD5 or CD7. TCR genes are usually rearranged. The most common translocations are t(7;14), t(11;14), inv(14), and t(14;14)—translocations that involve TCR genes.

Clinical Features

Peripheral T-cell lymphoma NOS[326] are aggressive NHLs, presenting with a median age of 65 years, with 69% of patients having stage III/IV disease. Both nodal and extranodal sites are common, including the skin, the liver, the spleen, and other viscera. B symptoms and pruritus are commonly seen. Laboratory abnormalities, including eosinophilia and hemophagocytic syndrome, are features of PTCL NOS.

Treatment

For PTCL NOS, most studies failed to show any advantage for regimens other than CHOP. A retrospective subset analysis of a phase 3 study in PTCL patients of CHOP versus CHOEP showed a significant improvement in EFS for PTCL patients younger than age 60 years with a normal LDH at diagnosis, but there was no difference in OS.[361] Various prognostic models for PTCL NOS have evolved, but generally, the IPI provides a reasonable stratification of outcome, with low-risk patients having a 55% 2-year OS and high-risk patients having a less than 15% 2-year OS.[361] ASCT has been applied to patients with PTCL NOS in first remission with approximately 50% 3- to 5-year PFS and OS. Given the generally unfavorable outcome for patients with PTCL NOS, clinical trials should be considered.

Recurrent disease is associated with very poor prognosis, with the median second PFS and OS after relapse of 4.6 and 6.7 months, respectively.[362] Conventional agents such as gemcitabine have limited activity.[363] Several FDA-approved drugs for relapsed PTCL, including the antifolate agent pralatrexate and HDAC inhibitors romidepsin and belinostat, all of which have a 25% to 30% RR with median durations of response of less than 18 months.[364,365] Nonmyeloablative alloSCT has a role for selected patients with 5-year OS and PFS of 50% and 40%, respectively, and nonrelapsed mortality of 12%.[366]

Angioimmunoblastic T-Cell Lymphoma

Angioimmunoblastic T-cell lymphoma (AITL) constitutes 4% of all NHLs and about 20% all T-cell NHLs.

Pathology and Genetics

Lymph nodes are diffusely effaced by a polymorphous population of lymphocytes of varying size, shape, and immunoblasts. Stains for CD21, CD23, and CD35 reveal an expanded network of follicular dendritic cells, which often surround tumor cells with moderately abundant clear cytoplasm. The neoplastic cells resemble normal CD4-positive follicular T cells, and in addition to expression of pan–T-cell markers such as CD3, often express CXCL13, PD-1, CD10, and BCL6. Immunoblasts in the background are often EBV-positive B cells, which expand in this disease and may give rise to secondary EBV-positive B-cell lymphomas. Trisomy 3 and/or 5 may occur.[367] Deep sequencing has revealed mutations in about 50% of cases in ten-eleven translocation 2 (*TET2*), an epigenetic modifier previously implicated in myelodysplastic syndromes.[368] Around 33% of PCTL NOS were also found to have *TET2* mutations in the same study; many of these tumors had some features reminiscent of AITL, suggesting that there is an overlap between these two disease categories.

Clinical Features

AITL presents in patients with a median age of 62 years. Often, there is acute onset of generalized lymphadenopathy, hepatomegaly, fever, B symptoms, skin rash with a lymphohistiocytic infiltrate, and autoimmune phenomenon, including polyarthritis, thyroid dysfunction, and hemolytic anemia. Laboratory study abnormalities include eosinophilia, polyclonal hypergammaglobulinemia, elevated serum LDH, anemia, and a positive Coombs test. Bone marrow involvement is common, with over 80% of patients having stage III or IV disease. The median survival ranges from 15 to 36 months, with patients dying of relapse, secondary EBV-positive DLBCL, or opportunistic infection.

Treatment

Up to one-third of patients with AITL can have spontaneous remissions or initial remissions to corticosteroids alone. AITL is approached similarly to PTCL NOS, with combination chemotherapy regimens such as CHOP and followed by autologous SCT in first remission is an option for younger patients based on phase 2 studies. For relapsed disease, the options are similar to PTCL NOS, except few responses to pralatrexate were seen.

Enteropathy-Associated T-Cell Lymphoma

Enteropathy-associated T-cell lymphoma (EATL) is a rare aggressive disease of intraepithelial T cells that is often associated with a history of gluten enteropathy.[370,371] The more common type 1 is associated with clinical or serologic evidence of celiac disease and HLADQA1*0501, DQB1*0201 genotype.[372] Treatment of celiac disease with a gluten-free diet prevents the development of lymphoma.[370] Type II EATL is not associated celiac disease and is now considered not to be an EATL.

Pathology

Two variants have been described: type I and type II. Type I EATL is grossly characterized by diffuse infiltration of the bowel wall by an atypical lymphoid infiltrate that often produces mucosal ulcerations, sometimes accompanied by tumorous masses. The morphology of the tumor cells varies, but often they are large and have anaplastic features. In cases associated with celiac sprue, adjacent mucosa may show a dense infiltrate of small intraepithelial lymphocytes associated with villous atrophy. These cells may have the same TCR rearrangement as the large tumor cell population, suggesting that they represent a precursor lesion to EATL that arises in the setting of long-standing celiac disease. Type II EATL is not associated with celiac disease and may represent a different entity.

Immunophenotype and Genetics

Type I EATL cells express CD3 and CD103, an integrin expressed on intestinal lymphocytes. The tumor cells may be CD4 positive (11%), CD8 positive (43%), or CD4/CD8 double negative, and some cases are CD30 positive as well. Type II EATL cells are positive for CD8 and CD56.[373] Of type I and II cases, 50% to 60% have amplifications of the 9q31.3 region. A distinct feature of type II EATL is amplification of *MYC* due to copy gains of chromosome 8q24.

Clinical Features and Therapy

Patients with EATL present with intestinal obstruction, perforation, and bleeding. In some patients, there is a brief history of gluten sensitivity or worsening gluten enteropathy. Uncommonly, there is extraintestinal disease with dissemination to the lungs or skin. The small bowel is the most common site of disease, with the stomach or colon affected less often, whereas other viscera, the lung, the skin, or soft tissues may also be involved.[371] These patients have a very poor prognosis, with a median survival of 10 months. Surgery for limited-stage disease cures a small number of patients. Intensive induction with combination chemotherapy, including high-dose methotrexate, and autologous SCT in first remission, may yield better outcomes than chemotherapy alone.[374]

Anaplastic Large-Cell Lymphoma

ALCL constitutes 2% of all NHLs, but is the third most common T-cell NHL. ALCL is more frequent in children, representing 10% of all pediatric lymphomas. It is a heterogeneous disease category with several molecular and clinicopathologic subtypes. One of these unusual forms arises within the breast in association with breast implants.[375]

Pathology

Several morphologic variants of ALCL are recognized. The most common (80%) are composed of large cells with round or horseshoe-shaped or embryoid nuclei with multiple (or single) prominent nucleoli, which are referred to as *hallmark* cells. These cells have abundant cytoplasm, which gives them an epithelioid or histiocyte-like appearance. The remaining morphologies, which are most commonly seen in children, are the small-cell, lymphohistiocytic, and monomorphic variants. Tumor cells may preferentially localize within the sinuses of lymph nodes, producing an appearance that can be mistaken for metastatic solid tumors.

Immunophenotype and Genetics

Virtually all cases are CD30 positive. Over 60% of cases express CD3, CD25, CD43, or CD45RO, and many cases are CD4 positive. Unlike classical HL, ALCL cells usually lack CD15. A minority do not express B- or T-cell antigens, and up to 40% of cases may fail to express the common leukocyte antigen (CD45). TCR genes are clonally rearranged in most cases, but some tumors (particularly those that fail to express T-cell markers) apparently lack TCR rearrangements. Rearrangements involving the *ALK* gene are present in 40% to 60% of cases, more commonly in children and younger adults. The most common rearrangement is the t(2;5), which fuses a portion of the nucleolar protein nucleophosmin-1 (*NPM1*) gene on chromosome 5q35 to a portion of *ALK* on chromosome 2p23.[376] The resulting fusion gene encodes a chimeric *NPM–ALK* fusion protein with constitutive tyrosine-kinase activity. Immunohistochemistry for ALK can be used to reliably identify cases associated with *ALK* gene rearrangements.

Clinical Features

ALCL encompasses at least three distinct clinicopathologic entities: primary systemic ALCL, ALK positive; primary systemic ALCL, ALK negative; and primary cutaneous ALCL. Systemic ALCL, regardless of ALK status, may present in lymph nodes or extranodal sites, including but not limited to the skin. Primary cutaneous ALCL is morphologically similar to systemic ALCL but lacks ALK expression or rearrangements, and is by definition restricted to the skin at diagnosis (see Chapter 40). ALCL has a male predominance, with a median age of 34 years for ALK-positive disease, and 58 years for ALK-negative disease.[377] Except for age, there is no difference in clinical presentations of ALK-positive and ALK-negative systemic disease. Patients with systemic disease often present with B symptoms, peripheral and retroperitoneal adenopathy, and skin involvement (25% of patients). Although marrow involvement is infrequent, 60% of patients have stage III or IV disease.

Treatment

Generally, ALCL has been treated with combination chemotherapy, largely CHOP. A subset analysis of the randomized CHOP versus CHOEP trial in patients less than age 60 years with normal LDH, found superior outcome with CHOEP (90% versus 55% OS).[361] Compared to other peripheral T-cell NHLs, ALCL has the highest 5-year OS, driven by the IPI score and the expression of ALK, with ALK-positive disease associated with a favorable prognosis,[378,379] with 8-year OS of 82% versus only 49% in ALK disease. The major impact of ALK expression was seen in patients age 40 years or greater.[380] For relapsed patients, options include SCT following reinduction therapy. The anti-CD30 antibody drug conjugate brentuximab vedotin (anti-CD30 monomethyl auristatin E [MMAE] antitubulin conjugate) is highly active,[381] with an overall RR of 86%, and a CR rate of 57%, with the median duration of CR of 13 months. Brentuximab is being examined in the initial treatment of ALCL. Crizotinib, an inhibitor of the ALK tyrosine kinase, has reported activity in relapsed disease.[382]

Hepatosplenic T-Cell Lymphoma

Hepatosplenic T-cell lymphoma is an extremely rare disease of cytotoxic T cells.

Pathology

The tumor cells infiltrate the red pulp of the spleen and liver sinusoids as well as the bone marrow, although this can be subtle. Cells are medium sized with round nuclei, moderately condensed chromatin, and moderately abundant pale cytoplasm.

Immunophenotype and Genetics

The tumor cells are CD2+, CD3+, variably CD8+, CD7+, and CD56+. In contrast to most PTCL, which generally express the αβ T-cell receptor, these tumors commonly express γδ T-cell receptor. Isochromosome 7q and trisomy 8 have been reported in many cases, and these tumors are genetically distinct from other PTCL.[383]

Clinical Features and Treatment

Hepatosplenic T-cell lymphoma is an extremely rare disease presenting in adolescents and young adults, with a male predominance. Features include marked hepatosplenomegaly, often with marrow involvement, and occasionally, peripheral blood involvement and pancytopenia.[384,385] Of patients, 10% to 20% occur in immunosuppressed, solid-organ allograft recipients and in patients with Crohn's disease on thiopurines.[386] This is an aggressive disease, which usually relapses after the initial response to chemotherapy. The median survival is 1 to 2 years, with rare patients being long-term survivors after alloSCT.

Subcutaneous Panniculitis-Like T-Cell Lymphoma

Subcutaneous panniculitis-like T-cell lymphoma is a rare T-cell NHL of cytotoxic CD8+ T cells presenting with subcutaneous nodules.[387] This entity represents less than 1% of all NHLs.

Pathology

The cellular infiltrates are found in the subcutaneous fat and generally spare the overlying skin. This consists of an infiltrate of small, medium, and large atypical lymphocytes that infiltrate fat lobules, often forming rims around individual adipocytes. Cells express CD3 and CD8, and are usually negative for CD4 and CD56. Cytotoxic granules containing granzyme B, T cell intercellular antigen 1 (TIA-1) and perforin are also present. Most cases express αβ TCRs, but a subset expresses γδ TCRs instead. Like other PTCLs, there is often an aberrant immunophenotype marked by loss of one or more T-cell antigens (e.g., CD2, CD5, CD7). Clonal T-cell receptor rearrangements are present, but no specific cytogenetic abnormalities for this disease have been reported.

Clinical Features

This disease affects females more than males, with an age ranging from 40 to 60 years. The disease is localized to the skin with extremely uncommon involvement of other sites, including lymph nodes or bone marrow. The disease can wax and wane, and many patients' disease behaves like cutaneous T-cell NHLs, with a 5-year OS of 82%. Hemophagocytic lymphohistiocytosis (HLH) is reported in 17% of patients, and is associated with much lower 5-year survival (46 versus 91%). Patients with HLH merit combination chemotherapy and should be considered for SCT.

Extranodal Natural Killer/T-Cell Lymphomas, Nasal Type

Extranodal NK/T-cell lymphoma, nasal type, is an extranodal lymphoma usually presenting in the upper aerodigestive tract with occasional extranodal sites. This is a malignancy of NK cells that is generally EBV positive, with some cases of cytotoxic T-cell origin. This disease is rare in the United States and Europe, but is much more common in Asia (Hong Kong) and native populations in Peru.[388]

Pathology

Extranodal NK/T-cell lymphoma, nasal type, has widely varying cytologic features, but usually consists of a proliferation of a mixture of small and atypical lymphoid cells. The most characteristic features are prominent vascular invasion associated with fibrinoid necrosis of vessels walls and infarction of surrounding tissues.[3,389] In touch preparations, cytoplasmic azurophilic granules may be seen in the neoplastic cells.

Immunophenotype and Genetics

The cells express CD2, CD56, and cytoplasmic CD3 and are generally negative for CD4, CD8, TCR, and surface CD3. The T-cell receptor and Ig genes are usually germ line. EBV genomes are present in virtually all cases. There is loss of heterozygosity at 6q and 13q, with frequent overexpression of p53 and/or TP53 mutations.

Clinical Features

The extranodal NK/T-cell lymphomas, nasal type are rare, typically presenting in males with an average age of 60 years. The vast majority of patients have localized disease with nasal obstruction and a destructive mass involving the nose sinuses and palate. Stage I disease is present in 81% of patients, and stage II disease in 17% of patients.[390] B symptoms are uncommon. Although uncommon, other extranasal sites include: the intestines (37%), the skin (26%), the testis (17%), the lung (14%), the eye or soft tissue (9% each), the adrenal gland (6%), the brain (6%), and the breast or tongue (3% each). Patients with extranasal disease have higher stage, elevated LDH, bulky disease, and a poor performance status. Extranasal disease is associated with a worse prognosis than the nasal subtype for both early and late stage disease.[390] A prognostic index for NK/T-cell lymphoma has been developed with the factors including B symptoms, stage III or IV disease, elevated LDH, and lymph node involvement.[391] CNS risk is increased in patients with three or four factors (10%) compared with less than 2% of those with one or two features.[392] The EBV viral load at diagnosis and end of therapy is predictive of PFS and OS.[393]

Treatment

Overall, patients with stage IE/IIE have a 5-year DFS of 59%. The 5-year OS and PFS for patients with stage IE disease is 78% and 63%, respectively, and for stage IIE, the OS and PFS is 46% and 40%, respectively. In this series, there was no difference between combined modality and RT alone.[390,395] For patients with stage IE/IIE, early use of radiotherapy (50 to 55 Gy) is critical to optimal treatment. This is usually delivered with IMRT, a technique that allows for a reduction of dose to critical organs such as the eyes. This technique often uses treatment planning that fuses the MRI with the planning CT scan for optimal delineation of the tumor volume. Patients who received initial treatment with RT followed by chemotherapy had superior CR and OS rates as compared to patients who received chemotherapy before RT. Patients with stage II to IV disease generally have a very poor prognosis with relapses in other extranodal sites. More recent studies suggest that combined modality treatment may yield more favorable results. Phase 2 trials of concurrent RT and weekly cisplatin followed by three cycles of etoposide, ifosfamide, cisplatin, and dexamethasone reported overall RR of 83% and 3-year PFS and OS of 85% and 86%, respectively.[396-399] For disseminated NK/T-cell lymphoma, only 30% of patients achieve a CR with CHOP chemotherapy with median OS of 4.3 months.[390] Regimens with L-asparaginase have shown promising results in relapsed disease.[400,401] The regimen SMILE (dexamethasone, methotrexate, ifosfamide, L-asparaginase, and etoposide) in disseminated disease has an ORR of 79%, with 45% CRs. The 1-year PFS and OS of 53% and 55%, respectively, have been reported.[402]

Adult T-Cell Leukemia/Lymphoma

ATLL is a highly aggressive disease that is associated with infection by the HTLV-1 in 100% of cases.[403-405] This virus is endemic in southern Japan, the Caribbean basin, western Africa, the Southeastern United States and northeast Iran. The virus predominantly spreads by breast milk, and may be transmitted through sexual exposure and/or blood transfusion. The disease has a long clinical latency period, suggesting that HTLV-1 may not be sufficient for disease. The risk of developing ATLL following infection with HTLV-1 is estimated to be 4%. HTLV-1 causes an ATLL-like disease in severe combined immune deficiency (SCID) mice.[406]

Pathology

Lymph nodes are diffusely effaced by an atypical lymphoid infiltrate that preferentially involves T-cell zones and the medulla. The most characteristic morphologic feature is seen in the peripheral blood, where the circulating tumor cells often have multilobated nuclear contours, referred to as a *sunflower* or *starburst* appearance.

Immunophenotype and Genetics

ATLL is a tumor of CD4+ T cell, expressing CD2, CD3, CD5, CD25, but lacking CD7. The uniformly high levels of CD25 and variable expression of the transcription factor FOXO1 has led to the suggestion that this may be a tumor of Tregs. Deletions at 6q, trisomy 3, and monosomy X and Y are common, but key genetic events associated with ATLL development are largely unknown.

Clinical Features

The median age of ATLL patients is 60 years, with a male predominance.[406,407] There are several variants of the disease: acute (60% of patients), lymphomatous (20% of patients), chronic (15% of patients), and smoldering (5% of patients), with median survivals of 6 months, 10 months, 24 months, and not yet reached, respectively.[408] The chronic form can evolve into the acute type. Patients present with bone marrow and peripheral blood involvement, high white blood cell count, hypercalcemia (due to parathyroid hormone [PTH]-related protein, transforming growth factor beta [TGF-β], and receptor activator of NF-κB [RANK] ligand), lytic bone lesions, lymphadenopathy, hepatosplenomegaly, skin lesions resembling cutaneous T-cell lymphoma, and interstitial pulmonary infiltrates. Opportunistic infections can also accompany the clinical presentation, including pneumocystis, cryptococcus meningitis, strongyloides, and disseminated herpes zoster.[409]

Therapy

ATLL is generally approached with intensive multiagent chemotherapy regimens.[410,411] Antiviral therapy with zidovudine and interferon-α should be considered upfront for the smoldering, chronic subtype. A retrospective analysis of 116 patients suggested an improved survival with interferon-α and zidovudine antiviral therapy for acute, chronic, and smoldering subtypes, whereas patients with the lymphomatous type experienced a better outcome with first-line chemotherapy.[411,412] For the acute leukemia lymphoma type, a phase 3 randomized trial of 118 patients[413] reported that an intensive regimen vincristine, cyclophosphamide, doxorubicin, and prednisone, VCAP; doxorubicin, ranimustine, and prednisone, AMP; and vindesine, etoposide, carboplatin, and prednisone, VECP (VCAP-AMP-VECP) had a significantly higher CR rate but no difference in overall RR than CHOP-14 with intrathecal methotrexate. The 3-year OS was 24% with VCAP-AMP-VECP, but only 13% with CHOP. Based on expression of the CCR4 chemokine receptor on ATLL cells, mogamulizumab, an anti-CCR4 mAb is being investigated in combination with chemotherapy.[414] With the poor results of chemotherapy, both myeloablative and reduced intensity alloSCT has been applied to ATLL, with limited success.[415-417]

Primary Central Nervous System Lymphoma

Primary CNS lymphoma is the subject of Chapter 41.

Central Nervous System Prophylaxis for Aggressive Lymphomas

Prophylaxis for the development of CNS disease in DLBCL is highly controversial. Several sites of disease, including the testis, the ovary, bone marrow, the breast, the epidural space, and paranasal sinuses, have been reported to be associated with a high risk of CNS dissemination. A high-intermediate or high IPI score and multiple extranodal sites are also risk factors. Patients with BCLU BL/DLBCL, as well as patients with *double-hit* cytogenetics, are at increased risk. In a retrospective analysis of aggressive NHLs, in the pre-rituximab era, the cumulative risk of CNS involvement was 2.8%. Intraparenchymal and intraspinal disease occurred in 66%, whereas isolated leptomeningeal disease was seen in only 26%. Eighty percent of CNS relapses occurred on or within 6 months of completing chemotherapy, suggesting a subclinical disease at diagnosis. In the current period of chemoimmunotherapy, it remains controversial if the addition of rituximab lowers the risk of CNS disease.[418] With the significant number of parenchymal relapses, intrathecal chemotherapy alone may be inadequate prophylaxis, making high-dose methotrexate a potentially more effective therapy. However, there is no compelling evidence that high-dose methotrexate is superior to the intrathecal route.

Lymphoma in Children

See Chapter 36 for a discussion of lymphomas in children.

Posttransplant Lymphoproliferative Disorders

Posttransplant lymphoproliferative disorders (PTLD) are a common and significant complication following solid organ transplantation, occurring in up to 10% of adult patients.[419] PTLD is less commonly seen after alloSCT. They constitute a heterogeneous collection of diagnoses ranging from early lesions, with reactive plasmacytic hyperplasia, to polymorphic PTLD, with polyclonal or monoclonal expansion of atypical lymphoid cells, to monomorphic PTLD, with lymphoma histopathology and immunophenotype.[332] They differ from nontransplant-related adult lymphomas in that they tend to be extranodal, high grade, and have an aggressive clinical course with a mortality often exceeding 50%.

PTLD following hematopoietic SCT is usually a malignancy of donor lymphoid cells, whereas PTLD following solid organ transplantation is traditionally thought to be of recipient origin in the majority of cases, although donor-derived cases have been reported and typically involve the grafted organ. In both PTLD following hematopoietic and solid organ transplantation, over 80% of PTLDs are of B-cell origin.[420] PTLD following solid organ transplantation can occur early, within the first year following transplant, or late, at 1 year or greater from transplantation. Early PTLD is much more common, with an incidence of 224 per 100,000 that falls to 54 per 100,000 by the second year. Over 90% of early onset B-cell PTLDs are EBV positive, whereas over 50% of late onset B-cell PTLD are EBV negative.[421] Immunosuppression following solid organ transplantation, however, results in a loss of EBV-specific cytotoxic T cells allowing for growth and acquisition of additional mutations in EBV-transformed B cells, such as alterations in MYC, BCL6, TP53, and DNA hypermethylation.[422]

EBV serologic status before transplant, as well as the degree and type of immunosuppression following transplant, are risks of developing PTLD. EBV-naïve patients pretransplant and younger patients have higher risk of PTLD.[423] The nature of immunosuppression is also related to risk. The use of anti–T-cell mAbs, tacrolimus, and multiple immunosuppressive agents are associated with increased risk.

The incidence of PTLD varies with the type of organ being transplanted; in adult patients, this ranges from 1% to 3% of kidney and liver transplants, from 1% to 6% of heart transplants, from 2% to 6% of heart–lung transplants, from 4% to 10% of lung transplants, and up to 20% of small bowel transplants.[424]

Antiviral agents have been studied in both the treatment and prophylaxis settings. For treatment, no study has demonstrated a clear benefit, although they may have some efficacy in early or polymorphic disease.[19] Antiviral therapy (ganciclovir) may decrease PTLD in high-risk EBV-seronegative patients.[425] The other strategy for early intervention is to monitor EBV viral load. EBV viral load has been shown to be significantly increased in patients who develop PTLD.[426] The use of a rising or increased viral load to alter clinical practice has been investigated following hematopoietic SCT, with a reduction in immunosuppression and/or preemptive therapy with rituximab or EBV cytotoxic T cells.[427] But this has not yet translated into studies investigating preemptive changes in clinical management in the solid organ transplant setting.

Pathology

The histologic appearance of PTLD is highly variable. The WHO classification system includes the following categories: (1) early lesions, reactive plasmacytic hyperplasia, and infectious mononucleosis-like; (2) polymorphic PTLD, infectious mononucleosis-like appearance with architectural effacement and tissue destruction; (3) monomorphic PTLD (classified according to lymphoma classification schemes), including DLBCL, BL, multiple myeloma, plasmacytoma, PTCL NOS, other types of T-cell lymphoma; and HL and Hodgkin's-like lymphomas.[44]

Clinical Presentation and Prognosis

PTLDs present as both nodal and extranodal disease. CNS involvement was reported in 22% of PTLDs. Other common extranodal sites include the lung and GI tract, which may be associated with a better prognosis. In solid organ transplants of the heart, lung, and liver, the allograft is reported to be the site of disease in 22% of cases. Survival statistics in PTLD are variable, owing to the heterogeneity of the diagnosis, ranging from early lesions to monomorphic PTLD, and to advances in therapy. Median 1-year and 5-year survival are approximately 50% to 60% and 30% to 40%, respectively, depending on the type of organ transplanted. Reported median OS is 20 to 30 months.[428,429] The IPI for aggressive NHLs has been applied to PTLD with limited utility. Other prognostic models for PTLD have been developed with risk factors being age ≥60 years, eastern cooperative oncology group (ECOG PS ≥2, and elevated LDH.[430] Low (zero risk factors), intermediate (one risk factor), and high-risk (two to three risk factors) groups had 2-year OS rates of 88%, 50%, and 0%, respectively.

Therapy

There are no established treatment recommendations for PTLD given the heterogeneity of the diagnosis, from pathology to prognosis, and the general lack of prospective, randomized studies in the field. As we have learned more about the varied natural history of the different diseases and their risk and prognostic factors, therapy can now be better tailored to the individual patient. For instance, a stepwise approach to therapy is often indicated for patients with either early lesions or polymorphic disease, starting with a reduction in immunosuppression with or without the addition of antiviral therapy, to single-agent rituximab, to chemoimmunotherapy if indicated. This typically involves a 25% to 50% reduction in cyclosporine and tacrolimus and discontinuation of azathioprine and mycophenolate mofetil.[431]

For patients with monomorphic disease, the initial reduction in immunosuppression is typically accompanied by the addition of rituximab with or without chemotherapy, depending on the aggressiveness and histopathology of the disease.[432] RRs to rituximab alone range from 44% to 79%.[433] The PFS and OS at a follow-up of 27.5 months in these studies range from 42% to 47%, respectively. Patients with higher risk, more aggressive monomorphic disease are treated with sequentially dosed rituximab followed by CHOP with encouraging results with an overall RR of 90% (68% complete).[434,435]

Antiviral therapy has been investigated in more resistant disease. The combination of arginine butyrate, an activator of latently infected lymphoma cells via the induction of EBV thymidine kinase, has been combined with ganciclovir with encouraging results in limited number of patients treated. SCT has anecdotal experience in refractory patients. EBV-specific allogeneic T-cell lines may also have a role in refractory disease.[436]

HIV–Associated Non-Hodgkin's Lymphoma

Aggressive NHLs are AIDS-defining malignancies. AIDS-related NHL occurs in three broad categories: systemic lymphoma, which represents about 85% of all lymphomas; primary CNS lymphoma, accounting for 15% of all lymphomas; and primary effusion or body cavity lymphomas, which are rare.[44] The breakdown of histologic subtypes includes DLBCL (75%); BL (20%); plasmablastic lymphoma (less than 5%); T-cell lymphoma (1% to 3%); and indolent B-cell lymphomas (less than 10%). About 30% of AIDS-related lymphomas have deregulation of the bcl-6 gene and a similar number have c-myc abnormalities. Approximately 60% of cases have abnormalities of p53.[437] The pathogenesis is analogous to PTLD, with EBV infection playing a major role in HIV-associated NHLs.[438] An HHV-8 infection is associated with primary effusion lymphoma.[5] The risk factors for developing lymphoma include depressed CD4 count, high HIV viral load, and a lack of effective antiretroviral therapy. Other risks include a lack of the CCR5-32 deletion.

Systemic AIDS-related NHLs are generally highly aggressive diseases.[439] Besides nodal disease, extranodal disease is exceedingly common, with GI tract, skin and soft tissues, liver, lung, heart, as well as bone marrow and CNS involvement (in 5% to 20% of cases). B symptoms are also common presenting symptoms.

Plasmablastic lymphoma is a rare subtype of large B-cell NHL.[440] The cells have plasmacytoid cytoplasmic features like plasma cells, but often have large nuclei with large single nucleoli. The malignant cells express plasma cell markers (e.g., CD38, CD138, MUM1) and often lack pan–B-cell markers (e.g., CD20, CD79a). This disease was originally described as oropharyngeal plasmablastic lymphomas that occur most frequently in HIV-positive individuals and are often EBV positive. An identical tumor can also occur in other immunodeficiency states. Plasmablastic lymphoma is a very aggressive disease with a poor prognosis.

Primary effusion lymphomas (PEL) present in fluid collections in the pleura, the peritoneum, or the pericardium, or, more rarely, in the CSF.[441] Solid tumor variants of PEL occur rarely in the GI tract. The PEL cells are large and pleomorphic, often lack CD20 and CD19, but may be CD79a+ and CD45+; they also often express CD30 and CD138. They are uniformly associated with Kaposi's sarcoma herpesvirus/HHV-8, and most tumors are coinfected with HHV-8 and EBV. Both plasmablastic lymphomas and PELs rarely occur in nonimmunocompromised hosts.

Presently, more than 50% of patients with AIDS-related lymphoma have long-term DFS. By histology, patients with HL have about a 70% long-term OS, patients with DLBCL and BL around 50%, and patients with primary CNS lymphoma the lowest at 20% to 25%.[351] Treatment for AIDS-related DLBCL with CD4 count that is 50 or greater should be CHOP-R. There is controversy concerning the inclusion of rituximab if the CD4 count is less than 50.[442] For plasmablastic lymphoma or if the Ki-67 staining is greater than 80%, we consider DA-EPOCH, adding rituximab if the patient is CD20 positive. Examination of the CSF is considered for all patients, as is prophylaxis against *Pneumocystis jiroveci* pneumonia, herpes zoster, and Candida as well as continuation of antiretroviral therapy, if tolerated. For BL histology, we consider CODOX-M/IVAC rather than CHOP-R.[443] Based on a recent report in both patients who are HIV positive and patients who are HIV negative, DA-EPOCH-R is an alternative choice.[356]

REFERENCES

1. Siegel R, Ma J, Zou Z, et al. Cancer statistics, 2014. *CA Cancer J Clin* 2014;64:9–29.
2. Kuppers R. Mechanisms of B-cell lymphoma pathogenesis. *Nat Rev Cancer* 2005;5:251–262.
3. Jaffe ES. Classification of natural killer (NK) cell and NK-like T-cell malignancies. *Blood* 1996;87:1207–1210.
4. Smith MR, Greene WC. Molecular biology of the type I human T-cell leukemia virus (HTLV-I) and adult T cell leukemia. *J Clin Invest* 1991;87:761–766.
5. Cesarman E, Chang Y, Moore PS, et al. Kaposi's sarcoma-associated herpesvirus-like DNA sequences in AIDS-related body-cavity-based lymphomas. *N Engl J Med* 1995;332:1186–1191.
6. Ulrickson M, Quesenberry CP Jr, Guo D, et al. Incidence of non-Hodgkin's lymphoma among individuals with chronic hepatitis B virus infection. *Hepatology* 2007;46:107–112.
7. Hussell T, Isaacson PG, Crabtree JE, et al. The response of cells from low-grade B-cell gastric lymphomas of mucosa-associated lymphoid tissue to Helicobacter pylori. *Lancet* 1993;342:571–574.
8. Saadoun D, Suarez F, Lefrere F, et al. Splenic lymphoma with villous lymphocytes, associated with type II cryoglobulinemia and HCV infection: a new entity? *Blood* 2005;105:74–76.
9. Husain A, Roberts D, Pro B, et al. Meta-analyses of the association between Chlamydia psittaci and ocular adnexal lymphoma and the response of ocular adnexal lymphoma to antibiotics. *Cancer* 2007;110:809–815.
10. Lecuit M, Abachin E, Martin A, et al. Immunoproliferative small intestinal disease associated with Campylobacter jejuni. *N Engl J Med* 2004;350:239–248.
11. Goodlad JR, Davidson MM, Hollowood K, et al. Borrelia burgdorferi-associated cutaneous marginal zone lymphoma: a clinicopathological study of two cases illustrating the temporal progression of B. burgdorferi-associated B-cell proliferation in the skin. *Histopathology* 2000;37:501–508.
12. Agopian J, Navarro JM, Gac AC, et al. Agricultural pesticide exposure and the molecular connection to lymphomagenesis. *J Exp Med* 2009;206:1473–1483.
13. Frumkin H. Agent Orange and cancer: an overview for clinicians. *CA Cancer J Clin* 2003;53:245–255.
14. Hardell L, Eriksson M. A case-control study of non-Hodgkin lymphoma and exposure to pesticides. *Cancer* 1999;85:1353–1360.
15. Chiu BC, Dave BJ, Blair A, et al. Agricultural pesticide use and risk of t(14;18)-defined subtypes of non-Hodgkin lymphoma. *Blood* 2006;108:1363–1369.
16. Rafnsson V. Risk of non-Hodgkin's lymphoma and exposure to hexachlorocyclohexane, a nested case-control study. *Eur J Cancer* 2006;42:2781–2785.
17. Persson B, Fredriksson M, Olsen K, et al. Some occupational exposures as risk factors for malignant lymphomas. *Cancer* 1993;72:1773–1778.
18. List AF, Greer JP, Cousar JB, et al. Non-Hodgkin's lymphoma after treatment of Hodgkin's disease: association with Epstein-Barr virus. *Ann Intern Med* 1986;105:668–673.
19. Starzl TE, Nalesnik MA, Porter KA, et al. Reversibility of lymphomas and lymphoproliferative lesions developing under cyclosporin-steroid therapy. *Lancet* 1984;1:583–587.
20. Ballerini P, Gaidano G, Gong JZ, et al. Multiple genetic lesions in acquired immunodeficiency syndrome-related non-Hodgkin's lymphoma. *Blood* 1993;81:166–176.
21. Smedby KE, Hjalgrim H, Askling J, et al. Autoimmune and chronic inflammatory disorders and risk of non-Hodgkin lymphoma by subtype. *J Natl Cancer Inst* 2006;98:51–60.
22. Saadoun D, Sellam J, Ghillani Dalbin P, et al. Increased risks of lymphoma and death among patients with non-hepatitis C virus-related mixed cryoglobulinemia. *Arch Intern Med* 2006;166:2101–2108.
23. Wang SS, Slager SL, Brennan P, et al. Family history of hematopoietic malignancies and risk of non-Hodgkin lymphoma (NHL): a pooled analysis of 10 211 cases and 11 905 controls from the International Lymphoma Epidemiology Consortium (InterLymph). *Blood* 2007;109:3479–3488.
24. Brown JR, Neuberg D, Phillips K, et al. Prevalence of familial malignancy in a prospectively screened cohort of patients with lymphoproliferative disorders. *Br J Haematol* 2008;143:361–368.
25. Orkin SH, Zon LI. Hematopoiesis: an evolving paradigm for stem cell biology. *Cell* 2008;132:631–644.
26. Busslinger M. Transcriptional control of early B cell development. *Annu Rev Immunol* 2004;22:55–79.
27. Chen J, Alt FW. Gene rearrangement and B-cell development. *Curr Opin Immunol* 1993;5:194–200.
28. Korsmeyer SJ, Hieter PA, Ravetch JV, et al. Developmental hierarchy of immunoglobulin gene rearrangements in human leukemic pre-B-cells. *Proc Natl Acad Sci U S A* 1981;78:7096–7100.
29. Shipp MA, Richardson NE, Sayre PH, et al. Molecular cloning of the common acute lymphoblastic leukemia antigen (CALLA) identifies a type II integral membrane protein. *Proc Natl Acad Sci U S A* 1988;85:4819–4823.
30. Martin F, Kearney JF. B1 cells: similarities and differences with other B cell subsets. *Curr Opin Immunol* 2001;13:195–201.
31. Campbell JJ, Butcher EC. Chemokines in tissue-specific and microenvironment-specific lymphocyte homing. *Curr Opin Immunol* 2000;12:336–341.
32. Calado DP, Sasaki Y, Godinho SA, et al. The cell-cycle regulator c-Myc is essential for the formation and maintenance of germinal centers. *Nat Immunol* 2012;13:1092–1100.
33. Dominguez-Sola D, Victora GD, Ying CY, et al. The proto-oncogene MYC is required for selection in the germinal center and cyclic reentry. *Nat Immunol* 2012;13:1083–1091.
34. Fukuda T, Yoshida T, Okada S, et al. Disruption of the Bcl6 gene results in an impaired germinal center formation. *J Exp Med* 1997;186:439–448.
35. Muramatsu M, Kinoshita K, Fagarasan S, et al. Class switch recombination and hypermutation require activation-induced cytidine deaminase (AID), a potential RNA editing enzyme. *Cell* 2000;102:553–563.
36. Tangye SG, Ma CS, Brink R, et al. The good, the bad and the ugly—TFH cells in human health and disease. *Nat Rev Immunol* 2013;13:412–426.
37. Radtke F, Fasnacht N, Macdonald HR. Notch signaling in the immune system. *Immunity* 2010;32:14–27.
38. Maillard I, Fang T, Pear WS. Regulation of lymphoid development, differentiation, and function by the Notch pathway. *Annu Rev Immunol* 2005;23:945–974.
39. Klein L, Hinterberger M, Wirnsberger G, et al. Antigen presentation in the thymus for positive selection and central tolerance induction. *Nat Rev Immunol* 2009;9:833–844.
40. Engel P, Gribben JG, Freeman GJ, et al. The B7-2 (B70) costimulatory molecule expressed by monocytes and activated B lymphocytes is the CD86 differentiation antigen. *Blood* 1994;84:1402–1407.
41. Delves PJ, Roitt IM. The immune system. Second of two parts. *N Engl J Med* 2000;343:108–117.
42. Delves PJ, Roitt IM. The immune system. First of two parts. *N Engl J Med* 2000;343:37–49.
43. Awasthi A, Kuchroo VK. Immunology. The yin and yang of follicular helper T cells. *Science* 2009;325:953–955.
44. Swerdlow SH, Campo E, Harris NL, et al., eds. *WHO Classification of Tumours of Haematopoietic and Lymphoid Tissues*. Lyon, France: IARC; 2008.
45. Harris NL, Jaffe ES, Stein H, et al. A revised European-American classification of lymphoid neoplasms: a proposal from the International Lymphoma Study Group. *Blood* 1994;84:1361–1392.

46. Rosenwald A, Wright G, Chan WC, et al. The use of molecular profiling to predict survival after chemotherapy for diffuse large-B-cell lymphoma. N Engl J Med 2002;346;1937–1947.
47. Pangalis GA, Vassilakopoulos TP, Boussiotis VA, et al. Clinical approach to lymphadenopathy. Semin Oncol 1993;20:570–582.
48. Mentzer SJ, Reilly JJ, Skarin AT, et al. Patterns of lung involvement by malignant lymphoma. Surgery 1993;113:507–514.
49. Elstrom R, Guan L, Baker G, et al. Utility of FDG-PET scanning in lymphoma by WHO classification. Blood 2003;101:3875–3876.
50. Schoder H, Noy A, Gonen M, et al. Intensity of 18fluorodeoxyglucose uptake in positron emission tomography distinguishes between indolent and aggressive non-Hodgkin's lymphoma. J Clin Oncol 2005;23:4643–4651.
51. Juweid ME, Wiseman GA, Vose JM, et al. Response assessment of aggressive non-Hodgkin's lymphoma by integrated International Workshop Criteria and fluorine-18-fluorodeoxyglucose positron emission tomography. J Clin Oncol 2005;23:4652–4661.
52. Zinzani PL, Fanti S, Battista G, et al. Predictive role of positron emission tomography (PET) in the outcome of lymphoma patients. Br J Cancer 2004;91:850–854.
53. Juweid ME, Stroobants S, Hoekstra OS, et al. Use of positron emission tomography for response assessment of lymphoma: consensus of the Imaging Subcommittee of International Harmonization Project in Lymphoma. J Clin Oncol 2007;25:571–578.
54. Rosenberg SA. Validity of the Ann Arbor staging classification for the non-Hodgkin's lymphomas. Cancer Treat Rep 1977;61:1023–1027.
55. A predictive model for aggressive non-Hodgkin's lymphoma. The International Non-Hodgkin's Lymphoma Prognostic Factors Project. N Engl J Med 1993;329:987–994.
56. Sehn LH, Berry B, Chhanabhai M, et al. The revised International Prognostic Index (R-IPI) is a better predictor of outcome than the standard IPI for patients with diffuse large B-cell lymphoma treated with R-CHOP. Blood 2007;109:1857–1861.
57. Solal-Celigny P, Roy P, Colombat P, et al. Follicular lymphoma international prognostic index. Blood 2004;104:1258–1265.
58. Hoster E, Dreyling M, Klapper W, et al. A new prognostic index (MIPI) for patients with advanced-stage mantle cell lymphoma. Blood 2008;111:558–565.
59. Gallamini A, Stelitano C, Calvi R, et al. Peripheral T-cell lymphoma unspecified (PTCL-U): a new prognostic model from a retrospective multicentric clinical study. Blood 2004;103:2474–2479.
60. Hans CP, Weisenburger DD, Greiner TC, et al. Confirmation of the molecular classification of diffuse large B-cell lymphoma by immunohistochemistry using a tissue microarray. Blood 2004;103:275–282.
61. Soslow RA, Baergen RN, Warnke RA. B-lineage lymphoblastic lymphoma is a clinicopathologic entity distinct from other histologically similar aggressive lymphomas with blastic morphology. Cancer 1999;85:2648–2654.
62. A clinical evaluation of the International Lymphoma Study Group classification of non-Hodgkin's lymphoma. The Non-Hodgkin's Lymphoma Classification Project. Blood 1997;89:3909–3918.
63. Armitage JO, Weisenburger DD. New approach to classifying non-Hodgkin's lymphomas: clinical features of the major histologic subtypes. Non-Hodgkin's Lymphoma Classification Project. J Clin Oncol 1998;16:2780–2795.
64. Harris NL, Jaffe ES, Diebold J, et al. World Health Organization classification of neoplastic diseases of the hematopoietic and lymphoid tissues: report of the Clinical Advisory Committee meeting-Airlie House, Virginia, November 1997. J Clin Oncol 1999;17:3835–3849.
65. Biagi JJ, Seymour JF. Insights into the molecular pathogenesis of follicular lymphoma arising from analysis of geographic variation. Blood 2002;99:4265–4275.
66. Ott G, Katzenberger T, Lohr A, et al. Cytomorphologic, immunohistochemical, and cytogenetic profiles of follicular lymphoma: 2 types of follicular lymphoma grade 3. Blood 2002;99:3806–3812.
67. Morin RD, Mendez-Lago M, Mungall AJ, et al. Frequent mutation of histone-modifying genes in non-Hodgkin lymphoma. Nature 2011;476:298–303.
68. Pasqualucci L, Trifonov V, Fabbri G, et al. Analysis of the coding genome of diffuse large B-cell lymphoma. Nat Genet 2011;43:830–837.
69. Kridel R, Sehn LH, Gascoyne RD. Pathogenesis of follicular lymphoma. J Clin Invest 2012;122:3424–3431.
70. Schmatz AI, Streubel B, Kretschmer-Chott E, et al. Primary follicular lymphoma of the duodenum is a distinct mucosal/submucosal variant of follicular lymphoma: a retrospective study of 63 cases. J Clin Oncol 2011;29:1445–1451.
71. Freedman AS. Biology and management of histologic transformation of indolent lymphoma. Hematology Am Soc Hematol Educ Program 2005:314–320.
72. Link BK, Maurer MJ, Nowakowski GS, et al. Rates and outcomes of follicular lymphoma transformation in the immunochemotherapy era: a report from the University of Iowa/MayoClinic Specialized Program of Research Excellence Molecular Epidemiology Resource. J Clin Oncol 2013;31:3272–3278.
73. Montoto S, Davies AJ, Matthews J, et al. Risk and clinical implications of transformation of follicular lymphoma to diffuse large B-cell lymphoma. J Clin Oncol 2007;25:2426–2433.
74. Relander T, Johnson NA, Farinha P, et al. Prognostic factors in follicular lymphoma. J Clin Oncol 2010;28:2902–2913.
75. Federico M, Bellei M, Marcheselli L, et al. Follicular lymphoma international prognostic index 2: a new prognostic index for follicular lymphoma developed by the international follicular lymphoma prognostic factor project. J Clin Oncol 2009;27:4555–4562.
76. Buske C, Hoster E, Dreyling M, et al. The Follicular Lymphoma International Prognostic Index (FLIPI) separates high-risk from intermediate- or low-risk patients with advanced-stage follicular lymphoma treated frontline with rituximab and the combination of cyclophosphamide, doxorubicin, vincristine, and prednisone (R-CHOP) with respect to treatment outcome. Blood 2006;108;1504–1508.
77. Wahlin BE, Yri OE, Kimby E, et al. Clinical significance of the WHO grades of follicular lymphoma in a population-based cohort of 505 patients with long follow-up times. Br J Haematol 2012;156:225–233.
78. Alvaro T, Lejeune M, Salvado MT, et al. Immunohistochemical patterns of reactive microenvironment are associated with clinicobiologic behavior in follicular lymphoma patients. J Clin Oncol 2006;24:5350–5357.
79. Canioni D, Salles G, Mounier N, et al. High numbers of tumor-associated macrophages have an adverse prognostic value that can be circumvented by rituximab in patients with follicular lymphoma enrolled onto the GELA-GOELAMS FL-2000 trial. J Clin Oncol 2008;26:440–446.
80. Carreras J, Lopez-Guillermo A, Fox BC, et al. High numbers of tumor-infiltrating FOXP3-positive regulatory T cells are associated with improved overall survival in follicular lymphoma. Blood 2006;108:2957–2964.
81. Dave SS, Wright G, Tan B, et al. Prediction of survival in follicular lymphoma based on molecular features of tumor-infiltrating immune cells. N Engl J Med 2004;351:2159–2169.
82. Farinha P, Masoudi H, Skinnider BF, et al. Analysis of multiple biomarkers shows that lymphoma-associated macrophage (LAM) content is an independent predictor of survival in follicular lymphoma (FL). Blood 2005;106:2169–2174.
83. Glas AM, Knoops L, Delahaye L, et al. Gene-expression and immunohistochemical study of specific T-cell subsets and accessory cell types in the transformation and prognosis of follicular lymphoma. J Clin Oncol 2007;25:390–398.
84. Klapper W, Hoster E, Rolver L, et al. Tumor sclerosis but not cell proliferation or malignancy grade is a prognostic marker in advanced-stage follicular lymphoma: the German Low Grade Lymphoma Study Group. J Clin Oncol 2007;25:3330–3336.
85. Kuppers R. Prognosis in follicular lymphoma—it's in the microenvironment. N Engl J Med 2004;351:2152–2153.
86. Lee AM, Clear AJ, Calaminici M, et al. Number of CD4+ cells and location of forkhead box protein P3-positive cells in diagnostic follicular lymphoma tissue microarrays correlates with outcome. J Clin Oncol 2006;24:5052–5059.
87. Wahlin BE, Sander B, Christensson B, et al. CD8+ T-cell content in diagnostic lymph node biopsies is predictive by flow cytometry is a predictor of survival in follicular lymphoma. Clin Cancer Res 2007;13:388–397.
88. Friedberg J, Huang J, Dillon H, et al. Initial therapeutic strategy in follicular lymphoma: an analysis from the National LymphoCare Study. J Clin Oncol 2006;24: 428s.
89. Guadagnolo BA, Li S, Neuberg D, et al. Long-term outcome and mortality trends in early-stage, Grade 1-2 follicular lymphoma treated with radiation therapy. Int J Radiat Oncol Biol Phys 2006;64:928–934.
90. Lowry L, Smith P, Qian W, et al. Reduced dose radiotherapy for local control in non-Hodgkin lymphoma: a randomised phase III trial. Radiother Oncol 2011;100:86–92.
91. Pugh TJ, Ballonoff A, Newman F, et al. Improved survival in patients with early stage low-grade follicular lymphoma treated with radiation: a Surveillance, Epidemiology, and End Results database analysis. Cancer 2010;116:3843–3851.
92. Kelsey SM, Newland AC, Hudson GV, et al. A British National Lymphoma Investigation randomised trial of single agent chlorambucil plus radiotherapy versus radiotherapy alone in low grade, localised non-Hodgkins lymphoma. Med Oncol 1994;11:19–25.
93. Friedberg JW, Byrtek M, Link BK, et al. Effectiveness of first-line management strategies for stage I follicular lymphoma: analysis of the National LymphoCare Study. J Clin Oncol 2012;30:3368–3375.
94. Advani R, Rosenberg SA, Horning SJ. Stage I and II follicular non-Hodgkin's lymphoma: long-term follow-up of no initial therapy. J Clin Oncol 2004;22:1454–1459.
95. Ardeshna KM, Smith P, Norton A, et al. Long-term effect of a watch and wait policy versus immediate systemic treatment for asymptomatic advanced-stage non-Hodgkin lymphoma: a randomised controlled trial. Lancet 2003;362:516–522.
96. Brice P, Bastion Y, Lepage E, et al. Comparison in low-tumor-burden follicular lymphomas between an initial no-treatment policy, prednimustine, or interferon alfa: a randomized study from the Groupe d'Etude des Lymphomes Folliculaires. Groupe d'Etude des Lymphomes de l'Adulte. J Clin Oncol 1997;15:1110–1117.
97. Solal-Celigny P, Bellei M, Marcheselli L, et al. Watchful waiting in low-tumor burden follicular lymphoma in the rituximab era: results of an F2-study database. J Clin Oncol 2012;30:3848–3853.
98. Ardeshna K, Smith P, Qian W, et al. An intergroup randomised trial of rituximab versus a watch and wait strategy in patients with stage II, III, IV, asymptomatic, non-bulky follicular lymphoma (grades 1, 2 and 3a). A preliminary analysis. Blood 2010;116:abstract 6.
99. Fisher RI, LeBlanc M, Press OW, et al. New treatment options have changed the survival of patients with follicular lymphoma. J Clin Oncol 2005;23:8447–8452.
100. Herold M, Haas A, Srock S, et al. Rituximab added to first-line mitoxantrone, chlorambucil, and prednisolone chemotherapy followed by interferon maintenance prolongs survival in patients with advanced follicular lymphoma: an East German Study Group Hematology and Oncology Study. J Clin Oncol 2007;25:1986–1992.

101. Hiddemann W, Kneba M, Dreyling M, et al. Frontline therapy with rituximab added to the combination of cyclophosphamide, doxorubicin, vincristine, and prednisone (CHOP) significantly improves the outcome for patients with advanced-stage follicular lymphoma compared with therapy with CHOP alone: results of a prospective randomized study of the German Low-Grade Lymphoma Study Group. *Blood* 2005;106:3725–3732.

102. Marcus R, Imrie K, Belch A, et al. CVP chemotherapy plus rituximab compared with CVP as first-line treatment for advanced follicular lymphoma. *Blood* 2005;105:1417–1423.

103. Marcus R, Imrie K, Solal-Celigny P, et al. Phase III study of R-CVP compared with cyclophosphamide, vincristine, and prednisone alone in patients with previously untreated advanced follicular lymphoma. *J Clin Oncol* 2008;26:4579–4586.

104. Salles G, Mounier N, de Guibert S, et al. Rituximab combined with chemotherapy and interferon in follicular lymphoma patients: results of the GELA-GOELAMS FL2000 study. *Blood* 2008;112:4824–4831.

105. Dupuis J, Berriolo-Riedinger A, Julian A, et al. Impact of [(18)F]fluorodeoxyglucose positron emission tomography response evaluation in patients with high-tumor burden follicular lymphoma treated with immunochemotherapy: a prospective study from the Groupe d'Etudes des Lymphomes de l'Adulte and GOELAMS. *J Clin Oncol* 2012;30:4317–4322.

106. Rummel MJ, Niederle N, Maschmeyer G, et al. Bendamustine plus rituximab versus CHOP plus rituximab as first-line treatment for patients with indolent and mantle-cell lymphomas: an open-label, multicentre, randomised, phase 3 non-inferiority trial. *Lancet* 2013;381:1203–1210.

107. Watanabe T, Tobinai K, Shibata T, et al. Phase II/III study of R-CHOP-21 versus R-CHOP-14 for untreated indolent B-cell non-Hodgkin's lymphoma: JCOG 0203 trial. *J Clin Oncol* 2011;29:3990–3998.

108. Czuczman MS, Koryzna A, Mohr A, et al. Rituximab in combination with fludarabine chemotherapy in low-grade or follicular lymphoma. *J Clin Oncol* 2005;23:694–704.

109. McLaughlin P, Hagemeister FB, Rodriguez MA, et al. Safety of fludarabine, mitoxantrone, and dexamethasone combined with rituximab in the treatment of stage IV indolent lymphoma. *Semin Oncol* 2000;27:37–41.

110. Federico M, Luminari S, Dondi A, et al. R CVP versus R-CHOP versus R-FM for the initial treatment of patients with advanced-stage follicular lymphoma: results of the FOLL05 trial conducted by the Fondazione Italiana Linfomi. *J Clin Oncol* 2013;31:1506–1513.

111. Colombat P, Salles G, Brousse N, et al. Rituximab (anti-CD20 monoclonal antibody) as single first-line therapy for patients with follicular lymphoma with a low tumor burden: clinical and molecular evaluation. *Blood* 2001;97:101–106.

112. Ghielmini M, Schmitz SF, Cogliatti SB, et al. Prolonged treatment with rituximab in patients with follicular lymphoma significantly increases event-free survival and response duration compared with the standard weekly × 4 schedule. *Blood* 2004;103:4416–4423.

113. Witzig TE, Vukov AM, Habermann TM, et al. Rituximab therapy for patients with newly diagnosed, advanced-stage, follicular grade I non-Hodgkin's lymphoma: a phase II trial in the North Central Cancer Treatment Group. *J Clin Oncol* 2005;23:1103–1108.

114. Martinelli G, Schmitz SF, Utiger U, et al. Long-term follow-up of patients with follicular lymphoma receiving single-agent rituximab at two different schedules in trial SAKK 35/98. *J Clin Oncol* 2010;28:4480–4484.

115. Hochster H, Weller E, Gascoyne RD, et al. Maintenance rituximab after cyclophosphamide, vincristine, and prednisone prolongs progression-free survival in advanced indolent lymphoma: results of the randomized phase III ECOG 1496 Study. *J Clin Oncol* 2009;27:1607–1614.

116. Salles G, Seymour JF, Offner F, et al. Rituximab maintenance for 2 years in patients with high tumour burden follicular lymphoma responding to rituximab plus chemotherapy (PRIMA): a phase 3, randomised controlled trial. *Lancet* 2011;377:42–51.

117. Kaminski MS, Tuck M, Estes J, et al. 131I-tositumomab therapy as initial treatment for follicular lymphoma. *N Engl J Med* 2005;352:441–449.

118. Scholz CW, Pinto A, Linkesch W, et al. (90)Yttrium-ibritumomab-tiuxetan as first-line treatment for follicular lymphoma: 30 months of follow-up data from an international multicenter phase II clinical trial. *J Clin Oncol* 2013;31:308–313.

119. Zinzani PL, Tani M, Pulsoni A, et al. Fludarabine and mitoxantrone followed by yttrium-90 ibritumomab tiuxetan in previously untreated patients with follicular non-Hodgkin lymphoma trial: a phase II non-randomised trial (FLUMIZ). *Lancet Oncol* 2008;9:352–358.

120. Jacobs SA, Swerdlow SH, Kant J, et al. Phase II trial of short-course CHOP-R followed by 90Y-ibritumomab tiuxetan and extended rituximab in previously untreated follicular lymphoma. *Clin Cancer Res* 2008;14:7088–7094.

121. Leonard JP, Coleman M, Kostakoglu L, et al. Abbreviated chemotherapy with fludarabine followed by tositumomab and iodine I 131 tositumomab for untreated follicular lymphoma. *J Clin Oncol* 2005;23:5696–5704.

122. Morschhauser F, Radford J, Van Hoof A, et al. Phase III trial of consolidation therapy with yttrium-90-ibritumomab tiuxetan compared with no additional therapy after first remission in advanced follicular lymphoma. *J Clin Oncol* 2008;26:5156–5164.

123. Press OW, Unger JM, Rimsza LM, et al. Phase III randomized intergroup trial of CHOP plus rituximab compared with CHOP chemotherapy plus (131)iodine-tositumomab for previously untreated follicular non-Hodgkin lymphoma: SWOG S0016. *J Clin Oncol* 2013;31:314–320.

124. Brown JR, Feng Y, Gribben JG, et al. Long-term survival after autologous bone marrow transplantation for follicular lymphoma in first remission. *Biol Blood Marrow Transplant* 2007;13:1057–1065.

125. Deconinck E, Foussard C, Milpied N, et al. High-dose therapy followed by autologous purged stem-cell transplantation and doxorubicin-based chemotherapy in patients with advanced follicular lymphoma: a randomized multicenter study by GOELAMS. *Blood* 2005;105:3817–3823.

126. Lenz G, Dreyling M, Schiegnitz E, et al. Myeloablative radiochemotherapy followed by autologous stem cell transplantation in first remission prolongs progression-free survival in follicular lymphoma: results of a prospective, randomized trial of the German Low-Grade Lymphoma Study Group. *Blood* 2004;104:2667–2674.

127. Sebban C, Mounier N, Brousse N, et al. Standard chemotherapy with interferon compared with CHOP followed by high-dose therapy with autologous stem cell transplantation in untreated patients with advanced follicular lymphoma: the GELF-94 randomized study from the Groupe d'Etude des Lymphomes de l'Adulte (GELA). *Blood* 2006;108:2540–2544.

128. Ladetto M, De Marco F, Benedetti F, et al. Prospective, multicenter randomized GITMO/IIL trial comparing intensive (R-HDS) versus conventional (CHOP-R) chemoimmunotherapy in high-risk follicular lymphoma at diagnosis: the superior disease control of R-HDS does not translate into an overall survival advantage. *Blood* 2008;111:4004–4013.

129. Gyan E, Foussard C, Bertrand P, et al. High-dose therapy followed by autologous purged stem cell transplantation and doxorubicin-based chemotherapy in patients with advanced follicular lymphoma: a randomized multicenter study by the GOELAMS with final results after a median follow-up of 9 years. *Blood* 2009;113:995–1001.

130. Al Khabori M, de Almeida JR, Guyatt GH, et al. Autologous stem cell transplantation in follicular lymphoma: a systematic review and meta-analysis. *J Natl Cancer Inst* 2012;104:18–28.

131. Davis TA, Grillo-Lopez AJ, White CA, et al. Rituximab anti-CD20 monoclonal antibody therapy in non-Hodgkin's lymphoma: safety and efficacy of re-treatment. *J Clin Oncol* 2000;18:3135–3143.

132. van Oers MH, Van Glabbeke M, Giurgea L, et al. Rituximab maintenance treatment of relapsed/resistant follicular non-Hodgkin's lymphoma: long-term outcome of the EORTC 20981 phase III randomized intergroup study. *J Clin Oncol* 2010;28:2853–2858.

133. Forstpointner R, Dreyling M, Repp R, et al. The addition of rituximab to a combination of fludarabine, cyclophosphamide, mitoxantrone (FCM) significantly increases the response rate and prolongs survival as compared with FCM alone in patients with relapsed and refractory follicular and mantle cell lymphoma: results of a prospective randomized study of the German Low-Grade Lymphoma Study Group. *Blood* 2004;104:3064–3071.

134. Friedberg JW, Cohen P, Chen L, et al. Bendamustine in patients with rituximab-refractory indolent and transformed non-Hodgkin's lymphoma: results from a phase II multicenter, single-agent study. *J Clin Oncol* 2008;26:204–210.

135. Robinson KS, Williams ME, van der Jagt RH, et al. Phase II multicenter study of bendamustine plus rituximab in patients with relapsed indolent B-cell and mantle cell non-Hodgkin's lymphoma. *J Clin Oncol* 2008;26:4473–4479.

136. Rummel MJ, Al-Batran SE, Kim SZ, et al. Bendamustine plus rituximab is effective and has a favorable toxicity profile in the treatment of mantle cell and low-grade non-Hodgkin's lymphoma. *J Clin Oncol* 2005;23:3383–3389.

137. Tam CS, Wolf M, Prince HM, et al. Fludarabine, cyclophosphamide, and rituximab for the treatment of patients with chronic lymphocytic leukemia or indolent non-Hodgkin lymphoma. *Cancer* 2006;106:2412–2420.

138. de Vos S, Goy A, Dakhil SR, et al. Multicenter randomized phase II study of weekly or twice-weekly bortezomib plus rituximab in patients with relapsed or refractory follicular or marginal-zone B-cell lymphoma. *J Clin Oncol* 2009;27:5023–5030.

139. Friedberg JW, Vose JM, Kelly JL, et al. The combination of bendamustine, bortezomib, and rituximab for patients with relapsed/refractory indolent and mantle cell non-Hodgkin lymphoma. *Blood* 2011;117:2807–2812.

140. Cheson BD. Radioimmunotherapy of non-Hodgkin lymphomas. *Blood* 2003;101:391–398.

141. Fisher RI, Kaminski MS, Wahl RL, et al. Tositumomab and iodine-131 tositumomab produces durable complete remissions in a subset of heavily pretreated patients with low-grade and transformed non-Hodgkin's lymphomas. *J Clin Oncol* 2005;23:7565–7573.

142. Witzig TE, Molina A, Gordon LI, et al. Long-term responses in patients with recurring or refractory B-cell non-Hodgkin lymphoma treated with yttrium 90 ibritumomab tiuxetan. *Cancer* 2007;109:1804–1810.

143. Witzig TE, Gordon LI, Cabanillas F, et al. Randomized controlled trial of yttrium-90-labeled ibritumomab tiuxetan radioimmunotherapy versus rituximab immunotherapy for patients with relapsed or refractory low-grade, follicular, or transformed B-cell non-Hodgkin's lymphoma. *J Clin Oncol* 2002;20:2453–2463.

144. Kaminski MS, Radford JA, Gregory SA, et al. Re-treatment with I-131 tositumomab in patients with non-Hodgkin's lymphoma who had previously responded to I-131 tositumomab. *J Clin Oncol* 2005;23:7985–7993.

145. Russo AL, Chen YH, Martin NE, et al. Low-dose involved-field radiation in the treatment of non-hodgkin lymphoma: predictors of response and treatment failure. *Int J Radiat Oncol Biol Phys* 2013;86:121–127.

146. Montoto S, Corradini P, Dreyling M, et al. Indications for hematopoietic stem cell transplantation in patients with follicular lymphoma: a consensus project of the EBMT-Lymphoma Working Party. *Haematologica* 2013;98:1014–1021.

147. Rohatiner AZ, Nadler L, Davies AJ, et al. Myeloablative therapy with autologous bone marrow transplantation for follicular lymphoma at the time of second or subsequent remission: long-term follow-up. *J Clin Oncol* 2007;25:2554–2559.

148. Bierman PJ, Vose JM, Anderson JR, et al. High-dose therapy with autologous hematopoietic rescue for follicular low-grade non-Hodgkin's lymphoma. *J Clin Oncol* 1997;15:445–450.
149. Cao TM, Horning S, Negrin RS, et al. High-dose therapy and autologous hematopoietic-cell transplantation for follicular lymphoma beyond first remission: the Stanford University experience. *Biol Blood Marrow Transplant* 2001;7:294–301.
150. Safar V, Gastinne T, Milpied N, et al. Very long term follow-up of autologous stem cell transplantation in follicular lymphoma: a retrospective single-institution experience. *Ann Oncol* 2008;19:183.
151. Bastion Y, Brice P, Haioun C, et al. Intensive therapy with peripheral blood progenitor cell transplantation in 60 patients with poor-prognosis follicular lymphoma. *Blood* 1995;86:3257–3262.
152. Schouten HC, Qian W, Kvaloy S, et al. High-dose therapy improves progression-free survival and survival in relapsed follicular non-Hodgkin's lymphoma: results from the randomized European CUP trial. *J Clin Oncol* 2003;21:3918–3927.
153. Pettengell R, Schmitz N, Gisselbrecht C, et al. Rituximab purging and/or maintenance in patients undergoing autologous transplantation for relapsed follicular lymphoma: a prospective randomized trial from the lymphoma working party of the European group for blood and marrow transplantation. *J Clin Oncol* 2013;31:1624–1630.
154. van Besien K, Loberiza FR Jr, Bajorunaite R, et al. Comparison of autologous and allogeneic hematopoietic stem cell transplantation for follicular lymphoma. *Blood* 2003;102:3521–3529.
155. Khouri IF, McLaughlin P, Saliba RM, et al. Eight-year experience with allogeneic stem cell transplantation for relapsed follicular lymphoma after nonmyeloablative conditioning with fludarabine, cyclophosphamide, and rituximab. *Blood* 2008;111:5530–5536.
156. Hari P, Carreras J, Zhang MJ, et al. Allogeneic transplants in follicular lymphoma: higher risk of disease progression after reduced-intensity compared to myeloablative conditioning. *Biol Blood Marrow Transplant* 2008;14:236–245.
157. Tomblyn MR, Ewell M, Bredeson C, et al. Autologous versus reduced-intensity allogeneic hematopoietic cell transplantation for patients with chemosensitive follicular non-Hodgkin lymphoma beyond first complete response or first partial response. *Biol Blood Marrow Transplant* 2011;17:1051–1057.
158. Evens AM, Vanderplas A, LaCasce AS, et al. Stem cell transplantation for follicular lymphoma relapsed/refractory after prior rituximab: a comprehensive analysis from the NCCN lymphoma outcomes project. *Cancer* 2013;119:3662–3671.
159. Montoto S, Fitzgibbon J. Transformation of indolent B-cell lymphomas. *J Clin Oncol* 2011;29:1827–1834.
160. Yuen AR, Kamel OW, Halpern J, et al. Long-term survival after histologic transformation of low-grade follicular lymphoma. *J Clin Oncol* 1995;13:1726–1733.
161. Leonard JP, Friedberg JW, Younes A, et al. A phase I/II study of galiximab (an anti-CD80 monoclonal antibody) in combination with rituximab for relapsed or refractory, follicular lymphoma. *Ann Oncol* 2007;18:1216–1223.
162. Bence-Bruckler I, Macdonald D, Stiff P, et al. A phase 2, double-blind, placebo-controlled trial of rituximab + galiximab vs rituximab + placebo in advanced follicular non-Hodgkin's lymphoma (NHL). *Blood* 2010;116:abstract 428.
163. Leonard JP, Schuster SJ, Emmanouilides C, et al. Durable complete responses from therapy with combined epratuzumab and rituximab: final results from an international multicenter, phase 2 study in recurrent, indolent, non-Hodgkin lymphoma. *Cancer* 2008;113:2714–2723.
164. Grant B, Leonard J, Johnson J, et al. Combination biologic therapy as initial treatment for follicular lymphoma: initial results from CALGB 50701—a phase II trial of extended induction epratuzumab (anti-CD22) and rituximab (anti-CD20). *Blood* 2010;116:abstract 427.
165. Fanale M, Assouline S, Kuruvilla J, et al. Phase IA/II, multicentre, open-label study of the CD40 antagonistic monoclonal antibody lucatumumab in adult patients with advanced non-Hodgkin or Hodgkin lymphoma. *Br J Haematol* 2014;164:258–265.
166. Hagenbeek A, Gadeberg O, Johnson P, et al. First clinical use of ofatumumab, a novel fully human anti-CD20 monoclonal antibody in relapsed or refractory follicular lymphoma: results of a phase 1/2 trial. *Blood* 2008;111:5486–5495.
167. Morschhauser F, Leonard JP, Fayad L, et al. Humanized anti-CD20 antibody, veltuzumab, in refractory/recurrent non-Hodgkin's lymphoma: phase I/II results. *J Clin Oncol* 2009;27:3346–3353.
168. Morschhauser F, Marlton P, Vitolo U, et al. Results of a phase I/II study of ocrelizumab, a fully humanized anti-CD20 mAb, in patients with relapsed/refractory follicular lymphoma. *Ann Oncol* 2010;21:1870–1876.
169. Salles GA, Morschhauser F, Solal-Celigny P, et al. Obinutuzumab (GA101) in patients with relapsed/refractory indolent non-Hodgkin lymphoma: results from the phase II GAUGUIN study. *J Clin Oncol* 2013;31:2920–2926.
170. Radford J, Davies A, Cartron G, et al. Obinutuzumab (GA101) plus CHOP or FC in relapsed/refractory follicular lymphoma: results of the GAUDI study (BO21000). *Blood* 2013;122:1137–1143.
171. Friedberg JW, Kelly JL, Neuberg D, et al. Phase II study of a TLR-9 agonist (1018 ISS) with rituximab in patients with relapsed or refractory follicular lymphoma. *Br J Haematol* 2009;146:282–291.
172. Friedberg JW. Treatment of follicular non-Hodgkin's lymphoma: the old and the new. *Semin Hematol* 2008;45:S2–S6.
173. Freedman A, Neelapu SS, Nichols C, et al. Placebo-controlled phase III trial of patient-specific immunotherapy with mitumprotimut-T and granulocyte-macrophage colony-stimulating factor after rituximab in patients with follicular lymphoma. *J Clin Oncol* 2009;27:3036–3043.
174. Schuster SJ, Neelapu SS, Gause BL, et al. Vaccination with patient-specific tumor derived antigen in first remission improves disease-free survival in follicular lymphoma. *J Clin Oncol* 2011;29:2787–2794.
175. Kahl B, Byrd J, Flinn I, et al. Clinical safety and activity in a phase 1 study of CAL-101, an isoform-selective inhibitor of phosphatidylinositol 3-kinase P110δ, in patients with relapsed or refractory non-Hodgkin lymphoma. *Blood* 2010;116:abstract 1777.
176. Fowler F, Porte Sharman J, Smith S, et al. The Btk Inhibitor, PCI-32765, induces durable responses with minimal toxicity in patients with relapsed/refractory B-cell malignancies: results from a phase I study. *Blood* 2010;116:abstract 964.
177. Friedberg JW, Sharman J, Sweetenham J, et al. Inhibition of Syk with fostamatinib disodium has significant clinical activity in non-Hodgkin lymphoma and chronic lymphocytic leukemia. *Blood* 2010;115:2578–2585.
178. Anderson JR, Vose JM, Bierman PJ, et al. Clinical features and prognosis of follicular large-cell lymphoma, a report from the Nebraska Lymphoma Study Group. *J Clin Oncol* 1993;11:218–224.
179. Hans CP, Weisenburger DD, Vose JM, et al. A significant diffuse component predicts for inferior survival in grade 3 follicular lymphoma, but cytologic subtypes do not predict survival. *Blood* 2003;101:2363–2367.
180. Rodriguez J, McLaughlin P, Hagemeister FB, et al. Follicular large cell lymphoma: an aggressive lymphoma that often presents with favorable prognostic features. *Blood* 1999;93:2202–2207.
181. Chau I, Jones R, Cunningham D, et al. Outcome of follicular lymphoma grade 3: is anthracycline necessary as front-line therapy? *Br J Cancer* 2003;89:36–42.
182. Shustik J, Quinn M, Connors JM, et al. Follicular non-Hodgkin lymphoma grades 3A and 3B have a similar outcome and appear incurable with anthracycline-based therapy. *Ann Oncol* 2011;22:1164–1169.
183. Murray F, Darzentas N, Hadzidimitriou A, et al. Stereotyped patterns of somatic hypermutation in subsets of patients with chronic lymphocytic leukemia: implications for the role of antigen selection in leukemogenesis. *Blood* 2008;111:1524–1533.
184. Rassenti LZ, Jain S, Keating MJ, et al. Relative value of ZAP-70, CD38, and immunoglobulin mutation status in predicting aggressive disease in chronic lymphocytic leukemia. *Blood* 2008;112:1923–1930.
185. Grever MR, Lucas DM, Dewald GW, et al. Comprehensive assessment of genetic and molecular features predicting outcome in patients with chronic lymphocytic leukemia: results from the US Intergroup Phase III Trial E2997. *J Clin Oncol* 2007;25:799–804.
186. Landau DA, Carter SL, Stojanov P, et al. Evolution and impact of subclonal mutations in chronic lymphocytic leukemia. *Cell* 2013;152:714–726.
187. Tsimberidou AM, Keating MJ. Richter syndrome: biology, incidence, and therapeutic strategies. *Cancer* 2005;103:216–228.
188. Vallisa D, Bernuzzi P, Arcaini L, et al. Role of anti-hepatitis C virus (HCV) treatment in HCV-related, low-grade, B-cell, non-Hodgkin's lymphoma: a multicenter Italian experience. *J Clin Oncol* 2005;23:468–473.
189. Giordano TP, Henderson L, Landgren O, et al. Risk of non-Hodgkin lymphoma and lymphoproliferative precursor diseases in US veterans with hepatitis C virus. *JAMA* 2007;297:2010–2017.
190. Vijay A, Gertz MA. Waldenstrom macroglobulinemia. *Blood* 2007;109:5096–5103.
191. Dimopoulos MA, Zervas C, Zomas A, et al. Treatment of Waldenstrom's macroglobulinemia with rituximab. *J Clin Oncol* 2002;20:2327–2333.
192. Dimopoulos MA, Anagnostopoulos A, Kyrtsonis MC, et al. Primary treatment of Waldenstrom macroglobulinemia with dexamethasone, rituximab, and cyclophosphamide. *J Clin Oncol* 2007;25:3344–3349.
193. Treon SP, Ioakimidis L, Soumerai JD, et al. Primary therapy of Waldenstrom macroglobulinemia with bortezomib, dexamethasone, and rituximab: WMCTG clinical trial 05-180. *J Clin Oncol* 2009;27:3830–3835.
194. Treon SP, Soumerai JD, Branagan AR, et al. Thalidomide and rituximab in Waldenstrom macroglobulinemia. *Blood* 2008;112:4452–4457.
195. Ansell SM, Kyle RA, Reeder CB, et al. Diagnosis and management of Waldenstrom macroglobulinemia: Mayo stratification of macroglobulinemia and risk-adapted therapy (mSMART) guidelines. *Mayo Clin Proc* 2010;85:824–833.
196. Nathwani BN, Drachenberg MR, Hernandez AM, et al. Nodal monocytoid B-cell lymphoma (nodal marginal-zone B-cell lymphoma). *Semin Hematol* 1999;36:128–138.
197. Isaacson PG. Mucosa-associated lymphoid tissue lymphoma. *Semin Hematol* 1999;36:139–147.
198. Rossi D, Trifonov V, Fangazio M, et al. The coding genome of splenic marginal zone lymphoma: activation of NOTCH2 and other pathways regulating marginal zone development. *J Exp Med* 2012;209:1537–1551.
199. Bain BJ, Catovsky D, Ewan PW. Acquired angioedema as the presenting feature of lymphoproliferative disorders of mature B-lymphocytes. *Cancer* 1993;72:3318–3322.
200. Arcaini L, Lazzarino M, Colombo N, et al. Splenic marginal zone lymphoma: a prognostic model for clinical use. *Blood* 2006;107:4643–4649.
201. Else M, Marin-Niebla A, de la Cruz F, et al. Rituximab, used alone or in combination, is superior to other treatment modalities in splenic marginal zone lymphoma. *Br J Haematol* 2012;159:322–328.
202. Kalpadakis C, Pangalis GA, Angelopoulou MK, et al. Treatment of splenic marginal zone lymphoma with rituximab monotherapy: progress report and comparison with splenectomy. *Oncologist* 2013;18:190–197.
203. Ambrosetti A, Zanotti R, Pattaro C, et al. Most cases of primary salivary mucosa-associated lymphoid tissue lymphoma are associated either with Sjoegren syndrome or hepatitis C virus infection. *Br J Haematol* 2004;126:43–49.

204. Ferreri AJ, Dolcetti R, Dognini GP, et al. Chlamydophila psittaci is viable and infectious in the conjunctiva and peripheral blood of patients with ocular adnexal lymphoma: results of a single-center prospective case-control study. Int J Cancer 2008;123:1089–1093.
205. Hussell T, Isaacson PG, Crabtree JE, et al. Helicobacter pylori-specific tumour-infiltrating T cells provide contact dependent help for the growth of malignant B cells in low-grade gastric lymphoma of mucosa-associated lymphoid tissue. J Pathol 1996;178:122–127.
206. Schollkopf C, Melbye M, Munksgaard L, et al. Borrelia infection and risk of non-Hodgkin lymphoma. Blood 2008;111:5524–5529.
207. Thieblemont C, Coiffier B. Management of marginal zone lymphomas. Curr Treat Options Oncol 2006;7:213–222.
208. Connor J, Ashton-Key M. Gastric and intestinal diffuse large B-cell lymphomas are clinically and immunophenotypically different. An immunohistochemical and clinical study. Histopathology 2007;51:697–703.
209. Jaso J, Chen L, Li S, et al. CD5-positive mucosa-associated lymphoid tissue (MALT) lymphoma: a clinicopathologic study of 14 cases. Hum Pathol 2012; 43:1436–1443.
210. Auer IA, Gascoyne RD, Connors JM, et al. t(11;18)(q21;q21) is the most common translocation in MALT lymphomas. Ann Oncol 1997;8:979–985.
211. Ott G, Katzenberger T, Greiner A, et al. The t(11;18)(q21;q21) chromosome translocation is a frequent and specific aberration in low-grade but not high-grade malignant non-Hodgkin's lymphomas of the mucosa-associated lymphoid tissue (MALT-) type. Cancer Res 1997;57:3944–3948.
212. Stoffel A, Chaurushiya M, Singh B, et al. Activation of NF-kappaB and inhibition of p53-mediated apoptosis by API2/mucosa-associated lymphoid tissue 1 fusions promote oncogenesis. Proc Natl Acad Sci U S A 2004;101:9079–9084.
213. Alpen B, Neubauer A, Dierlamm J, et al. Translocation t(11;18) absent in early gastric marginal zone B-cell lymphoma of MALT type responding to eradication of Helicobacter pylori infection. Blood 2000;95:4014–4015.
214. Bende RJ, Aarts WM, Riedl RG, et al. Among B cell non-Hodgkin's lymphomas, MALT lymphomas express a unique antibody repertoire with frequent rheumatoid factor reactivity. J Exp Med 2005;201:1229–1241.
215. Streubel B, Lamprecht A, Dierlamm J, et al. T(14;18)(q32;q21) involving IGH and MALT1 is a frequent chromosomal aberration in MALT lymphoma. Blood 2003;101:2335–2339.
216. Streubel B, Vinatzer U, Lamprecht A, et al. T(3;14)(p14.1;q32) involving IGH and FOXP1 is a novel recurrent chromosomal aberration in MALT lymphoma. Leukemia 2005;19:652–658.
217. Rinaldi A, Mian M, Chigrinova E, et al. Genome-wide DNA profiling of marginal zone lymphomas identifies subtype-specific lesions with an impact on the clinical outcome. Blood 2011;117:1595–1604.
218. Fiche M, Caprons F, Berger F, et al. Primary pulmonary non-Hodgkin's lymphomas. Histopathology 1995;26:529–537.
219. Wohrer S, Streubel B, Bartsch R, et al. Monoclonal immunoglobulin production is a frequent event in patients with mucosa-associated lymphoid tissue lymphoma. Clin Cancer Res 2004;10:7179–7181.
220. Raderer M, Wohrer S, Streubel B, et al. Assessment of disease dissemination in gastric compared with extragastric mucosa-associated lymphoid tissue lymphoma using extensive staging: a single-center experience. J Clin Oncol 2006;24:3136–3141.
221. Wundisch T, Thiede C, Morgner A, et al. Long-term follow-up of gastric MALT lymphoma after Helicobacter pylori eradication. J Clin Oncol 2005;23:8018–8024.
222. Chen LT, Lin JT, Tai JJ, et al. Long-term results of anti-Helicobacter pylori therapy in early-stage gastric high-grade transformed MALT lymphoma. J Natl Cancer Inst 2005;97:1345–1353.
223. Stathis A, Chini C, Bertoni F, et al. Long-term outcome following Helicobacter pylori eradication in a retrospective study of 105 patients with localized gastric marginal zone B-cell lymphoma of MALT type. Ann Oncol 2009;20:1086–1093.
224. Tsang RW, Gospodarowicz MK, Pintilie M, et al. Localized mucosa-associated lymphoid tissue lymphoma treated with radiation therapy has excellent clinical outcome. J Clin Oncol 2003;21:4157–4164.
225. Conconi A, Martinelli G, Thieblemont C, et al. Clinical activity of rituximab in extranodal marginal zone B-cell lymphoma of MALT type. Blood 2003;102:2741–2745.
226. Martinelli G, Laszlo D, Ferreri AJ, et al. Clinical activity of rituximab in gastric marginal zone non-Hodgkin's lymphoma resistant to or not eligible for anti-Helicobacter pylori therapy. J Clin Oncol 2005;23:1979–1983.
227. Uno T, Isobe K, Shikama N, et al. Radiotherapy for extranodal, marginal zone, B-cell lymphoma of mucosa-associated lymphoid tissue originating in the ocular adnexa: a multiinstitutional, retrospective review of 50 patients. Cancer 2003;98:865–871.
228. Govi S, Dolcetti R, Ponzoni M, et al. Final results of a multicenter phase II trial with translational elements to investigate the possible infective causes of ocular adnexal marginal zone B-cell lymphoma (OAMZL) with particular reference to chlamydia species and the efficacy of doxycycline as first-line lymphoma treatment (the IELSG#27 TRIAL). Blood 2011;118:a267.
229. Hammel P, Haioun C, Chaumette MT, et al. Efficacy of single-agent chemotherapy in low-grade B-cell mucosa-associated lymphoid tissue lymphoma with prominent gastric expression. J Clin Oncol 1995;13:2524–2529.
230. Brown JR, Friedberg JW, Feng Y, et al. A phase 2 study of concurrent fludarabine and rituximab for the treatment of marginal zone lymphomas. Br J Haematol 2009;145:741–748.

231. Walsh SH, Thorselius M, Johnson A, et al. Mutated VH genes and preferential VH3-21 use define new subsets of mantle cell lymphoma. Blood 2003;101:4047–4054.
232. Salaverria I, Royo C, Carvajal-Cuenca A, et al. CCND2 rearrangements are the most frequent genetic events in cyclin D1(-) mantle cell lymphoma. Blood 2013;121:1394–1402.
233. Salaverria I, Zettl A, Bea S, et al. Specific secondary genetic alterations in mantle cell lymphoma provide prognostic information independent of the gene expression-based proliferation signature. J Clin Oncol 2007;25:1216–1222.
234. Kridel R, Meissner B, Rogic S, et al. Whole transcriptome sequencing reveals recurrent NOTCH1 mutations in mantle cell lymphoma. Blood 2012;119:1963–1971.
235. Nygren L, Baumgartner Wennerholm S, Klimkowska M, et al. Prognostic role of SOX11 in a population-based cohort of mantle cell lymphoma. Blood 2012;119:4215–4223.
236. Romaguera JE, Medeiros LJ, Hagemeister FB, et al. Frequency of gastrointestinal involvement and its clinical significance in mantle cell lymphoma. Cancer 2003;97:586–591.
237. Martin P, Chadburn A, Christos P, et al. Outcome of deferred initial therapy in mantle-cell lymphoma. J Clin Oncol 2009;27:1209–1213.
238. Raty R, Franssila K, Jansson SE, et al. Predictive factors for blastoid transformation in the common variant of mantle cell lymphoma. Eur J Cancer 2003;39:321–329.
239. Geisler CH, Kolstad A, Laurell A, et al. The Mantle Cell Lymphoma International Prognostic Index (MIPI) is superior to the International Prognostic Index (IPI) in predicting survival following intensive first-line immunochemotherapy and autologous stem cell transplantation (ASCT). Blood 2010;115:1530–1533.
240. Determann O, Hoster E, Ott G, et al. Ki-67 predicts outcome in advanced-stage mantle cell lymphoma patients treated with anti-CD20 immunochemotherapy: results from randomized trials of the European MCL Network and the German Low Grade Lymphoma Study Group. Blood 2008;111:2385–2387.
241. Fernandez V, Salamero O, Espinet B, et al. Genomic and gene expression profiling defines indolent forms of mantle cell lymphoma. Cancer Res 2010;70:1408–1418.
242. Espinet B, Salaverria I, Bea S, et al. Incidence and prognostic impact of secondary cytogenetic aberrations in a series of 145 patients with mantle cell lymphoma. Genes Chromosomes Cancer 2010;49:439–451.
243. Fisher RI, Dahlberg S, Nathwani BN, et al. A clinical analysis of two indolent lymphoma entities: mantle cell lymphoma and marginal zone lymphoma (including the mucosa-associated lymphoid tissue and monocytoid B-cell subcategories): a Southwest Oncology Group study. Blood 1995;85:1075–1082.
244. Teodorovic I, Pittaluga S, Kluin-Nelemans JC, et al. Efficacy of four different regimens in 64 mantle-cell lymphoma cases: clinicopathologic comparison with 498 other non-Hodgkin's lymphoma subtypes. European Organization for the Research and Treatment of Cancer Lymphoma Cooperative Group. J Clin Oncol 1995;13:2819–2826.
245. Griffiths R, Mikhael J, Gleeson M, et al. Addition of rituximab to chemotherapy alone as first-line therapy improves overall survival in elderly patients with mantle cell lymphoma. Blood 2011;118:4808–4816.
246. Kluin-Nelemans HC, Hoster E, Hermine O, et al. Treatment of older patients with mantle-cell lymphoma. N Engl J Med 2012;367:520–531.
247. Romaguera JE, Fayad LE, Feng L, et al. Ten-year follow-up after intense chemoimmunotherapy with Rituximab-HyperCVAD alternating with rituximab-high dose methotrexate/cytarabine (R-MA) and without stem cell transplantation in patients with untreated aggressive mantle cell lymphoma. Br J Haematol 2010;150:200–208.
248. Bernstein SH, Epner E, Unger JM, et al. A phase II multicenter trial of hyperCVAD MTX/Ara-C and rituximab in patients with previously untreated mantle cell lymphoma; SWOG 0213. Ann Oncol 2013;24:1587–1593.
249. Merli F, Luminari S, Ilariucci F, et al. Rituximab plus HyperCVAD alternating with high dose cytarabine and methotrexate for the initial treatment of patients with mantle cell lymphoma, a multicentre trial from Gruppo Italiano Studio Linfomi. Br J Haematol 2012;156:346–353.
250. Dreyling M, Lenz G, Hoster E, et al. Early consolidation by myeloablative radiochemotherapy followed by autologous stem cell transplantation in first remission significantly prolongs progression-free survival in mantle-cell lymphoma: results of a prospective randomized trial of the European MCL Network. Blood 2005;105:2677–2684.
251. Geisler CH, Kolstad A, Laurell A, et al. Nordic MCL2 trial update: six-year follow-up after intensive immunochemotherapy for untreated mantle cell lymphoma followed by BEAM or BEAC + autologous stem-cell support: still very long survival but late relapses do occur. Br J Haematol 2012;158:355–362.
252. O'Connor OA, Moskowitz C, Portlock C, et al. Patients with chemotherapy-refractory mantle cell lymphoma experience high response rates and identical progression-free survivals compared with patients with relapsed disease following treatment with single agent bortezomib: results of a multicentre Phase 2 clinical trial. Br J Haematol 2009;145:34–39.
253. Witzig TE, Vose JM, Zinzani PL, et al. An international phase II trial of single-agent lenalidomide for relapsed or refractory aggressive B-cell non-Hodgkin's lymphoma. Ann Oncol 2011;22:1622–1627.
254. Eve HE, Carey S, Richardson SJ, et al. Single-agent lenalidomide in relapsed/refractory mantle cell lymphoma: results from a UK phase II study suggest activity and possible gender differences. Br J Haematol 2012;159:154–163.
255. Wang ML, Rule S, Martin P, et al. Targeting BTK with ibrutinib in relapsed or refractory mantle-cell lymphoma. N Engl J Med 2013;369:507–516.

256. Leonard JP, LaCasce AS, Smith MR, et al. Selective CDK4/6 inhibition with tumor responses by PD0332991 in patients with mantle cell lymphoma. Blood 2012;119:4597–4607.
257. Rosenbluth BD, Yahalom J. Highly effective local control and palliation of mantle cell lymphoma with involved-field radiation therapy (IFRT). Int J Radiat Oncol Biol Phys 2006;65:1185–1191.
258. Jacobsen E, Freedman A. An update on the role of high-dose therapy with autologous or allogeneic stem cell transplantation in mantle cell lymphoma. Curr Opin Oncol 2004;16:106–113.
259. Le Gouill S, Kroger N, Dhedin N, et al. Reduced-intensity conditioning allogeneic stem cell transplantation for relapsed/refractory mantle cell lymphoma: a multicenter experience. Ann Oncol 2012;23:2695–2703.
260. Abramson JS. T-cell/histiocyte-rich B cell lymphoma: biology, diagnosis, and management. Oncologist 2006;11:384–392.
261. Yamaguchi M, Seto M, Okamoto M, et al. De novo CD5+ diffuse large B-cell lymphoma: a clinicopathologic study of 109 patients. Blood 2002;99:815–821.
262. De Paepe P, Achten R, Verhoef G, et al. Large cleaved and immunoblastic lymphoma may represent two distinct clinicopathologic entities within the group of diffuse large B cell lymphomas. J Clin Oncol 2005;23:7060–7068.
263. Hu S, Xu-Monette ZY, Balasubramanyam A, et al. CD30 expression defines a novel subgroup of diffuse large B-cell lymphoma with favorable prognosis and distinct gene expression signature: a report from the International DLBCL Rituximab-CHOP Consortium Program Study. Blood 2013;121:2715–2724.
264. Kramer MH, Hermans J, Wijburg E, et al. Clinical relevance of BCL2, BCL6, and MYC rearrangements in diffuse large B-cell lymphoma. Blood 1998;92:3152–3162.
265. Lossos IS, Morgensztern D. Prognostic biomarkers in diffuse large B-cell lymphoma. J Clin Oncol 2006;24:995–1007.
266. Parekh S, Polo JM, Shaknovich R, et al. BCL6 programs lymphoma cells for survival and differentiation through distinct biochemical mechanisms. Blood 2007;110:2067–2074.
267. Huang JZ, Sanger WG, Greiner TC, et al. The t(14;18) defines a unique subset of diffuse large B-cell lymphoma with a germinal center B-cell gene expression profile. Blood 2002;99:2285–2290.
268. Ottensmeier CH, Stevenson FK. Isotype switch variants reveal clonally related subpopulations in diffuse large B cell lymphoma. Blood 2000;96:2550–2556.
269. Bea S, Zettl A, Wright G, et al. Diffuse large B-cell lymphoma subgroups have distinct genetic profiles that influence tumor biology and improve gene-expression-based survival prediction. Blood 2005;106:3183–3190.
270. Morin RD, Johnson NA, Severson TM, et al. Somatic mutations altering EZH2 (Tyr641) in follicular and diffuse large B-cell lymphomas of germinal-center origin. Nat Genet 2010;42:181–185.
271. Tam W, Gomez M, Chadburn A, et al. Mutational analysis of PRDM1 indicates a tumor-suppressor role in diffuse large B-cell lymphomas. Blood 2006; 107:4090–4100.
272. Davis RE, Ngo VN, Lenz G, et al. Chronic active B-cell-receptor signalling in diffuse large B-cell lymphoma. Nature 2010;463:88–92.
273. Aukema SM, Siebert R, Schuuring E, et al. Double-hit B-cell lymphomas. Blood 2011;117:2319–2331.
274. Barrans S, Crouch S, Smith A, et al. Rearrangement of MYC is associated with poor prognosis in patients with diffuse large B-cell lymphoma treated in the era of rituximab. J Clin Oncol 2010;28:3360–3365.
275. Stasik CJ, Nitta H, Zhang W, et al. Increased MYC gene copy number correlates with increased mRNA levels in diffuse large B-cell lymphoma. Haematologica 2010;95:597–603.
276. Lohr JG, Stojanov P, Lawrence MS, et al. Discovery and prioritization of somatic mutations in diffuse large B-cell lymphoma (DLBCL) by whole-exome sequencing. Proc Natl Acad Sci U S A 2012;109:3879–3884.
277. Shenoy PJ, Malik N, Nooka A, et al. Racial differences in the presentation and outcomes of diffuse large B-cell lymphoma in the United States. Cancer 2011;117:2530–2540.
278. Vitolo U, Chiappella A, Ferreri AJ, et al. First-line treatment for primary testicular diffuse large B-cell lymphoma with rituximab-CHOP, CNS prophylaxis, and contralateral testis irradiation: final results of an international phase II trial. J Clin Oncol 2011;29:2766–2772.
279. van Besien K, Ha CS, Murphy S, et al. Risk factors, treatment, and outcome of central nervous system recurrence in adults with intermediate-grade and immunoblastic lymphoma. Blood 1998;91:1178–1184.
280. Miller TP, Dahlberg S, Cassady JR, et al. Chemotherapy alone compared with chemotherapy plus radiotherapy for localized intermediate- and high-grade non-Hodgkin's lymphoma. N Engl J Med 1998;339:21–26.
281. Persky DO, Unger JM, Spier CM, et al. Phase II study of rituximab plus three cycles of CHOP and involved-field radiotherapy for patients with limited-stage aggressive B-cell lymphoma: Southwest Oncology Group study 0014. J Clin Oncol 2008;26:2258–2263.
282. Horning SJ, Weller E, Kim K, et al. Chemotherapy with or without radiotherapy in limited-stage diffuse aggressive non-Hodgkin's lymphoma: Eastern Cooperative Oncology Group study 1484. J Clin Oncol 2004;22:3032–3038.
283. Reyes F, Lepage E, Ganem G, et al. ACVBP versus CHOP plus radiotherapy for localized aggressive lymphoma. N Engl J Med 2005;352:1197–1205.
284. Bonnet C, Fillet G, Mounier N, et al. CHOP alone compared with CHOP plus radiotherapy for localized aggressive lymphoma in elderly patients: a study by the Groupe d'Etude des Lymphomes de l'Adulte. J Clin Oncol 2007; 25:787–792.
285. Pfreundschuh M, Trumper L, Osterborg A, et al. CHOP-like chemotherapy plus rituximab versus CHOP-like chemotherapy alone in young patients with good-prognosis diffuse large-B-cell lymphoma: a randomised controlled trial by the MabThera International Trial (MInT) Group. Lancet Oncol 2006;7: 379–391.
286. Coiffier B, Lepage E, Briere J, et al. CHOP chemotherapy plus rituximab compared with CHOP alone in elderly patients with diffuse large-B-cell lymphoma. N Engl J Med 2002;346:235–242.
287. Feugier P, Van Hoof A, Sebban C, et al. Long-term results of the R-CHOP study in the treatment of elderly patients with diffuse large B-cell lymphoma: a study by the Groupe d'Etude des Lymphomes de l'Adulte. J Clin Oncol 2005;23:4117–4126.
288. Habermann TM, Weller EA, Morrison VA, et al. Rituximab-CHOP versus CHOP alone or with maintenance rituximab in older patients with diffuse large B-cell lymphoma. J Clin Oncol 2006;24:3121–3127.
289. Pfreundschuh M, Schubert J, Ziepert M, et al. Six versus eight cycles of bi-weekly CHOP-14 with or without rituximab in elderly patients with aggressive CD20+ B-cell lymphomas: a randomised controlled trial (RICOVER-60). Lancet Oncol 2008;9:105–116.
290. Cunningham D, Hawkes EA, Jack A, et al. Rituximab plus cyclophosphamide, doxorubicin, vincristine, and prednisolone in patients with newly diagnosed diffuse large B-cell non-Hodgkin lymphoma: a phase 3 comparison of dose intensification with 14-day versus 21-day cycles. Lancet 2013;381:1817–1826.
291. Recher C, Coiffier B, Haioun C, et al. Intensified chemotherapy with ACVBP plus rituximab versus standard CHOP plus rituximab for the treatment of diffuse large B-cell lymphoma (LNH03-2B): an open-label randomised phase 3 trial. Lancet 2011;378:1858–1867.
292. Greb A, Bohlius J, Schiefer D, et al. High-dose chemotherapy with autologous stem cell transplantation in the first line treatment of aggressive non-Hodgkin lymphoma (NHL) in adults. Cochrane Database Syst Rev 2008;23(1): CD004024.
293. Schmitz N, Nickelsen M, Ziepert M, et al. Conventional chemotherapy (CHOEP-14) with rituximab or high-dose chemotherapy (MegaCHOEP) with rituximab for young, high-risk patients with aggressive B-cell lymphoma: an open-label, randomised, phase 3 trial (DSHNHL 2002-1). Lancet Oncol 2012;13:1250–1259.
294. Stiff PJ, Unger JM, Cook JR, et al. Autologous transplantation as consolidation for aggressive non-Hodgkin's lymphoma. N Engl J Med 2013;369:1681–1690.
295. Larouche JF, Berger F, Chassagne-Clement C, et al. Lymphoma recurrence 5 years or later following diffuse large B-cell lymphoma: clinical characteristics and outcome. J Clin Oncol 2010;28:2094–2100.
296. Philip T, Armitage JO, Spitzer G, et al. High-dose methotrexate as a single agent in treatment of non-Hodgkin's lymphoma. Am J Med 1984;77:845–850.
297. Ohmachi K, Niitsu N, Uchida T, et al. Multicenter phase II study of bendamustine plus rituximab in patients with relapsed or refractory diffuse large B-cell lymphoma. J Clin Oncol. 2013;31:2103–2109.
298. Ohmachi K, Ando K, Ogura M, et al. Multicenter phase II study of bendamustine for relapsed or refractory indolent B-cell non-Hodgkin lymphoma and mantle cell lymphoma. Cancer Sci 2010;101:2059–2064.
299. Ruan J, Martin P, Coleman M, et al. Durable responses with the metronomic rituximab and thalidomide plus prednisone, etoposide, procarbazine, and cyclophosphamide regimen in elderly patients with recurrent mantle cell lymphoma. Cancer 2010;116:2655–2664.
300. Gisselbrecht C, Glass B, Mounier N, et al. R-ICE versus R-DHAP in relapsed patients with CD20 diffuse large B-cell lymphoma (DLBCL) followed by autologous stem cell transplantation: CORAL study. J Clin Oncol 2009; 27:8509.
301. Gisselbrecht C, Glass B, Mounier N, et al. Salvage regimens with autologous transplantation for relapsed large B-cell lymphoma in the rituximab era. J Clin Oncol 2010;28:4184–4190.
302. Philip T, Armitage JO, Spitzer G, et al. High-dose therapy and autologous bone marrow transplantation after failure of conventional chemotherapy in adults with intermediate-grade or high-grade non-Hodgkin's lymphoma. N Engl J Med 1987;316:1493–1498.
303. Philip T, Guglielmi C, Hagenbeek A, et al. Autologous bone marrow transplantation as compared with salvage chemotherapy in relapses of chemotherapy-sensitive non-Hodgkin's lymphoma. N Engl J Med 1995;333:1540–1545.
304. Gisselbrecht C, Schmitz N, Mounier N, et al. Rituximab maintenance therapy after autologous stem cell transplantation in patients with relapsed CD20(+) diffuse large B-cell lymphoma: final analysis of the collaborative trial in relapsed aggressive lymphoma. J Clin Oncol 2013;31:1662–1668.
305. Reeder C, Gornet M, Habermann T, et al. A phase II trial of the oral mTOR inhibitor Everolimus (RAD001) in relapsed aggressive non-Hodgkin lymphoma (NHL). Blood 2007;110:121a.
306. Salit RB, Fowler DH, Wilson WH, et al. Dose-adjusted EPOCH-rituximab combined with fludarabine provides an effective bridge to reduced-intensity allogeneic hematopoietic stem-cell transplantation in patients with lymphoid malignancies. J Clin Oncol 2012;30:830–836.
307. van Kampen RJ, Canals C, Schouten HC, et al. Allogeneic stem-cell transplantation as salvage therapy for patients with diffuse large B-cell non-Hodgkin's lymphoma relapsing after an autologous stem-cell transplantation: an analysis of the European Group for Blood and Marrow Transplantation Registry. J Clin Oncol 2011;29:1342–1348.
308. Porter DL, Levine BL, Kalos M, et al. Chimeric antigen receptor-modified T cells in chronic lymphoid leukemia. N Engl J Med 2011;365:725–733.
309. Kalos M, Levine BL, Porter DL, et al. T cells with chimeric antigen receptors have potent antitumor effects and can establish memory in patients with advanced leukemia. Sci Transl Med 2011;3:95ra73.

310. Davila ML, Riviere I, Wang X, et al. Efficacy and toxicity management of 19-28z CAR T cell therapy in B cell acute lymphoblastic leukemia. Sci Transl Med 2014;6:224ra25.
311. Carpenito C, Milone MC, Hassan R, et al. Control of human T cells containing CD28 and CD137 domains. Proc Natl Acad Sci 2009;106:3360–3365.
312. Kochenderfer JN, Dudley ME, Kassim SH, et al. Effective treatment of chemotherapy-refractory diffuse large B-cell lymphoma with autologous T cells genetically-engineered to express an anti-CD19 chimeric antigen receptor. Blood 2013;122:a168
313. Ferreri AJ, Campo E, Seymour JF, et al. Intravascular lymphoma: clinical presentation, natural history, management and prognostic factors in a series of 38 cases, with special emphasis on the 'cutaneous variant'. Br J Haematol 2004;127:173–183.
314. Ponzoni M, Ferreri AJ, Campo E, et al. Definition, diagnosis, and management of intravascular large B-cell lymphoma: proposals and perspectives from an international consensus meeting. J Clin Oncol 2007;25:3168–3173.
315. Shimada K, Matsue K, Yamamoto K, et al. Retrospective analysis of intravascular large B-cell lymphoma treated with rituximab-containing chemotherapy as reported by the IVL study group in Japan. J Clin Oncol 2008;26:3189–3195.
316. Achten R, Verhoef G, Vanuytsel L, et al. T-cell/histiocyte-rich large B-cell lymphoma: a distinct clinicopathologic entity. J Clin Oncol 2002;20:1269–1277.
317. Dupuis J, Emile JF, Mounier N, et al. Prognostic significance of Epstein-Barr virus in nodal peripheral T-cell lymphoma, unspecified: A Groupe d'Etude des Lymphomes de l'Adulte (GELA) study. Blood 2006;108:4163–4169.
318. Montes-Moreno S, Odqvist L, Diaz-Perez JA, et al. EBV-positive diffuse large B-cell lymphoma of the elderly is an aggressive post-germinal center B-cell neoplasm characterized by prominent nuclear factor-kB activation. Mod Pathol 2012;25:968–982.
319. Laurent C, Do C, Gascoyne RD, et al. Anaplastic lymphoma kinase-positive diffuse large B-cell lymphoma: a rare clinicopathologic entity with poor prognosis. J Clin Oncol 2009;27:4211–4216.
320. Zucca E, Conconi A, Mughal TI, et al. Patterns of outcome and prognostic factors in primary large-cell lymphoma of the testis in a survey by the International Extranodal Lymphoma Study Group. J Clin Oncol 2003;21:20–27.
321. Thieblemont C, Coiffier B. Lymphoma in older patients. J Clin Oncol 2007;25:1916–1923.
322. Fields PA, Linch DC. Treatment of the elderly patient with diffuse large B cell lymphoma. Br J Haematol 2012;157:159–170.
323. Wunderer J, Smith S D, et al. Elderly and very elderly patients with diffuse large B-cell non-Hodgkin lymphoma: impact of functional status and co-morbidities on outcome. Br J Haematol 2012;156:196–204.
324. Mounier N, Heutte N, Thieblemont C, et al. Ten-year relative survival and causes of death in elderly patients treated with R-CHOP or CHOP in the GELA LNH-985 trial. Clin Lymphoma Myeloma Leuk 2012;12:151–154.
325. Peyrade F, Jardin F, Thieblemont C, et al. Attenuated immunochemotherapy regimen (R-miniCHOP) in elderly patients older than 80 years with diffuse large B-cell lymphoma: a multicentre, single-arm, phase 2 trial. Lancet Oncol 2011;12:460–468.
326. Weisenburger DD, Savage KJ, Harris NL, et al. Peripheral T-cell lymphoma, not otherwise specified: a report of 340 cases from the International Peripheral T-cell Lymphoma Project. Blood 2011;117:3402–3408.
327. van Besien K, Kelta M, Bahaguna P. Primary mediastinal B-cell lymphoma: a review of pathology and management. J Clin Oncol 2001;19:1855–1864.
328. Rodig SJ, Savage KJ, Nguyen V, et al. TRAF1 expression and c-Rel activation are useful adjuncts in distinguishing classical Hodgkin lymphoma from a subset of morphologically or immunophenotypically similar lymphomas. Am J Surg Pathol 2005;29:196–203.
329. Rosenwald A, Wright G, Leroy K, et al. Molecular diagnosis of primary mediastinal B cell lymphoma identifies a clinically favorable subgroup of diffuse large B cell lymphoma related to Hodgkin lymphoma. J Exp Med 2003;198:851–862.
330. Rieger M, Osterborg A, Pettengell R, et al. Primary mediastinal B-cell lymphoma treated with CHOP-like chemotherapy with or without rituximab: results of the Mabthera International Trial Group study. Ann Oncol 2011;22:664–670.
331. Dunleavy K, Pittaluga S, Maeda LS, et al. Dose-adjusted EPOCH-rituximab therapy in primary mediastinal B-cell lymphoma. N Engl J Med 2013;368:1408–1416.
332. Swerdlow SH, Campo E, Harris NL, et al. WHO Classification of Tumours of Haematopoietic and Lymphoid Tissues. Lyon, France: IARC Press; 2008.
333. Hummel M, Bentink S, Berger H, et al. A biologic definition of Burkitt's lymphoma from transcriptional and genomic profiling. N Engl J Med 2006;354:2419–2430.
334. Cobain E, Ahmadi T, Hoffman M, et al. B cell lymphoma, unclassifiable: survival advantage for aggressive therapy. Blood 2011;118:2689.
335. Lin P, Dickason TJ, Fayad LE, et al. Prognostic value of MYC rearrangement in cases of B-cell lymphoma, unclassifiable, with features intermediate between diffuse large B-cell lymphoma and Burkitt lymphoma. Cancer 2012;118:1566–1573.
336. Savage KJ, Johnson NA, Ben-Neriah S, et al. MYC gene rearrangements are associated with a poor prognosis in diffuse large B-cell lymphoma patients treated with R-CHOP chemotherapy. Blood 2009;114:3533–3537.
337. Johnson NA, Slack GW, Savage KJ, et al. Concurrent expression of MYC and BCL2 in diffuse large B-cell lymphoma treated with rituximab plus cyclophosphamide, doxorubicin, vincristine, and prednisone. J Clin Oncol 2012;30:3452–3459.
338. Corazzelli G, Frigeri F, Russo F, et al. RD-CODOX-M/IVAC with rituximab and intrathecal liposomal cytarabine in adult Burkitt lymphoma and 'unclassifiable' highly aggressive B-cell lymphoma. Br J Haematol 2012;156:234–244.

339. Dunleavy K, Pittaluga S, Wayne AS, et al. MYC + aggressive B-cell lymphomas: novel therapy of untreated Burkitt lymphoma (BL) and MYC+ diffuse large B cell lymphoma (DLBCL) with DA-EPOCH-R. Ann Oncol 2011;22:071a.
340. Savage KJ, Monti S, Kutok JL, et al. The molecular signature of mediastinal large B-cell lymphoma differs from that of other diffuse large B-cell lymphomas and shares features with classical Hodgkin lymphoma. Blood 2003;102:3871–3879.
341. Green MR, Monti S, Rodig SJ, et al. Integrative analysis reveals selective 9p24.1 amplification, increased PD-1 ligand expression, and further induction via JAK2 in nodular sclerosing Hodgkin lymphoma and primary mediastinal large B-cell lymphoma. Blood 2010;116:3268–3277.
342. Eberle FC, Rodriguez-Canales J, Wei L, et al. Methylation profiling of mediastinal gray zone lymphoma reveals a distinctive signature with elements shared by classical Hodgkin's lymphoma and primary mediastinal large B-cell lymphoma. Haematologica 2011;96:558–566.
343. Traverse-Glehen A, Pittaluga S, Gaulard P, et al. Mediastinal gray zone lymphoma: the missing link between classic Hodgkin's lymphoma and mediastinal large B-cell lymphoma. Am J Surg Pathol 2005;29:1411–1421.
344. Kolstad A, Nome O, Delabie J, et al. Standard CHOP-21 as first line therapy for elderly patients with Hodgkin's lymphoma. Leuk Lymphoma 2007;48:570–576.
345. Walewski J, Lampka E, Tajer J, et al. CHOP-21 for unfavorable Hodgkin's lymphoma. An exploratory study. Med Oncol 2010;27:262–267.
346. Aviles A, Neri N, Fernandez R, et al. Randomized clinical trial to assess the efficacy of radiotherapy in primary mediastinal large B-lymphoma. Int J Radiat Oncol Biol Phys 2012;83:1227–1231.
347. Klapproth K, Wirth T. Advances in the understanding of MYC-induced lymphomagenesis. Br J Haematol 2010;149:484–497.
348. Blum KA, Lozanski G, Byrd JC. Adult Burkitt leukemia and lymphoma. Blood 2004;104:3009–3020.
349. Dave SS, Fu K, Wright GW, et al. Molecular diagnosis of Burkitt's lymphoma. N Engl J Med 2006;354:2431–2442.
350. Harris NL, Horning SJ. Burkitt's lymphoma—the message from microarrays. N Engl J Med 2006;354:2495–2498.
351. Ribera JM, Garcia O, Grande C, et al. Dose-intensive chemotherapy including rituximab in Burkitt's leukemia or lymphoma regardless of human immunodeficiency virus infection status: final results of a phase 2 study (Burkimab). Cancer 2013;119:1660–1668.
352. Magrath I, Adde M, Shad A, et al. Adults and children with small non-cleaved-cell lymphoma have a similar excellent outcome when treated with the same chemotherapy regimen. J Clin Oncol 1996;14:925–934.
353. Lacasce A, Howard O, Lib S, et al. Modified magrath regimens for adults with Burkitt and Burkitt-like lymphomas: preserved efficacy with decreased toxicity. Leuk Lymphoma 2004;45:761–767.
354. Mead GM, Barrans SL, Qian W, et al. A prospective clinicopathological study of dose modified CODOX-M/IVAC in patients with sporadic Burkitt lymphoma defined using cytogenetic and immunophenotypic criteria (MRC/NCRI LY10 trial). Blood 2008;112:2248–2260.
355. Thomas DA, Faderl S, O'Brien S, et al. Chemoimmunotherapy with hyper-CVAD plus rituximab for the treatment of adult Burkitt and Burkitt-type lymphoma or acute lymphoblastic leukemia. Cancer 2006;106:1569–1580.
356. Dunleavy K, Pittaluga S, Shovlin M, et al. Low-intensity therapy in adults with Burkitt's lymphoma. N Engl J Med 2013;369:1915–1925.
357. Song KW, Barnett MJ, Gascoyne RD, et al. Haematopoietic stem cell transplantation as primary therapy of sporadic adult Burkitt lymphoma. Br J Haematol 2006;133:634–637.
358. Sweetenham JW, Pearce R, Taghipour G, et al. Adult Burkitt's and Burkitt-like non-Hodgkin's lymphoma—outcome for patients treated with high-dose therapy and autologous stem cell transplantation in first remission or at relapse: results from the European Group for Blood and Marrow Transplantation. J Clin Oncol 1996;14:2465–2472.
359. Rizvi MA, Evens AM, Tallman MS, et al. T-cell non-Hodgkin lymphoma. Blood 2006;107:1255–1264.
360. Jaffe ES, Harris NL, Vardiman J. Neoplasms of the Hematopoietic and Lymphoid Tissues. Lyon, France: IARC Press; 2001.
361. Schmitz N, Trumper L, Ziepert M, et al. Treatment and prognosis of mature T-cell and NK-cell lymphoma: an analysis of patients with T-cell lymphoma treated in studies of the German High-Grade Non-Hodgkin Lymphoma Study Group. Blood 2010;116:3418–3425.
362. Mak V, Hamm J, Chhanabhai M, et al. Survival of patients with peripheral T cell lymphoma after first relapse or progression: spectrum of disease and rare long-term survivors. J Clin Oncol 2013;31:1970–1976.
363. Zinzani PL, Venturini F, Stefoni V, et al. Gemcitabine as single agent in pretreated T-cell lymphoma patients: evaluation of the long-term outcome. Ann Oncol 2010;21:860–863.
364. Malik SM, Liu K, Qiang X, et al. Folotyn (pralatrexate injection) for the treatment of patients with relapsed or refractory peripheral T-cell lymphoma: U.S. Food and Drug Administration drug approval summary. Clin Cancer Res 2011;16:4921–4927.
365. Coiffier B, Pro B, Prince HM, et al. Results from a pivotal, open-label, phase II study of romidepsin in relapsed or refractory peripheral T-cell lymphoma after prior systemic therapy. J Clin Oncol 2012;30:631–636.
366. Dodero A, Spina F, Narni F, et al. Allogeneic transplantation following a reduced-intensity conditioning regimen in relapsed/refractory peripheral T-cell lymphomas: long-term remissions and response to donor lymphocyte infusions support the role of a graft-versus-lymphoma effect. Leukemia 2012;26(3):520–526.

367. Zhou Y, Attygalle AD, Chuang SS, et al. Angioimmunoblastic T-cell lymphomas with mutations in progress ... associated with EBV and HHV6B viral load. Br J Haematol 2007;138:44–53.
368. Lemonnier F, Couronne L, Parrens M, et al. Recurrent TET2 mutations in peripheral T-cell lymphomas correlate with TFH-like features and adverse clinical parameters. Blood 2012;120:1466–1469.
369. Federico M, Rudiger T, Bellei M, et al. Clinicopathologic characteristics of angioimmunoblastic T-cell lymphoma: analysis of the international peripheral T-cell lymphoma project. J Clin Oncol 2013;31:240–246.
370. Catassi C, Fabiani E, Corrao G, et al. Risk of non-Hodgkin lymphoma in celiac disease. JAMA 2002;287:1413–1419.
371. Gale J, Simmonds PD, Mead GM, et al. Enteropathy-type intestinal T-cell lymphoma: clinical features and treatment of 31 patients in a single center. J Clin Oncol 2000;18:795–803.
372. Delabie J, Holte H, Vose JM, et al. Enteropathy-associated T-cell lymphoma: clinical and histological findings from the international peripheral T-cell lymphoma project. Blood 2011;118:148–155.
373. Chan JK, Chan AC, Cheuk W, et al. Type II enteropathy-associated T-cell lymphoma: a distinct aggressive lymphoma with frequent gammadelta T-cell receptor expression. Am J Surg Pathol 2011;35:1557–1569.
374. Sieniawski M, Angamuthu N, Boyd K, et al. Evaluation of enteropathy-associated T-cell lymphoma comparing standard therapies with a novel regimen including autologous stem cell transplantation. Blood 2010;115:3664–3670.
375. de Jong D, Vasmel WL, de Boer JP, et al. Anaplastic large-cell lymphoma in women with breast implants. JAMA 2008;300:2030–2035.
376. Chiarle R, Voena C, Ambrogio C, et al. The anaplastic lymphoma kinase in the pathogenesis of cancer. Nat Rev Cancer 2008;8:11–23.
377. Savage KJ, Harris NL, Vose JM, et al. ALK- anaplastic large-cell lymphoma is clinically and immunophenotypically different from both ALK+ ALCL and peripheral T-cell lymphoma, not otherwise specified: report from the International Peripheral T-Cell Lymphoma Project. Blood 2008;111:5496–5504.
378. Sonnen R, Schmidt WP, Muller-Hermelink HK, et al. The International Prognostic Index determines the outcome of patients with nodal mature T-cell lymphomas. Br J Haematol 2005;129:366–372.
379. Gascoyne RD, Aoun P, Wu D, et al. Prognostic significance of anaplastic lymphoma kinase (ALK) protein expression in adults with anaplastic large cell lymphoma. Blood 1999;93:3913–3921.
380. Sibon D, Fournier M, Briere J, et al. Long-term outcome of adults with systemic anaplastic large-cell lymphoma treated within the Groupe d'Etude des Lymphomes de l'Adulte trials. J Clin Oncol 2012;30:3939–3946.
381. Pro B, Advani R, Brice P, et al. Brentuximab vedotin (SGN-35) in patients with relapsed or refractory systemic anaplastic large-cell lymphoma: results of a phase II study. J Clin Oncol 2012;30:2190–2196.
382. Gambacorti-Passerini C, Messa C, Pogliani EM. Crizotinib in anaplastic large-cell lymphoma. N Engl J Med 2011;364:775–776.
383. Miyazaki K, Yamaguchi M, Imai H, et al. Gene expression profiling of peripheral T-cell lymphoma including gammadelta T-cell lymphoma. Blood 2009;113:1071–1074.
384. Belhadj K, Reyes F, Farcet JP, et al. Hepatosplenic gammadelta T-cell lymphoma is a rare clinicopathologic entity with poor outcome: report on a series of 21 patients. Blood 2003;102:4261–4269.
385. Falchook GS, Vega F, Dang NH, et al. Hepatosplenic gamma-delta T-cell lymphoma: clinicopathological features and treatment. Ann Oncol 2009;20:1080–1085.
386. Kotlyar DS, Osterman MT, Diamond RH, et al. A systematic review of factors that contribute to hepatosplenic T-cell lymphoma in patients with inflammatory bowel disease. Clin Gastroenterol Hepatol 2011;9:36–41.
387. Willemze R, Jansen PM, Cerroni L, et al. Subcutaneous panniculitis-like T-cell lymphoma: definition, classification, and prognostic factors: an EORTC Cutaneous Lymphoma Group Study of 83 cases. Blood 2008;111:838–845.
388. Laurini JA, Perry AM, Boilesen E, et al. Classification of non-Hodgkin lymphoma in Central and South America: a review of 1028 cases. Blood 2012;120:4795–4801.
389. Chim CS, Ma SY, Au WY, et al. Primary nasal natural killer cell lymphoma: long-term treatment outcome and relationship with the International Prognostic Index. Blood 2004;103:216–221.
390. Au WY, Weisenburger DD, Intragumtornchai T, et al. Clinical differences between nasal and extranasal natural killer/T-cell lymphoma: a study of 136 cases from the International Peripheral T-Cell Lymphoma Project. Blood 2009;113:3931–3937.
391. Lee J, Suh C, Park YH, et al. Extranodal natural killer T-cell lymphoma, nasal-type: a prognostic model from a retrospective multicenter study. J Clin Oncol 2006;24:612–618.
392. Kim SJ, Oh SY, Hong JY, et al. When do we need central nervous system prophylaxis in patients with extranodal NK/T-cell lymphoma, nasal type? Ann Oncol 2010;21:1058–1063.
393. Wang ZY, Liu QF, Wang H, et al. Clinical implications of plasma Epstein-Barr virus DNA in early-stage extranodal nasal-type NK/T-cell lymphoma patients receiving primary radiotherapy. Blood 2012;120:2003–2010.
394. Huang MJ, Jiang Y, Liu WP, et al. Early or up-front radiotherapy improved survival of localized extranodal NK/T-cell lymphoma, nasal-type in the upper aerodigestive tract. Int J Radiat Oncol Biol Phys 2008;70:166–174.
395. Li YX, Liu QF, Fang H, et al. Variable clinical presentations of nasal and Waldeyer ring natural killer/T-cell lymphoma. Clin Cancer Res 2009;15:2905–2912.

396. Yamaguchi M, Tobinai K, Oguchi M, et al. Phase I/II study of concurrent chemoradiotherapy for localized nasal natural killer/T-cell lymphoma: Japan Clinical Oncology Group Study JCOG0211. J Clin Oncol 2009;27:5594–5600.
397. Kim SJ, Kim K, Kim BS, et al. Phase II trial of concurrent radiation and weekly cisplatin followed by VIPD chemotherapy in newly diagnosed, stage IE to IIE, nasal extranodal NK/T-Cell Lymphoma: Consortium for Improving Survival of Lymphoma study. J Clin Oncol 2009;27:6027–6032.
398. Yamaguchi M, Tobinai K, Oguchi M, et al. Concurrent chemoradiotherapy for localized nasal natural killer/T-cell lymphoma: an updated analysis of the Japan clinical oncology group study JCOG0211. J Clin Oncol 2012;30:4044–4046.
399. Wang H, Li YX, Wang WH, et al. Mild toxicity and favorable prognosis of high-dose and extended involved-field intensity modulated radiotherapy for patients with early-stage nasal NK/T-cell lymphoma. Int J Radiat Oncol Biol Phys 2012;82:1115–1121.
400. Yong W, Zheng W, Zhu J, et al. L-asparaginase in the treatment of refractory and relapsed extranodal NK/T-cell lymphoma, nasal type. Ann Hematol 2009;88:647–652.
401. Jaccard A, Gachard N, Marin B, et al. Efficacy of L-asparaginase with methotrexate and dexamethasone (AspaMetDex regimen) in patients with refractory or relapsing extranodal NK/T-cell lymphoma, a phase 2 study. Blood 2011;117:1834–1839.
402. Yamaguchi M, Kwong YL, Kim WS, et al. Phase II study of SMILE chemotherapy for newly diagnosed stage IV, relapsed, or refractory extranodal natural killer (NK)/T-cell lymphoma, nasal type: the NK-Cell Tumor Study Group study. J Clin Oncol 2011;29:4410–4416.
403. Uchiyama T, Yodoi J, Sagawa K, et al. Adult T-cell leukemia: clinical and hematologic features of 16 cases. Blood 1977;50:481–492.
404. Bunn PA Jr, Schechter GP, Jaffe E, et al. Clinical course of retrovirus-associated adult T-cell lymphoma in the United States. N Engl J Med 1983;309:257–264.
405. Tsukasaki K, Hermine O, Bazarbachi A, et al. Definition, prognostic factors, treatment, and response criteria of adult T-cell leukemia-lymphoma: a proposal from an international consensus meeting. J Clin Oncol 2009;27:453–459.
406. Banerjee P, Tripp A, Lairmore MD, et al. Adult T-cell leukemia/lymphoma development in HTLV-1-infected humanized SCID mice. Blood 2010;115:2640–2648.
407. Vose J, Armitage J, Weisenburger D. International peripheral T-cell and natural killer/T-cell lymphoma study: pathology findings and clinical outcomes. J Clin Oncol 2008;26:4124–4130.
408. Takasaki Y, Iwanaga M, Imaizumi Y, et al. Long-term study of indolent adult T-cell leukemia-lymphoma. Blood 2010;115:4337–4343.
409. Verdonck K, Gonzalez E, Van Dooren S, et al. Human T-lymphotropic virus 1: recent knowledge about an ancient infection. Lancet Infect Dis 2007;7:266–2681.
410. Yamada Y, Tomonaga M, Fukuda H, et al. A new G-CSF-supported combination chemotherapy, LSG15, for adult T-cell leukaemia-lymphoma: Japan Clinical Oncology Group Study 9303. Br J Haematol 2001;113:375–382.
411. Bazarbachi A, Suarez F, Fields P, et al. How I treat adult T-cell leukemia/lymphoma. Blood 2011;118:1736–1745.
412. Bazarbachi A, Plumelle Y, Carlos Ramos J, et al. Meta-analysis on the use of zidovudine and interferon-alfa in adult T-cell leukemia/lymphoma showing improved survival in the leukemic subtypes. J Clin Oncol 2010;28:4177–4183.
413. Tsukasaki K, Utsunomiya A, Fukuda H, et al. VCAP-AMP-VECP compared with biweekly CHOP for adult T-cell leukemia-lymphoma: Japan Clinical Oncology Group Study JCOG9801. J Clin Oncol 2007;25:5458–5464.
414. Tobinai K, Takahashi T, Akinaga S. Targeting chemokine receptor CCR4 in adult T-cell leukemia-lymphoma and other T-cell lymphomas. Curr Hematol Malig Rep. 2012;7:235–240.
415. Hishizawa M, Kanda J, Utsunomiya A, et al. Transplantation of allogeneic hematopoietic stem cells for adult T-cell leukemia: a nationwide retrospective study. Blood 2010;116:1369–1376.
416. Kanda J, Hishizawa M, Utsunomiya A, et al. Impact of graft-versus-host disease on outcomes after allogeneic hematopoietic cell transplantation for adult T-cell leukemia: a retrospective cohort study. Blood 2012;119:2141–2148.
417. Ishida T, Hishizawa M, Kato K, et al. Allogeneic hematopoietic stem cell transplantation for adult T-cell leukemia-lymphoma with special emphasis on preconditioning regimen: a nationwide retrospective study. Blood 2012;120:1734–1741.
418. Boehme V, Schmitz N, Zeynalova S, et al. CNS events in elderly patients with aggressive lymphoma treated with modern chemotherapy (CHOP-14) with or without rituximab: an analysis of patients treated in the RICOVER-60 trial of the German High-Grade Non-Hodgkin Lymphoma Study Group (DSHNHL). Blood 2009;113:3896–3902.
419. Opelz G, Dohler B. Lymphomas after solid organ transplantation: a collaborative transplant study report. Am J Transplant 2004;4:222–230.
420. Morrison VA, Dunn DL, Manivel JC, et al. Clinical characteristics of post-transplant lymphoproliferative disorders. Am J Med 1994;97:14–24.
421. Cohen JI. Epstein-Barr virus infection. N Engl J Med 2000;343:481–492.
422. Capello D, Rossi D, Gaidano G. Post-transplant lymphoproliferative disorders: molecular basis of disease histogenesis and pathogenesis. Hematol Oncol 2005;23:61–67.
423. Caillard S, Dharnidharka V, Agodoa L, et al. Posttransplant lymphoproliferative disorders after renal transplantation in the United States in era of modern immunosuppression. Transplantation 2005;80:1233–1243.
424. Taylor AL, Marcus R, Bradley JA. Post-transplant lymphoproliferative disorders (PTLD) after solid organ transplantation. Crit Rev Oncol Hematol 2005;56:155–167.

425. McDiarmid SV, Jordan S, Kim GS, et al. Prevention and preemptive therapy of postransplant lymphoproliferative disease in pediatric liver recipients. Transplantation 1998;66:1604–1611.
426. Riddler SA, Breinig MC, McKnight JL. Increased levels of circulating Epstein-Barr virus (EBV)-infected lymphocytes and decreased EBV nuclear antigen antibody responses are associated with the development of posttransplant lymphoproliferative disease in solid-organ transplant recipients. Blood 1994; 84(3):972–984.
427. Styczynski J, Einsele H, Gil L, et al. Outcome of treatment of Epstein-Barr virus-related post-transplant lymphoproliferative disorder in hematopoietic stem cell recipients: a comprehensive review of reported cases. Transpl Infect Dis 2009;11:383–392.
428. Leblond V, Dhedin N, Mamzer Bruneel MF, et al. Identification of prognostic factors in 61 patients with posttransplantation lymphoproliferative disorders. J Clin Oncol 2001;19(3):772–778.
429. Ghobrial IM, Habermann TM, Maurer MJ, et al. Prognostic analysis for survival in adult solid organ transplant recipients with post-transplantation lymphoproliferative disorders. J Clin Oncol 2005;23(30):7574–7582.
430. Choquet S, Oertel S, LeBlond V, et al. Rituximab in the management of post-transplantation lymphoproliferative disorder after solid organ transplantation: proceed with caution. Ann Hematol 2007;86:599–607.
431. Paya CV, Fung JJ, Nalesnik MA, et al. Epstein-Barr virus-induced posttransplant lymphoproliferative disorders. ASTS/ASTP EBV-PTLD Task Force and The Mayo Clinic Organized International Consensus Development Meeting. Transplantation 1999;68:1517–1525.
432. Parker A, Bowles K, Bradley JA, et al. Management of post-transplant lymphoproliferative disorder in adult solid organ transplant recipients–BCSH and BTS Guidelines. Br J Haematol 2010;149:693–705.
433. Evens AM, David KA, Helenowski I, et al. Multicenter analysis of 80 solid organ transplantation recipients with post-transplantation lymphoproliferative disease: outcomes and prognostic factors in the modern era. J Clin Oncol 2010;28:1038–1046.
434. Gonzalez-Barca E, Domingo-Domenech E, Capote FJ, et al. Prospective phase II trial of extended treatment with rituximab in patients with B-cell post-transplant lymphoproliferative disease. Haematologica 2007;92:1489–1494.
435. Trappe R, Oertel S, Leblond V, et al. Sequential treatment with rituximab followed by CHOP chemotherapy in adult B-cell post-transplant lymphoproliferative disorder (PTLD): the prospective international multicentre phase 2 PTLD-1 trial. Lancet Oncol 2012;13:196–206.
436. Bollard CM, Rooney CM, Heslop HE. T-cell therapy in the treatment of post-transplant lymphoproliferative disease. Nat Rev Clin Oncol 2012;9:510–519.
437. Gaidano G, Dalla-Favera R. Molecular pathogenesis of AIDS-related lymphomas. Adv Cancer Res 1995;67:113–153.
438. Ometto L, Menin C, Masiero S, et al. Molecular profile of Epstein-Barr virus in human immunodeficiency virus type 1-related lymphadenopathies and lymphomas. Blood 1997;90:313–322.
439. Knowles DM. Etiology and pathogenesis of AIDS-related non-Hodgkin's lymphoma. Hematol Oncol Clin North Am 2003;17:785–820.
440. Castillo JJ, Furman M, Beltran BE, et al. Human immunodeficiency virus-associated plasmablastic lymphoma: poor prognosis in the era of highly active antiretroviral therapy. Cancer 2012;118:5270–5277.
441. Simonelli C, Spina M, Cinelli R, et al. Clinical features and outcome of primary effusion lymphoma in HIV-infected patients: a single-institution study. J Clin Oncol 2003;21:3948–3954.
442. Barta SK, Xue X, Wang D, et al. Treatment factors affecting outcomes in HIV-associated non-Hodgkin lymphomas: a pooled analysis of 1546 patients. Blood 2013;122:3251–3262.
443. Rizzieri DA, Johnson JL, Niedzwiecki D, et al. Intensive chemotherapy with and without cranial radiation for Burkitt leukemia and lymphoma: final results of Cancer and Leukemia Group B Study 9251. Cancer 2004;100:1438–1448.

40 Cutaneous Lymphomas

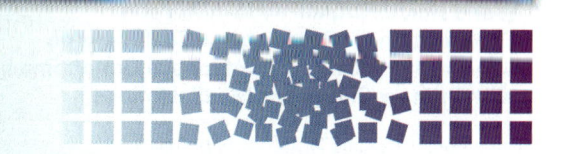

Francine M. Foss, Juliet F. Gibson, Richard L. Edelson, and Lynn D. Wilson

INTRODUCTION

The cutaneous lymphomas comprise a heterogeneous group of malignancies of both T and B lymphocytes that localize to the skin. According to Surveillance, Epidemiology, and End Results (SEER) data, the skin is the second most common site of extranodal non-Hodgkin's lymphoma, with an estimated annual incidence of 1:100,000.[1] The Dutch and Austrian Cutaneous Lymphoma registries report that more than 70% of all cutaneous lymphomas are of T-cell origin, and 22% are of B-cell origin.[2] The term *cutaneous T-cell lymphoma* (CTCL) was formally adopted in 1979 at a conference sponsored by the National Cancer Institute (NCI) to describe a heterogeneous group of malignant T-cell lymphomas with primary manifestations in the skin. The World Health Organization and European Organization for Research and Treatment of Cancer (WHO-EORTC) classification of primary cutaneous lymphomas (Table 40.1, 40.2) defines three groups of cutaneous lymphomas: the cutaneous T-cell and natural killer (NK) lymphomas, the cutaneous B-cell lymphomas, and the precursor hematologic neoplasms.[2]

Further subgrouping based on clinical outcomes has been proposed for the cutaneous T-cell entities.[2,3] The entities with indolent clinical behavior include mycosis fungoides (MF) and its variants, the cutaneous CD30+ entities, subcutaneous panniculitis-like T-cell lymphoma, and the primary cutaneous CD4+ small-/medium-sized pleomorphic T-cell lymphoma. Included in the aggressive group are Sézary syndrome (SS), the NK/T-cell disorders, gamma-delta positive disorders, CD8+ cutaneous diseases, and primary cutaneous peripheral T-cell lymphoma (PTCL). A similar classification for the cutaneous B-cell lymphomas has been proposed based on the histology (follicular or large cell type) and site of disease, with favorable outcomes seen in disease of the head or upper trunk and an unfavorable prognosis seen with either disseminated lesions or disease in the lower extremities (Table 40.3).

MYCOSIS FUNGOIDES AND THE SÉZARY SYNDROME

MF was first reported by Alibert in 1806 as a common epidermotropic lymphoma with an indolent evolution characterized by cutaneous lesions in the forms of patches, plaques, or skin tumors. In 1980, Bunn et al.[4] reported the presence of Sézary cells in the blood of patients with MF, and the Sézary syndrome (diffuse erythroderma, circulating Sézary cells, and involvement of lymph nodes and bone marrow) was thus identified.[5–7] The International Society of Cutaneous Lymphoma (ISCL) established criteria for the diagnosis of SS, which include an absolute Sézary count of at least 1,000 cells/mm³ in the blood, immunophenotypic abnormalities (expanded CD4+ populations and/or loss of antigens such as CD2, CD3, CD5, or CD4), or the presence of a T-cell clone in the blood.[8]

Epidemiology and Etiology

According to SEER data, the incidence of MF–CTCL had increased 3.2-fold between 1973 and 1984. The overall incidence rate is approximately 4 per 1 million, with an incidence of 1,500 cases per year. The actual incidence rate may be an order of magnitude higher, given possible underreporting and the difficulty and confusion in making the diagnosis. The incidence of MF rises with age such that the majority of patients are between 40 and 60 years. The disease is 2.2 times more common in men than in women, and incidence rates are somewhat higher in African Americans than in Caucasians.

One hypothesis regarding the etiology of MF/SS is that it may possibly represent a clonal evolution from a chronic antigenic stimulus. Associations with exposure to occupational chemicals or pesticides have been proposed but not definitely demonstrated in epidemiologic studies.[5,6] In other studies, an association with a *Chlamydia* infection of keratinocytes has been proposed, but data demonstrating *Chlamydia* proteins in affected skin lesions are equivocal.[9,10] The association between human T-cell leukemia virus (HTLV) type 1 infection and adult T-cell leukemia-lymphoma (ATLL) or Epstein-Barr virus in conjunction with nasal NK/T-cell lymphoma is not reflected in the epidemiology of MF–CTCL, but there are reports of the detection of HTLV-like viral particles in affected skin lesions and antibodies to HTLV-1 tax protein in patients with MF/SS.[11–14] These results suggest the association of perhaps a yet unknown retrovirus in some cases of MF/SS. Although there is no known geographical clustering and no evidence of maternal transmission of the disease, there are reports of multiple cases of MF/SS in a small number of families.

Pathobiology

The immunophenotypic profile of MF is one of clonal mature CD4+ CD45RO+ T cells with a marked homing capacity for the papillary dermis and epidermis. Some CTCL variants are CD8+ and different subtypes have distinct prognoses. Antigen loss is characteristic of the disease, with a loss of CD7, CD5, or CD2 and dim staining for CD3. Sézary cells express a TH2 phenotype, with secretion of interleukin (IL)-4, IL-5, IL-6, IL-10, and IL-13. The pruritus characteristic of the disease is related to secretion of IL-5 as well as other chemokines. One characteristic of the disease, even at its earliest stages, is profound immunosuppression with aberrant T-cell repertoires, cutaneous anergy, and increased susceptibility to bacterial and opportunistic infections.[15,16]

The homing to skin by CTCL cells appears to be mediated in part by expression of the surface glycoprotein cutaneous lymphoid antigen (CLA), an antigen whose expression is low or absent on normal infiltrating T cells.[17,18] CLA mediates binding to E-selectin on endothelial cells of cutaneous venules, thereby facilitating their exit from the circulation and into the skin. CLA is the physiologic ligand of endothelial cell E-selectin, a cell adhesion molecule

TABLE 40.1

World Health Organization–European Organisation for Research and Treatment of Cancer Classification of Cutaneous Lymphomas with Primary Cutaneous Manifestations

Cutaneous T-cell and NK-cell lymphomas
- Mycosis fungoides
- MF variants and subtypes
  - Folliculotropic MF
  - Pagetoid reticulosis
  - Granulomatous slack skin
- Sézary syndrome
- Adult T-cell leukemia/lymphoma
- Primary cutaneous CD30+ lymphoproliferative disorders
  - Primary cutaneous anaplastic large cell lymphoma
  - Lymphomatoid papulosis
- Subcutaneous panniculitis-like T-cell lymphoma
- Extranodal NK/T-cell lymphoma, nasal type
- Primary cutaneous peripheral T-cell lymphoma, unspecified
  - Primary cutaneous aggressive epidermotropic CD8+ T-cell lymphoma (provisional)
  - Cutaneous gamma/delta T cell lymphoma (provisional)
  - Primary cutaneous CD4+ small-/medium-sized pleomorphic T-cell lymphoma (provisional)

Cutaneous B-cell lymphomas
- Primary cutaneous marginal zone B-cell lymphoma
- Primary cutaneous follicle center lymphoma
- Primary cutaneous diffuse large B-cell lymphoma, leg type
- Primary cutaneous diffuse large B-cell lymphoma, other
  - Intravascular large B-cell lymphoma

Precursor hematologic neoplasm
- CD4+/CD56+ hematodermic neoplasm (blastic NK-cell lymphoma)

NK, natural killer; MF, mycosis fungoides.
From Willemze R, Jaffe ES, Burg G, et al. WHO-EORTC classification for cutaneous lymphomas. *Blood* 2005;105:3768–3785, with permission.

TABLE 40.2

Clinical Outcomes Based on World Health Organization–European Organisation for Research and Treatment of Cancer Classification for Cutaneous T-Cell Lymphomas

WHO–EORTC Classification	Frequency (%)	Disease-Specific 5-year Survival (%)
Indolent behavior		
Mycosis fungoides and its variants	50	88–100
Primary cutaneous ALCL	8	95
Lymphomatoid papulosis	12	100
Subcutaneous panniculitis like	1	82
Primary CD4+ small/medium pleomorphic	2	75
Aggressive behavior		
Sézary syndrome	3	24
NK/T nasal type	<1	–
Primary cutaneous CD8+ lymphoma	<1	18
Primary cutaneous gamma/delta T-cell lymphoma	<1	–
Primary cutaneous peripheral T-cell lymphoma unspecified	2	16

ALCL, anaplastic large-cell lymphoma.
From Willemze R, Jaffe ES, Burg G, et al. WHO-EORTC classification for cutaneous lymphomas. *Blood* 2005;105:3768–3785; Willemze R, Meijer CJ. Classification of cutaneous T-cell lymphoma: from Alibert to WHO-EORTC. *J Cutan Pathol* 2006;33:18–26, with permission.

expressed on the surface of endothelial cells of cutaneous venules during chronic inflammation.[19] Chemokine receptor CCR4 expressed by cells binds chemokine CCL17 that has adhered to the luminal side of the endothelium, facilitating T-cell leukocyte function antigen-1 binding to endothelial cell intracellular adhesion molecule-1 and fostering extravasation into the dermis.[4]

One of the most striking features of MF/SS is epidermotropism, or infiltration of the epidermis by malignant T cells.

TABLE 40.3

Cutaneous B-Cell Lymphoma Prognostic Index

CBCL-PI Group	Histology	Site	Overall Survival	Relative Survival	HR	95% CL	p
IA	Any indolent[a]	Any	81	94	1.0		
IB	Diffuse large B cell	Favorable[b]	72	86	1.3	0.99–1.7	0.06
II	Diffuse large B cell	Unfavorable[c]	48	60	2.1	1.6–2.7	<0.0001
	Immunoblastic diffuse large B cell	Favorable					
III	Immunoblastic diffuse large B cell	Unfavorable	27	34	4.5	2.8–7.2	<0.0001

Note: Model is adjusted for age; sex; race; year of diagnosis; confirmed B cell lineage; Surveillance, Epidemiology, and End Results historic stage; and treatment with radiation.
[a] Indolent histologies include follicular, marginal zone, small lymphocyte not otherwise specified, and lymphoplasmacytic.
[b] Favorable skin sites include the head/neck and arm.
[c] Unfavorable skin sites include the trunk, leg, and disseminated.
CBCL-PI, cutaneous B-cell lymphoma prognostic index; HR, hazard ratio; CL, confidence limit.
From Smith BD, Smith GL, Cooper DL, et al. The cutaneous B-cell lymphoma prognostic index: a novel prognostic index derived from a population-based registry. *J Clin Oncol* 2005;23:3390–3395.

The pathognomonic feature of MF is the Pautrier's microabscess, a collection of clonal malignant cells within the epidermis. The Pautrier's microabscesses may be a consequence of the expression of intracellular adhesion molecule 1 (ICAM 1) on keratinocytes. ICAM expression is induced by interferon (IFN), which is produced by infiltrating T cells and is a ligand for leukocyte function antigen-1.[20,21] In advanced disease or SS, the keratinocytes lose the ability to express ICAM-1 due to low levels of IFN-γ production, resulting in loss of epidermotropism.[21] Although specimens from early lesions of MF have lymphocytes in both the epidermis and dermis, clonality studies on dissected cells demonstrated that virtually all of the lymphocytes found in the epidermis belong to the malignant clone, whereas the dermis contains a predominance of inflammatory cells and nonmalignant lymphocytes.

Although there is no characteristic chromosomal translocation in patients with MF and SS, significant chromosomal instability is noted and losses on 1p, 10q, 13q, and 17p and gains of 4, 17q, and 18 are commonly observed.[22,23] Genetic instability is also evidenced by significant copy number alterations even in early disease.[24] Recent studies have shown a high prevalence of deletions or translocations involving a gene, NAV3, at 12q2, which has helicase-like activity and might therefore contribute to genomic instability.[25] Chromosomal amplification of JunB at 19p12 has also been detected in MF/SS and is thought to be contributory to the TH2 cytokine profile characteristic of Sézary cells.[26] In Lin et al.,[24] 21 regions of amplification and 42 regions of deletion were identified, with significant amplifications of 8q (MYC) and 17q (signal transducer and activator of transcription 3 [STAT3]) and deletions of 17p (TP53) and 10 (phosphatase and tension homologue [PTEN], FAS).[24]

DIAGNOSIS AND STAGING

The diagnosis of MF depends on both clinical and histopathologic criteria. The skin manifestations can be in the form of patches, plaques, erythroderma, cutaneous tumors, or ulcers. Early patch and plaque lesions may be indistinguishable from those of benign dermatoses, including psoriasis, eczema, large plaque parapsoriasis, or drug eruptions. The distribution of the lesions favors non–sun-exposed areas such as the *bathing trunk* distribution. An early diagnosis can be difficult and may rely on multiple biopsies obtained from different lesions over time. The ISCL has developed criteria for the diagnosis of early-stage MF that relies on clinical, histopathologic, immunopathologic, and molecular criteria[27] (Table 40.4). Of note, T-cell receptor clonality can be found in benign dermatoses and in lymphomatoid papulosis and pityriasis lichenoides (clonal dermatitis).[28,29] Long-term follow-up of patients with clonal dermatitis reveals a significant risk of progression to overt MF, suggesting careful follow-up.

Early lesions of MF may be asymptomatic, such as scaling erythematous macular eruptions often in sun-shielded areas (Fig. 40.1). A patch is defined as a lesion that is not elevated or indurated and that may be hyper- or hypopigmented. A plaque is raised or indurated and may be associated with scaling, crusting, or ulceration. A tumor is a lesion that is more than 1 cm with evidence of depth or vertical growth. Erythroderma is defined as diffuse erythema involving more than 80% of the skin surface with or without scaling.[8]

Painful and/or pruritic erythroderma may arise de novo or during any of the earlier described phases and is not always associated with frank T-cell leukemia (as in SS). Infrequently, MF presents with cutaneous tumor nodules in the absence of patches or plaques (as in *tumor d'emblée*). Patients may also present with or progress to involvement of visceral organs.

The Sézary Syndrome

The diagnostic criteria for SS are dependent on the presence of a circulating Sézary cell count of at least 1,000 cells/mm³. The phenotype is typically that of a mature, memory CD4+ T cell with a frequent loss of normal T-cell antigens (CD3, CD5, CD2, CD7, and CD26).[8] The CD4/CD8 ratio is elevated, usually more than 10, and a T-cell clone is detected in the blood by polymerase chain reaction (PCR). The presence of more than 1,000 Sézary cells/mm³ is not absolutely diagnostic of SS in the absence of other clinical features of the disease, because these cells may be seen in about 5% of patients with benign dermatoses manifested by erythroderma.[30,31] Histopathologic features in skin biopsies of patients with SS can be nonspecific, and there is a loss of epidermotropism in up to 70% of cases. Cytogenetic studies demonstrate unbalanced translocations and deletions, often involving 1p, 10q, 14q, and 15q, with evidence of clonal evolution and chromosomal instability over time.[32] A differential diagnosis includes viral or drug-induced exanthems, atopic dermatitis, or psoriasis.

Clinical features of the SS include extensive skin involvement with erythroderma, which may progress to lichenification, palmoplantar hyperkeratosis, and diffuse exfoliation. Skin edema, hypoalbuminemia due to insensible fluid loss related to impaired skin integument, and intense pruritus are frequently observed in patients with advanced disease. Lymphadenopathy, histopathologically effaced nodes, and bone marrow involvement are common. Significant immunosuppression occurs related to impaired T-helper function as well as T-cell repertoire skewing, leading to a high incidence of infections, particularly related to indwelling intravenous catheters. The overall prognosis is poor, with a median survival of 2 to 4 years.[33]

Staging and Prognosis of Mycosis Fungoides and the Sézary Syndrome

Staging systems for MF have been developed based on clinical features of skin involvement as well as infiltration of lymph nodes

TABLE 40.4

International Society for Cutaneous Lymphomas Algorithm for the Diagnosis of Early-Stage Mycosis Fungoides

Criteria	Major (2 Points)	Minor (1 Point)
Clinical		
Persistent and/or progressive patches and plaques plus	Any 2	Any 1
1. Non–sun exposed location		
2. Size/shape variation		
3. Poikiloderma		
Histopathologic		
Superficial lymphoid infiltrate plus	Both	Either
1. Epidermotropism		
2. Atypia		
Molecular/Biologic		
Clonal *TCR* gene rearrangement	–	Present
Immunopathologic		
1. CD2, 3, 5 <59% of T cells	–	Any 1
2. CD7 <10% of T cells		
3. Epidermal discordance from expression of CD2, 3, 5, and 7 on dermal T cells		

From Pimpinelli N, Olsen EA, Santucci M, et al. Defining early mycosis fungoides. *J Am Acad Dermatol* 2005;53:1053–1063, with permission.

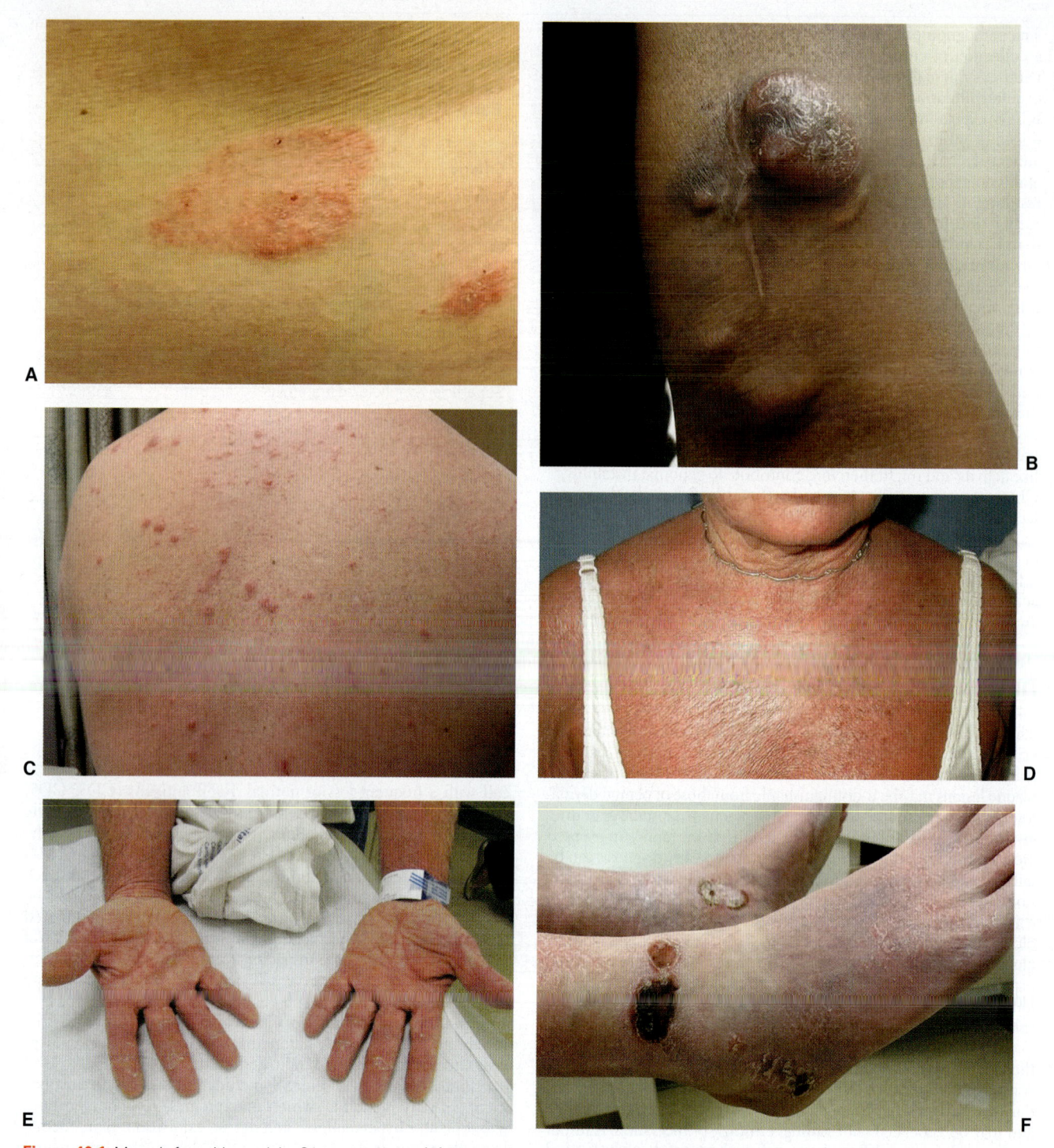

Figure 40.1 Mycosis fungoides and the Sézary syndrome. **(A)** Mycosis fungoides cutaneous plaque. **(B)** Cutaneous tumor. **(C)** Folliculotropic mycosis fungiodes. **(D)** Sézary syndrome with diffuse erythroderma. **(E)** Hyperkeratosis and involvement of palms with Sézary syndrome. **(F)** CD8+ cytotoxic T-cell lymphoma of the skin.

and viscera. Skin involvement is defined on the basis of the type of lesions and extent. T1 and T2 diseases are patches or plaques involving less than or more than 10% of the skin surface, respectively. T3 disease is the presence of at least one cutaneous tumor. T4 disease is erythroderma. Lymph node involvement has been classified based on the degree of infiltration with malignant cells. The dermatopathic node demonstrates typically many atypical lymphocytes in three to six cell clusters (LN2) or larger aggregates of atypical lymphocytes with nodal architecture preserved (LN3) clusters of T cells often with expansion of the parafollicular zones. LN4 nodes are effaced by tumor cells, and typically such effacement is by atypical lymphocytes or neoplastic cells.[5] T-cell receptor rearrangement (TCRR) is found in half of patients with LN3 nodes and rarely in those with LN2 histology.[34] Bone marrow involvement has been shown to have prognostic significance based on the degree of involvement, with cytologically atypical lymphoid aggregates and infiltrative disease associated with inferior survival.[35] In retrospective studies, bone marrow involvement was associated with blood involvement and advanced lymph node disease.[7,36–38]

TABLE 40.5
Staging Systems for Mycosis Fungoides

	MF Cooperative Group 1979[a]			ISCL Group 2007[b]				
Stage	T	N	M	Stage	T	N	M	B
IA	1	0	0	IA	1	0	0	0, 1
IB	2	0	0	IB	2	0	0	0, 1
IIA	1–2	1	0	II	1–2	1–2	0	0, 1
IIB	3	0, 1	0	IIB	3	0–2	0	0, 1
III	4	0, 1	0	III	4	0–2	0	0–1
				IIIA	4	0–2	0	0
				IIIB	4	0–2	0	1
IVA	1–4	2–3	0	IVA$_1$	1–4	0–2	0	2
IVB	1–4	2–3	1	IVA$_2$	1–4	3	0	0–2
				IVA$_3$		0–3	1	0–2

Note: T1 patches or plaques, <10% bovine serum albumin (BSA); T2 patches or plaques, >10% BSA; T3, cutaneous tumors; T4, erythroderma; N1 = LN 0–2; N2 = LN 3; N3 = LN 4; B0, <5% of lymphocytes are atypical; B1, >5% of lymphocytes are atypical; B2, >1,000 Sézary cells/mm^3 with positive clone.
[a] Data derived from Agar NS, Wedgeworth E, Crichton S, et al. Survival outcomes and prognostic factors in mycosis fungoides/Sezary syndrome: validation of the revised International Society for Cutaneous Lymphomas/European Organisation for Research and Treatment of Cancer staging proposal. *J Clin Oncol* 2010;28:4730–4739.
[b] Proposed modifications to the staging system by the International Society of Cutaneous Lymphoma (ISCL). Olsen F, Vonderheid E, Piminelli N, et al. Revisions to the staging and classification of mycosis fungoides and Sezary syndrome: a proposal of the International Society for Cutaneous Lymphomas (ISCL) and the cutaneous lymphoma task force of the European Organization of Research and Treatment of Cancer (EORTC). *Blood* 2007;110:1713.

The initial staging system for MF/SS was proposed by the MF Cooperative Group in 1979 and was based on skin involvement, palpable nodes, and visceral involvement.[39] More recently, the ISCL further stratifies patients based on the extent of blood involvement (Table 40.5).[40] In this new system, patients with significant blood involvement are identified in the erythroderma, or stage III group, and patients with stage IVA disease are further categorized based on the degree of lymph node and blood infiltration. Early stage (T1/T2) disease has been proposed to be divided into patch alone versus both patch and plaque disease. These changes have been validated by Agar et al.,[41] who analyzed the outcome of 1,502 MF/SS patients at their institution.

Overall outcome in MF/SS is correlated with clinical stage, and retrospective studies have identified the extent of skin involvement as well as visceral disease as the most important prognostic factors.[7,14,38] Patients with limited patch/plaque disease covering less than 10% of their skin surface have a prognosis indistinguishable from that of age-, sex-, and race-matched controls.[42] The 10-year disease-specific survival for patients with more extensive skin involvement with patches or plaques is 83%, whereas those with tumors or histologically documented lymph node involvement had survivals of 42% or 20%, respectively.[38] Patients with effaced lymph nodes or the presence of large cell transformation had a uniformly poor prognosis.[43,44] Other poor prognostic factors include blood involvement and loss of T-cell markers CD5 and CD7.[45] Even in patients with B0 disease, the presence of T-cell clonality has been shown to portend a worse prognosis.[41]

CLINICAL EVALUATION OF PATIENTS WITH CUTANEOUS LYMPHOMA

An initial evaluation should include a careful assessment of the number and distribution of each type of skin lesion. The Skin Weighted Assessment Tool divides the body surface into areas that are assigned a value based on the percent of total body surface area represented.[46] The observer then estimates the percent of each body area involved with disease based on the estimation that the palm of the hand is 1%. The involvement is weighted based on whether the lesions are patch, plaque, or tumor. The sum is the skin score, which can be recorded and monitored during therapy.

Skin biopsies at multiple sites may be necessary to establish the diagnosis because lesion morphology varies even for different lesions from the same patient and the quality and quantity of infiltrating cells may be affected by topical therapies, including topical steroids. In addition, most of the cells in the underlying, often much more impressive dermal infiltrate are nonneoplastic reactive CD4+ and CD8+ T lymphocytes. Features of pleomorphism and the presence of large cells should be noted. Transformation to a large cell phenotype in patients with MF/SS is associated with a poor prognosis. Immunophenotyping and molecular studies for TCRR should be performed on skin biopsies.

Laboratory studies should include flow cytometry to detect circulating neoplastic cells. In investigational settings, it is possible to use monoclonal antibodies directed against TCR-Vb families to detect and precisely quantitate the levels of circulating leukemia cells. In most instances, the level of circulating CTCL cells is actually much higher than estimated by less-sensitive techniques such as by evaluation of the peripheral smear for atypical cells.[21] In many patients, the expansion of the neoplastic T-cell clone is accompanied by depression of normal T cells to levels comparable with those observed in advanced AIDS. Such a de facto T-cell deficiency may both explain the susceptibility of erythrodermic CTCL patients to infection by bacterial, viral, and fungal pathogens and contribute to the progression of the disease, which is often held in check by host immune mechanisms.[47]

Flow cytometry should be performed with antibodies to the CD4, CD8, CD3, CD45RO, and CD26 antigens. The ratio of CD4+ to CD8+ cells is normally 0.5:3.5; elevations in this ratio correlate with total leukocyte count and with extent of skin disease in CTCL patients. An elevated ratio of CD4+ to CD8+

cells above 4.5:1.0 strongly suggests significant levels of circulating CTCL cells. Dual color staining with CD4 and other antigens can detect low or absent expression of CD3, CD7, or CD26 as a feature of Sézary cells.

Imaging studies (computed tomography scan or magnetic resonance imaging) are recommended at the initial evaluation, especially for those with advanced disease, as well as during follow-up, to detect enlargement of thoracic, abdominal, or pelvic nodes. Positron emission tomography has been performed for patients with CTCL, but there is not enough experience to reliably determine the sensitivity and specificity in cutaneous lymphoma.[48,49] Pathologically enlarged lymph nodes should be biopsied at the initial staging and subsequently if enlargement is detected on the physical examination or imaging studies because a proportion of patients with CTCL may have other lymphomas (B or T cell; e.g., Hodgkin's) concurrently. A bone marrow biopsy should be obtained in patients with advanced disease, including those with SS, as well as in patients with compromised hematologic function. Biopsies of visceral organs such as the liver should be dictated based on clinical indication or to confirm findings on imaging studies.

PRINCIPLES OF THERAPY OF MYCOSIS FUNGOIDES AND THE SÉZARY SYNDROME

Treatment approaches for MF/SS depend on the clinical stage of disease. Early-stage disease that is localized to the skin (patch or plaque disease) has an excellent chance of cure or long-term control with therapies directed to the skin alone. In contrast, tumor stage disease, extensive plaque stage disease that is refractory to topical therapies, and nodal or visceral disease can be palliated but rarely cured. Over the past 15 years, a number of novel agents have shown activity in MF/SS (Table 40.6). Because MF/SS is immunosuppressive and an immunologically responsive disease, initial therapies for many patients involve cutaneous and biologic approaches, which act directly on CTCL cells (e.g., they are directly cytotoxic) but also have indirect effects (e.g., alter the cutaneous environment) that may play a role in disease control.[50]

Skin-Directed Therapy

Skin-directed modalities include those for localized disease (radiotherapy, bexarotene, and carmustine) and those applicable to total skin therapy (topical chemotherapy with nitrogen mustard [NM], phototherapy, and total skin electron-beam therapy [TSEBT]; Table 10.6). All skin-directed therapies exert their primary effects on disease confined to the skin by inducing apoptosis of tumor cells and interfering with the local production of cytokines by epithelial and stromal cells necessary for neoplastic T-cell survival and proliferation.[51]

Approximately 7% of patients with stage I disease present with a solitary cutaneous lesion or several in proximity. Wilson et al.[52] found that the rate of clinical remission after local external-beam radiotherapy is very high (approximately 95%) in these patients and may be the treatment of choice. In one study, a total of 21 patients were treated with electron-beam radiation to a median dose of 20 Gy. With a median follow-up of 36 months, the actuarial disease-free survival rates at 5 and 10 years were 75% and 64%, respectively, with a local control rate of 83% at 10 years.

Topical Chemotherapies

Topical NM is one of the first treatments for cutaneous manifestations of MF. The NM liquid can be applied to the skin as an aqueous solution of 10 mg/dL or applied in an ointment base. Long-term effects include induction of second cutaneous malignancies (e.g., squamous cell carcinomas) and hyperpigmentation and hypopigmentation. Between 64% and 90% of NM-treated patients with T1 and T2 CTCL can achieve a complete response to therapy.

Topical Bexarotene Gel

Bexarotene (Targretin) is a novel RXR retinoid (retinoid X receptor) that has been shown to be effective both systemically and topically for patients with MF/SS. The overall response rate to topical bexarotene in clinical trials was 44%. The drug is not absorbed to any significant levels. The irritant dermatitis induced by the retinoid limits the use of the gel to patients with body surface area (BSA) of less than 15% because of discomfort. In many cases, topical bexarotene gel is used, alternating with topical steroids to minimize the irritant effect.

Phototherapy

Phototherapy has been effective for patients with MF/SS because keratinocytes are resistant to ultraviolet (UV) light–induced injuries, whereas lymphocytes are extremely sensitive to light in the form of either UVA (320 to 400 nm), UVB (290 to 320 nm), or narrow-band UVB (311 nm). Currently, narrow-band UVB is used most commonly because of the low risk of secondary skin neoplasms. Patients typically are treated three to four times per week for approximately 30 to 40 treatments to achieve a remission, and then treatment frequency is decreased to a maintenance schedule at weekly intervals. Broad-band UVB has the same treatment schedule.

Photochemotherapy with orally administered PUVA (ultraviolet A light with oral methoxypsoralen) has been an effective therapy for patients with patch and plaque stage MF. The intensity of the light and frequency of administration are titrated based on patient response and tolerability. Maintenance treatment is often necessary to prevent disease recurrence.

Combination Regimens Involving PUVA Photochemotherapy

Several well-conducted trials have assessed the role of PUVA in combination with various systemic agents, notably IFN-α and retinoids. Phase I and II studies of PUVA (three times weekly) combined with variable doses of IFN-α (maximum tolerated dose of 12 MU/m^2 three times weekly) in 39 patients with MF (all stages) and SS have reported an overall response rate of 100%.[53] The median duration of response (DOR) was 28 months, with a median survival of 62 months.

A randomized controlled trial compared PUVA (two to five times weekly) plus IFN-α (9 MU three times weekly) with IFN-α plus a retinoic acid receptor (RAR) retinoid, acitretin (25 to 50 mg per day), in 98 patients with a maximum duration of treatment in both groups of 48 weeks.[54] In 82 patients with stage I/II diseases, complete response rates were 70% in the PUVA/IFN group compared with 38% in the IFN/acitretin group. Time to response was 18.6 weeks in the PUVA/IFN group, compared with 21.8 weeks in the IFN/acitretin group.

Total Skin Electron-Beam Therapy

Total skin electron-beam therapy (TSEB) involves the use of electrons ranging in energy between 4 and 7 MeV applied homogeneously to the skin surface.[55] Structures below the deep dermis are relatively spared because most of the dose (80%) is typically administered within the first 10 mm of depth, and less than 5% beyond 20 mm depth. Generally, doses to skin target are in the range of 30 to 36 Gy. Blood and superficial lymph nodes may receive 20% to 40% of the skin surface dose, and this may be clinically important.

TSEBT may be administered as just one in a sequence of treatments for CTCL in a particular patient. For example, TSEBT

TABLE 40.6
Treatments for Mycosis Fungoides/Sézary Syndrome

Therapy	Response (%)	Toxicities
Topical Agents		
Mechlorethamine or carmustine	CRR Stage I: 76–86 Stage IIA: 55 Stage III: 22–49	Contact dermatitis, secondary cutaneous malignancies
Bexarotene	Stage IA–IIA: 21 CR, 42 PR	Contact dermatitis
Phototherapy		
UVB	CRR Stage IA/IB: 75–83	Erythema, pruritus
PUVA	CRR Stage IA: 79–88 Stage IB: 52–59 Stage IIA: 83 Stage III: 46	Nausea, phototoxic reactions, secondary cutaneous malignancies
PUVA plus IFN-α (1) vs. acitretin plus IFN-α (2)	CRR Stage I/II: 70 (1) vs. 38 (2)	Flulike symptoms
Immunotherapy		
IFN-α	ORR IA–IV: 40–80	Flulike syndrome, hematologic toxicity, nausea, fatigue
ECP	ORR III–IV: 31–86	Hypotension, fever
Radiotherapy		
Total skin electron-beam therapy	CRR Stage IA–IIA: 96 Stage IIB: 36 Stage III: 60	Secondary cutaneous malignancies, pigmentation, anhidrosis, pruritus, alopecia, xerosis, telangiectasia
Cytotoxic Chemotherapy		
EPOCH	ORR Stage IIB–IV: 80	Myelosuppression
Pentostatin	ORR Stage IIB: 75 Stage III: 58 Stage IV: 50	Lymphopenia
Fludarabine plus IFN-α	ORR Stage IIA–IVA: 58 Stage IVB: 40	Neutropenia
Gemcitabine	ORR Stage IIB/III: 70	Neutropenia
Pegylated liposomal doxorubicin	ORR Stage IA–IV: 88	Infusion-related events
Novel Targeted Strategies		
Bexarotene	ORR Stage IA/IIA: 20–67 Stage IIB–IV: 49	Hypertriglyceridemia hyperlipidemia, hypothyroidism
Vorinostat	ORR: 29 Stage IA/IIA: 20–31 Stage IIB–IV: 25–30	Diarrhea, nausea, vomiting, fatigue
Romidepsin	ORR: 34–38 Stage IB/IIA: 25–66 Stage IIB–IVA: 29–38	Nausea, vomiting, anorexia, diarrhea, headache, ageusia
Denileukin diftitox	Stage I/IIA: 37 Stage IIB–IV: 24 Stages II–IV (less heavily pretreated) 62	Flulike symptoms, infusion-related events, vascular leak syndrome

(continued)

TABLE 40.6

Treatments for Mycosis Fungoides/Sézary Syndrome *(continued)*

Therapy	Response (%)	Toxicities
Novel Targeted Strategies (continued)		
Denileukin diftitox + bexarotene	ORR: 72	Lymphopenia, leukopenia
Alemtuzumab	ORR III–IV: 86–100	Infusion reaction, immunosuppression
Zanolimumab	ORR: 56 IA–IIA: 34 IIB–IVB: 22	Low-grade infection, eczematous dermatitis
Mogamulizumab	ORR: 37 MF: 29 SS: 47	Infusion reaction, skin rash
Brentuximab vedotin	ORR: 71 MF: 50 LyP and pc-ALCL: 100	Peripheral neuropathy, drug rash, diarrhea, fatigue

CRR, complete response rate; CR, complete response; PR, partial response; UVB, ultraviolet B; PUVA, ultraviolet A light with oral methoxypsoralen; ORR, overall response rate; ECP, extracorporeal photochemotherapy; EPOCH, etoposide, vincristine, doxorubicin, cyclophosphamide, and prednisone; SS, Sézary syndrome; LyP, lymphomatoid papulosis; pc-ALCL, primary cutaneous anaplastic large-cell lymphoma.

is excellent treatment for patients with diffuse involvement with thick plaques or cutaneous tumors and is also suitable for patients with symptomatic erythroderma–T4 disease.[56] TSEBT is also an excellent alternative for patients with extensive patches or thin plaques refractory to PUVA or other skin-directed therapies.[57] Subsequently, TSEBT may be administered to a patient several times using a variety of dose schedules, as clinically required to help control progressive disease.

Clinical complete response rates for patients with T1 or T2 (patch or plaque) disease range from 71% to 98% and are higher in patients with less-extensive disease. Patients with T1 and T2 disease treated with TSEBT have disease-free and overall survivals of 50% to 65% and 80% to 90%, respectively, at 5 years, although patients with antecedent or coexisting lymphomatoid papulosis or alopecia mucinosa–follicular mucinosis appear to have a shorter disease-free survival after TSEBT than those who do not. Patients with more advanced T3 and T4 disease fare significantly worse, with 5-year disease-free and overall survivals of approximately 20% and 50%, respectively. However, those T3 patients with less than 10% of the total skin surface involved by CTCL have significantly better disease-free and overall survival after TSEBT than those with more extensive disease. For patients with erythrodermic MF (T4) who are managed with TSEBT alone (32 to 40 Gy), without concomitant or neoadjuvant therapy, the complete response rate is approximately 70%. The 5-year progression-free, cause-specific, and overall survivals are 26%, 52%, and 38%, respectively.[56] Based on data from Stanford lower dose TSEBT can also be considered. Overall response rates were in excess of 90% in those T2-T4 disease receiving 5–19 Gy. For those who received 1–<20 gy and 20 to <30 Gy, overall response was in excess of 95%.[58]

Palliation of adenopathy or visceral involvement in patients with N3 disease can be accomplished by the use of appropriate high-energy orthovoltage or megavoltage photons to doses of 20 to 30 Gy. Even 6 to 8 Gy in three fractions are sufficient (e.g., when combined with TSEBT). Combinations of TSEBT with total nodal radiation have been investigated. Although feasible, such combinations do not appear to prolong survival and may be associated with hematologic toxicities not observed with TSEBT alone.

TSEBT is well tolerated by most patients; acute sequelae either during or within the initial 6 months after treatment may include pruritus, desquamation, alopecia, epilation, hypohidrosis, xerosis, erythema, lower extremity edema, bullae of the feet, and onychoptosis. Chronic changes can include atrophy of the skin, telangiectasia, alopecia, hypohidrosis, and xerosis. Second malignancies such as squamous and basal cell carcinomas, as well as malignant melanomas, have been observed in patients treated with TSEBT, particularly in patients exposed to multiple therapies that are themselves known to be mutagenic, such as PUVA and mechlorethamine.[57,59]

For patients who suffer diffuse cutaneous recurrences after TSEBT not amenable to other skin-directed therapies, a second course of TSEBT is both feasible and worthwhile. At Yale University, a total of 14 patients have received two courses and 5 patients received three courses of TSEBT. The median total dose after these additional courses was 57 Gy, and 86% of the patients achieved a complete response after the second course, with a median disease-free interval of 11.5 months. The median dose was 36 Gy for the first course, 18 Gy for the second, and 12 Gy for the third.[60] A similar experience was reported from Stanford University, where 15 patients were identified who had been treated with a second course of TSEBT (median dose of 20 Gy), with a complete response rate of 40%.[61] Nine of these patients had a partial response to therapy, and the median total dose for the entire group was 56 Gy. In both series, repeat courses were relatively well tolerated, and sequelae were similar to those observed during and after the first course of therapy.

Combined and Sequential Therapy

The adjuvant use of PUVA after TSEBT in patients with T1 and T2 disease significantly decreased cutaneous relapse. Patients treated with adjuvant PUVA after TSEBT had a 5-year disease-free survival of 85%, compared with 50% for those not receiving PUVA ($p < 0.02$). The median disease-free survival for the T1 patients receiving adjuvant PUVA was not reached at 103 months, versus 66 months for the non-PUVA group ($p < 0.01$). For those with T2 disease, the disease-free survival figures were 60 and 20 months, respectively ($p < 0.03$).[62] Adjuvant topical NM also appears able to delay cutaneous recurrence after TSEBT. In 1999, Chinn et al.[63] from Stanford University showed that TSEBT with or without NM provided improved response rates compared with mustard alone for those patients with T2 and T3 level disease (76% versus 39%, $p < 0.03$ for T2; 44% versus 8%, $p < 0.05$ for T3).[63] For those with patch/plaque (T2), adjuvant mustard offered improved freedom from relapse after TSEBT compared with no adjuvant treatment. No significant survival differences were noted between the groups.

The combination of extracorporeal photochemotherapy (ECP) administered during and after TSEBT may improve survival ($p < 0.06$) for patients with T3 or T4 disease who have achieved a complete response to TSEBT; however, the group of treated patients was small, and the data are retrospective.[64] Wilson et al.[65] identified a significant improvement in cause-specific survival for erythrodermic patients (blood status both B0 and B1) treated with the combination of TSEBT and ECP compared with those not treated with ECP. The 2-year progression-free, cause-specific, and overall survivals for those receiving TSEBT/ECP were 66%, 100%, and 88%, respectively, compared with 36%, 69%, and 63%, respectively, for those not managed with the combination.

SYSTEMIC THERAPY FOR MYCOSIS FUNGOIDES AND THE SÉZARY SYNDROME

Biologic Therapies

IFN-α has been demonstrated in a number of studies to be a highly active agent in CTCL with response rates ranging from 40% to 80%.[66] Doses have ranged from 1 to 18 mU administered subcutaneously on a number of schedules, the most common being three times a week. IFN-γ has also demonstrated activity but is not as widely used. Constitutional symptoms and bone marrow suppression have limited aggressive and long-term use of interferons for many patients. Early studies with high-dose IL-2 has demonstrated activity in relapsed CTCL but with significant toxicity. In a recent study of intermediate-dose IL-2, 11 patients (median age, 60 years) with advanced or refractory CTCL underwent 8-week cycles of daily subcutaneous injections of 11 mIU, 4 days per week for 6 weeks, followed by 2 weeks off of therapy. This dose was well tolerated, and there were four partial responses, three of which were sustained.[67] IL-12 has also demonstrated activity in early and advanced MF. A phase 2 study demonstrated responses in 43% of the patients, with response durations ranging from 3 to 45 weeks.[68]

Extracorporeal Photochemotherapy

ECP, or photopheresis, involves a leukapheresis to isolate mononuclear cells that are exposed ex vivo to UVA in the presence of methoxypsoralen and then reinfused back into the patient. Methoxypsoralen incorporates into DNA and, in the presence of UV light, induces strand breaks and, subsequently, apoptosis. Circulating T cells and Sézary leukemia cells are more susceptible to UVA-induced apoptosis than are monocytes. The mechanism of action of ECP is believed to be related to the induction of apoptosis in clonal Sézary T cells, leading to uptake and processing of tumor antigens by immature dendritic cells generated from the effects of the ECP process on circulating monocytoid precursors.[69,70] The process of ECP has been shown to induce a cell-mediated antitumor response. Clinical improvement with ECP has been demonstrated in both patients with SS and in patients with tumor and plaque-stage CTCL.

In a study of ECP in erythrodermic CTCL, Edelson et al. demonstrated an overall response rate of 83%. Since then, studies have reported a range of overall response rates from 31% to 86% and vary in their definition of response (50% clearing or 25% clearing).[45,71–73] There is some evidence that ECP may be advantageous even in early stage disease (stage T1/T2) when there is any blood involvement.[74] Immune adjuvant therapies have been combined with ECP and have shortened the time to response.[75–78] Duvic et al.[79] compared treatment of stage III and IV MF/SS patients with ECP alone or ECP in combination with IFN-α, bexarotene, or granulocyte monocyte colony–stimulating factor and found a 57% response rate in the group undergoing combination therapy as compared to 40% in those undergoing ECP alone.

Bexarotene (Retinoid Therapy)

Bexarotene (Targretin) is an oral RXR-selective retinoid that has been shown to alter T-cell trafficking through downregulation of CCR4 and E-selectin.[81] It is active both topically and orally. In a clinical trial of heavily pretreated refractory CTCL, oral monotherapy with bexarotene had a response rate of 54% in early-stage and 45% in advanced-stage CTCL patients. The median response duration was 299 days with continuous dosing at a dose of 300 mg/m^2 per day, and responses occurred in all groups of patients (57% at stage IIB, 32% at stage III, 44% at stage IVA, and 40% at stage IVB) including those with large-cell transformation. Pruritus decreased significantly in the treated patients and led to overall improvement in quality-of-life indices.[82] The major toxicities of bexarotene included elevations in serum lipids and cholesterol and suppression of thyroid function.

Bexarotene combination therapy has been studied extensively but has yielded limited additional benefit. Straus et al.[83] demonstrated that bexarotene in combination with IFN-α-2b did not have an increased response rate as compared to bexarotene alone. In the EORTC task force's phase 3 randomized clinical trial investigating PUVA and bexarotene, there also was no significant difference between groups.[84] A phase 2 clinical trial (GEMBEX) of gemcitabine and bexarotene showed lower response rates than those for gemcitabine monotherapy. Another phase 2 trial investigating liposomal doxorubicin and bexarotene found no added benefit of bexarotene.[85] A clinical trial of pralatrexate and bexarotene is ongoing.

Histone Deacetylase Inhibitors

Histone deacetylase (HDAC) inhibitors modulate gene expression by inhibiting the deacetylation of histone proteins associated with DNA, thereby permitting expression of a number of genes. HDAC inhibition has been shown to induce histone acetylation, cell cycle arrest, and apoptosis in leukemia and lymphoma cell lines. The HDAC inhibitor romidepsin was tested in clinical trials at the NCI, and responses were seen in patients with T-cell lymphomas who received 14 mg/m^2 given intravenously on days 1, 8, and 15 of a 21-day cycle.[86] Two multicenter phase 2 trials of romidepsin have been completed and have led to U.S. Food and Drug Administration (FDA) approval for romidepsin in CTCL.[86,87] In these trials, the overall response rate in 167 patients with advanced or refractory CTCL was 35%, with 6% achieving a clinical complete response. The median response duration was 11 and 14 months in the NCI and the sponsor phase 2 studies, respectively. The most frequent adverse events (all grades) were nausea, constitutional symptoms, thrombocytopenia, and reversible ST-T segment changes.

Vorinostat (Zolinza, suberoylanilide hydroxamic acid), an orally bioavailable HDAC inhibitor, was explored in a phase 1/2 study and showed activity in CTCL.[88] In a subsequent phase 2 study, vorinostat administered at 400 mg daily was associated with a 29% response rate in 74 patients with refractory CTCL, including 61 with stage IIB or higher disease. The response durations ranged from 34 to 441+ days.[89] Overall, 32% of patients had relief of pruritus. Panobinostat is an oral HDAC inhibitor that has been shown to have activity in CTCL. Of 139 patients enrolled in a phase 2 trial of panobinostat 20 mg three times a week, the response rate was 17.3%.[91]

Denileukin Diftitox

Denileukin diftitox is a fusion protein consisting of the *IL-2* gene joined to the active and membrane-translocating domains of diphtheria toxin. In the pivotal trial that led to FDA approval of denileukin diftitox, the drug was administered at a dose of either 9 mg per kilogram or 18 mg per kilogram, for 5 days every 21 days, in 71 patients with relapsed or refractory CTCL.[92] The median number of prior therapies in this study was five. The overall response rate was similar for both dose groups and was 30% overall, with

10% complete responses (7 patients) and 20% partial responses (14 patients).[92] The median response duration was 6.9 months. The major toxicities included a reversible elevation of hepatic transaminases, a hypersensitivity syndrome associated with drug infusion, and a mild vascular leak syndrome, all of which were alleviated in part by steroid pretreatment.[93]

A randomized, placebo-controlled phase 3 trial has been completed comparing denileukin diftitox at doses of 9 and 18 ug per kilogram daily for 5 days on a 21 day schedule in patients with earlier stage CTCL who have had fewer prior therapies.[94] Of 144 patients treated, the overall response rates were 46%, 37%, and 15% for the 18 ug, 9 ug, and placebo arms, respectively. A combination study of bexarotene (75 to 300 mg) and denileukin diftitox (18 μg per kilogram for 3 days every 21 days)[95] reported an overall response rate of 70%, with four complete responses (35%) and four partial responses (35%). This study demonstrated that doses of bexarotene greater than 150 mg per day were capable of in vivo upregulation of CD25 (IL-2) expression and may enhance the efficacy of denileukin diftitox.

Monoclonal Antibodies

Alemtuzumab, a humanized monoclonal antibody that targets the CD52 antigen, has been shown to be active in relapsed or refractory T-cell lymphomas. Recent studies with lower doses of alemtuzumab (10 mg three times per week) have reported responses in 6 of 10 patients, including 2 complete responses and 4 partial responses, with minimal immunosuppression.[96,97]

Zanolimumab, a high-affinity, fully humanized monoclonal antibody that targets the CD4 receptor[98] It has shown promising results in patients with biopsy proven CD4+ CTCL, including 23 patients with advanced stage disease.[99] Partial remissions were reported in 16 of 36 (44%) evaluable patients overall, including 3 of 6 with advanced disease at 980 mg per week.

Mogamulizumab (KW-0761) is a humanized anti-CCR4 antibody that enhances antibody-dependent cellular cytotoxicity against malignant T cells. CCR4 has been shown to have increased expression in a subset of patients with MF.[100] The overall response rate in a phase 2 trial of mogamulizumab in relapsed/refractory CTCL patients was 37% (29% in MF, 47% in SS).[101] Phase 2 studies are ongoing in CTCL, PTCL, and ATLL.

Brentuximab vedotin is a CD30-targeted antibody conjugated to an auristatin (monomethyl auristatin E [MMAE]), an antitubulin agent. After binding to CD30, the molecule is internalized and MMAE is released and binds to tubulin, leading to cell cycle arrest. In a phase 2 open label trial of 48 patients with CD30+ lymphoproliferative disorders including lymphomatoid papulosis (LyP) and primary cutaneous anaplastic large-cell lymphoma (pc-ALCL) or CD30+ MF, brentuximab demonstrated an overall response rate of 71% (34 out of 48), with 35% of patients achieving a complete remission (17 out of 48). Interestingly, it showed a 50% overall response rate in MF irrespective of the level of CD30 expression.[102]

Cytotoxic Chemotherapy

Combination chemotherapy regimens have produced higher responses in patients with advanced refractory CTCL, but these responses have not been durable. A study of infusional EPOCH (etoposide, vincristine, doxorubicin, bolus cyclophosphamide, and oral prednisone) in advanced refractory CTCL demonstrated an overall response rate of 80% (12 patients), with 4 (27%) complete responses but a response duration of 8 months.[103] Treatment-related toxicity was significant with 61% of the patients experiencing grade 3/4 myelosuppression. Because of the high risk of infection and myelosuppression and modest response durations with combination chemotherapy, single-agent therapies are preferred except in patients who are refractory or who present with extensive adenopathy and/or visceral involvement and require immediate palliation.

Purine Analogs

Response rates up to 70% have been reported for single-agent pentostatin in refractory patients. Investigators at the M.D. Anderson Cancer Center reported a response rate of 56% for dose-escalated pentostatin (3 to 5 mg/m^2 per day for 3 days on a 21-day schedule) in 42 patients with CTCL.[104] The failure-free survival was 2.1 months. Grade 3/4 neutropenia occurred in 21% of patients. The incidence of infectious complications with pentostatin was initially high but was subsequently reduced by prophylactic trimethoprim and antiviral therapies. In a combination study of pentostatin at 4 mg/m^2 per day for 3 days with intermediate-dose IFN-α, the overall response rate was similar, but the median progression-free survival was improved to 13.1 months.[105]

Fludarabine and cladribine have demonstrated more modest single-agent activity in MF/SS. The combination of fludarabine with IFN-α had greater efficacy with an overall response rate of 51% (4 complete responses, 14 partial responses) with a median progression-free survival of 5.9 months and an overall survival of 19.6 months.[106] Similarly, a combination of fludarabine (18 mg/m^2) and cyclophosphamide (250 mg/m^2) for 3 days monthly was associated with a DOR of 10 months but with significant hematologic toxicity.[107]

Gemcitabine has demonstrated impressive clinical activity in advanced and refractory CTCL. In a study of chemotherapy-naïve patients treated with 1,200 mg/m^2, the response rate was 75%, with 22% complete response rate.[108]

Liposomal Doxorubicin

Pegylated liposomal doxorubicin is an active agent in Kaposi's sarcoma and has been shown to accumulate in involved skin lesions. In patients with advanced MF, response rates of 80% have been reported. In one small prospective multicenter study investigating liposomal doxorubicin monotherapy in 25 patients, 5 complete responses and 9 partial responses were reported.[109] In a larger phase 2 trial carried out at the EORTC of 49 patients with stage IIB, IVA, or IVB MF, 3 patients experienced a complete response and 17 experienced a partial response with a median duration of response of 6 months and a median time to progression of 7.4 months.[110] With the exception of infusion related events, liposomal doxorubicin was well tolerated with no grade 3 or 4 adverse events (AEs).

Pralatrexate

Pralatrexate is a promising new folate antagonist with activity in patients with T cell lymphoma that has been approved for patients with aggressive peripheral T-cell lymphoma and MF with large cell transformation. In preclinical studies, pralatrexate has been shown to be more potent than methotrexate.[111] In the PROPEL study, 111 patients with relapsed or refractory PTCL were treated with pralatrexate. The overall response rate was 29%, with a median duration of response of 10.1 months.[112] In an open label phase 1 clinical trial including 54 CTCL patients who failed at least one systemic therapy, pralatrexate was given at a dose of 15 mg/m^2 for 3 to 4 weeks, and the overall response rate was 41% (35% partial response, 6% complete response).[113] Grade 3/4 adverse events were mucositis and leukopenia. In patients with transformed MF in the PROPEL study, the overall response rate was 25% (n = 3), demonstrating efficacy in a group that is largely refractory to therapy.

Autologous and Allogeneic Bone Marrow Transplantation

Results with autologous stem cell transplantation have not been promising in patients with MF/SS. One major issue in many studies is eradication of disease prior to transplant, and most patients have undergone extensive prior therapy. Molina et al.[114] reported successful outcomes with donor transplants in six of eight refractory CTCL patients. All achieved a complete remission; however, two died from transplant-related complications. Paralkar[115] reported results using reduced intensity conditioning regimens in 12 refractory CTCL patients. Six patients (50%) achieved complete remission and the median duration of response was 22 months. In a retrospective analysis of allogeneic transplant for MF and SS, in a group of 60 patients where 44 underwent reduced intensity conditioning (RIC), patients with RIC had a 1- and 3-year overall survival of 73% and 63%, respectively, supporting a significant graft versus lymphoma effect.[116]

OTHER CUTANEOUS LYMPHOMAS

Primary CD30+ Lymphoproliferative Disorders

The primary CD30+ lymphomas comprise a spectrum of disease, with LyP being a clonal but nonmalignant variant and cutaneous ALCL (C-ALCL) resembling its systemic counterpart. Clinically and histopathologically, LyP and C-ALCL may be indistinguishable. The classic presentation of LyP is papular, papulonodular, or papulonecrotic skin lesions at different stages of development with a waxing and waning course. The lesions often disappear within 12 weeks and often leave a scar. The median patient age is 45 years, but the disease does occur in children; the male to female ratio is 1.5:1. Three histologic subtypes have been identified, all demonstrating large CD30+ cells with (type A) or without (type C) infiltrating inflammatory cells.[117] In some cases (type B), there is infiltration of the epidermis, similar to MF. Up to 60% of cases demonstrate clonality for T-cell receptor (TCR), but the (2:5) (p23;q35) translocation characteristic of alk+ ALCL is not present. Up to 20% of cases may be preceded by or follow another lymphoma, including MF, ALCL, or Hodgkin's lymphoma. For most patients, the prognosis is excellent, and the disease is managed either with no treatment, low doses of oral methotrexate, or PUVA. In a series of 118 isolated cases of LyP, only 4% of patients developed systemic lymphoma.

C-ALCL is similar to systemic ALCL except for the cutaneous presentation and the absence of systemic disease. All patients with C-ALCL should undergo careful staging to rule out systemic involvement before being classified as C-ALCL. Most patients present with solitary nodules, tumors, or ulcerating lesions that may spontaneously regress, but multifocal disease has been observed in up to 20% of patients. The histopathologic features of the disease include the presence of large, anaplastic cells that express CD30 antigen in more than 70% of the tumor cells. The tumor cells demonstrate clonality for TCRR, an activated CD4 phenotype with loss of other T-cell antigens and frequent expression of cytotoxic proteins (granzyme B, T-cell intracellular antigen-1 [TIA-1], perforin). The (2:5) (p23;q35) alk translocation that is frequently seen in systemic ALCL is uncommonly observed in C-ALCL. In addition, the systemic ALCL expresses epithelial membrane antigen, which is absent in C-ALCL. The overall prognosis is excellent and most patients are treated by surgical excision and/or local radiotherapy to the lesions. For recurrent disease, low doses of methotrexate or other cytotoxic agents may be used. A new family of humanized anti-CD30 antibodies has been developed and has shown efficacy in both systemic and cutaneous ALCL.

Subcutaneous Panniculitis-like T-Cell Lymphoma and Cutaneous Peripheral T-Cell Lymphoma Unspecified

Subcutaneous panniculitis-like T-cell lymphoma (SPTL) and cutaneous peripheral T-cell lymphomas have distinct clinicopathologic features and outcomes. SPTCL is comprised of two subtypes, the alpha/beta and the gamma/delta, and both are characterized by subcutaneous masses or flat plaques that mainly involve the legs but may be generalized. Often, patients present with B symptoms such as fever, fatigue, and weight loss. The WHO–EORTC classification has separated these phenotypes because of their disparate outcomes.[2] The alpha/beta SPTCL is characterized by subcutaneous infiltrates that spare the epidermis and dermis and rim individual fat cells. In early stages, the tumor cells may lack significant atypia and an inflammatory infiltrate may be present, leading to a diagnosis of inflammatory panniculitis. The phenotype of the malignant lymphocytes is CD3+, CD4−, and CD8+ with an expression of cytotoxic proteins. The outcome for the alpha/beta type of SPCL is excellent, with an 80% 5-year survival. Treatments include corticosteroids, single-agent chemotherapy, and radiotherapy. The cutaneous gamma/delta T-cell lymphomas are characterized by disseminated disease with frequent mucosal and extranodal involvement. Hemophagocytic syndrome may occur. Histopathologic features include involvement of the dermis, epidermis, and fat with rimming of fat globules and angioinvasion. The phenotype of the cells is CD3+, CD2+−, CD8+, and CD56+ beta F1− with a lack of expression of either CD4 or CD8. Most patients have a poor outcome despite aggressive chemotherapy, with a median survival of 15 months reported in one series of 33 patients.

Primary cutaneous PTCL unspecified is characterized by infiltration of the dermis by CD3+ CD4+ or CD3+ CD8+ pleomorphic small- and medium-sized cells, in many cases with an admixture of reactive lymphocytes. Most cases demonstrate a loss of T-cell markers and are CD30 negative and rarely CD56+. The clinical features are plaques or tumors, often on the face, neck, or upper trunk. The estimated 5-year survival of the CD4+ types is 80% and the preferred treatments are surgery, radiation, or single-agent chemotherapy. The CD8+ variants often express cytotoxic phenotypes (granzyme B+, perforin+, TIA-1+) and are characterized by ulcerative or necrotic tumor or plaques with frequent dissemination to visceral sites but rarely to lymph nodes. The median survival for this group of patients is 32 months despite aggressive systemic chemotherapy.

The Cutaneous Natural Killer Lymphomas

Extranodal NK/T-cell lymphoma is an Epstein-Barr virus–positive lymphoma with an NK or cytotoxic T-cell phenotype most commonly found in South America, South Asia, and Central America. The skin is the second most common site of involvement after the nasal cavity and sinuses. Skin manifestations include ulcerative or necrotic skin lesions characterized histopathologically by angiodestruction and extensive necrosis. The neoplastic cells express CD2, CD56, and cytotoxic proteins but lack surface CD3. The TCR is often germ line, and Epstein-Barr virus is almost always expressed. The median survival for disease presenting in the skin alone is 27 months, and 5 months for those presenting with other sites of disease.

Another variant of cutaneous NK lymphoma, the blastic NK lymphoma, has been recently reclassified by the WHO–EORTC as CD4+/CD56+ hematodermic neoplasm because recent studies have demonstrated a plasmacytoid dendritic cell derivation. This neoplasm commonly presents in the skin with solitary or multiple tumors or nodules. Most patients who present with skin involvement only rapidly develop widespread disease in multiple visceral sites. The infiltrates are CD4+ CD56+, and CD45RA+ cells, which lack CD3 and cytotoxic proteins and express CD123 and TCL 1, which are characteristic of plasmacytoid dendritic cells. The differential diagnosis is myelomonocytic or lymphocytic leukemia cutis, which can be distinguished by staining for myeloperoxidase and CD3, respectively. The skin biopsy is notable for a diffuse nonepidermotropic infiltration of the dermis by intermediate-sized blastlike cells with frequent mitoses. The prognosis is poor, with a median survival of 14 months. Initial therapy is often with acute myeloid leukemia type of regimens, which induce brief initial responses.

Cutaneous B-Cell Lymphoma

The primary cutaneous B-cell lymphomas (PCBCL) are 1.4 times more common in men than women, and more common in Caucasians.[118] The etiology of PCBCL is also unclear, and the pathogenesis not well understood, but *Borrelia* has been identified in a small percentage of patients presenting with PCBCL. For PCBCL, nodal classification systems have been used, but given the different natural history of such lesions, specific classification and prognostic systems are necessary. In addition to the WHO–EORTC classification system for both T- and B-cell cutaneous lymphomas, other prognostic systems have been developed that take the location and histology of the lesion into account.[119]

Types of Primary Cutaneous B-Cell Lymphomas

The histologic subtypes of PCBCLs include marginal zone, follicular center cell type, and diffuse large cell (see Table 40.1). Mucosa-associated lymphoid tissue can be found in a variety of anatomic locations, and marginal zone lymphoma of the skin is the cutaneous counterpart. Small lymphocytes and reactive germinal centers are frequently appreciated in conjunction with marginal zone cells. The expression of CD20, CD79, and, commonly, bcl-2 but not bcl-6 has been identified in addition to the identification of the *IHG* and *MLT* genes of chromosomes 14 and 18, respectively. Follicle center cell cutaneous lymphomas often spare the epidermis and may consist of centrocytes, germinal centers, and reactive T cells. A follicular pattern is common and the expression of CD20 and CD79 is often noted. The expression of bcl-2 and MUM-1 is typically absent. The t(14;18) translocation, which is often seen in the nodal counterpart, is absent in the cutaneous presentation.

Cutaneous plasmacytoma consists of a cutaneous infiltrate of plasma cells without bone marrow involvement. This presentation of PCBCL is quite rare and may present as papules, plaques, or tumors/nodules. Typically, the dermis is occupied by mononuclear cells, and amyloid deposition is often identified within the infiltrate. Immunoglobulins are often present, and cells may express CD38.

Diffuse large B-cell type is distinguished based on whether it occurs on the leg and whether it is intravascular type. Expression of CD20 and CD79 may be seen, and lesions identified on the lower extremity may express bcl-2, bcl-6, and MUM-1. Lesions that are found in other cutaneous locations may also express these markers, but more typically they are found on the lower extremities. Inactivation of p16 suppressor genes, additions for 18q and 7p, and loss of 6q may be noted with cutaneous diffuse large B-cell lymphoma.[120]

Treatment for PCBCL depends on the histopathologic subtype. More indolent forms of PCBCL, such as marginal zone or follicle center cell, tend to be bothersome to the patient, but rarely follow an aggressive clinical course. Radiotherapy, surgical excision, and observation are options for such patients. Radiotherapy for PCBCL is very much the same as that described for MF–CTCL. The technical aspects of the treatment delivery are quite similar, as are the side effects. Patients who present with diffuse large cell leg-type histology are typically treated more aggressively, given the relatively poor outcomes with radiotherapy alone. Combined modality therapy is often considered for this group of patients, and therapeutic courses tend to follow those used in nodal lymphomas of similar histology. If the histology is diffuse large cell, but not of the leg type, consideration can be given to the use of radiotherapy alone as the sole therapeutic modality. Rituximab has been used in the management of patients with PCBCL, and in those with widespread disease, but the evidence regarding efficacy and outcomes is anecdotal, and series are small. For patients with localized CBCL, the complete response rates approach 100%, with 5-year disease-free survivals of approximately 50%.[118,121–125]

REFERENCES

1. Groves FD, Linet MS, Travis LB, et al. Cancer surveillance series: non-Hodgkin's lymphoma incidence by histologic subtype in the United States from 1978 through 1995. *J Natl Cancer Inst* 2000;92:1240–1251.
2. Willemze R, Jaffe ES, Burg G, et al. WHO-EORTC classification for cutaneous lymphomas. *Blood* 2005;105:3768–3785.
3. Willemze R, Meijer CJ. Classification of cutaneous T-cell lymphoma: from Alibert to WHO-EORTC. *J Cutan Pathol* 2006;33:18–26.
4. Bunn PA Jr, Huberman MS, Whang-Peng J, et al. Prospective staging evaluation of patients with cutaneous T cell lymphomas. Demonstration of a high frequency of extracutaneous dissemination. *Ann Intern Med* 1980;93:223–230.
5. Sausville EA, Worsham GF, Matthews MJ, et al. Histologic assessment of lymph nodes in mycosis fungoides/Sezary syndrome (cutaneous T-cell lymphoma): clinical correlations and prognostic import of a new classification system. *Hum Pathol* 1985;16:1098–1109.
6. Schechter GP, Bunn PA, Fischmann AB, et al. Blood and lymph node T lymphocytes in cutaneous T cell lymphoma: evaluation by light microscopy. *Cancer Treat Rep* 1979;63:571–574.
7. Toro JR, Stoll HL Jr, Stomper PC, et al. Prognostic factors and evaluation of mycosis fungoides and Sezary syndrome. *J Am Acad Dermatol* 1997;37:58–67.
8. Vonderheid EC, Bernengo MG, Burg G, et al. Update on erythrodermic cutaneous T-cell lymphoma: report of the International Society for Cutaneous Lymphomas. *J Am Acad Dermatol* 2002;46:95–106.
9. Abrams JT, Balin BJ, Vonderheid EC. Association between Sezary T cell-activating factor, Chlamydia pneumoniae, and cutaneous T cell lymphoma. *Ann N Y Acad Sci* 2001;941:69–85.
10. Rossler MJ, Rappl G, Muche M, et al. No evidence of skin infection with Chlamydia pneumoniae in patients with cutaneous T cell lymphoma. *Clin Microbiol Infect* 2003;9:721–723.
11. Pancake BA, Wasset EH, Zucker-Franklin D. Demonstration of antibodies to human T-cell lymphotropic virus-I tax in patients with the cutaneous T-cell lymphoma, mycosis fungoides who are seronegative for antibodies to the structural proteins of the virus. *Blood* 1996;88:3004–3009.
12. Pancake BA, Zucker-Franklin D. The difficulty of detecting HTLV-1 proviral sequences in patients with mycosis fungoides. *J Acquir Immune Defic Syndr Hum Retrovirol* 1996;13:314–319.
13. Zucker-Franklin D, Coutavas EE, Rush MG, et al. Detection of human T-lymphotropic virus-like particles in cultures of peripheral blood lymphocytes from patients with mycosis fungoides. *Proc Natl Acad Sci U S A* 1991;88:7630–7634.
14. Zucker-Franklin D, Hooper WC, Evatt BL. Human lymphotropic retroviruses associated with mycosis fungoides: evidence that human T-cell lymphotropic virus type II (HTLV-II) as well as HTLV-I may play a role in the disease. *Blood* 1992;80:1537–1545.
15. Axelrod PI, Lorber B, Vonderheid EC. Infections complicating mycosis fungoides and Sezary syndrome. *JAMA* 1992;267:1354–1358.
16. Yawalkar N, Ferenczi K, Jones DA, et al. Profound loss of T-cell receptor repertoire complexity in cutaneous T-cell lymphoma. *Blood* 2003;102:4059–4066.
17. Girardi M, Heald PW, Wilson LD. The pathogenesis of mycosis fungoides. *N Engl J Med* 2004;350:1978–1988.
18. Picker LJ, Kishimoto TK, Smith CW, et al. ELAM-1 is an adhesion molecule for skin-homing T cells. *Nature* 1991;349:796–799.
19. Berg EL, Yoshino T, Rott LS, et al. The cutaneous lymphocyte antigen is a skin lymphocyte homing receptor for the vascular lectin endothelial cell-leukocyte adhesion molecule 1. *J Exp Med* 1991;174:1461–1466.
20. Nickoloff BJ, Griffiths CE. T lymphocytes and monocytes bind to keratinocytes in frozen sections of biopsy specimens of normal skin treated with gamma interferon. *J Am Acad Dermatol* 1989;20:736–743.
21. Nickoloff BJ, Griffiths CE, Baadsgaard O, et al. Markedly diminished epidermal keratinocyte expression of intercellular adhesion molecule-1 (ICAM-1) in Sezary syndrome. *JAMA* 1989;261:2217–2221.
22. Mao X, Orchard G, Lillington DM, et al. Amplification and overexpression of JUNB is associated with primary cutaneous T-cell lymphomas. *Blood* 2003;101:1513–1519.
23. Scarisbrick JJ, Woolford AJ, Russell-Jones R, et al. Loss of heterozygosity on 10q and microsatellite instability in advanced stages of primary cutaneous T-cell lymphoma and possible association with homozygous deletion of PTEN. *Blood* 2000;95:2937–2942.
24. Lin WM, Lewis JM, Filler RB, et al. Characterization of the DNA copy-number genome in the blood of cutaneous T cell lymphoma patients. *J Invest Dermatol* 2012;132:188–197.
25. Karenko L, Hahtola S, Paivinen S, et al. Primary cutaneous T-cell lymphomas show a deletion or translocation affecting NAV3, the human UNC-53 homologue. *Cancer Res* 2005;65:8101–8110.

26. Mao X, Lillington DM, Czepulkowski B, et al. Molecular cytogenetic characterization of Sezary syndrome. Genes Chromosomes Cancer 2003;36:250–260.
27. Pimpinelli N, Olsen EA, Santucci M, et al. Defining early mycosis fungoides. J Am Acad Dermatol 2005;57:1053–1063.
28. Simon M, Flaig MJ, Kind P, et al. Large plaque parapsoriasis: clinical and genotypic correlations. J Cutan Pathol 2000;27:57–60.
29. Wood GS, Tung RM, Haeffner AC, et al. Detection of clonal T-cell receptor gamma gene rearrangements in early mycosis fungoides/Sezary syndrome by polymerase chain reaction and denaturing gradient gel electrophoresis (PCR/DGGE). J Invest Dermatol 1994;103:34–41.
30. Duangurai K, Piamphongsant T, Himmungnan T. Sezary cell count in exfoliative dermatitis. Int J Dermatol 1988;27:248–252.
31. Duncan SC, Winkelmann RK. Circulating Sezary cells in hospitalized dermatology patients. Br J Dermatol 1978;99:171–178.
32. Mao X, Lillington D, Scarisbrick JJ, et al. Molecular cytogenetic analysis of cutaneous T-cell lymphomas: identification of common genetic alterations in Sezary syndrome and mycosis fungoides. Br J Dermatol 2002;147:464–475.
33. Scarisbrick JJ, Whittaker S, Evans AV, et al. Prognostic significance of tumor burden in the blood of patients with erythrodermic primary cutaneous T-cell lymphoma. Blood 2001;97:624–630.
34. Lynch JW Jr, Linoilla I, Sausville EA, et al. Prognostic implications of evaluation for lymph node involvement by T-cell antigen receptor gene rearrangement in mycosis fungoides. Blood 1992;79:3293–3299.
35. Graham SJ, Sharpe RW, Steinberg SM, et al. Prognostic implications of a bone marrow histopathologic classification system in mycosis fungoides and the Sezary syndrome. Cancer 1993;72:726–734.
36. Diamandidou E, Colome M, Fayad L, et al. Prognostic factor analysis in mycosis fungoides/Sezary syndrome. J Am Acad Dermatol 1999;40:914–924.
37. Salhany KE, Greer JP, Cousar JB, et al. Marrow involvement in cutaneous T-cell lymphoma. A clinicopathologic study of 60 cases. Am J Clin Pathol 1989;92:747–754.
38. Sausville EA, Eddy JL, Makuch RW, et al. Histopathologic staging at initial diagnosis of mycosis fungoides and the Sezary syndrome. Definition of three distinctive prognostic groups. Ann Intern Med 1988;109:372–382.
39. Bunn PA Jr, Lamberg SI. Report of the committee on staging and classification of cutaneous T-cell lymphomas. Cancer Treat Rep 1979;63:725–728.
40. Olsen E, Vonderheid E, Pimpinelli N, et al. Revisions to the staging and classification of mycosis fungoides and Sezary syndrome: a proposal of the International Society for Cutaneous Lymphomas (ISCL) and the cutaneous lymphoma task force of the European Organization of Research and Treatment of Cancer (EORTC). Blood 2007;110:1713–1722.
41. Agar NS, Wedgeworth E, Crichton S, et al. Survival outcomes and prognostic factors in mycosis fungoides/Sezary syndrome: validation of the revised International Society for Cutaneous Lymphomas/European Organisation for Research and Treatment of Cancer staging proposal. J Clin Oncol 2010;28:4730–4739.
42. Kim YH, Bishop K, Varghese A, et al. Prognostic factors in erythrodermic mycosis fungoides and the Sezary syndrome. Arch Dermatol 1995;131:1003–1008.
43. Diamandidou E, Colome-Grimmer M, Fayad L, et al. Transformation of mycosis fungoides/Sezary syndrome: clinical characteristics and prognosis. Blood 1998;92:1150–1159.
44. Dmitrovsky E, Matthews MJ, Bunn PA, et al. Cytologic transformation in cutaneous T cell lymphoma: a clinicopathologic entity associated with poor prognosis. J Clin Oncol 1987;5:208–215.
45. Olsen EA, Rook AH, Zic J, et al. Sezary syndrome: immunopathogenesis, literature review of therapeutic options, and recommendations for therapy by the United States Cutaneous Lymphoma Consortium (USCLC). J Am Acad Dermatol 2011;64:352–404.
46. Stevens SR, Ke MS, Parry EJ, et al. Quantifying skin disease burden in mycosis fungoides-type cutaneous T-cell lymphomas: the severity-weighted assessment tool (SWAT). Arch Dermatol 2002;138:42–48.
47. Dummer R, Heald PW, Nestle FO, et al. Sezary syndrome T-cell clones display T-helper 2 cytokines and express the accessory factor-1 (interferon-gamma receptor beta-chain). Blood 1996;88:1383–1389.
48. Kumar R, Xiu Y, Zhuang HM, et al. 18F-fluorodeoxyglucose-positron emission tomography in evaluation of primary cutaneous lymphoma. Br J Dermatol 2006;155:357–363.
49. Tsai EY, Taur A, Espinosa L, et al. Staging accuracy in mycosis fungoides and sezary syndrome using integrated positron emission tomography and computed tomography. Arch Dermatol 2006;142:577–584.
50. Kim YH, Liu HL, Mraz-Gernhard S, et al. Long-term outcome of 525 patients with mycosis fungoides and Sezary syndrome: clinical prognostic factors and risk for disease progression. Arch Dermatol 2003;139:857–866.
51. Dewey WC, Ling CC, Meyn RE. Radiation-induced apoptosis: relevance to radiotherapy. Int J Radiat Oncol Biol Phys 1995;33:781–796.
52. Wilson LD, Kacinski BM, Jones GW. Local superficial radiotherapy in the management of minimal stage IA cutaneous T-cell lymphoma (Mycosis Fungoides). Int J Radiat Oncol Biol Phys 1998;40:109–115.
53. Kuzel TM, Roenigk HH Jr, Samuelson E, et al. Effectiveness of interferon alfa-2a combined with phototherapy for mycosis fungoides and the Sezary syndrome. J Clin Oncol 1995;13:257–263.
54. Stadler R, Otte HG, Luger T, et al. Prospective randomized multicenter clinical trial on the use of interferon -2a plus acitretin versus interferon -2a plus PUVA in patients with cutaneous T-cell lymphoma stages I and II. Blood 1998;92:3578–3581.
55. Jones GW, Kacinski BM, Wilson LD, et al. Total skin electron radiation in the management of mycosis fungoides: Consensus of the European Organization for Research and Treatment of Cancer (EORTC) Cutaneous Lymphoma Project Group. J Am Acad Dermatol 2002;47:364–370.
56. Jones GW, Rosenthal D, Wilson LD. Total skin electron radiation for patients with erythrodermic cutaneous T-cell lymphoma (mycosis fungoides and the Sezary syndrome). Cancer 1999;85:1985–1995.
57. Jones G, Wilson LD, Fox-Goguen L. Total skin electron beam radiotherapy for patients who have mycosis fungoides. Hematol Oncol Clin North Am 2003;17:1421–1434.
58. Harrison C, Young J, Navi D, et al. Revisiting low dose total skin electron beam therapy in mycosis fungoides. Int J Radiant Oncol Biol Phys 2011;81:e651–e657.
59. Licata AG, Wilson LD, Braverman IM, et al. Malignant melanoma and other second cutaneous malignancies in cutaneous T-cell lymphoma. The influence of additional therapy after total skin electron beam radiation. Arch Dermatol 1995;131:432–435.
60. Wilson LD, Quiros PA, Kolenik SA, et al. Additional courses of total skin electron beam therapy in the treatment of patients with recurrent cutaneous T-cell lymphoma. J Am Acad Dermatol 1996;35:69–73.
61. Becker M, Hoppe RT, Knox SJ. Multiple courses of high-dose total skin electron beam therapy in the management of mycosis fungoides. Int J Radiat Oncol Biol Phys 1995;32:1445–1449.
62. Quiros PA, Jones GW, Kacinski BM, et al. Total skin electron beam therapy followed by adjuvant psoralen/ultraviolet-A light in the management of patients with T1 and T2 cutaneous T-cell lymphoma (mycosis fungoides). Int J Radiat Oncol Biol Phys 1997;38:1027–1035.
63. Chinn DM, Chow S, Kim YH, et al. Total skin electron beam therapy with or without adjuvant topical nitrogen mustard or nitrogen mustard alone as initial treatment of T2 and T3 mycosis fungoides. Int J Radiat Oncol Biol Phys 1999;43:951–958.
64. Wilson LD, Licata AL, Braverman IM, et al. Systemic chemotherapy and extracorporeal photochemotherapy for T3 and T4 cutaneous T-cell lymphoma patients who have achieved a complete response to total skin electron beam therapy. Int J Radiat Oncol Biol Phys 1995;32:987–995.
65. Wilson LD, Jones GW, Kim D, et al. Experience with total skin electron beam therapy in combination with extracorporeal photopheresis in the management of patients with erythrodermic (T4) mycosis fungoides. J Am Acad Dermatol 2000;43:54–60.
66. Olsen EA, Bunn PA. Interferon in the treatment of cutaneous T-cell lymphoma. Hematol Oncol Clin North Am 1995;9:1089–1107.
67. Foss FM, Higgins B. Intermediate dose interleukin-2 demonstrates activity in patients with relapsed or refractory cutaneous T-cell lymphoma. Blood 2004;104:2642.
68. Duvic M, Sherman ML, Wood GS, et al. A phase II open-label study of recombinant human interleukin-12 in patients with stage IA, IB, or IIA mycosis fungoides. J Am Acad Dermatol 2006;55:807–813.
69. Berger CL, Xu AL, Hanlon D, et al. Induction of human tumor-loaded dendritic cells. Int J Cancer 2001;91:438–447.
70. Girardi M, Berger C, Hanlon D, et al. Efficient tumor antigen loading of dendritic antigen presenting cells by transimmunization. Technol Cancer Res Treat 2002;1:65–69.
71. Knobler R, Duvic M, Querfeld C, et al. Long-term follow-up and survival of cutaneous T-cell lymphoma patients treated with extracorporeal photopheresis. Photodermatol Photoimmunol Photomed 2012;28:250–257.
72. Dani T, Knobler R. Extracorporeal photoimmunotherapy-photopheresis. Front Biosci (Landmark Ed) 2009;14:4769–4777.
73. Duvic M, Hester JP, Lemak NA. Photopheresis therapy for cutaneous T-cell lymphoma. J Am Acad Dermatol 1996;35:573–579.
74. Talpur R, Demierre MF, Geskin L, et al. Multicenter photopheresis intervention trial in early-stage mycosis fungoides. Clin Lymphoma Myeloma Leuk 2011;11:219–227.
75. Suchin KR, Cucchiara AJ, Gottleib SL, et al. Treatment of cutaneous T-cell lymphoma with combined immunomodulatory therapy: a 14-year experience at a single institution. Arch Dermatol 2002;138:1054–1060.
76. Talpur R, Ward S, Apisarnthanarax N, et al. Optimizing bexarotene therapy for cutaneous T-cell lymphoma. J Am Acad Dermatol 2002;47:672–684.
77. Bisaccia E, Gonzalez J, Palangio M, et al. Extracorporeal photochemotherapy alone or with adjuvant therapy in the treatment of cutaneous T-cell lymphoma: a 9-year retrospective study at a single institution. J Am Acad Dermatol 2000;43:263–271.
78. Tsirigotis P, Pappa V, Papageorgiou S, et al. Extracorporeal photopheresis in combination with bexarotene in the treatment of mycosis fungoides and Sezary syndrome. Br J Dermatol 2007;156:1379–1381.
79. Duvic M, Chiao N, Talpur R. Extracorporeal photopheresis for the treatment of cutaneous T-cell lymphoma. J Cutan Med Surg 2003;7:3–7.
80. Girardi M, Berger CL, Wilson LD, et al. Transimmunization for cutaneous T cell lymphoma: a Phase I study. Leuk Lymphoma 2006;47:1495–1503.
81. Richardson SK, Newton SB, Bach TL, et al. Bexarotene blunts malignant T-cell chemotaxis in Sezary syndrome: reduction of chemokine receptor 4-positive lymphocytes and decreased chemotaxis to thymus and activation-regulated chemokine. Am J Hematol 2007;82:792–797.

82. Duvic M, Hymes K, Heald P, et al. Bexarotene is effective and safe for treatment of refractory advanced-stage cutaneous T-cell lymphoma: multinational phase II-III trial results. *J Clin Oncol* 2001;19:2456–2471.
83. Straus DJ, Duvic M, Kuzel T, et al. Results of a phase II trial of oral bexarotene (Targretin) combined with interferon alfa-2b (Intron-A) for patients with cutaneous T-cell lymphoma. *Cancer* 2007;109:1799–1803.
84. Whittaker S, Ortiz P, Dummer R, et al. Efficacy and safety of bexarotene combined with psoralen-ultraviolet A (PUVA) compared with PUVA treatment alone in stage IB-IIA mycosis fungoides: final results from the EORTC Cutaneous Lymphoma Task Force phase III randomized clinical trial (NCT00056056). *Br J Dermatol* 2012;167:678–687.
85. Straus DJ, Duvic M, Horwitz SM, et al. Final results of phase II trial of doxorubicin HCl liposome injection followed by bexarotene in advanced cutaneous T-cell lymphoma. *Ann Oncol* 2014;25:206–210.
86. Piekarz RL, Frye R, Turner M, et al. Phase II multi-institutional trial of the histone deacetylase inhibitor romidepsin as monotherapy for patients with cutaneous T-cell lymphoma. *J Clin Oncol* 2009;27:5410–5417.
87. Whittaker SJ, Demierre MF, Kim EJ, et al. Final results from a multicenter, international, pivotal study of romidepsin in refractory cutaneous T-cell lymphoma. *J Clin Oncol* 2010;28:4485–4491.
88. Duvic M, Talpur R, Ni X, et al. Phase 2 trial of oral vorinostat (suberoylanilide hydroxamic acid, SAHA) for refractory cutaneous T-cell lymphoma (CTCL). *Blood* 2007;109:31–39.
89. Olsen EA, Kim YH, Kuzel TM, et al. Phase IIb multicenter trial of vorinostat in patients with persistent, progressive, or treatment refractory cutaneous T-cell lymphoma. *J Clin Oncol* 2007;25:3109–3115.
90. Pohlman B, Advani R, Duvic M, et al. Final results of a phase II trial of belinostat (PXD101) in patients with recurrent or refractory peripheral or cutaneous T-cell lymphoma. *Blood* 2009;Abstract 920.
91. Duvic M, Dummer R, Becker JC, et al. Panobinostat activity in both bexarotene-exposed and -naive patients with refractory cutaneous T-cell lymphoma: results of a phase II trial. *Eur J Cancer* 2013;49:386–394.
92. Olsen E, Duvic M, Frankel A, et al. Pivotal phase III trial of two dose levels of denileukin diftitox for the treatment of cutaneous T-cell lymphoma. *J Clin Oncol* 2001;19:376–388.
93. Foss FM, Bacha P, Osann KE, et al. Biological correlates of acute hypersensitivity events with DAB(389)IL-2 (denileukin diftitox, ONTAK) in cutaneous T-cell lymphoma: decrease in frequency and severity with steroid premedication. *Clin Lymphoma* 2001;1:298–302.
94. Negro-Vilar A, Prince H, Duvic M, et al. Efficacy and safety of denileukin diftitox (Dd) in cutaneous T-cell lymphoma (CTCL) patients: Integrated analysis of three large phase III trials. *J Clin Oncol* 2008;26:8551.
95. Foss F, Demierre MF, DiVenuti G. A phase-1 trial of bexarotene and denileukin diftitox in patients with relapsed or refractory cutaneous T-cell lymphoma. *Blood* 2005;106:454–457.
96. Kennedy GA, Seymour JF, Wolf M, et al. Treatment of patients with advanced mycosis fungoides and Sezary syndrome with alemtuzumab. *Eur J Haematol* 2003;71:250–256.
97. Lundin J, Hagberg H, Repp R, et al. Phase 2 study of alemtuzumab (anti-CD52 monoclonal antibody) in patients with advanced mycosis fungoides/Sezary syndrome. *Blood* 2003;101:4267–4272.
98. Rider DA, Havenith CE, de Ridder R, et al. A human CD4 monoclonal antibody for the treatment of T-cell lymphoma combines inhibition of T-cell signaling by a dual mechanism with potent Fc-dependent effector activity. *Cancer Res* 2007;67:9945–9953.
99. Kim YH, Duvic M, Obitz E, et al. Clinical efficacy of zanolimumab (HuMax-CD4): two phase 2 studies in refractory cutaneous T-cell lymphoma. *Blood* 2007;109:4655–4662.
100. Ishida T, Iida S, Akatsuka Y, et al. The CC chemokine receptor 4 as a novel specific molecular target for immunotherapy in adult T-Cell leukemia/lymphoma. *Clin Cancer Res* 2004;10:7529–7539.
101. Duvic M, Pinter-Brown L, Foss F, et al. Correlation of target molecule expression and overall response in refractory cutaneous T-cell lymphoma patients dosed with mogamulizumab (KW-0761), a monoclonal antibody directed against CC chemokine receptor type 4 (CCR4). *Blood* 2012;120.
102. Duvic M, Tetzlaff M, Clos A, et al. Phase II trial of brentuximab vedotin For CD30+ cutaneous T-cell lymphomas and lymphoproliferative disorders. *Blood* 2013;122:367.
103. Koizumi K, Sawada K, Nishio M, et al. Effective high-dose chemotherapy followed by autologous peripheral blood stem cell transplantation in a patient with the aggressive form of cytophagic histiocytic panniculitis. *Bone Marrow Transplant* 1997;20:171–173.
104. Kurzrock R, Pilat S, Duvic M. Pentostatin therapy of T-cell lymphomas with cutaneous manifestations. *J Clin Oncol* 1999;17:3117–3121.
105. Foss FM, Ihde DC, Breneman DL, et al. Phase II study of pentostatin and intermittent high-dose recombinant interferon alfa-2a in advanced mycosis fungoides/Sezary syndrome. *J Clin Oncol* 1992;10:1907–1913.
106. Foss FM, Ihde DC, Linnoila IR, et al. Phase II trial of fludarabine phosphate and interferon alfa-2a in advanced mycosis fungoides/Sezary syndrome. *J Clin Oncol* 1994;12:2051–2059.
107. Scarisbrick JJ, Child FJ, Clift A, et al. A trial of fludarabine and cyclophosphamide combination chemotherapy in the treatment of advanced refractory primary cutaneous T-cell lymphoma. *Br J Dermatol* 2001;144:1010–1015.
108. Marchi E, Alinari L, Tani M, et al. Gemcitabine as frontline treatment for cutaneous T-cell lymphoma: phase II study of 32 patients. *Cancer* 2005;104:2437–2441.
109. Quereux G, Marques S, Nguyen JM, et al. Prospective multicenter study of pegylated liposomal doxorubicin treatment in patients with advanced or refractory mycosis fungoides or Sezary syndrome. *Arch Dermatol* 2008;144:727–733.
110. Dummer R, Quaglino P, Becker JC, et al. Prospective international multicenter phase II trial of intravenous pegylated liposomal doxorubicin monochemotherapy in patients with stage IIB, IVA, or IVB advanced mycosis fungoides: final results from EORTC 21012. *J Clin Oncol* 2012;30:4091–4097.
111. Izbicka E, Diaz A, Streeper R, et al. Distinct mechanistic activity profile of pralatrexate in comparison to other antifolates in in vitro and in vivo models of human cancers. *Cancer Chemother Pharmacol* 2009;64:993–999.
112. O'Connor OA, Pro B, Pinter-Brown L, et al. Pralatrexate in patients with relapsed or refractory peripheral T-cell lymphoma: results from the pivotal PROPEL study. *J Clin Oncol* 2011;29:1182–1189.
113. Horwitz SM, Kim YH, Foss F, et al. Identification of an active, well-tolerated dose of pralatrexate in patients with relapsed or refractory cutaneous T-cell lymphoma. *Blood* 2012;119:4115–4122.
114. Molina A, Zain J, Arber DA, et al. Durable clinical, cytogenetic, and molecular remissions after allogeneic hematopoietic cell transplantation for refractory Sezary syndrome and mycosis fungoides. *J Clin Oncol* 2005;23:6163–6171.
115. Paralkar VR, Nasta SD, Morrissey K, et al. Allogeneic hematopoietic SCT for primary cutaneous T cell lymphomas. *Bone Marrow Transplant* 2012;47:940–945.
116. Duarte RF, Canals C, Onida F, et al. Allogeneic hematopoietic cell transplantation for patients with mycosis fungoides and Sezary syndrome: a retrospective analysis of the Lymphoma Working Party of the European Group for Blood and Marrow Transplantation. *J Clin Oncol* 2010;28:4492–4499.
117. Kadin ME. Pathobiology of CD30+ cutaneous T-cell lymphomas. *J Cutan Pathol* 2006;33:10–17.
118. Smith BD, Glusac EJ, McNiff JM, et al. Primary cutaneous B-cell lymphoma treated with radiotherapy: a comparison of the European Organization for Research and Treatment of Cancer and the WHO classification systems. *J Clin Oncol* 2004;22:634–639.
119. Smith BD, Smith GL, Cooper DL, et al. The cutaneous B-cell lymphoma prognostic index: a novel prognostic index derived from a population-based registry. *J Clin Oncol* 2005;23:3390–3395.
120. Child FJ, Scarisbrick JJ, Calonje E, et al. Inactivation of tumor suppressor genes p15(INK4b) and p16(INK4a) in primary cutaneous B cell lymphoma. *J Invest Dermatol* 2002;118:941–948.
121. Eich HT, Eich D, Micke O, et al. Long-term efficacy, curative potential, and prognostic factors of radiotherapy in primary cutaneous B-cell lymphoma. *Int J Radiat Oncol Biol Phys* 2003;55:899–906.
122. Kirova YM, Piedbois Y, Le Bourgeois JP. Radiotherapy in the management of cutaneous B-cell lymphoma. Our experience in 25 cases. *Radiother Oncol* 1999;52:15–18.
123. Piccinno R, Caccialanza M, Berti E. Dermatologic radiotherapy of primary cutaneous follicle center cell lymphoma. *Eur J Dermatol* 2003;13:49–52.
124. Piccinno R, Caccialanza M, Berti E, et al. Radiotherapy of cutaneous B cell lymphomas: our experience in 31 cases. *Int J Radiat Oncol Biol Phys* 1993;27:385–389.
125. Rijlaarsdam JU, Toonstra J, Meijer OW, et al. Treatment of primary cutaneous B-cell lymphomas of follicle center cell origin: a clinical follow-up study of 55 patients treated with radiotherapy or polychemotherapy. *J Clin Oncol* 1996;14:549–555.

41 Primary Central Nervous System Lymphoma

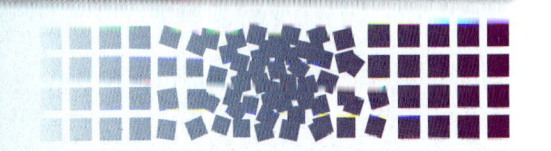

Tracy T. Batchelor

EPIDEMIOLOGY

Primary central nervous system lymphoma (PCNSL) is an extranodal non-Hodgkin lymphoma (NHL) confined to the brain, leptomeninges, eyes, or spinal cord. PCNSL accounts for approximately 2% of all primary central nervous system (CNS) tumors, with a median age of 65 years at diagnosis.[1] The annual incidence rate is 0.47 cases per 100,000 person-years.[1,2] Since 2000, there has been an increase in the overall incidence of PCNSL, especially in the elderly.

PATHOLOGY

Approximately 90% of PCNSL cases are diffuse large B-cell lymphomas (DLBCL), with the remainder consisting of T-cell lymphomas, poorly characterized low-grade lymphomas, or Burkitt lymphomas.[3] Primary CNS DLBCL is composed of centroblasts or immunoblasts clustered in the perivascular space, with reactive lymphocytes, macrophages, and activated microglial cells intermixed with the tumor cells. Most tumors express pan–B-cell markers, including CD19, CD20, CD22, and CD79a. The molecular mechanisms underlying transformation and localization to the CNS are poorly understood.[4] Limitations in molecular studies of PCNSL include the rarity of the disease and the limited availability of tissue because the diagnosis is most often made with stereotactic needle biopsy. Like systemic DLBCL, PCNSL harbors chromosomal translocations of the BCL6 gene, deletions in 6q, and aberrant somatic hypermutation in proto-oncogenes including MYC and PAX5. Inactivation of CDKN2A is also commonly observed in both entities. Also like DLBCL, PCNSL can be classified into three molecular subclasses by gene expression profiling: type 3 large B-cell lymphoma, germinal center B cell, and activated B-cell lymphoma. However, certain molecular features distinguish primary CNS DLBCL from systemic DLBCL. Gene expression profiles demonstrate that PCNSL is characterized by differential expression of genes related to adhesion and the extracellular matrix pathways, including MUM1, CXCL13, and CHI3L1. The ongoing somatic hypermutation with biased use of V_H gene segments that has been observed in PCNSL is suggestive of an antigen-dependent proliferation. These observations are consistent with the hypothesis that PCNSL is secondary to antigen-dependent activation of circulating B cells, which subsequently localize to the CNS by expression of various adhesion and extracellular matrix–related genes. However, further molecular studies to investigate the transforming events and the subsequent events responsible for CNS tropism in PCNSL are needed. Insights into the molecular pathogenesis of PCNSL may allow for the development of targeted therapeutic approaches for tumors.[4]

DIAGNOSIS AND PROGNOSTIC FACTORS

Neurocognitive symptoms are the most common presenting clinical features of PCNSL. The International PCNSL Collaborative Group (IPCG) has developed guidelines to determine the extent of disease.[5] A gadolinium-enhanced brain magnetic resonance imaging (MRI) scan is the most sensitive radiographic study for the detection of PCNSL (Fig. 41.1). Most PCNSL patients present with a single brain mass. The mass is typically isointense to hyperintense on T2-weighted MRI sequences and homogeneously enhancing on postcontrast images. The diagnosis of PCNSL is typically made by stereotactic brain biopsy, cerebrospinal fluid (CSF) analysis, or by analysis of vitreous aspirate in patients with ocular involvement. Given the possible delay in diagnosis and treatment with the latter two methods, prompt stereotactic biopsy is advised in almost all cases that are surgically accessible. Secondary CSF and ocular involvement occurs in approximately 15% to 20% and 5% to 20% of PCNSL patients, respectively. Presenting symptoms of ocular involvement include eye pain, blurred vision, and floaters.[6] B symptoms such as weight loss, fevers, and night sweats are infrequent in PCNSL. A thorough diagnostic evaluation is needed to establish the extent of the lymphoma and to confirm localization to the CNS. Physical examination should consist of a lymph node examination, a testicular examination in men, and a comprehensive neurologic examination. A lumbar puncture should be performed if not contraindicated, and CSF should be assessed by flow cytometry, cytology, and immunoglobulin heavy-chain gene rearrangement. Because extraneural disease must be excluded to establish a diagnosis of *primary* CNS lymphoma, CT or CT/positron-emission tomography (PET) scans of the chest, abdomen, and pelvis, and a bone marrow biopsy and aspirate should be performed to exclude occult systemic disease. Involvement of the optic nerve, retina, or vitreous humor should be excluded with a comprehensive eye evaluation by an ophthalmologist that includes a slit-lamp examination. Blood tests should include a complete blood count, a basic metabolic panel, serum lactate dehydrogenase, and HIV serology.[5]

Two prognostic scoring systems have been developed specifically for PCNSL.[7,8] In a retrospective review of 105 PCNSL patients, the International Extranodal Lymphoma Study Group (IELSG) identified age >60 years, Eastern Cooperative Oncology Group (ECOG) performance status >1, elevated serum lactate dehydrogenase (LDH) level, elevated CSF protein concentration, and involvement of deep regions of the brain as independent predictors of poor prognosis. In patients with 0 to 1 factors, 2 to 3 factors, and 4 to 5 factors, the 2-year survival proportions were 80%, 48%, and 15%, respectively. In another prognostic model, PCNSL patients were divided into three groups based on age and performance status: (1) <50 years old, (2) ≥50 years old with a Karnofsky Performance Scale (KPS) ≥70, and (3) ≥50 years old with a KPS <70. Based on these three divisions, significant differences in overall and failure-free survival were observed.

STAGING

There is no staging system that correlates with prognosis or response to treatment in PCNSL. However, because PCNSL is a

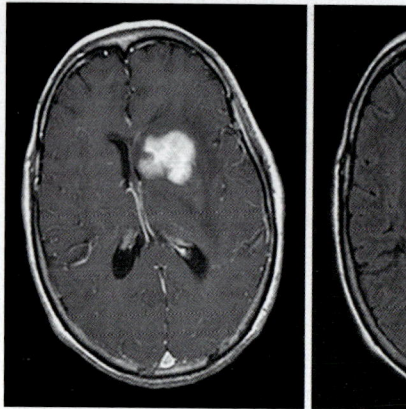

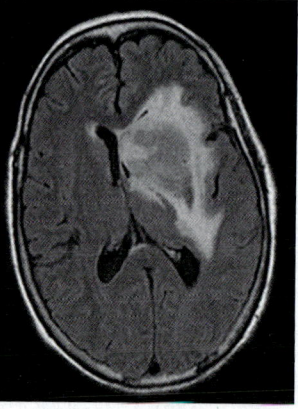

Figure 41.1 Magnetic resonance images from a patient with PCNSL. A T1-weighted, postcontrast, sequence (left) demonstrates intense, homogenous enhancement of the tumor in the region of the left caudate nuclear. A T2/fluid attenuated inversion recovery (FLAIR) sequence (right) demonstrates hyperintense signal surrounding the tumor, reflecting a vasogenic cerebral edema. (Courtesy of Priscilla Brastianos, MD.)

multicompartmental disease potentially involving the brain, spinal cord, eyes, and CSF, the IPCG recommends an extent of disease evaluation, as noted previously, which will enable clinicians to follow the response to therapy.[5]

TREATMENT

Defining a response to treatment in PCNSL requires an assessment of all sites involved by the disease. The IPCG has established response criteria that have been adopted into most prospective clinical trials (Table 41.1).[5]

Corticosteroids decrease tumor-associated edema and may result in partial radiographic regression of the tumor. An initial response to corticosteroids is associated with a favorable outcome in PCNSL.[9] However, after an initial response to corticosteroids, almost all patients quickly relapse. Corticosteroids should be avoided if possible prior to a biopsy, given the risk of disrupting cellular morphology, resulting in a nondiagnostic pathologic specimen.

Surgical resection is not part of the standard treatment approach for PCNSL given the multifocal nature of this tumor.[10] The role of neurosurgery in PCNSL is to establish a diagnosis via a stereotactic biopsy.

Standardized induction and consolidation treatment for PCNSL has yet to be defined. Historically, PCNSL was treated only with whole brain radiation (WBRT) at doses ranging from 36 to 45 Gy, which resulted not only in a high proportion of radiographic responses, but also in rapid relapse. In a multicenter, phase II trial, 41 patients were treated with WBRT to 40 Gy plus a 20 Gy tumor boost and achieved a median overall survival (OS) of only 12 months.[11] Given the lack of durable responses to radiation and the risk of neurotoxicity associated with this modality of therapy, WBRT alone is no longer a recommended treatment for most patients with PCNSL. Moreover, because PCNSL is an infiltrative, multifocal disease, focal radiation or radiosurgery is not recommended. The most effective treatment for PCNSL is intravenous, high-dose methotrexate (HD-MTX) at variable doses (1 to 8 g/m^2), typically utilized in combination with other chemotherapeutic agents and/or WBRT. However, there is no consensus on the optimal dose of HD-MTX or on the role of radiation in combination with methotrexate in the management of PCNSL. A number of randomized trials are ongoing to address these issues. Doses of methotrexate $\geq$ 3 g/m^2 result in therapeutic concentrations in the brain parenchyma and CSF, and when combined with WBRT, lead to more durable treatment responses.[12–14] In a phase II trial, 79 PCNSL patients were randomized to receive either HD-MTX (3.5 g/m^2, day 1) or HD-MTX (3.5 g/m^2, day 1) + cytarabine (2 g/m^2 twice per day, days 2 to 3). Each chemotherapy cycle was 21 days. All patients underwent consolidative WBRT after induction chemotherapy. The HD-MTX + cytarabine arm had a higher proportion of complete radiographic responses and a superior 3-year OS.[14] However, it is now widely recognized that there is a high incidence of neurotoxicity with combined modality treatment that includes WBRT.[15] The latter observation prompted studies utilizing *lower doses* of WBRT. In a

TABLE 41.1

International PCNSL Collaborative Group Consensus Guidelines for the Assessment of Response in PCNSL

Response	Brain Imaging	Steroid Dose	Ophthalmologic Examination	Cerebrospinal Fluid Cytology
Complete response	No contrast enhancing disease	None	Normal	Negative
Unconfirmed complete response	No contrast enhancing disease	Any	Normal	Negative
	Minimal enhancing disease	Any	Minor RPE abnormality	Negative
Partial response	50% decrease in enhancement	N/A	Normal or minor RPE abnormality	Negative
	No contrast enhancing disease	N/A	Decrease in vitreous cells or retinal infiltrate	Persistent or suspicious
Progressive disease	25% increase in enhancing disease	N/A	Recurrent or new disease	Recurrent or positive
	Any new site of disease			
Stable disease	All scenarios not covered by responses above			

RPE, retinal pigment epithelium.
Abrey LE, Batchelor TT, Ferreri AJ, et al. Report of an international workshop to standardize baseline evaluation and response criteria for primary CNS lymphoma. *J Clin Oncol* 2005;23:5034–5043.

multicenter, phase II study, no significant neurocognitive decline was observed after consolidative reduced dose WBRT (23.4 Gy) and cytarabine in patients who had achieved a complete response to induction chemotherapy including HD-MTX.[16] However, further study and longer neuropsychological follow-up of these patients is necessary to definitively assess the safety of this regimen because numerous studies have demonstrated the delayed neurotoxic effects of WBRT in the PCNSL population and the reduced risk of neurotoxicity in regimens consisting of chemotherapy alone.[17,18] Given the risk of clinical neurotoxicity, other studies have assessed whether WBRT can be *eliminated* from the initial management of PCNSL. In a multicenter, phase III trial, patients were randomized to receive HD-MTX–based chemotherapy with or without WBRT.[19] Five hundred and fifty-one patients were enrolled, of whom 318 were treated per protocol. The intent to treat analysis revealed that patients treated in the combined modality arm (chemotherapy + WBRT) achieved prolonged progression-free survival (PFS) but no improvement in OS, demonstrating that the elimination of WBRT from the treatment regimen did not compromise OS. This has led to deferral of WBRT and chemotherapy-alone approaches for newly diagnosed PCNSL patients. These approaches are based on a foundation of HD-MTX. Variable doses and schedules of HD-MTX have been utilized, but in general, doses ≥3 g/m^2 delivered as an initial bolus followed by an infusion over 3 hours administered every 10 to 21 days is recommended for optimal outcomes and adequate CSF concentrations.[20] Multiple, phase II studies have demonstrated the safety, efficacy, and relatively preserved cognition of HD-MTX–based chemotherapy regimens.[21,22] Moreover, longer duration of induction chemotherapy with HD-MTX (>six cycles) results in higher complete response proportions.[16,21]

Several first-generation chemotherapy regimens for PCNSL included intrathecal chemotherapy. However, a number of nonrandomized studies that included intrathecal chemotherapy did not improve outcomes in PCNSL relative to regimens that did not include intrathecal injections of chemotherapy.[23,24] Moreover, the ability to consistently achieve micromolar concentrations of MTX in the CSF at a dose of 8 g/m^2 has led to the elimination of intrathecal chemotherapy from most of the chemotherapy regimens currently in use. However, the question regarding the role of intrathecal chemotherapy in the management of PCNSL should ultimately be addressed in a randomized trial.

Rituximab, a chimeric monoclonal antibody targeting the CD20 antigen on B lymphocytes, is being incorporated in combination regimens for PCNSL. When rituximab is administered intravenously at doses of 375 to 800 mg/m^2, CSF levels from 0.1% to 4.4% of serum levels are achieved. Despite limited CSF penetration, radiographic responses have been observed in relapsed PCNSL patients treated with rituximab monotherapy, and this antibody has been incorporated into contemporary regimens for PCNSL.[25] In a cooperative group, phase II study, 44 PCNSL patients were treated with induction chemotherapy consisting of HD-MTX at 8 g/m^2 (day 1), rituximab at 375 mg/m^2 (day 3), and temozolomide at 150 mg/m^2 (days 7 through 11), all of which are drugs with demonstrated efficacy as monotherapy in PCNSL.[22] This induction chemotherapy was followed by consolidation chemotherapy consisting of intravenous etoposide 5 mg/kg as a continuous infusion over 96 hours and cytarabine at 2 g/m^2 every 12 hours for 8 doses. Of these patients, 68% achieved complete response, median PFS of the entire group was 4 years, and median OS was not observed at the time of publication. These results are comparable to any regimen that *includes* WBRT. It is noteworthy that PFS was shorter in PCNSL patients in whom chemotherapy was delayed >1 month after diagnosis compared to those patients who promptly initiated chemotherapy (3-year PFS of 20% versus 59%; p = 0.05). This observation highlights the importance of prompt biopsy and early initiation of chemotherapy in this patient population.

Given the limited durability of responses observed in many studies of PCNSL, there is increasing interest in high dose chemotherapy (HDT) followed by autologous stem cell transplantation (ASCT) as first-line, consolidative therapy for PCNSL. Conditioning regimens including thioTEPA have demonstrated the most encouraging results. In a multicenter, phase II study, 79 patients were treated with induction HD-MTX, cytarabine, rituximab, and thioTEPA, followed by carmustine and thioTEPA conditioning prior to ASCT. The overall radiographic response (ORR) was 91%, 2-year OS was 87%, and treatment-related deaths occurred in <10% of enrolled patients. The toxicities, mostly cytopenias, were manageable.[26] There are three ongoing, multicenter, randomized trials comparing the efficacy of consolidative HDT/ASCT versus chemotherapy or WBRT for newly diagnosed PCNSL (Table 41.2).

Treatment in the Elderly

Elderly patients account for more than half of all the subjects diagnosed with PCNSL.[27] The risk of neurotoxicity is highest in this population and, in general, chemotherapy alone is the preferred option for this subgroup. The majority of PCNSL patients >60 years of age develop clinical neurotoxicity after treatment with a WBRT-containing regimen, and some of these patients die of treatment-related complications, rather than recurrent disease.[28] Several studies have indicated that HD-MTX at doses of 3.5 to 8 g/m^2 is well tolerated in elderly patients with manageable grade 3 or 4 renal and hematologic toxicity.[29,30] In a multicenter, randomized, phase II trial of chemotherapy alone in elderly patients with PCNSL, 98 patients were randomized to receive three cycles of either MPV-A (methotrexate 3.5 g/m^2, days 1 and 15; procarbazine 100 mg/m^2, days 1 through 7; vincristine 1.4 mg/m^2, days 1 and 15) or MT (methotrexate 3.5 g/m^2, days 1 and 15; temozolomide 100 to 150 mg/m^2, days 1 through 5 and 15 through 19) with one additional cycle of cytarabine (3 g/m^2 per day for 2 consecutive days) in the MPV arm only. Although trends favored the MPV-A regimen over the simpler, less toxic MT regimen with respect to complete response rate, PFS, and OS, none of these differences reached statistical difference.[31] Subsequent studies suggest that the addition of rituximab to both MPV and MT could increase the radiographic response rate. Both of these chemotherapy regimens are options in elderly PCNSL patients.

Salvage Treatment

Despite high initial response rates with HD-MTX–based induction therapy, most patients with PCNSL relapse. Moreover, there is a small subset of patients who have HD-MTX–refractory disease. Prognosis of progressive or relapsed PCNSL is poor, with a limited number of prospective, phase II studies for guidance on management. Rechallenge with HD-MTX has been shown to be effective in patients who had previously responded to this agent. In a multicenter, retrospective study of 22 relapsed PCNSL patients, 91% had a radiographic response to the first salvage treatment with HD-MTX, and 100% to second salvage. The median OS from the first salvage was 61.9 months.[32] In a phase II trial of 43 patients with relapsed or refractory PCNSL, salvage therapy with high-dose cytarabine and etoposide was followed by HDT/ASCT with a conditioning regimen consisting of thioTEPA, busulfan, cyclophosphamide. There were 27 patients who ultimately proceeded to transplantation. Of 27 patients, 26 had a CR and the median PFS and OS in this group were 41.1 and 58.6 months, respectively.[33] In patients who were not initially treated with HDT/ASCT, this strategy remains an option. It is noteworthy that in a small series of patients with relapsed PCNSL after initial HDT/ASCT, a second autotransplantation was successful as salvage treatment.[34] Finally, WBRT in patients who have not received it as a part of their initial

TABLE 41.2

Randomized Trials in Primary Central Nervous System Lymphoma

Induction	Consolidation
Completed Trials	*Completed Trials*
Medical Research Council Phase II, n = 53 (stopped early) CHOP versus WBRT followed by CHOP[39] **IELSG 20 – NCT00210314** Phase II; n = 79, Ages 18–75 y Induction Arm 1: Methotrexate + Cytarabine → WBRT Induction Arm 2: Methotrexate → WBRT[14] **ANOCEF-GOELAMS – NCT00503594** Phase II, n = 95, age ≥60 y Arm 1: Methotrexate, procarbazine, vincristine, cytarabine Arm 2: Methotrexate, temozolomide[31]	**G-PCNSL-SG-1 – NCT00153530** Phase III, n = 551, age ≥18 y Arm 1: Methotrexate ± ifosfamide → WBRT Arm 2: Methotrexate ± ifosfamide[19]
Ongoing Trials	*Ongoing Trials*
IESLG 32 - NCT01011920 Phase II, n = 200, Ages 18–70 y Induction Arm 1: Methotrexate, cytarabine Induction Arm 2: Methotrexate, cytarabine, rituximab Induction Arm 3: Methotrexate, cytarabine, rituximab, thioTEPA **ALLG/HOVON – EudraCT 2009-014722-42** Phase III, n = 200, Ages 18–70 y Arm 1: Methotrexate, BCNU, teniposide, prednisone → Cytarabine, WBRT Arm 2: Methotrexate, BCNU, teniposide, prednisone → Cytarabine, WBRT	**IESLG 32 - NCT01011920** Phase II, n = 104, Ages 18–70 y Consolidation Arm 1: WBRT Consolidation Arm 1: HDT/ASCT **ANOCEF-GOELAMS - NCT00863460** Phase II, n = 100, Ages 18–60 y R-MBVP → Consolidation Arm 1: HDT/ASCT Consolidation Arm 2: WBRT **RTOG 1114 - NCT01399372** Phase II, n = 84, Age ≥18 y Methotrexate, procarbazine, vincristine, rituximab → Consolidation Arm 1: WBRT (lower dose) → cytarabine Consolidation Arm 2: Cytarabine **Alliance 51101 - NCT01511562** Phase II, n = 160, Ages 18–75 y Methotrexate, temozolomide, rituximab, cytarabine → Consolidation Arm 1: HDT/ASCT Consolidation Arm 2: Etoposide, cytarabine

CHOP, cyclophosphamide, hydroxydaunorubicin, oncovin (vincristine), prednisone; ANOCEF, Association des Neuro-Oncologue d'Expression Française; GOELAMS, Groupe Ouest Est d'Etude des Leucémies et Autres Maladies du Sang; G-PCNSL-SG, German Primary CNS Lymphoma Study Group; ALLG, Australasian Leukaemia and Lymphoma Group; HOVON, Stichting Hemato-Oncologie voor Volwassenen Nederland (Dutch-Belgian Cooperative Trial Group for Hematology Oncology); BCNU, bischloroethylnitrosourea; IELSG, International Extranodal Lymphoma Study Group; NCT, national clinical trial; R-MBVP, rituximab, methotrexate, BCNU, VP-16 (etoposide), prednisone; RTOG, Radiation Therapy Oncology Group.

treatment is an effective option in the relapsed PCNSL setting, although the risk of neurotoxicity remains.[35,36] Many clinicians reserve WBRT for those patients with chemotherapy-refractory disease or at the time of relapse. In a series of 27 relapsed or refractory PCNSL patients treated with WBRT (median dose: 36 Gy), 74% achieved an ORR and the median OS was 10.6 months. Delayed neurotoxicity rates of 15% were noted at doses >36 Gy, even in the setting of short survival.[35] Novel therapeutics currently under study for systemic DLBCL have entered early phase clinical trials in primary CNS DLBCL and include bendamustine, lenalidomide, pomalidomide, everolimus, and pemetrexed.[4]

Neurotoxicity

The most frequent complication in long-term PCNSL survivors is delayed neurotoxicity. The exact incidence of delayed neurotoxicity is unclear, because earlier studies did not systematically assess neurocognitive function with serial neuropsychological testing. The elderly are at highest risk for this complication, with nearly all patients over the age of 60 developing clinical neurotoxicity following combined modality therapy. Treatment with WBRT has been identified as the major risk factor for the development of late neurotoxicity. Common symptoms and signs include deficits in attention, memory, executive function, gait ataxia, and incontinence. These deficits have a detrimental impact on quality of life. Radiographic findings include periventricular white matter changes, ventricular enlargement, and cortical atrophy. Pathologic studies reveal demyelination, hippocampal neuronal loss, and large-vessel atherosclerosis.[37] Although the pathophysiology is unclear and likely multifactorial, damage to neural progenitor cells has been implicated to play an important role in radiation-related neurotoxicity.[38] Currently, there are no treatments to reverse these delayed neurotoxic effects. It is critical that serial neuropsychological assessments are incorporated into the management of patients with PCNSL, because cognitive outcome is a critical end point. The IPCG has developed an instrument for this purpose, which is composed of quality of life questionnaires and standardized neuropsychological tests that include an assessment of executive function, attention, memory, and psychomotor speed.[15]

REFERENCES

1. Dolecek TA, Propp JM, Stroup NE, et al. CBTRUS statistical report: primary brain and central nervous system tumors diagnosed in the United States in 2005–2009. *Neuro Oncol* 2012;14:v1–v49.
2. Villano JL, Koshy M, Shaikh H, et al. Age, gender, and racial differences in incidence and survival in primary CNS lymphoma. *Br J Cancer* 2011;105:1414–1418.
3. Swerdlow SH, Campo E, Harris NL, et al., eds. *WHO Classification of Tumours of the Haematopoietic and Lymphoid Tissues.* Lyon, France: International Agency for Research on Cancer; 2008.
4. Ponzoni M, Issa S, Batchelor TT, et al. Beyond high-dose methotrexate and brain radiotherapy: novel targets and agents for primary CNS lymphoma. *Ann Oncol* 2014;25:316–322.
5. Abrey LE, Batchelor TT, Ferreri AJ, et al. Report of an international workshop to standardize baseline evaluation and response criteria for primary CNS lymphoma. *J Clin Oncol* 2005;23:5034–5043.
6. Chan CC, Rubenstein JL, Coupland SE, et al. Primary vitreoretinal lymphoma: a report from an International Primary Central Nervous System Lymphoma Collaborative Group symposium. *Oncologist* 2011;16:1589–1599.
7. Ferreri AJ, Blay JY, Reni M, et al. Prognostic scoring system for primary CNS lymphomas: the International Extranodal Lymphoma Study Group experience. *J Clin Oncol* 2003;21:266–272.
8. Abrey LE, Ben-Porat L, Panageas KS, et al. Primary central nervous system lymphoma: the Memorial Sloan-Kettering Cancer Center prognostic model. *J Clin Oncol* 2006;24:5711–5715.
9. Mathew BS, Carson KA, Grossman SA. Initial response to glucocorticoids: a potentially important prognostic factor in patients with primary CNS lymphoma. *Cancer* 2006;15:383–387.
10. Bellinzona M, Roser F, Ostertag H, et al. Surgical removal of primary central nervous system lymphoma (PCNSL) presenting as space occupying lesions: a series of 33 cases. *Eur J Surg Oncol* 2005;31:100–105.
11. Nelson DF, Martz KL, Bonner H, et al. Non-Hodgkin's lymphoma of the brain: can high dose, large volume radiation therapy improve survival? Report on a prospective trial by the Radiation Therapy Oncology Group (RTOG): RTOG 8315. *Int J Radiat Oncol Biol Phys* 1992;23:9–17.
12. Glantz MJ, Cole BF, Recht L, et al. High-dose intravenous methotrexate for patients with nonleukemic leptomeningeal cancer: is intrathecal chemotherapy necessary? *J Clin Oncol* 1998;16:1561–1567.
13. DeAngelis LM, Seiferheld W, Schold SC, et al. Combination chemotherapy and radiotherapy for primary central nervous system lymphoma: Radiation Therapy Oncology Group Study 93-10. *J Clin Oncol* 2002;20:4643–4648.
14. Ferreri AJ, Reni M, Foppoli M, et al. High-dose cytarabine plus high-dose methotrexate versus high-dose methotrexate alone in patients with primary CNS lymphoma: a randomised phase 2 trial. *Lancet* 2009;374:1512–1520.
15. Correa DD, Maron L, Harder H, et al. Cognitive functions in primary central nervous system lymphoma: literature review and assessment guidelines. *Ann Oncol* 2007;18:1145–1151.
16. Morris PG, Correa DD, Yahalom J, et al. Rituximab, methotrexate, procarbazine and vincristine followed by consolidation reduced-dose whole-brain radiotherapy and cytarabine in newly diagnosed primary CNS lymphoma: final results and long-term outcome. *J Clin Oncol* 2013;31:3971–3979.
17. Doolittle ND, Korfel A, Lubow MA, et al. Long-term cognitive function, neuroimaging and quality of life in primary CNS lymphoma. *Neurology* 2013;81:84–92.
18. Juergens A, Pels H, Rogowski S, et al. Long-term survival with favorable cognitive outcome after chemotherapy in primary central nervous system lymphoma. *Ann Neurol* 2010;67:182–189.
19. Thiel E, Korfel A, Martus P, et al. High-dose methotrexate with or without whole brain radiotherapy for primary CNS lymphoma (G-PCNSL-SG-1): a phase 3, randomised, non-inferiority trial. *Lancet Oncol* 2010;11:1036–1047.
20. Ferreri AJ, Guerra E, Regazzi M, et al. Area under the curve of methotrexate and creatinine clearance are outcome-determining factors in primary CNS lymphomas. *Br J Cancer* 2004;90:353–358.
21. Batchelor T, Carson K, O'Neill A, et al. Treatment of primary CNS lymphoma with methotrexate and deferred radiotherapy: a report of NABTT 96-07. *J Clin Oncol* 2003;21:1044–1049.
22. Rubenstein JL, Hsi ED, Johnson JL, et al. Intensive chemotherapy and immunotherapy in patients with newly diagnosed primary CNS lymphoma: CALGB 50202 (Alliance 50202). *J Clin Oncol* 2013;31:3061–3068.
23. Khan RB, Shi W, Thaler HT, et al. Is intrathecal methotrexate necessary in the treatment of primary CNS lymphoma? *J Neurooncol* 2002;58:175–178.
24. Sierra Del Rio M, Ricard D, Houillier C, et al. Prophylactic intrathecal chemotherapy in primary CNS lymphoma. *J Neurooncol* 2012;106:143–146.
25. Batchelor TT, Grossman SA, Mikkelsen T, et al. Rituximab monotherapy for patients with recurrent primary CNS lymphoma. *Neurology* 2011;76:929–930.
26. Illerhaus G, Fritsch K, Egerer G, et al. Sequential high dose immunochemotherapy followed by autologous peripheral blood stem cell transplantation for patients with untreated primary central nervous system lymphoma—a multicentre study by the Collaborative PCNSL Study Group Freiburg. Presented at: 2012 American Society of Hematology Annual Meeting; 2012; Atlanta, GA.
27. Ostrom QT, Gittleman H, Farah P, et al. CBTRUS statistical report: primary brain and central nervous system tumors diagnosed in the United States 2006-2010. *Neuro-Oncol* 2013;14:ii1–ii56.
28. Nayak L, Batchelor TT. Recent advances in treatment of primary central nervous system lymphoma. *Curr Treat Options Oncol* 2013;14:539–552.
29. Jahnke K, Korfel A, Martus P, et al. High-dose methotrexate toxicity in elderly patients with primary central nervous system lymphoma. *Ann Oncol* 2005;16:445–449.
30. Zhu JJ, Gerstner ER, Engler DA, et al. High-dose methotrexate for elderly patients with primary CNS lymphoma. *Neuro Oncol* 2009;11:211–215.
31. Omuro A, Chinot O, Taillandier L, et al. Multicenter randomized phase II trial of methotrexate (MTX) and temozolomide (TMZ) versus MTX, procarbazine, vincristine, and cytarabine for primary CNS lymphoma (PCNSL) in the elderly: an Anocef and Goelams Intergroup study. Presented at: 2013 American Society of Clinical Oncology Annual Meeting; 2013; Chicago, IL.
32. Plotkin SR, Betensky RA, Hochberg FH, et al. Treatment of relapsed central nervous system lymphoma with high-dose methotrexate. *Clin Cancer Res* 2004;10:5643–5646.
33. Soussain C, Hoang-Xuan K, Taillandier L, et al. Intensive chemotherapy followed by hematopoietic stem-cell rescue for refractory and recurrent primary CNS and intraocular lymphoma: Societe Francaise de Greffe de Moelle Osseuse-Therapie Cellulaire. *J Clin Oncol* 2008;26:2512–2518.
34. Kasenda B, Schorb E, Fritsch K, et al. Primary CNS lymphoma—radiation-free salvage therapy by second autologous stem cell transplantation. *Biol Blood Marrow Transplant* 2011;17:281–283.
35. Nguyen PL, Chakravarti A, Finkelstein DM, et al. Results of whole-brain radiation as salvage of methotrexate failure for immunocompetent patients with primary CNS lymphoma. *J Clin Oncol* 2005;23:1507–1513.
36. Hottinger AF, DeAngelis LM, Yahalom J, et al. Salvage whole brain radiotherapy for recurrent or refractory primary CNS lymphoma. *Neurology* 2007;69:1178–1182.
37. Lai R, Abrey LE, Rosenblum MK, et al. Treatment-induced leukoencephalopathy in primary CNS lymphoma: a clinical and autopsy study. *Neurology* 2004;62:451–456.
38. Monje ML, Vogel H, Masek M, et al. Impaired hippocampal neurogenesis after treatment for central nervous system malignancies. *Ann Neurol* 2007;62:515–520.
39. Mead GM, Bleehen NM, Bullimore GA, et al. A medical research council randomized trial in patients with primary cerebral non-Hodgkin lymphoma: cerebral radiotherapy with and without cyclophosphamide, doxorubicin, vincristine, and prednisone chemotherapy. *Cancer* 2000;89:1359–1370.

Section 3 Leukemias and Plasma Cell Tumors

42 Molecular Biology of Acute Leukemias

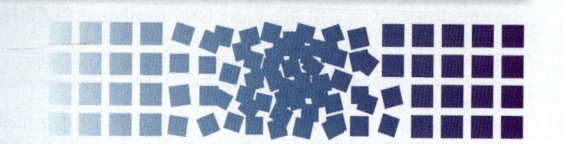

Glen D. Raffel and Jan Cerny

INTRODUCTION

Our understanding of the molecular genetics of acute leukemias has improved dramatically over the past decade. Fueled in part by the availability of the complete sequence of the human genome, more than 100 different mutations have been identified that can be causally implicated in the pathogenesis of acute leukemias (Table 42.1). At first glance, the plethora of mutations presents a discouraging prospect for the development of molecular-targeted therapies. However, far more mutations are identified than there are phenotypes of acute leukemia, and a theme is developed in this chapter that many of these mutations must target similar signal transduction or transcriptional pathways. Thus, it is plausible to consider therapeutic approaches that target these shared pathways of transformation. Although many mutations remain to be identified, those observed thus far have provided critical insights into the pathophysiology of leukemia and the development of novel therapeutic targets.

LEUKEMIC STEM CELL

An important emerging concept in the pathobiology of leukemia is the existence of a *leukemic stem cell*. In normal hematopoietic development, there is a rare population of hematopoietic stem cells that have self-renewal capacity and that give rise to multipotent hematopoietic progenitors. These multipotent myeloid or lymphoid progenitors do not have a self-renewal capacity but mature into normal terminally differentiated cells in the peripheral blood. It is hypothesized that there is a leukemic stem cell that has limitless self-renewal capacity and that gives rise to clonogenic leukemic progenitors that do not have self-renewal capacity but are incapable of normal hematopoietic differentiation. Hypothesized functional differences between the rare leukemic stem cells and the bulk of derived leukemic progeny such as increased quiescence or engagement within a protective niche are believed to provide an intrinsic chemoresistance.

The first convincing evidence in support of the existence of a leukemic stem cell was derived from experiments in which human leukemic cells were injected into immunodeficient nonobese diabetic mice with severe combined immunodeficiency disease (NOD-SCID) mice.[1,2] These data show that the resultant leukemias are derived from as few as 1:1000 to 1:10,000 cells, indicating that there is a rare population of human leukemic cells that have self-renewal capacity in this assay. These cells have similar immunophenotypes to normal self-renewing hematopoietic progenitors and suggest that the leukemogenic mutation occurs in a hematopoietic stem cell. In support of this hypothesis, clonal cytogenetic abnormalities, such as the t(9;22), have been detected in primitive hematopoietic progenitors such as CD34+CD38– cells.[3]

However, this paradigm has been recently challenged and revised. First, new protocols that enhance engraftment of human leukemia in the xenotransplant setting have been described, suggesting the importance of homing and the role of the microenvironment.[4] Data also show that it may be the leukemic oncogenes themselves that confer properties of self-renewal. In a murine system, transduction of the leukemia oncogenes mixed-lineage leukemia 1/eleven nineteen leukemia (*MLL/ENL*), monocytic leukemia zinc finger protein/transcriptional intermediary factor 2 (*MOZ/TIF2*) or *MLL/ALL1* fused gene from chromosome 9 protein (*AF9*) can confer properties of self-renewal to purified committed hematopoietic progenitors that have no capacity for self-renewal.[5,6] *HOX* family and *NOTCH* genes, frequent mutational targets in acute leukemia as discussed later in this chapter, have been found to have significant roles in hematopoietic stem cell self-renewal.[7] Secondary mutations may also enable activation of similar self-renewal pathways. For example, an analysis of cells from acute myeloid leukemia (AML) blast crisis in chronic myeloid leukemia (CML) shows a shift in the leukemic stem cell to an immunophenotype of a committed myeloid progenitor and concurrent nuclear localization of β-catenin, a process thought to increase stem cell self-renewal.[8] One of the major goals is the identification of transcriptional programs, genes, and pathways that confer limitless self-renewal and may be targets for therapeutic intervention.

ELUCIDATION OF GENETIC EVENTS IN ACUTE LEUKEMIA

The search for causative mutations in acute leukemia has accelerated in recent years due to the availability of new means for evaluating genome integrity in leukemic cells. The bulk of known translocations and deletions were found by analyzing conventionally stained chromosomal banding patterns of karyotypes. The classical karyotypic analysis is able to identify lesions with a resolution of 5 to 10 Mb. These include balanced reciprocal chromosomal translocations, such as t(8;21)(q22;q22) or t(15;17)(q22;q21); internal deletions of single chromosomes, such as 5q- or 7q-; gain or loss of whole chromosomes (+8 or −7); or chromosome inversions, such as inv(3), inv(16), or inv(8). Array-based technologies such as comparative genomic hybridization (CGH) and single-nucleotide polymorphism (SNP) arrays allow detailed (<35 kb) mapping of unbalanced insertions or deletions.[9,10] Array CGH determines DNA copy gain or loss by comparing the hybridization of sample DNA to a series of clones or oligonucleotides from regions throughout the genome bound to a chip with a normal reference DNA sample. SNP arrays differ in that oligomers of SNP sequences representing known alleles throughout the genome are used in the array to measure changes in expected genotype and copy number. Finally, low-cost high-throughput sequencing and

TABLE 42.1
Selected Examples of Cytogenetic and Molecular Abnormalities in Leukemia

Lesion	Genes Involved	Derivation of Abbreviation	Protein Characterization	Disease
Mutations Involving the Core-Binding Factors (CBFs)				
t(8;21)(q22;q22) AML1/ETO	ETO (CBFA2T1) (8q22) AML1 (RUNX1) (21q22)	Eight twenty-one Acute myeloid leukemia 1	Zinc finger protein α subunit of CBF complex	AML
inv(16)(p13q22) CBFβ/MYH11	MYH11 (SMMHC) (16p13) CBFB/CBFβ (16q22)	Myosin heavy chain 11 Core-binding factor-β	Smooth muscle myosin heavy chain β subunit of CBF complex	AML
t(3;21)(q26;q22) AML1/EVI1	EVI1 (3q26) AML1 (RUNX1) (21q22)	Ecotropic virus integration site 1 Acute myeloid leukemia 1	Multiple zinc fingers α subunit of CBF complex	MDS, AML CML-BC
t(12;21)(p13;q22) TEL/AML1	TEL (ETV6) (12p13) AML1 (RUNX1) (21q22)	Translocation ETS leukemia Acute myeloid leukemia 1	ETS-related transcription factor α subunit of CBF complex	ALL
AML1 deletion/truncation	AML1 (RUNX1)	Acute myeloid leukemia 1	α subunit of CBF complex	FDP/AML
Fusions Involving MLL				
t(4;11)(q21;q23) MLL/AF4	AF4 (4q21) MLL (11q23)	ALL1 fused chromosome 4 Mixed-lineage leukemia	Transactivator *Drosophila* trithorax homolog	ALL, AML
t(11;19)(q23;p13.3) MLL/ENL	MLL (11q23) ENL (19p13.3)	Mixed-lineage leukemia Eleven nineteen leukemia	*Drosophila* trithorax homolog Transcription factor	AML, ALL
t(9;11)(p22;q23) MLL/AF9	AF9 (9p22) MLL (11q23)	ALL1 fused chromosome 9 Mixed-lineage leukemia	Nuclear protein, ENL homology *Drosophila* trithorax homolog	AML, ALL
t(1;11)(q21;q23) MLL/AF1	AF1q (1q21) MLL (11q23)	ALL1 fused chromosome 1q Mixed-lineage leukemia	No homology to any known protein *Drosophila* trithorax homolog	AML
MLL partial tandem duplication	MLL (11q23)	Mixed-lineage leukemia	*Drosophila* trithorax homolog	AML
Fusions Involving RAR-α				
t(15;17)(q22;q12-21) PML/RARα	PML (15q21) RAR-α (17q21)	Promyelocytic leukemia Retinoic acid receptor-α	Zinc finger protein Retinoic acid receptor-α	APL
t(11;17)(q23;q21) PLZF/RARα	PLZF (11q23) RAR-α (17q21)	Promyelocytic leukemia zinc finger Retinoic acid receptor-α	Zinc finger protein Retinoic acid receptor-α	APL
T(5;17)(q32;q21) NPM1/RARα	NPM1 RAR-α (17q21)	Nucleophosmin Retinoic acid receptor-α	Chaperone Retinoic acid receptor-α	APL
Mutations Involving Lymphoid Differentiation Factors				
dic(9;12)(p13;p13) PAX5/TEL	PAX5 (9p13) TEL (ETV6) (12p13)	Paired box 5 Translocation ETS leukemia	Transcription factor Transcription factor	B-ALL
PAX5 loss of function	PAX5 (9p13)	Paired box 5	Transcription factor	B-ALL
EBF1 loss of function	EBF1	Early B-cell factor 1	Transcription factor	B-ALL
IKZF1 loss of function/DN	IKZF1	IKAROS family zinc finger 1	Transcription factor	B-ALL
LEF1 loss of function	LEF1	Lymphoid enhancer binding factor 1	Transcription factor	ALL
t(17;19)(q22;p13.3) TCF3/HLF	HLF (17q22) TCF3 (E2A) (19p13.3)	Hepatic leukemia factor Transcription factor 3	Leucine zipper bHLH transcription factor	B-ALL
Mutations Involving Hox Genes				
t(7;11)(p15;p15) NUP98/HOXA9	HOXA9 (7p15) NUP98 (11p15)	Homeobox A9 Nuclear pore 98	Homeobox protein Nucleoporin	AML/MDS AML
t(12;13)(p13;q12) TEL/CDX2	TEL (ETV6) CDX2	Ten-eleven translocation Caudal type homeobox 2	Transcription factor Homeobox protein	AML
t(1;19)(q23;p13) TCF3/PBX1	TCF3 (E2A) PBX1	Transcription factor 3 Pre–B-cell leukemia homeobox 1	Transcription factor Homeobox protein	B-ALL

(continued)

TABLE 42.1

Selected Examples of Cytogenetic and Molecular Abnormalities in Leukemia *(continued)*

Lesion	Genes Involved	Derivation of Abbreviation	Protein Characterization	Disease
Other Transcription Factors				
t(1;22)(p13;q13) OTT1/MAL	OTT1 (RBM15) (1p13) MAL (MKL1) (22q13)	One twenty-two Megakaryocytic acute leukemia	Spen homolog Serum response cofactor	AMKL
GATA1s truncation	GATA1	GATA binding protein 1	Transcription factor	AMKL
CEBPA truncation	CEBPA	CCAAT/enhancer binding protein-α	Transcription factor	AML
NOTCH1 PEST/HD point mutations	NOTCH1	Notch 1 (*Drosophila* wing phenotype)	Transcription factor	T-ALL
t(6;9)(p23;q34) DEK/NUP214	DEK (6p23) NUP214 (CAN) (9q34)	Not relevant to molecule Nuclear pore 214	Transcription factor Nucleoporin	AML
Translocations Involving the Immunoglobulin Enhancer Loci				
t(8;14)(q24;q32)	MYC (8q24) IGH (14q32)	Myelocytomatosis virus Immunoglobulin heavy chain	bHLH/bZIP transcription factor Ig heavy chain promoter	B-ALL
t(2;8)(p12;q24)	IGK (2p12) MYC (8q24)	Immunoglobulin κ-chain Myelocytomatosis virus	Igκ-chain promoter bHLH/bZIP transcription factor	B-ALL
t(8;22)(q24;q11)	MYC (8q24) IGL (22q11)	Myelocytomatosis virus Immunoglobulin λ-chain	bHLH/bZIP transcription factor Igλ-chain promoter	B-ALL
t(X;14)(p22;q32) & t(Y;14)(p11;q32)	IGH (14q32) CRLF2 (Xp22)/(Yp11)	Immunoglobulin heavy chain Cytokine receptor like 2	Ig heavy chain promoter Extracellular receptor	B-ALL
Translocations Involving the T-Cell Receptor Genes				
t(1;14)(p32;q11)	TAL1/SCL (1p32) TCRα/δ (14q11)	T cell acute leukemia 1/stem cell leukemia T-cell receptor-α/δ	bHLH transcription factor T-cell receptor promoter	T-ALL
t(1;7)(p32;q34)	TAL1/SCL (1p32) TCRβ (7q34)	T-cell acute leukemia 1/stem cell leukemia T-cell receptor-β	bHLH transcription factor T-cell receptor promoter	T-ALL
t(7;9)(q34;q34)	TCRβ (7q34) TAL2/SCL2 (9q34)	T-cell receptor-β T-cell acute leukemia 2/stem cell leukemia	T-cell receptor promoter bHLH transcription factor	T-ALL
t(7;19)(q34;p13)	TCRβ (7q34) LYL1 (19p13)	T-cell receptor-β Lymphoid leukemia 1	T-cell receptor promoter bHLH transcription factor	T-ALL
t(8;14)(q24;q11)	MYC (8q24) TCRα/δ (14q11)	Myelocytomatosis virus T-cell receptor-α/δ	bHLH/bZIP transcription factor T-cell receptor promoter	T-ALL
t(11;14)(p15;q11)	LMO1 (11p15) TCRα/δ (14q11)	LIM only 1 T-cell receptor-α/δ	Zinc finger T-cell receptor promoter	T-ALL
t(11;14)(p13;q11)	LMO2 (11p13) TCRα/δ (14q11)	LIM only 2 T-cell receptor-α/δ	Zinc finger T-cell receptor promoter	T-ALL
t(7;10)(q34;q24)	TCRβ (7q34) HOX11 (10q24)	T-cell receptor-β Homeobox 11	T-cell receptor promoter Homeobox gene	T-ALL
t(7;9)(q34;q34.3)	TCRβ (7q34) NOTCH1 (9q34.3)	T-cell receptor-β Notch 1 (drosophila wing)	T-cell receptor promoter Transcription factor	T-ALL
Receptors and Signaling Molecules				
t(9;22)(q34;q11) BCR/ABL1	BCR ABL1	Breakpoint cluster region c-Abl oncogene 1	S/T kinase, GTPase activating Nonreceptor tyrosine kinase	AML, ALL
FLT3 ITD and activating loop mutation	FLT3R	FMS-like tyrosine kinase	Receptor tyrosine kinase	AML
NRAS activating mutation	NRAS	Neuroblastoma rat sarcoma viral oncogene homolog	Small GTPase	AML, ALL
KRAS activating mutation	KRAS	Kirsten rat sarcoma viral oncogene homolog	Small GTPase	AML, ALL

(continued)

TABLE 42.1 Selected Examples of Cytogenetic and Molecular Abnormalities in Leukemia (continued)

Lesion	Genes Involved	Derivation of Abbreviation	Protein Characterization	Disease
Receptors and Signaling Molecules				
KIT activating mutation	KIT	v-Kit feline sarcoma viral oncoprotein	Receptor tyrosine kinase	AML
JAK2, JAK3 activating mutation	JAK2, JAK3	Janus kinase 2, 3	Nonreceptor tyrosine kinase	AMKL
MPL activating mutation	MPL	Myeloproliferative leukemia virus oncogene	Thrombopoietin receptor	AMKL
Epigenetic Modifiers				
inv8(p11q13)	MOZ	Monocytic leukemia zinc finger protein	K(lysine) acetyltransferase	AML
MOZ/TIF2	TIF2	Transcriptional intermediary factor 2	Nuclear receptor coactivator	
TET2 LOH4q24, loss of function	TET2	Ten-eleven translocation 2	Methylcytosine dioxygenase	AML, MDS, MPN
IDH1/2 activating mutation	IDH1/IDH2	Isocitrate dehydrogenase 1 and 2	Isocitrate dehydrogenase	AML, MDS, MPN
DNMT3 loss of function	DNMT3	DNA methyltransferase 3	Cytosine-5-methyltransferase	AML
EZH2 loss of function	EZH2	Enhancer of zeste homolog 2	Histone methyltransferase	MDS, MPN, AML
Tumor Suppressors				
WT1 loss of function	WT1	Wilms tumor 1	Transcriptional regulator	AML
TP53 deletion (–17p)	TP53	Tumor protein p53 kDa	Transcription factor	AML, ALL

AML, acute myeloid leukemia; CBF, core-binding factor; MDS, myelodysplastic syndrome; CML, chronic myeloid leukemia; ETS, E twenty-six retrovirus; ALL, acute lymphoblastic leukemia; ENL, eleven-nineteen leukemia; MLL, mixed-lineage leukemia; APL, acute promyelocytic leukemia; B-ALL, B lineage acute lymphoblastic leukemia; AMKL, acute megakaryocytic leukemia; bHLH, basic helix–loop–helix; T-ALL, T lineage acute lymphoblastic leukemia; bZIP, basic region/leucine zipper; Ig, immunoglobulin; LIM, Lin-11, Isl-2, Mec-3 homeodomain; MPN, myeloproliferative neoplasia; LOH, loss of heterozygosity.

---

microarray-based resequencing techniques have allowed for the identification of new somatic mutations at the single-nucleotide level and are making enormous inroads into the pathogenesis, prognosis, and classification of leukemias with *normal* cytogenetics. Worldwide initiatives to sequence large numbers of cancer genomes, including leukemia subtypes, are being coordinated and cataloged through the International Cancer Genome Consortium (http://www.icgc.org) and the Cancer Genome Atlas (TCGA) (https://tcga-data.nci.nih.gov/tcga).[12]

Although intensive effort has focused on chromosomal translocations in leukemia, in part because of their high frequency in various kinds of leukemia, it has become increasingly clear that point mutations play an important role in a spectrum of leukemias. Ongoing high-throughput sequencing initiatives have identified numerous solitary and recurring somatic point mutations within the various leukemic subtypes. The interpretation of this sequencing data requires the identification of *driver* versus *passenger* mutations. *Driver* mutations cause genetic alterations contributing to leukemic pathophysiology, whereas *passenger* mutations occur in leukemia cells and are propagated but are not etiologic to the disease.[13] It is, therefore, essential that newly discovered somatic mutations in leukemia undergo subsequent biologic validation through sequencing studies in an experimental model system.

MUTATIONS THAT TARGET CORE-BINDING FACTOR

Core-binding factor (CBF) is targeted by more than a dozen different chromosomal translocations in acute leukemias, including the t(8;21) or inv(16), observed in approximately 20% of AMLs, and the t(12;21), present in approximately 25% of patients with pediatric B-lineage acute lymphoblastic leukemia (ALL).[14] Adult patients with CBF leukemias have a favorable prognosis and the *translocation ETS leukemia (TEL)/AML1* fusion that is expressed as a consequence of t(12;21) in children confers a favorable prognosis among B-cell ALL.[15] CBF is a heterodimeric transcription factor composed of the AML1 (also known as RUNX1 or CBFA2) and CBFβ proteins that is critical for normal hematopoietic development. Loss of function of either subunit results in a complete lack of definitive hematopoiesis.[16,17] The AML1 subunit of CBF contacts DNA but only weakly transactivates target genes as a monomer. When bound to its heterodimeric partner CBFβ, which does not itself contact DNA, transactivation of CBF target genes is dramatically enhanced.[15,18,19] CBF transactivates a spectrum of target genes that are important in normal myeloid development, including transcription factors (e.g., *PU.1*, *CEBP/A* and *GATA1*), cytokines (e.g., granulocyte-macrophage colony-stimulating factor [GM-CSF]) and cytokine receptors (such as macrophage-colony stimulating factor [M-CSF] receptor), as well as in lymphoid development, such as the T-cell receptor beta (TCRβ) enhancer and the immunoglobulin (Ig) heavy-chain loci.[18–21] Because CBF targets genes that are important for normal hematopoietic development, a mutation or gene rearrangement that resulted in loss of function of either AML1 or CBFβ might be expected to impair hematopoietic differentiation.[15,18,19]

In addition to frequent involvement of *AML1* as a consequence of chromosomal translocations, it has been determined that loss-of-function mutations in *AML1* are responsible for the inherited leukemia syndrome familial platelet disorder with propensity to develop AML (FPD/AML).[22,23] Approximately 3% to 5% of sporadic cases of AML harbor loss-of-function mutations in *AML1*,[22,24] with a higher frequency in M0 AML (25%) and in AML or myelodysplastic syndrome (MDS) with trisomy 21. AML1 loss-of-function mutations are associated with poor rather than good prognosis subgroups such as acute myeloid leukemia 1/eight twenty-one (AML1/ETO); however, this may be a result of occurring in the context of myelodysplasia or mixed lineage leukemias.[19]

Compelling evidence has been shown that translocations that target CBF result in a loss of function through dominant negative inhibition. The AML1/ETO fusion associated with t(8;21) and the CBFβ/MYH11 (aka CBFβ/SMMHC) fusion associated with inv(16) are dominant negative inhibitors of CBF and impair hematopoietic differentiation. The expression of either the AML1/ETO or CBFβ/MYH11 fusion genes from their endogenous promoter in mice completely inhibits the function of the residual AML1 or CBFβ alleles, resulting in a lack of definitive hematopoiesis and resultant embryonic lethality.[16,17] The phenotype observed is the same as that seen in AML1–/– or CBFβ–/– mice, indicating that the AML1/ETO or CBFβ/MYH11 fusions, respectively, act as potent dominant negative inhibitors of the native proteins.[25,26] However, AML1/ETO and CBFβ/MYH11 have been shown to confer novel contributory gain-of-function effects beyond those involving CBF transcriptional targets. For example, AML1/ETO blocks the tumor suppressors p14ARF and nuclear factor 1 (NF1), whereas CBFβ/MYH11 blocks the expression of p15INK4B.[27,28] AML1/ETO downregulates DNA-repair genes, perhaps enhancing genomic instability.[29] Histone deacetylases (HDAC) and DNA-methyltransferases (DNMT) associated with AML1/ETO alter the epigenetic profile of normal and leukemic cells to generate global changes in gene expression, which may be integral to leukemogenesis. Respective inhibitors such as suberoylanilide hydroxamic acid (SAHA) and azacytidine may, therefore, have therapeutic value in CBF leukemias.[18]

Although the expression of AML1/ETO leads to alterations of gene expression and hematopoietic cell proliferation leukemia and confers the ability to serially replate in methylcellulose culture (a measure of self-renewal potential), this does not result in the development of leukemia in an animal model. However, co-expression of an alternatively spliced isoform of the AML1/ETO transcript, AML1/ETO9a, which includes an extra exon, exon 9a, of the ETO gene (AML1/ETO9a encodes a C-terminally truncated AML1-ETO protein of 575 amino acids) leads to a rapid development of leukemia in a mouse retroviral transduction-transplantation model.[32] The presence of AML1/ETO9a closely correlates with the presence of activating c-KIT mutations in humans, conferring a poor prognosis.[33] Similarly, the expression of CBFβ/MYH11 in adult hematopoietic cells results in leukemia only after a markedly prolonged latency; this latency can be shortened using mutagenesis strategies.[26] In summary, translocations that target CBF impair hematopoietic differentiation and confer certain properties of leukemic stem cells, such as the ability to serially replate, but are not sufficient to cause leukemia.

In pediatric B-ALL, 25% of cases have t(12;21)(p13;q13) in which the TEL (aka ETV6) gene translocates into AML1, thus allowing the production of a chimeric protein, TEL/AML1 (aka ETV6/RUNX1).[34,35] TEL is a transcriptional repressor mediated through associated HDACs and, like AML1, has requirements in fetal and definitive hematopoiesis.[30,34,36] TEL has 30 known fusion partners of different functional classes, including tyrosine kinases such as in TEL/platelet-derived growth factor receptor (PDGFR) and HOX genes such as in PAX5/TEL, although TEL/AML1 is the most common.[34] The fusion protein preserves the central repressor domain in TEL and contains almost the entire AML1 protein sequence. TEL/AML1 has the ability to bind to AML1 consensus sequences but now brings an HDAC-dependent repressor function to AML1-responsive promoter elements, thereby suppressing AML1 targets.[34] In addition, physiologic TEL function may be dysregulated by the fusion through heterodimerization via TEL helix–loop–helix domains.[34] TEL/AML1 is often found in conjunction with deletions in the pre-B receptor, VPREB, and the tumor suppressor gene, CDKN2A.[37]

CHROMOSOMAL TRANSLOCATIONS THAT TARGET THE RETINOIC ACID RECEPTOR ALPHA GENE

The empiric observation that all-trans-retinoic acid (ATRA) induces complete responses in patients with acute promyelocytic leukemia (APL) drove the subsequent cloning of the t(15;17)(q22;q21) fusion gene involving the RARα locus. Several groups demonstrated at approximately the same time that the RARα gene on chromosome 17 was fused to a novel partner that was eventually identified as the promyelocytic leukemia (PML) gene.[38–40] Two reciprocal fusion RNA species are produced as a consequence of the translocation, RARα/PML and PML/RARα. The PML/RAR-α fusion protein contains the zinc finger of PML fused to the DNA- and protein-binding domains of RAR-α. Several other chromosomal translocations target the RARα locus and are associated with an APL phenotype. The best studied of these is the promyelocytic leukemia zinc finger (PLZF/RAR-α) fusion, which also aberrantly recruits the nuclear corepressor complex. However, in contrast with the PML/RAR-α fusion, ATRA is not able to relieve corepression mediated by the PLZF/RAR-α fusion and thus is not effective in patients who harbor the t(11;17) associated with this fusion gene.[11]

The PML gene has a broad, although incompletely understood role in the homeostasis of cells in part as an organizing component of nuclear bodies (PML-NB) responsible for nuclear structure and shuttling.[41,43] Recently, an important independent cytoplasmic role for PML as a tumor suppressor has been uncovered, whereby PML localized to the contact points between the endoplasmic reticulum and mitochondrial-associated membranes controls calcium transport and apoptosis.[44] PML is essential for maintaining self-renewal in hematopoietic stem cells (HSC) as shown by a mouse knockout model of PML, which demonstrated increased proliferation and premature exhaustion in the HSC compartment.[45] The PML region of PML-RARα was also identified as the target for arsenic trioxide therapy. The binding of arsenic increases PML oligomerization followed by SUMOylation, which in turn, causes PML/RARα degradation.[46]

RARα possesses a DNA-binding domain, a hormone-binding domain, and a retinoid X receptor (RXR)–binding domain, all of which are included within the PML/RARα chimeric protein. RARα transactivates multiple genes involved in myeloid differentiation.[47] PML/RARα homodimers, enabled via a coiled coil domain in the PML portion, bind to RAR sites and repress genes important for granulocytic differentiation in part through HDAC and corepressor recruitment.[47] PML/RARα, however, does not have effects solely through dominant inhibition of RARα/RXR binding sites. PML/RARα was shown to have an extended repertoire of DNA consensus binding sites beyond those found for RARα.[48] PML/RARα appears to extensively modify histone-acetylation and methylation marks in expressing cells in an ATRA-dependent manner, likely through recruitment of HDACs and histone methyltransferases and demethylases within the PML-RARα complex.[48,49] Drug targeting of PML/RARα-associated epigenetic modifying proteins may, therefore, provide effective adjuncts to ATRA-based therapies.

The transforming properties of the PML/RARα fusion gene have been tested in murine models. Expression of PML/RAR-α in transgenic mice from promoters that direct expression to the promyelocyte compartment result in an APL-like phenotype.[50–52] However, there is approximately a 6-month lag before the development of leukemia, incomplete penetrance of approximately 15% to 30%, and acquired karyotypic abnormalities, all suggesting that second mutations are required for induction of leukemia.

In at least some cases, activating mutations in FLT3 may be the additional mutation required. ATRA is efficacious in leukemic animals expressing both PML/RARα and activated FLT3, and this model has allowed for the preclinical testing of newer agents such as arsenic trioxide.[53]

MUTATIONS THAT TARGET HOX FAMILY MEMBERS

HOX genes are homeodomain-containing transcription factors important in patterning in vertebrate development and in hematopoietic development.[54,55] HOX genes are clustered in four genomic loci HOXA-D, although additional *orphan* HOX genes occur elsewhere in the genome. Transactivation by HOX genes is potentiated by cofactors such as pre–B cell leukemia (PBX1) and myeloid ecotropic insertion site (Meis1). NUP98, a nuclear transport protein, is a fusion partner to at least eight different HOX genes in AML as well as numerous other genes.[56] HOX gene expression is tightly regulated during hematopoietic development. HOXA9, for example, is expressed in early hematopoietic progenitor cells but is downregulated during hematopoietic differentiation and is undetectable in terminally differentiated cells. The expression of NUP98/HOXA9 results in derepression of HOXA cluster genes, several of which promote HSC self-renewal.[54,56]

The contribution of the NUP98 moiety to leukemic transformation is not fully understood. NUP98 is normally a component of the nuclear pore complex and is constitutively and ubiquitously expressed. However, several lines of evidence suggest that NUP98 contributes more than a constitutively activated promoter. For example, NUP98 motifs known as FG repeats are critical for homo formation and may serve to recruit transcriptional coactivators, such as CBP/p300, to HOXA9 DNA-binding sites.[57] In murine models of leukemia, overexpression of HOXA9 alone is not sufficient to cause AML, but coexpression of HOXA9 with transcriptional cofactors, such as MEIS1, results in efficient induction of AML.[58] Thus, the NUP98 moiety in the context of the NUP98/HOXA9 fusion may serve multiple functions, including provision of an active promoter, and recruitment of transcriptional coactivators such as CBP/p300 that subserve the function of other cofactors such as MEIS1. Epidemiologic evidence that the NUP98 moiety contributes to leukemogenesis includes the observation that there are now a spectrum of fusion proteins involving components of the nuclear pore that are targeted by chromosomal translocations in acute leukemias. These include NUP98 and NUP214 fused to a diverse group of partners, including HOXA9 and HOXD13, and the DDX10, PMX1, DEK, and ABL1 genes, respectively.

Dysregulated HOX gene expression may be important in leukemias that do not directly target HOX family members. Several proteins that are upstream of HOX expression have been observed as fusion genes associated with AML, the most frequent of these are MLL gene rearrangements. More than 40 chromosomal translocations target MLL and result in fusions of MLL with a broad spectrum of partners. In addition, dysregulation of HOX genes by an enhancer effect, which occurs in t(7;10)(q34;q24), where the TCRβ translocates into the HOX11 locus, is an important contributor to T cell acute lymphoid leukemia (T-ALL) leukemogenesis.[59] However, a common biologic feature of all of these may be their ability to dysregulate HOX gene expression during hematopoietic development. For example, t(12;13) associated with AML results in the expression of high levels of CDX2 from the TEL locus.[60] CDX2 is a homeotic protein that regulates the expression of HOX family members in the colonic epithelium. As in hematopoietic development, HOX gene expression is highest in colonic stem cells in the colonic crypts and is downregulated with maturation. It has been shown that CDX2 and CDX4 can dysregulate HOX expression in hematopoietic progenitors and can result in leukemia.[58,60] Evidence to support this includes the ability of CDX2 to induce leukemia in murine retroviral transduction models.[58,60]

Taken together, these data indicate that the NUP98/HOXA9 fusion transforms hematopoietic progenitors in part through dysregulated overexpression and by transactivation mediated through the NUP98 transactivation domain that recruits CBP. However, like other gene rearrangements involving hematopoietic transcription factors, expression of NUP98/HOXA9 alone is not sufficient to cause leukemia. In murine bone marrow transplant models, NUP98/HOXA9 induces AML only after markedly prolonged latencies indicative of a requirement for second mutation. Coexpression of Meis1 or FLT3ITD with NUP98/HOXA9 in mice significantly shortens the latency; however, these mutations are not present in all human cases, suggesting that additional cooperating pathways exist.[61,62]

CHROMOSOMAL TRANSLOCATIONS THAT TARGET THE *MLL* GENE

The MLL locus is involved in more than 80 different chromosomal translocations with a remarkably diverse group of fusion partners[63,64] and are associated with mostly French-American-British (FAB) subtype M4 or M5, and fewer with M2 AML. Patients who have received prior chemotherapy for cancer and develop AML (therapy-related MDS/therapy-related AML [t-AML]) often have abnormalities in 11q23, especially those patients treated with topoisomerase inhibitors such as etoposide or topotecan. Chromosomal translocations involving band 11q23 result in the expression of a fusion gene containing amino-terminal MLL sequences fused to a wide variety of partners. There has been no common functional motif or activity ascribed to all partners; however, specific fusions may be associated with specific leukemic phenotypes. The MLL/AF4 fusion associated with t(4;11) is frequently observed in infant leukemias and is associated with an ALL phenotype in more than 90% of cases, whereas the MLL/AF9 fusion associated with the t(9;11) is almost exclusively associated with AML. Certain MLL fusion genes also have prognostic significance. For example, patients with t(9;11)(p22;q23) have a better outcome than those with other translocations involving 11q23.

The MLL gene encodes a large, ubiquitously expressed protein. The *Drosophila* protein trithorax, a homolog of MLL, regulates patterning and HOX gene expression during development. It has been hypothesized, in part based on these observations, that MLL might be required for maintenance of HOX gene expression.[65] Mice that have homozygous deficiency for MLL have an embryonic lethal phenotype at postconception day 10.5. Even heterozygous animals have developmental anomalies in the axial skeleton and hematopoietic deficits, including anemia.[66] Thus, as for other genes targeted by chromosomal translocations, MLL is important for normal hematopoietic development.

Major advances have been made recently regarding the mechanisms underlying MLL and MLL-fusion gene function. MLL binds a broad cohort of epigenetic regulators including bromodomain-containing 3 and 4 (BRD3 and BRD4); the H3K79 histone methyl transferase, DOT1; the lysine-specific demethylase, KDM1A; and the polycomb-repressive complex 2 (PRC2). Although MLL possesses a Su(var)3-9, enhancer-of-zeste and trithorax (SET) homology H3K4 histone methyl-transferase, it is not retained in MLL-fusion proteins. MLL and MLL fusions also require complex formation with menin (MEN1) and lens epithelium–derived growth factor (LEDGF) to be able to interact with DNA and activate target genes.[67,68] MLL fusions have been shown to affect transcriptional *poising* at target genes as part of a larger super elongation complex (SEC).[69] The control of RNA polymerase II elongation after recruitment to promoter sites provides an additional layer of regulation to target genes such as HOXA9.[69,70] MLL fusions also form a complex known as *DotCom*, which, via associated DOT1 activity, yields H3K79 di/trimethylation marks, thus altering expression at affected genes.[69] MLL-fusion/DotCom interaction allows binding and transcription at target genes of the

Wnt/β-catenin pathway via binding of nuclear-localized β-catenin. The Wnt pathway is essential for fetal HSC self-renewal, and aberrant activation of its downstream targets mediated by MLL-fusions is hypothesized to confer self-renewal properties to leukemic stem cells (LSCs).[71]

Although various MLL fusions have similar transforming properties in vitro, there are distinctive differences in disease penetrance and latency in the murine models depending on the fusion partner. It is possible that the MLL gene rearrangement may be critical for transformation, whereas the fusion partners confer properties related to disease phenotype. The long latency of disease in murine models supports the hypothesis that MLL fusions, like the PML/RAR-α and CBF-related fusion proteins, require second mutations to cause leukemia.

As noted previously in the section Leukemic Stem Cell, data indicate that certain MLL fusion genes may also confer properties of self-renewal to hematopoietic progenitors. MLL/ENL expression in common myeloid progenitors or granulocyte-monocyte progenitors in a murine system conferred properties of self-renewal, including the ability to serially replate in methylcellulose cultures and to engender a transplantable AML phenotype in recipient animals.[5] Similarly, in a mouse model of MLL/AF9 oncogene-induced leukemia, up to a quarter of the leukemic cells exhibited stem cell behavior.[72] Furthermore, the MLL/AF9-positive LSC are heterogeneous as they give rise to ALL when injected into immunodeficient mice. The same cells cause AML when injected into immunodeficient mice that are transgenic for the human genes stem cell factor (SCF), GM-CSF, and interleukin 3 (IL-3).[73] These data indicate that leukemogenic mutations may occur in cells that have no intrinsic self-renewal capacity and yet confer these properties by activation of specific transcriptional programs, which may be further modified by clues from the microenvironment.

MUTATION OF C/EBPα

C/EBPα is a 42-kDa hematopoietic transcription factor that is required for normal myeloid lineage differentiation and that inhibits proliferation.[74] C/EBPα is downregulated in 50% of AML, often through methylation of its promoter region.[75] Therefore, loss of C/EBPα function in leukemia likely impairs myeloid differentiation and removes a block on proliferation.[76] Two major types of C/EBPα point mutations have been described in AML—short frame-shifting mutations in the region encoding the amino-terminus, causing the expression of a shortened 30 kDa protein with dominant negative activity, and in-frame insertions or deletions in the region of the carboxy-terminus, which alter the DNA-binding or dimerization domains, causing a loss of function.[77] Two-thirds of C/EBPα-mutated leukemias have both N- and C-terminal mutations on each allele.[76] Although the bulk of C/EBPα mutations occur in patients with normal cytogenetics, overall and progression-free survival is more favorable; therefore, C/EBPα status is an important prognostic determinant.[78] In contrast to AML, 2% of pre–B-ALL has been shown to have an upregulation of C/EBPα or family members through enhancer effects of IgH locus translocation into the C/EBPα locus as seen in t(14;19)(q32;q13).[79,80]

MUTATION OF GATA-1

GATA-1 mutations are associated with a subset of acute megakaryocytic leukemias (AMKL) (FAB M7), in particular leukemias arising in patients with Down syndrome (constitutional trisomy 21).[81] GATA-1 is a transcription factor promoting erythroid and megakaryocytic development.[82,83] GATA-1 mutations result in the early termination of the full-length GATA-1 protein; however, translation of a short-form (GATA-1s) from an alternate initiation codon occurs. GATA-1s is theorized to function as either a hypomorphic or dominant negative allele, and dysregulation of GATA-1 pathways are thought to contribute to leukemogenesis.[84,85] GATA-1 mutations are often seen in a transient myeloproliferative disorder (TMD), which precedes Down syndrome–associated AMKL, suggesting that a GATA-1 mutation is an early event cooperating with germ-line trisomy 21.[84] GATA-1 mutations have been noted in Down syndrome fetal livers, and GATA-1s expression in a mouse model causes hyperproliferation of fetal liver megakaryocytes, supporting the hypothesis of an in utero origin of the disease.[86] Current efforts to identify the critical cooperating genes dysregulated in trisomy 21 are utilizing mouse models possessing trisomies syntenic with the 8.35-Mb Down syndrome critical region to identify candidate genes.[87]

t(1;22) TRANSLOCATION ASSOCIATED WITH INFANT AMKL

The t(1;22)(p13;q13) is associated with the majority of non–Down syndrome AMKL in infants and results in the expression of the OTT1/MAL (aka RBM15/MKL1) fusion gene.[88,89] OTT1 (RBM15) contains three amino-terminal RNA recognition motifs and a Spen paralog and ortholog C-terminal motif that is a transcriptional activator/repressor. Ott1 deletion in mice reveals multiple hematopoietic roles, including megakaryocyte growth and hematopoietic stem cell function.[90,91] The MAL (MKL1) gene is a Rho-GTPase–regulated cofactor for serum response factor (SRF) and controls megakaryocyte development.[92,93] A knockin mouse model expressing OTT1/MAL is able to recapitulate AMKL and demonstrated constitutive transcriptional activation from recombination signal binding protein for immunoglobulin kappa J (RBPJκ) binding sites, including Notch1 downstream targets, which is essential for its pathogenesis.[94]

MUTATIONS OF EPIGENETIC MODIFIERS

Several translocations associated with leukemia involve transcriptional coactivators and chromatin modifying proteins that have no apparent DNA-binding specificity. These include the mixed-lineage leukemia/ CREB-binding protein (MLL/CBP) and MOZ/CBP fusions that involve the transcriptional coactivator CBP and the MLL/p300 and MOZ/TIF2 fusions, which involve the coactivators p300 and TIF2, respectively.[95,96] Although TIF2 itself is not known to have histone acetylase transferase (HAT) activity, a hallmark of the coactivators CBP and p300, it has a well-characterized CBP interaction domain that serves to recruit CBP into a complex with MOZ/TIF2.[97] Thus, recruitment of CBP/p300 is a shared theme among this group of fusion genes.

The transcriptional targets and transformation properties of this class of fusion proteins are not fully understood. Transduction of MLL/CBP into primary murine bone marrow cells followed by transplantation results in a long-latency AML, suggesting the need for secondary mutations.[98] MOZ/TIF2 also results in leukemia in a similar model system. MOZ is a HAT protein that contains a nucleosome-binding domain and an acetyl–coenzyme A–binding catalytic domain. A mutational analysis shows that leukemogenic activity requires MOZ nucleosome-binding activity and CBP recruitment activity, but the MOZ HAT activity is dispensable. These data would be consistent with a CBP gain-of-function in which CBP is recruited to MOZ nucleosome-binding sites.[97] However, it has also been hypothesized that the leukemogenic potential of this class of fusions may be related to dominant negative interference with CBP/p300 or that the translocation leads to simple loss of function of CBP expressed from one allele. In support of this hypothesis, loss of a single allele of CBP/p300 in the human Rubinstein-Taybi syndrome increases predisposition to malignancies, including colon cancer and mice that are heterozygous for CBP that develop hematopoietic tumors.[99]

The *TET2* gene located on 4q24 belongs to the ten-eleven translocation (TET) family (*TET1, TET2, TET3*), which converts 5-methylcytosine (5-mC) to hydroxymethylcytosine (5-hmC), the initial step in DNA demethylation. Mutations of the *TET2* gene have been found in 8% to 27% of AML cases, in 20% to 25% of MDS cases, and in 4% to 13% of myeloproliferative neoplasms (MPN) cases. TET2 mutations are mono-allelic loss of function in most cases, including missense, frameshift, and nonsense mutations. The presence of the mutant *TET2* is associated with superior survival in MDS and inferior survival in AML and chronic myelomonocytic leukemia (CMML).[100] TET2 mutations are almost mutually exclusive with isocitrate dehydrogenase (IDH1/2) mutations, suggesting a similar epigenetic defect as IDH1/2 mutations.[101] In vivo, TET2 inactivation induced both myeloid and also lymphoid malignancies. The precise mechanisms and downstream effects of TET2 are as yet unknown.[102]

Mutations in the gene encoding *IDH1/2* functionally overlap with TET2 mutations, resulting in hypermethylation of leukemia cells, disruption of TET2 function, and impaired hematopoietic differentiation. IDH1 and IDH2 are nicotinamide adenine dinucleotide phosphate (NADP)-dependent IDHs that catalyze isocitrate to alpha-ketoglutarate (α-KG) in the tricarboxylic acid (TCA) cycle.[103] IDH1/2 mutations are detected in 15% to 33% of AML, mostly in normal karyotype AML, in 3.5% of MDS, in 2% to 5% of MPN, and also in glioma.[103] The mutations have been shown to exhibit a gain of function, leading to an aberrant accumulation of 2-hydroxyglutarate (2-HG). 2-HG is an oncometabolite, which inhibits an enzymatic activity of TET2 and stimulates hypoxia-inducible factor 1-alpha (HIF1α), leading to the initiation and promotion of cancer.[104] The impact of IDH mutations on the survival of AML patients is unclear. Some studies have observed no difference in outcome with respect to the IDH mutation status, whereas others have demonstrated a poor prognostic impact in certain AML subgroups.

Mammalian DNMTs catalyze the transfer of a methyl group onto the 5′-position of cytosine at CpG dinucleotides. DNMT3A and DNMT3B catalyze de novo DNA methylation, whereas DNMT1 is primarily responsible for maintenance methylation. Recurrent *DNMT3A* mutations at multiple sites were recently detected in a large cohort (22%) of patients with AML. Several different loss-of-function mutations have been found in all exons of DNMT3A, whereas a missense point mutation at amino acid R882, which decreases catalytic activity and DNA binding affinity, is most frequently identified.[105] DNMT3A-null hematopoietic stem cells have increased self-renewal capacity and lose their differentiation potential, which was accompanied by an aberrant methylation pattern implicated in leukemogenesis.[106] However, knockout of DNMT3A alone was not sufficient to initiate leukemia. DNMT3A mutations were reported to occur more frequently in AML with a normal karyotype and associated with FAB M5 morphology. The association with NPM1 and FLT3 mutations, unique DNA methylation and gene expression profiles, as well as unfavorable prognoses were observed in conjunction with *DNMT3A* mutations.[105]

EZH2 is a H3K27 methyltransferase, which is one of the components of PRC2, required for silencing target genes and maintaining the *stemness* in stem cells. EZH2 augments leukemogenesis by the inhibition of differentiation programs in leukemic stem cells.[107] EZH2 mutations were found 6% of MDS cases and in 3% to 13% of MPN cases, but rarely in AML.[108]

CHROMOSOMAL TRANSLOCATIONS THAT RESULT IN OVEREXPRESSION OF c-MYC

The chromosomal translocations described thus far result in the expression of aberrant fusion genes. Chromosomal translocations may also result in the overexpression of otherwise normal genes as a result of juxtaposition of a gene not normally expressed in adult hematopoietic tissues adjacent to an active promoter or enhancer. Most of those identified thus far involve the Ig or TCR enhancer loci, and thus most of these are associated with lymphoid malignancies; however, alternative mechanisms resulting in MYC overexpression have been shown to be important in AML or CML blast crisis.[109]

The prototypical example of juxtaposition of an Ig enhancer locus to an oncogene resulting in B-cell leukemia and lymphoma is the t(8;14)(q24;q32), resulting in overexpression of the MYC basic helix–loop–helix/basic region/leucine zipper (bHLH/bZIP) transcription factor on chromosome 8 due to juxtaposition to the Ig heavy-chain enhancer on chromosome 14.[110] Similar phenotypes ensue from juxtaposition to other Ig enhancers in the human genome, such as the Igκ locus on chromosome 2 or the Igλ locus on chromosome 22, and are characterized as B-ALL or lymphoma. Overexpression of MYC from Ig enhancers in murine models results in B-cell leukemias and lymphomas, confirming a central role for MYC overexpression in transformation. MYC is fully active as a transcription factor when heterodimerized with MAX. MAX is normally a homodimer, or a heterodimer complexed with MAD, which represses transcription. Overexpression of MYC is thought to shift the equilibrium in favor of an MYC-MAX homodimer that transactivates a wide range of target genes, including those involved in metabolism, cell cycle, and apoptosis and those contributing to leukemogenesis.[111]

CHROMOSOMAL TRANSLOCATIONS INVOLVING THE T-CELL RECEPTOR

T-cell leukemias are often associated with overexpression of a number of genes due to juxtaposition to the TCR enhancer loci (*TCRβ* at chromosome 7q34 or *TCRα/δ* at chromosome 14q11). Overexpression is thus associated with T-cell phenotypes, including T-cell ALL and lymphoma. For example, T-cell ALL may be associated with overexpression of bHLH family members that include T-cell acute leukemia 1/stem cell leukemia (TAL1/SCL), TAL2/SCL2, LYL1, homeo-box 11 (HOX11), HOX11L2, LIM only 2 (LMO2), LMO1, and MYC.[110,112] In addition to the minority of T-ALL cases with gene rearrangements involving these loci, it has been demonstrated that many patients without evident cytogenetic abnormalities overexpress TAL1, LMO2, HOX11, or HOX11L2.

POINT MUTATIONS IN ACUTE LEUKEMIA

Oncogenic RAS Mutations

Activating mutations in RAS may be associated with AML, ALL, and MDS, typically at codons 12, 13, or 61 in N- or K-RAS. The reported incidence varies widely between studies from 25% to 44%, and RAS mutations may confer a worse prognosis.[113,114] RAS mediates signals from upstream receptors through multiple downstream effectors including phosphoinositol 3′ kinase (PI3K) and the rapidly accelerated fibrosarcoma/mitogen activated protein kinase kinase/extracellular signal-regulated kinase (RAF/MEK/ERK) pathways.[114,115] Considerable effort has been devoted to developing small-molecule inhibitors of RAS activation, with a focus on prenylation inhibitors, including farnesyl transferase and geranylgeranylation inhibitors that preclude appropriate targeting of activated RAS to the plasma membrane.[115,116] Specifically targeting activated RAS mutants remains an attractive option, and prenyltransferase inhibitors appear to have activity in AML. However, clinical activity is not correlated with the presence of activating mutations in RAS or even with inhibition of the target farnesyl transferase itself.[116,117] Several possible interpretations can be made of these observations, including the possibility that

RAS is activated by mechanisms other than intrinsic point mutations (e.g., constitutively activated tyrosine kinases such as FLT3), that other proteins that are targets of prenylation are important in leukemia pathogenesis, or that farnesyl transferase inhibitors have off-target effects. Additional efforts have focused on inhibiting the downstream effectors instead including PI3K and RAF/MEK/MAPK.[115]

Activating Mutations in Tyrosine Kinases and Associated Receptors

The identification and characterization of activating mutations in hematopoietic tyrosine kinases has been one of the exciting developments in the pathogenesis of AML. Substantial evidence has been shown that chromosomal translocations that activate tyrosine kinases can contribute to the pathogenesis of CML and other MPNs. The most common of these is the *BCR/ABL* gene rearrangement, but other examples include the TEL/ABL, TEL/PDGFβR, TEL/Janus kinase 2 (JAK2), H4/PDGFβR, FIP1/PDGFβR, and rabaptin/PDGFβR fusion proteins. However, these fusion genes are only rarely encountered in AMLs. Approximately 1% to 2% of cases of de novo AML have the *BCR/abelson* (ABL) gene rearrangement, whereas *BCR/ABL* gene rearrangement is present in 20% to 30% of adult ALL[118] and in 2% to 3% of children with ALL.[119] The Philadelphia chromosome[120] is a translocation between the *ABL1* oncogene on the long arm of chromosome 9 and a breakpoint cluster region (BCR) on the long arm of chromosome 22, t(9;22), resulting in a fusion gene,[121] *BCR/ABL1*, that encodes an oncogenic protein with constitutively active tyrosine kinase activity. The molecular weight of this protein depends on the precise chromosome breakpoint. Most patients with ALL express a 190-kDa protein (p190), and the remainder express a 210-kDa oncoprotein (p210), which is also commonly found in CML. Although *BCR/ABL* may be necessary and sufficient for the development CML, this is not the case for Ph+ ALL. SRC kinases are required for the development of Ph+ ALL.[122] There are many additional epigenetic changes, copy number abnormalities, and mutations downstream of *BCR-ABL* that contribute to the very aggressive clinical course. In addition, very rare cases of disease progression from CML to AML are associated with the acquisition of second mutations such as the NUP98/HOXA9, AML1/ETO, or AML1/EVI1 rearrangement.

Point mutations in the tyrosine kinase activation loop and juxtamembrane (JM) mutations that activate *FLT3* and *c-KIT* receptor tyrosine kinases normally expressed on hematopoietic progenitors, have been identified in a significant proportion of AML cases. These findings may have important therapeutic implications with the demonstration of the efficacy of molecular targeting of the ABL kinase in BCR/ABL-positive CML and CML blast crisis with imatinib.[123] Activating mutations in *FLT3* have been reported in approximately 30% to 35% of cases of AML.[124] In 20% to 25% of cases, internal tandem duplications (ITD) within the JM domain result in constitutive activation of FLT3. These can range in size from a few to more than 50 amino acids and are always in frame. Because of the extensive variability in size and exact position of the repeats within the JM domain, it has been hypothesized that these mutations impair an autoinhibitory domain, resulting in constitutive kinase activation in the absence of ligand. In support of this, the crystallographic structure of FLT3 demonstrates a seven amino acid extension of the JM domain that intercalates into the catalytic domain, thereby precluding kinase activation.[125] It is likely that ITD mutations in this region would disrupt the structure of the autoinhibitory domain, resulting in kinase activation.

Large studies have confirmed the frequency of these mutations in adult and pediatric AML populations and that mutations in *FLT3* appear to confer a poor prognosis.[126-128] In an additional 5% to 10% of cases, so-called activating loop mutations occur near position D835 in the tyrosine kinase.[129] When these mutations (D835 position) develop during treatment with a FLT3 inhibitor, they confer resistance to this inhibitor.[130] High throughput sequencing of AML patient samples lacking known FLT3 mutations revealed nine novel acquired mutations resulting in amino acid changes within the extracellular, JM, and activation domains; however, only four of the nine changes were *driver* mutations capable of kinase activation and conferring growth factor independence, thus emphasizing the need for biologic validation of sequencing data.[131] *FLT3* mutations may occur in conjunction with known gene rearrangements, such as AML1/ETO, PML/RARα, CBFβ/MYH11, or MLL. Analogous activating loop mutations at position D816 have also been reported in *C-KIT* in approximately 5% of cases of AML. Activating mutations in the thrombopoietin receptor, MPLW515L, originally identified in myelofibrosis with myeloid metaplasia (MMM), and MPLT487A have been observed in both primary cases of AMKL and those secondary to MMM.[132-134]

The JAK1 through 3 family of nonreceptor tyrosine kinases, in addition to involvement in translocation-derived fusions such as TEL/JAK2, have been found to contain activating point mutations. JAK kinases are important signaling intermediaries of multiple hematopoietic cytokine receptors and downstream effectors such as signal transducer and activator of transcription (STAT) proteins.[135] JAKV617F, originally identified as a causative mutation in *polycythemia vera*, is also seen in 8% de novo AML and up to 77% of AML cases transformed from MPN.[136,137] Additional mutations in JAK2 and JAK3 have been isolated in AMKL.[134,138] Mutations in JAK1, 2, or 3 are found in approximately 11% of BCR/ABL-negative childhood acute lymphoid leukemia and were often concurrent with deletion of the IKAROS lymphoid specific transcription factor and the CDKN2A/B tumor suppressor.[139] Activating phosphorylation of STAT3 and STAT5a/b has been reported in a substantial proportion (44% to 76%) of AML patients[136] and confers a poor prognosis.[140,141]

A recently described subtype of precursor ALL is characterized by *cytokine receptor-like factor 2 (CRLF2)* alterations, which occur in about 5% to 7% of pediatric ALL, but in a significantly higher proportion of ALL with Down syndrome (~50%). Overexpression of *CRLF2* is associated with activation of the JAK-STAT pathway. The mechanism involves translocation of *CRLF2* and the *immunoglobulin heavy chain (IGH@)* locus or a deletion juxtaposing *CRLF2* with the *P2RY8* promoter. The P2RY8/CRLF2 fusion appears to be the most relevant prognostic factor independent of CRLF2 overexpression for poor outcome and high risk of relapse.[142]

As sequencing efforts continue, it is likely that the list of activating kinase mutations will continue to increase. Because kinases are proving to be relatively amenable to targeted therapy, the opportunities for treatment tailored to these activated kinases should likewise expand.

MUTATIONS IN TUMOR SUPPRESSOR GENES

The Wilms tumor gene was originally described as a tumor suppressor gene in patients with Wilms tumor, aniridia, genitourinary anomalies, and mental retardation (WAGR).[143] *WT1* is found in adult tumors from different origins, and these tumors arise in tissues that normally do not express *WT1*; therefore, it has been suggested that the expression of *WT1* might play an oncogenic role in these tumors.[144] *WT1* is located at the chromosome 11p and encodes for a transcription factor with N-terminal transcriptional regulatory domain and C-terminal zinc finger domain (exon 7 to 10). The expression of *WT1* inversely correlates with the degree of differentiation in the hematopoietic system because it is present in CD34+ cells and absent in mature leukocytes.[144,145] *WT1* functions as a potent transcription regulator of genes important for cell survival and cell differentiation. The disruption of WT1 function promotes stem cell proliferation and hampers differentiation.[144] Although the precise role of WT1 in normal and malignant hematopoiesis remains to be further elucidated, it seems to have a dual role in leukemia.[146]

The wild-type form of WT1 is highly (75% to 100%) expressed in a variety of acute leukemias.[147] Consistent with the function of an oncogene is the pattern of WT1 expression in CML, where low levels are found in the chronic phase, but are frequently increased in the accelerated and blast crisis phase.[148] High levels of WT1 in patients after chemotherapy is associated with a poor prognosis.

WT1 can act as a tumor suppressor in mice.[149] Mutation of the WT1 gene can be detected in approximately 10% of normal karyotype AMLs.[150,151] Mutations that cluster to exon 7 (mostly frameshift mutations resulting from insertions and deletions) and exon 9 (mostly substitutions) are associated with a poor clinical outcome.[151–153] These data are examples of WT1 as a tumor suppressor. On the other hand, a recent study analyzed mutations within the entire WT1 coding sequence in a very large cohort of young adults with normal karyotype AML. Contrary to the previous observations,[151–153] WT1 mutations had no prognostic impact.[154] The different results from these large studies could be explained by the variable biologic role of WT1 in AML, possible differences in therapy, and other patient characteristics. Therefore, it is desirable that testing for WT1 mutations becomes part of the risk assessment in future clinical trials to resolve these discrepancies.

TP53 is a tumor suppressor that induces cell-cycle arrest in a response to apoptotic cell death or DNA repair due to genotoxic substances, oncogenes, hypoxia, DNA damage, or ribonucleotide depletion.[155] Inactivation of TP53 plays an important role during neoplastic transformation in solid tumors and also during progression of hematologic malignancies.[156–158] Animal experiments suggest that the loss of one TP53 allele could be sufficient for tumorigenesis.[159] This could be relevant for the development of leukemia in patients with a single TP53 deletion. The loss of 17p in AML is often accompanied by a TP53 mutation resulting in a loss of heterozygosity.[160,161] Another possibility is the inactivation of downstream mediators of TP53, which affect not only cell-cycle arrest, but also DNA repair and apoptosis. Alternatively, overexpression of genes inhibiting or promoting degradation of TP53 can be considered—for instance, MDM2 gene amplifications have been detected in B-CLL.[162] TP53 deletion can be present as a loss of 17p as a part of a complex aberrant karyotype or as a single chromosomal aberration, both resulting in a poor clinical outcome.[163–166] The incidence of TP53 aberrations is high in AML with a complex aberrant karyotype (up to 70%),[163] but relatively rare in other AML groups (2% to 9%),[128,163,167] and TP53 mutations without cytogenetic alteration are a rare event.[161,168] Low-risk AML t(8;21) or inv(16) are not associated with TP53 deletion. There is significant positive association between TP53 deletion and other high-risk chromosomal aberrations such as del(5q) and monosomy 5 and 7.[20,166] Molecular risk factors FLT3-ITD and NPM1 mutation do not seem to cluster with the TP53 deletion in complex karyotype patients.[166] TP53-deleted cells have greater resistance to various conventional antileukemic drugs.[169] However, published data of multidrug-resistance gene expression showed a negative influence on therapy response in complex aberrant patients.[170] The association of TP53 deletion and MDR1 expression has been confirmed for CML, but not for AML.[171] Hence, an independent mechanism of resistance needs to be considered.[166] Taken together, TP53 deletion is a high-risk factor conveying a poor outcome, and further studies are necessary to provide and evaluate alternative therapies.

ACTIVATING MUTATIONS OF NOTCH

NOTCH1 is a component of an evolutionarily conserved pathway shown to direct T-cell lineage determination in early and late stages of lymphocyte development as well as play a role in hematopoietic stem cell self-renewal.[172,173] NOTCH1 is a heterodimeric transmembrane receptor. Ligand binding to NOTCH1 allows proteolytic cleavage of the heterodimerization domain (HD) by adamalysin (ADAM)-type protease and γ-secretase of the C-terminal intracellular domain (ICD), which then localizes to the nucleus to function as a transactivator. Involvement of NOTCH1 in T-ALL had been observed with the rare t(7;9)(q34;q34.3) in which translocation of TCRβ locus into the NOTCH1 gene results in the expression of the truncated, transcriptionally active ICD. A series of point mutations in NOTCH1 were identified in over half of all T-ALL cases.[112,174] These mutations clustered in two primary locations, the HD and the proline-, glutamate-, serine-, and threonine-rich (PEST) domain. The missense mutations within the HD domain make NOTCH1 more amenable to γ-secretase–mediated cleavage, thus enhancing activation. The PEST domain controls the rate of degradation of the activated ICN. PEST domain mutants are primarily small insertions/deletions into the reading frame, causing a deletion of all or part of the domain and extending the half-life of the activated ICN. An alternative mechanism for NOTCH1 activation are inactivating mutations of the F Box protein, FBXW7, which is a component of the ubiquitin ligase complex that targets the NOTCH1 ICN as well as MYC for degradation and which occurs in ~15% of T-ALL.[110,175]

Fortuitously, γ-secretase inhibitors (GSI) had already undergone significant clinical development due to the involvement of γ-secretase in processing the pathogenic β-amyloid peptide associated with Alzheimer's dementia. Initial clinical trials of GSIs in T-ALL have shown minimal effects on disease and significant gastrointestinal toxicity.[176] Use of GSIs in combination with agents affecting alternative pathways may provide synergism and improve efficacy. Treatment of a mouse model of T-ALL with GSIs and corticosteroids has demonstrated that GSIs are capable of abrogating corticosteroid resistance in established cell lines as well as limiting GSI-mediated gut toxicity.[177]

MUTATIONS ALTERING LOCALIZATION OF NPM1

Nucleophosmin (NPM1) encodes a protein that acts as a molecular chaperone between the nucleus and cytoplasm. It is involved in multiple cellular processes, including the regulation of TP53/ARF pathways, ribosome biogenesis, and the duplication of centrosomes.[178] NPM1 had been previously identified in acute leukemias as a translocation fusion partner with RAR and MLF as well as with ALK in anaplastic large cell lymphoma. Aberrant cytoplasmic localization of NPM1 has been observed in 25% to 30% of adult AML and is associated with point mutations within exon 12, which are hypothesized to enhance a nuclear export motif within the expressed protein.[179] The mechanism by which mutated NPM1 causes leukemia is not clear; however, the cytoplasmic localization of NPM1 is thought to be intrinsic to its altered function.[180] NPM1 mutations are found more frequently in AML with normal karyotypes (50% to 60%) and more apt to have FLT3-ITD mutations as well. Among normal cytogenetic AMLs, the presence of cytoplasmic NPM1 in the absence of the FLT3-ITD is associated with a more favorable prognosis.[180]

MUTATION OF LYMPHOID DEVELOPMENT GENES IN ACUTE LYMPHOID LEUKEMIA

An important mechanism underlying the pathogenesis of B-lineage ALL is the mutation of transcription factors essential for B-cell commitment and differentiation.[181] Due to the requirement of these factors for normal early to late precursor B development, the immunophenotypic stage most closely related to the leukemias, it is hypothesized that the loss of normal expression levels leads to a block in differentiation, a critical step in leukemogenesis.[182]

Although translocations involving these genes had been identified in a smaller percentage of B-cell ALLs, earlier, high-resolution SNP arrays and genomic sequencing of disease samples has actually demonstrated that frequent microdeletions and point mutations are extremely common.[181] PAX5 is a master regulator of B-cell development at the pro– and pre–B-cell stage, the immunophenotypic stage most closely related to many B-ALLs.[37] PAX5 is a DNA-binding protein capable of interaction with corepressors, chromatin remodeling proteins, and other transcription factors such as erythroblastosis virus E26 oncogene homolog-1 (ETS1) and myeloblastosis (MYB).[37] The dual role of PAX5 is to simultaneously transactivate downstream factors promoting B-cell development and repress genes of alternative lineages such as NOTCH1 and CSFR1.[183] Deletion of Pax5 in mice yields early B cells that are not completely committed to B differentiation and can be transdifferentiated through the use of cytokines into other lineages.[183] Several rare translocations have been identified involving PAX5, including dic(9;12)(p13;p13), generating the PAX5/ETV6 fusion protein, which functions as a dominant negative.[184] In actuality, 30% of B-ALLs possess monoallelic loss-of-function mutations when examined by sequencing.[182] How PAX5 haploinsufficiency contributes to B-ALL leukemogenesis is not entirely clear, and PAX5 mutational status does not appear to influence prognosis.[181]

IKAROS family members (IKZF1–3) are also frequently mutated in B-ALL.[185] IKZF1 is essential for hematopoietic stem cell function and lymphoid commitment.[186,187] IKZF1 possesses zinc finger domains important for DNA-binding domains and homo/heterodimerization. Like PAX5, IKZF1 both activates lymphoid-specific genes such as IL-7R and represses genes, such as PU.1, required for alternative lineages. The function of IKZF1 as a transcriptional activator may be modulated through inherent mechanisms of chromatin remodeling and transcriptional elongation.[188] Approximately 15% of pediatric B-ALL patients have deletions or point mutations in IKZF1 leading to loss of function or dominant negative activity and correlating with a poor prognosis.[185] Interestingly, IKZF1 mutations are more frequently associated with mutations in tyrosine kinases such as BCR/ABL1 and JAK2 and cytokine receptors such as IL7R and CRLF2.[37] Furthermore, IKZF1 mutations appear in 20% of lymphoid blast crises evolving from chronic myelogenous leukemia.[189]

Other recurrent mutations have been found, to a lesser frequency, in a large number of lymphoid-specific transcription factors, including, for example, E2A, encoded by the *transcription factor 3 (TCF3)* gene, EBF1, and LEF1. The most common mutation in TCF3 in B-ALL is the translocation, t(1;19)(q23;p13), encoding the fusion product, TCF3/PBX1, which is postulated to dysregulate both B-cell and HOX-associated pathways.[190] EBF1 has reported monoallelic loss-of-function mutations in B-ALL, whereas LEF1 has been observed with mono- and biallelic deletions in both T- and B- ALL.[182] The common feature of these genetic lesions are their requirement in normal lymphopoiesis, and deciphering the pathophysiologic effect of each mutation, particularly with regard to haploinsufficiency, will guide future therapeutic efforts.

MUTATIONAL COMPLEMENTATION GROUPS IN ACUTE LEUKEMIAS

Several lines of evidence indicate that more than one mutation is necessary for the pathogenesis of acute leukemia. First, there is evidence for the acquisition of additional cytogenetic abnormalities with disease progression from CML to AML (i.e., CML blast crisis). Published examples of progression in BCR/ABL-positive CML include the acquisition of t(3;21) *AML1/EVI1*, t(8;21) *AML1/ETO*, or t(7;11) *NUP98/HOXA9* gene rearrangements. Progression of chronic myelomonocytic leukemia to AML in a patient with the TEL/PDGFβR gene rearrangement was associated with acquisition of a t(8;21) *AML1/ETO* gene rearrangement.[191] Second, expression of the AML1/ETO or CBFβ/MYH11 fusion proteins in murine models is not sufficient to cause AML.[26,192] Chemical mutagens must be used in these contexts to generate second mutations that cause the AML phenotype. Third, evidence indicates that in some cases the TEL/AML1 gene rearrangement associated with pediatric ALL may be acquired in utero, but ALL does not develop until years later, indicating a requirement for a second mutation.[193] Fourth, AML develops in transgenic mice that express the PML/RAR-α fusion protein only after a long latency of 3 to 6 months, with incomplete penetrance, indicating a need for a second mutation.[50–52]

The genetic epidemiology of AML provides important clues to the nature of the collaborating mutations. One broad complementation group in AML is comprised of mutations that activate signal transduction pathways. These include activating mutations in FLT3, RAS, and KIT, and more rarely, the BCR/ABL and TEL/PDGFβR fusion associated with disease progression in CML. These can be viewed as a complementation group because, although they are collectively present in approximately 50% of cases of AML, they rarely, if ever, occur together in the same patient.

A second complementation group, typified by translocations involving hematopoietic transcription factors, includes AML1/ETO, CBFβ/SMMHC, PML/RARα, NUP98/HOXA9, MLL gene rearrangements, and MOZ/TIF2 and they are never observed together in the same leukemia. In general, this second class of mutations impair hematopoietic differentiation and may confer properties of self-renewal to the leukemic stem cell but are not sufficient to cause leukemia when expressed alone. However, one mutation from each of these two complementation groups often coexists in the same leukemia. For example, activating mutations in FLT3 or RAS have been observed in association with virtually all of the fusion genes in the second class described earlier.[194]

These findings suggest a hypothesis for pathogenesis of AML in which there are two broad classes of cooperating mutations (Fig. 42.1A).[194] One class, exemplified by activating mutations in FLT3 or RAS, confers either a proliferative or survival advantage, or both, to hematopoietic progenitors but do not affect differentiation. These mutations do not confer self-renewal capacity as assessed in part by the ability to serially replate in culture or to serially transplant disease in murine models.[195,196] A second class of mutations, exemplified by AML1/ETO, CBFβ/SMMHC, PML/RARα, NUP98/HOXA9, MLL gene rearrangements, and MOZ/TIF2 serve primarily to impair hematopoietic differentiation and confer properties of self-renewal. Together, these cooperating mutations induce the AML phenotype characterized by enhanced proliferative and survival advantage, impaired differentiation, and limitless self-renewal capacity. Although the two class model holds for a limited number of mutational combinations, it likely broadly simplifies the interplay between genetic lesions, because many have dual pleotropic effects on proliferation and differentiation.

Deeper insight into the cooperativity of different mutations has been aided by whole-genome or whole-exome sequencing of DNA samples. The Cancer Genome Atlas Consortium recently published the results of sequencing 200 individual AML samples along with matched epigenetic and RNA expression analysis.[12] Only an average of 13 coding mutations/genomes were uncovered, less than observed for most solid tumors. Mutations were grouped into the functional classes: transcription factor fusions, NPM1 related, tumor suppressors, DNA methylation related, signaling, chromatin modifying, myeloid transcription factor, cohesion complex, and spliceosome complex related. Certain mutational groups are mutually exclusive of each other, indicating possible convergent downstream pathways. For example, mutations in cohesion, spliceosome, signaling, and histone modification pathways do not usually occur in the same patient (Fig. 42.1B).[12,197] Experimental validation of these novel individual mutations alone or in conjunction with suspected cooperating lesions is an important focus to identify driver versus passenger mutations and clinical significance. In addition, sequencing of a population, which allows for the quantification of mutational frequency in subclones in consecutive patient samples during the diagnosis, treatment, and relapse, identifies the mutations important for leukemia, initiation, progression, and resistance.[198]

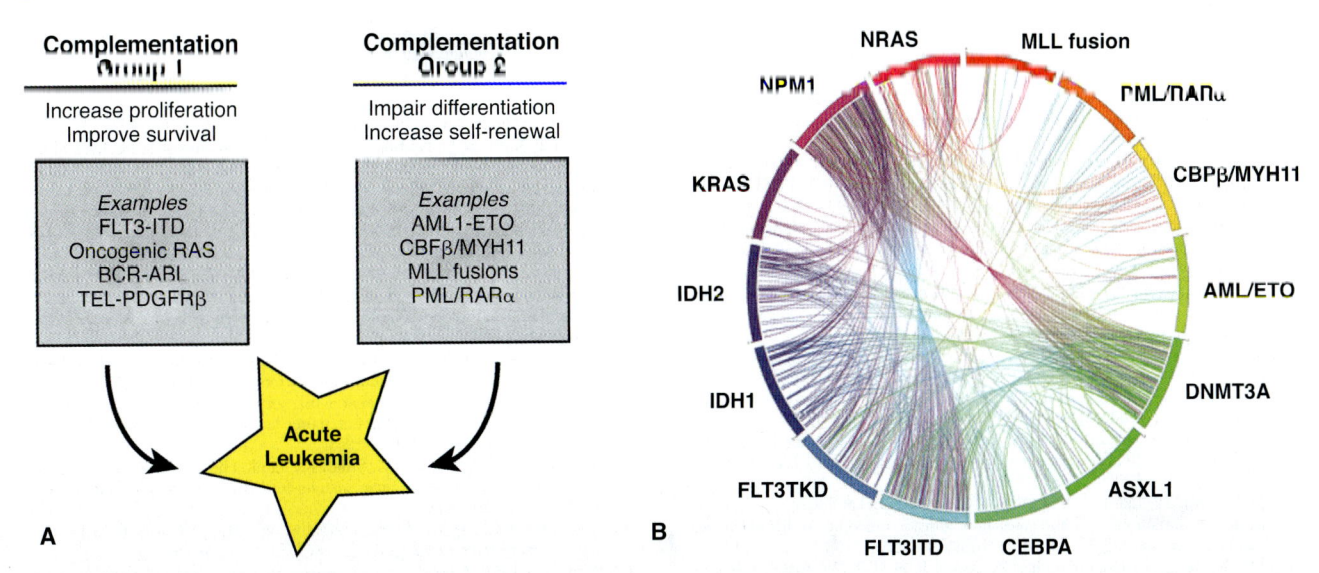

Figure 42.1 Cooperating mutations in acute leukemia. **A:** A classic model of leukemogenesis, composed of two broad complementation groups, is defined by a lack of concurrence of any two mutations in the same complementation group in the same patient. One group is characterized by activating mutations in signal transduction pathways. When expressed alone, these mutations confer a proliferative or survival advantage, or both, but do not affect differentiation. The second group is associated with impaired differentiation and the ability to confer properties of self-renewal to hematopoietic progenitors. Together, the complementation groups collaborate to engender the acute leukemia phenotype. **B:** Circos plot showing concurrent mutational groups in 498 cases of AML. Each connecting line represents simultaneous mutations in an AML sample and demonstrates the how high resolution analysis of AML genomes can establish complementation groups for recurrent mutations. (Modified from Sanders MA, Valk PJ. The evolving molecular genetic landscape in acute myeloid leukemia. *Curr Opin Hematol* 2013;20:79–85.)

CONCLUSION

The quest to elucidate the essential pathophysiologic changes involved in leukemogenesis has been accelerated with the usage of newer technologies, such as high resolution mapping and high throughput sequencing. It is now possible to identify specific molecular pathways complementing known recurrent translocations as well as gaining insight into the mechanisms underlying normal karyotype leukemias. Not only can these novel mutations be used for more accurate prognostication, but they can also provide an opportunity for drug development, targeting the essential pathways dysregulated in leukemia. As the availability of pathway-targeted therapeutics increases, interrogation of a patient's leukemia for alterations at the genomic level may allow for individualized therapy addressing the pathways responsible for leukemic cell survival, proliferation, and differentiation, which ideally would improve treatment efficacy and reduce therapy-related morbidity and mortality.

REFERENCES

1. Lapidot T, Sirard C, Vormoor J, et al. A cell initiating human acute myeloid leukaemia after transplantation into SCID mice. *Nature*. 1994;367:645–648.
2. Bonnet D, Dick JE. Human acute myeloid leukemia is organized as a hierarchy that originates from a primitive hematopoietic cell. *Nat Med* 1997;3:730–737.
3. Buss EC, Ho AD. Leukemia stem cells. *Int J Cancer* 2011;129:2328–2336.
4. Saito T, Chiba S, Ichikawa M, et al. Notch2 is preferentially expressed in mature B cells and indispensable for marginal zone B lineage development. *Immunity* 2003;18:675–685.
5. Cozzio A, Passegue E, Ayton PM, et al. Similar MLL-associated leukemias arising from self-renewing stem cells and short-lived myeloid progenitors. *Genes Dev* 2003;17:3029–3035.
6. Huntly BJ, Shigematsu H, Deguchi K, et al. MOZ-TIF2, but not BCR-ABL, confers properties of leukemic stem cells to committed murine hematopoietic progenitors. *Cancer Cell* 2004;6:587–596.
7. Huntly BJ, Gilliland DG. Leukaemia stem cells and the evolution of cancer-stem-cell research. *Nat Rev Cancer* 2005;5:311–321.
8. Jamieson CH, Ailles LE, Dylla SJ, et al. Granulocyte-macrophage progenitors as candidate leukemic stem cells in blast-crisis CML. *N Engl J Med* 2004;351:657–667.
9. Speicher MR, Carter NP. The new cytogenetics: blurring the boundaries with molecular biology. *Nat Rev Genet* 2005;6:782–792.
10. Feuk L, Carson AR, Scherer SW. Structural variation in the human genome. *Nat Rev Genet* 2006;7:85–97.
11. International Cancer Genome Consortium, Hudson TJ, Anderson W, et al. International network of cancer genome projects. *Nature* 2010;464:993–998.
12. Cancer Genome Atlas Research Network. Genomic and epigenomic landscapes of adult de novo acute myeloid leukemia. *N Engl J Med* 2013;368:2059–2074.
13. Stratton MR, Campbell PJ, Futreal PA. The cancer genome. *Nature* 2009;458:719–724.
14. Koschmieder S, Halmos B, Levantini E, et al. Dysregulation of the C/EBPalpha differentiation pathway in human cancer. *J Clin Oncol* 2009;27:619–628.
15. Speck NA, Gilliland DG. Core-binding factors in haematopoiesis and leukaemia. *Nat Rev Cancer* 2002;2:502–513.
16. Wang Q, Stacy T, Binder M, et al. Disruption of the Cbfa2 gene causes necrosis and hemorrhaging in the central nervous system and blocks definitive hematopoiesis. *Proc Natl Acad Sci U S A* 1996;93:3444–3449.
17. Okuda T, van Deursen J, Hiebert SW, et al. AML1, the target of multiple chromosomal translocations in human leukemia, is essential for normal fetal liver hematopoiesis. *Cell* 1996;84:321–330.
18. Goyama S, Mulloy JC. Molecular pathogenesis of core binding factor leukemia: current knowledge and future prospects. *Int J Hematol* 2011;94:126–133.
19. Ichikawa M, Yoshimi A, Nakagawa M, et al. A role for RUNX1 in hematopoiesis and myeloid leukemia. *Int J Hematol* 2013;97:726–734.
20. Vangala RK, Heiss-Neumann MS, Rangatia JS, et al. The myeloid master regulator transcription factor PU.1 is inactivated by AML1-ETO in t(8;21) myeloid leukemia. *Blood* 2003;101:270–277.
21. Choi Y, Elagib KE, Delehanty LL, et al. Erythroid inhibition by the leukemic fusion AML1-ETO is associated with impaired acetylation of the major erythroid transcription factor GATA-1. *Cancer Res* 2006;66:2990–2996.
22. Song WJ, Sullivan MG, Legare RD, et al. Haploinsufficiency of CBFA2 causes familial thrombocytopenia with propensity to develop acute myelogenous leukaemia. *Nat Genet* 1999;23:166–175.
23. Michaud J, Wu F, Osato M, et al. In vitro analyses of known and novel RUNX1/AML1 mutations in dominant familial platelet disorder with predisposition to acute myelogenous leukemia: implications for mechanisms of pathogenesis. *Blood* 2002;99:1364–1372.
24. Osato M, Asou N, Abdalla E, et al. Biallelic and heterozygous point mutations in the runt domain of the AML1/PEBP2alphaB gene associated with myeloblastic leukemias. *Blood* 1999;93:1817–1824.

25. Yergeau DA, Hetherington CJ, Wang Q, et al. Embryonic lethality and impairment of haematopoiesis in mice heterozygous for an AML1-ETO fusion gene. *Nat Genet* 1997;15:303–306.
26. Castilla LH, Garrett L, Adya N, et al. The fusion gene Cbfb-MYH11 blocks myeloid differentiation and predisposes mice to acute myelomonocytic leukaemia. *Nat Genet* 1999;23:144–146.
27. Linggi B, Muller-Tidow C, van de Locht L, et al. The t(8;21) fusion protein, AML1 ETO, specifically represses the transcription of the p14(ARF) tumor suppressor in acute myeloid leukemia. *Nat Med* 2002;8:743–750.
28. Markus J, Garin MT, Bies J, et al. Methylation-independent silencing of the tumor suppressor INK4b (p15) by CBFbeta-SMMHC in acute myelogenous leukemia with inv(16). *Cancer Res* 2007;67:992–1000.
29. Alcalay M, Meani N, Gelmetti V, et al. Acute myeloid leukemia fusion proteins deregulate genes involved in stem cell maintenance and DNA repair. *J Clin Invest* 2003;112:1751–1761.
30. Wang LC, Swat W, Fujiwara Y, et al. The TEL/ETV6 gene is required specifically for hematopoiesis in the bone marrow. *Genes Dev* 1998;12:2392–2402.
31. Liu S, Shen T, Huynh L, et al. Interplay of RUNX1/MTG8 and DNA methyltransferase 1 in acute myeloid leukemia. *Cancer Res* 2005;65:1277–1284.
32. Yan M, Ahn EY, Hiebert SW, et al. RUNX1/AML1 DNA-binding domain and ETO/MTG8 NHR2-dimerization domain are critical to AML1-ETO9a leukemogenesis. *Blood* 2009;113:883–886.
33. Jiao B, Wu CF, Liang Y, et al. AML1-ETO9a is correlated with C-KIT overexpression/mutations and indicates poor disease outcome in t(8;21) acute myeloid leukemia-M2. *Leukemia* 2009;23:1598–1604.
34. De Braekeleer E, Douet-Guilbert N, Morel F, et al. ETV6 fusion genes in hematological malignancies: a review. *Leuk Res* 2012;36:945–961.
35. Mullighan CG. Genomic characterization of childhood acute lymphoblastic leukemia. *Semin Hematol* 2013;50:314–324.
36. Wang LC, Kuo F, Fujiwara Y, et al. Yolk sac angiogenic defect and intra-embryonic apoptosis in mice lacking the Ets-related factor TEL. *Embo J* 1997;16:4374–4383.
37. Tijchon E, Havinga J, van Leeuwen FN, et al. B-lineage transcription factors and cooperating gene lesions required for leukemia development. *Leukemia* 2013;27:541–552.
38. Goddard AD, Borrow J, Freemont PS, et al. Characterization of a zinc finger gene disrupted by the t(15;17) in acute promyelocytic leukemia. *Science* 1991;254:1371–1374.
39. Kakizuka A, Miller WH Jr, Umesono K, et al. Chromosomal translocation t(15;17) in human acute promyclocytic leukemia fuses RAR alpha with a novel putative transcription factor, PML. *Cell* 1991;66:663–674.
40. de Thé H, Lavau C, Marchio A, et al. The PML-RAR alpha fusion mRNA generated by the t(15;17) translocation in acute promyelocytic leukemia encodes a functionally altered RAR. *Cell* 1991;66:675–684.
41. Zelent A, Guidez F, Melnick A, et al. Translocations of the RARalpha gene in acute promyelocytic leukemia. *Oncogene* 2001;20:7186–7203.
42. Li W, Rich T, Watson CJ. PML: a tumor suppressor that regulates cell fate in mammary gland. *Cell Cycle* 2009;8:2711–2717.
43. Carracedo A, Ito K, Pandolfi PP. The nuclear bodies inside out: PML conquers the cytoplasm. *Curr Opin Cell Biol* 2011;23:360–366.
44. Giorgi C, Ito K, Lin HK, et al. PML regulates apoptosis at endoplasmic reticulum by modulating calcium release. *Science* 2010;330:1247–1251.
45. Ito K, Bernardi R, Morotti A, et al. PML targeting eradicates quiescent leukemia-initiating cells. *Nature* 2008;453:1072–1078.
46. Zhang XW, Yan XJ, Zhou ZR, et al. Arsenic trioxide controls the fate of the PML-RARalpha oncoprotein by directly binding PML. *Science* 2010;328:240–243.
47. de Thé H, Chen Z. Acute promyelocytic leukaemia: novel insights into the mechanisms of cure. *Nat Rev Cancer* 2010;10:775–783.
48. Martens JH, Brinkman AB, Simmer F, et al. PML-RARalpha/RXR Alters the Epigenetic Landscape in Acute Promyelocytic Leukemia. *Cancer Cell* 2010;17:173–185.
49. Saeed S, Logie C, Stunnenberg HG, et al. Genome-wide functions of PML-RARalpha in acute promyelocytic leukaemia. *Br J Cancer* 2011;104:554–558.
50. Grisolano JL, Wesselschmidt RL, Pelicci PG, et al. Altered myeloid development and acute leukemia in transgenic mice expressing PML-RAR alpha under control of cathepsin G regulatory sequences. *Blood* 1997;89:376–387.
51. He LZ, Tribioli C, Rivi R, et al. Acute leukemia with promyelocytic features in PML/RARalpha transgenic mice. *Proc Natl Acad Sci U S A* 1997;94:5302–5307.
52. Brown D, Kogan S, Lagasse E, et al. A PMLRARalpha transgene initiates murine acute promyelocytic leukemia. *Proc Natl Acad Sci U S A* 1997;94:2551–2556.
53. Tallman MS, Nabhan C, Feusner JH, et al. Acute promyelocytic leukemia: evolving therapeutic strategies. *Blood* 2002;99:759–767.
54. Alharbi RA, Pettengell R, Pandha HS, et al. The role of HOX genes in normal hematopoiesis and acute leukemia. *Leukemia* 2013;27:1000–1008.
55. Abramovich C, Humphries RK. Hox regulation of normal and leukemic hematopoietic stem cells. *Curr Opin Hematol* 2005;12:210–216.
56. Gough SM, Slape CI, Aplan PD. NUP98 gene fusions and hematopoietic malignancies: common themes and new biologic insights. *Blood* 2011;118:6247–6257.
57. Kasper LH, Brindle PK, Schnabel CA, et al. CREB binding protein interacts with nucleoporin-specific FG repeats that activate transcription and mediate NUP98-HOXA9 oncogenicity. *Mol Cell Biol* 1999;19:764–776.
58. Bansal D, Scholl C, Frohling S, et al. Cdx4 dysregulates Hox gene expression and generates acute myeloid leukemia alone and in cooperation with Meis1a in a murine model. *Proc Natl Acad Sci U S A* 2006;103:16924–16929.

59. Hatano M, Roberts CW, Minden M, et al. Deregulation of a homeobox gene, HOX11, by the t(10;14) in T cell leukemia. *Science* 1991;253:79–82.
60. Rawat VP, Cusan M, Deshpande A, et al. Ectopic expression of the homeobox gene Cdx2 is the transforming event in a mouse model of t(12;13)(p13;q12) acute myeloid leukemia. *Proc Natl Acad Sci U S A* 2004;101:817–822.
61. Pineault N, Buske C, Feuring-Buske M, et al. Induction of acute myeloid leukemia in mice by the human leukemia-specific fusion gene NUP98-HOXD13 in concert with Meis1. *Blood* 2003;101:4529–4538.
62. Palmqvist L, Argiropoulos B, Pineault N, et al. The Flt3 receptor tyrosine kinase collaborates with NUP98-HOX fusions in acute myeloid leukemia. *Blood* 2006;108:1030–1036.
63. Eguchi M, Eguchi-Ishimae M, Greaves M. Molecular pathogenesis of MLL-associated leukemias. *Int J Hematol* 2005;82:9–20.
64. Slany RK. The molecular biology of mixed lineage leukemia. *Haematologica* 2009;94:984–993.
65. Ng RK, Kong CT, So CC, et al. Epigenetic dysregulation of leukemic Hox code in MLL-rearranged leukemia mouse model. *J Pathol* 2014;232:65–74.
66. Yu BD, Hanson RD, Hess JL, et al. MLL, a mammalian trithorax-group gene, functions as a transcriptional maintenance factor in morphogenesis. *Proc Natl Acad Sci U S A* 1998;95:10632–10636.
67. Yokoyama A, Somervaille TC, Smith KS, et al. The menin tumor suppressor protein is an essential oncogenic cofactor for MLL-associated leukemogenesis. *Cell* 2005;123:207–218.
68. Yokoyama A, Cleary ML. Menin critically links MLL proteins with LEDGF on cancer-associated target genes. *Cancer Cell* 2008;14:36–46.
69. Mohan M, Lin C, Guest E, et al. Licensed to elongate: a molecular mechanism for MLL-based leukaemogenesis. *Nat Rev Cancer* 2010;10:721–728.
70. Lin C, Smith ER, Takahashi H, et al. AFF4, a component of the ELL/P-TEFb elongation complex and a shared subunit of MLL chimeras, can link transcription elongation to leukemia. *Mol Cell* 2010;37:429–437.
71. Yeung J, Esposito MT, Gandillet A, et al. beta-Catenin mediates the establishment and drug resistance of MLL leukemic stem cells. *Cancer Cell* 2010;18:606–618.
72. Somervaille TC, Cleary ML. Identification and characterization of leukemia stem cells in murine MLL-AF9 acute myeloid leukemia. *Cancer Cell* 2006;10:257–268.
73. Wei J, Wunderlich M, Fox C, et al. Microenvironment determines lineage fate in a human model of MLL-AF9 leukemia. *Cancer Cell* 2008;13:483–495.
74. Wang X, Scott E, Sawyers CL, et al. C/EBPalpha bypasses granulocyte colony-stimulating factor signals to rapidly induce PU.1 gene expression, stimulate granulocytic differentiation, and limit proliferation in 32D cl3 myeloblasts. *Blood* 1999;94:560–571.
75. Hackanson B, Bennett KL, Brena RM, et al. Epigenetic modification of CCAAT/enhancer binding protein alpha expression in acute myeloid leukemia. *Cancer Res* 2008;68:3142–3151.
76. Paz-Priel I, Friedman A. C/EBPalpha dysregulation in AML and ALL. *Crit Rev Oncog* 2011;16:93–102.
77. Mueller BU, Pabst T. C/EBPalpha and the pathophysiology of acute myeloid leukemia. *Curr Opin Hematol* 2006;13:7–14.
78. Schlenk RF, Dohner K, Krauter J, et al. Mutations and treatment outcome in cytogenetically normal acute myeloid leukemia. *N Engl J Med* 2008;358:1909–1918.
79. Chapiro E, Russell L, Radford-Weiss I, et al. Overexpression of CEBPA resulting from the translocation t(14;19)(q32;q13) of human precursor B acute lymphoblastic leukemia. *Blood* 2006;108:3560–3563.
80. Akasaka T, Balasas T, Russell LJ, et al. Five members of the CEBP transcription factor family are targeted by recurrent IGH translocations in B-cell precursor acute lymphoblastic leukemia (BCP-ALL). *Blood* 2007;109:3451–3461.
81. Khan I, Malinge S, Crispino J. Myeloid leukemia in Down syndrome. *Crit Rev Oncog* 2011;16:25–36.
82. Crispino JD. GATA1 mutations in Down syndrome: implications for biology and diagnosis of children with transient myeloproliferative disorder and acute megakaryoblastic leukemia. *Pediatr Blood Cancer* 2005;44:40–44.
83. Bresnick EH, Katsumura KR, Lee HY, et al. Master regulatory GATA transcription factors: mechanistic principles and emerging links to hematologic malignancies. *Nucleic Acids Res* 2012;40:5819–5831.
84. Wechsler J, Greene M, McDevitt MA, et al. Acquired mutations in GATA1 in the megakaryoblastic leukemia of Down syndrome. *Nat Genet* 2002;32:148–152.
85. Malinge S, Izraeli S, Crispino JD. Insights into the manifestations, outcomes, and mechanisms of leukemogenesis in Down syndrome. *Blood* 2009;113:2619–2628.
86. Taub JW, Mundschau G, Ge Y, et al. Prenatal origin of GATA1 mutations may be an initiating step in the development of megakaryocytic leukemia in Down syndrome. *Blood* 2004;104:1588–1589.
87. Kirsammer G, Jilani S, Liu H, et al. Highly penetrant myeloproliferative disease in the Ts65Dn mouse model of Down syndrome. *Blood* 2008;111:767–775.
88. Ma Z, Morris SW, Valentine V, et al. Fusion of two novel genes, RBM15 and MKL1, in the t(1;22)(p13;q13) of acute megakaryoblastic leukemia. *Nat Genet* 2001;28:220–221.
89. Mercher T, Busson-Le Coniat M, Khac FN, et al. Recurrence of OTT-MAL fusion in t(1;22) of infant AML-M7. *Genes Chromosomes Cancer* 2002;33:22–28.
90. Raffel GD, Mercher T, Shigematsu H, et al. Ott1(Rbm15) has pleiotropic roles in hematopoietic development. *Proc Natl Acad Sci U S A* 2007;104:6001–6006.
91. Xiao N, Jani K, Morgan K, et al. Hematopoietic stem cells lacking Ott1 display aspects associated with aging and are unable to maintain quiescence during proliferative stress. *Blood* 2012;119:4898–4907.

97. Miralles F, Posern G, Zaromytidou AI, et al. Actin dynamics control SRF activity by regulation of its coactivator MAL. Cell 2003;113:329–342.
93. Smith EC, Teixeira AM, Chen RC, et al. Induction of megakaryocyte differentiation drives nuclear accumulation and transcriptional function of MKL1 via actin polymerization and RhoA activation. Blood 2013;121:1094–1101.
94. Mercher T, Raffel GD, Moore SA, et al. The OTT-MAL fusion oncogene activates RBPJ-mediated transcription and induces acute megakaryoblastic leukemia in a knockin mouse model. J Clin Invest 2009;119:852–864.
95. Taki T, Sako M, Tsuchida M, et al. The t(11;16)(q23;p13) translocation in myelodysplastic syndrome fuses the MLL gene to the CBP gene. Blood 1997;89:3945–3950.
96. Carapeti M, Aguiar RC, Goldman JM, et al. A novel fusion between MOZ and the nuclear receptor coactivator TIF2 in acute myeloid leukemia. Blood 1998;91:3127–3133.
97. Deguchi K, Ayton PM, Carapeti M, et al. MOZ-TIF2-induced acute myeloid leukemia requires the MOZ nucleosome binding motif and TIF2-mediated recruitment of CBP. Cancer Cell 2003;3:259–271.
98. Lavau C, Luo RT, Du C, et al. Retrovirus-mediated gene transfer of MLL-ELL transforms primary myeloid progenitors and causes acute myeloid leukemias in mice. Proc Natl Acad Sci U S A 2000;97:10984–10989.
99. Kung AL, Rebel VI, Bronson RT, et al. Gene dose-dependent control of hematopoiesis and hematologic tumor suppression by CBP. Genes Dev 2000;14:272–277.
100. Tefferi A. Novel mutations and their functional and clinical relevance in myeloproliferative neoplasms: JAK2, MPL, TET2, ASXL1, CBL, IDH and IKZF1. Leukemia 2010;24:1128–1138.
101. Patel JP, Gonen M, Figueroa ME, et al. Prognostic relevance of integrated genetic profiling in acute myeloid leukemia. N Engl J Med 2012;366:1079–1089.
102. Moran-Crusio K, Reavie L, Shih A, et al. Tet2 loss leads to increased hematopoietic stem cell self-renewal and myeloid transformation. Cancer Cell 2011;20:11–24.
103. Dang L, Jin S, Su SM. IDH mutations in glioma and acute myeloid leukemia. Trends Mol Med 2010;16:387–397.
104. Dang L, White DW, Gross S, et al. Cancer-associated IDH1 mutations produce 2-hydroxyglutarate. Nature 2009;462:739–744.
105. Ley TJ, Ding L, Walter MJ, et al. DNMT3A mutations in acute myeloid leukemia. N Engl J Med 2010;363:2424–2433.
106. Tadokoro Y, Ema H, Okano M, et al. De novo DNA methyltransferase is essential for self-renewal, but not for differentiation, in hematopoietic stem cells. J Exp Med 2007;204:715–722.
107. Tanaka S, Miyagi S, Sashida G, et al. Ezh2 augments leukemogenicity by reinforcing differentiation blockage in acute myeloid leukemia. Blood 2012;120:1107–1117.
108. Ernst T, Chase AJ, Score J, et al. Inactivating mutations of the histone methyltransferase gene EZH2 in myeloid disorders. Nat Genet 2010;42:722–726.
109. Delgado MD, Albajar M, Gomez-Casares MT, et al. MYC oncogene in myeloid neoplasias. Clin Transl Oncol 2013;15:87–94.
110. O'Neil J, Look AT. Mechanisms of transcription factor deregulation in lymphoid cell transformation. Oncogene 2007;26:6838–6849.
111. Dang CV. MYC on the path to cancer. Cell 2012;149:22–35.
112. Van Vlierberghe P, Ferrando A. The molecular basis of T cell acute lymphoblastic leukemia. J Clin Invest 2012;122:3398–3406.
113. Steelman LS, Franklin RA, Abrams SL, et al. Roles of the Ras/Raf/MEK/ERK pathway in leukemia therapy. Leukemia 2011;25:1080–1094.
114. Chung E, Kondo M. Role of Ras/Raf/MEK/ERK signaling in physiological hematopoiesis and leukemia development. Immunol Res 2011;49:248–268.
115. Takashima A, Faller DV. Targeting the RAS oncogene. Expert Opin Ther Targets 2013;17:507–531.
116. Lancet JE, Karp JE. Farnesyltransferase inhibitors in hematologic malignancies: new horizons in therapy. Blood 2003;102:3880–3889.
117. Braun BS, Shannon K. Targeting Ras in myeloid leukemias. Clin Cancer Res 2008;14:2249–2252.
118. Moorman AV, Harrison CJ, Buck GA, et al. Karyotype is an independent prognostic factor in adult acute lymphoblastic leukemia (ALL): analysis of cytogenetic data from patients treated on the Medical Research Council (MRC) UKALLXII/Eastern Cooperative Oncology Group (ECOG) 2993 trial. Blood 2007;109:3189–3197.
119. Jones LK, Saha V. Philadelphia positive acute lymphoblastic leukaemia of childhood. Br J Haematol 2005;130:489–500.
120. Nowell PC, Hungerford DA. Chromosome studies on normal and leukemic human leukocytes. J Natl Cancer Inst 1960;25:85–109.
121. Rowley JD. Letter: A new consistent chromosomal abnormality in chronic myelogenous leukaemia identified by quinacrine fluorescence and Giemsa staining. Nature 1973;243:290–293.
122. Hu Y, Liu Y, Pelletier S, et al. Requirement of Src kinases Lyn, Hck and Fgr for BCR-ABL1-induced B-lymphoblastic leukemia but not chronic myeloid leukemia. Nat Genet 2004;36:453–461.
123. Deininger M, Buchdunger E, Druker BJ. The development of imatinib as a therapeutic agent for chronic myeloid leukemia. Blood 2005;105:2640–2653.
124. Stirewalt DL, Radich JP. The role of FLT3 in haematopoietic malignancies. Nat Rev Cancer 2003;3:650–665.
125. Griffith J, Black J, Faerman C, et al. The structural basis for autoinhibition of FLT3 by the juxtamembrane domain. Mol Cell 2004;13:169–178.
126. Abu-Duhier FM, Goodeve AC, Wilson GA, et al. FLT3 internal tandem duplication mutations in adult acute myeloid leukaemia define a high-risk group. Br J Haematol 2000;111:190–195.

127. Kiyoi H, Naoe T, Nakano Y, et al. Prognostic implication of FLT3 and N-RAS gene mutations in acute myeloid leukemia. Blood 1999;93:3074–3080.
128. Meshinchi S, Woods WG, Stirewalt DL, et al. Prevalence and prognostic significance of Flt3 internal tandem duplication in pediatric acute myeloid leukemia. Blood 2001;97:89–94.
129. Griffin JD. Point mutations in the FLT3 gene in AML. Blood 2001;97:2193A–2193.
130. Kampa-Schittenhelm KM, Heinrich MC, Akmut F, et al. Quizartinib (AC220) is a potent second generation class III tyrosine kinase inhibitor that displays a distinct inhibition profile against mutant-FLT3, -PDGFRA and -KIT isoforms. Mol Cancer 2013;12:19.
131. Frohling S, Scholl C, Levine RL, et al. Identification of driver and passenger mutations of FLT3 by high-throughput DNA sequence analysis and functional assessment of candidate alleles. Cancer Cell 2007;12:501–513.
132. Pardanani AD, Levine RL, Lasho T, et al. MPL515 mutations in myeloproliferative and other myeloid disorders: a study of 1182 patients. Blood 2006;108:3472–3476.
133. Hussein K, Bock O, Theophile K, et al. MPLW515L mutation in acute megakaryoblastic leukaemia. Leukemia 2009;23:852–855.
134. Malinge S, Ragu C, Della-Valle V, et al. Activating mutations in human acute megakaryoblastic leukemia. Blood 2008;112:4220–4226.
135. Baker SJ, Rane SG, Reddy EP. Hematopoietic cytokine receptor signaling. Oncogene 2007;26:6724–6737.
136. Steensma DP, McClure RF, Karp JE, et al. JAK2 V617F is a rare finding in de novo acute myeloid leukemia, but STAT3 activation is common and remains unexplained. Leukemia 2006;20:971–978.
137. Frohling S, Lipka DB, Kayser S, et al. Rare occurrence of the JAK2 V617F mutation in AML subtypes M5, M6, and M7. Blood 2006;107:1242–1243.
138. Walters DK, Mercher T, Gu TL, et al. Activating alleles of JAK3 in acute megakaryoblastic leukemia. Cancer Cell 2006;10:65–75.
139. Mullighan CG, Zhang J, Harvey RC, et al. JAK mutations in high-risk childhood acute lymphoblastic leukemia. Proc Natl Acad Sci U S A 2009;106:9414–9418.
140. Benekli M, Xia Z, Donohue KA, et al. Constitutive activity of signal transducer and activator of transcription 3 protein in acute myeloid leukemia blasts is associated with short disease-free survival. Blood 2002;99:252–257.
141. Redell MS, Ruiz MJ, Gerbing RB, et al. FACS analysis of Stat3/5 signaling reveals sensitivity to G-CSF and IL-6 as a significant prognostic factor in pediatric AML: a Children's Oncology Group report. Blood 2013;121:1083–1093.
142. Palmi C, Vendramini E, Silvestri D, et al. Poor prognosis for P2RY8-CRLF2 fusion but not for CRLF2 over-expression in children with intermediate risk B-cell precursor acute lymphoblastic leukemia. Leukemia 2012;26:2245–2253.
143. Haber DA, Buckler AJ, Glaser T, et al. An internal deletion within an 11p13 zinc finger gene contributes to the development of Wilms' tumor. Cell 1990;61:1257–1269.
144. Hohenstein P, Hastie ND. The many facets of the Wilms' tumour gene, WT1. Hum Mol Genet 2006;15:R196–R201.
145. Baird PN, Simmons PJ. Expression of the Wilms' tumor gene (WT1) in normal hemopoiesis. Exp Hematol 1997;25:312–320.
146. Yang L, Han Y, Suarez Saiz F, et al. A tumor suppressor and oncogene: the WT1 story. Leukemia 2007;21:868–876.
147. Miyagi T, Ahuja H, Kubota T, et al. Expression of the candidate Wilm's tumor gene, WT1, in human leukemia cells. Leukemia 1993;7:970–977.
148. Miwa H, Beran M, Saunders GF. Expression of the Wilms' tumor gene (WT1) in human leukemias. Leukemia 1992;6:405–409.
149. Smith SI, Down M, Boyd AW, et al. Expression of the Wilms' tumor suppressor gene, WT1, reduces the tumorigenicity of the leukemic cell line M1 in C.B-17 scid/scid mice. Cancer Res 2000;60:808–814.
150. King-Underwood L, Renshaw J, Pritchard-Jones K. Mutations in the Wilms' tumor gene WT1 in leukemias. Blood 1996;87:2171–2179.
151. Summers K, Stevens J, Kakkas I, et al. Wilms' tumour 1 mutations are associated with FLT3-ITD and failure of standard induction chemotherapy in patients with normal karyotype AML. Leukemia 2007;21:550–551.
152. Virappane P, Gale R, Hills R, et al. Mutation of the Wilms' tumor 1 gene is a poor prognostic factor associated with chemotherapy resistance in normal karyotype acute myeloid leukemia: the United Kingdom Medical Research Council Adult Leukaemia Working Party. J Clin Oncol 2008;26:5429–5435.
153. Paschka P, Marcucci G, Ruppert AS, et al. Wilms' tumor 1 gene mutations independently predict poor outcome in adults with cytogenetically normal acute myeloid leukemia: a cancer and leukemia group B study. J Clin Oncol 2008;26:4595–4602.
154. Gaidzik VI, Schlenk RF, Moschny S, et al. Prognostic impact of WT1 mutations in cytogenetically normal acute myeloid leukemia: a study of the German-Austrian AML Study Group. Blood 2009;113:4505–4511.
155. Vousden KH, Lu X. Live or let die: the cell's response to p53. Nat Rev Cancer 2002;2:594–604.
156. Nakai H, Misawa S, Taniwaki M, et al. Prognostic significance of loss of a chromosome 17p and p53 gene mutations in blast crisis of chronic myelogenous leukaemia. Br J Haematol 1994;87:425–427.
157. Dohner H, Fischer K, Bentz M, et al. p53 gene deletion predicts for poor survival and non-response to therapy with purine analogs in chronic B-cell leukemias. Blood 1995;85:1580–1589.
158. Sander CA, Yano T, Clark HM, et al. p53 mutation is associated with progression in follicular lymphomas. Blood 1993;82:1994–2004.
159. Venkatachalam S, Shi YP, Jones SN, et al. Retention of wild-type p53 in tumors from p53 heterozygous mice: reduction of p53 dosage can promote cancer formation. Embo J 1998;17:4657–4667.

160. Herzog G, Lu-Hesselmann J, Zimmermann Y, et al. Microsatellite instability and p53 mutations are characteristic of subgroups of acute myeloid leukemia but independent events. *Haematologica* 2005;90:693–695.
161. Fenaux P, Jonveaux P, Quiquandon I, et al. P53 gene mutations in acute myeloid leukemia with 17p monosomy. *Blood* 1991;78:1652–1657.
162. Watanabe T, Hotta T, Ichikawa A, et al. The MDM2 oncogene overexpression in chronic lymphocytic leukemia and low-grade lymphoma of B-cell origin. *Blood* 1994;84:3158–3165.
163. Haferlach C, Dicker F, Herholz H, et al. Mutations of the TP53 gene in acute myeloid leukemia are strongly associated with a complex aberrant karyotype. *Leukemia* 2008;22:1539–1541.
164. Schoch C, Kern W, Kohlmann A, et al. Acute myeloid leukemia with a complex aberrant karyotype is a distinct biological entity characterized by genomic imbalances and a specific gene expression profile. *Genes Chromosomes Cancer* 2005;43:227–238.
165. van der Holt B, Breems DA, Berna Beverloo H, et al. Various distinctive cytogenetic abnormalities in patients with acute myeloid leukaemia aged 60 years and older express adverse prognostic value: results from a prospective clinical trial. *Br J Haematol* 2007;136:96–105.
166. Seifert H, Mohr B, Thiede C, et al. The prognostic impact of 17p (p53) deletion in 2272 adults with acute myeloid leukemia. *Leukemia* 2009;23:656–663.
167. Fenaux P, Preudhomme C, Quiquandon I, et al. Mutations of the P53 gene in acute myeloid leukaemia. *Br J Haematol* 1992;80:178–183.
168. Lai JL, Preudhomme C, Zandecki M, et al. Myelodysplastic syndromes and acute myeloid leukemia with 17p deletion. An entity characterized by specific dysgranulopoiesis and a high incidence of P53 mutations. *Leukemia* 1995;9:370–381.
169. Nahi H, Selivanova G, Lehmann S, et al. Mutated and non-mutated TP53 as targets in the treatment of leukaemia. *Br J Haematol* 2008;141:445–453.
170. Schaich M, Soucek S, Thiede C, et al. MDR1 and MRP1 gene expression are independent predictors for treatment outcome in adult acute myeloid leukaemia. *Br J Haematol* 2005;128:324–332.
171. Cavalcanti GB Jr, Vasconcelos FC, Pinto de Faria G, et al. Coexpression of p53 protein and MDR functional phenotype in leukemias: the predominant association in chronic myeloid leukemia. *Cytometry B Clin Cytom* 2004;61:1–8.
172. Radtke F, Wilson A, MacDonald HR. Notch signaling in hematopoiesis and lymphopoiesis: lessons from Drosophila. *Bioessays* 2005;27:1117–1128.
173. Pancewicz J, Nicot C. Current views on the role of Notch signaling and the pathogenesis of human leukemia. *BMC Cancer* 2011;11:502.
174. Weng AP, Ferrando AA, Lee W, et al. Activating mutations of NOTCH1 in human T cell acute lymphoblastic leukemia. *Science* 2004;306:269–271.
175. Thompson BJ, Buonamici S, Sulis ML, et al. The SCFFBW7 ubiquitin ligase complex as a tumor suppressor in T cell leukemia. *J Exp Med* 2007;204:1825–1835.
176. DeAngelo DJ, Stone JR, Silverman LB, et al. A phase I clinical Trial of the notch inhibitor MK-0752 in patients with T-cell acute lymphoblastic leukemia/lymphoma (T-ALL) and other leukemias. *ASCO Meeting Abstracts* 2006:6585.
177. Real PJ, Tosello V, Palomero T, et al. Gamma-secretase inhibitors reverse glucocorticoid resistance in T cell acute lymphoblastic leukemia. *Nat Med* 2009;15:50–58.
178. Federici L, Falini B. Nucleophosmin mutations in acute myeloid leukemia: a tale of protein unfolding and mislocalization. *Protein Sci* 2013;22:545–556.
179. Falini B, Mecucci C, Tiacci E, et al. Cytoplasmic nucleophosmin in acute myelogenous leukemia with a normal karyotype. *N Engl J Med* 2005;352:254–266.
180. Falini B, Nicoletti I, Martelli MF, et al. Acute myeloid leukemia carrying cytoplasmic/mutated nucleophosmin (NPMc+ AML): biologic and clinical features. *Blood* 2007;109:874–885.
181. Mullighan CG. Molecular genetics of B-precursor acute lymphoblastic leukemia. *J Clin Invest* 2012;122:3407–3415.
182. Mullighan CG, Goorha S, Radtke I, et al. Genome-wide analysis of genetic alterations in acute lymphoblastic leukaemia. *Nature* 2007;446:758–764.
183. Nutt SL, Heavey B, Rolink AG, et al. Commitment to the B-lymphoid lineage depends on the transcription factor Pax5. *Nature* 1999;401:556–562.
184. Kawamata N, Pennella MA, Woo JL, et al. Dominant-negative mechanism of leukemogenic PAX5 fusions. *Oncogene* 2012;31:966–977.
185. Mullighan CG, Su X, Zhang J, et al. Deletion of IKZF1 and prognosis in acute lymphoblastic leukemia. *N Engl J Med* 2009;360:470–480.
186. Georgopoulos K, Bigby M, Wang JH, et al. The Ikaros gene is required for the development of all lymphoid lineages. *Cell* 1994;79:143–156.
187. Merkenschlager M. Ikaros in immune receptor signaling, lymphocyte differentiation, and function. *FEBS Lett* 2010;584:4910–4914.
188. Bottardi S, Zmiri FA, Bourgoin V, et al. Ikaros interacts with P-TEFb and cooperates with GATA-1 to enhance transcription elongation. *Nucleic Acids Res* 2011;39:3505–3519.
189. Mullighan CG, Miller CB, Radtke I, et al. BCR-ABL1 lymphoblastic leukemia is characterized by the deletion of Ikaros. *Nature* 2008;453:110–114.
190. Lu Q, Kamps MP. Heterodimerization of Hox proteins with Pbx1 and oncoprotein E2a-Pbx1 generates unique DNA-binding specifities at nucleotides predicted to contact the N-terminal arm of the Hox homeodomain—demonstration of Hox-dependent targeting of E2a-Pbx1 in vivo. *Oncogene* 1997;14:75–83.
191. Golub TR, Barker GF, Lovett M, et al. Fusion of PDGF receptor beta to a novel ets-like gene, tel, in chronic myelomonocytic leukemia with t(5;12) chromosomal translocation. *Cell* 1994;77:307–316.
192. Higuchi M, O'Brien D, Kumaravelu P, et al. Expression of a conditional AML1-ETO oncogene bypasses embryonic lethality and establishes a murine model of human t(8;21) acute myeloid leukemia. *Cancer Cell* 2002;1:63–74.
193. Wiemels JL, Cazzaniga G, Daniotti M, et al. Prenatal origin of acute lymphoblastic leukaemia in children. *Lancet* 1999;354:1499–1503.
194. Gilliland DG. Molecular genetics of human leukemias: new insights into therapy. *Semin Hematol* 2002;39:6–11.
195. Kelly LM, Liu Q, Kutok JL, et al. FLT3 internal tandem duplication mutations associated with human acute myeloid leukemias induce myeloproliferative disease in a murine bone marrow transplant model. *Blood* 2002;99:310–318.
196. Chan IT, Kutok JL, Williams IR, et al. Conditional expression of oncogenic K-ras from its endogenous promoter induces a myeloproliferative disease. *J Clin Invest* 2004;113:528–538.
197. Sanders MA, Valk PJ. The evolving molecular genetic landscape in acute myeloid leukaemia. *Curr Opin Hematol* 2013;20:79–85.
198. Welch JS, Ley TJ, Link DC, et al. The origin and evolution of mutations in acute myeloid leukemia. *Cell* 2012;150:264–278.

43 Management of Acute Leukemias

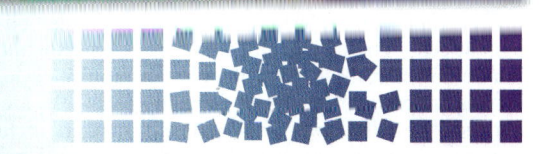

Partow Kebriaei, Marcos de Lima, Elihu H. Estey, and Richard Champlin

INTRODUCTION

Acute leukemias result from malignant transformation of immature hematopoietic cells followed by clonal proliferation and accumulation of the transformed cells. The pathogenesis of leukemia transformation is incompletely defined but is likely to be a multistep process.[1] Acute leukemias are characterized by aberrant differentiation and maturation of the malignant cells, with a maturation arrest and accumulation of leukemic blasts in the bone marrow. Acute leukemias are categorized according to their differentiation along the myeloid or lymphoid lineage. In 10% to 20% of patients, the leukemic cells have characteristics of both myeloid and lymphoid cells. Typically myeloid and lymphoid markers are found on the same cell. Less often, separate myeloid and lymphoid populations are present.

Hematopoietic cells are derived from stem cells and progenitors giving rise to the myeloid and lymphoid system. Stem cells have the fundamental properties of self-renewal and differentiation into distinct lineages. Hematopoietic stem cells and progenitors are resident in the bone marrow where they are supported and regulated through interactions with the local microenvironment. Leukemia likely develops after transformation of a hematopoietic stem cell or progenitor, which acquires stem cell–like properties of unlimited self-renewal.[2] The malignant stem cells represent a small fraction of the leukemia. The bulk of leukemic cells are the differentiated progeny that undergo limited maturation along the myeloid or lymphoid lineage. Leukemia chemotherapy must eradicate the disease while sparing normal hematopoietic stem cells. Treatments that eradicate the differentiated leukemia cells typically do not eradicate the malignant stem cells; consequently, relapse of the leukemia commonly occurs.[3] High-dose, stem cell–toxic therapies may be used if followed by hematopoietic stem cell transplantation (HSCT) to restore normal hematopoiesis, and HSCT is an important modality of treatment for acute leukemias. However, a significant antileukemia effect mediated by donor T and natural killer (NK) cells also plays an important role in allogeneic transplantation, particularly for acute myelogenous leukemia (AML). A better understanding of the biology of normal and malignant stem cells and the marrow microenvironment is required for development of more effective therapies.

Although the cause of acute leukemias is unknown, malignant transformation is unlikely to be the result of a single event. Rather, it is likely caused by the culmination of multiple processes that produce genetic damage secondary to physical or chemical exposure in susceptible progenitor cells. Genomic analyses indicate that AML has fewer mutations than all solid tumors studied to date, with an average of 13 coding mutations per patient, of which only an average of 5 (and on occasion as few as 2) are recurrently mutated (*driver*) mutations; among the latter aberrations in DNA (cytosine-5)-methyltransferase 3A (*DNMT3a*), isocitrate dehydrogenase (*IDH*), tet methylcytosine dioxygenase 2 (*TET2*), or nucleophosmin (*NPM1*) contribute to the establishment of a founding AML clone and in FMS-like tyrosine kinase 3 (*FLT3*) to progression to the clinically apparent disease. The nonrecurrent *passenger* mutations appear to represent mutations that occur during the life span of normal hematopoietic progenitors and are retained when a malignant mutation(s) occurs. Over time, subclones arise characterized by other mutations that contribute to resistance.[4,5] Leukemia may occur following exposure to a number of carcinogens, such as benzene or radiation exposure. Acute leukemias may occur following chemotherapy, such as alkylators or topoisomerase II inhibitors, or radiation therapy given for another malignancy.[6,7] These secondary leukemias typically have a high risk of cytogenetic abnormalities and have a poor prognosis. Other acquired factors include infectious agents and environmental toxins. Among infectious causes, the Epstein-Barr virus is associated with mature B-cell or Burkitt's acute lymphoblastic leukemia (ALL). Inherited genetic abnormalities that predispose to leukemia include ataxia telangiectasia, Down syndrome, and certain polymorphisms in Methylenetetrahydrofolate Reductase (*MTHFR*) (a gene involved in the folate metabolism).[8]

The presenting clinical symptoms are a result of bone marrow failure or the effects of tissue infiltration or circulating leukemia cells. Patients commonly complain of fatigue or spontaneous bleeding. Weight loss, fever, night sweats, and lethargy may also be present. Infections related to neutropenia may occur. Central nervous system (CNS) involvement is more common in ALL than AML. Bone and testicular involvement is also more commonly seen in ALL, and most commonly in children rather than adults.[9] On physical examination, pallor and signs associated with thrombocytopenia may be present, such as gingival bleeding, epistaxis, petechiae, ecchymoses, or fundal hemorrhages. Less commonly, generalized lymphadenopathy, hepatosplenomegaly, or dermal involvement by leukemia cutis may be present. T-lineage ALL may commonly present with a mediastinal mass.

The diagnosis of acute leukemias requires morphologic identification of malignant blasts in the blood and bone marrow.[10] This requires an evaluation of peripheral blood and bone marrow aspirate smears, phenotypic analysis of the blasts by cytochemical studies and flow cytometry, or immunohistochemistry with an appropriate panel of surface and cytoplasmic markers. Acute leukemias are classified according to their differentiation into the myeloid or lymphoid lineage, although some cases appear biphenotypic. The French–American–British Group (FAB) described a widely utilized classification system[11] that has been largely replaced by the World Health Organization's (WHO) classification system.[12] Cytospin slides made from cerebrospinal fluid (CSF) are used to diagnose CNS involvement. The current definition of CNS involvement used by the Children's Cancer Group (CCG) is greater than five white blood cells (WBC) per microliter of CSF plus unequivocal blasts identified on the cytospin.[13] However, the risk for CNS relapse and the need for additional CNS-directed therapy is controversial when there are less than WBC per microliter of CSF, but blasts are present. Some studies suggest that the presence of blasts, even in the absence of pleocytosis, requires additional CNS-directed therapy,[14] whereas others do not. A related concern is the prognostic significance of a traumatic lumbar puncture at diagnosis. Most studies concur that the presence of blasts in a traumatic lumbar puncture is associated with an inferior outcome.[15]

ACUTE MYELOGENOUS LEUKEMIA

AML is characterized by limited myeloid differentiation of the malignant cells. The malignant cells characteristically undergo maturation arrest at the level of the blast or promyelocyte, although varying proportions of mature hematopoietic cells are leukemia derived. The cells display myeloid specific markers, including Auer rods (aberrant primary granules), cytochemistry (Sudan black, myeloperoxidase, or nonspecific esterase), and cell surface antigens.[11] The WHO classification system's criterion for a diagnosis of AML is >20% blasts in marrow or blood, with patients having <20% blasts said most often to have a myelodysplastic syndrome (MDS). However, this distinction is purely arbitrary. And, indeed, the natural history of patients with 10% to 19% blasts (high-risk MDS) frequently bears more resemblance to that of AML than to that of patients with <10% blasts. Furthermore, the outcome of AML therapy is often similar in patients with high-risk MDS as in those with AML.

Management Options for Acute Myelogenous Leukemia

Broadly speaking, there are three management options for AML: supportive care only, supportive care plus standard anti-AML therapy, or supportive care plus investigational anti-AML therapy. When the disease was first systematically described 50 years ago, few patients lived more than 4 to 6 months after diagnosis. Today, with the advent of better antibiotics and transfusion practices, the natural history is almost certainly better, particularly in patients with WBC <25,000 to 50,000/μL. Nonetheless, it is safe to say that patients will, on average, lose >90% of their remaining life expectancy if given supportive care only. Furthermore, quality of life suffers dominated by time spent waiting for frequent transfusions and hospital admissions for infections, which ultimately lead to death. For these reasons, patients presenting to academic medical centers are generally interested in treatment beyond supportive care. This leads to a decision between standard and investigational therapies. The results of the latter are, by definition, unknown. It follows that the decision must rest on the likely outcome of standard therapy. The worse the outcome, the more likely appropriately informed patients select a clinical trial. Hence, the topic of prognostic factors with standard therapies is fundamental to the management of AML. Here, standard induction therapies will refer to (1) 3 days of an anthracycline, usually daunorubicin or idarubicin (days 1 through 3), plus 7 days of ara-C (100 to 200 mg/m^2 days 1 through 7), (2) decitabine or azacitidine, or (3) a lower dose of ara-C and standard postremission therapies of the previous, including ara-C at doses of 0.5 to 3.0 g/m^2.

Prognostic Factors in Acute Myelogenous Leukemia

There are two types of prognostic factors: those associated with treatment-related mortality (TRM) and those associated with resistance to therapy. Although there is considerable overlap between these two, TRM is often defined as death occurring within the first 28 days of initial therapy or occurring in patients in remission. Patients dying within the first 28 days appear to be a qualitatively distinct group. Resistance then may be considered as failure to enter remission despite not incurring TRM or as relapse from remission. Although considerable attention is often devoted to TRM and associated morbidity, there is little doubt that even in patients in their 70s, resistance is a more frequent cause of failure to enter complete remission (CR), and that relapse is at least threefold more common than death in CR.

Predictors of Treatment-Related Mortality

Although it is commonly believed that age is the principal covariate associated with TRM, Walter et al.[16] found that performance status is more important than age and that both interact with lower albumin and platelet count, higher creatinine, WBC and percentage of blood blasts, and secondary AML. These were all used to compute a TRM score following the use of 3+7 as given in the Southwest Oncology Group (SWOG) or higher doses of ara-C as given at M. D. Anderson Cancer Center (MDACC). As such, they defined a group of patients who might be candidates for *less intense* therapies. However, this possibility needs to account for decreasing TRM rates, as noted by Othus et al.[17] In SWOG, these declined from 18% in 1991 through 1995 to 3% in 2006 through 2009. Analogous figures at MDACC were 16% and 4%. The decline was independent of covariates such as those considered in the TRM score. The possibility that this reflected a tendency in recent years to give less intense drugs, such as azacitidine or decitabine rather than 3+7, to older patients at high risk of TRM who thus would be excluded from analyses seems unlikely because the same temporal trend in TRM was found in both younger and older patients; it seems improbable that the former were more likely to receive less intense therapy in recent years. Othus et al.'s data emphasize that the main problem in AML therapy is resistance. Hence, merely decreasing intensity is unlikely to result in improved outcomes unless efficacy is improved in parallel.

Predictors of Resistance to Standard Therapy

Cytogenetics. Various means to classify pretreatment AML cytogenetics have been proposed (Table 43.1 and 43.2), and generally separate patients into three to four distinct prognostic groups.

Favorable Group. The core binding factor (CBF)–related AMLs have the most favorable prognosis and constitute 10% to 15% of cases in patients under age 60 years.[18] CBFs regulate the transcription of genes involved in the differentiation of normal blasts into mature progeny. CBFs contain a β unit (*CBFB*, located on the long arm of chromosome 16) and an α unit, one of which is known as *RUNX1* (formerly *AML1* and located on chromosome 21). The CBF AMLs result from translocations involving *RUNX1* or *CBFB*. Specifically, in t(8;21) *RUNX1* is fused with *RUNX1T1* (formerly *ETO*) located on chromosome 8, whereas in inv(16), *CBFB* is linked with the *MYH11* gene located on the short arm of chromosome 16. These abnormal CBFs exert a *dominant negative* effect over normal CBFs, leading to differentiation block and, in the presence of other genetic aberrations that promote survival of the affected stem cells, to AML. It is important to distinguish deletion of the long arm of chromosome 16(del16q), which does not affect *CBFB*, from translocation between the two chromosome 16s, t(16;16), which is quite rare but does disrupt *CBFB* and, unlike del16q, behaves clinically like inv(16). Eighty-five percent of cases of inv(16) or t(8;21) AML are found in those under age 60 years. Although inv(16) is most frequently associated with the FAB subtype M4Eo, 40% of the 145 cases of inv(16) AML seen at MDACC over the past 25 years have had less than 5% eosinophils. Similarly, although t(8;21) AML is most often seen in the FAB subtype M2, 30% of the 124 cases at MDACC were seen in association with other FAB subtypes.

Inv(16) AML and t(8;21) AML differ in several ways. For example, t(8;21) tends to present with lower WBC counts and is frequently accompanied by the loss of a sex chromosome (particularly the Y) or a deletion (del) of the long arm (q) of chromosome 9(del9q), whereas inv(16) is often accompanied by trisomy (+) 22 (+22), +(8), or +(21). Although both inv(16) and t(8;21) are distinguished by CR rates of approximately 90% and long remissions and survival, inv(16) AML is more apt to respond once relapse occurs; as a result, patients with inv(16) tend to live longer

TABLE 43.1
Acute Myeloid Leukemia Prognostic Index

Group	NCRI (formerly MRC)	SWOG/ECOG	CALGB
Best	inv(16); t(8;21)	inv(16); t(8;21) w/o del (9q) or complex changes	inv(16); t(8;21)
Intermediate	Normal; 11q abnormalities[a]; +8; Others not in favorable or unfavorable groups	Normal; +8; Others not in favorable or unfavorable groups	Normal; t(9;11); +8 (for relapse); del(5q); Loss of 7q
Worst	−5/−7; Complex (≥5 chromosomes involved)	−5/−7; Complex (≥3 chromosomes involved); 11q abnormalities[a]; inv(3q); del(20q); t(6;9); abnormal 17p	Complex (≥3 chromosomes involved); −7; +8 (for survival); inv(3)

NCRI, National Cancer Research Institute; MRC, Medical Research Center; SWOG, Southwest Oncology Group; ECOG, Eastern Cooperative Oncology Group; CALGB, Cancer and Leukemia Group B.
[a] Patients with t(9;11) may fall into the intermediate group and patients with other 11q abnormalities into the unfavorable group.

than those with t(8;21). The prognosis of CBF AML is quite variable (although not as variable as normal karyotype AML). Thus, long-term remissions occur in only 25% to 30% of patients aged >65 years or with high levels of mutant tyrosine-protein kinase (C-KIT) alleles.[19]

Worst Group. There is some debate as to the placement of patients with other abnormal karyotypes. Thus, for example, both the Medical Research Council (MRC) and SWOG cytogenetic classification systems include patients with +8,−Y in an *intermediate* prognostic group together with normal cytogenetic (NC)-AML (see Table 43.1). However, although the MRC considers del20q or t(6;9) AML in its intermediate group, the SWOG places these in its *worst* group, and other differences exist (see Table 43.1). However, there is very little debate about the great bulk of patients in the worst group: those with monosomy of chromosome 5 (−5), and/or 7 (−7), deletions (del) of the long arms of chromosomes 5 (del 5q) or 7 (del 7q) and with abnormalities of 3q. Particularly poor prognoses have been associated with *complex* abnormalities involving at least three to four distinct changes. In the last 5 years, some of the prognostic import of complex cytogenetics has been attributed to an association with a *monosomal karyotype* (MK+) defined by the presence of two or more autosomal monosomies (i.e., not involving the X or Y chromosome) or by the presence of one autosomal monosomy and a structural change, which is a translocation but no addition. MK+ patients are largely incurable with standard therapy, with median survivals of approximately 6 months. Now it appears that alterations in the tumor suppressor gene TP53, located on the short arm(p) of chromosome 17, underlie the prognostic effect of MK.

TABLE 43.2
European Leukemia Net Classification System

Prognostic Group	Proportion of De Novo Patients in Group by Age <60 years, Age ≥60 years	Subsets
Favorable	41%, 20%	Inv (16), t(16;16), t(8;21); NC with NPM mutation (NPM+) but no FLT3 ITD (ITD−); NC with mutated CEBPA
Intermediate 1	18%, 19%	NPM− ITD−; NPM+ ITD+; NPM− ITD+
Intermediate 2	19%, 30%	Cytogenetic abnormalities (including t9;11) not considered best or worst
Adverse	22%, 31%	3q abnormalities, t(6;9), −7, −5, del 5q, abnormal 11q (other than t9;11), abnormal 17p, complex abnormalities

NC, normal cytogenetics; FLT3, FMS-like tyrosine kinase 3; ITD, internal tandem duplication; NPM, nucleophosmin; CEBPA, CCAAT enhancer binding protein alpha.

Intermediate Group. Criteria for intermediate cytogenetics differ (see Table 43.1). However, there is agreement that patients with NC-AML are the lynchpin of this group. NC-AML occurs in 25% to 40% of patients depending on age (less frequent with increasing age) and type of AML (less frequent with therapy related AML [t-AML]). As might be expected from the term *intermediate cytogenetics* and the frequency of NC-AML, NC-AML is associated with greater variation in outcome than any other single cytogenetic group.

NPM, FLT3 ITD, and CEBPA. Recent years have shown the ability of molecular biology to dissect this heterogeneity. Today, patients with NC-AML should routinely be tested for internal tandem duplications (ITD) in the *FLT3* gene, mutations in the nucleophosmin gene (*NPM1*), and in the CCAAT enhancer-binding protein alpha (*CEBPA*) gene. Most cost effectively, this would be done once a diagnosis of NC-AML is established (the prognostic relevance of *NPM*, *FLT3*, and *CEBPA* being less in other patients than in those with NC-AML), and *CEBPA* testing would only be carried out in patients who were negative for *FLT3*, *ITD*, and *NPM1*. NC-AML patients with *NPM1* mutations but without *FLT3* ITDs and patients with a double *CEBPA* mutation have a prognosis with standard therapy essentially equivalent to patients with best cytogenetics. In contrast, patients with *FLT3* ITDs have a prognosis more closely resembling that of patients with the worst cytogenetics. This has been codified in the widely employed four-group European Leukemia Net (ELN) Classification system (see Table 43.2). The system has been tested in patients with de novo AML that did not contribute to its development; treatment was standard. Each of the four groups were relevant in patients age < 60 years, whereas the two intermediate groups were difficult to distinguish prognostically in older patients.

Secondary AML. Although many studies detailing effects of various molecular markers include only patients with de novo AML, there is little doubt that t-AML or AML following a documented abnormality in blood count for 1 to 3 months before the diagnosis of AML, often called an antecedent hematologic disorder (AHD), is associated with resistance. T-AML and AML after an AHD are collectively known as secondary AML. The association between resistance and secondary AML is independent of the tendency of patients with secondary AML to have the worst group cytogenetics (see previously). The relative effects of an AHD and t-AML remain to be established, although it has been suggested that the latter is more important.

Age. Although much of the association between older age and resistance reflects an association with the worst group cytogenetics (see previously) and/or with secondary AML, age per se probably predisposes to resistance.

Mutations Other than NPM, FLT3 ITD, and CEBPA. The ability of cytogenetics, *NPM*, and *FLT3* ITD, along with older age and secondary AML to predict resistance has been studied using areas under receiver operating characteristic curves (AUC). An AUC of 1.0 indicates perfect prediction, an AUC of 0.5 is a coin flip (sensitivity = specificity), and an AUC of 0.6 to 0.69, 0.70 to 79, and 0.80 to 0.89 is often taken as denoting poor, fair, and good predictive ability, respectively. Walter et al.[16] defined resistance in several ways: (1) no CR despite no death within 28 days of starting therapy (TRM), (2) as in 1 plus relapse within 3 months, (3) as in 1 plus relapse within 6 months, and (4) as in 1 plus relapse within 1 year. They used data from 4,565 patients treated on trials of the national cooperative groups of the UK (MRC/National Cancer Research Institute [NCRI]) and the Netherlands (HOVON) and on trials of the SWOG and MDACC in the United States. Age, performance status, WBC count, secondary disease, cytogenetic risk, and *FLT3-ITD/NPM1* mutation status were each independently associated with failure to achieve CR despite no early death (*primary refractoriness*). However, the AUC of a bootstrap-corrected multivariate model predicting this outcome was only 0.78, indicating fair predictive ability. Removal of *FLT3*-ITD and *NPM1* information slightly decreased the AUC (0.76). The prediction of therapeutic resistance, defined as primary refractoriness or early treatment failure as indicated by short relapse-free survival (RFS), was more difficult, with AUCs for models predicting primary refractory disease or RFS of ≤3, ≤6, or ≤12 months of 0.75/0.73 (with/without inclusion of *FLT3*-ITD/*NPM1* data), 0.76/0.73, and 0.75/0.71, respectively.[16] These data indicate that our ability to forecast resistance based on routinely available clinical covariates is limited and argues for the integration of additional disease characteristics to optimize outcome projection in AML.

Minimal Residual Disease

Although the incorporation of the pretreatment molecular information described previously will likely improve prognostic accuracy, the information obtained posttreatment will almost certainly also be relevant. Of particular note are assessments of minimal residual disease (MRD) in patients in CR by standard criteria. Given that AML relapses in most patients, such patients presumably have residual AML (MRD) even in CR. Quantification of MRD would allow broad recommendations for postremission therapy. In particular, patients with low levels of MRD that remain stable or decrease might continue on their initial therapy. In contrast, therapy might be changed in patients with high or rising MRD levels, in an effort to possibly avert subsequent hematologic relapse. Because relapse can only be diagnosed when more than 5% blasts are present in the marrow, the sensitivity of morphologic examination of the marrow for the detection of relapse is only 1 in 20. In contrast, if 30 metaphases are examined, a cytogenetic examination has a sensitivity of 1 in 30, whereas fluorescence in situ hybridization (FISH) typically has a sensitivity of 1 in 500.

MRD can be determined by polymerase chain reaction (PCR) to detect (1) leukemia fusion genes (such as those characteristic of inv 16, t(8;21), or t(15;17)); (2) mutations (e.g., in *NPM1*); or (3) overexpression of genes such as Wilms tumor 1 (*WT1*). PCR techniques generally have sensitivities of 1 in 10 (−4). An MRD can also be examined by multiparameter flow cytometry (MPFC), which relies on the identification of patterns of cell surface antigens characteristic of the patient's AML. The sensitivity is 1 in 10 (−3)−10 (−4). Bucciano et al.[20] have shown that patients with good (inv 16, t(8;21)) or intermediate karyotypes who have MRD detected by MPFC (MRD+) at the end of postremission therapy have outcomes resembling those in patients with *FLT3* ITD+ or unfavorable karyotype AML. In turn, patients who are *FLT3* ITD+ but without MRD fare better than those who are *FLT3* ITD+ with MRD. In patients where both MPFC and PCR are applicable, data suggest PCR is more sensitive and specific. It remains to be established whether blood can be used rather than bone marrow, whether MRD should be assessed at multiple time points (e.g., CR, immediately after completion of post remission therapy and beyond), what levels of MRD should motivate a change in therapy and whether these levels are reproducible at different centers, and critically, whether a reduction in MRD will lead to better relapse-free or overall survival rather than MRD merely being a surrogate of refractory AML.

Treatment of Newly Diagnosed Acute Myelogenous Leukemia

Treatment of AML begins with induction chemotherapy, with the goal of achieving CR with a resolution of morphologically detectable disease and the restoration of normal blood counts. This is followed by postremission therapy to eradicate MRD. Both chemotherapy and HSCT have been utilized, and each approach has a major role in the treatment of this disease. An AML cure occurs in only a minority of patients with available forms of chemotherapy. HSCT has a greater antileukemia effect but is associated with higher TRM.

Regardless of a patient's age, the initial goal in treating AML is to produce a CR, defined as a marrow with less than 5% myeloblasts, a neutrophil count greater than 1,000/μL, and a platelet count greater than 100,000/μL.[21,22] When successful, induction therapy preferentially targets AML blasts, thus allowing normal blasts to resume control of hematopoiesis. Obtaining CR is critical because, at least in the past, only patients who do so have a chance of potential cure. An operational definition of potential cure is a remission lasting 2 to 3 years, after which the risk of relapse declines sharply to less than 10%.[23] Responses less than CR are now recognized: CRp for which the criteria are the same as CR except that the platelet count can be <100,000/μL, although platelet transfusions are not being given,[21] and CRi for which no blood count minima are specified, however, the marrow must be reasonably cellular (e.g., least 200 cells must be counted)[21] because if such were not the case, a CRi could be produced in any patient by simply rendering the marrow hypoplastic with high doses of cytotoxic chemotherapy. It remains unclear whether CRp or CRi will prolong survival to the same extent as CR.[24] It is known that CRp and CRi are more likely to be associated with MRD than CR.[25] However, following treatments where CR is perhaps more likely to be associated with MRD (e.g., after use of lower intensity treatments such as azacitidine or decitabine), there may be less value to obtaining a CR.

Prolongation of the initial response has traditionally entailed further chemotherapy, typically two to four courses of consolidation with or without subsequent prolonged lower dose *maintenance*. However, several randomized studies suggest that maintenance chemotherapy, although occasionally prolonging remissions, does not lengthen survival.[26] These results have spurred interest in development of new approaches. In particular, recent years have seen the advent of targeted therapy. Although, as described previously, successful chemotherapy is itself selectively toxic to AML blasts, targeted therapy is taken to mean therapy that, although perhaps less toxic to AML blasts than chemotherapy, is much less toxic than chemotherapy to normal blasts and to gastrointestinal epithelium, damage to which can lead to sepsis and death. However, as noted previously, the main problem in AML is overcoming resistance, even in patients in their 70s.[27,28] It is axiomatic that therapy depends on the prognosis. Accordingly, we will discuss induction and postremission therapy according to the patient's prognostic group with standard therapy, as determined by the ELN classification system (see Table 43.2) and within each group note modifications that might be made for patients whose prognosis might differ from that of the group as a whole (e.g., older patients). The focus will be on the choice between standard therapy, now including decitabine and azacitidine, which are widely used in the treatment of older patients, and investigational treatment.

European Leukemia Net Favorable Prognosis Patients

Remission induction should typically consist of 3 days (days 1 through 3) of drugs, such as daunorubicin or idarubicin, that interact with the enzyme topoisomerase 2 (topo II) and 7 days (days 1 through 7) of the pyrimidine analog cytarabine (ara-C) at 100 mg/m² daily; such combinations are called 3+7. A bone marrow aspiration is typically obtained approximately 14 days after the initiation of 3+7. If the marrow shows less than 10% blasts or is hypocellular, marrows are repeated, usually weekly, until it is clear that either a CR has occurred or that there has been a reappearance of AML, often best assessed using MPFC, which can distinguish an excess of normal blasts often seen during marrow recovery from chemotherapy from an excess of AML blasts.

Retreatment usually takes the form of either another course of 3+7, the administration of high dose ara-C, or of an investigational salvage regimen. SWOG data indicate a CR rate of 10% with a second course of 3+7, which compares favorably with previous investigational *salvage* regimens.[29,30] Furthermore, the SWOG analysis could not identify patients more or less likely to respond to a second 3+7 course.[29,30]

Two randomized trials have shown that a daily daunorubicin dose of 90 mg/m² in 3+7 is superior to a daily dose of 45 mg/m² in patients up to age 65 years, particularly in patients with CBF AML.[31,32] A French retrospective study suggested that 90 mg/m² might be superior to 60 mg/m² in patients with CBF AML.[33] The MRC/NCRI in the United Kingdom is currently randomizing patients between these two doses. Although a French trial suggests that idarubicin at 12 mg/m² daily for 3 days is superior to daunorubicin at 80 mg/m² daily for 3 days,[34] there have often been greater differences between separate randomized trials examining this issue than between daunorubicin and idarubicin in a given study. As a result, there is a consensus that these drugs are interchangeable in 3+7, with idarubicin (12 mg/m² daily, days 1 through 3) and daunorubicin (60 mg/m² daily, days 1 through 3) used most frequently.

The ara-C dose to be used during induction has also been the subject of debate.[35] The HOVON/SAKK group randomized 431 adults age <60 years to ara-C at a daily dose 200 mg/m² for 7 days (previously shown equivalent to 100 mg/m² daily for 7 days[36]) during cycle 1 of induction therapy and 1 g/m² twice daily on days 1 through 5 during cycle 2 of induction therapy and 429 similar patients to 1 g/m² every 12 hours on days 1 through 6 in cycle 1 and 2 g/m² twice daily on days 1, 2, 4, and 6 in cycle 2. Idarubicin 12 mg/m² daily for 3 days was given during cycle 1 and amsacrine, analogous to idarubicin/daunorubicin, was given during cycle 2.[5] Subsequently, patients with CBF AML in remission received 1 cycle of mitoxantrone + etoposide, whereas patients with other cytogenetic findings received an autologous or allogeneic transplant. With a median follow-up of 5 years, there was no difference between the two regimens in CR rate (80% to 82%) and, at 5 years, the cumulative incidences of relapse, relapse-free survival, event-free survival (34% to 35%), and overall survival (40% to 42%) were similar between the two regimens. Furthermore, there was no suggestion that any cytogenetic group benefited more from the higher dose ara-C regimen; in particular, 5-year survival rates were 64% to 67% in patients with CBF AML. The latter results seem equivalent to those using ara-C doses of 3 g/m² twice daily on days 1, 3, and 5 during postremission therapy as is often done in the United States. Othus et al. have recently not found an advantage in patients with NC-AML who were NPM+/FLT3 ITD negative according to whether they received during induction standard 3+7 (in SWOG) or idarubicin + ara-C at 1.5 g/m² daily for 3 to 4 days (at MDACC). Both groups received intermediate (1 g/m² per dose) and high (2 to 3 g/m² per dose) doses during postremission therapy.[37] The HOVON and SWOG/M. D. Anderson results seem to indicate that there is no benefit for intermediate- or high-dose ara-C during induction. However, as indicated by a randomized Cancer and Leukemia Group B (CALGB) study, there is a benefit for higher doses of ara-C during postremission therapy after 3+7 induction in CBF AML (3 g/m² twice daily on days 1, 3, and 5 versus 400 mg/m² or, particularly, 100 mg/m² daily for 5 days) or in NC-AML (with the 3 g/m² and 400 mg/m² doses being equivalent and both superior to the 100 mg/m²,[38] although as noted in MRC's AML 15 trial, the 3 g/m² dose can be replaced by 1.5 g/m².[39]

The duration of postremission therapy is also uncertain, although it seems that between two (based on HOVON data[5]) and four cycles (based on MRC/NCRI data[39]) are sufficient. It is likely that determinations of MRD (e.g., using PCR in CBF and NPM+/FLT3 ITD–negative AML[40,41]) will be important here. For example, in patients with CBF, AML MRC/NCRI randomized data suggest that a fifth cycle might be useful in patients who are MRD negative after the fourth cycle, but not in patients who are MRD positive after the fourth cycle. Patients who are MRD positive after the completion of planned postremission therapy might be candidates for further therapy. Given their low risk of relapse relative to the risk of nonrelapse mortality following allogeneic HSCT, a general consensus is that the average patient with CBF, NPM+/FLT3 ITD–negative AML, or CEBPA+ AML is not a candidate for HSCT in CR1,[42] although recent data suggest that HSCT is indicated in patients with double CEBPA mutations.[43]

There are clearly patients in the best prognosis group who have worse prognoses than the averages reported on trials. These include CBF AML patients age 60 to 65 years,[19] and those with high levels of mutant CKIT alleles.[19] Reduced-intensity HSCT is an alternative in the former. A randomized American–German trial is examining dasatinib in CBF AML based on the drug's ability to inhibit CKIT, which is mutated in 20% to 25% of these patients and overexpressed in others.[44] Finally, meta-analyses of several trials randomizing patients to 3+7+/− gemtuzumab ozogamicin (GO) 3 to 6 mg/m² once during remission induction have indicated unequivocal survival benefit due to a lower incidence of relapse in patients with CBF (and many with NC-AML) leading to attempts to reintroduce this drug into clinical practice.[45,46] Fludarabine as given in FLAG-ida therapy also appears to be useful as induction and postremission therapy in CBF AML.[39]

European Leukemia Net Intermediate 2 and Worst Prognosis Groups

Even patients age <60 years in the intermediate 2 group have 5-year survival rates of only 20% to 25% and median survivals of less than 2 years, recalling that the ELN prognostic system does not account for the unfavorable effect of secondary AML.[22] Hence, these patients, particularly those in the worst group, are considered prime candidates for clinical trials.[22] Although it is not unreasonable to use 3+7 for induction and to begin the trial once in CR, it is noteworthy that differences in induction therapy can affect relapse[45–47] and, accordingly, survival rates; furthermore, CR rates in the worst groups are generally <50%.[27] Here, we will describe therapies that, although not likely better than standard, are in common clinical use.

Dose Intensification

Generally, intensification of an ara-C dose (e.g., to 3 g/m² every 12 hours on days 1, 3, and 5) during postremission therapy has not improved outcomes in intermediate 2 or the worst patients,[38] or if improving it "statistically," it has improved it only minimally (e.g., $p = 0.02$, but from zero to only 13% 5-year survival in the HOVON trial).[5]

Clofarabine, Cladribine, and Fludarabine

The MRC/NCRI group has conducted two randomized trials involving clofarabine. Older patients considered fit for intensive therapy had similar outcomes whether given clofarabine + daunorubicin or daunorubicin + 10 days of standard dose ara-C.[48] Older patients not considered fit for intensive therapy had higher CR rates but similar survival when given clofarabine rather than low-dose ara-C.[49] A multicenter trial randomizing patients with relapsed AML also found higher CR rates but similar survival with clofarabine + high-dose ara C compared with high-dose ara-C alone, largely due to more TRM in the clofarabine arm.[50] The Polish Acute Leukemia Group reported longer survival in adults age <60 years with either de novo or secondary AML randomized to daunorubicin, ara-C (DA) + cladribine (DAC) rather than to standard induction DA.[4] In contrast, a randomized MRC/NCRI trial in adult patients age <60 years found that FLAG-ida given for induction and one postremission course was associated with longer event-free survival

and fewer relapses than daunorubicin + ara-C, although survival was similar due to more deaths in CR with FLAG-ida.[39]

Azacitidine and Decitabine

The majority of patients in the intermediate 2 and worst prognostic groups are aged >65 years. It is in these groups that azacitidine and decitabine have found greatest use. It is becoming apparent that results with these drugs used alone rival those with more intense therapies, at least in older patients. For example, Quintas-Cardama et al.[51] found similar overall survival (OS) among 557 patients aged >65 years given regimens generally containing ara-C at 1 to 2 g/m² daily and idarubicin or fludarabine +/− other agents and 114 patients given decitabine (n = 67) or azacitidine (n = 57) despite higher CR rates with the more intense therapies.[51] An international study randomizing 485 patients age >65 years, one-third of whom had the worst prognosis cytogenetics and one-third of whom had secondary AML, found median survivals of 7.7 months for decitabine at 20 mg/m² daily for 5 days versus 5.0 months for standard treatment (88% low-dose ara-C, 12% supportive care only).[52] A focus on whether the difference is statistically significant (p = 0.037) loses sight of the unsatisfactory results in both arms, with patients losing >90% of their normally remaining life expectancy. An analogous trial involving azacitidine leads to the same conclusion.[53] Thus, a fundamental question is whether results with either drug can be improved. One possibility is identifying patients more likely to respond either based on molecular characteristics or less active disease. Examples of the latter are patients in CR, although use of decitabine to delay relapse appears to have been unsuccessful,[54] or patients with MRD after HSCT.[55] A second possibility is combination with other active drugs. A combination of decitabine with deoxyguanosine (SGI-110) increases exposure to decitabine but has not obviously improved outcomes to date.[56] More fundamentally, it remains unclear whether azacitidine or decitabine, although known as hypomethylating agents, actually exert their effects via hypomethylation.[57]

Gemtuzumab Ozogamicin

In contrast to its utility in patients with CBF AML, meta-analyses have not indicated a role for this drug in combination in ELN intermediate 2 and the worst prognosis patients.[45]

Hematopoietic Stem Cell Transplantation

It is generally recommended that patients in ELN intermediate 2 or the worst prognosis groups receive HSCT in CR1 as detailed in the transplant section that follows.

ELN Intermediate 1 Prognosis Group

Here, the decision between the relatively standard approaches discussed for the favorable group and the emphasis on clinical trials stressed in the last section is more difficult. It is perhaps, at times, best to defer this decision to the patient; experience suggests that given the same prognostic data following use of standard therapies, some patients will prefer these, whereas others prefer a trial. Here, the need for new prognostic information is most acute and there might be great use in incorporating posttreatment information into the decision; examples include time or courses to CR,[58] achievement of CRp/CRi rather than CR,[24] or MRD measured by MPFC[20] or PCR for NPM1[41] or WT1.[59] The use of FLAG-ida might be considered because its ability to decrease high relapse rates relative to CBF AML, might justify the increased incidence of death in CR associated with its use.[39] Transplantation in CR1 is often suggested, although it is possible that, provided CR rates after relapse are in the 50% range (much more likely than in the ELN intermediate 2 and the worst groups), a strategy of delaying HSCT until the second CR may be reasonable.[60]

Although their prognosis is, on average, worse than others in the ELN intermediate 1 group, patients with *FLT3* ITDs are currently included in this group (see Table 43.2). They often present with a high WBC count, usually have NC-AML, although t(6;9) AML is very specific for *FLT3* ITDs, and, although having CR rates similar to others with NC-AML, are prone to relapse.[61] The abnormal tyrosine kinase activity associated with *FLT3* ITDs can be inhibited by various drugs (tyrosine-kinase inhibitors [TKI]). Used alone, *FLT3* inhibitors have limited activity in relapsed/refractory AML, with quizartinib being the most effective, producing *composite CR* rates of about 50%, with >90% of the responses being CRi rather than CR or CRp. However, this response rate has allowed 25% to 35% of patients given quizartinib to subsequently receive HSCT.[62] It is uncertain whether the failure of count recovery, and hence, the lack of CRs reflects concomitant quizartinib-induced inhibition of *CKIT* or the presence of other aberrations in the blasts that are not affected by *FLT3* inhibitors. However, the latter possibility has motivated the addition of chemotherapy to quizartinib.[63] Sorafenib, a commercially available *FLT3* inhibitor, has been combined with 3+7 and compared with 3+7 alone in two randomized studies. In patients aged >60 years the combination produced only increased toxicity,[64] but in younger patients, it was associated with longer event-free but not overall survival. In neither study were effects different in patients with or without *FLT3* ITDs,[65] indicating that sorafenib's relevant mechanism of action may be independent of *FLT3* inhibition and perhaps prefiguring a more general use of chemotherapy–sorafenib combinations. Even quizartinib, presumed to be a much more selective *FLT3* inhibitor than sorafenib, may also have activity in patients without *FLT3* ITDs.[62] As predicted by various genomic studies, resistance to quizartinib is associated with the emergence of new subclones: In the case of quizartinib these contain *FLT3* point mutations whose abnormal TK activity might be decreased by crenolanib, another *FLT3* inhibitor.[66] Although it is generally accepted that patients with FLT3 ITDs should receive HSCT in CR1, *FLT3* ITDs predict for relapse even after HSCT. Accordingly, another potential role for quizartinib, and by extension other targeted agents, is the prevention of relapse after HSCT or even in patients who cannot receive HSCT.

Summary of Treatment Recommendations

Patients with favorable prognoses as specified by the ELN[22] can be treated with standard therapy emphasizing higher doses of ara-C post-CR (HiDAC), although it remains unknown if the same is true in patients considered at best risk based on *NPM1+/ FLT3* ITD–status rather than cytogenetics. Older patients with CBF AML and CBF patients with multiple alleles affected by *CKIT* mutations have worse prognoses than average CBF and thus might be candidates for (reduced intensity) HSCT or for clinical trials with dasatinib. The choice of 3+7 rather than a clinical trial for induction in the ELN intermediate 1 group depends on whether patients see their prognosis with the former as good enough to be reluctant to undertake a clinical trial, which might produce a worse outcome. FLAG-ida might be useful as induction and postremission therapy in the intermediate 1 and CBF groups and the availability of gemtuzumab ozogamicin (GO) as part of induction therapy would be useful because the drug clearly prolongs survival in CBF and in many intermediate 1 patients.[16] In contrast, CR rates are often <50% in the ELN intermediate 2 and adverse groups with standard therapy making a clinical trial particularly important, recalling that the choice of induction therapy can affect the relapse rate. The general consensus is that patients in the intermediate 1, 2, and adverse groups should receive HSCT in the first CR. Results with HSCT are still sufficiently poor that clinical trials involving new transplant preparative regimens or the means to prevent post-HSCT relapse should be considered in these groups, as discussed later in this chapter. Given that many older patients will fall into the intermediate 2 or the worst ELN prognostic categories and have particularly poor outcomes with standard therapy, most such patients are candidates for clinical trials, as suggested by both ELN[22] and National Comprehensive Cancer Network (NCCN)[67] guidelines. It is important to recall that the major cause of treatment failure in older patients is resistance to therapy, not TRM. Thus, the use of less intense therapy is appropriate only if the chosen therapy is plausibly more effective, and not merely less toxic, than standard therapy. These recommendations are summarized in Table 43.3. Regardless of specific recommendations, any choice of therapy in older patients must refer to the observations of Sekeres et al.[68] that 74% of older patients estimated that their chances of cure with 3+7 were at least 50%; in contrast, 85% of their physicians estimated this chance to be less than 10%. Although the most plausible cause of this discrepancy is a patient's natural tendency to hope for a favorable outcome, there may also be gaps in communication between physicians and patients.

Acute Promyelocytic Leukemia

Acute promyelocytic leukemia (APL) has a unique pathophysiology and requires special considerations for treatment. In more than 95% of cases, APL results from a chromosomal translocation, t(15;17). This translocation results in a fusion protein

TABLE 43.3

Treatment Recommendations According to European Leukemia Net Prognostic Group

ELN Group (see Table 43.2)	Induction	Postremission	Other Considerations
Best	3+7; consider FLAG-ida if CBF	1 cycle of idarubicin + ara-C 1g/m² BID × 5 days; then 1–3 cycles with ara-C as above; consider 1 cycle FLAG-ida particularly if CBF	(a) Dose reductions if treatment-related mortality (TRM) scores > 10–20 and clinical trials if TRM scores > 20; (b) Reduced-intensity HSCT for older CBF patients or those with high levels of CKIT mutation; (c) Trials of dasatinib for the latter
Intermediate 1	3+7, FLAG-ida, or clinical trial	If high level FLT3 ITD HSCT in CR1 using related donor or unrelated donor; if not, using related donor or postremission therapy as in ELN best group	If high level FLT3 ITD (a) clinical trial combining 3+7 and newer FLT3 inhibitors quizartinib, crenolanib, or (b) 3+7 + sorafenib if age <60 years
Intermediate 2 or worst	Clinical trial	HSCT in CR1 using related or unrelated donors	(a) Trials testing means to decrease relapse post-HSCT (b) Supportive care only if TRM score > 20–30

PML/retinoic acid receptor alpha (RARα), the gene for *PML* being located on chromosome 15 and the gene for *RARα* on chromosome 17. The PML-RARα protein, an aberrant form of the normal RAR, recruits corepressor complexes that inhibit transcription of genes involved in promyelocytic differentiation.[69] Predictors of APL in patients with AML are younger age, Hispanic ethnicity, and obesity.[70] Although it typically has a distinctive morphology characterized by abnormal granules and multiple Auer rods, a microgranular variant exists. The possibility of this variant must be borne in mind in patients who present without morphologically typical APL but with the coagulopathy that is the clinical hallmark of the disease. The diagnosis of APL requires proof of the PML-RARα rearrangement. Although this can be obtained by demonstration of the presence of t(15;17), at least 2 to 3 days are required for test results. Immediate confirmation of the diagnosis can be made by using immunohistochemistry to demonstrate an abnormal pattern of anti-PML antibody nuclear staining consequent to the formation of PML-RARα (the PML oncogenic domains test). If doubt remains about the diagnosis, all-transretinoic acid (ATRA) should be added to 3+7.[69]

APL is very sensitive to daunorubicin or idarubicin and is uniquely sensitive to ATRA and arsenic trioxide. The responsiveness to the anthracyclines may reflect the absence of multidrug resistance gene (*MDR1*) in APL cells,[71] whereas pharmacologic doses of ATRA release corepressor complexes and lead to degradation of PML-RARα.[69] For many years, the initial treatment of APL has consisted of idarubicin 12 mg/m^2 daily for 4 to 5 days and ATRA 45 mg/m^2 until CR (AIDA regimen).[69] Use of transfusions to maintain the platelet count above 30,000/μL, serum fibrinogen above 150 mg/mL, and the international normalized ratio (INR) below 1.5 is mandatory. Ten percent to 25% of patients will develop the APL differentiation syndrome (APLDS) characterized by fever, weight gain/edema, pleural effusions, and pulmonary infiltrates; the WBC is often elevated. Steroids (e.g., methylprednisolone 45 mg intravenous (IV) daily with subsequent tapering) are effective for the treatment of APLDS. The principal prognostic factor in untreated APL is initial WBC. Patients with WBC less than 10,000/μL will have CR rates greater than 90% with idarubicin plus ATRA, whereas patients with higher WBC counts will have CR rates of 80% to 85%. Almost all patients who fail to achieve CR die, which is usually related to bleeding in the brain or lung before treatment begins or in the first few days thereafter. Once in CR, patients typically receive three courses of consolidation with idarubicin 12 mg/m^2 daily for 3 days and ATRA 45 mg/m^2 daily on a 2-week on, 2-week off basis. With this treatment, at least 90% of patients should test negative using PCR to detect residual PML-RARα transcripts after completion of consolidation therapy; patients who are not have a 50% chance of relapse versus 5% for patients who are PCR negative. The former should receive arsenic trioxide (ATO) with or without GO[72] and an allogeneic stem cell transplant if these measures do not produce PCR negativity. Although many protocols omit ara-C, allowing for the administration of higher doses of idarubicin or daunorubicin, a French trial found superior results in patients randomized to receive ara-C in addition to ATRA and daunorubicin.[73] It has been suggested, however, that this outcome reflected the use of relatively low doses of daunorubicin.

Recent developments have highlighted the use of ATO for newly diagnosed rather than purely for relapsed APL. The use of ATO during consolidation in patients treated with AIDA has largely obviated the need for maintenance therapy.[74] After demonstration by Estey et al.[75] that ATRA + ATO could be used without the addition of chemotherapy to cure patients presenting with WBC <10,000/μL, LoCoco et al.[75] randomized patients age less than 70 years old with WBC <10,000/μL between ATRA/idarubicin (AIDA) as conventionally given and ATO/ATRA as described by Estey et al.[75] With a median follow-up of 34 months, 2-year event-free survival was 87% with AIDA and 96% with ATO + ATRA ($p = 0.02$ for superiority) and 2-year survival was also better with ATO + ATRA ($p = 0.02$).[76] Fever, prolonged myelosuppression, and early deaths were more common with AIDA and clinically insignificant hepatotoxicity with ATO + ATRA. It is likely that ATO + ATRA will become the new standard for treatment of APL with WBC <10,000/μL. The relapse rate appears so low that there is probably no need to routinely monitor patients with PCR testing. Similarly, Australasian Leukemia Study Group data suggest that the addition of ATO to AIDA induction will improve outcomes in patients presenting with WBC >10,000/μL.[77] In these patients, however, PCR monitoring in CR probably remains necessary for 2 years. Attention in APL currently focuses on the discrepancy between results, such as those described previously, in academic centers and the poorer results noted in population-based studies[78]; it has been proposed that the initiation of ATRA upon suspicion of a diagnosis of APL might reduce this discrepancy.[78]

Salvage Therapy

Salvage therapy refers to treatment given for relapsed AML or AML that has never gone into CR (primary refractory). As usual, it is critical to assess a patient's chance for success following the administration of standard salvage therapy, using regimens such as FLAG + ida or mitoxantrone + etoposide + ara-C (2 g/m^2 daily for 5 days) (MEC). A principal predictor of response to first salvage therapy is the duration of first remission; this has been true even when the therapy used for salvage contained no drugs used initially. As is often the case, consideration of several covariates to assess prognosis is useful.[79] Data presented in the section on transplantation suggest that HSCT should be the first option for such patients, although the possibility of selection bias contributing to results with HSCT needs to be kept in mind. There is also uncertainty as to whether those patients in whom a donor is available should receive investigational chemotherapy before HSCT. If HSCT is unavailable or while a search for a donor is ongoing, patients should receive investigational treatments, including or not including conventional agents.

Hematopoietic Stem Cell Transplantation for Acute Myelogenous Leukemia

Stem cell transplantation provides the possibility of cure for a significant fraction of patients with AML. The approach utilizes a preparative regimen of chemotherapy or radiation with the goal of eradicating the leukemia and providing sufficient immunosuppression of the recipient to prevent rejection of the transplant. There is also an allogeneic graft-versus-leukemia (GVL) effect in which donor T and NK cells act to eradicate malignant cells that survive the preparative regimen.[80] Autologous transplants can be done. Patients initially have their own hematopoietic cells collected and cryopreserved; these cells are then reinfused after high-dose therapy to restore hematopoiesis. Improvements in supportive care, histocompatibility, and tissue matching and development of less toxic preparative regimens have all increased the likelihood of success with autologous or allogeneic transplantation. This section reviews the role of HSCT in the treatment of AML in adults.

Prognostic Factors and Indications for Transplant

Outcomes of HSCT are improved if the transplant is performed earlier in the disease course, preferably in CR, due to less chemo refractoriness and the lower likelihood of infections or chemotherapy-related side effects. The major prognosticator is disease status at transplant (Fig. 43.1). Prognostics of patients in CR are significantly better than for those with active disease at the time of HSCT. Similarly, most of the covariates discussed in the previous paragraphs retain their influence in the setting of HSCT, such as cytogenetics and FLT3 mutational status (Fig. 43.2).[81] Secondary

Figure 43.1 Disease status at transplantation is the major determinant of survival after allogeneic hematopoietic stem cell transplantation (HSCT) for acute myelogenous leukemia (AML). Leukemia-free survival (LFS) of 773 AML patients (379 were in first complete remission and 394 had active disease at HSCT) who underwent first allogeneic HSCT using matched related, matched unrelated, and mismatched donors between 2001 through 2012. Three-year LFS were 52.2% and 15.6% for CR1 and active disease patients, respectively. (Data courtesy of Dr. Betul Oran.)

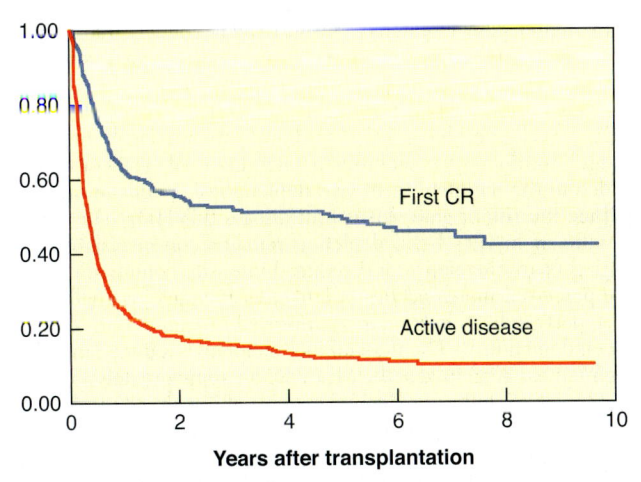

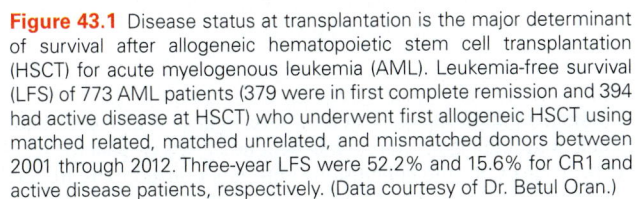

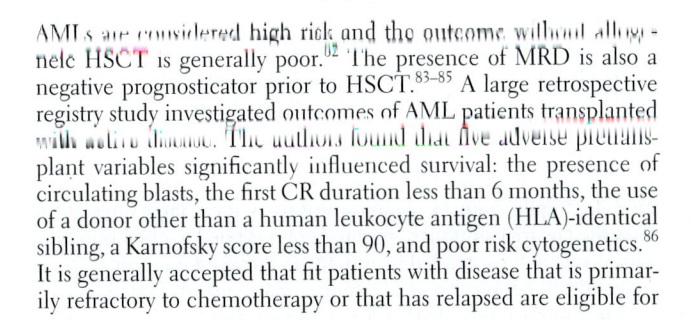

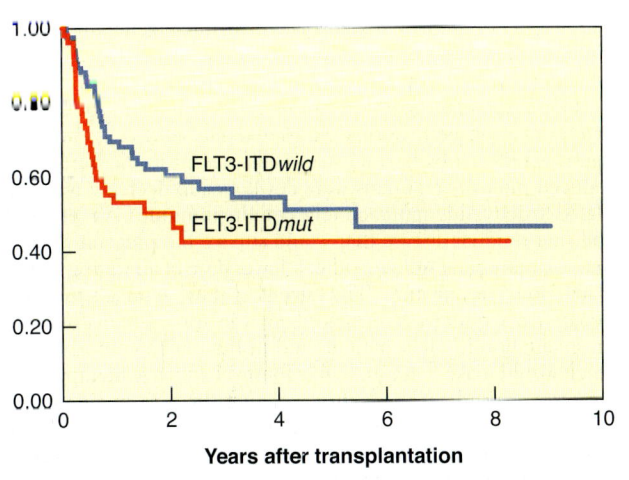

Figure 43.2 The influence of FLT3-ITD mutational status on survival is illustrated here. Leukemia-free survival of 227 AML patients that underwent first allogeneic hematopoietic stem cell transplantation (HSCT) in first complete remission and FLT3-ITD mutation at diagnosis were evaluable. Donors included matched related, matched unrelated, and mismatched. Three-year LFS after HSCT were 56.9% and 42.6% for patient with FLT3-ITDwild and FLT3-ITDmut at diagnosis, respectively. (Data courtesy of Dr. Betul Oran.)

AMLs are considered high risk and the outcome without allogeneic HSCT is generally poor.[82] The presence of MRD is also a negative prognosticator prior to HSCT.[83–85] A large retrospective registry study investigated outcomes of AML patients transplanted with active disease. The authors found that five adverse pretransplant variables significantly influenced survival: the presence of circulating blasts, the first CR duration less than 6 months, the use of a donor other than a human leukocyte antigen (HLA)-identical sibling, a Karnofsky score less than 90, and poor risk cytogenetics.[86] It is generally accepted that fit patients with disease that is primarily refractory to chemotherapy or that has relapsed are eligible for allogeneic or autologous HSCT, as will be discussed. There is, however, controversy surrounding HSCT in first CR. Table 43.4 lists indications for allogeneic HSCT in AML.

Preparative Regimens and Regimen Intensity

The preparative regimen (chemotherapy with or without radiation therapy that precedes the infusion of hematopoietic progenitor cells) provides treatment for AML and the necessary immunosuppression to prevent graft rejection of an allogeneic transplant. Preparative regimens may be chemotherapy or total body irra-

TABLE 43.4
Indications for Allogeneic Transplant in Acute Myelogenous Leukemia

Disease Stage	Cytogenetics[a]	Mutations
First remission	Diploid: presence of mutations may dictate decision to transplant	FLT3 ITD FLT3 TKD NPM with FLT3 or ERG mutation MLL PTD Overexpression of BAALC Overexpression of ERG
First remission	Complex; del 5, del 7	
First remission, age > 50–55 years	Diploid cytogenetics: controversial	
First remission, therapy-related or secondary disease[b]	All eligible	All eligible
Primary induction failure	All eligible	All eligible
Second or subsequent remission	All eligible	All eligible
Relapsed, active disease	All eligible	All eligible

ITD, internal tandem duplication; NPM, nucleophosmin; ETS-related gene; FLT3, FMS-like tyrosine kinase 3; TDK, tyrosine-kinase domain.
[a] There is variability in the definition of high-risk cytogenetics depending on the classification used. There is also some controversy surrounding the influence of chromosomal abnormalities involving the MLL gene located at 11q23, such as in t(9;11), t(6;11), and t(11;19). Some authors will classify patients with these abnormalities as intermediate-risk disease, as opposed to granting them high-risk status. Presence of 9q and 11q abnormalities may also place patients in first complete remission in a higher than desired risk of relapse.
[b] Secondary disease: preceding myelodysplastic syndrome or chemo- or radiation-therapy induced.

diation (TBI) based. A myeloablative regimen generally causes cessation of normal marrow function to a degree that requires autologous or allogeneic hematopoietic cell transplant. Hematopoietic transplantation allows for the use of stem cell toxic agents, which eradicate both normal and leukemic stem cells; hematopoiesis is restored by normal stem cells present in the transplant. Reduced intensity regimens were developed to decrease regimen related toxicity; this approach relies on the immune GVL effect to eradicate residual disease that would survive the preparative regimen. Conditioning utilizes either a lower dose of alkylating agents or low doses of radiation. The advent of these reduced intensity preparative regimens has allowed for the use of hematopoietic transplantation in older patients and in those with comorbidities, which would make them ineligible for myeloablative therapy. This has been an important advance, because the peak incidence of AML is in the 6th and 7th decades of life. Still, there is controversy regarding which patients should receive myeloablative versus reduced-intensity preparative regimens. The safety of myeloablative regimens is improving, and their use for *fit* patients aged 55 to 65 years is now an attainable goal. Randomized clinical trials will be necessary to resolve this question of regimen choice and intensity. It is recommended that older patients with AML be treated within clinical trials.

Myeloablative Regimens. The most commonly used myeloablative regimens are cyclophosphamide-TBI (Cy-TBI),[87] busulfan-cyclophosphamide (BuCy),[88] and, more recently, busulfan and fludarabine.[89] The development of BuCy as an alternative to TBI-containing regimens led to ongoing debates as to which conditioning regimen is the best for the treatment of myeloid leukemia with HSCT. Two randomized studies were performed. The Nordic group compared Cy-TBI to BuCy in a heterogeneous group of patients with AML, lymphoid malignancies, and CML receiving allogeneic HSCT.[90] Results indicated improved Disease free survival (DFS) among advanced stage disease patients treated with Cy-TBI, along with an increased rate of long-term complications for recipients of BuCy. Similarly, Blaise et al.[91] studied young patients with AML in first CRs and concluded that Cy-TBI and allogeneic HSCT produced better disease-free and overall survival than BuCy. The major pitfall of these reports is the use of the oral busulfan formulation, which results in unpredictable plasma levels. The Center for International Bone Marrow Transplant Research (CIBMTR) compared the use of oral or intravenous (IV) BuCy and Cy-TBI in 1,230 AML patients who received allogeneic transplantation in first remission. There was less nonrelapse mortality and relapse 1 year after transplant, and improved leukemia free survival (LFS) in recipients of IV busulfan compared to TBI regimens.[92] A prospective cohort study tested the hypothesis of noninferiority of survival after IV busulfan ablative regimens, compared to TBI-based regimens for myeloid leukemia patients (n = 1,025 versus n = 458, respectively). Two-year probability of survival was better after IV busulfan treatment (56% versus 48%; $p = 0.03$).[93] Another retrospective registry analysis performed with the European Cooperative Group for Bone Marrow Transplantation (EBMT) database found IV BuCy to lead to similar outcomes to CyTBI for the treatment of AML in first CRs.[94] Exchanging cyclophosphamide for the nucleoside analog fludarabine may increase the safety margin of the regimen.[95] Fludarabine appears to increase alkylator-induced cell killing by inhibiting DNA-damage repair and is highly immunosuppressive. A preparative regimen using fludarabine and single daily dosing of IV busulfan has been studied in multiple centers and appears to be effective and potentially less toxic than the commonly used BuCy regimen.

Reduced Intensity Conditioning Regimens. Given the relative insensitivity of AML to the GVL effect, chemotherapy or radiation intensity is an important component of HSCT. There is a trade-off between nonrelapse mortality (NRM) and dose intensity, which may negate the decrease in relapse rates associated with higher dose regimens. The CIBMTR collects information on most transplants performed in North America. The most commonly used reduced-intensity regimens (for all indications) as reported to the CIBMTR are fludarabine combined with low-dose TBI,[96] cyclophosphamide,[97] busulfan,[98] melphalan,[99] or other drugs. Antithymocyte globulin or alemtuzumab are commonly added to the regimen for in vivo depletion of T cells in order to reduce the risk of graft versus host disease (GVHD). The use of in vitro or in vivo T-cell depletion remains controversial in the setting of myeloablative and reduced-intensity conditioning, but the perceived increased risk of leukemia relapse[100] is challenged by reports indicating similar or improved outcomes with ex vivo T-cell depletion.[101] The fludarabine–melphalan reduced-intensity regimen has been used at the MDACC for approximately 15 years, and long-term follow-up demonstrates its ability to induce durable disease control in a significant fraction of AML patients.[102] Likewise, the Seattle group experience of treating AML in first CRs (median age of 59 years) with a nonmyeloablative, low-dose TBI-based regimen achieved a low TRM rate.[103]

Transplants for AML in First Complete Remission. Although multiple phase 2 studies have indicated that both allogeneic and autologous transplants benefit subsets of patients with AML in first CRs, the conclusions from randomized trials are less clear.[104–107] The majority of studies indicate that allogeneic and autologous transplants are associated with lower relapse rates but also with higher mortality rates in CR (especially allogeneic HSCT). Nonrelapse mortality (death of all causes for patients in CRs) traditionally has reduced the benefit of less relapses after allogeneic HSCT, and most randomized studies did not show statistically significant advantage in survival (Table 43.5). The debate is far from resolved, given that newer preparative regimens (as discussed previously) and improvements in supportive care are reducing nonrelapse mortality significantly. A common feature of these large clinical trials is the fact that, although most patients assigned to chemotherapy will complete the intended treatment, a significant minority of those assigned will not receive an allogeneic or autologous HSCT.

Most studies indicate that the use of consolidation chemotherapy prior to myeloablative or reduced intensity allogeneic HSCT in first remission does not influence survival after transplant.[108] In the autologous HSCT setting, however, another retrospective registry analysis concluded that consolidation may improve transplant outcomes. Leukemia-free and overall survival rates were improved for those who received consolidation, but the number of consolidation cycles (one versus two) and the cytarabine dose did not significantly affect transplantation outcomes.[109]

The European Organization of Research and Treatment of Cancer—Leukemia Group/ Gruppo Italiano Malattie EMatologiche dell'Adulto (EORTC-LG/GIMEMA) AML-10 trial set out to compare autologous and allogeneic HSCT for patients in first CRs.[107] After one course of consolidation chemotherapy, patients younger than 46 years with an HLA-identical sibling donor were assigned to undergo allogeneic HSCT, whereas all others were to undergo autologous HSCT. In the donor group, 68.9% received an allogeneic HSCT, whereas in the no-donor subset, an autologous transplant was performed in 55.8% of those eligible. DFS was improved in the former group, whereas the death rate in first CR was decreased in the latter (17.4% versus 5.3%). OS was similar, but DFS was improved for patients with poor prognosis cytogenetics after allogeneic HSCT, especially for patients aged 15 to 35 years. Instead, however, the MRC study indicated an advantage in survival for allogeneic transplanted recipients with intermediate-risk disease.[105] In both the EORTC/GIMENA AML-8 and the MRC AML-10 trials, the relapse-free survival was improved with autologous HSCT when compared to chemotherapy alone, without an OS benefit. The likelihood of achieving another remission after relapse was higher in the chemotherapy arms, which led to the similar survival.

TABLE 43.5
Acute Myeloid Leukemia in First Complete Remission: Studies Comparing Allogeneic and Autologous Hematopoietic Stem Cell Transplantation to Chemotherapy

Clinical Study/Type (Ref.)	No. of Patients and Age	Treatment Assignment	Proportion Completing Assigned Treatment	Risk of Relapse	Actuarial Progression-Free Survival	Preparative Regimen	Treatment-related Mortality	Actuarial Survival
United Kingdom Medical Research Council Acute Myeloid Leukemia 10 trial Prospective, genetic randomization[252]	N = 1,602 in CR1 <56 years Tissue typed = n = 1,063	Donor n = 419 No donor n = 868	61% (n = 257) (allogeneic HSCT) 93% (chemotherapy) 66% (autologous HSCT)	Donor vs. no donor 36% vs. 52% (p = 0.001) Auto vs. chemo only 37% vs. 58% (p = 0.0007)	Benefit for allogeneic HSCT in intermediate risk cytogenetics 51% vs. 39% (p = 0.004)	Cy-TBI for both autologous and allogeneic HSCT (BuCy in 43 patients)	Donor: allogeneic = 24% Chemo = 11% No donor: autologous[a] = 12% Chemo = 8%	Donor × no donor 55% × 50% (p = 0.1) Benefit for allogeneic HSCT in intermediate risk cytogenetics 55% × 44% (p = 0.02) Autologous × chemo 7-year: 57% × 45% (p = 0.2)
The European Organisation for Research and Treatment of Cancer Leukemia Group and Gruppo Italiano Malattie Ematologiche dell' Adulto (EORTC-LG/GIMEMA) Prospective, genetic randomization[107]	N = 734 in CR1 that received a single intensive consolidation chemotherapy <46 years	Donor n = 293 No donor n = 441	55.8% (autologous HSCT) 68.9% (allogeneic HSCT)	Donor vs. no donor 30% vs. 52% (p <0.0001) Poor risk cytogenetics:43% vs. 18% (p = NS)	4-year donor vs. no donor 52% vs. 42% (p = 0.44)	Cy-TBI or BuCy	Death in CR1: Donor × no donor 17% × 5% (p <0.0001)	Donor × no donor 58% × 51% (p = 0.18)
Dutch-Belgian Hemato-Oncology Cooperative Group (HOVON) and the Swiss Group for Cancer Research (SAKK) Retrospective analysis of three prospective studies conducted from 1987 to 2004. Genetic randomization[111]	N = 1,032 patients in CR after two chemotherapy cycles Consolidation: either third cycle of chemotherapy, auto or allo-HSCT Age <55 years Median follow-up from diagnosis is 63 months	Donor n = 326 patients (32%) No donor n = 706 (68%)	82% (n = 268) (allogeneic HSCT) 28% (n = 165) (autologous HSCT) No donor group: 8% received allogeneic HSCT from other donors, 65% went to receive a 3rd chemo cycle	Donor vs. no donor 32% vs. 59% (p <0.001) Reduction in risk of relapse was observed in all cytogenetics categories, including poor risk group	Donor vs. no donor 48% vs. 27%, HR 0.7, 95% CI, 0.55–0.84 (p <.001) Improved DFS was observed in all cytogenetics categories, but was only significant in the intermediate and poor risk groups Age ≤40 years (HR 0.59, 95% CI, 0.46–0.77; p <0.001) Age >40 years: HR 0.83, 95% CI, 0.64–1.07; p = NS)	BuCy	Death in CR1: Donor × no donor 21% × 4% (p <0.001)	Donor × no donor 4-year survival 54% × 45% HR 0.35, CI 0.70–1.03; p = 0.09

NS, not statistically significant; HR, hazard ratio; CI, confidence interval; CR, complete remission; DFS, disease-free survival; HSCT, hematopoietic stem cell transplant; Cy-TB, cyclophosphamide and total-body irradiation; BuCy, busulfan and cyclophosphamide.
[a]Two patients died after unrelated donor transplant.

Jourdan et al.[110] reported the long-term follow-up results of four studies investigating postremission consolidation strategies conducted by the Bordeaux Grenoble Marseille Toulouse (BGMT) cooperative group in Europe. The donor group (i.e., with the HLA-identical sibling) comprised 182 patients (38% of those who had achieved a first CR); allogeneic HSCT was performed in 171 patients (94%). The no-donor group had 290 patients, of which 62% received an autologous HSCT. The intent-to-treat analysis (donor versus no donor) showed a statistically nonsignificant advantage in overall 10-year survival probability of 51% versus 43% for the donor group. Patients were stratified using the covariates WBC count at diagnosis, the FAB subtype, the cytogenetic risk, and the number of induction courses to achieve a CR. An intermediate risk group benefited from allogeneic HSCT, with longer survival, whereas small numbers precluded definitive conclusions in other subgroups.

Cornelissen et al.[111] updated the follow-up and consolidated the results of three consecutive studies sponsored by the Dutch-Belgian Hemato-Oncology Cooperative Group (HOVON) and the Swiss Group for Cancer Research (SAKK) between 1987 and 2004. These studies investigated myeloablative allogeneic HSCT for young patients with AML in first CR, comparing results in patients with a transplant donor identified versus those with no donor who received conventional chemotherapy. Subsets of patients in the no-donor subgroup were eligible to receive autologous HSCT. The initial sample size was 2,287 patients. Patients younger than 55 years, without FAB M3 disease, who achieved a first CR after a maximum of two cycles of chemotherapy and then received consolidation treatment were considered eligible for allogeneic HSCT (n = 1,032, 45% of the cohort). The donor group comprised 326 patients (32%), and the no-donor group comprised 599 patients (58%). In the donor group, 82% went on to an allogeneic transplant. Patients in the donor group had fewer relapses and longer DFS. Patients with a donor younger than 40 years of age and with an intermediate- or poor-risk profile had statistically significantly improved DFS.

It is likely that some subsets of patients in first CR will benefit more from HSCT than others. Patients older than 55 years have an extremely poor outcome with conventional chemotherapy. Historically, they have not been eligible for myeloablative allogeneic transplantation because of concern for toxicities, but this group may benefit from nonmyeloablative allogeneic HSCT. A feasibility study demonstrated a marked improvement in relapse-free survival with nonablative allogeneic transplants in elderly patients with AML in first CR compared to patients without a donor who received standard chemotherapy.[112] The incorporation of comorbidity indexes to estimate NRM risk have contributed to patient selection as well, and the proportion of patients ultimately receiving allogeneic HSCT is increasing, especially in reference centers.[113,114]

High-dose ara-C–containing chemotherapy regimens, on the other hand, have improved the outcome of young patients, particularly for patients with good risk cytogenetics (t[8;21] and inv16); the consensus is to not perform allogeneic HSCT in these patients while in first CR. An HLA-compatible family donor (an HLA-identical sibling or a one-antigen mismatch relative) is available in less than 35% of the cases. Unrelated donor transplants that are HLA matched using high resolution methods for the HLA-A, -B, -C, and -DR loci fare comparably with matched sibling donors.[115] Interestingly, in the unrelated donor setting, it is possible that donor-derived NK cell reactivity could reduce relapse rates. A study of 1,277 patients with AML that received unrelated donor HSCT indicated that the activating KIR2DS1 gene provided an HLA-C–dependent prevention of relapse, whereas the donor KIR3DS1 gene was correlated with reduced mortality. This information may guide donor choice aiming at relapse prevention.[116]

Autologous HSCT has been proposed and extensively investigated as an option for first CR consolidation (see Table 43.5). The role of autologous HSCT in first CR, however, remains controversial. Phase 2 and 3 studies demonstrate that some subgroups of AML patients may benefit from autologous HSCT, with a reduction in relapse and improvement in leukemia-free survival. Patients with unfavorable cytogenetics do not appear to benefit, and allogeneic transplant is their preferred option. AML patients, however, are very often poor mobilizers of stem cells, possibly due to AML and treatment-related changes on the normal stem cell pool. Reinfusion of leukemia stem cells contained in the autologous graft is a possibility, and gene marking studies have demonstrated that malignant cells contained in the autograft may contribute to systemic relapse.[117] *Purging* describes the various ex vivo procedures that have been used to eliminate these residual leukemic cells from the graft.[118] Preclinical studies have suggested that this strategy significantly reduces the number of clonogenic progenitors. Chemotherapeutic agents have been extensively used for ex vivo purging, but none of the purging techniques have been tested in a randomized fashion, and conclusive evidence of a benefit for purged grafts is lacking.

Most studies of autologous HSCT enrolled patients younger than 50 years old. However, autologous HSCT transplants have also been investigated for patients older than 60 years. The EORTC-GIMEMA AML-13 trial proposed the collection of peripheral blood stem cells after induction therapy with mitoxantrone, cytarabine, and etoposide (MICE) with or without G-CSF, and consolidation chemotherapy with idarubicin, cytarabine, and etoposide (mini-ICE). Patients aged 61 to 70 years with good performance status were eligible. Of 61 patients, 54 (88%) had peripheral blood stem cells harvested, but only 35 patients received autologous HSCT (57%). The 3-year disease-free and overall survival rates were 21% and 32%, respectively. The authors considered this a negative study that exemplified the limitations of dose intensification for patients with AML in this age range.[119] An updated analysis of the multicenter European AML96 trial (n = 586 patients) suggested a role for autologous transplants for AML in first CR. Patients were to be consolidated with allogeneic or autologous transplantation, or with chemotherapy. Patient risk was estimated based on age, percentage of CD34-positive blasts, FLT3-ITD mutant–to–wild-type ratio, cytogenetic risk, and de novo or secondary AML. Allogeneic improved survival in the favorable subgroup, and autologous transplants improved survival in the intermediate-risk group.[120] It is possible that new molecularly defined subgroups of AML patients in first CR might benefit from autologous transplantation, but clear recommendations will have to await analysis of larger patient cohorts and/or historic databases and correlative samples.[43]

A meta-analysis of 24 trials comparing chemotherapy to autologous and allogeneic HSCT that involved 6,007 patients (3,638 patients with cytogenetics information), remission-free survival benefit was observed for poor-risk (hazard ratio [HR], 0.69; 95% confidence interval [CI], 0.57 to 0.84) and intermediate-risk AML (HR, 0.76; 95% CI, 0.68 to 0.85) but not for good-risk disease (HR 1.06; 95% CI, 0.80 to 1.42). Similar results were obtained in the OS analysis. Allogeneic HSCT improved survival for poor-risk (HR 0.73; 95% CI, 0.59 to 0.90) and intermediate-risk AML (HR 0.83; 95% CI, 0.74 to 0.93) but not for good-risk AML (HR 1.07; 95% CI, 0.83 to 1.38). The use of autologous HSCT was not associated with improved outcomes.[121] Therefore, considering that TRM has decreased substantially in the context of allogeneic HSCT, this approach is considered in all adult patients up to age 75 years in first CR who do not have good risk cytogenetics if a sibling or a molecularly matched unrelated donor (HLA-A, -B, -C, -DRB1, -DQB1) is available (see Table 43.5). The decision to proceed to HSCT in first CR should take into account disease and patient-related factors, as well as donor source and expected TRM. It has been proposed that allogeneic HSCT should be considered in situations where DFS is expected to be improved by at least 10%.[122]

Transplantation for Acute Myelogenous Leukemia in Relapse and Primary Induction Failure. Outcomes of relapsing AML patients are influenced to a large extent by the duration of the first CR. First remissions shorter than 6 months and failure to achieve a CR with initial therapy (primary induction failure) are associated with a likelihood of CR of less than 10% to 20%. Patients relapsing within the first year of remission that fail to respond to the first salvage attempt are, for practical purposes, incurable with standard chemotherapy regimens. Autologous HSCT has been used to treat relapsed and refractory patients, but with poor results. Allogeneic HSCT is considered the treatment of choice for AML in primary induction failure or beyond the first CR, resulting in long-term disease-free survival in 20% to 40% of patients.[123] Results of allogeneic and autologous HSCT are generally better if performed in the second CR as opposed to during an active relapse. However, results were comparable in patients in early relapse versus second remission if one can proceed promptly with HSCT.[124]

Armistead et al,[125] performed a retrospective review to evaluate all relapsed AML patients treated at MDACC between 1995 and 2004. Median age was 58 years, and 59% of the patients had poor risk cytogenetics. After removing patients who died from their initial salvage therapy or who received a stem cell transplant as their first salvage regimen, the survival outcomes from 490 patients (130 of whom were transplanted) were analyzed. This cohort was divided into the 113 patients who achieved a second CR and the 377 who did not. In both groups, the patients who underwent allogeneic HSCT had a statistically significant survival benefit compared to those who did not. In patients who achieved a second CR, 2-year overall survival was 45% versus 20% for patients who did not undergo transplant after achieving a second CR ($p = 0.005$). For the relapsed refractory group, 2-year OS in the transplant cohort was 13% versus zero for the nontransplanted patients ($p < 0.001$).[125]

The value of salvage chemotherapy prior to transplant is controversial. As indicated previously, patients in second CR have a better prognosis after HSCT than those transplanted in relapse in most studies. On the other hand, early and more indolent relapses should probably be treated with allogeneic transplantation as soon as possible, assuming that an acceptable donor is readily available. A patient who had a remission duration of 6 months or less is unlikely to enter second remission with chemotherapy, which may be needed, however, given the speed of progression or other problems that may preclude allogeneic HSCT in a timely fashion. Patients transplanted in second CR will have long-term disease control in 20% to 60% of the cases with HSCT, whereas patients transplanted in primary induction failure will benefit in 10% to 30% of the cases. The cure rate for patients in first and subsequent relapses is in the 10% to 30% range and, as expected, refractory relapses comprise the worse subgroup.

Alternative Donor Transplantation. As discussed previously, many patients lack an HLA-compatible related or unrelated donor. It is often necessary to proceed to transplantation urgently, and unrelated donor searches typically require several months to identify a donor. Therefore, alternative approaches have been studied, including unrelated umbilical cord blood (CB) transplants or related haploidentical grafts.

Cord blood is a rich source of hematopoietic stem cells for transplantation. The number of cells is approximately 1 log fewer than in a typical bone marrow harvest, but CB transplants are associated with less severe GVHD. This has allowed for the successful use of cord blood transplants from donors mismatched for up to two of the HLA-A and -B (intermediate resolution) and -DR loci (high-resolution typing). As the number of transplants reported to the international registries increases, the importance of high-resolution typing for class I HLA genes is also becoming clearer.[126] Given the lower cell dose, cord blood transplants are associated with slower engraftment, particularly in adults. Results of retrospective studies are similar to those with unrelated donor bone marrow transplants in selected patient populations.[127,128] Although outcomes are better in pediatric patients, cord blood transplants have been used successfully in patients in the 6th and 7th decades of life.[129,130]

A variety of approaches are under investigation aiming at expediting CB engraftment in adults, including ex vivo expansion.[131,132] Individuals inherit one HLA haplotype from each parent, in almost all patients will have a haploidentical relative available. Haploidentical transplants are associated with a high risk of graft rejection and GVHD. The *classic* approach utilized extensive ex vivo T-lymphocyte depletion in order to prevent GVHD. Engraftment is enhanced by transplantation of large numbers of CD34+ cells. This labor-intensive approach is linked to delayed immune recovery posttransplant.[133] Another approach is the use of T-cell replete hematopoietic stem cell grafts followed by two doses of posttransplant cyclophosphamide, with or without additional immunosuppression.[134] There is increasing preclinical and clinical evidence that NK cells mediate a potent antileukemia effect. Donor versus host NK-cell reactivity can thus be predicted by KIR gene expression in the donor and the absence of inhibitory KIR ligands in the recipient (HLA BW4 and C alleles). AML patients who receive haploidentical HSCT in which donor NK cells were predicted to be alloreactive had significantly lower relapse rates and improved leukemia-free survival.[135]

Treatment and Prevention of Relapse after Allogeneic Transplantation. AML recurrence is a major cause of treatment failure. A reduction of early TRM, leading to higher overall survivorship rates, and transplantation of patients at high risk for relapse have led to an increase in the number of recurrences after allogeneic HSCT. There is no homogeneity or consensus regarding treatment of this difficult clinical scenario. Donor lymphocyte infusion, second transplant, chemotherapy, and immunosuppression withdrawal are commonly used with low success rates. CR duration after HSCT is a major determinant of salvage success, as is response to treatment of relapse.[136] The biology of disease relapse is complex, and this is an area of active basic and clinical research.[137,138] The prevention of relapse may include immunologic or pharmacologic interventions, such as the use of leukemia-specific cytotoxic T lymphocytes or the maintenance of remission with 5-azacitidine or other drugs, such as FLT3 inhibitors for patients harboring the mutation. Low-dose azacitidine maintenance of remission is currently under investigation in a randomized trial.[55,139–143]

ACUTE LYMPHOBLASTIC LEUKEMIA

ALL is a heterogeneous disease with distinct biologic and prognostic groupings. Considerable progress has been made in understanding the biology of ALL, which has led to more precise disease prognostication and treatment strategies tailored to specific disease subgroups. This has resulted in dramatic improvements in the outcomes of children with ALL, with cure rates up to 80%. The therapeutic approach for adult ALL is modeled on pediatric regimens, and although initial remission rates range between 80% to 90%, only 25% to 50% of adults achieve long-term disease-free survival. This stark difference in outcome for adults as compared to children has been variously attributed to the greater incidence of adverse cytogenetic subgroups found in adults and possibly poorer tolerance and compliance of adults with intensive therapies required for the successful treatment of ALL. Continued research into the biology of this heterogeneous disease and further development of targeted therapies used in a risk-stratified manner will hopefully lead to comparable survival rates in the near future.

Epidemiology

ALL accounts for approximately 20% of acute leukemias in adults, with increasing incidence above 50 years of age. The incidence of ALL is more common in Caucasians compared with African Americans, with an age-adjusted overall incidence in the United States of 1.5 per 100,000 in Caucasians and 0.8 per 100,000 in African Americans.[144] A higher incidence of ALL has been reported in industrialized countries and urban areas. Finally, ALL is slightly more common among men than among women (1.3 to 1.0).

Diagnosis and Evaluation

Historically, the FAB classification system distinguished three subtypes of ALL based on cell morphology.[11] L1 lymphoblasts, which were small to intermediate in size, were the most common, followed by L2, which defined slightly larger sized blasts, and finally L3, which defined large blasts, described as having a *starry sky* appearance, which were seen in Burkitt's leukemia or lymphoma. This classification system has been replaced by the WHO system, which is based on immunophenotypic, cytogenetic, and molecular information, and consequently provides more precise and clinically relevant disease subgroupings.[12]

Of all cases of ALL, 85% are of B-cell lineage, and the most common form is the precursor B phenotype (also called common precursor-B ALL or early precursor-B ALL); these cells express a B-cell immunophenotype (CD19, CD22), TdT, cytoplasmic CD79A, CD34, CD10 (CALLA), and lack cytoplasmic μ and surface immunoglobulin (sIg). It is found frequently in patients with the Philadelphia chromosome, t(9;22)(q34;q11). A less common type, termed pro-B ALL, lacks CD10 expression and may represent an earlier level of B-cell maturation. Mature B-cell lineage ALL has the immunophenotype of mature B cells with sIg expression and is seen with Burkitt's leukemia or lymphoma. T-lineage ALL accounts for 15% to 20% of cases. This common thymocyte type expresses pan T-cell markers, CD2, cytoplasmic CD3 (cCD3), CD7, CD5, and distinctively shows coexpression of CD4 and CD8 and expression of CD1a. A more primitive type called *prothymocyte* or *immature thymocyte* type has TdT, cCD3, and variable expression of CD5, CD2, and CD7, but lacks CD4, CD8, and CD1a.

More recently, using molecular profiling, a distinct subset within the immature thymocyte group has been identified as early T-cell precursor (ETP) with very poor prognosis.[145] These leukemias express one or more myeloid or stem cell markers (CD117, CD34, HLA-DR, CD13, CD33, CD11b, or CD65) in addition to the immature thymocyte markers.[145] The mature T-lineage phenotype expresses the pan T-cell markers, variable TdT, but lacks CD1a.

Cytogenetic and Molecular Abnormalities

Specific and well-characterized recurring chromosomal abnormalities facilitate diagnosis, confirm subtype classification, and have major prognostic value for treatment planning. Abnormalities in chromosome number or structure are found in approximately 90% of children and 70% of adult ALL patients.[146–150] Differences in the frequency at which good- and poor-risk prognosis cytogenetic abnormalities occur in children versus adults may partially explain the differences in treatment outcomes between childhood and adult ALL. These cytogenetic abnormalities are acquired somatic mutations that frequently result from translocations of chromosomal DNA and lead to new aberrant protein products presumed to be responsible for the cellular dysregulation that leads to the malignant state. Deletions or loss of DNA may eliminate genes that have tumor suppressor functions. Gains of additional chromosomes may lead to gene dosage effects that provide transformed cells with survival advantages. As in AML, cytogenetic abnormalities in ALL define unique prognostic groups, as listed in Table 43.6.

Molecular methods are increasingly used to better understand the genetic consequences of these cytogenetic abnormalities intrinsic to the pathophysiology of ALL, as well as to refine prognosis and identify novel therapeutic targets in ALL. Quantitative reverse transcription polymerase chain reaction technology (RT-PCR) allows for quantification of MRD, which is an independent

TABLE 43.6
Common Karyotypic Abnormalities in Pediatric and Acute Lymphoblastic Leukemia

Phenotype	Karyotype	Genes Involved	Function of Fusion Protein	Frequency (%) in ALL Children	Frequency (%) in ALL Adults	Overall Survival (%) at 3–5 Years Children	Overall Survival (%) at 3–5 Years Adults
Pro B	t(4;11)(q21;q23)	MLL, AF4	Alters HOX gene expression	5–8	3–6	<10	10–24
Pre-B	t(1;19)(q23;p13)	E2A, PBX1	Transcription factor; induction of cell differentiation arrest	5–6	1–3	70–80	30–60
B lineage	t(9;22)(q34;q11)	BCR, ABL	Tyrosine kinase	2–3	15–36	30–80[a]	45–75[a]
B lineage	t(12;21)(p13;q22) or del 12p	ETV6-RUNX1	Alters HOX gene expression	20–25	1–3	85–90	40
T lineage	14q11, 7q35, 7p14-15	Translocation of oncogenes to T-cell receptor genes	Overexpression of respective proteins	40–50	<5	65–75	30–60
B or T lineage	t(8;14), t(8;22), t(2;8)	c-MYC	MYC overexpression	2–5	3–7	75–85	20–45
B or T lineage	del 9p/9p abnormality	MTAP, CDKN2, CDKN2B	Tumor suppressor genes	10	<10	60	40–60
B or T lineage	del 6q	?	Tumor suppressor genes?	5	<10	>70	30–40
B or T lineage	<45 chromosomes			5–7	4–10	25–50	10–20
B or T lineage	>50 chromosomes			25–38	2–10	80–90	40–50

[a]These results include the use of imatinib with average 3-year follow-up.

prognostic factor in both pediatric and adult ALL.[151,152] High-resolution genomic profiling has revealed distinct gene-expression patterns in subtypes of ALL, which may be used to yield insights into the biology of ALL and identify new therapeutic targets[157-159] as well as further refine disease-risk stratification[160,161] and identify genetic markers associated with drug sensitivity and resistance pathways.[162] For example, alterations in the lymphoid transcription factor gene IKZF1 (IKAROS), are present in 70% of patients with BCR-ABL ALL, and some patients without the BCR-ABL translocation; both the BCR-ABL–positive and BCR-ABL–negative patients behave similarly with poor outcome.[163] Importantly, patients with the IKAROS gene profile harbor novel kinase-activating mutations[164] and xenograft models show evidence for response to TKIs.[165] Additionally, activating NOTCH1 mutations are present in up to 50% of T-ALL cases, and the signaling pathways and target genes responsible for Notch1-induced neoplastic transformation are currently under investigation; the nuclear factor kappa B (NF-κB) pathway appears to be one of the major mediators, suggesting that the use of gamma-secretase inhibitors used in combination with NF-κB inhibitors, such as bortezomib, may have synergistic effects.[166]

Mechanisms for drug resistance are also affected by pharmacogenomics, which is the study of how genetic variation among individuals contributes to interindividual differences in efficacy and toxicity of drugs.[167,168,169] For example, hyperdiploid cells accumulate more methotrexate polyglutamates because they possess extra copies of the gene-encoding reduced folate carrier, an active transporter of methotrexate.[170] Associations also have been identified between germ-line genetic characteristics (genes that encode drug-metabolizing enzymes, transporters, and drug targets) and drug metabolism and sensitivity to chemotherapy. Rocha et al.[171] studied 16 genetic polymorphisms that affected the pharmacodynamics of antileukemic agents and observed that, among 130 children with high-risk disease, the glutathione S-transferase μ1 (GSTM1) nonnull genotype was associated with a higher risk of recurrence, which was increased further by the thymidylate synthetase (TYMS) 3/3 genotype.

Finally, epigenetic changes, including hypermethylation of tumor-suppressor genes or microRNA genes, and hypomethylation of oncogenes have been identified in up to 80% of patients with ALL,[172,173] and insights into these mechanisms provide another area for therapeutic development.[174]

Therapy for Acute Lymphoblastic Leukemia

Treatment for adult ALL is modeled on therapy developed for childhood ALL and consists of remission induction, consolidation, and maintenance therapy and CNS prophylaxis, using a risk-stratified approach. Selecting therapy based on patient- and disease-specific prognostic factors has led to a significant improvement in outcomes for childhood ALL, and the adoption of this approach for adults has had a similarly favorable impact.

Prognostic Factors and Risk Assessment

Classic evaluations of prognostic features in adult ALL have led to five widely accepted features: age, WBC count, leukemic cell immunophenotype, cytogenetic subtype, and time to achieve CR.[175] The presence of recurring molecular abnormalities and detection of MRD are more recently used prognostic features based on increasing data supporting their predictive value (Table 43.7).[176] The presence of any of these features portends a high risk for relapse following standard ALL therapy, and the remaining patients are considered standard risk. Up to 75% of adults with ALL are considered to be poor-risk patients, with an expected DFS rate of 25%, and 25% of adults with ALL constitute standard-risk patients, with a projected DFS rate of greater than 50%.[177] Age, WBC count, and treatment response during induction therapy remain classic prognostic features.

TABLE 43.7

Unfavorable Prognostic Features in Adult Acute Lymphoblastic Leukemia

Characteristic	High-Risk Factor(s)
Clinical Factors	
Age	>35 years
Leukocytosis	>30 × 10⁹/L (B lineage); >100 × 10⁹/L (T lineage)
Immunophenotype	Early T-cell precursor
Karyotype	t(9;22)(q24;q11.2), t(4;11)(q21;q23), t(8;14)(q24.1;q32), complex, low hypodiploidy
Molecular profile	IKZF1, CRLF2, TP53, LYL1
Treatment Related	
Therapy response	Time to morphologic CR >4 weeks
	Persistent MRD

CR, complete response; MRD, minimal residual disease.

Age is a continuous variable with OS, decreasing with increasing age; OS ranges from 34% to 57% for patients younger than 30 years compared with only 15% to 17% for patients older than 50 years.[178] A high WBC count is also a continuous variable; generally, a WBC count greater than 30,000/μL or 50,000/μL for B-lineage ALL and greater than 100,000/μL for T-lineage ALL predict for poor prognosis. Of note, while an increased WBC count holds prognostic significance independently as a measure of tumor burden, a high WBC count may be also associated with increased risk of complications during induction therapy, increased risk of CNS relapse, and association with poor-risk cytogenetic subgroups (e.g., t[4;11] and t[9;22]). Finally, the achievement of CR and time to CR after induction therapy carry significant prognostic implications, with patients who require more than 4 weeks to achieve a CR having a lower likelihood of being cured. The emergence of MRD monitoring provides an even more accurate assessment of disease response. In contrast to children, a decrease in MRD burden occurs more slowly in adults.[151] In general, the presence of MRD, defined as 10^{-4} at any time after the start of consolidation is associated with an increased relapse risk, and the predictive value increases at later time points.[151] Patel et al.[152] prospectively analyzed MRD samples following induction, consolidation, and maintenance of 161 patients with non–T-lineage, Ph negative, ALL treated on the international MRC UKALL XII/ECOG 2993 trial. MRD status best discriminated outcome after 10 weeks of therapy, when the relative risk of relapse was 8.95-fold higher in MRD-positive patients and the 5-year relapse-free survival was 15% compared to 71% in MRD-negative patients. The predictive value of MRD depends on the technical quality of the assay and the frequency of monitoring. There is not yet consensus on the clinically relevant time points to measure MRD or the standard methodology to measure MRD.

Specific cytogenetic abnormalities have a major impact on prognosis. The presence of the Ph chromosome and t(4;11)(q21;q23) has been associated with inferior survival in multiple large series.[150,177,179] Additionally, the presence of the t(8;14)(q24.1;q32) complex karyotype, defined as *five or more chromosomal abnormalities or low hypodiploidy or near triploidy*, was noted to result in poor survival in the analysis of patients treated on the UKALL XII/ECOG 2993 trial; in contrast, the presence of hyperdiploidy or del(9p) indicated a good prognosis.[179] Of note, the t(8;14) associated with a mature B ALL phenotype has a poor prognosis when treated with standard ALL regimens. However, modified ALL regimens, incorporating

CD20-targeted therapy, now result in significantly better survival for this group.[180] Similarly, although the Ph chromosome has traditionally been considered a marker of high-risk disease, the outcome for this subset of patients has greatly changed with the incorporation of TKIs into classic ALL therapy. Reports from studies incorporating TKI into their regimens show a greater proportion achieving CR and MRD negativity, and thus suggesting a better prognosis.[181–183] Finally, patients with early T-cell precursor ALL form a distinct subset of patients with T lineage with inferior CR rates and increased rates of relapse.[145]

Remission Induction

In the remission-induction phase of therapy, the goals are to eradicate 99% of the initial tumor burden and to restore normal hematopoiesis and performance status. Current induction regimens for adults consist of at least a glucocorticoid (prednisone, prednisolone, or dexamethasone), vincristine, and an anthracycline, with expected remission rates of 72% to 92% and a median remission duration of 18 months (Table 43.8). Dexamethasone has replaced prednisone based on better in vitro antileukemic activity and higher drug levels in the CSF.[184] The German multicenter study group for ALL (GMALL) noted decreased early mortality when dexamethasone was given in an interrupted schedule rather than continuously.[185] The most commonly used anthracycline is daunorubicin, and attempts have been made to increase the dosage, with no clear benefit noted, possibly due to the increased hematologic toxicity.[186] Intensification of the induction regimen has been attempted with the addition of cyclophosphamide, asparaginase, or cytarabine. Although no clear improvement in CR rates have been noted,[187,188] remission duration may be improved in some ALL subtypes (e.g., cytarabine in T-ALL, cyclophosphamide in mature B ALL). Additionally, treatment intensification specifically for patients in the adolescent age range (e.g., 15 to 20 years old) appears to result in better outcomes with survival rates nearing those of pediatric patients.[189] The use of targeted therapies during induction (e.g., rituximab for mature B ALL and imatinib for Ph + ALL) has improved CR rates for these subtypes of ALL. Finally, supportive care is of great importance during this period. Treatment-related early deaths occur in up to 10% of patients, and significant comorbidities, such fungal infections, occur as a consequence of prolonged cytopenia. The use of growth factors lessens the regimen-induced myelosuppression and may allow for the timely administration of treatment. In a randomized trial, the use of G-CSF during induction was associated with faster recovery of neutrophils and decreased hospital stay.[190] In the G-CSF treated group, the CR rate was higher (90% versus 81%; $p = 0.10$), and the rate of induction deaths was lower (4% versus 11%; $p = 0.04$).

Consolidation Therapy

Once in remission, the consolidation is administered at a relatively higher level of intensity in efforts to further reduce the leukemic burden and decrease the likelihood of relapse. Consolidation may include rotational consolidation programs, modified induction regimens, or HSCT. Most regimens include methotrexate, cytarabine, cyclophosphamide, and asparaginase. But it is difficult to compare regimens as the number and schedule of the chemotherapy agents used vary. Results from the UKALL XA, GIMEMA ALL 0288, and PETHEMA (Programa para el Estudio de la Terapéutica en Hemopatía Maligna) ALL-89 multicenter randomized trials failed to demonstrate a benefit for intensification in terms of prolonging OS and DFS.[186,191,192] However, more recent nonrandomized studies and regimens using a risk-adapted strategy indicate that intensive consolidation may improve outcome.

In the CALGB 8811 study, the induction course consisted of a five-drug combination and was followed by early and late intensification courses with eight drugs.[193] This regimen improved the median duration of CR and median survival to 29 and 36 months, respectively—considerably better than results with earlier trials.[193] A dose-intense regimen of hyperfractionated cyclophosphamide, vincristine, doxorubicin, and dexamethasone (hyper-CVAD), alternating with high doses of cytarabine and methotrexate, led to significantly higher CR rates and survival ($p < 0.01$)[187] when compared to the less-intense vincristine, doxorubicin, dexamethasone (VAD) regimen,[194] with an OS of 38% at 5 years.

Finally, the GMALL 05/93 study intensified consolidation in a subtype-specific manner. High-dose methotrexate was used in standard-risk B-lineage ALL, high-dose methotrexate, and

TABLE 43.8
Selected Prospective Trials in Adult Acute Lymphoblastic Leukemia

Study (Ref.)	Year	N	Median Age (Range)	SCT	CR (%)	Early Death (%)	Survival (%)
CALGB 8811, USA[193]	1995	197	32 (16–80)	—	85	9	50 (3 yr)
CALGB 9111, USA[190]	1998	198	35 (16–83)	Ph+	82	8	43 (3 yr)
LALA 87, France[197]	2000	572	33 (15–60)	D	76	9	27 (10 yr)
GMALL 05/93, Germany[195]	2001	1,163	35 (15–65)	R	83	NR	35 (5 yr)
JALSG-ALL93, Japan[201]	2002	263	31 (15–59)	D	78	6	33 (6 yr)
GIMEMA 0288, Italy[186]	2002	778	28 (12–60)	—	82	11	27 (9 yr)
M. D. Anderson Cancer Center, USA[253]	2004	288	40 (15–92)	Ph+	92	5	38 (5 yr)
EORTC ALL-3, Europe[202]	2004	340	33 (14–79)	D	74	NR	36 (6 yr)
LALA 94, France[198]	2004	922	33 (15–55)	R	84	5	36 (5 yr)
Pethema ALL-93, Spain[203]	2005	222	27 (15–50)	HR	82	6	34 (5 yr)
MRC XII/ECOG E 2993, UK-USA[199]	2008	1,913	31 (15–65)	D	91	NR	39 (5 yr)
HOVON, Netherlands[200]	2009	433	29 (15–55)	D	89	7	40 (5 yr)

SCT, stem cell transplant; HSCT, hematopoietic stem cell transplantation; ALL, acute lymphoblastic leukemia; Ph+, HSCT in Philadelphia–positive ALL; D, prospective HSCT in all patients with donor; R, HSCT according to prospective risk model; HR, prospective HSCT in high-risk patients only; NR, not reported.
[a] Median survival in months.

high-dose cytarabine in high-risk B-linage ALL, and cyclophosphamide and cytarabine in T-linage ALL. The CR rate was 87% in standard risk patients, with a 5-year OS of 55%.[195] Intensified induction and consolidation improved the CR and DFS rates in a subset of high-risk patients with the pro–B ALL immunophenotype, in whom a continuous CR rate of 41% was achieved as compared to 19% for the others.[195]

Hematopoietic Stem Cell Transplantation for Acute Lymphoblastic Leukemia in First Remission

Allogeneic hematopoietic transplantation has a major role in the treatment of ALL, particularly in patients who have recurrent disease or high-risk features (NCCN guidelines). The role of allogeneic HSCT for ALL patients in first CR is controversial. A review of a number of small, phase 2 trials in high-risk adult ALL who underwent allogeneic HSCT in first CR suggests a higher DFS when compared with historic controls based on conventional chemotherapy, ranging broadly from 21% to 71%.[196] Several multicenter, randomized, prospective studies have been conducted (see Table 43.8). To minimize patient selection bias, these trials employed a "genetic" randomization method, offering allogeneic HSCT in first CR to all patients with a sibling donor and chemotherapy or autologous HSCT to patients without a donor. Results were then analyzed using intent-to-treat methods that compared patients with or without donors.

The multicenter French study group Leucemie Aigue Lymphoblastique de l'Adulte completed two large studies between 1986 and 1991 (LALA-87)[197] and 1994 and 2002 (LALA-94).[198] Using an intent-to-treat analysis, a significant DFS and OS benefit was observed for allogeneic HSCT in high-risk patients in both trials. High-risk was defined as having one or more of the following factors: presence of the Ph chromosome, null ALL, age older than 35 years, WBC count greater than 30×10^9/L, or time to CR greater than 4 weeks. The international MRC UKALL XII/ECOG E2993 trial also noted significantly improved survival (53% versus 45%) for patients who received an allogeneic HSCT in first CR as compared to chemotherapy or autologous HSCT.[199] However, in contrast to the LALA studies, this advantage was confined to the standard-risk patient subset (OS 63% versus 51%) due to the high TRM observed in the high-risk group (39%) as compared to the standard-risk group (20%). Of note, high risk in this study was defined as age older than 35 years or a high WBC (greater than 30,000 for B-lineage or greater than 100,000 for T-ALL); Ph+ patients were excluded in this analysis. Similarly, the advantage of SCT was confined to standard-risk ALL in a similar study by the Dutch Cooperative Trials group.[200] In contrast to these studies, no survival advantage was noted for allogeneic HSCT in first CR in three other multicenter, prospective studies.[201–203] In the EORTC ALL-3 trial, although the donor group had a lower relapse rate (38% versus 56%; $p = 0.001$), it also had a higher cumulative incidence of death in CR (23% versus 7%; $p = 0.0004$), resulting in similar survival rates (41% versus 39%).[202] Finally, no survival advantage has ever been shown for autologous HSCT as compared to chemotherapy for patients who do not have a matched related donor.[197–199,202,203]

In addition to the transplant donor, the transplant preparative regimen, source of stem cells, and immunosuppression prophylaxis all impact treatment outcome. TBI remains the standard backbone for myeloablative ALL transplant preparative regimens. The most widely used regimen remains the combination of TBI and cyclophosphamide, although a retrospective analysis of registry data from the CIBMTR suggests that the combination of TBI and etoposide may afford better survival for patients in second CR when compared to cyclophosphamide and TBI.[204] Nonradiation-containing regimens, most commonly busulfan and cyclophosphamide, have been investigated in hopes of decreasing radiation-related complications, with no significant differences noted in outcome.[205,206]

As illustrated in the MRC UKALL XII/ECOG 2993 study, an increasing TRM rate with age compromises the antileukemia benefit for older patients.[199] Because the incidence of ALL increases in adults over age 50 years, transplant approaches with reduced TRM are needed. Reduced-intensity preparative regimens are under evaluation with a goal to reduce toxicity.

The EBMT reported results from the largest series of 97 adult patients with ALL treated with reduced-intensity conditioning (RIC) HSCT and confirmed the benefit of RIC for patients in remission, with a 2-year OS of 52% versus 27% for patients transplanted with advanced disease.[207] Smaller studies have corroborated the benefit for RIC transplantation for older patients with early stage ALL.[208–210] Marks et al.[206] compared transplant conditioning regimen intensity, myeloablative versus RIC, within the limitations of a retrospective analysis in patients with Ph-ALL receiving an allogeneic HSCT in first CR and second CR. Although regimen intensity did not impact TRM or relapse risk in a multivariate analysis, a significantly older patient population was able to tolerate RIC versus myeloablative conditioning (median age 45 years versus 28 years; $p < 0.001$). Thus, RIC merits further investigation in prospective studies.

Maintenance Therapy

Maintenance therapy is administered to patients in remission after consolidation therapy at a low level of intensity, but for a protracted period of time. It has experienced the least modification over time. It consists of a backbone of daily 6-mercaptopurine, weekly methotrexate, and monthly pulses of vincristine and prednisone, generally administered for 2 to 3 years.[211] Attempts to omit maintenance, or shorten its duration to 12 to 18 months, have led to inferior results.[179] However, maintenance therapy is not necessary in mature B ALL, in which a high cure rate is achieved with short-term, dose-intense regimens. The best maintenance regimen for Ph+ patients is not clear but should include a TKI, and is also recommended after transplant,[212] although the duration post-SCT is not clear. Many investigators recommend maintaining the WBC count below 3,000/μL during maintenance. Transaminitis is commonly observed during this period and appears to be caused by the methylated metabolites of mercaptopurine. It is not necessary to alter the regimen because of liver enzyme elevation, because the transaminitis promptly resolves with completion of therapy.

Central Nervous System Prophylaxis

CNS prophylaxis can consist of intrathecal (IT) chemotherapy (methotrexate, cytarabine, corticosteroids), high-dose systemic chemotherapy (methotrexate, cytarabine, L-asparaginase), and CNS irradiation. Despite aggressive systemic therapy, the CNS remains a sanctuary site, and without specific meningeal-directed therapy, CNS disease will develop in up to 50% of adult patients.[14] Risk factors for CNS disease include elevated WBC or lactate dehydrogenase (LDH) at diagnosis, traumatic lumbar puncture, and T-lineage ALL phenotypes. Although some trials still rely on CNS irradiation, most treatment regimens are adopting a risk-adapted approach[213] and attempting to omit CNS irradiation[175] due to its many acute and late complications, including endocrinopathy, neurocognitive deficits, and secondary cancers.

Treatment of Specific Acute Lymphoblastic Leukemia Subgroups

Philadelphia Chromosome–Positive Acute Lymphoblastic Leukemia

Historically, patients with Ph+ ALL have had a poor prognosis, with long-term DFS rates of 10% to 20%.[214] Allogeneic transplantation from a related or unrelated donor was widely used for consolidation, with 30% to 65% long-term survival for patients receiving HSCT in first CR.[215-217] Beyond first remission, HSCT was curative in only a small fraction of patients, with DFS ranging between 5% and 17%.[218]

However, the development of potent TKI of the tyrosine kinase activity of the BCR-ABL fusion product, resulting from the Philadelphia chromosome translocation, has revolutionized therapy for Ph-associated leukemias. Imatinib mesylate was the first TKI to demonstrate significant activity in patients with CML and Ph+ ALL,[219] although response duration in Ph+ ALL was short, with a median time to progression and median OS of 2.2 and 4.9 months, respectively. However, synergistic effects have been observed in vitro when imatinib has been combined with commonly used chemotherapy agents, and a number of studies have investigated the benefit of concurrent or sequential administration of imatinib with chemotherapy. Results from these trials suggest that the incorporation of imatinib into standard ALL therapy results in significantly improved remission induction rates, more patients being able to receive transplant in first remission, and ultimately, better OS rates ranging from 52% to 78%.[181-183,220] Whether consolidation with HSCT in first CR will remain the standard of care for these patients will depend on the durability of the remission inductions, which is currently under investigation. Long-term follow-up of the GRAAPH-2003 study, which incorporated imatinib into its remission and consolidation treatment, resulted in a 50% 4-year OS for patients receiving allogeneic SCT compared with 33% at for those not transplanted.[221] A national multicenter trial is currently in progress in which patients with Ph+ ALL were prospectively randomized to continued chemotherapy or allogeneic transplant in an effort to determine the best route of consolidation for these patients.

The role of imatinib in the treatment of elderly patients with Ph+ ALL is of particular interest. This is a group with a historically poor outcome due to poor tolerance of the standard chemotherapy regimens and disease resistance. Several trials have examined various approaches in this population. Use of imatinib and methylprednisolone alternated with chemotherapy improved the CR rate and OS at 1 year in 30 patients older than 55 years as compared to historical controls (72% versus 29% and 66% versus 44%, respectively).[222] More impressive was a 100% CR noted among 29 patients, with median age 60 years, ranging from 61 to 83 years, who were treated with a combination of imatinib and prednisone only. The median survival from diagnosis was 20 months.[223] Finally, Ottmann et al.[224] conducted a randomized trial of imatinib monotherapy versus standard induction therapy followed by imatinib plus standard consolidation chemotherapy for all patients. Fifty-five patients with a median age of 67 years were treated. The imatinib-treated arm had a significantly higher CR rate (96% versus 50%) with less regimen-related toxicity as compared to the standard induction arm; however, there was no significant difference in OS between the two arms (42% at 2 years).

The development of resistance to imatinib has led to the search for alternative, second-generation TKI such as dasatinib and nilotinib.[225,226] Dasatinib is a dual Src and Abl kinase inhibitor that has shown significant activity in patients with imatinib-resistant disease.[227-229] The significant activity of dasatinib has prompted investigation of its use in front-line regimens. Early response rates suggest a higher and faster rate of molecular remissions when compared to imatinib.[230,231]

Mature B-Lineage Acute Lymphoblastic Leukemia

Treatment of Burkitt's leukemia or lymphoma with the conventional ALL regimens have been disappointing. Short-duration, intensive regimens that maintain serum drug concentrations and minimize treatment delays have demonstrated the greatest efficacy in this disease, mainly due to its high-growth fraction.[232] These regimens incorporate strategies such as the use of fractionated cyclophosphamide, alternation of non–cross-resistant cytotoxic agents between treatment cycles, and aggressive CNS prophylaxis.[233] More recently, the addition of the anti-CD20 monoclonal antibody rituximab has further improved the outcome of patients with Burkitt's leukemia or lymphoma. Thomas et al.[234] administered rituximab in addition to the hyper-CVAD regimen and reported a CR rate of 86%, with 3-year OS of 89%. This was significantly better than the 19% 3-year survival reported for hyper-CVAD alone.

T-Cell Acute Lymphoblastic Leukemia and T-Lymphoblastic Lymphoma

The survival of patients with T-cell ALL and T-lymphoblastic lymphoma (T-LBL) has improved significantly using the regimens designed for ALL, with OS ranging from 50% to 70%.[235] Use of mediastinal radiation given after chemotherapy appears to reduce mediastinal relapse. A proportion of patients with relapsed disease can achieve a second CR and long-term survival with allogeneic stem cell transplant. Compared to patients with B-lineage ALL, the spectrum of genetic abnormalities in T-cell ALL is less well characterized; FISH or PCR testing is required to detect the higher rate of cryptic chromosomal translocations and gene mutations in T-cell ALL. Subset analysis of T-cell ALL patients treated on the MRC/UKALL trial revealed complex cytogenetics, CD13 positivity, and CD1a negativity to be associated with poorer outcome.[236] Greater understanding of the molecular pathogenesis of this subset of ALL has led to the development of novel therapies, such as nelarabine and forodesine,[237] developed specifically towards neoplastic T cells, and gamma-secretase and TKIs developed specifically toward aberrant pathways.[156,158] In CALGB study 19801, 26 patients with relapsed T-cell ALL received nelarabine at 1.5 g/m² per day on days 1, 3, and 5 repeated every 22 days, with a median number of two courses administered.[238] A relatively high CR rate of 31% was noted in this heavily treated group of patients, suggesting that nelarabine induces cytotoxicity through therapeutic pathways different from that of currently used standard drugs. Furthermore, the median DFS was 20 weeks, which should allow sufficient time for a select group of patients with a preserved performance status to proceed to transplant (approximately one-third of patients progressed to transplant in this study). These findings were corroborated in a recent German study in which 126 patients with relapsed/refractory T-ALL or LBL received single-agent nelarabine and 36% of patients achieved CR. Eighty percent of the patients in CR subsequently received SCT, with a 3-year OS of 31% for the transplanted patients.[239] The most common nonhematologic toxicity noted in the study was reversible peripheral sensory and motor neuropathy.[238] Nelarabine is also being combined with standard combination chemotherapy to improve long-term outcome in higher risk T-ALL.[240] Unfortunately, many of the commonly used agents for ALL therapy, such as vincristine and methotrexate, also have neuropathic toxicities, so nelarabine use remains limited. Newer strategies, including long continuous infusions of nelarabine, are currently being explored to reduce dose-limiting neurotoxicity.

Treatment of Primary Refractory or Relapsed Adult Acute Lymphoblastic Leukemia

Most current induction regimens obtain complete responses in 72% to 92% of newly diagnosed patients. Early deaths account for some of the induction failures, but in most studies, 5% to 10% of patients have disease that is resistant to the remission induction regimen. These patients often have poor prognostic factors at presentation, and additional attempts at induction chemotherapy may be unsuccessful. Several studies suggest that patients with an HLA-identical sibling benefit if they proceed directly to allogeneic transplantation without undergoing a second attempt at induction therapy.[173,241] In the largest of these studies, approximately 35% of these patients with primary refractory disease became long-term disease-free survivors.[242]

In addition to primary refractory patients, 60% to 70% of patients who achieve a complete response eventually relapse. Numerous regimens have been reported in the setting of relapsed ALL. These can be divided into two main groups: those that repeat the regimens used for newly diagnosed patients and those that involve high-dose, typically cytarabine-based regimens, with no superior reinduction therapy identified. Cytarabine has been used in combination with L-asparaginase, anthracyclines, or mitoxantrone, with responses as high as 72%.[243,244] However, these are transient, short-lived responses, and allogeneic HSCT remains the most effective modality for achieving durable remissions for patients in or beyond second CR. Two large multicenter trials have best characterized prognosis and outcome following relapse. The outcome of 609 adults with relapsed ALL, all of whom were previously treated on the MRC UKALL12/ECOG 2993 study, was investigated.[245] The survival at 5 years after relapse was 7%. Factors predicting a good outcome after salvage therapy were young age (OS 12% for patients older than 20 years versus 3% for patients older than 50 years) and duration of first remission greater than 2 years (OS 11% versus 5%). When survival was evaluated based on treatment strategy, survival following HSCT ranged from 15% to 23% depending on donor type (15% for autograft, 16% for matched unrelated donor, 23% for matched related donor), and was significantly better than chemotherapy only at 4% ($p < 0.00005$).[245] Oriol et al.[246] reported on the outcome of 263 adults with relapsed ALL, all of whom were previously treated on four consecutive PETHEMA trials with similar induction therapies. OS at 5 years was 10%. Factors predicting a good outcome were identical to the prior study: age less than 30 years (OS 21% versus 10%) and duration of first remission greater than 2 years (OS 36% versus 17%). Forty-five percent of patients achieved a second remission, with better outcomes noted in the group who then proceeded to transplant. The best outcome was noted for patients younger than 30 years old with a long first remission duration transplanted in second CR, with an OS of 38% at 5 years. TRM was higher for patients who had received a prior transplant during first remission (TRM 45% versus 23%), but there was no difference in OS. Similar long-term leukemia-free survival rates of 14% to 43% have been reported from other small series for patients who received HSCT in second CR. As expected, the primary cause of failure is relapse (greater than 50%).

CNS relapse occurs in approximately 2% to 10% of patients who have received appropriate prophylaxis. In the majority of patients, concurrent bone marrow relapse can be documented. Occasionally, CNS relapse may occur without demonstrable systemic relapse; however, this event almost always predicts subsequent bone marrow relapse, and patients with isolated CNS relapse should first receive CNS-directed therapy and then systemic reinduction chemotherapy. Long-term outcome is poor, with zero to 6% OS at 4 years.[245] Intensive treatment, with a combination of intrathecal or radiotherapy and systemic chemotherapy, followed by consolidation with HSCT may improve results.

Several new agents are being investigated in the treatment of acute lymphoblastic leukemia. Among the more successful approaches has been the use of novel monoclonal antibodies alone and in combination with chemotherapy. The anti-CD20 monoclonal antibody rituximab has already been successfully implemented in the treatment of CD20+ and Burkitt's leukemia. A new anti-CD20 antibody, ofatumumab is currently under investigation. Inotuzumab ozogamicin, a novel anti-CD22 antibody conjugated to calicheamicin is also being developed in the treatment of B-ALL and has shown promise. In a phase 2 study of 49 patients with relapsed and refractory B-ALL with a median age of 36 years, the OR rate was 57%.[247] Further single-agent and combination studies are ongoing. A novel T cell engaging CD19/CD3 bispecific antibody, blinatumomab, has also shown impressive activity in patients with previously treated ALL. In a phase 2 trial of blinatumomab in patients with MRD or persistent disease after induction/consolidation for B-ALL, 16 out of 21 (76%) patients became MRD negative, with a relapse-free survival of 78% at a median of 405 days.[248] Further studies of blinatumomab in the relapsed setting are ongoing. Further investigation into the genetic basis of ALL continues to uncover pathogenic driver mutations and activated signaling pathways that could potentially be therapeutically targeted.[249] Finally, cellular therapy in the form of T-cell therapy is showing great promise in patients with advanced ALL. Patients with multiply-relapsed ALL are showing dramatic responses to treatment with chimeric antigen receptor–modified, CD19-directed T-cell therapy.[250] This approach is being used as a bridge to transplant,[251] and has been evaluated in the adjuvant setting in the form of a preemptive donor lymphocyte infusion (DLI).[252]

REFERENCES

1. Fialkow PJ, Janssen J, Bartram CR. Clonal remissions in acute nonlymphocytic leukemia: evidence for a multistep pathogenesis of the malignancy. *Blood* 1991;77:1415–1417.
2. Reya T, Morrison SJ, Clarke MF, et al. Stem cells, cancer, and cancer stem cells. *Nature* 2001;414:105–111.
3. Jones RJ, Matsui W. Cancer stem cells: from bench to bedside. *Biol Blood Marrow Transplant* 2007;13:47–52.
4. Holowiecki J, Grosicki S, Giebel S, et al. Cladribine, but not fludarabine, added to daunorubicin and cytarabine during induction prolongs survival of patients with acute myeloid leukemia: a multicenter, randomized phase III study. *J Clin Oncol* 2012;30:2441–2448.
5. Lowenberg B, Pabst T, Vellenga E, et al. Cytarabine dose for acute myeloid leukemia. *N Engl J Med* 2011;364:1027–1036.
6. Pui CH, Ribeiro RC, Hancock ML, et al. Acute myeloid leukemia in children treated with epipodophyllotoxins for acute lymphoblastic leukemia. *N Engl J Med* 1991;325:1682–1687.
7. Armitage JO, Carbone PP, Connors JM, et al. Treatment-related myelodysplasia and acute leukemia in non-Hodgkin's lymphoma patients. *J Clin Oncol* 2003;21:897–906.
8. Andersen MK, Christiansen DH, Jensen BA, et al. Therapy-related acute lymphoblastic leukaemia with MLL rearrangements following DNA topoisomerase II inhibitors, an increasing problem: report on two new cases and review of the literature since 1992. *Br J Haematol* 2001;114:539–543.
9. Stoffel TJ, Nesbit ME, Levitt SH. Extramedullary involvement of the testes in childhood leukemia. *Cancer* 1975;35:1203–1211.
10. Cheson BD, Cassileth PA, Head DR, et al. Report of the National Cancer Institute-sponsored workshop on definitions of diagnosis and response in acute myeloid leukemia. *J Clin Oncol* 1990;8:813–819.
11. Bennett J, Catovsky D, Daniel MT, et al. The morphological classification of acute lymphoblastic leukaemia: concordance among observers and clinical correlations. *Br J Haematol* 1981;47:553–561.
12. Harris NL, Jaffe ES, Diebold J, et al. World Health Organization classification of neoplastic diseases of the hematopoietic and lymphoid tissues: report of the Clinical Advisory Committee meeting-Airlie House, Virginia, November 1997. *J Clin Oncol* 1999;17:3835–3849.
13. Mastrangelo R, Poplack D, Bleyer A, et al. Report and recommendations of the rome workshop concerning poor-prognosis acute lymphoblastic leukemia in children: biologic bases for staging, stratification, and treatment. *Med Pediatr Oncol* 1986;14:191–194.
14. Mahmoud HH, Rivera GK, Hancock ML, et al. Low leukocyte counts with blast cells in cerebrospinal fluid of children with newly diagnosed acute lymphoblastic leukemia. *N Engl J Med* 1993;329:314–319.
15. Bürger B, Zimmermann M, Mann G, et al. Diagnostic cerebrospinal fluid examination in children with acute lymphoblastic leukemia: significance of low leukocyte counts with blasts or traumatic lumbar puncture. *J Clin Oncol* 2003;21:184–188.

16. Walter RB, Othus M, Borthakur G, et al. Prediction of early death after induction therapy for newly diagnosed acute myeloid leukemia with pretreatment risk scores: a novel paradigm for treatment assignment. *J Clin Oncol* 2011;29:4417–4423.
17. Othus M, Kantarjian H, Petersdorf S, et al. Declining rates of treatment-related mortality in patients with newly diagnosed AML given 'intense' induction regimens: a report from SWOG and MD Anderson. *Leukemia* 2014;28:289–292.
18. Downing JR. The core-binding factor leukemias: lessons learned from murine models. *Curr Opin Genet Dev* 2003;13:48–54.
19. Appelbaum FR, Kopecky KJ, Tallman MS, et al. The clinical spectrum of adult acute myeloid leukaemia associated with core binding factor translocations. *Br J Haematol* 2006;135:165–173.
20. Buccisano F, Maurillo L, Spagnoli A, et al. Cytogenetic and molecular diagnostic characterization combined to postconsolidation minimal residual disease assessment by flow cytometry improves risk stratification in adult acute myeloid leukemia. *Blood* 2010;116:2295–2303.
21. Cheson BD, Bennett JM, Kopecky KJ, et al. Revised recommendations of the international working group for diagnosis, standardization of response criteria, treatment outcomes, and reporting standards for therapeutic trials in acute myeloid leukemia. *J Clin Oncol* 2003;21:4642–4649.
22. Dohner H, Estey EH, Amadori S, et al. Diagnosis and management of acute myeloid leukemia in adults: recommendations from an international expert panel, on behalf of the European LeukemiaNet. *Blood* 2010;115:453–474.
23. de Lima M, Strom SS, Keating M, et al. Implications of potential cure in acute myelogenous leukemia: development of subsequent cancer and return to work. *Blood* 1997;90:4719–4724.
24. Walter RB, Kantarjian HM, Huang X, et al. Effect of complete remission and responses less than complete remission on survival in acute myeloid leukemia: a combined Eastern Cooperative Oncology Group, Southwest Oncology Group, and M. D. Anderson Cancer Center Study. *J Clin Oncol* 2010;28:1766–1771.
25. Chen X, Xie H, Bohm C, et al. The relation of clinical response and minimal residual disease and their prognostic impact on outcome in acute myeloid leukemia. *ASH Annual Meeting Abstracts* 2012;120:1418.
26. Büchner T, Hiddemann W, Berdel WE, et al. 6-Thioguanine, cytarabine, and daunorubicin (TAD) and high-dose cytarabine and mitoxantrone (HAM) for induction, TAD for consolidation, and either prolonged maintenance by reduced monthly TAD or TAD/HAM/TAD and one course of intensive consolidation by sequential HAM in adult patients at all ages with de novo acute myeloid leukemia (AML): a randomized trial of the German AML Cooperative Group. *J Clin Oncol* 2003;21:4496–4504.
27. Appelbaum FR, Gundacker H, Head DR, et al. Age and acute myeloid leukemia. *Blood* 2006;107:3481–3485.
28. Yanada M, Garcia-Manero G, Borthakur G, et al. Relapse and death during first remission in acute myeloid leukemia. *Haematologica* 2008;93:633–634.
29. Sudipto M, Sekeres MA, Godwin J, et al. Prediction of CR on reinduction in patients with newly diagnosed acute myeloid leukemia given intensive induction regimens: a report from SWOG and Cleveland Clinic. *Blood* 2013;122:3924.
30. Appelbaum FR, Petersdorf S, Erba HP, et al. Evaluation of which patients get a second course of 3+7 on cooperative group trials for newly diagnosed acute myeloid leukemia: a report from SWOG. *Blood* 2013;122:3925.
31. Fernandez HF, Sun Z, Yao X, et al. Anthracycline dose intensification in acute myeloid leukemia. *N Engl J Med* 2009;361:1249–1259.
32. Löwenberg B, Ossenkoppele GJ, van Putten W, et al. High-dose daunorubicin in older patients with acute myeloid leukemia. *N Engl J Med* 2009;361:1235–1248.
33. Bertoli S, Delabesse E, Mozziconacci M-J, et al. Impact of anthracycline dose intensification on minimal residual disease and outcome of core binding factors acute myeloid leukemias. *Blood* 2013;122:2681.
34. Gardin C, Chevret S, Pautas C, et al. Superior long-term outcome with idarubicin compared with high-dose daunorubicin in patients with acute myeloid leukemia age 50 years and older. *J Clin Oncol* 2013;31:321–327.
35. Löwenberg B. Sense and nonsense of high-dose cytarabine for acute myeloid leukemia. *Blood* 2013;121:26–28.
36. Dillman R, Davis R, Green M, et al. A comparative study of two different doses of cytarabine for acute myeloid leukemia: a phase III trial of Cancer and Leukemia Group B. *Blood* 1991;78:2520–2526.
37. Othus M, Faderl SH, Stirewalt DL, et al. Impact of cytarabine dose in the induction regimen on the outcome of patients with newly diagnosed acute myeloid leukemia with or without NPM1 and/Or FLT3 mutations: a SWOG and MD Anderson Cancer Center Report. *Blood* 2013;122:2686.
38. Bloomfield CD, Lawrence D, Byrd JC, et al. Frequency of prolonged remission duration after high-dose cytarabine intensification in acute myeloid leukemia varies by cytogenetic subtype. *Cancer Res* 1998;58:4173–4179.
39. Burnett AK, Russell NH, Hills RK, et al. Optimization of chemotherapy for younger patients with acute myeloid leukemia: results of the medical research council AML15 trial. *J Clin Oncol* 2013;31:3360–3368.
40. Yin JA, O'Brien MA, Hills RK, et al. Minimal residual disease monitoring by quantitative RT PCR in core binding factor AML allows risk stratification and predicts relapse: results of the United Kingdom MRC AML-15 trial. *Blood* 2012;120:2826–2835.
41. Schnittger S, Kern W, Tschulik C, et al. Minimal residual disease levels assessed by NPM1 mutation-specific RQ-PCR provide important prognostic information in AML. *Blood* 2009;114:2220–2231.
42. Koreth J, Schlenk R, Kopecky KJ, et al. Allogeneic stem cell transplantation for acute myeloid leukemia in first complete remission: systematic review and meta-analysis of prospective clinical trials. *JAMA* 2009;301:2349–2361.
43. Schlenk RF, Taskesen E, van Norden Y, et al. The value of allogeneic and autologous hematopoietic stem cell transplantation in prognostically favorable acute myeloid leukemia with double mutant CEBPA. *Blood* 2013;122:1576–1582.
44. Geyer S, Zhao J, Caroll AJ, et al. Adding the KIT inhibitor dasatinib (DAS) to standard induction and consolidation therapy for newly diagnosed patients (pts) with core binding factor (CBF) acute myeloid leukemia (AML): initial results of the CALGB 10801 (Alliance) study. *Blood* 2013;122:357.
45. Petersdorf S, Estey EH, Othus M, et al. The addition of gemtuzumab ozogamicin (GO) to induction chemotherapy reduces relapse and improves survival in patients without adverse risk karyotype: results of an individual patient meta-analysis of the five randomised trials. *Blood* 2013;122:356.
46. Ravandi F, Estey EH, Appelbaum FR, et al. Gemtuzumab ozogamicin: time to resurrect? *J Clin Oncol* 2012;30:3921–3923.
47. Woods W, Kobrinsky N, Buckley J, et al. Timed-sequential induction therapy improves postremission outcome in acute myeloid leukemia: a report from the Children's Cancer Group. *Blood* 1996;87:4979–4989.
48. Burnett AK, Russell NH, Kell J, et al. A comparison of daunorubicin/Ara-C (DA) versus daunorubicin/clofarabine (DClo) and two versus three courses of total treatment for older patients with AML and high risk MDS: results of the UK NCRI AML16 trial. *ASH Annual Meeting Abstracts* 2012;120:892.
49. Burnett AK, Russell NH, Hunter AE, et al. Clofarabine doubles the response rate in older patients with acute myeloid leukemia but does not improve survival. *Blood* 2013;122:1384–94.
50. Faderl S, Wetzler M, Rizzieri D, et al. Clofarabine plus cytarabine compared with cytarabine alone in older patients with relapsed or refractory acute myelogenous leukemia: results from the CLASSIC I Trial. *J Clin Oncol* 2012;30:2492–2499.
51. Quintas-Cardama A, Ravandi F, Liu-Dumlao T, et al. Epigenetic therapy is associated with similar survival compared with intensive chemotherapy in older patients with newly diagnosed acute myeloid leukemia. *Blood* 2012;120:4840–4845.
52. Kantarjian HM, Thomas XG, Dmoszynska A, et al. Multicenter, randomized, open-label, phase III trial of decitabine versus patient choice, with physician advice, of either supportive care or low-dose cytarabine for the treatment of older patients with newly diagnosed acute myeloid leukemia. *J Clin Oncol* 2012;30:2670–2677.
53. Fenaux P, Mufti GJ, Hellstrom-Lindberg E, et al. Azacitidine prolongs overall survival compared with conventional care regimens in elderly patients with low bone marrow blast count acute myeloid leukemia. *J Clin Oncol* 2010;28:562–569.
54. Boumber Y, Kantarjian H, Jorgensen J, et al. A randomized study of decitabine versus conventional care for maintenance therapy in patients with acute myeloid leukemia in complete remission. *Leukemia* 2012;26:2428–2431.
55. de Lima M, Giralt S, Thall PF, et al. Maintenance therapy with low-dose azacitidine after allogeneic hematopoietic stem cell transplantation for recurrent acute myelogenous leukemia or myelodysplastic syndrome: a dose and schedule finding study. *Cancer* 2010;116:5420–5431.
56. Jabbour E, Yee K, Kropf P, et al. First clinical results of a randomized phase 2 study of SCI-110, a novel subcutaneous (SQ) hypomethylating agent (HMA), in adult patients with acute myeloid leukemia (AML). *Blood* 2013;122:497.
57. Estey EH. Epigenetics in clinical practice: the examples of azacitidine and decitabine in myelodysplasia and acute myeloid leukemia. *Leukemia* 2013;27:1803–1812.
58. Estey EH, Shen Y, Thall PF. Effect of time to complete remission on subsequent survival and disease-free survival time in AML, RAEB-t, and RAEB. *Blood* 2000;95:72–77.
59. Cilloni D, Renneville A, Hermitte F, et al. Real-time quantitative polymerase chain reaction detection of minimal residual disease by standardized WT1 assay to enhance risk stratification in acute myeloid leukemia: a European LeukemiaNet study. *J Clin Oncol* 2009;27:5195–5201.
60. Burnett AK, Goldstone A, Hills RK, et al. Curability of patients with acute myeloid leukemia who did not undergo transplantation in first remission. *J Clin Oncol* 2013;31(10):1293–301.
61. Gale RE, Green C, Allen C, et al. The impact of FLT3 internal tandem duplication mutant level, number, size, and interaction with NPM1 mutations in a large cohort of young adult patients with acute myeloid leukemia. *Blood* 2008;111:2776–2784.
62. Cortes JE, Kantarjian H, Foran JM, et al. Phase I study of quizartinib administered daily to patients with relapsed or refractory acute myeloid leukemia irrespective of FMS-like tyrosine kinase 3-internal tandem duplication status. *J Clin Oncol* 2013;31:3681–3687.
63. Foran JM, Pratz KW, Trone D, et al. Results of a phase 1 study of quizartinib (AC220, ASP2689) in combination with induction and consolidation chemotherapy in younger patients with newly diagnosed acute myeloid leukemia. *Blood* 2013;122:623.
64. Serve H, Krug U, Wagner R, et al. Sorafenib in combination with intensive chemotherapy in elderly patients with acute myeloid leukemia: results from a randomized, placebo-controlled trial. *J Clin Oncol* 2013;31:3110–3118.
65. Rollig C, Muller-Tidow C, Huttmann A, et al. Sorafenib versus placebo in addition to standard therapy in adult patients >=60 years with newly diagnosed acute myeloid leukemia: results from the randomized-controlled soraml trial. *ASH Annual Meeting Abstracts* 2012;120:144.

66. Galanis A, Ma H, Rajkhowa T, et al. Crenolanib is a potent inhibitor of FLT3 with activity against resistance-conferring point mutants. *Blood* 2014;123:94–100.
67. O'Donnell MR, Tallman MS, Abboud GN, et al. Acute myeloid leukemia, version 2.2013. *J Natl Compr Canc Netw* 2013;11:1047–1055.
68. Sekeres MA, Stone RM, Zahrieh D, et al. Decision-making and quality of life in older adults with acute myeloid leukemia or advanced myelodysplastic syndrome. *Leukemia* 2004;18:809–816.
69. Sanz MA, Grimwade D, Tallman MS, et al. Management of acute promyelocytic leukemia: recommendations from an expert panel on behalf of the European LeukemiaNet. *Blood* 2009;113:1875–1891.
70. Estey E, Thall P, Kantarjian H, et al. Association between increased body mass index and a diagnosis of acute promyelocytic leukemia in patients with acute myeloid leukemia. *Leukemia* 1997;11:1661–1664.
71. Paietta E, Andersen J, Racevskis J, et al. Significantly lower P-glycoprotein expression in acute promyelocytic leukemia than in other types of acute myeloid leukemia: immunological, molecular and functional analyses. *Leukemia* 1994;8:968–973.
72. Lo-Coco F, Cimino G, Breccia M, et al. Gemtuzumab ozogamicin (Mylotarg) as a single agent for molecularly relapsed acute promyelocytic leukemia. *Blood* 2004;104:1995–1999.
73. Ades L, Chevret S, Raffoux E, et al. Long-term follow-up of European APL 2000 trial, evaluating the role of cytarabine combined with ATRA and Daunorubicin in the treatment of nonelderly APL patients. *Am J Hematol* 2013;88:556–559.
74. Powell BL, Moser B, Stock W, et al. Arsenic trioxide improves event-free and overall survival for adults with acute promyelocytic leukemia: North American Leukemia Intergroup Study C9710. *Blood* 2010;116:3751–3757.
75. Estey E, Garcia-Manero G, Ferrajoli A, et al. Use of all-trans retinoic acid plus arsenic trioxide as an alternative to chemotherapy in untreated acute promyelocytic leukemia. *Blood* 2006;107:3469–3473.
76. Lo-Coco F, Avvisati G, Vignetti M, et al. Retinoic acid and arsenic trioxide for acute promyelocytic leukemia. *N Engl J Med* 2013;369:111–121.
77. Iland HJ, Bradstock K, Supple SG, et al. All-trans-retinoic acid, idarubicin, and IV arsenic trioxide as initial therapy in acute promyelocytic leukemia (APML4). *Blood* 2012;120:1570–1580.
78. Park JH, Qiao B, Panageas KS, et al. Early death rate in acute promyelocytic leukemia remains high despite all-trans retinoic acid. *Blood* 2011;118:1248–1254.
79. Breems DA, Van Putten WL, Huijgens PC, et al. Prognostic index for adult patients with acute myeloid leukemia in first relapse. *J Clin Oncol* 2005;23:1969–1978.
80. Horowitz MM, Gale RP, Sondel PM, et al. Graft versus leukemia reactions after bone marrow transplantation. *Blood* 1990;75:555–562.
81. Schlenk RF, Döhner K, Krauter J, et al. Mutations and treatment outcome in cytogenetically normal acute myeloid leukemia. *N Engl J Med* 2008;358:1909–1918.
82. Litzow MR, Tarima S, Pérez WS, et al. Allogeneic transplantation for therapy-related myelodysplastic syndrome and acute myeloid leukemia. *Blood* 2010;115:1850–1857.
83. Walter RB, Gooley TA, Wood BL, et al. Impact of pretransplantation minimal residual disease, as detected by multiparametric flow cytometry, on outcome of myeloablative hematopoietic cell transplantation for acute myeloid leukemia. *J Clin Oncol* 2011;29:1190–1197.
84. Ustun C, Wiseman AC, Defor TE, et al. Achieving stringent CR is essential before reduced-intensity conditioning allogeneic hematopoietic cell transplantation in AML. *Bone Marrow Transplant* 2013;48:1415–1420.
85. Walter RB, Buckley SA, Pagel JM, et al. Significance of minimal residual disease before myeloablative allogeneic hematopoietic cell transplantation for AML in first and second complete remission. *Blood* 2013;122:1813–1821.
86. Duval M, Klein JP, He W, et al. Hematopoietic stem-cell transplantation for acute leukemia in relapse or primary induction failure. *J Clin Oncol* 2010;28:3730–3738.
87. Thomas ED, Buckner CD, Banaji M, et al. One hundred patients with acute leukemia treated by chemotherapy, total body irradiation, and allogeneic marrow transplantation. *Blood* 1977;49:511–533.
88. Santos GW, Tutschka PJ, Brookmeyer R, et al. Marrow transplantation for acute nonlymphocytic leukemia after treatment with busulfan and cyclophosphamide. *N Engl J Med* 1983;309:1347–1353.
89. Andersson BS, de Lima M, Thall PF, et al. Once daily i.v. busulfan and fludarabine (i.v. Bu-Flu) compares favorably with i.v. busulfan and cyclophosphamide (i.v. BuCy2) as pretransplant conditioning therapy in AML/MDS. *Biol Blood Marrow Transplant* 2008;14:672–684.
90. Ringden O, Remberger M, Ruutu T, et al. Increased risk of chronic graft-versus-host disease, obstructive bronchiolitis, and alopecia with busulfan versus total body irradiation: long-term results of a randomized trial in allogeneic marrow recipients with leukemia. *Blood* 1999;93:2196–2201.
91. Blaise D, Maraninchi D, Michallet M, et al. Long-term follow-up of a randomized trial comparing the combination of cyclophosphamide with total body irradiation or busulfan as conditioning regimen for patients receiving HLA-identical marrow grafts for acute myeloblastic leukemia in first complete remission. *Blood* 2001;97:3669–3671.
92. Copelan EA, Hamilton BK, Avalos B, et al. Better leukemia-free and overall survival in AML in first remission following cyclophosphamide in combination with busulfan compared with TBI. *Blood* 2013;122:3863–3870.
93. Bredeson C, Lerademacher J, Kato K, et al. Prospective cohort study comparing intravenous busulfan to total body irradiation in hematopoietic cell transplantation. *Blood* 2013;122:3871–3878.
94. Nagler A, Rocha V, Labopin M, et al. Allogeneic hematopoietic stem-cell transplantation for acute myeloid leukemia in remission: comparison of intravenous busulfan plus cyclophosphamide (Cy) versus total body irradiation plus Cy as conditioning regimen—a report from the acute leukemia working party of the European group for blood and marrow transplantation. *J Clin Oncol* 2013;31:3549–3556.
95. de Lima M, Anagnostopoulos A, Munsell M, et al. Nonablative versus reduced-intensity conditioning regimens in the treatment of acute myeloid leukemia and high-risk myclodysplastic syndrome: dose is relevant for long-term disease control after allogeneic hematopoietic stem cell transplantation. *Blood* 2004;104:865–872.
96. Baron F, Maris MB, Sandmaier BM, et al. Graft-versus-tumor effects after allogeneic hematopoietic cell transplantation with nonmyeloablative conditioning. *J Clin Oncol* 2005;23:1993–2003.
97. Childs R, Clave E, Contentin N, et al. Engraftment kinetics after nonmyeloablative allogeneic peripheral blood stem cell transplantation: full donor T-cell chimerism precedes alloimmune responses. *Blood* 1999;94:3234–3241.
98. Slavin S, Nagler A, Naparstek E, et al. Nonmyeloablative stem cell transplantation and cell therapy as an alternative to conventional bone marrow transplantation with lethal cytoreduction for the treatment of malignant and nonmalignant hematologic diseases. *Blood* 1998;91:756–763.
99. Giralt S, Thall PF, Khouri I, et al. Melphalan and purine analog–containing preparative regimens: reduced-intensity conditioning for patients with hematologic malignancies undergoing allogeneic progenitor cell transplantation. *Blood* 2001;97:631–637.
100. Kottaridis PD, Milligan DW, Chopra R, et al. In vivo CAMPATH-1H prevents graft-versus-host disease following nonmyeloablative stem cell transplantation. *Blood* 2000;96:2419–2425.
101. Bayraktar UD, de Lima M, Saliba RM, et al. Ex vivo T cell-depleted versus unmodified allografts in patients with acute myeloid leukemia in first complete remission. *Biol Blood Marrow Transplant* 2013;19:898–903.
102. Oran B, Giralt S, Saliba R, et al. Allogeneic hematopoietic stem cell transplantation for the treatment of high-risk acute myelogenous leukemia and myelodysplastic syndrome using reduced-intensity conditioning with fludarabine and melphalan. *Biol Blood Marrow Transplant* 2007;13:454–462.
103. Feinstein LC, Sandmaier BM, Hegenbart U, et al. Non-myeloablative allografting from human leucocyte antigen-identical sibling donors for treatment of acute myeloid leukaemia in first complete remission. *Br J Haematol* 2003;120:281–288.
104. Cassileth PA, Harrington DP, Appelbaum FR, et al. Chemotherapy compared with autologous or allogeneic bone marrow transplantation in the management of acute myeloid leukemia in first remission. *N Engl J Med* 1998;339:1649–1656.
105. Burnett AK, Wheatley K, Goldstone AH, et al. The value of allogeneic bone marrow transplant in patients with acute myeloid leukaemia at differing risk of relapse: results of the UK MRC AML 10 trial. *Br J Haematol* 2002;118:385–400.
106. Zittoun RA, Mandelli F, Willemze R, et al. Autologous or allogeneic bone marrow transplantation compared with intensive chemotherapy in acute myelogenous leukemia. European Organization for Research and Treatment of Cancer (EORTC) and the Gruppo Italiano Malattie Ematologiche Maligne dell'Adulto (GIMEMA) Leukemia Cooperative Groups. *N Engl J Med* 1995;332:217–223.
107. Suciu S, Mandelli F, de Witte T, et al. Allogeneic compared with autologous stem cell transplantation in the treatment of patients younger than 46 years with acute myeloid leukemia (AML) in first complete remission (CR1): an intention-to-treat analysis of the EORTC/GIMEMAAML-10 trial. *Blood* 2003;102:1232–1240.
108. Warlick ED, Paulson K, Brazauskas R, et al. Effect of postremission therapy before reduced-intensity conditioning allogeneic transplantation for acute myeloid leukemia in first complete remission. *Biol Blood Marrow Transplant* 2014;20:202–208.
109. Tallman MS, Pérez WS, Lazarus HM, et al. Pretransplantation consolidation chemotherapy decreases leukemia relapse after autologous blood and bone marrow transplants for acute myelogenous leukemia in first remission. *Biol Blood Marrow Transplant* 2006;12:204–216.
110. Jourdan E, Boiron JM, Dastugue N, et al. Early allogeneic stem-cell transplantation for young adults with acute myeloblastic leukemia in first complete remission: an intent-to-treat long-term analysis of the BGMT experience. *J Clin Oncol* 2005;23:7676–7684.
111. Cornelissen JJ, van Putten WL, Verdonck LF, et al. Results of a HOVON/SAKK donor versus no-donor analysis of myeloablative HLA-identical sibling stem cell transplantation in first remission acute myeloid leukemia in young and middle-aged adults: benefits for whom? *Blood* 2007;109:3658–3666.
112. Estey E, de Lima M, Tibes R, et al. Prospective feasibility analysis of reduced-intensity conditioning (RIC) regimens for hematopoietic stem cell transplantation (HSCT) in elderly patients with acute myeloid leukemia (AML) and high-risk myelodysplastic syndrome (MDS). *Blood* 2007;109:1395–1400.
113. Sorror ML, Appelbaum FR. Risk assessment before allogeneic hematopoietic cell transplantation for older adults with acute myeloid leukemia. *Expert Rev Hematol* 2013;6:547–562.
114. Mawad R, Gooley TA, Sandhu V, et al. Frequency of allogeneic hematopoietic cell transplantation among patients with high- or intermediate-risk acute myeloid leukemia in first complete remission. *J Clin Oncol* 2013;31:3883–3888.

115. Flomenberg N, Baxter-Lowe LA, Confer D, et al. Impact of HLA class I and class II high-resolution matching on outcomes of unrelated donor bone marrow transplantation: HLA-C mismatching is associated with a strong adverse effect on transplantation outcome. *Blood* 2004;104:1923–1930.
116. Venstrom JM, Pittari G, Gooley TA, et al. HLA-C-dependent prevention of leukemia relapse by donor activating KIR2DS1. *N Engl J Med* 2012;367:805–816.
117. Brenner M, Krance R, Heslop HE, et al. Assessment of the efficacy of purging by using gene marked autologous marrow transplantation for children with AML in first complete remission. St. Jude Children's Research Hospital, Memphis, Tennessee. *Human gene therapy* 1994;5:481–499.
118. Champlin R. Purging: the separation of normal from malignant cells for autologous transplantation. *Transfusion* 1996;36:910–918.
119. Miller CB, Rowlings PA, Zhang MJ, et al. The effect of graft purging with 4-hydroperoxycyclophosphamide in autologous bone marrow transplantation for acute myelogenous leukemia. *Exp Hematol* 2001;29:1336–1346.
120. Pfirrmann M, Ehninger G, Thiede C, et al. Prediction of post-remission survival in acute myeloid leukaemia: a post-hoc analysis of the AML96 trial. *Lancet Oncol* 2012;13:207–214.
121. Koreth J, Schlenk R, Kopecky KJ, et al. Allogeneic stem cell transplantation for acute myeloid leukemia in first complete remission. *JAMA* 2009;301:2349–2361.
122. Cornelissen JJ, Gratwohl A, Schlenk RF, et al. The European LeukemiaNet AML Working Party consensus statement on allogeneic HSCT for patients with AML in remission: an integrated-risk adapted approach. *Nat Rev Clin Oncol* 2012;9:579–90.
123. Forman SJ, Schmidt G, Nademanee A, et al. Allogeneic bone marrow transplantation as therapy for primary induction failure for patients with acute leukemia. *J Clin Oncol* 1991;9:1570–1574.
124. Appelbaum FR, Clift R, Buckner CD, et al. Allogeneic marrow transplantation for acute nonlymphoblastic leukemia after first relapse. *Blood* 1983;61:949–953.
125. Armistead PM, de Lima M, Pierce S, et al. Quantifying the survival benefit for allogeneic hematopoietic stem cell transplantation in relapsed acute myelogenous leukemia. *Biol Blood Marrow Transplant* 2009;15:1431–1438.
126. Eapen M, Klein JP, Ruggeri A, et al. Impact of allele-level HLA matching on outcomes after myeloablative single unit umbilical cord blood transplantation for hematologic malignancy. *Blood* 2014;123:133–140.
127. Rocha V, Labopin M, Sanz G, et al. Transplants of umbilical-cord blood or bone marrow from unrelated donors in adults with acute leukemia. *N Engl J Med* 2004;351:2276–2285.
128. Peffault de Latour R, Brunstein CG, Porcher R, et al. Similar overall survival using sibling, unrelated, and cord blood grafts after reduced-intensity conditioning for older patients with acute myelogenous leukemia. *Biol Blood Marrow Transplant* 2013;19:1355–1360.
129. Majhail NS, Brunstein CG, Tomblyn M, et al. Reduced-intensity allogeneic transplant in patients older than 55 years: unrelated umbilical cord blood is safe and effective for patients without a matched related donor. *Biol Blood Marrow Transplant* 2008;14:282–289.
130. Eapen M, Klein JP, Sanz GF, et al. Effect of donor-recipient HLA matching at HLA A, B, C, and DRB1 on outcomes after umbilical-cord blood transplantation for leukaemia and myelodysplastic syndrome: a retrospective analysis. *Lancet Oncol* 2011;12:1214–1221.
131. Metheny L, Caimi P, de Lima M. Cord blood transplantation: can we make it better? *Front Oncol* 2013;3:238.
132. de Lima M, McNiece I, Robinson SN, et al. Cord-blood engraftment with ex vivo mesenchymal-cell coculture. *N Engl J Med* 2012;367:2305–2315.
133. Aversa F, Tabilio A, Velardi A, et al. Treatment of high-risk acute leukemia with T-cell–depleted stem cells from related donors with one fully mismatched HLA haplotype. *N Engl J Med* 1998;339:1186–1193.
134. Luznik L, Fuchs EJ. High-dose, post-transplantation cyclophosphamide to promote graft-host tolerance after allogeneic hematopoietic stem cell transplantation. *Immunol Res* 2010;47:65–77.
135. Ruggeri L, Capanni M, Mancusi A, et al. Natural killer cell alloreactivity in haploidentical hematopoietic stem cell transplantation. *Int J Hematol* 2005;81:13–17.
136. Oran B, Giralt S, Couriel D, et al. Treatment of AML and MDS relapsing after reduced-intensity conditioning and allogeneic hematopoietic stem cell transplantation. *Leukemia* 2007;21:2540–2544.
137. Vago L, Perna SK, Zanussi M, et al. Loss of mismatched HLA in leukemia after stem-cell transplantation. *N Engl J Med* 2009;361:478–488.
138. Cairo MS, Jordan CT, Maley CC, et al. NCI first international workshop on the biology, prevention, and treatment of relapse after allogeneic hematopoietic stem cell transplantation: report from the committee on the biological considerations of hematological relapse following allogeneic stem cell transplantation unrelated to graft-versus-tumor effects: state of the science. *Biol Blood Marrow Transplant* 2010;16:709–728.
139. Goodyear OC, Dennis M, Jilani NY, et al. Azacitidine augments expansion of regulatory T cells after allogeneic stem cell transplantation in patients with acute myeloid leukemia (AML). *Blood* 2012;119:3361–3369.
140. Bashir Q, William BM, Garcia-Manero G, et al. Epigenetic therapy in allogeneic hematopoietic stem cell transplantation. *Rev Bras Hematol Hemoter* 2013;35:126–133.
141. Gress RE, Miller JS, Battiwalla M, et al. Proceedings from the National Cancer Institute's Second International Workshop on the Biology, Prevention, and Treatment of Relapse after Hematopoietic Stem Cell Transplantation: Part I. Biology of relapse after transplantation. *Biol Blood Marrow Transplant* 2013;19:1537–1545.

142. Hourigan CS, McCarthy P, de Lima M. Back to the future! The evolving role of maintenance therapy after hematopoietic stem cell transplantation. *Biol Blood Marrow Transplant* 2014;20:154–163.
143. de Lima M, Porter DL, Battiwalla M, et al. Proceedings from the National Cancer Institute's Second International Workshop on the Biology, Prevention, and Treatment of Relapse after Hematopoietic Stem Cell Transplantation: Part III. Prevention and Treatment of Relapse after Allogeneic Transplantation. *Biol Blood Marrow Transplant* 2014;20:4–13.
144. Hoelzer D, Gökbuget N. Recent approaches in acute lymphoblastic leukemia in adults. *Crit Rev Oncol Hematol* 2000;36:49–58.
145. Coustan-Smith E, Mullighan CG, Onciu M, et al. Early T-cell precursor leukaemia: a subtype of very high-risk acute lymphoblastic leukaemia. *Lancet Oncol* 2009;10:147–156.
146. Faderl S, Kantarjian HM, Talpaz M, et al. Clinical significance of cytogenetic abnormalities in adult acute lymphoblastic leukemia. *Blood* 1998;91:3995–4019.
147. Szczepański T, Harrison CJ, van Dongen JJ. Genetic aberrations in paediatric acute leukaemias and implications for management of patients. *Lancet Oncol* 2010;11:880–889.
148. Moorman AV, Chilton L, Wilkinson J, et al. A population-based cytogenetic study of adults with acute lymphoblastic leukemia. *Blood* 2010;115:206–214.
149. Moorman AV, Harrison CJ, Buck GA, et al. Karyotype is an independent prognostic factor in adult acute lymphoblastic leukemia (ALL): analysis of cytogenetic data from patients treated on the Medical Research Council (MRC) UKALLXII/Eastern Cooperative Oncology Group (ECOG) 2993 trial. *Blood* 2007;109:3189–3197.
150. Moorman AV, Ensor HM, Richards SM, et al. Prognostic effect of chromosomal abnormalities in childhood B-cell precursor acute lymphoblastic leukaemia: results from the UK Medical Research Council ALL97/99 randomised trial. *Lancet Oncol* 2010;11:429–438.
151. Brüggemann M, Raff T, Flohr T, et al. Clinical significance of minimal residual disease quantification in adult patients with standard-risk acute lymphoblastic leukemia. *Blood* 2006;107:1116–1123.
152. Patel B, Rai L, Buck G, et al. Minimal residual disease is a significant predictor of treatment failure in non T-lineage adult acute lymphoblastic leukaemia: final results of the international trial UKALL XII/ECOG2993. *Br J Haematol* 2010;148:80–89.
153. Ebert BL, Golub TR. Genomic approaches to hematologic malignancies. *Blood* 2004;104:923–932.
154. Fine BM, Stanulla M, Schrappe M, et al. Gene expression patterns associated with recurrent chromosomal translocations in acute lymphoblastic leukemia. *Blood* 2004;103:1043–1049.
155. Mullighan CG, Goorha S, Radtke I, et al. Genome-wide analysis of genetic alterations in acute lymphoblastic leukaemia. *Nature* 2007;446:758–764.
156. Vilimas T, Mascarenhas J, Palomero T, et al. Targeting the NF-kappaB signaling pathway in Notch1-induced T-cell leukemia. *Nat Med* 2007;13:70–77.
157. Hagemeijer A, Graux C. ABL1 rearrangements in T-Cell acute lymphoblastic leukemia. *Genes Chromosomes Cancer* 2010;49:299–308.
158. Graux C, Cools J, Melotte C, et al. Fusion of NUP214 to ABL1 on amplified episomes in T-cell acute lymphoblastic leukemia. *Nat Genet* 2004;36:1084–1089.
159. Grabher C, Harald von Boehmer A. Notch 1 activation in the molecular pathogenesis of T-cell acute lymphoblastic leukaemia. *Nat Rev Cancer* 2006;6:347–359.
160. Mullighan CG, Su X, Zhang J, et al. Deletion of IKZF1 and prognosis in acute lymphoblastic leukemia. *N Engl J Med* 2009;360:470–480.
161. Tsutsumi S, Taketani T, Nishimura K, et al. Two distinct gene expression signatures in pediatric acute lymphoblastic leukemia with MLL rearrangements. *Cancer Res* 2003;63:4882–4887.
162. Holleman A, Cheok MH, den Boer ML, et al. Gene-expression patterns in drug-resistant acute lymphoblastic leukemia cells and response to treatment. *N Engl J Med* 2004;351:533–542.
163. Mullighan CG, Miller CB, Radtke I, et al. BCR-ABL1 lymphoblastic leukaemia is characterized by the deletion of Ikaros. *Nature* 2008;453:110–114.
164. Roberts KG, Morin RD, Zhang J, et al. Genetic alterations activating kinase and cytokine receptor signaling in high-risk acute lymphoblastic leukemia. *Cancer Cell* 2012;22:153–166.
165. Maude SL, Tasian SK, Vincent T, et al. Targeting JAK1/2 and mTOR in murine xenograft models of Ph-like acute lymphoblastic leukemia. *Blood* 2012;120:3510–3518.
166. Koyama D, Kikuchi J, Hiraoka N, et al. Proteasome inhibitors exert cytotoxicity and increase chemosensitivity via transcriptional repression of Notch1 in T-cell acute lymphoblastic leukemia. *Leukemia* 2014;28:1216–1226.
167. Yang JJ, Cheng C, Yang W, et al. Genome-wide interrogation of germline genetic variation associated with treatment response in childhood acute lymphoblastic leukemia. *JAMA* 2009;301:393–403.
168. Evans WE, Relling MV. Moving towards individualized medicine with pharmacogenomics. *Nature* 2004;429:464–468.
169. Relling MV, Ramsey LB. Pharmacogenomics of acute lymphoid leukemia: new insights into treatment toxicity and efficacy. *Hematology Am Soc Hematol Educ Program* 2013;2013:126–130.
170. Belkov VM, Krynetski EY, Schuetz JD, et al. Reduced folate carrier expression in acute lymphoblastic leukemia: a mechanism for ploidy but not lineage differences in methotrexate accumulation. *Blood* 1999;93:1643–1650.
171. Rocha JC, Cheng C, Liu W, et al. Pharmacogenetics of outcome in children with acute lymphoblastic leukemia. *Blood* 2005;105:4752–4758.

172. Garcia-Manero G, Yang H, Kuang SQ, et al. Epigenetics of acute lymphocytic leukemia. *Semin Hematol* 2009;46:24–32.
173. Roman-Gomez J, Agirre X, Jimenez-Velasco A, et al. Epigenetic regulation of microRNAs in acute lymphoblastic leukemia. *J Clin Oncol* 2009;27:1316–1322.
174. Geng H, Brennan S, Milne TA, et al. Integrative epigenomic analysis identifies biomarkers and therapeutic targets in adult B-acute lymphoblastic leukemia. *Cancer Discov* 2012;2:1004–1023.
175. Pui CH, Evans WE. Treatment of acute lymphoblastic leukemia. *N Engl J Med* 2006;354:166–178.
176. Rowe JM. Prognostic factors in adult acute lymphoblastic leukaemia. *Br J Haematol* 2010;150:389–405.
177. Gökbuget N, Hoelzer D. Treatment of adult acute lymphoblastic leukemia. *ASH Education Program Book* 2006;2006:133–141.
178. Pui CH, Evans WE. Acute lymphoblastic leukemia. *N Engl J Med* 1998;339:605–615.
179. Czuczman MS, Dodge RK, Stewart CC, et al. Value of immunophenotype in intensively treated adult acute lymphoblastic leukemia: cancer and leukemia Group B study 8364. *Blood* 1999;93:3931–3939.
180. Thomas DA, O'Brien S, Kantarjian HM. Monoclonal antibody therapy with rituximab for acute lymphoblastic leukemia. *Hematol Oncol Clin North Am* 2009;23:949–971.
181. Yanada M, Takeuchi J, Sugiura I, et al. High complete remission rate and promising outcome by combination of Imatinib and chemotherapy for newly diagnosed BCR-ABL–Positive acute lymphoblastic leukemia: a phase II study by the Japan Adult Leukemia Study Group. *J Clin Oncol* 2006;24:460–466.
182. Thomas DA, Faderl S, Cortes J, et al. Treatment of Philadelphia chromosome–positive acute lymphocytic leukemia with hyper-CVAD and imatinib mesylate. *Blood* 2004;103:4396–4407.
183. de Labarthe A, Rousselot P, Huguet-Rigal F, et al. Imatinib combined with induction or consolidation chemotherapy in patients with de novo Philadelphia chromosome–positive acute lymphoblastic leukemia: results of the GRAAPH-2003 study. *Blood* 2007;109:1408–1413.
184. Rowe JM, Buck G, Burnett AK, et al. Induction therapy for adults with acute lymphoblastic leukemia: results of more than 1500 patients from the international ALL trial: MRC UKALL XII/ECOG E2993. *Blood* 2005;106:3760–3767.
185. Gökbuget N, Baur K-H, Beck J, et al. Dexamethasone Dose and Schedule Significantly Influences Remission Rate and Toxicity of Induction Therapy in Adult Acute Lymphoblastic Leukemia (ALL): Results of the GMALL Pilot Trial 06/99. *Blood* 2005;106:1832–1832.
186. Annino L, Vegna ML, Camera A, et al. Treatment of adult acute lymphoblastic leukemia (ALL): long-term follow-up of the GIMEMA ALL 0288 randomized study. *Blood* 2002;99:863–871.
187. Kantarjian HM, O'Brien S, Smith TL, et al. Results of treatment with hyper-CVAD, a dose-intensive regimen, in adult acute lymphocytic leukemia. *J Clin Oncol* 2000;18:547–561.
188. Hallbook H, Simonsson B, Ahlgren T, et al. High-dose cytarabine in upfront therapy for adult patients with acute lymphoblastic leukaemia. *Br J Haematol* 2002;118:748–754.
189. DeAngelo DJ. The treatment of adolescents and young adults with acute lymphoblastic leukemia. *ASH Education Program Book* 2005;2005:123–130.
190. Larson RA, Dodge RK, Linker CA, et al. A randomized controlled trial of filgrastim during remission induction and consolidation chemotherapy for adults with acute lymphoblastic leukemia: CALGB study 9111. *Blood* 1998;92:1556–1564.
191. Ribera JM, Ortega JJ, Oriol A, et al. Late intensification chemotherapy has not improved the results of intensive chemotherapy in adult acute lymphoblastic leukemia. Results of a prospective multicenter randomized trial (PETHEMA ALL-89). Spanish Society of Hematology. *Haematologica* 1998;83:222–230.
192. Durrant I, Grant Prentice H, Richards S. Intensification of treatment for adults with acute lymphoblastic leukaemia: results of UK Medical Research Council randomized trial UKALL XA. *Br J Haematol* 1997;99:84–92.
193. Larson RA, Dodge R, Burns C, et al. A five-drug remission induction regimen with intensive consolidation for adults with acute lymphoblastic leukemia: cancer and leukemia group B study 8811. *Blood* 1995;85:2025–2037.
194. Kantarjian HM, Walters RS, Keating MJ, et al. Experience with vincristine, doxorubicin, and dexamethasone (VAD) chemotherapy in adults with refractory acute lymphocytic leukemia. *Cancer* 1989;64:16–22.
195. Gökbuget N, Arnold R, Buechner T, et al. Intensification of induction and consolidation improves only subgroups of adult ALL: Analysis of 1200 patients in GMALL study 05/93. *Blood* 2001;98:802a.
196. Chao NJ, Forman SJ, Schmidt GM, et al. Allogeneic bone marrow transplantation for high-risk acute lymphoblastic leukemia during first complete remission. *Blood* 1991;78:1923–1927.
197. Thiebaut A, Vernant JP, Degos L, et al. Adult acute lymphocytic leukemia study testing chemotherapy and autologous and allogeneic transplantation: a follow-up report of the French protocol LALA 87. *Hematol Oncol Clin North Am* 2000;14:1353–1366.
198. Thomas X, Boiron JM, Huguet F, et al. Outcome of treatment in adults with acute lymphoblastic leukemia: analysis of the LALA-94 trial. *J Clin Oncol* 2004;22:4075–4086.
199. Goldstone AH, Richards SM, Lazarus HM, et al. In adults with standard-risk acute lymphoblastic leukemia, the greatest benefit is achieved from a matched sibling allogeneic transplantation in first complete remission, and an autologous transplantation is less effective than conventional consolidation/maintenance chemotherapy in all patients: final results of the International ALL Trial (MRC UKALL XII/ECOG E2993). *Blood* 2008;111:1827–1833.
200. Cornelissen JJ, van der Holt B, Verhoef GE, et al. Myeloablative allogeneic versus autologous stem cell transplantation in adult patients with acute lymphoblastic leukemia in first remission: a prospective sibling donor versus no-donor comparison. *Blood* 2009;113:1375–1382.
201. Takeuchi J, Kyo T, Naito K, et al. Induction therapy by frequent administration of doxorubicin with four other drugs, followed by intensive consolidation and maintenance therapy for adult acute lymphoblastic leukemia: the JALSG-ALL93 study. *Leukemia* 2002;16:1259–1266.
202. Labar B, Suciu S, Zittoun R, et al. Allogeneic stem cell transplantation in acute lymphoblastic leukemia and non-Hodgkin's lymphoma for patients < or = 50 years old in first complete remission: results of the EORTC ALL-3 trial. *Haematologica* 2004;89:809–817.
203. Ribera JM, Oriol A, Bethencourt C, et al. Comparison of intensive chemotherapy, allogeneic or autologous stem cell transplantation as post-remission treatment for adult patients with high-risk acute lymphoblastic leukemia. Results of the PETHEMA ALL-93 trial. *Haematologica* 2005;90:1346–1356.
204. Marks DI, Forman SJ, Blume KG, et al. A comparison of cyclophosphamide and total body irradiation with etoposide and total body irradiation as conditioning regimens for patients undergoing sibling allografting for acute lymphoblastic leukemia in first or second complete remission. *Biol Blood Marrow Transplant* 2006;12:438–453.
205. Blume KG, Kopecky KJ, Henslee-Downey JP, et al. A prospective randomized comparison of total body irradiation-etoposide versus busulfan-cyclophosphamide as preparatory regimens for bone marrow transplantation in patients with leukemia who were not in first remission: a Southwest Oncology Group study. *Blood* 1993;81:2187–2193.
206. Marks DI, Wang T, Pérez WS, et al. The outcome of full-intensity and reduced intensity conditioning matched sibling or unrelated donor transplantation in adults with Philadelphia chromosome–negative acute lymphoblastic leukemia in first and second complete remission. *Blood* 2010;116:366–374.
207. Mohty M, Labopin M, Tabrizzi R, et al. Reduced intensity conditioning allogeneic stem cell transplantation for adult patients with acute lymphoblastic leukemia: a retrospective study from the European Group for Blood and Marrow Transplantation. *Haematologica* 2008;93:303–306.
208. Stein AS, Palmer JM, O'Donnell MR, et al. Reduced-intensity conditioning followed by peripheral blood stem cell transplantation for adult patients with high-risk acute lymphoblastic leukemia. *Biol Blood Marrow Transplant* 2009;15:1407–1414.
209. Hamaki T, Kami M, Kanda Y, et al. Reduced-intensity stem-cell transplantation for adult acute lymphoblastic leukemia: a retrospective study of 33 patients. *Bone Marrow Transplant* 2005;35:549–556.
210. Martino R, Giralt S, Caballero MD, et al. Allogeneic hematopoietic stem cell transplantation with reduced-intensity conditioning in acute lymphoblastic leukemia: a feasibility study. *Haematologica* 2003;88:555–560.
211. Aricó M, Baruchel A, Bertrand Y, et al. The seventh international childhood acute lymphoblastic leukemia workshop report: Palermo, Italy, January 29–30, 2005. *Leukemia* 2005;19:1145–1152.
212. Pfeifer H, Wassmann B, Bethge W, et al. Randomized comparison of prophylactic and minimal residual disease-triggered imatinib after allogeneic stem cell transplantation for BCR-ABL1-positive acute lymphoblastic leukemia. *Leukemia* 2013;27:1254–1262.
213. Cortes J, O'Brien SM, Pierce S, et al. The value of high-dose systemic chemotherapy and intrathecal therapy for central nervous system prophylaxis in different risk groups of adult acute lymphoblastic leukemia. *Blood* 1995;86:2091–2097.
214. Wetzler M, Dodge RK, Mrozek K, et al. Prospective karyotype analysis in adult acute lymphoblastic leukemia: the cancer and leukemia Group B experience. *Blood* 1999;93:3983–3993.
215. Laport GG, Alvarnas JC, Palmer JM, et al. Long-term remission of Philadelphia chromosome–positive acute lymphoblastic leukemia after allogeneic hematopoietic cell transplantation from matched sibling donors: a 20-year experience with the fractionated total body irradiation–etoposide regimen. *Blood* 2008;112:903–909.
216. Snyder D, Nademanee A, O'Donnell M, et al. Long-term follow-up of 23 patients with Philadelphia chromosome-positive acute lymphoblastic leukemia treated with allogeneic bone marrow transplant in first complete remission. *Leukemia* 1999;13:2053–2058.
217. Fielding AK, Rowe JM, Richards SM, et al. Prospective outcome data on 267 unselected adult patients with Philadelphia chromosome–positive acute lymphoblastic leukemia confirms superiority of allogeneic transplantation over chemotherapy in the pre-imatinib era: results from the International ALL Trial MRC UKALLXII/ECOG2993. *Blood* 2009;113:4489–4496.
218. Cornelissen JJ, Carston M, Kollman C, et al. Unrelated marrow transplantation for adult patients with poor-risk acute lymphoblastic leukemia: strong graft-versus-leukemia effect and risk factors determining outcome. *Blood* 2001;97:1572–1577.
219. Ottmann OG, Druker BJ, Sawyers CL, et al. A phase 2 study of imatinib in patients with relapsed or refractory Philadelphia chromosome–positive acute lymphoid leukemias. *Blood* 2002;100:1965–1971.

220. Lee S, Kim YJ, Min CK, et al. The effect of first-line imatinib interim therapy on the outcome of allogeneic stem cell transplantation in adults with newly diagnosed Philadelphia chromosome–positive acute lymphoblastic leukemia. *Blood* 2005;105:3449–3457.
221. Tanguy-Schmidt A, Rousselot P, Chalandon Y, et al. Long-term follow-up of the imatinib GRAAPH-2003 study in newly diagnosed patients with de novo Philadelphia chromosome-positive acute lymphoblastic leukemia: a GRAALL study. *Biol Blood Marrow Transplant* 2013;19:150–155.
222. Delannoy A, Delabesse E, Lheritier V, et al. Imatinib and methylprednisolone alternated with chemotherapy improve the outcome of elderly patients with Philadelphia-positive acute lymphoblastic leukemia: results of the GRAALL AFR09 study. *Leukemia* 2006;20:1526–1532.
223. Vignetti M, Fazi P, Cimino G, et al. Imatinib plus steroids induces complete remissions and prolonged survival in elderly Philadelphia chromosome–positive patients with acute lymphoblastic leukemia without additional chemotherapy: results of the Gruppo Italiano Malattie Ematologiche dell'Adulto (GIMEMA) LAL0201-B protocol. *Blood* 2007;109:3676–3678.
224. Ottmann OG, Wassmann B, Pfeifer H, et al. Imatinib compared with chemotherapy as front-line treatment of elderly patients with Philadelphia chromosome-positive acute lymphoblastic leukemia (Ph+ ALL). *Cancer* 2007;109:2068–2076.
225. Talpaz M, Shah NP, Kantarjian H, et al. Dasatinib in imatinib-resistant Philadelphia chromosome–positive leukemias. *N Engl J Med* 2006;354:2531–2541.
226. Kantarjian H, Giles F, Wunderle L, et al. Nilotinib in imatinib-resistant CML and Philadelphia chromosome–positive ALL. *N Engl J Med* 2006;354:2542–2551.
227. Cortes J, Rousselot P, Kim DW, et al. Dasatinib induces complete hematologic and cytogenetic responses in patients with imatinib-resistant or-intolerant chronic myeloid leukemia in blast crisis. *Blood* 2007;109:3207–3213.
228. Ottmann O, Dombret H, Martinelli G, et al. Dasatinib induces rapid hematologic and cytogenetic responses in adult patients with Philadelphia chromosome positive acute lymphoblastic leukemia with resistance or intolerance to imatinib: interim results of a phase 2 study. *Blood* 2007;110:2309–2315.
229. Lilly MB, Ottmann OG, Shah NP, et al. Dasatinib 140 mg once daily versus 70 mg twice daily in patients with Ph-positive acute lymphoblastic leukemia who failed imatinib: results from a phase 3 study. *Am J Hematol* 2010;85:164–170.
230. Ravandi F, O'Brien S, Thomas D, et al. First report of phase 2 study of dasatinib with hyper-CVAD for the frontline treatment of patients with Philadelphia chromosome–positive (Ph+) acute lymphoblastic leukemia. *Blood* 2010;116:2070–2077.
231. Ravandi F, Jorgensen JL, Thomas DA, et al. Detection of MRD may predict the outcome of patients with Philadelphia chromosome-positive ALL treated with tyrosine kinase inhibitors plus chemotherapy. *Blood* 2013;122:1214–1221.
232. Blum KA, Lozanski G, Byrd JC. Adult Burkitt leukemia and lymphoma. *Blood* 2004;104:3009–3020.
233. Rizzieri DA, Johnson JL, Niedzwiecki D, et al. Intensive chemotherapy with and without cranial radiation for Burkitt leukemia and lymphoma: final results of Cancer and Leukemia Group B Study 9251. *Cancer* 2004;100:1438–1448.
234. Thomas DA, Faderl S, O'Brien S, et al. Chemoimmunotherapy with hyper-CVAD plus rituximab for the treatment of adult Burkitt and Burkitt-type lymphoma or acute lymphoblastic leukemia. *Cancer* 2006;106:1569–1580.
235. Vitale A, Guarini A, Ariola C, et al. Adult T-cell acute lymphoblastic leukemia: biologic profile at presentation and correlation with response to induction treatment in patients enrolled in the GIMEMA LAL 0496 protocol. *Blood* 2006;107:473–479.
236. Marks DI, Paietta EM, Moorman AV, et al. T-cell acute lymphoblastic leukemia in adults: clinical features, immunophenotype, cytogenetics, and outcome from the large randomized prospective trial (UKALL XII/ECOG 2993). *Blood* 2009;114:5136–5145.
237. Ravandi F, Gandhi V. Novel purine nucleoside analogues for T-cell-lineage acute lymphoblastic leukaemia and lymphoma. *Expert Opin Investig Drugs* 2006;15:1601–1613.
238. DeAngelo DJ, Yu D, Johnson JL, et al. Nelarabine induces complete remissions in adults with relapsed or refractory T-lineage acute lymphoblastic leukemia or lymphoblastic lymphoma: Cancer and Leukemia Group B study 19801. *Blood* 2007;109:5136–5142.
239. Gokbuget N, Basara N, Baurmann H, et al. High single-drug activity of nelarabine in relapsed T-lymphoblastic leukemia/lymphoma offers curative option with subsequent stem cell transplantation. *Blood* 2011;118:3504–3511.
240. Dunsmore KP, Devidas M, Linda SB, et al. Pilot study of nelarabine in combination with intensive chemotherapy in high-risk T-cell acute lymphoblastic leukemia: a report from the Children's Oncology Group. *J Clin Oncol* 2012;30:2753–2759.
241. Terwey T, Massenkeil G, Tamm I, et al. Allogeneic SCT in refractory or relapsed adult ALL is effective without prior reinduction chemotherapy. *Bone Marrow Transplant* 2008;42:791–798.
242. Biggs JC, Horowitz MM, Gale RP, et al. Bone marrow transplants may cure patients with acute leukemia never achieving remission with chemotherapy. *Blood* 1992;80:1090–1093.
243. Capizzi RL, Poole M, Cooper MR, et al. Treatment of poor risk acute leukemia with sequential high-dose ARA-C and asparaginase. *Blood* 1984;63:694–700.
244. Kantarjian HM, Walters RL, Keating MJ, et al. Mitoxantrone and high-dose cytosine arabinoside for the treatment of refractory acute lymphocytic leukemia. *Cancer* 1990;65:5–8.
245. Fielding AK, Richards SM, Chopra R, et al. Outcome of 609 adults after relapse of acute lymphoblastic leukemia (ALL); an MRC UKALL12/ECOG 2993 study. *Blood* 2007;109:944–950.
246. Oriol A, Vives S, Hernández-Rivas JM, et al. Outcome after relapse of acute lymphoblastic leukemia in adult patients included in four consecutive risk-adapted trials by the PETHEMA Study Group. *Haematologica* 2010;95:589–596.
247. Kantarjian H, Thomas D, Jorgensen J, et al. Inotuzumab ozogamicin, an anti-CD22-calecheamicin conjugate, for refractory and relapsed acute lymphocytic leukaemia: a phase 2 study. *Lancet Oncol* 2012;13:403–411.
248. Topp MS, Kufer P, Gokbuget N, et al. Targeted therapy with the T-cell-engaging antibody blinatumomab of chemotherapy-refractory minimal residual disease in B-lineage acute lymphoblastic leukemia patients results in high response rate and prolonged leukemia-free survival. *J Clin Oncol* 2011;29:2493–2498.
249. Zhang J, Ding L, Holmfeldt L, et al. The genetic basis of early T-cell precursor acute lymphoblastic leukaemia. *Nature* 2012;481:157–163.
250. Grupp SA, Kalos M, Barrett D, et al. Chimeric antigen receptor-modified T cells for acute lymphoid leukemia. *N Engl J Med* 2013;368:1509–1518.
251. Brentjens RJ, Davila ML, Riviere I, et al. CD19-targeted T cells rapidly induce molecular remissions in adults with chemotherapy-refractory acute lymphoblastic leukemia. *Sci Transl Med* 2013;5:177ra38.
252. Kebriaei P, Huls H, Singh H, et al. First clinical trials employing *Sleeping Beauty* gene transfer system and artificial antigen presenting cells to generate and infuse t cells expressing CD19-specific chimeric antigen receptor. *ASH Annual Meeting Abstracts* 2013:166a.
253. Burnett AK, Goldstone AH, Stevens RM, et al. Randomised comparison of addition of autologous bone-marrow transplantation to intensive chemotherapy for acute myeloid leukaemia in first remission: results of MRC AML 10 trial. UK Medical Research Council Adult and Children's Leukaemia Working Parties. *Lancet* 1998;351:700–708.

44 Molecular Biology of Chronic Leukemias

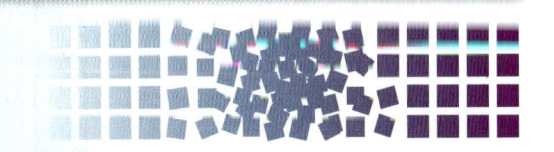

James S. Blachly*, Christopher A. Eide*, John C. Byrd, and Anupriya Agarwal

INTRODUCTION

Chronic myeloid leukemia (CML) and chronic lymphocytic leukemia (CLL) are very different diseases and yet share important clinical features. Both are usually diagnosed in an indolent stage characterized by the expansion of differentiating cells that can last for several, sometimes many years. In both, the acquisition of additional mutations promotes progression to advanced therapy-refractory disease and both are incurable with currently available drug therapy. In this chapter, we will discuss the key pathogenetic mechanisms of CML and CLL, with an emphasis on recent data and potential therapeutic implications.

CHRONIC MYELOID LEUKEMIA

CML is caused by the constitutively active tyrosine kinase BCR-ABL1 generated as the result of a reciprocal translocation between chromosomes 9 and 22. The annual incidence of CML is 1.3 to 1.5 per 10^5, with a slight male preponderance, but no significant differences across ethnicities. The only established CML risk factor is exposure to ionizing radiation, evident from studies in survivors of the nuclear explosions in Japan and patients exposed to Thorotrast or radiotherapy. During the initial chronic phase (CP), cellular differentiation and function are largely maintained, therapy is effective, and mortality is low. Without effective treatment, the disease invariably progresses to a rapidly fatal blastic phase (BP) of myeloid or lymphoid nature.

Pathogenesis

The first cases of what was probably CML were described by Bennett and Virchow in the mid 1840s. In 1960, Philadelphia cytogeneticists Nowell and Hungerford[1] described a "minute" chromosome 22 in CML cells that became known as the Philadelphia (Ph) chromosome. In 1973, the work of another cytogeneticist, Janet Rowley,[2] revealed that this abnormality is, in fact, the result of a reciprocal translocation between chromosomes 9 and 22 (t[9;22] [q34;q11]). The genes juxtaposed by the translocation were subsequently identified as *ABL1* (Abelson) on 9q34 and breakpoint cluster region (*BCR*) on chromosome 22q11 (Fig. 44.1A). As a result of the (9;22) translocation, the *BCR-ABL1* fusion gene is formed on the derivative of chromosome 22 (22q−, Ph), whereas the reciprocal *ABL1-BCR* resides on the derivative of 9q+. A series of seminal studies demonstrated that the constitutive tyrosine kinase activity of BCR-ABL1 is required for cellular transformation and that the clinical disease was reproducible in a murine model.[3] According to the World Health Organization, the presence of *BCR-ABL1* in the context of a myeloproliferative neoplasm is diagnostic of CML, although the translocation is also found in a subset of patients with acute lymphoblastic leukemia (ALL) and rare cases of acute myeloid leukemia (AML).

*Share equal contribution.

Molecular Anatomy of the BCR-ABL1 Junction

The breakpoints within *ABL1* occur upstream of exon 1b, downstream of exon 1a, or more frequently, between the two. Regardless of the exact breakpoint location, splicing of the primary transcript yields an mRNA in which *BCR* sequences are fused to *ABL1* exon a2. Breakpoints within *BCR* localize to one of three breakpoint cluster regions. More than 90% of CML patients and one-third of Ph+ ALL patients express the 210-kDa isoform of BCR-ABL1, in which the break occurs in the 5.8-kb major breakpoint cluster region (M-*bcr*), which spans exons e12-e16 (formerly b1-b5). Alternative splicing gives rise to either b2a2 (e13a2) or b3a2 (e14a2) transcripts,[4] which are mutually exclusive and present in 36% and 64% of patients, respectively. Patients with b3a2 rearrangements are, on average, older than patients with b2a2 transcripts and have elevated platelet levels.[5] The remainder of Ph+ ALL patients and rare CML cases harbor breakpoints further upstream in the 54.4-kb minor breakpoint cluster region (m-*bcr*), generating an e1a2 transcript that is translated into p190$^{BCR-ABL1}$.[6] A third breakpoint downstream of exon 19 in the micro breakpoint cluster region (μ-*bcr*) gives rise to an e19a2 *BCR-ABL1* mRNA and p230$^{BCR-ABL1}$ and is associated with neutrophilia. The reciprocal *ABL1-BCR* transcript, although detectable in approximately two-thirds of patients, does not seem to play any significant role in pathogenesis.[7]

Functional Domains of BCR-ABL1 and Kinase Activation

p210$^{BCR-ABL1}$ contains several distinct domains (Fig. 44.1B).[8] The N-terminal coiled-coil domain of BCR allows BCR-ABL1 dimerization, which is critical for kinase activation. The p210$^{BCR-ABL1}$ protein also retains the serine/threonine kinase and Rho guanine nucleotide exchange factor homology (Rho-GEF) domains of BCR, which are deleted in p190$^{BCR-ABL1}$, which may explain differences in disease phenotype associated with the two variants. In contrast to BCR, the ABL1 sequence is almost completely retained, including SRC homology domains 2 and 3, the tyrosine–kinase domain, a proline-rich sequence, and a large C terminus with nuclear localization signal, DNA-binding, and actin-binding domains. The N-terminal "cap" region of ABL1, which is lost in the BCR-ABL1 fusion, negatively regulates kinase activity by binding to a hydrophobic pocket at the base of the kinase domain, which, in the 1b isoform, is mediated by N-terminal myristoylation.

Signal Transduction

Numerous substrates and binding partners of BCR-ABL1 have been identified (see Fig. 44.1B) that contribute to increased proliferation, decreased apoptosis, defective adhesion to bone marrow stroma, and genetic instability.[9] Because a comprehensive review of the multiple implicated pathways is beyond the scope of this chapter, we will focus on those for which strong evidence supports a rate-limiting role in disease pathogenesis.

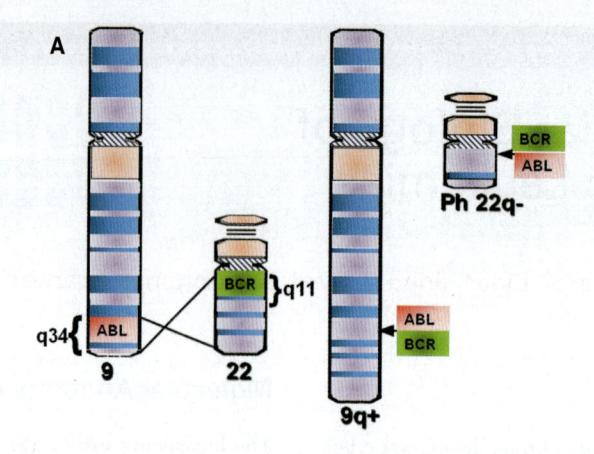

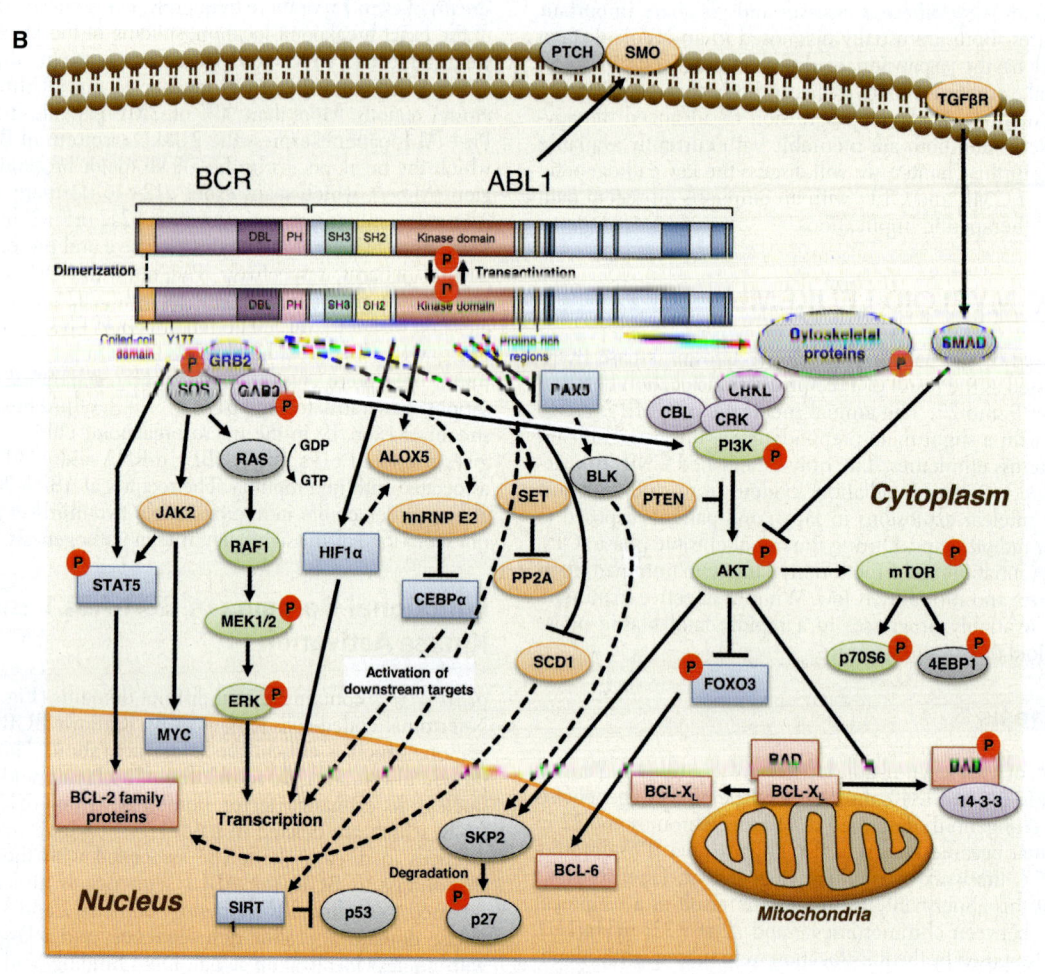

Figure 44.1 **(A)** A Schematic representation of the t(9;22)(q34;q11) translocation that creates the Philadelphia (Ph) chromosome. The *ABL1* and *BCR* genes reside on the long arms of chromosome 9 and 22, respectively. As a result of the (9;22) translocation, the *BCR ABL1* gene is formed on the derivative of chromosome of 22 (22q−, Ph chromosome), whereas the reciprocal *ABL1-BCR* resides on the derivative of 9q+. **(B)** The BCR-ABL1 domain structure and simplified representation of molecular signaling pathways activated in CML cells. Following dimerization of BCR-ABL1, autophosphorylation generates docking sites on BCR-ABL1 that facilitate interaction with intermediary adapter proteins *(purple)* such as GRB2. CRKL and CBL are also direct substrates of BCR-ABL1 that are part of a multimeric complex. These BCR-ABL1–dependent signaling complexes in turn lead to activation of multiple pathways whose net result is enhanced survival, inhibition of apoptosis, and perturbation of cell adhesion and migration. A subset of these pathways and their constituent transcription factors *(blue)*, serine/threonine-specific kinases *(green)*, and apoptosis-related proteins *(red)* are shown. Also included are a few pathways that have been more recently implicated in CML stem cell maintenance and BCR-ABL1–mediated disease transformation *(orange)*. However, it is important to note that this is a simplified diagram and that many more associations between BCR-ABL1 and signaling proteins have been reported. DBL, diffuse poorly-differentiated B-cell lymphoma; SH3, Src homology 3; SH2, Src homology 2; GRB2, growth factor receptor-bound protein 2; SOS, son of sevenless; PI3K, phosphatidylinositol-3 kinase; JAK2, janus kinase; RAS-GTP, rat sarcoma-guanosine triphosphate; RAS-GDP, rat sarcoma-guanosine diphosphate; hnRNP E2, heterogeneous nuclear ribonucleoprotein E2; AKT, RAC alpha serine/threonine protein kinase; mTOR, mammalian target of rapamycin; STAT5, signal transducer and activator of transcription 5; MEK1/2, mitogen-activated protein kinase 1/2; CEBPa, CCAAT/enhancer binding protein alpha; PP2A, protein phosphatase 2A; ERK, extracellular signal-regulated kinase; FOXO3, forhead O transcription factor; SKP2, S-phase kinase-associated protein 2; BAD, BCL2-associated agonist of cell death.

Phosphatidylinositol-3 Kinase

Phosphatidylinositol 3 kinase (PI3K) is activated by autophosphorylation of tyrosine 177, which generates a high-affinity docking site for the GRB2 adapter, which in turn recruits GAB2 into a complex that activates PI3K. Consistent with a critical role of the Y177/GRB2/GAB2 axis, a mutation of this critical tyrosine to phenylalanine or a lack of GAB2 abrogates myeloid leukemia.[10] An alternative pathway of PI3K activation is a complex formation between its p85 regulatory subunit, CBL, and CrkL, which bind to the SH2 and proline-rich domains of BCR-ABL1.[11] PI3K activates the serine/threonine kinase AKT, which suppresses the activity of the forkhead O transcription factors (FOXO), thereby promoting survival.[12] Additionally, PI3K enhances cell proliferation by promoting proteasomal degradation of p27 through upregulation of S-phase kinase-associated protein 2 (SKP2), the F-Box recognition protein of the SCF^{SKP2} E3 ubiquitin ligase.[13] Another important outlet of PI3K signaling is the AKT-dependent activation of mammalian target of rapamycin (mTOR), which enhances protein translation and cell proliferation.[14]

Rat Sarcoma/Mitogen-Activated Protein Kinase Pathways

GRB2-mediated recruitment and activation of son of sevenless (SOS) promotes exchange of guanosine triphosphate (GTP) for GDP on rat sarcoma (RAS).[15] GTP-RAS activates mitogen-activated protein kinase (MAPK), promoting proliferation. Signaling from RAS to MAPK involves the serine/threonine kinase RAF-1[16] and ras-related C3 botulinum toxin substrate (RAC), another GTP–GDP exchange factor.[17] A crucial role for the latter is supported by the fact that a lack of RAC1/2 delays BCR-ABL1–driven leukemia in a murine model.

Janus Kinase/Signal Transducer and Activator of Transcription Pathway

BCR-ABL1 activates signal transducer and activator of transcription 5 (STAT5) through direct phosphorylation or indirectly through phosphorylation by hematopoietic cell kinase (HCK), a SRC family kinase, or janus kinase 2 (JAK2).[18] Active STAT5 induces the transcription of antiapoptotic proteins like myeloid cell leukemia 1 (MCL-1) and B-cell lymphoma-extra large (Bcl-xL).[19] JAK2 has been shown to play a central role in the cytokine signaling machinery that enables survival of CML stem cells in the presence of BCR-ABL1 tyrosine kinase inhibitors. Recent studies have also shown that the complete lack of STAT5 abrogates both myeloid and lymphoid leukemogenesis, implicating it as a potential target for the elimination leukemic stem cells.[20–22]

Cytoskeletal Proteins

BCR-ABL1 phosphorylates several proteins involved in adhesion and migration, including focal adhesion kinase (FAK), paxillin, p130 CrK-associated substrate (p130CAS), and human enhancer of filamentation 1 (HEF1). This and the activation of RAS[23] are thought to impair integrin-mediated adhesion of CML progenitors to stroma and the extracellular matrix, causing premature circulation as well as abnormal proliferation of Ph+ progenitors.[24] A novel adaptor protein pathway in which BCR-ABL1 interaction with Grb2-related adaptor downstream of Shc (GADS)/SH2 domain containing leukocyte protein of 76kDa (SLP-76)/non-catalytic region of tyrosine kinase adaptor protein 1 (NCK1) regulates the actin cytoskeleton and nonapoptotic membrane blebbing was also recently described.[25]

DNA Repair

BCR-ABL1 impairs DNA damage surveillance by various mechanisms. For example, BCR-ABL1 has been shown to suppress checkpoint kinase 1 (CHK1) through the inhibition of ataxia telangiectasia and Rad3-related protein (ATR)[26] or the downregulation of breast cancer 1, early onset (BRCA1), a substrate of ataxia telangiectasia mutated (ATM).[27] Nonhomologous end joining and homologous recombination, both critical double strand break repair pathways, are defective in CML. BCR-ABL1 also upregulates RAD51, inducing rapid but low-fidelity double strand break repairs on challenge with cytotoxic agents and inducing reactive oxygen species (ROS) that promote chronic oxidative DNA damage, double-strand breaks, and point mutations. It has been demonstrated that BCR-ABL1 kinase inhibits the activity of uracil-DNA glycosylase (UNG2), which leads to the accumulation of uracil derivatives in genomic DNA and contributes to increased point mutations.[28] Lastly, telomere length decreases with disease progression from CP to BP.[29]

Although significant progress has been made to understand the extraordinary complexity of CML biology, a complete picture is still elusive. To overcome the limitations of investigating single pathways, quantitative proteomics[30] and whole transcriptome analyses[31] are being used to establish a comprehensive picture of BCR-ABL1 signaling. These results suggest that cellular processes in CML, rather than relying on a single pathway, use integrated networks to fully realize their leukemogenic potential.

Murine Models of Chronic Myeloid Leukemia

The most commonly used murine model of CML is the retroviral expression of BCR-ABL1 in bone marrow followed by transplantation into lethally irradiated syngeneic recipients, which develop a CML-like myeloproliferative neoplasm.[32] Recently, an inducible transgenic mouse model has been developed, in which conditional BCR-ABL1 expression is under the control of the three enhancers of the murine stem cell leukemia (SCL) gene. This model serves as a promising new tool for studying leukemogenic mechanisms in hematopoietic stem cells during disease initiation and progression.[33] Lastly, xenograft models use various strains of immunodeficient mice for engraftment of primary CML cells.[34] A limitation of xenograft models is low engraftment of CML CP cells, probably because of their compromised interactions with the microenvironment as a result of species differences in cytokines and adhesion molecules. Promising results have been obtained by injecting CML cells directly into the livers of newborn mice.[35]

Chronic Myeloid Leukemia Stem Cells

The origin of CML in a pluripotent hematopoietic stem cell (HSC) was elegantly demonstrated in the late 1970s.[36] BCR-ABL1 does not confer self-renewal, implying that it must be acquired by an HSC already endowed with this capacity.[37] For unknown reasons, the main cellular expansion occurs in the progenitor cell compartment, while, at least initially, the majority of HSCs are Ph negative.[38] Serial xenograft studies have shown that CML leukemia stem cells (LSC) reside within the quiescent CD34+38− fraction of bone marrow cells. Significant progress has recently been made by the identification of the interleukin 1 (IL-1) receptor–associated protein (IL-1RAP) as a surface marker specifically expressed on CD34+38− CML LSC.[39] Several genes were shown to have a critical role for LSC maintenance in CML, including promyelocytic leukemia (PML),[40] Rac2 GTPase,[41] smoothened (SMO)/hedgehog (Hh),[42] Wnt/β-catenin,[43,44] phosphatase and tensin homolog (PTEN),[45] hypoxia-inducible factor 1 (HIF-1),[46] B lymphoid kinase (BLK),[47] stearoyl-CoA desaturase1 (SCD1),[48] transforming growth factor beta (TGF-β), and FOXO3a.[12] Additionally, BCL6 was reported to be required for the maintenance of LSCs in CML and contribute to drug resistance.[49] BCL6 expression in these cells is regulated in a PTEN/AKT/FOXO-dependent manner. Recently, an interesting new role of lipid metabolism has emerged in CML stem cell maintenance due to the increased expression of arachidonate 5-lipoxygenase (ALOX5). Alox5 knockout mice fail to develop CML, suggesting a critical role of ALOX5 in CML leukemogenesis.[50] Sirtuin 1 (SIRT1), a nicotinamide adenine dinucleotide–dependent protein deacetylase that promotes cell survival under metabolic, oxidative, and genotoxic stresses through deacetylation of multiple substrates including p53, Ku70, and FOXO, is also transcriptionally activated by BCR-ABL1. SIRT1 knockdown or inhibition by a small-molecule inhibitor effectively suppresses the development of CML-like myeloproliferative disease in mice.[51] Importantly, it has been shown that CML stem cell survival may be independent of BCR-ABL1 kinase activity.[52] A number of studies further suggest that the bone marrow microenvironment provides survival signals to LSCs by involving a number of mechanisms such as chemokine (C-X-C motif) receptor 4 (CXCR4)/stromal cell-derived factor 1 (SDF-1),[53,54] N-cadherin, and Wnt/β-catenin.[55] However, the fact that many of these genes are also critical for maintenance and self-renewal of normal HSCs may be an obstacle to exploiting them as therapeutic targets.

Progression to Blastic Phase

Disease progression is believed to be due to the accumulation of molecular abnormalities that lead to a loss of terminal differentiation capacity of the leukemic clone, which continues to depend on BCR-ABL1 activity. BCR-ABL1 mRNA and protein levels are higher in CML-BP than in CP cells, including CD34+ granulocyte macrophage progenitors (GMP), which are expanded in BP.[56] One of the mechanisms that enhances BCR-ABL1 activity in BP is inactivation of the phosphatase protein phosphatase 2A (PP2A) through upregulation of SET.[57,58] Constitutive BCR-ABL1 activity has also been shown to perturb the CML transcriptome,[59] resulting in altered expression of genes implicated in BP (e.g., preferentially expressed antigen in melanoma [PRAME], myeloid zinc finger 1 [MZF1], ecotropic virus integration site 1 [EVI-1], Wilms tumor 1 [WT1], and JUN-B). Interestingly, a six-gene signature (NIN1/RPN12 binding protein 1 homolog [S. cerevisiae] [NOB1], DEAD [Asp-Glu-Ala-Asp] box polypeptide 47 [DDX47], immunoglobulin superfamily member 2 [IGSF2], lymphotoxin beta receptor 4 [LTBR4], scavenger receptor class B, member 1 [SCARB1], and solute carrier family 25 member A [SLC25A3]) was recently found to accurately discriminate early from late CP, CP from AP, and CP from BP[60]; however, the biologic role of these genes in disease progression is still unknown.

CML-BP patients also harbor various additional genetic lesions such as additional chromosomes, gene insertions and deletions, and/or point mutations. A deep-sequencing study of a small cohort of CML-BP patients detected mutations in 76.9% of cases.[61] The most common mutations (other than those in the BCR-ABL1 kinase domain) occur at the loci of the runt-related transcription factor (RUNX1),[62] the additional sex combs like 1 (ASXL1), WT1, and the tumor suppressor gene TP53[63] in myeloid BP and in cyclin-dependent kinase inhibitor 2A/2B (CDKN2A/B), and the Ikaros transcription factor (IKZF1) in lymphoid BP.[64]

The most striking feature of BP, the loss of differentiation capacity, suggests that the function of key myeloid transcription factors must be compromised. Occasionally, the differentiation block can be ascribed to mutations that result in the formation of dominant-negative transcription factors such as runt-related transcription factor 1- ecotropic virus integration site 1 (AML1-EVI-1) or nucleoporin 98kDa-homeobox A9 (NUP98-HOXA9), which block differentiation or favor preferential growth of immature precursors.[65,66] Isolated cases of myeloid transformation have been associated with the acquisition of core binding factor mutations typical of AML. A more universal mechanism appears to be the BCR-ABL1–induced downregulation of CCAAT/enhancer binding protein-α (CEBPα) through the stabilization of the translational regulator heterogeneous nuclear ribonucleoprotein E2 (hnRNP E2), which is low or undetectable in CP but readily detectable in CML-BP.[67]

Aberrant Wnt/β-catenin activation cooperates with interferon-regulatory factor 8 (Irf8)[68] to contribute to CML progression by conferring self-renewal capacity to GMPs.[69] The acquisition of self-renewal by GMPs is expected to greatly increase the pool of LSCs in BP. Recently, a crucial role of the RNA-binding protein Musashi2 (MSI2) was shown in CML progression to BP, where MSI2 represses the expression of Numb, a protein that impairs the development and propagation of BP.[70] Interestingly, expression microarray studies have implicated a few genes such as β-catenin not only in disease progression, but also in resistance to tyrosine–kinase inhibitors, supporting the view that drug resistance and disease progression share a common genetic basis.[71] This has implications for prognostication as well as for the development of strategies to prevent progression and overcome resistance.

Conclusions

BCR-ABL1 orchestrates an integrated network of signaling pathways that upend the physiologic control of proliferation, cell death, DNA repair, and microenvironment interaction and lead to the clinical phenotype of CML. Cooperation with additional genetic events that accumulate over time inevitably leads to BP and drug resistance. Although significant progress has been made toward understanding transformation and disease progression, much remains to be learned. Efforts toward determining the molecular pathways critical for the maintenance of these cells, and to develop better and faster techniques to differentiate the LSC from the normal HSC, have been intensified in the last decade. The availability of genomewide scanning tools has undoubtedly accelerated this process. This knowledge has been used to design new strategies to target LSCs and hopefully lead to the discovery of new therapeutic targets to eliminate CML stem cells, overcome drug resistance unless effective therapy is initiated early on, and improve the prognosis of patients whose disease has progressed on therapy.

CHRONIC LYMPHOCYTIC LEUKEMIA

CLL is one of the most common leukemias in adults and has a relatively consistent immunophenotype, including dim surface immunoglobulin expression, CD19, CD20, CD23, along with the pan T-cell marker CD5.[72] The impact on overall survival in both young and elderly patients with CLL is substantial: patients diagnosed under the age of 50 have a median expected life span of 12.3 years, compared to 31.2 years in an age-matched control group.[73] Although younger patients have poor outcomes and shortened survival with CLL, several studies have also identified elderly patients as a high-risk group for poor survival following treatment.[74–77] A subset of CLL patients have indolent disease for many years and do not require therapy. Improving our understanding of the origin, biology, and progression of CLL will improve risk stratification and will help identify new treatments for this disease.

Origin of Chronic Lymphocytic Leukemia

The identification of a normal B-cell counterpart remains controversial.[78–80] Unlike most other B-cell lymphomas and leukemias (with the notable exception of mantle cell lymphoma), CLL coexpresses typical mature B-cell markers with CD5. This prompted many to hypothesize that CLL may be derived from CD5+ B cells whose immunoglobulin (Ig) V$_H$ is unmutated. However, the overall phenotype of CLL with expression of CD5, CD23, and CD19, and low levels of surface IgM or IgD is not observed in any normal B-cell counterpart. Additionally, investigators identified that approximately 40% of CLL cases have an unmutated IGHV locus, whereas the remainder are mutated.[81,82] These two groups were also shown to have distinct clinical features, prompting the hypothesis that CLL may represent two distinct diseases.[81,82]

In contrast, two seminal articles examining gene expression profiling in CLL and normal B cells provided findings suggesting that CLL is in fact one disease with a common CLL gene signature.[83,84] The first, by Klein et al.,[83] examined mRNA profiles derived from IGHV unmutated, IGHV mutated, and normal B cells from different stages of differentiation. An unsupervised analysis of gene expression profiles demonstrated that IGHV mutated and unmutated CLL cases were not distinguished in any manner among a common profile typical of CLL. This CLL profile in the majority of samples most resembled postgerminal center memory B cells and lacked any similarity to naïve B cells, CD5+ B cells, or germinal center centroblasts. A supervised analysis of IGHV-unmutated and -mutated CLL did, however, demonstrate distinct genes that could separate these two clinical subsets of CLL.

A second article, published concurrently by Rosenwald et al.,[84] demonstrated similar findings of a common CLL profile described by Klein et al., as compared with other normal B cells and B-cell malignancies. In particular, the CLL gene phenotype was not shared by CD5+ normal B cells, thereby providing corroborating evidence that this is likely not the CLL cell of origin. In an unsupervised analysis of CLL samples, IGHV-unmutated and -mutated samples were intermingled. However, a supervised analysis of IGHV-unmutated and -mutated CLL again identified a number of genes differentially expressed in the former group related to B-cell receptor signaling and proliferation. In particular, ZAP70 (zeta-chain associated protein kinase) was overexpressed in IGHV-unmutated CLL as compared with IGHV-mutated CLL.[85-88]

Subsequent studies have suggested that ZAP-70 expression may partly explain why IGHV-unmutated CLL patients show more B-cell receptor signaling activity upon ligation of the B-cell receptor.[89-91] Multiple studies confirming both the clinical prognostic significance of IGHV mutational status and/or ZAP-70 expression have subsequently been reported. IGHV status and/or ZAP70 represent very strong independent variables in predicting early disease progression, treatment remission duration, and survival of CLL patients. The variability in direct measurement of ZAP-70 among investigators has limited the application of this biomarker clinically, but more recently, ZAP70 methylation status has been demonstrated to be a clinically relevant surrogate.[92] In the future, the assessment of methylation may supplant the direct measurement of ZAP-70.

Chromosomal Abnormalities in the Pathogenesis of Chronic Lymphocytic Leukemia

In CLL, conventional metaphase cytogenetics can identify chromosomal aberrations in only 20% to 50% of cases because of the low in vitro mitotic activity of CLL tumor cells.[93] Early unstimulated metaphase karyotype studies of CLL demonstrated abnormalities, including trisomy 12, deletions at 13q14, structural aberrations of 14q32, and deletions of 11q, 17p, and 6q in descending frequency of occurrence.[94] In addition, complex karyotype (three or more abnormalities) occurs in approximately 15% of patients and was noted in these early studies to predict for rapid disease progression, Richter's transformation, and inferior survival.[95-97] A stimulated metaphase analysis has also been reported with the identification of translocations in 33 of 96 patients (34%) that were both balanced and unbalanced, which is associated with significantly shorter median time from diagnosis to requiring therapy and overall survival.[98] Subsequent comparative genomic hybridization (CGH) and global single nucleotide polymorphism (SNP) array studies in CLL have confirmed these and other chromosomal deletions in CLL.[99-101] Increasing aberrations in these same studies of CGH or SNP arrays have been associated with more aggressive disease.

Given the limitation of standard or stimulated karyotype analysis, interphase cytogenetics of known abnormalities are used to identify common, clinically significant aberrations in CLL. The largest study of interphase cytogenetics resulted in improved sensitivity to detect partial trisomies (12q12, 3q27, 8q24), deletions (13q14, 11q22-23, 6q21, 6q27, 17p13), and translocations (band 14q32) in more than 80% of all cases. In a large study of 325 patients by Dölmer et al.,[102] a hierarchical model consisting of five genetic subgroups was constructed on the basis of regression analysis of CLL patients with chromosomal aberrations. The patients with a 17p deletion had a median survival time of 32 months and the shortest treatment-free interval (TFI) of 9 months, whereas patients with an 11q deletion followed closely with 79 months and 13 months, respectively.[102] The favorable 13q14 deletion group had a long TFI of 92 months and a median survival of 133 months, whereas the group without detectable chromosomal anomalies and those with trisomy 12 fell into the intermediate group with median survival of 111 and 114 months, respectively. Their TFI was 33 and 49 months, respectively. Based on this pivotal study, CLL patients are prioritized in a hierarchical order (deletion 17p13 > deletion 11q22-q23 > trisomy 12 > no aberration > deletion 13q14).[102] Interestingly, patients with high-risk interphase cytogenetics or other complex abnormalities almost always have IGHV unmutated or ZAP-70–positive CLL.[103]

The frequency of recurrent deletions in CLL suggests the possibility of unique tumor suppressor genes in these lost regions. In particular, attention to coding genes within the 13q14 region failed to identify a viable tumor suppressor gene candidate for many years of investigation to the frustration of multiple investigators. However, in 2002, Croce and colleagues[104] identified miR-15 and miR-16, two noncoding microRNAs, in the deleted region of 13q14. MicroRNAs range in size from 21 to 25 nucleotides and represent a newly recognized class of gene products whose function is to silence genes through binding to the 3′-untranslated region of specific genes to inhibit translation. When near compatible hybridization of the noncoding RNA exists, RNA transcription can also be antagonized. This same group later showed that miR-16 regulates the expression of bcl-2, which is overexpressed in CLL and other B-cell lymphoproliferative disorders.[105] Multiple different studies have associated specific miR expression with rapid disease progression, fludarabine resistance, and poor prognosis. In addition, miR-34a has been directly related to the adverse outcome associated with p53 dysfunction.[106,107] At the time of writing this chapter, several reports are coming forth in CLL and other types of cancer about the role of miRs in cell-to-cell communication via exosomes. Further study of miRs in CLL is under way to elucidate their full role in the pathogenesis and progression of CLL. In addition, other conserved, larger noncoding RNAs with different siRNA and epigenetic silencing roles have been recently identified to have a significant role in CLL.

Recurrent Mutations in Chronic Lymphocytic Leukemia

Several groups have recently used next-generation sequencing to demonstrate a number of recurrent mutations in CLL, including known and novel mutations in over two dozen genes with functions as diverse as cell cycle control (ATM, TP53), histones (HISTH1E), inflammation (MYD88, DDX3X, MAPK1), Notch signaling (FBXW7, NOTCH1), general signal transduction (BRAF, KRAS, PRKD3), gene transcription (SMARCA2, NFKBIE), and RNA processing (SF3B1, XPO1).[108-111] These mutations are seen in select genetic subtypes—for instance, NOTCH1 in patients with trisomy 12,[112] MyD88 among IGHV-mutated patients,[110] and SF3B1 in del(11q22.3) patients.[108] Although the disease potential of alterations in, for example, TP53, ATM, or even the very rare BRAF mutation may be clear, the pathogenesis of most of these recurrently mutated genes or pathways remain yet to be worked out and is a promising area for investigation, particularly if experimental therapeutics could be targeted to patients according to their specific genomic alterations. Additionally, several of these genes, including NOTCH1[110,113] and SF3B1,[108] also appear to impact the prognosis of CLL, providing justification for potentially assessing mutational status to predict disease outcome.

Progression of Chronic Lymphocytic Leukemia: The Role of Genomic Instability and Clonal Evolution

Several studies have been examined for features associated with clonal evolution and have noted this to be more frequent in patients with *IGHV*-unmutated status[114] or those expressing the surrogate marker for *IGHV*-mutational status, ZAP-70.[115] In another study, patients with long telomere length were more likely to have *IGHV*-mutated disease and del(13q14), whereas those with del(11q22.3), del(17p13.1), complex karyotype (more than abnormalities), and *IGHV*-unmutated disease were likely to have extended telomeres.[116] Furthermore, one small study suggested long telomere length among patients with *IGHV*-unmutated disease could identify patients with an expected extended progression-free survival.[117] More recently, Landau et al.[118] examined the role of intratumoral heterogeneity and the presence of subclonal driver mutations in the progression of CLL. Using sequencing and copy number analysis at multiple time points, early events (del(13q), +12, *MYD88* mutation) could be delineated from later events (e.g., *SF3B1*, *TP53* mutation), and the development of mutations or expansion in preexisting subclones could be related to the administration of chemotherapy. In addition, the presence of subclonal driver mutations early in the disease was an independent adverse prognostic factor. The contributions of telomere length, global hypomethylation, and subclonal driver mutations' clonal expansion to CLL progression still require further study.

Chronic Lymphocytic Leukemia and Proliferation

For decades, CLL was viewed as a nonproliferating leukemia driven solely by disrupted apoptosis and extended tumor cell survival. This paradigm was, in part, perpetuated based on the nonproliferating blood compartment. However, it has been recognized that, as with normal B cells, CLL cell proliferation likely occurs in sites where microenvironment stimulation can occur, such as the lymph node and bone marrow. In such sites, proliferation centers are observed with a high proportion of dividing CLL cells that are often surrounded by either T cells or accessory stromal cells capable of providing cytokine costimulation.[119,120] In patients, all body compartments can now be accurately measured with the oral intake of heavy water, and the birth rate of CLL tumor cells can thereby be assessed in vivo.[121] These studies have demonstrated a broad range of proliferation of CLL cells, varying by disease state and *IGHV*-mutational status.[122,123] As one might expect, this proliferation rate identified through heavy water studies in CLL was shown to be predictive of disease progression. Collectively, these studies have at least partially discredited the theory that CLL is purely an accumulative disease and have focused the study on specific body compartments that have very different biologic features of proliferation.

Chronic Lymphocytic Leukemia and Disrupted Apoptosis

Because the normal counterpart to CLL is unknown, it is quite difficult to directly compare differences in spontaneous apoptosis. However, several studies derived from CLL do provide evidence that apoptosis is disrupted. Despite the rarity of *BCL2* gene rearrangement in CLL, overexpression of *BCL2* mRNA and Bcl-2 protein is common and has been shown to contribute to both disrupted spontaneous apoptosis and also ex vivo drug resistance.[124-128] Similarly, other antiapoptotic Bcl-2 family member proteins including MCL-1, A1, and Bcl-xL have also been shown to be elevated either in resting CLL or in CLL cells exposed to soluble and contact factors present in the microenvironment; these factors also contribute to drug resistance.[129-131]

Finally, a host of transcription factors involving the nuclear factor kappa B (NF-κB),[132] WNT,[133] Hedgehog,[134] and JAK/STAT[135] signaling pathway have been shown to be constitutively active and also to contribute to disrupted apoptosis and drug resistance in CLL. In particular, differential activation of NF-κB in CLL[136-140] versus normal resting B cells, its prognostic significance[141-143] with respect to predicting outcome, and also its positive role in regulating many of the antiapoptotic genes upregulated in CLL has generated particular interest.

B-Cell Receptor Signaling in Chronic Lymphocytic Leukemia

The identification of the divergent natural history of CLL based on *IGHV*-mutational status, ZAP-70 expression, and associated enhanced B-cell receptor signaling has raised interest in this pathway's role in the pathogenesis of CLL.[89-91,144] Why the BCR is constitutively active in CLL is not yet clear, but current theories include stimulation by self- or ubiquitous environmental antigens as well as tonic BCR self-transactivation. Downstream, activation of the proximal lyn and syk kinases, and Bruton's tyrosine kinase (BTK), in turn, has been demonstrated in CLL.[145-149] Additionally, increased activity of the PI3K pathway has been reported.[150-152] Complementing this, a study demonstrated that mature memory B-cell development was, in great part, dependent on the PI3K pathway.[152] A study of the isoform-specific inhibitor of PI3K-δ demonstrated that much of the survival protection generated by the microenvironment from stromal cells, cytokines (CD40L, IL-6, tumor necrosis factor alpha [TNF-α]), and fibronectin contact is mediated via PI3K-δ isoform signaling.[153] Moving inhibitors of B-cell receptor kinase pathway inhibitors into clinical trials has been of great interest. Here, syk, PI3K-δ isoform inhibitors, and BTK inhibitors have demonstrated dramatic and often rapid clinical responses with relatively favorable toxicity profile in CLL patients.[154] The success of such therapeutics further emphasizes the importance of BCR signaling in the pathogenesis of CLL.

Conclusion

Data concerning the pathogenesis of CLL continue to accumulate. Emerging from such work is the importance of epigenetics in the progression of CLL from normal B cells, the presence of recurrent genetic mutations, and the critical role of enhanced B-cell receptor signaling. Mouse models have demonstrated the importance of NF-κB, Bcl-2, Tcl1, and loss of miR-15, miR-16, and *DLEU2* in the pathogenesis of CLL. The application of these principles (e.g., ibrutinib to quench tonic BCR signaling) in human trials is already yielding dramatic changes in the treatment of patients with CLL.[154] It is likely that current investigations, combined with whole-transcriptome sequencing, global proteomic assessment, and miR profiling, will lead to further advances in risk stratification and treatments for CLL.

ACKNOWLEDGMENTS

We thank Dr. Michael Deininger to help us in preparation of the 9th edition of this chapter, which served as a scaffold for the 10th edition.

REFERENCES

1. Nowell PC, Hungerford DA. Chromosome studies on normal and leukemic human leukocytes. *J Natl Cancer Inst* 1960;25;85–109.
2. Rowley JD. Letter: A new consistent chromosomal abnormality in chronic myelogenous leukaemia identified by quinacrine fluorescence and Giemsa staining. *Nature* 1973;243:290–293.
3. Daley GQ, Van Etten RA, Baltimore D. Induction of chronic myelogenous leukemia in mice by the P210bcr/abl gene of the Philadelphia chromosome. *Science* 1990;247:824–830.
4. Groffen J, Stephenson JR, Heisterkamp N, et al. Philadelphia chromosomal breakpoints are clustered within a limited region, bcr, on chromosome 22. *Cell* 1984;36:93–99.
5. Bennour A, Ouahchi I, Achour B, et al. Analysis of the clinico-hematological relevance of the breakpoint location within M-BCR in chronic myeloid leukemia. *Med Oncol* 2013;30:348
6. Melo JV. The diversity of BCR-ABL fusion proteins and their relationship to leukemia phenotype. *Blood* 1996;88:2375–2384.
7. Melo JV, Gordon DE, Cross NC, et al. The ABL BCR fusion gene is expressed in chronic myeloid leukemia. *Blood* 1993;81:158–165.
8. Hantschel O, Superti-Furga G. Regulation of the c-Abl and Bcr-Abl tyrosine kinases. *Nat Rev Mol Cell Biol* 2004;5:33–44.
9. Quintás-Cardama A, Cortes J. Molecular biology of bcr-abl1-positive chronic myeloid leukemia. *Blood* 2009;113:1619–1630.
10. Sattler M, Mohi MG, Pride YB, et al. Critical role for Gab2 in transformation by BCR/ABL. *Cancer Cell* 2002;1:479–492.
11. Gaston I, Johnson KJ, Oda T, et al. Coexistence of phosphotyrosine-dependent and -independent interactions between Cbl and Bcr-Abl. *Exp Hematol* 2004;32:113–121.
12. Naka K, Hoshii T, Muraguchi T, et al. TGF-beta-FOXO signalling maintains leukaemia-initiating cells in chronic myeloid leukaemia. *Nature* 2010;463:676–680.
13. Agarwal A, Bumm TG, Corbin AS, et al. Absence of SKP2 expression attenuates BCR-ABL-induced myeloproliferative disease. *Blood* 2008;112:1960–1970.
14. Markova B, Albers C, Breitenbuecher F, et al. Novel pathway in Bcr-Abl signal transduction involves Akt-independent PLC-gamma1-driven activation of mTOR/p70S6 kinase pathway. *Oncogene* 2010;29:739–751.
15. Kardinal C, Konkol B, Lin H, et al. Chronic myelogenous leukemia blast cell proliferation is inhibited by peptides that disrupt Grb2-SoS complexes. *Blood* 2001;98:1773–1781.
16. Salomoni P, Wasik MA, Riedel RF, et al. Expression of constitutively active Raf-1 in the mitochondria restores antiapoptotic and leukemogenic potential of a transformation-deficient BCR/ABL mutant. *J Exp Med* 1998;187:1995–2007.
17. Thomas EK, Cancelas JA, Zheng Y, et al. Rac GTPases as key regulators of p210-BCR-ABL-dependent leukemogenesis. *Leukemia* 2008;22:898–904.
18. Ilaria RL Jr, Van Etten RA. P210 and P190(BCR/ABL) induce the tyrosine phosphorylation and DNA binding activity of multiple specific STAT family members. *J Biol Chem* 1996;271:31704–31710.
19. Klejman A, Schreiner SJ, Nieborowska-Skorska M, et al. The Src family kinase Hck couples BCR/ABL to STAT5 activation in myeloid leukemia cells. *EMBO J* 2002;21:5766–5774.
20. Hoelbl A, Schuster C, Kovacic B, et al. Stat5 is indispensable for the maintenance of bcr/abl-positive leukaemia. *EMBO Mol Med* 2010;2:98–110.
21. Walz C, Ahmed W, Lazarides K, et al. Essential role for Stat5a/b in myeloproliferative neoplasms induced by BCR-ABL1 and JAK2(V617F) in mice. *Blood* 2012;119:3550–3560.
22. Warsch W, Walz C, Sexl V. JAK of all trades: JAK2-STAT5 as novel therapeutic targets in BCR-ABL1+ chronic myeloid leukemia. *Blood* 2013;122:2167–2175.
23. Verfaillie CM, Hurley R, Zhao RC, et al. Pathophysiology of CML: do defects in integrin function contribute to the premature circulation and massive expansion of the BCR/ABL positive clone? *J Lab Clin Med* 1997;129:584–591.
24. Ramaraj P, Singh H, Niu N, et al. Effect of mutational inactivation of tyrosine kinase activity on BCR/ABL-induced abnormalities in cell growth and adhesion in human hematopoietic progenitors. *Cancer Res* 2004;64:5322–5331.
25. Preisinger C, Kolch W. The Bcr-Abl kinase regulates the actin cytoskeleton via a GADS/Slp-76/Nck1 adaptor protein pathway. *Cell Signal* 2010;22:848–856.
26. Melo JV, Barnes DJ. Chronic myeloid leukaemia as a model of disease evolution in human cancer. *Nat Rev Cancer* 2007;7:441–453.
27. Risch HA, McLaughlin JR, Cole DE, et al. Population BRCA1 and BRCA2 mutation frequencies and cancer penetrances: a kin-cohort study in Ontario, Canada. *J Natl Cancer Inst* 2006;98:1694–1706.
28. Slupianek A, Falinski R, Znojek P, et al. BCR-ABL1 kinase inhibits uracil DNA glycosylase UNG2 to enhance oxidative DNA damage and stimulate genomic instability. *Leukemia* 2013;27:629–634.
29. Koptyra M, Falinski R, Nowicki MO, et al. BCR/ABL kinase induces self-mutagenesis via reactive oxygen species to encode imatinib resistance. *Blood* 2006;108:319–327.
30. Brehme M, Hantschel O, Colinge J, et al. Charting the molecular network of the drug target Bcr-Abl. *Proc Natl Acad Sci U S A* 2009;106:7414–7419.
31. Gerber JM, Gucwa JL, Esopi D, et al. Genome-wide comparison of the transcriptomes of highly enriched normal and chronic myeloid leukemia stem and progenitor cell populations. *Oncotarget* 2013;4:715–728.
32. Pear WS, Miller JP, Xu L, et al. Efficient and rapid induction of a chronic myelogenous leukemia-like myeloproliferative disease in mice receiving P210 bcr/abl-transduced bone marrow. *Blood* 1998;92:3780–3792.
33. Koschmieder S, Göttgens B, Zhang P, et al. Inducible chronic phase of myeloid leukemia with expansion of hematopoietic stem cells in a transgenic model of BCR-ABL leukemogenesis. *Blood* 2005;105:324–334.
34. Agliano A, Martin-Padura I, Mancuso P, et al. Human acute leukemia cells injected in NOD/LtSz-scid/IL-2Rgamma null mice generate a faster and more efficient disease compared to other NOD/scid-related strains. *Int J Cancer* 2008;123:2222–2227.
35. Abrahamsson AE, Geron I, Gotlib J, et al. Glycogen synthase kinase 3beta missplicing contributes to leukemia stem cell generation. *Proc Natl Acad Sci U S A* 2009;106:3925–3929.
36. Fialkow PJ, Jacobson RJ, Papayannopoulou T. Chronic myelocytic leukemia: clonal origin in a stem cell common to the granulocyte, erythrocyte, platelet and monocyte/macrophage. *Am J Med* 1977;63:125–130.
37. Huntly BJ, Shigematsu H, Deguchi K, et al. MOZ-TIF2, but not BCR-ABL, confers properties of leukemic stem cells to committed murine hematopoietic progenitors. *Cancer Cell* 2004;6:587–596.
38. Petzer AL, Eaves CJ, Barnett MJ, et al. Selective expansion of primitive normal hematopoietic cells in cytokine-supplemented cultures of purified cells from patients with chronic myeloid leukemia. *Blood* 1997;90:64–69.
39. Jaras M, Johnels P, Hansen N, et al. Isolation and killing of candidate chronic myeloid leukemia stem cells by antibody targeting of IL-1 receptor accessory protein. *Proc Natl Acad Sci U S A* 2010;107:16280–16285.
40. Ito K, Bernardi R, Morotti A, et al. PML targeting eradicates quiescent leukaemia-initiating cells. *Nature* 2008;453:1072–1078.
41. Sengupta A, Arnett J, Dunn S, et al. Rac2 GTPase deficiency depletes BCR-ABL+ leukemic stem cells and progenitors in vivo. *Blood* 2010;116:81–84.
42. Zhao C, Chen A, Jamieson CH, et al. Hedgehog signalling is essential for maintenance of cancer stem cells in myeloid leukaemia. *Nature* 2009;458:776–779.
43. Zhao C, Blum J, Chen A, et al. Loss of beta-catenin impairs the renewal of normal and CML stem cells in vivo. *Cancer Cell* 2007;12:528–541.
44. Jamieson CH, Ailles LE, Dylla SJ, et al. Granulocyte-macrophage progenitors as candidate leukemic stem cells in blast-crisis CML. *N Engl J Med* 2004;351:657–667.
45. Ferri C, Bianchini M, Bengio R, et al. Expression of LYN and PTEN genes in chronic myeloid leukemia and their importance in therapeutic strategy. *Blood Cells Mol Dis* 2014;52:121–125.
46. Zhang H, Li H, Xi HS, et al. HIF1alpha is required for survival maintenance of chronic myeloid leukemia stem cells. *Blood* 2012;119:2595–2607.
47. Zhang H, Peng C, Hu Y, et al. The Blk pathway functions as a tumor suppressor in chronic myeloid leukemia stem cells. *Nat Genet* 2012;44:861–871.
48. Zhang H, Li H, Ho N, et al. Scd1 plays a tumor-suppressive role in survival of leukemia stem cells and the development of chronic myeloid leukemia. *Mol Cell Biol* 2012;32:1776–1787.
49. Hurtz C, Hatzi K, Cerchietti L, et al. BCL6-mediated repression of p53 is critical for leukemia stem cell survival in chronic myeloid leukemia. *J Exp Med* 2011;208:2163–2174.
50. Chen Y, Hu Y, Zhang H, et al. Loss of the Alox5 gene impairs leukemia stem cells and prevents chronic myeloid leukemia. *Nat Genet* 2009;41:783–792.
51. Li L, Wang L, Li L, et al. Activation of p53 by SIRT1 inhibition enhances elimination of CML leukemia stem cells in combination with imatinib. *Cancer Cell* 2012;21:266–281.
52. Corbin AS, Agarwal A, Loriaux M, et al. Human chronic myeloid leukemia stem cells are insensitive to imatinib despite inhibition of BCR-ABL activity. *J Clin Invest* 2011;121:396–409.
53. Agarwal A, Fleischman AG, Petersen CL, et al. Effects of plerixafor in combination with BCR-ABL kinase inhibition in a murine model of CML. *Blood* 2012;120:2658–2668.
54. Agarwal A, O'Hare T, Deininger MW. CXCR4 antagonists for the treatment of CML. In: Fruehauf S, Zeller WJ, Calandra G, eds. *Novel Developments in Stem Cell Mobilization: Focus on CXCR4.* New York: Springer; 2012: 351–367.
55. Zhang B, Li M, McDonald T, et al. Microenvironmental protection of CML stem and progenitor cells from tyrosine kinase inhibitors through N-cadherin and Wnt-beta-catenin signaling. *Blood* 2013;121:1824–1838.
56. Barnes DJ, Schultheis B, Adedeji S, et al. Dose-dependent effects of Bcr-Abl in cell line models of different stages of chronic myeloid leukemia. *Oncogene* 2005;24:6432–6440.
57. Perrotti D, Neviani P. ReSETting PP2A tumour suppressor activity in blast crisis and imatinib-resistant chronic myelogenous leukaemia. *Br J Cancer* 2006;95:775–781.
58. Agarwal A, MacKenzie R, Oddo J, et al. A novel SET antagonist (OP449) is cytotoxic to CML cells, including the highly-resistant BCR-ABLT315I mutant, and demonstrates enhanced efficacy in combination with ABL tyrosine kinase inhibitors. *Am Soc Hematol* 2011;118:3757.
59. Radich JP, Dai H, Mao M, et al. Gene expression changes associated with progression and response in chronic myeloid leukemia. *Proc Natl Acad Sci U S A* 2006;103:2794–2799.

60. Oehler VG, Yeung KY, Choi YE, et al. The derivation of diagnostic markers of chronic myeloid leukemia progression from microarray data. *Blood* 2009;114:3292–3298.
61. Grossmann V, Kohlmann A, Zenger M, et al. A deep-sequencing study of chronic myeloid leukemia patients in blast crisis (BC-CML) detects mutations in 76.9% of cases. *Leukemia* 2011;25:557–560.
62. Zhao LJ, Wang YY, Li G, et al. Functional features of RUNX1 mutants in acute transformation of chronic myeloid leukemia and their contribution to inducing murine full-blown leukemia. *Blood* 2012;119:2873–2882.
63. Sailaja K, Rao VR, Yadav S, et al. Intronic SNPs of TP53 gene in chronic myeloid leukemia: Impact on drug response. *J Nat Sci Biol Med* 2012;3:182–185.
64. Mullighan CG, Miller CB, Radtke I, et al. BCR-ABL1 lymphoblastic leukaemia is characterized by the deletion of Ikaros. *Nature* 2008;453:110–114.
65. Dash AB, Williams IR, Kutok JL, et al. A murine model of CML blast crisis induced by cooperation between BCR/ABL and NUP98/HOXA9. *Proc Natl Acad Sci U S A* 2002;99:7622–7627.
66. Nucifora G, Birn DJ, Espinosa R 3rd, et al. Involvement of the AML1 gene in the t(3;21) in therapy-related leukemia and in chronic myeloid leukemia in blast crisis. *Blood* 1993;81:2728–2734.
67. Chang JS, Santhanam R, Trotta R, et al. High levels of the BCR/ABL oncoprotein are required for the MAPK-hnRNP-E2 dependent suppression of C/EBPalpha-driven myeloid differentiation. *Blood* 2007;110:994–1003.
68. Scheller M, Schonheit J, Zimmermann K, et al. Cross talk between Wnt/beta-catenin and Irf8 in leukemia progression and drug resistance. *J Exp Med* 2013;210:2239–2256.
69. Jamieson CH, Ailles LE, Dylla SJ, et al. Granulocyte-macrophage progenitors as candidate leukemic stem cells in blast-crisis CML. *N Engl J Med* 2004;351:657–667.
70. Ito T, Kwon HY, Zimdahl B, et al. Regulation of myeloid leukaemia by the cell-fate determinant Musashi. *Nature* 2010;466:765–768.
71. McWeeney SK, Pemberton LC, Loriaux MM, et al. A gene expression signature of CD34+ cells to predict major cytogenetic response in chronic-phase chronic myeloid leukemia patients treated with imatinib. *Blood* 2010;115:315–325.
72. Matutes E, Wotherspoon A, Catovsky D. Differential diagnosis in chronic lymphocytic leukaemia. *Best Pract Res Clin Haematol* 2007;20:367–384.
73. Montserrat E, Gomis F, Vallespi T, et al. Presenting features and prognosis of chronic lymphocytic leukemia in younger adults. *Blood* 1991;78:1545–1551.
74. Eichhorst B, Goede V, Hallek M. Treatment of elderly patients with chronic lymphocytic leukemia. *Leuk Lymphoma* 2009;50:171–178.
75. Keating MJ, O'Brien S, Albitar M, et al. Early results of a chemoimmunotherapy regimen of fludarabine, cyclophosphamide, and rituximab as initial therapy for chronic lymphocytic leukemia. *J Clin Oncol* 2005;23:4079–4088.
76. Wierda W, O'Brien S, Wen S, et al. Chemoimmunotherapy with fludarabine, cyclophosphamide, and rituximab for relapsed and refractory chronic lymphocytic leukemia. *J Clin Oncol* 2005;23:4070–4078.
77. Wierda W, O'Brien S, Faderl S, et al. A retrospective comparison of three sequential groups of patients with Recurrent/Refractory chronic lymphocytic leukemia treated with fludarabine-based regimens. *Cancer* 2006;106:337–345.
78. Ghia P, Scielzo C, Frenquelli M, et al. From normal to clonal B cells: chronic lymphocytic leukemia (CLL) at the crossroad between neoplasia and autoimmunity. *Autoimmun Rev* 2007;7:127–131.
79. Caligaris-Cappio F, Ghia P. The normal counterpart to the chronic lymphocytic leukemia B cell. *Best Pract Res Clin Haematol*. 2007;20:385–397.
80. Oppezzo P, Magnac C, Bianchi S, et al. Do CLL B cells correspond to naive or memory B-lymphocytes? Evidence for an active Ig switch unrelated to phenotype expression and Ig mutational pattern in B-CLL cells. *Leukemia* 2002;16:2438–2446.
81. Hamblin TJ, Davis Z, Gardiner A, et al. Unmutated Ig V(H) genes are associated with a more aggressive form of chronic lymphocytic leukemia. *Blood* 1999;94:1848–1854.
82. Damle RN, Wasil T, Fais F, et al. Ig V gene mutation status and CD38 expression as novel prognostic indicators in chronic lymphocytic leukemia. *Blood* 1999;94:1840–1847.
83. Klein U, Tu Y, Stolovitzky GA, et al. Gene expression profiling of B cell chronic lymphocytic leukemia reveals a homogeneous phenotype related to memory B cells. *J Exp Med* 2001;194:1625–1638.
84. Rosenwald A, Alizadeh AA, Widhopf G, et al. Relation of gene expression phenotype to immunoglobulin mutation genotype in B cell chronic lymphocytic leukemia. *J Exp Med* 2001;194:1639–1647.
85. Orchard JA, Ibbotson RE, Davis Z, et al. ZAP-70 expression and prognosis in chronic lymphocytic leukaemia. *Lancet* 2004;363:105–111.
86. Wiestner A, Rosenwald A, Barry TS, et al. ZAP-70 expression identifies a chronic lymphocytic leukemia subtype with unmutated immunoglobulin genes, inferior clinical outcome, and distinct gene expression profile. *Blood* 2003;101:4944–4951.
87. Rassenti LZ, Huynh L, Toy TL, et al. ZAP-70 compared with immunoglobulin heavy-chain gene mutation status as a predictor of disease progression in chronic lymphocytic leukemia. *N Engl J Med* 2004;351:893–901.
88. Crespo M, Bosch F, Villamor N, et al. ZAP-70 expression as a surrogate for immunoglobulin-variable-region mutations in chronic lymphocytic leukemia. *N Engl J Med* 2003;348:1764–1775.
89. Chen L, Apgar J, Huynh L, et al. ZAP-70 directly enhances IgM signaling in chronic lymphocytic leukemia. *Blood* 2005;105:2036–2041.
90. Gobessi S, Laurenti L, Longo PG, et al. ZAP-70 enhances B-cell-receptor signaling despite absent or inefficient tyrosine kinase activation in chronic lymphocytic leukemia and lymphoma B cells. *Blood* 2007;109:2032–2039.
91. Chen L, Huynh L, Apgar J, et al. ZAP-70 enhances IgM signaling independent of its kinase activity in chronic lymphocytic leukemia. *Blood* 2008;111:2685–2692.
92. Claus R, Lucas DM, Stilgenbauer S, et al. Quantitative DNA methylation analysis identifies a single CpG dinucleotide important for ZAP-70 expression and predictive of prognosis in chronic lymphocytic leukemia. *J Clin Oncol* 2012;30:2483–2491.
93. Juliusson G, Gahrton G. Chromosome aberrations in B-cell chronic lymphocytic leukemia. Pathogenetic and clinical implications. *Cancer Genet Cytogenet* 1990;45:143–160.
94. Juliusson G, Merup M. Cytogenetics in chronic lymphocytic leukemia. *Semin Oncol* 1998;25:19–26.
95. Oscier DG, Stevens J, Hamblin TJ, et al. Correlation of chromosome abnormalities with laboratory features and clinical course in B-cell chronic lymphocytic leukaemia. *Br J Haematol* 1990;76:352–358.
96. Oscier DG, Stevens J, Hamblin TJ, et al. Prognostic factors in stage A0 B-cell chronic lymphocytic leukaemia. *Br J Haematol* 1990;76:348–351.
97. Juliusson G, Oscier DG, Fitchett M, et al. Prognostic subgroups in B-cell chronic lymphocytic leukemia defined by specific chromosomal abnormalities. *N Engl J Med* 1990;323:720–724.
98. Mayr C, Speicher MR, Kofler DM, et al. Chromosomal translocations are associated with poor prognosis in chronic lymphocytic leukemia. *Blood* 2006;107:742–751.
99. Kujawski L, Ouillette P, Erba H, et al. Genomic complexity identifies patients with aggressive chronic lymphocytic leukemia. *Blood* 2008;112:1993–2003.
100. Pfeifer D, Pantic M, Skatulla I, et al. Genome-wide analysis of DNA copy number changes and LOH in CLL using high-density SNP arrays. *Blood* 2007;109:1202–1210.
101. Schwaenen C, Nessling M, Wessendorf S, et al. Automated array-based genomic profiling in chronic lymphocytic leukemia: development of a clinical tool and discovery of recurrent genomic alterations. *Proc Natl Acad Sci U S A* 2004;101:1039–1044.
102. Döhner H, Stilgenbauer S, Benner A, et al. Genomic aberrations and survival in chronic lymphocytic leukemia. *N Engl J Med* 2000;343:1910–1916.
103. Kröber A, Seiler T, Benner A, et al. V(H) mutation status, CD38 expression level, genomic aberrations, and survival in chronic lymphocytic leukemia. *Blood* 2002;100:1410–1416.
104. Calin GA, Dumitru CD, Shimizu M, et al. Frequent deletions and downregulation of micro-RNA genes miR15 and miR16 at 13q14 in chronic lymphocytic leukemia. *Proc Natl Acad Sci U S A* 2002;99:15524–15529.
105. Cimmino A, Calin GA, Fabbri M, et al. miR-15 and miR-16 induce apoptosis by targeting BCL2. *Proc Natl Acad Sci U S A* 2005;102:13944–13949.
106. Fabbri M, Bottoni A, Shimizu M, et al. Association of a microRNA/TP53 feedback circuitry with pathogenesis and outcome of B-cell chronic lymphocytic leukemia. *JAMA* 2011;305:59–67.
107. Zenz T, Habe S, Denzel T, et al. Detailed analysis of p53 pathway defects in fludarabine-refractory chronic lymphocytic leukemia (CLL): dissecting the contribution of 17p deletion, TP53 mutation, p53-p21 dysfunction, and miR34a in a prospective clinical trial. *Blood* 2009;114:2589–2597.
108. Wang L, Lawrence MS, Wan Y, et al. SF3B1 and other novel cancer genes in chronic lymphocytic leukemia. *N Engl J Med* 2011;365:2497–2506.
109. Fabbri G, Rasi S, Rossi D, et al. Analysis of the chronic lymphocytic leukemia coding genome: role of NOTCH1 mutational activation. *J Exp Med* 2011;208:1389–1401.
110. Puente XS, Pinyol M, Quesada V, et al. Whole-genome sequencing identifies recurrent mutations in chronic lymphocytic leukaemia. *Nature* 2011;475:101–105.
111. Doménech E, Gómez-López G, Gzlez-Peña D, et al. New mutations in chronic lymphocytic leukemia identified by target enrichment and deep sequencing. *PLoS One* 2012;7:e38158.
112. Balatti V, Bottoni A, Palamarchuk A, et al. NOTCH1 mutations in CLL associated with trisomy 12. *Blood* 2012;119:329–331.
113. Rossi D, Rasi S, Fabbri G, et al. Mutations of NOTCH1 are an independent predictor of survival in chronic lymphocytic leukemia. *Blood* 2012;119:521–529.
114. Stilgenbauer S, Sander S, Bullinger L, et al. Clonal evolution in chronic lymphocytic leukemia: acquisition of high-risk genomic aberrations associated with unmutated VH, resistance to therapy, and short survival. *Haematologica* 2007;92:1242–1245.
115. Shanafelt TD, Witzig TE, Fink SR, et al. Prospective evaluation of clonal evolution during long-term follow-up of patients with untreated early-stage chronic lymphocytic leukemia. *J Clin Oncol* 2006;24:4634–4641.
116. Roos G, Kröber A, Grabowski P, et al. Short telomeres are associated with genetic complexity, high-risk genomic aberrations, and short survival in chronic lymphocytic leukemia. *Blood* 2008;111:2246–2252.
117. Ricca I, Rocci A, Drandi D, et al. Telomere length identifies two different prognostic subgroups among VH-unmutated B-cell chronic lymphocytic leukemia patients. *Leukemia* 2007;21:697–705.
118. Landau Dan A, Carter Scott L, Stojanov P, et al. Evolution and impact of subclonal mutations in chronic lymphocytic leukemia. *Cell* 2013;152:714–726.
119. Giné E, Martinez A, Villamor N, et al. Expanded and highly active proliferation centers identify a histological subtype of chronic lymphocytic leukemia ("accelerated" chronic lymphocytic leukemia) with aggressive clinical behavior. *Haematologica* 2010;95:1526–1533.

120. Bonato M, Pittaluga S, Tierens A, et al. Lymph node histology in typical and atypical chronic lymphocytic leukemia. Am J Surg Pathol 1998;22:49–56.
121. Hayes GM, Busch R, Voogt J, et al. Isolation of malignant B cells from patients with chronic lymphocytic leukemia (CLL) for analysis of cell proliferation: validation of a simplified method suitable for multi-center clinical studies. Leuk Res 2010;34:809–815.
122. Calissano C, Damle RN, Hayes G, et al. In vivo intraclonal and interclonal kinetic heterogeneity in B-cell chronic lymphocytic leukemia. Blood 2009;114:4832–4842.
123. Messmer BT, Messmer D, Allen SL, et al. In vivo measurements document the dynamic cellular kinetics of chronic lymphocytic leukemia B cells. J Clin Invest 2005;115:755–764.
124. Hanada M, Delia D, Aiello A, et al. bcl-2 gene hypomethylation and high-level expression in B-cell chronic lymphocytic leukemia. Blood 1993;82:1820–1828.
125. Dancescu M, Rubio-Trujillo M, Biron G, et al. Interleukin 4 protects chronic lymphocytic leukemic B cells from death by apoptosis and upregulates Bcl-2 expression. J Exp Med 1992;176:1319–1326.
126. McConkey DJ, Chandra J, Wright S, et al. Apoptosis sensitivity in chronic lymphocytic leukemia is determined by endogenous endonuclease content and relative expression of BCL-2 and BAX. J Immunol 1996;156:2624–2630.
127. Pepper C, Bentley P, Hoy T. Regulation of clinical chemoresistance by bcl-2 and bax oncoproteins in B-cell chronic lymphocytic leukaemia. Br J Haematol 1996;95:513–517.
128. Robertson LE, Plunkett W, McConnell K, et al. Bcl-2 expression in chronic lymphocytic leukemia and its correlation with the induction of apoptosis and clinical outcome. Leukemia 1996;10:456–459.
129. Vogler M, Butterworth M, Majid A, et al. Concurrent up-regulation of BCL-XL and BCL2A1 induces approximately 1000-fold resistance to ABT-737 in chronic lymphocytic leukemia. Blood 2009;113:4403–4413.
130. Smit LA, Hallaert DY, Spijker R, et al. Differential Noxa/Mcl-1 balance in peripheral versus lymph node chronic lymphocytic leukemia cells correlates with survival capacity. Blood 2007;109:1660–1668.
131. Pedersen IM, Kitada S, Leoni LM, et al. Protection of CLL B cells by a follicular dendritic cell line is dependent on induction of Mcl-1. Blood 2002;100:1795–1801.
132. Furman RR, Asgary Z, Mascarenhas JO, et al. Modulation of NF-kappa B activity and apoptosis in chronic lymphocytic leukemia B cells. J Immunol 2000;164:2200–2206.
133. Lu D, Zhao Y, Tawatao R, et al. Activation of the Wnt signaling pathway in chronic lymphocytic leukemia. Proc Natl Acad Sci U S A 2004;101:3118–3123.
134. Hegde GV, Peterson KJ, Emanuel K, et al. Hedgehog-induced survival of B-cell chronic lymphocytic leukemia cells in a stromal cell microenvironment: a potential new therapeutic target. Mol Cancer Res 2008;6:1928–1936.
135. Frank DA, Mahajan S, Ritz J. B lymphocytes from patients with chronic lymphocytic leukemia contain signal transducer and activator of transcription (STAT) 1 and STAT3 constitutively phosphorylated on serine residues. J Clin Invest 1997;100:3140–3148.
136. Chen SS, Raval A, Johnson AJ, et al. Epigenetic changes during disease progression in a murine model of human chronic lymphocytic leukemia. Proc Natl Acad Sci U S A 2009;106:13433–13438.
137. Pekarsky Y, Palamarchuk A, Maximov V, et al. Tcl1 functions as a transcriptional regulator and is directly involved in the pathogenesis of CLL. Proc Natl Acad Sci U S A 2008;105:19643–19648.
138. Nishio M, Endo T, Tsukada N, et al. Nurselike cells express BAFF and APRIL, which can promote survival of chronic lymphocytic leukemia cells via a paracrine pathway distinct from that of SDF-1alpha. Blood 2005;106:1012–1020.
139. Munzert G, Kirchner D, Stobbe H, et al. Tumor necrosis factor receptor-associated factor 1 gene overexpression in B-cell chronic lymphocytic leukemia: analysis of NF-kappa B/Rel regulated inhibitors of apoptosis. Blood 2002;100:3749–3756.
140. Bernal A, Pastore RD, Asgary Z, et al. Survival of leukemic B cells promoted by engagement of the antigen receptor. Blood 2001;98:3050–3057.
141. Hewamana S, Lin TT, Rowntree C, et al. Rel a is an independent biomarker of clinical outcome in chronic lymphocytic leukemia. J Clin Oncol 2009;27:763–769.
142. Hewamana S, Lin TT, Jenkins C, et al. The novel nuclear factor-kappa B inhibitor LC-1 is equipotent in poor prognostic subsets of chronic lymphocytic leukemia and shows strong synergy with fludarabine. Clin Cancer Res 2008;14:8102–8111.
143. Hewamana S, Alghazal S, Lin TT, et al. The NF-kappa B subunit Rel A is associated with in vitro survival and clinical disease progression in chronic lymphocytic leukemia and represents a promising therapeutic target. Blood 2008;111:4681–4689.
144. Chen L, Widhopf G, Huynh L, et al. Expression of ZAP-70 is associated with increased B-cell receptor signaling in chronic lymphocytic leukemia. Blood 2002;100:4609–4614.
145. Buchner M, Fuchs S, Prinz G, et al. Spleen tyrosine kinase is overexpressed and represents a potential therapeutic target in chronic lymphocytic leukemia. Cancer Res 2009;69:5424–5432.
146. Trentin L, Frasson M, Donella-Deana A, et al. Geldanamycin-induced Lyn dissociation from aberrant Hsp90-stabilized cytosolic complex is an early event in apoptotic mechanisms in B-chronic lymphocytic leukemia. Blood 2008;112:4665–4674.
147. Quiroga MP, Balakrishnan K, Kurtova AV, et al. B-cell antigen receptor signaling enhances chronic lymphocytic leukemia cell migration and survival: specific targeting with a novel spleen tyrosine kinase inhibitor, R406. Blood 2009;114:1029–1037.
148. Herman SE, Barr PM, McAuley EM, et al. Fostamatinib inhibits B-cell receptor signaling, cellular activation and tumor proliferation in patients with relapsed and refractory chronic lymphocytic leukemia. Leukemia 2013;27:1769–1773.
149. Herman SE, Gordon AL, Hertlein E, et al. Bruton tyrosine kinase represents a promising therapeutic target for treatment of chronic lymphocytic leukemia and is effectively targeted by PCI-32765. Blood 2011;117:6287–6296.
150. Cuni S, Pérez-Aciego P, Pérez-Chacón G, et al. A sustained activation of PI3K/NF-kappa B pathway is critical for the survival of chronic lymphocytic leukemia B cells. Leukemia 2004;18:1391–1400.
151. Ringshausen I, Schneller F, Bogner C, et al. Constitutively activated phosphatidylinositol-3 kinase (PI-3K) is involved in the defect of apoptosis in B-CLL: association with protein kinase Cdelta. Blood 2002;100:3741–3748.
152. Srinivasan L, Sasaki Y, Calado DP, et al. PI3 kinase signals BCR-dependent mature B cell survival. Cell 2009;139:573–586.
153. Herman SE, Gordon AL, Wagner AJ, et al. Phosphatidylinositol 3-kinase-δ inhibitor CAL-101 shows promising preclinical activity in chronic lymphocytic leukemia by antagonizing intrinsic and extrinsic cellular survival signals. Blood 2010;116:2078–2088.
154. Byrd JC, Furman RR, Coutre SE, et al. Targeting BTK with ibrutinib in relapsed Chronic lymphocytic leukemia. N Engl J Med 2013;369:32–42.

45 Chronic Myelogenous Leukemia

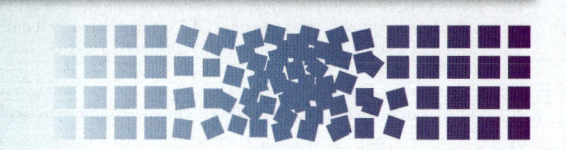

Brian J. Druker and David Marin

INTRODUCTION

Chronic myelogenous leukemia (CML; also called *chronic myeloid leukemia*) is a clonal hematopoietic disorder caused by an acquired genetic defect in a pluripotent stem cell. CML is a bi- or triphasic illness, with most patients diagnosed in a relatively indolent chronic or stable phase that is characterized by excessive numbers of myeloid lineage cells that fully mature. The disease has the capacity to progress to a more aggressive leukemia as a malignant clone loses the capacity for terminal differentiation. This more aggressive or advanced phase can be further subdivided into an accelerated phase and a blastic phase, with the blastic phase being akin to an acute leukemia and having a dismal prognosis.[1]

CML has become a paradigm for targeted drug development based on an understanding of the molecular pathogenesis of a disease. A series of discoveries led to the recognition that the BCR-ABL protein, which results from a reciprocal translocation involving chromosomes 9 and 22, has a central role in the pathogenesis of CML. The BCR-ABL protein functions as a constitutively activated tyrosine kinase and this knowledge led to the development of imatinib (Gleevec, Glivec), a drug that specifically inhibits the BCR-ABL tyrosine kinase.[2] Other tyrosine-kinase inhibitors (TKI) with improved potency have been developed, and BCR-ABL TKIs are now the standard therapy for newly diagnosed patients with CML. Allogeneic hematopoietic cell transplantation (HCT), which was the preferred therapy prior to the advent of targeted therapy, is now reserved for patients with resistance to TKIs or for patients with advanced phase disease.

EPIDEMIOLOGY

CML accounts for approximately 15% of all leukemias, with 4,000 to 5,000 new cases diagnosed in the United States annually. The incidence of CML is 1.6 to 2.0 cases per 100,000 persons per year, and the incidence is similar in all countries worldwide.[3] Although CML occurs in all age groups, its incidence increases with each decade of life, making it mainly a disease of adults. According to the Surveillance, Epidemiology, and End Results (SEER) program, the median age at diagnosis is 66 years, which is much higher than that reported in single-institutional series and clinical trials.[3] The disease has a slight male predominance (2.2:1.3).[3]

The only known risk factor for the development of CML is exposure to radiation at high doses. This is evident from studies of survivors of the atom bomb explosions in Japan in 1945 and from follow-ups of patients treated with radiation for ankylosing spondylitis and cervical cancer.[4-6] No known association has been found between CML and infectious agents or chemical exposures, and no familial predisposition has been implicated in CML.

PATHOGENESIS

The discovery of the Philadelphia (Ph) chromosome in 1960 made CML the first human neoplasm to be characterized by a consistent cytogenetic marker.[7] In 1973, the Ph chromosome, a shortened chromosome 22 (22q-), was shown to be the result of a balanced, reciprocal translocation between the long arms of chromosomes 9 and 22, t(9;22) (q34;q11) (Fig. 45.1).[8] In the 1980s, the *BCR-ABL* chimeric gene and protein formed as a result of the (9;22) translocation was characterized and its central role in the pathogenesis of CML was established.[9,10] The Ph chromosome and *BCR-ABL* are found in cells of the myeloid, erythroid, and megakaryocytic lineages, some B cells, and a small proportion of T cells, but not in other cells of the body, establishing CML as a clonal disorder that originates in a pluripotent hematopoietic stem cell.

The (9;22) translocation transposes the *ABL* (Abelson) proto-oncogene from chromosome 9 into a relatively small, 5.8-kb genomic region on chromosome 22 named the *breakpoint cluster region (bcr)*.[11] Although the genomic breakpoints in the *ABL* gene are highly variable, they almost always occur upstream of the second exon (a2), resulting in translocation of all but exon 1 of *ABL*. Two slightly different chimeric *BCR-ABL* genes are present in most patients with CML, depending on the precise location of the breakpoint in the *BCR* gene. Breaks can occur between exon e13 (also known as b2) and exon e14 (b3), yielding an e13a2 fusion messenger RNA (mRNA), whereas a break occurring between exons 14 and 15 produces an e14a2 fusion mRNA (Fig. 45.2).[9] In the majority of patients, either e13a2 or e14a2 transcripts are present, but occasionally, patients have both transcripts in their leukemia cells. Although the e14a2 mRNA encodes a BCR-ABL protein that is 25 amino acids larger than that encoded by the e13a2 transcript, both are referred to as p210BCR-ABL. Patients with e13a2 or e14a2 transcripts have similar prognoses. In 5% of the patients, the breakpoint occurs in other regions of the BCR gene resulting in the so-called *rare transcripts*; these transcripts have the same biological activity as the more common ones.[1,9] It is important, however, to identify patients harboring these rare transcripts because molecular monitoring may otherwise prove impossible.

The BCR-ABL fusion protein resides in the cytoplasm and has constitutive tyrosine kinase activity compared to the tightly regulated activity of the normal *ABL* product (p145).[12,13] The BCR-ABL tyrosine kinase binds to and phosphorylates numerous intracellular proteins. The net effect of this is to induce all of the phenotypic abnormalities observed in patients with CML.[9] These include increased proliferation or decreased apoptosis of hematopoietic stem or progenitor cells leading to a massive increase in myeloid cell numbers and the premature release of immature myeloid cells into the circulation, postulated to be due to a defect in adherence of myeloid progenitors to marrow stroma and genetic instability resulting in disease progression. Despite the complexity of BCR-ABL signal transduction, all of the transforming functions of BCR-ABL depend on its tyrosine kinase activity, making this disease an ideal candidate for therapy directed against this activity.

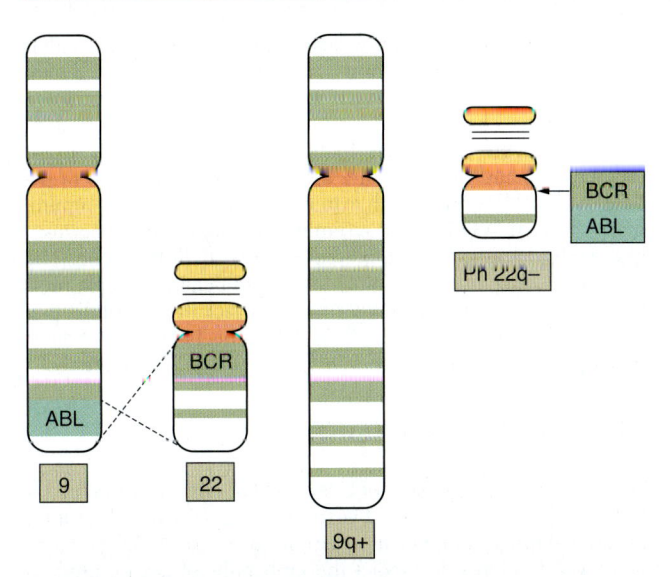

Figure 45.1 Diagrammatic representation of the formation of the Philadelphia (Ph) chromosome. The normal chromosomes 9 and 22 are shown, along with the derivative chromosomes 9q+ and 22q− (Ph). The approximate positions of the normal *ABL* gene at 9q34 and *BCR* at 22q11 and the *BCR-ABL* fusion gene formed as a result of the translocation are shown.

DIAGNOSIS

Clinical Manifestations

Of patients with CML, 90% are diagnosed in the chronic or stable phase. Of patients in older studies, 10% to 20% and as many as 50% in more recent series present without symptoms and are diagnosed as a result of finding an elevated white blood count on routine blood sampling. The most common presenting symptoms of CML are related to anemia, splenomegaly, and increased cell turnover. These symptoms include fatigue, left upper quadrant pain, abdominal distention or discomfort, early satiety, weight loss, and night sweats.[14]

Occasionally, patients may present with a hyperviscosity syndrome, which requires leukapheresis, with manifestations such as stroke, priapism, stupor, or visual changes caused by retinal hemorrhage. The most common physical finding is splenomegaly, its magnitude correlating with the degree of leukocytosis. Ecchymoses are frequently observed, but spontaneous bleeding is uncommon. A lymphadenopathy is not usually seen in the chronic phase.

Laboratory Tests

Peripheral Blood and Bone Marrow

The diagnosis of CML is frequently suspected from an examination of the peripheral blood and bone marrow. The white blood cell (WBC) count in the chronic phase of CML usually exceeds 50×10^9/L at the time of diagnosis and can range up to 800×10^9/L. During the chronic phase, leukemic WBCs differentiate and function normally. The peripheral blood smear shows a full spectrum of myeloid cells from blasts to neutrophils, with blasts comprising less than 15% and usually less than 5% of the WBC differential. Basophilia is invariably present, and its absence should prompt consideration of other myeloproliferative disorders. Eosinophilia is also commonly present. The majority of patients have thrombocytosis and, on occasion, the platelet count may be more than 1000×10^9/L. Most patients with CML have a normochromic, normocytic anemia that is inversely proportional to the degree of leukocytosis.

The bone marrow in patients with chronic phase CML is markedly hypercellular, with a predominance of myeloid cells with full maturation. Blasts are fewer than 15% and most commonly fewer than 5%, and basophilia is also present. Megakaryocytes are usually increased in number, are characteristically small, are hypo- or monolobated, and have a tendency to cluster. Erythroid hypoplasia is frequently present and may seem exaggerated because of the increased myeloid-to-erythroid ratio. Erythroid precursors are otherwise morphologically unremarkable. Reticulin fibrosis is usually absent or mild but may become more prominent with disease progression.[15]

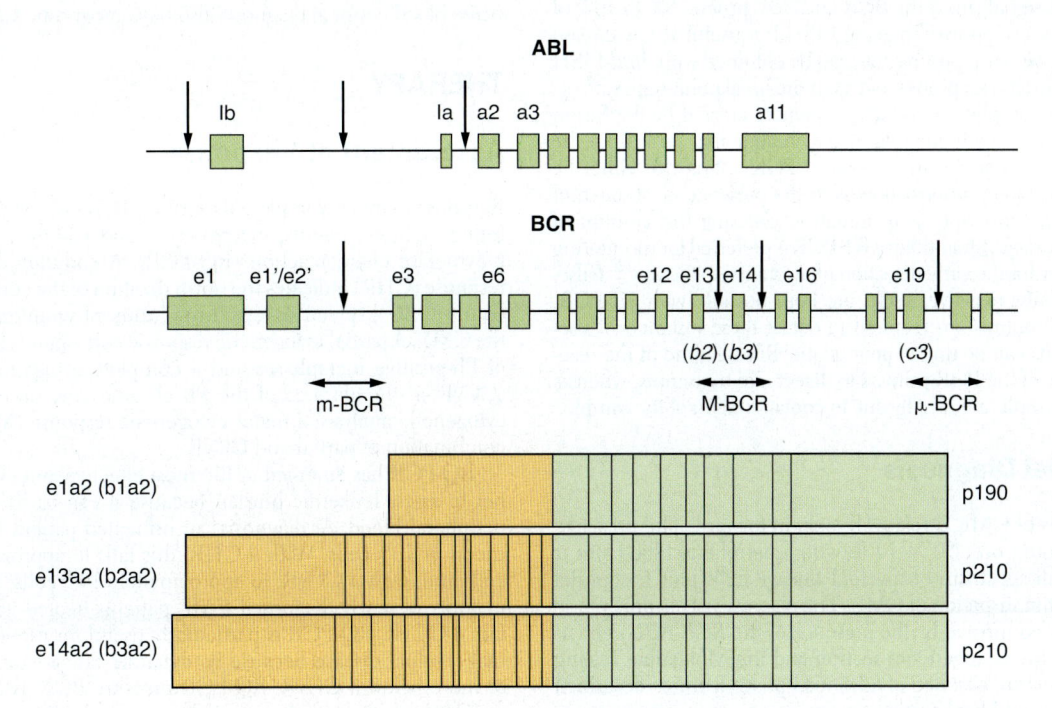

Figure 45.2 Schematic representation of the genomic structure of the normal *ABL* and *BCR* genes (*top*) and various fusion transcripts generated by the different *BCR-ABL* fusion genes (*bottom*). The b2a2 or the b3a2 transcript is found in the majority of patients with chronic myelogenous leukemia. See text for details.

Cytogenetics

A cytogenetic analysis of 20 bone marrow metaphases has been the standard method to detect the Ph chromosome, which is present in the majority of cells at diagnosis. Although most patients have a typical t(9;22)(q34;q11), approximately 5% have variant translocations that have no impact on prognosis.[16] These variant translocations may be simple, involving chromosome 22 and a chromosome other than chromosome 9, or they may be complex, involving one or more other chromosomes in addition to chromosomes 9 and 22.[17] Clonal cytogenetic abnormalities in addition to the Ph chromosome are present at diagnosis in approximately 5% of patients diagnosed in chronic phase.[18,19] The most common are duplication of the Ph chromosome and trisomy 8, iso-17q, and trisomy 19.[18,19] These abnormalities have only a small adverse prognostic impact when identified at diagnosis.[19]

Molecular Testing

The diagnosis of CML requires the presence of BCR-ABL. In 95% of patients, its presence can be inferred by the detection of the Ph chromosome using standard cytogenetics. Another 5% of patients with a hematologic picture resembling CML who lack a detectable Ph chromosome will have a BCR-ABL fusion gene detectable by fluorescence in situ hybridization (FISH) or reverse transcription–polymerase chain reaction (RT-PCR). These Ph chromosome–negative, BCR-ABL–positive patients have a clinical course that is indistinguishable from that of Ph chromosome positive, BCR-ABL–positive patients.[20] Patients with a hematologic picture resembling CML, but who are Ph chromosome negative and BCR-ABL negative, are classified within the myeloproliferative neoplasm group.[21] Some of these patients have mutations in the SETBP1[22] or CSF3R[23] genes, whereas others remain genetically unclassified.

FISH detects the colocalization of large, fluorescently labeled genomic probes specific to the BCR and ABL genes. FISH can be performed on metaphase or interphase cells and on peripheral blood. At diagnosis, when typically 90% of cells are BCR-ABL positive, FISH is a highly accurate diagnostic test, because false-negative results are uncommon.[24] However, because of the random colocalization of the signals from the BCR and ABL probes, 8% to 10% of normal cells score positive, making FISH less useful at low disease burdens. A lower false-positive rate can be obtained with dual-FISH (D-FISH), which uses probes that span the breakpoint region.[25]

RT-PCR to amplify the unique sequences created by the fusion of BCR and ABL is a highly sensitive technique that is ideal for the detection of minimal residual disease.[24] PCR testing can either be qualitative, providing information as to the presence or absence of the BCR-ABL transcript, or quantitative, assessing the amount of BCR-ABL message. Quantitative RT-PCR is preferred for monitoring and may allow for the early detection of resistance to therapy.[26] False-positive and false-negative results are both possible with RT-PCR, and rigorous controls are required to detect these instances. False-negative results can be due to poor quality RNA, failure of the reaction or failure of the PCR primers to detect rare transcripts, whereas false-positive results are usually due to contamination of the sample.

Differential Diagnosis

The diagnosis of CML is relatively straight forward. The presence of a WBC count over 50×10^9/L with a peripheral blood smear showing a full spectrum of myeloid lineage cells plus basophilia should raise the suspicion of CML. The diagnosis of chronic phase CML can be confirmed by the presence of the BCR-ABL gene as described in the Cytogenetics section and the Molecular Testing section and by the absence of advanced phase features described later in Advanced Phase Disease.

The main differential diagnosis includes a leukemoid reaction and other myeloproliferative neoplasms. In patients with a leukemoid reaction, which is typically seen in patients with underlying infections, the WBC count is usually less than 50×10^9/L and the peripheral blood smear consists predominantly of segmented neutrophils and bands, often with toxic granulations. Less mature myeloid cells are rarely seen; there is no basophilia; and the Ph chromosome and BCR-ABL are absent. Approximately 5% of patients with CML present with extreme thrombocytosis and a minimally elevated WBC count, resembling essential thrombocytosis, but are distinguished by the presence of the BCR-ABL gene. The differential diagnosis with other myeloproliferative neoplasm is relatively easy because the latter frequently lack the basophilia that is seen with CML and lack the BCR-ABL gene, but may have other molecular abnormalities such as SETBP1 or CSF3R mutations.

PROGNOSTIC FACTORS

Historically, the progression of CML to blast crisis occurred in 5% to 10% of patients in the first 2 years after diagnosis and, thereafter, the annual progression rate increased from 20% to 25%. The Sokal score was developed to predict the probability of disease progression, but this and a variety of other factors are now being used to predict the probability of optimal response to therapy. The Sokal score was developed to predict the probability of disease progression.[27] Despite it being developed in a pre-TKI era and as a predictor for disease progression, it has been found useful to predict the probability of achieving an optimal response to imatinib.[28,29]; however, it has been less useful for predicting responses to newer TKIs.[30,31] The Sokal score is a numerical value that is calculated from a complex equation that takes into account four factors at diagnosis: the percentage of blasts in peripheral blood, platelet count, spleen size (centimeters below the costal margin) and age of the patient.[27] Patients then were divided according to their individual numerical value into three risk groups: low, intermediate, and high, risk of progression, with median survivals of 5, 4, and 3 years, respectively. Many of these patients received therapies not currently in use, such as busulfan and hydroxyurea; however, the Sokal score remains useful to predict the response of patients treated with imatinib, but less so with newer TKIs.[28,31] Other variables closely related with the Sokal score such as hemoglobin and white blood count at diagnosis also have prognostic value.[29,32,33]

THERAPY

Assessment of Response

Response to therapy in patients with CML is assessed by the monitoring of blood counts, cytogenetics, and real-time quantitative polymerase chain reaction (RQ-PCR). A complete hematologic response (CHR) indicates the normalization of the complete blood count (CBC), spleen size, and resolution of symptoms related to the CML. A partial cytogenetic response corresponds to 1% to 35% of Ph-positive metaphases and a complete cytogenetic response (CCyR) is the absence of the Ph chromosome on conventional cytogenetic analysis; a major cytogenetic response (MCyR) is the combination of partial and CCyR.

RQ-PCR has emerged as the most effective and efficient manner to assess leukemic burden because it can easily be done on peripheral blood. At diagnosis, an untreated patient may have in excess of 10^{12} cells. With a CHR, this falls to approximately 10^{11} cells and, with a CCyR, to approximately 10^{10} cells. Because the majority of newly diagnosed CML patients treated with TKIs obtain a CCyR, RQ-PCR is particularly useful for monitoring minimal residual disease because its dynamic range extends two-logs or more below a CCyR. RQ-PCR measure BCR-ABL transcripts in relation to a control gene such as normal ABL or GUSB, and can be expressed as the absolute ratio or as log reductions from the 100% value. In an attempt to introduce some level of uniformity, many laboratories are using the International Scale (IS), whereby values are *corrected* to those obtained in a reference laboratory.[34] It is generally accepted that CCyR corresponds to an approximately 2-log reduction in transcript levels or 1% IS.[35] Major molecular response (MR3) is defined as a 3-log reduction in transcript levels or 0.1% IS, and this should correspond to a leukemia burden of approximately 10^9 cells. Similarly, MR4 is defined as a 4-log reduction (0.01% IS, or 10^8 leukemic cells). A complete molecular response (CMR) is generally defined as the absence of detectable BCR-ABL transcripts, a status that depends on the technology and criteria for negativity employed, with the limits of technology being somewhere between MR4 and MR5.

Treatment of Chronic Phase Disease

BCR-ABL TKIs are the standard frontline therapy for newly diagnosed patients with chronic phase CML. Hydroxyurea, a well-tolerated oral agent that inhibits DNA synthesis by inhibiting ribonucleotide reductase, remains in use as an initial therapy to control blood counts pending definitive diagnosis and therapy. Allogeneic HCT, although curative, is typically reserved for patients with resistance to TKI therapy or in the management of advanced phase disease due to its morbidity and mortality. Interferon-α, a previous mainstay of therapy, has been supplanted by TKIs, and has been used with variable results in clinical trials attempting to improve molecular responses to TKIs.

BCR-ABL Tyrosine-Kinase Inhibitors

BCR-ABL TKIs inhibit the BCR-ABL tyrosine kinase by competing with ATP binding to the kinase. The first drug of this class was imatinib, which rapidly became the treatment of choice for patients with chronic phase CML after it was approved by the U.S. Food and Drug Administration (FDA) in 2001.[2] Today, imatinib, nilotinib, dasatinib, bosutinib and ponatinib are licensed for use in CML. They differ in their respective affinity for the ABL-binding pocket—for example, imatinib has a BCR ABL IC50 of 221 nM, whereas ponatinib has an IC50 of 0.37 nM and respective half-lives, ranging from 13 hours for imatinib to 4 hours for dasatinib. They also differ in their ability to inhibit other tyrosine kinases, with ponatinib, dasatinib, and bosutinib being the most promiscuous, whereas imatinib and nilotinib are the most specific. Other kinases inhibited by imatinib and nilotinib include the platelet-derived growth factor receptors KIT, and ARG (*ABL*-related gene), whereas the other drugs inhibit SRC family members amongst many others. These differences explain, at least in part, the different toxicity profiles of the various drugs.[36–40] Despite that, it is possible to define a drug class side effect profile that includes myelosuppression, fatigue, gastrointestinal disturbances, hepatotoxicity, myalgias, arthralgias, and skin rashes.[41] All five drugs can cause these side effects, but the relative frequency of the individual side effect differs for each drug. Common toxicities observed are listed in Table 45.1.

TABLE 45.1

Comparison of Side Effects (All Grades) Reported in More Than 10% of the Patients Between Imatinib 400 mg Per Day, Nilotinib 300 mg Twice Per Day, Dasatinib 100 mg Per Day, and Bosutinib 500 mg Per Day

Side Effect	Imatinib	Alternative TKI	Clinical Trial
Peripheral edema	14	5	ENESTnd (Nilotinib)
	38	11	DASISION (Dasatinib)
	38	11	BELA (Bosutinib)
Pleural effusion	Rare	Rare	ENESTnd (Nilotinib)
	0	14	DASISION (Dasatinib)
	Rare	Rare	BELA (Bosutinib)
Skin rash	11	31	ENESTnd (Nilotinib)
	17	11	DASISION (Dasatinib)
	15	20	BELA (Bosutinib)
Nausea	31	11	ENESTnd (Nilotinib)
	23	10	DASISION (Dasatinib)
	35	31	BELA (Bosutinib)
Vomiting	14	5	ENESTnd (Nilotinib)
	10	5	DASISION (Dasatinib)
	13	32	BELA (Bosutinib)
Diarrhea	21	8	ENESTnd (Nilotinib)
	21	19	DASISION (Dasatinib)
	21	68	BELA (Bosutinib)
Fatigue	8	11	ENESTnd (Nilotinib)
	11	9	DASISION (Dasatinib)
	12	11	BELA (Bosutinib)
Musculoskeletal pain or muscle spasm	24	7	ENESTnd (Nilotinib)
	39	22	DASISION (Dasatinib)
	20	2	BELA (Bosutinib)
Headache	8	14	ENESTnd (Nilotinib)
	11	13	DASISION (Dasatinib)
	8	10	BELA (Bosutinib)

Based on data from the ENESTnd, DASISION, and BELA trials.[50,51,61,110,111]

Imatinib

With over 15 years of experience and hundreds of thousands of patients using imatinib as first-line therapy, the side effects are well understood and there are no apparent long-term safety concerns. Approximately 70% of patients that receive imatinib as first-line therapy will achieve CCyR by 12 months, and 80% will have done so by 5 years.[28,29] The 8-year survival for 553 patients treated with imatinib as part of a randomized trial comparing imatinib to interferon plus Ara-C was 85%, or 93% if only CML-related deaths were considered. This high survival rate has been confirmed in additional single-center studies.[42] Imatinib is given once daily, normally with food (in order to prevent nausea). The current standard dose of imatinib is 400 mg per day. Several randomized studies comparing 400 mg per day to 800 mg per day in newly diagnosed patients revealed more rapid responses with the higher doses; however, one-third of patients required dose reduction due to greater toxicity. With longer follow-up, the response rates to 400 mg per day and higher doses are similar. Progression-free survival (PFS) was not impacted by the higher doses, although a recent study from Germany has suggested that deeper molecular remissions that are more frequently obtained with higher doses of imatinib may translate into a trend toward improved PFS.[43–45]

Nilotinib

Nilotinib is a BCR-ABL inhibitor that was rationally designed to be more potent and selective than imatinib. Until recently, it had been used as a second-line agent at a dose of 400 mg twice daily. At this dose, it induces CCyR in 30% to 40% of the patients who are resistant to imatinib, and most interestingly, there is no cross-intolerance with imatinib.[46–48] Nilotinib obtained a license for first-line use in 2010. The first-line dose is 300 mg twice daily. Nilotinib is administered twice daily in a fasting state because food increases absorption and may lead to increased side effects, particularly the prolongation of Qtc intervals. Overall, nilotinib is well tolerated and causes less nausea, myalgia, arthralgia, and fluid retention than imatinib. On the other hand, it produces skin rashes or pruritus in the majority of patients; in most cases, these can be easily controlled with antihistamines. Nilotinib induces hyperglycemia in approximately 40% of patients; it also causes increases in cholesterol and triglyceride levels. Hepatotoxicity is frequent, although this is normally limited to mild increases in transaminases that do not require action. A severe toxic hepatitis occurs rarely. Similarly, nilotinib causes an increase in the bilirubin level in the majority of patients, but this seldom necessitates any modification of therapy. Nilotinib has also been associated with progressive peripheral arterial occlusive disease,[49] although the incidence of this complication is not yet clear.

Dasatinib

Dasatinib is a multitarget kinase inhibitor that is more than 300 times more potent than imatinib in inhibiting the BCR-ABL oncoprotein in vitro.[50,51] As with nilotinib, most of the experience to date has been using dasatinib in patients who are resistant to imatinib. Initially, dasatinib was used at a dose of 70 mg twice daily due to its short half-life, but a large randomized study comparing several schedules of dasatinib in patients with imatinib resistance showed that 100 mg once daily was equally efficacious to the 70 mg twice daily or 140 mg once daily schedules, but with significantly less toxicity for chronic phase patients.[52] Dasatinib induces CCyR in 30% to 40% of patients with imatinib resistance.[48,53,54] Dasatinib was also approved for first-line use in chronic phase CML patients at a dose of 100 mg per day. Dasatinib is generally well tolerated. Pleural effusions are the main complication of dasatinib therapy. Most studies report an incidence below 25%, although rates as high as 54% have been reported.[51,55–58] Pleural effusions can occur at any time during therapy and often recur despite a dose reduction. Diagnostic thoracocentesis is not usually required and, in practice, the effusion nearly always resolves on discontinuing the drug. Resolution of the pleural effusion can be accelerated by using 0.5 mg per kilogram of prednisolone for 1 or 2 weeks. Dasatinib has been associated with pulmonary hypertension. The incidence of this complication is not clearly established, and it may be at least partially reversible on discontinuation of the drug.[59]

Bosutinib

Bosutinib is a dual SRC and ABL TKI, which is currently licensed only for second-line use. Similarly to nilotinib and dasatinib, bosutinib induces CCyR in 30% to 40% of the patients who are resistant to at least one prior TKI therapy.[60] Bosutinib has also been evaluated in newly diagnosed patients, but it did not meet its primary endpoint of improved rates of CCyR at 1 year.[61] The drug is well tolerated. Its main side effect is diarrhea, which can easily be managed symptomatically.[60–62] Bosutinib has also been found to cause pleural effusions and pulmonary hypertension, although the incidence of both complications appears to be lower than with dasatinib.

Ponatinib

Ponatinib is the latest addition to the TKI armamentarium. It has been licensed for the management of patients who are resistant to at least two prior TKIs or who harbor the kinase domain mutation T315I. This mutation confers resistance to all the other TKIs discussed in this chapter. The peculiar chemical structure of ponatinib allows it to overcome the steric hindrance caused by the substitution of a threonine by isoleucine in position 315 of the kinase domain.[63] The efficacy of ponatinib has been explored in the PACE study where approximately 200 chronic phase patients who were resistant or intolerant to either dasatinib or nilotinib (the majority of these patients had failed at least three prior TKI lines) and 64 chronic phase patients with the T315I mutation were treated with 45 mg daily. The CCyR rate was 46% with a higher response rate in patients with the T315I mutation.[64–66] The main side effects are skin rash, pancreatitis, and hepatotoxicity. Various cardiac, cerebral, and peripheral vascular thrombotic events have been reported in patients on ponatinib. These have occurred in up to 27% of patients treated with ponatinib and have included fatal myocardial infarction and stroke. These vascular side effects led to the early termination of the phase 3 trial comparing ponatinib with imatinib as frontline therapy and a recommendation that lower doses of ponatinib be used—30 mg in patients initially and 15 mg after patients achieve a MR3. To date, strategies combining ponatinib with antithrombotic agents have not been formally reported.

Choice of Initial Therapy for the Newly Diagnosed Patient in Chronic Phase

Imatinib, nilotinib, and dasatinib are licensed for first-line use. Four randomized studies have been conducted comparing imatinib to newer TKIs, one each comparing imatinib to nilotinib or bosutinib, and two comparing imatinib to dasatinib. Data from these studies are summarized in Table 45.2. A few generalities emerge from these studies. All therapies are extremely effective with excellent PFS. The newer, more potent TKIs induce faster cytogenetic and molecular responses, but in only the imatinib versus nilotinib study has this translated into a significant difference in PFS at 3 years. In the other studies, there was either

TABLE 45.2

Comparison of the Efficacy Profiles of Imatinib, Nilotinib, Dasatinib, and Bosutinib as Front-line Therapy for Chronic Phase Patients Using Results of the Randomized Trials Comparing Nilotinib 300 mg Twice Daily Versus Imatinib 400 mg Daily (Enestnd),[110,111] Dasatinib 100 mg Once Daily Versus Imatinib 400 mg Daily (Dasision),[30,31] Dasatinib 100 mg Daily Versus Imatinib 400 mg Daily (North America Cooperative Group),[112] and Bosutinib 500 mg Once Daily Versus Imatinib 400 mg Once Daily (Bela)[61]

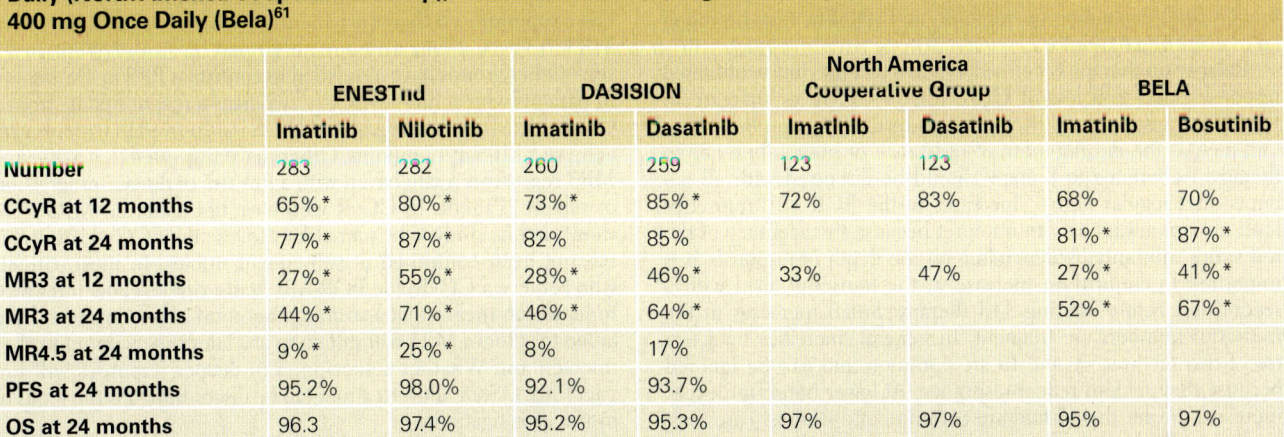

	ENESTnd		DASISION		North America Cooperative Group		BELA	
	Imatinib	Nilotinib	Imatinib	Dasatinib	Imatinib	Dasatinib	Imatinib	Bosutinib
Number	283	282	260	259	123	123		
CCyR at 12 months	65%*	80%*	73%*	85%*	72%	83%	68%	70%
CCyR at 24 months	77%*	87%*	82%	85%			81%*	87%*
MR3 at 12 months	27%*	55%*	28%*	46%*	33%	47%	27%*	41%*
MR3 at 24 months	44%*	71%*	46%*	64%*			52%*	67%*
MR4.5 at 24 months	9%*	25%*	8%	17%				
PFS at 24 months	95.2%	98.0%	92.1%	93.7%				
OS at 24 months	96.3	97.4%	95.2%	95.3%	97% (at 3 years)	97% (at 3 years)	95%	97%
Patients still on therapy at 24 months	67%	74%	75%	77%			71%*	63%*

The rates of response (CCyR, MR3, and MR4.5) are given as cumulative incidences. Progression free-survival (PFS) and overall survival (OS) are expressed as 2-year probabilities. Patients still on therapy at 24 months are expressed as proportions. Asterisks indicate that the difference is statistically significant (p <0.05).

---

no difference or a trend to improved PFS, but no studies have shown a significant difference in overall survival (OS). With most relapses on imatinib occuring in the first 3 years, it is unlikely that additional follow-up will lead to significant changes in this data.

Imatinib is still the first-line TKI for many clinicians because its long-term side effect profile is well understood. Further, in most health systems, it is significantly cheaper than dasatinib or nilotinib. The main arguments in favor of using nilotinib or dasatinib as first-line therapies are that they induce deep molecular responses in a higher proportion of patients and that this may impact PFS. With optimal responses to imatinib being highly dependent on the Sokal score, it would be reasonable to choose nilotinib or dasatinib for patients with higher risk Sokal scores.

Another consideration for the selection of initial therapy is comorbid conditions based on the side effect profiles described in Table 45.1. For example, nilotinib can increase the glucose level and serum lipids in a significant proportion of patients; therefore, clinicians may want to avoid nilotinib when treating a patient with diabetes or a dyslipidemia. Similarly, it has been suggested that patients with cardiovascular risk factors should not receive nilotinib because of the risk of developing peripheral arterial occlusive disease. It also should be avoided in patients with a history of pancreatitis. Dasatinib has been shown to inhibit platelet function and has been associated with hemorrhages, so one would favor the use of other TKIs in patients with platelet or clotting disorders. Patients of advanced age and patients with a history of autoimmune disease have a higher risk of developing pleural effusions on dasatinib. Other patients with preexisting pulmonary disease should not receive dasatinib because of the risk of developing pleural effusions, although there is no evidence that patients with pulmonary disease are more likely to develop pleural effusions. The major limitation of this strategy is that it only can be used in the proportion of patients with the relevant comorbidities. In addition, there are no specific circumstances where imatinib should be avoided in preference to other TKIs.

Management of Chronic Phase Patients on Tyrosine Kinase Inhibitor Therapy

TKI therapy can be started as soon as the definitive diagnosis of CML is made. Hydroxyurea may be used to control the peripheral counts while awaiting the results of diagnostic testing. Hydroxyurea can be stopped as soon as patients start on TKI therapy or may be continued for 1 or 2 weeks in cases where the WBC or platelet count is very high. Concomitant therapy with allopurinol is recommended until the WBC is consistently in the normal range. Tumor lysis syndrome is exceedingly rare even in patients with advanced phase disease. After initiating therapy, the WBC count should begin to fall within the first 2 weeks and usually normalizes within 6 weeks. The normalization of the platelet count is commonly delayed by 1 to 3 weeks.[28,67] Myelosuppression occurs in about 10% to 25% of patients. It may occur at any time, but it is more frequent within the first 2 to 6 weeks. Patients should have complete blood counts checked weekly to every other week during the first 2 months of therapy. In the absence of significant myelosuppression, the frequency of hematologic monitoring can be reduced. It is advisable to monitor electrolytes, calcium, magnesium levels, and hepatic and renal function at the same time as the CBC because liver toxicity, hypocalcemia, hypomagnesia, and changes in electrolytes levels are relatively common. Nonhematologic toxicity is normally managed with supportive measures or by interrupting the TKI therapy until resolution of side effects and then by the reintroduction the TKI at the same or at a reduced dose depending on the nature and the severity of the specific side effects. Because there is very little cross-intolerance between the various TKIs, it is advisable to switch TKIs for potentially dangerous or recurrent side effects with the exception of myelosuppression, which is more likely related to the underlying disease.

Bone marrow cytogenetics should be monitored every 6 months until a complete cytogenetic response CCyR is obtained. Some advocate for a marrow at 3 months, but the prognostic significance of this is less clear. With the wider availability of RQ-PCR standardized to the IS, RQ-PCR may replace the necessity of performing marrows. RQ-PCR for BCR-ABL transcripts should be performed every 3 months on peripheral blood for at least the first 2 years on therapy and, depending on response and stability, may be monitored every 4 to 6 months.

Relapse on therapy is defined as a loss of a previously obtained response, such as a loss of CHR, loss of CCyR, or increase in RQ-PCR transcript level. Relapses can be due to a number of factors such as the development of resistance or poor adherence to therapy. Adherence to therapy should be discussed with all patients on a regular basis.[33] Increases in the BCR-ABL transcript level are not always easy to interpret because the accuracy of the test varies substantially depending on the depth of response. It is important to confirm an increase in the transcript level with a second test before altering TKI therapy. Small increases in the transcript numbers are frequent. In general, increases by a factor of two or three on the IS are common and can be ignored because they seldom reflect resistance. At lower transcript levels, increases greater than 5-fold are common and in most cases can be dismissed. The magnitude of the increases is more critical than the loss of MR3, MR4, or CMR, which do not have clinical relevance. Repeated increases beyond interassay variability or confirmed increases consistent with loss of CCyR are should to be taken seriously.

Prognostic Landmarks on Therapy

Patient responses are normally assessed at 3, 6, and 12 months. Failure to achieve a CHR at 3 months is rare, and these patients have a poor prognosis.[68] Cytogenetic and molecular response have been evaluated for prognostic significance. One of the most widely accepted landmarks is the achievement of a CCyR at 12 months,[28,29,48,69–72] and many other parameters are based on the likelihood of obtaining this response. For example, for patients who do not achieve an MCyR by 6 months, the chances of obtaining a CCyR at 12 months is 50% or less.[29,68]

Another parameter that is gaining acceptance as having prognostic significance is the BCR-ABL transcript ratio at 3 months. Several studies have shown that patients with a BCR-ABL transcript ratio greater than 10% on the IS have a significantly higher PFS and lower cumulative incidence of CCyR and deep molecular responses (MR3 or higher).[42,73] Similar results have been obtained for patients treated with dasatinib or nilotinib.[48] One possible limitation to the use of this parameter is the lack of availability of standardized molecular testing.

A third parameter that has been analyzed for prognostic significance is the achievement of a MR3. An analysis of the phase 3 randomized clinical trial comparing imatinib to interferon-α plus Ara-C reported that patients who had achieved MR3 by 12 months had a superior PFS than the patients who were in CCyR but not in MR3.[74] These results were not confirmed by a subsequent analysis.[28] Other groups have also failed to confirm a PFS or OS benefit in patients who achieve MR3,[68,75] whereas a recent update from a German CML study suggested that OS is improved in patients who achieve a MR3 at 12 months. Others have suggested that achieving MR3 represents a safe haven with a low risk of disease progression or relapse. Patients in CCyR who have not achieved MR3 were shown in one study to be more likely to lose their CCyR,[68] but this has not been confirmed in subsequent studies. In most patients who achieve a CCyR, the BCR-ABL transcript level declines over time, which means that a sizable proportion of patients who have failed to achieve MR3 will still do so at a later time without further intervention. Whether achieving even deeper responses will impact PFS, OS, or allow treatment to be discontinued is the focus of future investigations.

Management of Hematologic Toxicity on Tyrosine Kinase Inhibitors

Grade 3 or 4 myelosuppression is relatively common at the onset of TKI therapy and probably reflects the elimination of hematopoiesis from Ph chromosome–positive stem cells before Ph-negative hematopoiesis can be adequately expanded. In the randomized studies comparing imatinib to nilotinib and imatinib to dasatinib, it appears that dasatinib is the most myelosuppressive, followed by imatinib, with nilotinib at 300 mg twice daily being the least myelosuppressive (Table 45.3). Even with nilotinib at 300 mg twice per day, 10% of patients will develop grade 3 or 4 myelosuppression. Although dasatinib may suppress normal hematopoiesis, the suppression of normal hematopoiesis by imatinib and nilotinib is relatively minimal; thus, dose reductions of imatinib and nilotinib are unlikely to expedite the recovery of normal blood counts. In the case of imatinib, doses lower than 300 mg per day may allow for the emergence of resistant leukemic clones, but the minimum adequate doses of dasatinib and nilotinib have not been established. For chronic phase patients, treatment should only be interrupted for an absolute neutrophil count of less than $1.0 \times 10^9/L$ and a platelet count less than $50 \times 10^9/L$. These parameters can

TABLE 45.3

Comparison of Grade 3/4 Myelosuppression Between Imatinib 400 mg Per Day, Nilotinib 300 mg Twice Per Day, Dasatinib 100 mg Per Day, and Bosutinib 500 mg Per Day

	Percentage (%) Imatinib	Alternative TKI	Clinical Trial
Anemia	5	3	ENESTnd (Nilotinib)
	8	11	DASISION (Dasatinib)
	7	6	BELA (Bosutinib)
Neutropenia	20	12	ENESTnd (Nilotinib)
	21	24	DASISION (Dasatinib)
	24	11	BELA (Bosutinib)
Thrombocytopenia	9	10	ENESTnd (Nilotinib)
	11	19	DASISION (Dasatinib)
	14	14	BELA (Bosutinib)

Based on data from the ENESTnd, DASISION, and BELA trials.[50,51,61,111,112]

be modified for patients with more advanced disease. The use of myeloid or erythroid growth factors while continuing therapy with imatinib appears to be safe. For patients with recurrent myelosuppression, the ability to obtain optimal responses may be compromised; thus, these patients may be candidates for more aggressive therapy. Recurrent pancytopenia is associated with primary cytogenetic resistance in spite of dose reduction or change of TKI therapy. This cohort of patients has a poor prognosis. One possible explanation for this phenomenon is that hematologic toxicity is linked to a lack of an expandable Ph-negative stem cell population that can restore effective Ph-negative hematopoiesis, and; therefore, these patients are intrinsically unable to respond adequately to TKI therapy.[29,30]

Management of Primary Treatment Resistance or Relapse

A loss of disease control in the first 5 years of therapy occurs in approximately 15% of chronic phase patients treated with imatinib. Point mutations in the BCR-ABL kinase domain that render the kinase less sensitive to imatinib are observed in approximately 40% of patients who relapse on therapy, but only in a minority of patients with primary resistance (defined as an inability to reach the landmarks defined in Prognostic Landmarks on Therapy). Regardless, all patients being considered for a change in therapy should have the ABL kinase domain sequenced because this may influence the choice of therapy. The point mutations that mediate resistance are scattered throughout the ABL kinase domain and disrupt critical contact points between imatinib and the BCR-ABL protein or induce structural alterations that prevent TKI binding.[2,76] Other mechanisms of resistance include BCR-ABL amplification, drug affinity, and BCR-ABL–independent mechanisms, such as clonal evolution.[77]

Given that the majority of patients who relapse have disease that remains dependent on the BCR-ABL kinase, it was logical to develop novel agents that inhibit imatinib-resistant mutations. As noted previously, dasatinib, nilotinib, bosutinib, and ponatinib were initially developed for patients with imatinib resistance or intolerance. All of these compounds inhibit the majority of imatinib-resistant mutations other than T315I, which is only inhibited by ponatinib.[36,37,78,79] The potency of the various drugs against kinase mutations varies. Some mutations are less sensitive to nilotinib (Y253H, E255K/V, and F359V/C), whereas others are less sensitive to dasatinib (F317L and V299L), bosutinib (F317L and V299L), or ponatinib (E255V).[80] T315I is the most common mutation that emerges in patients with resistance to dasatinib, bosutinib, and nilotinib, but this is rare (<2%) in patients not exposed to these drugs. Highly drug resistant compound mutations have been seen on occasion.[81]

If a patient becomes resistant or intolerant to a first-line therapy, second-line therapy should be started without delay. Patients who require second-line therapy because of nonhematologic toxicity and those with secondary cytogenetic resistance (loss of CCyR) to first-line TKI therapy have a 50% to 90% probability of achieving stable CCyR on second-line therapy.[31,48] Patients with primary cytogenetic resistance, particularly when associated with recurrent pancytopenia, constitute a poor risk group.[42,48] There are no randomized studies comparing the efficacy of the various drugs, and the various single-arm phase 2 studies report similar efficacy for all the drugs. Importantly, most of the published experience is based on the use of nilotinib, dasatinib, and bosutinib in patients who have failed imatinib. Limited data exists on the efficacy of these drugs on patients who have failed nilotinib or dasatinib. None exists on the use of imatinib after failure of other TKIs. The choice of second-line therapy may be guided by mutational analysis or potential toxicities. Once the new therapy is started, patients receiving second-line therapy should be managed and assessed for response as described in the first-line section. Responses to second-line TKIs are as durable as first line responses; therefore, responding patients do not necessarily need to be considered for allogeneic HCT.[48]

Hematopoietic Cell Transplantation

Until 1999, CML was the leading indication for allogeneic HCT, but with the widespread availability of imatinib and the other TKIs, HCT rates for CML have fallen.[82] However, the proportion of patients with advanced stage CML who proceed to HCT has increased.[83] HCT remains an effective therapy for patients who are resistant to TKIs and remain in chronic phase and for patients with advanced phase disease whose leukemia can be restored to the chronic phase.

If transplantation is performed with myeloablative conditioning during chronic phase using an HLA-identical sibling donor, 5-year survival rates are 60% to 80%, with a 10-year disease-free survival of 50% to 60%, and a 20-year survival of 38%.[84] Survival estimates roughly halve as the disease progresses from chronic phase to accelerated phase to blast crisis. For younger patients, HCT performed using unrelated donors yields results similar to those obtained with HLA-matched siblings.[85]

Reduced-intensity conditioning regimens, otherwise known as *nonmyeloablative regimens*, emphasize immunosuppression rather than myeloablation to facilitate engraftment, and can be performed in the outpatient setting. The cure relies on immune reconstitution from the donor, with or without additional lymphocyte infusions, to eradicate residual disease. Common preparative regimens include combinations of fludarabine, busulfan, low-dose total body irradiation, T-cell antibodies, and other immunosuppressive drugs. The reduced-intensity conditioning regimens avoid the high early mortality associated with myeloablative conditioning and prolonged neutropenia. Reduced intensity conditioning have shown to be superior to myeloablative HCT in patients over 60 years of age.[86] However, infections and acute and chronic graft versus host disease remain significant problems. Disease-free survival ranges from 40% to 85% at 3 to 5 years.[87,88] Imatinib has been used after HCT for prophylaxis against relapse. Small studies suggest that imatinib can be safely administered from the time of engraftment through the first post-HCT year in patients at high risk of post-transplant relapse.[89,90] Dasatinib and nilotinib post-HCT have also been used in a small number of patients.[91] These small numbers do not allow for an assessment of the effectiveness of this approach in increasing long-term disease-free survival rates.

Relapse after HCT is a common problem, particularly if T-cell depletion is used. Imatinib as the initial treatment for patients who relapse into the chronic phase after allogeneic HCT restores CMR in 83% of patients in molecular relapse and 58% of those in cytogenetic relapse.[92] Approximately 10% to 25% of patients attaining complete molecular remissions are able to discontinue imatinib after 6 to 24 months and remain in remission, whereas the others require either reinstitution of imatinib or donor lymphocyte infusions.[93] Lower and less durable responses to imatinib are seen in patients relapsing into the accelerated phase or blast crisis.[94] Early studies with dasatinib and nilotinib confirm their efficacy in this situation, but the number of patients studied is too small to draw firm conclusions.[91,95] Patients who relapse cytogenetically or hematologically into the chronic phase can also be treated with donor lymphocyte infusions, with 60% to 80% achieving durable remissions and a 5-year disease-free survival rate of approximately 50%.[96–98] In contrast, patients in the accelerated phase and blast crisis are much less responsive to immune manipulations. The risks of donor lymphocyte infusions are significant and result in a treatment-related mortality of 8% to 20%.[99] To date, formal comparison of donor lymphocyte infusions versus TKIs has been undertaken. In addition, strategies need to be developed for using TKIs plus donor lymphocyte infusions for the treatment of relapse after HCT.

ADVANCED PHASE DISEASE

The transformation to advanced phase typically occurs gradually, with the disease becoming more difficult to control with medical therapy. In other patients, the disease transforms abruptly into an acute leukemia, also known as *blast crisis*. Approximately 65% of patients evolve to blast crisis with myeloid lineage blasts; 30% have blasts of pre–B-lymphoid origin; and 5% have undifferentiated or T-cell blasts. On occasion, an isolated blast phase of extramedullary origin may occur while the patient's blood and marrow still meet the criteria for chronic phase disease.

The intermediate period, during which the patient is no longer in the chronic phase but is not yet in blastic transformation, has been termed the *accelerated phase*. Currently accepted criteria for accelerated phase include: (1) progressive splenomegaly and myelofibrosis; (2) bone marrow or peripheral blood blasts ≥15% but <30%; (3) bone marrow or peripheral blood blasts plus promyelocytes ≥30%; (4) bone marrow or peripheral blood basophils ≥20%; (5) platelet count <100 × 10^9/L unrelated to therapy; and (6) clonal evolution in a Ph-chromosome–positive clone.[100] The blastic phase is defined as bone marrow or peripheral blood blast ≥30% or the presence of extramedullary blast infiltrates.

Clonal cytogenetic abnormalities besides a single Ph chromosome may be acquired in patients with CML as their disease progresses, and up to 80% of patients with overt blastic transformation have additional cytogenetic abnormalities. The molecular basis of disease progression is poorly defined, but point mutations or deletions in the *p53* tumor suppressor gene have been observed in up to 33% of patients with myeloid blast crisis, and as many as 50% of patients with lymphoid transformation show a homozygous deletion in the *p16* tumor suppressor gene.[101]

Therapy of Advanced Phase Disease

The prognosis for patients in advanced phase remains poor. Although TKIs induce CCyR in 10% to 45% of patients treated with these drugs, remissions are typically short lasting.[102,103] For example, dasatinib as monotherapy for patients in blast crisis induces a CCyR in 20% to 40% of the patients,[103,104] but a majority of the patients relapse within 1 year, and the median survival is 8 months.[103] Conventional chemotherapy regimens such as a combination of fludarabine, cytarabine, idarubicin and filgrastim (FLAG-IDA) can induce CCyR in 30% to 40% of patients who have progressed to the blastic phase, but again, the majority of patients relapse within 6 months, and the survival is poor.[105] Currently, the standard therapy for patients who present with blast crisis or who have progressed to this phase on TKI therapy consists of two or three courses of conventional acute leukemia-like chemotherapy or a TKI in monotherapy followed by stem cell transplantation in eligible patients. With this approach, only 20% of the patients are alive at 5 years[84] (<20% at 2 years for patients who are not candidates for allogeneic HCT[105]). Because TKIs have been used successfully in combination with conventional chemotherapy for the therapy of Ph-positive acute lymphoblastic leukemia (ALL),[106] clinical trials are currently exploring the combination of chemotherapy with TKIs for patients in blast crisis.

The accelerated phase is a heterogeneous entity, and there are no large studies dissecting the prognosis of patients according to the different accelerated phase criteria. Most investigators consider patients in the accelerated phase due to a high percentage of blasts to have a similar prognosis to patients in the blastic phase. One of the major limitations of TKI therapy in accelerated phase patients is that the majority of these patients have also already received a TKI. Dasatinib induces a 20% to 30% CCyR rate in patients who have progressed to the accelerated phase on imatinib.[107] Because relapses in these patients are common, HCT should remain a consideration for eligible patients whose disease can be returned to the chronic phase and for patients who fail to achieve an MCyR by 3 months or a CCyR by 6 months.

FUTURE DIRECTIONS

There are now numerous treatment options available for patients with CML. While long-term disease control appears possible with current therapies, disease is not eradicated. Therefore, the most critical area for future development is minimal residual disease. Although the molecular basis of disease persistence is poorly understood, studies of the mechanism are ongoing. Meanwhile, a variety of therapies based on the manipulation of the immunologic system and signal transduction pathways are being investigated for their ability to impact CML stem cells, although it is not clear that it is necessary to eradicate every CML stem cell in order to achieve a cure. Several groups have discontinued imatinib in patients with a consistently negative RQ-PCR for BCR-ABL transcripts using a sensitive assay (>4.5 logs). In these studies, up to 40% of patients have maintained their PCR undetectable status with the majority of molecular relapses occurring within the first 6 months off of therapy.[108,109] With newer TKIs potentially achieving deeper molecular remissions, studies have commenced on the discontinuation of these drugs to see if a larger percentage of patients can discontinue therapy. If a larger percentage of patients achieve a molecular remission and a similar or greater percentage are able to discontinue therapy, the goal of achieving molecular remission may become a goal of treatment guidelines.

REFERENCES

1. Goldman JM, Melo JV. Chronic myeloid leukemia—advances in biology and new approaches to treatment. *N Engl J Med* 2003;349:1451–1464.
2. Druker BJ. Translation of the Philadelphia chromosome into therapy for CML. *Blood* 2008;112:4808–4817.
3. Rohrbacher M, Hasford J. Epidemiology of chronic myeloid leukaemia (CML). *Best Pract Res Clin Haematol* 2009;22:295–302.
4. Brown WM, Doll R. Mortality from cancer and other causes after radiotherapy for ankylosing spondylitis. *Br Med J* 1965;5474:1327–1332.
5. Curtis RE, Boice JD Jr, Stovall M, et al. Relationship of leukemia risk to radiation dose following cancer of the uterine corpus. *J Natl Cancer Inst* 1994;86:1315–1324.
6. Kato H, Schull WJ. Studies of the mortality of A-bomb survivors. 7. Mortality, 1950-1978: Part I. Cancer mortality. *Radiat Res* 1982;90:395–432.
7. Nowell PC, Hungerford DA. A minute chromosome in human chronic granulocytic leukemia. *Science* 1960;132:1497.
8. Rowley JD. A new consistent chromosomal abnormality in chronic myelogenous leukaemia identified by quinacrine fluorescence and Giemsa staining. *Nature* 1973;243:290–293.
9. Deininger MW, Goldman JM, Melo JV. The molecular biology of chronic myeloid leukemia. *Blood* 2000;96:3343–3356.
10. de Klein A, van Kessel AG, Grosveld G, et al. A cellular oncogene is translocated to the Philadelphia chromosome in chronic myelocytic leukaemia. *Nature* 1982;300:765–767.
11. Groffen J, Stephenson JR, Heisterkamp N, et al. Philadelphia chromosomal breakpoints are clustered within a limited region, bcr, on chromosome 22. *Cell* 1984;36:93–99.
12. Konopka JB, Watanabe SM, Witte ON. An alteration of the human c-abl protein in K562 leukemia cells unmasks associated tyrosine kinase activity. *Cell* 1984;37:1035–1042.
13. Lugo TG, Pendergast AM, Muller AJ, et al. Tyrosine kinase activity and transformation potency of bcr-abl oncogene products. *Science* 1990;247:1079–1082.
14. Savage DG, Szydlo RM, Goldman JM. Clinical features at diagnosis in 430 patients with chronic myeloid leukaemia seen at a referral centre over a 16-year period. *Br J Haematol* 1997;96:111–116.
15. Vardiman JW, Pierre RV, Thiele J, et al. Chronic myelogenous leukaemia. In: Jaffe SE, Harris NL, Stein H, et al, eds. *World Health Organization Classification of Tumours. Pathology and Genetics of Tumours of Haematopoietic and Lymphoid Tissues*. Lyon: IARC Press; 2001: 20–26.

16. El-Zimaity MM, Kantarjian H, Talpaz M, et al. Results of imatinib mesylate therapy in chronic myelogenous leukaemia with variant Philadelphia chromosome. Br J Haematol 2004;125:187–195.
17. Mitelman F. The cytogenetic scenario of chronic myeloid leukemia. Leuk Lymphoma 1993;11:11–15.
18. Luatti S, Castagnetti F, Marzocchi G, et al. Additional chromosomal abnormalities in Philadelphia-positive clone: adverse prognostic influence on front-line imatinib therapy: a GIMEMA Working Party on CML analysis. Blood 2012;120:761–767.
19. Fabarius A, Leitner A, Hochhaus A, et al. Impact of additional cytogenetic aberrations at diagnosis on prognosis of CML: long-term observation of 1151 patients from the randomized CML Study IV. Blood 2011;118:6760–6768.
20. Cortes JE, Talpaz M, Beran M, et al. Philadelphia chromosome-negative chronic myelogenous leukemia with rearrangement of the breakpoint cluster region. Long-term follow-up results. Cancer 1995;75:464–470.
21. Kurzrock R, Bueso-Ramos CE, Kantarjian H, et al. BCR rearrangement-negative chronic myelogenous leukemia revisited. J Clin Oncol 2001;19:2915–2926.
22. Piazza R, Valletta S, Winkelmann N, et al. Recurrent SETBP1 mutations in atypical chronic myeloid leukemia. Nat Genet 2013;45:18–24.
23. Maxson JE, Gotlib J, Pollyea DA, et al. Oncogenic CSF3R mutations in chronic neutrophilic leukemia and atypical CML. N Engl J Med 2013;368:1781–1790.
24. Wang YL, Bagg A, Pear W, et al. Chronic myelogenous leukemia: laboratory diagnosis and monitoring. Genes Chromosomes Cancer 2001;32:97–111.
25. DeWald GW, Wyatt WA, Juneau AL, et al. Highly sensitive fluorescence in situ hybridization method to detect double BCR/ABL fusion and monitor response to therapy in chronic myeloid leukemia. Blood 1998;91:3357–3365.
26. Cross NC. Quantitative PCR techniques and applications. Br J Haematol 1995;89:693–697.
27. Sokal JE, Cox EB, Baccarani M, et al. Prognostic discrimination in "good-risk" chronic granulocytic leukemia. Blood 1984;63:789–799.
28. Druker B, Guilhot F, O'Brien S, et al. Five-year follow-up of imatinib therapy for newly diagnosed chronic myelogenous leukemia in chronic-phase shows sustained responses and high overall survival. N Engl J Med 2006;355:2408–2417.
29. de Lavallade H, Apperley JF, Khorashad JS, et al. Imatinib for newly diagnosed patients with chronic myeloid leukemia: incidences of sustained responses in an intention to treat analysis. J Clin Oncol 2008;26:3358–3363.
30. Marin D, Marktel S, Bua M, et al. Prognostic factors for patients with chronic myeloid leukaemia in chronic phase treated with imatinib mesylate after failure of interferon alfa. Leukemia 2003;17:1448–1453.
31. Milojkovic D, Nicholson E, Apperley JF, et al. Early prediction of success or failure using second generation tyrosine kinase inhibitors for chronic myeloid leukemia. Haematologica 2010;92:224–231.
32. Sokal JE, Baccarani M, Tura S, et al. Prognostic discrimination among younger patients with chronic granulocytic leukemia: relevance to bone marrow transplantation. Blood 1985;66:1352–1357.
33. Marin D, Bazeos A, Mahon FX, et al. Adherence is the critical factor for achieving molecular responses in chronic myeloid leukemia patients who achieve complete cytogenetic responses on imatinib. J Clin Oncol 2010;24:2381–2388.
34. Cross NC, White HE, Muller MC, et al. Standardized definitions of molecular response in chronic myeloid leukemia. Leukemia 2012;26:2172–2175.
35. Lin F, Chase A, Bungey J, et al. Correlation between the proportion of Philadelphia chromosome-positive metaphase cells and levels of BCR-ABL mRNA in chronic myeloid leukaemia. Genes Chromosomes Cancer 1995;13:110–114.
36. Weisberg E, Manley PW, Breitenstein W, et al. Characterization of AMN107, a selective inhibitor of native and mutant Bcr-Abl. Cancer Cell 2005;7:129–141.
37. O'Hare T, Shakespeare WC, Zhu X, et al. AP24534, a pan-BCR-ABL inhibitor for chronic myeloid leukemia, potently inhibits the T315I mutant and overcomes mutation-based resistance. Cancer Cell 2009;16:401–412.
38. Remsing Rix LL, Rix U, Colinge J, et al. Global target profile of the kinase inhibitor bosutinib in primary chronic myeloid leukemia cells. Leukemia 2009;23:477–485.
39. Manley PW, Stiefl N, Cowan-Jacob SW, et al. Structural resemblances and comparisons of the relative pharmacological properties of imatinib and nilotinib. Bioorg Med Chem 2010;18:6977–6986.
40. Manley PW, Cowan-Jacob SW, Mestan J. Advances in the structural biology, design and clinical development of Bcr-Abl kinase inhibitors for the treatment of chronic myeloid leukaemia. Biochim Biophys Acta 2005;1754:3–13.
41. Marin D. Initial choice of therapy among plenty for newly diagnosed chronic myeloid leukemia. Hematology Am Soc Hematol Educ Program 2012;2012:115–121.
42. Marin D, Ibrahim AR, Lucas CM, et al. Assessment of BCR-ABL1 transcript levels at 3 months is the only requirement for predicting outcome for patients with chronic myeloid leukemia treated with tyrosine kinase inhibitors. J Clin Oncol 2012;30:232–238.
43. Cortes JE, Baccarani M, Guilhot F, et al. Phase III, randomized, open-label study of daily imatinib mesylate 400 mg versus 800 mg in patients with newly diagnosed, previously untreated chronic myeloid leukemia in chronic phase using molecular end points: tyrosine kinase inhibitor optimization and selectivity study. J Clin Oncol 2010;28:424–430.
44. Baccarani M, Rosti G, Castagnetti F, et al. Comparison of imatinib 400 mg and 800 mg daily in the front-line treatment of high-risk, Philadelphia-positive chronic myeloid leukemia: a European LeukemiaNet Study. Blood 2009;113:4497–4504.
45. Hehlmann R, Müller MC, Lauseker M, et al. Deep molecular response is reached by the majority of patients treated with imatinib, predicts survival, and is achieved more quickly by optimized high dose imatinib: results from the randomized CML Study IV. J Clin Oncol 2014;32:415–423.
46. Kantarjian H, Giles F, Wunderle L, et al. Nilotinib in imatinib-resistant CML and Philadelphia chromosome-positive ALL. N Engl J Med 2006;354:2542–2551.
47. Kantarjian HM, Giles FJ, Bhalla KN, et al. Nilotinib is effective in patients with chronic myeloid leukemia in chronic phase after imatinib resistance or intolerance: 24-month follow-up results. Blood 2011;117:1141–1145.
48. Milojkovic D, Apperley JF, Gerrard G, et al. Responses to second line tyrosine kinase inhibitors are durable: an intention to treat analysis in chronic myeloid leukemia patients. Blood 2012;119:1838–1843.
49. Aichberger KJ, Herndlhofer S, Schernthaner GH, et al. Progressive peripheral arterial occlusive disease and other vascular events during nilotinib therapy in CML. Am J Hematol 2012;86:533–539.
50. Kantarjian H, Shah NP, Hochhaus A, et al. Dasatinib versus imatinib in newly diagnosed chronic-phase chronic myeloid leukemia. N Engl J Med 2010;362:2260–2270.
51. Kantarjian HM, Shah NP, Cortes JE, et al. Dasatinib or imatinib in newly diagnosed chronic-phase chronic myeloid leukemia: 2-year follow-up from a randomized phase 3 trial (DASISION). Blood 2012;119:1123–1129.
52. Shah NP, Kantarjian HM, Kim DW, et al. Intermittent target inhibition with dasatinib 100 mg once daily preserves efficacy and improves tolerability in imatinib-resistant and -intolerant chronic-phase chronic myeloid leukemia. J Clin Oncol 2008;26:3204–3212.
53. Talpaz M, Shah NP, Kantarjian H, et al. Dasatinib in imatinib-resistant Philadelphia chromosome-positive leukemias. N Engl J Med 2006;354:2531–2541.
54. Shah NP, Kim DW, Kantarjian H, et al. Potent, transient inhibition of BCR-ABL with dasatinib 100 mg daily achieves rapid and durable cytogenetic responses and high transformation-free survival rates in chronic phase chronic myeloid leukemia patients with resistance, suboptimal response or intolerance to imatinib. Haematologica 2010;95:232–240.
55. de Lavallade H, Punnialingam S, Milojkovic D, et al. Pleural effusions in patients with chronic myeloid leukaemia treated with dasatinib may have an immune-mediated pathogenesis. Br J Haematol 2008;141:743–747.
56. Quintas-Cardama A, Kantarjian H, O'Brien S, et al. Pleural effusion in patients with chronic myelogenous leukemia treated with dasatinib after imatinib failure. J Clin Oncol 2007;25:3908–3914.
57. Kim D, Goh HG, Kim SH, et al. Long-term pattern of pleural effusion from chronic myeloid leukemia patients in second-line dasatinib therapy. Int J Hematol 2011;94:361–371.
58. Porkka K, Khoury HJ, Paquette RL, et al. Dasatinib 100 mg once daily minimizes the occurrence of pleural effusion in patients with chronic myeloid leukemia in chronic phase and efficacy is unaffected in patients who develop pleural effusion. Cancer 2010;116:377–386.
59. Montani D, Bergot E, Gunther S, et al. Pulmonary Arterial Hypertension in Patients Treated by Dasatinib. Circulation 2012;125:2128–2137.
60. Cortes JE, Kantarjian HM, Brummendorf TH, et al. Safety and efficacy of bosutinib (SKI-606) in chronic phase Philadelphia chromosome positive CML patients with resistance or intolerance to imatinib. Blood 2011;118:4567–4576.
61. Cortes JE, Kim DW, Kantarjian HM, et al. Bosutinib versus imatinib in newly diagnosed chronic-phase chronic myeloid leukemia: results from the BELA trial. J Clin Oncol 2012;30:3486–3492.
62. Cortes JE, Maru A, Souza CAAD, et al. Bosutinib versus imatinib in newly diagnosed chronic phase chronic myeloid leukemia - BELA Trial: 24-month follow-up. ASH Annual Meeting Abstracts 2011;118:455.
63. Cortes JE, Kantarjian H, Shah NP, et al. Ponatinib in refractory Philadelphia chromosome-positive leukemias. N Engl J Med 2012;367:2075–2088.
64. Kantarjian HM, Kim DW, Pinilla-Ibarz J, et al. Efficacy and safety of ponatinib in patients with accelerated phase or blast phase chronic myeloid leukemia (AP-CML or BP-CML) or Philadelphia chromosome-positive acute lymphoblastic leukemia (Ph+ALL): 12-month follow-up of the PACE Trial. ASH Annual Meeting Abstracts 2012;120:915.
65. Deininger MW, Cortes JE, Kantarjian HM, et al. Long-term anti-leukemic activity of ponatinib in patients with Philadelphia chromosome-positive leukemia: updated results from an ongoing phase 1 study. ASH Annual Meeting Abstracts 2012;120:3743.
66. Cortes JE, Kim DW, Pinilla-Ibarz J, et al. A pivotal phase 2 trial of ponatinib in patients with chronic myeloid leukemia (CML) and Philadelphia chromosome-positive acute lymphoblastic leukemia (Ph+ALL) resistant or intolerant to dasatinib or nilotinib, or with the T315I BCR-ABL mutation: 12-month follow-up of the PACE trial. ASH Annual Meeting Abstracts 2012;120:163.
67. O'Brien SG, Guilhot F, Larson RA, et al. Imatinib compared with interferon and low-dose cytarabine for newly diagnosed chronic-phase chronic myeloid leukemia. N Engl J Med 2003;348:994–1004.
68. Marin D, Milojkovic D, Olavarria E, et al. European LeukemiaNet criteria for failure or sub-optimal response reliably identify patients with CML in early chronic phase treated with imatinib whose eventual outcome is poor. Blood 2008;112:4437–4444.

69. Bonifazi F, de Vivo A, Rosti G, et al. Chronic myeloid leukemia and interferon-alpha: a study of complete cytogenetic responders. *Blood* 2001;98:3074–3081.
70. Ibrahim AR, Clark RE, Holyoake TL, et al. Second generation tyrosine kinase inhibitors improve the survival of patients with chronic myeloid leukemia who have failed imatinib therapy. *Haematologica* 2011;96:1779–1782.
71. Jabbour E, Kantarjian H, O'Brien S, et al. The achievement of an early complete cytogenetic response is a major determinant for outcome in patients with early chronic phase chronic myeloid leukemia treated with tyrosine kinase inhibitors. *Blood* 2011;118:4541–4546.
72. Quintas-Cardama A, Kantarjian H, Jones D, et al. Delayed achievement of cytogenetic and molecular response is associated with increased risk of progression among patients with chronic myeloid leukemia in early chronic phase receiving high-dose or standard-dose imatinib therapy. *Blood* 2009;113:6315–6321.
73. Hanfstein B, Muller MC, Hehlmann R, et al. Early molecular and cytogenetic response is predictive for long-term progression-free and overall survival in chronic myeloid leukemia (CML). *Leukemia* 2012;26:2096–2112.
74. Hughes TP, Kaeda J, Branford S, et al. Frequency of major molecular responses to imatinib or interferon alfa plus cytarabine in newly diagnosed chronic myeloid leukemia. *N Engl J Med* 2003;349:1423–1432.
75. Kantarjian HM, Talpaz M, O'Brien S, et al. Survival benefit with imatinib mesylate versus Interferon-a-based regimens in newly diagnosed chronic phase chronic myelogenous leukemia. *Blood* 2006;108:1835–1840.
76. Shah N, Nicoll J, Nagar B, et al. Multiple BCR-ABL kinase domain mutations confer polyclonal resistance to the tyrosine kinase inhibitor imatinib (STI571) in chronic phase and blast crisis chronic myeloid leukemia. *Cancer Cell* 2002;2:117–223.
77. Apperley JF. Part I: Mechanisms of resistance to imatinib in chronic myeloid leukaemia. *Lancet Oncol* 2007;8:1018–1029.
78. Shah NP, Tran C, Lee FY, et al. Overriding imatinib resistance with a novel ABL kinase inhibitor. *Science* 2004;305:399–401.
79. O'Hare T, Walters DK, Stoffregen EP, et al. In vitro activity of Bcr-Abl inhibitors AMN107 and BMS-354825 against clinically relevant imatinib-resistant Abl kinase domain mutants. *Cancer Res* 2005;65:4500–4505.
80. Redaelli S, Mologni L, Rostagno R, et al. Three novel patient-derived BCR/ABL mutants show different sensitivity to second and third generation tyrosine kinase inhibitors. *Am J Hematol* 2012;87:E125–E128.
81. Shah NP, Skaggs BJ, Branford S, et al. Sequential ABL kinase inhibitor therapy selects for compound drug-resistant BCR-ABL mutations with altered oncogenic potency. *J Clin Invest* 2007;117:2562–2569.
82. Gratwohl A, Schwendener A, Baldomero H, et al. Changes in the use of hematopoietic stem cell transplantation: a model for diffusion of medical technology. *Haematologica* 2010;95:637–643.
83. Giralt SA, Arora M, Goldman JM, et al. Impact of imatinib therapy on the use of allogeneic haematopoietic progenitor cell transplantation for the treatment of chronic myeloid leukaemia. *Br J Haematol* 2007;137:461–467.
84. Pavlu J, Szydlo RM, Goldman JM, et al. Three decades of transplantation for chronic myeloid leukemia: what have we learned? *Blood* 2011;117:755–763.
85. Weisdorf DJ, Anasetti C, Antin JH, et al. Allogeneic bone marrow transplantation for chronic myelogenous leukemia: comparative analysis of unrelated versus matched sibling donor transplantation. *Blood* 2002;99:1971–1977.
86. Warlick E, Ahn KW, Pedersen TL, et al. Reduced intensity conditioning is superior to nonmyeloablative conditioning for older chronic myelogenous leukemia patients undergoing hematopoietic cell transplant during the tyrosine kinase inhibitor era. *Blood* 2012;119:4083–4090.
87. Crawley C, Szydlo R, Lalancette M, et al. Outcomes of reduced-intensity transplantation for chronic myeloid leukemia: an analysis of prognostic factors from the Chronic Leukemia Working Party of the EBMT. *Blood* 2005;106:2969–2976.
88. Or R, Shapira MY, Resnick I, et al. Nonmyeloablative allogeneic stem cell transplantation for the treatment of chronic myeloid leukemia in first chronic phase. *Blood* 2003;101:441–445.
89. Olavarria E, Siddique S, Griffiths MJ, et al. Posttransplantation imatinib as a strategy to postpone the requirement for immunotherapy in patients undergoing reduced-intensity allografts for chronic myeloid leukemia. *Blood* 2007;110:4614–4617.
90. Carpenter PA, Snyder DS, Flowers ME, et al. Prophylactic administration of imatinib after hematopoietic cell transplantation for high-risk Philadelphia chromosome-positive leukemia. *Blood* 2007;109:2791–2793.
91. Klyuchnikov E, Schafhausen P, Kroger N, et al. Second-generation tyrosine kinase inhibitors in the post-transplant period in patients with chronic myeloid leukemia or Philadelphia-positive acute lymphoblastic leukemia. *Acta Haematol* 2009;122:6–10.
92. Hess G, Bunjes D, Siegert W, et al. Sustained complete molecular remissions after treatment with imatinib-mesylate in patients with failure after allogeneic stem cell transplantation for chronic myelogenous leukemia: results of a prospective phase II open-label multicenter study. *J Clin Oncol* 2005;23:7583–7593.
93. Weisser M, Tischer J, Schnittger S, et al. A comparison of donor lymphocyte infusions or imatinib mesylate for patients with chronic myelogenous leukemia who have relapsed after allogeneic stem cell transplantation. *Haematologica* 2006;91:663–666.
94. Olavarria E, Ottmann OG, Deininger M, et al. Response to imatinib in patients who relapse after allogeneic stem cell transplantation for chronic myeloid leukemia. *Leukemia* 2003;17:1707–1712.
95. Wright MP, Shepherd JD, Barnett MJ, et al. Response to tyrosine kinase inhibitor therapy in patients with chronic myelogenous leukemia relapsing in chronic and advanced phase following allogeneic hematopoietic stem cell transplantation. *Biol Blood Marrow Transplant* 2010;16:639–646.
96. Cummins M, Cwynarski K, Marktel S, et al. Management of chronic myeloid leukaemia in relapse following donor lymphocyte infusion induced remission: a retrospective study of the Clinical Trials Committee of the British Society of Blood & Marrow Transplantation (BSBMT). *Bone Marrow Transplant* 2005;36:1065–1069.
97. Porter DL, Collins RH Jr, Shpilberg O, et al. Long-term follow-up of patients who achieved complete remission after donor leukocyte infusions. *Biol Blood Marrow Transplant* 1999;5:253–261.
98. Dazzi F, Szydlo RM, Cross NC, et al. Durability of responses following donor lymphocyte infusions for patients who relapse after allogeneic stem cell transplantation for chronic myeloid leukemia. *Blood* 2000;96:2712–2716.
99. Simula MP, Marktel S, Fozza C, et al. Response to donor lymphocyte infusions for chronic myeloid leukemia is dose-dependent: the importance of escalating the cell dose to maximize therapeutic efficacy. *Leukemia* 2007;21:943–948.
100. Kantarjian HM, Dixon D, Keating MJ, et al. Characteristics of accelerated disease in chronic myelogenous leukemia. *Cancer* 1988;61:1441–1446.
101. Calabretta B, Perrotti D. The biology of CML blast crisis. *Blood* 2004;103:4010–4022.
102. Druker BJ, Sawyers CL, Kantarjian H, et al. Activity of a specific inhibitor of the BCR-ABL tyrosine kinase in the blast crisis of chronic myeloid leukemia and acute lymphoblastic leukemia with the Philadelphia chromosome. *N Engl J Med* 2001;344:1038–1042.
103. Saglio G, Hochhaus A, Goh YT, et al. Dasatinib in imatinib-resistant or imatinib-intolerant chronic myeloid leukemia in blast phase after 2 years of follow-up in a phase 3 study: efficacy and tolerability of 140 milligrams once daily and 70 milligrams twice daily. *Cancer* 2010;116:3852–3861.
104. Cortes J, Rousselot P, Kim DW, et al. Dasatinib induces complete hematologic and cytogenetic responses in patients with imatinib-resistant or -intolerant chronic myeloid leukemia in blast crisis. *Blood* 2007;109:3207–3213.
105. Wadhwa J, Szydlo RM, Apperley JF, et al. Factors affecting duration of survival after onset of blastic transformation of chronic myeloid leukemia. *Blood* 2002;99:2304–2309.
106. Rea D, Legros L, Raffoux E, et al. High-dose imatinib mesylate combined with vincristine and dexamethasone (DIV regimen) as induction therapy in patients with resistant Philadelphia-positive acute lymphoblastic leukemia and lymphoid blast crisis of chronic myeloid leukemia. *Leukemia* 2006;20:400–403.
107. Kantarjian H, Cortes J, Kim DW, et al. Phase 3 study of dasatinib 140 mg once daily versus 70 mg twice daily in patients with chronic myeloid leukemia in accelerated phase resistant or intolerant to imatinib: 15-month median follow-up. *Blood* 2009;113:6322–6329.
108. Rousselot P, Huguet F, Rea D, et al. Imatinib mesylate discontinuation in patients with chronic myelogenous leukemia in complete molecular remission for more than 2 years. *Blood* 2007;109:58–60.
109. Mahon FX, Rea D, Guilhot J, et al. Discontinuation of imatinib in patients with chronic myeloid leukaemia who have maintained complete molecular remission for at least 2 years: the prospective, multicentre Stop Imatinib (STIM) trial. *Lancet Oncol* 2010;11:1029–1035.
110. Saglio G, Kim DW, Issaragrisil S, et al. Nilotinib versus imatinib for newly diagnosed chronic myeloid leukemia. *N Engl J Med* 2010;362:2251–2259.
111. Kantarjian HM, Hochhaus A, Saglio G, et al. Nilotinib versus imatinib for the treatment of patients with newly diagnosed chronic phase, Philadelphia chromosome-positive, chronic myeloid leukaemia: 24-month minimum follow-up of the phase 3 randomised ENESTnd trial. *Lancet Oncol* 2011;12:841–851.
112. Radich JP, Kopecky KJ, Appelbaum FR, et al. A randomized trial of dasatinib 100 mg versus imatinib 400 mg in newly diagnosed chronic-phase chronic myeloid leukemia. *Blood* 2012;120:3898–3905.

46 Chronic Lymphocytic Leukemias

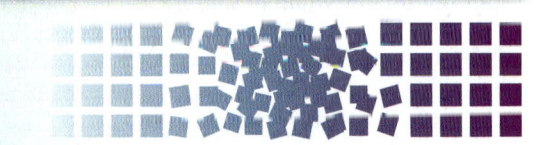

William G. Wierda and Susan M. O'Brien

INTRODUCTION

Chronic lymphocytic leukemia (CLL) is a monoclonal hematopoietic disorder characterized by progressive expansion of B lymphocytes. These small, mature-appearing lymphocytes accumulate in the blood, bone marrow, lymph nodes, liver, and spleen. CLL is the most common leukemia in the Western world, accounting for 25% to 30% of all adult leukemias.[1]

The estimated number of new CLL cases for 2014 was 15,720, with 9,100 men and 6,620 women affected; the median age at diagnosis was 72 years, and incidence increases with increasing age. During the same year, the estimated number of deaths was 4,600, with 2,800 men and 1,800 women; the median age at death was 79.[2,3] The majority of patients have significant comorbidities, which are associated with advanced age. As a result, they tend to have health, geographic, and access limitations. Patients with CLL seen at academic centers and enrolled in clinical trials tend to be younger, with a median age of 58 to 62 years, thereby limiting the ability to generalize results from such trials to community practice.

In Asian countries, CLL represents only 5% of leukemias, with T-cell phenotype predominating. Geographic and ethnic differences in incidence are most likely the result of genetic factors, as Japanese who settled in Hawaii do not have a higher incidence of CLL than native Japanese.[4] Population studies did not link CLL diagnosis to known occupational or environmental risk factors.[5] CLL has a strong familial aggregation, with a two- to seven-fold higher prevalence among family clusters than in the general population.[6]

MOLECULAR BIOLOGY

Immunophenotype

Clonality of CLL is confirmed by restricted expression of either kappa or lambda immunoglobulin light chain on the cell surface membrane.[1] Immunoglobulin gene rearrangement and usage is clonal; therefore, the CLL cells possess a unique idiotypic specificity and often have cytogenetic or molecular abnormalities.[7] With the use of sensitive techniques, monoclonal immunoglobulin can be detected in the serum of some patients, although only 5% to 10% of patients produce large enough quantities to be detected by serum electrophoresis. CLL cells express the B-cell markers CD19, CD20, CD21, CD23, and CD24; most CLL cells are also positive for major histocompatibility complex class II (DR and DQ), Fc receptors, and have receptors for mouse erythrocytes (Table 46.1).[8] Some surface markers that are usually found on normal B cells, including CD22, are infrequently found on CLL cells. CLL cells characteristically express CD5, an antigen normally found on T cells. Small numbers of normal polyclonal B cells can express CD5 and are predominantly in fetal circulation or in tonsils of normal adults. They usually are not detected in peripheral blood using standard immunophenotyping techniques.

Unexpectedly, as high as 3.5% of otherwise normal individuals over age 40 may harbor a population of clonal (by light chain analysis) CD5+/19+/23+ B cells.[9] These asymptomatic individuals do not have an absolute lymphocytosis, lymphadenopathy, or other clinical evidence of CLL and are referred to as having monoclonal B lymphocytosis (MBL). Furthermore, as many as 13% of family members of patients with familial CLL harbor a population of cells with an immunophenotype consistent with CLL, but do not fulfill CLL diagnostic criteria. Therefore, the prevalence of a monoclonal lymphoproliferative process is potentially much higher than previously appreciated. It is estimated that the rate of progression from MBL to CLL is 1 to 2% per year.[10] Currently, there is no indication to perform screening for MBL.

Immunoglobulin Heavy Chain Variable Gene (*IGHV*) Mutation Status

Because CD5+ B cells are found in fetal spleen and because surface immunoglobulin D is present on cells that have not encountered antigen in the germinal center, it was long thought that CLL cells were derived from naïve B cells. Normal B-cell development involves an antigen-independent phase and an antigen-dependent phase. During the antigen-independent phase, B cells undergo rearrangement of the V, D, and J genes in the bone marrow. Somatic mutation of the heavy- and light-chain variable gene occurs after encounter with antigen in the germinal center. Somatic mutation has occurred when there is <98% sequence homology with the germline gene. The figure of 98% is used because polymorphisms may account for lesser degrees of disparity.[11]

In the 1990s, data emerged that a significant percentage of patients had mutation of the immunoglobulin heavy chain variable gene (*IGHV*) in their CLL cells. Subsequently, it was confirmed that approximately 50% of patients have a mutated *IGHV* and that this provided prognostic information; patients with an unmutated *IGHV* have significantly shorter survival.[12,13] Characterization of the *IGHV* sequence is labor-intensive and has not been readily exportable to clinical laboratories. Thus, correlates with mutation status that may be more easily identified may be more accessible. A correlation between expression of CD38 and lack of somatic mutation was described.[12] Although the correlation is significant and the presence of CD38, irrespective of mutation status, is associated with inferior survival, a significant minority of patients have mutated *IGHV* and yet express CD38, and vice versa. These patients may have an intermediate prognosis. Also, there is variation in CD38 expression over time and by disease site (e.g., blood versus bone marrow) in some patients.

It was hypothesized that as patients with CLL can be segregated into two distinct prognostic categories based on *IGHV* mutation status, CLL may represent two separate disease entities, one derived from a naïve B cell that expressed unmutated *IGHV* and the other derived from a memory B cell that had been exposed to antigen and displayed a mutated *IGHV*. This hypothesis has been examined using gene expression profiling.[14] Investigators found that

TABLE 46.1
Immunophenotyping in Chronic B-Cell Leukemias

Disease	sIg	CD5	CD23	FMC7	CD22	CD79b	CD10
CLL	Weak	++	++	–/+	Weak/–	Weak/–	–
B-PLL	Strong	–/+	–/+	++	+	++	–
HCL	Strong	–	–	++	++	+	–
SLVL	Strong	–/+	–/+	++	++	++	–
FL	Strong	–	–	++	++	++	++
MCL	Strong	++	–/+	++	++	++	–/+

sIg, surface immunoglobulin; CLL, chronic lymphocytic leukemia; +, present; –, not present; B-PLL, B-cell prolymphocytic leukemia; HCL, hairy cell leukemia; SLVL, splenic lymphoma with villous lymphocytes; FL, follicular lymphoma; MCL, mantle cell lymphoma.

mutated and unmutated CLLs show a common gene expression pattern that is clearly distinguishable from that of other lymphomas, as well as normal B cells. Nevertheless, although the overall profile was similar, there were differentially expressed genes between the two groups. The gene that was most differentially expressed in one series was zeta-associated protein 70 (ZAP-70), with unmutated cases having significant expression of ZAP-70. Interestingly, ZAP-70 is normally found in T cells, where it functions as an intracellular signal–transduction molecule for the T-cell receptor. It was subsequently shown that ligation of the B-cell receptor (BCR) in CLL cells that expressed ZAP-70 produced greater tyrosine phosphorylation of cytosolic proteins than did stimulation of CLL cells that did not express ZAP-70; therefore, it may function in activating CLL cells. Expression of ZAP-70 was analyzed in 56 patients with CLL and was correlated with mutational status, disease progression, and survival in retrospective analyses (Fig. 46.1).[15]

Molecular Abnormalities

Conventional chromosome banding identified cytogenetic abnormalities in 40% to 50% of CLL cases; trisomy 12 was most common. This technique is hampered by the low mitotic activity of CLL cells. Fluorescence in situ hybridization (FISH), using genomic DNA probes to detect aberrations in interphase

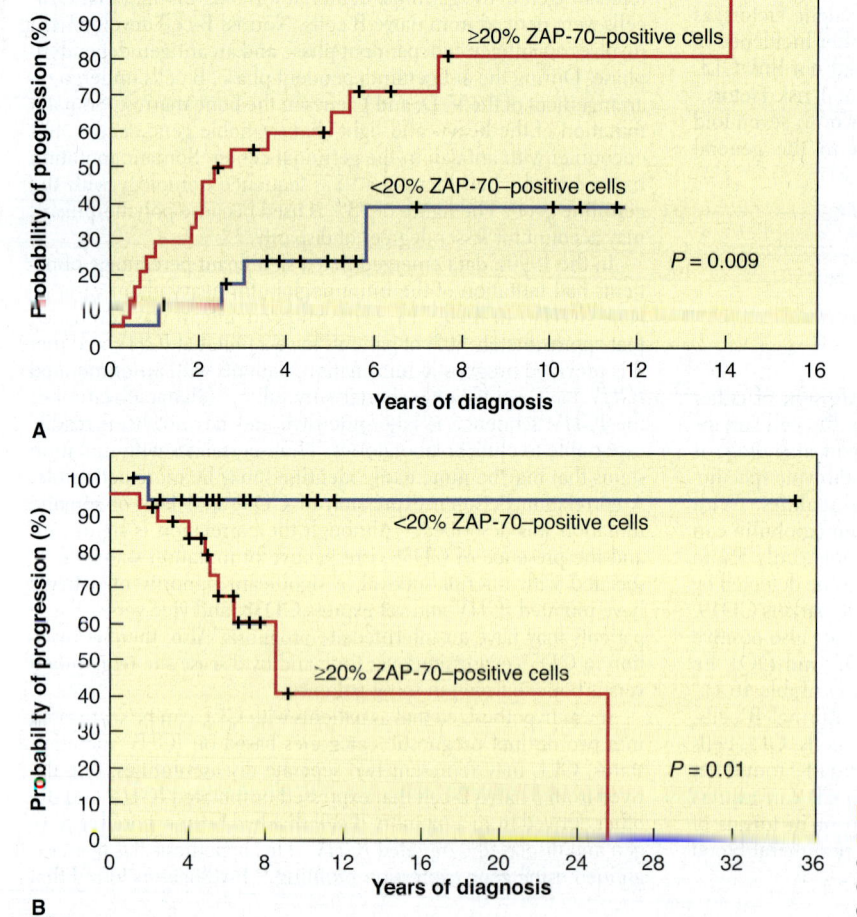

Figure 46.1 Kaplan-Meier estimates of the actuarial risk of disease progression (A) and the likelihood of survival (B) among patients with Binet stage A chronic lymphocytic leukemia, according to the level of expression of zeta-associated protein 70 (ZAP-70).

cells, enhanced the ability to detect molecular abnormalities in CLL. FISH has shown molecular abnormalities in over 80% of CLL cases.

Deletion 13q [del(13q)] is the most common genetic aberration in CLL; it is found by FISH as a sole abnormality in 55% of cases, followed by 11q deletion (18%) [del(11q)], 12q trisomy (16%), and 17p deletion (7%) [del(17p)]. Prognosis in CLL has been correlated with the presence of these chromosomal abnormalities. When divided into five hierarchical prognostic categories in order of highest risk—del(17p), del(11q), 12q trisomy, no abnormalities, and del(13q) (sole abnormality)—the survival times were 32 months, 79 months, 114 months, 111 months, and 133 months, respectively. Patients with del(17p) or del(11q) had more advanced disease with extensive lymphadenopathy. With hierarchical categorization, patients are assigned according to their highest-risk abnormality, including when multiple abnormalities are present. Clonal evolution can occur over time, particularly in the setting of cytotoxic treatment; therefore, repeated FISH assessment is important with changes in clinical status, such as in patients needing retreatment.

The frequency of del(13q) led to a search for a potentially new tumor suppressor gene in that location. At least eight genes were identified and screened for alterations at the DNA or RNA level, or both, but studies failed to find consistent involvement of any of those genes. However, two potentially relevant microRNA (miR) genes, miR15 and miR16, were identified in the critical minimal deleted region of del(13q) and were noted to be deleted or downregulated in more than two-thirds of all CLL cases.[16] MicroRNAs are nontranslated small RNAs that function to regulate gene expression. Both miR15 and miR16 negatively regulate BCL-2 transcript levels; the absence of miR15 and miR16 in cases with del(13q) may lead to Bcl-2 overexpression and resultant resistance to apoptosis.

Whole-exome sequencing of CLL cases identified mutated genes that may contribute to the pathogenesis and biology of the disease.[17–19] The frequency of mutated genes appears notably lower than the occurrence of cytogenetic abnormalities noted by FISH. Mutations are mostly private, and frequencies vary significantly by the patient population being characterized (e.g., untreated versus relapsed or refractory CLL). It is therefore unlikely that there is a single driver mutation that accounts for the disease. Indeed, the limited number of cases sequenced, the diversity in prior treatments among cases, and the relatively low frequency of mutations likely relate to the diversity in reported mutations. Consistently reported genes reported as mutated, albeit at low frequency, include NOTCH1, SF3B1, TP53, MYD88, XPO1, and ATM. Some of these mutations have been associated with clinical outcome such as TP53, SF3B1, NOTCH1, ATM, and BIRC3.[18–20] Some mutations may result in decreased protein level or function, others may result in activation or increased protein levels, depending on the gene and mutation. Serial sampling of individual patients for whole-exome sequencing is leading to insights into diversities in clonal evolution and an appreciation for how different treatments may impact the emergence, frequency, and type of mutations and loss of others through the course of a patient's disease.[21–23]

IMMUNE ABNORMALITIES

CLL cells disrupt immune function in patients with CLL. The most prominent manifestation of immune dysfunction is the increased risk and frequency of infections. Many patients with CLL succumb to infection or ineffectively treated autoimmunity. The treatments used for CLL, such as purine analogues, further immunosuppress patients and put them at increased risk for opportunistic infections and may exacerbate or unmask autoimmunity.

Early in the disease, in untreated CLL, the absolute number of T cells is increased with inversion of the T helper–T suppressor cell ratio.[24,25] The CD4 to CD8 ratio continues to drop with disease progression or after therapy with nucleoside analogues or alemtuzumab. Qualitative functional assessment of T cells has been inconclusive. Normal and decreased CD4-cell function has been reported. Similarly, decreased, normal, or excessive CD8 cell function has been reported. Others have shown that T-cell functions may be impaired by immunosuppressive factors produced by CLL cells.[24] Hypogammaglobulinemia is a common and progressive immune defect in patients with CLL and is another factor that increases the risk for infection. The pathogenesis of hypogammaglobulinemia in CLL is poorly understood. Impaired B-cell function and regulatory abnormalities of T cells, including the reversal of the normal helper–suppressor cell ratio, may play roles. In addition, CLL-derived natural killer (NK) cells have been shown to suppress immunoglobulin secretion by normal B cells in vitro.

DIAGNOSIS

The International Workshop on CLL (IWCLL) in 2008[26] updated the National Cancer Institute Working Group 1996 guidelines[27] for diagnostic criteria and treatment for CLL.

International Workshop on Chronic Lymphocytic Leukemia Revised Diagnostic Criteria

1. A blood monoclonal B lymphocyte count $>5 \times 10^9$/L, with <55% of the cells being atypical (prolymphocytes).
2. B-lymphocyte monoclonality should be demonstrated with cells expressing B-cell surface antigens (CD19, CD20, CD23), low-density surface immunoglobulin (M or D), and CD5.

A monoclonal B cell count $>5 \times 10^9$/L was specified to distinguish CLL from small lymphocytic lymphoma in patients with palpable lymph nodes or splenomegaly. However, it is arguable as to whether that distinction is clinically relevant. Bone marrow aspirate typically shows >30% lymphocytes, with flow cytometry confirming monoclonality in the CD19/CD20/CD23/CD5+ population; however, diagnosis may be made solely on blood.

Other B-cell malignancies may also present with increased circulating lymphoid cells and should be differentiated from CLL. The diseases that may be confused with CLL are prolymphocytic leukemia (PLL), the leukemic phase of non-Hodgkin's lymphoma (mantle cell lymphoma, follicular lymphoma, or splenic lymphoma with circulating villous lymphocytes), and hairy cell leukemia (HCL). Immunophenotyping is helpful in differentiating these disorders (Figs. 46.2, 46.3, and 46.4; see Table 46.1).

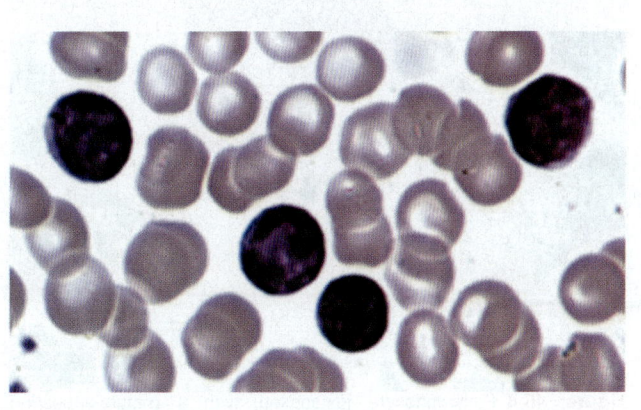

Figure 46.2 Chronic lymphocytic leukemia. Peripheral smear showing mature-appearing lymphocytes.

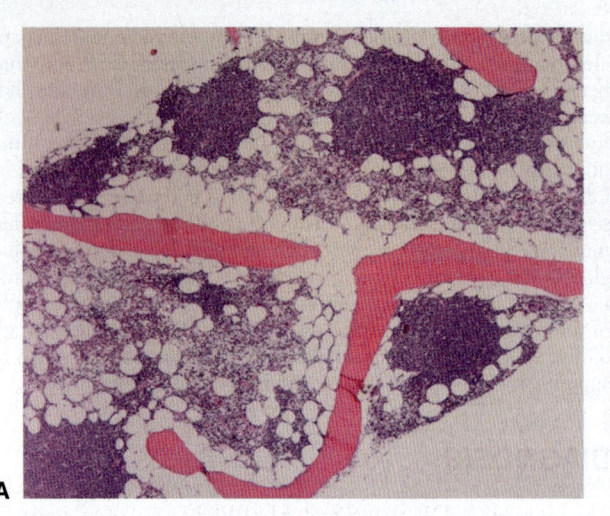

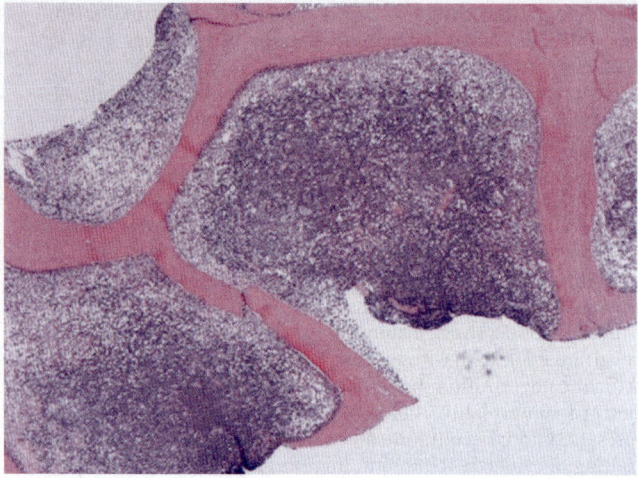

Figure 46.3 Chronic lymphocytic leukemia. Bone marrow infiltration may range from nodular/focal (**A**) to diffuse (**B**).

Clinical Manifestations

The majority of individuals diagnosed with CLL are asymptomatic and initially identified on routine blood count. Some patients remain asymptomatic for a long period of time. In patients presenting with symptoms, the most common is fatigue, which is generally mild. Sometimes, enlarged lymph nodes or the development of an infection is the initial manifestation of disease. Bacterial infections, such as pneumonia, are more common in patients who present with advanced-stage disease. Infections secondary to opportunistic organisms, particularly herpes zoster, may occur. Exaggerated skin reaction to a bee sting or an insect bite (Wells' syndrome) is frequent in CLL. In contrast to the situation in lymphoma, fever in the absence of infection is rare in CLL. Lymph nodes, when enlarged, are usually discrete, freely movable, and nontender. Splenomegaly may occur, but massive splenomegaly is usually seen in patients with advanced disease. Splenic infarction is rare. Hepatomegaly occurs less frequently than splenomegaly. Skin involvement occurs in <5% of cases. Leptomeningeal leukemia is rare and, if present, is usually seen in patients with refractory disease. Malignant pleural effusions are also rare, and when present, are associated with aggressive disease and poor prognosis.

Laboratory Findings

Absolute lymphocyte counts range from 5×10^9/L to over 500×10^9/L. Leukostasis is uncommon in CLL, probably because of the small size and pliability of the leukemia cells. The lymphocyte count usually increases over time, but fluctuations in the absolute lymphocyte count of untreated patients may occur, particularly in the setting of infection. The lymphocytes are typically small and mature appearing, but there may be variations in cell morphology, with some lymphocytes being larger or atypical, whereas others may be plasmacytoid or cleaved or there may be prolymphocytes. Ruptured lymphocytes or "smudge" cells are commonly seen in the peripheral smear, reflecting fragility and distortion during preparation of the peripheral smear on the glass slide. Marrow infiltration by lymphocytes is universal, affecting from 30% to 100% of the cellularity, with overall increased marrow cellularity. The patterns of lymphoid infiltration of the marrow seen in biopsy specimens include nodular, interstitial, diffuse, or a combination. Patients with diffuse infiltration typically have advanced disease and a worse prognosis. Nodular and interstitial or "nondiffuse" patterns are associated with less advanced disease and better outcome.

Anemia (hemoglobin <11 g/dl) and thrombocytopenia (platelet count $<100 \times 10^9$/L) are found in a minority of patients at diagnosis but develop with disease progression. A positive direct antiglobulin (Coombs') test is seen in approximately 25% of cases, but overt autoimmune hemolytic anemia (AIHA) occurs less frequently. The incidence of a positive Coombs' test increases significantly with clinical stage.[28] Immune thrombocytopenia is usually diagnosed on the basis of a low platelet count in the presence of adequate numbers of megakaryocytes in the bone marrow. Neutropenia may also be encountered. These cytopenias may be the result of bone marrow failure due to "packed" marrow by CLL or occur as a result of an immune-mediated process or hypersplenism. Hypogammaglobulinemia occurs in approximately 50% of patients with CLL. At diagnosis, it may be noted in <10% of patients, but its incidence increases significantly with disease progression. Usually, all three immunoglobin classes (G, A, and M) are decreased, but in some patients, only one or two may be low. Significant hypogammaglobulinemia and neutropenia potentially result in increased susceptibility to bacterial infections.

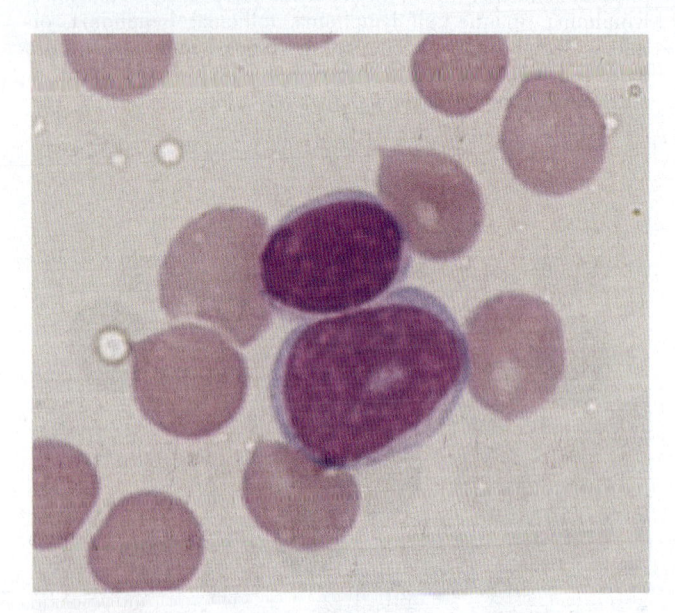

Figure 46.4 Prolymphocyte juxtaposed with a mature-appearing lymphocyte. Note larger size, less-condensed chromatin, and prominent nucleolus.

Autoimmune Complications

When autoantibodies occur in CLL, they are usually targeted against hematopoietic cells, resulting in AIHA, immune thrombocytopenia, immune-mediated granulocytopenia, or pure red cell aplasia; AIHA is the most frequent.[29] The autoantibodies are typically polyclonal and usually immunoglobulin G, indicating that they are not produced by the leukemic clone.[30] The severity of the autoimmune phenomenon does not necessarily correlate with the severity of CLL, and such events may develop in patients whose disease is responding to therapy. Prednisone is the most commonly used treatment for autoimmune complications, with high initial response rates. It is usually given at a dose of 1 mg/kg orally and tapered once a response is noted. Relapses are not uncommon. Cyclosporin A is another effective therapy and can produce good results, even in steroid-refractory patients.[31] CD20 and CD52 monoclonal antibodies (mAb) rituximab and alemtuzumab have been used alone or in combination with chemotherapy in some patients in whom standard therapy fails.[32,33] Splenectomy is also a viable therapeutic option for refractory cases.[28,34]

Staging

The clinical course for individuals with CLL is variable; survival times range from 2 to over 20 years from diagnosis. In 1975, Rai et al.[35] developed a staging system consisting of five stages (Rai 0 to IV) based on Dameshek's model of orderly disease progression in CLL (Table 46.2). The Rai staging system was later modified into a three-stage system: low-risk (Rai 0), intermediate-risk (Rai I, II), and high-risk (Rai III, IV). A similar staging system was developed in Europe by Binet et al.[36] Both classifications reflect bulk of disease and extent of marrow compromise (i.e., anemia, thrombocytopenia). Both staging systems have been recognized as simple and reliable predictors of survival (see Table 46.2). Although most patients in the high-risk group (Rai III, IV; Binet C) have a progressive clinical course and shortened survival, the course of the disease is not uniform. Patients in the low- and intermediate-risk groups may have an indolent disease course that spans years or even decades, or the course may be progressive and associated with a shortened survival. Thus, it is helpful to have prognostic factors associated with clinical outcomes particularly for the low-risk group. Several prognostic factors have been associated with shortened survival in CLL. These include a short lymphocyte doubling time (<6 months), a diffuse pattern of bone marrow infiltration, advanced age and male gender, abnormal karyotype, high serum levels of β_2-microglobulin and soluble CD23, and a CLL-PLL category (11% to 54% prolymphocytes in the blood).[37] Newer prognostic factors in CLL include *IGHV* mutation status, expression of CD38 and ZAP-70, and gene mutations. A prognostic model integrating cytogenetic abnormalities identified by FISH with mutated *NOTCH1*, *SF3B1*, *BIRC3*, and *TP53* was proposed as a dynamic prognostic algorithm for overall survival (OS).[20]

TREATMENT AND RESPONSE CRITERIA

An unusual feature of CLL compared to other leukemias is that making the diagnosis is not necessarily an indication to initiate treatment. This is true for several reasons. CLL is a disease of the older population; it may be diagnosed in an asymptomatic patient and have a prolonged course; CLL is not curable with current standard treatment approaches; and a survival advantage was not demonstrated in clinical trials of early intervention. Given that the majority of patients are older than 70 years, may have serious comorbid conditions associated with aging, and may have indolent disease, a significant fraction of patients will die of other causes and may never require therapy for their CLL.

The IWCLL revised criteria for active disease, an indication to initiate treatment,[26] include constitutional symptoms attributable to CLL: weight loss (>10% of baseline weight within the preceding 6 months), extreme fatigue (Eastern Cooperative Oncology Group performance status 2 or higher), fever (temperature higher than 38°C or 100.5°F for at least 2 weeks) or night sweats without evidence of infection; evidence of progressive bone marrow failure characterized by the development of or worsening of anemia, thrombocytopenia, or both; AIHA or autoimmune thrombocytopenia, or both, poorly responsive to corticosteroid therapy; massive (>6 cm below the left costal margin) or progressive splenomegaly; massive (>10 cm in longest diameter) or progressive lymphadenopathy; and progressive lymphocytosis defined as an increase in the absolute lymphocyte count by 50% over a 2-month period, or a doubling time predicted to be <6 months. Hypogammaglobulinemia or monoclonal gammopathy alone are not sufficient criteria to initiate therapy.

Several European groups conducted trials in the 1980s to evaluate whether immediate treatment in patients with early stage disease could improve survival.[38] These large randomized trials of immediate chlorambucil (CLB) therapy versus watch-and-wait were consistent in showing no survival benefit with early treatment. However, given significantly better current therapies, this question has been raised again. A limitation of randomizing all early stage patients is that approximately one-third of them may never require therapy for their disease, thus reducing the potential benefit of early treatment. Furthermore, the discovery of prognostic factors that identify early stage patients with a high likelihood of developing progressive disease may allow for randomized trials to more directly address this question of the benefit of early treatment.

The response criteria published in 1988[39] by the National Cancer Institute Working Group on CLL were revised in 1996[27] and most recently updated by the IWCLL (Table 46.3).[26] Updated recommendations made were that patients treated on clinical trial have

TABLE 46.2
Staging of Chronic Lymphocytic Leukemia

Rai Stage	Modified Rai Stage	Description	Binet Stage	Description
0	Low risk	Lymphocytosis only	A	Two or fewer lymphoid-bearing areas
I	Intermediate risk	Lymphocytosis and lymphadenopathy	B	Three or more lymphoid-bearing areas
II	Intermediate risk	Lymphocytosis and splenomegaly with/without lymphadenopathy	—	—
III	High risk	Lymphocytosis and anemia (hemoglobin, <11 g/dl)	C	Anemia (hemoglobin, <10 g/dl) or thrombocytopenia (platelets, 100 × 10⁶/dl)
IV	High risk	Lymphocytosis and thrombocytopenia (platelets, <100 × 10⁶/dl)		

TABLE 46.3

2008 International Workshop on Chronic Lymphocytic Leukemia Revised National Cancer Institute–Sponsored Working Group Response Criteria for Chronic Lymphocytic Leukemia

Parameter[a]	CR (all required)	PR
Lymphocytes	≤4,000/μl[b]	≥50% ↓[c]
LNs	No palpable disease (LN <1.5 cm)[d]	≥50% ↓[c]
Splenomegaly	None	≥50% ↓[c]
Hepatomegaly	None	≥50% ↓[c]
Bone marrow	<30% lymphocytes, no nodules[e]	NA
Constitutional symptoms	None	Variable
Neutrophils	≥1,500/μl	≥1,500/μl or ≥50% improvement[f]
Platelets	>100,000/μl	>100,000/μl or ≥50% improvement[f]
Hemoglobin	>11 g/dl (untransfused)	>11 g/dl or ≥50% improvement[f]

CR, complete response; PR, partial response; ↓, decrease; LN, lymph node; NA, not applicable.
[a] Assessed at least 2 months after completion of therapy.
[b] Include minimal residual disease assessed for clinical trials with reported sensitivity of method.
[c] Must achieve at least two parameters.
[d] Computed tomography scan of chest, abdomen, and pelvis desired for patients to confirm for patients on clinical trial.
[e] Less than 30% lymphocytes in marrow with residual nodules should have immunohistochemistry to characterize nodules.
[f] Must achieve at least one parameter.

evaluation of the blood or bone marrow by sensitive tests for minimal residual disease (MRD) such as multicolor flow cytometry or allele-specific polymerase chain reaction (PCR) for the IGHV gene and have confirmation of nodal response by computed tomography scan. In some patients who achieve complete remission by IWCLL criteria, one or both of these methods can demonstrate residual disease, referred to as MRD. Patients free of MRD following treatment have a longer remission duration and longer survival.[40,41] Therefore, in addition to improving complete remission rates, investigators are focusing on eliminating MRD to improve treatment outcomes.

A sensitive four-color flow cytometry assay was developed to differentiate CLL cells (CD5/CD19 with CD20/CD38, CD81/CD22, and CD79b/CD43) from normal B cells.[42] The assay can detect one CLL cell in 10^4 to 10^5 leukocytes. PCR techniques can also be used to assess MRD. Consensus primers for IGHV can be used in 70% to 80% of patients and may detect 1 in 10^4 residual cells. Allele-specific oligonucleotide primers generated for individual patients are more sensitive, detecting 1 in 10^5 CLL cells. Development of quantitative PCR techniques may aid in following patients over time but are technically complicated and therefore not available for routine clinical use.

Alkylating Agent-Based Treatments

For decades, the mainstay of therapy for CLL was alkylating agents, CLB and cyclophosphamide (CTX). These alkylating agents were given with or without corticosteroids. Various doses and schedules of oral CLB have been used. CLB is usually administered for several months, and the dose is adjusted to avoid its primary toxicity, myelosuppression. The overall response rate with either CLB or CTX monotherapy is approximately 40% to 60%, with 3% to 5% complete remission. Alkylating agents were combined with steroids to improve response rates.[43] Alkylating agent–based combinations have also included an anthracycline. No superior alkylating-agent combination has been identified.

Purine Analogues

Purine analogues, including fludarabine monophosphate, 2-chlorodeoxyadenosine (2-CdA), and pentostatin (deoxycoformycin), all have activity in treating patients with CLL.[43]

In a phase 2 trial conducted at MD Anderson Cancer Center, fludarabine was given at a dose of 30 mg/m² per day for 5 days every 4 weeks. A response rate of 59% was observed in 68 previously treated patients, while 17 achieved complete remission. A subsequent study explored the combination of fludarabine and prednisone. Response rates were identical to those seen with fludarabine monotherapy, but the addition of prednisone was associated with increased incidence of Pneumocystis jiroveci and Listeria monocytogenes infections. The major side effects associated with fludarabine were myelosuppression and immunosuppression, with low CD4 counts lasting for many months to years after completion of treatment.[43]

Single-arm studies evaluated fludarabine in previously untreated patients. Overall response rates were higher at 70% to 80%, and complete remission was seen in 10% to 25%.[43] An oral formulation of fludarabine was evaluated in relapsed patients with CLL. Seventy-eight patients received oral fludarabine 40 mg/m² per day for 5 days every 4 weeks for six to eight courses. The overall response rate was 51%, which was almost identical to prior trials using the intravenous formulation as a salvage regimen. Furthermore, oral fludarabine was used in the first-line Leukemia Research Foundation CLL4 trial[44] comparing fludarabine plus CTX versus fludarabine versus CLB, demonstrating efficacy and tolerability with the oral formulation, which is now approved by the US Food and Drug Administration (FDA).

Comparative Studies

A randomized European trial compared six courses of fludarabine versus six courses of CTX, doxorubicin, and prednisone (CAP) in 196 patients with Binet stage B or C CLL (Table 46.4).[45] In previously treated patients, a significantly higher overall response rate was observed with fludarabine compared to CAP. In previously untreated patients (see Table 46.4), the response rates with fludarabine were similar to those with CAP, but the duration of response was significantly longer with fludarabine. The French Cooperative Group on CLL randomized nearly 1,000 previously untreated patients to one of three treatment regimens: fludarabine, CTX, doxorubicin, prednisone, and vincristine, or CAP.[46] Higher overall response rate and longer time to progression were seen with fludarabine. Infection rates were similar, but extramedullary toxicity was less with fludarabine.

TABLE 46.4
Randomized Trials of Monotherapy or Alkylating Agent–Based Combinations as Initial Treatment for Chronic Lymphocytic Leukemia

Study (Ref.)	Agent	No. of Patients	CR (%)	OR (%)	Median RD	Median OS (mo)
Leporrier et al.[46]	Fludarabine vs.	341	40	71	32 mo (TTP)	69
	CAP vs.	240	15	58	28 mo (TTP)	70
	CHOP	357	30	72	30 mo (TTP)	67
Rai et al.[47]	Fludarabine + chlorambucil vs.	123	20	61	NR	55
	Fludarabine vs.	170	20	63	25 mo (TTP)	66
	Chlorambucil	181	4	37	14 mo (TTP)	56
Johnson et al.[45]	Fludarabine vs.	52	23	71	NR	60% at 4 y
	CAP	48	17	60	7	60% at 4 y
GCLLSG CLL5[49,a]	Fludarabine vs.	87	7	72	19 (PFS)	46
	Chlorambucil	98	0	51	18 (PFS)	64
Knauf et al.[50]	Bendamustine vs.	162	31	68	21.6 (PFS)	NR
	Chlorambucil	157	2	31	8.3 (PFS)	NR
Hillmen et al.[76]	Alemtuzumab vs.	149	24	83	14.6	NR
	Chlorambucil	148	2	55	11.7	NR

CR, complete remission; OR, overall response; RD, remission duration; OS, overall survival; CAP, cyclophosphamide, doxorubicin, prednisone; CHOP, cyclophosphamide, doxorubicin, prednisone, vincristine; TTP, time-to-progression; NR, not reached; GCLLSG, German Chronic Lymphocytic Leukemia Study Group; PFS, progression-free survival.
[a] Age 65 years and older.

Results from an Intergroup trial with 509 previously untreated patients with CLL showed significantly higher complete and overall remission rates in patients treated with fludarabine versus those given CLB (see Table 46.4).[47] A third arm, fludarabine plus CLB, was closed early because of infection-related toxicity. Crossover was allowed for patients with no response or relapse. Half the patients who failed to respond to CLB responded to fludarabine, including a 14% complete remission rate. In contrast, only 7% of patients who failed to respond to fludarabine achieved partial response with CLB. Although longer response duration and improved progression-free survival (PFS) were noted in patients treated with fludarabine, no difference in OS was found between the two groups in the initial report. However, updated data, with significantly longer follow-up, reported improved OS for patients treated initially with fludarabine; this difference in the survival curves emerged after 6 years follow-up.[48] The German CLL Study Group (GCLLSG) CLL5 evaluated fludarabine versus CLB monotherapy as initial treatment for patients older than 65 years (see Table 46.4).[49] Surprisingly, while treatment with fludarabine was associated with superior complete (7% versus 0%) and overall (72% versus 51%) response rates, there was no associated improvement in PFS or OS for these "elderly" patients. Thus, standard first-line treatment of the elderly does not require fludarabine.

Bendamustine has a benzimidazole (purinelike) ring structure with an alkylating group and has potent alkylating agent activity, inducing intra- and interstrand DNA crosslinks. Bendamustine was compared to CLB in a randomized phase 3 trial for previously untreated patients with CLL (see Table 46.4).[50] Treatment with bendamustine was associated with superior PFS (21.6 months versus 8.3 months), and complete (31% versus 2%) and overall (68% versus 31%) response rates; this was the basis for FDA approval of this agent. Myelosuppression was mild but more frequent with bendamustine; this did not result in an increased infection rate.

Fludarabine inhibits excision repair of DNA interstrand crosslinks induced by CTX, thereby potentiating activity and providing a rationale for combining these agents.[51] Phase 2 trials, which combined fludarabine and CTX (FC), suggested increased efficacy compared to that seen in historical patients treated with fludarabine monotherapy.[52–54] Three large randomized trials evaluated the efficacy of FC versus fludarabine monotherapy in previously untreated patients (Table 46.5). In the GCLLSG CLL4 trial, previously untreated patients younger than 65 with indications for treatment were randomized to receive six courses of FC or fludarabine.[55] The U.S. Intergroup E2997 trial[56] randomized previously untreated patients to receive FC or fludarabine and the UK Leukemia Research Foundation CLL4 trial[44] randomized patients to FC, fludarabine, or CLB in a 1:1:2 randomization. All three trials demonstrated superior PFS with FC treatment over fludarabine or CLB, and this was associated with superior complete and overall response rates. There was more myelosuppression with the combination, yet there was no difference in the incidence of infections in any of the trials. None of these trials showed a difference in OS with the follow-up available. Patients with del(17p) were confirmed to be high-risk with lower response rates and shorter survival compared to patients with other chromosome abnormalities, regardless of treatment. Patients with del(11q) were high-risk, but there appeared to be a large benefit for those patients treated with an alkylating agent combined with fludarabine. Patients with an unmutated *IGHV* gene had similar response rates to those with a mutated *IGHV*; however, their PFS and OS was shorter for those with an unmutated *IGHV* gene.

Cladribine (2-CdA) and pentostatin (2-deoxycoformyin) have activity in treating CLL.[57] There are no head-to-head comparisons available for purine analogue monotherapy. The large randomized Polish Adult Leukemia Group (PALG)-CLL2 trial compared cladribine monotherapy, cladribine with CTX, versus cladribine with CTX and mitoxantrone (CMC) as initial therapy and demonstrated a higher complete response rate for CMC compared to the other treatments (see Table 46.5).[58] Neutropenia was more common with CMC, as was infection. There were no significant differences in PFS or OS rates among the three arms. The PALG-CLL3 phase 3 trial demonstrated equivalent efficacy with cladribine

TABLE 46.5
Randomized Trials of Purine Analog Monotherapy Versus Combinations as Initial Treatment for Chronic Lymphocytic Leukemia

Study (Ref.)	Agent	No. of Patients	CR (%)	OR (%)	Median PFS (mo)
GCLLSG CLL4[55]	FC vs.	164	24	95	48
	Fludarabine	164	7	83	20
E2997[56]	FC vs.	137	23	74	32
	Fludarabine	132	6	60	19
LRF CLL4[44]	FC vs.	196	38	94	43
	Fludarabine vs.	194	15	80	23
	Chlorambucil	387	7	72	20
PALG CLL2[58]	CMC vs.	151	36	80	24
	CC vs.	162	29	83	22
	Cladribine	166	21	77	24
PALG CLL3[59]	CC vs.	211	47	88	28
	FC	212	46	82	27

CR, complete remission; OR, overall response; PFS, median progression-free survival; GCLLSG, German Chronic Lymphocytic Leukemia Study Group; FC, fludarabine + cyclophosphamide; LRF, Leukemia Research Foundation; PALG, Polish Adult Leukemia Group; CMC, cladribine + mitoxantrone + cyclophosphamide; CC, cladribine + cyclophosphamide.

with CTX and FC for previously untreated patients with CLL (see Table 46.5).[59] Patients with del(17p) had poor outcomes with either treatment.

Monoclonal Antibodies

Alemtuzumab is a humanized mAb targeting CD52, an antigen that is highly expressed on CLL cells and normal T and B lymphocytes. Alemtuzumab was originally approved by the FDA based on the pivotal trial that demonstrated monotherapy activity in fludarabine-refractory patients with CLL (Table 46.6).[60–74] Complete and partial remissions were noted in 2% and 31% of 93 treated patients, respectively; 55 (59%) had stable disease. Similar results were reported in a trial with a similar patient population treated with the same dose and duration of alemtuzumab administered subcutaneously.[75] Subcutaneous administration eliminates the infusion-related side effects, although local injection site reactions occur. Alemtuzumab was very effective at eliminating disease in the peripheral blood and bone marrow; bulky lymphadenopathy was less effectively treated, a pattern observed in other studies with alemtuzumab. The T-cell suppression that occurred with this agent has been concerning. As a consequence, a significant incidence of infections (including cytomegalovirus reactivation) is associated with therapy. Antibacterial and antiviral prophylaxis should always be used with alemtuzumab. Other studies confirmed the activity of alemtuzumab in less heavily pretreated patients (see Table 46.6). A randomized first-line trial demonstrated superior PFS associated with alemtuzumab monotherapy compared to CLB, as well as higher complete and overall response rates (see Table 46.4).[76]

The mechanism of action for alemtuzumab is independent of p53. TP53 is a gene deleted in patients who have loss of chromosome 17p. Loss of p53 function by deletion or mutation confers resistance to treatment with standard chemotherapy such as CLB and purine analogues. Alemtuzumab was reported to have activity in patients with leukemia cells that lack p53 function.[77] Despite treatment with alemtuzumab, patients with del(17p) have short remission duration and OS. Alemtuzumab was also combined with high-dose methylprednisolone for previously treated and treatment-naïve patients with better results, although there is concern for immunosuppression and risk for infection (see Table 46.6).

Rituximab is a chimeric immunoglobulin G1 (IgG1) mAb; CD20 is expressed on malignant and normal B cells.[78] Relatively low levels of CD20 are expressed on CLL cells compared to normal B or neoplastic B cells of other lymphomas. In addition, circulating CD20 was demonstrated in the plasma of patients with CLL; this may inhibit the capacity of rituximab to bind to CLL cells, resulting in rapid clearance and negatively affecting pharmacokinetics.[79] Rituximab binds to the large-loop domain of CD20 and mediates antileukemic activity predominantly through antibody-dependent cellular cytotoxicity and complement-dependent cytotoxicity (CDC) (type I CD20 mAb). Standard-dose rituximab monotherapy has limited activity in treating CLL (see Table 46.6). Dose-intense[80] and dose-dense[81] rituximab monotherapy increased efficacy (see Table 46.6). In addition, greater efficacy was seen when rituximab was used as first-line therapy (see Table 46.6).[82] Maintenance rituximab is not routine practice for patients with CLL.

The primary toxicity seen with rituximab is usually with the initial infusion and is predominantly fever and chills. These symptoms are generally mild to moderate, subside with completion or discontinuation of the infusion, and abate with subsequent infusions. Although normal B cells are also targeted by rituximab, trials to date have shown no significant decrease in immunoglobulin levels, and infection rates are low.

Rituximab was combined with alemtuzumab based on the rationale of targeting two distinct antigens expressed on CLL cells as well as the differential effectiveness by disease site; rituximab has activity in treating lymph node disease, and alemtuzumab is highly effective at clearing blood and bone marrow. Efficacy and tolerability were demonstrated in both untreated and previously treated CLL (see Table 46.6). In addition, rituximab was combined with high-dose methylprednisolone in an active regimen for untreated and previously treated patients (see Table 46.6). Immunosuppression was seen with this combination, owing to the use of high-dose steroids, and was effectively managed with prophylactic antibiotics.

Ofatumumab is a fully human immunoglobulin G1 CD20 mAb that binds to an epitope encompassing both large- and small-loop domains of CD20 and is highly effective at CDC (type I CD20 mAb). Ofatumumab monotherapy was first evaluated in phase 1 and 2 trials of escalating doses of four weekly infusions

TABLE 46.6
Monoclonal Antibody–Based Therapy for Chronic Lymphocytic Leukemia

Study (Ref.)	Monoclonal Antibody	Prior Rx	No. Patients Evaluable	CR (%)	OR (%)	Median PFS (mo)
Alemtuzumab						
Keating et al.[60]	30 mg IV TIW × 12 wk	Yes[a]	93	2	33	9
Osterborg et al.[61]	30 mg IV TIW × 12 wk	Yes	29	4	42	12
Rai et al.[62]	30 mg IV TIW × 16 wk	Yes	24	0	33	19.6
Ferrajoli et al.[63]	30 mg IV TIW × 12 wk	Yes	42	5	31	NA
Moreton et al.[40]	30 mg IV TIW × 16 wk	Yes	91	35	54	NA
Lundin et al.[64]	30 mg SC TIW × 18 wk	No	41	19	87	NR
Stilgenbauer et al.[75]	30 mg SC TIW × 12 wk	Yes[a]	103	4	34	7.7
NCRI-CLL206[65]	30 mg IV TIW × 16 wk + HDMP 1 gm/m² daily × 5, c1–4	No/Yes[b]	39	36	85	11.8
Rituximab						
McLaughlin et al.[66]	375 mg/m² IV weekly × 4	Yes	30	0	13	NA
Huhn et al.[67]	375 mg/m² IV weekly × 4	Yes	28	0	25	5
O'Brien et al.[80,c]	500–825 mg/m² IV weekly × 4	Yes	24	0	21	—
	1,000–1,500 mg/m² IV weekly × 4	Yes	7	0	43	8
	2,250 mg/m² IV weekly × 4	Yes	8	0	75	
Byrd et al.[81,d]	375 mg/m² IV TIW × 4 wk	No/Yes	29	4	52	11
Hainsworth[68]	375 mg/m² IV weekly × 4 then q 6 mo for 2 y	No	43	0	69	19
Ferrajoli[69]	375 mg/m² IV weekly × 4 + GM-CSF 25 mcg SC TIW × 8	Yes	118	9	65	NA
Castro et al.[70]	375 mg/m² IV weekly × 4 + HDMP 1 gm/m² d1–5	Yes	14	36	93	15
Bowen et al.[71]	375 mg/m² IV weekly × 4 + HDMP 1 gm/m² d1–5	Yes	37	22	78	21
Castro et al.[72]	375 mg/m² IV weekly × 4 + HDMP 1 gm/m² d1–3	No	28	32	96	30
Alemtuzumab + Rituximab						
Faderl et al.[73]	A-30 mg IV TIW × 4 wk + R-375 mg/m² IV weekly × 4	Yes	48	8	52	6
Zent et al.[74]	A-30 mg SC TIW × 4 wk + R-375 mg/m² IV weekly × 4	No	30	37	90	12.5
Ofatumumab						
Coiffier et al.[83]	2,000 mg IV weekly × 4	Yes	26	0	50	NA
Wierda et al.[84]	2,000 mg IV weekly × 8, then monthly × 4	FA-ref	59	0	58	5.7
		BF-ref	79	1	47	5.9

Rx, treatment; CR, complete remission; OR, overall response; PFS, progression-free survival; IV, intravenous; TIW, thrice weekly; NA, not available; SC, subcutaneous; NR, not reached; NCRI, National Cancer Research Institute; HDMP, high-dose methylprednisolone; GM-CSF, granulocyte macrophage–colony-stimulating factor; FA-ref, refractory to both fludarabine and alemtuzumab; BF-ref, refractory to fludarabine with bulky (>5 cm) adenopathy.
[a] Fludarabine refractory.
[b] All patients had del(17p).
[c] Dose-intense regimen.
[d] Dose-dense regimen.

(see Table 46.6).[83] The pivotal trial that led to FDA approval of ofatumumab enrolled patients who were refractory to fludarabine and alemtuzumab (FA-ref) as well as fludarabine-refractory patients with bulky (>5 cm) lymph nodes (and therefore poor candidates for treatment with alemtuzumab) (BF-ref); regulatory approval was based on outcome for the FA-ref group. Patients received ofatumumab 2,000 mg intravenously weekly for 8 weeks, then monthly for 4 months. The overall response rate was 58% and 47% for the FA-ref and BF-ref group, respectively. The median PFS and OS were 5.7 months and 13.7 months, respectively, in the FA-ref and 5.9 months and 15.4 months, respectively, in the BF-ref group, representing clinical benefit for these patients compared to historic outcomes with available treatment (see Table 46.6).[84] First infusion-associated toxicity was most common and effectively managed with premedication. Infection was seen, but expected in these highly refractory, heavily pretreated patients. Response rates, median survival, and adverse effects were similar between rituximab-treated, rituximab-refractory, and rituximab-naïve patients.[85]

Chemoimmunotherapy

In vitro data demonstrate synergy between fludarabine and rituximab. Rituximab downmodulates levels of the antiapoptotic protein bcl-2 and may sensitize leukemia cells to fludarabine-induced apoptosis. Furthermore, fludarabine downmodulates expression of complement-resistance proteins, CD46, CD55, and CD59 on malignant B cells and renders them more susceptible to rituximab-induced CDC. The randomized phase 2 multi-institutional Cancer and Leukemia Group B (CALGB) 9712 trial evaluated the activity of concurrent versus sequential fludarabine and rituximab as first-line treatment (Table 46.7).[86–90] All patients in this study

TABLE 46.7
Chemoimmunotherapy for Patients with Chronic Lymphocytic Leukemia

Study (Ref.)	Treatment	Prior Rx	No. Evaluable	CR (%)	OR (%)	Median PFS (mo)
FluCam[87]	F: 30 mg/m² IV d1–3, c1–6 A: 30 mg IV d1–3, c1–6	Yes	36	30	83	13 (TTP)
Mauro et al.[88]	F: 30 mg/m² IV d1–3, c1–4 A: 30 mg IV d1–3, c1–4	No (Age ≤60)	45	24	76	3-y PFS 42.5%
Elter et al.[107]	Randomized (phase 3) F: 25 mg/m² IV d1–5, c1–6 vs. F: 30 mg/m² IV d1–3, c1–6 A: 30 mg IV d1–3, c1–6	Yes Yes	167 168	4 13	75 82	17 24
Hillmen et al.[89]	Chl: 10 mg/m²/d PO d1–7, c1–6 R: 375–500 mg/m² IV d1, c1–6	No	100	10	84	24
Foa et al.[90]	Chl: 8 mg/m²/d PO d1–7, c1–8 R: 375–500 mg/m² IV d1, c3–8 Maintenance: R: 375 mg/m² IV q 8 wk × 12	No (Age >65)	85	17	82	35
GCLLSG CLL11[108]	Randomized (phase 3) Chl: 0.5 mg/kg PO d1,15, c1–6 vs. Chl: 0.5 mg/kg PO d1,15, c1–6 R: 375–500 mg/m² IV d1, c1–6 vs. Chl: 0.5 mg/kg PO d1,15, c1–6 Ob: 1000 mg IV d1,8,15, c1; d1, c2–6	(CIRS >6) No No No	118 330 333	0 7 21	31 65 78	11 15 27
CALGB 9712[06]	Randomized (phase 2) Concurrent F: 25 mg/m² IV d1–5, c1–6 R: 375 mg/m² IV d1,4, c1; d1, c2–6 2 mo observation then R: 375 mg/m² IV weekly × 4 vs. Sequential F: 25 mg/m² IV d1–5, c1–6 2 mo observation then R: 375 mg/m² IV weekly × 4	No No	51 53	47 28	90 77	2-y PFS 70% 2-y PFS 70%
MDACC-FCR[92–95]	F: 25 mg/m² IV d2–4, c1; d1–3, c2–6 C: 250 mg/m² IV d2–4, c1; d1–3, c2–6 R: 375–500 mg/m² IV d1, c1–6	No[92,94] Yes[93,95]	300 177	72 25	95 73	80 28
Foon et al.[101]	F: 20 mg/m² IV d2–4, c1; d2–3, c2–6 C: 150 mg/m² IV d2–4, c1; d2–3, c2–6 R: 375 mg/m² IV d1, c1; 500 mg/m² d14, c1; 500 mg/m² d1, c2–6; then 500 mg/m² q 3 mo	No	63	73	94	70
Bosch et al.[98]	F: 25 mg/m² IV d1–3, c1–6 C: 250 mg/m² IV d1–3, c1–6 M: 6 mg/m² IV d1, c1–6 R: 375–500 mg/m² IV d1, c1–6	No	71	83	90	NR
Faderl et al.[99]	F: 25 mg/m² IV d2–4, c1; d1–3, c2–6 C: 250 mg/m² IV d2–4, c1; d1–3, c2–6 M: 6 mg/m² IV d1, c1–6 R: 375–500 mg/m² IV d1, c1–6	No	30	83	96	NR
Hillmen et al.[100]	Randomized (phase 2) F: 24 mg/m²/d PO d1–5, c1–6 C: 150 mg/m²/d PO d1–5, c1–6 M: 6 mg/m² IV d1, c1–6 vs. F: 24 mg/m²/d PO d1–5, c1–6 C: 150 mg/m²/d PO d1–5, c1–6 M: 6 mg/m² IV d1, c1–6 R: 375–500 mg/m² IV d1, c1–6	Yes Yes	26 26	8 15	58 65	18 18
Kay et al.[103]	P: 2 mg/m² IV d1, c1–6 C: 600 mg/m² IV d1, c1–6 R: 375 mg/m² IV d1, c2–6	No	64	41	91	33

(continued)

TABLE 46.7
Chemoimmunotherapy for Patients with Chronic Lymphocytic Leukemia (continued)

Study (Ref.)	Treatment	Prior Rx	No. Evaluable	CR (%)	OR (%)	Median PFS (mo)
Shanafelt et al.[104]	P: 2 mg/m² IV d1, c1–6 C: 600 mg/m² IV d1, c1–6 Of: 300–1,000 mg IV d1, c1–6	No	48	46	96	NR
Lamanna et al.[102]	P: 4 mg/m² IV d1, c1–6 C: 600 mg/m² IV d1, c1–6 R: 375 mg/m² IV d1, c2–6	Yes	32	25	75	40 (TTF)
Fischer et al.[106]	B: 70 mg/m² IV d1,2, c1–6 R: 375–500 mg/m² IV d1, c1–6	Yes	78	9	59	14 (EFS)
Fischer et al.[105]	B: 90 mg/m² IV d1,2, c1–6 R: 375–500 mg/m² IV d1, c1–6	No	117	23	88	34 (EFS)
GCLLSG CLL8[96]	Randomized (phase 3) F: 25 mg/m² IV d2–4, c1; d1–3, c2–6 C: 250 mg/m² IV d2–4, c1; d1–3, c2–6 R: 375–500 mg/m² IV d1, c1–6 vs. F: 25 mg/m² IV d2–4, c1; d1–3, c2–6 C: 250 mg/m² IV d2–4, c1; d1–3, c2–6	(CIRS ≤6) No No	409 408	44 22	90 80	52 33
REACH[97]	Randomized (phase 3) F: 25 mg/m² IV d2–4, c1; d1–3, c2–6 C: 250 mg/m² IV d2–4, c1; d1–3, c2–6 R: 375–500 mg/m² IV d1, c1–6 vs. F: 25 mg/m² IV d1–3, c1–6 C: 250 mg/m² IV d1–3, c1–6	Yes Yes	276 276	24 13	70 60	30.6 20.6

Rx, treatment; CR, complete remission; OR, overall response; PFS, progression-free survival; F, fludarabine; IV, intravenous; c, course; A, alemtuzumab; TTP, time to progression; Chl, chlorambucil; R, rituximab; PO, by mouth; GCLLSG, German Chronic Lymphocytic Leukemia Study Group; Ob, obinutuzumab; CIRS, cumulative illness rating scale; CALGB, Cancer and Leukemia Group B; MDACC, MD Anderson Cancer Center; C, cyclophosphamide; M, mitoxantrone; NR, not reported; P, pentostatin; Of, ofatumumab; TTF, time to treatment failure; B, bendamustine; EFS, event-free survival.

---

received rituximab; the concurrent group received 2.5 times the cumulative dose given to the sequential group. This trial achieved the primary end point of demonstrating a significantly higher complete remission rate of 47% in the concurrent group versus 28% in the sequential group. The overall response rate and PFS were not significantly different between the two groups. Shorter PFS was noted for patients with unmutated *IGHV*; shorter PFS and OS were noted for patients with del(17p) or del(11q) by FISH. Notably, the incidence of grade 3 to 4 neutropenia was higher in patients who received concurrent fludarabine and rituximab (77%), compared to sequential (41%) treatment. No significant difference was seen in the incidence of infection between the two arms. Subsequently, an analysis comparing patients treated on the CALGB 9712 trial versus a historical group of patients treated first-line with fludarabine monotherapy in the randomized CALGB 9011 trial (no rituximab) demonstrated a statistically significantly higher complete remission rate, overall response rate, 2-year disease-free survival, and 2-year OS, favoring patients who received fludarabine and rituximab.[91]

The combination of fludarabine, CTX, and rituximab (FCR) was initially evaluated in phase 2 trials in previously treated and chemotherapy-naive patients with CLL (see Table 46.7).[92–95] In 300 previously untreated patients with CLL, the complete remission rate with FCR was 72% and the overall response rate was 95%, with most patients having no detectable disease by two-color flow cytometry evaluation of the bone marrow at the end of therapy.[92] Over 40% of complete responders tested were free of disease in the bone marrow by PCR for *IGHV*. This was the highest response rate reported for any regimen in previously untreated patients with CLL. The estimated median PFS was 80 months.

The GCLLSG CLL8 trial was a randomized multicenter phase 3 clinical trial of FCR versus FC for previously untreated patients (see Table 46.7).[96] This trial clearly demonstrated superior median PFS associated with FCR (52 months) versus FC (33 months) as well as superior complete and overall response rates at 44% and 95% versus 22% and 88%, respectively. FCR treatment was also associated with a higher incidence of grade 3 or 4 neutropenia (33.7% versus 21%; $p < 0.0001$); however, there was no difference in the incidence of grade 3 or 4 infection (18.8% versus 14.9%; $p = 0.14$). Most importantly, this trial demonstrated superior OS associated with first-line treatment with FCR (84% alive) versus FC (79% alive) at 38 months ($p = 0.01$). The largest benefit was seen for patients with Binet stage A and B disease and patients younger than 70.

The REACH trial was an international randomized phase 3 trial with identical treatment arms as CLL8 and enrolled previously treated patients (see Table 46.7).[97] Eligible patients could only have had one prior treatment that did not include rituximab or FC. The conclusions of this trial were consistent with those of CLL8: superior PFS associated with superior complete and overall response rate for FCR versus FC. Thus far, no difference in OS between treatment arms has been observed in the REACH trial.

Efforts to improve the efficacy of the FCR regimen have included adding mitoxantrone to the regimen in clinical trial (see Table 46.7).[98–100] There was no evidence that this addition produced a marked improvement over FCR. In addition, in an effort to reduce the myelosuppression of FCR and make the regimen more tolerable, a phase 2 trial was conducted with reduced doses of fludarabine and CTX and with the addition of maintenance rituximab, referred to as "FCR-lite" (see Table 46.7).[101] Impressive response rates, with a high complete response rate of 73%, and durable remissions were reported. Rituximab or ofatumumab was combined with pentostatin and CTX for previously treated and chemotherapy-naive patients with CLL (see Table 46.7).[102–104] Both studies demonstrated that this regimen was active and well tolerated; the most common toxicity was myelosuppression, and nausea and vomiting were the most common nonhematologic toxicities.

Results from a variety of clinical trials with chemoimmunotherapy regimens for CLL and non-Hodgkin's lymphomas generally indicate synergy between the mAbs and chemotherapy. Indeed, rituximab was also combined with bendamustine and evaluated in phase 2 trials for previously treated and chemotherapy-naïve patients with CLL (see Table 46.7).[105,106] Efficacy and tolerability were demonstrated with this regimen. Furthermore, fludarabine was combined with alemtuzumab for untreated and previously treated patients with CLL; superior efficacy over fludarabine monotherapy and safety were also demonstrated for this combination (see Table 46.7). In a randomized phase 3 trial of previously treated patients with CLL, fludarabine plus alemtuzumab prolonged PFS and OS, albeit with an increase in serious adverse events in the combination treatment group.[107]

Older (age ≥65 years) individuals and those with comorbidities have difficulty tolerating regimens that are more myelosuppressive such as FC or FCR. Furthermore, a randomized trial did not show benefit with fludarabine in first-line treatment for these individuals. Therefore, there have been several clinical trials combining CLB with a CD20 mAb aimed at developing an active and effective chemoimmunotherapy regimen that could be tolerated by this population, with less myelosuppression (see Table 46.7). CLB was combined with rituximab, giving encouraging preliminary results. Obinutuzumab is a type II CD20 mAb, resulting in potent direct induction of apoptosis, and is glycoengineered to enhance antibody-dependent cellular cytotoxicity. The GCLLSG conducted a three-arm, phase 3 trial (CLL11) of CLB monotherapy versus CLB with rituximab versus CLB with obinutuzumab (see Table 46.7).[108] This trial demonstrated superior PFS and OS with obinutuzumab and CLB over CLB monotherapy and demonstrated superior PFS with obinutuzumab over rituximab when combined with CLB. Treatment was well tolerated in these patients with comorbidities, and these trial results led the FDA to approve of obinutuzumab in this setting.

Eliminating Minimal Residual Disease

The clinical benefit of eliminating MRD was suggested in a report of 91 previously treated patients with CLL who received alemtuzumab; 20% had eradication of MRD in the blood and bone marrow evaluated by four-color flow cytometry.[40] MRD-free status was associated with longer PFS and OS. Clinical trials focused on prospectively evaluating the impact of eliminating MRD on PFS and OS are ongoing.

For patients with residual disease after purine analogue–based therapy, the marrow is the usual site of involvement. Because alemtuzumab has significant activity in clearing blood and bone marrow, it was evaluated in trials to eliminate MRD following chemotherapy.[109,110] These studies demonstrated the ability to improve responses and achieve MRD-free status in a percentage of patients treated with alemtuzumab, with anticipated associated risk for infection. However, studies reported unacceptable toxicity with this strategy.[111–113]

B-Cell Signaling Pathway Inhibitors for Treatment of Chronic Lymphocytic Leukemia

CLL cells receive stimulation, including growth and survival signals, from the microenvironment of bone marrow, lymph nodes, and spleen. The microenvironment provides signals directing CLL cell proliferation and survival through binding and ligation of surface receptors and soluble factors such as cytokines and chemokines. Bruton's tyrosine kinase (BTK) has emerged as a central intracellular signal transduction molecule in CLL cell interactions with the microenvironment and for survival.[114] BTK is a central molecule in signal transduction for the BCR as well as CD19, CD38, CD40, CXCR4 chemokine receptor, tumor necrosis factor receptors, and toll-like receptors. BCR signaling and interaction of CLL cells with the microenvironment involve complex biochemical cascades and protein interactions for intracellular signaling. Other key signal transduction molecules include phosphoinositide 3-kinase (PI3K) and spleen tyrosine kinase. These molecules are being targeted for inhibition with small molecules as a therapeutic strategy. The furthest along in clinical development is ibrutinib, an orally administered irreversible inhibitor of BTK recently approved by the FDA for patients with relapsed CLL. Idelalisib is an oral reversible inhibitor of PI3K, and there are spleen tyrosine kinase inhibitors in clinical development.

Bruton's Tyrosine Kinase Inhibitors

X-linked agammaglobulinemia results from mutation in BTK, leading to lack of mature B cells. BTK is essential in the Akt, extracellular signal-regulated protein kinase, and nuclear factor-κB signaling pathways of B cells. BTK inhibition occurs following covalent binding of ibrutinib to cysteine-481. Preclinical studies with ibrutinib demonstrated inhibition of BCR-stimulated activation of nuclear factor-κB and extracellular signal-regulated protein kinase, resulting in death of malignant B cells; antitumor activity was also seen in animal models of B-cell malignancies. A phase 1/2 clinical trial was reported with ibrutinib administered to 85 previously treated patients with CLL demonstrating durable disease control with continuous 420 mg or 840 mg daily monotherapy.[115] There were no dose-limiting toxicities, and target inhibition was associated with clinical reductions in tumor bulk. There was not a difference in activity between the two dose levels, 420 mg once daily is the recommended dose. The overall response rate was 71% (2 complete responses; 58 partial responses) by standard response criteria. Similar responses were noted across risk categories, including for high-risk del(17p), heavily pretreated, and advanced-stage disease. Best response was typically achieved by 1 year on treatment, with lymph node responses occurring rapidly, and lymphocytosis requiring longer time to improve. Most patients had transiently increased lymphocytosis upon initiating treatment, which likely represents egress of leukemia cells from lymph nodes and other protective niches. The 2-year PFS rate was 75% and OS rate was 83%, indicating durable responses with limited follow-up. Grade 3–4 treatment-related toxicity was rare. The most common toxicity was diarrhea, occurring in 49% of patients, 95% of which were grade 1–2. Ibrutinib monotherapy was evaluated as first-line treatment in 31 patients 65 years old or older.[116] The most common toxicities were diarrhea and nausea, occurring in 68% and 48% of patients, respectively; nearly all were grade 1–2. This was a very well-tolerated treatment, and the overall response rate was 71%, with 13% complete response and 58% partial response, with durable remissions although limited follow-up.

Ibrutinib was evaluated against ofatumumab monotherapy in 391 patients with relapsed CLL in an international randomized phase 3 clinical trial.[117,118] Treatment consisted of either ibrutinib 420 mg orally daily until progression or ofatumumab 300 mg first dose then 2,000 mg for seven weekly followed by four monthly doses. The primary end point was reached with an impressive improvement in PFS for ibrutinib (ibrutinib hazard ratio = 0.22; $p < 0.001$), with a relatively short overall median follow-up time of 9.4 months. Remarkably, there was a significant improvement in OS for those patients treated with ibrutinib (hazard ratio for death = 0.43; $p = 0.005$). Similarly improved outcomes were seen for high-risk patients, including those with del(17p) and those with fludarabine-refractory CLL. Diarrhea, fatigue, fever, and nausea were the most commonly reported adverse effects experienced by the patients treated with ibrutinib and were mild. According to early reports, mechanisms of ibrutinib resistance appear to include mutation of BTK at cysteine-481 (C481S) and gain-of-function mutations in PLCγ2, a signaling molecule immediately downstream of BTK.[119]

Phosphoinositide 3-Kinase Inhibitor

There are four class I PI3K isoforms, PI3K delta is expressed by leukocytes and participates in B cell development, signaling, and survival. PI3K mediates downstream signaling for the BCR as well as CXCR4, CD40, and CD49d. Idelalisib is an orally bioavailable, reversible small molecule inhibitor of p110δ of the PI3K complex; it produces no significant inhibition of other class I isoforms and no significant off-target inhibition of PI3K class II or III isoforms, mammalian target of rapamycin, or DNA protein kinases.

A phase 1 trial of idelalisib was conducted in relapsed and refractory patients with low-grade lymphoproliferative diseases, including CLL.[120] Idelalisib was well tolerated; elevated liver enzymes was the most frequent toxicity, and treatment resulted in a 30% response rate in relapsed patients with CLL.[120] There was rapid and marked reduction in lymph node size and an initial increase followed by decrease in circulating leukemia cells, indicating an initial redistribution of cells followed by cell death. A phase 3 clinical trial evaluated the activity of idelalisib in combination with rituximab versus rituximab with placebo as treatment for patients with relapsed CLL in 220 frail individuals with comorbidities or cytopenias.[121] Idelalisib 150 mg was dosed twice daily continuously in 110 patients. Rituximab was administered to all patients at 375 mg/m² first dose, 500 mg/m² every 2 weeks for four doses, then every 4 weeks for three doses (eight total doses). This trial demonstrated superior efficacy for combined idelalisib and rituximab over rituximab and placebo with a hazard ratio for PFS of 0.15 ($p < 0.001$) and hazard ratio for OS of 0.28 ($p = 0.02$), serious adverse events occurred in 40% and 35%, respectively this led to FDA approval of the combination.

NEW AND NOVEL TREATMENTS FOR CHRONIC LYMPHOCYTIC LEUKEMIA

A number of new therapeutic approaches are under development for patients with CLL. Important novel strategies or novel targets and pathways include targeting Bcl-2 family members for inhibition with BH3-mimetics, immune-modulating agents such as lenalidomide, and cellular therapy strategies.

Bcl-2 Inhibitors

CLL cells express high levels of antiapoptotic proteins of the Bcl-2 family, rendering them long-lived and resistant to senescence and death. Small molecule inhibitors of Bcl-2 family members are in therapeutic development. Navitoclax (ABT-263) is an orally administered small molecule inhibitor of Bcl-2, Bcl-w, and Bcl-xL. In vitro treatment of CLL cells with navitoclax induced cell death. A phase 1/2 trial of orally administered navitoclax was conducted and generated promising results. The majority of patients treated in the study had >50% reduction in leukemia counts, and some patients experienced reduction in lymph node size.[122] The dose-limiting toxicity was thrombocytopenia secondary to accelerated platelet senescence from inhibition of Bcl-xL in platelets. Given this activity, ABT-199 was designed as a molecule with greater affinity for Bcl-2 and reduced affinity for Bcl-xL.[123] A phase 1 trial is ongoing with ABT-199 monotherapy[124] and in combination with CD20 mAb.

Immunemodulation

Lenalidomide, a thalidomide analogue, has immunemodulatory and antiangiogenic activities. The mechanisms of action and effects on the microenvironment are not well understood. Lenalidomide monotherapy was initially studied in relapsed CLL. Phase 2 clinical trials in relapsed or refractory patients with CLL evaluated continuous and interrupted (21 of 28 days) administration of up to 25 mg daily and reported overall response rates of 32% to 47% with 7% to 9% achieving complete remission, including patients who achieved MRD-free status.[125,126] Furthermore, responses were noted in patients with high-risk features including del(11q) and del(17p). Subsequently, trials evaluated first-line monotherapy, demonstrating tolerability, good responses, and durable disease control.[127,128] In a study of 60 symptomatic patients with untreated CLL age 65 years or older, lenalidomide at an initial dose of 5 mg/d (and titrated up) was well tolerated and resulted in a 65% response rate.[128,129] Improvement in hypogammaglobulinemia and T-cell counts were noted in this setting, suggesting immune restoration. Subsequently, lenalidomide was evaluated in combination with rituximab for previously treated CLL.[130] The addition of CD20 mAb appeared to improve outcomes compared to monotherapy for relapsed disease.

Lenalidomide safety and toxicity concerns have been tumor lysis syndrome and tumor flare reaction, which occur upon initiation of treatment, as well as myelosuppression, which can be dose-limiting and occurs while patients are on treatment. Tumor lysis syndrome and tumor flare reaction have been minimized by initiating lenalidomide at low dose (2.5 mg to 5 mg daily), and by initiating CD20 mAb prior to lenalidomide in patients receiving the combination. Lenalidomide remains a promising agent with unique properties and is being studied earlier in treatment, in combinations and as maintenance therapy in CLL.

Cellular Therapy for Chronic Lymphocytic Leukemia

Chimeric Antigen Receptor–Bearing T-Cell Therapy

Immune-based cellular therapy takes advantage of the ability of the immune system to seek out and eliminate malignant cells in the body. It potentially provides a mechanism of surveillance to prevent recurrence of disease. Allogeneic stem cell transplant is a form of immune cellular therapy, which is curative for some patients with CLL. Another strategy of immune cellular therapy is being developed, based on T-cell expression of chimeric antigen receptors (CARs).[131-134] CARs are engineered immune receptors introduced ex vivo into T cells, usually autologous, that redirect these cells to react against CLL cells. Graft-versus-host reactions are avoided with autologous T cells, while inducing and enhancing a graft-versus-leukemia effect. The CAR is a recombinant protein composed of an antigen-binding domain derived from single-chain immunoglobulin variable genes, hinge-stalk-transmembrane domain, derived on CD8, constant domain of immunoglobulin or other molecule, and intracellular signaling domains derived from CD3ζ and costimulatory domains derived from CD28 and/or CD137. The engineered gene is transduced into autologous T cells and expressed on the surface where it can bind to target antigen and induce T-cell activation, cytokine production, proliferation, and killing of cells expressing the target antigen. CD19 is expressed by malignant B cells, including CLL, as well as normal B cells and has been targeted with CARs. On-target effects include a leukemia-specific reaction as well as elimination of normal B cells, resulting in hypogammaglobulinemia. While very robust treatment effects were reported, including durable complete remissions, infusion-related side effects, and more notably, cytokine-release syndrome have been challenging. Hypogammaglobulinemia has inspired a search for better and more specific leukemia-associated or leukemia-specific antigens. This strategy is in early phase trials and appears promising.

Allogeneic Stem Cell Transplantation

Myeloablative allogeneic stem cell transplantation was not a viable option in CLL in the past because of the prohibitive toxicity of this approach in older patients. Autologous bone marrow transplantation has been evaluated for CLL,[135,136] but does not appear to have a role. Reduced-intensity conditioning has made allogeneic stem cell transplant (allo-SCT) available for significantly more patients with CLL. While allo-SCT was associated with long-term remissions and possible cure, there is patient selection and reporting bias in these data. Early data with nonmyeloablative allogeneic transplant indicated almost universal engraftment, although the development of chimerism was slower than with myeloablative transplants. Patients with sensitive disease who were transplanted had a better outcome than those who had resistant disease.[137] Long-term follow-up data have been reported showing a 5-year OS rate of 50%.[138,139] Notably, immune manipulation by withdrawal of immunosuppression or donor lymphocyte infusions enhanced clinical responses, indicating that CLL is a disease vulnerable to immune-mediated elimination and control. A 6-year OS rate of 58% was reported in a series of 90 previously treated patients who underwent reduced-intensity conditioning and allo-SCT, with an event-free survival of 38% for the same period.[140] Furthermore, no association was noted between the presence of mutations in TP53, SF3B1, or NOTCH1 and OS or EFS, indicating efficacy for patients with high-risk features. Smaller series reported similar outcomes.[141–143] A single-center retrospective study of outcomes for individuals with relapsed CLL who had a matched allogeneic donor versus no donor showed improved survival for individuals who had a matched donor in landmark analysis starting 3 months after donor search was initiated. These data indicate that allo-SCT may improve survival for patients with relapsed high-risk CLL.[144]

Splenectomy

Studies suggest hematologic and survival benefits from splenectomy in patients with CLL. Splenectomy may be beneficial in individuals with immune-mediated cytopenias such as AIHA and immune thrombocytopenia purpura after corticosteroid failure or in improving blood counts in patients with hypersplenism. In a study from MD Anderson Cancer Center,[34] perioperative mortality among 55 patients was 9%, mostly related to poor preoperative performance status. Improvements in the platelet count, neutrophil count, and hemoglobin occurred in 81%, 59%, and 33% of patients, respectively. Among patients with Rai stage IV disease, a trend for improved survival was observed using case-control analysis.

Therapeutic Considerations for Specific Problems in Patients with Chronic Lymphocytic Leukemia

The most common cause of morbidity in patients with CLL is infection. Because hypogammaglobulinemia is a contributing factor to patients' increased susceptibility to infections, a randomized double-blind study evaluated the use of intravenous immunoglobulin, 400 mg/kg, versus placebo given every 3 weeks for 1 year to 84 patients with CLL.[145,146] A significant reduction in bacterial infections was seen in the group treated with intravenous immunoglobulin, but no statistically significant difference was observed in the number of life-threatening infections or nonbacterial infections. Because of the high cost of this therapy, monthly intravenous immunoglobulin therapy is best used in patients with hypogammaglobulinemia who experience repeated bacterial infections.[147,148]

SECOND MALIGNANCIES AND TRANSFORMATION

Approximately 25% of patients with CLL develop second neoplasms, the most common being skin cancer. Second neoplasm is the cause of death in 7% to 10% of patients. In approximately 2% to 6% of patients, CLL may evolve into a high-grade lymphoma of the diffuse large-cell type (Richter's transformation); less commonly Hodgkin's histology is diagnosed. Richter's transformation may arise from the original CLL clone, and its onset is heralded by fever, weight loss, a rising lactate dehydrogenase, and an asymmetric rapid lymph node enlargement.[149] Because the lymphoma may be patchy, a gallium or positron emission tomography scan, usually negative in CLL, may aid in identifying a "hot" lymph node that can be targeted for biopsy. Transformation must be diagnosed by histology. The prognosis of Richter's transformation is poor, with a median survival of only 6 months. Prolymphocytic transformation develops in approximately 2% to 5% of patients with CLL. This transformation is different immunophenotypically and clinically from primary or de novo PLL. Secondary PLL is marked by development of refractory anemia and thrombocytopenia, progressive splenomegaly, and an increase in the percentage of prolymphocytes to >30% of the leukemia cells. As with Richter's transformation, PLL transformation portends a poor prognosis despite aggressive therapy.

Therapy-related myeloid neoplasia (myelodysplasia or acute myeloid leukemia) is also a concern in CLL. In long-term follow-up of the US Intergroup Study E2997, 4.7% of patients developed therapy-related myeloid neoplasia at a median of 5 years from initial therapy.[150]

PROLYMPHOCYTIC LEUKEMIA

PLL is characterized by a high number of circulating prolymphocytes, splenomegaly, minimal lymphadenopathy, and a median survival of <3 years. This leukemia can be present at diagnosis or evolve from CLL.[151] Prolymphocytes are larger and less homogeneous than CLL cells and have abundant clear cytoplasm, clumped chromatin, and a prominent nucleolus. Prolymphocytes can be of either B- or T-cell type. B-PLL cells usually do not express CD5 but stain strongly for surface immunoglobulin and FMC7 (see Table 46.1). In 20% of cases of PLL, T-cell markers are expressed.

Splenectomy and lymphomalike regimens have been used to treat PLL without much success. Nucleoside analogue–based regimens appear to be the most effective, and alemtuzumab has shown promising activity in T-PLL.[152]

LARGE GRANULAR LYMPHOCYTE LEUKEMIA

Large granular lymphocytes (LGLs) are larger than normal lymphocytes and contain azurophilic granules in their cytoplasm. LGLs comprise 10% to 15% of peripheral blood mononuclear cells and are predominantly of NK-cell phenotype, a smaller fraction being of T-cell phenotype. There are generally four lymphoproliferative disorders of LGL: reactive/transient LGL expansion, chronic LGL lymphocytosis, indolent LGL leukemia, and aggressive LGL leukemia.[153] Clonal expansion of LGL can be of NK-cell or T-cell phenotype; the T-cell phenotype comprises 80% of LGL leukemias. T-LGL cells have a CD3+/CD57+/CD56− immunophenotype, and NK-LGL express CD3−/CD56+/CD57−. Clonality in T-LGL leukemia may be established by T-cell receptor gene rearrangement studies. T-LGL leukemia is usually indolent. Patients present with cytopenias, including neutropenia with accompanying infections, pure red cell aplasia, thrombocytopenia, and anemia. Serologic abnormalities, such as the presence of rheumatoid factor or antinuclear antibody, or both, hypergammaglobulinemia, and high β_2-microglobin are frequent. A small percentage of LGL leukemias have a more aggressive course, and these cases tend to have an NK-cell phenotype. Because lymphocyte counts are usually not elevated, diagnosis requires a high degree of suspicion and a careful examination of the peripheral blood smear and bone marrow. Although the disease may be indolent, most patients require treatment for cytopenias. Various therapies, including low-dose methotrexate (10 mg/m² orally once weekly), cyclosporine (3 mg/kg orally every 12 hours), or CTX (100 mg orally daily) with or without oral prednisone (1 mg/kg orally daily) have all been effective. Complete remissions may be seen in up to 50% of cases. Lymphoma-type regimens, such as CTX, doxorubicin, prednisone, and vincristine, have not been effective for aggressive disease.

HAIRY CELL LEUKEMIA

HCL is a rare B-cell lymphoproliferative disorder that affects adults and represents 2% of all leukemias. It has a marked preponderance in men. Most patients have cytopenias; splenomegaly is also frequent.[154] Hairy cells can be seen in the peripheral blood, but at low frequency, and therefore are easily missed. These cells are twice as large as normal lymphocytes, with the nuclei showing a loose chromatin pattern and villi-like cytoplasmic projections (best viewed under phase contrast microscopy). Hairy cells infiltrate the bone marrow in an interstitial or focal pattern, with clear zones in between cells ("fried egg appearance"). Marrow reticulin is increased, and aspirates may result in a dry tap. Immunophenotypic analysis of hairy cells shows the presence of CD19, CD20, CD22, CD25, and CD103 and, in contrast to CLL, hairy cells are negative for CD5 and CD23. Hairy cells also stain strongly for surface immunoglobulin and FMC7. Use of the CD103 antibody, which stains tartrate-resistant acid phosphatase, has obviated the need for cytochemical staining for tartrate-resistant acid phosphatase.

The BRAF V600E mutation was recently found to be present in all patients with HCL, a finding that is likely to have an impact on the diagnosis and possibly the treatment of this disease.[155,156] Vemurafenib is a BRAF inhibitor[157] currently in clinical trials as therapy for relapsed or refractory HCL.

HCL has no staging system. For many years, the only effective therapy was splenectomy.

Treatments for Hairy Cell Leukemia

Nucleoside Analogues

Pentostatin (2′ deoxycoformycin) and cladribine (2-CdA) are the nucleoside analogues that are the mainstay of treatment of HCL.[158] Pentostatin is administered at 4 mg/m² every 2 weeks until maximum response, and cladribine is given at 0.1 mg/kg per day as a continuous intravenous infusion for 7 days; the same total dose can be administered as a 2-hour infusion over 5 days. Because cladribine involves a single course of therapy and produces remission rates comparable to those of pentostatin, cladribine is used more frequently in the United States for the treatment of HCL. Multiple series have reported high response rates, with patients remaining in remission for many years. The majority of relapsed patients achieve second remission when retreated with pentostatin or cladribine. The choice of agent may depend on the duration of the first remission: if <3 years, an alternate agent should be used; if >5 years, the same agent may be given. The role of interferon-alpha is currently limited to patients who are unresponsive to nucleoside analogues.

Monoclonal Antibody-Drug Conjugate

A percentage of patients may relapse with cladribine-resistant disease. In addition, 10% to 20% of patients have a variant form of HCL with high numbers of circulating hairy cells and a poor response to nucleoside analogues. Classic and variant hairy cells strongly express CD22, a B-cell adhesion molecule. Data suggest marked efficacy of a recombinant immunotoxin, BL22, in the treatment of chemotherapy-resistant HCL.[159] This immunotoxin contains the variable domain of the anti-CD22 mAb RFB4, which is fused to a fragment of *Pseudomonas* exotoxin called *PE38* that lacks the domain necessary for cell binding and contains only the domain responsible for cell death. The phase 1 trial of BL22 included 16 cladribine-resistant patients with HCL; 11 achieved complete remission and 2 partial remissions were reported. Side effects included transient hypoalbuminemia, elevated aminotransferase levels and in 2 of 16 patients, a reversible hemolytic-uremic syndrome developed. A phase 2 trial was conducted with BL22 in 36 patients with relapsed or refractory HCL.[160] Overall, 47% achieved complete response and 25% partial response; 2 (6%) patients experienced reversible hemolytic uremic syndrome. Patients with smaller spleen were more likely to achieve complete response. Neutralizing antibodies were identified in four (11%) patients, which prevented retreatment. Moxetumomab pasudotox (HA22 or CAT-8015) is derived from BL22, selected for high-affinity for CD22. A phase 1 trial of moxetumomab pasudotox was performed in 28 patients with chemotherapy-resistant HCL.[161] Doses included 5 mcg/kg to 50 mcg/kg intravenously every other day for three doses for each course, with up to 16 courses repeated every 4 weeks. The median number of courses given was four, and no dose-limiting toxicity was observed up to the highest dose tested. The overall response rate was 86% and 46% achieved CR; these responses were durable.

REFERENCES

1. O'Brien S, del Giglio A, Keating M. Advances in the biology and treatment of B-cell chronic lymphocytic leukemia. *Blood* 1955;85:307–318.
2. Jemal A, Siegel R, Xu J, et al. Cancer statistics, 2010. *CA Cancer J Clin* 2010;60:277–300.
3. Siegel R, Ma J, Zou Z, et al. Cancer statistics, 2014. *CA Cancer J Clin* 2014;64:9–29.
4. Yanagihara ET, Blaisdell RK, Hayashi T, et al. Malignant lymphoma in Hawaii-Japanese: a retrospective morphologic survey. *Hematol Oncol* 1989;7:219–232.
5. Preston DL, Kusumi S, Tomonaga M, et al. Cancer incidence in atomic bomb survivors. Part III. Leukemia, lymphoma and multiple myeloma, 1950–1987. *Radiat Res* 1994;137:S68–S97.
6. Houlston RS, Catovsky D, Yuille MR. Genetic susceptibility to chronic lymphocytic leukemia. *Leukemia* 2002;16:1008–1014.
7. Dohner H, Stilgenbauer S, Dohner K, et al. Chromosome aberrations in B-cell chronic lymphocytic leukemia: reassessment based on molecular cytogenetic analysis. *J Mol Med* 1999;77:266–281.
8. Geisler CH, Larsen JK, Hansen NE, et al. Prognostic importance of flow cytometric immunophenotyping of 540 consecutive patients with B-cell chronic lymphocytic leukemia. *Blood* 1991;78:1795–1802.
9. Rawstron AC, Green MJ, Kuzmicki A, et al. Monoclonal B lymphocytes with the characteristics of "indolent" chronic lymphocytic leukemia are present in 3.5% of adults with normal blood counts. *Blood* 2002;100:635–639.
10. Rawstron AC, Bennett FL, O'Connor SJ, et al. Monoclonal B-cell lymphocytosis and chronic lymphocytic leukemia. *N Engl J Med* 2008;359:575–583.
11. Naylor M, Capra JD. Mutational status of Ig V(H) genes provides clinically valuable information in B-cell chronic lymphocytic leukemia. *Blood* 1999;94:1837–1839.
12. Damle RN, Wasil T, Fais F, et al. Ig V gene mutation status and CD38 expression as novel prognostic indicators in chronic lymphocytic leukemia. *Blood* 1999;94:1840–1847.
13. Hamblin TJ, Davis Z, Gardiner A, et al. Unmutated Ig V(H) genes are associated with a more aggressive form of chronic lymphocytic leukemia. *Blood* 1999;94:1848–1854.
14. Rosenwald A, Alizadeh AA, Widhopf G, et al. Relation of gene expression phenotype to immunoglobulin mutation genotype in B cell chronic lymphocytic leukemia. *J Exp Med* 2001;194:1639–1647.
15. Crespo M, Bosch F, Villamor N, et al. ZAP-70 expression as a surrogate for immunoglobulin-variable-region mutations in chronic lymphocytic leukemia. *N Engl J Med* 2003;348:1764–1775.
16. Calin GA, Dumitru CD, Shimizu M, et al. Frequent deletions and down-regulation of micro-RNA genes miR15 and miR16 at 13q14 in chronic lymphocytic leukemia. *Proc Natl Acad Sci U S A* 2002;99:15524–15529.
17. Puente XS, Pinyol M, Quesada V, et al. Whole-genome sequencing identifies recurrent mutations in chronic lymphocytic leukaemia. *Nature* 2011;475:101–105.
18. Quesada V, Conde L, Villamor N, et al. Exome sequencing identifies recurrent mutations of the splicing factor SF3B1 gene in chronic lymphocytic leukemia. *Nat Genet* 2012;44:47–52.

19. Wang L, Lawrence MS, Wan Y, et al. SF3B1 and other novel cancer genes in chronic lymphocytic leukemia. N Engl J Med 2011;365:2497–2506.
20. Rossi D, Rasi S, Spina V, et al. Integrated mutational and cytogenetic analysis identifies new prognostic subgroups in chronic lymphocytic leukemia. Blood 2013;121:1403–1412.
21. Landau DA, Carter SL, Stojanov P, et al. Evolution and impact of subclonal mutations in chronic lymphocytic leukemia. Cell 2013;152:714–726.
22. Ouillette P, Saiya-Cork K, Seymour E, et al. Clonal evolution, genomic drivers, and effects of therapy in chronic lymphocytic leukemia. Clin Cancer Res 2013;19:2893–2904.
23. Schuh A, Becq J, Humphray S, et al. Monitoring chronic lymphocytic leukemia progression by whole genome sequencing reveals heterogeneous clonal evolution patterns. Blood 2012;120:4191–4196.
24. Decker T, Flohr T, Trautmann P, et al. Role of accessory cells in cytokine production by T cells in chronic B-cell lymphocytic leukemia. Blood 1995;86:1115–1123.
25. Scrivener S, Goddard RV, Kaminski ER, et al. Abnormal T-cell function in B-cell chronic lymphocytic leukaemia. Leuk Lymphoma 2003;44:383–389.
26. Hallek M, Cheson BD, Catovsky D, et al. Guidelines for the diagnosis and treatment of chronic lymphocytic leukemia: a report from the International Workshop on Chronic Lymphocytic Leukemia updating the National Cancer Institute-Working Group 1996 guidelines. Blood 2008;111:5446–5456.
27. Cheson BD, Bennett JM, Grever M, et al. National Cancer Institute-sponsored Working Group guidelines for chronic lymphocytic leukemia: revised guidelines for diagnosis and treatment. Blood 1996;87:4990–4997.
28. Mauro FR, Foa R, Cerretti R, et al. Autoimmune hemolytic anemia in chronic lymphocytic leukemia: clinical, therapeutic, and prognostic features. Blood 2000;95:2786–2792.
29. Diehl LF, Ketchum LH. Autoimmune disease and chronic lymphocytic leukemia: autoimmune hemolytic anemia, pure red cell aplasia, and autoimmune thrombocytopenia. Semin Oncol 1998;25:80–97.
30. Kipps TJ, Carson DA. Autoantibodies in chronic lymphocytic leukemia and related systemic autoimmune diseases. Blood 1993;81:2475–2487.
31. Cortes J, O'Brien S, Loscertales J, et al. Cyclosporin A for the treatment of cytopenia associated with chronic lymphocytic leukemia. Cancer 2001;92:2016–2022.
32. Gupta N, Kavuru S, Patel D, et al. Rituximab-based chemotherapy for steroid-refractory autoimmune hemolytic anemia of chronic lymphocytic leukemia. Leukemia 2002;16:2092–2095.
33. Kaufman M, Limpin SA, Driscoll N, et al. A combination of rituximab, cyclophosphamide and dexamethasone effectively treats immune cytopenias of chronic lymphocytic leukemia. Leuk Lymphoma 2009;50:892–899.
34. Seymour JF, Cusack JD, Lerner SA, et al. Case/control study of the role of splenectomy in chronic lymphocytic leukemia. J Clin Oncol 1997;15:52–60.
35. Rai KR, Sawitsky A, Cronkite EP, et al. Clinical staging of chronic lymphocytic leukemia. Blood 1975;46:219–234.
36. Binet JL, Auquier A, Dighiero G, et al. A new prognostic classification of chronic lymphocytic leukemia derived from a multivariate survival analysis. Cancer 1981;48:198–206.
37. Zwiebel JA, Cheson BD. Chronic lymphocytic leukemia: staging and prognostic factors. Semin Oncol 1998;25:42–59.
38. CLL Trialists' Collaborative Group. Chemotherapeutic options in chronic lymphocytic leukemia: a meta-analysis of the randomized trials. J Natl Cancer Inst 1999;91:861–868.
39. Cheson BD, Bennett JM, Rai KR, et al. Guidelines for clinical protocols for chronic lymphocytic leukemia: recommendations of the National Cancer Institute-sponsored working group. Am J Hematol 1988;29:152–163.
40. Moreton P, Kennedy B, Lucas G, et al. Eradication of minimal residual disease in B-cell chronic lymphocytic leukemia after alemtuzumab therapy is associated with prolonged survival. J Clin Oncol 2005;23:2971–2979.
41. Bottcher S, Ritgen M, Fischer K, et al. Minimal residual disease quantification is an independent predictor of progression-free and overall survival in chronic lymphocytic leukemia: a multivariate analysis from the randomized GCLLSG CLL8 trial. J Clin Oncol 2012;30:980–988.
42. Rawstron AC, Villamor N, Ritgen M, et al. International standardized approach for flow cytometric residual disease monitoring in chronic lymphocytic leukaemia. Leukemia 2007;21:956–964.
43. Robak T, Kasznicki M. Alkylating agents and nucleoside analogues in the treatment of B cell chronic lymphocytic leukemia. Leukemia 2002;16:1015–1027.
44. Catovsky D, Richards S, Matutes E, et al. Assessment of fludarabine plus cyclophosphamide for patients with chronic lymphocytic leukaemia (the LRF CLL4 Trial): a randomised controlled trial. Lancet 2007;370:230–239.
45. Johnson S, Smith AG, Loffler H, et al. Multicentre prospective randomised trial of fludarabine versus cyclophosphamide, doxorubicin, and prednisone (CAP) for treatment of advanced-stage chronic lymphocytic leukaemia. The French Cooperative Group on CLL. Lancet 1996;347:1432–1438.
46. Leporrier M, Chevret S, Cazin B, et al. Randomized comparison of fludarabine, CAP, and ChOP in 938 previously untreated stage B and C chronic lymphocytic leukemia patients. Blood 2001;98:2319–2325.
47. Rai KR, Peterson BL, Appelbaum FR, et al. Fludarabine compared with chlorambucil as primary therapy for chronic lymphocytic leukemia. N Engl J Med 2000;343:1750–1757.
48. Rai KR, Peterson BL, Appelbaum FR, et al. Long-term survival analysis of the North American Intergroup study C9011 comparing fludarabine (F) and chlorambucil (C) in previously untreated patients with chronic lymphocytic leukemia (CLL). Blood 2009;114:Abstr 536.

49. Eichhorst BF, Busch R, Stilgenbauer S, et al. First-line therapy with fludarabine compared with chlorambucil does not result in a major benefit for elderly patients with advanced chronic lymphocytic leukemia. Blood 2009;114:3382–3391.
50. Knauf WU, Lissichkov T, Aldaoud A, et al. Phase III randomized study of bendamustine compared with chlorambucil in previously untreated patients with chronic lymphocytic leukemia. J Clin Oncol 2009;27:4378–4384.
51. Yamauchi T, Nowak BJ, Keating MJ, et al. DNA repair initiated in chronic lymphocytic leukemia lymphocytes by 4-hydroperoxycyclophosphamide is inhibited by fludarabine and clofarabine. Clin Cancer Res 2001;7:3580–3589.
52. Flinn IW, Byrd JC, Morrison C, et al. Fludarabine and cyclophosphamide with filgrastim support in patients with previously untreated indolent lymphoid malignancies. Blood 2000;96:71–75.
53. Hallek M, Schmitt B, Wilhelm M, et al. Fludarabine plus cyclophosphamide is an efficient treatment for advanced chronic lymphocytic leukaemia (CLL): results of a phase II study of the German CLL Study Group. Br J Haematol 2001;114:342–348.
54. O'Brien SM, Kantarjian HM, Cortes J, et al. Results of the fludarabine and cyclophosphamide combination regimen in chronic lymphocytic leukemia. J Clin Oncol 2001;19:1414–1420.
55. Eichhorst BF, Busch R, Hopfinger G, et al. Fludarabine plus cyclophosphamide versus fludarabine alone in first-line therapy of younger patients with chronic lymphocytic leukemia. Blood 2006;107:885–891.
56. Flinn IW, Neuberg DS, Grever MR, et al. Phase III trial of fludarabine plus cyclophosphamide compared with fludarabine for patients with previously untreated chronic lymphocytic leukemia: US Intergroup Trial E2997. J Clin Oncol 2007;25:793–798.
57. Robak T, Blonski JZ, Kasznicki M, et al. Cladribine with or without prednisone in the treatment of previously treated and untreated B-cell chronic lymphocytic leukaemia - updated results of the multicentre study of 378 patients. Br J Haematol 2000;108:357–368.
58. Robak T, Blonski JZ, Gora-Tybor J, et al. Cladribine alone and in combination with cyclophosphamide or cyclophosphamide plus mitoxantrone in the treatment of progressive chronic lymphocytic leukemia: report of a prospective, multicenter, randomized trial of the Polish Adult Leukemia Group (PALG CLL2). Blood 2006;108:473–479.
59. Robak T, Jamroziak K, Gora-Tybor J, et al. Comparison of cladribine plus cyclophosphamide with fludarabine plus cyclophosphamide as first line therapy for chronic lymphocytic leukemia: a phase III randomized study by the Polish Adult Leukemia Group (PALG-CLL3 Study). J Clin Oncol 2010;28:1863–1869.
60. Keating MJ, Flinn I, Jain V, et al. Therapeutic role of alemtuzumab (Campath-1H) in patients who have failed fludarabine: results of a large international study. Blood 2002;99:3554–3561.
61. Osterborg A, Dyer MJ, Bunjes D, et al. Phase II multicenter study of human CD52 antibody in previously treated chronic lymphocytic leukemia. European Study Group of CAMPATH-1H Treatment in Chronic Lymphocytic Leukemia. J Clin Oncol 1997;15:1567–1574.
62. Rai KR, Freter CE, Mercier RJ, et al. Alemtuzumab in previously treated chronic lymphocytic leukemia patients who also had received fludarabine. J Clin Oncol 2002;20:3891–3897.
63. Ferrajoli A, O'Brien SM, Cortes JE, et al. Phase II study of alemtuzumab in chronic lymphoproliferative disorders. Cancer 2003;98:773–778.
64. Lundin J, Kimby E, Bjorkholm M, et al. Phase II trial of subcutaneous anti-CD52 monoclonal antibody alemtuzumab (Campath-1H) as first-line treatment for patients with B-cell chronic lymphocytic leukemia (B-CLL). Blood 2002;100:768–773.
65. Pettitt AR, Jackson R, Carruthers S, et al. Alemtuzumab in combination with methylprednisolone is a highly effective induction regimen for patients with chronic lymphocytic leukemia and deletion of TP53: final results of the national cancer research institute CLL206 trial. J Clin Oncol 2012;30:1647–1655.
66. McLaughlin P, Grillo-Lopez AJ, Link BK, et al. Rituximab chimeric anti-CD20 monoclonal antibody therapy for relapsed indolent lymphoma: half of patients respond to a four-dose treatment program. J Clin Oncol 1998;16:2825–2833.
67. Huhn D, von Schilling C, Wilhelm M, et al. Rituximab therapy of patients with B-cell chronic lymphocytic leukemia. Blood 2001;98:1326–1331.
68. Hainsworth JD. Prolonging remission with rituximab maintenance therapy. Semin Oncol 2004;31:17–21.
69. Ferrajoli A. Incorporating the use of GM-CSF in the treatment of chronic lymphocytic leukemia. Leuk Lymphoma 2009;50:514–516.
70. Castro JE, Sandoval-Sus JD, Bole J, et al. Rituximab in combination with high-dose methylprednisolone for the treatment of fludarabine refractory high-risk chronic lymphocytic leukemia. Leukemia 2008;22:2048–2053.
71. Bowen DA, Call TG, Jenkins GD, et al. Methylprednisolone-rituximab is an effective salvage therapy for patients with relapsed chronic lymphocytic leukemia including those with unfavorable cytogenetic features. Leuk Lymphoma 2007;48:2412–2417.
72. Castro JE, James DF, Sandoval-Sus JD, et al. Rituximab in combination with high-dose methylprednisolone for the treatment of chronic lymphocytic leukemia. Leukemia 2009;23:1779–1789.
73. Faderl S, Thomas DA, O'Brien S, et al. Experience with alemtuzumab plus rituximab in patients with relapsed and refractory lymphoid malignancies. Blood 2003;101:3413–3415.
74. Zent CS, Call TG, Shanafelt TD, et al. Early treatment of high-risk chronic lymphocytic leukemia with alemtuzumab and rituximab. Cancer 2008;113:2110–2118.

75. Stilgenbauer S, Zenz T, Winkler D, et al. Subcutaneous alemtuzumab in fludarabine-refractory chronic lymphocytic leukemia: clinical results and prognostic marker analyses from the CLL2H study of the German Chronic Lymphocytic Leukemia Study Group. *J Clin Oncol* 2009;27:3994–4001.
76. Hillmen P, Skotnicki AB, Robak T, et al. Alemtuzumab compared with chlorambucil as first-line therapy for chronic lymphocytic leukemia. *J Clin Oncol* 2007;25:5616–5623.
77. Lozanski G, Heerema NA, Flinn IW, et al. Alemtuzumab is an effective therapy for chronic lymphocytic leukemia with p53 mutations and deletions. *Blood* 2004;103:3278–3281.
78. Avivi I, Robinson S, Goldstone A. Clinical use of rituximab in haematological malignancies. *Br J Cancer* 2003;89:1389–1394.
79. Manshouri T, Do KA, Wang X, et al. Circulating CD20 is detectable in the plasma of patients with chronic lymphocytic leukemia and is of prognostic significance. *Blood* 2003;101:2507–2513.
80. O'Brien SM, Kantarjian H, Thomas DA, et al. Rituximab dose escalation trial in chronic lymphocytic leukemia. *J Clin Oncol* 2001;19:2165–2170.
81. Byrd JC, Murphy T, Howard RS, et al. Rituximab using a thrice weekly dosing schedule in B-cell chronic lymphocytic leukemia and small lymphocytic lymphoma demonstrates clinical activity and acceptable toxicity. *J Clin Oncol* 2001;19:2153–2164.
82. Hainsworth JD, Litchy S, Barton JH, et al. Single-agent rituximab as first-line and maintenance treatment for patients with chronic lymphocytic leukemia or small lymphocytic lymphoma: a phase II trial of the Minnie Pearl Cancer Research Network. *J Clin Oncol* 2003;21:1746–1751.
83. Coiffier B, Lepretre S, Pedersen LM, et al. Safety and efficacy of ofatumumab, a fully human monoclonal anti-CD20 antibody, in patients with relapsed or refractory B-cell chronic lymphocytic leukemia: a phase 1–2 study. *Blood* 2008;111:1094–1100.
84. Wierda WG, Kipps TJ, Mayer J, et al. Ofatumumab as single-agent CD20 immunotherapy in fludarabine-refractory chronic lymphocytic leukemia. *J Clin Oncol* 2010;28:1749–1755.
85. Wierda WG, Padmanabhan S, Chan GW, et al. Ofatumumab is active in patients with fludarabine-refractory CLL irrespective of prior rituximab: results from the phase 2 international study. *Blood* 2011;118:5126–5129.
86. Byrd JC, Peterson BL, Morrison VA, et al. Randomized phase 2 study of fludarabine with concurrent versus sequential treatment with rituximab in symptomatic, untreated patients with B-cell chronic lymphocytic leukemia: results from Cancer and Leukemia Group B 9712 (CALGB 9712). *Blood* 2003;101:6–14.
87. Elter T, Borchmann P, Schulz H, et al. Fludarabine in combination with alemtuzumab is effective and feasible in patients with relapsed or refractory B-cell chronic lymphocytic leukemia: results of a phase II trial. *J Clin Oncol* 2005;23:7024–7031.
88. Mauro FR, Molica S, Laurenti L, et al. Fludarabine plus alemtuzumab (FA) front-line treatment in young patients with chronic lymphocytic leukemia (CLL) and an adverse biologic profile. *Leuk Res* 2014;38:198–203.
89. Hillmen P, Gribben JG, Follows GA, et al. Rituximab plus chlorambucil as first-line treatment for chronic lymphocytic leukemia: Final analysis of an open-label phase II study. *J Clin Oncol* 2014;32:1236–1241.
90. Foa R, Del Giudice I, Cuneo A, et al. Chlorambucil plus rituximab with or without maintenance rituximab as first-line treatment for elderly chronic lymphocytic leukemia patients. *Am J Hematol* 2014;89:480–486.
91. Byrd JC, Rai K, Peterson BL, et al. Addition of rituximab to fludarabine may prolong progression-free survival and overall survival in patients with previously untreated chronic lymphocytic leukemia: an updated retrospective comparative analysis of CALGB 9712 and CALGB 9011. *Blood* 2005;105:49–53.
92. Keating MJ, O'Brien S, Albitar M, et al. Early results of a chemoimmunotherapy regimen of fludarabine, cyclophosphamide, and rituximab as initial therapy for chronic lymphocytic leukemia. *J Clin Oncol* 2005;23:4079–4088.
93. Wierda W, O'Brien S, Wen S, et al. Chemoimmunotherapy with fludarabine, cyclophosphamide, and rituximab for relapsed and refractory chronic lymphocytic leukemia. *J Clin Oncol* 2005;23:4070–4078.
94. Tam CS, O'Brien S, Wierda W, et al. Long-term results of the fludarabine, cyclophosphamide, and rituximab regimen as initial therapy of chronic lymphocytic leukemia. *Blood* 2008;112:975–980.
95. Badoux XC, Keating MJ, Wang X, et al. Fludarabine, cyclophosphamide, and rituximab chemoimmunotherapy is highly effective treatment for relapsed patients with CLL. *Blood* 2011;117:3016–3024.
96. Hallek M, Fischer K, Fingerle-Rowson G, et al. Addition of rituximab to fludarabine and cyclophosphamide in patients with chronic lymphocytic leukaemia: a randomised, open-label, phase 3 trial. *Lancet* 2010;376:1164–1174.
97. Robak T, Dmoszynska A, Solal-Celigny P, et al. Rituximab plus fludarabine and cyclophosphamide prolongs progression-free survival compared with fludarabine and cyclophosphamide alone in previously untreated chronic lymphocytic leukemia. *J Clin Oncol* 2010;28:1756–1765.
98. Bosch F, Abrisqueta P, Villamor N, et al. Rituximab, fludarabine, cyclophosphamide, and mitoxantrone: a new, highly active chemoimmunotherapy regimen for chronic lymphocytic leukemia. *J Clin Oncol* 2009;27:4578–4584.
99. Faderl S, Wierda W, O'Brien S, et al. Fludarabine, cyclophosphamide, mitoxantrone plus rituximab (FCM-R) in frontline CLL <70 years. *Leuk Res* 2010;34:284–288.
100. Hillmen P, Cohen DR, Cocks K, et al. A randomized phase II trial of fludarabine, cyclophosphamide and mitoxantrone (FCM) with or without rituximab in previously treated chronic lymphocytic leukaemia. *Br J Haematol* 2011;152:570–578.
101. Foon KA, Mehta D, Lentzsch S, et al. Long-term results of chemoimmunotherapy with low-dose fludarabine, cyclophosphamide and high-dose rituximab as initial treatment for patients with chronic lymphocytic leukemia. *Blood* 2012;119:3184–3185.
102. Lamanna N, Kalaycio M, Maslak P, et al. Pentostatin, cyclophosphamide, and rituximab is an active, well-tolerated regimen for patients with previously treated chronic lymphocytic leukemia. *J Clin Oncol* 2006;24:1575–1581.
103. Kay NE, Geyer SM, Call TG, et al. Combination chemoimmunotherapy with pentostatin, cyclophosphamide, and rituximab shows significant clinical activity with low accompanying toxicity in previously untreated B chronic lymphocytic leukemia. *Blood* 2007;109:405–411.
104. Shanafelt T, Lanasa MC, Call TG, et al. Ofatumumab-based chemoimmunotherapy is effective and well tolerated in patients with previously untreated chronic lymphocytic leukemia (CLL). *Cancer* 2013;119:3788–3796.
105. Fischer K, Cramer P, Busch R, et al. Bendamustine in combination with rituximab for previously untreated patients with chronic lymphocytic leukemia: a multicenter phase II trial of the German Chronic Lymphocytic Leukemia Study Group. *J Clin Oncol* 2012;30:3209–3216.
106. Fischer K, Cramer P, Busch R, et al. Bendamustine combined with rituximab in patients with relapsed and/or refractory chronic lymphocytic leukemia: a multicenter phase II trial of the German Chronic Lymphocytic Leukemia Study Group. *J Clin Oncol* 2011;29:3559–3566.
107. Elter T, Gercheva-Kyuchukova L, Pylylpenko H, et al. Fludarabine plus alemtuzumab versus fludarabine alone in patients with previously treated chronic lymphocytic leukaemia: a randomised phase 3 trial. *Lancet Oncol* 2011;12:1204–1213.
108. Goede V, Fischer K, Busch R, et al. Obinutuzumab plus chlorambucil in patients with CLL and coexisting conditions. *N Engl J Med* 2014;370:1101–1110.
109. Montillo M, Tedeschi A, Miqueleiz S, et al. Alemtuzumab as consolidation after a response to fludarabine is effective in purging residual disease in patients with chronic lymphocytic leukemia. *J Clin Oncol* 2006;24:2337–2342.
110. O'Brien SM, Kantarjian HM, Thomas DA, et al. Alemtuzumab as treatment for residual disease after chemotherapy in patients with chronic lymphocytic leukemia. *Cancer* 2003;98:2657–2663.
111. Lin TS, Donohue KA, Byrd JC, et al. Consolidation therapy with subcutaneous alemtuzumab after fludarabine and rituximab induction therapy for previously untreated chronic lymphocytic leukemia: final analysis of CALGB 10101. *J Clin Oncol* 2010;28:4500–4506.
112. Schweighofer CD, Ritgen M, Eichhorst BF, et al. Consolidation with alemtuzumab improves progression-free survival in patients with chronic lymphocytic leukemia (CLL) in first remission: long-term follow-up of a randomized phase III trial of the German CLL Study Group (GCLLSG). *Br J Haematol* 2009;144:95–98.
113. Jones JA, Ruppert AS, Zhao W, et al. Patients with chronic lymphocytic leukemia with high-risk genomic features have inferior outcome on successive Cancer and Leukemia Group B trials with alemtuzumab consolidation: subgroup analysis from CALGB 19901 and CALGB 10101. *Leuk Lymphoma* 2013;54:2654–2659.
114. Ponader S, Burger JA. Bruton's tyrosine kinase: from X-linked agammaglobulinemia toward targeted therapy for B-cell malignancies. *J Clin Oncol* 2014;32:1830–1839.
115. Byrd JC, Furman RR, Coutre SE, et al. Targeting BTK with ibrutinib in relapsed chronic lymphocytic leukemia. *N Engl J Med* 2013;369:32–42.
116. O'Brien S, Furman RR, Coutre SE, et al. Ibrutinib as initial therapy for elderly patients with chronic lymphocytic leukaemia or small lymphocytic lymphoma: an open-label, multicentre, phase 1b/2 trial. *Lancet Oncol* 2014;15:48–58.
117. Byrd JC, Brown JR, O'Brien S, et al. Ibrutinib versus ofatumumab in previously treated chronic lymphoid leukemia. *N Engl J Med* 2014;371:213–223.
118. Byrd JC, Brown JR, O'Brien SM, et al. Randomized comparison of ibrutinib versus ofatumumab in relapsed or refractory (R/R) chronic lymphocytic leukemia/small lymphocytic lymphoma: Results from the phase III RESONATE trial. *J Clin Oncol* 2014;32:Abstr LBA7008.
119. Woyach JA, Furman RR, Liu TM, et al. Resistance mechanisms for the Bruton's tyrosine kinase inhibitor ibrutinib. *N Engl J Med* 2014;370:2286–2294.
120. Brown JR, Byrd JC, Coutre SE, et al. Idelalisib, an inhibitor of phosphatidylinositol 3 kinase p110delta, for relapsed/refractory chronic lymphocytic leukemia. *Blood* 2014;123:3390–3397.
121. Furman RR, Sharman JP, Coutre SE. Idelalisib and rituximab in relapsed chronic lymphocytic leukemia. *N Engl J Med* 2014;370:997–1007.
122. Roberts AW, Seymour JF, Brown JR, et al. Substantial susceptibility of chronic lymphocytic leukemia to BCL2 inhibition: results of a phase I study of navitoclax in patients with relapsed or refractory disease. *J Clin Oncol* 2012;30:488–496.
123. Souers AJ, Leverson JD, Boghaert ER, et al. ABT-199, a potent and selective BCL-2 inhibitor, achieves antitumor activity while sparing platelets. *Nat Med* 2013;19:202–208.
124. Seymour JF, Davids MS, Pagel JM, et al. Bcl-2 inhibitor ABT-199 (GDC-0199) monotherapy shows anti-tumor activity including complete remissions in high-risk relapsed/refractory (R/R) chronic lymphocytic leukemia (CLL) and small lymphocytic lymphoma (SLL). *Blood* 2013;122:Abstr 872.
125. Chanan-Khan A, Miller KC, Musial L, et al. Clinical efficacy of lenalidomide in patients with relapsed or refractory chronic lymphocytic leukemia: results of a phase II study. *J Clin Oncol* 2006;24:5343–5349.

126. Ferrajoli A, Lee BN, Schlette EJ, et al. Lenalidomide induces complete and partial remissions in patients with relapsed and refractory chronic lymphocytic leukemia. *Blood* 2008;111:5291–5297.
127. Chen CI, Bergsagel PL, Paul H, et al. Single-agent lenalidomide in the treatment of previously untreated chronic lymphocytic leukemia. *J Clin Oncol* 2011;29:1175–1181.
128. Badoux XC, Keating MJ, Wen S, et al. Lenalidomide as initial therapy of elderly patients with chronic lymphocytic leukemia. *Blood* 2011;118:3489–3498.
129. Strati P, Keating MJ, Wierda WG, et al. Lenalidomide induces long-lasting responses in elderly patients with chronic lymphocytic leukemia. *Blood* 2013;122:734–737.
130. Badoux XC, Keating MJ, Wen S, et al. Phase II study of lenalidomide and rituximab as salvage therapy for patients with relapsed or refractory chronic lymphocytic leukemia. *J Clin Oncol* 2013;31:584–591.
131. Brentjens RJ, Riviere I, Park JH, et al. Safety and persistence of adoptively transferred autologous CD19-targeted T cells in patients with relapsed or chemotherapy refractory B-cell leukemias. *Blood* 2011;118:4817–4828.
132. Grupp SA, Kalos M, Barrett D, et al. Chimeric antigen receptor-modified T cells for acute lymphoid leukemia. *N Engl J Med* 2013;368:1509–1518.
133. Kalos M, Levine BL, Porter DL, et al. T cells with chimeric antigen receptors have potent antitumor effects and can establish memory in patients with advanced leukemia. *Sci Transl Med* 2011;3:95ra73.
134. Porter DL, Levine BL, Kalos M, et al. Chimeric antigen receptor-modified T cells in chronic lymphoid leukemia. *N Engl J Med* 2011;365:725–733.
135. Dreger P, Montserrat E. Autologous and allogeneic stem cell transplantation for chronic lymphocytic leukemia. *Leukemia* 2002;16:985–992.
136. van Besien K, Keralavarma B, Devine S, et al. Allogeneic and autologous transplantation for chronic lymphocytic leukemia. *Leukemia* 2001;15:1317–1325.
137. Dreger P, Brand R, Hansz J, et al. Treatment-related mortality and graft-versus-leukemia activity after allogeneic stem cell transplantation for chronic lymphocytic leukemia using intensity-reduced conditioning. *Leukemia* 2003;17:841–848.
138. Sorror ML, Storer BE, Sandmaier BM, et al. Five-year follow-up of patients with advanced chronic lymphocytic leukemia treated with allogeneic hematopoietic cell transplantation after nonmyeloablative conditioning. *J Clin Oncol* 2008;26:4912–4920.
139. Khouri IF, Bassett R, Poindexter N, et al. Nonmyeloablative allogeneic stem cell transplantation in relapsed/refractory chronic lymphocytic leukemia: long-term follow-up, prognostic factors, and effect of human leukocyte histocompatibility antigen subtype on outcome. *Cancer* 2011;117:4679–4688.
140. Dreger P, Schnaiter A, Zenz T, et al. TP53, SF3B1, and NOTCH1 mutations and outcome of allotransplantation for chronic lymphocytic leukemia: six-year follow-up of the GCLLSG CLL3X trial. *Blood* 2013;121:3284–3288.
141. Brown JR, Kim HT, Li S, et al. Predictors of improved progression-free survival after nonmyeloablative allogeneic stem cell transplantation for advanced chronic lymphocytic leukemia. *Biol Blood Marrow Transplant* 2006;12:1056–1064.
142. Michallet M, Socie G, Mohty M, et al. Rituximab, fludarabine, and total body irradiation as conditioning regimen before allogeneic hematopoietic stem cell transplantation for advanced chronic lymphocytic leukemia: long-term prospective multicenter study. *Exp Hematol* 2013;41:127–133.
143. Richardson SE, Khan I, Rawstron A, et al. Risk-stratified adoptive cellular therapy following allogeneic hematopoietic stem cell transplantation for advanced chronic lymphocytic leukaemia. *Br J Haematol* 2013;160:640–648.
144. Herth I, Dietrich S, Benner A, et al. The impact of allogeneic stem cell transplantation on the natural course of poor-risk chronic lymphocytic leukemia as defined by the EBMT consensus criteria: a retrospective donor versus no donor comparison. *Ann Oncol* 2014;25:200–206.
145. Boughton BJ, Jackson N, Lim S, et al. Randomized trial of intravenous immunoglobulin prophylaxis for patients with chronic lymphocytic leukaemia and secondary hypogammaglobulinaemia. *Clin Lab Haematol* 1995;17:75–80.
146. Molica S, Musto P, Chiurazzi F, et al. Prophylaxis against infections with low-dose intravenous immunoglobulins (IVIG) in chronic lymphocytic leukemia. Results of a crossover study. *Haematologica* 1996;81:121–126.
147. Griffiths H, Brennan V, Lea J, et al. Crossover study of immunoglobulin replacement therapy in patients with low-grade B-cell tumors. *Blood* 1989;73:366–368.
148. Raanani P, Gafter-Gvili A, Paul M, et al. Immunoglobulin prophylaxis in chronic lymphocytic leukemia and multiple myeloma: systematic review and meta-analysis. *Leuk Lymphoma* 2009;50:764–772.
149. Giles FJ, O'Brien SM, Keating MJ. Chronic lymphocytic leukemia in (Richter's) transformation. *Semin Oncol* 1998;25:117–125.
150. Smith MR, Neuberg D, Flinn IW, et al. Incidence of therapy-related myeloid neoplasia after initial therapy for chronic lymphocytic leukemia with fludarabine-cyclophosphamide versus fludarabine: long-term follow-up of US Intergroup Study E2997. *Blood* 2011;118:3525–3527.
151. Hercher C, Robain M, Davi F, et al. A multicentric study of 41 cases of B-prolymphocytic leukemia: two evolutive forms. *Leuk Lymphoma* 2001;42:981–987.
152. Cao TM, Coutre SE. T-cell prolymphocytic leukemia: update and focus on alemtuzumab (Campath-1H). *Hematology* 2003;8:1–6.
153. Lamy T, Loughran TP Jr. Clinical features of large granular lymphocyte leukemia. *Semin Hematol* 2003;40:185–195.
154. Allsup DJ, Cawley JC. The diagnosis and treatment of hairy-cell leukaemia. *Blood Rev* 2002;16:255–262.
155. Arcaini L, Zibellini S, Boveri E, et al. The BRAF V600E mutation in hairy cell leukemia and other mature B-cell neoplasms. *Blood* 2012;119:188–191.
156. Tiacci E, Trifonov V, Schiavoni G, et al. BRAF mutations in hairy-cell leukemia. *N Engl J Med* 2011;364:2305–2315.
157. Dietrich S, Glimm H, Andrulis M, et al. BRAF inhibition in refractory hairy-cell leukemia. *N Engl J Med* 2012;366:2038–2040.
158. Mey U, Strehl J, Gorschluter M, et al. Advances in the treatment of hairy-cell leukaemia. *Lancet Oncol* 2003;4:86–94.
159. Kreitman RJ, Wilson WH, Bergeron K, et al. Efficacy of the anti-CD22 recombinant immunotoxin BL22 in chemotherapy-resistant hairy-cell leukemia. *N Engl J Med* 2001;345:241–247.
160. Kreitman RJ, Stetler-Stevenson M, Margulies I, et al. Phase II trial of recombinant immunotoxin RFB4(dsFv)-PE38 (BL22) in patients with hairy cell leukemia. *J Clin Oncol* 2009;27:2983–2990.
161. Kreitman RJ, Tallman MS, Robak T, et al. Phase I trial of anti-CD22 recombinant immunotoxin moxetumomab pasudotox (CAT-8015 or HA22) in patients with hairy cell leukemia. *J Clin Oncol* 2012;30:1822–1828.

47 Myelodysplastic Syndromes

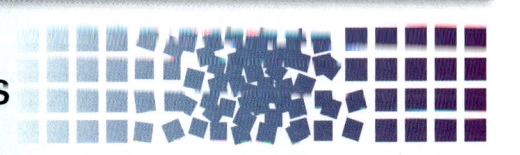

Rami S. Komrokji, Eric Padron, and Alan F. List

INTRODUCTION

The myelodysplastic syndromes (MDS) represent a spectrum of hematopoietic stem cell malignancies that share morphologic features of dysplasia, ineffective hematopoiesis, and a risk for leukemia evolution. The hallmark of early disease is accelerated apoptosis and proliferation of bone marrow precursors that drives increased marrow cellularity and peripheral cytopenias. In advanced disease, increasing maturation impairment is accompanied by the acquisition of survival signals that leads to increasing proportions of myeloblasts. MDS are clonal stem cell neoplasms that arise from interplay of genetic and epigenetics events with altered microenvironmental pressures that are senescence dependent. Although the risk of progression to acute myeloid leukemia (AML) varies, the majority of patients succumb to complications related to cytopenias.[1]

HISTORICAL PERSPECTIVE

The description of MDS dates back to early 1900s when reference was first made to a group of patients with a form of anemia refractory to available treatments. The term *anemia pseudoaplastica* was one of the earliest descriptions of MDS.[2] In the late 1940s, it was thought that the disease progresses to leukemia and, hence, the term *preleukemia* was applied.[3] The definition was expanded to include peripheral blood descriptors such as neutropenia and thrombocytopenia in the early 1950s.[4] The French-American-British (FAB) group coined the term *myelodysplastic syndromes* in a series of proposals on acute leukemias in 1976 and later expanded the FAB classification in 1980s.[5,6] The original FAB classification included only two categories: refractory anemia with excess blasts (RAEB) and chronic myelomonocytic leukemia (CMML), to which others were added in 1982. In 1997, the International Prognostic Scoring System (IPSS) was introduced.[7] Under the auspices of the World Health Organization (WHO), the pathologic classification of MDS was refined and later revised in 2008.[1,8,9] New prognostic models were later introduced, such as the WHO Prognostic Scoring System (WPSS), the Global M.D. Anderson Risk Model, the Lower Risk M.D. Anderson Model, and more recently, the revised-IPSS (IPSS-R).[10–13]

Recent years witnessed an acceleration in understanding the disease biology and associated molecular genetics events. Today, molecular abnormalities are demonstrable in more than 80% of MDS patients. Finally, in the past decade, three medications were approved specifically for the treatment of MDS: azacitidine, decitabine, and lenalidomide.

EPIDEMIOLOGY

MDS is one of the most common hematologic malignancies. According to the Surveillance, Epidemiology, and End Results (SEER): the United States cancer surveillance program 2006 to 2010 statistics, the age-adjusted incidence rate of MDS was 4.8 per 100,000 and 0.4 per 100,000 for CMML.[14] MDS was more common in males (6.5 per 100,000) than in females (3.7 per 100,000). MDS is a disease of the elderly (median age at diagnosis is 72 years); the incidence rate was highest among 80 years and older (20 per 100,000).[14] SEER/North American Association of Central Cancer Registries (NAACCR) reported a similar MDS annual age-adjusted incidence rate of 3.27 per 100,000.[15] The incidence rate among the Medicare population (age >65 years) was 162 per 100,000, which translates to approximately 45,000 newly diagnosed cases per year.[16] Recent data suggest a high rate of uncaptured MDS cases among hospital cancer registries.[17] The incidence of MDS reported from Europe is similar to that observed in the United States, ranging from 3.2 to 8.1 per 100,000.[18] Interestingly, a lower incidence, younger age, and different spectrum of pathologic subtypes have been reported in Asia.[19]

ETIOLOGY

For the vast majority of cases, senescence per se is the highest risk factor for MDS development. Familial/genetic predisposition contributes to a small proportion of MDS cases.[20] There is an increased risk of MDS among inherited bone marrow failure syndromes (BMFS), such as Fanconi anemia, dyskeratosis congenita, severe congenital neutropenia, and Shwachman–Diamond syndrome.[20] Familial cases of MDS beyond BMFS are well recognized and molecularly distinct. Two important familial syndromes are the familial platelet disorder with a propensity to myeloid malignancy, arising from an autosomal-dominant *RUNX-1* germ-line gene mutation that results in thrombocytopenia with a corresponding frequency of MDS/AML in carriers that approaches 50%[21] and familial MDS/AML with *GATA2* mutation, which is also autosomal dominant but with variable penetrance.[22]

Benzene exposure is a well-recognized environmental exposure linked to AML/MDS.[23] The risk of MDS but not AML was increased among petroleum distribution workers at relatively lower levels of exposure in a dose-dependent manner.[24] Cigarette smoking had also been associated with an increased risk of developing MDS. In a meta-analysis, current and former smokers had increased risks of MDS, with an odds ratio (OR) of 1.81 (95% confidence interval [CI], 1.24 to 2.66) and 1.67 (95% CI, 1.42 to 1.96), respectively.[25] A population-based study from Sweden suggested that a prior history of infection (OR, 1.3; 95% CI, 1.1 to 1.5) or autoimmune disease (OR 2.1-fold; 95% CI, 1.7 to 2.6) significantly increased the probability of developing MDS.[26]

A case-control study was conducted to investigate associations between lifestyle characteristics and MDS risk.[27] A family history of hematopoietic cancer (OR = 1.92), smoking (OR = 1.65), and exposure to agricultural chemicals (OR = 4.55) or solvents (OR = 2.05) were associated with MDS. The highest risk was among smokers exposed to solvents/agricultural chemicals (OR = 3.22).

In the context of successful chemotherapeutic treatment of other hematologic malignancies and solid tumors, a growing percentage of MDS cases are considered secondary or arising from prior radiation or chemotherapy. Treatment-related MDS (t-MDS) accounts for 10% to 20% of all MDS cases. It is generally characterized by a high rate of unfavorable cytogenetics and poor outcome. Chemotherapy and, to a lesser extent, radiotherapy are associated with an increased risk of developing AML/MDS.[28,29] The risk of t-MDS varies from less than 1% (adjuvant breast cancer chemotherapy studies) to 15% (heavily treated lymphoma patients). Two types of t-MDS are recognized: Type I is related to alkylating agent exposure where MDS occurs after a latency period of 3 to 5 years in which monosomy 5 or 7 are cytogenetic characteristics of the disease; and type II t-MDS is related to treatment with topoisomerase II inhibitors, which generally arises after a short interval from chemotherapy exposure and rapidly progresses to AML. Chromosome 11q23 abnormalities that involve the MLL gene are characteristic of this type.[30] Radiation-related MDS have a prognosis similar to de novo MDS.[31]

PATHOLOGY

The diagnosis of MDS requires the presence of persistent cytopenia(s) in the absence of hematinic deficiencies such as vitamin B12 or folic acid, and one of the following: (1) demonstration of cytologic dysplasia in ≥10% of cells in a given lineage, (2) demonstration of increased myeloblasts (5% to 19%) (Fig. 47.1),[32] or (3) a specific cytogenetic abnormality detected in the setting of sustained unexplained cytopenia ("presumptive MDS" by WHO 2008 criteria). In certain cases, the diagnosis of MDS can be made without clear evidence of morphologic dysplasia, such as CMML if monocytes are persistently elevated.

A 500-cell count differential is recommended, with exclusion of lymphocytes and plasma cells. Cytologic dysplasia must exceed 10% of cells in any lineage and the percentage of myeloblasts calculated. If the absolute percentage of erythroid precursors is 50% or greater, the percentage of myeloblasts is estimated among nonerythroid precursors. Iron stains are essential to address the percentage of ring sideroblasts. The bone marrow core biopsy could complement the bone marrow aspirate in several aspects,[30] namely, cellularity, dysmegakaryopoiesis, and identifying clusters of abnormal localization of immature precursors (ALIP), which are immature cells/myeloblasts or promyelocytes that are displaced from the paratrabecular area to the intertrabecular areas often corresponding to the vascular niche. In addition, the reticulin stain provides information regarding medullary fibrosis, which can add prognostic information.[33,34]

The French-British-American Classification

The original FAB classification (Table 47.1) included only two of the subtypes.[5] In 1982, a revision to the FAB classification expanded that to five subgroups: refractory anemia (RA), refractory anemia with ring sideroblasts (RARS), RAEB, RAEB in transformation (RAEB-t), and CMML.[6]

The World Health Organization Classification

The WHO classification was proposed to address some of the FAB shortcomings.[35,36] WHO distinguishes between single lineage and multilineage dysplasia: Categories of refractory cytopenia with multilineage dysplasia (RCMD) and RCMD with ring sideroblasts (RCMD-RS) were added, capturing those cases with dysplastic changes in either myeloid or megakaryocytic lineages in addition to erythroid dysplasia. The 5q- syndrome was recognized as a distinct subset, with an isolated cytogenetic abnormality involving del(5q) and less than 5% myeloblasts. RAEB was divided into RAEB I with 5% to 9% blasts and RAEB II with 10% to 19% blasts.[35,37] RAEB-t was omitted and the blast threshold for AML diagnosis lowered to 20% rather than 30%.[35,37,38] Finally, WHO recognizes MDS/myeloproliferative neoplasms (MPN). This includes diseases such as CMML, juvenile myelomonocytic leukemia (JMML), and atypical chronic myeloid leukemia (aCML).[35,37,38] CMML is further classified based on the percentage of bone marrow blasts, where CMML type 1 includes 0% to 4% blasts and/or promonocytes on peripheral blood or <10% in the bone marrow, and type 2 includes 5% to 19% blasts and promonocytes in the peripheral blood or <20% in the bone marrow.[8]

The WHO classification was revised in 2008,[39,40] adding the category of refractory cytopenia with unilineage dysplasia (RCUD) that include RA, refractory neutropenia (RN) and refractory thrombocytopenia (RT). The patients may have a corresponding cytopenia but not pancytopenia. Patients with pancytopenia and unilineage dysplasia, patients with no overt dysplasia but cytogenetic evidence of MDS, and cases of RCUD or RCMD with peripheral blood (PB) blasts of 1% are categorized as MDS unclassified (MDS-U). RAEB-1 includes 2% to 4 % peripheral blood blasts and RAEB-II includes 5% to 19% peripheral blood blasts. The presence of Auer rods regardless of blast percentage qualifies as RAEB-II or CMML-2.[41] A provisional entity of refractory anemia with ring sideroblasts and thrombocytosis (RARS-T) was proposed in which there is a sustained thrombocytosis of 450,000/mm^3 or greater.[42] Up to 50% of RARS-T patients harbor a gain-of-function mutation involving the Janus kinase 2 (JAK2) gene. A subset of patients with CMML and eosinophilia with accompanying genetic abnormalities involving the platelet-derived growth factor receptor alpha (PDGFRα) or PDGFRβ were reclassified as myeloid neoplasms with eosinophilia.[43]

Hypocellular MDS (or hypoplastic MDS) is not recognized as a distinct entity with the WHO classification. It accounts for 10% to 20% of MDS cases. The challenge on diagnosis is to distinguish those cases from aplastic anemia.[44] Although not part of the WHO classification, the term idiopathic cytopenia of unknown significance (ICUS) was proposed for those cases with persistent cytopenia(s) unrelated to nutritional deficiency that have dysplasia in less than 10% of cells in any lineage and that lack cytogenetic abnormalities. Many of those patients may develop MDS over time. Whether the latter cases can be distinguished a priori by the presence of gene mutations is under investigation. Some cases may also demonstrate dysplasia below the 10% WHO cutoff with no cytopenia, referred to as idiopathic dysplasia of unknown significance (IDUS).[45]

PATHOGENESIS

MDS is a clonal disease driven by acquisition and expansion of genetic alterations (Fig. 47.2). The clonal nature of many MDS cases was first apparent by the conventional metaphase karyotype analysis. Studies leveraging restriction fragment length polymorphisms (RFLP) of X-chromosome genes in females, single nucleotide polymorphism (SNP) arrays, and glucose-6-phosphate dehydrogenase (G6PD) analyses confirmed that hematopoiesis is clonal across all subtypes of MDS.[46-49] The two most comprehensive studies demonstrating the frequency and nature of chromosome abnormalities in MDS confirmed that approximately 50% of patients with MDS harbor a chromosome abnormality.[50,51] The most common recurrent abnormalities were del(5q) (30%), −7 or 7q− (21%), and +8 (16%). Deletion of genes encoded within the commonly deleted region (CDR) of human del(5q) MDS is sufficient to induce an MDS phenotype, indicating that these recurrent genetic lesions are critical to the development of the disease.[52]

In addition to large chromosomal deletions or duplications, DNA sequencing technology has uncovered gene mutations that aggregate within pathways previously unrecognized to be important in MDS pathogenesis. These include mutations predicted to result in deregulation of genes involved in signaling pathways and epigenetic control, RNA splicing, and transcription factors.[53]

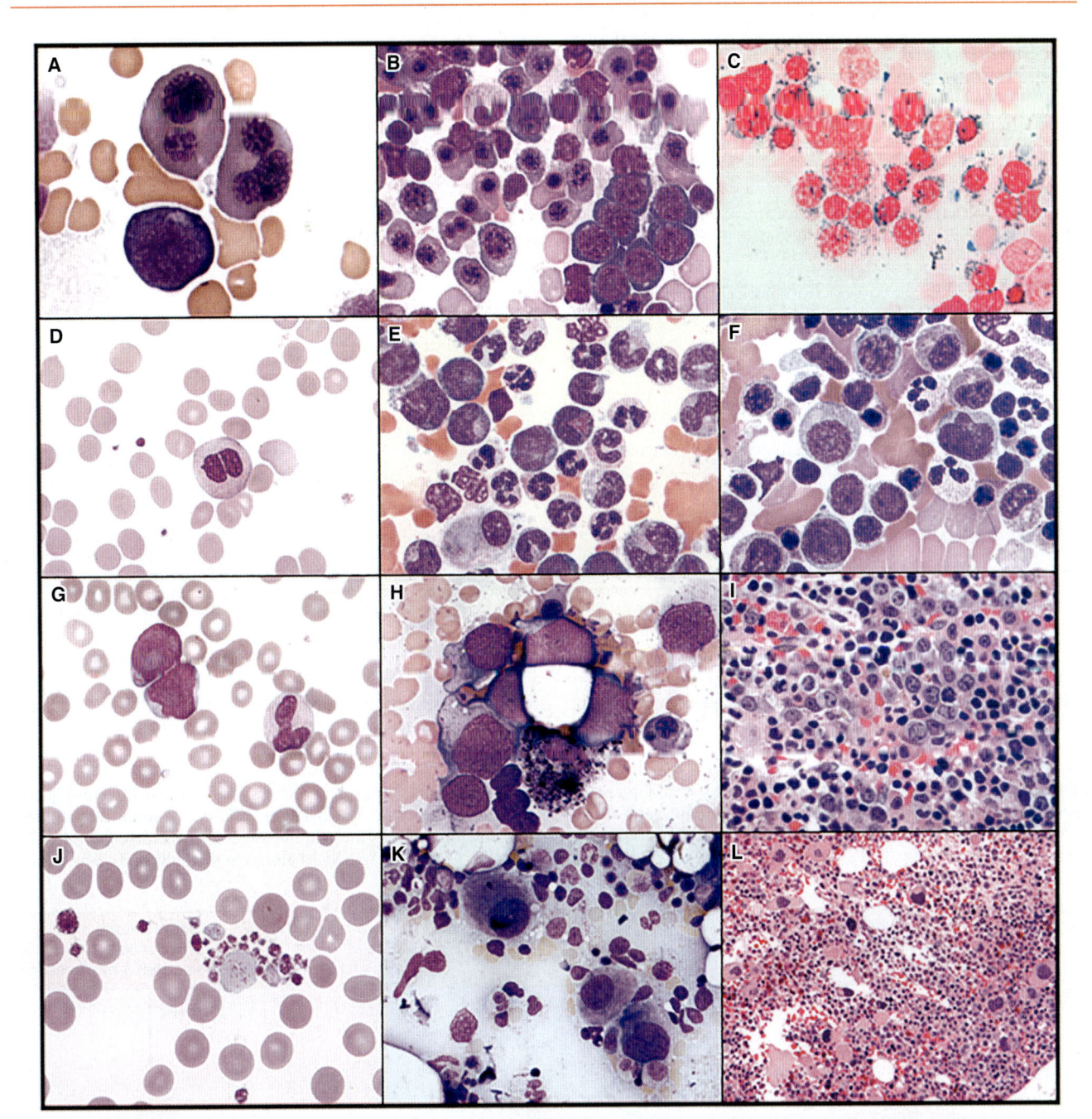

Figure 47.1 Morphologic findings of myelodysplasia in peripheral blood and bone marrow. **A:** Erythroid precursors displaying cytoplasmic to nuclear maturation asynchrony and multinucleation in bone marrow aspirate smear (Wright Giemsa stain). **B:** Bone marrow aspirate with erythroid hyperplasia, left shifted and megaloblastoid maturation, occasional nuclear budding and binucleation (Wright Giemsa strain). **C:** Numerous ringed-sideroblasts are highlighted by Prussian-blue iron stain in bone marrow aspirate. **D:** Circulating granulocytes showing pseudo-Pelger-Huet change with hyposegmentation and hypogranulation in cytoplasm in peripheral blood smear (May-Grünwald-Giemsa stain). **E:** Abnormal distribution of cytoplasmic granules or patch loss of granules in eosinophilic precursors as well as abnormal lobation of neutrophils are present in the peripheral blood of a MDS patient (May-Grünwald-Giemsa stain). **F:** Predominant myeloid dysplasia including marked hypogranulation, cytoplasmic to nuclear maturation asynchrony with increased immature precursors/myeloblasts noted in bone marrow aspirate (Wright Giemsa stain). **G:** Circulating blasts with round to oval nucleus, lacy chromatin, one to more than one very prominent nucleoli and a small amount of cytoplasm are identified in peripheral blood smear (May-Grünwald-Giemsa stain). There is a single Auer rod noted in the cytoplasm of one blast, and a background of hypogranulated granulocytes is present (May-Grünwald-Giemsa stain). **H:** Bone marrow aspirate containing small to large blasts with fine chromatin, visible to prominent nucleoli and scant to some amount of basophilic cytoplasm admixed with dysplastic polychromatic normoblasts showing nuclear budding (Wright Giemsa stain). **I:** Bone marrow core biopsy showing non–paratrabecular-located immature myeloid precursors in cluster; abnormal localization of immature precursors (ALIPs) (hematoxylin and eosin [H&E] stain). **J:** Dysplastic platelets displaying variable in size and shape including giant hypogranulated platelets. **K:** Medium-sized megakaryocytes with single lobated nucleus characterized in 5q- syndrome, subtype of myelodysplastic syndrome. **L:** Representative bone marrow core biopsy of 5q- syndrome with moderately increased in single or hypolobated megakaryocytes (H&E stain).

TABLE 47.1
Gene Mutations in MDS

FAB	WHO	WHO 2008	Dysplasia	BM Blast (%)	PB Blasts (%)
RA	RA MDS-U RCMD Del(5q) MDS	RCUD RA RN, RT RCMD Isolated del(5q) MDS-U	Erythroid Nonerythroid Erythroid + other Erythroid + mega Unilineage + pancytopenia or RCMD/RCUD with 1% PB blasts	<5 <5 <5 <5 <5	<1 <1 <1 <1 1
RARS	RARS RCMD-RS	RARS RCMD-RS	Erythroid only Erythroid + other (all >15% ring sideroblasts)	<5 <5	<1 <1
RAEB	RAEB-1 RAEB-2	RAEB-1 RAEB-2	>1 lineage >1 lineage	5–9 10–19	2–4[a] 5–19[a] Auer rods[a]
RAEB-t	AML	AML	Myeloid + other	>20	
CMML	MDS/MPD CMML JMML aCML MDS/MPD-U	MDS/MPN CMML JMML BCR/Abl neg CML MDS/MPD-U	Variable >1 × 10⁹/L monocytosis	<20	

BM, bone marrow; PB, peripheral blood; RA, refractory anemia; MDS-U, MDS unclassified; RCMD, refractory cytopenia with multilineage dysplasia; RCUD, refractory cytopenia with unilineage dysplasia; RN, refractory anemia; RT, refractory thrombocytopenia; mega, megakaryocyte; RARS, refractory anemia with ring sideroblasts; RCMD-RS, RCMD with ring sideroblasts; RAEB-t, RAEB in transformation; MPD, myeloproliferative disease; JMML, juvenile myelomonocytic leukemia; MPD-U, MPD unclassified; CML, chronic myeloid leukemia.
[a] Diagnosis and Classification of MDS.

Mutations are common in MDS, because targeted sequencing of select genes can identify at least one event (average: three events per sample) in approximately 80% of cases.[54] Although there are no MDS-defining mutations, a *genomic fingerprint*, which is characteristic of MDS is materializing as a result of several large-scale gene sequencing efforts. Among the most common gene mutations in MDS is that involving the gene, ten-eleven-translocation-2 (*TET2*).[55] Inactivating *TET2* mutations, which disrupt TET2 enzymatic activity, are frequently observed in MDS. TET2 catalyzes the conversion of methyl cytosine to hydroxymethylcytosine (5-hmC), thereby inducing subsequent DNA demethylation and the release of epigenetic repression.[56] Patients with *TET2* gene mutations have lower DNA levels of 5-hmC with consequent increased genomic methylation. Other commonly mutated epigenetic modifiers include the associated sex-linked combs like 1 (*ASLX1*) gene.[57–60] ASXL1 belongs to the polycomb gene family

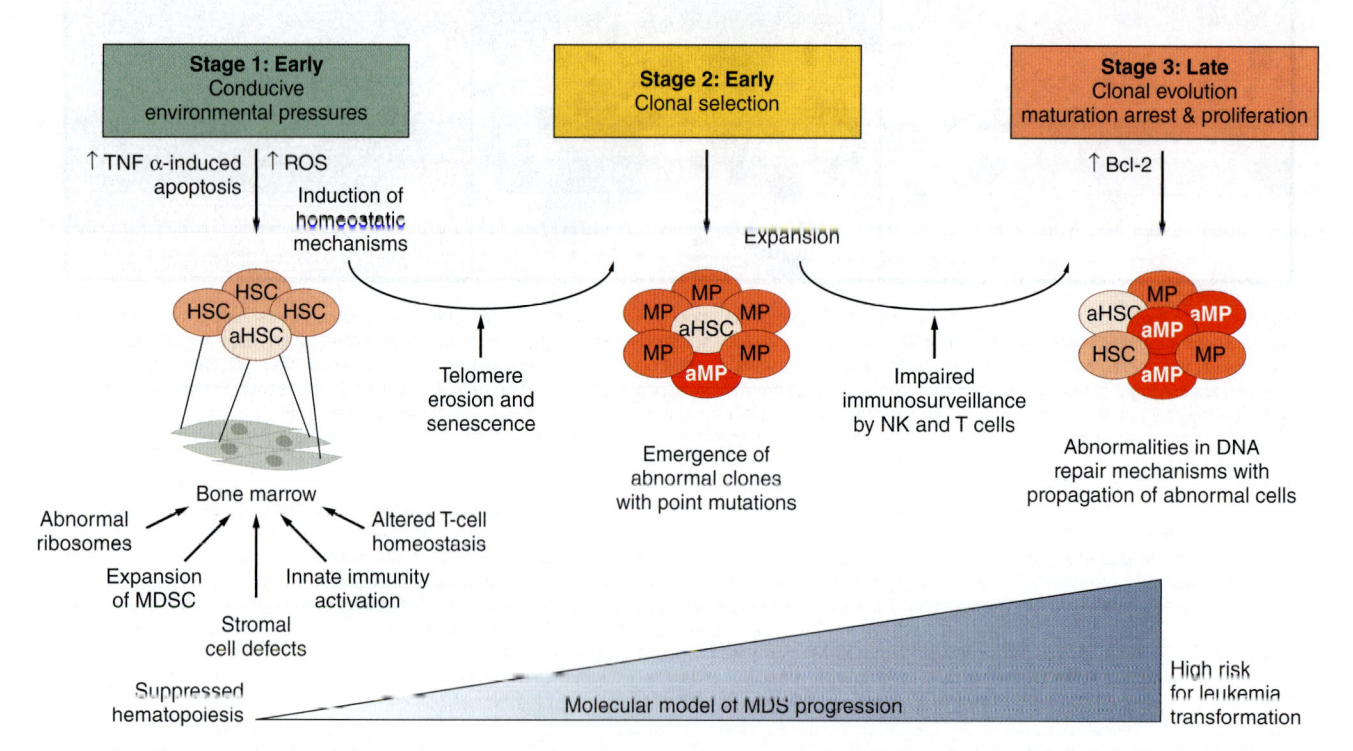

Figure 47.2 Model of MDS progression. TNFα, tumor necrosis factor alpha; HSC, hematopoietic stem cell; aHSC, abnormal hematopoietic stem cell; MDSC, myeloid derived suppressor cells; MP, myeloid progenitors; aMP, abnormal myeloid progenitor; NK, natural killer. (Modified from Epling-Burnette PK, List AF. Advancements in the molecular pathogenesis of myelodysplastic syndrome. *Curr Opin Hematol* 2009;16:70–76.)

and is an essential component of chromatin remodeling through its interaction with the polycomb repressive complex 2 (PRC2).[61,62] Deletion and conditional knock-in murine models for both TET2 and ASXL1 demonstrate that these lesions are sufficient to induce a myeloid neoplasm akin to MDS.[61,63,64]

Next-generation sequencing of MDS genomes recently identified genes involved in the regulation of alternative gene splicing.[65] Subsequent studies have shown that they are among the most common gene mutations in MDS.[53,54] They appear to occur early in disease pathogenesis, alter RNA splicing, and are prognostically relevant.[66–68] Interestingly, the two most common mutations involving the splicing factor 3b subunit 1 (SF3B1) and serine/arginine-rich splicing factor 2 (SRSF2) genes have strong phenotypic linkage with ringed sideroblasts and monocyte expansion (CMML), respectively.[67,69]

Lastly, the specific type and number of gene mutations directly impacts clinical behavior and risk of progression to AML. Elegant work using whole-genome sequencing to reconstruct the clonal architecture of MDS cases that transform to AML at sequential time points demonstrates that this transformation is associated with the acquisition and expansion of distinct genetic events.[70] Emerging data, however, suggest that these events do not display complete fidelity. That is, the same genetic events can be responsible for disease initiation, and therefore, disease founding in one case while representing a secondary event in another case with the same diagnosis. Collectively, these and other gene mutations described in Table 47.2 demonstrate that distinct genetic events can result in MDS and are likely the major drivers of the disease and its behavior.

Dysregulation of Immunity as a Driver in MDS

The environmental cues that are conducive to emergence of the genetic events that lead to MDS are unknown. Bone marrow stromal alterations have been implicated, but an intriguing emerging hypothesis that immune dysregulation and associated chronic inflammatory changes may be a critical environmental pressure in MDS pathogenesis. Clinical and laboratory evidence suggests that both adaptive and innate immunity is altered and potentially contributory to MDS pathogenesis. It is this inflammation that could represent the nidus for mutational acquisition in some patients, or these inflammatory changes are induced by an expanded clone. A recent population-based study demonstrated a strong linkage between chronic immune stimulation and autoimmune disorders with MDS predisposition.[26] Several studies confirmed the higher than expected association between MDS and autoimmune disease.[26,71–73]

Impaired T-cell homeostasis and early senescence is a feature of patients with MDS.[74] Indeed, up to 50% of T cells are clonal and even more appear to have intrinsic defects in telomerase function, perhaps accounting for their premature senescence.[75,76] In addition to expansion and senescence, the T-cell receptor (TCR) repertoire appears to be augmented and hematopoietic inhibitory capacity appears to be increased.[77] Lastly, T-cell characteristics can mark clinical parameters in MDS. For instance, the expansion of effector memory T-regulator cells (T_{regs}) is associated anemia and increased blast percentage, and represents an unfavorable prognostic biomarker.[78]

Activation of innate immunity with consequent nuclear factor kappa B (NF-κB) induction contributes to the inflammatory microenvironment in MDS.[79,80] Haplodeficiency of two microRNA genes, miR-145 and miR-146a, located within the distal commonly deleted region of chromosome 5q at 5q32, results in constitutive activation of Toll-like receptor (TLR) signaling in del(5q) MDS. Toll-interleukin 1 receptor domain–containing adapter protein (TIRAP) and tumor necrosis factor receptor–associated factor-6 (TRAF6), which encode key intermediates involved in the MyD88-dependent TLR-signaling pathway, are targets of miR-145 and miR-146a, thereby upregulating their expression with allelic insufficiency. Myeloid-derived suppressor cells (MDSC), potent effectors of innate immunity, are recently recognized as critical cellular effectors involved in the pathogenesis of MDS. MDSCs are markedly expanded in the bone marrow of MDS patients and promote ineffective hematopoiesis. These MDSCs are genetically distinct from the MDS clone, overproduce hematopoietic suppressive cytokines, and also act as potent effectors of apoptosis that target autologous hematopoietic progenitors. MDSC expansion is driven by excess generation of the proinflammatory molecule S100A9, which is a ligand for TLR4. Moreover, a transgenic S100A9 mouse model phenocopies human MDS, displaying bone marrow accumulation of MDSC accompanied by progressive age-dependent multilineage cytopenias and cytologic dysplasia.[81]

The 5q Minus Syndrome

The hematologic and pathologic phenotype of the 5q- syndrome is now recognized to be a product of haploinsufficiency of several genes located within the CDR at 5q32.[82] Among 40 genes residing in the CDR, only inactivation of RPS14 impaired erythroblast proliferation and viability, whereas corresponding overexpression of RPS14 was sufficient to rescue erythropoiesis in primary del(5q) MDS specimens.[83] Haploinsufficiency for RPS14 disrupts ribosome assembly, leading to nucleolar stress and sequestration of the human homolog of the mouse double minute 2 protein (MDM2) by free ribosomal proteins, thereby triggering its degradation and p53 stabilization.[84] A murine model of the human 5q− syndrome generated by allelic deletion of the genes in the human CDR showed that p53 inactivation rescues the hematologic features.[52] Gene dosage of two dual specificity phosphatases encoded within or adjacent to the proximal CDR at 5q31 (i.e., cell division cycle 25C [Cdc25C] and protein phosphatases 2A catalytic domain alpha [PP2Aca]), underlies the selective suppression of del(5q) clones.[85]

CLINICAL PRESENTATION

The most common clinical presentation of MDS is sustained and progressive cytopenia with corresponding symptoms and complications. Macrocytic anemia is the most common hematologic

TABLE 47.2
Spectrum of Genetic Alterations in Myelodysplastic Syndromes

Gene Symbol	Molecular Pathway Affected	Incidence in MDS (%)
ASXL1	Epigenetics	20–25
TET2	Epigenetics	30–35
IDH2	Epigenetics	1–5
EZH2	Epigenetics	5
DNMT3a	Epigenetics	10–15
BCOR	Epigenetics	1–5
STAG2	Cohesin	5–10
TP53	Genome stability	5
SRSF2	Splicing	15–20
U2AF1	Splicing	5–10
ZRSR2	Splicing	5–10
SF3B1	Splicing	30–35
NRAS	Signaling	1–5
CBL	Signaling	5
RUNX1	Signaling	10
JAK2	Signaling	5

feature, mandating the exclusion of common causes of anemia and nutritional deficiencies. In one analysis, MDS was the fifth most common cause of anemia in elderly patients after iron deficiency, bleeding, renal insufficiency, and anemia of chronic disease.[30,86] Thrombocytopenia and/or platelet dysfunction are common in MDS patients, with an overall prevalence ranging from 40% to 65%. Thrombocytopenia is more common in higher risk diseases, but occurs in lower risk patients and can be exacerbated by therapy. The frequency of hemorrhagic death ranges from 14% to 24%.[87] Bleeding can occur even in the absence of thrombocytopenia attributable to platelet dysfunction as evidenced by a prolonged bleeding time corresponding to an increase in atypical megakaryocytes.[88]

Among all patients with MDS, over one-third will undergo transformation into AML. In the remaining patients, the majority will succumb to infection, in part from neutropenia, iron overload, and granulocyte dysfunction illustrated by impaired phagocytic adhesion, chemotaxis, and microcidal killing.[89] Bacterial pneumonias and skin abscesses are most common, but unusual/opportunistic infections such as disseminated *Mycobacterium avium-intracellulare*,[90] *Aeromonas hydrophila* endocarditis,[91] bacterial thyroiditis,[92] and Epstein-Barr virus hepatitis may arise.[92]

MDS patients can also manifest a wide range of autoimmune phenomena such as cutaneous vasculitis, polymyalgia rheumatica, necrotizing panniculitis, Coombs-positive autoimmune hemolytic anemia, sweet syndrome, and an seronegative arthritis.[93–96]

In patients with MDS/MPN such as CMML, hepatosplenomegaly, lymphadenopathy, and pleural effusion are manifestations attributed to the proliferative nature of this group.[97] In patients with RARS-T, the risk of thrombotic events is similar to essential thrombocytosis.[98]

RISK ASSESSMENT AND PROGNOSIS

Risk stratification and prognostic assessment represent a critical first step in the management of MDS (Table 47.3). It provides useful information for the patients as to "the disease forecast" and, more importantly, allows physicians to tailor therapy accordingly. For patients with a higher risk, the goal of therapy is to alter the natural history of the disease and to extend survival. The goal of therapy in lower risk MDS is to alleviate symptomatic cytopenias using treatments that may restore effective hematopoiesis and lessen associated complications. The prognosis will depend on the inherent disease's specific features and host-related features. Risk models in MDS are constructed by incorporating several validated prognostic variables in a weighted scoring system, permitting patients to be divided into defined risk groups.

The International Prognostic Scoring System

The IPSS remains the most widely used staging system in MDS.[7] It has been embraced by community oncologists, adopted in clinical trials, and forms the basis of determining the time table for allogeneic hematopoietic cell transplantation in decision models. However, IPSS has several shortcomings. It was not developed as a dynamic system. It does not account for severity of cytopenias, and it overlooks two-thirds of the cytogenetic abnormalities encountered. Moreover, the IPSS is not applicable to patients with MDS/MPN or t-MDS.

The Revised IPSS

The IPSS-R was proposed as a refinement to adjust for those deficiencies of the original IPSS.[13] The major changes include the incorporation of less common karyotype abnormalities, the prognostic relevance of which was discerned from the larger patient cohort, and the weighing of the severity of each lineage of cytopenia. Several groups have validated the new prognostic system.[99,100]

The Global M.D. Anderson Scoring System

The Global M.D. Anderson Scoring System (MDAS) incorporates host factors such as age and performance status,[11] as well as anemia, transfusion burden, karyotype, and most importantly, the severity of thrombocytopenia. It captures the prognostic impact of leukocytosis for MDS/MPN. This model further refines IPSS. The MDAS upstaged 25% of patients to a higher risk category.[101] It can be applied for MDS/MPN cases, as well as t-MDS.

Other risk models that had been utilized and validated include the *Lower Risk M.D. Anderson Scoring System* (LR-MDAS),[102] and the *WPSS*, which is more widely used in Europe.[10] For MDS/MPN subtypes, only the MDAS, discussed previously, can be applied. Several other models have been developed specifically for CMML (Table 47.4).

Five gene mutations independently predicted overall survival in a large cohort of MDS patients after adjusting for age and IPSS score.[103] These five genes include mutations involving *TP53* (hazard ratio [HR], 2.48), *EZH2* (HR, 2.13), *ETV6* (HR, 2.04), *RUNX1* (HR, 1.47), and *ASXL1* (HR, 1.38). In lower risk MDS, *EZH2*, *NRAS*, and *ASXL1* gene mutations upstaged 21% of low/intermediate 1 (int-1) IPSS risk MDS patients.[104] Only the *EZH2* mutation provided additional risk discrimination to upstage 8% of the patients classified by LR-MDAS.[104]

The causes of death in MDS include AML transformation in 30% to 40% of all patients (10% to 20% of lower risk MDS patients), whereas the vast majority, unfortunately, succumb due to complications secondary to the disease, namely infection and bleeding.[105] Other important prognostic factors in MDS include red blood cell (RBC) transfusion dependence[106] and elevated serum ferritin >1,000 ng/mL, which is associated with both inferior overall survival and time to AML transformation.[107] Bone marrow fibrosis in MDS is typically associated with a higher risk disease, increased myeloblasts, or complex cytogenetics, and worse outcome. Patients with bone marrow fibrosis are often categorized morphologically as MDS-U or MDS with fibrosis (MDS-F).[34]

Patients with MDS often suffer from other medical comorbidities that may impact survival, affect performance status, and limit therapeutic options. Using the ACE-27 comorbidity index, the median survival was 31.8, 16.8, 15.2, and 9.7 months for those with none, mild, moderate, and severe comorbidities, respectively ($p < 0.001$). A prognostic model including age, IPSS, and comorbidity score predicted median survival.[108] The Italian group added further refinement by developing an MDS-specific comorbidity index (MDS-CI). Cardiac disease, moderate to severe liver disease, severe pulmonary disease, renal disease, and history of solid tumors were found to independently affect the risk of nonleukemic death, whereas diabetes and cerebrovascular disease did not.[109]

MANAGEMENT OF MYELODYSPLASTIC SYNDROMES

Erythropoiesis-Stimulating Agents

More than 90% of MDS patients have anemia, and 30% to 50% are transfusion dependent.[110] Erythropoiesis-stimulating agents (ESA) are the most widely used treatment for anemia in lower risk MDS; more than 50% of newly diagnosed and established patients in the United States receive ESA. Response rates range from 15% to 20% in unselected patients receiving doses equivalent to 40,000 to 60,000 U of epoetin alpha weekly.[111] Treatment lasting 8 to 12 weeks provides an adequate trial to assess ESA responsiveness, with median duration of responses ranging from 12 to 24 months.[112] Case-matching studies suggest a survival advantage among erythroid responders.[112] Darbepoetin is at least as effective as epoetin alfa.[113] Patient selection improves response probability to ESAs and conserves resources. Using a simple model based on

TABLE 47.3
Risk Stratification Models in Myelodysplastic Syndromes

IPSS		
Variable		**Score**
Bone Marrow Blasts (%)		
<5		0
5–10		0.5
11–20		1.5
21–30		2.0
Karyotype[a]		
Good		0
Intermediate		0.5
Poor		1.0
Cytopenia[c]		
0/1		0
2/3		0.5

Risk Group	Sum Score	OS (y)
Low	0	5.7
Int-1	0.5–1	3.5
Int-2	1.5–2.0	1.1
High	≥2.5	0.4

IPSS-R		
Variable		**Score**
Bone Marrow Blasts (%)		
<2		0
>2–<5		1
5–10		2
>10		3
Karyotype[b]		
Very Good		0
Good		1
Intermediate		2
Poor		3
Very poor		4
Hgb ≥ 10 g/dL		0
8–<10 g/dL		1
<8 g/dL		1.5
ANC ≤0.8		0.5
Platelets ≥100		0
50–100		0.5
<50		1

Risk Group	Sum Score	OS (y)
Very good	0–2	8.8
Good	3–5	5.3
Int	6–7	3.0
Poor	8–9	1.6
Very poor	10–18	0.8

WPSS		
Variable		**Score**
WHO Category		
RA, RARS, Del(5q)		0
RCMD, RCMD-RS		1
RAEB-I		2
RAEB-II		3
Karyotype[a]		
Good		0
Intermediate		1
Poor		2.0
Transfusion[d]		
Yes		1
No		0

Risk Group	Sum Score	OS (mos)
Very Low	0	141
Low	1	66
Intermediate	2	48
High	3–4	26
Very High	5–6	9

Global MDAS		
Variable		**Score**
PS >2		2
Age (y)		
50–64		1
≥65		2
Platelets (× 10⁹/L)		
<30		3
30–49		2
50–199		1
Hgb <12 g/dL		2
BM blasts (%)		
5–10		1
11–29		2
WBC >20 × 10⁹/L		2
Karyotype		
Chromosome 7 Abn or complex ≥3 Abns		3
Transfusion		1

Risk Group	Sum Score	OS (mos)
Low	0–4	54
Int-1	5–6	25
Int-2	7–8	14
High	≥9	6

LR-MDAS		
Variable		**Score**
Unfavorable cytogenetics[e]		2
Age ≥60 y		2
Hb <10 g/dL		1
Plt <50 × 10⁹/L		2
50–200 × 10⁹/L		1
BM blasts ≥4%		1

Risk Group	Sum Score	OS (mos)
Cat-1	0–2	80
Cat-2	3–4	27
Cat-3	≥5	14

MDAS, M.D. Anderson Scoring System; LR-MDAS, Lower Risk M.D. Anderson Scoring System; Hb, hemoglobin; Plt, platelet; BM, bone marrow; Hgb, hemoglobin; WBC, white blood cell count; ANC, absolute neutrophil count; Abn, abnormality.

[a] Good is normal, −Y, del(5q), del(20q). Intermediate is other karyotypic abnormalities. Poor is complex (≥three abnormalities) or chromosome 7 abnormalities.
[b] Very good −Y, del(11q). Good is normal, single del(5q), del(12p), del(20q), or double including del(5q). Intermediate includes single cell(7q), +8, I(17q), +19, or any double not including del(5q). Poor includes der(3q), monosomy 7, double including −7/7q, or three abnormalities. Very poor is more than three abnormalities.
[c] Hb <10 g/dL, ANC <1,800/μL; platelets <100,000/μL.
[d] RBC transfusion dependence was defined as having at least one RBC transfusion every 8 weeks over a period of 4 mo.
[e] In this analysis, diploid and 5q were favorable cytogenetics, all others were considered as unfavorable cytogenetics.

TABLE 47.4
Prognostic Models in Chronic Myelomonocytic Leukemia

Score	Blast	IMP	NOC	DOC	LDH	Karyotype	Lymph	WBC	PS	Age	Mol
Bournemouth[a]	x		x								
Dusseldorf[b]	x		x		x						
IPSS[7]	x		x			x					
MDAPS[c]	x	x						x			
Spanish[d]	x					x		x			
MDASC[e]	x			x		x		x	x	x	
IPSS-R[13]	x			x		x				x	
Mayo[f]		x		x				x			
GFM[68]				x				x		x	x

Blast, myeloblast and promonocyte percentage in the bone marrow; IMP, immature myeloid precursor (represent the sum of peripheral blasts, promyelocytes, myelocytes, and metamyelocytes); NOC, number of cytopenias; DOC, duration of cytopenias; LDH, lactate dehydrogenase; lymph, lymphocyte count; WBC, white blood cell count; PS, Eastern Cooperative Oncology Group performance status; Mol, molecular profiling; MDAPS, MD Anderson Score from Prognostication in CMML; MDASC, Global MD Anderson Scoring System; GFM, Groupe Francias des Myelodysplasia.

[a] Worsley A, Oscier DG, Stevens J, et al. Prognostic features of chronic myelomonocytic leukaemia: a modified Bournemouth score gives the best prediction of survival. *Br J Haematol* 1988;68:17–21.
[b] Aul C, Gattermann N, Heyll A, et al. Primary myelodysplastic syndromes: analysis of prognostic factors in 235 patients and proposals for an improved scoring system. *Leukemia* 1992;6:52–59.
[c] Onida F, Kantarjian HM, Smith TL, et al. Prognostic factors and scoring systems in chronic myelomonocytic leukemia: a retrospective analysis of 213 patients. *Blood* 2002;99:840–849.
[d] Such E, Germing U, Malcovati L, et al. Development and validation of a prognostic scoring system for patients with chronic myelomonocytic leukemia. *Blood* 2013;121:3005–3015.
[e] Kantarjian H, O'Brien S, Ravandi F, et al. Proposal for a new risk model in myelodysplastic syndrome that accounts for events not considered in the original International Prognostic Scoring System. *Cancer* 2008;113:1351–1361.
[f] Patnaik MM, Padron E, Laborde RR, et al. Mayo prognostic model for WHO-defined chronic myelomonocytic leukemia: ASXL1 and spliceosome component mutations and outcomes. *Leukemia* 2013;27:1504–1510.

pretreatment endogenous serum erythropoietin (EPO) concentration (<100, 100 to 500, or >500 U per liter) and RBC transfusion burden (< or ≥2 U per month one would distinguish three response categories: high probability of erythroid response (74%), intermediate (23%), and low (7%).[114]

Lenalidomide

Lenalidomide is approved by the U.S. Food and Drug Administration (FDA) for the treatment of transfusion-dependent anemia in lower risk MDS patients with a chromosome 5q deletion (del[5q]) with or without additional cytogenetic abnormalities. In the lenalidomide registration (MDS-003) phase II clinical trial, the overall transfusion response rate was 76%, with 67% achieving transfusion independence.[115] The median time to response was 4.6 weeks, accompanied by a median rise in hemoglobin (Hgb) of 5.4 g/dL. Median duration of response exceeded 2 years and is longer in patients with isolate del(5q). Lenalidomide was administered at a dose of 10 mg daily either continuously or for 21 days every 4 weeks. Cytogenetic response and hematologic improvement were the strongest independent covariates for overall survival (OS) (HR, 5.295; p <0.001).[116,117] Recent studies indicate that TP53 gene mutations are demonstrable in approximately 20% of del(5q) MDS patients, expand over time, and are associated with a higher risk of disease progression and a lower frequency of cytogenetic response to lenalidomide.[118–120]

The most commonly observed adverse event was early myelosuppression, generally occurring in the first 8 weeks of treatment (62%). More than half of the patients (55%) experienced neutropenia, and 44% had thrombocytopenia. Dose reduction or treatment interruption for hematologic adverse events was necessary in the majority (84%) of patients. The median time to first dose reduction was 22 days. At week 24, only 32% of patients were receiving a 10-mg dose. Early cytopenias with lenalidomide treatment correlated with the probability of achieving RBC transfusion independence.[121] Non–hematologic-adverse events include dry skin, rash and pruritus, itching of the scalp, and diarrhea. Hypothyroidism has been reported in approximately 7% of patients.[122,123] Patients with renal insufficiency were excluded. In such patients, it is prudent to adjust the dosage based on creatinine clearance given the renal excretion of lenalidomide.[124] The incidence of venous thromboembolic events (VTE) in MDS patients treated with lenalidomide monotherapy was low, with VTE reported in 3% of the del(5q) patients.

A subsequent phase III, placebo-controlled study (MDS-004) compared two different doses and schedules of lenalidomide in the same del(5q) MDS population.[125] Two hundred and five patients were randomized to receive treatment with either lenalidomide 10 mg daily for 21 days every 4 weeks, continuous treatment with lenalidomide 5 mg daily, or placebo. The rates of sustained transfusion independence (>24 weeks) were 53.6%, 33.3%, and 6%, respectively (p <0.001). Cytogenetic response rates were also highest in the 10-mg arm. The median rise in hemoglobin was highest in patients treated with the 10-mg lenalidomide dose. No difference was observed in the frequency or magnitude of myelosuppression between the two lenalidomide doses, nor was there a difference in the rate of AML transformation.

The use of lenalidomide in lower risk non-del(5q) MDS was explored in a phase II study (MDS-002), which enrolled 214 non-del(5q) patients.[126] Based on the International Working Group 2000 (IWG 2000) response criteria, 26% patients achieved transfusion independence. Median rise in hemoglobin was 3.2 g/dL, and median duration of response was 41 weeks. Attempts to improve the activity of lenalidomide in non-del(5q) patients include biomarker-guided patient selection and combination strategies with an ESA.[127,128] Preliminary results of a randomized phase II clinical trial comparing lenalidomide to a lenalidomide/ESA combination yielded higher erythroid response rates with the combination treatment: 23% versus 40%, respectively (p = 0.043).

Lenalidomide's mechanism of action in MDS is karyotype specific. In del(5q) MDS, lenalidomide relieves p53 arrest by stabilizing MDM2 to permit cell cycle reentry by inhibiting the haplodeficient PP2A. The resulting hyperphosphorylation of inhibitory serine/threonine residues on MDM2 suppresses its autologous ubiquitination, thereby stabilizing the protein and, in turn, promoting the proteasomal degradation of p53.[84] In non-del(5q) MDS, lenalidomide enhances erythroid receptor signaling. The inhibition of PP2A promotes coalescence of lipid rafts with attendant incorporation of the erythropoietin receptor along with its signaling intermediates to yield a more efficient receptor signaling platform.[129]

The use of lenalidomide in higher risk MDS patients remains investigational. Several studies reported modest response rates and rates of transfusion independence.[130–132] A high rate of complete response have been reported when combining azacitidine and lenalidomide in higher risk MDS in a phase I/II trial, which is the subject of an ongoing intergroup randomized phase II clinical study.[133] Use of lenalidomide in the treatment of MDS/MPN subtypes is often extrapolated from its use in MDS. Nonproliferative lower risk CMML patients were included in the studies summarized previously. Anecdotal case reports suggest lenalidomide activity in patient with the RARS-T subtype.[134]

Azanucleosides

Azacitidine and decitabine are azanucleoside analogs with varied capacity to act as hypomethylating agents (HMA) to reverse epigenetic gene repression. Covalent bonds formed between deoxycytidine nucleotides and DNA methyltransferase deplete the enzyme and, as a consequence, promotes demethylation of silenced genes. These agents also are cytotoxic as DNA interactive nucleoside analogs and, in the case of azacitidine, which is incorporated largely into RNA, by inhibiting RNA translation and protein synthesis.

Azacitidine was the first FDA-approved drug for the treatment of all FAB MDS subtypes.[135] The overall CR+partial response (PR) rate was 23% (CR, 7%; PR, 16%), with a corresponding extension in median time to AML transformation from 12 to 21 months. The subsequent AZA-001 trial was the first study to demonstrate a survival advantage for any treatment in higher risks MDS.[136] Patients with intermediate 2 (Int-2) or high-risk MDS (n = 358) were randomized to treatment with either azacitidine or conventional care regimens (CCR) that included either best supportive care (BSC) alone, low-dose cytarabine, or intensive AML-type induction chemotherapy. The median OS was significantly extended in the azacitidine group compared to CCR: 24.5 months versus 15 months, respectively (p = 0.0001). AML progression was delayed by more than 14 months with the azacitidine treatment. Hematologic response rates also favored azacitidine, with 45% achieving RBC transfusion independence compared to 11% with CCR. The OS benefit with azacitidine treatment extended to those patients with AML according to the WHO classification (myeloblasts: 20% to 30%). A landmark analysis at cycle four revealed that patients who achieve hematologic improvement (HI) or better response according to IWG criteria experienced a survival advantage.[137] The probability of HI response, and therefore the potential for survival improvement, diminish with time, reaching less than 15% after 6 months of treatment.[138] Poor-risk cytogenetics, increased myeloblasts, and prior treatment with low-dose cytarabine are predictive variables for a lower response rate.[139] The loss of function mutations involving the TET2 gene is associated with a higher rate of response to azacitidine.[140] In lower risk MDS, nearly 50% of patients achieve HI and/or RBC transfusion independence (TI). The HI rate with treatment with a 5-day regimen appears equivalent to 5-2-2 or 5-2-5 regimens with less toxicity; however, its impact, if any, on OS is unknown.[141]

Decitabine was FDA approved based on a phase III trial in the United States comparing 15 mg/m² intravenously (IV) administered over 3 hours every 8 hours for 3 consecutive days to BSC in patients with INT-1, -2, and HR MDS.[142] The overall response rate was 30% with decitabine (9% CR, 8% PR, and 13% HI). Kantarjian et al.[143] compared three decitabine schedules using a reduced cumulative dosing schedule in a similar population. This study identified 20 mg/m² IV daily for 5 days as the preferred schedule, where the CR rate was 39%. The ADOPT trial was a multicenter validation study involving 99 MDS patients treated with the 20 mg/m² 5-day regimen; the study reported 17% CR with a corresponding median OS of 19.4 month.[144] A subsequent phase III study compared the effects of the FDA-approved decitabine regimen to supportive care in Int-2 and high-risk MDS.[145] The OS and the median time to AML transformation or death were not significantly different from the supportive care (SC) arm.

Outcomes after azanucleoside failure is poor, with median OS ranging from 4 to 8 months, and a 12-month survival of approximately 30%.[146–148] CR rates with standard intensive chemotherapy are 20% or less. Treatment of patients who fail azanucleosides represent an unmet need. Recent data suggest that outcomes are poor after azanucleoside failure in lower risk MDS as well.[149]

Small numbers of MDS/MPN patients, namely CMML, were included in the original azanucleoside clinical trials. Large retrospective series suggest similar response rates, but probably an inferior effect on OS. Splenomegaly and leukocytosis are predictors for worse outcomes among CMML patients treated with azacitidine.[150]

Immunosuppressive Therapy

HI is observed in approximately one-third of unselected MDS patients treated with antithymocyte globulin (ATG) with or without cyclosporine. Age is the strongest covariate for hematologic response. In a multivariate analysis age, the duration of RBC TD and the presence of a human leukocyte antigen DR15 were independent response variables.[151] Other retrospective studies identified bone marrow hypocellularity and the presence of a paroxysmal nocturnal hemoglobinuria clone as covariates for response to immunosuppressive therapy (IST). Rabbit ATG offers comparable effectiveness in treating MDS patients.[152] Alemtuzumab was reported to yield high response rates in preselected patients with the previously described features associated with the probability for response to IST.[153]

Allogeneic Hematopoietic Cell Transplantation

Allogeneic hematopoietic cell transplantation (AHCT) remains the only known curative treatment for patients with MDS. Unfortunately, the majority of MDS patients are not candidates for the procedure due to advanced age or comorbidities, and the procedure itself carries significant morbidity and mortality. With the decision of Medicare to provide coverage with evidence development for the AHCT in MDS patients in 2008, the number of procedures performed in the United States for patients with MDS, particularly those older than 60 years, has significantly increased over the past decade.

Using a markovian decision analysis model, early AHCT is recommended for higher risk MDS patients to maximize survival potential, whereas for lower risk patients, delaying AHCT until disease progression is a strategy that offered best overall survival.[154] A subsequent decision model in the azanucleoside era utilizing data from reduced intensity AHCT and predominantly in elderly patients (60 to 70 years) confirmed the recommendation of early AHCT for higher risk MDS and delayed AHCT for those with a lower risk.[155] No randomized controlled trials, evaluating AHCT versus nontransplant strategies, are available.

The most important predictors of outcome after AHCT are disease status (myeloblasts >5% and poor risk cytogenetics), but not age.[156] A study reported experience involving 1,333 MDS patients >50 years (449 patients >60 years) who underwent HCT. Four-year OS estimates for the 50 to 60 year olds and the <60 years cohort was 34% and 27%, respectively.

The question of therapy prior to AHCT remains controversial. Earlier studies did not show a convincing advantage for induction chemotherapy prior to AHCT; however, those studies were not randomized and were subject to selection bias by treating higher risk patients with chemotherapy. Among patients who receive intensive chemotherapy, those who achieved CR prior to AHCT had a better outcome. A phase II study evaluated 265 consecutive patients who received an AHCT. There was no difference in 3-year OS whether patients received azacitidine, intensive chemotherapy, or azacitidine preceded or followed by intensive chemotherapy (55% versus 48% versus 32%, respectively; $p = 0.07$).[157] Azanucleosides may also play a role as a maintenance strategy post-HCT. de Lima et al.[158] demonstrated that maintenance therapy with low-dose azacitidine (32 mg/m² for four cycles) is feasible in the post-AHCT setting for recurrent AML or MDS. This strategy is the subject of a prospective randomized clinical trial.[158] An analysis of 435 patients with higher risk MDS who had failed treatment with azanucleosides showed that patients who proceeded to AHCT or investigational agents had better survival compared to those offered supportive care or conventional chemotherapy, whether a low or an intensive dose.[147]

Iron Chelation Therapy

Several groups reported that iron overload and elevated serum ferritin in MDS patients is associated with inferior OS and higher rate of leukemia evolution.[107] Nonrandomized studies suggest that iron chelation therapy (ICT) impacts outcomes in lower risk MDS.[159,160] Two studies showed that the oral iron chelator deferasirox (Exjade) effectively lowered serum ferritin and labile plasma iron concentration in lower risk MDS.[161,162] Adverse effects from deferasirox may include renal failure, diarrhea, hepatic failure, and gastrointestinal hemorrhage. Deferasirox is contraindicated in patients with a creatinine clearance less than 40 mL per minute, higher risk MDS patients, and in patients with platelet count less than 50×10^9/L. Deferiprone (Ferriprox) is another oral iron chelator approved in the United States. The adverse effect of greatest concern is agranulocytosis, but it has less renal toxicity.[163] The MDS foundation recommends the consideration of ICT in transfusion-dependent lower risk MDS patients with serum ferritin persistently >1,000 ng/mL, whereas the National Comprehensive Cancer Network (NCCN) guidelines use a >2,500 ng/mL threshold. An ongoing randomized phase III, placebo-controlled study (TELESTO) is intended to address the potential clinical benefit of deferasirox chelation therapy.

How Do I Treat MDS Patients?

The first step in the management of MDS requires confirming the diagnosis, which in many instances, may require a hematopathologist's experienced eyes.[164] After establishing a diagnosis, risk stratification is critical for management decisions. We complement the standard IPSS risk model by newer clinical risk models such as IPSS-R and MDAS (or CMML-specific models in cases of CMML), and a molecular profile to more precisely delineate the disease risk category.[7,11,13,165]

For higher risk patients, we initiate treatment with azacitidine 75 mg/m² SC for 7 days every 28 days and assess patients for hematopoeitic stem cell transplant (HCT) in the absence of major comorbidities and a good performance status.[155] For patients who do not proceed to AHCT, we continue treatment until disease progression or loss of response. The response to azacitidine is evaluated after 4 to 6 cycles. If the disease is stable or better, treatment is continued. Experience from the AZA-001 trial tells us that hematologic improvement is predictive for improved overall survival.[136,166] In patients with baseline thrombocytopenia and neutropenia, we do not delay therapy or reduce dose, but rather provide more focused supportive care with close hematologic monitoring. We avoid the use of granulocyte-colony stimulating factor (G-CSF) or GM-CSF except in the setting of febrile neutropenia. Combination strategies adding to the backbone of azacitidine are being explored in clinical trials such as the combinations with lenalidomide, vorinostat, or pracinostat.[167–169] Crossing over to the alternate azanucleoside is generally minimally effective.[170] We consider a clinical trial or AHCT for those patients after azanucleoside failure.[147] Several agents are under investigation in patients after azanucleoside failure. A phase III trial with rigosertib, a multikinase inhibitor, recently completed accrual.[171] In cases of secondary AML, response rates to standard 3 + 7 induction chemotherapy is disappointing, with short OS. In this setting, we offer patients intensive chemotherapy, preferably in the context of a clinical trial such as the phase III randomized study comparing CPX-351 (liposomal formulation of a 5:1 molar ratio of cytarabine and daunorubicin), which demonstrated promising efficacy in a phase II randomized study.[172] Outside the context of a clinical trial, we favor the use the cladribine, cytarabine, G-CSF, and mitoxantrone (CLAG-M) regimen for induction in secondary AML after azacitidine failure, for which we previously reported a >50% complete response rate.[173]

In lower risk MDS, anemia remains the most common indication for therapy. In patients with a low endogenous serum erythropoietin level (<500 mU/mL) and low transfusion burden, we begin treatment with an ESA. An 8- to 12-week minimum trial of epoetin alfa is started at a dose of 40,000 to 60,000 U weekly or darbepoetin alfa dose equivalence as sufficient. In the absence of response, and particularly for patients with RARS, we consider the addition of G-CSF.[111] Subsequent treatment alternatives are guided by the type and severity of additional cytopenias, and include lenalidomide or azacitidine. For non-del(5q) lower risk MDS, lenalidomide may be considered in patients with isolated anemia and adequate platelets and neutrophils.[126] Use of lenalidomide prior to azanucleosides may yield higher response rates.[174] Lenalidomide in combination with ESA is currently under investigation with promising higher responses than lenalidomide alone.[127,128] Azacitidine is also used for lower risk MDS patients. We commonly use azacitidine at a dose of 75 mg/m² for 5 days in lower risk patients.[141] For MDS patients younger than 60 years of age with a short duration of transfusion dependence, a cluster of differentiation 4 cells (CD4):CD8 ratio <2.0 or those with trisomy 8, immunosuppressive therapy is a reasonable treatment strategy. For lower risk MDS patients with thrombocytopenia or neutropenia, particularly if the goal of treatment is to improve thrombocytopenia, azanucleosides are the treatment of choice or IST if there is a high chance of response. In del(5q) lower risk MDS patients who either failed or are not a candidate for treatment with an ESA, lenalidomide is the treatment of choice in the presence of adequate neutrophil and platelet counts.[115] Lenalidomide is administered daily at a dose of 10 mg orally. Complete blood counts are monitored weekly during the first 8 weeks. The vast majority of patients will need dose interruption after 2 to 3 weeks, with resumption of lenalidomide treatment upon hematologic recovery at the next lower dose level. In selected patients with lower risk MDS who are younger and who have no major comorbidities, AHCT may be discussed after failure of standard therapy. In our opinion, clinical trials remain the standard of care for treating MDS patients and should be considered whenever available.

REFERENCES

1. Vardiman JW, Thiele J, Arber DA, et al. The 2008 revision of the World Health Organization (WHO) classification of myeloid neoplasms and acute leukemia: rationale and important changes. *Blood* 2009;114:937–951.
2. Luzzatto A. Sull anemia grave megaloblastica senza reporto ematologico corrispondente (anemia pseudoaplastica). *Riv Veneta di sc Med Venezia* 1907;47:193–212.
3. Hamilton-Paterson JL. Pre-leukemia anemia. *Acta Hematologica* 1949;2:309–316.
4. Block M, Jacobson LO, Bethard WF. Preleukemic acute human leukemia. *JAMA* 1953;152:1018–1028.
5. Bennett JM, Catovsky D, Daniel MT, et al. Proposals for the classification of the acute leukaemias. French-American-British (FAB) co-operative group. *Br J Haematol* 1976;33:451–458.
6. Bennett JM, Catovsky D, Daniel MT, et al. Proposals for the classification of the myelodysplastic syndromes. *Br J Haematol* 1982;51:189–199.
7. Greenberg P, Cox C, LeBeau MM, et al. International scoring system for evaluating prognosis in myelodysplastic syndromes. *Blood* 1997;89:2079–2088.
8. Bennett JM, Brunning RD, Vardiman JW. Myelodysplastic syndromes: from French-American-British to World Health Organization: a commentary. *Blood* 2002;99:3074–3075.
9. Harris NL, Jaffe ES, Diebold J, et al. World Health Organization classification of neoplastic diseases of the hematopoietic and lymphoid tissues: report of the Clinical Advisory Committee meeting—Airlie House, Virginia, November 1997. *J Clin Oncol* 1999;17:3835–3849.
10. Malcovati L, Germing U, Kuendgen A, et al. Time-dependent prognostic scoring system for predicting survival and leukemic evolution in myelodysplastic syndromes. *J Clin Oncol* 2007;25:3503–3510.
11. Kantarjian H, O'Brien S, Ravandi F, et al. Proposal for a new risk model in myelodysplastic syndrome that accounts for events not considered in the original International Prognostic Scoring System. *Cancer* 2008;113:1351–1361.
12. Garcia Manero G, Shan J, Faderl S, et al. A prognostic score for patients with lower risk myelodysplastic syndrome. *Leukemia* 2008;22:538–543.
13. Greenberg PL, Tuechler H, Schanz J, et al. Revised International Prognostic Scoring System for myelodysplastic syndromes. *Blood* 2012;120:2454–2465.
14. Ma X, Does M, Raza A, et al. Myelodysplastic syndromes: incidence and survival in the United States. *Cancer* 2007;109:1536–1542.
15. Rollison DE, Howlader N, Smith MT, et al. Epidemiology of myelodysplastic syndromes and chronic myeloproliferative disorders in the United States, 2001-2003, using data from the NAACCR and SEER programs. *Blood* 2008;112:45–52.
16. Goldberg SL, Chen E, Corral M, et al. Incidence and clinical complications of myelodysplastic syndromes among United States Medicare beneficiaries. *J Clin Oncol* 2010;28:2847–2852.
17. Cogle CR, Iannacone MR, Yu D, et al. High rate of uncaptured myelodysplastic syndrome cases and an improved method of case ascertainment. *Leuk Res* 2014;38:71–75.
18. Strom SS, Vélez-Bravo V, Estey EH. Epidemiology of myelodysplastic syndromes. *Semin Hematol* 2008;45:8–13.
19. Komrokji R. Myelodysplastic syndromes: a view from where the sun rises and where the sun sets. *Leuk Res* 2006;30:1067–1068.
20. Churpek JE, Lorenz R, Nedumgottil S, et al. Proposal for the clinical detection and management of patients and their family members with familial myelodysplastic syndrome/acute leukemia predisposition syndromes. *Leuk Lymphoma* 2013;54:28–35.
21. Liew E, Owen C. Familial myelodysplastic syndromes: a review of the literature. *Haematologica* 2011;96:1536–1542.
22. Ostergaard P, Simpson MA, Connell FC, et al. Mutations in GATA2 cause primary lymphedema associated with a predisposition to acute myeloid leukemia (Emberger syndrome). *Nat Genet* 2011;43:929–931.
23. International Agency for Research on Cancer. IARC Monographs. *Chemical Agents and Related Occupations, Volume F. A Review of Human Carcinogens.* Lyon: IARC; 2012.
24. Schnatter AR, Glass DC, Tang G, et al. Myelodysplastic syndrome and benzene exposure among petroleum workers: an international pooled analysis. *J Natl Cancer Inst* 2012;104:1724–1737.
25. Tong H, Hu C, Yin X, et al. A meta-analysis of the relationship between cigarette smoking and incidence of myelodysplastic syndromes. *PLoS One* 2013;8:e67537.
26. Kristinsson SY, Björkholm M, Hultcrantz M, et al. Chronic immune stimulation might act as a trigger for the development of acute myeloid leukemia or myelodysplastic syndromes. *J Clin Oncol* 2011;29:2897–2903.
27. Strom SS, Gu Y, Gruschkus SK, et al. Risk factors of myelodysplastic syndromes: a case-control study. *Leukemia* 2005;19:1912–1918.
28. Park DJ, Koeffler HP. Therapy-related myelodysplastic syndromes. *Semin Hematol* 1996;33:256–273.
29. Smith SM, Le Beau MM, Huo D, et al. Clinical-cytogenetic associations in 306 patients with therapy-related myelodysplasia and myeloid leukemia: the University of Chicago series. *Blood* 2003;102:43–52.
30. Bennett JM, Komrokji R, Kouides P. The myelodysplastic syndromes. In: Abeloff MD, Armitage JO, Niederhuber JE, Kastan MB, eds., *Clinical Oncology*. 3rd ed. New York: Churchill Livingstone; 2004: 2849–2881.
31. Nardi V, Winkfield KM, Ok CY, et al. Acute myeloid leukemia and myelodysplastic syndromes after radiation therapy are similar to de novo disease and differ from other therapy-related myeloid neoplasms. *J Clin Oncol* 2012;30:2340–2347.
32. Valent P, Horny HP, Bennett JM, et al. Definitions and standards in the diagnosis and treatment of the myelodysplastic syndromes: Consensus statements and report from a working conference. *Leuk Res* 2007;31:727–736.
33. Malcovati L, Della Porta MG, Cazzola M. Predicting survival and leukemic evolution in patients with myelodysplastic syndrome. *Haematologica* 2006;91:1588–1590.
34. Della Porta MG, Malcovati L, Boveri E, et al. Clinical relevance of bone marrow fibrosis and CD34-positive cell clusters in primary myelodysplastic syndromes. *J Clin Oncol* 2009;27:754–762.
35. Bennett JM. World Health Organization classification of the acute leukemias and myelodysplastic syndrome. *Int J Hematol* 2000;72:131–133.
36. Komrokji R, Bennett J. What is "WHO"? Myelodysplastic syndromes classification. *Clinical Leukemia* 2008;2:20–27. http://www.ncbi.nlm.nih.gov/pubmed/20425325.
37. Komrokji R, Bennett JM. The myelodysplastic syndromes: classification and prognosis. *Curr Hematol Rep* 2003;2:179–185.
38. Vardiman JW, Harris NL, Brunning RD. The World Health Organization (WHO) classification of the myeloid neoplasms. *Blood* 2002;100:2292–2302.
39. Brunning RD, Orazi A, Germing U. Myelodysplastic Syndromes/neoplasms overview. In: Swerdlow SH, Campo E, Harris NL, Jaffe ES, eds., *WHO Classification of Tumours of Haematopoietic and Lymphoid Tissues*, 4th ed. Lyon: IARC; 2008: 88–93.
40. Komrokji R, Bennett JM. What Is "WHO"?: Myelodysplastic Syndrome Classification and Prognosis. ASCO Educational Book: 2009;413–419. http://www.ncbi.nlm.nih.gov/pubmed/20425325.
41. Orazi A, Brunning RD, Hasserjian RP. Refractory anemia with excess blasts. In: Swerdlow SH, Campo E, Harris NL, Jaffe ES, eds., *WHO Classification of Tumours of Haematopoietic and Lymphoid Tissues*, 4th ed. Lyon: IARC; 2008: 100–101.
42. Vardiman JW, Bennett JM, Bain BJ. Myelodysplastic/myeloproliferative neoplasm, unclassifiable. In: Swerdlow SH, Campo E, Harris NL, Jaffe ES, eds., *WHO Classification of Tumours of Haematopoietic and Lymphoid Tissues*, 4th ed. Lyon: IARC; 2008: 85–86.
43. Orazi A, Bennett JM, Germing U. Chronic myelomonocytic leukemia. In: Swerdlow SH, Campo E, Harris NL, Jaffe ES, eds., *WHO Classification of Tumours of Haematopoietic and Lymphoid Tissues*, 4th ed. Lyon: IARC; 2008: 76–79.
44. Young NS, Calado RT, Scheinberg P. Current concepts in the pathophysiology and treatment of aplastic anemia. *Blood* 2006;108:2509–2519.
45. Steensma D. Dysplasia has a differential diagnosis: distinguishing genuine myelodysplastic syndromes (MDS) from mimics, imitators, copycats and impostors. *Curr Hematol Malig Rep* 2012;7:310–320.
46. Tsukamoto N, Morita K, Maehara T, et al. Clonality in myelodysplastic syndromes: demonstration of pluripotent stem cell origin using X-linked restriction fragment length polymorphisms. *Br J Haematol* 1993;83:589–594.
47. Anastasi J, Feng J, Le Beau MM, et al. Cytogenetic clonality in myelodysplastic syndromes studied with fluorescence in situ hybridization: lineage, response to growth factor therapy, and clone expansion. *Blood* 1993;81:1580–1585.
48. Abrahamson G, Boultwood J, Madden J, et al. Clonality of cell populations in refractory anaemia using combined approach of gene loss and X-linked restriction fragment length polymorphism-methylation analyses. *Br J Haematol* 1991;79:550–555.
49. Janssen JW, Buschle M, Layton M, et al. Clonal analysis of myelodysplastic syndromes: evidence of multipotent stem cell origin. *Blood* 1989;73:248–254.
50. Schanz J, Steidl C, Fonatsch C, et al. Coalesced multicentric analysis of 2,351 patients with myelodysplastic syndromes indicates an underestimation of poor-risk cytogenetics of myelodysplastic syndromes in the international prognostic scoring system. *J Clin Oncol* 2011;29:1963–1970.
51. Haase D, Germing U, Schanz J, et al. New insights into the prognostic impact of the karyotype in MDS and correlation with subtypes: evidence from a core dataset of 2124 patients. *Blood* 2007;110:4385–4395.
52. Barlow JL, Drynan LF, Hewett DR, et al. A p53-dependent mechanism underlies macrocytic anemia in a mouse model of human 5q- syndrome. *Nat Med* 2010;16:59–66.
53. Papaemmanuil E, Gerstung M, Malcovati L, et al. Clinical and biological implications of driver mutations in myelodysplastic syndromes. *Blood* 2013;122:3616–3627.
54. Haferlach T, Nagata Y, Grossmann V, et al. Landscape of genetic lesions in 944 patients with myelodysplastic syndromes. *Leukemia* 2014;28:241–247.
55. Delhommeau F, Dupont S, Della Valle V, et al. Mutation in TET2 in myeloid cancers. *N Engl J Med* 2009;360:2289–2301.
56. Ko M, Huang Y, Jankowska AM, et al. Impaired hydroxylation of 5-methylcytosine in myeloid cancers with mutant TET2. *Nature* 2010;468:839–843.
57. Grossmann V, Kohlmann A, Eder C, et al. Analyses of 81 chronic myelomonocytic leukemia (CMML) for EZH2, TET2, ASXL1, CBL, KRAS, NRAS, RUNX1, IDH1, IDH2, and NPM1 revealed mutations in 86.4% of all patients with TET2 and EZH2 being of high prognostic relevance. ASH Annual Meeting Abstracts 2010;116:296. http://www.ncbi.nlm.nih.gov/pubmed/20425325.
58. Gelsi-Boyer V, Trouplin V, Adelaide J, et al. Mutations of polycomb-associated gene ASXL1 in myelodysplastic syndromes and chronic myelomonocytic leukaemia. *Br J Haematol* 2009;145:788–800.
59. Bejar R, Stevenson K, Abdel-Wahab O, et al. Clinical effect of point mutations in myelodysplastic syndromes. *N Engl J Med* 2011;364:2496–2506.

60. Jankowska AM, Makishima H, Tiu RV, et al. Mutational spectrum analysis of chronic myelomonocytic leukemia includes genes associated with epigenetic regulation: UTX, EZH2, and DNMT3A. Blood 2011;118:3932–3941.
61. Abdel-Wahab O, Adli M, LaFave LM, et al. ASXL1 mutations promote myeloid transformation through loss of PRC2-mediated gene repression. Cancer Cell 2012;22:180–193.
62. Dey A, Seshasayee D, Noubade R, et al. Loss of the tumor suppressor BAP1 causes myeloid transformation. Science 2012;337:1541–1546.
63. Abdel-Wahab O, Gao J, Adli M, et al. Deletion of Asxl1 results in myelodysplasia and severe developmental defects in vivo. J Exp Med 2013;210:2641–2659.
64. Li Z, Cai X, Cai CL, et al. Deletion of Tet2 in mice leads to dysregulated hematopoietic stem cells and subsequent development of myeloid malignancies. Blood 2011;118:4509–4518.
65. Yoshida K, Sanada M, Shiraishi Y, et al. Frequent pathway mutations of splicing machinery in myelodysplasia. Nature 2011;478:64–69.
66. Wu SJ, Kuo YY, Hou HA, et al. The clinical implication of SRSF2 mutation in patients with myelodysplastic syndrome and its stability during disease evolution. Blood 2012;120:3106–3111.
67. Meggendorfer M, Roller A, Haferlach T, et al. SRSF2 mutations in 275 cases with chronic myelomonocytic leukemia (CMML). Blood 2012;120:3080–3088.
68. Itzykson R, Kosmider O, Renneville A, et al. Prognostic score including gene mutations in chronic myelomonocytic leukemia. J Clin Oncol 2013;31:2428–2436.
69. Papaemmanuil E, Cazzola M, Boultwood J, et al. Somatic SF3B1 mutation in myelodysplasia with ring sideroblasts. N Engl J Med 2011;365:1384–1395.
70. Walter MJ, Shen D, Ding L, et al. Clonal architecture of secondary acute myeloid leukemia. N Engl J Med 2012;366:1090–1098.
71. Miller JS, Arthur DC, Litz CE, et al. Myelodysplastic syndrome after autologous bone marrow transplantation: an additional late complication of curative cancer therapy. Blood 1994;83:3780–3786.
72. Kulasekararaj AG, Al Ali NH, Kordasti SY, et al. Characteristics and outcome of myelodysplastic syndromes (MDS) patients with autoimmune diseases. Blood 2013;122:746. http://www.ncbi.nlm.nih.gov/pubmed/20425325.
73. Tabata R, Tabata C, Okamoto T, et al. Autoimmune pancreatitis associated with myelodysplastic syndrome. Int Arch Allergy Immunol 2010;151:168–172.
74. Zou JX, Rollison DE, Boulware D, et al. Altered naive and memory CD4+ T-cell homeostasis and immunosenescence characterize younger patients with myelodysplastic syndrome. Leukemia 2009;23:1288–1296.
75. Epling-Burnette PK, Painter JS, Rollison DE, et al. Prevalence and clinical association of clonal T-cell expansions in myelodysplastic syndrome. Leukemia 2007;21:659–667.
76. Yang L, Mailloux A, Rollison DE, et al. Naive T-cells in myelodysplastic syndrome display intrinsic human telomerase reverse transcriptase (hTERT) deficiency. Leukemia 2013;27:897–906.
77. Fozza C, Contini S, Galleu A, et al. Patients with myelodysplastic syndromes display several T-cell expansions, which are mostly polyclonal in the CD4(+) subset and oligoclonal in the CD8(+) subset. Exp Hematol 2009;37:947–955.
78. Mailloux AW, Sugimori C, Komrokji RS, et al. Expansion of effector memory regulatory T cells represents a novel prognostic factor in lower risk myelodysplastic syndrome. J Immunol 2012;189:3198–3208.
79. Wei Y, Dimicoli S, Bueso-Ramos C, et al. Toll-like receptor alterations in myelodysplastic syndrome. Leukemia 2013;27:1832–1840.
80. Dimicoli S, Wei Y, Bueso-Ramos C, et al. Overexpression of the toll-like receptor (TLR) signaling adaptor MYD88, but lack of genetic mutation, in myelodysplastic syndromes. PLoS One 2013;8:e71120.
81. Chen X, Eksioglu EA, Zhou J, et al. Induction of myelodysplasia by myeloid-derived suppressor cells. J Clin Invest 2013;123:4595–4611.
82. Boultwood J, Fidler C, Strickson AJ, et al. Narrowing and genomic annotation of the commonly deleted region of the 5q- syndrome. Blood 2002;99:4638–4641.
83. Ebert BL, Pretz J, Bosco J, et al. Identification of RPS14 as a 5q- syndrome gene by RNA interference screen. Nature 2008;451:335–339.
84. Wei S, Chen X, McGraw K, et al. Lenalidomide promotes p53 degradation by inhibiting MDM2 auto-ubiquitination in myelodysplastic syndrome with chromosome 5q deletion. Oncogene 2013;32:1110–1120.
85. Wei S, Chen X, Rocha K, et al. A critical role for phosphatase haplodeficiency in the selective suppression of deletion 5q MDS by lenalidomide. Proc Natl Acad Sci U S A 2009;106:12974–12979.
86. Rosing JL, Komrokji RS, Margolin EG. Anemia in elderly hospitalized veterans: prevalence, causes, and clinical impact. ASH Annual Meeting Abstracts 2005;106:3756. http://www.ncbi.nlm.nih.gov/pubmed/20425325.
87. Kantarjian H, Giles F, List A, et al. The incidence and impact of thrombocytopenia in myelodysplastic syndromes. Cancer 2007;109:1705–1714.
88. Raman BK, Van Slyck EJ, Riddle J, et al. Platelet function and structure in myeloproliferative disease, myelodysplastic syndrome, and secondary thrombocytosis. Am J Clin Pathol 1989;91:647–655.
89. Boogaerts MA, Nelissen V, Roelant C, et al. Blood neutrophil function in primary myelodysplastic syndromes. Br J Haematol 1983;55:217–227.
90. Tsukada H, Chou T, Ishizuka Y, et al. Disseminated Mycobacterium avium-intracellulare infection in a patient with myelodysplastic syndrome (refractory anemia). Am J Hematol 1994;45:325–329.
91. Ong KR, Sordillo E, Frankel E. Unusual case of Aeromonas hydrophila endocarditis. J Clin Microbiol 1991;29:1056–1057.
92. Pomeroy C, Oken MM, Rydell RE, et al. Infection in the myelodysplastic syndromes. Am J Med 1991;90:338–344.
93. Al Ustwani O, Ford LA, Sait SJ, et al. Myelodysplastic syndromes and autoimmune diseases—case series and review of literature. Leuk Res 2013;37:894–899.
94. Fain O, Braun T, Stirnemann J, et al. [Systemic and autoimmune manifestations in myelodysplastic syndromes]. Rev Med Interne 2011;32:552–559.
95. Enright H, Miller W. Autoimmune phenomena in patients with myelodysplastic syndromes. Leuk Lymphoma 1997;24:483–489.
96. Sanz C, Cervantes F, Pereira A, et al. [Coombs-positive autoimmune hemolytic anemia as a striking initial manifestation of myelodysplastic syndromes]. Sangre (Barc) 1990;35:329.
97. Parikh SA, Tefferi A. Chronic myelomonocytic leukemia: 2013 update on diagnosis, risk stratification, and management. Am J Hematol 2013;88:967–974.
98. Malcovati L, Della Porta MG, Pietra D, et al. Molecular and clinical features of refractory anemia with ringed sideroblasts associated with marked thrombocytosis. Blood 2009;114:3538–3545.
99. Mishra A, Corrales-Yepez M, Ali NA, et al. Validation of the revised International Prognostic Scoring System in treated patients with myelodysplastic syndromes. Am J Hematol 2013;88:566–570.
100. Sekeres MA, Elson P, Tiu RV, et al. Validating the lower-risk MD Anderson Prognostic Scoring System (LR-PSS) and the Revised International Prognostic Scoring System (IPSS-R) for patients with myelodysplastic syndromes. ASH Annual Meeting Abstracts 2011;118:(abstract 1720).
101. Komrokji RS, Corrales-Yepez M, Al Ali N, et al. Validation of the MD Anderson Prognostic Risk Model for patients with myelodysplastic syndrome. Cancer 2012;118(10):2659–2664.
102. Garcia-Manero G, Shan J, Faderl S, et al. A prognostic score for patients with lower risk myelodysplastic syndrome. Leukemia 2007;22:538–543.
103. Bejar R, Stevenson K, Abdel-Wahab O, et al. Clinical effect of point mutations in myelodysplastic syndromes. N Engl J Med 2011;364(26):2496–2506.
104. Bejar R, Stevenson KE, Caughey BA, et al. Validation of a prognostic model and the impact of mutations in patients with lower-risk myelodysplastic syndromes. J Clin Oncol 2012;30(27):3376–3382.
105. Dayyani F, Conley AP, Strom SS, et al. Cause of death in patients with lower-risk myelodysplastic syndrome. Cancer 2010;116:2174–2179.
106. Malcovati L, Porta MG, Pascutto C, et al. Prognostic factors and life expectancy in myelodysplastic syndromes classified according to WHO criteria: a basis for clinical decision making. J Clin Oncol 2005;23:7594–7603.
107. Sanz G, Nomdedeu B, Such E, et al. Independent impact of iron overload and transfusion dependency on survival and leukemic evolution in patients with myelodysplastic syndrome. ASH Annual Meeting Abstracts 2008;112: (abstract 640).
108. Naqvi K, Garcia-Manero G, Sardesai S, et al. Association of comorbidities with overall survival in myelodysplastic syndrome: development of a prognostic model. J Clin Oncol 2011;29(16):2240–2246.
109. Della Porta MG, Malcovati L, Strupp C, et al. Risk stratification based on both disease status and extra-hematologic comorbidities in patients with myelodysplastic syndrome. Haematologica 2011;96(3):441–449.
110. Bennett JM. Consensus statement on iron overload in myelodysplastic syndromes. Am J Hematol 2008;83:858–861.
111. Hellstrom-Lindberg E. Efficacy of erythropoietin in the myelodysplastic syndromes: a meta-analysis of 205 patients from 17 studies. Br J Haematol 1995;89:67–71.
112. Jadersten M, Malcovati L, Dybedal I, et al. Erythropoietin and granulocyte-colony stimulating factor treatment associated with improved survival in myelodysplastic syndrome. J Clin Oncol 2008;26:3607–3613.
113. Moyo V, Lefebvre P, Duh MS, et al. Erythropoiesis-stimulating agents in the treatment of anemia in myelodysplastic syndromes: a meta-analysis. Ann Hematol 2008;87:527–536.
114. Hellstrom-Lindberg E, Gulbrandsen N, Lindberg G, et al. A validated decision model for treating the anaemia of myelodysplastic syndromes with erythropoietin + granulocyte colony-stimulating factor: significant effects on quality of life. Br J Haematol 2003;120:1037–1046.
115. List A, Dewald G, Bennett J, et al. Lenalidomide in the myelodysplastic syndrome with chromosome 5q deletion. N Engl J Med 2006;355:1456–1465.
116. List A, Dewald G, Bennett J, et al. Cytogenetic response to lenalidomide is associated with improved survival in patients with chromosome 5q deletion. Leuk Res 2007;31:s38.
117. Gohring G, Giagounidis A, Busche G, et al. Patients with del(5q) MDS who fail to achieve sustained erythroid or cytogenetic remission after treatment with lenalidomide have an increased risk for clonal evolution and AML progression. Ann Hematol 2010;89(4):365–374.
118. Kulasekararaj AG, Smith AE, Mian SA, et al. TP53 mutations in myelodysplastic syndrome are strongly correlated with aberrations of chromosome 5, and correlate with adverse prognosis. Br J Haematol 2013;160:660–672.
119. Jadersten M, Saft L, Smith A, et al. TP53 mutations in low-risk myelodysplastic syndromes with del(5q) predict disease progression. J Clin Oncol 2011;29:1971–1979.
120. Bally C, Ades L, Renneville A, et al. Incidence and prognostic value of TP53 mutations in lower risk MDS with Del 5q. ASH Annual Meeting Abstracts 2012;120:(abstract 2809).
121. Sekeres MA, Maciejewski JP, Giagounidis AA, et al. Relationship of treatment-related cytopenias and response to lenalidomide in patients with lower-risk myelodysplastic syndromes. J Clin Oncol 2008;26:5943–5949.
122. Giagounidis A, Fenaux P, Mufti GJ, et al. Practical recommendations on the use of lenalidomide in the management of myelodysplastic syndromes. Ann Hematol 2008;87:345–352.
123. Komrokji R, Giagounidis A. Lenalidomide therapy in MDS. In: Steensma DP, ed., Myelodysplastic Syndromes: Pathobiology and Clinical Management, 2nd ed. London, Informa Health Care; 2008: 457–483.

124. Chen N, Lau H, Kong L, et al. Pharmacokinetics of lenalidomide in subjects with various degrees of renal impairment and in subjects on hemodialysis. *J Clin Pharmacol* 2007;47:1466–1475.
125. Fenaux P, Giagounidis A, Selleslag D, et al. A randomized phase 3 study of lenalidomide versus placebo in RBC transfusion-dependent patients with low-/intermediate-1-risk myelodysplastic syndromes with del5q. *Blood* 2011;118:3765–3776.
126. Raza A, Reeves JA, Feldman EJ, et al. Phase 2 study of lenalidomide in transfusion-dependent, low-risk, and intermediate-1 risk myelodysplastic syndromes with karyotypes other than deletion 5q. *Blood* 2008;111:86–93.
127. Komrokji RS, Lancet JE, Swern AS, et al. Combined treatment with lenalidomide and epoetin alfa in lower-risk patients with myelodysplastic syndrome. *Blood* 2012;120(17):3419–3424.
128. Toma A, Chevret S, Kosmider O, et al. A randomized study of lenalidomide (LEN) with or without EPO in RBC transfusion dependent (TD) IPSS low and int-1 (lower risk) myelodysplastic syndromes (MDS) without del 5q resistant to EPO. *ASCO Meeting Abstracts* 2013;31:(abstract 7002).
129. List AF, Estes M, Williams A, et al. Lenalidomide (CC-5013; revlimid(R)) promotes erythropoiesis in myelodysplastic syndromes (MDS) by CD45 protein tyrosine phosphatase (PTP) inhibition. *ASH Annual Meeting Abstracts* 2006;108:(abstract 1360).
130. Burcheri S, Prebet T, Beyne-Rauzy O, et al. Lenalidomide (LEN) in INT 2 and high risk MDS with DEL 5q. Interim results of a phase II trial by the GFM. *ASH Annual Meeting Abstracts* 2007;110:(abstract 820).
131. Mollgard L, Nilsson L, Kjeldsen L, et al. Lenalidomide in high-risk myelodysplastic syndrome and acute myeloid leukemia with chromosome 5 abnormalities. *ASH Annual Meeting Abstracts* 2009;114:(abstract 115).
132. Vij R, Nelson A, Uy GL, et al. A phase II study of high dose lenalidomide as initial therapy for acute myeloid leukemia in patients >60 years old. *ASH Annual Meeting Abstracts* 2009;114:(abstract 842).
133. Sekeres MA, Tiu RV, Komrokji R, et al. Phase 2 study of the lenalidomide and azacitidine combination in patients with higher-risk myelodysplastic syndromes. *Blood* 2012;120:4945–4951.
134. Huls G, Mulder AB, Rosati S, et al. Efficacy of single-agent lenalidomide in patients with JAK2 (V617F) mutated refractory anemia with ring sideroblasts and thrombocytosis. *Blood* 2010;116:100–102.
135. Silverman LR, Demakos EP, Peterson BL, et al. Randomized controlled trial of azacitidine in patients with the myelodysplastic syndrome: a study of the cancer and leukemia group B. *J Clin Oncol* 2002;20:2429–2440.
136. Fenaux P, Mufti GJ, Hellstrom-Lindberg E, et al. Efficacy of azacitidine compared with that of conventional care regimens in the treatment of higher-risk myelodysplastic syndromes: a randomised, open-label, phase III study. *Lancet Oncol* 2009;10:223–232.
137. List AF, Fenaux P, Mufti GJ, et al. Effect of azacitidine (AZA) on overall survival in higher-risk myelodysplastic syndromes (MDS) without complete remission. *ASCO Meeting Abstracts* 2008;26:(abstract 7006).
138. Gore S, Fenaux P, Santini V, et al. Time-dependent decision analysis: Stable disease in azacitidine (AZA)-treated patients (pts) with higher-risk MDS. *ASCO Meeting Abstracts* 2010;28:(abstract 6503).
139. Itzykson R, Thepot S, Quesnel B, et al. Prognostic factors for response and overall survival in 282 patients with higher-risk myelodysplastic syndromes treated with azacitidine. *Blood* 2011;117(2):403–411.
140. Itzykson R, Kosmider O, Cluzeau T, et al. Presence of TET2 mutation predicts a higher response rate to azacitidine in MDS and AML post MDS. *ASH Annual Meeting Abstracts* 2010;116:(abstract 439).
141. Lyons RM, Cosgriff TM, Modi SS, et al. Hematologic response to three alternative dosing schedules of azacitidine in patients with myelodysplastic syndromes. *J Clin Oncol* 2009;27:1850–1856.
142. Kantarjian HM, O'Brien S, Shan J, et al. Update of the decitabine experience in higher risk myelodysplastic syndrome and analysis of prognostic factors associated with outcome. *Cancer* 2007;109:265–273.
143. Kantarjian H, Oki Y, Garcia-Manero G, et al. Results of a randomized study of 3 schedules of low-dose decitabine in higher-risk myelodysplastic syndrome and chronic myelomonocytic leukemia. *Blood* 2007;109:52–57.
144. Steensma DP, Baer MR, Slack JL, et al. Multicenter study of decitabine administered daily for 5 days every 4 weeks to adults with myelodysplastic syndromes: the alternative dosing for outpatient treatment (ADOPT) trial. *J Clin Oncol* 2009;27:3842–3848.
145. Lubbert M, Suciu S, Baila L, et al. Low-dose decitabine versus best supportive care in elderly patients with intermediate- or high-risk myelodysplastic syndrome (MDS) ineligible for intensive chemotherapy: final results of the randomized phase III study of the European Organisation for Research and Treatment of Cancer Leukemia Group and the German MDS Study Group. *J Clin Oncol* 2011;29:1987–1996.
146. Jabbour E, Garcia-Manero G, Batty N, et al. Outcome of patients with myelodysplastic syndrome after failure of decitabine therapy. *Cancer* 2010;116:3830–3834.
147. Prebet T, Gore SD, Esterni B, et al. Outcome of high-risk myelodysplastic syndrome after azacitidine treatment failure. *J Clin Oncol* 2011;29:3322–3327.
148. Duong VH, Lin K, Reljic T, et al. Poor outcome of patients with myelodysplastic syndrome after azacitidine treatment failure. *Clin Lymphoma Myeloma Leuk* 2013;13:711–715.
149. Jabbour E, Garcia-Manero G, Xiao L, et al. Outcome Of patients (pts) with low and intermediate-1 risk myelodysplastic syndrome (MDS) after hypomethylating agent (HMA) failure. *Blood* 2013;122:388.
150. Ades L, Sekeres MA, Wolfromm A, et al. Predictive factors of response and survival among chronic myelomonocytic leukemia patients treated with azacitidine. *Leuk Res* 2013;37:609–613.
151. Sloand EM, Wu CO, Greenberg P, et al. Factors affecting response and survival in patients with myelodysplasia treated with immunosuppressive therapy. *J Clin Oncol* 2008;26:2505–2511.
152. Komrokji RS, Mailloux AW, Chen DT, et al. A phase 2 multicenter rabbit antithymocyte globulin trial in patients with myelodysplastic syndromes identifying a novel model for response prediction. *Haematologica* 2014;99(7):1176–1183.
153. Sloand EM, Olnes MJ, Shenoy A, et al. Alemtuzumab treatment of intermediate-1 myelodysplasia patients is associated with sustained improvement in blood counts and cytogenetic remissions. *J Clin Oncol* 2010;28(35):5166–5173.
154. Cutler CS, Lee SJ, Greenberg P, et al. A decision analysis of allogeneic bone marrow transplantation for the myelodysplastic syndromes: delayed transplantation for low-risk myelodysplasia is associated with improved outcome. *Blood* 2004;104:579–585.
155. Koreth J, Pidala J, Perez WS, et al. Role of reduced-intensity conditioning allogeneic hematopoietic stem-cell transplantation in older patients with de novo myelodysplastic syndromes: an international collaborative decision analysis. *J Clin Oncol* 2013;31:2662–2670.
156. Lim Z, Brand R, Martino R, et al. Allogeneic hematopoietic stem-cell transplantation for patients 50 years or older with myelodysplastic syndromes or secondary acute myeloid leukemia. *J Clin Oncol* 2010;28(3):405–411.
157. Damaj G, Duhamel A, Robin M, et al. Impact of azacitidine before allogeneic stem-cell transplantation for myelodysplastic syndromes: a study by the Société Française de Greffe de Moelle et de Thérapie-Cellulaire and the Groupe-Francophone des Myélodysplasies. *J Clin Oncol* 2012;30(36):4533–4540.
158. de Lima M, Giralt S, Thall PF, et al. Maintenance therapy with low-dose azacitidine after allogeneic hematopoietic stem cell transplantation for recurrent acute myelogenous leukemia or myelodysplastic syndrome: a dose and schedule finding study. *Cancer* 2010;116:5420–5431.
159. Leitch HA. Improving clinical outcome in patients with myelodysplastic syndrome and iron overload using iron chelation therapy. *Leuk Res* 2007;31:S7–S9.
160. Rose C, Brechignac S, Vassilief D, et al. Does iron chelation therapy improve survival in regularly transfused lower risk MDS patients? A multicenter study by the GFM (Groupe Francophone des Myélodysplasies). *Leuk Res* 2010;34:864–870.
161. List AF, Baer MR, Steensma D, et al. Deferasirox (ICL670; Exjade(R)) reduces serum ferritin (SF) and labile plasma iron (LPI) in patients with myelodysplastic syndromes (MDS). *ASH Annual Meeting Abstracts* 2007;110:(abstract 1470).
162. Gattermann N, Schmid M, Porta MD, et al. Efficacy and safety of deferasirox (Exjade(R)) during 1 year of treatment in transfusion-dependent patients with myelodysplastic syndromes: results from EPIC Trial. *ASH Annual Meeting Abstracts* 2008;112:(abstract 633).
163. Cermak J, Jonasova A, Vondrakova J, et al. Efficacy and safety of administration of oral iron chelator deferiprone in patients with early myelodysplastic syndrome. *Hemoglobin* 2011;35:217–227.
164. Naqvi K, Jabbour E, Bueso-Ramos C, et al. Implications of discrepancy in morphologic diagnosis of myelodysplastic syndrome between referral and tertiary care centers. *Blood* 2011;118:4690–4693.
165. Padron E, Ali NHA, Peker D, et al. A comparison of prognostic models for chronic myelomonocytic leukemia (CMML) in the era of hypomethylating agents. *ASH Annual Meeting Abstracts* 2012;120:(abstract 1695).
166. Gore SD, Fenaux P, Santini V, et al. A multivariate analysis of the relationship between response and survival among patients with higher-risk myelodysplastic syndromes treated within azacitidine or conventional care regimens in the randomized AZA-001 trial. *Haematologica* 2013;98:1067–1072.
167. Sekeres MA, Gundacker H, Lancet J, et al. A phase 2 study of lenalidomide monotherapy in patients with deletion 5q acute myeloid leukemia: Southwest Oncology Group Study S0605. *Blood* 2011;118(3):523–528.
168. Silverman LR, Verma A, Odchimar-Reissig R, et al. A phase I/II study of vorinostat, an oral histone deacetylase inhibitor, in combination with azacitidine in patients with the myelodysplastic syndrome (MDS) and acute myeloid leukemia (AML). Initial results of the phase I trial: A New York Cancer Consortium. *ASCO Meeting Abstracts* 2008;26:(abstract 7000).
169. Quintas-Cardama A, Kantarjian HM, Ravandi F, et al. Very high rates of clinical and cytogenetic response with the combination of the histone deacetylase inhibitor pracinostat (SB939) and 5-azacitidine in high-risk myelodysplastic syndrome. *ASH Annual Meeting Abstracts* 2012;120:(abstract 3821).
170. Komrokji RS, Apuri S, Al Ali N, et al. Evidence for selective benefit of sequential treatment with azanucleosides in patients with myelodysplastic syndromes (MDS). *ASCO Meeting Abstracts* 2013;31:7113.
171. Raza A, Greenberg PL, Olnes MJ, et al. Final phase I/II results of rigosertib (ON 01910.Na) hematological effects in patients with myelodysplastic syndrome and correlation with overall survival. *ASH Annual Meeting Abstracts* 2013;118:(abstract 3822).
172. Lancet JE, Cortes JE, Hogge DE, et al. Phase 2B randomized study of CPX-351 vs. cytarabine (CYT) + daunorubicin (DNR) (7 + 3 regimen) in newly diagnosed AML patients aged 60-75. *ASH Annual Meeting Abstracts* 2010;116:(abstract 655).
173. Jaglal MV, Duong VH, Bello CM, et al. Cladribine, cytarabine, filgrastim, and mitoxantrone (CLAG-M) compared to standard induction in acute myeloid leukemia from myelodysplastic syndrome after azanucleoside failure. *Leuk Res* 2013;38:443–446.
174. Komrokji R, Corrales-Yepez MG, Al Ali NH, et al. Lenalidomide treatment for lower risk non-deletion 5q myelodysplastic syndromes patients yields higher response rates when used prior to azanucleosides. *Blood* 2013;122:1507.

48 Plasma Cell Neoplasms

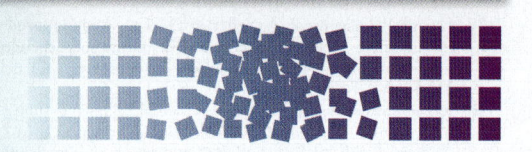

Nikhil C. Munshi and Kenneth C. Anderson

INTRODUCTION

Plasma cell neoplasms represent a spectrum of diseases characterized by clonal proliferation and the accumulation of immunoglobulin-producing terminally differentiated B cells. The spectrum includes clinically benign common conditions, such as monoclonal gammopathy of unknown significance (MGUS), as well as rare disorders such as Castleman's disease and α heavy chain disease; indolent conditions such as Waldenström's macroglobulinemia; the more common malignant entity, plasma cell myeloma; and a more aggressive form, plasma cell leukemia, with circulating malignant plasma cells in the blood. All of these disorders share common features of plasma cell morphology, production of immunoglobulin molecules, and immune dysfunction. A plasma cell neoplasm is considered to originate from a single B cell, with resultant monoclonal protein secretion that characterizes its type. Occasional oligoclonal or polyclonal protein abnormalities are observed in conditions such as Castleman's disease.

There are five major classes of immunoglobulin (Ig) synthesized by normal B cells and plasma cells: IgG, IgA, IgM, IgD, and IgE. The dysfunctional plasma cells secrete one of these intact immunoglobulin molecules; however, there may be a discrepancy in the production of the heavy and light chains leading to an imbalance with an excess of κ or λ light chain that is excreted in the urine (Bence Jones proteinuria), or in some instances, a production of only excess κ or λ light chain molecules. Occasionally, plasma cells do not secrete any paraproteins (nonsecretory type myeloma); however, they usually have cytoplasmic immunoglobulin and produce low levels of immunoglobulins undetectable by current methods. Although myeloma can be associated with any of the immunoglobulin subtypes, the IgM type is predominately associated with other malignant conditions such as Waldenström's macroglobulinemia and chronic lymphocytic leukemia (CLL).

HISTORY

The earliest evidence of myeloma has been reported from Egyptian mummies; however, the first published clinical description of the disease was reported in 1850 in England. A patient, Thomas Alexander McBean, presented to Dr. William Macintrye of London in 1845 with symptoms of episodic fatigue, diffuse bone pain, and urinary frequency. The urinalysis detected a urinary protein with a peculiar heat property, and McIntyre called it *mollities and fragilitas ossium* due to the patient's bony symptoms.[1] Later that year, Dr. Henry Bence Jones also tested urine specimens provided by Macintyre and corroborated the heat properties of urinary light chains. Bence Jones thought that the protein was the *hydrated deuteroxide of albumin* (now called Bence Jones proteins) and published his findings several years before Macintyre published his case report.[2] After the patient died in 1846, a surgeon, Dr. John Dalrymple, examined several bones, and his gross and microscopic observations are consistent with morphology of myeloma cells.

The term *multiple myeloma* was coined by Rustizky in 1873 following his independent observation in a similar patient with multiple bone lesions. Kahler, in 1889, published a review on this condition and the disease became known, particularly in Europe, as Kahler's disease.[3] Ellinger, in 1899, described the increased serum proteins and sedimentation rate in myeloma. In 1900, Wright described the involvement of plasma cells in this neoplasm and, for the first time, he described roentgenographic abnormalities in myeloma, which to date remain a hallmark of this disease.

The development of bone marrow aspiration in 1929,[4] electrophoresis to separate serum proteins in 1937,[5] and a later report of a specific spike in the γ globulin region, enhanced the diagnosis and understanding of myeloma. Identification of the heavy and light chains in the monoclonal protein by immunoelectrophoresis was described by Grabar in 1953, confirming the monoclonality of immunoglobulin in this disease. Other developments in recent times include understanding of the role of the bone marrow microenvironment in myeloma cell growth, survival, and development of drug resistance through cell–cell interactions and activation of cytokine networks.[6,7] The significance of chromosomal translocations in myeloma pathobiology, and more recently, the use of gene expression profiling and whole genome sequencing, are providing insights into the molecular pathogenesis of the disease.

No effective systemic therapy existed before 1947, when urethane was reported to show an effect in a few patients. However, a subsequent randomized trial indicated that the survival of patients receiving urethane was inferior to that observed with a placebo.[8] The first successful use of chemotherapeutic agent in myeloma was reported in 1958 by Blokhin and colleagues with the use of a racemic mixture of D-and L-phenylalanine mustards (Sarcolysine). Subsequently, the D- and L- isomers of phenylalanine mustard were tested separately, and the antimyeloma activity was found to reside in the L-isomer, melphalan. In 1962, Bergsagel and colleagues from the Southwest Oncology Group reported remissions in about one-third of myeloma patients treated with melphalan.[9] The administration of high doses of glucocorticoid was first reported to induce remissions in relapsing or refractory myeloma in 1967.[10] The use of melphalan in combination with prednisone was then studied extensively.[11] The role of high-dose therapy was investigated by McElwain in 1983, and the addition of bone marrow and, subsequently, stem cell transplantation improved safety and allowed for further dose escalation.[12] In the last 10 years, an elucidation of the genomic changes driving the disease process, coupled with improved understanding of the role of the bone marrow microenvironment in myeloma biology and the development of drug resistance, has led to the identification of novel targets and directed agents including immunomodulatory drugs, thalidomide, lenalidomide, and pomalidomide; proteasome inhibitors, bortezomib and carfilzomib; inhibitors directed at histone deacetylases, phosphoinositide 3-kinase (PI3K)/Akt signaling; as well as antibodies targeting CS1, CD138, and CD38.

EPIDEMIOLOGY

According to the most recent data from the Surveillance, Epidemiology, and End Results (SEER) program, multiple myeloma (MM) is a relatively uncommon malignancy in the United States, representing 1.4% of all malignancies in Caucasians and 2.0% in African Americans. Among hematologic malignancies, it constitutes 10% of the tumors and ranks as the second most frequently occurring hematologic cancer in the United States after non-Hodgkin's lymphoma. The prevalence of myeloma in the United States in 2011 was over 83,367 and estimated new cases in 2014 are approximately 24,050; 11,090 patients are expected to die from myeloma in 2014. The disease is more common in men and has an average annual age-adjusted (1970 US standard) incidence rate per 100,000 among Caucasians of 7.2 in men and 4.3 in women, whereas for African Americans, the incidence is 14.7 in men and 10.5 in women. The increased incidence in African Americans is not explained by factors such as social or economic condition, household size, or family income.[13] A study in the African population from Ghana has demonstrated an incidence of MGUS similar to the African American population, possibly implicating genetic risk factors.[14] The incidence rates for other ethnic groups including Asian/Pacific islanders, American Indians, and Alaskan natives are also lower relative to US Caucasians. The Chinese and Japanese populations similarly have a lower incidence than Caucasians. A recent survey of MGUS in 12,481 US patients showed significantly higher (p <0.001) prevalence of MGUS in African Americans (5.7%) compared with Caucasians (2.3%) (p = 0.001) or Hispanics (1.8%).[15] The incidence of multiple myeloma has slowly increased in the US Caucasian population since 1970; however, the incidence among African Americans has increased more prominently during the 1970s to 1990s. These observed differences in the prevalence have not been associated with any difference in the disease characteristics, response to therapy, and prognosis of myeloma worldwide.

The incidence of myeloma and other plasma cell disorders increases with advancing age. The median age at diagnosis is 69 years. The mortality pattern also closely follows the incidence curves for age distribution, with a median age at death of 75 years. The proportion of patients surviving at 5 years in 2010 was 45%. As seen in Figure 48.1, fewer than 2% of patients are younger than 40 years, whereas almost 50% patients are older than 70 years. A similar age distribution is also observed in other related plasma cell disorders including MGUS and Waldenström's macroglobulinemia.

ETIOLOGY

Environmental Exposure

Exposure to ionizing radiation is the strongest single factor linked to an increased risk of multiple myeloma.[16] This has been documented in atomic bomb survivors who have a five times greater incidence than a control group with a latent period of approximately 20 years from exposure.[17] People exposed to low levels of radiation also demonstrate an increased incidence of myeloma, including radiologists, employees in the nuclear industry, or those handling radioactive materials. An association between exposure to various chemicals and the risk of multiple myeloma remains ill defined. Exposure to metals, especially nickel; agricultural chemicals; benzene and petroleum products; other aromatic hydrocarbons; agent orange; and silicon have been considered as potential risk factors.[16,18–20] In contrast, alcohol and tobacco consumption has not been clearly linked to myeloma. Among medications, only mineral oil used as a laxative has been reported to be associated with an increased risk of multiple myeloma in some patients.[21,22]

Hereditary and genetic factors may predispose patients to myeloma development.[23,24] Among 37 families with at least two family members who had myeloma, occurrence among siblings was reported in 25 of the families. However, direct genetic linkage has not been established. Myeloma risk also appears to be enhanced by the presence of HLA-Cw2 in both African American and Caucasian populations. In a study in 917 Ghanaian men, the prevalence of MGUS was twice that in Caucasian men, implicating race related genetic susceptibility in the higher rates of MGUS in African populations.[14] More recently, high throughput genomic studies have identified various novel genomic changes in myeloma with significant clinical implications. A meta-analysis of two genome-wide association studies in myeloma (N = 1,661) showed that the t(11;14)(q13;q32) translocation, in which CCND1 is placed under the control of the immunoglobulin heavy chain enhancer, was strongly associated with the CCND1 c.870G>A polymorphism (p = $7.96 \times 10[-11]$), suggesting a model where a specific chromosomal translocation is associated with a constitutive genetic factor.[25] Recently, Genome Wide Association Studies (GWAS) have identified common single nucleotide polymorphisms (SNP) at 2p23.3(rs6746082), 3p22.1(rs1052501), 3q26.2(rs10936599), 6p21.33(rs2285803), 7p15.3(rs4487645), 17p11.2(rs4273077), and 22q13.1(rs877529) to influence MM risk; the same SNPs were also evaluated for MGUS risk and four of these SNPs (rs1052501,

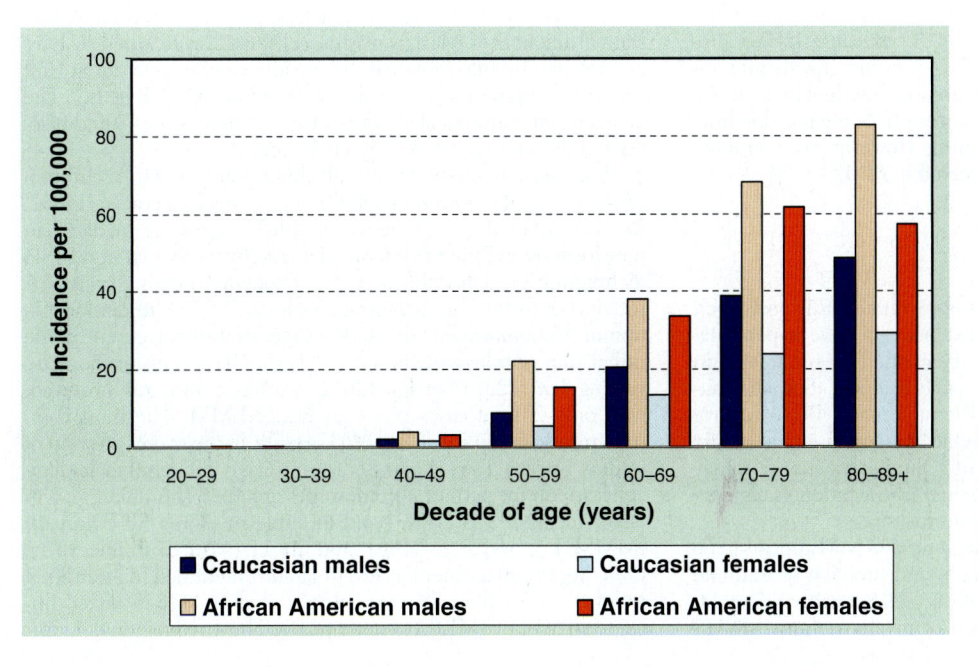

Figure 48.1 Multiple myeloma averages for age-, sex-, and race-specific incidence per 100,000 in United States, 1996 to 2000. An increase in incidence is noted with advancing age, and a higher incidence is observed in males than females and in the African American than in the Caucasian population.

rs2285803, rs4487645, and rs4273077) independently also influenced the development of MGUS. Collectively, these data support the view that genetic variation predisposes one to MGUS, thereby influencing the risk of developing MM.[26]

MGUS has been considered to be a premalignant condition; however, the rate of conversion to myeloma remains extremely low and is often associated with additional genetic changes.[27,28] Repeated infections or antigenic stimulation of the plasma cell compartment has also been proposed as a possible predisposing condition for developing myeloma. In one interesting patient report in the literature, a prior therapy with horse antiserum against tetanus led to a subsequent development of MGUS that lasted for 3 decades before conversion to MM. At the time of myeloma diagnosis, the serum IgG component was found to react specifically against horse α-2 macroglobulin.[29] This report suggests an initial antigen-driven stimulation of monoclonal protein-producing plasma cells, which eventually became malignant after acquiring additional genetic alterations. MGUS has been observed in mice dependent on strain of mice, age, preexisting immune status, and antigenic stimulation. MGUS has been associated with immune disorders and infectious diseases. In one report of 57 patients with MGUS who had undergone an evaluation for *Helicobacter pylori* infection for various gastrointestinal (GI) symptoms, 39 (68%) had evidence of *H. pylori* infection and 11 of these 39 patients (28%) had normalization of the serum paraproteins following eradication of this infection.[30] Seroprevalence of *H. pylori*, however, has not been consistently correlated with MGUS.[31] Development of MGUS has also been reported with T-cell deficiency disorders as in AIDS.[32] Importantly, a recent study indicates that the diagnosis of symptomatic MM is always preceded by MGUS by 2 or more years.[33]

Although epidemiologic studies have not been able to conclusively establish an association between MM and infectious or autoimmune diseases, a recent retrospective cohort study in US veterans demonstrated significantly elevated risks of MM in patients with a history of autoimmune, infectious, and inflammatory disorders. Risks for MGUS were generally of similar magnitude. These results indicate that various types of immune-mediated conditions might act as triggers for MM/MGUS development.[34] Although an initial report suggested the presence of the human herpes virus 8 (HHV8; Kaposi's sarcoma herpes virus) in the bone marrow dendritic cells of the majority of patients with MM,[35] analogous to its association with other lymphoproliferative diseases such as Castleman's disease,[36] body-cavity lymphoma,[37] and Kaposi's sarcoma,[38] other investigators have failed to identify HHV8 in myeloma cells or dendritic cells from various sources including mobilized peripheral blood stem cells.[39–42] Because HHV8 produces unique gene products, including possible growth promoting factors for myeloma such as analogs of interleukin 6 (IL-6), insulin-like growth factor 1 (IGF-1), and an IL-8, the possible linkage of HHV8 to myeloma was intriguing. However, even antibodies against HHV8 have not been observed in MM.[43]

PATHOGENESIS

MM is a germinal center–derived tumor with a mainly postswitch B-cell phenotype characterized by extensive Ig gene hypermutation in a pattern suggesting antigen selection. This is reflected in the exceedingly rare occurrence of IgM myeloma. Somatic mutations of other loci, such as B-cell lymphoma 6 (BCL-6), have also been reported in myeloma B cells, along with characteristic immunoglobulin gene rearrangement.[44] Similar mechanisms may be affecting other cell-cycle control genes whose products regulate cell proliferation and malignant transformation.

As in most malignancies, the pathogenesis of MM appears to be associated with dysregulated expression and function of multiple key cellular genes controlling apoptosis, cell growth, and proliferation. Understanding the evolution of myeloma from MGUS has provided a background for a multistep process involving alterations in various oncogenes and tumor suppressor genes.[45] In one study, the presence of 14q32 abnormalities were reported in patients with MGUS, and the addition of chromosome 13 change was associated with a transformation to overt MM.[46] This led to a theory that a subset of myeloma may derive from prior MGUS with a high incidence of monosomy 13, versus a second group of de novo myeloma in which other genetic abnormalities may be involved.[46] However, two recent reports suggest that all myelomas are preceded by MGUS[33,47] and that a small subset of MGUS carry del(13) along with t(4;14), which is not associated with an increased rate of progression to myeloma.[48,49] In one study in patients with smoldering myeloma, high-risk chromosomal aberrations (del(17p13), t(4;14), and +1q21) were observed in 35.9% of patients and predicted adverse prognostic factors for the progression to active myeloma, independent of tumor mass. Moreover, hyperdiploidy, which in myeloma is considered to be a low-risk feature, was present in 43.3% of smoldering and indolent multiple myeloma (SMM) patients and was an adverse prognostic factor.[50]

Myeloma occurs not only in humans, but also in mice, canines, and hamsters. In fact, genetic susceptibility to plasma cell tumors has been demonstrated in an inbred strain of mice. A common factor in various species has been the prevalence of endogenous retroviruses.[51,52] Animal models are now providing a basis for understanding the role of activation of oncogenes and tumor suppressor genes, cytokines, and the role of the bone marrow microenvironment in promoting and sustaining myeloma cell growth.

Cytogenetic and Molecular Genetic Alterations

Myeloma karyotypes are complex, with an average of 11 numeric and structural abnormalities per cell.[53] The relative incidence of gain or loss of various chromosomes with involved p and q arms are shown in Figure 48.2. The low proliferative activity of the tumor cells and possible clonal evolution have been obstacles to the identification of specific chromosomal and molecular changes in myeloma. The frequency and complexity of the chromosomal aberrations increases with advanced disease, and is uniformly abnormal in plasma cell leukemia. The detection of a complex karyotype predicts for poor prognosis. The newer techniques of multicolor fluorescent in situ hybridization (FISH) and spectral karyotyping, along with refined G-banding techniques, have identified many nonrandom changes in a large number of patients.[54–56] Using these techniques, over 90% of patients have involvement of at least one chromosome. A substantial fraction of MGUS plasma cells are also reported to have aneuploidy. By FISH analysis, the incidence of trisomy for at least one chromosome was reported in over 40% of MGUS cells.[57] The characteristic numerical abnormalities are monosomy 13 and trisomies of chromosome 3, 5, 7, 9, 11, 15, and 19.

The most frequent structural abnormality involves chromosome 1 and the immunoglobulin heavy chain gene at 14q32. By conventional cytogenetics, the 14q32 region is involved in translocation in 20% to 40% of cases, and by molecular and FISH techniques it is detectable at higher frequency, ranging from 50% in MGUS to 90% in advanced myeloma.[53,58,59] The demonstration of this abnormality in MGUS suggests its involvement in the initial step of transformation.[46,60,61] Light-chain translocations involving Igλ (22q11) or Igκ (2p12) are less commonly observed, with only 20% of cases even in advanced MM. The most common translocation involving 14q32 results in the overexpression of cyclins D1 (on 11q13) and D3 (on 6p21).[58,62] The other biologically important partner chromosomes are 4p16 (fibroblast growth factor receptor 3 [FGFR3] and multiple myeloma SET domain [MMSET]), 16q23 (c-MAF), and 20q11 (MAFB) (Table 48.1). Other recurrent partner loci less frequently identified include 8q24 (c-myc) in less than 5% cases, 18q21 (bcl-2), (11q23 mixed lineage leukemia 1 [MLL-1]), and 6p21.1. The 4p16 region contains

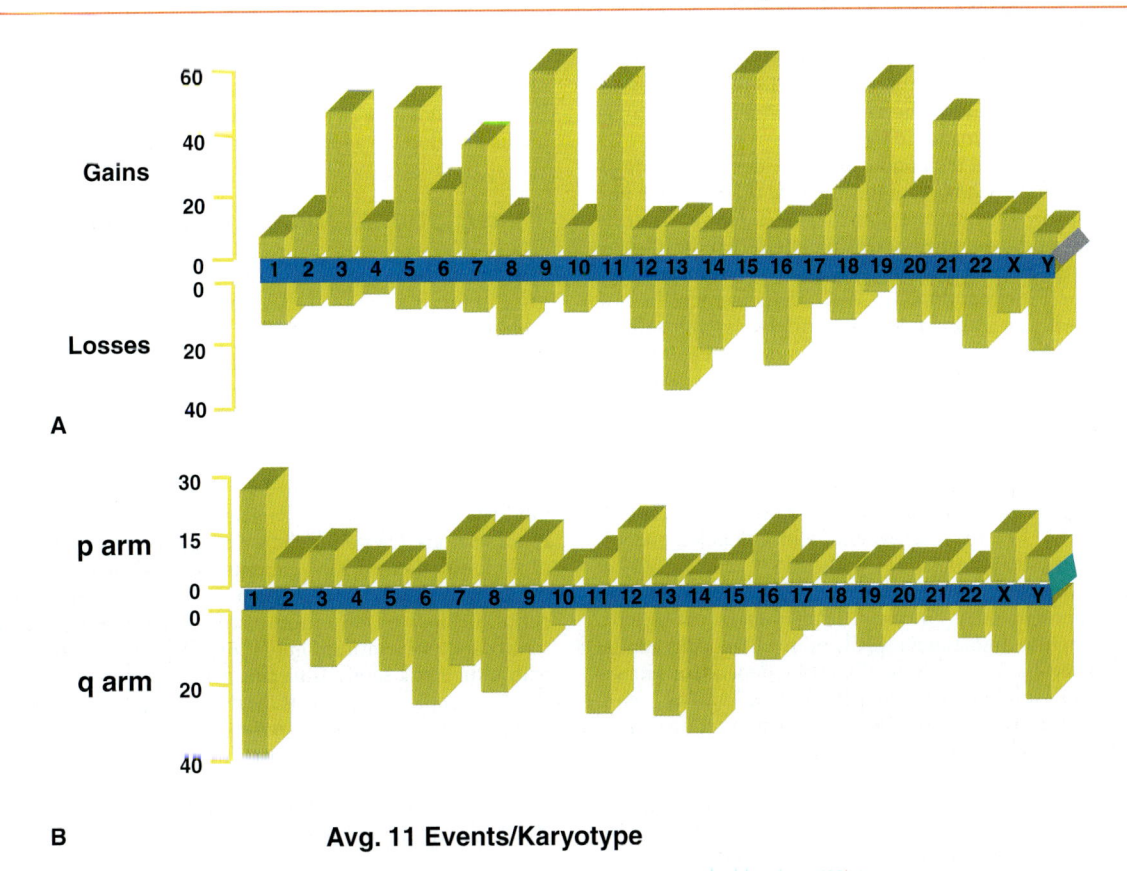

Figure 48.2 Summary karyotypic abnormalities in 158 patients with evaluable abnormal cytogenetics from a study of 492 patients demonstrating *chromosomal chaos*. **A:** Numeric changes with trisomies (gain) and monosomies (loss). **B:** Structural changes involving the short (p) and long (q) arm. (Courtesy of J. R. Sawyer.)

FGFR3 and MMSET genes. FGFR3 and its activating mutations trigger mitogen-activated protein (MAP) kinase signaling and growth of myeloma cells.[63] Mutated FGFR3 also confers resistance to caspase 3–related apoptosis.[64–66] This translocation also activates the *MMSET* gene, a homolog of *MLL1*, which is also independently involved in 11q23 translocation. With the enhanced sensitivity of spectral karyotyping, a nonrandom involvement of t(14:16) (q32:q22-23) has been described. A molecular analysis of the locus at chromosome 16q22 shows fusion of the immunoglobulin heavy chain with the sequence near the c-MAF oncogene, a b-ZIP transcription factor.[67] Additionally, translocation partners t(9;14) involving the paired box gene 5 (PAX-5) and t(6;14) involving interferon regulatory factor 4 (IRF4) gene have been described.[68,69] In the majority of cases, however, the translocating

TABLE 48.1
Recurrent Chromosomal Aberrations

Nonimmunoglobulin Sites for Illegitimate Switch Recombination in Multiple Myeloma

Chromosome	Frequency % Patients	Gene(s)	Function
11q13	30	Cyclin D1	Induces growth
4p16	25	FGFR3, MMSET	Growth factor
8q24	5	c-myc	Growth/apoptosis
16q23	1	c-maf	Transcription factor
6p25	<1	IRF4 transcription factor	Differentiation and growth
9p13	1	PAX-5	Transcription factor
20q12	1	MAFB	Transcription factor
18q21	1	Bcl-2	Antiapoptosis
Structural Chromosomal Aberrations			
del 17p13	15	p53 ?	
del 13	40–55	?	
Hypodiploidy	20–30	–	
Hyperdiploidy	45–50	–	

partner chromosome locus is not yet identified. Although 14q32 is one of the common translocations, its role in myeloma pathogenesis remains unclear due to the variety of partner chromosomes involved and its lack of prognostic significance.

Standard cytogenetics techniques did not identify rearrangements involving 8q24, which contains the c-MYC oncogene and is commonly involved in murine plasmacytoma. However, FISH analyses in one study identified karyotypic abnormalities that involve c-MYC in 45% cases of advanced myeloma.[70] Another study using interphase FISH confirmed c-MYC rearrangement in 15% of MM cases, with increasing frequency correlating with severity of disease. Interestingly, c-myc involvement is heterogeneous, suggesting its role in the evolution of disease.[71] Changes in c-MYC in the form of either abnormal size transcript or high level of expression have been reported in a majority of patients in one study.[72,73]

A deletion of chromosome 13 or 13q arm identified by conventional karyotyping confers a poor prognosis, even after high-dose therapy.[74] Using the RB1 gene as a probe, a FISH analysis reveals RB1 deletion in >40% of these patients.[75] In a detailed analysis of the 13q chromosome using an 11 probe FISH panel, >80% of 50 patients showed molecular deletions, with 13q14 representing a critical region most frequently involved.[76] Additionally, constitutive phosphorylation of retinoblastoma (pRB) in myeloma cells can be further enhanced by IL-6.[77] Cyclin D, cyclin-dependent kinases (CDK), and CDK inhibitors p15 and p16 (ink), p21 and p27 (cip), and p57 (kip), have also been investigated in myeloma due to their effect on pRB phosphorylation. Abnormalities in p16 and p15 have been reported in 75% and 67% of myeloma patients, respectively, suggesting an important defect in the pRB regulatory pathway.[78–80]

Mutations involving Ras are observed in about 30% of newly diagnosed MM patients, and are more frequently observed following progressive disease. Activating mutations of the ras oncogenes may also result in growth factor independence and the suppression of apoptosis in MM. One of the commonly altered genes in many malignancies is p53. In myeloma, abnormalities in p53 are detected in less than 10% of patients with early stage disease.[81,82]; however, p53 abnormalities represent an important late event associated with progression to an aggressive form of the disease. A study of p53 gene mutations in 52 patients with myeloma showed 7 of 52 patients to have p53 abnormalities, all with a clinically advanced and aggressive acute/leukemic stage of MM.[81] Murine double minute 2 (MDM2), an important inhibitor of p53 function, is overexpressed in the majority of myeloma cell lines; however, increased MDM2 expression is infrequently observed in primary myeloma cells.[83]

An important antiapoptotic gene, BCL-2, is uniformly overexpressed in low-grade non-Hodgkin's lymphoma. In this family of genes, BCL-2 and BCL-XL are antiapoptotic genes, whereas BAX, BAD, and BCL$_{XS}$ are proapoptotic genes. A balance between these genes determines cell survival. The t(14:18) translocation involving the BCL-2 gene is quite rare (2% to 3%) in myeloma. However, numerous myeloma cells lines as well as primary cells, express high levels of BCL-2.[84,85] Its relationship to development of drug resistance, as well as radiation resistance in myeloma cells is also well described.[86,87] One study in 63 patients showed a significant correlation between BCL-2 expression and resistance to therapy with interferon, but not melphalan and prednisone.[88] The association of BCL-2 expression with prognosis remains controversial, as one small study failed to show a correlation with short survival. BCL-XL is upregulated in myeloma cells as a consequence of IL-6–induced activation of signal transducers and activators of transcription 3 (STAT-3).[89] It confers a drug-resistant phenotype and, in conjunction with bcl-2, leads to increased genetic instability. Mcl-1, another antiapoptotic gene, is overexpressed in MM and is upregulated by IL-6. Its overexpression mediates potent resistance to apoptosis, and conversely, its downregulation by antisense oligonucleotide triggers apoptosis. Finally, Bcl-6 expression in MM cells is induced by its interaction with BMSC and is modulated, at least in part, via Janus kinase (JAK)/STAT-3 and canonical nuclear factor kappa B (NF-κB) pathways, and targeting Bcl-6, either directly or via these cascades, inhibits MM cell growth in the bone marrow (BM) milieu.[90]

High telomerase activity has also been demonstrated in myeloma cells, relative to normal cells and other malignant cell lines.[91] Telomerase activity confers growth and survival in MM, and is therefore an additional target for therapeutic intervention.

Transcriptional and Genomic Studies

Gene expression profiling, as well as studies focused on relative gains or loss of genomic DNA, have provided both prognostic and therapeutic information in MM. Molecular diagnostic tools and novel therapeutics now offer the potential for more accurate prognosis and personalized treatment.

The expression profiling studies in MM have provided insight into the progression of MGUS to MM, and provided the basis to predict outcome, as well as to identify potential therapeutic targets.[45] Expression studies have identified subtypes within the nonhyperdiploid group associated with specific chromosomal translocations.[92] A comprehensive expression profiling the survey of uniformly treated MM patients has identified 70 genes predictive of early disease-related death. Interestingly, one-third of these genes are located on chromosome 1, confirming the potential significance of chromosome 1 in MM pathobiology.[93] Patients with a high risk score using this gene signature had significantly shorter complete response (CR) duration (20% patients at 3 years) compared to those patients without such high risk features (60% at 5 years). A multivariate discriminant analysis identified a 17-gene signature that performed as well as the 70-gene model. A second large study by the Intergroupe Francophone du Myélome (IFM) group studied gene expression profiles in 182 newly diagnosed patients and developed a 15-gene model to calculate a risk score associated with overall survival. In this study, the high-risk group had an overexpression of cell cycle progression and its surveillance-related genes, whereas a hyperdiploid signature and heterogeneous gene expression characterized low-risk patients. Overall survival at 3 years in the low-risk group was 91% versus only 47% in the high-risk group, and these results were independent of traditional prognostic factors.[94] In a recent study in 320 newly diagnosed myeloma patients from the Dutch–Belgian/German HOVON-65/GMMG-HD4 trial, gene expression profiling identified a 92-gene signature and 10 subgroups in MM, which may represent unique diagnostic entities with potential novel therapeutic targets.[95] Additional expression profile studies have begun to define subtypes of myeloma with different prognostic significance following various therapies. An apparent lack of uniformity in the genes identified by these investigations suggests that therapy-related factors may determine the influence of different classes of genes in MM. Based on cytogenetics as well as expression data, cyclin D dysregulation occurs in the early pathogenesis of MM.

A high-resolution analysis of recurrent copy number alterations, coupled with expression analyses in MM cell lines and primary MM cells using array comparative genomic hybridization (aCGH), has identified distinct genomic subtypes. Additionally, this study has defined 87 discrete minimal common regions that have identified gene candidates for targeted drug discovery, improved the understanding of MM initiation and progression, and improved the prediction of clinical outcomes (Fig. 48.3). A high-density, SNP array analysis of myeloma cells from 192 newly diagnosed patients identified genomic copy number alteration in 98% of patients.[96] Amplifications in 1q and deletions in 1p, 12p, 14q, 16q, and 22q were the most frequent lesions associated with adverse prognosis, whereas amplifications of chromosomes 5, 9, 11, 15, and 19 were linked to a favorable prognosis. Amp(1q23.3), amp(5q31.3), and del(12p13.31) have been identified in a multivariate analysis to be independent prognostic factors. This prognostic model was validated in an independent validation cohort of 273 patients with myeloma, and identified patients with amp(5q31.3) alone and low serum beta-2-M to have an excellent prognosis (5-year overall survival, 87%) versus patients with del(12p13.31)

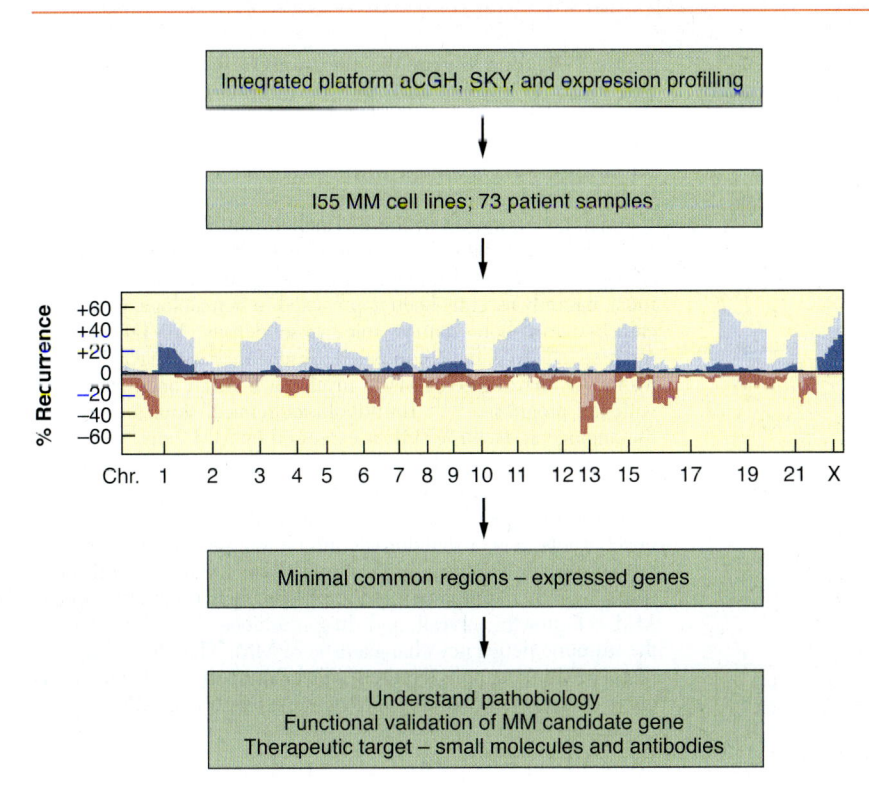

Figure 48.3 An array-based comparative genomic hybridization analysis evaluating 55 cell lines and 73 patient samples identified recurrent areas of gains and losses in multiple myeloma (MM) with the potential for understanding biology and validating target genes, which will then be potential therapeutic targets.

alone or amp(5q31.3) and del(12p13.31) and high serum beta-2-M with a poor outcome (5-year overall survival, 20%).

Epigenetic changes modulating myeloma cell growth and survival genes are also reported. For example, methylation of *p16*, a negative cell cycle regulator, is common and reported to be an early event even in MGUS. However, p16 methylation was not predictive of overall survival in a single large cohort study. The acetyl-lysine recognition domains (bromodomains) of putative coactivator proteins have been shown to play a significant role in transcriptional initiation and elongation as well as chromatin-dependent signal transduction. The bromodomain and extra-terminal (BET) bromodomain proteins have been identified as regulatory factors for c-Myc expression in myeloma, and their inhibition induces antiproliferative effects associated with cell-cycle arrest and cellular senescence in both in vitro and in vivo models.[97] A recent global methylation analysis (N = 159) of purified myeloma cells has identified prognostically important, epigenetically inactivated tumor suppressor genes. In this analysis, the combination of DNA methylation and gene expression profile identified hypermethylated GPX3, RBP1, SPARC, and TGFBI genes to be associated with significantly shorter overall survival, independent of other high-risk features such as International Staging System (ISS) stage or adverse cytogenetics.[98]

A role of microRNAs (miR) and potential therapeutic targeting of multiple mRNAs has recently been described in myeloma. miRNA expression profiling of MM and MGUS cells compared to normal donor plasma cells identified the overexpression of miR-21, miR-106b, and miR-181a and b in MM and MGUS samples, as well as selective upregulation of miR-32 and miR-17-92 in MM, but not in MGUS.[99] Another study analyzed the expression level of miRs and the gene expression profile in 60 newly diagnosed myeloma patients, and identified significantly dysregulated miRs expression in cytogenetically distinct subtypes.[100] The putative targets and their function are now being defined (e.g., miR-192, 194, and 215), which are downregulated in a subset of newly diagnosed myeloma, are transcriptionally activated by p53 and then modulate MDM2 expression. In addition, miR-192 and 215 target the IGF pathway, prevent the enhanced migration of plasma cells into bone marrow, and are positive regulators of p53, suggesting that their downregulation plays a key role in myeloma pathogenesis.[101] Recently, a role for miR-21,[102] miR-29,[103] and miR-34a[104] in supporting myeloma cell growth and survival have been defined, suggesting their potential as novel therapeutic targets.

Mutational changes in myeloma have now been evaluated using whole genome sequencing. An initial report using massively parallel sequencing of 38 tumor genomes and their comparison to matched normal DNAs identified several new oncogenic mechanisms based on the pattern of somatic mutations across the data set. These include mutations of genes involved in protein translation (seen in nearly half of the patients), histone methylation, and blood coagulation as well as NF-κB signaling, evidenced by mutations in 11 members of the NF-κB pathway.[105]

Using high-resolution SNP arrays (N = 24), clonal content and evolution was evaluated in myeloma. This analysis suggested selection and growth of genetically distinct subclones, which were not initially competitive against the dominant population but survived following therapy, with new acquired anomalies and subsequent outgrowth. These data point to the need to target and eradicate even a minor clone.[106] Recently, whole exome sequencing, copy number profiling, and a cytogenetics analysis performed in 84 myeloma samples have identified new candidate genes, including truncations of SP140, Lymphotoxin-beta (LTB), roundabout, axon guidance receptor, homolog 1 (ROBO1), and clustered missense mutations in early growth response protein 1 (EGR1). A further analysis revealed a complex subclonal structure including subclonal driver mutations. Serial sampling was performed in 15 patients, which revealed diverse patterns of clonal evolution: linear evolution, differential clonal response, and branching evolution. Diverse processes contributing to the mutational repertoire including kataegis and somatic hypermutation have been identified, and their relative contribution changed over time. This study demonstrates that the myeloma genome is heterogeneous, with clonal diversity at diagnosis and further evolution over time.[107]

Microenvironment and Cell Signaling

Myeloma cells express adhesion molecules that mediate interaction with the microenvironment, including both bone marrow stromal cell elements and extracellular matrix proteins (Table 48.2). These adhesion molecules mediate both homotypic and heterotypic adhesion. Adhesion not only plays a role in migration and

TABLE 48.2

Adhesion Molecule Expression on Normal Plasma Cells, Multiple Myeloma, and Plasma Cell Leukemia Cells

Adhesion Molecule	Normal Plasma Cell	MM Cell	PCL Cell
CD11a	+	−	−
CD11b	−	−	+
CD44	+	+	+
CD54	+	+	+
CD56	−	+	−
CD58	−	+	ND
LFA-1	−	−/+	+
VLA-4	+	+	ND
VLA-5	−	+	−
MPC-1	+	+	−
RHAMM	−	+	−/+
Syndecan-1	+	+	−
Surface Molecules			
CD19	+	−	−
CD28	−	−	+
CD38	+	+	+
CD40	+	+	+[a]
CD45	+	−[b]	−

PCL, plasma cell leukemia.
[a] CD40 expression is enhanced on PCL cells relative to normal plasma cells and MM cells.
[b] CD45 on immature myeloma cells.

localization of myeloma cells in the bone marrow, but also induces tumor cell growth and survival. For example, syndecan-1, a cell surface transmembrane heparan sulfate proteoglycan present on MM cells, interacts with type I collagen, and regulates growth of MM cells; it also mediates increased osteoclast activity.[108,109] Elevated levels of syndecan-1 shed into serum correlate with increased tumor mass, decreased matrix metalloproteinase-9 activity in the serum, and a poor prognosis.[108]

The BM microenvironment consists of a variety of cell types including stromal cells (BMSC), endothelial cells, osteoclasts, osteoblasts, as well as immune cells. The physical interaction between myeloma cells and these cells in the BM milieu plays a crucial role in MM pathogenesis both by direct adhesion-mediated signaling, as well as by secretion of factors such as IL-6, IGF-1, vascular endothelial growth factor (VEGF), B-cell activating factor (BAFF), fibroblast growth factor (FGF), stromal cell–derived factor (SDF) 1α, and tumor necrosis factor alpha (TNF-α), which mediate tumor cell growth, survival, drug resistance, and migration.[110–114] These interactions lead to the activation of several proliferative/antiapoptotic signaling cascades in MM cells: PI3K/Akt, Ras/Raf/mitogen-activated protein kinase (MAPK) kinase (MEK)/extracellular signal-related kinase (ERK), JAK2/ STAT-3, and NF-κB pathways. These pathways lead to MM cell growth, survival, antiapoptosis, migration, and development of drug resistance. Additionally, adhesion as well as cytokines secreted from MM cells and accessory cells in turn further augment cytokine secretion from these cells.

Activation of NF-κB has been noted in myeloma cells, especially following their interaction with BMSC. A number of abnormalities contributing to the dysregulation of NF-κB and constitutive activation of the noncanonical NF-κB pathway have recently been described.[115] Elevated expression of NF-κB-inducing kinase (NIK) due to genomic alterations or protein stabilization, and inactivating mutations of TNF receptor-associated factor 3 (TRAF3) able to trigger both classical and alternative NF-κB pathways have been reported.[116] These alterations activating the NF-κB pathway may allow MM cells to achieve autonomy from the bone marrow microenvironment.[117]

Each accessory cell in the BM milieu contributes differently to the overall effect of the microenvironment. The biologic and clinical relevance of increased angiogenesis, although established in solid tumors, has only recently been appreciated in hematologic malignancies. Increased bone marrow microvessel density (MVD) has been reported in MM patients compared to individuals with MGUS.[118–120] Moreover, the degree of MVD myeloma BM has been correlated with the prognosis.[121,122] Immunohistochemical studies show that the angiogenic factor VEGF is expressed by MM cells.[123] Hepatocyte growth factor, which also promotes angiogenesis, is increased in the serum of myeloma patients and predicts for poor outcome, especially in patients with increased β2 microglobulin levels.[124] Finally, novel agents such as thalidomide inhibit angiogenesis and can also overcome drug resistance in myeloma. Plasmacytoid dendritic cells (pDC), another component of the BM microenvironment, support MM cell growth, survival, and drug resistance, as well as mediate the immune deficiency characteristic of MM. Therefore, targeting pDC–MM interactions represent a therapeutic strategy to both overcome drug resistance and restore immune function in MM.[125]

Role of Cytokines

Myeloma cells and BMSCs produce cytokines including IL-6,[110] IGF-1,[111] VEGF,[112] SDF-1,[113] TNF-α,[111] TGF-β,[126] IL-17,[127] and others that mediate tumor cell growth, survival, antiapoptosis, migration, and the development of drug resistance.

Interleukin 6

IL-6 is an essential growth and survival factor for myeloma. The IL-6 receptor expressed by myeloma cells is composed of two polypeptide components: the α chain (gp80, IL-6Rα) and the signal transducing β chain (gp130). The gp130 component is shared by a family of cytokines including oncostatin M and leukemia inhibitory factor. The interaction of IL-6 with its receptor activates Ras/RAF/MEK/ERK, JAK/STAT, and PI3K/Akt signaling pathways, mediating growth, survival, and drug resistance (Fig. 48.4). IL-6 is mainly produced by stromal cells following the binding of myeloma cells and is also triggered by other cytokines including TNF-α,[111] IL-1β VEGF, and IL-17 in the BM milieu.[112] IL-6 mediates both autocrine and paracrine growth of myeloma cells. It increases the proportion of cells in S phase, prevents apoptosis of malignant plasma cells, and confers resistance to antitumor agents such as dexamethasone (Dex). Soluble IL-6Rα, shed by myeloma cells into the serum, can amplify the response of myeloma cells to IL-6; both high serum IL-6Rα levels and high serum IL-6 levels portend a poor prognosis. IL-6 and soluble IL-6Rα also mediate enhanced bone resorption by osteoclasts. To date, IL-6 has been targeted therapeutically using antibodies specific for IL-6 or its receptor. However, these treatment approaches have produced only transient responses in a small number of patients.

Insulin-like Growth Factor 1

IGF-1 is a growth and survival factor for human MM, which activates PI3K and MAPK signaling pathways mediating proliferation and antiapoptosis.[128,129] It induces more potent protection against Dex than does IL-6. IGF-1 upregulates FLICE-like inhibitory protein (FLIP), X-linked inhibitor of apoptosis (XIAP), and Bcl-2-related protein A1 (A1/Bfl1),[128] and increases telomerase activity, thereby further enhancing tumor cell growth and survival.[130] IGF-1 also mediates the adhesion and migration of myeloma cells via β1-integrin.[114] These studies have identified IGF-1 as a novel therapeutic target; both antibodies and small molecule inhibitors against IGF-1 have been investigated in preclinical studies.

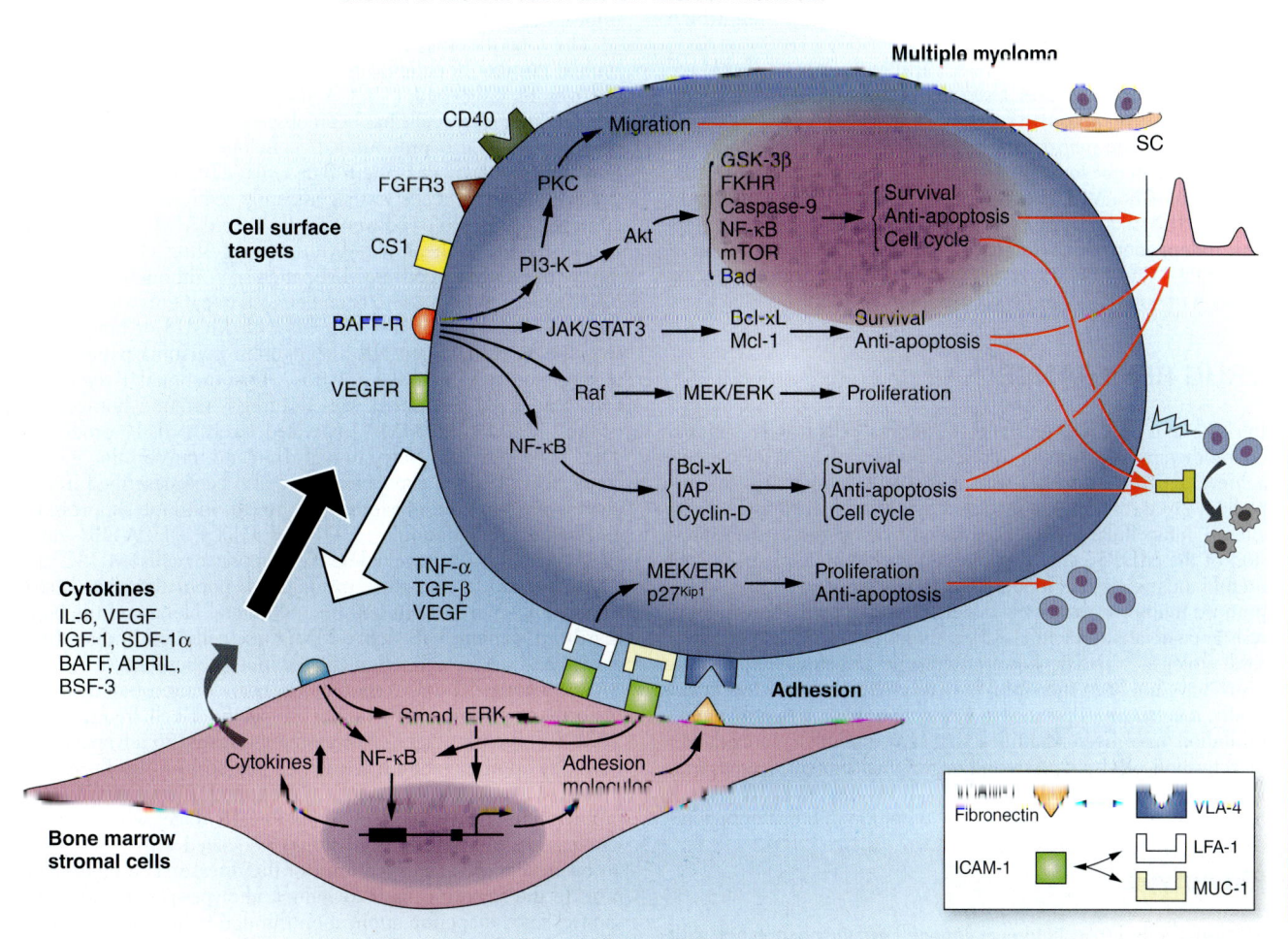

Figure 48.4 The interaction and adhesion of multiple myeloma (MM) cells to the bone marrow (BM) stromal cells (BMSCs) leads to adhesion- and cytokine-mediated signaling. MM cell binding to BMSCs induces the activation of p42/44 mitogen-activated protein kinase (MAPK) and nuclear factor kappa B (NF-κB) in BMSCs. The activation of NF-κB upregulates adhesion molecules on BMSCs. Cytokines secreted through this interaction includes interleukin-6 (IL-6) secretion, tumor necrosis factor α (TNF-α), and vascular endothelial growth factor (VEGF) to activate the main signaling pathways (p42/44 MAPK, Janus kinase (JAK)/signal transducer and activator of transcription 3 (STAT3) and/or phosphatidylinositol 3-kinase (PI3K)/Akt and their downstream targets, which triggers MM cell growth, survival, and migration.
The RAS/RAF/MAPK kinase (MEK)/MAPK pathway mediates the proliferation of MM. JAK/STAT3 along with upregulation of BCL-X$_L$ and MCL1 mediates survival. PI3K/Akt through downstream activation of BAD and NF-κB, and/or inactivation of caspase-9 mediates antiapoptosis. NF-κB and forkhead in rhabdomyosarcoma (FKHR) modulate cyclin D and KIP1, thereby regulating cell-cycle progression. Signaling through PI3K induces downstream protein kinase C (PKC) activity and MM cell migration. ICAM1; intercellular adhesion molecule 1; LFA1, lymphocyte function–associated antigen 1; muc1, mucin 1; VCAM1, vascular cell adhesion molecule 1; VLA4, very-late antigen 4; IGF1, insulin-like growth factor-1; IL, interleukin; SDF-1α, stromal-cell-derived factor-1α. (Adapted from Hideshima T, Mitsiades C, Tonon G, et al. Understanding multiple myeloma pathogenesis in the bone marrow to identify new therapeutic targets. *Nat Rev Cancer* 2007;7:585.)

Vascular Endothelial Growth Factor

VEGF has only modest proliferative effects on myeloma cells; however, it plays a more important role in triggering tumor cell migration and angiogenesis.[131,132] Its production in the BM milieu is upregulated both by myeloma cell adhesion to BMSCs and by IL-6.[133] Because it is a specific endothelial cell mitogen, elevated levels in myeloma may account, at least in part, for increased angiogenesis.[123] Myeloma cells express fms-related tyrosine kinase 1 (FLT1), and VEGF triggers its phosphorylation and activation of downstream MEK and protein kinase C (PKC) signaling. These data have provided the preclinical rationale to evaluate VEGF as a therapeutic target. Although PTK787, a potent inhibitor of VEGF receptor, has shown antimyeloma activity in vitro,[134] it has not shown clinical activity.

Other Cytokines

TNF-α is secreted by myeloma cells and does not have any significant direct effect on myeloma cell growth and survival; however, it induces the secretion of IL-6 by BMSCs. It is also a strong inducer of NF-κB activation, thereby upregulating adhesion molecules, with resultant binding of myeloma cells to BM and cell adhesion–mediated drug resistance (CAMDR). Although specific antibody inhibitors of TNF-α have not shown a clinical response, thalidomide and its immunomodulatpry drug (IMiD) analogs have potent anti-TNF-α activity and can overcome CAMDR.

SDF-1 is expressed by BMSCs, and its receptor CXCR4 is expressed by myeloma cells. It induces only a minimal proliferative effect; however, it plays a more important role mediating migration.

TGF-β is produced by MM cells and induces the secretion of IL-6 by BMSCs; it also contributes to immunosuppression, which is characteristic of myeloma.

Increased serum levels of IL-17, IL-21, IL-22, and IL-23, the proinflammatory cytokines associated with Th17 cells, are also observed in myeloma. IL-17 promotes myeloma cell growth and adhesion to bone marrow stromal cells, as well as contributes to bone disease in myeloma. In combination with IL-22, it also inhibits the production of Th1-mediated cytokines including interferon gamma (IFN-γ).[135] IL-21 induces proliferation and inhibits apoptosis independent of IL-6 signaling. It triggers phosphorylation of Jak1, Stat3, and Erk1/2 (p44/42 MAPK). TNF-α upregulates expression of both IL-21 and IL-21 receptor (IL-21R).

DRUG RESISTANCE

Intrinsic and acquired resistance of plasma cells to conventional chemotherapy is common, and as a result, only 50% of patients achieve a partial response, with few complete responses to melphalan. Drug resistance is mediated by several mechanisms.[136] An altered intracellular drug concentration may be due to overexpression of the MDR1 gene, encoding for P-glycoprotein, an integral membrane protein that functions as an ATP-dependent drug efflux pump, a multidrug resistance–associated protein (MRP), and a lung resistance–related protein (LRP), a member of the class of major vault proteins.[137] To date, however, strategies targeting these mechanisms have not been successful in overcoming drug resistance. Recently, mechanisms operative in inducing resistance to proteasome inhibition have been identified that have included upregulation or activation of Hsp90, Akt, and aggresomal protein degradation. Downregulation of Cereblon or lack of degradation of IKZF1 or 3 has been shown to mediate resistance to immunomodulatory agents.

Phenotype

Myeloma cells display heterogeneous cell surface phenotypes, with differences both between different patients and within the same patient at different disease stages. In general, all myeloma cells express high levels of CD38, with immature plasma cells additionally expressing CD45 and the IL-6 receptor.[138–140] More mature myeloma cells do not express CD45 and lack IL-6 receptor expression.[141] A subpopulation of myeloma cells may also express CD10, CD56, or CD49e (very late activation antigen 5 [VLA5]).[141–143] CD28 expression is associated with more aggressive disease[144]; CD20 expression is present on 20% to 30% of myeloma patients, and can be further upregulated with IFN-α.[145] The identity of the myeloma stem cell still remains an enigma. B cells expressing CD19 and CD11b can be induced to mature on stromal cells into monotypic plasma cells, suggesting that this cellular compartment may contain myeloma cell progenitors.[146,147] Using allele-specific oligonucleotide polymerase chain reaction (PCR) and the severe combined immunodeficiency (SCID)-hu model, the myeloma stem cell will be better defined in the future. These cell surface characteristics have also allowed for the development of eight color flow cytometries to measure minimal residual disease.

Immune Status

Myeloma patients present with suppressed immune function due to a variety of factors. Most significant is the suppression of uninvolved immunoglobulins (e.g., in patients with IgG myeloma, there is suppression of serum IgA and IgM levels).[148] The factors causing this suppression include a direct effect of monoclonal immunoglobulin, increased soluble Fc receptor or Fc expressing cells, suppression of helper cell functions, monoclonal Ig, and macrophage-related factors that affect B-cell maturation to plasma cells.[149] The recovery of uninvolved immunoglobulins to normal levels following effective therapy has been associated with both improved survival and protection from infectious complications.

The total T-cell count may be decreased; however, in a substantial number of patients, it may be normal, with no significant changes in CD8 cells.[150–152] A stage-dependent suppression of natural killer (NK) cells has been observed.[153] Deficiency of CD4 helper cells is also pronounced.[154] In one study, the proliferation and frequency of Epstein Barr virus (EBV)- and influenza A (inf A)- specific T cells was significantly reduced in a cohort of 24 newly diagnosed or conventionally treated MM patients when compared with 19 healthy individuals, suggesting an impaired response of CD8+ T cells in MM patients.[155] Although a defect in NK T-cell function has also been detected in patients with progressive myeloma compared to patients with MGUS or nonprogressive disease,[156] invariant NK T cells from myeloma patients can be activated and expanded in vitro.[157] Dysfunctional T regulatory cells have been associated with disturbed immune homeostasis in both MGUS and MM.[158] Elevated levels of IL-17 producing Th17 cells, possibly related to high IL-6 and transforming growth factor beta (TGF-β) expression, have also been described in myeloma, and promote myeloma cell growth, immune suppression, and osteoclast function.[135] CD11b(+)CD14(−)HLA-DR(−/low)CD33(+)CD15(+) myeloid-derived suppressor cells (MDSC) are a heterogeneous, immature myeloid cell population that is also significantly increased in both the peripheral blood and the bone marrow of patients with active MM; these cells both induce MM growth and suppress T-cell–mediated immune responses.[159]

Anti-idiotype T-cell response has been demonstrated in the majority of patients, with higher Id specific T cell frequency in MGUS and early stages of myeloma compared to advanced disease.[160] This observation supports the hypothesis that a protective immunologic response plays an important role in controlling the proliferation of the malignant clone in early stages of the disease, whereas loss of immune regulation is associated with evolution to an overt or more aggressive form of the disease. These data also provide the scientific basis to induce idiotype-specific T-cell responses for therapeutic application through either vaccination in vivo or the production of idiotype- or myeloma-specific cytotoxic T lymphocytes (CTL) in vitro.[161]

Murine Models

Three different models of murine myeloma have been described to study myeloma pathogenesis. In an inbred C57BL/Ka strain of mice, 16% spontaneously developed monoclonal gammopathies without tumor formation by 2 years.[51,52,162] In another model, BALB/c mice with a low spontaneous incidence of monoclonal gammopathies, the induction of plasmacytoma or myeloma is observed after the intraperitoneal injection of mineral oil or pristane.[51] Plasmacytomas, which develop within the oil, or other foreign body–mediated granulomas and lymphoplasmacytic infiltration can be blocked by the administration of indomethacin and accelerated by subsequent infection of the mice with Abelson's virus. Interestingly, however, the C57BL/Ka strain, with a high incidence of spontaneous monoclonal gammopathies, is relatively resistant to the induction of plasmacytoma by mineral oil. Plasmacytoma progression is associated with the dysregulated expression of c-myc as a result of translocation analogous to t(8;14) in humans. These plasmacytomas produce IgA immunoglobulins, and a growth factor present in the peritoneal fluid has been confirmed to be IL-6. Additionally, when animals are raised in a germ-free environment, the incidence of myeloma after mineral oil stimulation is markedly reduced, whereas that of other lymphoid neoplasms increases.[51] These studies suggest an important role of immune stimulation in myeloma development. A third model uses subcutaneous growth of murine plasmacytoma cell lines such as MOPC11 in immunocompetent mice, which allows for the study of immune modulation.

Human myeloma cell lines can grow and disseminate in a SCID mouse model, providing a unique opportunity to study this disease in an in vivo setting.[161] The introduction of fetal human bone into SCID mice (SCID-hu) has allowed for the engraftment and proliferation of the stromal cell–dependent human myeloma cell line[164] as well as primary human myeloma cells[165,166] in >80% mice and the monitoring of tumor burden by the detection of human myeloma–specific protein (soluble IL-6 receptor) or human Ig and light chains in murine blood samples, respectively. In this murine model of primary human disease, the fetal bone undergoes osteoporotic and osteolytic change as a consequence of clonotypic plasma cell proliferation and production of human cytokines. This model provides a unique opportunity to study the importance of stromal cell–myeloma cell interactions, as well as genetic and molecular mechanisms critical for myeloma growth and dissemination in vivo, and may provide clues to the origin of myeloma stem cells, thereby providing the opportunity to evaluate new treatment approaches targeting the myeloma cell and its microenvironment and bone disease in myeloma. A transgenic Eu-directed X-box Binding Protein-1 (XBP-1) spliced isoform mouse model has been generated in which mice develop features of MGUS and progress to MM.[167] XBP-1 is a transcription factor that is required for plasma cell differentiation, which is expressed at high levels in MM cells versus normal plasma cells.[168] This model provides a unique opportunity to study the biology of human myeloma and assess novel therapies in vivo. Recently, conditional MYC transgene expression has been demonstrated in Vk*MYC mice, which eventually develop an indolent multiple myeloma with features characteristic of human disease. This model serves to highlight the role of myc in myeloma and provides a unique animal model to test therapeutic or preventative strategies in myeloma.[169]

CLINICAL MANIFESTATIONS

Patients with MM may be entirely asymptomatic and diagnosed on routine blood work or may present with a myriad of symptoms such as hematologic manifestations, bone-related problems, infections, various organ dysfunctions, neurologic complaints, or bleeding tendencies (Table 48.3). These signs and symptoms result from direct tumor involvement in BM or extramedullary plasmacytomas, the effect of the protein produced by the tumor cells deposited in various organs, the production of cytokines by the tumor cells or by the BM microenvironment, and effects on the immune system.

TABLE 48.3
Clinical Features of Multiple Myeloma

Symptoms	Common Cause
Bone pain	Pathologic fracture
Easy fatigue	Anemia, high serum IL-6, therapy
Nausea and vomiting	Renal failure, hypercalcemia
Recurrent infections	Low uninvolved Ig, T cell dysfunction, therapy
Paraplegia	Cord compression
Confusion and CNS symptoms	Hyperviscosity or hypercalcemia
Peripheral neuropathy	Nerve compression, amyloidosis, POEMS, immune-mediated effects, therapy induced

CNS, central nervous system; Ig, immunoglobulin; POEMS, polyneuropathy, organomegaly, endocrinopathy, monoclonal gammopathy, and skin changes.

Anemia

A normochromic normocytic anemia is usually observed in myeloma patients due to tumor cell involvement of the marrow as well as inadequate erythropoietin responsiveness. The suppressive effects of various cytokines on erythropoiesis and the effect of renal dysfunction on erythropoietin production are also contributing factors. High immunoglobulin levels exacerbate the anemia due to dilutional effects. Anemia gives rise to fatigue, weakness, and occasionally, shortness of breath. Erythropoietin (Epo) administration is, therefore, an important supportive care therapy for patients with symptomatic anemia. In one study, improvement in hemoglobin by more than 2 g per deciliter was observed in 60% of treated patients, and responses were more frequent in patients with low Epo levels than in patients with normal or high levels (72% versus 20%).

Renal Failure

Nephropathy is one of the serious adverse complications that can be observed at the time of clinical presentation. The etiology of renal failure can be multifactorial. The most common cause is the development of light chain tubular casts leading to interstitial nephritis (myeloma kidney).[170] Another common cause of renal dysfunction is hypercalcemia leading to osmotic diuresis, volume depletion, and prerenal azotemia. Other modes of kidney involvement in myeloma include light chain deposition disease, which is more commonly associated with kappa light chain proteins and impaired glomerular filtration, AL amyloidosis, which is more frequently associated with lambda light chain (especially lambda light chain subtype VI) and may have an initial presentation as nephrotic range proteinuria; and renal calcium deposition, leading to interstitial nephritis.[171–173] The presence of lambda light chains in the urine is also more commonly associated with myeloma kidney. Bence Jones proteins bind to a common peptide segment of Tom-Horsfall glycoprotein to promote heterotypic aggregation and deposition in the kidney.[174] Additional factors exacerbating renal failure in myeloma patients include the use of nonsteroidal anti-inflammatory drugs for pain control, hyperuricemia, nephrotoxic chemotherapeutic agents, intravenous contrast for radiographic studies, bisphosphonate therapy, as well as calcium deposition and stones in the kidney. The proteinuria observed in patients with amyloidosis is more often nonspecific, which can help to differentiate it from typical myeloma-related kidney disease characterized by excessive light chain excretion.[175] Pathologic renal changes similar to human myeloma–related nephropathy develop in IL-6 transgenic mice expressing IL-6 under metallothionein-1 promoter, indicating a relationship between constitutive high IL-6 expression in the liver, dysproteinemia and long acute-phase response, and renal changes.[176]

Hypercalcemia and Bone Disease

The mechanism of bone abnormalities in myeloma, especially destruction, is an unbalanced process of increased osteoclast activity and suppressed osteoblast activity. These changes are due to an increase in osteoclast-activating factors produced predominantly by the BM microenvironment and also by myeloma cells.[177,178] These factors include IL-1β, TNF-β (lymphotoxin), IL-6, and macrophage inflammatory proteins-1 (MIP-1) alpha.[179–182] The receptor activator of nuclear factor kappa B ligand (RANKL) plays an important role in osteoclast differentiation via its receptor located on the osteoclast membrane. A member of the TNF family, it was originally described as a factor secreted by T cells, which induces maturation of dendritic cells. RANKL is also secreted by stromal cells and osteoblasts and induces differentiation and maturation of osteoclast progenitors. Moreover, its production is elicited by factors such as parathyroid hormone (PTH), PTH-related peptide (PTHrP), and OAFs.[178,183] Osteoprotegerin (OPG) acts as a decoy receptor for RANKL,[184,185] and has been implicated in the development of bone changes in myeloma. Additionally, a recently identified soluble factor produced by myeloma cells, DKK-1, inhibits osteoblast activity and is being therapeutically targeted.[186,187] Similarly, activin A, a TGF-β family member that induces osteolysis by inhibiting osteoblast differentiation via SMAD2-dependent distal-less homeobox-5 downregulation, is now being targeted therapeutically.[188]

All of these factors contribute to the development of osteoporosis and lytic bone lesions. Radiographic findings of such destruction are shown in Figure 48.5. These bone changes frequently involve the vertebral column and result in compression fractures, lytic bone lesions, and related pain.

A new onset of back pain or other bone pain is a frequent presenting symptom in myeloma patients. Changes in the cytokine milieu and bone destruction may also lead to the development of hypercalcemia, which is observed in approximately 25% of patients at some stage of the disease. Symptoms of high calcium include mental status changes, lethargy, constipation, and vomiting. High paraprotein levels, low albumin levels, or both are commonly observed in patients with myeloma, and require measurement of ionized calcium. Hypercalcemia may also contribute to renal failure and should, therefore, be considered an oncologic emergency requiring prompt intervention.

Infections

Myeloma patients are at risk for developing recurrent bacterial infections due to deficiencies in both humoral and cellular immunity.[149,189,190] Various factors including high monoclonal immunoglobulin levels, soluble Fc receptor in serum, and TGF-β lead to the suppression of B-cell function, which in turn leads to depressed uninvolved immunoglobulins.[126,191] This impairment in the patients' ability to mount humoral responses predisposes patients to infections with bacteria that are ordinarily opsonized by antibodies against bacterial antigens. Patients also have profound T-cell dysfunction due to various immunosuppressive cytokines such as TGF-β and IL-6 secreted by the microenvironment and fas ligand, which is present on the membrane of myeloma cells. Additional causes of immune suppression include programmed death-ligand 1 (PD-L1) and programmed cell death protein 1 (PD-1) expression on MM cells and MM T cells, respectively, as well as increased T-regulatory cells in MM. The therapy for myeloma, especially high-dose corticosteroids, increases infection-related risks in these patients. Therapy with bortezomib is also associated with a higher frequency of herpes zoster.[192] The highest risk of infection is within the first 2 months of initiation of therapy, as well as in patients with renal failure and in those with relapsed and refractory disease. Recurrent bacterial, fungal, and viral infections in myeloma require prompt diagnosis and treatment with additional prophylactic measures while receiving immunosuppressive therapy. Infections are an important cause of morbidity and the most common cause of death in patients with myeloma.[193]

Neurologic Symptoms

The most common cause of neurologic abnormalities is related to a tumor mass effect, especially compression of the spinal cord or cranial or spinal nerves. This may present as motor or, less frequently, sensory neuropathy. An interesting constellation of symptoms described as POEMS syndrome (polyneuropathy, organomegaly, endocrinopathy, monoclonal gammopathy, and skin changes) is observed in osteosclerotic myeloma with prominent

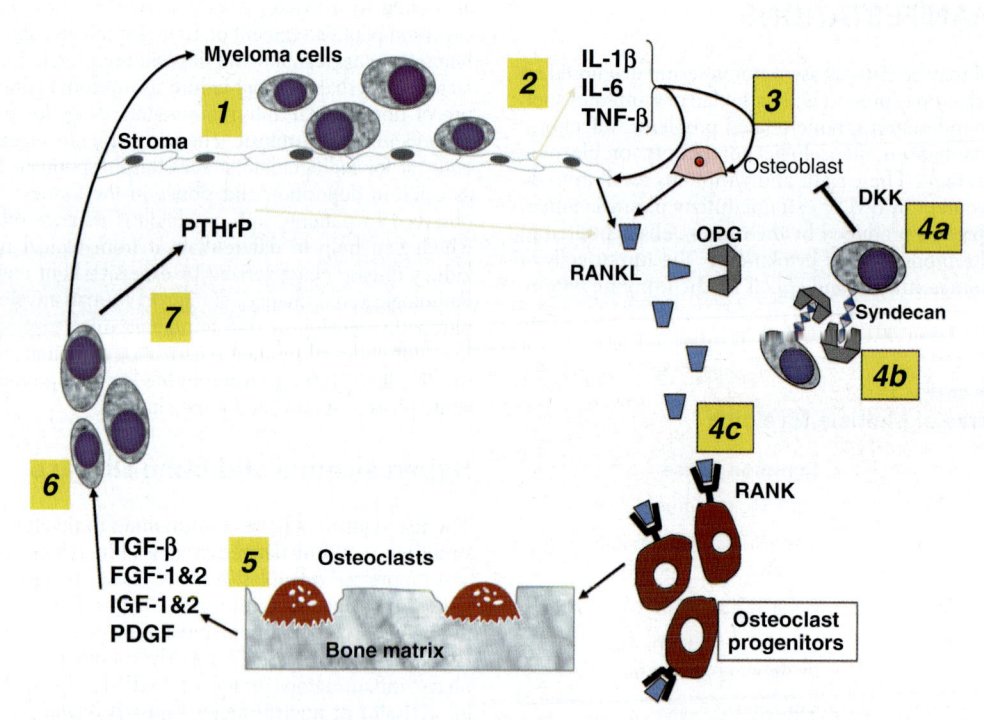

Figure 48.5 The biology of bone destruction in multiple myeloma (MM): **1.** MM cells adhere to stroma. **2.** Stromal cells secrete osteoclast activating factors (OAFs). **3.** OAFs elicit stroma and osteoblasts to secrete receptor activator of NF-κB ligand (RANKL). **4a.** DKK-1 produced by myeloma cells blocks osteoblast activity. **4b.** RANKL is blocked by osteoprotegerin (OPG); OPG levels are reduced in MM due to syndecan trapping OPG. **4c.** Excess RANKL is available to stimulate osteoclast differentiation and maturation. **5.** Increased osteoclastic activity leads to increased cytokine release from the bone matrix. **6.** These cytokines stimulate MM cell growth, which increases process number 1. **7.** These cytokines also cause a release of parathyroid hormone–related protein (PTHrP) from MM cells, which activate stromal cells to secrete additional RANKL. TGF, tumor growth factor; FGF, fibroblast growth factor; IGF, insulin-like growth factor; PDGF, platelet-derived growth factor; IL, interleukin; TNF, tumor necrosis factor.

sensory neuropathy.[194–197] The biologic and cellular basis of these manifestations is not yet well understood. Additionally, neurologic symptoms may occur as a consequence of hypercalcemia or hyperviscosity. Leptomeningeal involvement in myeloma with manifestations involving the central nervous system (CNS) has been described, usually in the late phase of the disease and associated with high-risk chromosomal abnormalities, plasmablastic morphology, and extramedullary manifestations.[198,199] Paraneoplastic CNS syndromes have also been described, possibly related to an immune mechanism directed at proteins present in the CNS, including the cerebellum. Peripheral neuropathy in myeloma may be due to an infiltrative process associated with the deposition of amyloid protein in the paraneural or *vasa nervorum*; due to a metabolic abnormality such as hypercalcemia, uremia, or hyperviscosity; or mediated by an autoimmune process or cytokines.[200] Peripheral neuropathy is also observed in patients with MGUS and more frequently associated with IgM paraprotein. More recently, peripheral neuropathy has been observed frequently with therapeutics, including thalidomide and bortezomib, especially with their prolonged use.

Hyperviscosity

The M components in myeloma can cause hyperviscosity and compromise circulation when the serum immunoglobulin levels exceed certain levels. The incidence is highest in Waldenström's macroglobulinemia with IgM, followed by IgA myeloma (25% patients), and is least common in IgG myeloma (<10% patients).[201–203] It can also be observed when immunoglobulins have a self-aggregating property leading to increased viscosity—for example, the IgG3 subclass is more commonly associated with hyperviscosity.[204] The syndrome is usually observed when serum viscosity exceeds 4.0 centipoise (cP) units relative to normal serum and manifests with circulatory compromise involving the CNS, the kidneys, and the lungs; it may also be associated with bleeding complications. Due to varying characteristics of idiotypes, the same level of increased viscosity may produce different severities of symptoms in individual patients. A high level of suspicion for this syndrome is important in any patient with paraproteinemia and either mental status changes or pulmonary distress, because prompt plasmapheresis can alleviate symptoms and avoid irreversible organ damage.

Coagulopathy

Myeloma patients may acquire coagulation abnormalities related to a high level of paraprotein interfering with the normal coagulation cascade or exhibit specific antibody activity leading to a clinical syndrome similar to acquired deficiency of factor VIII.[205,206] Additional factors, such as thrombosis in capillary circulation associated with hyperviscosity and anoxia, may lead to coagulation-related complications in 15% of patients with IgG myeloma and in more than 33% of patients with IgA myeloma. Although platelet counts are not suppressed in the early stages of myeloma, functional abnormalities of platelets have been described and may also contribute to bleeding.

Acquired activated protein C resistance is reported as a common single transitory baseline coagulation abnormality associated with venous thrombo embolism (VTE) in myeloma patients.[207] Additionally, patients may also present in a hypercoagulable state related to acquired deficiencies in protein S, or lupus anticoagulants leading to thromboembolic complications.[208] The fab fragment of the myeloma protein binds to fibrin and may prevent its aggregation.[209] Factor X deficiency is reported in patients with systemic AL amyloidosis[210]; however, an inhibitor has not been demonstrated in vitro to account for this manifestation.

Therapy may also increase the hypercoagulable state in myeloma. An increased incidence of deep venous thrombosis (12% to 24%) is observed in patients taking thalidomide and lenalidomide, especially along with dexamethasone or other combination chemotherapies. In one study, 12 out of 50 patients (24%) receiving thalidomide developed deep vein thrombosis (DVT), compared to 2 out of 50 (4%) patients receiving identical therapy without thalidomide.[211] Activated protein C resistance in the absence of factor V Leiden mutation and high serum homocysteine levels are associated with an increased risk of thrombotic complications with thalidomide.[212]

Extramedullary Disease

Extramedullary disease manifestations are uncommon in patients with myeloma at presentation. However, such manifestations have been observed more frequently in the setting of advanced stage disease or relapse following allogeneic transplantation. In a large study of 1,965 patients, primary extramedullary plasmacytoma was detected in 66 patients and secondary plasmacytoma was detected in 35 patients. The most common sites for extramedullary disease at diagnosis were the skin and soft tissues, whereas liver involvement was most prominent at relapse or progression. Extramedullary involvement may be suspected in patients who have more aggressive features of myeloma, including high lactate dehydrogenase levels, immunoblastic morphology, high tumor cell labeling index, and complex karyotypic features.[213] In the 70- and 80-gene risk models, it is associated with high-risk features and shorter survival.[214]

Diagnosis

As myeloma patients present with a variety of symptoms not specific to the disease, the diagnosis of myeloma is quite often delayed. An older patient with a new onset of unexplained back pain or bone pain, recurrent infection, anemia, or renal insufficiency should be screened for myeloma. Additional findings, including hyperproteinemia or proteinuria, anemia, hypoalbuminemia, low immunoglobulin levels, or marked elevation of erythrocyte sedimentation rate, should prompt for a further complete evaluation for a diagnosis of plasma cell myeloma.

The first step in the evaluation includes tests to confirm the presence, type, and quantity of monoclonal protein, as well as the detection and quantification of clonal plasma cells (Table 48.4). The second component to differentiate MGUS, SMM versus symptomatic myeloma is to identify end organ damage by performing a hemogram to detect anemia, a complete skeletal radiographic survey to detect bone lesions, and a chemistry profile to detect renal dysfunction and hypercalcemia. The diagnostic criteria for MGUS, SMM, and active MM are shown in Table 48.5.[215] A third component in the investigative workup involves an evaluation of prognostic variables including markers of tumor burden, genomic profiles, and therapy-related changes. Guidelines by the International Myeloma Workshop and National Comprehensive Cancer Center Network summarizes the standard investigative workup in myeloma.[216,217]

Protein Electrophoresis

Among patients with myeloma, 70% have IgG, 20% have IgA, and 5% to 10% have production of monoclonal light chains only. A small proportion (less than 1%) of patients produce monoclonal IgD, IgE, IgM, or have nonsecretory myeloma. The suppression of uninvolved immunoglobulins (e.g., IgM and IgA in IgG myeloma) is present in a majority of the patients at diagnosis. Suppression of all three major classes of immunoglobulins should raise the possibility that the patient may have light chain–only disease, IgD or IgE myeloma, or nonsecretory disease. Patients producing intact immunoglobulin can also have excess light chain production and excretion in the urine (Fig. 48.6). The distribution of κ and λ light chains in the majority of myeloma cases is similar, except in

TABLE 48.4
Patient Evaluation

Presence and Characterization of Monoclonal Protein
- Serum protein electrophoresis
- Quantitative immunoglobulin
- 24-hour urine: total protein and Bence Jones protein
- Immunofixation of urine and serum
- Serum free light chain and ratio

Detection of Clonal Plasma Cells
- Bone Marrow
- Aspirate and biopsy
  - Histology
  - Clonality by immunostaining: kappa/lambda
  - Flow cytometry
  - Cytogenetics and fluorescent in situ hybridization (FISH)

Laboratory Evaluation
- Chemistry panel (renal, calcium, albumin, uric acid, LDH)
- Beta-2 microglobulin, C-reactive protein

Radiologic Evaluation
- Skeletal Survey
- MRI with STIR Images
- Bone densitometry

Evaluation of Prognostic Factors
- Cytogenetics (metaphase karyotype and FISH)
- Serum B2 microglobulin and serum albumin
- Serum lactate dehydrogenase

Specialized Studies for Selected Patients
- Abdominal fat pad or rectal biopsy for amyloid
- Solitary lytic lesion biopsy
- Serum viscosity if IgM component or high IgA levels or serum M-component >7 g/dL
- Immunofixation for IgD or IgE in select cases

MRI, magnetic resonance imaging; STIR, short tau inversion recovery; CBC, complete blood cell count; LDH, lactate dehydrogenase; Ig, immunoglobulin.

IgD myeloma in which the λ light chain is more common. Currently, there is no difference in therapeutic approach between the different types of myeloma; however, patients with IgA myeloma, despite a higher initial response rate, have inferior survival.

Myeloma plasma cells usually produce a single, abnormal, and unique monoclonal antibody with a constant isotype and light-chain restriction. Rare occurrences of biclonal and triclonal cases have been reported at the time of diagnosis.[218] Occurrence of isotype switch and the appearance of abnormal protein bands have been reported in myeloma patients after treatment, especially high-dose therapy,[219] which appears to be related to the recovery of normal immunoglobulin production rather than alteration in disease biology. This change is also associated with improved survival. Occasionally, patients with initial intact Ig production relapse with only Bence Jones proteinuria (light chain escape) or nonsecretory disease, and this change has been correlated with more aggressive disease.[220]

A further analysis of a unique variable region in the myeloma-related idiotype (e.g., CDRIII) provides information on the monoclonal nature of the protein and also provides a tool to investigate minimal residual disease.[221]

Serum Free Light and Heavy/Light Chain

The measurement of serum free light chain (FLC) concentration has become an important tool to diagnose and follow the disease process, including response to therapy. It is especially useful in patients with light chain–only disease, oligo or nonsecretory myeloma, renal disease, amyloidosis, and as a prognostic marker, in MGUS and SMM, where an abnormal kappa/lambda free light chain ratio predicts a higher likelihood of progression to active myeloma.[222–226] Recently, a novel heavy/light chain (HLC) assay has been developed to quantitate the different light chain types of each immunoglobulin class (e.g., IgGκ, IgGλ, IgAκ, and IgAλ), which has been applied for both response assessments[227] and for prognostication.[228] For example, in a study where both HLC and FLC testing was utilized in 156 patients with IgG or IgA myeloma, the HLC ratio identified the presence of disease in 8 out of 31 patients with CR by conventional criteria.

Bone Marrow Examination

Various degrees of BM infiltration are observed in myeloma, with the majority of patients having an excess number of plasma cells. The pattern of BM involvement (diffuse versus nodular) is important, because patients with nodular disease seem to have poorer outcomes (in contrast to CLL).[229] The morphology of the plasma cell seems to be an important factor determining the severity of the disease. This is based on a histologic examination (Bartl grade) in which grade I suggests a slow growing disease, whereas grade III represents plasmablastic disease with an aggressive course.[230] There is also an increased incidence of cytogenetic abnormalities in patients with higher grade disease. Plasma cells contain cytoplasmic immunoglobulins with a constant heavy and light chain, which can be evaluated by a flow cytometric analysis or immunohistochemical staining of plasma cells.[231] When coupled with DNA staining using propidium iodide, a two-parameter analysis can detect changes in DNA content in myeloma cells (Fig. 48.7). DNA aneuploidy is observed in the BM of more than 80% patients, suggesting the existence of chromosomal abnormalities in the majority of patients.[231] This analysis also provides an objective marker to evaluate the response to therapy and to distinguish reactive from clonal plasmacytosis, especially in nonsecretory disease. A hypodiploid tumor cell has also been associated with refractoriness to standard-dose therapy.

Radiographic Evaluation

The radiographic survey of bone still remains a standard diagnostic evaluation, which shows osteopenia in an early phase of the disease and lytic punched out lesions associated with increasing tumor burden (Fig. 48.8). Osteosclerotic lesions are observed in POEMS syndrome.[194,196] Due to the predominant osteoclastic activity with osteoblastic inactivity, bone scans are seldom positive and are therefore not useful in the diagnosis of MM.

As demineralization of bone (osteoporosis) is one of the common manifestations of myeloma, measurement of bone mineral density (BMD) by dual-energy X-ray absorptiometry (DEXA) is an important evaluation at diagnosis.[232] In a study of 66 patients at diagnosis, the majority of the patients had decreased BMD with lumbar mean BMD value (Z score) 1.21 to 1.13. Following standard-dose therapy, lumbar BMD increased by 0.7%, whereas, in a group treated with high-dose therapy, the improvement was by 4.6% (p = 0.02).[233] Similar improvements in BMD have also been noted in patients undergoing high-dose therapy with the addition of bisphosphonates.[234] Differential effects of pamidronate on cortical and cancellous bone have been described in patients with myeloma undergoing autotransplants.[233,234]

TABLE 48.5
Diagnostic Criteria for Multiple Myeloma, Myeloma Variants, and Monoclonal Gammopathy of Unknown Significance

Monoclonal Gammopathy of Undetermined Significance (MGUS) or Monoclonal Gammopathy, Unattributed/Unassociated (MG[u])
M protein in serum <30 g/L
Bone marrow clonal plasma cells <10%
No evidence of other B-cell proliferative disorders
No myeloma related organ or tissue impairment (no end organ damage, including bone lesions)
Asymptomatic Myeloma (Smoldering Myeloma)
M protein in serum >30 g/L and/or
Bone marrow clonal plasma cell ≥10%
No related organ or tissue impairment (no end organ damage, including bone lesions) or symptoms
Symptomatic Multiple Myeloma
M protein in serum and/or urine*
Bone marrow (clonal) plasma cells* or plasmacytoma
Related organ or tissue impairment (end organ damage, including bone lesions)
*If flow cytometry is performed, most plasma cells (>90%) will show a neoplastic phenotype.
Solitary Plasmacytoma of Bone
No M protein in serum and/or urine*
Single area of bone destruction due to clonal plasma cells
Bone marrow not consistent with multiple myeloma
Normal skeletal survey (and MRI of spine and pelvis if done)
No related organ or tissue impairment (no end organ damage other than solitary bone lesion)*
*A small M component may sometimes be present
Nonsecretory Myeloma
No M protein in serum and/or urine with immunofixation
Bone marrow clonal plasmacytosis ≥10% or plasmacytoma
Related organ or tissue impairment (end organ damage, including bone lesions)
Extramedullary Plasmacytoma
No M protein in serum and/or urine*
Extramedullary tumor of clonal plasma cells
Normal bone marrow
Normal skeletal survey
No related organ or tissue impairment (end organ damage including bone lesions)
*A small M component may sometimes be present.
Multiple Solitary Plasmacytomas (± Recurrent)
No M protein in serum and/or urine*
More than one localized area of bone destruction or extramedullary tumor of clonal plasma cells, which may be recurrent
Normal bone marrow
Normal skeletal survey and MRI of spine and pelvis if done
No related organ or tissue impairment (no end organ damage other than the localized bone lesions)
*A small M component may sometimes be present.
Myeloma-Related Organ or Tissue Impairment (End Organ Damage) (ROTI)
Calcium levels increased: serum calcium >0–25 mmol/L above the upper limit of normal or >2–75 mmol/L
Renal insufficiency: creatinine >173 mmol/L
Anemia: hemoglobin 2 g/dL below the lower limit of normal or hemoglobin <10 g/dL
Bone lesions: lytic lesions or osteoporosis with compression fractures (MRI or CT may clarify)
Other: symptomatic hyperviscosity, amyloidosis, recurrent bacterial infections (more than two episodes in 12 months)

MRI, magnetic resonance imaging; CT, computed tomography.

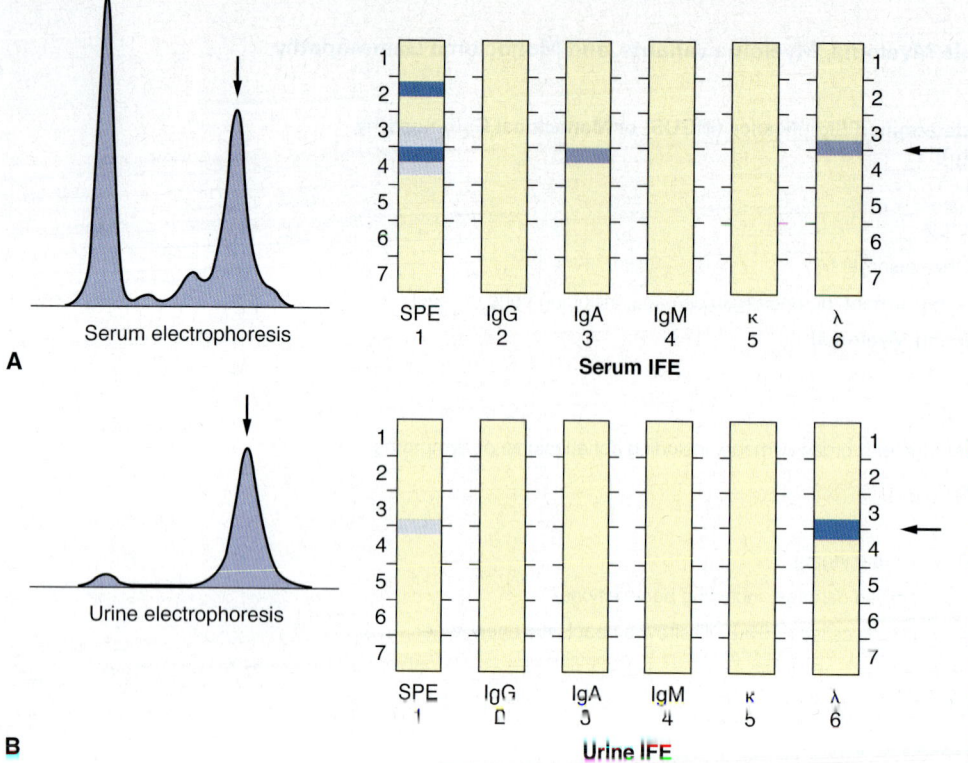

Figure 48.6 A: Serum (*top*) and urine (*bottom*) protein electrophoresis showing abnormal monoclonal protein bands (*arrow*). Quantitation of the M protein is performed by nephelometric measurement of the band. **B:** Identification of serum (*top*) and urine (*bottom*) M component by immunofixation technique. The labels indicate the specificity of the antiserum used in developing the immunofixation pattern. The top is IgA-γ in serum and the bottom is free γ light chain in urine.

Magnetic resonance imaging (MRI) of bone marrow provides a better assessment of tumor burden. More than 95% of myeloma patients have MRI abnormalities: one-third each have diffuse involvement of the bone marrow, focal lesions, or heterogeneous focal and diffused marrow involvement (Fig. 48.9A). Because myeloma is a macrofocal disease, random BM sampling may not be diagnostic or predictive of disease status, and MRI short tau inversion recovery images (STIR) may provide a better assessment of bone marrow involvement in myeloma.[235–237] An MRI of the spine and pelvis is required in all patients with a solitary plasmacytoma and SMM, both to detect occult lesions and to predict progression. In symptomatic myeloma, an MRI can be considered as a

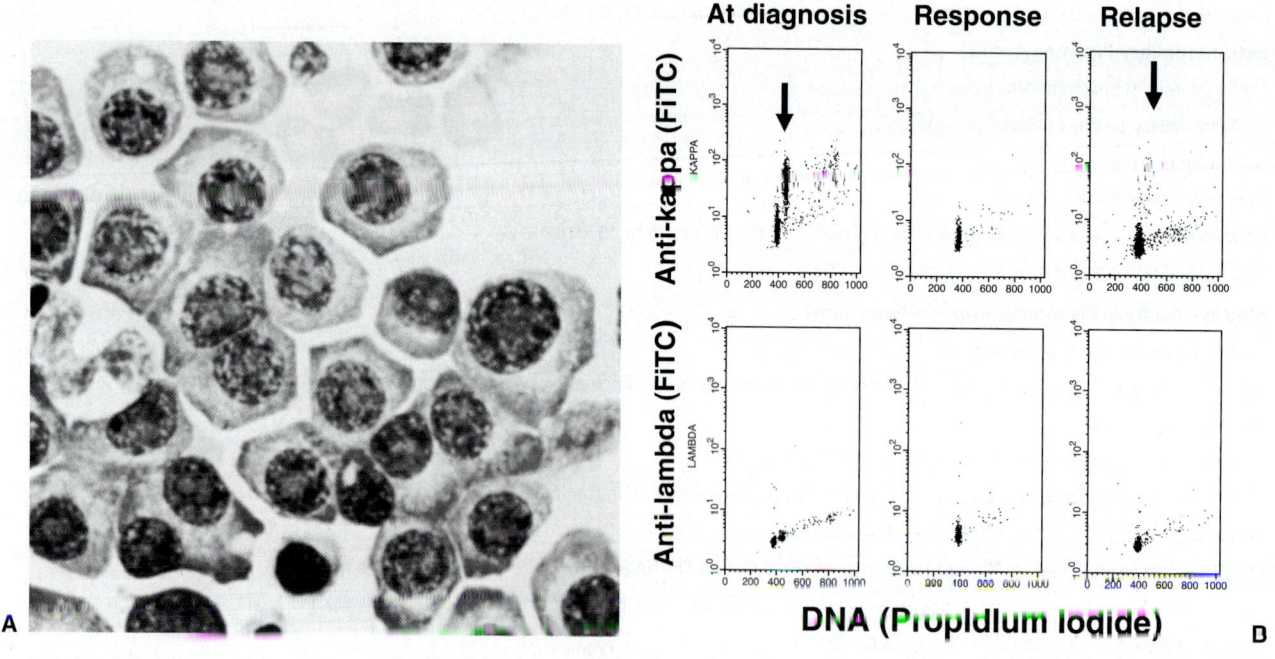

Figure 48.7 A: Bone marrow plasma cells in a patient with IgG myeloma showing neoplastic plasma cells at various stages of differentiation. **B:** Two parameter flow cytometry of DNA content of bone marrow cells; abscissa (propidium iodide) and cytoplasmic immunoglobulin (ordinate, anti-κ or anti-γ fluorescein isothiocyanate [FITC]). At diagnosis, approximately 45% hyperdiploid tumor cells show κ light chain restriction (*left panel*); at the time of maximal response, no hyperdiploid light chain restricted cells are seen (*middle panel*); at the time of early relapse, the reappearance of small hyperdiploid and κ light chain restricted population (<1%) is indicative of reemergence of small number of clonal cells, which may not yet be apparent on cytological examination of the bone marrow (*right panel*). A population of κ restricted but diploid cell population (*small arrow*) may represent a second clone.

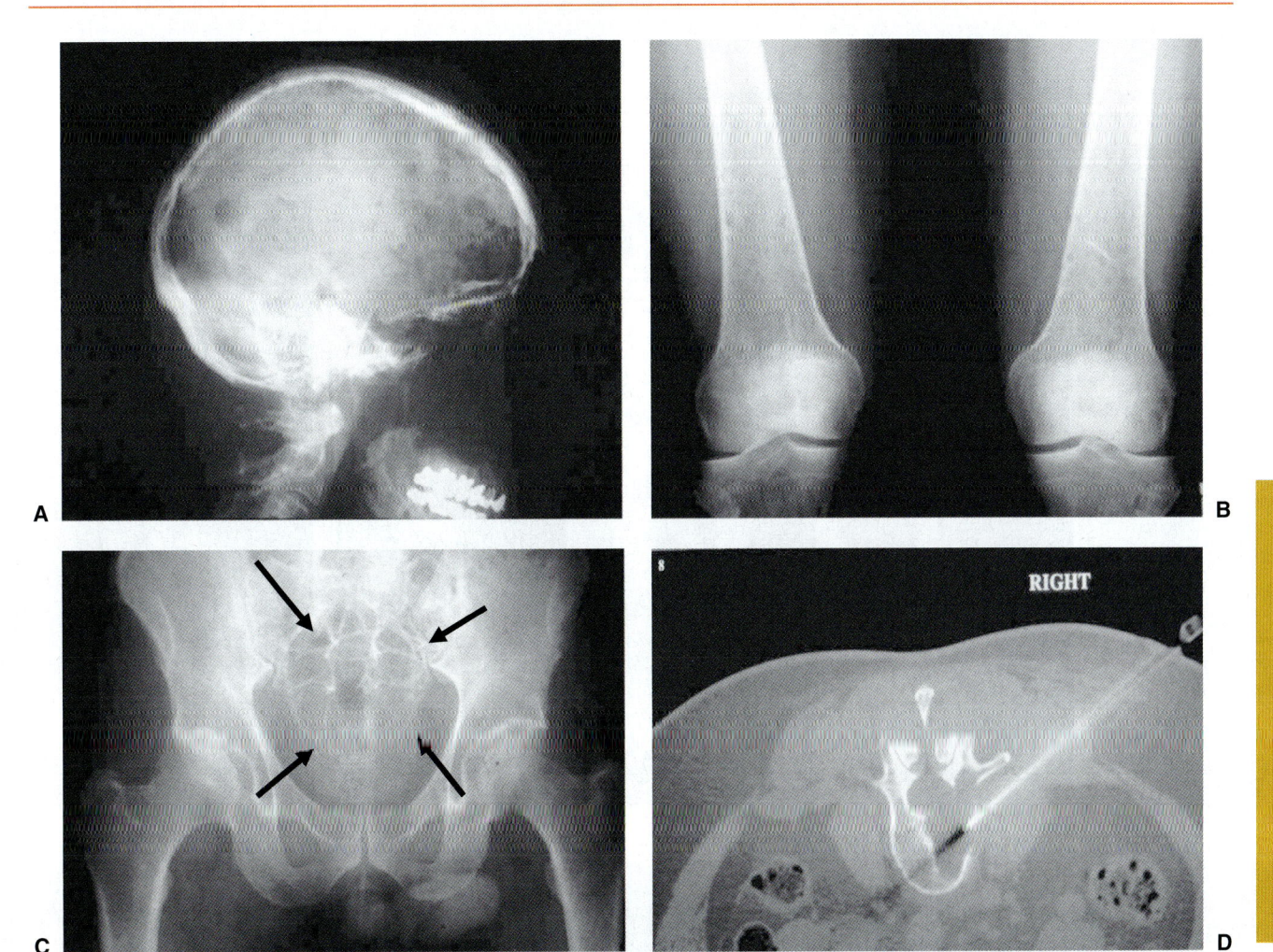

Figure 48.8 Typical skeletal changes on roentgenogram. **A:** Example of "punched-out" lytic lesions in skull. **B:** Small lytic lesions in the left femur. **C:** Large lytic lesion in sacrum. **D:** Fine-needle aspiration biopsy of the vertebral lesion. (Courtesy of Hemendra Shah.)

routine evaluation to detect unsuspected focal lesions and plasmacytomas involving the spine and pelvis, to define patterns of bone marrow involvement (i.e., diffuse pattern or a high number of focal lesions), to obtain a detailed evaluation of a painful area of the skeleton, and to investigate suspicion of cord compression.[238,239] A focal marrow plasmacytoma can be further analyzed through computerized tomography (CT)-guided fine needle aspiration (see Fig. 48.8), allowing for cytologic diagnosis. With effective therapy, the MRI pattern may change (Fig. 48.9B): Diffuse involvement of the marrow may evolve into focal disease, and normalization of MRI abnormalities may provide a better definition of complete responses.[237] Positron-emission tomography (PET) scanning has also been evaluated in a small number of studies and may provide a better functional definition of lesions observed on MRI or CT scans, as well as allowing for the selection of lesions for biopsy.[237,240] The PET–CT scan is utilized for the detection of extraosseous soft tissue masses, as well as for the evaluation of rib and appendicular bone lesions. A combination of PET–CT and MRI scans may improve the diagnostic accuracy for solitary plasmacytoma.[238] A recent study has identified the independent predictive value of baseline fludeoxyglucose (FDG)-PET/CT and of FDG suppression before high-dose therapy.[241]

Differential Diagnosis

In the presence of end organ damage associated with monoclonal protein and clonal plasma cells in bone marrow, the distinction of active myeloma from SMM and MGUS can be readily established (see Table 48.5). Patients with nonsecretory myeloma are diagnosed based on marrow plasmacytosis and the presence of bone lesions. MRI abnormalities and CT- or MRI-guided fine-needle aspiration biopsy of involved anatomic sites are important for the follow-up of the disease.

The diagnosis of solitary plasmacytoma of bone or soft tissue requires intense investigation to rule out systemic disease. Bone marrow examination in a true solitary lesion is normal, with no evidence of a clonal cell population. An MRI evaluation for myelomatous involvement of the BM helps detect early lesions before their detection by standard roentgenographic examination. The detection of such lesions and cytologic confirmation through CT- or MRI-guided fine-needle aspiration biopsy may help confirm a solitary plasmacytoma and its genetic makeup. In an individual with MGUS, such detection may change the diagnosis to solitary plasmacytoma or MM. It is important to note that patients with MGUS or solitary plasmacytoma seldom have suppression of uninvolved immunoglobulins. Conventional cytogenetic results are usually normal in MGUS; however, monoclonal plasma cells in some individuals with MGUS may be aneuploidy, and chromosomal abnormalities including IgH translocations and chromosome 13 deletions of unclear prognostic significance have been reported in MGUS.

Besides plasma cell neoplasms, various other conditions can present with monoclonal immunoglobulin secretion. These conditions include other B-cell neoplasms including CLL and B-cell non-Hodgkin's lymphoma; autoimmune conditions such as cold

	A	B	C	D
T1				
STIR				
A	Heterogeneous	Focal	Diffuse	Normal

B Pretherapy hyperintense marrow   Posttherapy hypointense marrow

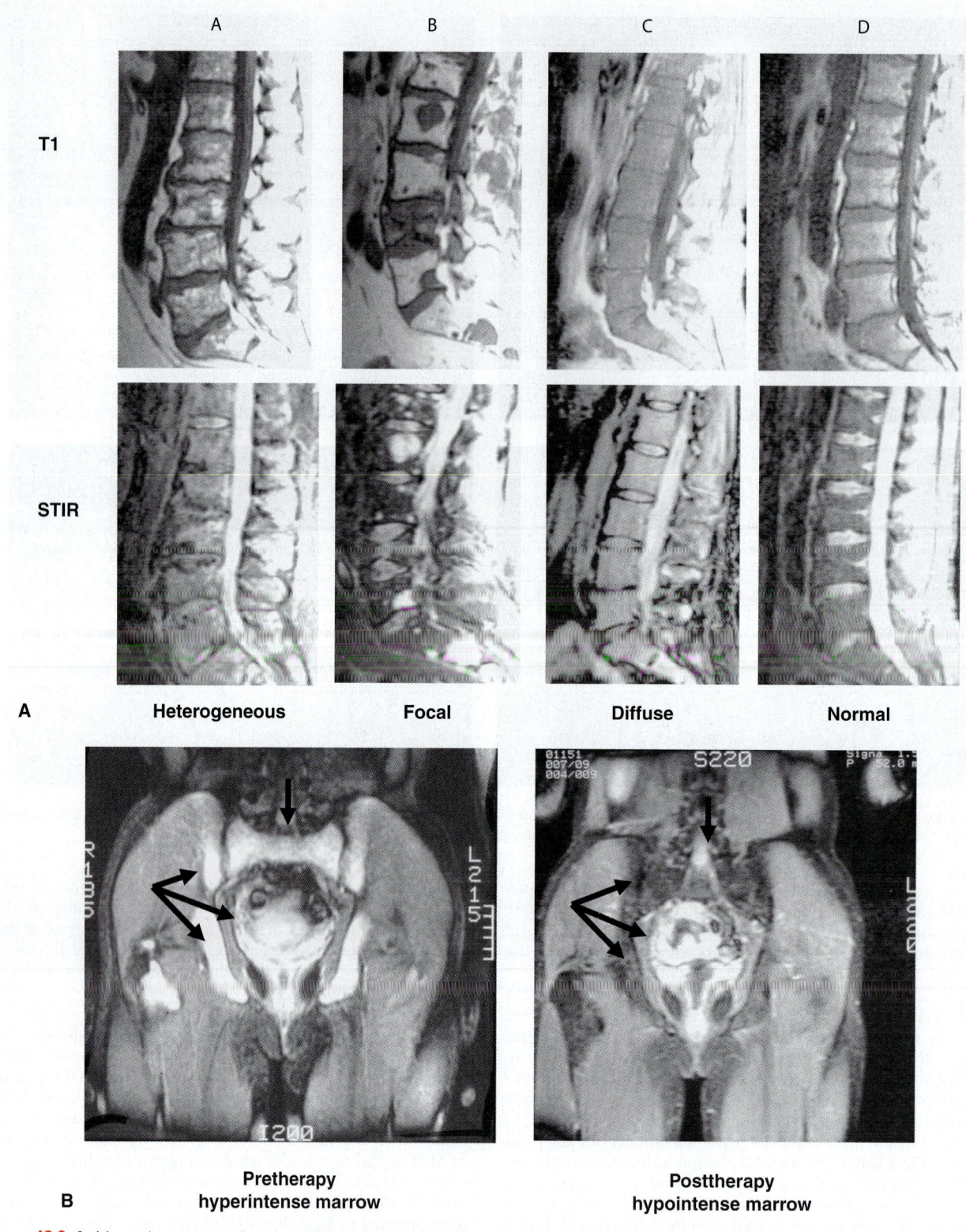

Figure 48.9 **A:** Magnetic resonance imaging (MRI) pattern in multiple myeloma at diagnosis: T1-weighted and STIR (short inversion-time inversion recovery) imaging shows approximately one-third of patients each presenting with heterogeneous pattern (*panel 1*), focal plasmacytoma lesions (*panel 2*), or diffuse homogeneous hyperintense marrow pattern (*panel 3*). Hyperintensity of marrow on STIR image is suggestive of uniform marrow involvement by myeloma. Few patients have a hypointense and homogenous pattern also seen in normal individuals (*panel 4*). **B:** The hyperintense marrow pattern suggestive of extensive marrow involvement pretherapy (*left, arrows*) changes to hypointense pattern following complete response and normalization of marrow (*right, arrows*); fine-needle aspiration examination in 73 patients with MRI focal disease showed a tumor in 93%, indicating that minimal response focal lesions in myeloma represent a tumor.

agglutinin diseases, mixed cryoglobulinemia, hypergammaglobulinemia, and Sjögren's syndrome; inflammatory or storage diseases such as lichen myxedema, Gaucher's disease, sarcoidosis, and cirrhosis; and rarely, other malignancies such as chronic myeloid leukemia as well as colon, breast, or prostate cancer.

Protein deposition disease involving various organs requires additional special diagnostic procedures. Deposition of amyloid protein (amyloidosis) can be clinically suspected based on macroglossia, vascular fragility (raccoon's eyes, periorbital subcutaneous hemorrhages), carpal tunnel syndrome, organomegaly, nephropathy, and cardiomegaly with arrhythmia. The detection of Congo red-positive amyloid with classic apple-green birefringence when visualized under polarized light in perivascular areas and subcutaneous fat, as well as bone marrow or rectal biopsy specimens, are diagnostic of AL amyloid. Electrocardiography may reveal low voltage, and an echocardiographic evaluation shows thickening of the interventricular septum or classic speckled pattern in the myocardium. Endomyocardial biopsy may establish the diagnosis of cardiac amyloid, which is usually associated with elevated serum brain natriuretic peptide (BNP) levels. Another manifestation of amyloid deposition includes autonomic dysfunction due to amyloid deposition in the vasa nervorum of the autonomic nerves, leading to orthostatic hypotension. Amyloid deposition in adrenal glands leads to hypoadrenalism; in the spleen, it may lead to hyposplenism with thrombocytosis; in the liver, it may be suspected based on elevated alkaline phosphatase and γ-glutamyl transpeptidase; and in the gastrointestinal tract, it may lead to malabsorption syndrome. Renal dysfunction must be further investigated with a renal biopsy, because light chain cast nephropathy or light chain deposition disease may be reversible following aggressive therapy, whereas deposition of amyloid requires a different therapeutic approach. As the deposition of immunoglobulin and light chain can mimic many manifestations of AL amyloid, an immunofluorescence analysis of unfixed tissue is important for a diagnosis.

Staging and Risk Assessment

Following the diagnostic investigation, more detailed cellular and molecular studies are required to stage myeloma and evaluate prognostic variables that determine the patient's probable outcome.

Patients with MM have variable disease courses, with survival ranging from less than 1 year with high-risk aggressive disease to more than 10 years with indolent presentation or sensitive disease. Various characteristics have been identified to predict the possible course of the disease. An evaluation of prognostic factors is important to define therapeutic strategies, permit comparison of clinical trial results, and predict life expectancy after diagnosis. The current risk stratification is applicable to newly diagnosed patients using parameters obtained at the diagnosis. On relapse, there is often an acquisition of additional or new risk features in which case patients should be reclassified as having high-risk disease. As shown in Table 48.6, prognostic factors are related to the tumor burden, the intrinsic property of the tumor, host and microenvironmental influences, and treatment/intervention-related factors.

A clinical staging system for MM using a standard laboratory measurement was developed by Durie and Salmon, which was predictive of clinical outcomes after standard-dose chemotherapy.[242] However, this staging system is not predictive of outcomes in patients undergoing high-dose chemotherapy as well as novel agents-based therapy and is no longer used clinically.

β2-microglobulin (β2M) has been identified as one of the most consistent predictors of survival in plasma cell myeloma. β2M, the light chain gene of the class I histocompatibility antigens expressed on the surface of all nucleated cells, is shed into the blood. Its renal excretion explains its elevation in renal failure. In MM, β2M, therefore, reflects both tumor burden and renal function.[243,244] High β2M (>2.5 mg per liter) levels carry a poor prognosis for treatment with both standard-dose and high-dose therapy.[245] The combination of serum β2M along with serum albumin has been proposed as a three-stage ISS (Table 48.7). Although this system predicts for outcome following both high-dose therapy as well as novel agents-based treatment, it lacks consideration of tumor biology–related factors, such as cytogenetics or molecular markers.

Cytogenetics

Because the myeloma cell represents a mature differentiated cell with low proliferative activity, cytogenetic abnormalities are not frequently detected. Abnormalities are observed in only one-third of the patients at the time of diagnosis; however, a repeated analysis increases the yield to almost one-half of patients. The normal karyotypic pattern observed in the remaining half most likely originates from dividing normal hematopoietic cells.[53]

Cytogenetic abnormalities have been identified as a major prognostic factor in plasma cell myeloma. Although the detection

TABLE 48.6

Prognostic Variable

Tumor-Burden Related Factors

β-2 microglobulin

>3 lytic bone lesions

Hemoglobin

Serum calcium

Tumor-Biology Related Factors

Cytogenetic/FISH abnormality (t(4;14), t(14;16), del17p-); hypodiploidy

Gene expression profile pattern

Plasma cell labeling index

Bartl grade

Mitotic activity

IgA myeloma

C-reactive protein (CRP)

LDH

Soluble IL-6 receptor

Renal failure

Tumor Microenvironment-Related Factors

Bone marrow microvessel density

Serum syndecan-1 levels

MMP-9 levels

Soluble CD16

Treatment-Related Factors

Tandem transplant

Achieving complete response or very good partial response

Patient-Related Factors

Age

Albumin

Performance status

Other organ problems not related to myeloma or amyloid deposits

Ig, immunoglobulin; LDH, lactate dehydrogenase; MMP-9, Matrix metallopeptidase 9.

TABLE 48.7
International Staging System

Stage	Criteria	Median Survival (mo)
I	Serum β_2 microglobulin <3.5 mg/L Serum albumin ≥3.5 g/dL	62
II	Not stage I or III	44
III	Serum β_2 microglobulin ≥5.5 mg/L	29

There are two categories for stage II: serum β_2 microglobulin <3.5 mg/L but serum albumin <3.5 g/dL; or serum β_2 microglobulin 3.5 to <5.5 mg/L irrespective of the serum albumin level.

of any cytogenetic abnormality is considered to suggest a higher risk disease, the specific abnormalities considered as poor risk are cytogenetically detected chromosomal 13 or 13q deletion and detection by FISH of t(4;14); t(14;16) and del17p. Del13 or 13q- detected only by FISH and in the absence of other abnormality does not carry significantly higher risk, whereas t(11;14) does not predict superior outcome. The cytogenetic and interphase FISH analysis has identified numeric aberrations involving trisomies of chromosomes 3, 5, 7, 9, 11, 15, 19, and 21, which predict for favorable outcomes.[55] Limited studies have shown that 1q34+, and del1p may have clinical significance as a poor risk feature. Importantly, both bortezomib and lenalidomide are able to overcome adverse outcomes associated with chromosome 13 deletion and, to a lesser extent, t(4;14).[246]

Other independent factors associated with poor prognosis include elevated C-reactive protein (CRP), elevated serum lactate dehydrogenase (LDH) with extramedullary disease, serum IL-6, serum soluble IL-6 receptor, and IgA isotype.[247] Because CRP levels reflect IL-6 activity and elevated CRP levels can be associated with acute-phase reactions including inflammation and infections, the predictive value of elevated CRP in myeloma is important only when other possible causes for its elevation are ruled out. BM plasmacytosis reflects tumor burden, but does not predict survival. Peripheral blood monoclonal plasma cells predict for survival in myeloma: In a study of 254 patients, blood monoclonal plasma cell counts ≥4% in 57% patients were associated with a median survival of 2.4 years compared with 4.4 years in patients with less than 4% circulating plasma cells.[248]

Among the various other disease biology–related variables, plasma cell proliferation rate, as measured by the labeling index (LI), is a valuable prognostic factor: Early in the disease, the proportion of myeloma cells in the cell cycle is small; bromodeoxyuridine or tritiated thymidine methods show a median of 1% cycling cells at the diagnosis. With progressive disease, the LI increases, suggesting a more proliferative phenotype. The LI has important prognostic significance, because patients with more than 1% cells in the S-phase in BM have worse outcomes[231,249,250]; however, the lack of standardized reproducible methods to measure the LI has limited its use as a prognostic marker. One study combining β2M and LI identified a low-risk group with both parameters low, an intermediate-risk group with one parameter high, and a high-risk group with both parameters high to have median survivals of 71 months, 40 months, and 15 months, respectively.[250] Additional tumor-related factors predictive of inferior survival include an increased soluble IL-6 receptor level, elevated serum LDH with extramedullary disease, and increased tumor cell mitotic activity (greater than 1 per high power field).

Among the microenvironment-related factors, BM MVD has been identified as an important prognosticator. High MVD in BM (≥4 per high power field) at the diagnosis confers shorter event-free survival (EFS; 2.7 versus 4.3 years; $p = 0.03$) and overall survival (OS; 7.9+ versus 4.3 years; $p = 0.006$) after high-dose chemotherapy.[251] An increased level of serum syndecan-1, as well as reduced levels of soluble CD16, have been described to portend a poor prognosis.[252]

Among therapy- and intervention-related prognostic factors, the type of response and length of response to prior therapy are additional risk stratification criteria; progression while on therapy and a short duration of response to prior therapy are poor risk features. The speed of response does not suggest poor overall outcomes with newer agents.

The risk stratification is applicable to newly diagnosed patients. However, the myeloma cell can acquire new changes over time, acquiring the same genomic abnormalities at relapse that are predictive of poor outcomes at diagnosis. Thus, in good-risk patients, it is necessary to evaluate for high-risk features at relapse. There is also a consensus that the high-risk features will change in the future, with the introduction of other new agents or possibly new combinations.[253]

An analysis of genome-wide copy number alterations (CNA) in 192 newly diagnosed, uniformly treated patients with MM using high-density SNP array suggested global genomic instability in MM.[96] One of three distinct patterns of CNAs are present in 98% of cases. A multivariate analysis identified a prognostic model that includes amp(1q23.3), amp(5q31.3), and del(12p13.31) as the most powerful independent adverse markers ($p <0.0001$). The availability of larger scale expression profiling data in uniformly treated patient populations has provided the basis for RNA-based prognostic classification systems.[92] Three large studies have evaluated the prognostic significance of gene expression profiling to identify poor-risk patient populations: the UAMS 70-gene model,[93] the 15-gene IFM model,[94] and the 97-gene HOVON model.[95] Interestingly, these studies identified patients with a short survival, but were not designed to select patients with very good risk. It is intriguing that none of these models share common genes, highlighting the redundancy in the genes and pathways that control growth, proliferation, and survival; differences in the treatment used to define the patient population; and the complexity of tumor cell biology. These initial attempts at molecular classification and prognostication will need further validation and incorporation into more commonly available methods for larger application. Moreover, the high-risk features identified previously are highly dependent on the therapeutic intervention used. For example, the newer biologically based therapies such as lenalidomide and bortezomib are able to overcome drug resistance, and some traditional adverse prognostic factors are no longer predictive of survival. Additional molecular studies with FISH analysis, as well as proteomic and genomic analyses, including SNP, may identify future uniformly applicable prognostic systems.

TREATMENT

The therapeutic intervention in plasma cell disorders is dependent on the presenting condition. For example, individuals with the diagnosis of MGUS do not require immediate treatment. Patients with solitary plasmacytomas can be treated with local therapy only, whereas those with indolent asymptomatic myeloma can smolder for a long period of time prior to becoming symptomatic and requiring treatment.

Solitary Plasmacytoma

Solitary plasmacytoma requires specialized techniques for accurate staging, including a CT scan and MRI to exclude more disseminated disease. Solitary plasmacytomas of the bone involve vertebral bodies in one-third of patients and frequently affect men (70%) at a younger age (median 56 years).[254] A monoclonal protein in the serum is observed in 24% to 54% of patients, but no detectable monoclonal protein is observed, even on immunofixation, in the remaining cases. Extramedullary plasmacytomas are diagnosed less frequently and require a workup including MRI and PET scanning to rule out additional sites or disseminated disease. The optimal therapy for true solitary plasmacytoma is curative dose (4,000 to 5,000 cGy) radiotherapy.[255,256] With this dose, local tumor recurrence rates have been less than 10%; 30% of patients with solitary osseous plasmacytomas versus more than 70% of patients with solitary extramedullary plasmacytomas achieve long disease-free survival.[257,258] Monoclonal protein disappears after radiotherapy in 25% to 50% of patients, suggesting a possible eradication of the disease, conversely, the reappearance of monoclonal protein predicts for recurrence of the disease. With better staging using MRI, true solitary plasmacytoma of bone can be cured in a high proportion of patients.

Monoclonal Gammopathy of Unknown Significance and Smoldering Myeloma

Patents with MGUS or smoldering myeloma have a low tumor mass and indolent disease course presenting without specific symptoms. Such patients do not have end organ damage. In patients with indolent light chain disease, Bence Jones proteinuria does not exceed >10 g per day. About 1% patients with MGUS per year progress to symptomatic myeloma. Non-IgG subtype, abnormal kappa/lambda free light chain ratio, and serum M protein more than 1.5 g per deciliter are associated with higher incidences of progression from MGUS to myeloma. Patients with none of these risk features have a 5% chance of progression, whereas those with all three features have a 60% chance of progression to myeloma in 20 years. The features responsible for the higher risk of progression from smoldering myeloma to active MM are bone marrow plasmacytosis >30%, abnormal kappa/lambda free light chain ratio, and serum M protein >30 g per liter (3.0 g per deciliter). Patients with all three adverse features have a nearly 50% chance of progression in 2 years.[259,260] Typically, patients with MGUS require no therapy. Similarly, patients with smoldering myeloma are also not treated routinely until disease progression or the appearance of end organ damage, such as the development of bone lesions or anemia. However, ongoing clinical trials have focused on evaluating the role of early intervention to prevent the progression of smoldering to symptomatic myeloma. For example, an evaluation of thalidomide in 31 patients with indolent myeloma showed responses in 66% of patients, with the potential to delay the progression to symptomatic disease.[261] In a recent phase 3 randomized, open-label, trial, 119 high-risk smoldering myeloma patients were assigned to treatment (lenalidomide at a dose of 25 mg per day on days 1 to 21, plus dexamethasone at a dose of 20 mg per day on days 1 to 4 and days 12 to 15, at 4-week intervals for nine cycles) or observation.[262] Patients in the treatment group received a maintenance regimen (lenalidomide at a dose of 10 mg per day on days 1 to 21 of each 28-day cycle for 2 years) after completing induction treatment. After the induction phase, a partial response or better was achieved in 79% of patients in the treatment group, which increased to 90% during the maintenance phase. With a median follow-up of 40 months, the median time to progression was significantly longer in the treatment group compared to the observation group (median not reached versus 21 months, respectively; p < 0.001). Importantly, the 3-year overall survival rate was also significantly higher in the treatment compared to the control group (94% versus 80%; p = 0.03). The treatment was well tolerated. This study for the first time suggests that an early intervention in patients with high-risk smoldering myeloma may provide survival benefit. However, further investigations are necessary to establish an optimal patient population and directed intervention that may help with the prevention of progression of SMM to active MM and may prolong overall survival.

Symptomatic Multiple Myeloma

Standard-Dose Conventional Therapy

Oral melphalan and prednisone was the first successful combination chemotherapy for myeloma; subsequently, various other single agents and combinations, as well as high-dose chemotherapy regimens, have been investigated and reported to have significant antimyeloma activity.

Melphalan and Prednisone. Treatment with oral melphalan and prednisone (MP) achieves a partial response (PR) in 50% to 60% of patients, with 3% to 5% of patients achieving a CR, and provides symptomatic relief as well as tumor mass reduction.[263] The median response duration is 18 months, and OS is 24 to 36 months. The absorption of oral melphalan is unpredictable, requiring its ingestion on an empty stomach and an increase in dose if the patient does not develop cytopenia.[264] With the availability of an intravenous formulation, dose and pharmacokinetics are now predictable. Frequent complications after MP therapy include the development of cytopenia and, with chronic administration, myelodysplastic changes in the marrow. MP in any combination should not be used as induction therapy in patients eligible for high-dose therapy and stem cell transplant because melphalan damages stem cells and compromises the ability to mobilize adequate numbers of stem cells. As described as follows, MP is now combined with one of the novel agents.

VAD and Alkylating Agent-Based Combinations. Various chemotherapeutic combinations have been investigated in myeloma, including vincristine (V), cyclophosphamide (C), BCNU (B), melphalan (M), adriamycin (A), and prednisone (P). Commonly used combinations in the past include VBMCP or VMCP/VBAP.[265,266] These combinations are no longer utilized. Similarly, high-dose dexamethasone (40 mg orally on days 1 through 4, 9 through 12, and 17 through 20) in combination with 24-hour continuous infusion of vincristine (0.25 mg/m^2) and adriamycin (9 mg/m^2) (VAD) for 4 days[267] was once a preferred induction regimen achieving a nearly 50% response rate; however, with the availability of novel agent-based combinations, VAD is no longer used as an induction regimen.[268] Although effective, high-dose dexamethasone used in various dosages (20 to 40 mg) and schedules (once a week, 4 days every 2 weeks to a 4 days on and 4 days off regimen) have been associated with predisposition to systemic infections, as well as insomnia, hyperactivity, hyperglycemia, and psychiatric problems. An Eastern Co-operative Oncology Group study suggests that dexamethasone once a week in combination with lenalidomide may be less toxic and more effective than a high-dose dexamethasone regimen.[269] Glucocorticoids downregulate IL-6 production and induce apoptosis in vitro; conversely, myeloma cells can be rescued from glucocorticoid-mediated killing by the addition of IL-6 to in vitro cultures or by coculturing them with bone marrow stromal cells, which are a source of IL-6 in vivo.

Interferon. Interferon causes direct growth inhibition, as well as antiangiogenic and immunomodulatory activity. Although it has been one of the most investigated agents in myeloma especially in maintenance settings, it has not demonstrated significant beneficial effects.[270,271] A meta-analysis of eight trials involving 929 patients showed prolongation of relapse-free survival by 7 months and OS by 5 months in patients receiving IFN. However, a large US intergroup study failed to show a benefit of IFN maintenance after high-dose therapy.[272] IFN is associated with flulike symptoms, weight loss, impotence, depression, mental status changes, and cytopenias; in addition, its prolonged use has been associated with inability to mobilize stem cells, therefore, it is no longer utilized.

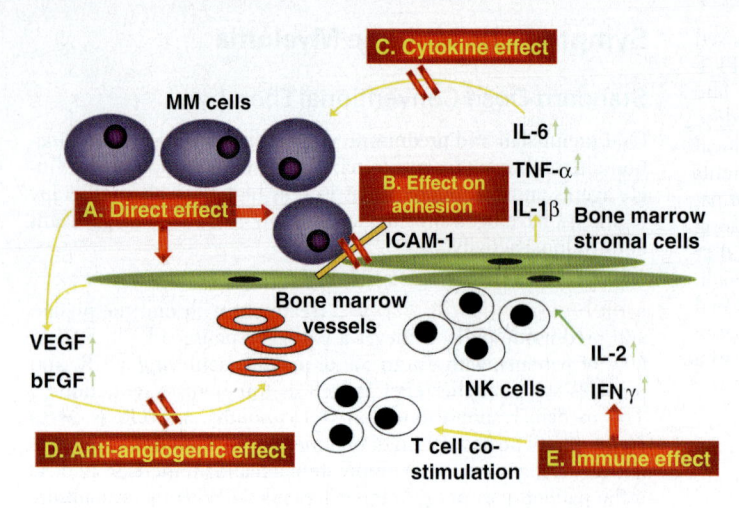

Figure 48.10 Potential mechanisms of action of thalidomide and its analogs. **A:** Direct effect on the myeloma cells. **B:** Inhibition of MM cell–BMSC adhesion. **C:** Inhibition of cytokine production in the microenvironment. **D:** Antiangiogenic effects through inhibition of the proangiogenic cytokines. **E:** Modulation of immune function, especially NK cells and T cells. MM, multiple myeloma; BMSC, bone marrow stromal cells; ICAM, intracellular adhesion molecule; IL, interleukin; TNF, tumor necrosis factor; VEGF, vascular endothelial growth factor; bFGF, basic fibroblast growth factor; IFN, interferon; NK, natural killer.

Radiation Therapy

Radiation therapy was considered the mainstay of treatment for myeloma prior to the availability of chemotherapeutic options. However, with more effective therapy, the role of radiation has now been limited.[273] A definitive role remains in patients with solitary bone and extramedullary plasmacytoma. Importantly, patients with solitary bone plasmacytoma treated with definitive radiation therapy (4,000 to 5,000 cGy) have progression-free survival of 30%, compared to 70% in those with extramedullary plasmacytomas.[255–258,274] The indication for radiation therapy in MM remains palliation in cases of impending pathologic fracture and to treat spinal cord compression. In patients with bone pain or symptomatic soft tissue masses, radiation is only considered when patients have failed chemotherapeutic options.[275,276] Radiation to BM-containing areas, such as the pelvic bone, should be used judiciously if there is a need for the collection of stem cells. The dose of palliative radiation therapy ranges from 1,500 to 2,500 cGy. Studies to date have failed to show any benefit of hemibody radiation in MM. However, total body radiation has been used prior to allogeneic and autologous transplantation. More recent studies have demonstrated that total body radiation does not provide additional cytoreductive potential; moreover, when combined with high-dose melphalan conditioning, it increases treatment-related morbidity and mortality, as well as delays immune recovery compared to high dose melphalan alone. Recent studies with nonmyeloablative regimens followed by allogeneic stem cell transplantation use low-dose radiation and achieve adequate engraftment, avoiding myeloablation and attendant toxicity of total body irradiation.

Novel Biologically Based Agents

Novel therapeutic agents specifically targeting the mechanisms whereby myeloma cells grow and survive in the BM milieu can overcome resistance to standard-dose and high-dose therapies. The immunomodulatory agents thalidomide and its analog lenalidomide, as well as the proteasome inhibitor bortezomib, are agents that have demonstrated efficacy in both relapsed and newly diagnosed myeloma and have now been integrated into standard algorithms for myeloma management.

Thalidomide. The initial rationale for use of thalidomide in myeloma was its known antiangiogenic activity, coupled with reports of increased angiogenesis in MM BM. Further investigations have shown that besides their direct effect on MM cells, thalidomide and other immunomodulatory agents (lenalidomide and pomalidomide) abrogate the adhesion of MM cells to BMSCs and block the secretion of MM growth and survival factors such as IL-6, TNF-α, VEGF, and FGF triggered by the binding of MM cells to BMSCs.[277] Additionally, these agents significantly modulate immune responses by expanding the number and function of NK cells, improving DC function, and enhancing T-cell function by providing T-cell costimulatory signals through the B7-CD28 pathway.[277] Importantly, two recent studies have shown that lenalidomide binds to cereblon (CRBN), the substrate-recognition subunit of a ubiquitin ligase complex. This in turn leads to specific ubiquitination and, subsequently, degradation of two related transcription factors, Ikaros family zinc finger 1 (IKZF1) and Aiolos IKZF3, with essential roles in B- and T-cell differentiation, as well as myeloma cell survival (Fig. 48.10).[278,279] A glutamine residue within the second zinc finger of IKZF1 and IKZF3 seems to provide the specificity of this interaction, because its absence in the highly homologous Ikaros family members IKZF2 and IKZF4 makes them resistant to lenalidomide. Importantly, the expression of IKZF1 or IKZF3 mutants lacking the key glutamine residue in the CRBN degron sequence or knockdown of CRBN conferred lenalidomide resistance. These results now provide a unique molecular understanding of lenalidomide activity, as a single agent or in combination.

Thalidomide was initially evaluated in a phase 2 study in 169 posttransplant-relapsed MM patients in incremental doses of 200 mg to 800 mg. A partial response was observed in 26% patients, with an overall response rate of 34%.[280,281] Subsequently, the efficacy of thalidomide alone and in combination has been confirmed in several phase 2 and 3 studies in MM (Table 48.8A). In combination with dexamethasone, it achieved >50% responses in relapsed MM patients and 70% responses in newly diagnosed patients. Additional combinations of thalidomide with MP have improved overall response, as well as both EFS and OS, in newly diagnosed patients over the age of 65 years (Table 48.8B). The major toxicities of thalidomide are somnolence, constipation, and neurologic symptoms, including neuropathy, fatigue, and DVT.[211] Due to the significant risk of DVT and pulmonary embolism when thalidomide is used in combination with dexamethasone, a prophylaxis against clotting is warranted in all patients. Although aspirin has been used as prophylaxis in patients at a low risk of DVT, either standard-dose Coumadin or low–molecular-weight heparin is indicated in patients at a higher risk of DVT.[282]

Lenalidomide. Lenalidomide, a more potent analog of thalidomide, in a phase 1 clinical trial, achieved at least a minimal response (at least a 25% reduction in paraproteins) in 15 of 24 (63%) patients, including in 11 patients who had received prior thalidomide.[283] A subsequent randomized study in patients with at least one prior therapy of lenalidomide and dexamethasone versus dexamethasone alone achieved PR or better rate (61% versus 20%; p <0.001); CR rate (14% versus 0.6%; p <0.001); a median time to progression (11.1 months versus 4.7 months;

TABLE 48.8A
Thalidomide Regimens in Relapsed/Refractory Multiple Myeloma

Study	Phase	N	Regimen	Media # of Prior Tx	Median TTP (mo)	CR/VGPR (%)	CR + PR (%)	Reference
Singhal	II	84	Thal	N/R	3.0 (EFS)	17	25	N Engl J Med 1999
Barlogie	II	169	Thal	N/R	~5 (EFS)	20	30	Blood 2001
Palumbo	II	77	Thal + Dex	2	12	18	41	Haematol 2001
Dimopoulos	II	44	Thal + Dex	3	4.2	30	55	Ann Oncol 2001
Terpos	II	50	MD-T	2	21.2	10 (CR)	62	Hematologica 2006

Tx, treatment; TTP, time to progression; CR, complete response; VGPR, very good partial response; PR, partial response; Thal, thalidomide; N/R, not reported; EFS, event-free survival; Dex, dexamethasone; MD-T, melphalan, dex, thalidomide.

p <0.001); and median overall survival (29.6 versus 20.2 months; p <0.001). In newly diagnosed patients, lenalidomide combined with dexamethasone achieves PR or better in over 90% of patients.[284] A similar study in Europe had almost identical results. Recently, lenalidomide and low-dose dexamethasone (Rd) versus melphalan, prednisone, and thalidomide (MPT) have been compared in a multicenter, open-label, phase 3 trial in newly diagnosed transplant-ineligible MM patients ≥65 years of age. A total of 1,623 patients (median age, 73 years) were randomized to one of three arms: Rd in 28-day cycles until disease progression (Arm A); Rd in 28-day cycles for 72 weeks (18 cycles, Arm B); or MPT in 42-day cycles for 72 weeks (12 cycles, Arm C). Overall response was 75%, 72%, and 62%, for Arms A, B, and C, respectively (p <0.00001). Continuous treatment with Rd (Arm A) had a 28% reduction in the risk of progression or death (hazard ratio [HR] = 0.72; p = 0.00006), with a 22% reduction in risk of death in favor of Arm A versus Arm C (HR = 0.78; p = 0.01685). All other secondary end points also showed an improvement in favor of Arm A versus Arm C; DOR (HR = 0.63; p <0.00001), and PFS2 (HR = 0.78; p = 0.0051). In Arm A versus Arm C grade 3/4 neutropenia was 28% versus 45% and neuropathy 5% versus 15%. This study establishes Rd with continuous treatment until progression as a standard of care in newly diagnosed MM in older individuals.[285] Tables 48.9A and B list selected major studies demonstrating the activity of lenalidomide in both relapsed and newly diagnosed myeloma. Importantly, no significant somnolence, constipation, or neuropathy is observed with lenalidomide. However, myelosuppression was the dose-limiting toxicity and requires monitoring during therapy. Similar to thalidomide, it is associated with an increased incidence of DVT and requires concurrent prophylactic measures for its prevention.[202] Due to its renal excretion, a dose modification is necessary when used in patients with renal dysfunction.

Bortezomib. Bortezomib is the first-in-class proteasome inhibitor originally used in MM due to its blockade of NF-κB activation and related paracrine IL-6 production by BMSCs. Bortezomib has been subsequently demonstrated to act directly on MM cells to induce apoptosis through both caspase 8 and 9 activation, to overcome the protective effects of IL-6, and to add to the anti-MM

TABLE 48.8B
Thalidomide Regimens in Newly Diagnosed Multiple Myeloma

Study	Phase	N	Regimen	CR/VGPR (%)	CR + PR (%)	1-yr Survival (%)	Reference
Rajkumar (Mayo)	II	50	Thal + Dex	N/R	64	N/R	JCO 2002
Cavo	II	71	Thal + Dex	17	66	N/R	Hematologica 2004
Rajkumar, E1A00	III	103	Thal + Dex	4 (CR)	63	80	JCO 2006
Rajkumar, MM003	III	470	Thal + Dex	44	69	80	ASH 2006
Palumbo	III	129	MP-T	36	76	87	Lancet 2006
Facon	III	124	MP-T	50	81	88	ASCO 2006
Barlogie	III	323	TT2 + Thal	69	83	92	N Engl J Med 2006
Goldschmidt	III	203	TAD	7	80	N/R	ASH 2005
Wang	II	36	Thal + Bort + Dex (VTD)	19	92	N/R	ASH 2005

CR, complete response; VGPR, very good partial response; PR, partial response; Thal, thalidomide; Dex, dexamethasone; N/R, not reported; MP-T, melphalan, prednisone, thalidomide; TT2, total therapy 2; TAD, thalidomide, adriamycin, dex; Bort, bortezomib.

TABLE 48.9A
Lenalidomide Regimens in Relapsed/Refractory Multiple Myeloma

Study	Phase	N	Regimen	Median # of Prior Tx	Median TTP (mo)	CR/VGPR (%)	CR + PR (%)	Reference
Richardson	I/II	24	Len	3	N/R	13	30	*Blood* 2002
Richardson	II	102	Len	>3	4.6	4	17	*Blood* 2006
Weber	III	171	Len + Dex	3	11.1	13	59	*ASCO* 2006
Dimopoulos	III	176	Len + Dex	3	11.3	15	59	*ASCO* 2006
Richardson	I	36	Len + Bort	5	N/R	6	39	*ASH* 2006
Richardson	I/II	28	Len + Bort + Dex	5	N/R	6	31	*ASH* 2006
Baz	I/II	52	Len + DVD (Len + PLD + Bort)	3	12	29	75	*Ann Oncol* 2006

Tx, treatment; TTP, time to progress; CR, complete response; VGPR, very good PR; PR, partial response; Len, lenalidomide; N/R, not reported; Dex, dexamethasone; Bort, bortezomib PLD, liposomal doxorubicin.

effects of Dex. Importantly, it acts in the microenvironment to inhibit the binding of MM cells to BMSCs, the secretion of MM growth promoting cytokines, and BM angiogenesis.[286–289] Based on its efficacy and safety profile in a phase 1 study, a multicenter phase 2 trial in 193 evaluable patients showed a 35% PR or greater response.[290] The median duration of response was 12 months, and the median OS was 16 months. Grade 3 adverse events included thrombocytopenia (28%), fatigue (12%), peripheral neuropathy (12%), and neutropenia (11%). The addition of Dex in this study improved responses in 19% patients, confirming synergism between these two agents. A subsequent randomized study in 669 patients with relapsed myeloma comparing bortezomib versus Dex reported a higher response rate (38% versus 18% respectively; p <0.001), a longer time to progression (6.22 months versus 3.49 months, respectively; p <0.001), and a longer survival (1-year survival rate 80% versus 66%, respectively; p = 0.003).[291] Tables 48.10A and B list selected major studies demonstrating its activity in both relapsed and newly diagnosed myeloma. In a randomized multicenter international study, the combination of bortezomib and pegylated liposomal doxorubicin was shown to be superior to bortezomib alone for both overall response (50% versus 42% respectively; p = 0.05) and time to progression (9.3 months versus 6.5 months respectively; p <0.0001), leading to U.S. Food and Drug Administration (FDA) approval of this combination in relapsed MM.[292] Bortezomib has been shown to overcome the adverse outcome associated with t(4;14),[293] can be given safely in patients with renal failure,[294] and improves osteoblastic activity.[295] The major toxicities include fatigue, diarrhea, reversible thrombocytopenia, and peripheral neuropathy. In a randomized phase 3 study of 222 relapsed MM patients, the subcutaneous administration of bortezomib was compared with traditional intravenous administration. overall response rates (ORR) after four cycles was 42% in both groups, and no significant differences in time to progression (median 10.4 months versus 9.4 months; p = 0.387) and 1-year OS (72.6% versus 76.7%; p = 0.504) were observed. Importantly, toxicity profiles were improved with the subcutaneous versus intravenous administration, including peripheral neuropathy of any grade (38% versus 53%; p = 0.044) and grade 2 or worse (24% versus 41%; p = 0.012), making subcutaneous administration a preferred route of administration.[296]

Induction Therapy in the Newly Diagnosed Patient

Decision about the induction regimen and its dose and schedule in newly diagnosed MM is partly influenced by the patient's age and comorbidities. Importantly, in a transplant-eligible patient, alkylating agents should be avoided because these agents may compromise stem cell collection. In newly diagnosed patients, thalidomide and dexamethasone have been demonstrated to be superior to dexamethasone alone (ORR 63% versus 41%, respectively; p = 0.0017).[297] Based on this data, thalidomide and dexamethasone is approved by the FDA as an induction regimen. With the availability of lenalidomide and bortezomib, alternative combinations have been investigated and are now preferred. The Southwest Oncology Group (SWOG) compared lenalidomide plus dexamethasone (LD) (n = 97) to placebo plus high-dose

TABLE 48.9B
Lenalidomide Regimens in Newly Diagnosed Multiple Myeloma

Study	Phase	N	Regimen	CR/VGPR (%)	CR + PR (%)	1-yr Survival Rate (%)	Reference
Rajkumar; Lacy	II	34	Len + Dex	56	91	90	*Blood* 2005
Niesvizky	II	42	Len + Dex + clarithro	51	94	86	*ASCO* 2006
Rajkumar, E4A03 Arm A	III	223	Len + standard-dose Dex	N/A	N/A	87	*Lancet Oncol.* 2007
Rajkumar, E4A03 Arm B	III	222	Len + low-dose Dex	N/A	N/A	96	*Lancet Oncol.* 2007
Palumbo	I/II	21	Len + MP (MP-R)	48	81	100	*EHA* 2007

CR, complete response; VGPR, very good PR; PR, partial response; Len, lenalidomide; Dex, dexamethasone; clarithro, clarithromycin; N/A, not available; MP, melphalan, prednisone; MP-R, MP+lenalidomide.

TABLE 48.10A
Bortezomib Regimens in Relapsed/Refractory Multiple Myeloma

Study	Phase	N	Regimen	Median # of Prior Tx	Median TTP (mo)	CR/VGPR (%)	CR + PR (%)	Reference
Richardson	II	188	Bort	>3	~7	10	27	N Engl J Med 2003
Richardson	III	333	Bort	2	6.2	4	43	N Engl J Med 2005
Richardson	I/II	28	Len + Bort + Dex	5	N/R	6	31	ASH 2006
Harrousseau	III	324	Bort + PLD	≥2	9.3	36	48	ASH 2006; ASCO 2007
Terpos	II	53	VMDT (Bort + Mel + Thal + Dex)	2	9.5	37	60	ASH 2006
Palumbo	I/II	30	Bort + MPT (VMPT)	3	N/R	43	67	ASH 2006

Tx, treatment; TTP, time to progress; CR, complete response; VGPR, verygood PR; PR, partial response; Bort, bortizomib; Len, lenalidomide; N/R, not reported; Dex, dexamethasone; Mel, melphalan; PLD, liposomal doxorubicin; Thal, thalidomide; VMDT, bortezomib, melphalan, dex, thalidomide; MPT, melphalan, prednisone, thalidomide.

dexamethasone (D) (n = 95) in newly diagnosed myeloma in a randomized study.[298] Overall response rate and 1-year progression-free survival were superior with LD (78% versus 48%; p <0.001 and 78% versus 52%; p = 0.002, respectively), whereas 1-year OS was similar (94% versus 88%; p = 0.25). Toxicities were more pronounced with LD (neutropenia grade 3 to 4: 21% versus 5%; p ≤0.001 and DVT despite aspirin prophylaxis: 23.5% versus 5%; p ≤0.001). A randomized study performed by ECOG compared lenalidomide at 25 mg daily for 3 weeks out of 4 along with high-dose Dex (40 mg days 1 through 4, 9 through 12, and 17 through 20) versus lenalidomide with low-dose Dex (40 mg once a week).[269] With 445 patients randomized, 79% patients receiving high-dose and 68% patients on low-dose dexamethasone had CR or PR within four cycles (p = 0.008). However, OS at 1 year was 96% versus 87% in favor of the low-dose dexamethasone group (p = 0.0002); and toxicity was also higher in the high-dose versus low-dose dexamethasone group (any grade 3 or 4 toxicity 52% versus 35%, respectively, p = 0.0001; early mortality 5.4% versus 0.5% respectively, p = 0.003 and DVT 26% versus 12% respectively, p = 0.0003). Bortezomib-containing regimens have also been evaluated in newly diagnosed patients. Jagannath et al.[299] have reported 18% CR and 88% overall response rates in a phase 2 study using a combination of bortezomib and Dex in newly diagnosed patients.

The IFM group has randomized 242 newly diagnosed patients to VAD or bortezomib plus dexamethasone (VD) followed by dexamethasone, cyclophosphamide, etoposide, cis-platinum (DCEP) consolidation and autologous stem-cell transplantation.[300] CR/nCR (15% versus 6%), at least VGPR (38% versus 15%), and over all response (79% versus 63%) rates after four cycles of induction therapy were significantly higher with VD compared to VAD. Interestingly, the superior response after induction also translated into significantly improved response after transplant with CR/nCR (35% versus 18%) and at least VGPR (54% versus 37%) rates in favor of VD compared to the VAD group. Median progression-free survival (PFS) was 36.0 months versus 29.7 months (p = 0.064) with VD versus VAD. The incidence of severe adverse events appeared similar between the groups. A short-term bortezomib induction has been reported to improve outcomes of patients with t(4;14) but not del(17p).[301] The recently approved proteasome inhibitor carfilzomib has also been evaluated in newly diagnosed patients. In combination with lenalidomide and dexamethasone, it achieves 94% overall response and 80% CR/nCR after 12 cycles. In a phase 1/2 study in patients with newly diagnosed MM (n = 53) after a median of 12 cycles of carfilzomib, lenalidomide, dexamethasone (CRd) (range, 1 to 25), 62% patients achieved at least a near CR and 42% stringent CR. In 36 patients completing eight

TABLE 48.10B
Bortezomib Regimens in Newly Diagnosed Multiple Myeloma

Study	Phase	N	Regimen	CR/VGPR (%)	CR + PR (%)	1-yr Survival (%)	Reference
Richardson	II	63	Bort	10	40	N/R	ASCO 2006
Jagannath	II	48	Bort ± Dex	19	90	80	BrJH 2005
Harousseau	II	48	Bort + Dex	31	66	N/R	Haem 2006
Harousseau	III	79	Bort + Dex	43	82	N/R	ASH 2006
Rosinol	II	40	Alternating Bort/Dex	22	64	N/R	ASCO 2007
Mateos	I/II	60	MP-V	43	89	87	Blood 2006
Oakervee	II	21	PAD	29	95	N/R	BrJH 2005
Orlowski	II	29	Bort + PLD	28	79	N/R	ASH 2006
Barlogie	II	303	TT3 with Bort	80	90	92	ASCO 2007

CR, complete response; VGPR, very good PR; PR, partial response; Bort (V), bortizomib; Dex (D), dexamethasone; N/R, not reported; Thal (T), thalidomide; MP, melphalan, prednisone; PAD, bortezomib, adriamycin, dex; PLD, liposomal doxorubicin; TT3, total therapy 3.

or more cycles, 78% patients reached at least a near CR and 61% achieved a stringent CR. With a median follow-up of 13 months (range, 4 to 25 months), the 24-month PFS estimate was 92%. Thus, CRd is well tolerated with exceptional response rates.[302]

With the success of two-drug combinations, three-drug combinations have been investigated with demonstrated high response rates. Bortezomib and dexamethasone have been combined with thalidomide (VTD: CR 32%, VGPR: 62%, and ORR: 94%), doxorubicin (VDD CR/nCR: 31%, VGPR: 42%, and ORR: 83%), cyclophosphamide[303] (VCD CR/nCR: 39%, VGPR: 61%, and ORR: 88%), and lenalidomide[304] (VRD CR/nCR: 52%, VGPR: 74%, and PR: 100%). A four-drug combination combining VRD with cyclophosphamide has not shown a clear benefit. These novel agent combinations have progressively improved both frequency and depth of responses in newly diagnosed patients with myeloma (Fig. 48.11).

For patients who are not transplant candidates, the same regimen described previously can be utilized. In addition, MP in combination with novel agents has significantly improved outcomes. Five randomized studies have compared MP with thalidomide (MPT) versus MP (Table 48.11) and demonstrated both superior overall response and complete response rate, as well as event-free survival (four out of five studies) and OS (two out of five studies), suggesting MPT as an active regimen in this patient population. The combination of bortezomib with MP (VMP) has been compared with MP in a randomized study,[305] which demonstrated superior CR and PR rates for the VMP regimen (71% versus 35% and 30% versus 4% respectively; $p < 0.001$). The time to progression for the VMP group was 24.0 months, as compared with 16.6 months for the MP cohort ($p < 0.001$). The combination of lenalidomide with MP followed by lenalidomide maintenance (MPRR) has been compared with MP and demonstrated higher response rates (CR 18% versus 5% and ORR 76% versus 49%; $p < 0.001$) and PFS (not reached versus 13.2 months; $p = 0.002$). A four-drug combination combining MPT with bortezomib has not shown significant further improvements.

High-Dose Therapy with Peripheral Blood Stem Cell Support

To overcome resistance to standard-dose therapy, a pilot study by the late Tim McElwain and his colleagues at the Royal Marsden Hospital evaluated the role of melphalan dose escalation (140 mg/m^2). They reported complete remissions in refractory patients[12]; however, treatment-related mortality was high due to BM toxicity. Bone marrow support in subsequent studies improved the treatment-related mortality, and dose escalation of melphalan to 200 mg/m^2 further improved response.

Transplant in Newly Diagnosed Patients

The initial demonstration of activity of high-dose melphalan therapy lead to series of evaluations of the role of high-dose therapy with stem cell support in myeloma. These studies reported complete remissions in up to 50% of patients, with prolongation of EFS and OS to more than 3 years and more than 5 to 6 years, respectively.[306–310]

The superiority of high-dose chemotherapy with autologous BM support was confirmed in a randomized trial conducted by IFM. The response rate (≥50% reduction in myeloma protein) in 100 patients receiving high-dose therapy (Mel-140 + TBI) was 81% (22% complete remission) compared with 57% (5% complete

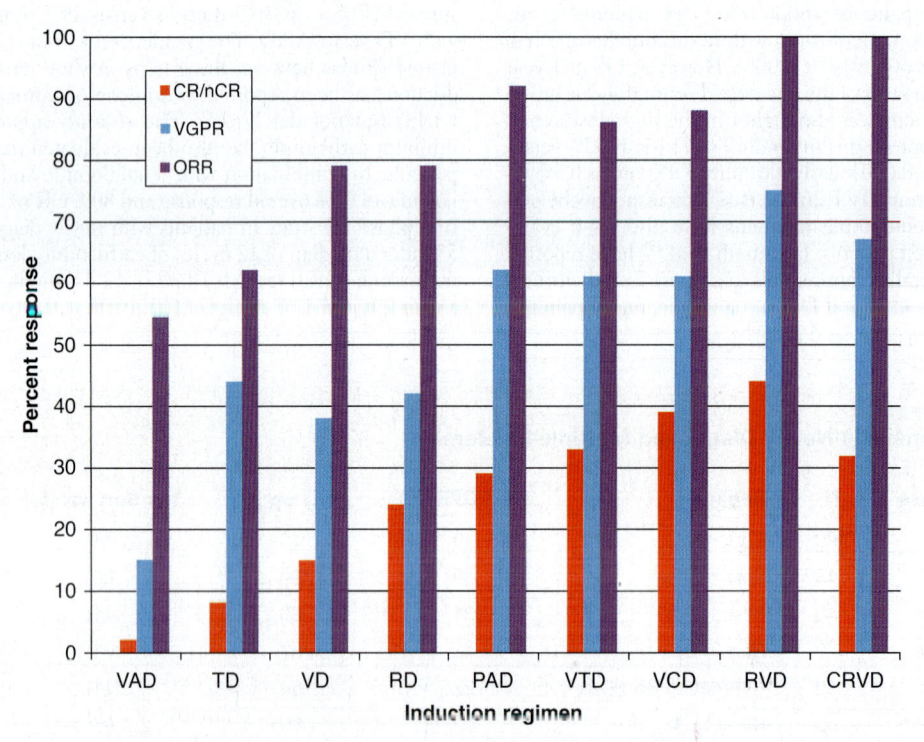

Figure 48.11 Progressive improvement in response to combination therapies incorporating newer agents. The nCR/CR, VGPR, and ORR rates following induction therapy of newly diagnosed multiple myeloma patients is plotted for common novel agent combinations selected from larger phase III and II studies and compared with VAD regimen. VAD, vincristine, adriamycin, and dexamethasone; T, thalidomide; D, dexamethasone; R, Lenalidomide; P, bortezomib; V, bortezomib (except in VAD); A, adriamycin; C, cyclophosphamide. CR/nCR, complete response/near CR; VGPR, very good partial response; ORR, overall response rate.

TABLE 48.11
Randomized Studies Comparing Mp-Related Regimens: Results

Authors/Study	Regimen	Complete Response	Partial Response	PFS (median months)	OS (median months)
Palumbo et al./GIMEMA[402]	MPT vs MP	16% vs 4% (p <0.001)	69% vs 48% (p <0.0001)	21.8 vs 14.5 (p = 0.0004)	45 vs 47.6 (p value NS)
Facon et al./IFM 99-06[403]	MPT vs MP	13% vs 2% (p = 0.0008)	76% vs 35% (p <0.0001)	27.5 vs 18 (p <0.0001)	51.5 vs 33 (p = 0.006)
Hulin et al./IFM 01-01[404]	MPT vs MP	7% vs 1% (p <0.001)	62% vs 31% (p <0.001)	24 vs 18.5 (p = 0.001)	44 vs 29 (p = 0.028)
Wijermans et al./HOVON[405]	MPT vs MP	2% vs 2%	66% vs 45% (p <0.001)	13 vs 9 (p <0.001)	40 vs 32 (p = 0.05)
Waage et al./NMSG[406]	MPT vs MP	—	57% vs 40% (p <0.0001)	15 vs 14 (p value NS)	29 vs 32 (p value NS)
San Miguel et al./VISTA[305]	MPV vs MP	30% vs 4% (p <0.001)	71% vs 35% (p <0.001)	24 vs 16.6[a] (p <0.001)	Not reached vs 43
Palumbo et al.[407]	MPRR vs MP	18% vs 5% (p <0.001)	77% vs 49% (p <0.001)	Not reached vs 13 (p = 0.002)	Not reached

MP, melphalan, prednisone; PFS, progression-free survival; OS, overall survival; NS, significant difference.
[a] TTP, time to progression.

remission) in a similar number of patients receiving standard-dose chemotherapy consisting of VMCP (vincristine, melphalan, cyclophosphamide, and prednisone) alternating with a BVAP (carmustine, vincristine, doxorubicin, and prednisone) regimen (p < 0.001). Significantly longer event-free (median, 28 versus 18 months) and overall (median, 57 versus 42 months) survivals were reported after high-dose therapy (Fig. 48.12). The projected 5-year EFS and OS were 28% and 52% after high-dose therapy compared to 10% and 12% following standard-dose therapy, respectively.[311]

A similar response and survival benefit has been reported from the Medical Research Council (MRC)-VII trial, which randomized 407 patients to either standard-dose chemotherapy or HDT with transplantation.[312] A Spanish trial of 164 patients treated with HDT versus conventional therapy also showed a superior CR rate in the HDT arm, with a trend for prolonged EFS and OS in the HDT arm (Table 48.12).[313] In contrast, the Myelome Autogreffe Group (MAG) trial by Fermand et al.[314] in 190 newly diagnosed MM patients failed to show superiority of HDT. The US intergroup study, which randomized patients between HDT versus conventional therapy followed by delayed HDT at relapse, failed to show superiority of HDT for either achievement of CR or OS; EFS benefit was modest (1 months) in the high-dose therapy cohort.[277] A meta-analysis combining nine studies comprising 2,411 patients reported a combined hazard of death with HDT of 0.92 (95% confidence interval [CI], 0.74 to 1.13) and a combined hazard of progression with HDT of 0.75 (95% CI, 0.59 to 0.96). The analysis of the randomized data indicated PFS benefit, but not OS benefit, for HDT with single autologous transplantation in multiple myeloma.[315]

Although the responses to induction therapy have now significantly improved with the use of novel agent combination therapies (see Fig. 48.11), some recent studies have indicated that HDT is able to further improve the depth of response (Fig. 48.13). These observations have raised questions about the role of HDT in newly diagnosed patients with myeloma receiving novel agent

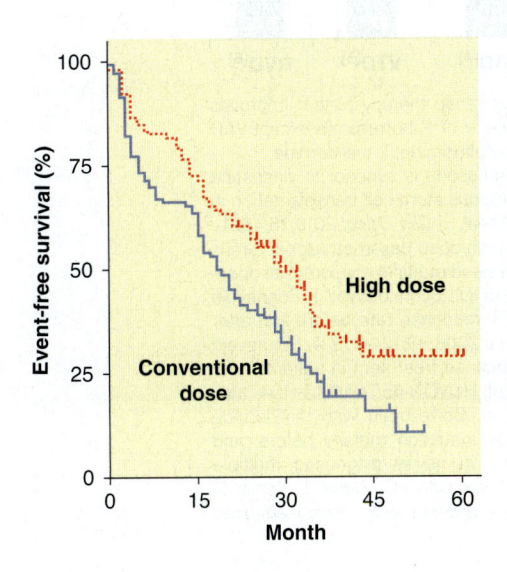

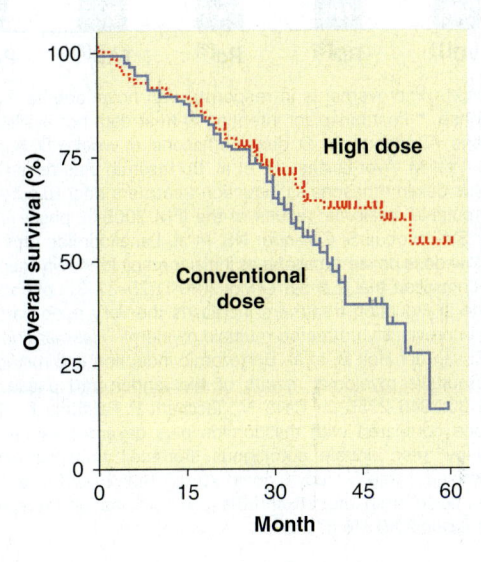

Figure 48.12 Comparative trials of high-dose therapy (HDT) versus standard-dose chemotherapy (SDT). IFM-90 (Intergroupe Francais de Myeloma) randomized trial with 100 patients accrued to each arm comparing SDT with VMCP-VBAP and HDT with melphalan 140 mg/m² plus total body irradiation (800 cGy). Higher complete remission rates and significantly longer event-free and overall survival were noted with HDT. (From Harousseau JL, Attal M, Divine M, et al. Autologous stem cell transplantation after first remission induction treatment in multiple myeloma. A report of the French Registry on Autologous Transplantation in Multiple Myeloma. *Stem Cells* 1995;13:132–139, with permission.)

TABLE 48.12
Results of Large Randomized Study Comparing Standard Dose Therapy Versus High-Dose Therapy

Authors		No. of Patients (n)	CR (%)	EFS (median months)	OS (median months)
Attal et al.[311]	Conventional	100	5[b]	18[b]	37[b]
	HDT	100	22	27	52
Fermand et al.[314]	Conventional	96	–	18.7[b]	50.4[a]
	HDT	94	–	24.3	55.3
Blade et al.[313]	Conventional	83	11[b]	34.3[b]	66.9[a]
	HDT	81	30	42.5	67.4
Child et al.[312]	Conventional	200	8.5[b]	19.6[b]	42.3[b]
	HDT	201	44	31.6	54.8
Barlogie et al.[272]	Conventional	255	15[a]	21[a]	53[a]
	HDT	261	17	25	58

CR, complete remission; EFS, event-free survival; OS, overall survival; HDT, high-dose therapy.
[a] No significant difference.
[b] Significant difference.

combination therapy. Two recent studies have reconfirmed the role of high-dose therapy in myeloma. In one study, patients received four cycles of lenalidomide and dexamethasone and were then randomized to either Cytoxan, lenalidomide, and dexamethasone (CRD) for six cycles or HDT with melphalan 200 mg/m² (Mel200) with transplant. PFS with Mel200 was significantly longer than after CRD: 27 months versus not reached (p = 0.012). A second study compared MPR versus Mel200 after R/d induction therapy and reported superior PFS (24 versus 30 months respectively (p <0.0001) with a trend in improved 5-year OS, 62 versus 71% (p = 0.27) in favor of Mel200. An ongoing study is evaluating the role of transplant in patients receiving RVD combination.

Tandem Transplants

Attempts to further improve the results of autotransplantation have included intensification with tandem transplants. Harousseau et al.[316] were the first to report feasibility of tandem autologous BM transplantation, with a 69% CR rate in a small select group of patients. Barlogie et al.[317] investigated a sequential non–cross-resistant

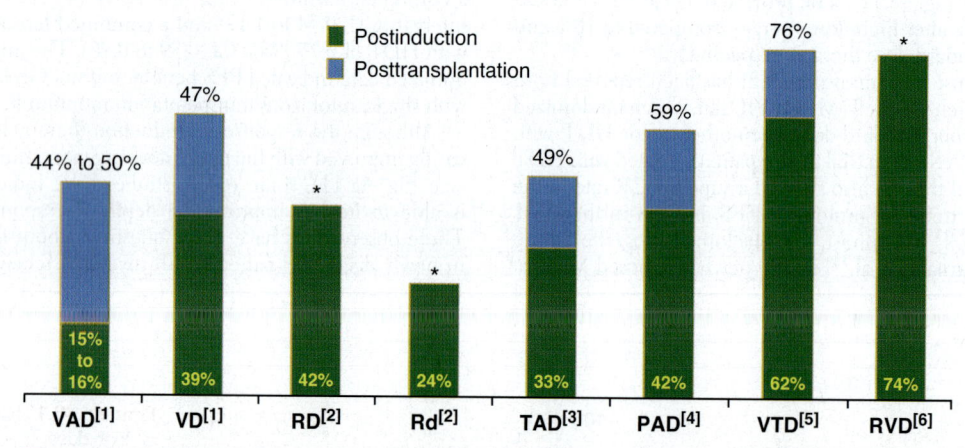

Figure 48.13 Despite improvements in response with novel agents, high-dose therapy further improves the depth of response. * Posttransplant intention-to-treat data not available. V or P, bortezomib except VAD where V is vincristine; A, Adriamycin; D, dexamethasone; d, weekly D; R, lenalidomide; T, thalidomide.
1. Harousseau JL, Attal M, Avet-Loiseau H, et al. Bortezomib plus dexamethasone is superior to vincristine plus doxorubicin plus dexamethasone as induction treatment prior to autologous stem-cell transplantation in newly diagnosed multiple myeloma: results of the IFM 2005-01 phase III trial. *J Clin Oncol* 2010;28:4621–4629. 2. Rajkumar SV, Jacobus S, Callander NS, et al. Lenalidomide plus high-dose dexamethasone versus lenalidomide plus low-dose dexamethasone as initial therapy for newly diagnosed multiple myeloma: an open-label randomised controlled trial. *Lancet Oncol* 2010;11:29–37. 3. Lokhorst HM, Schmidt-Wolf I, Sonneveld P, et al. Thalidomide in induction treatment increases the very good partial response rate before and after high-dose therapy in previously untreated multiple myeloma. *Haematologica* 2008;93:124–127. 4. Sonneveld P, Schmidt-Wolf IG, van der Holt B, et al. Bortezomib induction and maintenance treatment in patients with newly diagnosed multiple myeloma: results of the randomized phase III HOVON 65/ GMMG HD4 trial. *J Clin Oncol* 2012;30:2946–2955. 5. Cavo M, Tacchetti P, Patriarca F, et al. Bortezomib with thalidomide plus dexamethasone compared with thalidomide plus dexamethasone as induction therapy before, and consolidation therapy after, double autologous stem-cell transplantation in newly diagnosed multiple myeloma: a randomised phase 3 study. *Lancet* 2010;376:2075–2085. 6. Richardson PG, Weller E, Lonial S, et al. Lenalidomide, bortezomib, and dexamethasone combination therapy in patients with newly diagnosed multiple myeloma. *Blood* 2010;116:679–686.

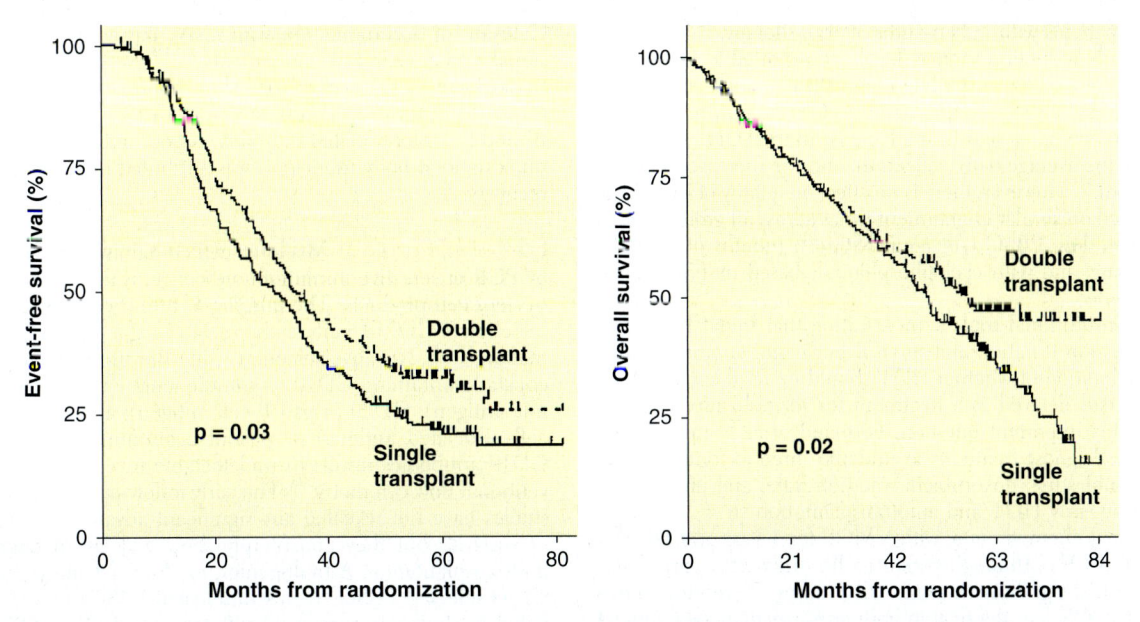

Figure 48.14 Comparative trial of single versus double high-dose therapy (HDT). IFM 94 trial with 399 patients randomized to a single HDT with melphalan 140 mg/m² plus total body irradiation (800 cGy) versus first HDT with melphalan 140 mg/m² and subsequent second HDT with melphalan 140 mg/m² plus total body irradiation (800 cGy). Superior event-free and overall survival was noted with double HDT. (From Attal M, Harousseau JL, Facon T, et al. Single versus double autologous stem-cell transplantation for multiple myeloma. *N Engl J Med* 2003;349:2495–2502, with permission.)

remission induction regimen followed by tandem autologous transplantations (*total therapy*) in 231 newly diagnosed patients. 41% of patients achieved CR after two transplants, and the median EFS and OS times were 43 months and 68 months, respectively.

Attal et al.[245] (IFM-94) reported a randomized comparison of single HDT (melphalan [140 mg/m²] and TBI [8 Gy]) versus double HDT (melphalan [200 mg/m²], followed by melphalan [140 mg/m²] and TBI [8 Gy]) in 399 newly diagnosed patients. This study reported no significant improvement in CR or very good PR rate between the two arms (42% versus 50% respectively; p = 0.10); however, there was a significant improvement in the double HDT arm in probability of EFS at 7 years (10% versus 20%; p = 0.03) and estimated OS at 7 years (21% versus 42%; p = 0.01) (Fig. 48.14). A similar study by the Dutch-Belgian Hematology-Oncology Cooperative Group (HOVON) (n = 255) showed a superior CR rate (13 versus 28%) and EFS (20 versus 22 months) in favor of tandem transplants; however, it failed to show OS benefit. The MAG (n = 193) and Bologna (n = 178) trials, with a median follow-up of 27 to 30 months, have not yet shown a significant benefit for tandem transplantation (Table 48.13).

Various factors need special consideration in the management of myeloma with high-dose chemotherapy. These factors include a source of stem cells, the conditioning regimen, the timing of transplant, and tumor-cell purging.

Timing of High-Dose Therapy. To obtain high-quality hematopoietic stem cells, the ideal timing for stem cell collection is early in the course of the induction treatment. The ability to collect adequate stem cells (≥2 × 10⁶ CD34+ cells per kilogram) in patients with less than 12 months of prior therapy is 86% compared

TABLE 48.13

Single Versus Double ASCT for Newly Diagnosed Multiple Myeloma

Study	ASCT	No. of Patients	CR (%)[a]	Median EFS (mo)	Median OS (mo)
Attal et al.[245] (IFM94)	Single	199	42[b] (p = NS)	25 (p = 0.03)	48 (p = 0.01)
	Double	200	50[b]	30	58
Fermand et al.[314] (MAG95)	Single	94	42[a] (p = NS)	No difference	No difference
	Double	99	37[a]		
Sonneveld et al.[408] (HOVON24)	Single	148	13 (p = 0.002)	20 (p = 0.02)	55 (p = NS)
	Double	155	28	22	50
Cavo et al.[409] (Bologna 96)	Single	115	35 (p = NS)	Significant prolongation of EFS with double SCT	59 (p = NS)
	Double	113	48		73

ASCT, autologous stem cell transplantation; CR, complete remission; EFS, event-free survival; OS, overall survival; SCT, stem cell transplant.
[a] CR + minimum residual disease.
[b] CR + VGPR.

to 48% in patients with >24 months of prior therapy.[318] Prolonged lenalidomide induction therapy has been reported to affect stem cell mobilization. Patients undergoing PBSC mobilization with granulocyte-colony stimulating factor (G-CSF) following lenalidomide induction had a significant decrease in total CD34 (+) cells collected, the average daily collection, and the increased number of aphereses.[319] However, there is no effect on quality of PBSC collected based on similar engraftment times across all groups. Based on these studies, PBSC collection within 6 months of lenalidomide therapy and with cyclophosphamide-based mobilization is recommended.[320,321]

Multi-institutional trials demonstrating that initial HDT prolongs remission duration and survival but is not curative has led to the exploration of whether HDT should be used early after diagnosis versus delayed as a treatment for relapsed myeloma. To evaluate this important question, Fermand et al.[314] randomized 185 newly diagnosed patients to undergo three to four cycles of VAMP (vinblastine, doxorubicin, methotrexate, and prednisone) followed by early HDT and autotransplantation (n = 91) versus conventional chemotherapy with VMCP for 1 year and HDT at relapse (n = 94). Although patients who underwent early transplantation had significantly longer EFS times (39 months versus 13 months), OS was identical in both arms (median, 64.6 and 64 months). Importantly, the time without symptoms and toxicity analysis reflecting quality of life (mean, 27.8 versus 22.3 months) showed superior results for the early HDT arm (Table 48.14). Vesole et al.[322] have confirmed effectiveness of high-dose chemotherapy as a salvage therapy achieving EFS and OS times of 21 and >43 months, respectively, in 135 patients with advanced refractory MM. In this study, patients with primary unresponsive disease had superior outcomes to patients with resistant relapse (progression on last-salvage chemotherapy) with EFS of 37 months versus 17 months, respectively (p = 0.0004), and OS of 43 months versus 21 months, respectively (p = 0.0003). Gertz et al.,[323] from the Mayo clinic, have also reported a similar experience in 64 patients undergoing elective delayed transplant at the time of progression following standard therapy. Finally, the Intergroup trial in the United States randomizing patients to up-front high-dose therapy or standard therapy with high-dose therapy as a salvage treatment also confirms a similar modest EFS benefit for early versus late transplants.[272]

High-Dose Regimen. High-dose melphalan (140 to 200 mg/m^2), with or without total body irradiation, is the most common conditioning regimen used in myeloma.[324–326] Melphalan's predominant myelotoxicity and metabolism independent of renal function is ideal for MM patients who commonly have renal function abnormalities. Melphalan seems to be superior to thioTEPA when given with total body irradiation, with patients achieving longer relapse-free and overall survival duration.[326] A combination regimen containing high-dose carboplatin with etoposide and Cytoxan, or a combination with CBV, has achieved only occasional responses in resistant patients.[327,328] No regimen has shown marked superiority over others. The addition of TBI has not been shown to improve cytoreduction and, in fact, increases morbidity and treatment-related mortality. A poor outcome in one study utilizing total body irradiation was attributed to delayed immune recovery.

Stem Cell Purging. Myeloma cell contamination, as evaluated by PCR or sensitive immunofluorescence, is universally observed in stem cell products. The purging of tumor cells by the positive selection of CD34+ cells leads to a 3 to 5 log reduction in contamination.[329,330] Negative selection using the monoclonal antibody cocktail containing CD10 (common acute lymphoblastic leukemia antigen); CD20 (a pan B-cell antigen); and PCA-1 (plasma cell–associated antigen) or peanut agglutinin (PNA) and anti-CD19 antibodies results in undetectable myeloma cells by conventional flow cytometry.[309] The early follow-up results from these studies have not revealed any significant advantage in responses or survival, but they consistently show a delay in engraftment posttransplantation. A multicenter, randomized study comparing CD34-selected PBSCs versus unselected PBSCs in 131 patients failed to show any significant difference in EFS or OS time.[331] Even when cells were purged using FACS sorting of very early hematopoietic stem cells (CD34$^+$, Thy1$^+$, and Lin), relapses were frequent and patients had delayed hematopoietic engraftment and suppressed immune status for prolonged periods of time.[332,333] Due to these data, emphasis is now on strategies to improve responses to HDT, rather than on purging autografts.

Hematopoietic Stem Cell Source. Mobilized PBSCs provide for more rapid engraftment compared to BM. Myeloma patients with less than 1 year of prior therapy had faster granulocyte and platelet recovery after peripheral blood stem cell transplants compared with BM autografts.[334] The duration of prior chemotherapy, especially with stem-cell–damaging agents (melphalan, BCNU, and high-doses of cyclophosphamide) along with radiation to BM-containing areas, significantly affects the ability to procure adequate quantities of PBSCs and engraftment kinetics posttransplant.[335] After mobilization with cyclophosphamide and GM-CSF, normal PBSCs are mobilized during the first 3 days of leukapheresis, whereas peak levels of contaminating myeloma cells are present on subsequent days. These myeloma cells show a higher LI and a more immature phenotype (CD19$^+$).[336]

Management of Older Patients

Unlike in the past, melphalan and prednisone is no longer a standard of care for older adults with myeloma. The two- and three-drug combinations of novel agents described previously for newly diagnosed patients remains an important option. In this age group, which most of the time is not considered eligible for transplant, the combination of bortezomib, or lenalidomide, or both with dexamethasone is considered the preferred option. However, MP in combination with these novel agents also achieves high levels of response and can be considered an alternative (see Fig. 48.11). A recent study showing superiority and decreased secondary malignancy risk of continuous Rd combination over MPT suggests that future utilization of MP based therapy will decrease in newly diagnosed older individuals with myeloma. To manage toxicity, the dose of therapeutic agents, including dexamethasone, needs to be reduced in patients >75 years of age.[337] The presence of comorbidities, frailty, and disabilities needs to be assessed and considered in the selection of agents and dose modifications.[338] As the incidence of myeloma increases with age, the role of HDT has also been evaluated in patients >65 years old. Older age does not impact stem cell mobilization or engraftment.[339] The feasibility and efficacy of HDT with PBSC transplant has been evaluated

TABLE 48.14
Stem Cell Transplantation as Upfront Versus Rescue Treatment: Results of a Randomized Study

	Early Transplant N = 91	Late Transplant N = 94
CR	19%	5%
Med EFS	39 mo	13 mo
Med OS	64.6 mo	64 mo
TWISTT	27.8 mo	22.3 mo

Note: Median f/u 50 months.
CR, complete remission; EFS, event free survival; TWISTT, time without symptoms or treatment toxicity.
[a] Significant difference.

in patients 70 years old (median age, 72 years of age; range, 70 to 83 years of age) treated with melphalan (200 mg/m² or 140 mg/m²).[340] Of note, treatment-related mortality was higher (16%) in the initial 25 patients receiving melphalan at 200 mg/m². CR was achieved in 27% patients, but median CR duration was only 1.5 years, with 3-year EFS and OS rates projected at 20% and 31%, respectively. Although this study confirms the feasibility of HDT in older patients with MM, it also indicates a higher risk in this patient population. High response rates using the novel agent combinations are decreasing the consideration of HDT in this elderly population.

Management of Patients with Renal Dysfunction

One-third of patients with overt MM present with renal insufficiency. With hydration, control of hypercalcemia, and effective therapy, it is reversible in 50% cases. Renal dysfunction of <6 months duration and the rapid initiation of therapy with a reduction in monoclonal protein are associated with a higher likelihood of improvement in renal function. Improved renal function is observed mainly in patients with light chain cast nephropathy and light chain deposition disease; therefore, renal biopsy is used to identify these reversible conditions and the need for aggressive treatment. A number of agents can be safely used in patients with renal dysfunction. This includes steroids, melphalan,[341] cyclophosphamide, bortezomib,[294,342] and thalidomide. Ease of administration, limited toxicity, and effectiveness make these novel agents the primary modes of therapy for myeloma patients with renal failure. In one retrospective analysis, 24 patients on dialysis were treated with bortezomib or bortezomib-based combinations. Of 20 patients with available response data, 75% patients achieved at least PRs, with 30% patients achieving CRs + near CRs. One patient was spared dialysis, and three other patients became independent of dialysis following bortezomib-based treatment.[294,342] Lenalidomide has predominant renal excretion and requires dose modification if used in patients with renal failure based on creatinine clearance.[342] However, pomalidomide can be safely administered in these patients. Because the pharmacokinetics of melphalan are unaltered by renal failure, such patients have been previously considered as potential candidates for high-dose therapy.[341] In one study, high-dose melphalan and PBSC transplantation was used to treat 81 patients with MM and renal dysfunction (creatinine >2 mg per deciliter).[343] Although renal failure had no impact on the quality of stem cell collection and/or engraftment, treatment-related mortality rates were 6% and 13% after the first and second autologous SCTs, respectively, and melphalan at 200 mg/m² caused excessive toxicity. Complete remission was achieved in 31 patients (38%) after tandem SCT, and the probabilities of EFS and OS at 3 years were 48% and 55%, respectively. Dose reduction and close monitoring are therefore needed to ensure the safety of the procedure, and the role of transplantation in the setting of renal failure remains investigational.

Maintenance Therapy

Despite improvements in remission rates, there is no clear plateau in the survival curves following conventional or HDT. Although the proportion of patients achieving complete responses has increased, all patients eventually relapse. Various maintenance therapies have been evaluated in MM in an effort to sustain remission. IFN-α is the most widely evaluated agent as maintenance therapy; however, randomized studies have only demonstrated modest improvements in EFS and OS times (5 to 12 months) in patients achieving remission with standard-dose therapy, and its role following HDT has not been confirmed.[344] Low-dose prednisone administered on alternate days has prolonged remission duration following standard-dose therapy in a single randomized study.[345] In the last few years, many studies have evaluated novel agent-based maintenance regimens (Table 48.15). Attal and his

TABLE 48.15

Randomized Studies Comparing Maintenance Therapy in Myeloma

Authors/Study	Regimen	PFS (median months)	OS (median months)
Spencer et al.[410]	Control vs thalidomide/prednisone	23 vs 42 (p <0.001)	75 vs 86 (p = 0.004)
Barlogie et al.[411]	Control vs thalidomide	44% vs 57% (p = 0.01)[a]	Not reached
Attal et al.[346]	Control vs thalidomide + pamidronate	36 vs 52 (p = 0.009)	77 vs 87 (p = 0.04)
Attal et al.[347]	Control vs lenalidomide	24 vs Not reached (p <0.0001)	80% vs 88%[b]
Palumbo et al.[348]	MPRR vs MPR	Not reached vs 13.2 (p = 0.002)	Not reached
McCarthy et al.[349]	Control vs lenalidomide	Not reached vs 25.5 (p <0.001)[c]	Not reached
Mateos et al.[351]	VP vs VT	32 vs 24 (p = 0.01)	Not reached

PFS, progression-free survival; OS, overall survival; NA, not accessed; M, melphalan; P, prednisone; R, lenalidomide; RR, lenalidomide with maintenance; V, bortezomib; T, thalidomide.
[a] Five-year PFS rates.
[b] Survival after 3 years.
[c] TTP, time to progression.

colleagues from the IFM group reported improved probability of EFS and OS at 3 years in patients receiving thalidomide and pamidronate compared to the patient cohorts receiving either pamidronate alone or no maintenance therapy following high-dose therapy (PFS 52%, 37%, and 36%, respectively; p <0.009; OS 87%, 74%, and 77%, respectively; p <0.04).[346] In this study, patients had not received thalidomide prior to its evaluation as maintenance therapy, and the benefit was observed in those patients who had further evidence of response to thalidomide. The prolonged use of thalidomide leads to the development of neuropathy, and more recently, lenalidomide, which has a more favorable toxicity profile, has been evaluated as maintenance therapy in the dose of 10 to 15 mg daily for 21 out of a 28-day cycle in three different studies: two posttransplantations and one following standard-dose MPR therapy.[347–349] All three studies show clear evidence of benefit, evidenced by the prolongation of PFS. One of the studies (CALGB 100104) has now shown OS benefit with lenalidomide maintenance, whereas two other studies with limited follow-ups are yet to observe an OS improvement. Importantly, all three studies show a small increased incidence of second primary malignancy in the arms receiving lenalidomide compared to placebo. This has prompted a careful evaluation and discussion with the patient of the benefit of lenalidomide maintenance. Because of its significant benefit, lenalidomide is considered the standard of care for maintenance therapy in myeloma. The HOVON trial has compared vincristine, adriamycin, and dexamethasone induction followed by high-dose melphalan and transplantation with Velcade maintenance versus Velcade, adriamycin, and dexamethasone induction high-dose melphalan and transplantation followed by thalidomide maintenance. With a 5-year follow-up, there is a PFS and OS benefit in the Velcade arm, including patients with high-risk (p17 deleted) MM.[350] In the nontransplant population, a recent study has also highlighted the use of a Velcade-based maintenance regimen especially in combination with low-dose thalidomide.[351] Additional immune manipulations, such as idiotype vaccinations, protein-pulsed dendritic cell-based vaccinations, dendritic cell–MM cell fusion vaccinations, and/or PD-1 checkpoint blockades are all strategies under evaluation as maintenance treatments to prolong EFS and OS in patients with myeloma.[352,353]

Minimal Residual Disease

Due to improvements in therapies, higher frequencies and depth of responses are being observed. There is emerging data that patients achieving CRs have superior survival outcomes compared to those achieving partial responses or no responses. This has now led to the investigation of methods to refine CR definition. The current definition includes the absence of paraprotein in the urine and serum by immunofixation and the disappearance of clonal plasma cells in the bone marrow using cytologic examination; stringent CR in addition requires normalization of the kappa/lambda free light chain ratio. The newer sensitive seven-color flow cytometric immunophenotypic assays can detect 1 clonal cell in 10^4 normal cells, and a molecular method that incorporates allele-specific oligonucleotide PCR (ASO-PCR) can detect up to 1 clonal cell in 10^{5-6} normal cells, each enhancing the ability to detect greater depth of response. To obviate the need for patient-specific customization, a sequencing-based molecular method is now being developed that identifies clonal gene rearrangements using consensus primers to universally amplify rearranged IgH and k gene segments, followed by high-throughput sequencing to quantify these rearrangements in follow-up minimal residual disease (MRD) samples.[354] In early studies using multiparameter flow cytometry, the prognostic value of MRD was assessed: in 378 patients after induction therapy and at day 100 after autologous stem cell transplantation (ASCT) and in 245 patients at the end of induction therapy in nontransplant patients. In patients undergoing ASCT, the absence of MRD at day 100 after ASCT was highly predictive of a favorable outcome (PFS, p <0.001; OS, p = 0.0183), including in patients achieving immunofixation-negative CR (p = 0.0068). An MRD assessment after induction therapy in the non–intensive-pathway patients was not predictive of outcome (PFS, p = 0.1). This and other emerging data highlight the need to measure and achieve molecular CR in myeloma.[355] Similarly, in a study using a multiparameter flow cytometry method to detect MRD in 241 patients in CR at day +100 after ASCT, the detection of persistent MRD after ASCT was the only independent factor (HR, 8.0; p = 0.005), besides high-risk cytogenetics, that predicted for unsustained CR and a poor outcome.[356]

Allogeneic Transplantation

Syngeneic Transplantation

Bensinger et al.[357] have reported their experience with 11 patients receiving syngeneic transplants: Five patients achieved CR and three achieved PR, with one patient from both groups alive at 9 and 15 years after transplantation, respectively. A larger experience from the European bone marrow transplant (EBMT) Registry compared 25 patients undergoing syngeneic transplants with 125 case-matched patients undergoing autotransplantation or allogeneic transplantation.[358] The complete remission rate was not significantly different between the three grafts (twin: 68%, autologous: 48%, and allogeneic: 58%). However, patients undergoing syngeneic transplantation had significantly superior median survival time compared with autologous (72 months versus 25 months; p = 0.009) or allogeneic (72 months versus 16 months; p = 0.008) transplant recipients.

Allogeneic Transplantation

Allogeneic transplantation has remained a difficult procedure in myeloma. An elder age population with limited donor availability coupled with frequent renal impairment has restricted the use of

TABLE 48.16

Studies of Allogeneic Transplantation for Newly Diagnosed Myeloma

Authors	No. of Patients	TRM (%)	CR (%)	OS (actuarial, months)	EFS (actuarial, months)
Gahrton et al.	162	41	44	28% at 84	45% at 60
Bensinger et al.	80	44	36	20% at 54	24% at 54
Alyea et al.	61[a]	5	28	40% at 36	20% at 38

TRM, treatment-related mortality; CR, complete remission; OS, overall survival; EFS, event-free survival.
[a] T-cell depleted.

matched sibling transplantation in MM. Additionally, almost 50% 1-year mortality has limited use of this procedure to only a high-risk patient population. Importantly, the allogeneic graft versus myeloma (GVM) effect may result in a favorable long-term outcome after allogeneic transplantation. Results of three large studies are listed in Table 48.16. A retrospective analysis of a case-matched analysis of EBMT registry data compared 189 patients receiving allografts with an equal number of patients from the same time period receiving autotransplants. This study showed a superior median survival outcome for patients undergoing autotransplants compared to allogeneic transplants (34 versus 18 months, respectively).[359] The 1-year treatment-related mortality was significantly higher following allogeneic transplantation (41% with allotransplants and 13% with autotransplants). However, patients undergoing allogeneic transplantation and surviving the 1st year had a tendency for better PFS and OS.

A very low transplant-related mortality of 10% has been reported from a single-center experience from the Dana-Farber Cancer Institute due to the selective depletion of CD6+ T cells as the sole form of a graft versus host disease (GvHD) prophylaxis.[360] However, the median PFS time was 12 months, and the median OS time was 22 months, a result inferior to their previous experience of autologous transplantation. Case-matched comparative studies from other single institutions have also failed to show a survival advantage for allotransplants.[361]

Donor Lymphocyte Infusions

A GVM effect has been demonstrated by the induction of CR with donor lymphocyte infusion (DLI) following relapse after allogeneic transplantation.[362] In a large study, Lokhorst et al.[363] have reported 6 CR and 8 PR following DLI in 27 patients after allotransplant. Five of these patients remained disease free >30 months after DLI. However, DLI was associated with acute GvHD in 55% and chronic GvHD in 26% of patients. Five patients experienced BM aplasia, which was fatal in two cases. A similar DLI experience has been reported by Salama et al.[364] Several strategies have been explored to reduce GvHD after DLI,[365,366] including lowering the number of T cells infused, the selective depletion of CD8+ T cells, and the use of herpes simplex virus (HSV) thymidine kinase gene transduction of DLI to allow for use of ganciclovir to deplete T cells if significant GvHD develops. Immunizing donors with an idiotype vaccine may allow for the selective transfer of T cells specific for GVM without increasing the incidence of GvHD.

Nonmyeloablative Transplants

Studies in a canine model showed that a nonmyeloablative dose of TBI could lead to successful engraftment when used in conjunction with a combination of cyclosporine and

TABLE 48.17
Representative Studies of Miniallogeneic Transplantation in Myeloma

Authors	Conditioning	No. of Patients	TRM at 1 year (%)	Response (%)	Acute Grade II–IV GVHD (%)	Chronic Extensive GVHD (%)	PFS/EFS/DFS	OS
Lee et al.[412]	Mel or Mel/TBI/Flu	45	36	CR 64	36	36	3-y EFS 13%	Median 14 mo 2 y 74%
Maloney et al.[370]	PBSCT + TBI/MMF/Cyc	54	7	CR 57 PR 26	39	46	2-y PFS 55%	18 mo 78%
Bruno et al.[371]	PBSCT + TBI/MMF/Cyc	58	7	CR 55 PR 31	43	36	Median 43 mo	Median >46 mo

TRM, treatment-related mortality; GVHD, graft versus host disease; PFS, progression free survival; EFS, event-free survival; DFS, disease-free survival; OS, overall survival; Mel, melphalan; TBI, total body irradiation; Flu, fludarabine; CR, complete response; PR, partial response; PBSCT, peripheral blood stem cell transplant; Cyc, cyclosporine.

mycophenolate mofetil.[367] This animal experience, coupled with reduced day 100 transplant-related mortality in pilot studies in patients, has allowed for allogeneic-matched sibling transplantation in patients who were otherwise considered poor risk for the standard allogeneic preparative regimen. Results from larger published studies evaluating nonmyeloablative regimens with allogeneic transplantation are listed in Table 48.17. Badros et al.[369] first reported on 31 patients undergoing allogeneic transplants following nonmyeloablative conditioning with melphalan (100 mg/m²). Transplant-related mortality in the first 120 days was low (10%). Nineteen (61%) patients achieved CR or near CR; however, acute GvHD developed in 18 patients (58%), and chronic GvHD was seen in 10 patients (35%).[368] Giralt et al.[369] have used reduced intensity conditioning with fludarabine and melphalan in 16 patients; successful engraftment was observed in all patients; however, the 100-day mortality rate was 20% and the 1-year mortality rate was 40%, with only six patients alive after a median follow-up period of 15 months. Maloney et al.[370] have evaluated the combination of initial autotransplantation for tumor cytoreduction followed by nonmyeloablative matched-sibling transplantation in 54 patients. The treatment was performed in an outpatient setting with a low 100-day mortality (2%). The overall response rate was 83%, with 53% achieving CRs. With a median follow-up of 552 days after allografting, OS is 78%. However, GvHD continues to be a problem; 38% of patients developed acute GvHD and 46% developing chronic GvHD requiring therapy.

In a more recent clinical study, 162 consecutive patients with newly diagnosed myeloma who were less than 65 years of age received induction therapy with VAD, followed by either nonmyeloablative total-body irradiation and stem cells from the HLA-identical sibling after an initial autograft (n = 80) or two consecutive myeloablative doses of melphalan, each of which was followed by autologous stem-cell rescue if an HLA-identical donor was not available (n = 82). After a median follow-up of 45 months (range, 21 to 90), the median OS (80 months versus 54 months; p = 0.01) and event-free survival (35 months versus 29 months; p = 0.02) were longer in the patients with HLA-identical siblings than in the patients without HLA-identical siblings. Treatment-related mortality did not differ significantly between the two groups, (p = 0.09) but disease-related mortality was significantly higher in the double-autologous transplant group (43% versus 7%; p <0.001). The cumulative incidence rates of > grades I and grade IV GvHD were 43% and 4%, respectively. These results suggest a role for allografting, especially in patients with high-risk disease where improvement in long-term outcome has been limited.[371] Although the early clinical results with nonmyeloablative transplants are encouraging, this strategy is associated with significant morbidity due to acute and chronic GvHD and a mortality rate of 10% to 20% at 1 year. Another study by Risonol et al.[372] reported on 110 patients with MM undergoing ASCT, who either received a second ASCT (85 patients) or a reduced-intensity conditioning allograft (allo-RIC; 25 patients), depending on the HLA-matched sibling donor availability. Although there was a trend toward a longer PFS (median, 31 months versus not reached; p = 0.08) in favor of allo-RIC, it was associated with a trend toward a higher transplantation-related mortality (16% versus 5%; p = 0.07), and there was no statistical difference in event-free survival and overall survivals.[372] It should, therefore, only be utilized in the context of clinical trials attempting to improve patient outcome by both enhancing efficacy and reducing toxicity.[373] The CTN most recently compared single autografts followed by nonmyeloablative allografts if a matched donor was available versus a second autograft in the absence of an appropriate donor and found that the outcome was similar in both arms.[374] Due to attendant toxicity in all allografting studies, including nonmyeloablative regimens, allotransplant is recommended primarily in the context of a clinical trial to exploit the graft versus MM immune effect while avoiding attendant toxicity.

Bisphosphonates

The second- and third-generation bisphosphonates, pamidronate and zoledronate, reduce skeletal complications and bone pain in myeloma (Table 48.18).[375,376] Their mechanism of action includes the downregulation of osteoclast activity, decreased IL-6 production, the activation of gamma/delta T cells with antimyeloma activity, and the induction of apoptosis of osteoclasts through the inhibition of farnesyl and geranylgeranyl transferase activity.[377,378] Besides reducing bone-related problems, the continued administration of pamidronate over 21 months showed some survival advantage (21 versus 14 months; p = 0.041) in patients receiving salvage chemotherapy and pamidronate versus chemotherapy alone.[375,379] In vitro cytotoxic effects of bisphosphonates have been observed in myeloma cell lines[380,381] and patient cells in vitro, as well as in patient tumor specimens in the SCID-hu in vivo model. Preliminary reports of pamidronate administered alone frequently (every 2 weeks) have shown a response or delay in disease progression in occasional patients.[382] Pamidronate 90 mg and zoledronic acid 4 mg are equipotent in reducing bone-related problems in myeloma; the infusion time for zoledronic acid is 15 minutes compared to 1 to 2 hours for pamidronate.

The role of zoledronic acid was confirmed by the MRC Myeloma IX study, in which 1960 patients were randomized to

TABLE 48.18
Summary of Published Placebo-Controlled Trials of Bisphosphonates in Patients with Multiple Myeloma

	Belch et al.[413]	Lahtinen et al.[414]	Berenson et al.[375]
No. of Evaluable Patients	166	336	377
Bisphosphonate Therapy	Etidronate 5 mg/kg daily (oral)	Clodronate 2.4 g/d (oral) for 24 months	Pamidronate 90 mg (IV q 4 weeks × 9 cycles)
Lytic Bone Lesions	0	+	0
Pathologic Fractures	0	0	+
Radiation Therapy	NA	NA	+
Bone Pain	0	0	+
Hypercalcemia	0	0	+
Survival	−	0	+

0, no effect; +, beneficial effect; −, negative effect; NA, not assessed.

intravenous zoledronic acid or oral clodronic acid (1,600 mg per day). There was a significantly lower incidence of skeletal-related events with zoledronic acid (77% versus 11%, respectively; p = 0.0004) both in patients with and without bone lesions at baseline.[383] The results of this study support the early use of zoledronic acid in newly diagnosed MM, irrespective of bone disease status. A further analysis of this data suggested that its continued use beyond 2 years was beneficial. Interestingly, the study also showed that zoledronic acid reduced mortality by 16% versus clodronic acid (p = 0.0118), and extended median OS by 5.5 months (50.0 months versus 44.5 months; p = 0.04). Zoledronic acid also significantly improved PFS by 12% (95% CI, 2 to 20) versus clodronic acid (p = 0.0179), for the first time confirming antimyeloma activity of bisphosphonates. Rates of complete, very good partial, or partial response did not differ significantly between the zoledronic acid and clodronic acid groups.[384] Patients on long-term bisphosphonates should be monitored for development of renal toxicity. Renal dysfunction induced by pamidronate affects mainly tubules and manifests first as proteinuria followed by a rise in creatinine, whereas zoledronic acid affects glomeruli and manifests as a rise in creatinine without proteinuria. Even mild renal dysfunction requires bisphosphonate dose adjustment, and renal effects of bisphosphonates can be partly prevented by extending the duration of infusion. Osteonecrosis of the jaw (ONJ) is another complication of prolonged bisphosphonate therapy, which is observed in patients with dental procedures and in relationship to dental infection. In one study, 11 of 292 patients with MM (3.8%) had ONJ.[385] There is also some association between prolonged use and development of ONJ. Due to the increased detection of this complication, a prophylactic dental checkup and follow-up is recommended. After 2 years of administration, the frequency of administration of bisphosphonate may be modified in patients achieving VGPR or CR.[386] In a large phase 3 study, the antimyeloma activity of zoledronic acid has been described. Multiple agents directed at novel bone-directed targets are under investigation. The efficacy of denosumab, a RANKL-targeting antibody, has been confirmed in a phase 3 study in myeloma and breast cancer. An antibody targeting DKK-1 (BHQ-880), which improves osteoblastic activity, and a chimeric protein targeting activin A (ACE-011), are currently under evaluation in phase 1/2 clinical studies.

Therapy in Relapsed Patients

The options and therapeutic strategies for relapsed MM patients depend on the induction regimen used and whether the patients have undergone high-dose therapy and stem cell transplant. With the availability of multiple novel agents that have been approved for clinical use in MM— bortezomib, lenalidomide/dexamethasone, bortezomib and liposomal doxorubicin, pomalidomide, and carfilzomib—the choice will partly depend on the agent or combination not used as an induction and on the presence of existing toxicity such as neuropathy, cytopenias, or DVT.

The results of the international randomized phase III trial of bortezomib (1.3 mg/m^2 intravenously [IV] on days 1, 4, 8, and 11 every 3 weeks for eight cycles) have demonstrated its superiority over dexamethasone alone (40 mg by mouth [PO] on days 1 through 4, 9 through 12, and 17 through 20 every 5 weeks for four cycles) in terms of response rates (38% versus 18%, respectively; p <0.001), median time to progression (6.22 months versus 3.49 months respectively; p <0.001) and survival (1-year survival 80% versus 66%, respectively; p = 0.003) in 669 relapsed patients with MM who had received one to three prior therapies.[291] Another open label study has further confirmed the ability of added dexamethasone to improve response in relapsed patients. Various combinations of bortezomib with other agents such as doxorubicin, cyclophosphamide, and melphalan have been used to treat patients with MM, and results of larger representative studies are shown in Table 48.10B. For example, a randomized phase 3 multicenter international study has confirmed that the combination of bortezomib and pegylated liposomal doxorubicin is superior to bortezomib alone for both overall response (50% versus 42% respectively; p = 0.05), and time to progression (9.3 months versus 6.5 months, respectively; p <0.0001) in relapsed MM patients. Additionally, a combination of oral cyclophosphamide, dexamethasone, and bortezomib in 50 patients with relapsed/refractory MM has been reported to achieve ORR in 88% of patients, with a median event-free survival of 10 months and median overall survival not yet reached. The broader clinical benefit of other regimens remains to be determined.

Lenalidomide has been evaluated in two large phase 3 studies comparing it in combination with dexamethasone to high-dose dexamethasone and placebo. The combination of lenalidomide and dexamethasone showed significant advantages in the response rate (CR + PR: 56% versus 24%, respectively; p <0.001) and in time to progression (14 versus 5 months, respectively; p <0.01), as well as OS (30 versus 20 months, respectively; p <0.01). Lenalidomide was equally active in patients with or without previous exposure to bortezomib or thalidomide. However, lenalidomide in combination with high-dose dexamethasone had significantly higher rates of DVT (14% versus 5%, respectively; p <0.01). Lenalidomide has also been assessed in combination with bortezomib and dexamethasone in a phase 1/2 trial in patients with relapsed or refractory MM.

A pilot phase 1/2 study in relapsed refractory myeloma has evaluated the combination of lenalidomide and bortezomib in 38 patients. A 61% minimal response or better was observed, and 83% patients achieved stable disease or better when dexamethasone was added, including patients whose MM was resistant to either agent alone. Thalidomide has also been an active agent, both alone and in combination with dexamethasone in relapsed patients (see Table 48.8B). Although lenalidomide activity has been demonstrated in patients relapsing after thalidomide, it is unclear whether patients relapsing after lenalidomide will respond to thalidomide. A combination of bortezomib (1.0 to

1.3 mg/m²), thalidomide (50 to 200 mg per day) and dexamethasone (40 mg for 4 days) has been evaluated by Zangari et al.; In 83 patients with relapsed/refractory disease (over 70% patients having previously received thalidomide), 80% overall response with 16% CRs was reported. In relapsed MM, the combination of conventional chemotherapy not previously used with or without novel agents can be effective. Four-drug combinations, such as DCEP (dexamethasone, cyclophosphamide, etoposide, and cis-platinum), have been reported to achieve high response rates in relapsed patients, especially with aggressive disease. A regimen incorporating thalidomide + adriamycin with DCEP (DTPACE) for relapsed/refractory MM (n = 236) prior to HDT/SCT achieved 32% PR after two cycles of DTPACE, with 16% attaining a CR or nCR.[387]

A number of newer agents have been investigated in relapsed and/or refractory myeloma. In 2013, two novel agents, carfilzomib and pomalidomide, have been approved by the FDA for use in relapsed/refractory patients with myeloma. Carfilzomib, a second-generation proteasome inhibitor that selectively and irreversibly binds its target, has demonstrated single-agent and combination activity in relapsed and refractory patients with MM. In patients with relapsed MM after ≥ two previous therapies including bortezomib and an immunomodulatory agent and refractory to the last treatment (n = 42), the best ORR was 16.7%, and the median duration of response was 7.2 months.[388] In another phase 2, open-label, multicenter clinical trial (n = 35), patients with relapsed and/or refractory MM following one to three prior therapies including at least one bortezomib-based regimen, the best ORR was 17.1%, the median duration of response was >10.6 months, and the median time to progression was 4.6 months.[389] In an expanded single-arm phase 2 study, patients received single-agent carfilzomib 20 mg/m² intravenously twice weekly for 3 of 4 weeks in cycle 1, then 27 mg/m² for ≤12 cycles. In this study, 95% of 266 patients were refractory to their last therapy and 80% refractory or intolerant to both bortezomib and lenalidomide. In this study, ORR was 23.7%, with a median duration of response of 7.8 months, and median OS was 15.6 months.[390] Based on results of these studies, carfilzomib is now FDA approved for the treatment of relapsed myeloma. In another study in 129 bortezomib-naïve patients with relapsed MM, ORR was 42.4% in Cohort 1 and 52.2% in Cohort 2, in which patients received an increased dose of 27 mg/m² after the first cycle.[391] A low incidence of peripheral neuropathy (17.1% overall; one grade 3; no grade 4) was observed in these bortezomib-naïve patients. Notably, in all studies, peripheral neuropathy and neuropathy-related AEs were generally mild and infrequent. An analysis of response and survival data from the PX-171-03 study (n = 229) identified 62 patients (27.1%) with high-risk cytogenetics profiles (del 17p13, t[4;14] or t[14;16] by FISH or deletion 13 or hypodiploidy by metaphase cytogenetics) versus 167 patients (72.9%) with standard risk. Overall response was comparable between these two groups (25.8% versus 24.6%, respectively), but there was a trend in high-risk patients for a shorter median duration of response (5.6 months versus 8.3 months, respectively) and OS (9.3 months versus 19.0 months, respectively; p = 0.0003). This study suggests that single-agent carfilzomib is efficacious and has the potential to at least partially overcome the impact of high-risk cytogenetics in heavily pretreated MM.[392]

Pomalidomide, a more potent immunomodulatory drug, has demonstrated activity even in patients with MM resistant to lenalidomide. Pomalidomide at doses of 2 or 4 mg per day with weekly dexamethasone at 40 mg has demonstrated excellent activity in patients with MM. A phase 2 study (n = 35) confirmed responses in the 2-mg cohort (14% VGPR, 11% PR, and 23% MR), with an overall response rate (ORR) of 49%; and in the 4-mg cohort (3% CR, 9% VGPR, 17% PR and 14% MR), with an ORR of 43%. Overall survival at 6 months was 78% and 67% in the 2- and 4-mg cohort, respectively. Myelosuppression was the most common toxicity.[393] In another study (n = 60), pomalidomide 2 mg daily with Dex 40 mg orally on days 1, 8, 15, and 22 of each cycle in relapsed or refractory MM achieved a 63% response, including 5% CR and 28% VGPR. Responses were observed in 40% patients with lenalidomide-refractory MM. The median PFS was 11.6 months.[394] A phase 1 dose-escalation study determined the maximum tolerated dose (MTD) of oral pomalidomide 4 mg to be administered on days 1 to 21 of each 28-day cycle in patients with relapsed and refractory MM, with Dex added if no response occurred after four cycles. Among the 38 patients enrolled (including 22 with added dexamethasone), 42% achieved a minimal response or better, 21% achieved a partial response or better, and 3% achieved a complete response. The median duration of response, PFS, and OS were 4.6, 4.6, and 18.3 months, respectively.[395] IFM conducted a phase 2 randomized study comparing pomalidomide (4 mg) on days 1 to 21 (n = 43) or continuously (n = 41) over a 28-day cycle, plus dexamethasone given weekly, and reported similar response rates (35% versus 34%); time to progression (5.8 versus 4.8 months) and OS (14.9 versus 14.8 months); along with a similar toxicity profile, primarily myelosuppression, in both groups.[396] These studies have established pomalidomide 4 mg per day on days 1 to 21 of a 28-day cycle with 40-mg weekly dexamethasone as a standard for future studies. A phase 3, multicenter, randomized, open-label study of pomalidomide in combination with low-dose demonstrated a significant PFS and OS advantage over dexamethasone alone in patients with relapsed/refractory MM.[397] In a recent phase 1 study combining pomalidomide with bortezomib and dexamethasone in patients with relapsed/refractory MM showed 73% ORR and 27% VGPR, in patients who had previously received both bortezomib and lenalidomide, including 73% patients whose disease progressed on lenalidomide.[398]

Based on preclinical synergistic activity and phase 2 studies showing the ability of HDAC inhibitors (vorinostat and panobinostat) to overcome bortezomib resistance, ongoing phase 3 studies comparing bortezomib with combination of bortezomib with vorinostat and with panobinostat have been completed. Although increased responses were noted in relapsed MM treated with bortezomib and vorinostat versus vorinostat, alone, the PFS advantage was only one month, with treatment limited by diarrhea, thrombocytopenia, and fatigue.[399] The more selective HDAC inhibitor rocilinostat has been combined with bortezomib, as well as with lenalidomide/dexamethasone[400] and has achieved responses with a more favorable side effect profile. The combination of bortezomib and Akt inhibitor perifosine is able to overcome bortezomib resistance.[401] Finally, an antibody targeting CS-1 cell surface molecule (elotuzumab) has been shown to achieve over 80% response when combined with lenalidomide/dexamethasone in relapsed MM, and anti-CD38 monoclonal antibodies (daratumumab) are similarly achieving responses, even in high-risk relapsed MM.

Other Potential Agents and Future Direction

Both in vitro systems and in vivo animal models have been developed to characterize mechanisms of MM cell homing to BM, as well as factors (MM cell–BM stromal cell interactions, cytokines, angiogenesis) promoting MM cell growth, survival, drug resistance, and migration in the BM milieu. These model systems have allowed for the development of several promising biologically based therapies including the previously mentioned anti-CS1 antibody elotuzumab, the anti-CD38 antibody daratumumab, the HDAC6 inhibitor rocilinostat, as well as heat shock protein 90 inhibitor (AUY 922) and telomerase inhibitor GRN 163L, among many others (Fig. 48.15). Detailed oncogenomic studies are identifying novel targets and pathways operative in myeloma, and ongoing studies are determining mechanisms of action of novel agents at a gene and protein level in order to provide the framework for rational combination clinical trials that will overcome drug resistance and improve patient outcomes.

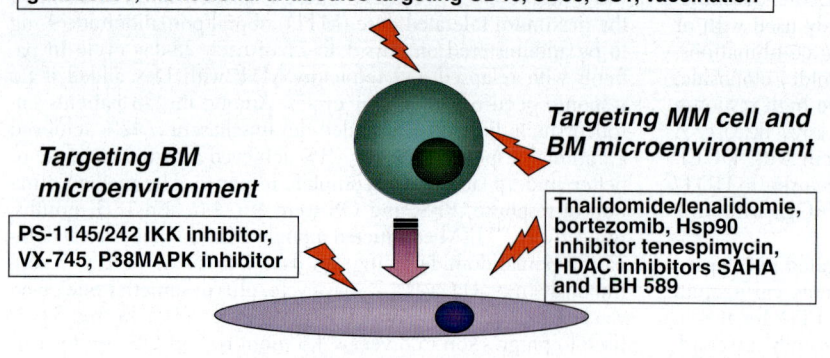

Figure 48.15 Novel therapies in preclinical or clinical development targeting the myeloma cells or their microenvironment or both.

REFERENCES

1. Macintyre W. Case of mollities and fragilitas ossium, accompanied with urine strongly charged with animal matter. *Med Chir Trans* 1859;33:211–232.
2. Bence J. On a new substance occurring in the urine of a patient with mollities and fragilits ossium. *Phil Trans R Soc Lond* 1848;55:673.
3. Kahler O. Zur Symptomatologie des multiplen Myeloms; beobachtung von Albumosurie. *Prag Med Wochnschr* 1889;14-33.
4. Arinkin M. The intravitale Untersuchungs-Methodik des Knochenmarks. *Folia Haematol (Leipz)* 1929;38:233.
5. Tiselius A. Electrophoresis of serum globulin. II. Electrophoretic analysis of normal and immune sera. *Biochem J* 1937;31:1464–1477.
6. Chauhan D, Uchiyama H, Akbarali Y, et al. Multiple myeloma cell adhesion-induced interleukin-6 expression in bone marrow stromal cells involves activation of NF-kappa B. *Blood* 1996;87:1104–1112.
7. Chauhan D, Anderson KC. *Cytokines and Signal Transduction in Multiple Myeloma* (4th ed.). Cambridge, UK: Cambridge University Press; 2001.
8. Holland JR, Hosley H, Scharlau C, et al. A controlled trial of urethane treatment in multiple myeloma. *Blood* 1966;27:328–342.
9. Bergsagel D. Evaluation of new chemotherapeutic agents in the treatment of multiple myeloma. IV. L-Phenylalanine mustard (NSC-8806). *Cancer Chemother Rep* 1962;21:87–99.
10. Salmon SE, Shadduck RK, Schilling A. Intermittent high-dose prednisone (NSC-10023) therapy for multiple myeloma. *Cancer Chemother Rep* 1967;51:179–187.
11. Alexanian R, Bonnet J, Gehan E, et al. Combination chemotherapy for multiple myeloma. *Cancer* 1972;30:382–389.
12. McElwain T, Powles R. High-dose intravenous melphalan for plasma-cell leukemia and myeloma. *Lancet* 1983;1:822–824.
13. Cohen HJ, Crawford J, Rao MK, et al. Racial differences in the prevalence of monoclonal gammopathy in a community-based sample of the elderly. *Am J Med* 1998;104:439–444.
14. Landgren O, Katzmann JA, Hsing AW, et al. Prevalence of monoclonal gammopathy of undetermined significance among men in Ghana. *Mayo Clin Proc* 2007;82:1468–1473.
15. Landgren O, Graubard BI, Katzmann JA, et al. Racial disparities in the prevalence of monoclonal gammopathies: a population-based study of 12 482 persons from the National Health and Nutritional Examination Survey. *Leukemia* 2014;28:1537–1542.
16. Riedel DA, Pottern LM. The epidemiology of multiple myeloma. *Hematol Oncol Clin North Am* 1992;6:225–247.
17. Ichimaru M, Ishimaru T, Mikami M, et al. Multiple myeloma among atomic bomb survivors in Hiroshima and Nagasaki, 1950-76: relationship to radiation dose absorbed by marrow. *J Natl Cancer Inst* 1982;69:323–328.
18. Bergsagel DE, Wong O, Bergsagel PL, et al. Benzene and multiple myeloma: appraisal of the scientific evidence. *Blood* 1999;94:1174–1182.
19. Lundberg I, Milatou-Smith R. Mortality and cancer incidence among Swedish paint industry workers with long-term exposure to organic solvents. *Scandinavian J Work Environ Health* 1998;24:270–275.
20. Salmon SE, Kyle RA. Silicone gels, induction of plasma cell tumors, and genetic susceptibility in mice: a call for epidemiologic investigation of women with silicone breast implants. *J Natl Cancer Inst* 1994;86:1040–1041.
21. Doody MM, Linet MS, Glass AG, et al. Risks of non-Hodgkin's lymphoma, multiple myeloma, and leukemia associated with common medications. *Epidemiology* 1996;7:131–139.
22. Linet MS, Harlow SD, McLaughlin JK. A case-control study of multiple myeloma in whites: chronic antigenic stimulation, occupation, and drug use. *Cancer Res* 1987;47:2978–2981.
23. Brown LM, Linet MS, Greenberg RS, et al. Multiple myeloma and family history of cancer among blacks and whites in the U.S. *Cancer* 1999;85:2385–2390.
24. Grosbois B, Jego P, Attal M, et al. Familial multiple myeloma: report of fifteen families. *Br J Haematol* 1999;105:768–770.
25. Weinhold N, Johnson DC, Chubb D, et al. The CCND1 c.870G>A polymorphism is a risk factor for t(11;14)(q13;q32) multiple myeloma. *Nat Genet* 2013;45:522–525.
26. Weinhold N, Johnson DC, Rawstron AC, et al. Inherited genetic susceptibility to monoclonal gammopathy of unknown significance. *Blood* 2014;124:
27. Kyle RA, Therneau TM, Rajkumar SV, et al. A long-term study of prognosis in monoclonal gammopathy of undetermined significance. *N Engl J Med* 2002;346:564–569.
28. Avet-Loiseau H, Facon T, Daviet A, et al. 14q32 translocations and monosomy 13 observed in monoclonal gammopathy of undetermined significance delineate a multistep process for the oncogenesis of multiple myeloma. Intergroupe Francophone du Myelome. *Cancer Res* 1999;59:4546–4550.
29. Seligmann M, Sassy C, Chevalier A. A human IgG myeloma protein with anti-2 macroglobulin antibody activity. *J Immunol* 1973;110:85–90.
30. Malik AA, Ganti AK, Potti A, et al. Role of Helicobacter pylori infection in the incidence and clinical course of monoclonal gammopathy of undetermined significance. *Am J Gastroenterol* 2002;97:1371–1374.
31. Rajkumar SV, Kyle RA, Plevak MF, et al. Helicobacter pylori infection and monoclonal gammopathy of undetermined significance. *Br J Haematol* 2002;119:706–708.
32. Konrad RJ, Kricka LJ, Goodman DB, et al. Brief report: myeloma-associated paraprotein directed against the HIV-1 p24 antigen in an HIV-1-seropositive patient. *N Engl J Med* 1993;328:1817–1819.
33. Landgren O, Kyle RA, Pfeiffer RM, et al. Monoclonal gammopathy of undetermined significance (MGUS) consistently precedes multiple myeloma: a prospective study. *Blood* 2009;113:5412–5417.
34. Brown LM, Gridley G, Check D, et al. Risk of multiple myeloma and monoclonal gammopathy of undetermined significance among white and black male United States veterans with prior autoimmune, infectious, inflammatory, and allergic disorders. *Blood* 2008;111:3388–3394.
35. Rettig MB, Ma HJ, Vescio RA, et al. Kaposi's sarcoma-associated herpesvirus infection of bone marrow dendritic cells from multiple myeloma patients [see comments]. *Science* 1997;276:1851–1854.
36. Soulier J, Grollet L, Oksenhendler E, et al. Kaposi's sarcoma-associated herpesvirus-like DNA sequences in multicentric Castleman's disease [see comments]. *Blood* 1995;86:1276–1280.
37. Said W, Chien K, Takeuchi S, et al. Kaposi's sarcoma-associated herpesvirus (KSHV or HHV8) in primary effusion lymphoma: ultrastructural demonstration of herpesvirus in lymphoma cells. *Blood* 1996;87:4937–4943.
38. Schalling M, Ekman M, Kaaya EE, et al. A role for a new herpes virus (KSHV) in different forms of Kaposi's sarcoma. *Nat Med* 1995;1:707–708.
39. Cull GM, Carter GI, Timms JM, et al. Low incidence of human herpesvirus 8 in stem cell collections from myeloma patients. *Bone Marrow Transplant* 1999;23:759–761.
40. Tarte K, Chang Y, Klein B. Kaposi's sarcoma-associated herpesvirus and multiple myeloma: lack of criteria for causality. *Blood* 1999;93:3159–3163.
41. Yi Q, Ekman M, Anton D, et al. Blood dendritic cells from myeloma patients are not infected with Kaposi's sarcoma-associated herpesvirus (KSHV/HHV-8). *Blood* 1998;92:402–404.
42. Tarte K, Olsen SJ, Yang Lu Z, et al. Clinical-grade functional dendritic cells from patients with multiple myeloma are not infected with Kaposi's sarcoma-associated herpesvirus. *Blood* 1998;91:1852–1857.

43. Brander C, Raje N, O'Connor PG, et al. Absence of biologically important Kaposi sarcoma associated herpesvirus gene products and virus-specific cellular immune responses in multiple myeloma. *Blood* 2002;100:648–700.
44. Sahota SS, Davis Z, Hamblin T, et al. Discordant somatic mutation of immunoglobulin variable region genes and bcl-6 genes in chronic lymphocytic leukemia. *Blood* 1999;94:662a.
45. Davies FE, Dring AM, Li C, et al. Insights into the multistep transformation of MGUS to myeloma using microarray expression analysis. *Blood* 2003;102:4504–4511.
46. Avet-Loiseau H, Li JY, Morineau N, et al. Monosomy 13 is associated with the transition of monoclonal gammopathy of undetermined significance to multiple myeloma. Intergroupe Francophone du Myelome. *Blood* 1999;94:2583–2589.
47. Weiss BM, Abadie J, Verma P, et al. A monoclonal gammopathy precedes multiple myeloma in most patients. *Blood* 2009;113:5418–5422.
48. Fonseca R, Bailey RJ, Ahmann GJ, et al. Genomic abnormalities in monoclonal gammopathy of undetermined significance. *Blood* 2002;100:1417–1424.
49. Kaufmann H, Ackermann J, Baldia C, et al. Both IGH translocations and chromosome 13q deletions are early events in monoclonal gammopathy of undetermined significance and do not evolve during transition to multiple myeloma. *Leukemia* 2004;18:1879–1882.
50. Neben K, Jauch A, Hielscher T, et al. Progression in smoldering myeloma is independently determined by the chromosomal abnormalities del(17p), t(4;14), gain 1q, hyperdiploidy, and tumor load. *J Clin Oncol* 2013;31:4325–4332.
51. Potter M. Experimental plasmacytomagenesis in mice. *Hematol Oncol Clin North Am* 1997;11:323–347.
52. Radl J. Multiple myeloma and related disorders. Lessons from an animal model. *Pathol Biol (Paris)* 1999;47:109–114.
53. Sawyer J, Waldron J, Jagannath S, et al. Cytogenetics findings in 200 patients with multiple myeloma. *Cancer Genet Cytogenet* 1995;82:41–49.
54. Sawyer JR, Lukacs JL, Thomas EL, et al. Multicolour spectral karyotyping identifies new translocations and a recurring pathway for chromosome loss in multiple myeloma. *Br J Haematol* 2001;112:167–174.
55. Perez-Simon JA, Garcia-Sanz R, Tabernero MD, et al. Prognostic value of numerical chromosome aberrations in multiple myeloma: a FISH analysis of 15 different chromosomes. *Blood* 1998;91:3366–3371.
56. Rasillo A, Tabernero MD, Sanchez ML, et al. Fluorescence in situ hybridization analysis of aneuploidization patterns in monoclonal gammopathy of undetermined significance versus multiple myeloma and plasma cell leukemia. *Cancer* 2003;97:601–609.
57. Chng WJ, Van Wier SA, Ahmann GJ, et al. A validated FISH trisomy index demonstrates the hyperdiploid and nonhyperdiploid dichotomy in MGUS. *Blood* 2005;106:2156–2161.
58. Hallek M, Bergsagel LP, Anderson KD. Multiple myeloma: increasing evidence for a multistep transformation process. *Blood* 1998;91:3–21.
59. Dewald GW, Kyle RA, Hicks GA, et al. The clinical significance of cytogenetic studies in 100 patients with multiple myeloma, plasma cell leukemia, or amyloidosis. *Blood* 1985;66:380–390.
60. Drach J, Angerler J, Schuster J, et al. Interphase fluorescence in situ hybridization identifies chromosomal abnormalities in plasma cells from patients with monoclonal gammopathy of undetermined significance. *Blood* 1995;86:3915–3921.
61. Hayman SR, Bailey RJ, Jalal SM, et al. Translocations involving the immunoglobulin heavy-chain locus are possible early genetic events in patients with primary systemic amyloidosis. *Blood* 2001;98:2266–2268.
62. Chesi M, Bergsagel PL, Brents LA, et al. Dysregulation of cyclin D1 by translocation into an IgH gamma switch region in two multiple myeloma cell lines [see comments]. *Blood* 1996;88:674–681.
63. Hart KC, Robertson SC, Kanemitsu MY, et al. Transformation and Stat activation by derivatives of FGFR1, FGFR3, and FGFR4. *Oncogene* 2000;19:3309–3320.
64. Chesi M, Nardini E, Brents LA, et al. Frequent translocation t(4;14)(p16.3;q32.3) in multiple myeloma is associated with increased expression and activating mutations of fibroblast growth factor receptor 3. *Nat Genet* 1997;16:260–264.
65. Chesi M, Brents LA, Ely SA, et al. Activated fibroblast growth factor receptor 3 is an oncogene that contributes to tumor progression in multiple myeloma. *Blood* 2001;97:729–736.
66. Plowright EE, Li Z, Bergsagel PL, et al. Ectopic expression of fibroblast growth factor receptor 3 promotes myeloma cell proliferation and prevents apoptosis. *Blood* 2000;95:992–998.
67. Chesi M, Bergsagel PL, Shonukan OO, et al. Frequent dysregulation of the c-maf proto-oncogene at 16q23 by translocation to an Ig locus in multiple myeloma. *Blood* 1998;91:4457–4463.
68. Iida S, Rao PH, Butler M, et al. Deregulation of MUM1/IRF4 by chromosomal translocation in multiple myeloma. *Nat Genet* 1997;17:226–230.
69. Mahmoud MS, Huang N, Nobuyoshi M, et al. Altered expression of Pax-5 gene in human myeloma cells. *Blood* 1996;87:4311–4315.
70. Shou Y, Martelli ML, Gabrea A, et al. Diverse karyotypic abnormalities of the c-myc locus associated with c-myc dysregulation and tumor progression in multiple myeloma. *Proc Natl Acad Sci U S A* 2000;97:228–233.
71. Avet-Loiseau H, Gerson F, Magrangeas F, et al. Rearrangements of the c-myc oncogene are present in 15% of primary human multiple myeloma tumors. *Blood* 2001;98:3082–3086.
72. Selvanayagam P, Blick M, Narni F, et al. Alteration and abnormal expression of the c-myc oncogene in human multiple myeloma. *Blood* 1988;71:30–35.
73. Greil R, Fasching B, Loidl P, et al. Expression of the C-Myc proto-oncogene in multiple myeloma and chronic lymphocytic leukemia: an in situ analysis. *Blood* 1991;78:180–191.
74. Tricot G, Sawyer JR, Jaganath S, et al. Poor prognosis in multiple myeloma is associated only with partial or complete deletion of chromosome 13 or abnormalities involving 11q and not with other karyotype abnormalities. *Blood* 1995;86:4250–4256.
75. Dao DD, Sawyer JR, Epstein J, et al. Deletion on of the retinoblastoma gene on multiple myeloma. *Leukemia* 1994;8:1280–1284.
76. Shaughnessy J, Barlogie B. Chromosome 13 deletion in myeloma. *Curr Top Microbiol Immunol* 1999;246:199–203.
77. Urashima M, Ogata A, Chauhan D, et al. Interleukin-6 promotes multiple myeloma cell growth via phosphorylation of retinoblastoma protein. *Blood* 1996;88:2219–2227.
78. Ng MH, Chung YF, Lo KW, et al. Frequent hypermethylation of p16 and p15 genes in multiple myeloma. *Blood* 1997;89:2500–2506.
79. Urashima M, Teoh G, Ogata A, et al. Characterization of p16(INK4A) expression in multiple myeloma and plasma cell leukemia. *Clin Cancer Res* 1997;3:2173–2179.
80. Kawano MM, Mahmoud MS, Ishikawa H. Cyclin D1 and p16INK4A are preferentially expressed in immature and mature myeloma cells, respectively. *Br J Haematol* 1997;99:131–138.
81. Neri A, Baldini L, Trecca D, et al. p53 gene mutations in multiple myeloma are associated with advanced forms of malignancy. *Blood* 1993;81:128–135.
82. Portier M, Moles JP, Mazars GR, et al. p53 and RAS gene mutations in multiple myeloma. *Oncogene* 1992;7:2539–2543.
83. Teoh G, Urashima M, Ogata A, et al. MDM2 protein overexpression promotes proliferation and survival of multiple myeloma cells. *Blood* 1997;90:1982–1992.
84. Pettersson M, Jernberg-Wiklund H, Larsson LG, et al. Expression if the Bcl-2 gene in human multiple myeloma cell lines and normal plasma cells. *Blood* 1992;79:495–502.
85. Puthier D, Pellat-Deceunynck C, Barille S, et al. Differential expression of Bcl-2 in human plasma cell disorders according to proliferation status and malignancy. *Leukemia* 1999;13:289–294.
86. Gazitt Y, Fey V, Thomas C, et al. Bcl-2 overexpression is associated with resistance to dexamethasone, but not melphalan, in multiple myeloma cells. *Int J Oncol* 1998;13:397–405.
87. Iyer R, Ding L, Batchu RB, et al. Antisense p53 transduction leads to overexpression of bcl-2 and dexamethasone resistance in multiple myeloma. *Leuk Res* 2003;27:73–78.
88. Sangfelt O, Osterborg A, Grander D, et al. Response to interferon therapy in patients with multiple myeloma correlates with expression of the Bcl-2 oncoprotein. *Int J Cancer* 1995;63:190–192.
89. Catlett-Falcone R, Landowski TH, Oshiro MM, et al. Constitutive activation of Stat3 signaling confers resistance to apoptosis in human U266 myeloma cells. *Immunity* 1999;10:105–115.
90. Hideshima T, Mitsiades C, Ikeda H, et al. A proto-oncogene BCL6 is up-regulated in the bone marrow microenvironment in multiple myeloma cells. *Blood* 2010;115:3772–3775.
91. Shammas MA, Shmookler Reis RJ, Akiyama M, et al. Telomerase inhibition and cell growth arrest by G-quadruplex interactive agent in multiple myeloma. *Mol Cancer Ther* 2003;2:825–833.
92. Bergsagel DE, Kuehl M, Zhan F, et al. Cyclin D dysregulation: an early and unifying pathogenic event in multiple myeloma. *Blood* 2005;106:296–303.
93. Shaughnessy JD Jr, Zhan F, Burington BE, et al. A validated gene expression model of high-risk multiple myeloma is defined by deregulated expression of genes mapping to chromosome 1. *Blood* 2007;109:2276–2284.
94. Decaux O, Lode L, Magrangeas F, et al. Prediction of survival in multiple myeloma based on gene expression profiles reveals cell cycle and chromosomal instability signatures in high-risk patients and hyperdiploid signatures in low-risk patients: a study of the Intergroupe Francophone du Myelome. *J Clin Oncol* 2008;26:4798–4805.
95. Broyl A, Hose D, Lokhorst H, et al. Gene expression profiling for molecular classification of multiple myeloma in newly diagnosed patients. *Blood* 2010;116:2543–2553.
96. Avet-Loiseau H, Li C, Magrangeas F, et al. Prognostic significance of copy-number alterations in multiple myeloma. *J Clin Oncol* 2009;27:4585–4590.
97. Delmore JE, Issa GC, Lemieux ME, et al. BET bromodomain inhibition as a therapeutic strategy to target c-Myc. *Cell* 2011;146:904–917.
98. Kaiser MF, Johnson DC, Wu P, et al. Global methylation analysis identifies prognostically important epigenetically inactivated tumor suppressor genes in multiple myeloma. *Blood* 2013;122:219–226.
99. Pichiorri F, Suh SS, Ladetto M, et al. MicroRNAs regulate critical genes associated with multiple myeloma pathogenesis. *Proc Natl Acad Sci U S A* 2008;105:12885–12890.
100. Gutierrez NC, Sarasquete ME, Misiewicz-Krzeminska I, et al. Deregulation of microRNA expression in the different genetic subtypes of multiple myeloma and correlation with gene expression profiling. *Leukemia* 2010;24:629–637.
101. Pichiorri F, Suh SS, Rocci A, et al. Downregulation of p53-inducible microRNAs 192, 194, and 215 impairs the p53/MDM2 autoregulatory loop in multiple myeloma development. *Cancer Cell* 2008;18:367–381.
102. Leone E, Morelli E, Di Martino MT, et al. Targeting miR-21 inhibits in vitro and in vivo multiple myeloma cell growth. *Clin Cancer Res* 2013;19:2096–2106.
103. Amodio N, Bellizzi D, Leotta M, et al. miR-29b induces SOCS-1 expression by promoter demethylation and negatively regulates migration of multiple myeloma and endothelial cells. *Cell Cycle* 2013;12:3650–3662.

104. Di Martino MT, Leone E, Amodio N, et al. Synthetic miR-34a mimics as a novel therapeutic agent for multiple myeloma: in vitro and in vivo evidence. *Clin Cancer Res* 2012;18:6260–6270.
105. Chapman MA, Lawrence MS, Keats JJ, et al. Initial genome sequencing and analysis of multiple myeloma. *Nature* 2011;471:467–472.
106. Magrangeas F, Avet-Loiseau H, Gouraud W, et al. Minor clone provides a reservoir for relapse in multiple myeloma. *Leukemia* 2013;27:473–481.
107. Bolli N, Avet-Loiseau H, Wedge DC, et al. Heterogeneity of genomic evolution and mutational profiles in multiple myeloma. *Nat Commun* 2014;5:2997.
108. Dhodapkar MV, Kelly T, Theus A, et al. Elevated levels of shed syndecan-1 correlate with tumour mass and decreased matrix metalloproteinase-9 activity in the serum of patients with multiple myeloma [published erratum appears in Br J Haematol 1998 May;101(2):398]. *Br J Haematol* 1997;99:368–371.
109. Yang Y, Yaccoby S, Liu W, et al. Soluble syndecan-1 promotes growth of myeloma tumors in vivo. *Blood* 2002;100:610–617.
110. Chauhan D, Uchiyama H, Urashima M, et al. Regulation of interleukin-6 in multiple myeloma and bone marrow stromal cells. *Stem Cells* 1995;15:35–39.
111. Hideshima T, Chauhan D, Schlossman R, et al. The role of Tumor necrosis factor a in the pathophysiology of human multiple myeloma: therapeutic applications. *Oncogene* 2001;20:4519–4527.
112. Dankar B, Padro T, Leo R, et al. Vascular endothelial growth factor and interleukin-6 in paracrine tumor-stromal cell interactions in multiple myeloma. *Blood* 2000;95:2630–2636.
113. Hideshima T, Chauhan D, Hayashi T, et al. The biological sequelae of stromal cell-derived factor-1alpha in multiple myeloma. *Mol Cancer Ther* 2002;1:539–544.
114. Tai YT, Podar K, Catley L, et al. Insulin-like growth factor-1 induces adhesion and migration in human multiple myeloma cells via activation of beta1-integrin and phosphatidylinositol 3'-kinase/AKT signaling. *Cancer Res* 2003;63:5850–5858.
115. Keats JJ, Fonseca R, Chesi M, et al. Promiscuous mutations activate the non-canonical NF kappaB pathway in multiple myeloma. *Cancer Cell* 2007;12:131–144.
116. Annunziata CM, Davis RE, Demchenko Y, et al. Frequent engagement of the classical and alternative NF-kappaB pathways by diverse genetic abnormalities in multiple myeloma. *Cancer Cell* 2007;12:115–130.
117. Demchenko YN, Glebov OK, Zingone A, et al. Classical and/or alternative NF-kappaB pathway activation in multiple myeloma. *Blood* 2010;115:3541–3552.
118. Vacca A, Ribatti D, Roncali L, et al. Bone marrow angiogenesis and progression in multiple myeloma. *Br J Haematol* 1994;87:503–508.
119. Rajkumar SV, Fonseca R, Witzig TE, et al. Bone marrow angiogenesis in patients achieving complete response after stem cell transplantation for multiple myeloma. *Leukemia* 1999;13:469–472.
120. Rajkumar SV, Mesa RA, Fonseca R, et al. Bone marrow angiogenesis in 400 patients with monoclonal gammopathy of undetermined significance, multiple myeloma, and primary amyloidosis. *Clin Cancer Res* 2002;8:2210–2216.
121. Munshi NC, Wilson C. Increased bone marrow microvessel density in newly diagnosed multiple myeloma carries a poor prognosis. *Semin Oncol* 2001;28:565–569.
122. Kumar S, Fonseca R, Dispenzieri A, et al. Bone marrow angiogenesis in multiple myeloma: effect of therapy. *Br J Haematol* 2002;119:665–671.
123. Bellamy WT, Richter L, Frutiger Y, et al. Expression of vascular endothelial growth factor and its receptors in hematopoietic malignancies. *Cancer Res* 1999;59:728–733.
124. Seidel C, Borset M, Turesson I, et al. Elevated serum concentrations of hepatocyte growth factor in patients with multiple myeloma. The Nordic Myeloma Study Group. *Blood* 1998;91:806–812.
125. Chauhan D, Singh AV, Brahmandam M, et al. Functional interaction of plasmacytoid dendritic cells with multiple myeloma cells: a therapeutic target. *Cancer Cell* 2009;16:309–323.
126. Urashima M, Ogata A, Chauhan D, et al. Transforming growth factor-beta1: differential effects on multiple myeloma versus normal B cells. *Blood* 1996;87:1928–1938.
127. Brenne AT, Baade Ro T, Waage A, et al. Interleukin-21 is a growth and survival factor for human myeloma cells. *Blood* 2002;99:3756–3762.
128. Mitsiades CS, Mitsiades N, Poulaki V, et al. Activation of NF-kappaB and upregulation of intracellular anti-apoptotic proteins via the IGF-1/Akt signaling in human multiple myeloma cells: therapeutic implications. *Oncogene* 2002;21:5673–5683.
129. Qiang YW, Kopantzev E, Rudikoff S. Insulinlike growth factor-I signaling in multiple myeloma: downstream elements, functional correlates, and pathway cross-talk. *Blood* 2002;99:4138–4146.
130. Akiyama M, Hideshima T, Hayashi T, et al. Cytokines modulate telomerase activity in a human multiple myeloma cell line. *Cancer Res* 2002;62:3876–3882.
131. Podar K, Tai YT, Davies FE, et al. Vascular endothelial growth factor triggers signaling cascades mediating multiple myeloma cell growth and migration. *Blood* 2001;98:428–435.
132. Podar K, Tai YT, Lin BK, et al. Vascular endothelial growth factor-induced migration of multiple myeloma cells is associated with beta 1 integrin- and phosphatidylinositol 3-kinase-dependent PKC alpha activation. *J Biol Chem* 2002;277:7875–7881.
133. Gupta D, Treon SP, Shima Y, et al. Adherence of multiple myeloma cells to bone marrow stromal cells upregulates vascular endothelial growth factor secretion: therapeutic applications. *Leukemia* 2001;15:1950–1961.
134. Lin B, Podar K, Gupta D, et al. The vascular endothelial growth factor receptor tyrosine kinase inhibitor PTK787/ZK222584 inhibits growth and migration of multiple myeloma cells in the bone marrow microenvironment. *Cancer Res* 2002;62:5019–5026.
135. Prabhala RH, Pelluru D, Fulciniti M, et al. Elevated IL-17 produced by TH17 cells promotes myeloma cell growth and inhibits immune function in multiple myeloma. *Blood* 2010;115:5385–5392.
136. Gieseler F, Nussler V. Cellular resistance mechanisms with impact on the therapy of multiple myeloma. *Leukemia* 1998;12:1009–1012.
137. Raaijmakers HG, Izquierdo MA, Lokhorst HM, et al. Lung-resistance-related protein expression is a negative predictive factor for response to conventional low but not to intensified dose alkylating chemotherapy in multiple myeloma. *Blood* 1998;91:1029–1036.
138. Pilarski LM, Jensen GS. Monoclonal circulating B cells in multiple myeloma. A continuously differentiating, possibly invasive, population as defined by expression of CD45 isoforms and adhesion molecules. *Hematol Oncol Clin North Am* 1992;6:297–322.
139. Jensen GS, Mant MJ, Belch AJ, et al. Selective expression of CD45 isoforms defines CALLA+ monoclonal B-lineage cells in peripheral blood from myeloma patients as late stage B cells. *Blood* 1991;78:711–719.
140. Hata H, Xiao HQ, Petrucci MT, et al. Interleukin-6 gene expression in multiple myeloma: a characteristic of immature myeloma cells. *Blood* 1993;81:3357–3364.
141. Kawano MM, Huang N, Harada H, et al. Identification of immature and mature myeloma cells in the bone marrow of human myelomas. *Blood* 1993;82:564–570.
142. Epstein J, Barlogie B, Katzmann J, et al. Phenotypic heterogeneity in aneuploid multiple myeloma indicates pre-B cell involvement. *Blood* 1988;71:861–865.
143. Kawano MM, Mahmoud MS, Huang N, et al. High proportions of VLA-5-immature myeloma cells correlated well with poor response to treatment in multiple myeloma. *Br J Haematol* 1995;91:860–864.
144. Robillard N, Jego G, Pellat-Deceunynck C, et al. CD28, a marker associated with tumoral expansion in multiple myeloma. *Clin Cancer Res* 1998;4:1521–1526.
145. Treon SP, Shima Y, Preffer FI, et al. Treatment of plasma cell dyscrasias by antibody-mediated immunotherapy. *Semin Oncol* 1999;26:97–106.
146. Thomas X, Xiao HQ, Chang R, et al. Circulating B lymphocytes in multiple myeloma patients contain an autocrine IL-6 driven pre-myeloma cell population. *Curr Top Microbiol Immunol* 1995;182:201–207.
147. Matsui W, Huff CA, Wang Q, et al. Characterization of clonogenic multiple myeloma cells. *Blood* 2004;103:2332–2336.
148. Pilarski LM, Andrews EJ, Mant MJ, et al. Humoral immune deficiency in multiple myeloma patients due to compromised B-cell function. *J Clin Immunol* 1986;6:491–501.
149. Munshi NC. Immunoregulatory mechanisms in multiple myeloma. *Hematol Oncol Clin North Am* 1997;11:51–69.
150. Ludwig H, Fritz E. [Lymphocyte subpopulations in multiple myeloma. Shift in the helper/suppressor cell relation]. *Acta Medica Austriaca* 1982;9:215–220.
151. Mellstedt H, Holm G, Pettersson D, et al. T cells in monoclonal gammopathies. *Scand J Haematol* 1982;29:57–64.
152. Mills KH, Cawley JC. Abnormal monoclonal antibody-defined helper/suppressor T-cell subpopulations in multiple myeloma: relationship to treatment and clinical stage. *Br J Haematol* 1983;53:271–275.
153. Osterborg A, Nilsson B, Bjorkholm M, et al. Natural killer cell activity in monoclonal gammopathies: relation to disease activity. *Eur J Haematol* 1990;45:153–157.
154. Pilarski LM, Mant MJ, Ruether BA, et al. Abnormal clonogenic potential of T cells from multiple myeloma patients. *Blood* 1985;66:1266–1271.
155. Maecker B, Anderson KS, von Bergwelt-Baildon MS, et al. Viral antigen-specific CD8+ T-cell responses are impaired in multiple myeloma. *Br J Haematol* 2003;121:842–848.
156. Dhodapkar MV, Geller MD, Chang DH, et al. A reversible defect in natural killer T cell function characterizes the progression of premalignant to malignant multiple myeloma. *J Exp Med* 2003;197:1667–1676.
157. Song W, van der Vliet HJ, Tai YT, et al. Generation of antitumor invariant natural killer T cell lines in multiple myeloma and promotion of their functions via lenalidomide: a strategy for immunotherapy. *Clin Cancer Res* 2008;14:6955–6962.
158. Prabhala RH, Neri P, Bae JE, et al. Dysfunctional T regulatory cells in multiple myeloma. *Blood* 2006;107:301–304.
159. Gorgun GT, Whitehill G, Anderson JL, et al. Tumor-promoting immune-suppressive myeloid-derived suppressor cells in the multiple myeloma microenvironment in humans. *Blood* 2013;121:2975–2987.
160. Yi Q, Osterborg A, Bergenbrant S, et al. Idiotype-reactive T-cell subsets and tumor load in monoclonal gammopathies. *Blood* 1995;86:3043–3049.
161. Yi Q, Osterborg A. Idiotype-specific T cells in multiple myeloma: targets for an immunotherapeutic intervention? *Med Oncol* 1996;13:1–7.
162. Radl J, Croese JW, Zurcher C, et al. Animal model of human disease. Multiple myeloma. *Am J Pathol* 1988;132:593–597.
163. Feo-Zuppardi FJ, Taylor CW, Iwato K, et al. Long-term engraftment of fresh human myeloma cells in SCID mice. *Blood* 1992;80:2843–2850.
164. Tassone P, Neri P, Carrasco DR, et al. A clinically relevant SCID-hu in vivo model of human multiple myeloma. *Blood* 2005;106:713–716.
165. Urashima M, Chen BP, Chen S, et al. The development of a model for the homing of multiple myeloma cells to human bone marrow. *Blood* 1997;90:754–765.

166. Yaccoby S, Barlogie B, Epstein J. Primary myeloma cells growing in SCID-hu mice: a model for studying the biology and treatment of myeloma and its manifestations. *Blood* 1998;92:2908–2913.
167. Carrasco DR, Sukhdeo K, Protopopova M, et al. The differentiation and stress response factor XBP-1 drives multiple myeloma pathogenesis. *Cancer Cell* 2007;11:349–360.
168. Iwakoshi NN, Lee AH, Vallabhajosyula P, et al. Plasma cell differentiation and the unfolded protein response intersect at the transcription factor XBP-1. *Nat Immunol* 2003;4:321–329.
169. Chesi M, Robbiani DF, Sebag M, et al. AID-dependent activation of a MYC transgene induces multiple myeloma in a conditional mouse model of postgerminal center malignancies. *Cancer Cell* 2008;13:167–180.
170. Solomon A, Weiss DT, Kattine AA. Nephrotoxic potential of Bence Jones proteins [see comments]. *N Engl J Med* 1991;324:1845–1851.
171. Khamlichi AA, Rocca A, Touchard G, et al. Role of light chain variable region in myeloma with light chain deposition disease: evidence from an experimental model. *Blood* 1995;86:3655–3659.
172. Pozzi C, Fogazzi GB, Banfi G, et al. Renal disease and patient survival in light chain deposition disease. *Clin Nephrol* 1995;43:281–287.
173. Clark AD, Shetty A, Soutar R. Renal failure and multiple myeloma: pathogenesis and treatment of renal failure and management of underlying myeloma. *Blood Rev* 1999;13:79–90.
174. Huang ZQ, Sanders PW. Localization of a single binding site for immunoglobulin light chains on human Tamm-Horsfall glycoprotein. *J Clin Invest* 1997;99:732–736.
175. Kyle RA, Greipp PR. Amyloidosis (AL): clinical and laboratory features in 229 cases. *Mayo Clin Proc* 1983;58:665–583.
176. Fattori E, Della Rocca C, Costa P, et al. Development of progressive kidney damage and myeloma kidney in interleukin-6 transgenic mice. *Blood* 1994;83:2570–2579.
177. Mundy GR, Raisz LG, Cooper RA, et al. Evidence for the secretion of an osteoclast stimulating factor in myeloma. *N Engl J Med* 1974;291:1041–1046.
178. Roodman GD. Mechanisms of bone lesions in multiple myeloma and lymphoma. *Cancer* 1997;80:1557–1563.
179. Bataille R, Manolagas SC, Berenson JR. Pathogenesis and management of bone lesions in multiple myeloma. *Hematol Oncol Clin North Am* 1997;11:349–361.
180. Cozzolino F, Torcia M, Aldinucci D, et al. Production of interleukin-1 by bone marrow myeloma cells. *Blood* 1989;74:380–387.
181. Garrett R, Durie B, Nedwin G, et al. Production of lymphotoxin, a bone resorbing cytokine, by cultured human myeloma cells. *N Engl J Med* 1987;317:526–532.
182. Oba Y, Lee JW, Ehrlich LA, et al. MIP-1alpha utilizes both CCR1 and CCR5 to induce osteoclast formation and increase adhesion of myeloma cells to marrow stromal cells. *Exp Hematol* 2005;33:272–278.
183. Tricot G. New Insights into role of microenvironment in multiple myeloma. *Lancet* 2000;355:248–250.
184. Lacey DL, Timms E, Tan HL, et al. Osteoprotegerin ligand is a cytokine that regulates osteoclast differentiation and activation. *Cell* 1998;93:165–176.
185. Simonet WS, Lacey DL, Dunstan CR, et al. Osteoprotegerin: a novel secreted protein involved in the regulation of bone density [see comments]. *Cell* 1997;89:309–319.
186. Tian E, Zhan F, Walker R, et al. The role of the Wnt-signaling antagonist DKK1 in the development of osteolytic lesions in multiple myeloma. *N Engl J Med* 2003;349:2483–2494.
187. Fulciniti M, Tassone P, Hideshima T, et al. Anti-DKK1 mAb (BHQ880) as a potential therapeutic agent for multiple myeloma. *Blood* 2009;114:371–379.
188. Vallet S, Mukherjee S, Vaghela N, et al. Activin A promotes multiple myeloma-induced osteolysis and is a promising target for myeloma bone disease. *Proc Natl Acad Sci U S A* 2010;107:5124–5129.
189. Broder S, Humphrey R, Durm M, et al. Impaired synthesis of polyclonal (non-paraprotein) immunoglobulins by circulating lymphocytes from patients with multiple myeloma Role of suppressor cells. *N Engl J Med* 1975;293:887–892.
190. Jacobson DR, Zolla-Pazner S. Immunosuppression and infection in multiple myeloma. *Semin Oncol* 1986;13:282–290.
191. Cook G, Campbell JD, Carr CE, et al. Transforming growth factor beta from multiple myeloma cells inhibits proliferation and IL-2 responsiveness in T lymphocytes. *J Leukoc Biol* 1999;66:981–988.
192. Wu KL, van Wieringen W, Vellenga E, et al. Analysis of the efficacy and toxicity of bortezomib for treatment of relapsed or refractory multiple myeloma in community practice. *Haematologica* 2005;90:996–997.
193. Paradisi F, Corti G, Cinelli R. Infections in multiple myeloma. *Infect Dis Clin North Am* 2001;15:373–384, vii–viii.
194. Soubrier MJ, Dubost JJ, Sauvezie BJM. Syndrome at FSGoP. POEMS syndrome: a study of 25 cases and a review of the literature. *Am J Med* 1994;97:543–553.
195. Lacy MQ, Gertz MA, Hanson CA, et al. Multiple myeloma associated with diffuse osteosclerotic bone lesions: a clinical entity distinct from osteosclerotic myeloma (POEMS syndrome). *Am J Hematol* 1997;56:288–293.
196. Miralles GD, O'Fallon JR, Talley NJ. Plasma-cell dyscrasia with polyneuropathy. The spectrum of POEMS syndrome. *N Engl J Med* 1992;327:1919–1923.
197. Waldenstrom JG, Adner A, Gydell K, et al. Osteosclerotic "plasmocytoma" with polyneuropathy, hypertrichosis and diabetes. *Acta Medica Scandinavica* 1978;203(4):297–303.
198. Leifer D, Grabowski T, Simonian N, et al. Leptomeningeal myelomatosis presenting with mental status changes and other neurologic findings. *Cancer* 1992;70:1899–1904.
199. Fassas AB, Muwalla F, Berryman T, et al. Myeloma of the central nervous system association with high-risk chromosomal abnormalities, plasmablastic morphology and extramedullary manifestations. *Br J Haematol* 2002;117:103–108.
200. Dispenzieri A, Kyle RA. Neurological aspects of multiple myeloma and related disorders. *Best Pract Res Clin Haematol* 2005;18:673–688.
201. Pruzanski W, Watt JG. Serum viscosity and hyperviscosity syndrome in IgG multiple myeloma. Report on 10 patients and a review of the literature. *Ann Intern Med* 1972;77:853–860.
202. Preston FE, Cooke KB, Foster ME, et al. Myelomatosis and the hyperviscosity syndrome. *Br J Haematol* 1978;38:517–530.
203. Chandy KG, Stockley RA, Leonard RC, et al. Relationship between serum viscosity and intravascular IgA polymer concentration in IgA myeloma. *Clin Exp Immunol* 1981;46:653–661.
204. Capra JD, Kunkel HG. Aggregation of gamma-G3 proteins: relevance to the hyperviscosity syndrome. *J Clin Invest* 1970;49:610–621.
205. Perkins HA, MacKenzie MR, Fudenberg HH. Hemostatic defects in dysproteinemias. *Blood* 1970;35:695–707.
206. Lackner H. Hemostatic abnormalities associated with dysproteinemias. *Semin Hematol* 1973;10(2):125–133.
207. Elice F, Fink L, Tricot G, et al. Acquired resistance to activated protein C (aAPCR) in multiple myeloma is a transitory abnormality associated with an increased risk of venous thromboembolism. *Br J Haematol* 2006;134:399–405.
208. Deitcher SR, Erban JK, Limentani SA. Acquired free protein S deficiency associated with multiple myeloma: a case report. *Am J Hematol* 1996;51:319–323.
209. Coleman M, Vigliano EM, Weksler ME, et al. Inhibition of fibrin monomer polymerization by lambda myeloma globulins. *Blood* 1972;39:210–223.
210. Furie B, Greene E, Furie BC. Syndrome of acquired factor X deficiency and systemic amyloidosis in vivo studies of the metabolic fate of factor X. *N Engl J Med* 1977;297:81–85.
211. Zangari M, Anaissie E, Barlogie B, et al. Increased risk of deep-vein thrombosis in patients with multiple myeloma receiving thalidomide and chemotherapy. *Blood* 2001;98:1614–1615.
212. Zangari M, Saghafifar F, Anaissie E, et al. Activated protein C resistance in the absence of factor V Leiden mutation is a common finding in multiple myeloma and is associated with an increased risk of thrombotic complications. *Blood Coagul Fibrinolysis* 2002;13:187–192.
213. Barlogie B, Smallwood L, Smith T, et al. High serum levels of lactic dehydrogenase identify a high-grade lymphoma-like myeloma. *Ann Intern Med* 1989;110:521–525.
214. Usmani SZ, Heuck C, Mitchell A, et al. Extramedullary disease portends poor prognosis in multiple myeloma and is over-represented in high-risk disease even in the era of novel agents. *Haematologica* 2012;97:1761–1767.
215. International Myeloma Working Group. Criteria for the classification of monoclonal gammopathies, multiple myeloma and related disorders: a report of the International Myeloma Working Group. *Br J Haematol* 2003;121:749–757.
216. Dimopoulos M, Kyle R, Fermand JP, et al. Consensus recommendations for standard investigative workup: report of the International Myeloma Workshop Consensus Panel 3. *Blood* 2011;117:4701–4705.
217. Anderson K. Multiple myeloma: advances reported in 2013 are useful in the clinic. *J Natl Compr Canc Netw* 2014;12(5 Suppl):808–811.
218. Pizzolato M, Bragantini G, Bresciani P, et al. IgG1-kappa biclonal gammopathy associated with multiple myeloma suggests a regulatory mechanism. *Br J Haematol* 1998;102:503–508.
219. Zent CS, Wilson CS, Tricot G, et al. Oligoclonal protein bands and Ig isotype switching in multiple myeloma treated with high-dose therapy and hematopoietic cell transplantation. *Blood* 1998;91:3518–3523.
220. Kozuru M, Uike N, Takahira H, et al. Immunoglobulin class switch from IgA1 to IgG2 and simultaneous association with Bence Jones proteinuria in the escape phase in a myeloma patient treated with interferon alpha. *Br J Haematol* 1997;98:114–118.
221. Martinez-Lopez J, Lahuerta JJ, Pepin F, et al. Prognostic value of deep sequencing method for minimal residual disease detection in multiple myeloma. *Blood* 2014;123:3073–3079.
222. Rajkumar SV, Kyle RA, Therneau TM, et al. Serum free light chain ratio is an independent risk factor for progression in monoclonal gammopathy of undetermined significance. *Blood* 2005;106:812–817.
223. Dispenzieri A, Lacy MQ, Katzmann JA, et al. Absolute values of immunoglobulin free light chains are prognostic in patients with primary systemic amyloidosis undergoing peripheral blood stem cell transplantation. *Blood* 2006;107:3378–3383.
224. Mead GP, Carr-Smith HD, Drayson MT, et al. Serum free light chains for monitoring multiple myeloma. *Br J Haematol* 2004;126:348–354.
225. Shaw GR. Nonsecretory plasma cell myeloma—becoming even more rare with serum free light-chain assay: a brief review. *Arch Pathol Lab Med* 2006;130:1212–1215.
226. van Rhee F, Bolejack V, Hollmig K, et al. High serum free-light chain levels and their rapid reduction in response to therapy define an aggressive multiple myeloma subtype with poor prognosis. *Blood* 2007;110:827–832.
227. Ludwig H, Milosavljevic D, Zojer N, et al. Immunoglobulin heavy/light chain ratios improve paraprotein detection and monitoring, identify residual disease and correlate with survival in multiple myeloma patients. *Leukemia* 2013;27:213–219.
228. Bradwell A, Harding S, Fourrier N, et al. Prognostic utility of intact immunoglobulin Ig'kappa/Ig'lambda ratios in multiple myeloma patients. *Leukemia* 2013;27:202–207.

229. Barlogie B, Gale RP. Multiple myeloma and chronic lymphocytic leukemia: commonalities and differences in biology and therapy. *Leuk Lymph* 1991:27–32.
230. Bartl R, Frisch B. Clinical significance of bone marrow biopsy and plasma cell morphology in MM and MGUS. *Pathol Biol (Paris)* 1999;47:158–168.
231. Barlogie B, Alexanian R, Pershouse M, et al. Cytoplasmic immunoglobulin content in multiple myeloma. *J Clin Invest* 1985;76:765–769
232. Mariette X, Khalifa P, Ravaud P, et al. Bone densitometry in patients with multiple myeloma [see comments]. *Am J Med* 1992;93:595–598.
233. Mariette X, Bergot C, Ravaud P, et al. Evolution of bone densitometry in patients with myeloma treated with conventional or intensive therapy. *Cancer* 1995;76:1559–1563.
234. Chodimella U, Dhodapkar M, Weinstein R, et al. Differential effects of pamidronate (PAM) on cortical and cancellous bone in patients with myeloma (MM) undergoing autotransplants (AT). *Proc ASCO* 1998;10.
235. Moulopoulos LA, Dimopoulos MA, Smith T, et al. Prognostic significance of magnetic resonance imaging in patients with asymptomatic multiple myeloma. *J Clin Oncol* 1995;13:251–256.
236. Vande Berg BC, Lecouvet FE, Michaux L, et al. Magnetic resonance imaging of the bone marrow in hematological malignancies. *Eur Radiol* 1998;8:1335–1344.
237. Walker R, Barlogie B, Haessler J, et al. Magnetic resonance imaging in multiple myeloma: diagnostic and clinical implications. *J Clin Oncol* 2007;25:1121–1128.
238. Bartel TB, Haessler J, Brown TL, et al. F18-fluorodeoxyglucose positron emission tomography in the context of other imaging techniques and prognostic factors in multiple myeloma. *Blood* 2009;114:2068–2076.
239. Dimopoulos M, Terpos E, Comenzo RL, et al. International myeloma working group consensus statement and guidelines regarding the current role of imaging techniques in the diagnosis and monitoring of multiple myeloma. *Leukemia* 2009;23:1545–1556.
240. el-Shirbiny AM, Yeung H, Imbriaco M, et al. Technetium-99m-MIBI versus fluorine-18-FDG in diffuse multiple myeloma. *J Nucl Med* 1997;38:1208–1210.
241. Zamagni E, Nanni C, Patriarca F, et al. A prospective comparison of 18F-fluorodeoxyglucose positron emission tomography-computed tomography, magnetic resonance imaging and whole-body planar radiographs in the assessment of bone disease in newly diagnosed multiple myeloma. *Haematologica* 2007;92:50-55.
242. Durie B, Salmon S. Clinical staging system for myeloma. Correlation of measured myeloma cell mass with presenting clinical features, response to treatment, and survival. *Cancer* 1975;36:842–854.
243. Child JA, Norfolk DR, Cooper EH. Serum beta 2-microglobulin in myelomatosis [letter]. *Br J Haematol* 1986;63:406–407.
244. Garewal H, Durie BG, Kyle RA, et al. Serum beta 2–microglobulin in the initial staging and subsequent monitoring of monoclonal plasma cell disorders. *J Clin Oncol* 1984;2:51–57.
245. Attal M, Harousseau JL, Facon T, et al. Single versus double autologous stem-cell transplantation for multiple myeloma. *N Engl J Med* 2003;349:2495–2502.
246. Avet-Loiseau H, Daviet A, Brigaudeau C, et al. Cytogenetic, interphase, and multicolor fluorescence in situ hybridization analyses in primary plasma cell leukemia: a study of 40 patients at diagnosis, on behalf of the Intergroupe Francophone du Myelome and the Groupe Francais de Cytogenetique Hematologique. *Blood* 2001;97:822–825.
247. Vesole DH, Tricot G, Jagannath S, et al. Autotransplants in multiple myeloma: what have we learned? *Blood* 1996;88:838–847.
248. Witzig TE, Gertz MA, Lust JA, et al. Peripheral blood monoclonal plasma cells as a predictor of survival in patients with multiple myeloma [see comments]. *Blood* 1996;88:1780–1787.
249. Witzig TE, Gonchoroff NJ, Katzmann JA, et al. Peripheral blood B cell labeling indices are a measure of disease activity in patients with monoclonal gammopathies. *J Clin Oncol* 1988;6:1041–1046.
250. Greipp PR, Lust JA, O'Fallon WM, et al. Plasma cell labeling index and beta 2-microglobulin predict survival independent of thymidine kinase and C-reactive protein in multiple myeloma [see comments]. *Blood* 1993;81:3382–3387.
251. Munshi N, Wilson C, Penn J, et al. Angiogenesis in newly diagnosed multiple myeloma (MM): poor prognosis with increased microvessel density (MVD) in bone marrow biopsies (BMBX). *Blood* 1998;92:98a.
252. Mathiot C, Galon J, Tartour E, et al. Soluble CD16 in plasma cell dyscrasias. *Leuk Lymph* 1999;32:467–474.
253. Munshi NC, Anderson KC, Bergsagel PL, et al. Consensus recommendations for risk stratification in multiple myeloma: report of the International Myeloma Workshop Consensus Panel 2. *Blood* 2011;117:4696–4700.
254. Dimopoulos MA, Moulopoulos A, Delasalle K, et al. Solitary plasmacytoma of bone and asymptomatic multiple myeloma. *Hematol Oncol Clin North Am* 1992;6:359–369.
255. Mill WB, Griffith R. The role of radiation therapy in the management of plasma cell tumors. *Cancer* 1980;45:647–652.
256. Liebross RH, Ha CS, Cox JD, et al. Solitary bone plasmacytoma: outcome and prognostic factors following radiotherapy. *Int J Radiat Oncol Biol Phys* 1998;41:1063–1067.
257. Corwin J, Lindberg RD. Solitary plasmacytoma of bone vs. extramedullary plasmacytoma. *Cancer* 1979;43:1007–1013.
258. Woodruff RK, Malpas JS, White FE. Solitary plasmacytoma. II: Solitary plasmacytoma of bone. *Cancer* 1979;43:2344–2347.
259. Kyle RA, Remstein ED, Therneau TM, et al. Clinical course and prognosis of smoldering (asymptomatic) multiple myeloma. *N Engl J Med* 2007;356:2582–2590.
260. Dispenzieri A, Kyle RA, Katzmann JA, et al. Immunoglobulin free light chain ratio is an independent risk factor for progression of smoldering (asymptomatic) multiple myeloma. *Blood* 2008;111:785–789.
261. Rajkumar SV, Gertz MA, Lacy MQ, et al. Thalidomide as initial therapy for early-stage myeloma. *Leukemia* 2003;17:775–779.
262. Mateos MV, San Miguel JF. Treatment for high-risk smoldering myeloma. *N Engl J Med* 2013;369:1764–1765.
263. Bergsagel DE, Sprague CC, Austin C, et al. Evaluation of new chemotherapeutic agents in the treatment of myeloma IV: phenylalaine mustard. *Cancer Chemother Rep*. 1962;21:87.
264. Alexanian R, Haut A, Khan AU, et al. Treatment for multiple myeloma. Combination chemotherapy with different melphalan dose regimens. *JAMA* 1969;208:1680–1685.
265. Boccadoro M, Marmont F, Tribalto M, et al. Multiple myeloma: VMCP/VBAP alternating combination chemotherapy is not superior to melphalan and prednisone even in high-risk patients. *J Clin Oncol* 1991;9:444–448.
266. Palva IP, Ahrenberg P, Ala Harja K, et al. Intensive chemotherapy with combinations containing anthracyclines for refractory and relapsing multiple myeloma. Finnish Leukaemia Group. *Eur J Haematol* 1990;44:121–124.
267. Barlogie B, Smith L, Alexanian R. Effective treatment of advanced multiple myeloma refractory to alkylating agents. *N Engl J Med* 1984;310:1353–1356.
268. Cavo M, Zamagni E, Tosi P, et al. Superiority of thalidomide and dexamethasone over vincristine-doxorubicindexamethasone (VAD) as primary therapy in preparation for autologous transplantation for multiple myeloma. *Blood* 2005;106:35–39.
269. Rajkumar SV, Jacobus S, Callander NS, et al. Lenalidomide plus high-dose dexamethasone versus lenalidomide plus low-dose dexamethasone as initial therapy for newly diagnosed multiple myeloma: an open-label randomised controlled trial. *Lancet Oncol* 2010;11:29–37.
270. Mandelli F, Avvisati F, Amadori S, et al. Maintenance treatment with recombinant interferon alfa-2b in patients with multiple myeloma responding to conventional induction chemotherapy. *N Engl J Med* 1990;322:1430–1434.
271. Gisslinger H. Interferon alpha in the therapy of multiple myeloma. *Leukemia* 1997;11:S52–S56.
272. Barlogie B, Kyle RA, Anderson KC, et al. Standard chemotherapy compared with high dose chemoradiotherapy for multiple myeloma: final results of phase III US Intergroup Trial S9321. *J Clin Oncol* 2006;24:929–936.
273. Hu K, Yahalom J. Radiotherapy in the management of plasma cell tumors. *Oncology* 2000;14:101–111.
274. Woodruff RK, Whittle JM, Malpas JS. Solitary plasmacytoma. I: Extramedullary soft tissue plasmacytoma. *Cancer* 1979;43:2340–2343.
275. Wallington M, Mendis S, Premawardhana U, et al. Local control and survival in spinal cord compression from lymphoma and myeloma. *Radiother Oncol* 1997;42:43–47.
276. Rowell NP, Tobias JS. The role of radiotherapy in the management of multiple myeloma. *Blood Rev* 1991;5:84–89.
277. Raje N, Anderson K. Thalidomide—a revival story [editorial; comment]. *New Engl J Med* 1999;341:1606–1609.
278. Kronke J, Udeshi ND, Narla A, et al. Lenalidomide causes selective degradation of IKZF1 and IKZF3 in multiple myeloma cells. *Science* 2014;343:301–305.
279. Lu G, Middleton RE, Sun H, et al. The myeloma drug lenalidomide promotes the cereblon-dependent destruction of Ikaros proteins. *Science* 2014;343:305–309.
280. Barlogie B, Desikan R, Eddlemon P, et al. Extended survival in advanced and refractory multiple myeloma after single-agent thalidomide: identification of prognostic factors in a phase 2 study of 169 patients. *Blood* 2001;98:492–494.
281. Singhal S, Mehta J, Desikan R, et al. Antitumor activity of thalidomide in refractory multiple myeloma [see comments]. *N Engl J Med* 1999;341:1565–1571.
282. Palumbo A, Rajkumar SV, Dimopoulos MA, et al. Prevention of thalidomide- and lenalidomide-associated thrombosis in myeloma. *Leukemia* 2008;22:414–423.
283. Richardson PG, Schlossman RL, Weller E, et al. Immunomodulatory drug CC-5013 overcomes drug resistance and is well tolerated in patients with relapsed multiple myeloma. *Blood* 2002;100:3063–3067.
284. Weber DM, Chen C, Niesvizky R, et al. Lenalidomide plus dexamethasone for relapsed multiple myeloma in North America. *N Engl J Med* 2007;357:2133–2142.
285. Benboubker L, Dimopoulos MA, Dispenzieri A, et al. Lenalidomide and dexamethasone in transplant-ineligible patients with myeloma. *N Engl J Med* 2014;371:906–917.
286. Hideshima T, Anderson KC. Molecular mechanisms of novel therapeutic approaches for multiple myeloma. *Nat Rev Cancer* 2002;2:927–937.
287. Mitsiades N, Mitsiades CS, Poulaki V, et al. Biologic sequelae of nuclear factor-κB blockade in multiple myeloma: therapeutic applications. *Blood* 2002;99:4079–4086.
288. Hideshima T, Richardson P, Chauhan D, et al. The proteasome inhibitor PS-341 inhibits growth, induces apoptosis, and overcomes drug resistance in human multiple myeloma cells. *Cancer Res* 2001;61:3071–3076.
289. Mitsiades N, Mitsiades CS, Poulaki V, et al. Molecular sequelae of proteasome inhibition in human multiple myeloma cells. *Proc Natl Acad Sci U S A* 2002;99:14374–14379.
290. Richardson PG, Barlogie B, Berenson J, et al. A phase 2 study of bortezomib in relapsed, refractory myeloma. *N Engl J Med* 2003;348:2609–2617.
291. Richardson PG, Sonneveld P, Schuster MW, et al. Bortezomib or high-dose dexamethasone for relapsed multiple myeloma. *N Engl J Med* 2005;352:2487–2498.
292. Orlowski RZ, Zhuang SH, Parckh T, et al. The combination of pegylated liposomal doxorubicin and bortezomib significantly improves time to progression of patients with relapsed/refractory multiple myeloma compared with bortezomib alone: results from a planned interim analysis of a randomized phase III study. *Blood* 2006,108:404a.

293. Jagannath S, Richardson PG, Sonneveld P, et al. Bortezomib appears to overcome the poor prognosis conferred by chromosome 13 deletion in phase 2 and 3 trials. *Leukemia* 2007;21:151–157.
294. Chanan-Khan AA, Kaufman JL, Mehta J, et al. Activity and safety of bortezomib in multiple myeloma patients with advanced renal failure: a multicenter retrospective study. *Blood* 2007;109:2604–2606.
295. Zangari M, Esseltine D, Lee CK, et al. Response to bortezomib is associated to osteoblastic activation in patients with multiple myeloma. *Br J Haematol* 2005;131:71–73.
296. Moreau P, Pylypenko H, Grosicki S, et al. Subcutaneous versus intravenous administration of bortezomib in patients with relapsed multiple myeloma: a randomised, phase 3, non-inferiority study. *Lancet Oncol* 2011;12:431–440.
297. Rajkumar SV, Blood E, Vesole D, et al. Phase III clinical trial of thalidomide plus dexamethasone compared with dexamethasone alone in newly diagnosed multiple myeloma: a clinical trial coordinated by the Eastern Cooperative Oncology Group. *J Clin Oncol* 2006;24:431–436.
298. Zonder JA, Crowley J, Hussein MA, et al. Lenalidomide and high-dose dexamethasone compared with dexamethasone as initial therapy for multiple myeloma: a randomized Southwest Oncology Group trial (S0232). *Blood* 2010;116:5838–5841.
299. Jagannath S, Barlogie B, Berenson J, et al. A phase 2 study of two doses of bortezomib in relapsed or refractory myeloma. *Br J Haematol* 2004;127:165–172.
300. Harousseau JL, Attal M, Avet-Loiseau H, et al. Bortezomib plus dexamethasone is superior to vincristine plus doxorubicin plus dexamethasone as induction treatment prior to autologous stem-cell transplantation in newly diagnosed multiple myeloma: results of the IFM 2005-01 phase III trial. *J Clin Oncol* 2010;28:4621–4629.
301. Avet-Loiseau H, Leleu X, Roussel M, et al. Bortezomib plus dexamethasone induction improves outcome of patients with t(4;14) myeloma but not outcome of patients with del(17p). *J Clin Oncol* 2010;28:4630–4634.
302. Jakubowiak AJ, Dytfeld D, Griffith KA, et al. A phase 1/2 study of carfilzomib in combination with lenalidomide and low-dose dexamethasone as a frontline treatment for multiple myeloma. *Blood* 2012;120:1801–1809.
303. Reeder CB, Reece DE, Kukreti V, et al. Cyclophosphamide, bortezomib and dexamethasone induction for newly diagnosed multiple myeloma: high response rates in a phase II clinical trial. *Leukemia* 2009;23:1337–1341.
304. Richardson PG, Weller E, Lonial S, et al. Lenalidomide, bortezomib, and dexamethasone combination therapy in patients with newly diagnosed multiple myeloma. *Blood* 2010;116:679–686.
305. San Miguel JF, Schlag R, Khuageva NK, et al. Bortezomib plus melphalan and prednisone for initial treatment of multiple myeloma. *N Engl J Med* 2008;359:906–917.
306. Cunningham D, Paz-Ares L, Milan S, et al. High-dose melphalan and autologous bone marrow transplantation as consolidation in previously untreated myeloma. *J Clin Oncol* 1994;12:759–763.
307. Bensinger WI, Rowley SD, Demirer T, et al. High-dose therapy followed by autologous hematopoietic stem-cell infusion for patients with multiple myeloma. *J Clin Oncol* 1996;14:1447–1456.
308. Fermand JP, Ravaud P, Chevret S, et al. High-dose therapy and autologous blood stem cell transplantation in multiple myeloma: preliminary results of a randomized trial involving 167 patients. *Stem Cells* 1995;13:156–159.
309. Anderson KC, Andersen J, Soiffer R, et al. Monoclonal antibody-purged bone marrow transplantation therapy for multiple myeloma. *Blood* 1993;82:2568–2576.
310. Harousseau JL, Attal M, Divine M, et al. Autologous stem cell transplantation after first remission induction treatment in multiple myeloma. A report of the French Registry on Autologous Transplantation in Multiple Myeloma. *Stem Cells* 1995;13:132–139.
311. Attal M, Harousseau JL, Stoppa AM, et al. A prospective, randomized trial of autologous bone marrow transplantation and chemotherapy in multiple myeloma. Intergroupe Francais du Myelome. *N Engl J Med* 1996;335:91–97.
312. Child JA, Morgan GJ, Davies FE, et al. High-dose chemotherapy with hematopoietic stem-cell rescue for multiple myeloma. *N Engl J Med* 2003;348:1875–1883.
313. Blade J, Surenda A, Diaz-Mediavilla J, et al. High-dose therapy autotransplantation/intensification vs continued conventional chemotherapy in multiple myeloma patients responding to initial treatment chemotherapy. Results of a prospective randomized trial from the Spanish Cooperative group PETHEMA. *Blood* 2001;98:815a.
314. Fermand JP, Ravaud P, Chevret S, et al. High-dose therapy and autologous peripheral blood stem cell transplantation in multiple myeloma: up-front or rescue treatment? Results of a multicenter sequential randomized clinical trial. *Blood* 1998;92:3131–3136.
315. Koreth J, Cutler CS, Djulbegovic B, et al. High-dose therapy with single autologous transplantation versus chemotherapy for newly diagnosed multiple myeloma: A systematic review and meta-analysis of randomized controlled trials. *Biol Blood Marrow Transplant* 2007;13:183–196.
316. Harousseau JL, Milpied N, Laporte JP, et al. Double-intensive therapy in high-risk multiple myeloma. *Blood* 1992;79:2827–2833.
317. Barlogie B, Jagannath S, Desikan KR, et al. Total therapy with tandem transplants for newly diagnosed multiple myeloma. *Blood* 1999;93:55–65.
318. Tricot G, Jagannath S, Vesole D, et al. Peripheral blood stem cell transplant for multiple myeloma: identification of favorable variables for rapid engraftment in 225 patients. *Blood* 1995;85:588.
319. Kumar S, Dispenzieri A, Lacy MQ, et al. Impact of lenalidomide therapy on stem cell mobilization and engraftment post-peripheral blood stem cell transplantation in patients with newly diagnosed multiple myeloma. *Leukemia* 2007;21:2035–2042.
320. Mark T, Stern J, Furst JR, et al. Stem cell mobilization with cyclophosphamide overcomes the suppressive effect of lenalidomide therapy on stem cell collection in multiple myeloma. *Biol Blood Marrow Transplant* 2008;14:795–798.
321. Kumar S, Giralt S, Stadtmauer EA, et al. Mobilization in myeloma revisited: IMWG consensus perspective on stem cell collection following initial therapy with thalidomide-, lenalidomide-, or bortezomib-containing regimens. *Blood* 2009;114:1729–1735.
322. Vesole DH, Barlogie B, Jagannath S, et al. High dose therapy for refractory multiple myeloma: improved prognosis with better supportive care and double transplants. *Blood* 1994;84:950–956.
323. Gertz MA, Lacy MQ, Inwards DJ, et al. Early harvest and late transplantation as an effective therapeutic strategy in multiple myeloma. *Bone Marrow Transplant* 1999;23:221–226.
324. Barlogie B, Dicke KA, Alexanian R. High dose melphalan for refractory myeloma—the M.D. Anderson experience. *Hematol Oncol* 1988;6:167–172.
325. Desikan KR, Fassas A, Siegel D, et al. Superior outcome with melphalan 200 mg/m^2 (MEL 200) for scheduled second autotransplant compared to MEL+TBI or CTX for myeloma (MM) in pre-tx-2 PR. *Blood* 1997;90:231a.
326. Jagannath S, Barlogie B. Autologous bone marrow transplantation for multiple myeloma. *Hematol Oncol Clin North Am* 1992;6:437–449
327. Fermand JP, Levy Y, Gerota J, et al. Treatment of aggressive multiple myeloma by high-dose chemotherapy and total body irradiation followed by blood stem cells autologous graft. *Blood* 1989;73:20–23.
328. Ventura GJ, Barlogie B, Hester JP, et al. High dose cyclophosphamide, BCNU and VP-16 with autologous blood cell support for refractory multiple myeloma. *Bone Marrow Transplant* 1990;5:265–268.
329. Vescio RA, Hong CH, Cao J, et al. The hematopoietic stem cell antigen, CD34, is not expressed on the malignant cells in multiple myeloma. *Blood* 1994;84:3283–3290.
330. Schiller G, Vescio R, Freytes C, et al. Transplantation of CD34+ peripheral blood progenitor cells after high-dose chemotherapy for patients with advanced multiple myeloma. *Blood* 1995;86:390–397.
331. Stewart AK, Vescio R, Schiller G, et al. Purging of autologous peripheral-blood stem cells using CD34 selection does not improve overall or progression-free survival after high dose chemotherapy for multiple myeloma: results of a multicenter randomized controlled trial. *J Clin Oncol* 2001;19:3771–3779.
332. Gazitt Y, Reading CC, Hoffman R, et al. Purified CD34+Lin-Thy+ stem cells do not contain clonal myeloma cells. *Blood* 1995;86:381–389.
333. Tricot G, Gazitt Y, Leemhuis T, et al. Collection, tumor contamination, and engraftment kinetics of highly purified hematopoietic progenitor cells to support high dose therapy in multiple myeloma. *Blood* 1998;91:4489–4495.
334. Harousseau JL, Attal M, Divine M, et al. Comparison of autologous bone marrow transplantation and peripheral blood stem cell transplantation after first remission induction treatment in multiple myeloma. *Bone Marrow Transplant* 1995;15:963–969.
335. Tricot G, Jagannath S, Vesole D, et al. Peripheral blood stem cell transplants for multiple myeloma: identification of favorable variables for rapid engraftment in 225 patients. *Blood* 1995;85:588–596.
336. Gazitt Y, Tian E, Barlogie B, et al. Differential mobilization of myeloma cells and normal hematopoietic stem cells in multiple myeloma after treatment with cyclophosphamide and granulocyte-macrophage colony-stimulating factor. *Blood* 1996;87:805–811.
337. Palumbo A, Anderson K. Multiple myeloma. *N Engl J Med* 2011;364:1046–1060.
338. Palumbo A, Rajkumar SV, San Miguel JF, et al. International Myeloma Working Group consensus statement for the management, treatment, and supportive care of patients with myeloma not eligible for standard autologous stem-cell transplantation. *J Clin Oncol* 2014;32:587–600.
339. Siegel DS, Desikan KR, Mehta J, et al. Age is not a prognostic variable with autotransplants for multiple myeloma. *Blood* 1999;93:51–54.
340. Badros A, Barlogie B, Siegel E, et al. Autologous stem cell transplantation in elderly multiple myeloma patients over the age of 70 years. *Br J Haematol* 2001;114:600–607.
341. Tricot G, Alberts DS, Johnson C, et al. Safety of autotransplants with high-dose melphalan in renal failure: a pharmacokinetic and toxicity study. *Clin Cancer Res* 1996;2:947–952.
342. Dimopoulos MA, Terpos E, Chanan-Khan A, et al. Renal impairment in patients with multiple myeloma: a consensus statement on behalf of the International Myeloma Working Group. *J Clin Oncol* 2010;30:4976–4984.
343. Badros A, Barlogie B, Siegel E, et al. Results of autologous stem cell transplant in multiple myeloma patients with renal failure. *Br J Haematol* 2001;114:822–829.
344. Browman G, Bergsagel D, Sicheri D, et al. Randomized trial of interferon maintenance in multiple myeloma: a study of the National Cancer Institute of Canada Clinical Trials Group. *J Clin Oncol* 1995;13:2354–2360.
345. Berenson JR, Crowley JJ, Grogan TM, et al. Maintenance therapy with alternate-day prednisone improves survival in multiple myeloma patients. *Blood* 2002;99:3163–3168.
346. Attal M, Harousseau JL, Leyvraz S, et al. Maintenance therapy with thalidomide improves survival in patients with multiple myeloma. *Blood* 2006;108:3289–3294.
347. Attal M, Lauwers-Cances V, Marit G, et al. Lenalidomide maintenance after stem-cell transplantation for multiple myeloma. *N Engl J Med* 2012;366:1782–1791.
348. McCarthy PL, Owzar K, Hofmeister CC, et al. Lenalidomide after stem-cell transplantation for multiple myeloma. *N Engl J Med* 2012;366:1770–1781.

349. Palumbo A, Hajek R, Delforge M, et al. Continuous lenalidomide treatment for newly diagnosed multiple myeloma. *N Engl J Med* 2012;366:1759–1769.
350. Sonneveld P, Schmidt-Wolf IG, van der Holt B, et al. Bortezomib induction and maintenance treatment in patients with newly diagnosed multiple myeloma: results of the randomized phase III HOVON-65/ GMMG-HD4 trial. *J Clin Oncol* 2012;30:2946–2955.
351. Mateos MV, Oriol A, Martinez-Lopez J, et al. Bortezomib, melphalan, and prednisone versus bortezomib, thalidomide, and prednisone as induction therapy followed by maintenance treatment with bortezomib and thalidomide versus bortezomib and prednisone in elderly patients with untreated multiple myeloma: a randomised trial. *Lancet Oncol* 2010;11: 934–941.
352. Rosenblatt J, Vasir B, Uhl L, et al. Vaccination with dendritic cell/tumor fusion cells results in cellular and humoral antitumor immune responses in patients with multiple myeloma. *Blood* 2011;117:393–402.
353. Rosenblatt J, Avivi I, Vasir B, et al. Vaccination with dendritic cell/tumor fusions following autologous stem cell transplant induces immunologic and clinical responses in multiple myeloma patients. *Clin Cancer Res* 2013;19: 3640–3648.
354. Munshi NC, Anderson KC. Minimal residual disease in multiple myeloma. *J Clin Oncol* 2013;31:2523–2526.
355. Rawstron AC, Child JA, de Tute RM, et al. Minimal residual disease assessed by multiparameter flow cytometry in multiple myeloma: impact on outcome in the Medical Research Council Myeloma IX Study. *J Clin Oncol* 2013;31: 2540–2547.
356. Paiva B, Gutierrez NC, Rosinol L, et al. High-risk cytogenetics and persistent minimal residual disease by multiparameter flow cytometry predict unsustained complete response after autologous stem cell transplantation in multiple myeloma. *Blood* 2012;119:687–691.
357. Bensinger WI, Demirer T, Buckner CD, et al. Syngeneic marrow transplantation in patients with multiple myeloma. *Bone Marrow Transplant* 1996;18: 527–531.
358. Gahrton G, Svensson H, Bjorkstrand B, et al. Syngeneic transplantation in multiple myeloma—a case matched comparison with autologous and allogeneic transplantation. *Bone Marrow Transplant* 1999;24:741–745.
359. Bjorkstrand B, Ljungman P, Svensson H, et al. Allogenic bone marrow transplantation versus autologous stem cell transplantation in multiple myeloma, a retrospective case matched study from the European Group for Blood and Marrow Transplantation. *Blood* 1996;88:4711–4718.
360. Alyea EP, Anderson KC. Allotransplantation for multiple myeloma. *Cancer J* 2001;7:166–174.
361. Mehta J, Tricot G, Jagannath S, et al. Salvage autologous or allogeneic transplantation for multiple myeloma refractory to or relapsing after a first-line autograft? *Bone Marrow Transplant* 1998;21:887–892.
362. Tricot G, Vesole DH, Jagannath S, et al. Graft-versus-myeloma effect: proof of principle. *Blood* 1996;87:1196–1198.
363. Lokhorst HM, Schattenberg A, Cornelissen JJ, et al. Donor lymphocyte infusions for relapsed multiple myeloma after allogeneic stem-cell transplantation: predictive factors for response and long-term outcome. *Blood* 2000;18:3031–3037.
364. Salama M, Nevill T, Marcellus D, et al. Donor leukocyte infusions for multiple myeloma. *Bone Marrow Transplant* 2000;26:1179–1184.
365. Munshi NC, Govindarajan R, Drake R, et al. Thymidine kinase (TK) gene-transduced human lymphocytes can be highly purified, remain fully functional and are killed efficiently with ganciclovir. *Blood* 1997;89:1334–1340.
366. Soiffer RJ, Alyea EP, Hochberg E, et al. Randomized trial of CD8+ T-cell depletion in the prevention of graft-versus-host disease associated with donor lymphocyte infusion. *Biol Blood Marrow Transplant* 2002;8:625–632.
367. Storb R, Yu C, Zaucha JM, et al. Stable mixed hematopoietic chimerism in dogs given donor antigen, CTLA4Ig, and 100 cGy total body irradiation before and pharmacologic immunosuppression after marrow transplant. *Blood* 1999;94:2523–2529.
368. Badros A, Barlogie B, Siegel E, et al. Improved outcome of allogeneic transplantation in high-risk multiple myeloma patients after nonmyeloablative conditioning. *J Clin Oncol* 2002;20:1295–1303.
369. Giralt S, Aleman A, Anagnostopoulos A, et al. Fludarabine/melphalan conditioning for allogeneic transplantation in patients with multiple myeloma. *Bone Marrow Transplant* 2002;30:367–373.
370. Maloney DG, Molina AJ, Sahebi F, et al. Allografting with nonmyeloablative conditioning following cytoreductive autografts for the treatment of patients with multiple myeloma. *Blood* 2003;102:3447–3454.
371. Bruno B, Rotta M, Patriarca F, et al. A comparison of allografting with autografting for newly diagnosed myeloma. *N Engl J Med* 2007;356:1110–1120.
372. Rosinol L, Perez-Simon JA, Sureda A, et al. A prospective PETHEMA study of tandem autologous transplantation versus autograft followed by reduced-intensity conditioning allogeneic transplantation in newly diagnosed multiple myeloma. *Blood* 2008;112:3591–3593.
373. Lokhorst H, Einsele H, Vesole D, et al. International Myeloma Working Group consensus statement regarding the current status of allogeneic stem-cell transplantation for multiple myeloma. *J Clin Oncol* 2010;28:4521–4530.
374. Krishnan A, Pasquini MC, Logan B, et al. Autologous haemopoietic stem-cell transplantation followed by allogeneic or autologous haemopoietic stem-cell transplantation in patients with multiple myeloma (BMT CTN 0102): a phase 3 biological assignment trial. *Lancet Oncol* 2011;12:1195–1203.
375. Berenson JR, Lichtenstein A, Porter L, et al. Efficacy of pamidronate in reducing skeletal events in patients with advanced multiple myeloma. *N Engl J Med* 1996;334:488–493.
376. Apperley JF, Croucher PI. Bisphosphonates in multiple myeloma. *Pathol Biol (Paris)* 1999;47:178–181.
377. Berenson JR, Lipton A. Bisphosphonates in the treatment of malignant bone disease. *Ann Rev Med* 1999;50:237–248.
378. Shipman CM, Croucher PI, Russell RG, et al. The bisphosphonate incadronate (YM175) causes apoptosis of human myeloma cells in vitro by inhibiting the mevalonate pathway. *Cancer Res* 1998;58:5294–5297.
379. Berenson JR, Lichtenstein A, Porter L, et al. Long-term pamidronate treatment of advanced multiple myeloma patients reduces skeletal events. Myeloma Aredia Study Group. *J Clin Oncol* 1998;16:593–602.
380. Aparicio A, Gardner A, Tu Y, et al. In vitro cytoreductive effects on multiple myeloma cells induced by bisphosphonates. *Leukemia* 1998;12: 220–229.
381. Shipman CM, Rogers MJ, Apperley JF, et al. Anti-tumour activity of bisphosphonates in human myeloma cells. *Leuk Lymph* 1998;32:129–138.
382. Dhodapkar MV, Singh J, Mehta J, et al. Anti-myeloma activity of pamidronate in vivo. *Br J Haematol* 1998;103:530–532.
383. Morgan GJ, Child JA, Gregory WM, et al. Effects of zoledronic acid versus clodronic acid on skeletal morbidity in patients with newly diagnosed multiple myeloma (MRC Myeloma IX): secondary outcomes from a randomised controlled trial. *Lancet Oncol* 2011;12:743–752.
384. Morgan GJ, Davies FE, Gregory WM, et al. First-line treatment with zoledronic acid as compared with clodronic acid in multiple myeloma (MRC Myeloma IX): a randomised controlled trial. *Lancet* 2010;376:1989–1999.
385. Wang EP, Kaban LB, Strewler GJ, et al. Incidence of osteonecrosis of the jaw in patients with multiple myeloma and breast or prostate cancer on intravenous bisphosphonate therapy. *J Oral Maxillofac Surg* 2007;65:1328–1331.
386. Kyle RA, Yee GC, Somerfield MR, et al. American Society of Clinical Oncology 2007 clinical practice guideline update on the role of bisphosphonates in multiple myeloma. *J Clin Oncol* 2007;25:2464–2472.
387. Lee CK, Barlogie B, Munshi N, et al. DTPACE: an effective, novel combination chemotherapy with thalidomide for previously treated patients with myeloma. *J Clin Oncol* 2003;21:2732–2739.
388. Jagannath S, Vij R, Stewart AK, et al. An open-label single-arm pilot phase II study (PX-171-003-A0) of low-dose, single-agent carfilzomib in patients with relapsed and refractory multiple myeloma. *Clin Lymphoma Myeloma Leuk* 2012;12:310–318.
389. Vij R, Siegel DS, Jagannath S, et al. An open-label, single-arm, phase 2 study of single-agent carfilzomib in patients with relapsed and/or refractory multiple myeloma who have been previously treated with bortezomib. *Br J Haematol* 2012;158:739–748.
390. Siegel DS, Martin T, Wang M, et al. A phase 2 study of single-agent carfilzomib (PX-171-003-A1) in patients with relapsed and refractory multiple myeloma. *Blood* 2012;120:2817–2825.
391. Vij R, Wang M, Kaufman JL, et al. An open-label, single-arm, phase 2 (PX-171-004) study of single-agent carfilzomib in bortezomib-naive patients with relapsed and/or refractory multiple myeloma. *Blood* 2012;119: 5661–5670.
392. Jakubowiak AJ, Siegel DS, Martin T, et al. Treatment outcomes in patients with relapsed and refractory multiple myeloma and high-risk cytogenetics receiving single-agent carfilzomib in the PX-171-003-A1 study. *Leukemia* 2013;27: 2351–2356.
393. Lacy MQ, Allred JB, Gertz MA, et al. Pomalidomide plus low-dose dexamethasone in myeloma refractory to both bortezomib and lenalidomide: comparison of 2 dosing strategies in dual-refractory disease. *Blood* 2011;118:2970–2975.
394. Lacy MQ, Hayman SR, Gertz MA, et al. Pomalidomide (CC4047) plus low-dose dexamethasone as therapy for relapsed multiple myeloma. *J Clin Oncol* 2009;27:5008–5014.
395. Richardson PG, Siegel D, Baz R, et al. Phase 1 study of pomalidomide MTD, safety, and efficacy in patients with refractory multiple myeloma who have received lenalidomide and bortezomib. *Blood* 2013;121:1961–1967.
396. Leleu X, Attal M, Arnulf B, et al. Pomalidomide plus low-dose dexamethasone is active and well tolerated in bortezomib and lenalidomide-refractory multiple myeloma: Intergroupe Francophone du Myelome 2009-02. *Blood* 2013;121:1968–1975.
397. San Miguel J, Weisel K, Moreau P, et al. Pomalidomide plus low-dose dexamethasone versus high-dose dexamethasone alone for patients with relapsed and refractory multiple myeloma (MM-003): a randomised, open-label, phase 3 trial. *Lancet Oncol* 2013;14:1055–1066.
398. Richardson PG, Hofmeister CG, Siegel D, et al. MM-005: A Phase 1 Trial Of Pomalidomide, Bortezomib, and Low-Dose Dexamethasone (PVD) In Relapsed and/Or Refractory Multiple Myeloma (RRMM). *Blood* 2013;122:1969. [ePub ahead of Print].
399. Dimopoulos M, Siegel DS, Lonial S, et al. Vorinostat or placebo in combination with bortezomib in patients with multiple myeloma (VANTAGE 088): a multicentre, randomised, double-blind study. *Lancet Oncol* 2013;14: 1129–1140.
400. Santo L, Hideshima T, Kung AL, et al. Preclinical activity, pharmacodynamic, and pharmacokinetic properties of a selective HDAC6 inhibitor, ACY-1215, in combination with bortezomib in multiple myeloma. *Blood* 2012;119: 2579–2589.
401. Richardson PG, Eng C, Kolesar J, et al. Perifosine, an oral, anti-cancer agent and inhibitor of the Akt pathway: mechanistic actions, pharmacodynamics, pharmacokinetics, and clinical activity. *Expert Opin Drug Metab Toxicol* 2012;8:623–633.

402. Palumbo A, Bringhen S, Caravita T, et al. Oral melphalan and prednisone chemotherapy plus thalidomide compared with melphalan and prednisone alone in elderly patients with multiple myeloma: randomised controlled trial. *Lancet* 2006;367:825–831.
403. Facon T, Mary JY, Hulin C, et al. Melphalan and prednisone plus thalidomide versus melphalan and prednisone alone or reduced-intensity autologous stem cell transplantation in elderly patients with multiple myeloma (IFM 99-06): a randomised trial. *Lancet* 2007;370:1209–1218.
404. Hulin C, Facon T, Rodon P, et al. Efficacy of melphalan and prednisone plus thalidomide in patients older than 75 years with newly diagnosed multiple myeloma: IFM 01/01 trial. *J Clin Oncol* 2009;27:3664–3670.
405. Wijermans P, Schaafsma M, Termorshuizen F, et al. Phase III study of the value of thalidomide added to melphalan plus prednisone in elderly patients with newly diagnosed multiple myeloma: the HOVON 49 study. *J Clin Oncol* 2010;28:3160–3166.
406. Waage A, Gimsing P, Fayers P, et al. Melphalan and prednisone plus thalidomide or placebo in elderly patients with multiple myeloma. *Blood* 2010;116:1405–1412.
407. Sonneveld P, van der Holt B, Segeren CM, et al. Intermediate-dose melphalan compared with myeloablative treatment in multiple myeloma: long-term follow-up of the Dutch Cooperative Group HOVON 24 trial. *Haematologica* 2007;92:928–935.
408. Cavo M, Tosi P, Zamagni E, et al. Prospective, randomized study of single compared with double autologous stem cell transplantation for multiple myeloma: Bologna 96 clinical study. *J Clin Oncol* 2007;25:2434–2441.
409. Spencer A, Prince HM, Roberts AW, et al. Consolidation therapy with low-dose thalidomide and prednisolone prolongs the survival of multiple myeloma patients undergoing a single autologous stem-cell transplantation procedure. *J Clin Oncol* 2009;27:1788–1793.
410. Barlogie B, Tricot G, Anaissie E, et al. Thalidomide and hematopoietic-cell transplantation for multiple myeloma. *N Engl J Med* 2006;354:1021–1030.
411. Lee CK, Badros A, Barlogie B, et al. Prognostic factors in allogeneic transplantation for patients with high-risk multiple myeloma after reduced intensity conditioning. *Exp Hematol* 2003;31:73–80.
412. Lee CK, Badros A, Barlogie B, et al. Prognostic factors in allogeneic transplantation for patients with high-risk multiple myeloma after reduced intensity conditioning. *Exp Hematol* 2003;31:73–80.
413. Belch AR, Bergsagel DE, Wilson K, et al. Effect of daily etidronate on the osteolysis of multiple myeloma. *J Clin Oncol* 1991;9:1397–1402.
414. Lahtinen R, Laakso M, Palva I, et al. Randomised, placebo-controlled multicentre trial of clodronate in multiple myeloma. Finnish Leukaemia Group. *Lancet* 1992;340:1049–1052.

INDEX

Note: Page locators followed by *f* and *t* indicate figure and table, respectively.

A

A20 protein, 4
Abarelix, 309
ABC transporter polymorphisms, 248
ABC-DLBCL, 457*f*
Aberrant somatic hypermutation (ASHM), 450, 452
Abiraterone acetate, 191*t*, 297*t*, 299*t*, 303*t*, 310
ABL gene, 599*f*
ABL kinase inhibitors, 255
Absorption, 186
ABVD regimen
  for advanced-stage Hodgkin's lymphoma, 480, 481*t*, 482
AC220, 261
Acquired immunodeficiency syndrome (AIDS)
  malignancies associated with. *See also* Human immunodeficiency virus (HIV)
Acrolein, 209
Activating point mutations, 452
Activation-induced cytidine deaminase (AID), 449
Active immunization, 174
Acute leukemias. *See also specific leukemia*
  cooperating mutations in, 560, 561*f*
  genetic events in, 550, 551*t*–552*t*, 553
  management of, 566–583
  point mutations in, 557–558
Acute lymphoblastic leukemia (ALL), 577–583
  BCR-ABL fusion gene in, 598
  clinical trials with adults, 580*t*
  CNS prophylaxis, 581
  consolidation therapy, 580
  cytogenetics, 578–579
  diagnosis, 578
  epidemiology, 577–578
  imatinib trials, 582
  incidence, 436
  lymphoid antigen in blasts, 438
  lymphoid development in, 559–560
  maintenance therapy, 581
  mature B-lineage, 582
  pediatric
    CNS involvement, 438, 439*t*
    diagnosis, 438*t*
    karyotypic abnormalities, 579*t*
    prognostic factors, 437*t*, 439–441
    relapsed, 441
    remission, 441
    survival trends, 437*f*
    treatment, 439–442
  Ph chromosome in, 580–581, 598
  Philadelphia chromosome–positive, 581
  prognosis, 579–580, 580*t*
  relapsed/refractory, 583
  remission induction, 580

  T-cell, 582
  T-lineage, 440
Acute megakaryoblastic leukemia (AMKL), 556
Acute myelogenous leukemia (AML)
  BCR-ABL fusion gene in, 598
  cooperating mutations in, 560
  cytogenetic classification, 566–567, 567*t*
  FLT3 inhibitors in, 260–261
  genetic heterogeneity in, 567–568
  hematopoietic cell transplantation and, 572, 573–578
  histology, 436
  isocitrate dehydrogenase mutations in, 264
  minimal residual disease, 569
  newly diagnosed, 568
  pediatric
    description of, 437*t*, 441–442
    survival trends, 437*f*
  prognosis for, 441–442, 566
  relapse of, after allogeneic stem cell transplantation, 579
  salvage therapy, 572
  secondary, 568
  survival, 573*f*
  transplants
    in first remission, 581
    in relapse, 576
  treatment of, 566, 568
  whole-genome analysis, 6–7
Acute myeloid leukemia (AML). *See* Acute myelogenous leukemia (AML)
Acute promyelocytic leukemia (APL), 571–572
Acute promyelocytic leukemia differentiation syndrome (APLDS), 572
ADAM (a disintegrin and metalloproteinase) family proteins, 4
ADAMTS (ADAMs with thrombospondin domains), 4
Adducts, DNA, 98
Adenomatous polyposis coli (APC)
  workup algorithm for, 378*f*
Adenopathy, 538
Adenosine triphosphatase-binding cassette (ABC), 248
Adjuvant therapy
  for breast cancer, 162
  for head and neck cancer, 162
  for lung cancer, 162
Adoptive cell therapy (ACT), 19, 174–176, 175*f*
Ado-trastuzumab emtansine, 247*t*, 251, 292, 295*t*, 296*t*, 330*t*, 334
Adult T cell leukemia/lymphoma (ATLL), 82, 460–461, 520, 531
Advanced-stage Hodgkin's lymphoma
  chemotherapy for, 480–482
  consolidation radiotherapy, 482

  description of, 478–479
  initial therapy for, 480–482
  International Prognostic Score, 479
  positron-emission tomography–directed approaches for, 482
  prognostic factors in, 479
Afatinib, 256*t*, 296*t*
AG014699, 285
Age/aging
  mycosis fungoides and, 531
  pharmacokinetics affected by, 189
AIB1 (amplified in breast cancer 1), 303
AKT1, 48*t*
AKT2, 48*t*
AKT3, 48*t*
Alcohol
  dietary consumption of, 111–112
Alemtuzumab (Campath-1H), 330*t*, 333
  for chronic lymphocytic leukemia, 616–617
  for mycosis fungoides with Sézary syndrome, 538*t*, 540
ALK inhibitors, 260
Alkyl sulfonates
  classification of, 203
  clinical pharmacology of, 205*t*
  therapeutic uses of, 205*t*
  toxicities, 205*t*
Alkylating agents, 203–212
  bladder toxicity associated with, 208
  chemistry, 203
  for chronic lymphocytic leukemia, 614, 615*t*
  classification of, 203–207
  clinically useful, 205*t*–207*t*
  conjugates with steroids, 210
  doses and schedules, 206*t*–207*t*
  gonadal toxicity associated with, 208
  high-dose therapy with, 210
  immunosuppression caused by, 210
  for multiple myeloma, 659
  perspectives, 203
  pharmacodynamics of, 207–208
  pharmacokinetics of, 207–208
  renal toxicity associated with, 208
  therapeutic uses of, 208–209
  toxicities of, 209–210
Alkylating reactions, 203
Allele-specific polymerase chain reaction, 53*t*, 54
Allergic reactions, 210
Allogeneic hematopoietic stem cell transplantation (alloHSCT)
  for chronic lymphocytic leukemia, 621–622
  for Hodgkin's lymphoma, 487
  T-cell gene therapy with, 181
  umbilical cord blood cells, 487
All-*trans*-retinoic acid, 554–555

682

Index

Alopecia
 toxicity of alkylating agents, 210
 vinca alkaloids and, 251
Alopecia mucinosa, 538
Alpha-Fetoprotein (AFP)
 liver cancer and, 417
 serial levels of, 343–344
Altretamine, 205t
American Cancer Society guidelines, 119
American Society of Clinical Oncology (ASCO), 344
Aminoglutethimide, 306
Aminoimidazole carboxamide (AICAR) formyltransferase, 223
Aminopterin, 223. See also Antifolates
AML1-EVI-1 transcription factor, 592
AML1 gene. See RUNX1 gene
AML1/ETO fusion gene, 554
β-Amyloid peptide, gamma-secretase and, 559
Analytic validity, 47
Analytical studies
 classification of, 131f
 epidemiologic, 130–133
Anaplastic astrocytomas, 3
Anaplastic large cell lymphoma (ALCL), 461–462, 518–519
Anaplastic lymphoma kinase, 48t, 355
Anaplastic oligodendrogliomas, 3
Anastrozole (ATAC), 303t, 306–307
Androgen receptor
 super antagonists of, 303t
Androgens, 303t. See also specific androgens
Anemia
 clofarabine and, 231
 in myelodysplastic syndromes, 636
 normochromic normocytic, 649
Ang1, 320
Ang2, 320
Angiogenesis, 29–30
 angiogenic switch, 317
 in breast cancer, 90
 combination therapies, 324
 endogenous inhibitors of, 317–318
 inflammation's role in, 90–91
 inhibitors of, 317–318
  drug development of, 318–320
  drugs with secondary action as, 320t
  examples of, 318t
 process of, 317–318
 regulation of, 317
 tumor, 324
Angiogenic switch, 317
Angioimmunoblastic T-cell lymphoma (AITL), 461, 517–518
Angiopoietin inhibitors, 320
Angiostatin, 317, 318
Animal models
 chemical carcinogenesis and, 96–97
 of chronic myelogenous leukemia, 591
 of multiple myeloma, 648–649
 of proteasome inhibitor activity, 280
Anthracenediones, 240
Anthracyclines
 bevacizumab with, 334
 cardiac toxicities, 240
 description of, 238
Antiandrogens
 description of, 309–310

Antiangiogenic therapy
 agents used in, 317–325, 319t, 320t, 320–324
 biomarkers of, 324
 clinical utility, 320–326
 modes of action, 318–319
 rationale for, 318
 resistance to, 325
Antibodies
 bispecific, 332
 cell-mediated cytotoxicity and, 331–332
 humanized, 329
 modified, 329
 monoclonal. See Monoclonal antibodies
 size of, tumor targeting and, 331
 solid tumors treated with, 333
 tumor targeting using, 331
 unconjugated, 331f, 331–332
Antibody–drug conjugates, 332
Anti-CD19 chimeric antigen receptors, 179–181
Anticonvulsants
 for hot flashes, 302
Anti–cytotoxic T lymphocyte antigen 4 blocking antibodies, 172–173
Antidepressants
 for hot flashes, 302
 for smoking cessation, 359
Antidiuretic hormone
 syndrome of inappropriate secretion of. See Syndrome of inappropriate secretion of antidiuretic hormone (SIADH)
Antifolates, 223–225
 clinical pharmacology, 223–225
 mechanism of action, 223
 mechanism of resistance, 223
Anti-infectives, 400
Anti-inflammatory drugs
 as cancer risk–reducing agents, 394–395
Antimetabolites, 223–231
 radiation sensitivity and, 152
Antimicrotubule agents, 245–252, 246f, 247t
Antioxidant micronutrients, 388–392, 391t
Anti–programmed death 1, 173
Anti–programmed death ligand 1, 173
Anti-VEGFR2 monoclonal antibody, 324
APC. See Adenomatous polyposis coli (APC)
Apoptosis
 resisting of, 27
 triggering of, 27
ARID5B gene, 436
Aristolochic acid, 98–99, 99f
Aromatase inhibitors, 397
 cancer treatment with, 303t
 use of, 306–308
Aromatic amines, 98
Artemis protein, 148
Asbestos
 cellular responses to, 107–108
 damage induction mechanisms, 107
 lung cancer and, 108
 mesothelioma and, 108
 reactive oxygen species induced by, 107
 tissue responses to, 107–108
L-Asparaginase
 characteristics of, 294t
 description of, 290–291
Aspirin
 inhibition of MTX excretion, 223

Asthenia, 229
Ataxia-telangiectasia
 ionizing radiation and, 103
Ataxia-telangiectasia and RAD3 related (ATR) kinase, 146
Ataxia-telangiectasia mutated (ATM) kinase, 145–147
ATM gene, 453
ATR kinase, 146
Auristatins, 251
Aurora kinase inhibitors, 251–252
Autophagocytosis, 104
Autophagy, 27
Axitinib, 256t, 261, 298t, 319t, 323
Azacitidine, 570, 635
5-Azacitidine (5AC), 270–271, 271t, 273
Azacytosine nucleosides, 270–271
Aza-epothilone B, 250–251. See also Ixabepilone
Azanucleosides, for myelodysplastic syndromes, 635
AZD6244, 259
Aziridines, 203–204
Aziridinium ions, 211

B

B vitamins, 392–393
BAP1 gene, 4
Basal cell carcinoma (BCC)
 ultraviolet radiation and, 106
Base excision repair (BER)
 description of, 115, 785
B/Cdk1, activation of, 147
B-cell(s)
 development of, 496–498, 497f
 differentiation of, 496–498
 marginal zone, 508
 monocytoid, 508
 origin of, 449
B-cell leukemias
 chronic lymphocytic leukemia, 506
 description of, 557
B-cell lymphomas, 4, 334–335, 515–516
B-cell neoplasms, 499t, 499–501
B-cell non-Hodgkin lymphoma, 85
B-cell receptors (BCRs), 449, 594
BCL-2, 621, 644
BCL6, 449, 454
BCL2L12, 10
BCNU. See Carmustine (BCNU)
BCR gene structure, 599f
BCR-ABL1, 591
BCR-ABL fusion gene, 255, 598
BCR/ABL gene rearrangement, 558
BCR-ABL kinase
 in chronic myelogenous leukemia pathogenesis, 598
 DNA repair impaired by, 591
 domain structure, 590f
 function of, 598
 imatinib resistance and, 605
 protein phosphorylation by, 591
 T315I mutation, 264
BCR-ABL tyrosine-kinase inhibitors, 601
BEACOPP regimen, for advanced-stage Hodgkin's lymphoma, 480–482, 481t
Beclin-1 gene, 27
Beclin-1 protein, 27

Belinostat (PXD101), 271t
Bence Jones proteins, 649
Bendamustine, 211–212, 615
Benzamides, 272
Benzene, 627
Benzodiazepines, 210
Berries, 401t
Beta-carotene, 116, 388–389, 391
Bethesda system, 380t
Bevacizumab (Avastin)
　binding of, 332
　characteristics of, 330t
　clinical utility, 320–321
　combination therapies using, 321
　dosages, 319t
　for glioblastoma multiforme, 321
　indications, 297t, 319t
　mechanism of action, 334
　specificity of, 261
Bexarotene, 536, 537t, 539
BI-2536, 252
Biases
　definition of, 133
　in epidemiologic studies, 133
　sources of, 133
Bicalutamide
　dosage, 303t
　pharmacology, 309
　tolerability of, 309
Bilateral salpingo-oophorectomy (BSO), 430
Binding-site barrier hypothesis, 331
Bioavailability, 186
Biochemical cure, 377
Biological agents. See also specific agents
　for mycosis fungoides with Sézary syndrome, 539
Biomarkers, 342–344
　chromosomal translocations as, 47
　description of, 97–98
　mutations as, 50
　response criteria for, 343t
Bis-aceto-amine-dichloro-cyclohexylamine platinum IV. See Satraplatin
Bischloroethylamines. See Nitrogen mustards
Bischloroethylnitrosourea, 209
Bisphosphonates
　adverse effects, 672
　mechanism of action, 399
　for multiple myeloma, 671–672, 672t
Blastic NK lymphoma, 541
Bleomycin
　adverse effects
　　pulmonary toxicity, 291
　characteristics of, 294t
　description of, 291
　for Hodgkin lymphoma, 291
　pneumonitis caused by, 291
BLIMP1 gene inactivation, 456
Blinatumomab, 332
BMS-247550. See Ixabepilone
Body mass index, 124
Bone marrow
　biology of, 496
　microenvironments, 644–645, 647f
　monitoring of, 603–604
　multiple myeloma and, 647f
　myeloma infiltration of, 652, 654f
　toxicity of alkylating agents, 209

Bone marrow transplant (BMT)
　allogeneic, 670t
　miniallogeneic, 671t
　for mycosis fungoides with Sézary syndrome, 540–541
Bone marrow-derived cells, 29–30
Bone metastases
　multiple myeloma and, 649–650
Bone sarcomas. See also specific sarcoma
Bortezomib (Velcade)
　antiangiogenic properties of, 318
　approval of, 279
　clinical activity, 280–281
　combination therapy using, 281
　for mantle cell lymphoma, 281
　for multiple myeloma, 281, 318, 640, 661–662, 663t, 672–673
　preclinical development, 280
　therapeutic use of, 280t
　toxicity, 280–281
Bosutinib, 256t, 297t, 602
Brachytherapy
　isotopes for, 159, 159t
　treatment with, 159–160
BRAF kinase
　mutations, 258–260
BRAF mutations, 48t
　in colorectal cancer, 18f
　KRAS mutations and, 13
　melanoma, 190f
Brain tumors
　radiation tolerance, 163t
　treatment planning, 158f
Brain stem
　radiation tolerance, 163f
BRCA
　breast cancer risk and, 368
　PARP inhibitors and, 286, 288
BRCA1
　carriers of, 372–373
　DNA repair and, 285–286
　female carriers of, 429–430
　Jewish ancestry and, 426
BRCA1/2
　ovarian cancer and, 430
BRCA2
　carriers of, 372–373
　DNA repair and, 285–286
　female carriers of, 429–430
　genetic counseling in, 428
　Jewish ancestry and, 426
BRCA1 protein
　down-regulation of, 591
　Rad51 loading and, 148
BRCA2 protein
　ovarian cancer and, 372
Breakage-fusion-bridge, 28
Breakpoint cluster region (bcr), 598
Breast cancer
　adjuvant therapy, 162
　angiogenesis in, 90
　bevacizumab for, 334
　BRCA1 and, 429–430
　BRCA2 and, 429–430
　CEA overexpression, 169
　diet and, 112, 115
　ductal carcinoma in situ, 414
　early-stage, 410
　fiber and, 115

　fruit consumption and, 114
　genetic mutations
　　BRCA1, 429–430
　　BRCA2, 429–430
　HER2-expressing, 302–303
　high-risk patients, 368–369
　incidence of, 140–141
　metastatic disease
　　capecitabine for, 227
　mortality rates, 141
　obesity and, 123–124, 140
　pathologic complete response in, 342
　physical activity and, 123–124
　PIK3CA mutations in, 3, 258
　prevention of, 393
　screening for, 410–415
　　breast density, 414
　　clinical breast examination, 410
　　ductal carcinoma in situ, 414
　　effectiveness of, 410, 412
　　harms of, 414
　　in high-risk women, 414
　　mammography, 140, 410, 412, 414
　　mortality benefits of, 410
　　recommendations, 411t, 414–415
　　self-examination, 410
　　in women age 40 to 49, 412, 414
　soy products and, 116
　tamoxifen for, 141, 200, 302, 396
　taxanes in
　　mTOR inhibitors, 267
　　taxanes in, 245
　　trastuzumab, 333
　vegetable consumption and, 114
　vitamin D for prevention of, 393
BReast CAncer genes. See BRCA
Breast density, 414
Bremsstrahlung x-rays, 153
Brentuximab vedotin, 247t, 299t, 330t, 335, 482, 485t, 488–489, 538t, 540
Bruton's tyrosine kinase inhibitors, 620
B-UNC/BL/DLBCL, 515–516
Bupropion (Wellbutrin, Zyban), 359
Burkitt lymphoma, 516–517
　cell of origin, 453
　Epstein-Barr virus and, 78
　genetic lesions in, 453–454
　pediatric, 444
　Plasmodium falciparum and, 78
Busulfan (Myleran)
　adverse effects, 205t
　in chronic myelogenous leukemia treatment, 203, 600
　clinical pharmacology of, 205t
　doses and schedules, 206t
　neurotoxicity, 210
　therapeutic uses of, 205t
bZIP factor, 81

C

CA-125, 343
　ovarian cancer and, 418, 430
　use in response evaluation, 343
Cabazitaxel
　development of, 245
　dosages, 247t
　formulation of, 245
　indications, 247t, 299t
　toxicity, 247t

Cabozantinib, 256t, 260, 297t, 319t, 323
Caenorhabditis elegans, 2
Calcium, 115, 393
cAMP response element-binding protein/
    activating transcription factor, 81
Camptothecins, 234–235
  conjugates and analogs, 236–237
Cancer
  immunotherapies, 170t, 170–181
  viral-associated antigens, 170
Cancer approval endpoints, 344, 345f
Cancer cells
  cell-to-cell signaling pathways, 39f
  description of, 35, 38–41
  endothelial cells, 36
  fibroblasts, 35–36
  genetic heterogeneity of, 41
  immune inflammatory cells, 36–37
  pericytes, 36
  progenitor cells, 37
  stem cells, 37–38
Cancer epigenome, 267
Cancer genes, 2–20
  discovery of, 2–4
  drug resistance and, 19–20
  identification of, 2
  landscapes, 12f, 14f, 15–16
  mutations of, 2
  pathway oriented models, 11–13
  project networks, 13–15
  somatic alteration classes, 10–11
  somatic alterations per tumor, 5
  taxonomy of tumors, 16–19
Cancer Genome Atlas, 14, 258
Cancer outcomes research, 133–134
Cancer risk–reducing agents
  anti-infectives, 400
  anti-inflammatory drugs, 394–395
  aromatase inhibitors, 397
  biochemical prescreening assays, 385
  biomarkers as targets of, 387, 388t
  bisphosphonates, 399
  clinical development of, 386–388
  defining of, 384
  developmental phases of, 387–388
  diet-derived natural products, 400
  difluoromethylornithine, 398, 399t
  identification of, 384
  in vitro efficacy models, 385–386
  metformin, 399–400
  micronutrients, 388–394. *See also*
    Micronutrients
  multiagent approaches to, 400
  preclinical development of, 384–386
  selective estrogen receptor modulators, 395–397, 396t
  signal transduction modifiers, 398–400
  statins, 398–399
  5α-steroid reductase inhibitors, 397–398
Cancer stem cells, 40–41
Cancer surveillance systems, 138
Cancer-associated fibroblasts, 35–36
Cancer/germ-line antigens, 167–169
Cancer/testes antigens, 167–169, 168f
Canfosfamide, 211
Capecitabine
  clinical pharmacology, 227
  description, 227
  docetaxel and, 227
  dosages, 224t
  radiation sensitivity and, 152
  therapeutic uses, 224t
  toxicities, 224t, 227
Capillaries. *See also* Angiogenesis
Carbohydrates, 117
Carbonium ion structure, 204f
Carboplatin
  doses and schedules, 206t
  toxicities, 214
Carcinoembryonic antigen (CEA)
  overexpression of, 169
Carcinogenesis
  models of, 386t–387t
  molecular biomarkers of, 385f
  toxicity of alkylating agents, 209–210
  tumor microenvironment and, 37–38
Carcinogens
  chemical, 95–99, 96t
  in tobacco, 66–69, 67t–69t
CARD11 mutations, 456
Carfilzomib
  clinical trials, 279
  combination chemotherapy, 282
  development of, 281–282
  indications for, 298t
  preclinical development, 280–281
  therapeutic use of, 280t
C-arm linear accelerator, 154f
Carmustine (BCNU)
  adverse effects, 205t
  clinical pharmacology, 205t
  doses and schedules, 206t
  for mycosis fungoides with Sézary syndrome, 535, 537t
  therapeutic uses, 205t
Carotenoids, 116, 388–392
Case-cohort studies, 132
Case-control studies, 110
  advantages of, 132
  classification of, 131f
  controls for, 132
  description of, 132–133
  prospective, 132
Case-crossover studies, 132
Caspase recruitment domain (CARD), 456
Castleman disease, 640
Catharanthus roseus G. Don., 249
Cathepsin B, 90
Causality, judgment of, 132
Caveolin-1, 90
CBFB gene, 566
CCI-779. *See* Temsirolimus
CD38, 609
CD19 antibodies, 179, 332
CD20 antibodies, 332
CD30 antigen, 541
CD33 antigen, 332
CD4+ T cells
  mutated gene products recognized by, 169–170
  self-antigen recognition, 169–170
CD8+ T cells
  mutated gene products recognized by, 169–170
  self-antigen recognition, 169–170
CDC45, checkpoint pathways and, 145
CDC25A phosphatase, 145
CDC25C, 147
CDH1 gene
  description of, 30
  mutations
    in diffuse gastric cancer, 370–372
    screening criteria, 371
CDK4
  characteristics of, 48t
CDK8, 48t
CDKN2A gene
  ALL and, 436
  characteristics of, 48t
  function of, 268
  inactivation of, 453
CDKN2B
  function of, 268
CEBPA, 567
CEBPE gene, 436, 556
Cell cycle
  effects of radiation on, 151
Cell death. *See also* Apoptosis
  delayed reproductive, 149
  ionizing radiation-induced, 104
  microtubule inhibitors as cause of, 246
  necrotic, 27
  resisting of, 26–27
  ultraviolet light as cause of, 106
Cell senescence, 25–26
Cell transfer therapy, 175t, 178t
Cell-free circulating DNA, 18
Cell-mediated cytotoxicity, 331f, 331–332
Cell-to-cell signaling pathways, 39f
Celsus, Aulus Cornelius, 88
Central nervous system
  aggressive lymphoma prophylaxis, 520
Centrocytes (CC), 449, 503
CEP-18770
  clinical trials, 279
  therapeutic use of, 280t
Cephalon. *See* Bendamustine
Cephalosporins, 223
Ceritinib, 256t
Cervical cancer
  human papillomavirus and, 167, 417
  locally advanced, 161
  prevention of, 167
  screening for, 411t, 417–418
Cervix, 392
Cetuximab (Erbitux)
  binding of, 332
  characteristics of, 330t
  indications for, 298t
  mechanism of action, 333–334
  radiation sensitivity and, 152
  for squamous cell carcinoma, 164
Chance, epidemiologic findings and, 133
Checkpoint kinases, 145, 591
Checkpoint pathways, DNA damage and, 145–147
Chemical carcinogens, 95–99, 96t
Chemokine ligands, 532
Chemokine receptors, 532
Chemoprevention, 384
Chemoradiotherapy. *See also* Chemotherapy; Radiation therapy; *specific cancers*
Chemotherapy. *See also specific agents; specific regimens*
  for adult T-cell leukemia/lymphoma, 82
  adverse effects of
    pulmonary toxicity. *See* Pulmonary toxicity

Chemotherapy (Continued)
  L-asparaginase, 290–291, 294t
  cytotoxic, 540
  dihydropyrimidine dehydrogenase, 200
  drug interactions, 190–191
  genotype-guided, 197t
  hematologic malignancies secondary to, 483
  for Hodgkin's lymphoma
    advanced-stage, 480–482
    early-stage, 477–478
  homoharringtonine, 290
  omacetaxine, 290
  pharmacogenomics of, 199–201
  proteasome inhibitors, 279–282
  taxanes in, 245
  thiopurine methyltransferase, 199–200
  tumor response to, 196
Children. See also Pediatric patients
  presymptomatic testing in, 388
  solid tumors in, 5
Chimeric antigen receptor–bearing T-cell therapy, for chronic lymphocytic leukemia, 621
Chimeric antigen receptors
  anti-CD19, 179–181
  description of, 179
  hematologic antigens targeted by, 181
CHK1
  development of, 147
  inhibitors of, 147
Chlamydophila psittaci, 432–433
Chlorambucil
  clinical pharmacology, 205t
  stability of, 207
  therapeutic uses, 205t
  toxicities, 205t
Chloroethyl diazohydroxide, 204f
Chloroethyl nitrosoureas, 204f, 207
Chlorozotocin, 207
CHOP regimen
  rituximab with, 334
Chromatin, in gene regulation, 269–270
Chromatin immunoprecipitation with sequencing, 60
Chromoplexy, 9
Chromosomal translocation, 47, 451f, 451–452, 498–499, 499t
Chromosome 4, 148f
Chromothripsis, 9
Chronic B-cell leukemia, 610t
Chronic granulocytic leukemia. See Chronic myelogenous leukemia (CML)
Chronic leukemia, 589–594. See also specific leukemia
Chronic lymphocytic leukemia (CLL)
  adenopathy regression in, 180f
  autoimmune complications, 613
  B cell, 500, 506
  B-cell receptor signaling in, 594
  cell of origin, 458
  chromosomal abnormalities in, 593
  clinical manifestations, 612
  diagnosis, 611–613
  disrupted apoptosis in, 594
  epigenetic silencing in, 593
  fludarabine-refractory, ofatumumab for, 335
  genetic lesions, 458–459
  histology, 611f–612f
  immune abnormalities, 611
  immunoglobulin heavy chain variable gene mutation status in, 609
  immunophenotype, 609
  laboratory findings, 612
  molecular abnormalities in, 609–610
  molecular biology of, 609–611
  origin of, 592–593
  pathogenesis of, 593
  progression of, 593–594
  proliferation, 593
  recurrent mutations in, 593
  residual disease, 620
  response criteria, 614t
  risk of progression, 610f
  second malignancies, 622
  staging, 613, 613t
  treatment of
    alemtuzumab, 335
    allogeneic stem cell transplantation, 621–622
    B-cell signaling pathway inhibitors for, 620
    Bcl-2 inhibitors, 621
    cellular therapy, 621–622
    chemoimmunotherapy, 617–618, 618t–619t
    chimeric antigen receptor–bearing T-cell therapy, 621
    modalities for, 613–622, 616t
    monoclonal antibodies, 616, 617t
    ofatumumab, 335
    phosphoinositide 3-kinase inhibitor, 621
Chronic myelogenous leukemia (CML), 591–606
  advanced phase disease, 606
  animal models of, 591
  BCR-ABL
    domain structure, 590f
    functional domains of, 589
    signal transduction, 589–591
    transcripts, 589
    translocation, 255
    tyrosine-kinase inhibitors, 601
  blastic phase, 592
  busulfan for, 203
  clinical course, 600
  cytogenetics, 600
  diagnosis, 599–600
  differential diagnosis of, 600
  epidemiology, 598
  hematopoietic cell transplantation for, 605
  imatinib for
    BCR-ABL kinase inhibitors and, 263
    description of, 255, 605
  laboratory tests, 599–600
  molecular biology of, 591–594
  molecular testing, 600
  murine models of, 591
  pathogenesis of, 589, 598
  pathway-directed therapy for, 196
  peripheral blood and bone marrow tests in, 599–600
  prognosis, 600
  stem cells and, 591–592
  translocations in, 255, 257
  treatment of, 600–601
Chronic myelomonocytic leukemia, 634t
Chronic transforming retroviruses, 81
CI-994, 271t
Cigarettes. See Smoking; Tobacco
Cilengitide, 320
Circulating tumor cells, 344
Circulating tumor DNA, 344
Cis-diamminecyclobutanedicarboxylate platinum (II). See Carboplatin
Cis-diamminedichloroplatinum (II). See Cisplatin
Cisplatin
  clinical pharmacology, 219
  doses and schedules, 206t
  for ovarian cancer, 214
  radiation sensitivity and, 152
  routes of administration, 220
  for testicular cancer, 214
  toxicities, 214, 220
CLA. See Cutaneous lymphoid antigen (CLA)
Cladribine (2-CdA)
  for acute myelogenous leukemia, 570
  for chronic lymphocytic leukemia, 615
  clinical pharmacology, 231
  description, 231
  dosages, 225t
  for hairy cell leukemia, 623
  mechanism of action, 230–231
  mechanism of resistance, 231
  for mycosis fungoides with Sézary syndrome, 540
  resistance to, 332
  therapeutic usages, 225t
  toxicities, 225t, 231
Class-switch recombination (CSR), 449
Clearance, 187
Clinical benefit response (CBR), 342
Clinical Laboratory Improvement Amendments of 1988, 50
Clinical response, assessment of, 339–349
Clinical trials
  clinical response assessment, 339–349
Clinical utility, 47
Clinical validity, 47
Clofarabine
  for AML, 570
  clinical pharmacology, 231
  description, 231
  dosages, 225t
  mechanism of action, 231
  mechanism of resistance, 231
  therapeutic usages, 225t
  toxicities, 225t, 231
Clonal cells, 47
Clonal dermatitis, 533
Clonal evolution, 593–594
Clonazepam, 210
Cluster designations (CD), 497t
c-myc, 444
Coagulopathies, 651
Cockayne syndrome, 105
Cognate kinase inhibitor, 255
Cohort studies, 110–111
  ambidirectional, 131
  classification of, 131f
  description of, 131–132
  prospective, 131
  retrospective, 131
COLO 829, 11f
Colon
  cancer of. See Colorectal cancer
  micronutrients efficacy in, 392
  radiation tolerance, 163f
Colon adenomas, 125
Colonoscopy, 415
Colorectal adenomas, 114–115

Colorectal cancer. *See also* Rectal cancer
  CEA overexpression, 169
  dietary fat and, 112–113
  dietary fiber and, 114
  fruit consumption and, 113
  genome landscape, 12f
  hereditary nonpolyposis. *See also* Lynch syndrome
  hormone replacement therapy and, 139
  incidence of
    trends in, 139–140
  KRAS mutations in, 16
  Lynch syndrome and, 380–381
  meat intake and, 115
  obesity and, 125
  physical activity and, 124–125
  PIK3CA mutations in, 3, 258
  screening for, 411t, 415–416
    colonoscopy, 415
    computed tomography colonoscopy, 415–416
    fecal occult blood testing, 415
    flexible sigmoidoscopy, 415
    in high-risk patients, 416
    recommendations, 416, 416t
  syndromes associated with, 380t
  testing guidelines, 380t
  treated, somatic mutations in, 18f
  treatment of
    bevacizumab, 334
    cetuximab, 333–334
    oxaliplatin, 214
    panitumumab, 334
  vegetable consumption and, 113
Combined modality toxicity, 162
Community-based interventions, 131f
Companion diagnostics, 255, 342
Comparative genomic hybridization, 34, 49
  in chronic lymphocytic leukemia, 593
Complementary and alternative medicine (CAM)
  drug interactions, 191
Complementary determining regions (CDR), 329
Complement-dependent cytotoxicity, 332
Compton scattering, 153, 156
Computed tomography (CT)
  colonoscopy, 415–416
  planning RT treatment and, 155, 158f
Concomitant boost, 162
Confidence intervals, 133
Confidentiality, genetic testing and, 431
Confounding, 133
Consolidation therapy, ALL, 581
Contact inhibition, 26
COPP regimen, for advanced-stage Hodgkin's lymphoma, 481t
Copy number gains, 452
Copy number variation, 49
Core-binding factor (CBF), 553–554
Cowden syndrome
  pathogenesis of, 374
CpG islands, 268–269
CRC. *See* Colorectal cancer
Crizotinib, 256t, 260, 296t, 298t
CRLX101, 236
Cross-sectional studies
  classification of, 131f
  description of, 130–131
Cryptotethya crypta, 228

β-Cryptoxanthin, 388
ctDNA, 19
CTLA-4. *See* Cytotoxic T lymphocyte-associated antigen 4 (CTLA-4)
Cumulative incidence ratios, 131
Curcumin, 401t
Current smoking, 353
Cutaneous B-cell lymphoma (CBCL)
  classification of, 542
  incidence, 542
  prognostic index, 532t
Cutaneous CD30+ anaplastic large cell lymphoma (C-ALCL), 541
Cutaneous lymphoid antigen (CLA), 531
Cutaneous lymphomas, 531–542, 533t, 535
Cutaneous peripheral T-cell lymphoma (PTL), 541
Cutaneous plasmacytoma, 542
Cutaneous T-cell lymphoma (CTCL), 342, 462. *See also* Cutaneous lymphomas
Cyclic tetrapeptides, 272
Cyclins
  D
  cyclin D1, 453
Cyclophosphamide (Cytoxan)
  activation of, 208, 208f
  adverse effects
    cardiotoxicity, 210
    hemorrhagic cystitis, 209
  clinical pharmacology, 205t
  detoxification of, 208f
  doses and schedules, 206t
  metabolism of, 208f
  for multiple myeloma, 672–673
  for mycosis fungoides with Sézary syndrome, 540
  stability of, 207
  synthesis of, 211
  therapeutic uses, 205t
  toxicities, 205t
CYLD gene, 4
CYP3A, 305
CYP3A4
  docetaxel metabolism by, 247
  paclitaxel metabolism by, 246
CYP3A5, docetaxel metabolism by, 247
CYP2B6, 208
CYP2C8, 246
CYP2D6 gene
  inhibition of, 304–305
Cytarabine (ara-C)
  catabolism of, 228
  clinical pharmacology, 228
  description, 228
  dosages, 224t
  mechanism of action, 228
  mechanism of resistance, 228
  therapeutic uses, 224t
  toxicities, 224t, 228
Cytidine deaminase, 271
Cytochrome C, 27
Cytochrome P450
  targeted therapies using, 211
Cytochrome P-450 19, 306
Cytochrome P45017 alpha inhibitors, 303t
Cytochrome P450 2D6, 200–201
Cytosine, methylation, 267
Cytotoxic agents. *See also* Chemotherapy
Cytotoxic chemotherapy, 540

Cytotoxic T lymphocyte-associated antigen 4 (CTLA-4)
  description of, 172
  mechanism of action, 173f
Cytotoxic T lymphocytes (CTL), 33, 167

D

Dabrafenib, 256t, 296t
Dacarbazine
  activation of, 208
  clinical pharmacology, 205t
  doses and schedules, 206t
  therapeutic uses, 205t
  toxicities, 205t
Dactinomycin
  description of, 240–241
Dairy products, 115, 118
Darbepoetin alfa, 632
Dasatinib (Sprycel)
  adverse effects, 602–603
  for ALL, 582
  for chronic myelogenous leukemia, 263, 264, 602, 604–606
  food effects on, 191t
  imatinib compared with, 601t
  indications, 256t, 299t
Daunorubicin, 238–239, 239t
Decitabine
  for acute myelogenous leukemia, 570
  dosage, 271
  for MDS, 271, 635
Degarelix
  characteristics of, 309
  dosage, 303t, 309
  efficacy of, 309
Degradome, human, 3
Delanzomib, 279, 280, 280t
Delayed reproductive cell death, 149
Demethylating agents, 267–275
Denileukin diftitox, 537t, 538t, 539–540
Denosumab (Prolia)
  characteristics of, 330t
  indications for, 296t, 298t, 334
2′-Deoxy-5-azacytidine, 270, 271t
Deoxyepothilone B, 251
Depression, brain cancer and, 130–131
Depth-dose curves, 156, 156f–157f
Dermatofibrosarcoma protuberans (DFSP)
  translocations in, 257–258
Descriptive studies, 130, 131f
Desmoid tumors
  in FAP, 379
Deubiquitinating enzymes (DUB), 4
Dexamethasone
  for multiple myeloma, 666, 668–669, 672–673
  for myelomas, 659–664
Diet
  alcohol consumption in, 111–112
  assessment of, 111
  breast cancer and, 112
  calcium in, 115
  after cancer diagnosis, 117
  carbohydrates, 117
  carotenoids in, 116
  colorectal cancer and, 112–113
  dairy products in, 115
  in early life phases, 117
  energy and, 111
  epidemiologic studies of, 118

Diet (Continued)
  fat intake, 112–113
  folate in, 116
  fruits, 113–114
  methodologic challenges for studying, 110–114
  milk consumption in, 115, 118
  prostate cancer and, 113
  recommendations for, 119
  red meat, 115
  selenium in, 116
  soy products in, 116–117
  vegetables, 113–114
  vegetarian, 117
Dietary fiber, 114–115
Dietary patterns, 117
Diet-derived natural products, 400
Diethylstilbestrol (DES), 311
Diffuse gastric cancer (DGC), 369t, 370f
Diffuse large B-cell lymphomas (DLBCL), 511–514, 542, 545
  cell of origin, 455
  genetic lesions in, 455–458, 456f
  rituximab for, 334–335
Diffusion-mediated hypoxia, 151
Difluoromethylornithine, 398, 399t, 400
Digitoxin, tamoxifen interaction with, 305
Dihydrofolate reductase (DHFR), 223
Dihydropyrimidine dehydrogenase (DPD)
  description of, 200
Diphtheria toxin, denileukin diftitox from, 539
Direct angiogenesis inhibitor, 320
Direct-to-consumer (DTC) marketing, 368
Direct-to-consumer genetic testing, 432
Discoidin domain-containing receptor 2, 48t
Disposition, 186–187
Distribution, 186
DM1, 251
DNA
  ionizing radiation damage to, 102–103
  platination of, 216
DNA adducts, 98
DNA damage
  H2AX staining, 146f
  linear energy transfer and, 146f
  radiation induced, 145–148
  unfaithful restitution, 148
DNA hypermethylation, 91
DNA methylation, 268–269
DNA methyltransferases (DNMTs)
  description of, 268
  inhibitors of, 270–271
DNA mismatch repair
  genes involved in, 374
DNA polymerases, 148
DNA repair, 285
  BRCA mutations and, 285–286
  faulty, 148
  homologous recombination in, 147f, 148
  nonhomologous end joining, 147f, 147–148
  PARP inhibitors and, 285
  types of, 148
DNA sequencing, 25
DNMT3A gene, 7, 270
DNMT3b, 270
Dll4-Notch signaling system, 318
Docetaxel (Taxotere)
  adverse effects, 247t, 249
  approval of, 245

capecitabine and, 227
clinical pharmacology, 247
dosages, 247t
drug interactions, 248
identification of, 245
indications, 247t
mechanisms of action, 245–246
radiation sensitivity and, 152
Dose proportionality, 187
Dose-calculation algorithms, 156–157
Double-strand breaks, 285. See also DNA repair
Doxorubicin (Adriamycin)
  alopecia and, 210
  characteristics of, 239t
  description of, 238
  indications for, 297t
  liposomal, 238, 672
  pegylated, 281
  pegylated liposomal
    characteristics of, 239t
    for mycosis fungoides with Sézary syndrome, 537t, 540
  toxicities of, 238
Driver mutations, 47
"Driver" mutations, 13
Drosophila melanogaster, 2
Drug development, 339–349
Drug interactions, 190–191
Drug maytansinoid-1, 251
Drug resistance
  after alkylating agents, 211
  cancer genomics and, 19–20
  in plasma cells, 648–649
  to tyrosine kinase inhibitors, 605
Ductal carcinoma in situ (DCIS)
  description of, 414
Dynamic instability, microtubule, 245
Dysmorphology, screening, 428

E
E7 protein, 76
Early-stage Hodgkin's lymphoma
  chemotherapy for, 477–478
  clinical trials for, 479t
  combined modality therapy for, 477
  criteria for, 476t
  description of, 476
  involved node irradiation therapy for, 477
  prognostic features of, 476
  radiation therapy for, 476–477
EBF1 mutations, 560
E-Cadherin gene, 371f
Echinoderm microtubule-associated protein like 4 (EML4) gene. See EML4-ALK fusion gene
Ecologic studies, 110, 130
Eculizumab, 298t
E2F family, checkpoint pathways and, 145
Effect modification, 133
Effect modifiers, 133
EGFR gene
  mutations
    drug resistance and, 19
    in lung adenocarcinoma, 256–257
Elderly
  Hodgkin's lymphoma in, 483
  non-Hodgkin's lymphoma in, 515
  primary central nervous system lymphomas in, 547

Electromagnetic fields, 107
Electronic cigarettes, 352
Elimination, 186
Elimination rate constant, 187
EML4-ALK fusion gene
  description of, 260
  translocations, 10, 16
Endocrine tumors
  thyroid cancer. See Thyroid cancer
Endogenous base damage, 285
Endometrial cancer
  hereditary
    prophylactic surgery, 372–373
  obesity and, 125
  PIK3CA mutations in, 3, 258
  prophylactic surgery in, 373–374
  screening for, 419
  tamoxifen and, 302
Endostatin, angiogenesis inhibition by, 318
Endothelial cells, 36
Endothelial monocyte-activating polypeptide II, 90
Endoxifen, 303–305
Energy, 111
Energy metabolism, 32
Energy restriction, 111
Entecavir, 83
Enteropathy-associated T-cell lymphoma (EATL), 518
Entinostat, 271t, 272, 273
Environmental exposures
  multiple myeloma and, 641–642
  non-Hodgkin's lymphoma and, 495
Enzalutamide, 297t, 303t, 310
Ephedra, 192t
Epidemiology
  methods
    case-control studies, 132–133
    cohort studies, 131–132
    cross-sectional studies, 130–131
    ecologic studies, 130
    interpretation of findings, 133
    study design, 131f
    types of studies, 130
  molecular, 97, 134–136
Epidermal growth factor receptor (EGFR)
  description of, 48t
  radiation synergy with, 164, 164f
  smoking and, 355
Epidermodysplasia verruciformis, 76
Epidermotropism, 532
Epigenetic changes, 267–268, 268f
Epigenetic silencing, 16
Epigenetics, 91–92
  description of, 267
  DNA methyltransferase inhibitors, 273
Epipodophyllotoxins, 241
Epirubicin
  description of, 239–240
Epithelial-to-mesenchymal transition, 26, 30
EPO906. See Epothilone B
EPOCH regimen, 540
Epothilone B, 251
Epothilone D. See Deoxyepothilone B
Epothilones, 251
Epstein-Barr virus (EBV)
  Burkitt's lymphoma and, 78
  carcinomas associated with, 79
  characteristics of, 74t

classic Hodgkin's lymphoma and, 474
extranodal NK/T-cell lymphoma and, 541
history of, 78
Hodgkin's lymphoma and, 474
leukemias and, 565
life cycle of, 78
lymphoid cancers, 79
lymphomas induced by, 443
nasal NK/T-cell lymphoma and, 531
non-Hodgkin's lymphoma and, 452
prevention of, 79
treatment of, 79
ERBB2 gene
characteristics of, 48t, 90
Eribulin mesylate, 299t
Erlotinib (Tarceva)
clinical development of, 257
food effects on, 191t
indications, 256t, 296t
for non–small-cell lung cancer, 19
radiation sensitivity and, 152
Error, sources of, 133
Erythroderma, 533
Erythropoiesis-stimulating agents (ESA)
for myelodysplastic syndromes, 632, 634
Erythropoietin
radiotherapy and, 151
Erythropoietin receptor, 48t
Esophageal adenocarcinoma (EAC), 126
Esophageal cancer
locally advanced, 161
screening for, 416
Esophagus
micronutrients efficacy in, 392
radiation tolerance, 163f
Essential thrombocytosis, 258
Estradiol, 303t, 311
Estramustine phosphate
description of, 247t, 251
structure of, 210
Estrogen(s). See also Estradiol
cancer treatment with, 303t
use of, 311
Estrogen receptor (ER)
downregulator, 303t
Etaracizumab (Abegrin), 320
Ethylenediaminetetraacetic acid, 51
Ethyleneimines, 205t
Etiologic studies, 131f
Etirinotecan pegol, 237
ETO gene. See RUNX1T1 gene
Etoposide (VP-16)
characteristics of, 239, 241
doses and schedules, 206t
for mycosis fungoides with Sézary syndrome, 540
Evaluation criteria, 340t–341t
Everolimus (RAD001, Afinitor)
approved indications, 256t
cancer therapy with, 320, 323–324
description of, 293, 295t
dosages, 319t
food effects on, 191t
indications, 297t, 298t, 319t
mTOR inhibition by, 261
safety profile of, 293
Exemestane, 306
breast cancer risk reduction, 397
characteristics of, 307–308
dosage, 303t

pharmacology, 308
side effects, 308
Exercise. See also Physical activity
Exomes, 4–5
Experimental studies
classification of, 131f
epidemiologic, 130
Exposure odds ratio, 132
External beam radiation therapy (EBRT)
treatment with, 158–159
Extracorporeal phototherapy (ECP), 539
Extramedullary plasmacytomas, 651
Extranodal marginal zone lymphoma, 509–510
Extranodal natural killer/T-cell lymphoma, 519–520
Eye
uveal melanomas, 4
EZH2 mutations, 455

F

Fab domains, 329
Fadrozole, 306
FAK protein, 591
Fallopian tube cancer, 372
Familial adenomatous polyposis (FAP)
desmoids in, 379
extracolonic features of, 379
prophylactic surgery in, 377–380
workup algorithm for, 378f
Familial breast cancer/ovarian cancer syndrome, 369t
Familial cylindromatosis, 4
Family history
cancer clustering, 428
genetic counseling and, 427–428
Fanconi anemia (FA)
family history in, 427
FAP. See Familial adenomatous polyposis
Fat intake, 112–113
Fatigue
radiation-induced, 163
FCR regimen, 619–620
FcγR, 331–332
Fecal occult blood testing, 415
Feedback-controlled dosing, 192–193
Fenretinide, 390–391
Fiber, dietary, 114–115
Fibroblast growth factor receptor 1, 48t
Fibroblast growth factors (FGFs)
basic, angiogenesis and, 318
Fibroblasts, cancer-associated, 35–36
Fine-needle aspiration (FNA)
of myeloma lesions, 655f
First-pass effect, 186
FISH testing, 600
Flexible sigmoidoscopy, for colorectal cancer, 415
FLT3, 567t
FLT3 gene, 48t, 557–558
FLT inhibitors, 260–261, 571
Fludarabine
for acute myelogenous leukemia, 570
adverse effects, 225t, 230
for chronic lymphocytic leukemia, 614–617, 619–620
clinical pharmacology, 230
description, 230
dosages, 225t
mechanism of action, 230
mechanism of resistance, 230

for mycosis fungoides with Sézary syndrome, 537t, 540
therapeutic uses, 225t
Fluorescent in situ hybridization, 53t, 57–58, 58f
Fluorodeoxyglucose-positron emission tomography, 342
Fluoropyrimidines
biomodulation of, 226–227
clinical pharmacology, 226
mechanism of action, 225–226
mechanism of resistance, 226
toxicity, 226
5-Fluoropyrimidines, 225–228
5-Fluorouracil (5-FU)
dosages, 224t
mechanism of action, 225–226
radiation sensitivity and, 152
therapeutic uses, 224t
toxicities, 224t
Fluoxymesterone
dosage, 303t, 310
pharmacology, 310–311
toxicities, 310
Flutamide
dosage, 303t, 309
toxicity of, 309
Folate, 116
FOLFOX regimen
bevacizumab with, for colorectal cancer, 321
Folic acid, 116, 392–393
Follicular lymphoma, 502t, 503–507, 506
advanced, 504
cell of origin, 454
clinical features of, 504
early-stage, 504
genetic lesions in, 455
immunophenotype of, 503–504
pathology of, 503
prognosis for, 504
relapsed, 505–506
rituximab for, 334
treatment of, 504–505
Follicular mucinosis, 538
Follow-up, in cohort design studies, 132
Folylpolyglutamyl synthetase (FPGS), 223
Forest plots, 347
Forkhead O transcription factors (FOXO), 591
Former smoking, 353
Formestane, 306
Fractionation, 162
Fragment analysis, 53t, 55, 56f
Free radicals, 145
Fruits, 113–114
Fulvestrant
dosage, 303t
pharmacology, 306
structure of, 306f
use of, 306

G

G1 phase, 145
G2 phase
arrest of, 147
checkpoint pathways and, 145, 147
Gabapentin
for hot flashes, 302
Galeterone, 310
Gallbladder cancer
description of, 126

GAP1 phase. *See* G1 phase
GAP2 phase. *See* G2 phase
Gardasil, 76
Gastrectomy
 prophylactic, 371–372
Gastric cancer. *See also* Stomach cancer
 breast cancer risk in, 369t
 inheritance of, 370f
 screening for, 417
Gastroesophageal junction cancer, 245
Gastrointestinal cancers
 cytokines in, 89
Gastrointestinal stromal tumors (GIST)
 kinase inhibitors in, 255
GATA-1 point mutations, 556
Gefitinib (Iressa)
 approved indications, 256t
 clinical development of, 257
 food effects on, 191t
 for non–small-cell lung cancer, 19
Gemcitabine
 clinical pharmacology, 229
 description, 229
 dosages, 224t
 mechanism of action, 229
 mechanism of resistance, 229
 for mycosis fungoides with Sézary syndrome, 537t, 540
 radiation sensitivity and, 152
 therapeutic uses, 224t
 toxicities, 224t, 229
Gemtuzumab ozogamicin (Mylotarg)
 for AML, 571
 characteristics of, 330t
 description of, 251
 use of, 332
Gender
 mycosis fungoides and, 531
Gene amplification, 47
Gene expression profiling
 in chronic lymphocytic leukemia, 592
 overexpression of gene products, 169
Gene products, 169
Gene silencing
 description of, 267–268
 reversal of layers, 270
Gene–environment interactions, 134
Genes, patents on, 432
Genetic counseling, 426–432
 candidates for, 426–427
 components of, 427–430
 counselors, 427t
 DNA testing, 428–429
 follow-up after, 430
 indications for, 427t
 issues in
  confidentiality, 431
  discrimination, 431–432
  insurance, 431–432
  psychosocial, 430–431
 presymptomatic testing and, 431
 reproductive issues, 432
 risk assessment and, 428
 surveillance options and, 429–430
Genetic epidemiology, 135
Genetic Information Nondiscrimination Act, 368
Genetic polymorphism, 97
Genetic susceptibility, 97

Genetic testing
 categories of results, 429
 direct-to-consumer, 432
 patents on genes, 432
Genome analyses, 15t, 20
Genome instability and mutation, 33–34
Genome-wide association studies (GWAS), 134–135
Genomewide gene expression profiling, 198–199
Genomic instability
 CCL progression and, 593–594
Genomic microarrays, 54t, 60–61
Genomics, 16, 92
Genotoxic carcinogens, 95–96
Genotype-guided cancer chemotherapy, 197t
Genotypic markers, 135
Germinal centers, 449–450, 503
Germ-line antigens, 167–169
Gimatecan, 237
Ginger (*Zingiber officinale*), 401t
Ginkgo, 192t
Ginseng (*Panax ginseng, P. quinquefolius*), 192t
Glasgow Prognostic Score, 89
Glioblastoma(s)
 genomic analysis of, 264
 isocitrate dehydrogenase mutations in, 264
 PIK3CA mutations in, 3
Global M. D. Anderson Scoring System, 632
Glucocorticoids. *See also specific agents*
Glutathione-S-transferase pi, 211
Glycinamide ribonucleotide (GAR) formyltransferase, 223
Glycolytic fueling, 32
Gonadotropin-releasing hormone (GnRH)
 analogues
  characteristics, 308
  pharmacology, 308–309
 antagonists, 303t
  mechanism of action, 309
  pharmacology, 309
Goserelin, 303t, 308–309, 309
Graft versus host disease (GVHD)
 after hematopoietic cell transplantation, 605
Graft-versus-leukemia, 487, 572
Graft versus myeloma effect, 670
Green fluorescent protein, 37
Green tea (*Camellia sinensis*), 192t, 401t
Grey zone lymphoma, 515
Growth kinetics, 349
Growth rate constants, 348f, 349
Growth suppressors, 26
G1/S interface, 145, 147
Guardian of the genome, 34
Gynecomastia, 309

H

Hair. *See also* Alopecia
Hairy cell leukemia, 623
Hallmarks, of cancer
 angiogenesis induction, 29–30
 characteristics that facilitate, 33–35
 energy metabolism, 32
 evading growth suppressors, 26
 evading immune destruction, 32–33
 invasion, 30–32
 metastasis, 30–32
 overview of, 24
 proliferative signaling, 24–26
 replicative immortality, 28–29

 resisting cell death, 26–29
 therapeutic targeting of, 41–42, 42f
 tumor-promoting inflammation, 34–35
Hand-foot syndrome, 225
Haploidentical transplantation, 577
HapMap, 2
H2AX
 checkpoint pathways and, 145
 staining of, 146f
Hazard ratios, 347
Head and neck cancer. *See* Head and neck squamous cell carcinoma (HNSCC)
Head and neck squamous cell carcinoma (HNSCC)
 adjuvant therapy, 162
 cetuximab for, 333
 locally advanced, 161
 treatment of, 245
Health insurance
 discrimination in, 431–432
 genetic testing and, 431–432
Heart
 radiation tolerance, 163f
HEF1 protein, 591
Helical tomotherapy, 155, 155f
Helicobacter pylori
 MALT lymphoma and, 458
 non-Hodgkin's lymphoma and, 452–453
 stomach cancer and, 142
 treatment of, 400
Hellers Hirschowitz/Lichtscope, 5, 6t, 7f
Hematologic malignancies. *See also specific cancers*
 lymphocyte genetic modification to treat, 178–179, 179t
 rituximab for, 334–335
Hematopoietic cell transplantation (HCT). *See also* Hematopoietic stem cell transplantation (HSCT)
 allogeneic
  T-cell gene therapy in, 181
  umbilical cord blood cells, 487
 in CML, 605
 CML relapse after, 605
Hematopoietic cells, 565
Hematopoietic stem cell transplantation (HSCT)
 in acute lymphoblastic leukemia, 501–502
 for acute myelogenous leukemia, 571, 572–577
 allogeneic, 574–576, 575t
 for AML, 575t
 autologous, 574–576, 575t
 for acute myeloid leukemia, 574–576
 for follicular lymphoma, 505–506
 for Hodgkin's lymphoma, 483–484
 conditioning regimens, 574
 in older patients, 581–582
 stem cell sources, 668
Hematopoietic stem cells, chronic myeloid leukemia and, 591
Hemorrhagic cystitis, 209
Hepatitis B virus
 characteristics of, 74t, 83
 management of, 83
Hepatitis C virus
 B-cell non-Hodgkin lymphoma and, 85
 characteristics of, 74t, 83–84
 non-Hodgkin's lymphoma and, 452
 reactivation of, 84

Hepatitis viruses
  B. *See* Hepatitis B virus
  C. *See* Hepatitis C virus
  description of, 83
  hepatocellular carcinoma induced by, 84
  malignancies associated with, 84–85
  pathogenesis of, 84
Hepatocellular carcinoma (HCC). *See also* Liver cancer
  hepatitis viruses and, 84
  PIK3CA mutations in, 3
  treatment of
    sorafenib, 322
Hepatosplenic T-cell lymphoma, 519
Hereditary cancer syndromes
  genetic counseling in, 427*t*
  list of, 369*t*
  surgery's role in prevention of, 368–381
Hereditary diffuse gastric cancer (HDGC), 369*t*, 370*f*
Hereditary nonpolyposis colorectal cancer (HNPCC). *See also* Lynch syndrome
Heredity, molecular epidemiology and, 135
HER2/neu. *See* ERBB2
Her-2/neu, 169
Herpes simplex virus
  Kaposi's sarcoma, 79–80
HES/FIP1L1-PDGFR-α, 257
Heterocyclic amines, 98
HIF. *See* Hypoxia-inducible factor (HIF)
High linear energy transfer, 145
Highly active antiretroviral therapy, 175–176
High-resolution melting curve analysis, 55–56, 56*f*
Hills, 11
Histone deacetylase inhibitors
  cyclic tetrapeptides, 272
  description of, 267–275
  for Hodgkin's lymphoma, 489
  for mycosis fungoides with Sézary syndrome, 539–540
  small chain fatty acids, 272
  types of, 272
Histone methyltransferases, 269
Histones, DNA methylation and, 269–270
HIV-associated malignancies
  Hodgkin's lymphoma, 475–476
HMG-CoA reductase inhibitors, 398
Hodgkin lymphoma (HL)
  advanced-stage
    chemotherapy for, 480–482
    consolidation radiotherapy, 482
    description of, 478–479
    initial therapy for, 480–482
    International Prognostic Score, 479
    positron-emission tomography–directed approaches for, 482
    prognostic factors in, 479
  biology of, 469
  cell lineage in, 469, 470*t*
  cells of origin in, 462, 469, 470*t*
  classic
    differential diagnosis of, 475
    Epstein-Barr virus and, 474
    microenvironment of, 473–474
    morphology of, 472–473
    phenotype of, 473
    Reed-Sternberg cells associated with, 469, 472, 474*f*
    classification of, 470*f*
  differential diagnosis of, 474–476
  early-stage
    chemotherapy for, 477–478
    clinical trials for, 479*t*
    combined modality therapy for, 477
    criteria for, 476*t*
    description of, 476
    involved node irradiation therapy for, 477
    prognostic features of, 476
    radiation therapy for, 476–477
  in elderly patients, 483
  genetic lesions in, 462
  HIV-associated, 475–476
  lymphocyte-predominant cells in, 469, 471
  mediastinal gray zone lymphoma, 475
  molecular markers in, 470*t*
  nodular lymphocyte-predominant
    differential diagnosis of, 474–475
    lymphocyte-predominant cells, 469, 471
    microenvironment for, 471–472
    morphology of, 470, 471*t*
    patterns of, 472*f*
    phenotype of, 471
    T-cell/histiocyte-rich large B-cell lymphoma versus, 474
  pathology of, 470–474
  pediatric, 442*t*, 444–445
  in pregnancy, 483
  Reed-Sternberg cells, 469, 472, 474*f*
  refractory, salvage chemotherapy for, 484, 485*t*–486*t*
  relapsed
    brentuximab vedotin for, 488–489
    salvage chemotherapy for, 484, 485*t*–486*t*
  TNFAIP3 mutation in, 4
  treatment of
    chemotherapy, 477–478, 480–484, 485*t*–486*t*
    combined modality therapy, 477
    complications of, 483
    consolidation radiotherapy, 482
    FDG-PET in response assessment, 484, 486
    histone deacetylase inhibitors, 489
    investigational agents, 489
    novel agents used in, 482–483
    PI3K/AKT/mTOR pathway inhibitors, 489
    radiation therapy, 476–477, 482
    response-adapted, 478
    salvage chemotherapy, 484, 485*t*–486*t*
      allogeneic, 487–488
      autologous, 483–486
      radiation after, 487
      relapse after, 488–489
      second transplant, 488
Holliday junctions, 148
Homoharringtonine, 290
Homologous recombination (HR), 285
Homologous recombination repair (HRR), 147*f*, 148
Hormonal therapy. *See also* Hormone replacement therapy (HRT)
  in cancer, 303*t*
  endocrine manipulation, 302–312
Hormone replacement therapy (HRT)
  colorectal cancer and, 139
Hospice, for pediatric patients, 445
Host–environment interactions, 136
Hot flashes
  management of, 302, 311
  tamoxifen and, 302

HOX transcription factor family, 555
HRAS, 48*t*
Human chorionic gonadotropin (hCG), 343–344
Human Genome Project, 2
Human herpesvirus-8 (HHV-8)
  description of, 452–453
  Kaposi's sarcoma and, 79
  non-Hodgkin's lymphoma and, 495
Human immunodeficiency virus (HIV)
  lymphomas associated with, 521–522
  non-Hodgkin's lymphoma and
    cell of origin, 460
    description of, 452
    genetic lesions, 460
Human papillomavirus (HPV)
  cancers associated with
    antigens in, 170
    cervical, 417
    E5 oncogene expression of, 76
    genomes of, 75
    history of, 75
    HPV16
      description of, 75
    HPV18, 75
    nonmelanoma skin cancer, 76
    oropharyngeal cancer, 76
    testing for, 417
    tissue tropism, 75–76
    types of, 75
    vaccines, 76
      cervical cancer prevention and, 143, 167, 418
      description of, 418
Human T-cell leukemia virus type 1 (HTLV-1)
  adult T-cell leukemia/lymphoma and, 531
  characteristics of, 74*t*
  epidemiology of, 81
  etiology, 495
  malignancies associated with, 82–83
  molecular biology of, 81–82
  non-Hodgkin's lymphoma and, 452
Human telomerase reverse transcriptase (hTERT), 169
Humoral hypercalcemia of malignancy. *See also* Hypercalcemia
Hydroxamic acids, 272
4-Hydroxytamoxifen. *See* Tamoxifen
Hydroxyurea, 600–601, 603
25-Hydroxyvitamin D, 115
Hyperbaric oxygen (HBO) therapy, 151
Hypercalcemia
  multiple myeloma and, 649–650
Hypereosinophilic syndrome (HES)
  description of, 257
  FIP1L1-PDGFR-α translocation, 257
Hyperfractionation, 162
Hyperviscosity, 651
Hyperviscosity syndrome, 599
Hypocellular myelodysplastic syndromes, 628
Hypofractionation, 162
Hypoxia
  acute, 151
  chronic, 151
  diffusion-mediated, 151
  oxygen consumption and, 151
  prognostic value of, 151
  transient, 151
Hypoxia-inducible factor (HIF), 261, 317–318
Hysterectomy, 373, 430

I

Ibritumomab tiuxetan (Zevalin), 330t, 333
Ibrutinib, 296t, 620
Idarubicin, 240
Idelalisib, 256t, 263
IDH1, 5, 6
IDH2, 5
Ifosfamide
  activation of, 208
  adverse effects
    hemorrhagic cystitis, 209
    neurotoxicity, 210
  clinical pharmacology, 205t
  doses and schedules, 207t
  synthesis of, 211
  therapeutic uses, 205t
  toxicities, 205t
IKAROS mutations, 560
IKK-α, 91
IKZF1 gene, 436
Illumina HiSeq 2000, 6t
Image-guided radiation therapy (IGRT)
  systems used in, 155–156
Imatinib mesylate (Gleevec, Glivec)
  approved indications, 256t
  for chronic myelogenous leukemia, 20, 255, 602
  dasatinib compared with, 601t
  dosage, 602
  food effects on, 191t
  for hypereosinophilic syndrome, 257
  mechanism of action, 598
  nilotinib compared with, 601t
  resistance to, 582, 605
  side effects, 602–603
Immonium ions, 204f
Immune inflammatory cells, 36–37
Immunoconjugates, 332
Immunocytokine conjugates, 332
Immunoglobulin receptors, 331–332
Immunoglobulins (Igs)
  description of, 329
  functional domains of, 329
  structure of, 329
Immunosuppression
  from alkylating agents, 210
  for myelodysplastic syndromes, 635
Immunotherapy, 167–181
  active immunization approaches, 174
  adoptive cell transfer, 174–176, 175f
  anti–cytotoxic T lymphocyte antigen 4 blocking antibodies, 172–173
  antigens in viral-associated cancers, 170
  approaches to, 170t
  cancer/germ-line antigens, 167–169
  checkpoint inhibitors, 172–173
  chimeric antigen receptors
    anti-CD19, 179–181
    description of, 179
    hematologic antigens targeted by, 181
  gene products, 169
  interleukin-2, 171
  melanocyte differentiation antigens, 169
  tumor antigens, 167–170
Immunotoxins, 332
Incidence, trends in, 138–143, 140t
Incidence density ratios, 131
Indels, 10

Indirect angiogenesis inhibitor, 320
Individual-based therapy, 131f
Induction chemotherapy. *See also*
  Chemotherapy; Hematopoietic stem cell transplantation (HSCT);
  specific regimens
Infections. *See also specific infections*
  in lymphomas, 452–453
  multiple myeloma and, 650
Inflammation
  in angiogenesis, 90–91
  in cancer diagnosis, 92
  description of, 88
  epigenetics and, 91–92
  genomics and, 92
  in invasion, 90
  in metastasis, 91
  molecular basis of, 88
  origins of, 89f
  in proliferation, 90
  in survival, 89
  targeted therapies and, 92
  transcription factors, 89
  in transformation, 88–89
  word origin of, 88
Inflammatory cells, 31
Information bias, 133
Informed consent, 409
Insulin-like growth factor 1 (IGF-1)
  myeloma cells and, 646
Integrins
  β-4, 320
  description of, 320
Intensity-modulated radiation therapy (IMRT)
  beam intensity patterns, 155
  isodose distribution, 159f
  treatment planning, 158
Interaction, 133
Interferon(s)
  for follicular lymphoma, 511
  for multiple myeloma, 659
Interferon-α
  bevacizumab with, 321
  in chronic myelogenous leukemia treatment, 601
  for mycosis fungoides with Sézary syndrome, 537t, 539
Interferon regulatory factor 4/multiple myeloma oncogene 1, 469
Interleukin(s)
  IL-2, 171
    description of, 171
    immune stimulation with, 167
    for metastatic melanoma, 171–172
    for metastatic renal cell cancer, 171
    for mycosis fungoides with Sézary syndrome, 539
    safe administration of, 172
    toxicities, 172
  IL-5, 531
  IL-6
    myeloma cells and, 646
    radiation toxicity and, 163
  IL-7, 48t
  IL-12
    for mycosis fungoides with Sézary syndrome, 539
  IL-17, 646, 648
  IL-21, 646, 648

  IL-22, 648
  IL-23, 648
International Cancer Genome Consortium (ICGC), 14–15, 258
International Prognostic Index, 502t
International Prognostic Scoring System, 479, 632
International Working Group (IWG), 342
Interstitial pneumonitis, 209
Intraepithelial neoplasias, 388t
Intraocular melanoma. *See* Uveal melanomas
Intravascular large B-cell lymphomas, 514
Ionizing radiation (IR). *See also* Radiation; Radiation therapy
  cancer risks associated with, 104–105
  cell cycle effects, 151
  cell death caused by, 104
  cell survival and, 149–150
  cellular responses of, 103–105
  damage induction mechanisms, 102–103, 103f
  definition of, 102
  DNA damage caused by, 102–103, 146f
  dose-rate effects, 150–151
  linear energy transfer, 102
  non-Hodgkin's lymphoma and, 495
  protein damage caused by, 103
  radon, 104
  second primary cancers caused by, 104–105
  threshold doses, 149
IPASS study, 257
Ipilimumab, 173
Iressa. *See* Gefitinib
Irinotecan
  cetuximab plus, 333
  description of, 235
  toxicities associated with, 235
Iron chelation therapy, for myelodysplastic syndromes, 636
Isocitrate dehydrogenase (IDH)
  IDH1 mutations and, 6
  mutations
    in AML, 264
    in glioblastoma, 264
Isodose distributions, 159f
Isotopes, radioactive, 159
Ispinesib, 252
ITD, 567
Ixabepilone
  characteristics of, 251
  dosages, 247t
  indications, 247t
  toxicity, 247t
Ixazomib, 279, 280t, 282

J

JAK1, 48t
JAK2, 48t
JAK3, 48t
Janus kinase 2 (JAK2)
  mutations in
    essential thrombocytosis, 258
    myelofibrosis, 258
    polycythemia vera and, 258
    V617F mutations in, 258
Janus kinase (JAK), 591
Japanese arrowroot, 192t
Jewish ancestry, 426. *See also* Race/ethnicity
JM216. *See* Satraplatin
Juvenile myelomonocytic leukemia (JMML), 442

K

Kahler disease. *See* Multiple myeloma
Kaplan-Meier plots, 316-347
Kaposi's sarcoma
  characteristics of, 74t
  clinical manifestations of, 80f
  herpesvirus, 79-80
  lymphoproliferative disorders caused by, 80
Kataegis, 9
Kava-kava, 192t
Ketoconazole, 190
Kidney
  radiation tolerance, 163f
  toxicity of alkylating agents, 209
Kidney cancer. *See also* Renal cell carcinoma
  kinase inhibitors for, 261
  obesity and, 126
Kinase inhibitors
  as anticancer drugs, 255-264
  approved, 256t
  combinations of, 263-264
  early successes with, 255-256
  resistance to, 263-264
  role in cancer medicine, 264
Kinases, cancers driven by, 258
Kinesin spindle protein (KSP, EG5), 252
KIT
  characterization of, 48t
KRAS
  description of, 48t
  mutations
    BRAF mutations and, 15
    in colorectal cancer, 16, 18f
    in pancreatic cancer, 16
Ku heterodimer, 147-148

L

Lambrolizumab, 173
Langerhans cells, 106
Lapatinib
  approved indications, 256t
  for breast cancer, 227
  description of, 197
  food effects on, 191t
Large B-cell lymphomas, 514
Large granular lymphocytes (LGLs), 622-623
Laromustine, 211
Laryngeal cancer
  radiation therapy, 161
LBH589, 271t, 272-273. *See also* Panobinostat (LBH589)
LEF1 mutations, 560
Lenalidomide (Revlimid)
  adverse effects of, 634
  in cancer therapy, 318
  characteristics of, 294
  in chronic lymphocytic leukemia, 621
  mechanism of action, 634-635
  for multiple myeloma, 640, 661t, 663-664, 666, 668-669, 672-673
  for myelodysplastic syndromes, 634-636
  for myelomas, 659-661
  with thalidomide, 294, 335
Length bias, 408, 409f
Letrozole, 306
  characteristics, 307
  dosage, 303t
  structure of, 307f
Leukapheresis, 539

Leukemia(s). *See also* specific leukemia
  acute. *See also* specific leukemia
    cooperating mutations in, 560, 561f
    genetic events in, 550, 551t-552t, 553
    management of, 565-583
    point mutations in, 557-558
  cytogenetic abnormalities, 551t-553t
  molecular abnormalities, 551t-553t
  pediatric, 436-445
    diagnosis, 438
    genetics of, 436-438
Leukemia oncogene transduction, in a murine system, 550
Leukemic stem cells (LSCs)
  chronic myeloid leukemia and, 591-592
  concept of, 550
Leuprolide
  dosage, 303t, 308
  potency of, 308
  route of administration, 308
Levetiracetam, 210
Lewis Y antigen, 181
Life/APG's SOLiD3, 5
Life/APG's SOLiD 5500xl, 6t, 7f
Li-Fraumeni syndrome
  breast cancer risk and, 369t
  genes linked to, 369t
  pathogenesis of, 374
Linear accelerator x-ray beam production, 155f
Linear energy transfer (LET), 102, 146f
Linear-quadratic model, 104
Linitis plastica, 370. *See also* Diffuse gastric cancer (DGC)
Liposomal doxorubicin (DaunoXome), 238. *See also* Doxorubicin
Liquid biopsies, 19
Liver cancer. *See also* Hepatocellular carcinoma (HCC)
  radiation tolerance, 163f
  screening for, 417
Liver disease, radiation-induced, 163
lncRNA, 9
Lobular carcinoma in situ (LCIS), 368
Long-term care, 445
Lorazepam
  for busulfan-induced seizures, 210
Loss of function mutations, 50
Loss of heterozygosity analysis, 59
Louis-Bar syndrome, 369t
Low linear energy transfer, 145
Low-dose computerized tomography, for lung cancer screening, 419-420
Lung
  alkylating agent toxicity, 210
  micronutrient efficacy in, 389-390
  radiation tolerance, 163f
Lung cancer. *See also* Non-small-cell lung cancer; Small cell lung cancer
  adjuvant therapy, 162
  asbestos and, 108
  EGFR mutations in, 256-257
  fruit consumption and, 114
  incidence of, 138-139
  locally advanced, 161
  low-dose computerized tomography screening for, 419-420
  obesity and, 127
  physical activity and, 127

  screening for, 411t, 419-420
  squamous carcinoma, 16
  vegetable consumption and, 114
Lung resistance-related protein (LRP), 648
Luteinizing hormone releasing hormone (LHRH)
  description of, 303t
Lymph nodes
  biology of, 496
Lymphocytes
  adoptive cell therapy for, 176-178
  radiation killing of, 163
Lymphoid cells, 497t, 498
Lymphoid neoplasms, 496-498, 499-501
  genetic abnormalities, 499t
  genetic studies, 503-504
  immunophenotyping, 498
Lymphomas. *See also* Hodgkin lymphoma; Non-Hodgkin lymphoma; specific lymphoma
  cells of origin, 449-451
  cutaneous, 531-542
  genetic lesions in, 451-453
  IWG criteria for, 342
  molecular biology of, 449-462
  pediatric, 442-445
  primary effusion, 80
Lymphoplasmacytic lymphoma, 507-508
Lymphoproliferative disorders, Kaposi's sarcoma and, 80
Lynch syndrome. *See also* Hereditary nonpolyposis colorectal cancer (HNPCC)
  prophylactic surgery in, 373-374, 380-381
  surveillance procedures, 430
  total abdominal colectomy in, 381t

M

Macrophages
  cytotoxicity of, 331
  tumor-associated, 91
MAGE-1, 167
MAGE-A1 antigen, 168f
MAGE-A3 antigen, 168, 168f
MAGEA12 antigen, 168
Magnetic resonance imaging (MRI)
  radiation therapy planning using, 157, 158f
Major histocompatibility complex (MHC)
  molecules, 167, 168f
Major molecular response (MMR), 602, 604
Malignant melanoma, 7. *See also* Melanoma(s)
MALT lymphoma
  cell or origin, 458
  genetic lesions in, 458
Mammalian target of rapamycin (mTOR)
  activation of, 25, 591
  inhibitors of, 261
    for breast cancer, 263
    description of, 323
    for Hodgkin's lymphoma, 489
    indications for use of, 263
    for tuberous sclerosis, 263
Mammalian target of rapamycin-associated protein complexes (mTORC)
  pathway, 262f
Mammography, 140, 410, 412, 414
Mantle cell lymphoma (MCL), 510-511
  bortezomib for, 281
  cell of origin, 453

Mantle cell lymphoma (MCL) (*Continued*)
  genetic lesions in, 453
  treatment of
    mTOR inhibitors, 292–293
    proteasome inhibitors in, 281
Marginal zone lymphoma
  description of, 508
  extranodal, 509–510
Marizomib, 280, 280*t*
MART-1 antigen, 169
MART-1 gene, 169
Mastectomy
  prophylactic, 368–370
Matrix metalloproteinases (MMP)
  inhibitors of, 320
  MMP-9, 29
Mature B-cell neoplasms, 503
Maytansinoids, 251
MBD2, 270
MCC. *See* Merkel cell carcinoma
MDM2 gene
  amplifications, 559
  description of, 48*t*
MDR1 antagonists, 572
MDR1 gene, 648
Meat, 115
Mechlorethamine
  clinical pharmacology, 205*t*
  for mycosis fungoides with Sézary syndrome, 537*t*
  stability of, 207
  therapeutic uses, 205*t*
  toxicities, 205*t*
Mediastinal B-cell lymphomas, 475
Mediastinal gray zone lymphoma, 475
Mediastinal large B-cell lymphoma, 515
Medroxyprogesterone acetate (MPA)
  dosage, 311
  pharmacology, 311–312
  route of administration, 303*t*
  tamoxifen interaction with, 305
  toxicities, 311
Medullary thyroid carcinoma (MTC)
  hereditary, 431
  MEN-2 and, 374–377
  RET mutations in, 375*t*
  sporadic, 375*t*
  vandetanib for, 322
Medulloblastoma
  PIK3CA mutations in, 3
Megestrol acetate
  dosage, 311
  for hot flashes, 302
  pharmacology, 311–312
  route of administration, 303*t*
  toxicities, 311
Melan-A, 169
Melanocyte differentiation antigens (MDA), 169
Melanocytes, 169
Melanoma(s). *See also* Malignant melanoma; Skin cancer
  BRAF mutant, 16, 258–260
  gene mutations in, 4
  incidence of, 142
  metastatic disease
    complete response to treatment, 172*f*
    interleukin-2 therapy for, 171–172
  T cells reactive to, 167
  ultraviolet light and, 106
  uveal
    BAP1 mutation in, 4
    description of, 4
Melphalan (Alkeran)
  administration of, 207
  characteristics of, 207
  clinical pharmacology, 205*t*
  doses and schedules, 207*t*
  high-dose therapy, 665*f*, 665–669
  for multiple myeloma, 640, 659, 667*f*, 672
  therapeutic uses, 205*t*
  toxicities, 205*t*
Meningiomas
  in neurofibromatosis type 2
2-Mercaptoethane sulfonate (MESNA), 209
6-Mercaptopurine (6-MP)
  description, 230
  dosages, 225*t*
  metabolic pathways, 230
  therapeutic uses, 225*t*
  toxicities, 225*t*
Merkel cell carcinoma (MCC)
  clinical features of, 77*f*
  transcriptome of, 10
Merkel cell polyomavirus, 74*t*, 77–78
Mesenchymal stem cells, 30
Mesotheliomas
  description of, 108
MET, 48*t*
Meta-analyses
  epidemiology methods, 134
Metastases
  bone
    multiple myeloma and, 649–650
  as cancer hallmark, 30–33
  dissemination, 31
  inflammation's role in, 91
  phases of, 31–32
  stromal cells in, 30–31
Metatypical carcinomas. *See also* Basal cell carcinoma (BCC)
Metformin, 399–400
Methotrexate (MTX)
  adverse effects, 224*t*, 225
    gastrointestinal, 225
    myelosuppression, 225
  bioavailability, 223
  dosages, 224*t*
  drug interactions, 250
  efficacy of, 223
  excretion, 223
  inhibition of, 223
  for mycosis fungoides with Sézary syndrome, 540
  therapeutic uses, 224*t*
Methylation analysis, 58–59
Methylation-sensitive multiplex ligation-dependent probe amplification, 58–59
Methylcholanthrene (MCA), 167
Methylenetetrahydrofolate reductase, 116
Methylmelamines, 205*t*
4-(Methylnitrosamino)-1-(3-pyridyl)-1-butanone, 66, 69
Metronomic chemotherapy, 324
MGCD-0103, 271*t*
MGMT gene, 207
Microenvironment, of tumor
  angiogenesis targeting through, 320
  cancer-associated fibroblasts, 35–36
  cell-to-cell signaling pathways, 39*f*
  coevolution of, in carcinogenesis, 37–38, 40*f*
  description of, 35
  endothelial cells, 36
  heterotypic signaling in, 37
  immune inflammatory cells, 36–37
  oxygen levels in, 151
  pericytes, 36
  progenitor cells, 37
  stem cells, 37
Micrometastases, 31
Micronutrients
  antioxidant, 388–392, 391*t*
  B vitamins, 392–393
  calcium, 393
  as cancer risk–reducing agents, 388–394
  carotenoids, 388–392
  definition of, 388
  folic acid, 392–393
  retinoids, 388–392, 390*t*
  summary of, 393–394
  vitamin D, 393
MicroRNAs, 42, 268
  miR15, 593
  miR16, 593
Microsatellite instability analysis, 59
Microtubular antagonists
  auristatins, 251
  estramustine phosphate, 251
  maytansinoids, 251
  mechanisms of resistance to, 252
Microtubule inhibitors, 252
Microtubule-associated proteins (MAP), 252
Microtubules, 245
Microwave radiation, 106–107
Midostaurin, 261
Migrant studies, 110
Milk consumption, 115, 118
Minimal residual disease, 438, 568, 620, 670
Misclassification, epidemiologic studies, 133
Mismatch repair
  DNA
    genes involved in, 374
Mitogen-activated protein kinase (MAPK) pathway, 259*f*
Mitotic motor protein inhibitors, 251–252
Mitoxantrone
  characteristics of, 239*t*
MLL fusion genes, 555–556
MLL/AF9 fusion gene, 550, 555–556
MLL/ENL fusion gene, 550
MLN 2238, 280*t*
MLN 9708, 280*t*
MMAE, 251
Mogamulizumab, 538*t*, 540
Molecular diagnostics
  allele specific polymerase chain reaction, 53*t*, 54
  expression panels, 61
  fluorescent in situ hybridization, 53*t*, 57–58, 58*f*
  fragment analysis, 53*t*, 55, 56*f*
  genomic microarrays, 54*t*, 60–61
  high-resolution melting curve analysis, 55–56, 56*f*
  laboratory, 50
  loss of heterozygosity analysis, 59
  methylation analysis, 58–59
  microsatellite instability analysis, 59
  next-generation sequencing, 59–60, 60*f*–61*f*

oncology applications of, 47–50
polymerase chain reaction, 52
pyrosequencing, 53t, 57
real-time polymerase chain reaction, 52–54, 53t
reverse transcriptase polymerase chain reaction, 53t, 54–55, 55f
Sanger sequencing, 53t, 56–57, 57f
single nucleotide extension assay, 53t, 57
specimen for, 51, 134
testing process of, 51–52
Molecular epidemiology, 97, 134–136
Molecular markers, 135
Monoclonal antibodies, 329–335. *See also* Specific antibodies; Specific antigens
  altered signal transduction and, 332
  anti-VEGFR2, 324
  bispecific, 332
  for chronic lymphocytic leukemia, 616
  complement-dependent cytotoxicity and, 332
  engineering of, 329
  immunoconjugate strategies, 332
  immunocytokine conjugates, 332
  immunotoxins and, 332
  for mycosis fungoides with Sézary syndrome, 540
  naming rules, 330t
  radioimmunoconjugates, 333
Monoclonal gammopathy of unknown significance (MGUS), 640–642, 659
Monocytes, 91, 331
Monocytoid B cells, 508
Monomethyl auristatin E, 251
Monte Carlo techniques, 157
MOPP regimen
  for advanced-stage Hodgkin's lymphoma, 480
Mortality/mortality rates
  breast cancer, 141
  prostate cancer, 141–142
  smoking effects on, 353–354
  trends in, 138–143
Motesanib, 260
Mountains, 11
MOZ/CBP fusion protein, 556
MP regimen, 665t
MPL, 48t
MPT regimen, 665t
MRN complex, 145, 146f
MS-275. *See* Entinostat
MTC. *See* Medullary thyroid carcinoma (MTC)
MTHFR gene, 565
mTOR. *See* Mammalian target of rapamycin (mTOR)
Mucosa-associated lymphoid tissue (MALT), 496, 508. *See also* MALT lymphoma
Mucositis
  paclitaxel and, 248
Multicentric Castleman disease (MCD), 80
Multidrug resistance–associated protein (MRP), 648
Multileaf collimator shaping, 154–155
Multiple endocrine neoplasia
  RET mutations in, 376f
  type 2
    gene carriers, 374–375
Multiple myeloma (MM)
  adhesion molecules in, 645–646
  alkylating agents for, 659

allogeneic transplantation for, 670
bone destruction in, 650f
cell phenotypes, 618
clinical manifestations, 649–658
combination therapies, 664f
cytogenetics of, 642–644, 657–658
cytokines in, 646–648
diagnosis, 649t, 651, 653t
differential diagnosis of, 655, 657
donor lymphocyte infusions for, 670
epidemiology, 641
etiology, 641–642
free light chain in, 652
genomic studies, 644–645
heavy/light chain in, 652
immune status, 648
incidence, 641f
karyotypic abnormalities, 643f
microenvironment, 645–646
minimal residual disease, 670
molecular alterations in, 642–644
MRI pattern, 656f
murine models, 648–649
neurologic symptoms of, 650–651
pathogenesis, 641–648
prognostic variables, 657, 657t
radiographic evaluation of, 652–655
relapsed, 672–673
risk assessments, 657
skeletal changes, 655f
skeletal involvement, 655f
staging of, 657, 658t
switch recombination in, 643t
terminology, 640
transcriptional studies, 644–645
treatment of, 658–674
  maintenance therapy, 669t, 669–670
  novel therapies, 673
  in older patients, 668–669
Multivariate logistic regression models, 131
MYC gene
  in Burkitt's lymphoma, 79
  overexpression, 557
  translocations, 454
Mycosis fungoides, Sézary syndrome and, 531–532
  chemotherapies for, 536
  diagnosis of, 533, 534f, 535t
  epidemiology of, 531
  etiology of, 531
  pathobiology of, 531–532
  prognosis, 533–534
  staging, 533–534, 533–535, 536t
  systemic treatment of, 539–541
  treatment of, 535–541, 537t–538t
Myelodysplastic syndromes (MDS)
  anemia associated with, 636
  benzene exposure and, 627
  bone marrow failure and, 627
  clinical presentation of, 631–632
  definition of, 627
  epidemiology of, 627
  etiology of, 627–628
  flow cytometry, 438
  French-British-American classification of, 628
  Global M.D. Anderson Scoring System, 632
  history of, 627
  hypocellular, 628
  immunity dysregulation as driver in, 631

International Prognostic Scoring System for, 632
morphologic findings in, 629f
mutations associated with, 630
next-generation sequencing of, 631
pathogenesis of, 628–631
pathology of, 628
pediatric, 436
prognosis for, 632
progression of, 630f
5q minus syndrome, 631
risk assessment of, 632
risk stratification models in, 633t
treatment of
  5AC in, 271
  allogeneic hematopoietic cell transplantation, 635–636
  azanucleosides, 635
  decitabine, 271, 635
  decitabine in, 271
  erythropoiesis-stimulating agents, 632, 634
  immunosuppressive therapy, 635
  iron chelation, 636
  lenalidomide, 634–636
World Health Organization classification of, 628
Myelofibrosis, 258
Myelomas
  first report of, 640
  metastatic disease, 123t
  multiple. *See* Multiple myeloma
  smoldering, 659
Myeloproliferative disorders, 258
Myelosuppression
  bone marrow monitoring for, 603–604
  cladribine and, 231
  clofarabine and, 231
  gemcitabine and, 229
MYH11 gene, 566
MYH-associated polyposis (MAP), 377–380
Myofibroblasts, 35

N

Nab-paclitaxel, 246, 248
Nanoparticles, 108
National Health and Nutrition Examination Survey (NHANES), 130
National Oncology Association, 356
Natural killer cells (NK cells), 331, 498
Nausea and vomiting
  alkylating agents and, 209
  radiation-induced, 163
NAV3 gene deletions, 532
Navitoclax (ABT-263), 621
Nbs1 protein, 145
Neck. *See also* Head and neck squamous cell carcinoma
  squamous cell carcinoma of. *See* Head and neck squamous cell carcinoma
Necrotic cell death, 27
Negative predictive value, 407
Negative-feedback mechanisms, 25
Nephropathy, multiple myeloma and, 649
Neutropenia, 247, 248–249
  clofarabine and, 231
  vinblastine and, 250
Never smoking, 353
Next-generation sequencing
  description of, 51t, 59–60, 60f–61f

Nicotinamide, 151
Nicotine, 352
Nicotine replacement therapy, for smoking cessation, 359, 360t
Nicotinic acetylcholine receptors, 69
Nijmegen breakage syndrome
 checkpoint pathways and, 145
Nilotinib (Tasigna)
 for ALL, 582
 approved indications, 256t
 for chronic myelogenous leukemia, 263, 602, 604–605
 food effects on, 191t
 imatinib compared with, 601t
 resistance to, 605
 side effects, 602–603
Nilutamide, 310
 dosage, 303t
Nitrogen mustards
 characteristics of, 204, 207
 clinical pharmacology, 205t
 metabolism of, 204f
 metabolites of, 203
 for mycosis fungoides with Sézary syndrome, 535
 structure of, 204f
 therapeutic uses, 205t
 toxicities, 205t
Nitrosoureas
 characteristics of, 207
 clinical pharmacology, 205t
 mechanisms of action, 208
 metabolism of, 204f
 metabolites of, 203
 therapeutic uses, 205t
 toxicities, 205t
Nivolumab, 173
NK lymphomas, 541
NK/T-cell lymphomas, 541
N-nitrosamine, 98
NNK. See 4-(Methylnitrosamino)-1-(3-pyridyl)-1-butanone
Nodal marginal zone B-cell lymphoma, 508
Nodular lymphocyte-predominant Hodgkin's lymphoma (NLPHL)
 differential diagnosis of, 474–475
 lymphocyte-predominant cells, 469, 471
 microenvironment for, 471–472
 morphology of, 470, 471t
 patterns of, 472f
 pediatric, 445
 phenotype of, 471
 T-cell/histiocyte-rich large B-cell lymphoma versus, 474
Noncoding RNAs, 9, 268
Non-Hodgkin lymphoma (NHL), 495–522
 alemtuzumab for, 335
 BCL-2 overexpression in, 644
 diagnosis of, 501
 diseases associated with, 495, 496t
 environmental exposures and, 495
 epidemiology, 495
 etiology, 495
 genetic lesions, 451–453
 HIV-related
  cell of origin, 460
  genetic lesions, 460
 management of, 501–503
 molecular pathogenesis, 453–460

obesity and, 126
pediatric, 442t, 442–444, 443t
prognosis for, 502, 502t
restaging, 507
rituximab for, 334
staging, 502t, 502–503
T-cell, 460–462
tositumomab for, 333
Nonhomologous end joining (NHEJ), 147f, 147–148, 285
Nonisocentric miniature linac robotic delivery systems, 155
Nonmyeloablative regimens, 605
Non–small-cell lung cancer (NSCLC). See also Lung cancer
 bevacizumab for, 334
 cetuximab for, 334
 EML4-ALK translocations in, 10, 16
 treatment of
  resistance to, 19
  taxanes in, 245
Nonsteroidal anti-inflammatory drugs (NSAIDs)
 as cancer risk–reducing drugs, 394–395
 clinical trials of, 395t
 inhibition of MTX excretion, 223
NOTCH1, 559
NOTCH1, 49t, 579
NOTCH2, 49t
NPI-0052, 279
 clinical trials, 279
 therapeutic use of, 280t
NPM, 567
NPM1 gene, 559
NRAS, 19, 48t
Nucleophilic substitution reactions, 203
Nucleoside analogues, for hairy cell leukemia, 623
Nucleotide excision repair (NER), 105
Nucleotide substitutions, 10
NUP98/HOXA9 fusion protein, 555, 592
NuRD, 270
NY-ESO-1 antigen, 168, 168f

O

Obesity
 breast cancer and, 123–124, 140
 cancer risk and, 123
 colorectal cancer and, 125
 description of, 111, 123
 endometrial cancer and, 125
 esophageal adenocarcinoma and, 126
 kidney cancer and, 126
 lung cancer and, 127
 non-Hodgkin lymphoma and, 126
 ovarian cancer and, 127
 pancreatic cancer and, 126
 prostate cancer and, 127
Obinutuzumab, 296t
Observational studies
 classification of, 131f
 epidemiologic, 130
Ocrelizumab, 332
Octreotide
 description, 312
 dosage, 312
 pharmacology, 312
 routes of administration, 303t
 tolerability, 312

Odds ratio, 133
Ofatumumab (Arzerra), 330t, 335, 616–617
Olaparib, 286
Omacetaxine, 290, 297t
Omega-3 fatty acids
 characteristics of, 401t
 description of, 400
ON01910, 252
Oncogene(s). See also specific oncogene
 glycolytic fueling, 32
 mutations, 2
 rearrangements, 498–499
 sources of, 50
Oncogene addiction, 255
Oncogene viruses
 description of, 73, 75
 Epstein-Barr virus. See Epstein-Barr virus
 papillomaviruses, 75–76
 types of, 74t
 virology of, 73, 75
Oncotype DX 21 gene assay, 303
ONX 0912, 280t
Oprozomib, 279–281, 280t
Oropharyngeal cancer, 76
Orteronel, 310
Osteonecrosis of the jaw (ONJ), 672
Osteoprotegerin (OPG), 649
OTT1/MAL fusion gene, 556
Outcomes
 clinical responses, 339–349
 evaluation criteria, 340t–341t
Ovarian cancer
 asymptomatic patients, 343
 BRCA1/2, 430
 hereditary, prophylactic surgery, 372–373
 obesity and, 127
 physical activity and, 127
 screening for, 412t, 418–419
 surveillance procedures, 430
 treatment of, 245
Overall response rate (ORR), 344
Overall survival (OS)
 response evaluation using, 346, 347f
 stable disease and, 344
Overdiagnosis, 408
Oxaliplatin
 chemistry of, 215
 for colorectal cancer, 215
Oxazaphosphorines, 209
Oxygen, radiosensitization and, 151
Oxygen effect, 102

P

p58.2, 169
p16 gene
 promoter hypermethylation and, 268
p53 gene
 angiogenesis and, 318
p53 protein, 104
Pacific Biosciences PacBio RS, 5, 6t
Paclitaxel (Taxol)
 albumin-bound
  dosages, 247t
  formulation of, 246
  indications, 247t
  toxicity, 247t, 248
 approval of, 245
 bevacizumab with, 321, 334
 clinical pharmacology, 246

Index

dosages, 247t
  systemic exposure and, 187
drug interactions, 248
identification of, 245
indications, 247t, 296t
mechanisms of action, 245–246
nanoparticle albumin-bound, 246, 248. See also Nab-paclitaxel
radiation sensitivity and, 152
toxicity, 247t, 248
Palliative care
  for pediatric patients, 445
Pan-Cancer initiative, 15
Pancreas
  cancer of. See Pancreatic cancer
Pancreatic cancer
  gemcitabine-based treatment, 152
  KRAS mutations, 16
  obesity and, 126
  screening for, 417
  signaling pathways, 12f
Panitumumab (Vectibix)
  binding of, 332
  characteristics of, 330t
  mechanism of action, 334
Panobinostat (LBH589), 272–273, 539, 673
Papanicolaou (Pap) smears
  cervical cancer screening using, 417
  cytologic terminology for, 417
  description of, 417
Papillomaviridae, 75
Papillomaviruses, 75–76. See also Human papillomaviruses (HPVs)
Parafollicular cells
  description of, 508
Paroxetine (Paxil)
  for hot flashes, 302
Passenger mutations, 13, 47
Patched-1, 264
Patents, on genes, 432
Patupilone. See Epothilone B
Pautrier's microabscess, 532
PAX5 mutations, 560
Paxillin, 591
Pazopanib (Votrient)
  description of, 322
  dosages, 319t
  indications, 256t, 298t, 319t
  VEGFR inhibition by, 261
$p210^{BCR-ABL1}$, 589, 598
p53BP1 protein, 145
p130CAS, 591
PCBCL. See Primary cutaneous B-cell lymphomas
PD-1, 173
PD325901, 259
PDGFRA, 48t
PDGFRB, 48t
Pediatric patients. See also Children
  acute lymphoblastic leukemia, 436, 579t
  leukemias/lymphomas, 436–445
    palliative care, 445
    supportive care, 445
  lymphomas, 442–445
  presymptomatic testing in, 431
  solid tumors in, 5
  supportive care, 445
Pegylated liposomal doxorubicin (Doxil). See also Doxorubicin, liposomal

Pemetrexed (Alimta)
  clinical pharmacology, 223
  description of, 223
  dosages, 224t
  therapeutic uses, 224t
  toxicities, 224t
    hand-foot syndrome, 225
    mucositis, 225
    myelosuppression, 225
    rashes, 225
Pentostatin
  for chronic lymphocytic leukemia, 614–615
  for hairy cell leukemia, 623
  for mycosis fungoides with Sézary syndrome, 537t, 540
Pericytes, 29, 36
Peripheral blood stem cell support, 665–669
Peripheral neuropathy
  description of, 293
Peripheral T-cell lymphoma (PTCLs), 461, 517
Peritoneal serous carcinoma, 373
Pertuzumab, 298t, 330t, 333
Pertuzumab injection, 296t
Peutz-Jeghers syndrome
  breast cancer risk in, 369t
  genetics of, 369t
PF-02341066 (crizotinib), 260
Pharmacodynamics
  description of, 186, 188, 188t
  dose adaptation using, 192–193
  variability in, 187–192
Pharmacogenomics
  of chemotherapy drug toxicity, 199–201
  therapy guided by, 196
  tumor response, 196–199
Pharmacokinetics
  absorption, 186
  age and, 188
  of alkylating agents, 207–208
  body size and composition effects on, 188
  disease effects on, 189
  disposition, 186–187
  distribution, 186
  dose-adaptation using, 192–193
  dose proportionality, 187
  drug interactions and, 190–191
  elimination, 186
  gender effects on, 190
  hepatic impairment effects on, 190
  inherited genetic factors effect on, 191–192
  pathophysiologic changes that affect, 189–190
  renal impairment effects on, 189–190
  serum proteins effect on, 190
  variability in, 187–192
Phenotypic markers, 135
Phenylalanine mustards (Sarcolysine), 640
Phenytoin
  tamoxifen interaction with, 305
  toxicities, 210
Philadelphia chromosome, 440, 589, 590f, 598
  acute lymphoblastic leukemia positive for, 582
  formation of, 599f
Phosphatase and tensin homolog on chromosome 10. See also Cowden syndrome

Phosphatase mutations, 3
Phosphatidylinositol 3-kinase pathway
  activation of, 591
  direct targeting of, 263
  feedback inhibition of, 262f
  inhibitors of, 263
  mutations in, 263
Phosphatidylinositol 3-kinase (PI3K) gene family, 3
Photochemotherapy, 539
Photoimmunosuppression, 106
Photon beams, 153–156
Photons
  interactions of, 153
  therapeutic use of, 160
Photopheresis, 539
Phototherapy, 536, 537t, 539
Physical activity. See also Exercise
  breast cancer and, 123–124
  cancer risk and, 123
  colorectal cancer and, 124–125
  definition of, 123
  endometrial cancer and, 125
  esophageal adenocarcinoma and, 126
  lung cancer and, 127
  ovarian cancer and, 127
  prostate cancer and, 126–127
  renal cell carcinoma and, 126
PI3K/AKT/mTOR pathway inhibitors, 489
PIK3CA mutations
  in colorectal cancer, 18f
  description of, 48t, 198
  in endometrial cancer, 258
  somatic, 3
  tumors expressing, 258
PIK3R1, 48t, 263
PIK3R2, 48t
$p15^{INK4B}$ gene, 274
Placental growth factor, angiogenesis and, 317
Plasma cell leukemias, 645f
Plasma cell neoplasms, 640–674
  history of, 640
  multiple myeloma. See Multiple myeloma
Plasma cells, 508
Plasmablastic lymphoma (PBL), 521–522
Plasmacytomas, solitary, 658–659
Platelet-derived growth factor (PDGF)
  angiogenesis and, 317
  description of, 36
  PDGF-α, 257
Platelet-derived growth factor receptors (PDGFRs), 258
Platinum agents
  analogues of, 214–221
  chemistry of, 214
  radiation sensitivity and, 152
PLCO Cancer Screening Trial, 421
PLX4032, 19
  antitumor response, 20
  for BRAF mutant melanoma, 259
PML/RARα fusion gene, 554–555
Pneumonitis
  bleomycin-induced, 291
  radiation-induced, 163
POEMS syndrome, 650
Point mutations
  in acute leukemias, 557–558
  C/EBPα gene, 556
  GATA-1 gene, 556

Pol proteins, 81
Poliovirus receptor-related 2 (PVRL2) gene, 461
Pololike kinase inhibitors, 251–252
Polonator G.007, 5, 6t
Poly(ADP-ribose) polymerase, 285–288
  in clinical development, 287t
  clinical results, 286
  development of, 285
  DNA repair pathways, 285
  inhibitors of
    BRCA mutation and, 286, 288
    synthetic lethality of, 286
  radiation sensitivity and, 153
  resistance to, 287–288
  for sporadic tumors, 287
  treatment using, 286, 430
Polyamines, 398
Polycyclic aromatic hydrocarbons
  description of, 66, 98
Polycythemia vera, 258, 558
Polymerase chain reaction, 52
Polymorphism, 50
Polyomaviruses
  history of, 77
  Merkel cell, 77–78
Pomalidomide, 294, 295t, 296t, 672–673
Ponatinib, 256t, 607
Pooled analyses, 134
Population attributable risks, 131
Positive predictive value, 402
Positron emission tomography (PET)
  of advanced-disease Hodgkin's lymphoma, 482
  radiation therapy planning using, 157, 158f
Posttransplant lymphoproliferative disorder (PTLD), 520–521
PR-047, 280t. See also ONX 0912
PR-171. See Carfilzomib
Pralatrexate, 223. See also Antifolates
  clinical pharmacology, 225
  dosages, 224t
  for mycosis fungoides with Sézary syndrome, 540
  therapeutic uses, 224t
  toxicities, 224t, 225
PRAME gene, 169
Pravastatin, 398
Precursor B-cell neoplasms, 503
Precursor T-cell neoplasms, 503
Prednimustine, 210
Prednisone. See also EPOCH regimen; MOPP regimen
  for multiple myeloma, 659, 669t
  for mycosis fungoides with Sézary syndrome, 540
Pregnancy
  Hodgkin's lymphoma during, 483
Presymptomatic testing, 431
Primary central nervous system lymphoma (PCNSL)
  description of, 520
  diagnosis of, 545
  diffuse large B-cell lymphomas, 545
  in elderly, 547
  epidemiology of, 545
  magnetic resonance imaging of, 546f
  neurotoxicity associated with, 548
  pathology of, 545
  prognostic factors for, 545

salvage treatment for, 547–548
scoring systems for, 545
staging of, 545–546
treatment of, 546t, 546–548
whole brain radiation therapy for, 546
Primary cutaneous B-cell lymphomas (PCBCL), 542
Primary effusion lymphoma (PEL), 80, 522
Probability odds, 131
Probenecid, 223
Procarbazine (Matulane)
  characteristics of, 295t
  description of, 291
  myelosuppression caused by, 291
Prodrug therapies, 211
Progenitor cells, 37
Progestational agents, 303t
Programmed cell death. See Apoptosis
Programmed cell death protein 1, 355
Progression-free survival (PFS)
  as endpoint, 346f
  response evaluation using, 344, 347f, 348f
Proliferative signaling, 24–26
Prolymphocytes, 612f
Prolymphocytic leukemia (PLL), 622
Promiscuous translocations, 451
Promyelocytic leukemia (PML), 335, 554–555
Prostaglandins, 394
Prostate cancer
  biomarkers of. See also Prostate-specific antigen
  castration-resistant
    survival rates in, 174f
  diet and, 113
  incidence of, 141–142
  mortality rates, 141–142
  obesity and, 127
  physical activity and, 126–127
  screening for, 420–422
  TMPRSS2–ERG translocations, 10
  treatment of
    cabazitaxel for, 249
    mortality rates and, 421
    radiotherapy, 161
Prostate gland
  micronutrients efficacy in, 392
Prostate-specific antigen
  screening programs, 420–422
  serial levels of, 343
Proteasome inhibitors
  biomarkers for, 281
  chemical classes of, 279
  in chemotherapy, 279–282
  synthetic
    antitumor activity, 280
    preclinical pharmacology of, 279–280
Proteasomes, 280t
Protein electrophoresis, 651–652, 654f
Proteinase K, 51
Protooncogenes
  alteration of, 452
Psychosocial issues
  genetic counseling and, 430–431
PTCH1, 48t
PTEN gene, 48t
  chromosome 1- deletions and, 652
  mutations, 263
  negative feedback, 25
PTEN hamartoma syndrome, 369t

PTEN protein, in colorectal cancer, 18f
Pulmonary fibrosis, 209
Pulmonary toxicity, chemotherapy-induced
  bleomycin, 291
Purines
  analogues of, 540, 614
PUVA, 536–539, 537t
$p21^{WAF1/CIP1}$ gene, 145
PX-171-004, 282
PXD101. See Belinostat (PXD101)
Pyrosequencing, 53t, 57

Q

5q minus syndrome, 631
Quality of life (QOL)
  response evaluation using, 348
Quizartinib, 261

R

Race/ethnicity
  acute leukemias and, 436
  hereditary cancer syndromes and, 427t
  mycosis fungoides and, 531
RAD001. See Everolimus
RAD51
  BRCA1 and loading of, 148
  function of, 285–286
  upregulation of, 591
Rad54, 148
Radiation. See also Ionizing radiation; Radiation therapy
  adverse effects of, 162–163
  cell survival and, 149f, 149–150
  multiple myeloma and, 641
  of normal tissue, 149f
  physics of, 153–157
  responses to, 150–152
  sensitization to, 152–153
  tolerance doses, 163f
  toxicity of, 162
  tumor oxygenation and, 151
  types of, 160–161
Radiation oncology
  biologic aspects of, 145–150
  principles of, 145–164
  treatment intent, 161–162
  treatment planning, 157–158
Radiation recall, 238
Radiation therapy
  anticancer agents with, 164
  clinical applications of, 160–161
  for early-stage Hodgkin's lymphoma, 476–477
  fractionated, 150–152, 162
  for Hodgkin's lymphoma, 476–477
  late effects of, 163
  for multiple myeloma, 660
  for mycosis fungoides with Sézary syndrome, 537f
  for prostate cancer, 161
  sensitization to, 151
Radiation-induced pneumonitis
  description of, 163
Radical prostatectomy. See also Prostate cancer
Radical scavengers, 102
Radioactive isotopes, 159
Radiofrequency radiation, 106–107
Radioimmunoconjugates, 333
Radium, 296t
Radon, 104

Index

Rad3-related mediated cell cycle checkpoints, 105–106
Raloxifene
  for breast cancer, 141
  description of, 396
  dosage, 303t
  efficacy of, 305
  pharmacology, 305–306
Ramucirumab, 324
Randomized clinical trials, 111, 409, 413t
Rapalogs, 261, 263
Rapamycin, 261. See also Sirolimus
Ras, 644
RAS gene
  description of, 25
  mutations, 557–558
RAS/MAP kinase, 263, 591
RAS–RAF–MEK–ERK signaling pathway, 259f
Rate ratios, 131
RB protein, 26
Reactive oxygen species, 107
Real-time polymerase chain reaction, 52–54, 53t
Reassortment, after radiation, 150–151
RecA, 148
Recent smoking, 353
RECIST 1.0 guidelines, 339–341, 341f
Rectal cancer. See also Colorectal cancer
Rectum
  micronutrients efficacy in, 392
  radiation tolerance, 163f
Red meat, 115
Reed-Sternberg cells, 467, 469, 474f
Regorafenib, 297t, 319t, 323
Reimbursement, 431–432
Rejection responses, 167
Renal cell carcinoma (RCC). See also Kidney cancer
  cDNA screening, 169
  everolimus for, 323
  metastatic
    complete response to treatment, 172f
    interleukin-2 therapy for, 171
  physical activity and, 126
  sorafenib for, 322
Renal failure
  description of, 649
  multiple myeloma treatment, 669
Reoxygenation, 151
Replicative senescence, 28
Replicons, initiation failure, 145
Repopulation
  accelerated, 162
  after radiation, 150
Response Evaluation Criteria in Solid Tumors (RECIST), 339
  evaluation criteria, 340t–341t
  WHO criteria compared with, 341f
Resveratrol, 401t
RET
  mutations of
    description of, 49t
    genotype-phenotype correlations, 375
    in medullary thyroid carcinoma, 375t
    in MEN, 376f
    risk-reducing thyroidectomy in, 375–376, 377f
  studies of, 260
RET tyrosine-kinase receptors, 260
Retina, tamoxifen toxicity of, 302

Retinoic acid receptor alpha gene, 554–555
Retinoid X receptor–selective retinoids, 390
Retinoids
  as cancer risk–reducing agents, 388–392, 390t
  for mycosis fungoides with Sézary syndrome, 539
Retrospective studies, 131
Retroviruses
  animal, 81–82
  chronic transforming, 81
  classification of, 81
  endogenous, 81
  exogenous, 81
  HTLV-1 and, 495
Reverse transcriptase polymerase chain reaction, 53t, 54–55, 55f
Revlimid. See Lenalidomide
Ring sideroblasts and thrombocytosis, 628
Risk ratio, 131
Risk-reducing bilateral salpingo-oophorectomy (RRSO)
  complications of, 373
  ovarian cancer and, 372–373
  studies of, 372
Risk-reducing thyroidectomy, 375–376, 377f
Rituximab (Rituxan)
  characteristics of, 330t
  CHOP regimen with, 334
  for chronic lymphocytic leukemia, 616–617, 619–621
  for follicular lymphoma, 504–507
  function of, 332
  for hematologic malignancies, 334–335
  for PCBCLs, 542
  for primary central nervous system lymphomas, 547
  response rates, 211
RNA-sequencing, 59–60
Roche, 5, 6t, 7f
Rogletimide, 306
Romidepsin
  characteristics of, 271t
  description of, 272
  HDAC inhibition by, 273
  for mycosis fungoides with Sézary syndrome, 539
ROS1, 49t
RUNX1 gene, 553–554, 566
RUNX1T1 gene, 566
Ruxolitinib, 256t, 298t

S

S-1, 227
S phase
  arrest of, 145
  checkpoint pathways and, 145–147
S-adenosylmethionine, 116
Salinosporamide A, 279, 280t
Salpingo-oophorectomy
  prophylactic, 368–381
  risk-reducing bilateral, 372–373
Sample sizes
  in epidemiologic studies, 133
Sanger sequencing, 4–5, 53t, 56–57, 57f
Sarcomas. See also Bone sarcomas; specific sarcoma
Satraplatin, 216
SB-715992. See Ispinesib

Screening
  for breast cancer, 410–415
    breast density, 111
    clinical breast examination, 410
    ductal carcinoma in situ, 414
    effectiveness of, 410, 412
    harms of, 414
    in high-risk women, 414
    mammography, 140, 410, 412, 414
    mortality benefits of, 410
    recommendations, 411t, 414–415
    self-examination, 410
    in women age 40 to 49, 412, 414
  for cervical cancer, 411t, 417–418
  for colorectal cancer, 411t, 415–416
    colonoscopy, 415
    computed tomography colonoscopy, 415–416
    fecal occult blood testing, 415
    flexible sigmoidoscopy, 415
    in high-risk patients, 416
    recommendations, 416, 416t
  for dysmorphology, 428
  for endometrial cancer, 419
  for esophageal cancer, 416
  for gastric cancer, 417
  guidelines and recommendations for, 410–415
  for liver cancer, 417
  for lung cancer, 411t, 419–420
  for ovarian cancer, 412t, 418–419
  for pancreatic cancer, 417
  Papanicolaou (Pap) smear
    cervical cancer screening using, 417
    cytologic terminology for, 417
    description of, 417
  for prostate cancer, 420–422
  for skin cancer, 412t, 422
  trends in, 138, 139t
Screening tests
  assessment of, 407–409
  informed consent for, 409
  length bias, 408, 409f
  negative predictive value, 407
  outcomes of, 409
  overdiagnosis, 408
  performance characteristics of, 407, 408t
  positive predictive value, 407, 407t
  randomized trials, 409
  results of, 407–409
Secondary primary cancers
  after alkylating agents, 209
  ionizing radiation as cause of, 104
  prevention of, 389–390
  smoking effects on, 355
  topoisomerase inhibitors as cause of, 241
Second-generation sequencing, 6–9
Seizures, alkylating agent induced, 210
E-Selectin, 531
Selection biases, in epidemiologic studies, 133
Selective estrogen receptor modulators (SERM)
  cancer treatment with, 303t
  treatment using, 302–306
Selective estrogen receptor modulators, 395–397, 396t
Selenium, 116
Self-antigens, 170
Sequencing platforms, 5, 6t

SEREX (serological analysis of recombinant cDNA expression) libraries, 167
Serological analysis of recombinant cDNA expression, 167
Serous cancer, 373
Serum amyloid A, 89
Sézary syndrome
  immunosuppression in, 533
  mycosis fungoides and, 531–532
  staging, 533–534
SG110, 271t
Shrinking field technique, 161
SIFT algorithm, 13
Sigmoidoscopy, flexible, 415
Signal transducer and activator of transcription (STAT) pathway
  in chronic myeloid leukemia, 591
  STAT5 activation of, 591
Signal transduction modifiers, 398–400
Signet ring cell cancer. See Diffuse gastric cancer (DGC)
Simvastatin, 398
Single nucleotide extension assay, 53t, 57
Single-molecule–targeted therapy, 19
Single-nucleotide polymorphisms (SNP). See also Specific genes
  in chronic lymphocytic leukemia, 593
  epidemiology methods, 134–135
  HapMap, 2
Single-strand DNA breaks, 187
Sinus bradycardia, 248
Sirolimus (rapamycin)
  approved indications, 256t
  description of, 292–293
SIRT1, 270
Skin
  retinoids application to, 390
Skin cancer. See also Malignant melanoma; Melanoma(s)
  nonmelanoma
    description of, 76
    screening for, 412t, 422
Skin Weighted Assessment Tool, 535
Small cell lung cancer (SCLC). See also Lung cancer
Small chain fatty acids, 272
Small intestine
  radiation tolerance, 163f
Small lymphocytic leukemia (SLL), 507
SMO (smoothened) gene, 48t
Smokeless tobacco, 66
Smoking. See also Tobacco
  cancer recurrence and, 354
  cancer treatment toxicity and, 354–355
  epidermal growth factor receptor and, 355
  global rates of, 64
  human papilloma virus and, 355
  mortality affected by, 353–354
  National Oncology Association statements on, 356
  second primary cancer risks, 355
Smoking cessation
  algorithm for, 357f
  assistance with, 358
  future considerations for, 362–363
  implementation of, 356–358
  interventions for, 360–361
  model treatment programs for, 361–362, 362t
  nicotine replacement therapy for, 359, 360t
  pharmacologic treatment for, 359–360, 360t
  resources for, 358t
  strategies for, 359t
  support during, 361
Smoldering adult T-cell leukemia/lymphoma, 82
Smoldering myeloma, 659
Smoothened gene, 48t
S_N2 alkylation reactions, 203
SNDX-275. See Entinostat
Sodium phenylbutyrate, 272
Sofosbuvir, 84
Sokal scores, 600
Solitary plasmacytoma, 655, 658–659
Somatic analysis, 199
Somatic hypermutation (SHM), 450
Somatostatin analogs
  cancer treatment with, 303t
Sorafenib (Nexavar)
  adverse effects of, 322
  for BRAF mutant melanoma, 258–260
  clinical utility, 321–322
  dosages, 319t
  food effects on, 191t
  indications, 256t, 296t, 319t
  off-target activities of, 261
  for thyroid cancer, 260
Sorangium cellulosum, 251
Soy products, 116–117
Spatial additivity, 161
Specimens, 51, 134
Spinal cord
  radiation tolerance, 163f
Spleen, 496
Splenectomy
  in chronic lymphocytic leukemia, 622
Splenic marginal zone lymphoma, 508–509
Split-dose repair (SDR), 150–151
Squamous cell carcinomas (SCCs)
  head and neck. See Head and neck squamous cell carcinoma
  lung, 16
  ultraviolet light and, 106
St. John's wort (*Hypericum perforatum*), 192t
Stable disease (SD), 344
STAT1, 48t
STAT3, 48t
Stathmin overexpression, 252
Stem cell(s), 37–38, 40–41
Stem cell purging, 668
Stem cell transplantation (SCT). See also Hematopoietic cell transplantation (HCT)
  allogeneic
    for Hodgkin's lymphoma, 487
    T-cell gene therapy with, 181
    umbilical cord blood cells, 487, 577
  autologous
    for follicular lymphoma, 505–506
    for Hodgkin's lymphoma, 483–484
  in chronic lymphocytic leukemia, 621–622
Steroid receptor RNA activator, 9
5α-Steroid reductase inhibitors, 397–398
Steroids, alkylating agent conjugated with, 210
STI571. See Imatinib
STK11, 374
Stomach
  micronutrients efficacy in, 392
  radiation tolerance, 163f

Stomach cancer. See also Gastric cancer
  dietary fiber and, 115
  fruit consumption and, 113–114
  vegetable consumption and, 113–114
Streptozotocin
  clinical pharmacology, 205t
  design of, 207
  doses and schedules, 207t
  therapeutic uses, 205t
  toxicities, 205t
Stromal cell–derived factor-1 (SDF-1), 646–647
Stromal cells, 30–31
Study designs
  case-cohort studies, 133
  case-control studies, 132–133
  case-crossover studies, 132
  cohort studies, 132
  evaluation of findings, 133
  in molecular epidemiology, 134
Subcutaneous panniculitis-like T-cell lymphoma, 519, 541
Subependymal giant-cell astrocytomas, 263
Suicide genes, 181
Sunitinib
  for cancer therapy, 322
  dosages, 319t
  food effects on, 191t
  indications, 256t, 296t, 319t
  off-target activities of, 261
Surgery. See also Specific procedures
Surveillance, in genetic counseling, 430
Syndrome of inappropriate secretion of antidiuretic hormone (SIADH)
  vinca alkaloids and, 251
Synthetic lethality, 286, 288
Synthetic phase. See S phase

T

T-cell receptor complexes, 167, 168f
t(1;22) translocations, 556
Tamoxifen
  for breast cancer, 141, 200, 396
  carcinogenic potential of, 303
  dosage, 302, 302t
  drug interactions, 305
  mechanism of action, 302
  metabolism of, 304f
  pharmacokinetics of, 303
  pharmacology of, 302–305
  resistance to, 302–303
  toxicities, 302, 397
Targeted therapies. See also specific cancer; specific therapies
  inflammation and, 92
Taxanes, 245–249. See also specific drug
  bevacizumab with, 335
  mechanism of action, 245–246
  radiation sensitivity and, 152
Taxus brevifolia, 245
T cell(s)
  in allogeneic hematopoietic stem cell transplantation, 181
  CD4+
    mutated gene products recognized by, 169–170
    self-antigen recognition, 169–170

CD8+
　mutated gene products recognized by, 169–170
　self-antigen recognition, 169–170
　development of, 497f, 498
　differentiation of, 498
　genetic modification of
　　for adoptive cell transfer, 176–178
　　for hematologic malignancies, 178–179, 179t
　normal development of, 451
T-cell acute lymphoblastic leukemia (T-ALL), 559
T-cell antigen receptors, 514
T-cell histiocyte-rich large B-cell lymphoma, 514
T cell leukemias, 557
T-cell lymphomas
　classification of, 541
　non-Hodgkin's, 460–462
　subcutaneous panniculitis-like, 541
T-cell receptor rearrangement (TCRR), 533
T-cell receptors (TCRs), 533, 557
T-cell/histiocyte-rich large B-cell lymphoma, 474
TCL1 gene, 594
Teachable moment, 353
Telbivudine, 83
TEL/JAK2 fusion proteins, 558
Telomerase
　delayed activation of, 28–29
　description of, 28
　transient deficiency of, 28
Telomerase reverse transcriptase, 9
TEL-PDGFR-β, 257
Temozolomide (TMZ)
　clinical pharmacology, 205t
　doses and schedules, 207t
　mechanism of action, 204
　PARP inhibitors and, 285
　therapeutic uses, 205t
　toxicities, 205t
Temsirolimus (Torisel)
　approved indications, 256t
　cancer therapy with, 324
　description of, 292–293, 295t
　dosages, 319t
　indications, 319t
　mTOR inhibition by, 261
Teniposide, 239t, 241
Teratogenesis, 209–210
Terminally ill patients
　TERT-CLPTM1L, 135
Tesetaxel, 248
Testicular cancer
　cisplatin for, 214
Testicular diffuse large B-cell lymphoma, 514–515
TET2 gene, 557
Thalidomide (Thalomid)
　antiangiogenic properties of, 318, 320
　in cancer therapy, 318
　description of, 293–294, 295t
　lenalidomide and, 294, 335
　for multiple myeloma, 640, 660f, 661t, 663–664, 669–670, 672–673
　for myelomas, 659–661
6-Thioguanine (6-TG)
　description, 229
　dosages, 225t
　therapeutic uses, 225t
　toxicities, 225t
Thiopurine methyltransferase, 47, 199–200

6-Thiopurine methyltransferase (TPMT), 230
6-Thiopurines
　clinical pharmacology, 230
　description, 229–230
　mechanism of action, 229
　mechanism of resistance, 229–230
　toxicities, 230
Thiotepa, 204
　clinical pharmacology, 205t
　doses and schedules, 207t
　therapeutic uses, 205t
　toxicities, 205t
Thrombocytopenia
　clofarabine and, 231
Thrombospondin-1 (TSP-1)
　angiogenesis inhibition by, 318, 320
　description of, 29
Thymidylate synthase (TS), 223
Thymus
　biology of, 496
Thyroid cancers
　incidence of, 142–143
　tyrosine kinase inhibitors for, 260
Thyroidectomy
　risk-reducing, 375–376, 377f
Tie-2 receptor, 320
Time to treatment failure, 344
Titanium dioxide, 108
Tivozanib, 261
T315I, 605
TMPRSS-ETS, 47
TMPRSS2-ERG fusion, 10
TNFAIP3 gene, 4, 456
Tobacco. See also Smoking
　cancer caused by, 69, 70t
　cancer patient's use of, 353
　carcinogens in, 66–69, 67t–69t
　control policies for, 64
　deaths caused by, 64
　dependence on, 352
　epidemiology of, 64–66
　mortality effects of, 353–354
　nicotine in, 352
　polycyclic aromatic hydrocarbons in, 66
　prevalence of, 352–353
　products with, evolution of, 65–66
　smokeless, 66
　use behaviors for, 65
Tom-Horsfall glycoprotein, 649
Topoisomerase(s)
　biochemical characteristics of, 233
　classification of, 233
　cleavage complexes of, 233
　as interfacial poisons, 233–235
　mechanisms of, 233
Topoisomerase inhibitors
　camptothecin, 234
　classification of, 234t
　cytotoxic mechanisms of, 235
　I
　　camptothecin, 234–237
　　classification of, 234t
　　in development, 237t
　　irinotecan, 235, 236f
　　mechanism of action, 234
　　noncamptothecin, 238
　　topotecan, 236, 237t
　II. See also Anthracyclines
　　for acute lymphoblastic leukemia, 565

　anthracenediones, 240
　classification of, 234t
　dactinomycin, 240–241
　daunorubicin, 238–239
　doxorubicin. See Doxorubicin
　epipodophyllotoxins, 241
　epirubicin, 239–240
　etoposide. See Etoposide
　idarubicin, 240
　mechanism of action, 234
　secondary primary leukemias, 241
　teniposide, 241
Topotecan
　description of, 236, 237t
TOR complex 1, 261
Toremifene, 305
　dosage, 303t
　pharmacology, 305
Tositumomab (Bexxar), 330t, 333
Total abdominal colectomy, 381t
Total skin electron-beam therapy, 536–538
TP53 gene
　description of, 26
　histology of, 373f
　inactivation of, 559
　loss of
　　in Burkitt lymphoma, 454
　　in mantle cell lymphoma, 453
TRAF3, 281
Trametinib, 256t, 296t
Transformation, inflammation's role in, 88–89
Transforming growth factor-β
　angiogenesis and, 317
　antiproliferative effects of, 26
　myeloma cells and, 648
　radiation toxicity and, 162
Trans-3'-hydroxycotinine, 65
Transient myeloproliferative disease, 438
Transient transaminasemia, 229
Transvaginal ultrasound (TVUS), 418–419
Trastuzumab (Herceptin)
　characteristics of, 330t
　indications for, 299t
　mechanism of action, 333
Treadmilling, microtubule, 245
Treanda, 212
Trends, cancer
　future, predicting of, 143
　in incidence, 138–143, 140t
　in mortality, 138–143
　in risk factors, 138, 139t
　in screening, 138, 139t
　understanding of, 138
Triazines, 204
　clinical pharmacology, 205t
　therapeutic uses, 205t
　toxicities, 205t
Trimethoprim, 540
Trithorax, 555
TRP-1, 169
TRP-2, 169
Tuberous sclerosis
　mTOR inhibitors for, 263
Tuberous sclerosis complex 1, 263
Tubulin
　isotypes, 249, 252
　polymerization of, 245
Tumor(s). See also specific tumor
　genetic complexity of, 5

Tumor(s) (*Continued*)
  microenvironment of
    angiogenesis targeting through, 320
    cancer-associated fibroblasts, 35–36
    cell-to-cell signaling pathways, 39f
    coevolution of, in carcinogenesis, 37–38, 40f
    description of, 35
    endothelial cells, 36
    heterotypic signaling in, 37
    immune inflammatory cells, 36–37
    oxygen levels in, 151
    pericytes, 36
    progenitor cells, 37
    stem cells, 37
Tumor antigens, 167–170
  categories of, 169–170
  characteristics, 331
  glycosylation, 331
  half-life/clearance rate, 331
Tumor density, CT-based, 342
Tumor necrosis factors
  TNF-α
    myeloma cells and, 646–648
    radiation toxicity and, 163
Tumor oxygenation, 151
Tumor progression, 3f
Tumor suppressor genes
  inactivation of, 452, 453
  mutations, 2, 558, 559
Tumorigenesis
  research timeline, 1f
Tumor-infiltrating lymphocytes
  culture of, 169
Tumor-promoting inflammation, 34–35
Tumstatin, 318
Tyrosine-kinase inhibitors
  BCR-ABL, 601
  Bruton's, 620
  in chronic myelogenous leukemia treatment, 601–605
  description of, 321–322
  hematologic toxicity caused by, 604
  management of patients receiving, 603–604
  pre-HCT in CML, 605
Tyrosine kinases, 558
Tyrosine kinase domain, 3

U

Ubiquitin-proteasome pathway, 279
UGT1A1, 235
Ultraviolet light
  cancer risks associated with, 106
  cell death caused by, 106
  cell membrane receptor activation, 106
  cellular responses to, 105, 105f
  damage induction mechanisms of, 105
  description of, 102
  nonmelanoma skin cancer and, 106
  photoimmunosuppression, 106
  Rad3-related mediated cell cycle checkpoints, 105–106
  translesion DNA synthesis, 105
Ultraviolet radiation (UVR)
  for mycosis fungoides with Sézary syndrome, 539
Umbilical cord blood transplantation, 487, 577
Urethane, 640
Urinary bladder
  toxicity of alkylating agents, 209

Urothelial cancers
  human carcinogens and, 98–99
Uterine cancers
  description of, 430
Uterine sarcomas
  after tamoxifen therapy, 302
Uveal melanomas
  description of, 4

V

Vaccines
  cancer, 174, 174t
  for follicular lymphoma, 506–507
  HPV, 167
VAD regimen, 659, 664, 664f
Valproic acid (VPA)
  description of, 272
  dose range, 271t
  HDAC inhibition by, 272
  routes of administration, 271t
  target of, 271t
Vandetanib, 256t, 260, 299t, 319t, 322
Vanillylmandelic acid (VMA), 408
Varenicline, 359
Vascular endothelial growth factor
  angiogenesis and, 318
  antibodies to, 151
  anti-VEGF therapy, 320–321
  forms of, 320
  myeloma cells and, 646–648
  as proangiogenic growth factor, 320
  secretion, 261
Vascular endothelial growth factor-A, 29
Vascular endothelial growth factor inhibitors, 261
Vascular endothelial growth factor-2 receptor, 178
Vasohibin, 318
VBM regimen, for advanced-stage Hodgkin's lymphoma, 481t
VBMCP regimen, 659
V(D)J rejoining, 148
Vegetables, 113–114
Vegetarian diet, 117
Vemurafenib, 256t, 299t
Venlafaxine (Effexor)
  for hot flashes, 302
VEPEMB regimen, for advanced-stage Hodgkin's lymphoma, 481t
Villous lymphocytes, 508
Vinblastine (VBL)
  dosages, 247t
  indications, 247t
  mechanism of action, 250
  toxicities, 247t, 251
Vinca alkaloids
  clinical pharmacology, 249
  drug interactions, 250
  mechanism of action, 249
  overview, 249
  radiation sensitivity and, 153
  toxicity, 250–251
Vincristine (VCR)
  alopecia and, 210
  dosages, 247t
  indications, 247t, 297t
  mechanism of action, 249–250
  radiation sensitivity and, 153
  toxicity, 247t, 250–251

Vinflunine, 250
Vinorelbine (VRL)
  dosages, 247t
  mechanism of action, 250
  toxicities, 247t, 250–251
Viral-associated cancers, 170
Viral-mediated gene delivery, 176
Virtual colonoscopy, 415–416
Viruses. *See specific virus*
Viruslike particles (VLP), 170
Vismodegib, 191t, 292, 295t, 298t
Vitamin C, 389
Vitamin D, 393
  colorectal cancer and, 115
Vitamin D receptors, 115–116
Vitamin E
  food sources of, 389
VMCP/VBAP regimen, 659
Volume of distribution, 186
Vomiting. *See* Nausea and vomiting
Von Hippel Lindau *(VHL)* gene, 261
Vorinostat
  characteristics of, 271t
  food effects on, 191t
  for multiple myeloma, 673
  for mycosis fungoides with Sézary syndrome, 537t, 539
  pharmacodynamics of, 273
Vorozole, 306

W

Waldenström's macroglobulinemia
  description of, 640, 651
Warburg effect, 32
Warfarin, 305
Waterfall plots, 348f, 348–349
Wells' syndrome, 612
White blood cells, count after TKIs, 603
Whole-exome analysis, 9–10
Whole-genome analysis, 6–9
Wilms tumor, aniridia, genitourinary anomalies, and mental retardation (WAGR), 558
World Health Organization (WHO)
  classification systems, 499–501, 500t
  evaluation criteria, 340t–341t
  RECIST criteria compared with, 341f
  treatment response criteria, 339
WT1 gene
  mutations, in acute leukemias, 558

X

Xanthine oxidase, 230
XELOX regimen, 227
X-linked agammaglobulinemia, 620
XRCC4/DNA ligase IV complex, 148

Y

Yttrium microspheres, 161

Z

Zanolimumab, 538t, 540
ZAP-70
  chronic lymphocytic leukemia and, 593, 610
  description of, 593–594
  expression, 593–594
Ziv-aflibercept, 297t, 319t, 321
ZK-EPO, 251